Nutrition in the Prevention and Treatment of Disease

Third Edition

ELSEVIER *science & technology books*

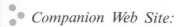

Companion Web Site:

http://booksite.elsevier.com/9780123918840

Nutrition in the Prevention and Treatment of Disease
Ann M. Coulston, Carol J. Boushey and Mario G. Ferruzzi, Editors

Resources for Professors:

- All figures from the book available as both Power Point slides and .jpeg files

TOOLS FOR ALL YOUR TEACHING NEEDS
textbooks.elsevier.com

ACADEMIC PRESS

Nutrition in the Prevention and Treatment of Disease

Third Edition

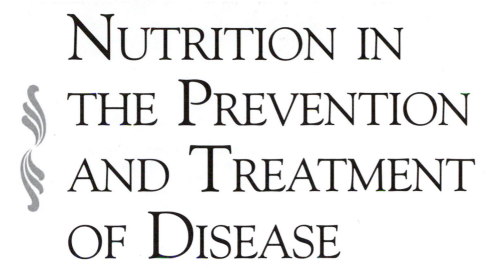

Edited by

Ann M. Coulston, MS, RD, FADA
Nutrition Consultant, Santa Fe, NM

Carol J. Boushey, PHD, MPH, RD
University of Hawaii Cancer Center, Honolulu, HI

Mario G. Ferruzzi, PHD
Purdue University, West Lafayette, IN

ELSEVIER

AMSTERDAM • BOSTON • HEIDELBERG • LONDON
NEW YORK • OXFORD • PARIS • SAN DIEGO
SAN FRANCISCO • SINGAPORE • SYDNEY • TOKYO
Academic Press is an imprint of Elsevier

Academic Press is an imprint of Elsevier
32 Jamestown Road, London NW1 7BY, UK
225 Wyman Street, Waltham, MA 02451, USA
525 B Street, Suite 1800, San Diego, CA 92101-4495, USA

First edition 2001
Second edition 2008

Notice

No responsibility is assumed by the publisher for any injury and/or damage to persons or property as a matter of products liability, negligence or otherwise, or from any use or operation of any methods, products, instructions or ideas contained in the material herein. Because of rapid advances in the medical sciences, in particular, independent verification of diagnoses and drug dosages should be made

Medicine is an ever-changing field. Standard safety precautions must be followed, but as new research and clinical experience broaden our knowledge, changes in treatment and drug therapy may become necessary or appropriate. Readers are advised to check the most current product information provided by the manufacturer of each drug to be administered to verify the recommended dose, the method and duration of administrations, and contraindications. It is the responsibility of the treating physician, relying on experience and knowledge of the patient, to determine dosages and the best treatment for each individual patient. Neither the publisher nor the authors assume any liability for any injury and/or damage to persons or property arising from this publication.

British Library Cataloguing-in-Publication Data
A catalogue record for this book is available from the British Library

Library of Congress Cataloging-in-Publication Data
A catalog record for this book is available from the Library of Congress

ISBN : 978-0-12-391884-0

For information on all Academic Press publications
visit our website at www.store.elsevier.com

Typeset by MPS Limited, Chennai, India

1006903463

Printed and bound in United States of America
12 13 14 15   10 9 8 7 6 5 4 3 2 1

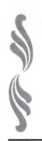

Contents

2

NUTRITION FOR HEALTH MAINTAINENCE, PREVENTION, AND DISEASE-SPECIFIC TREATMENT

Part A: Food and Nutrition Intake for Health

Contributors

Merlin W. Ariefdjohan, PhD   Purdue University, West Lafayette, IN

Marion Taylor Baer, PhD, MS, RD   Department of Community Health Sciences, School of Public Health, University of California at Los Angeles, Los Angeles, CA

Jennifer L. Barnes, BS   University of Illinois at Urbana-Champaign, Urbana, IL

Bryan C. Batch, MD   Division of Endocrinology, Metabolism and Nutrition, Duke University Medical Center, Durham, NC

Sinead Ni Bhriain, BSc   Trinity College, University of Dublin, and Dublin Institute of Technology, Dublin, Ireland

Carol J. Boushey, PhD, MPH, RD   University of Hawaii Cancer Center, Honolulu, HI

Anne Bradford Harris, PhD, MPH, RD   University of Wisconsin-Madison, Madison, WI

Onikia N. Brown-Esters, PhD, RD   Purdue University, West Lafayette, IN

Lora E. Burke, PhD, MPH, FAHA, FAAN   University of Pittsburgh School of Nursing and Graduate School of Public Health, Pittsburgh, PA

Lisa Cadmus-Bertram, PhD   Department of Family and Preventive Medicine, University of California at San Diego, La Jolla, CA

Mona S. Calvo, PhD   Center for Food Safety and Applied Nutrition, U.S. Food and Drug Administration, Laurel, MD

Sara C. Campbell, PhD   Rutgers, The State University of New Jersey, New Brunswick, NJ

Rebecca B. Costello, PhD   Office of Dietary Supplements, National Institutes of Health, Bethesda, MD

Gemma Casadesus, PhD   Case Western Reserve University, Cleveland, OH

Amanda J. Cross, PhD   National Cancer Institute, National Institutes of Health, Department of Health and Human Services, Rockville, MD

Linda M. Delahanty, MS, RD   Massachusetts General Hospital Diabetes Center, Boston, MA

James P. DeLany, PhD   Department of Medicine, University of Pittsburgh, Pittsburgh, PA

Wendy Demark-Wahnefried, PhD, RD   Department of Nutrition Sciences, and UAB Comprehensive Cancer Center, University of Alabama at Birmingham, Birmingham, AL

Maria Duarte-Gardea, PhD, RD   The University of Texas at El Paso, El Paso, TX

Johanna T. Dwyer, DSc, RD   Office of Dietary Supplements, National Institutes of Health, Bethesda, MD

Mario G. Ferruzzi, PhD   Purdue University, West Lafayette, IN

Janis S. Fisler, PhD   Department of Nutrition, University of California at Davis, Davis, CA

Claire K. Fleming, BA   HealthPartners Research Foundation, Minneapolis, MN

Michael Flock, BSc   Pennsylvania State University, University Park, PA

Jo L. Freudenheim, PhD, RD   Department of Social and Preventive Medicine, School of Public Health and Health Professions, University at Buffalo, The State University of New York, Buffalo, NY

Rachel A. Froehlich, MS, RD, CSSD, LDN   University of Pittsburgh School of Nursing, Pittsburgh, PA

Daniel D. Gallaher, PhD   Department of Food Science and Nutrition, University of Minnesota, St. Paul, MN

Karen Glanz, PhD, MPH   University of Pennsylvania, Philadelphia, PA

Réjeanne Gougeon, BSc, MSc, PhD   McGill University, Crabtree Laboratory, Montreal, Canada

Martha Guevara-Cruz, MD, PhD, USDA, HNRCA At Tufts University, Boston, MA and Department of Fisiologia de la Nutricion, Instituto Nacional de Ciencias Medicas y Nutricion, México

Robert P. Heaney, MD   John A. Creighton University Professor, Creighton University, Omaha, NE

Joan M. Heins, MS, RD, LD, CDE   Washington University School of Medicine, St. Louis, MO

Holly Herrington, MS, RD   Center for Lifestyle Medicine, Northwestern University Feinberg School of Medicine, Chicago, IL

Steve Hertzler, PhD   Abbott Laboratories, Ross Products Division, Columbus, OH

James O. Hill, PhD   University of Colorado, Anschutz Medical Campus, Denver, CO

Kathleen M. Hill, PhD, RD   Purdue University, West Lafayette, IN

Karry A. Jackson, MS   Purdue University, West Lafayette, IN

Rachel K. Johnson, PhD, MPH, RD   The University of Vermont, Burlington, VT

James A. Joseph, PhD, USDA, HNRCA   At Tufts University, Boston, MA

Deborah A. Kerr, PhD, Msc, Grad Dip Diet, Bsc, APD School of Public Health, Curtin University, Perth, Western Australia

Gyo-Nam Kim, PhD   Department of Food Science, Purdue University, West Lafayette, IN

Kee-Hong Kim, PhD   Department of Food Science, Purdue University, West Lafayette, IN

Laurence N. Kolonel, MD, PhD   University of Hawaii Cancer Center, Honolulu, HI

Penny Kris-Etherton, PhD, RD   Pennsylvania State University, University Park, PA

Alan R. Kristal, PhD   Cancer Prevention Program, Fred Hutchinson Cancer Research Center, Seattle, WA

Robert F. Kushner, MD   Division of General Internal Medicine, Northwestern University Feinberg School of Medicine, Chicago, IL

HuiChuan J. Lai, PhD, RD   Departments of Nutritional Sciences, Pediatrics, and Biostatistics and Medical Informatics, University of Wisconsin, Madison, WI

Johanna W. Lampe, PhD, RD   Fred Hutchinson Cancer Research Center, Seattle, WA

Ki Won Lee, PhD   Department of Agricultural Biotechnology, Seoul National University, Seoul, Republic of Korea

Pao-Hwa Lin, PhD   Department of Medicine, Nephrology Division, Duke University Medical Center, Durham, NC

Robert Marcus, MD   Department of Medicine, Stanford University School of Medicine, Stanford, CA

Julie A. Mares, PhD   Department of Ophthalmology and Visual Sciences, University of Wisconsin–Madison, Madison, WI

Richard Mattes, MPH, PhD, RD   Department of Nutrition Science, Purdue University, West Lafayette, IN

Kristin J. Meyers, PhD, Scientist,   Department of Ophthalmology and Visual Sciences, University of Wisconsin–Madison, Madison, WI

Amy E. Millen, PhD, Assistant Professor,   Department of Social and Preventive Medicine, School of Public Health and Health Professions, University at Buffalo, The State University of New York, Buffalo, NY

Kris M. Mogensen, MS, RD, LDN, CNSC Department of Nutrition, Brigham and Women's Hospital, Boston, MA

Suzanne P. Murphy, PhD, RD   University of Hawaii Cancer Center, Honolulu, HI

Andrew P. Neilson, BS, PhD   Virginia Polytechnic Institute and State University, Blacksburg, VA

Mihai D. Niculescu, MD, PhD   University of North Carolina at Chapel Hill, Chapel Hill, NC

Beth Ogata, MS, RD   Division of Genetics and Development, University of Washington, Center on Human Development and Disability, Seattle, WA

Nicholas J. Ollberding, PhD, MS   Department of Health Studies, University of Chicago, Chicago, IL

Jose M. Ordovas, PhD, USDA, HNRCA   At Tufts University, Boston, MA

Song-Yi Park, PhD   University of Hawaii Cancer Center, Honolulu, HI

Ruth E. Patterson, PhD   Department of Family and Preventive Medicine, University of California at San Diego, La Jolla, CA

George Perry, PhD   University of Texas at San Antonio, San Antonio, TX

Michelle Pietzak, MD   University of Southern California Keck School of Medicine, Los Angeles, CA

Susan M. Pilch, PhD, MLS   National Institutes of Health Library, Bethesda, MD

Kim Robien, PhD, RD, CSO, FADA   Division of Epidemiology and and Community Health, and Masonic Cancer Center, University of Minnesota, Minneapolis, MN

Cheryl L. Rock, PhD, RD   Department of Family and Preventive Medicine, and Cancer Prevention and Control Program, University of California at San Diego, La Jolla, CA

Alison M. Roeder, BA   HealthPartners Research Foundation, Minneapolis, MN

Sarah Roller   Kelley Drye & Warren LLP, Washington, DC

Edward Saltzman, MD, USDA, HNRCA   At Tufts University, Boston, MA

Dennis A. Savaiano, PhD   Purdue University, West Lafayette, IN

TusaRebecca E. Schap, PhD, RD   Purdue University, West Lafayette, IN

Helen M. Seagle, MS, RD   Children's Hospital of Colorado, Anschutz Medical Campus, Denver, CO

Harold E. Seifried, PhD, DABT   National Cancer Institute, Rockville, MD

Meghan M. Senso, MS   HealthPartners Research Foundation, Minneapolis, MN

Nancy E. Sherwood, PhD   HealthPartners Research Foundation, Minneapolis, MN

Barbara Shukitt-Hale, PhD, USDA, HNRCA   At Tufts University, Boston, MA

Ann Skulas-Ray, PhD   Pennsylvania State University, University Park, PA

Mark A. Smith, PhD   Case Western Reserve University, Cleveland, OH

Linda G. Snetselaar, LD, PhD, RD   Department of Epidemiology, University of Iowa, Iowa City, IA

Fabrizis L. Suarez, PhD   Abbott Laboratories, Ross Products Division, Columbus, OH

Amy F. Subar, PhD, MPH, RD   National Cancer Institute, Bethesda, MD

Carol West Suitor, MS, DSc   Nutrition Consultant, Winooski, VT

Laura P. Svetkey, MD, MHS   Department of Medicine, Nephrology Division, Duke University Medical Center, Durham, NC

Sze-Yen Tan, PhD, MSc, APD   Department of Nutrition Science, Purdue University, West Lafayette, IN

Kelly A. Tappenden, PhD, RD   University of Illinois at Urbana-Champaign, Urbana, IL

Frances E. Thompson, BS, BS, MPH, PhD   National Cancer Institute, Bethesda, MD

Cristine M. Trahms, MS, RD   Division of Genetics and Development, University of Washington, Center on Human Development and Disability, Seattle, WA

Sabrina P. Trudo, PhD, RD   Department of Food Science and Nutrition, University of Minnesota, St. Paul, MN

Craig H. Warden, PhD   Department of Pediatrics, Rowe Program in Genetics and Section of Neurobiology, Physiology, and Behavior, University of California at Davis, Davis, CA

Connie M. Weaver, PhD   Purdue University, West Lafayette, IN

Susan J. Whiting, BSc, MSc, PhD   College of Pharmacy and Nutrition, University of Saskatchewan, Saskatoon, Saskatchewan, Canada

Holly R. Wyatt, MD   University of Colorado, Anschutz Medical Campus, Denver, CO

Judith Wylie-Rosett, EdD, RD   Albert Einstein College of Medicine, Bronx, NY

Zhumin Zhang, PhD   Department of Nutritional Sciences, University of Wisconsin, Madison, WI

Yaguang Zheng, MSN   University of Pittsburgh School of Nursing, Pittsburgh, PA

Preface

Our purpose in creating this text is to provide a compilation of current knowledge in clinical nutrition and an overview of the rationale and science base of its application to practice in the prevention and treatment of disease. The first section addresses basic principles and concepts that are central to clinical nutrition research methodology. Because nutrition information is gathered from a variety of study designs, research methodology, epidemiology, and intervention studies are reviewed, coupled with data analysis, intervention techniques, and application of behavioral principles to nutrition intervention. The use of biomarkers to monitor nutrition intervention is an example of a rapidly expanding field in research methodology. Throughout these chapters, new areas of study are discussed with the perspective that the application of the scientific method is by definition an evolutionary process. Specific examples, drawn from recently published reports, bring the principles to life.

The second section covers areas of study that contribute to knowledge in clinical nutrition, including disease-relevant biochemistry, metabolism, dietary factors within tissues and cells, and attitudes about food and the eating patterns and behaviors of targeted individuals or groups. This section presents a rich array of topics that cover areas of general interest and nutrition guidelines.

New to the third edition is a section on dietary bioactive compounds for health, which explores bioactive components present in edible plants of particular interest for the prevention of disease. Their widespread use has the potential to impact human health on the population level. Uses of these compounds are explored in cognition, eye disease, and obesity. Also, physiological factors that enhance digestion, absorption, and metabolism bring a greater understanding of bioactives to overall health.

Clinical nutrition is the aspect of nutrition science that is related to the development, progression, or management of disease, as differentiated from the issues of normal requirements, cellular functions, and activities. Interventions range from efforts to maintain health during short-term illness to optimization of health status in individuals at risk for or diagnosed with chronic diseases and to major nutritional and dietary modifications as specific or adjuvant treatments for disease. The first condition addressed is the ever-growing concern with overweight and obesity. As with many of the following disease groups, this grouping begins with a chapter on the genetics of human obesity and moves on to issues related to treatment, the role of physical activity, nutrient-related considerations, childhood and adolescent issues, and environmental queues controlling energy intake. New to the obesity section is a chapter on the management of patients who have undergone surgical treatment for obesity.

Cardiovascular disease, also a condition closely related to nutrition, is summarized in three chapters that examine genetic considerations, lipid disorders, and hypertension. Closely related to obesity and cardiovascular disease is diabetes mellitus. It is interesting how many of the clinical nutrition areas interrelate: Obesity is a risk factor for cardiovascular disease and diabetes, whereas diabetes is an independent risk factor for cardiovascular disease. Dietary intake or nutritional status may be altered as a result of disease or by the treatment modalities that are used, such as surgical treatments or medical management strategies, including prescription medications. The altered needs must be met by dietary or nutrition interventions in order to prevent malnutrition and the associated consequences that contribute to morbidity and mortality.

Nutrition intervention can be a critical component of disease prevention, an important aspect of disease management, or the primary treatment for disease. This is exemplified by the chapters dealing with cancer, beginning again with a discussion of the genetic components, followed by a discussion of malignancies that have connections to nutrition and specific nutrients. Gastrointestinal diseases, especially the newer knowledge about diet and microflora of the gastrointestinal tract, demonstrate the importance of food choices in disease prevention, treatment, and management. The bone health chapters cover three important topics linked by the nutrients calcium and vitamin D and tell an important story of the value of early nutrition on health in later years.

Generating and analyzing data that summarize dietary intake and its association with disease are valuable tasks in treating disease and developing disease prevention strategies. Well-founded medical nutrition therapies can minimize disease development and related complications. Providing scientifically sound, creative, and effective nutrition interventions is challenging and rewarding. We plan to update our knowledge and its application through future editions of this text.

Ann M. Coulston
Carol J. Boushey
Mario G. Ferruzzi

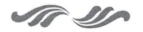

RESEARCH METHODOLOGY

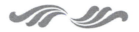

ASSESSMENT METHODS FOR RESEARCH AND PRACTICE

PART A

ASSESSMENT METHODS FOR
RESEARCH AND PRACTICE

1

Dietary Assessment Methodology

Frances E. Thompson, Amy F. Subar

National Cancer Institute, Bethesda, Maryland

I INTRODUCTION

This chapter is a revision of the similarly named chapter in the 2008 [1] and 2001 [2] editions of this book, which itself was based on the "Dietary Assessment Resource Manual" [3] by Frances E. Thompson and Tim Byers, adapted with permission from the *Journal of Nutrition*. Dietary assessment encompasses food supply and production at the national level, food purchases at the household level, and food consumption at the individual level. This review focuses only on individual-level food intake assessment. It is intended to serve as a resource for those who wish to assess diet in a research study, for example, to describe the intakes of a population, using individual measurements for group-level analysis. This chapter does not cover clinical assessment of individuals for individual counseling. The first section reviews major dietary assessment methods, their advantages and disadvantages, and validity. The next sections describe which dietary assessment methods are most appropriate for different types of studies and for various types of populations. Finally, specific issues that relate to all methods are discussed. The intent of this chapter is to contribute to an understanding of various dietary assessment methods so that the most appropriate method for a particular need is chosen.

II DIETARY ASSESSMENT METHODS

A Dietary Records

In the dietary record approach, the respondent records the foods and beverages and the amounts of each consumed over one or more days. Ideally, the recording is done at the time of the eating occasion in order to avoid reliance on memory. The amounts consumed may be measured, using a scale or household measures (e.g., cups or tablespoons), or estimated, using models, pictures, or no aid. If multiple days are recorded, they are usually consecutive, and no more than 7 days are included. Recording periods of more than 4 consecutive days are usually unsatisfactory, as reported intakes decrease [4] due to respondent fatigue, and individuals who do comply may differ systematically from those who do not. Because the foods and amounts consumed on consecutive days of reporting may be related (e.g., leftovers and eating more one day and less the next day), it may be advantageous to collect nonconsecutive single-day records in order to increase representativeness of the individual's diet.

To complete a dietary record, each respondent must be trained in the level of detail required to adequately describe the foods and amounts consumed, including the name of the food (brand name, if possible), preparation methods, recipes for food mixtures, and portion sizes. In some studies, this is enhanced if the investigator contacts the respondent and reviews the report after 1 day of recording. At the end of the recording period, a trained interviewer should review the records with the respondent to clarify entries and to probe for forgotten foods. Dietary records also can be recorded by someone other than the subject, such as parents reporting for their children.

The dietary record method has the potential for providing quantitatively accurate information on food consumed during the recording period [5]. By recording foods as they are consumed, the problem of omission may be lessened and the foods more fully described. Furthermore, the measurement of amounts of food consumed at each occasion should provide more accurate portion sizes than if the respondents were recalling portion sizes of foods previously eaten.

Nutrition in the Prevention and Treatment of Disease, Third Edition.
DOI: http://dx.doi.org/10.1016/B978-0-12-391884-0.00001-9

Although intake data using dietary records are typically collected in an open-ended form, close-ended forms have also been developed [6–12]. These forms consist of listings of food groups; the respondent indicates whether that food group has been consumed. In format, these "checklist" forms resemble food frequency questionnaires (FFQs) (see Section II.C). Unlike FFQs, which generally query about intake over a specified time period such as the past year or month, checklists are intended to be filled out concurrently, with actual intake or at the end of a day for that day's intake. A checklist can be developed to assess particular "core foods" that contribute substantially to intakes of some nutrients [13], and it also has been used to track food contaminants [14]. Portion size can also be asked, either in an open-ended manner or in categories.

A potential disadvantage of the dietary record method is that it is subject to bias both in the selection of the sample and in the sample's completion of the number of days recorded. Dietary record keeping requires that respondents or respondent proxies be both motivated and literate (if done on paper), which can potentially limit the method's use in some population groups (e.g., low literacy, recent immigrants, children, and some elderly groups). The requirements for cooperation in keeping records can limit who will respond, compromising the generalizability of the findings from the dietary records to the broader population from which the study sample was drawn. Research indicates that incomplete records increase significantly as more days of records are kept, and the validity of the collected information decreases in the later days of a 7-day recording period, in contrast to collected information in the earlier days [4]. Part of this decrease may occur because many respondents develop the practice of filling out the record retrospectively rather than concurrently. When respondents record only once per day, the record method becomes similar to the 24-hour dietary recall in terms of relying on memory rather than concurrent recording.

An important disadvantage of this method is that recording foods as they are being eaten can affect both the types of food chosen and the quantities consumed [15–17]. The knowledge that foods and amounts must be recorded and the demanding task of doing it may alter the dietary behaviors the tool is intended to measure [18]. This effect is a weakness when the aim is to measure typical dietary behaviors. However, when the aim is to enhance awareness of dietary behaviors and change them, as in some intervention studies, this effect can be seen as an advantage [19]. Recording, by itself, is an effective weight loss technique [20,21]. Recent interest in "real-time" assessment [22] has led to the development and testing of a dietary intake self-monitoring system delivered through a mobile phone that enables concurrent recording and immediate, automated feedback. A pilot study testing this approach found improved self-monitoring and adherence to dietary goals [19]. A later study found more frequent weight loss in those using electronic self-monitoring than in those using traditional paper-and-pencil dietary records [23].

A third disadvantage is that unless dietary records are collected electronically, the data can be burdensome to code and can lead to high personnel costs. Dietary assessment software that allows for easier data entry using common spellings of foods can save considerable time in data coding. Even with high-quality data entry, maintaining overall quality control for dietary records can be difficult because information often is not recorded consistently from respondent to respondent, nor are different coders consistent in their coding decisions. This highlights the need for training of both the respondents and the coders.

Several approaches using a variety of technological advances have been used to allow easier data capture. These include programs for recording food intake, delivered on the Internet [24], a CD-ROM [25], a personal digital assistant [9,26,27], which have now been replaced by mobile phones with cameras [28,29]. A computer-administered instrument illustrates the potential benefits of technology, particularly for low-literacy groups. With this approach, the respondent selects the food consumed and the appropriate portion size through food photographs on the computer screen [25,30]; this can be done using touch-screen technology [31]. A smart phone can be coupled with a camera that photographs foods selected [32]; this approach requires before and after pictures of a consumption event and training of the participant in how to consistently take pictures, using a standard reference object and a specific angle. Wearable cameras have been developed, which can continuously take pictures or videos, lessening the burden on the respondent and potentially allaying some reactivity (i.e., changes in the respondent's behavior that are caused by the instrument) [33,34].

Processing of the image information for all these methods is not yet fully developed. The images that illustrate the beginning of the consumption event and its completion must be selected, the food has to be identified, and the mathematical properties of the food image need to be quantified in order to develop an accurate estimate of the food's volume. However, if the foods and volumes can be accurately derived, they can be linked to appropriate databases (see Section V.E), dramatically reducing the burden of coding.

Respondent burden and reactivity bias may be less pronounced for the hybrid method of the "checklist" [35] because checking off a food item is easier than recording a complete description of the food [36], and the costs of data processing can be minimal, especially if the form is machine scannable. Checklists are often developed to assess particular foods that contribute substantially to intakes of some nutrients. However, as the comprehensiveness of the nutrients to be assessed increases, the length of the form also increases, and it becomes more burdensome to complete at each eating occasion. The checklist method may be most appropriate in settings with limited diets, such as institutional settings or in impoverished households, or for assessment of a limited set of foods or nutrients.

Many studies in selected small samples of adults indicate that reported energy and protein intakes on dietary records are underestimated in the range of 4–37% compared to energy expenditure as measured by doubly labeled water or protein intake as measured by urinary nitrogen [20,37–50]. Because of these findings, the dietary record is considered an imperfect gold standard. Underreporting on dietary records is probably a result of the combined effects of incomplete recording and the impact of the recording process on dietary choices leading to undereating, and thus not typical of usual intake [20,46,51,52]. The highest levels of underreporting on dietary records have been found among individuals with high body mass index (BMI) [39,41,42,53–55], particularly women [39,41,42,50,56–58]. This effect, however, may be due, in part, to the fact that overweight individuals are more likely to be dieting on any given individual day [59]. These relationships between underreporting and BMI and sex have also been found among elderly individuals [60]. Other research shows that demographic or psychological indices such as education, employment, social desirability, body image, or dietary restraint also may be important factors related to underreporting on diet records [39,46,57,58,61–63]. The research evidence for the psychosocial factors related to energy misreporting is reviewed in Mauer et al. [52]. A few studies suggest that underreporters compared to others have reported intakes that are lower in absolute intake of most nutrients [54], higher in percentage of energy from protein [54,58], and lower in percentage of energy as carbohydrate [54,58,64,65] and in percentage of energy from fat [65]. Correspondingly, underreporters may report lower intakes of desserts, sweet baked goods, butter, and alcoholic beverages [54,65] but more grains, meats, salads, and vegetables [54]. Some research has examined the validity of food checklists relative to accelerometry [66] or, more commonly, complete dietary records [10,11,36], 24-hour dietary recalls [13], dietary history [67], and biological markers [67].

An evaluation study of the 7-day precoded food diary used in the Danish National Survey of Dietary Habits and Physical Activity 2000–2002 reported that energy intake was underestimated by 12% compared to accelerometer [66].

Some approaches have been suggested to overcome underreporting in the dietary record approach. These include enhanced training of respondents and incorporating psychosocial questions known to be related to underreporting in order to estimate the level of underreporting [52]. Another approach is to calibrate dietary records to doubly labeled water or urinary nitrogen, biological indicators of energy expenditure and protein intake, respectively, including covariates of sex, weight, and height, to more accurately predict individuals' energy and protein intake [68]. This approach was applied to a subcohort of the Women's Health Initiative. Calibration equations that included BMI, age, and ethnicity explained much more of the variation in the energy and protein biomarkers than did simple calibration, for example, 45% vs. 8% for energy [55]. Further research is needed to test this approach and to develop and test other ideas.

B 24-Hour Dietary Recall

In the 24-hour dietary recall, the respondent is asked to remember and report all the foods and beverages consumed in the preceding 24 hours or in the preceding day. The recall typically is conducted by interview, in person or by telephone [69,70], either computer-assisted [71] or using a paper-and-pencil form, although self-administered electronic administration has recently become available [72–76]. When interviewer-administered, well-trained interviewers are crucial because much of the dietary information is collected by asking probing questions. Ideally, interviewers would be dietitians with education in foods and nutrition; however, non-nutritionists who have been trained in the use of a standardized instrument can be effective. All interviewers should be knowledgeable about foods available in the marketplace and about preparation practices, including prevalent regional or ethnic foods.

The interview is often structured, usually with specific probes, to help the respondent remember all foods consumed throughout the day. An early study found that respondents with interviewer probing reported 25% higher dietary intakes than did respondents without interviewer probing [77]. Probing is especially useful in collecting necessary details, such as how foods were prepared. It is also useful in recovering many items not originally reported, such as common additions to foods (e.g., butter on toast) and eating occasions not originally reported (e.g., snacks and beverage breaks). However, interviewers should be provided with standardized neutral probing questions so as to avoid leading the respondent to specific answers when the respondent really does not know or remember.

The current state-of-the-art 24-hour dietary recall instrument is the U.S. Department of Agriculture's (USDA) Automated Multiple-Pass Method (AMPM) [78,79], which is used in the U.S. National Health and Nutrition Examination Survey (NHANES), this country's only nationally representative dietary survey. In the AMPM, intake is reviewed more than once in an effort to retrieve forgotten eating occasions and foods. It consists of (1) an initial "quick list," in which the respondent reports all the foods and beverages consumed, without interruption from the interviewer; (2) a forgotten foods list of nine food categories commonly omitted in 24-hour recall reporting; (3) time and occasion, in which the time each eating occasion began and what the respondent would call it are reported; (4) a detail pass, in which probing questions ask for more detailed information about the food and the portion size, in addition to review of the eating occasions and times between the eating occasions; and (5) final review, in which any other item not already reported is asked [78,79]. In addition, research at USDA allowed development of the Food Model Booklet [80], a portion size booklet used in the NHANES in order to facilitate more accurate portion size estimation. A 24-hour recall interview using the multiple-pass approach typically requires between 30 and 45 minutes.

A quality control system to minimize error and increase reliability of interviewing and coding 24-hour recalls is essential. Such a system should include a detailed protocol for administration, training, and retraining sessions for interviewers; duplicate collection and coding of some of the recalls throughout the study period; and the use of a computerized database system for nutrient analysis. One study evaluated the marginal gains in accuracy of the estimates of mean and variance with increasing levels of quality control [81], and the authors recommended that the extent of quality control procedures adopted for a particular study should be carefully considered in light of that study's desired accuracy and precision and its resource constraints.

There are many advantages to the 24-hour recall. When an interviewer administers the tool and records the responses, literacy of the respondent is not required. However, for self-administered versions, literacy can be a constraint. Because of the immediacy of the recall period, respondents are generally able to recall most of their dietary intake. Because there is relatively little burden on the respondents, those who agree to give 24-hour dietary recalls are more likely to be representative of the population than are those who agree to keep food records. Thus, the 24-hour recall method is useful across a wide range of populations. In addition, interviewers can be trained to capture the detail necessary so that new foods reported can be researched later by the coding staff and coded appropriately. Finally, in contrast to record methods, dietary recalls occur after the food has been consumed, so there is less potential for the assessment method to interfere with dietary behavior.

Computerized data collection software systems are currently available in most developed countries, allowing direct coding of most foods reported during the interview. This is highly efficient with respect to processing dietary data, minimizing missing data, and standardizing interviews [82,83]. If direct coding of the interview is done, methods for the interviewer to easily enter those foods not found in the system should be available, and these methods should be reinforced by interviewer training and quality control procedures.

Another technological advance in 24-hour dietary recall methodology is the development of automated self-administered data collection systems [72,74–76,84–88]. These systems vary in the number of foods in their databases, the approach to asking about portion size, and their inclusion of probes regarding details of foods consumed and possible additions. The web-based Automated Self-Administered 24-hour dietary recall (ASA) developed at the National Cancer Institute (NCI) [72,87,88] allows respondents to complete a dietary recall with the aid of multimedia visual cues, prompts, and an animated character versus standard methods that require a trained interviewer. The system uses the most current USDA survey database [89] and includes many elements of the AMPM 24-hour interview developed by USDA [78] and currently used in the NHANES. Portion sizes are asked using digital photographs depicting up to eight sizes [88]. The instrument is freely available for use by researchers, clinicians, and educators. Such web-based tools allow researchers to economically collect high-quality dietary data in large-scale nutrition research. One study indicates that differences between interviewer- and self-administered recalls are minimal among adolescents [76]. Other studies are underway to evaluate differences between interviewer- and web-based self-administered recalls.

The main weakness of the 24-hour recall approach is that individuals may not report their food consumption accurately for various reasons related to knowledge, memory, and the interview situation. These cognitive influences are discussed in more detail in Section V.A.

A potential limitation is that multiple days of recalls may be needed. Whereas a single 24-hour recall can be used to describe the average dietary intake of a population, multiple days of recalls are needed to model estimates of the population's usual intake distributions and their relationships with other factors (see Section V.G).

The validity of the 24-hour dietary recall has been studied by comparing respondents' reports of intake either with intakes unobtrusively recorded/weighed by trained observers or with biological markers. Numerous observational studies of the effectiveness of the 24-hour recall have been conducted with children (see Section IV.B). In some studies with adults, group mean nutrient estimates from 24-hour recalls have been found to be similar to observed intakes [4,90], although respondents with lower observed intakes have tended to overreport and those with higher observed intakes have tended to underreport their intakes [90]. One observational study found energy underreporting during a self-selected eating period in both men and women, similar underreporting during a controlled diet period in men, and accurate reporting during a controlled diet period in women; underestimates of portion sizes accounted for much of the underreporting [91]. Studies with biological markers such as doubly labeled water and urinary nitrogen generally have found underreporting using 24-hour dietary recalls for energy in the range of 3–34% [25,40,75,79,92–98], with the largest two studies in adults using a multiple-pass method showing average underreporting to be between 12 and 23% [79,95]. For protein, underreporting tends to be in the range of 11–28% [92,95,96,98–102]. However, underreporting is not always found. Some have found overreporting of energy from 24-hour dietary recalls compared to doubly labeled water in proxy reports for young children and adolescents [103,104]. In addition, it is likely that the commonly reported phenomenon of underreporting in Western countries may not occur in all cultures; for example, Harrison et al. [105] reported that 24-hour recalls collected from Egyptian women were well within expected amounts. Finally, in many studies, energy adjustment has been found to reduce error. For example, for protein density (i.e., percentage energy from protein), 24-hour dietary recalls conducted in the large biomarker studies were in close agreement or somewhat higher compared to a biomarker-based measure [55,95,96].

In past national dietary surveys using multiple-pass methods, data suggested that underreporting may have affected up to 15% of all 24-hour recalls [106,107]. Underreporters compared to non-underreporters tended to report fewer numbers of foods, fewer mentions of foods consumed, and smaller portion sizes across a wide range of food groups and tended to report more frequent intakes of low-fat/diet foods and less frequent intakes of fat added to foods [106]. As was found for records, factors such as obesity, gender, social desirability, restrained eating, education, literacy, perceived health status, and race/ethnicity have been shown in various studies to be related to underreporting in recalls [46,55,59,61,79,93,101,106–110].

C Food Frequency

The food frequency approach [111,112] asks respondents to report their usual frequency of consumption of each food from a list of foods for a specific period. Information is collected on frequency, but little detail is collected on other characteristics of the foods as eaten, such as the methods of cooking, or the combinations of foods in meals. Many FFQs also incorporate portion size questions or specify portion sizes as part of each question. Overall nutrient intake estimates are derived by summing, over all foods, the products of the reported frequency of each food by the amount of nutrient in a specified (or assumed) serving of that food to produce an estimated daily intake of nutrients, dietary constituents, and food groups. In most cases, the purpose of an FFQ is to obtain a crude estimate of total intakes over a designated time period.

There are many FFQ instruments, and many continue to be adapted and developed for different populations and purposes. Among those evaluated and commonly used are the Block Questionnaires [113–123], the Fred Hutchinson Cancer Research Center Food Frequency Questionnaire [124,125], the Harvard University Food Frequency Questionnaires or Willett Questionnaires [111,121–123,126–133], and the NCI's Diet History Questionnaire [95,123,134,135], which was designed with an emphasis on cognitive ease for respondents [136–138]. Throughout the years, population-specific FFQs have been developed. Examples include FFQs designed to capture diets of Latinos, Native Americans [139–143], African Americans [144], Hispanics [145,146], native Hawaiians, and Asian ethnic groups living in Hawaii [147,148]. FFQs have been developed throughout the world, such as those for countries participating in the European Prospective Investigation into Cancer and Nutrition (EPIC) [45,149–154] and for Australia [155,156], Belgium [157], France [158], Germany [159], Norway [160], Japan [161,162], Korea [163], and the United Kingdom [164]. An FFQ-like instrument, called the Oxford WebQ, has been developed for large-scale epidemiologic research [165]. Like an FFQ, this instrument includes a comprehensive list of foods and portions, but the participant is asked to report whether the foods listed were consumed the previous day. Such instruments, like 24-hour dietary recalls, are meant to be administered at multiple time points in a study. Evaluation of this tool showed moderate correlations (average $r = 0.6$) with interviewer-administered recalls for the same day [165]—values slightly higher than those generally obtained when full-length FFQs that query intake during the past year are evaluated against interviewer-administered recalls. "Brief" FFQs that assess a limited number of dietary exposures are discussed in the next section. Because of the number of FFQs available, investigators need to carefully consider which best suits their research needs.

The appropriateness of the food list is crucial in the food frequency method [114]. The entire breadth of an individual's diet, which includes many different foods, brands, and preparation practices, cannot be fully captured with a finite food list. Obtaining accurate reports for foods eaten both as single items and in mixtures is particularly problematic. FFQs can ask the respondent either to report a combined frequency for a particular food eaten both alone and in mixtures or to report separate frequencies for each food use. (For example, one could ask about beans eaten alone and in mixtures, or one could ask separate questions about refried beans, bean soups, beans in burritos, and so on.) The first approach is cognitively complex for the respondent, but the second approach may lead to double counting (e.g., burritos with beans may be reported as both beans and as a Mexican mixture). Often, FFQs will include similar foods in a single question (e.g., beef, pork, or lamb). However, such grouping can create a cognitively complex question (e.g., for someone who often eats beef and occasionally eats pork and lamb). Differences in definitions of the food items asked may also be problematic; for example, rice is judged to be a vegetable by many nonacculturated Hispanics, a judgment not shared in other race/ethnic groups [166]. Finally, when a group of foods is asked as a single question, assumptions about the relative frequencies of intake of the foods constituting the group are made in the assignment of values in the nutrient database. These assumptions are generally based on information from an external study population (such as from a national survey sample) even though true eating patterns may differ considerably across population subgroups and over time.

Each quantitative FFQ must be associated with a database to allow estimation of nutrient intakes for an assumed or reported portion size of each food queried. For example, the FFQ item of macaroni and cheese encompasses a wide variety of different recipes with different nutrient composition, yet the FFQ database must have a single nutrient composition profile. There are several approaches to constructing such a database [111]. One approach uses quantitative dietary intake information from the target population to define the typical nutrient density of a particular food group category. For example, for the food group macaroni and cheese, all reports of the individual food codes reported in a population survey can be collected, and a mean or median nutrient composition (by portion size if necessary) can be estimated. Values can also be calculated by gender and age. Dietary analyses software, specific to each FFQ, is then used to compute nutrient intakes for individual respondents. These analyses are available commercially for the Block, Willett, and Hutchinson FFQs, and they are publicly available for the NCI FFQ.

In pursuit of improving the validity of the FFQ, investigators have addressed a variety of frequency questionnaire design issues, such as length, closed- versus open-ended response categories, portion size, seasonality, and time frame. Frequency instruments designed to assess total diet generally list more than 100 individual line items, many with additional portion size questions, requiring 30–60 minutes to complete. This raises concern about length and its effect on response rates. Although respondent burden is a factor in obtaining reasonable response rates for studies in general, a few studies have shown this not to be a decisive factor for FFQs [137,167–171]. This tension between length and specificity highlights the difficult issue of how to define a closed-ended list of foods for a food frequency instrument. The increasing use of optically scanned or web-based instruments has necessitated the use of closed-ended response categories, forcing a loss in specificity [172].

Although the amounts consumed by individuals are considered an important component in estimating dietary intakes, it is controversial as to whether or not portion size questions should be included on FFQs. Frequency has been found to be a greater contributor than serving size to the variance in intake of most foods [173]; therefore, some prefer to use FFQs without the additional respondent burden of reporting serving sizes [111]. Others cite small improvements in the performance of FFQs that ask the respondents to report a usual serving size for each food [116,118]. Some incorporate portion size and frequency into one question, asking how often a particular portion of the food is consumed [111]. Although some research has been conducted to determine the best ways to ask about portion size on FFQs [136,174,175], the marginal benefit of such information in a particular study may depend on the study objective and population characteristics.

Another design issue is the time frame about which intake is queried. Many instruments inquire about usual intakes during the past year [114,127], but it is possible to ask about the past week or month [176], depending on specific research situations. Even when intake during the past year is asked, some studies have indicated that the season in which the questionnaire is administered has an influence on reporting during the entire year [177,178].

Finally, analytical decisions are required in how food frequency data are processed. In research applications in which there are no automated quality checks to ensure that all questions are asked, decisions about how to handle missing data are needed. In particular, in self-administered situations, there are usually many initial frequency questions that are not answered. One approach is to assign null values because some research indicates that respondents selectively omit answering questions about foods they seldom or never eat [179,180]. Another approach is the imputation of frequency values for those not providing valid answers. Only a few studies have addressed this issue [181,182], and it is currently unclear whether imputation is an advance in FFQ analyses.

Strengths of the FFQ approach are that it is inexpensive to administer and process and it asks about the respondent's usual intake of foods over an extended period of time. Unlike other methods, the FFQ can be used to circumvent recent changes in diet (e.g., changes due to disease) by obtaining information about individuals' diets as recalled about a prior time period. Retrospective reports about diet nearly always use a food frequency approach. Food frequency responses are used to rank individuals according to their usual consumption of nutrients, foods, or groups of foods. Nearly all food frequency instruments are designed to be self-administered, require 30—60 minutes to complete depending on the instrument and the respondent, and most are either optically scanned paper versions or automated to be administered electronically [113,124,139,183—185]. Because the costs of data collection and processing and the respondent burden have traditionally been much lower for FFQs than for multiple diet records or recalls, FFQs have been a common way to estimate usual dietary intake in large epidemiological studies.

The major limitation of the food frequency method is that it contains a substantial amount of measurement error [55,95—98,135]. Many details of dietary intake are not measured, and the quantification of intake is not as accurate as with recalls or records. Inaccuracies result from an incomplete listing of all possible foods and from errors in frequency and usual serving size estimations. The estimation tasks required for a FFQ are complex and difficult [186]. As a result, the scale for nutrient intake estimates from a FFQ may be shifted considerably, yielding inaccurate estimates of the average intake for the group. Research suggests that longer food frequency lists may overestimate, whereas shorter lists may underestimate, intake of fruits and vegetables [187], but it is unclear whether or how this applies to nutrients and other food groups.

Portion size of foods consumed is difficult for respondents to evaluate and is thus problematic for all assessment instruments (see Section V.D). However, the inaccuracies involved in respondents attempting to estimate usual portion size in FFQs may be even greater because a respondent is asked to estimate an average for foods that may have highly variable portion sizes across eating occasions [188].

Because of the error inherent in the food frequency approach, it is generally considered inappropriate to use FFQ data to estimate quantitative parameters, such as the mean and variance, of a population's usual dietary intake [127,189—193]. Although some FFQs seem to produce estimates of population average intakes that are reasonable [155,159,189], different FFQs will perform in often unpredictable ways in different populations, so the levels of nutrient intakes estimated by FFQs should best be regarded as only approximations [190]. FFQ data are usually energy adjusted and then used for ranking subjects according to food or nutrient intake rather than for estimating absolute levels of intake, and they are used widely in case—control or cohort studies to assess the association between dietary intake and disease risk [194—196]. For estimating relative risks, the degree of misclassification of subjects is more important than is the quantitative scale on which the ranking is made [197].

The definitive validity study for a food frequency-based estimate of long-term usual diet would require nonintrusive observation of the respondent's total diet over a long time. Such studies are not possible in free-living populations. One early feeding study, with three defined 6-week feeding cycles (in which all intakes were known), showed some significant differences in known absolute nutrient intakes compared to the Willett FFQ for several fat components, mostly in the direction of underestimation by the FFQ [198]. The most practical approach to examining the concordance of food frequency responses and usual diet is to use multiple food recalls or records over a period as an indicator of usual diet. This approach has been used in many studies examining various FFQs (see [199] for register of such studies). In these studies, the correlations between the methods for most foods and nutrients are in the range of 0.4—0.7. However, recalls and records cannot be considered as accurate reference instruments because they suffer from mistakes that may be correlated with errors in the FFQs, and they may not represent the time period of interest. Biomarkers that do represent usual intake without bias are available for energy (doubly labeled water) [200] and protein (urinary nitrogen) [201]. Validation studies of various FFQs using these biomarkers have found large discrepancies with self-reported absolute energy intake [40,46,49,55,75,92,94—98] and protein intake [44,45,55,92,95,96,98,154,202—205], usually in the direction of underreporting. Correlations of FFQs and the biomarkers have ranged from 0.1 to 0.5 for energy [40,75,92,95,96,98] and from 0.2 to 0.5 for protein [44,45,92,95,96,98,154,202—205]. A few studies show that correlations between a biomarker for protein density constructed from both urinary nitrogen and doubly labeled water and self-reported protein density on an FFQ (kcal of protein as a percentage of total kcal) are higher than correlations between urinary nitrogen and FFQ-reported absolute protein intake [96,98,135], indicating that energy adjustment may alleviate some of the error inherent in food frequency instruments. Various statistical methods employing measurement error models and energy adjustment are used not only to assess the validity of FFQs but also to adjust estimates of relative risks for disease outcomes [55,206—216]. However, analyses indicate that correlations between an FFQ and a reference instrument, such as the 24-hour recall, may be overestimated because of correlated errors [55,96,135]. Furthermore, a few analyses comparing relative risk estimation from FFQs to dietary records [217,218] in prospective cohort studies indicate that observed relationships are severely attenuated, thereby obscuring associations that might exist, but such findings are not consistent [219]. Accordingly, some epidemiologists have suggested that the error in FFQs is a serious enough problem that alternative means (e.g., food records or 24-hour recalls) of collecting dietary data in large-scale prospective studies should be considered [220—222]. It has also been suggested that FFQ data might be combined with recall or record data to improve estimated intakes [222—224].

D Brief Dietary Assessment Instruments

Many brief dietary assessment instruments, also known as "screeners," have been developed. These instruments can be useful in situations that do not require either assessment of the total diet or quantitative accuracy in dietary estimates. For example, a brief diet assessment of some specific dietary components may be used to triage large numbers of individuals into groups to allow more focused attention on those at greatest need for intervention or education. Measurement of dietary intake, even if imprecise, can also serve to activate interest in the respondent, which in turn can facilitate nutrition education. These brief instruments may therefore have utility in clinical settings or in situations in which health promotion and

health education is the goal. In the intervention setting, brief instruments focused on specific aspects of a dietary intervention also have been used to track changes in diet. However, because of concern that responses to questions of intake that directly evolve from intervention messages may be biased [225] and that these instruments lack sensitivity to detect change [226], this use is not recommended. Brief instruments of specific dietary components such as fruits and vegetables are used for population surveillance at the state or local level, for example, in the Centers for Disease Control and Prevention's (CDC) Behavioral Risk Factor Surveillance System (BRFSS) [227] and the California Health Interview Survey (CHIS) [228] (see Section III.A). Brief instruments have also been used to examine relationships between some specific aspects of diet and other exposures, such as in the National Health Interview Survey (NHIS) [229]. Finally, some groups suggest the use of short screeners to evaluate the effectiveness of policy initiatives [228,230].

Brief instruments can be simplified or targeted FFQs, questionnaires that focus on specific eating behaviors other than the frequency of intake of specific foods, or daily checklists. Complete FFQs typically contain 100 or more food items to capture the range of foods contributing to the many different nutrients in the diet. If an investigator is interested only in estimating the intake of a single nutrient or food group, however, then far fewer foods need to be assessed. Often, only 15—30 foods might be required to account for most of the intake of a particular nutrient [231,232].

Numerous short questionnaires using a food frequency approach have been developed and compared with multiple days of dietary records, 24-hour recalls, complete FFQs, and/or biological indicators of diet. Single-exposure abbreviated FFQs have been developed and tested for a wide range of nutrients and other dietary components. The NCI has developed a Register of Validated Short Dietary Assessment Instruments [233], which contains descriptive information about short instruments and their validation studies and publications, as well as copies of the instruments when available. To be included, publications were required to be in English language peer-reviewed journals and published in January 1998 or later. Currently, the register includes 103 instruments assessing more than 25 dietary factors. Instruments from 29 different countries have been registered. Instruments in the register may be searched by dietary factors, questionnaire format, and number of questions. Descriptive information about the validation study includes the reference tool, the study population (age, sex, and race/ethnicity), and the geographical location. Much of the focus in brief instrument development has been on fruits and vegetables and on fats.

1 Brief Instruments Assessing Fruit and Vegetable Intake

Food frequency-type instruments to measure fruit and vegetable consumption range from including a single overall question to 45 or more individual questions [234–238]. An early 7-item tool developed by the NCI and private grantees for the NCI's 5 A Day for Better Health Program effort was used widely in the United States [239–241]. This tool was similar to one used in CDC's BRFSS [227,242,243]. Validation studies of the BRFSS and 5 A Day brief instruments, or "screeners," to assess fruit and vegetable intake suggested that without portion size adjustments, they often underestimated actual intake [234,239,243–245]. Using cognitive interviewing findings (see Section V.A), the NCI revised the tool, including adding portion size questions; some studies indicate improved performance [246] and utility in surveillance studies. However, its performance in community interventions was mixed. In six of eight site/sex comparisons, fruit and vegetable consumption was significantly overestimated relative to results from multiple 24-hour recalls [247]. More important, the screener indicated a change in consumption in both men and women when none was seen with the 24-hour recalls [248]. Using cognitive testing and expert guidance, the CDC has developed a new fruit and vegetable screener [249] that assesses intake of all forms of fruit and subgroups of vegetables that are particularly relevant to 2010 Dietary Guidelines for Americans [250]. Portion size, although not asked, will be estimated from external data about portion sizes reported by sex/age groups.

2 Brief Instruments Assessing Fat Intake

A fat screener, originally developed by Block [251] and currently composed of 17 items [113], was designed to account for most of the intake of fat using information about sources of fat intake in the U.S. population. The fat screener was used as an initial screen for high fat intake in the Women's Health Trial [251], and in the BRFSS for nutritional surveillance [252]. However, the screener did not perform well in Hispanic women [252]. A similar fat screener substantially overestimated percentage energy from fat and was only modestly correlated ($r = 0.36$) with multiple 24-hour recalls in a sample of medical students [253]. In samples of men participating in intervention trials, the screener was not as precise [226] or as sensitive [254] as complete FFQs. In addition, the screener did not reflect differences observed from 24-hour recalls among different demographic groups, possibly because the screener did not include all of the high-fat foods that contribute to differences in fat intake [226].

The MEDFICTS (meats, eggs, dairy, fried foods, fat in baked goods, convenience foods, fats added at the table, and snacks) questionnaire, initially developed to assess adherence to low total fat (≤30% energy from fat) and saturated fat diets [255], asks about frequency of intake and portion size of 20 individual foods that are major food sources of fat and saturated fat in the U.S. diet. Its initial evaluation showed high correlations with dietary records [255]. In additional cross-sectional studies, the MEDFICTS underestimated percentage calories from fat; it was effective in identifying very high-fat intakes but was not effective in identifying moderately high-fat diets [256] or correctly identifying low-fat diets [257]. The number of mixtures reported on an FFQ (e.g., pizza and macaroni and cheese), which were not specifically included in the MEDFICTS tool, was negatively related to its predictive ability [257]. In a longitudinal setting, positive changes in the MEDFICTS score have been correlated with improvements in serum lipids and waist circumference among cardiac rehabilitation patients [258]. In a large ethnically diverse population, MEDFICTS and the Block Health Habits and History Questionnaire, a food frequency questionnaire, were poorly correlated. Although the accuracy of MEDFICTS differed little among age or race/ethnicity groups, its specificity to correctly identify nonadherence to the prescribed diet was significantly worse for women than for men [259].

Other fat screeners have been developed to preserve the between-person variability of intake [260–262]—that is, to focus on the fat sources that most distinguish differences in fat intake among individuals or groups. A 20-item screener developed and tested at the German site of EPIC correlated with 7-day dietary records ($r = 0.84$) and a complete FFQ ($r = 0.82$) [260,261]. A 16-item percentage energy from fat screener had a correlation of 0.6 with 24-hour recalls in an older U.S. population [262]. However, its performance in intervention studies of adults was variable [263].

Often, dietary fat reduction interventions are designed to target specific food preparation or consumption behaviors rather than frequency of consuming specific foods. Such behaviors might include trimming the fat from red meats, removing the skin from chicken, or choosing low-fat dairy products. Many questionnaires have been developed in various populations to measure these types of dietary behaviors [252,264–271], and many have been found to correlate with fat intake estimated from other more detailed dietary instruments [272,273] or with blood lipids [268,274,275]. In addition, some studies have found that changes in dietary behavior scores have correlated with changes in blood lipids [269,274,276]. The Kristal Food Habits Questionnaire, also called the Eating Behaviors Questionnaire, was originally developed in 1990 [277]. It measures five dimensions of fat-related behavior: avoid fat as a spread or flavoring, substitute low-fat foods, modify meats, replace high-fat foods with fruits and vegetables, and replace high-fat foods with lower fat alternatives. The instrument has been updated and modified for use in different settings and populations [275,278,279]. A modification tested in African American adolescent girls had a relatively low correlation ($r = 0.31$) with multiple 24-hour recalls [280]. In another modification developed for African American women [281], a subset of 30 items from the SisterTalk Food Habits Questionnaire correlated with change in BMI ($r = -0.35$) as strongly as did the original 91 items ($r = -0.36$) [282].

3 Brief Multifactor Instruments

Recognizing the utility of assessing a few dimensions of diet simultaneously, several multifactor short instruments have been developed and evaluated, often combining fruits and vegetables with dietary fiber and/or fat components [16,283–287]. Others assess additional components of the diet. For example, Prime-Screen is composed of 18 FFQ items asking about consumption of fruits and vegetables, whole and low-fat dairy products, whole grains, fish and red meat, and sources of saturated and trans fatty acids; 7 items ask about supplement intake. The average correlation with estimates from a full FFQ over 18 food groups was 0.6 and over 13 nutrients was also 0.6 [288]. The 5-Factor Screener used in the 2005 NHIS Cancer Control Supplement assessed fruits and vegetables, fiber, added sugar, calcium, and dairy servings [289], and the dietary screener used in the 2005 CHIS assessed fruits and vegetables and added sugars [290]. The dietary screener administered in the 2009–2010 NHANES included 28 items addressing consumption of fruits and vegetables, whole grains, added sugars, dairy, fiber, calcium, red meats, and processed meats [291]. This screener was also used in the 2010 NHIS Cancer Control Supplement.

Some multicomponent behavioral questionnaires have also been developed. The Kristal Food Habits Questionnaire was expanded not only to measure the five fat factors described previously but also to measure three factors related to fiber: consumption of cereals and grains, consumption of fruits and vegetables, and substitution of high-fiber for low-fiber foods [292]. This fat- and fiber-related eating behavior questionnaire correlated with food frequency measures of percentage energy from fat (0.53) and fiber (0.50) among participants from a health maintenance organization in Seattle, Washington [292]. Schlundt et al. [293] developed a 51-item Eating Behavior Patterns Questionnaire targeted at assessing fat and fiber consumption among African American women. Newly incorporated in this

questionnaire were questions to reflect emotional eating and impulsive snacking.

Some instruments combine aspects of food frequency and behavioral questions to assess multiple dietary patterns. For example, the Rapid Eating and Activity Assessment for Patients is composed of 27 items assessing consumption of whole grains, calcium-rich foods, fruits and vegetables, fats, sugary beverages and foods, sodium, and alcohol. When compared to dietary records, correlations were 0.49 with the Healthy Eating Index (HEI) [294], a measure of overall diet quality, and moderately high (range of $r = 0.33 - 0.55$) for HEI subscores of fat, saturated fat, cholesterol, fruit, and meats. Correlations for other HEI subscores for sodium, grains, vegetables, and dairy products were low (range of $r = 0.03 - 0.27$) [295].

Because the cognitive processes for answering food frequency-type questions can be complex, some attempts have been made to reduce the respondent burden by creating brief instruments with questions that require only "yes–no" answers. Kristal et al. [296] developed another questionnaire to assess total fat, saturated fat, fiber, and percentage energy from fat that is composed of 44 food items for which respondents are asked whether they eat the items at a specified frequency. A simple index based on the number of "yes" responses was found to correlate well with diet as measured by 4-day dietary records and with FFQs assessing total diet [296]. This same "yes–no" approach to questioning for a food list has also been used as a modification of the 24-hour recall [297]. These "targeted" 24-hour recall instruments aim to assess particular foods, not the whole diet [67,298–300]. They present a precoded close-ended food list and ask whether the respondent ate each food on the previous day; portion size questions may also be asked. For example, a web-administered checklist has been developed to measure the Dietary Approaches to a Stop Hypertension diet. It includes a listing of foods grouped into 11 categories, and it includes serving size information [301].

4 Limitations of Brief Instruments

The brevity of these instruments and their correspondence with dietary intake as estimated by more extensive methods create a seductive option for investigators who would like to measure dietary intake at a low cost. Although brief instruments have many applications, they have several limitations. First, they do not capture information about the entire diet. Most measures are not quantitatively meaningful and, therefore, estimates of dietary intake for the population usually cannot be made. Even when measures aim to provide estimates of total intake, the estimates are not precise and have large measurement error. Finally, the specific dietary behaviors found to correlate with dietary intake in a particular population may not correlate similarly in another population or even in the same population at another time period. For example, behavioral questionnaires developed and tested in middle-class, middle-aged U.S. women [277] were found to perform very differently when applied to Canadian male manual laborers [302], to a low-income, low-education adult Canadian population [303], and to participants in a worksite intervention program in Nevada [304]. Similarly, a screener developed to assess fast-food and beverage consumption in a primarily white, adolescent population [305] was not useful in an overweight Latina adolescent population [306]. Investigators should carefully consider the needs of their study and their own population's dietary patterns before choosing an "off-the-shelf" instrument designed to briefly measure either food frequency or specific dietary behaviors.

E Diet History

The term *diet history* is used in many ways. In the most general sense, a dietary history is any dietary assessment that asks the respondent to report about past diet. Originally, as coined by Burke, the term *dietary history* referred to the collection of information not only about the frequency of intake of various foods but also about the typical makeup of meals [307,308]. Many now imprecisely use the term dietary history to refer to the food frequency method of dietary assessment. However, several investigators have developed diet history instruments that provide information about usual food intake patterns beyond simply food frequency data [309–312]. Some of these instruments characterize foods in much more detail than is allowed in food frequency lists (e.g., preparation methods and foods eaten in combination), and some of these instruments ask about foods consumed at every meal [311,313]. The term diet history is therefore probably best reserved for dietary assessment methods that are designed to ascertain a person's usual food intake in which many details about characteristics of foods as usually consumed are assessed in addition to the frequency and amount of food intake.

The Burke diet history included three elements: a detailed interview about usual pattern of eating, a food list asking for amount and frequency usually eaten, and a 3-day dietary record [307,308]. The detailed interview (which sometimes includes a 24-hour recall) is the central feature of the Burke dietary history, with the food frequency checklist and the 3-day diet record used as cross-checks of the history. The original Burke diet history, which requires administration by an interviewer, has not often been exactly reproduced because of the effort and expertise involved in capturing and coding the information. However, many variations of the Burke method have been developed and used in a variety of settings [309–312,314–318]. These variations attempt to ascertain the usual eating patterns for an extended period of time, including type, frequency, and amount of foods consumed; many include a cross-check feature [319,320].

Some diet history instruments have been automated and adapted for self-administration, sometimes with audio, thus eliminating the need for an interviewer to ask the questions [31,311,321]. Other diet histories have been automated but still continue to be administered by an interviewer [322,323]. Short-term recalls or records are often used for validation or calibration rather than as a part of the tool.

The major strength of the diet history method is its assessment of meal patterns and details of food intake rather than intakes for a short period of time (as in records or recalls) or only frequency of food consumption. Details of the means of preparation of foods can be helpful in better characterizing nutrient intake (e.g., frying vs. baking), as well as exposure to other factors in foods (e.g., charcoal broiling). When the information is collected separately for each meal, analyses of the joint effects of foods eaten together are possible (e.g., effects on iron absorption of concurrent intake of tea or foods containing vitamin C). Although a meal-based approach often requires more time from the respondent than does a food-based approach, it may provide more cognitive support for the recall process. For example, the respondent may be better able to report total bread consumption by reporting bread as consumed at each meal.

A weakness of the approach is that respondents are asked to make many judgments about both the usual foods consumed and the amounts of those foods eaten. These subjective tasks may be difficult for many respondents. Burke cautioned that nutrient intakes estimated from these data should be interpreted as relative rather than absolute. All of these limitations are also shared with the food frequency method. The meal-based approach is not useful for individuals who have no particular eating pattern and may be of limited use for individuals who "graze" (i.e., eat throughout the day rather than at defined mealtimes). The approach, when conducted by interviewers, requires trained nutrition professionals and is thus costly. Finally, the diet history as a method is not well standardized, and thus methods differ from each other and are difficult to reproduce, making comparisons across studies difficult.

Relative to other assessment approaches, few validation studies of diet history questionnaires using biological markers as a basis of comparison have been conducted. The studies found that reported mean energy intakes using the diet history approach in selected small samples of adults were underestimated in the range of 2−23% compared to energy expenditure as measured by doubly labeled water [324−327]. Generally, underreporting of protein, compared to urinary nitrogen, was less than that for energy and only sometimes significantly different [325,327−329]. These results have also been seen in children [330], adolescents [331,332], and the elderly [310]. Because of small sample sizes in these studies, few were able to examine characteristics related to underreporting, and their results were mixed, with some finding more underreporting with higher BMI [329,330] and others finding no relationship [310,326,333]. Although the diet history approach was extensively used as the main study instrument in European cohorts initiated in the 1990s, the approach is seldom used now in new cohort studies as other approaches have evolved. The approach is sometimes used as a reference instrument [334−336].

F Blended Instruments

Better understanding of various instruments' strengths and weaknesses has led to creative blending of approaches with the goal of maximizing the strengths of each instrument. For example, a record-assisted 24-hour recall has been used in several studies with children [337,338]. The child keeps notes of what he or she has eaten and then uses these notes as memory prompts in a later 24-hour recall. Several researchers have combined elements of a 24-hour recall and FFQ, often to assess specific dietary components. For example, in one assessment of fruits and vegetables, a limited set of questions is asked about the previous day's intake and the information is combined with usual frequency of consumption of common fruits and vegetables [17,339]. Similarly, the Nutritionist Five Collection Form combines a 2-day dietary recall with food frequency questions [340]. Thompson et al. [341] combined information from a series of daily checklists (i.e., precoded record) with frequency reports from an FFQ to form checklist-adjusted estimates of intake. In a validation study of this approach, validity improved for energy and protein but was unchanged for protein density [341].

A recent advance is the development of statistical methods that seek to better estimate usual intake of episodically consumed foods. A two-part statistical model developed by NCI uses information from two or more 24-hour recalls, allowing for the inclusion of daily frequency estimates derived from a food propensity questionnaire (a frequency questionnaire that does not ask about portion size), as well as other potentially contributing characteristics (e.g., age and race/ethnicity), as covariates [342]. Frequency information contributes to the model by providing additional information about an individual's propensity to consume a food—information not available from only a few recalls. The recalls, however, provide information about the nature and amount of the food consumed. A similar approach has been used in EPIC, which combined information from two non-consecutive 24-hour recalls with a food propensity questionnaire to identify those who do not consume each food [100]. Such methods are used to better measure usual intakes (see Section V.G).

Another statistical advance is the demonstration of enhanced accuracy and statistical power of combining 24-hour recall reports and biomarkers to estimate associations between diet and disease [343]. Carroll et al. [222] explored the number of days of 24-hour recall required to estimate associations between diet and disease in a cohort study and whether an FFQ, in addition, is beneficial. They concluded that for most nutrients and foods, 4 non-consecutive days of 24-hour recall report is optimal. The combination of FFQ and multiple 24-hour recalls was superior in estimating some nutrients and foods, especially for episodically consumed foods.

Developing hybrid instruments as well as developing new analytical techniques that combine information from different assessment methods may hold great promise for furthering our ability to accurately assess diets.

Table 1.1 summarizes the important characteristics of the main self-report dietary assessment methods.

III DIETARY ASSESSMENT IN DIFFERENT STUDY DESIGNS

The choice of the most appropriate dietary assessment method for a specific research question requires careful consideration. The primary research question must be clearly formed, and questions of secondary interest should be recognized as such. Projects can fail to achieve their primary goal because of too much attention to secondary goals. The choice of the most appropriate dietary assessment tool depends on many factors. Questions that must be answered in evaluating which dietary assessment tool is most appropriate for a particular research need include the following [195]: (1) Is information needed about foods, nutrients, other food components, or specific dietary behaviors? (2) Is the focus of the research question on describing intakes using estimates of average intake, and does it also require distributional information? (3) Is the focus of the research question on describing relationships between diet and health outcomes? (4) Is absolute or

TABLE 1.1 Comparison of Self-Report Dietary Assessment Methods by Important Characteristics

	Dietary record	24-hour recall	FFQ	Diet history	Screener
Type of information attainable					
Detailed information about foods consumed	X	X		X	
General information about food groups consumed			X		X
Meal-specific details	X	X		X	
Scope of information sought					
Total diet	X	X	X	X	
Specific components					X
Time frame asked					
Short term (e.g., yesterday, today)	X	X		X	
Long term (e.g., last month, last year)			X	X	X
Adaptable for diet in distant past					
Yes			X	X	X
No	X	X			
Cognitive requirements					
Measurement or estimated recording of foods and drinks as they are consumed	X				
Memory of recent consumption		X		X	
Ability to make judgments of long-term diet			X	X	X
Potential for reactivity					
High	X				
Low		X	X	X	X
Time required to complete					
<15 minutes					X
>20 minutes	X	X	X	X	
Suitable for cross-cultural comparisons without instrument adaptation					
Yes	X	X		X	
No			X	X	X

relative intake needed? (5) What level of accuracy and precision is needed? (6) What time period is of interest? (7) What are the research constraints in terms of money, interview time, staff, and respondent characteristics?

A Cross-Sectional Surveys

One of the most common types of population-level studies is the cross-sectional survey, a set of measurements of a population at a particular point in time. Such data can be collected solely to describe a particular population's intake. Alternatively, data can be used for surveillance at the national, state, and local levels as the basis for assessing risk of deficiency, toxicity, and overconsumption; to evaluate adherence to dietary guidelines and public health programs; and to develop food and nutrition policy. Cross-sectional data also may be used for examining associations between current diet and other factors including health. However, caution must be applied in examining many chronic diseases believed to be associated with past diet because the currently measured diet is not necessarily

related to past diet. Any of the dietary instruments discussed in this chapter can be used in cross-sectional studies. Some of the instruments, such as the 24-hour recall, are appropriate when the study purpose requires quantitative estimates of intake. Others, such as FFQs or behavioral indicators, are appropriate when qualitative estimates are sufficient—for example, frequency of consuming soda and frequency of eating from fast-food restaurants.

When measurements are collected on a sample at two or more times, the data can be used for purposes of monitoring dietary trends. To assess trends in intakes over time, it would be ideal for the dietary surveillance data collection methods, sampling procedures, and food composition databases to be similar from survey to survey. As a practical matter, however, this is difficult, and the benefits of trend analysis may not outweigh the benefits of improving the methods over time. The dietary assessment method used consistently throughout the years in U.S. national dietary surveillance is the interviewer-administered 24-hour recall. However, recall methodology has improved over time based on cognitive research, the addition of multiple interviewing passes, standardization of probes, automation of the interview, and automation of the coding.

Another issue that affects the assessment of trends over time is changes in the nutrient or food grouping databases and specification of default foods. Changes in the food supply are reflected in additions or subtractions to food composition databases, whereas changes in consumption trends may lead to subsequent reassignment of default codes for foods not fully specified in 24-hour recalls or records (e.g., when type of milk is not specified, the default code is now 2% milk as opposed to whole milk in the past). Food composition databases, too, are modified over time because of true changes in food composition, improved analytic methods for particular nutrients, or inclusion of information for new dietary components. Reflecting true changes over time is especially beneficial in trend analysis.

Since 1999, the major cross-sectional surveillance survey in the United States has been the NHANES [344]. This survey is conducted by the National Center for Health Statistics. The dietary component of the survey, called "What We Eat in America" [71], consists of 24-hour recalls collected using the USDA's AMPM (see Section II.B). The USDA also processes and analyzes the data. The 24-hour recalls in NHANES query the intake of dietary supplements as well as foods and beverages. In NHANES 2003–2004, 2005–2006, 2007–2008, and 2009–2010, two 24-hour dietary recalls were conducted, allowing for estimation not only of average usual intake but also of the distributions of usual intake of the dietary components (see Section V.G).

NHANES provides high-quality dietary intake data at the national level, but these data are of limited use for state and local researchers planning and evaluating their programs and policies [345]. Collection of state and local data is often constrained by lack of resources or interview time, leading to the frequent use of less expensive brief instruments. For example, the CDC has used telephone-administered screeners to periodically assess fruit and vegetable intake within the BRFSS [249]. The California Department of Public Health, in its California Dietary Practices Survey, has assessed dietary practices among adults biennially since 1989 [346]. The California Health Interview Survey used telephone-administered screeners to assess fruit and vegetable intake in 2001, 2005, and 2009 [228].

B Case–Control (Retrospective) Studies

A case–control study design classifies individuals with regard to current disease status (as cases or controls) and relates this to past (retrospective) exposures. For dietary exposure, the period of interest could be either the recent past (e.g., the year before diagnosis) or the distant past (e.g., 10 years ago or in childhood). Because of the need for information about diet before the onset of disease, dietary assessment methods that focus on current behavior, such as the 24-hour recall, are not useful in retrospective studies. The food frequency and diet history methods are well suited for assessing past diet and are therefore the only viable choices for case–control (retrospective) studies.

In any food frequency or diet history interview, the respondent is not asked to recall specific memories of each eating occasion but, rather, to respond on the basis of general perceptions of how frequently he or she ate a food. In case–control studies, the relevant period is often the year before the diagnosis of a disease or onset of symptoms or at particular life stages, such as adolescence and childhood. Thus, in assessing past diet, an additional requirement is to orient the respondent to the appropriate period.

The validity of recalled diet from the distant past is difficult to assess because definitive recovery biomarker information (doubly labeled water or urinary nitrogen) is not available for large samples from long ago. Instead, relative validity and long-term reproducibility of various FFQs have been assessed in various populations by asking participants from past dietary studies to recall their diet from that earlier time [347,348]. These studies have found that correlations between past and current reports about the past vary by nutrient and by food group [111,349], with higher correspondence for very frequently consumed and rarely consumed foods compared to that for foods consumed moderately often [349,350]. Evidence suggests that correspondence between past and recalled past decreases with the length of time between reports [347]. In particular, retrospective reports of diet in adolescence after long recall periods (i.e., >30 years) have shown little correspondence with the original reports [351]. Maternal reports about diets of their children in early childhood or adolescence have also shown low correspondence with the original reports [352,353].

Correspondence of retrospective diet reports with the diet as measured in the original study has usually been greater than the correspondence of current diet with past diet. This observation implies that if diet from years in the past is of interest, it is usually preferable to ask respondents to recall it than to simply consider current diet as a proxy for past diet. Nonetheless, the current diets of respondents may affect their retrospective reports about past diets. In particular, retrospective diet reports from seriously ill individuals may be biased by recent dietary changes [347,354]. Studies of groups in whom diet was previously measured indicate no consistent differences in the accuracy of retrospective reporting between those who recently became ill and others [355,356].

C Cohort (Prospective) Studies

In a cohort study design, exposures of interest are assessed at baseline in a group (cohort) of people and disease outcomes occurring over time (prospectively) are then related to the baseline exposure levels. In prospective dietary studies, dietary status at baseline is measured and related to later incidence of disease. For many chronic diseases, large numbers of individuals need to be followed for years before enough new cases with that disease accrue for statistical analyses. A broad assessment of diet is usually desirable in prospective studies because many dietary exposures and many disease end points will ultimately be investigated and areas of interest may not even be recognized at the beginning of a cohort study.

In order to relate diet at baseline to the eventual occurrence of disease, a measure of the usual intake of foods (see Section V.G) by study subjects is needed. Although a single 24-hour recall or a dietary record for a single day would not adequately characterize the usual diet of individual study subjects in a cohort study, such information could be later analyzed at the group level for contrasting the average dietary intakes of subsequent cases with those who did not acquire the disease. Typically, researchers are interested in estimating additional parameters, and therefore, 24-hour recalls or dietary records, if used, may require multiple administrations. Multiple dietary recalls, multiple records, diet histories, and food frequency methods have all been used effectively in prospective studies. Cost and logistic issues tend to favor food frequency methods because many prospective studies require thousands of respondents. However, because of concern about significant measurement error and attenuation attributed to the FFQ [217,220,221,357−360], other approaches are being considered. One approach is the use of automated self-administered 24-hour recall instruments (see Section II.B). Another approach is collecting multiple days of dietary records at baseline, with later coding and analysis of records for those respondents selected for analysis, using a nested case−control design [361,362]. Incorporating emerging technological advances in administering dietary records, such as using mobile phones, increases the feasibility of such approaches in prospective studies.

If using an FFQ in the cohort, it is desirable to include multiple recalls or records in subsamples of the population (preferably before beginning the study) to construct or modify the food frequency instrument and to calibrate it (see Section V.B). Information on the foods consumed could be used to ensure that the questionnaire includes the major food sources of key nutrients, with appropriate portion size categories. Because the diets of individuals change over time, it is desirable to measure diet throughout the follow-up period rather than just at baseline. If diet is measured repeatedly over years, repeated calibration is also desirable. Information from calibration studies can be used for three purposes: to give design information, such as the sample size needed [197]; to relate values from the food frequency tool (or a brief food list thus derived) to values from the recalls/records [214]; and to determine the degree of attenuation/measurement error in the estimates of association observed in the study (e.g., between diet and disease) [209,212,214,216,363−367] (see Section V.B).

D Intervention Studies

Intervention studies range from relatively small, highly controlled, clinical studies of targeted participants to large trials of population groups. Intervention studies may use dietary assessment for two purposes: (1) initial screening for inclusion (or exclusion) into the study and (2) measurement of dietary changes resulting from the intervention. Not all intervention trials require initial screening. For those that do, screening can be performed using very detailed instruments or less burdensome instruments. For example, food frequency instruments were used in the Women's Health Trial [251] and in the Women's Health Initiative Dietary Modification Trial [368] to identify groups with high fat intake and thus determine eligibility.

The need for careful planning and formative research in designing useful community intervention trials has been described [369]. A critical element is the existence of evidence that a particular intervention would create a measureable change in a particular group and setting. Measurement of the effects of a dietary intervention requires a valid measure of change from baseline to the conclusion of the intervention period. Often, post-intervention diet is also measured to assess the durability of any dietary change. Some work has been done to examine the validity of methods to measure dietary change in individuals or in populations [279,370]. Researchers have found that dietary records and scheduled 24-hour recalls were associated with changed eating behavior during the recording days and had less correspondence with biological measures [371], expected weight change [372], and increased underreporting [373]. One study using dietary screeners and a reference measure of multiple non-consecutive unannounced 24-hour recalls found that the change in fruit and vegetable intake was overestimated relative to the control group [248]; however, in the same study, the screener and the 24-hour recalls were consistent in finding no change in percentage energy from fat in the two groups [374]. Because of resource constraints, large intervention studies have often relied on less precise measures of diet, including FFQs and brief instruments. However, resource constraints may be less relevant with the availability of automated self-administered 24-hour recall instruments and less burdensome dietary records.

Intentional behavior change is a complex and sequential phenomenon, as has been shown for tobacco cessation [375], and this is also true for dietary change [376]. Measurement of specific dietary behaviors in addition to, or even in place of, dietary intake could be considered in intervention evaluations when the nature of the intervention involves education about specific behaviors. If, for instance, a community-wide campaign to choose low-fat dairy products were to be evaluated, food selection and shopping behaviors specific to choosing those items could be measured. The effects of educational interventions might also be assessed by measuring knowledge, attitudes, beliefs, barriers, and perceptions of readiness for dietary change, although the reliability of these types of questions has not been well assessed.

Whether an intervention is targeting individuals or the entire population, repeated measures of diet among study subjects can reflect reporting bias in the direction of the change being promoted [370]. Although not intending to be deceptive, some respondents may tend to report what they think investigators want to hear. Social desirability [377] and social approval [378] biases can be measured and the resulting scales incorporated into intervention analyses. Because of their greater subjectivity, behavioral questions, screeners, and the food frequency method may be more susceptible to social desirability biases than the 24-hour recall method [69,225]. On the other hand, greater awareness of diet and enhanced reporting skills because of the intervention may enhance the accuracy of reports [379]. Dietary records and scheduled 24-hour recalls are vulnerable to reactivity. If assessment is by 24-hour recalls, unannounced administration would avoid reactivity but possibly at the expense of participation. Because self-reports of diet are subject to bias in the context of an intervention study [370], an independent assessment of dietary change should be considered. For example, food availability and/or sales in worksite cafeterias, school cafeterias, or vending machines could be monitored. One such method useful in community-wide interventions is monitoring food sales [380]. Often, cooperation can be obtained from food retailers [381]. However, because the number of food items may be large, it may be possible to monitor only a small number, and the large effects on sales of day-to-day

pricing fluctuations should be carefully considered. Another method to consider is measuring changes in biomarkers of diet, such as serum carotenoids [379,382] or serum cholesterol [383], in the population. Consistency of changes in self-reported diet and appropriate biomarkers provides further evidence for real changes in the diet. See Chapters 10 and 11 for more in-depth discussions of the evaluation of diet in nutrition interventions and use of biomarkers in intervention studies respectively.

Table 1.2 summarizes the dietary methods commonly used in different study designs.

IV DIETARY ASSESSMENT IN SPECIAL POPULATIONS

A Respondents Unable to Self-Report

In many situations, respondents are unavailable or unable to report about their diets. For example, in case—control studies, surrogate reports may be obtained for cases who have died or who are too ill to interview. Although the accuracy of surrogate reports has not been examined using the reference biomarkers of doubly labeled water or urinary nitrogen, the comparability of reports by surrogates and subjects has been studied with the goal that surrogate information might be used interchangeably with information provided by subjects [384]. Common sense indicates that individuals who know most about a subject's lifestyle would make the best surrogate reporters [385]. Adult siblings provide the best information about a subject's early life, and spouses or children provide the best information about a subject's adult life. When food frequency instruments are used, the level of agreement between subject and surrogate reports of diet varies with the food and possibly with other variables, such as number of shared meals, interview situation, case status, and sex of the surrogate reporter. Mean frequencies of use computed for individual foods and food groups between surrogate reporters and subject

TABLE 1.2 Dietary Assessment Methods Commonly Used in Different Study Designs

Study design	Methods
Cross-sectional	24-Hour recall, FFQ, brief instruments
Case—control (retrospective)	FFQ, diet history
Cohort (prospective)	FFQ, diet history, 24-hour recall, dietary record
Intervention	FFQ, brief instruments, 24-hour recall

reporters tend to be similar [386–388], but agreement is much lower when detailed categories of frequency are compared. Several studies have shown that agreement is better for alcoholic beverages, coffee, and tea than for foods.

When subjects themselves report intakes in the extremes of a distribution, their surrogates seldom report intakes in the opposite extreme, although the surrogates tend to report intakes in the middle of the distribution [389]. This may limit the usefulness of surrogate information for individual-level analyses that rely on proper ranking. Furthermore, the quality of surrogate reports between spouses of deceased subjects and spouses of surviving subjects may differ substantially [390]. Thus far, however, little evidence suggests that dietary intakes are systematically overreported or underreported depending on the case status of the subject [391–393]. Nonetheless, use of surrogate respondents should be minimized for obtaining dietary information in analytical studies. When used, analyses excluding the surrogate reports should be done to examine the sensitivity of the reported associations to possible errors or biases in the surrogate reports. If planning a study using surrogate reports, the sample size should be inflated to account for a higher incidence of missing data, the inability to recruit surrogates for some number of cases, and the reduced precision of dietary estimates.

B Ethnic Populations

The widespread use of many ethnic foods in the United States throughout the population and the increasing diversity of the population have broadened the food composition databases and food lists used for the general population. Nonetheless, special modifications may be needed in the content of dietary assessment methods when the study population is composed of individuals whose cuisine or cooking practices are not mainstream [394]. If the method requires an interview, interviewers of the same ethnic or cultural background are preferable so that dietary information can be more effectively communicated. If dietary information is to be quantified into nutrient estimates, examination of the nutrient composition database is necessary to ascertain whether ethnic foods are included and whether those foods and their various preparation methods represent those consumed by the target population [395]. It is also necessary to examine the recipes and assumptions underlying the nutrient composition of certain ethnic foods. Some very different foods may be called the same name, or identical foods may be called by different names [396,397]. For these reasons, it may be necessary to obtain detailed recipe information for all ethnic mixtures reported.

To examine the suitability of the initial database, preliminary information about typical diets should be collected from individuals in the ethnic groups. This information could come from recalls or records with accompanying interviews or from focus group interviews. These interviews should focus on the foods eaten and the ways in which foods are prepared in that culture. Recipes and alternative names of the same food should be collected, and field interviewers should be familiarized with the results of these focus groups. Recipes and food names that are relatively uniform should be included in the nutrient composition database. Even with these modifications, it may be preferable for the field interviewers to collect detailed descriptions of ethnic foods reported rather than to directly code these foods using preselected lists most common in computer-assisted methods. This would prevent the detail of food choice and preparation from being lost by a priori coding.

USDA continues to incorporate new foods into the National Nutrient Database for Standard Reference (SR) (see Section V.E). For example, approximately 200 foods identified as Native American or Alaskan Native have been incorporated into the SR24 and also are available in the University of Minnesota Nutrient Database System. If a newly reported food is not available in the food composition database being used, a default code that is thought to closely mirror the nutrient composition of the new food can be used.

Use of FFQs developed for the majority population may be suboptimal for many individuals with ethnic eating patterns. Many members of ethnic groups consume both foods common in the mainstream culture and foods that are specific to their own ethnic group. Modification of the existing food list can be accomplished through expert judgment, qualitative interviews with the target population, and/or examination of the frequency of reported foods in the population from a set of dietary records or recalls. FFQs for Navajos [398], Alaska Natives [399], Chinese Americans [400], individuals in northern India [401], Hispanics [146,402], Israelis [403], and African Americans in the southern United States [404] have been developed using these approaches.

In addition to the food list, however, there are other important issues to consider when adapting existing FFQs for use in other populations. The relative intake of different foods within a food group line item may differ, thus requiring a change in the nutrient database associated with each line item. For example, Latino populations may consume more tropical fruit nectars and less apple and grape juice than the general U.S. population and therefore would require a different nutrient composition standard for juices. In addition, the portion sizes generally used may differ [405]. For example, rice may be consumed in larger quantities in Latino and Asian populations; the amount attributed to a large portion for the general population may be substantially lower than the amount typically consumed by Latino and Asian populations. Adaptation of an existing FFQ considering all of these factors has been done for an elderly Puerto Rican population [406], for white and African American adults in the Lower Mississippi Delta [407], and for the Hawaii–Los Angeles Multiethnic Cohort Study [408]. The Southern Community Cohort Study incorporated both race/ethnicity and geographic region into its FFQ database [409].

With some ethnic populations, it may be preferable to administer an FFQ using an interviewer rather than self-administration because literacy and language barriers may limit participation in the study as well as quality of response. In addition, portion size models, which interviewers can bring to a home interview, may be preferable to portion size pictures available in a self-administered instrument [399].

The NCI Dietary Calibration/Validation Studies Register [199] can be used to search for studies using FFQs in specific race/ethnicity groups. Performance of FFQs varies across ethnic groups [410]. Questionnaires aimed at allowing comparison of intakes across multiple cultures have been developed. Although some studies have found no appreciable validity differences across various race/ethnicity groups [259], most have found validity differences [145,406,408,411–413]. Understanding these validity differences is crucial to the appropriate interpretation of study results.

C Children

Assessing the diets of children is considered to be even more challenging than assessing the diets of adults. Children tend to have diets that are highly variable from day to day, and their food habits can change rapidly. Younger children are less able to recall, estimate, and cooperate in usual dietary assessment procedures; so much information by necessity has to be obtained by surrogate reporters. Although they are more able to report, adolescents may be less interested in giving accurate reports. Baranowski and Domel [414] have posited a cognitive model of how children report dietary information.

Dietary assessment in children and adolescents has been discussed and reviewed [415–422]. The 24-hour recall, dietary records (including precoded checklists [10]), dietary histories, FFQs, brief instruments [423–425], and blended instruments such as a dietary record-assisted 24-hour recall [337] have all been used to assess children's intakes. The use of direct observation of children's diets has also been used extensively, most often as a reference

method to compare with self-reported instruments [426,427]. As predicted from Baranowski and Domel's model, it has been found that children's estimates of portion size have large errors [428], and they are less able than adults to estimate portion sizes [429] (see Section V.D). Overall, the consensus seems to be that the characteristics of different age groups call for the use of different assessment approaches.

For preschool-aged children, information is obtained from surrogates, usually the primary caretaker(s), who may typically be a parent or an external caregiver. If information is obtained only from one surrogate reporter, the reports are likely to be less complete. Even for periods when the caregiver and child are together, foods tend to be underestimated [430]. A "consensus" recall method, in which the child and parents report as a group on a 24-hour recall, has been shown to give more accurate information than a recall from either parent or child alone [431]. Sobo and Rock [432] describe such interviews and suggest tips for interviewers to maximize data accuracy.

For older children, extensive research has been conducted on the 24-hour recall approach [433]. Baxter et al. [434] found that among fourth graders, 24-hour recall improves as the time between reporting and eating decreases, and meal-specific intrusions (i.e., reports of foods not consumed) are fewer in an open format interview than in a time-forward format interview (i.e., beginning at the earliest meal in the time period and working forward to the next meal). These intrusions are often associated with additional intrusions at the same meal [434]. Because accuracy of recall is greater when the time between eating and reporting is shorter, there will be differential error by meal; meals further away (e.g., at the beginning of the 24-hour recall period) will have substantially more error [435,436].

To make 24-hour recalls more feasible, self-administered automated 24-hour recall tools have been developed and tested for children [85]. An interviewer-administered 24-hour recall and a self-administered 24-hour recall using the Food Intake Recording Software System (FIRSSt) were compared to unobtrusive observations in fourth graders. Compared to observed intake, the interviewer-administered 24-hour recall was associated with a 59% match, 17% intrusion, and 24% omission rates, whereas the automated recall was associated with a 46% match, 24% intrusion, and 30% omission rates [85]. Baranowski et al. are developing a second-generation version of the FIRSSt with tailored food lists and prompts [437,438].

Other self-administered web-based tools have been developed for school-age children and adolescents. The Web-Span, developed in Canada, includes a dietary component [439,440] and has been used in school-age children and adolescents in school. When two non-consecutive days of Web-SPAN were compared with 3-day records, reported energy intake was significantly higher on the Web-SPAN than on the records; correlations between the two methods ranged from 0.24 to 0.40 [440]. The Synchronized Nutrition and Activity Program (SNAP), a web-based program, directs children to report the previous day's food intake by ticking the number of times they consumed each of 40 foods and nine drinks. However, compared to a 24-hour recall for the same period, SNAP generally underestimated counts of the foods assessed, and the accuracy decreased with increasing counts [441].

New technology has also been incorporated into other dietary assessment approaches. Williamson *et al.* [442] developed and tested digital photography in school cafeterias. This observation method consists of standardized photography of the food selected before the meal and the plate waste following the meal. Using reference portions of measured quantities of the foods, expert judgment is used to estimate the amount of each food consumed [442].

Another approach that has been taken with school-age children is a blended instrument, the record assisted 24-hour recall, in which the children record only the names of foods and beverages consumed throughout a 24-hour period. This information serves as a cue for the later 24-hour recall interview. The European Food Consumption Validation Project, a consortium of 13 institutes from 11 European countries, provisionally recommended a similar approach—a food recording booklet for foods eaten away from home—for schoolchildren 7–14 years old. Studies examining the validity of this approach have had mixed results [337,338,443].

Adaptation of food frequency instruments originally developed for adults requires consideration of the instrument itself (food list, question wording and format, and portion size categories) and the database for converting responses to nutrient intakes. Food frequency instruments, some web administered, have been developed and tested for use in child and adolescent populations [7,184,444–446]. A web-based food behavioral questionnaire underestimated the intake of middle-school children compared to a multiple-pass 24-hour recall [447]. Generally, correlations between food frequency type instruments and more precise reference instruments have been lower in child and adolescent populations than in adult populations. New technology-based methods, such as disposable cameras, mobile phones with cameras [28], and smart phones, are being developed for collecting records and may be particularly useful among adolescents, who prefer these methods to traditional methods [448].

For school-age children and adolescents, there is no consensus of which dietary assessment method is most accurate. The choice of which instrument to use may depend on the study objectives and study design factors, all of which will influence the appropriateness and feasibility of different approaches [449].

D Elderly

Measuring diets among the elderly can, but does not necessarily, present special challenges [450–452]. Both recall and food frequency techniques are inappropriate if memory or cognitive functioning is impaired. Similarly, self-administered tools may be inappropriate if physical disabilities such as poor vision are present. Interviewer administration is difficult when hearing problems are present [452]. Direct observation in institutional care facilities [450] or shelf inventories for elders who live at home can be useful. Even when cognitive integrity is not impaired, several factors can affect the assessment of diet among the elderly. Because of the frequency of chronic illness in this age group, it is more probable that special diets (e.g., low sodium, low fat, and high fiber) would have been recommended. Such recommendations could not only affect actual dietary intake but also bias reporting because individuals may report what they should eat rather than what they do eat. Alternatively, respondents on special diets may be more aware of their diets and may more accurately report them. When dentition is poor, the interviewer should probe regarding foods that are prepared or consumed in different ways. Relative to other age groups, the elderly are more apt to take multiple types of nutritional supplements [453], which present special problems in dietary assessment (see Chapter 2). Because of the concern of malnutrition among the elderly, specific instruments to detect risk of malnutrition, such as the Nutrition Screening Initiative in the United States [454,455], the Australian Nutrition Screening Initiative [456], the Mini Nutritional Assessment [457], the Geriatric Nutritional Risk Index [458], and the Simplified Nutritional Appetite Questionnaire [459], have been developed.

Some researchers have suggested that the short-term memory required for the 24-hour recall may be more difficult for the elderly, who are more adept at long-term memory [450]. However, interviewers conducting a FFQ among elderly respondents noted difficulty in maintaining interest and concentration, whereas these issues were not found during the more engaging 24-hour recall interview [451].

Validation studies using doubly labeled water and/or urinary biomarkers among the elderly are limited [40,460–462]. Generally, energy underreporting has been found to be positively related to elevated BMI and lower education, similar to younger populations.

However, in the NIH-funded Health, Aging, and Body Composition Study cohort, Shahar *et al.* [462] found that a substantial portion of elderly reporters were undereaters, losing more than 2% of their weight over a year.

Adaptations of standard dietary assessment methods have been suggested and evaluated, including using memory strategies, notifying the respondent prior to the dietary interview [463], combining methods [464], and adapting existing instruments [465]. Specific adaptations that have been made in elderly populations include the use of household measures rather than pictures to portray portion size for sight-impaired respondents [451] and tailoring the food list and portion sizes to be characteristic of the elderly rather than all adults in food frequency questionnaires and their related databases [466].

Some have suggested including measures of cognitive function within a study to aid the interpretation of results, but one such study found no relationship between the cognitive functioning score and the validity of a food frequency questionnaire [467].

The variability in functional status among the elderly suggests the need for a flexible approach in assessing dietary intake. Mixed mode design in survey research [468] has certain advantages with regard to enhancing coverage and decreasing nonresponse, but it may cause other biases [469].

Table 1.3 summarizes optimal assessment strategies for special populations.

V SELECTED ISSUES IN DIETARY ASSESSMENT METHODS

A Cognitive Testing Research Related to Dietary Assessment

Nearly all studies using dietary information about subjects rely on the subjects' own reports of their diets. Because such reports are based on complex cognitive processes, it is important to understand and take advantage of what is known about how respondents remember dietary information and how that information is retrieved and reported to the investigator. The need for and importance of such considerations in the assessment of diet has been discussed by several investigators [347,414,470–472], and research using cognitive testing methods in dietary assessment has been reported [12,136,230,246,295,313,471,473–477]. A thorough description of cognitive interviewing methods is found in Willis [478].

Specific and generic memories of diet are distinctly different. Specific memory relies on particular memories about episodes of eating and drinking, whereas

TABLE 1.3 Optimal Strategies for Special Populations

Special population	Optimal strategies
Respondents unable to self-report	Use the best-informed surrogate.
	Analyze the effect of potential bias on study results.
Ethnic populations	Use interviewers of same ethnic background.
	Use nutrient composition database reflective of foods consumed.
	For FFQs, use an appropriate food list and nutrient composition database.
Children	For young children, use caretakers in conjunction with the child.
	For older children and adolescents, blended instrument and other creative ways of engagement and motivation may work best.
	For FFQs, use an appropriate food list and portion size categories.
Elderly	Assess any special considerations, including: memory, special diets, dentition, use of supplements, etc., and adapt methods accordingly.

generic memory relies on general knowledge about typical diet. A 24-hour recall relies primarily on specific memory of all actual events in the very recent past, whereas a FFQ that directs a respondent to report the usual frequency of eating a food during the previous year relies primarily on generic memory. As the time between the behavior and the report increases, respondents may rely more on generic memory and less on specific memory [471].

Investigators can do several things to enhance retrieval and improve reporting of diet. Research indicates that the amount of dietary information retrieved from memory can be enhanced by the context in which the instrument is administered and by use of specific memory cues and probes. For example, for a 24-hour recall, foods that were not initially reported by the respondent can be recovered by interviewer probes. The effectiveness of these probes is well-established and is therefore part of the interviewing protocol for all standardized high-quality 24-hour recalls, including those administered in the NHANES. Probes can be useful in improving generic memory too, when subjects are asked to report their usual diets from periods in the past [347,472]. Such probes can feature questions about past living situations and related eating habits.

The way in which questions are asked can affect responses. Certain characteristics of the interviewing situation may affect the social desirability of particular responses for foods viewed as "good" or "bad." For example, the presence of other family members during the dietary interview may increase social desirability bias, especially for certain items such as alcoholic beverages. An interview in a health setting, such as a clinic, may also increase social desirability bias in reporting about foods that were previously proscribed or recommended in that setting. In all instances, interviewers should be trained to refrain from either positive or negative feedback and should repeatedly encourage subjects to accurately report all foods.

B Validation/Calibration Studies

It is important and desirable that any new dietary assessment method be validated or calibrated against more established methods [213,214,216,479]. Furthermore, even if an instrument has been evaluated, its proposed use in a different population may warrant additional validation research in that population. The purpose of such studies is to better understand how the method works in the particular research setting and to use that information to better interpret results from the overall study. For example, before a new FFQ or brief assessment questionnaire is used in the main study, it should be evaluated in a validation/calibration study that compares the questionnaire to another more detailed dietary assessment method, such as 24-hour recalls or dietary records, obtained from the same individuals and, preferably, to biological markers such as doubly labeled water or urinary nitrogen. The NCI maintains a register of validation/calibration studies and publications on the web [199].

Validation studies yield information about how well the new method is measuring what it is intended to measure, and calibration studies use the same information to relate (calibrate) the new method to a reference method using a regression model. Validation/calibration studies are challenging because of the difficulty and expense in collecting independent dietary information. Some researchers have used observational techniques to establish true dietary intake [109,430,480,481]. Others have used laboratory measures such as the 24-hour urine collection to measure protein, sodium, and potassium intakes and the doubly labeled water technique to measure energy expenditure, using it as a gold standard for energy intake when subjects are in energy balance [39–45,93,154,202,203,205,482,483]. However, the high cost of this latter technique can make it impractical for most studies. The overall validity of energy intake estimates from the dietary assessment can be roughly checked by comparing weight data to reported energy intakes, in conjunction with the use of equations to estimate basal metabolic rate [42,54,57,58,62,64,107,108,482,484,485].

The validation process can address the accuracy of reports for specific foods. Many studies using observers to accurately assess foods and amounts consumed relative to reported intakes have characterized reporting errors as intrusions and exclusions in the foods reported and erroneous portion size reports [486]. The granularity of this misreporting can be used to understand and potentially remedy errors in reporting. NCI will conduct an evaluation of its ASA24 instrument in an observational feeding study to examine food-specific reporting errors.

Because they are relatively expensive to conduct, validation/calibration studies are done on subsamples of the total study sample. However, the subsample should be sufficiently large to estimate the relationship between the study instrument and a reference method with reasonable precision. Increasing the numbers of individuals sampled and decreasing the number of repeat measures per individual (e.g., two non-consecutive 24-hour recalls on 100 people rather than four recalls on 50 people) often can help to increase precision without extra cost [487]. As often as possible, the subsample should be chosen randomly.

The subsequent analyses quantify the relationship between the new method and the reference method, and the resulting statistics can be used for a variety of purposes. Because, in most cases, the reference method (usually dietary records or 24-hour recalls) is itself imperfect and subject to within-person error (day-to-day variability), measures such as correlation coefficients may underestimate the level of agreement with the actual usual intake. This phenomenon, referred to as "attenuation bias," can be addressed through the use of measurement error models that allow for within-person error in the reference instrument, resulting in estimates that more nearly reflect the correlation between the diet measure and true diet [365,488]. The corrected correlation coefficients also give guidance with regard to the sample size required in a study because the less precise the diet measure, the more individuals will be needed to attain the desired statistical power [488]. The estimated regression relationship between the new method and the reference method can also be used to adjust the relationships between diet and outcome as assessed in the larger study [197]. For example, the mean amounts of foods or nutrients, and their distributions, as estimated by a brief method, can be adjusted according to the calibration study results [489]. In addition, methods to adjust estimates of the relationships measured in studies (e.g., the relative risk of disease for subjects with high nutrient intake compared to those with low intake) have been described [209,210,365,490,491]. Many of these adjustments require the assumption that the reference method is unbiased [209,363]. However, much evidence indicates that, at least for some nutrients, the reported intakes from recalls and records are biased in a manner correlated with the tool of interest (e.g., an FFQ) [135], violating this assumption. Violation of this assumption would lead to overestimates of validity. For these reasons, researchers have sometimes used biomarkers such as urinary nitrogen and doubly labeled water as reference measures, that have been shown in feeding studies to be unbiased measures of intake. Currently, only a few such biomarkers are known. Another area in need of further study is the effect of measurement error in a multivariate context because most research thus far has been limited to the effect on univariate relationships [212,216,492,493].

C Mode of Administration

Instruments may be interviewer-administered or self-administered. Interviewer-administered questionnaires may be in person or by telephone. A self-administered instrument may be completed on paper or electronically. All of these modes are currently used for dietary assessment.

For interviewer-administered instruments, telephone administration is less costly than in-person administration. However, concern is increasing about response rates in telephone surveys, given the public's distaste for prevalent telemarketing, technology that allows for the screening of calls, the increase in the proportion of the population (especially young adults [494]) who use only wireless telephones, and the general resistance of the public to engage in telephone interviews. For these reasons, response rates obtained using random digit dialing techniques have been dropping.

Despite these difficulties, many surveys and studies do collect dietary data over the telephone. For example, BRFSS [249] and the California Health Interview Survey [228] both include dietary screeners. NHANES [344] administers an initial 24-hour recall at the examination site and a second 24-hour recall later by telephone. For 24-hour recalls collected by telephone, the difficulty of reporting serving sizes can be eased by mailing picture booklets or other portion size estimation aids to participants before the interview. Many studies have evaluated the comparability of data from telephone versus in-person 24-hour recall interviews. Several have found substantial but imperfect agreement between dietary data collected by telephone and that estimated by other methods, including face-to-face interviews [70,495–497] or observed intakes [498].

Godwin *et al.* [499] and Yanek *et al.* [500] examined the accuracy of portion size estimates for known quantities of foods consumed that were assessed by telephone and by in-person interviews. Both estimates were found to be similarly accurate.

Self-administration is less costly than interviewer-administration. In addition, self-administered surveys tend to minimize social desirability bias [501]. However, self-administration may not be feasible for segments of the population who have low literacy levels or limited motivation. Thus, selection bias is a potential problem.

Web-administered questionnaires have cost advantages and have become popular as the penetrance of the Internet increases. However, it is estimated that only 69% of households in the United States had Internet access in 2009 [502]. Various FFQs [183], dietary history questionnaires [503], screeners [291,504], and 24-hour recall instruments [72,85,439] have been developed for web administration. In general, it has been found that initial response rates for web questionnaires are substantially lower than those for mailed or telephone interviewer questionnaires [505]. One study conducted in Sweden found a lower initial response rate to a web questionnaire compared to a mailed printed questionnaire but greater compliance in answering follow-up questions over the web [506]. Web-administered questionnaires may be more effective than telephone interviewer-administered questionnaires for the presentation of complex questions that are better processed visually than aurally by respondents and that can be answered at a pace set by the respondent rather than by the interviewer [507]. Beasley *et al.* [508] found that the responses to questions about diet on a web-administered FFQ were not significantly different from responses on a paper version of the same questionnaire. Dietary assessment with wireless phones is also an area of great potential. As these new modes of administration become more prevalent, it will be important to examine comparability with in-person and telephone-administered modes, as well as the potential for self-selection biases.

D Estimation of Portion Size

Research has shown that untrained individuals have difficulty in estimating portion sizes of foods, both when examining displayed foods and when reporting about foods previously consumed [88,429,437,499,509–525]. One study indicates that literacy, but not numeracy, is an important factor in an individual's ability to accurately estimate portions size [526]. Furthermore, respondents appear to be relatively insensitive to changes made in portion size amounts shown in reference categories asked on

FFQs [527]. Portion sizes of foods that are commonly bought and/or consumed in defined units (e.g., bread by the slice, pieces of fruit, and beverages in cans or bottles) may be more easily reported than amorphous foods (e.g., steak, lettuce, and pasta) or poured liquids [88,524]. Other studies indicate that small portion sizes tend to be overestimated and large portion sizes underestimated [511,523,528].

Aids are commonly used to help respondents estimate portion size. The NHANES, What We Eat in America, uses an extensive set of three-dimensional models for an initial in-person 24-hour dietary recall; respondents are then given a Food Model Booklet developed by the USDA [80] along with a limited number of three-dimensional models (e.g., measuring cups and spoons) for recalls collected by telephone. The accuracy of reporting using either models or household measures can be improved with training [529–532], but the effects deteriorate with time [533]. Studies that have compared three-dimensional food models to two-dimensional photographs in adults have shown that there is little difference in the reporting accuracy between methods [428,499,534,535]. One study in children, however, showed that using food models resulted in somewhat larger error than using digital images [521]. With the increased use of technology in dietary assessment, photographs and digital food images in multiple portion sizes are being tested. Studies have investigated the effects of a number of portion pictures, the size of picture, and concurrent versus sequential display on the accuracy of reports [88,437,520]. Such studies indicate preferences by respondents but generally little difference in accuracy. In one study, however, accuracy was higher when more portion size choices were offered [88]. An emerging use of digital technology removes respondent judgments of portion size, instead relying on digital photography of foods taken before and after consumption. Computer software is then used to both identify foods and estimate the amount consumed [536,537].

E Choice of Nutrient and Food Database

It is necessary to use a nutrient composition database when dietary data are to be converted to nutrient intake data. Typically, such a database includes the description of the food, a food code, and the nutrient composition per 100 grams of the food. The number of foods and nutrients included varies with the database. Research on nutrients, other dietary components, and foods is ongoing, and there is constant interest in updating current values and providing new values for a variety of dietary components of interest.

Some values in nutrient databases are obtained from laboratory analysis; however, because of the high cost of laboratory analyses, many values are estimated based on conversion factors or other knowledge about the food [538]. In addition, accepted analytical methods are not yet available for some nutrients of interest [539], analytical quality of the information varies with the nutrient [539,540], and the variances or ranges of nutrient composition of individual foods are in most cases unknown but are known to be large for some nutrients [541]. Rapid growth in the food processing sector and the global nature of the food supply add further challenges to estimating the mean and variability in the nutrient composition of foods eaten in a specific locale.

One of the USDA's primary missions is to provide nutrient composition data for foods in the U.S. food supply, accounting for various types of preparation [542]. Information about the USDA's nutrient composition databases is available at the USDA's Nutrient Data Laboratory home page [543]. The USDA produces and maintains the Nutrient Database for Standard Reference (SR). New releases are issued yearly; these include information on new foods and revised information on already included foods, and they identify foods deleted from the previous version of the database. The most recent release, SR24, includes information on up to 146 food components for more than 7900 foods [544], and it is available online.

Interest in nutrients and food components potentially associated with diseases has led the USDA to develop specialized databases for a smaller number of foods, such as flavonoids, proanthocyanidins, choline, and fluoride [545]. A separate database developed by the USDA Food Surveys Research Group—the Food and Nutrient Database for Dietary Studies (FNDDS)—is used by many investigators in analyses of foods reported in NHANES' What We Eat in America dietary recalls and is based on nutrient values in the USDA SR database [89].

Nutrient composition data are also compiled by a number of other countries, and the International Network of Food Data Systems maintains an international directory of nutrient composition tables [546]. Combining different food composition databases across countries poses comparability challenges, however. The European Food Information Resource [547] was formed to support the harmonization of food composition data among the European nations. The International Nutrient Databank Directory, an online compendium developed by the National Nutrient Databank Conference, provides information about the data included in a variety of databases, national reference databases, and specialized databases developed for software applications, such as the date the database was most recently updated, the number of nutrients provided for each food, and the completeness of the nutrient data for all foods listed [548].

In addition to nutrient databases, databases that can relate dietary intake to dietary guidance have been developed in the United States [549,550]. The USDA Food Patterns provide quantities of foods to consume from specific food groups in order to attain a diet consistent with the guidelines at a variety of calorie levels [551]. Just as FNDDS provides a nutrient profile for each food, the Food Patterns Equivalents Database (FPED) provides food group data for each food in FNDDS in order to allow assessment of the intake in terms of these Food Patterns. The FPED contains 32 food group components (e.g., dairy, fruits, and vegetables) and provides the amount of each food group per 100 grams of each food [552].

Other databases are available in the United States for use in analyzing dietary records and 24-hour recalls, but most are based fundamentally on the USDA SR database, often with added foods and specific brand names. One prominent such database is the University of Minnesota's Nutrition Coordinating Center's (NCC) Food and Nutrient Database [553]. This database includes information on 162 nutrients, nutrient ratios, and other food components for more than 18,000 foods, including 8000 brand-name products. The NCC is constantly updating its database to reflect values in the latest release of the USDA SR.

One limitation in all nutrient databases is the variability in the nutrient content of foods within a food category and the volatility of nutrient composition in manufactured foods. Recent changes in the sodium and fatty acid composition of manufactured foods, for example, illustrate the difficulty in maintaining accurate nutrient composition databases [554]. Obviously, a key consideration is how the database is maintained and supported.

Estimates of nutrient intake from 24-hour recalls and dietary records are often affected by the nutrient composition database that is used to process the data [555–557]. Inherent differences in the database used for analysis include factors such as the number of food items included in the database, how recently nutrient data were updated, and the number of missing or imputed nutrient composition values. Therefore, before choosing a nutrient composition database, a prime factor to consider is the completeness and accuracy of the data for the nutrients of interest. For some purposes, it may be useful to choose a database in which each nutrient value for each food also contains a code for the quality of the data (e.g., analytical value, calculated value, imputed value, or missing). Investigators need to be aware that a value of zero is assigned to missing values in some databases, whereas for other databases, the number of nutrients provided for each food may fluctuate depending on whether or not a value is missing, and for others all unknown values may be imputed.

The nutrient database should also include weight/volume equivalency information for each food item. Many foods are reported in volumetric measures (e.g., 1 cup) and must be converted to weight in grams in order to apply nutrient values. The number of common mixtures (e.g., spaghetti with sauce) available in the database is another important factor. If the study requires the precision of nutrient estimates, then procedures for calculating the nutrients in various mixtures must be developed and incorporated into nutrient composition calculations.

Developing a nutrient database for an FFQ presents additional challenges [558] because each item on the FFQ represents a food grouping rather than an individual food item. Various approaches that rely on 24-hour recall data, either from a national population sample or from a sample similar to the target population, have been used [114,138,559]. Generally, individual foods reported on 24-hour recalls are grouped into FFQ food groupings, and a composite nutrient profile for each food grouping is estimated based on the individual foods' relative consumption in the population. For this approach to be effective, the 24-hour recall data must be representative of the population for whom the FFQ is designed and connected to a trustworthy nutrient database.

F Choice of Dietary Analysis Software

Data processing of 24-hour recalls and dietary record requires creating a file that includes a food code and an amount consumed for each food reported. Computer software then links the nutrient composition of each food on the separate nutrient composition database file, converts the amount reported to multiples of 100 g, multiplies by that factor, stores that information, and sums across all foods for each nutrient for each individual for each day of intake. Many software packages have been developed that include both a nutrient composition database and software to convert individual responses to specific foods and, ultimately, to nutrients. A listing of many commercial dietary analysis software products has been compiled [548].

Software should be chosen on the basis of the research needs, the level of detail necessary, the quality of the nutrient composition database, and the hardware and software requirements [560]. If precise nutrient information is required, it is important that the system be able to expand to incorporate information about newer foods in the marketplace and to integrate detailed information about food preparation by processing recipe information (e.g., the ingredients and cooking steps for homemade stew). Sometimes the study purpose requires analysis of dietary data to derive intake estimates not only for nutrients but also for food groups (e.g., fruits and vegetables), food components other than standard nutrients (e.g., nitrites), or food characteristics (e.g., fried foods). These additional requirements limit the choice of appropriate software.

The semi-automated food coding system used for NHANES is USDA's Dietary Intake System, consisting of the AMPM for collecting food intakes; the Post-Interview Processing System, which translates the AMPM data and provides initial food coding; and the Survey Net food coding system for the final coding of the intake data [83]. Survey Net is a network dietary coding system that provides online coding, recipe modification and development, data editing and management, and nutrient analysis of dietary data; multiple users can use the software to manage their survey activities. It is available to government agencies and the general public only through special arrangement with the USDA. A similar program is available in a commercial software program called the Food Intake Analysis System [561], which is available from the University of Texas School of Public Health.

Many diet history and food frequency instruments have also been automated. Users of these software packages should be aware of the source of information in the nutrient database and the assumptions about the nutrient content of each food item listed in the questionnaire.

G Estimating Usual Intakes of Nutrients and Foods

In theory, usual intake is defined as the long-term average intake of a food or nutrient. The concept of long-term average daily intake, or "usual intake," is important because dietary recommendations are intended to be met over time and diet—health hypotheses are based on dietary intakes over the long term. Consequently, it is the usual intake that is often of most interest to policymakers (when they want to know the proportion of the population at or below a certain level of intake) or to researchers (when they want to examine relationships between diet and health). However, until recently, sophisticated efforts to capture this concept have been limited at best.

For estimates of mean usual intake in the population, data from a single day of recall or record can be used. Multiple days of recalls and records are needed to estimate the distribution of intakes. However, simple averages of intakes from these instruments across a few days do not adequately represent individuals' usual intake [562] because of the large day-to-day variability of individuals' diets. Distributions generated from averaging only a few days of data are generally substantially

wider than those of true usual intakes, thereby overestimating the proportion of the population above or below a certain cut point. Sophisticated methods based on statistical modeling have evolved for this purpose [562,563]. These methods rely on a minimum of two administrations of 24-hour recalls or dietary records to capture day-to-day variation, although more administrations are better.

For clinical assessment of an individual's intake, researchers have found that averaging as many as 7—14 days of 24-hour recalls may be required to adequately approximate an individual's usual intake for most nutrients and food groups [564—567]. However, for assessing relationships between usual diet and health outcomes in a population, a minimum of only 2 days is required. Data from FFQs, 24-hour recalls, and dietary records have all been used to estimate usual intake. FFQs are limited in their ability to estimate usual intake well and are known to contain a substantial amount of measurement error (see Section II.C) [55,75,95—98,135]. Dietary recalls or records, which also contain error, provide rich detail about types of foods and amounts consumed over short time periods, and they can be used in diet—disease research if usual intakes are estimated through statistical modeling.

Statistical modeling mitigates some of the limitations of having only a few days of intake by analytically estimating and removing the effects of day-to-day variation in dietary intake [562]. The earliest efforts at statistical modeling of the usual intake were developed by the Institute of Medicine [568] for nutrients, most of which are consumed nearly every day by most everyone, and then extended and updated for nutrients or foods that are more episodically consumed (e.g., dark green vegetables) by researchers at Iowa State University [569—571]. Others have developed usual intake models as well [223,572—575]. The NCI model uses a minimum of two 24-hour recalls to estimate intake of both nutrients and episodically consumed foods. This model as well as others [223] allow for covariates such as sex, age, race/ethnicity, or information from a FFQ to supplement the model [574]. The use of frequency information from a FFQ as a covariate in a statistical model designed to estimate usual intakes is novel. One study using the NCI method showed that including FFQ data as covariate in modeling usual intakes from 24-hour recalls increased precision for assessing the relationship of a highly episodically consumed food, fish, with blood mercury levels [224]. Modeling usual intakes to assess relationships to health outcomes by combining data from a few 24-hour recalls with an FFQ has been shown to provide better estimates compared to a single FFQ or a few 24-hour recalls alone [222,223,342]. The NCI Measurement Error Webinar Series [576] provides a thorough discussion of dietary measurement error, including usual intake estimation.

Acknowledgments

We gratefully acknowledge the contributions of Susan M. Krebs-Smith, Rachel Ballard-Barbash, Kevin Dodd, Thea Zimmerman, Tom Baranowski, and Gordon B. Willis in reviewing and editing portions of this chapter. We also thank Penny Randall-Levy for invaluable research assistance and Anne Rodgers for expert editorial assistance.

References

[1] A.M. Coulston, C.J. Boushey, Nutrition in the Prevention and Treatment of Disease, Elsevier, San Diego, 2008.

[2] F.E. Thompson, A.F. Subar, Dietary assessment methodology, in: A.M. Coulston, C.L. Rock, E.R. Monsen (Eds), Nutrition in the Prevention and Treatment of Disease, Academic Press, San Diego, 2001.

[3] F.E. Thompson, T. Byers, Dietary assessment resource manual, J. Nutr. 124 (1994) 2245S–2317S.

[4] M. Gersovitz, J.P. Madden, H. Smiciklas-Wright, Validity of the 24-hr dietary recall and seven-day record for group comparisons, J. Am. Diet. Assoc. 73 (1978) 48–55.

[5] R.S. Gibson, Principles of Nutritional Assessment, Oxford University Press, New York, 2005.

[6] N.E. Johnson, C.T. Sempos, P.J. Elmer, J.K. Allington, M.E. Matthews, Development of a dietary intake monitoring system for nursing homes, J. Am. Diet. Assoc. 80 (1982) 549–557.

[7] J. Hammond, M. Nelson, S. Chinn, R.J. Rona, Validation of a food frequency questionnaire for assessing dietary intake in a study of coronary heart disease risk factors in children, Eur. J. Clin. Nutr. 47 (1993) 242–250.

[8] N.E. Johnson, S. Nitzke, D.L. VandeBerg, A reporting system for nutrient adequacy, Fam. Consum. Sci. Res. J. 2 (1974) 210–221.

[9] M.J. Kretsch, A.K. Fong, Validity and reproducibility of a new computerized dietary assessment method: effects of gender and educational level, Nutr. Res. 13 (1993) 133–146.

[10] I.T. Lillegaard, E.B. Loken, L.F. Andersen, Relative validation of a pre-coded food diary among children, under-reporting varies with reporting day and time of the day, Eur. J. Clin. Nutr. 61 (2007) 61–68.

[11] R.R. Couris, G.R. Tataronis, S.L. Booth, G.E. Dallal, J.B. Blumberg, J.T. Dwyer, Development of a self-assessment instrument to determine daily intake and variability of dietary vitamin K, J. Am. Coll. Nutr. 19 (2000) 801–807.

[12] F.E. Thompson, A.F. Subar, C.C. Brown, A.F. Smith, C.O. Sharbaugh, J.B. Jobe, et al., Cognitive research enhances accuracy of food frequency questionnaire reports: results of an experimental validation study, J. Am. Diet. Assoc. 102 (2002) 212–225.

[13] K.W. Smith, D.M. Hoelscher, L.A. Lytle, J.T. Dwyer, T.A. Nicklas, M.M. Zive, et al., Reliability and validity of the Child and Adolescent Trial for Cardiovascular Health (CATCH) Food Checklist: a self-report instrument to measure fat and sodium intake by middle school students, J. Am. Diet. Assoc. 101 (2001) 635–647.

[14] D.L. MacIntosh, C. Kabiru, K.A. Scanlon, P.B. Ryan, Longitudinal investigation of exposure to arsenic, cadmium, chromium and lead via beverage consumption, J. Expo. Anal. Environ. Epidemiol. 10 (2000) 196–205.

[15] S.M. Rebro, R.E. Patterson, A.R. Kristal, C.L. Cheney, The effect of keeping food records on eating patterns, J. Am. Diet. Assoc. 98 (1998) 1163–1165.

[16] L.F. Andersen, L. Johansson, K. Solvoll, Usefulness of a short food frequency questionnaire for screening of low intake of fruit and vegetable and for intake of fat, Eur. J. Public Health 12 (2002) 208–213.

[17] A.G. Kristjansdottir, L.F. Andersen, J. Haraldsdottir, M.D. de Almeida, I. Thorsdottir, Validity of a questionnaire to assess fruit and vegetable intake in adults, Eur. J. Clin. Nutr. 60 (2006) 408–415.

[18] N. Vuckovic, C. Ritenbaugh, D.L. Taren, M. Tobar, A qualitative study of participants' experiences with dietary assessment, J. Am. Diet. Assoc. 100 (2000) 1023–1028.

[19] K. Glanz, S. Murphy, J. Moylan, D. Evensen, J.D. Curb, Improving dietary self-monitoring and adherence with hand-held computers: a pilot study, Am. J. Health Promot. 20 (2006) 165–170.

[20] A.H. Goris, M.S. Westerterp-Plantenga, K.R. Westerterp, Undereating and underrecording of habitual food intake in obese men: selective underreporting of fat intake, Am. J. Clin. Nutr. 71 (2000) 130–134.

[21] J.F. Hollis, C.M. Gullion, V.J. Stevens, P.J. Brantley, L.J. Appel, J.D. Ard, et al., Weight loss during the intensive intervention phase of the weight-loss maintenance trial, Am. J. Prev. Med. 35 (2008) 118–126.

[22] K. Glanz, S. Murphy, Dietary assessment and monitoring in real time, in: A.A. Stone, S. Schiffman, A.A. Atienza, L. Nebeling (Eds), The Science of Real-Time Data Capture: Self-Reports in Health Research, Oxford University Press, New York, 2007, pp. 151–168.

[23] L.E. Burke, M.B. Conroy, S.M. Sereika, O.U. Elci, M.A. Styn, S.D. Acharya, et al., The effect of electronic self-monitoring on weight loss and dietary intake: a randomized behavioral weight loss trial, Obesity. (Silver. Spring) 19 (2011) 338–344.

[24] U.S. Department of Agriculture, MyPyramid Tracker, Center for Nutrition Policy and Promotion, U.S. Department of Agriculture, 2007. Available at <http://www.mypyramidtracker.gov>.

[25] J. Di Noia, I.R. Contento, S.P. Schinke, Criterion validity of the Healthy Eating Self-monitoring Tool (HEST) for black adolescents, J. Am. Diet. Assoc. 107 (2007) 321–324.

[26] J. Beasley, W.T. Riley, J. Jean-Mary, Accuracy of a PDA-based dietary assessment program, Nutrition 21 (2005) 672–677.

[27] S. Kikunaga, T. Tin, G. Ishibashi, D.H. Wang, S. Kira, The application of a handheld personal digital assistant with camera and mobile phone card (Wellnavi) to the general population in a dietary survey, J. Nutr. Sci. Vitaminol. (Tokyo) 53 (2007) 109–116.

[28] B.L. Six, T.E. Schap, F.M. Zhu, A. Mariappan, M. Bosch, E.J. Delp, et al., Evidence-based development of a mobile telephone food record, J. Am. Diet. Assoc. 110 (2010) 74–79.

[29] R. Weiss, P.J. Stumbo, A. Divakaran, Automatic food documentation and volume computation using digital imaging and electronic transmission, J. Am. Diet. Assoc. 110 (2010) 42–44.

[30] J. Di Noia, I.R. Contento, Criterion validity and user acceptability of a CD-ROM-mediated food record for measuring fruit and vegetable consumption among black adolescents, Public Health Nutr. 12 (2009) 3–11.

[31] M.A. Murtaugh, K.N. Ma, T. Greene, D. Redwood, S. Edwards, J. Johnson, et al., Validation of a dietary history questionnaire for American Indian and Alaska Native people, Ethn. Dis. 20 (2010) 429–436.

[32] D.H. Wang, M. Kogashiwa, S. Kira, Development of a new instrument for evaluating individuals' dietary intakes, J. Am. Diet. Assoc. 106 (2006) 1588–1593.

[33] L. Arab, A. Winter, Automated camera-phone experience with the frequency of imaging necessary to capture diet, J. Am. Diet. Assoc. 110 (2010) 1238–1241.

[34] M. Sun, J.D. Fernstrom, W. Jia, S.A. Hackworth, N. Yao, Y. Li, et al., A wearable electronic system for objective dietary assessment, J. Am. Diet. Assoc. 110 (2010) 45–47.

[35] S.I. Kirkpatrick, D. Midthune, K.W. Dodd, N. Potischman, A.F. Subar, F.E. Thompson, Reactivity and its association with body

mass index across days on food checklists, J. Acad. Nutr. Diet. 112 (2012) 110−118.

[36] B. Holmes, K. Dick, M. Nelson, A comparison of four dietary assessment methods in materially deprived households in England, Public Health Nutr. 11 (2008) 444−456.

[37] J. Trabulsi, D.A. Schoeller, Evaluation of dietary assessment instruments against doubly labeled water, a biomarker of habitual energy intake, Am. J. Physiol. Endocrinol. Metab. 281 (2001) E891−E899.

[38] R.J. Hill, P.S. Davies, The validity of self-reported energy intake as determined using the doubly labelled water technique, Br. J. Nutr. 85 (2001) 415−430.

[39] D.L. Taren, M. Tobar, A. Hill, W. Howell, C. Shisslak, I. Bell, et al., The association of energy intake bias with psychological scores of women, Eur. J. Clin. Nutr. 53 (1999) 570−578.

[40] A.L. Sawaya, K. Tucker, R. Tsay, W. Willett, E. Saltzman, G.E. Dallal, et al., Evaluation of four methods for determining energy intake in young and older women: comparison with doubly labeled water measurements of total energy expenditure, Am. J. Clin. Nutr. 63 (1996) 491−499.

[41] A.E. Black, A.M. Prentice, G.R. Goldberg, S.A. Jebb, S.A. Bingham, M.B. Livingstone, et al., Measurements of total energy expenditure provide insights into the validity of dietary measurements of energy intake, J. Am. Diet. Assoc. 93 (1993) 572−579.

[42] A.E. Black, S.A. Bingham, G. Johansson, W.A. Coward, Validation of dietary intakes of protein and energy against 24 hour urinary N and DLW energy expenditure in middle-aged women, retired men and post-obese subjects: comparisons with validation against presumed energy requirements, Eur. J. Clin. Nutr. 51 (1997) 405−413.

[43] L.J. Martin, W. Su, P.J. Jones, G.A. Lockwood, D.L. Tritchler, N. F. Boyd, Comparison of energy intakes determined by food records and doubly labeled water in women participating in a dietary-intervention trial, Am. J. Clin. Nutr. 63 (1996) 483−490.

[44] E. Rothenberg, Validation of the food frequency questionnaire with the 4-day record method and analysis of 24-h urinary nitrogen, Eur. J. Clin. Nutr. 48 (1994) 725−735.

[45] S.A. Bingham, C. Gill, A. Welch, A. Cassidy, S.A. Runswick, S. Oakes, et al., Validation of dietary assessment methods in the UK arm of EPIC using weighed records, and 24-hour urinary nitrogen and potassium and serum vitamin C and carotenoids as biomarkers, Int. J. Epidemiol. 26 (1997) S137−S151.

[46] G.P. Bathalon, K.L. Tucker, N.P. Hays, A.G. Vinken, A.S. Greenberg, M.A. McCrory, et al., Psychological measures of eating behavior and the accuracy of 3 common dietary assessment methods in healthy postmenopausal women, Am. J. Clin. Nutr. 71 (2000) 739−745.

[47] J.L. Seale, W.V. Rumpler, Comparison of energy expenditure measurements by diet records, energy intake balance, doubly labeled water and room calorimetry, Eur. J. Clin. Nutr. 51 (1997) 856−863.

[48] J.L. Seale, G. Klein, J. Friedmann, G.L. Jensen, D.C. Mitchell, H. Smiciklas-Wright, Energy expenditure measured by doubly labeled water, activity recall, and diet records in the rural elderly, Nutrition 18 (2002) 568−573.

[49] S. Mahabir, D.J. Baer, C. Giffen, A. Subar, W. Campbell, T.J. Hartman, et al., Calorie intake misreporting by diet record and food frequency questionnaire compared to doubly labeled water among postmenopausal women, Eur. J. Clin. Nutr. 60 (2006) 561−565.

[50] K. Poslusna, J. Ruprich, J.H. de Vries, M. Jakubikova, P. van't Veer, Misreporting of energy and micronutrient intake estimated by food records and 24 hour recalls, control and adjustment methods in practice, Br. J. Nutr. 101 (2009) S73−S85.

[51] K.R. Westerterp, A.H. Goris, Validity of the assessment of dietary intake: problems of misreporting, Curr. Opin. Clin. Nutr. Metab. Care 5 (2002) 489−493.

[52] J. Maurer, D.L. Taren, P.J. Teixeira, C.A. Thomson, T.G. Lohman, S.B. Going, et al., The psychosocial and behavioral characteristics related to energy misreporting, Nutr. Rev. 64 (2006) 53−66.

[53] S.W. Lichtman, K. Pisarska, E.R. Berman, M. Pestone, H. Dowling, E. Offenbacher, et al., Discrepancy between self-reported and actual caloric intake and exercise in obese subjects, N. Engl. J. Med. 327 (1992) 1893−1898.

[54] J.A. Pryer, M. Vrijheid, R. Nichols, M. Kiggins, P. Elliott, Who are the "low energy reporters" in the dietary and nutritional survey of British adults? Int. J. Epidemiol. 26 (1997) 146−154.

[55] R.L. Prentice, Y. Mossavar-Rahmani, Y. Huang, H.L. Van, S.A. Beresford, B. Caan, et al., Evaluation and comparison of food records, recalls, and frequencies for energy and protein assessment by using recovery biomarkers, Am. J. Epidemiol. 174 (2011) 591−603.

[56] R.K. Johnson, M.I. Goran, E.T. Poehlman, Correlates of over- and underreporting of energy intake in healthy older men and women, Am. J. Clin. Nutr. 59 (1994) 1286−1290.

[57] T. Hirvonen, S. Mannisto, E. Roos, P. Pietinen, Increasing prevalence of underreporting does not necessarily distort dietary surveys, Eur. J. Clin. Nutr. 51 (1997) 297−301.

[58] L. Lafay, A. Basdevant, M.A. Charles, M. Vray, B. Balkau, J.M. Borys, et al., Determinants and nature of dietary underreporting in a free-living population: the Fleurbaix Laventie Ville Sante (FLVS) Study, Int. J. Obes. Relat. Metab. Disord. 21 (1997) 567−573.

[59] R. Ballard-Barbash, I. Graubard, S.M. Krebs-Smith, A. Schatzkin, F.E. Thompson, Contribution of dieting to the inverse association between energy intake and body mass index, Eur. J. Clin. Nutr. 50 (1996) 98−106.

[60] C. Bazelmans, C. Matthys, S. De Henauw, M. Dramaix, M. Kornitzer, G. De Backer, et al., Predictors of misreporting in an elderly population: the "Quality of life after 65" study, Public Health Nutr. 10 (2007) 185−191.

[61] J.R. Hebert, L. Clemow, L. Pbert, I.S. Ockene, J.K. Ockene, Social desirability bias in dietary self-report may compromise the validity of dietary intake measures, Int. J. Epidemiol. 24 (1995) 389−398.

[62] D.D. Stallone, E.J. Brunner, S.A. Bingham, M.G. Marmot, Dietary assessment in Whitehall II: the influence of reporting bias on apparent socioeconomic variation in nutrient intakes, Eur. J. Clin. Nutr. 51 (1997) 815−825.

[63] C.M. Champagne, G.A. Bray, A.A. Kurtz, J.B. Monteiro, E. Tucker, J. Volaufova, et al., Energy intake and energy expenditure: a controlled study comparing dietitians and non-dietitians, J. Am. Diet. Assoc. 102 (2002) 1428−1432.

[64] I. Kortzinger, A. Bierwag, M. Mast, M.J. Muller, Dietary underreporting: validity of dietary measurements of energy intake using a 7-day dietary record and a diet history in non-obese subjects, Ann. Nutr. Metab. 41 (1997) 37−44.

[65] L. Lafay, L. Mennen, A. Basdevant, M.A. Charles, J.M. Borys, E. Eschwege, et al., Does energy intake underreporting involve all kinds of food or only specific food items? Results from the Fleurbaix Laventie Ville Sante (FLVS) study, Int. J. Obes. Relat. Metab. Disord. 24 (2000) 1500−1506.

[66] A. Biltoft-Jensen, J. Matthiessen, L.B. Rasmussen, S. Fagt, M.V. Groth, O. Hels, Validation of the Danish 7-day pre-coded food diary among adults: energy intake v. energy expenditure and recording length, Br. J. Nutr. 102 (2009) 1838−1846.

[67] S.J. Zhou, M.J. Schilling, M. Makrides, Evaluation of an iron specific checklist for the assessment of dietary iron intake in pregnant and postpartum women, Nutrition 21 (2005) 908−913.

[68] J.L. Seale, Predicting total energy expenditure from self-reported dietary records and physical characteristics in adult and elderly men and women, Am. J. Clin. Nutr. 76 (2002) 529–534.

[69] I.M. Buzzard, C.L. Faucett, R.W. Jeffery, L. McBane, P. McGovern, J.S. Baxter, et al., Monitoring dietary change in a low-fat diet intervention study: advantages of using 24-hour dietary recalls vs food records, J. Am. Diet. Assoc. 96 (1996) 574–579.

[70] P.H. Casey, S.L. Goolsby, S.Y. Lensing, B.P. Perloff, M.L. Bogle, The use of telephone interview methodology to obtain 24-hour dietary recalls, J. Am. Diet. Assoc. 99 (1999) 1406–1411.

[71] U.S. Department of Agriculture, What We Eat in America, Agricultural Research Service, U.S. Department of Agriculture, 2010. Available at: <http://www.ars.usda.gov/Services/docs.htm?docid = 13793>.

[72] National Cancer Institute, ASA24 Automated Self-Administered 24-Hour Recall, Applied Research Program, National Cancer Institute, 2011. Available at: <http://riskfactor.cancer.gov/tools/instruments/asa24>.

[73] J.F. Sallis, N. Owen, Ecological models of health behavior, in: K. Glanz, B.K. Rimer, F.M. Lewis (Eds), Health Behavior and Health Education: Theory, Research, and Practice, third ed., Jossey-Bass, San Francisco, 2002, pp. 462–484.

[74] L. Arab, K. Wesseling-Perry, P. Jardack, J. Henry, A. Winter, Eight self-administered 24-hour dietary recalls using the Internet are feasible in African Americans and Whites: the energetics study, J. Am. Diet. Assoc. 110 (2010) 857–864.

[75] L. Arab, C.H. Tseng, A. Ang, P. Jardack, Validity of a multipass, web-based, 24-hour self-administered recall for assessment of total energy intake in blacks and whites, Am. J. Epidemiol. 174 (2011) 1256–1265.

[76] C.A. Vereecken, M. Covents, W. Sichert-Hellert, J.M. Alvira, D. C. Le, H.S. De, et al., Development and evaluation of a self-administered computerized 24-h dietary recall method for adolescents in Europe, Int. J. Obes. (London) 32 (2008) S26–S34.

[77] V.A. Campbell, M.L. Dodds, Collecting dietary information from groups of older people, J. Am. Diet. Assoc. 51 (1967) 29–33.

[78] N. Raper, B. Perloff, L. Ingwersen, L. Steinfeldt, J. Anand, An overview of USDA's dietary intake data system, J. Food Compost. Anal. 17 (2004) 545–555.

[79] A.J. Moshfegh, D.G. Rhodes, D.J. Baer, T. Murayi, J.C. Clemens, W.V. Rumpler, et al., The U.S. Department of Agriculture Automated Multiple-Pass Method reduces bias in the collection of energy intakes, Am. J. Clin. Nutr. 88 (2008) 324–332.

[80] J. McBride, Was it a slab, a slice, or a sliver? High-tech innovations take food survey to new level, Agric. Res. 49 (2001) 4–7.

[81] K.W. Cullen, K. Watson, J.H. Himes, T. Baranowski, J. Rochon, M. Waclawiw, et al., Evaluation of quality control procedures for 24-h dietary recalls: results from the Girls Health Enrichment Multisite Studies, Prev. Med. 38 (2004) S14–S23.

[82] Y.C. Probst, L.C. Tapsell, Overview of computerized dietary assessment programs for research and practice in nutrition education, J. Nutr. Educ. Behav. 37 (2005) 20–26.

[83] U.S. Department of Agriculture, USDA Automated Multiple-Pass Method, Agricultural Research Service, U.S. Department of Agriculture, 2010. Available at: <http://www.ars.usda.gov/Services/docs.htm?docid=7710>.

[84] L.I. Mennen, S. Bertrais, P. Galan, N. Arnault, G. Potier de Couray, S. Hercberg, The use of computerised 24 h dietary recalls in the French SU.VI.MAX Study: number of recalls required, Eur. J. Clin. Nutr. 56 (2002) 659–665.

[85] T. Baranowski, N. Islam, J. Baranowski, K.W. Cullen, D. Myres, T. Marsh, et al., The food intake recording software system is valid among fourth-grade children, J. Am. Diet. Assoc. 102 (2002) 380–385.

[86] C.A. Vereecken, M. Covents, C. Matthys, L. Maes, Young adolescents' nutrition assessment on computer (YANA-C), Eur. J. Clin. Nutr. 59 (2005) 658–667.

[87] A.F. Subar, F.E. Thompson, N. Potischman, B.H. Forsyth, R. Buday, D. Richards, et al., Formative research of a quick list for an automated self-administered 24-hour dietary recall, J. Am. Diet. Assoc. 107 (2007) 1002–1007.

[88] A.F. Subar, J. Crafts, T.P. Zimmerman, M. Wilson, B. Mittl, N.G. Islam, et al., Assessment of the accuracy of portion size reports using computer-based food photography aids in the development of an automated self-administered 24-hour recall, J. Am. Diet. Assoc. 110 (2010) 55–64.

[89] U.S. Department of Agriculture, Food and Nutrient Database for Dietary Studies, Agricultural Research Service, U.S. Department of Agriculture, 2010. Available at: <http://www.ars.usda.gov/Services/docs.htm?docid = 12089>.

[90] J.P. Madden, S.J. Goodman, H.A. Guthrie, Validity of the 24-hr recall. Analysis of data obtained from elderly subjects, J. Am. Diet. Assoc. 68 (1976) 143–147.

[91] S.S. Jonnalagadda, D.C. Mitchell, H. Smiciklas-Wright, K.B. Meaker, N. Van Heel, W. Karmally, et al., Accuracy of energy intake data estimated by a multiple-pass, 24-hour dietary recall technique, J. Am. Diet. Assoc. 100 (2000) 303–308.

[92] A. Kroke, K. Klipstein-Grobusch, S. Voss, J. Moseneder, F. Thielecke, R. Noack, et al., Validation of a self-administered food-frequency questionnaire administered in the European Prospective Investigation into Cancer and Nutrition (EPIC) Study: comparison of energy, protein, and macronutrient intakes estimated with the doubly labeled water, urinary nitrogen, and repeated 24-h dietary recall methods, Am. J. Clin. Nutr. 70 (1999) 439–447.

[93] R.K. Johnson, R.P. Soultanakis, D.E. Matthews, Literacy and body fatness are associated with underreporting of energy intake in U.S. low-income women using the multiple-pass 24-hour recall: a doubly labeled water study, J. Am. Diet. Assoc. 98 (1998) 1136–1140.

[94] J.R. Hebert, C.B. Ebbeling, C.E. Matthews, T.G. Hurley, Y. Ma, S. Druker, et al., Systematic errors in middle-aged women's estimates of energy intake: comparing three self-report measures to total energy expenditure from doubly labeled water, Ann. Epidemiol. 12 (2002) 577–586.

[95] A.F. Subar, V. Kipnis, R.P. Troiano, D. Midthune, D.A. Schoeller, S. Bingham, et al., Using intake biomarkers to evaluate the extent of dietary misreporting in a large sample of adults: the OPEN study, Am. J. Epidemiol. 158 (2003) 1–13.

[96] S.R. Preis, D. Spiegelman, B.B. Zhao, A. Moshfegh, D.J. Baer, W. C. Willett, Application of a repeat-measure biomarker measurement error model to 2 validation studies: examination of the effect of within-person variation in biomarker measurements, Am. J. Epidemiol. 173 (2011) 683–694.

[97] F.B. Scagliusi, E. Ferriolli, K. Pfrimer, C. Laureano, C.S. Cunha, B. Gualano, et al., Underreporting of energy intake in Brazilian women varies according to dietary assessment: a cross-sectional study using doubly labeled water, J. Am. Diet. Assoc. 108 (2008) 2031–2040.

[98] M.L. Neuhouser, L. Tinker, P.A. Shaw, D. Schoeller, S.A. Bingham, L.V. Horn, et al., Use of recovery biomarkers to calibrate nutrient consumption self-reports in the Women's Health Initiative, Am. J. Epidemiol. 167 (2008) 1247–1259.

[99] N. Slimani, S. Bingham, S. Runswick, P. Ferrari, N.E. Day, A.A. Welch, et al., Group level validation of protein intakes estimated by 24-hour diet recall and dietary questionnaires against 24-hour urinary nitrogen in the European Prospective Investigation into Cancer and Nutrition (EPIC) calibration study, Cancer Epidemiol. Biomarkers Prev. 12 (2003) 784–795.

[100] S.P. Crispim, A. Geelen, J.H. de Vries, H. Freisling, O.W. Souverein, P.J. Hulshof, et al., Bias in protein and potassium intake collected with 24-h recalls (EPIC-Soft) is rather comparable across European populations, Eur. J. Nutr. (2011).

[101] H. Freisling, M.M. van Bakel, C. Biessy, A.M. May, G. Byrnes, T. Norat, et al., Dietary reporting errors on 24 h recalls and dietary questionnaires are associated with BMI across six European countries as evaluated with recovery biomarkers for protein and potassium intake, Br. J. Nutr. 107 (2012) 910–920.

[102] S.P. Crispim, J.H. de Vries, A. Geelen, O.W. Souverein, P.J. Hulshof, L. Lafay, et al., Two non-consecutive 24 h recalls using EPIC-Soft software are sufficiently valid for comparing protein and potassium intake between five European centres: results from the European Food Consumption Validation (EFCOVAL) study, Br. J. Nutr. 105 (2011) 447–458.

[103] C. Montgomery, J.J. Reilly, D.M. Jackson, L.A. Kelly, C. Slater, J.Y. Paton, et al., Validation of energy intake by 24-hour multiple pass recall: comparison with total energy expenditure in children aged 5–7 years, Br. J. Nutr. 93 (2005) 671–676.

[104] B. Bokhof, A.E. Buyken, C. Dogan, A. Karaboga, J. Kaiser, A. Sonntag, et al., Validation of protein and potassium intakes assessed from 24 h recalls against levels estimated from 24 h urine samples in children and adolescents of Turkish descent living in Germany: results from the EVET! Study, Public Health Nutr. 15 (2012) 640–647.

[105] G.G. Harrison, O.M. Galal, N. Ibrahim, A. Khorshid, A. Stormer, J. Leslie, et al., Underreporting of food intake by dietary recall is not universal: a comparison of data from Egyptian and American women, J. Nutr. 130 (2000) 2049–2054.

[106] S.M. Krebs-Smith, B.I. Graubard, L.L. Kahle, A.F. Subar, L.E. Cleveland, R. Ballard-Barbash, Low energy reporters vs others: a comparison of reported food intakes, Eur. J. Clin. Nutr. 54 (2000) 281–287.

[107] R.R. Briefel, M.A. McDowell, K. Alaimo, C.R. Caughman, A.L. Bischof, M.D. Carroll, et al., Total energy intake of the U.S. population: the third National Health and Nutrition Examination Survey, 1988–1991, Am. J. Clin. Nutr. 62 (1995) 1072S–1080S.

[108] R.C. Klesges, L.H. Eck, J.W. Ray, Who underreports dietary intake in a dietary recall? Evidence from the Second National Health and Nutrition Examination Survey, J. Consult. Clin. Psychol. 63 (1995) 438–444.

[109] S.D. Poppitt, D. Swann, A.E. Black, A.M. Prentice, Assessment of selective under-reporting of food intake by both obese and non-obese women in a metabolic facility, Int. J. Obes. Relat. Metab. Disord. 22 (1998) 303–311.

[110] J.A. Tooze, A.F. Subar, F.E. Thompson, R. Troiano, A. Schatzkin, V. Kipnis, Psychosocial predictors of energy underreporting in a large doubly labeled water study, Am. J. Clin. Nutr. 79 (2004) 795–804.

[111] W.C. Willett, Nutritional Epidemiology, Oxford University Press, New York, 1998.

[112] S.N. Zulkifli, S.M. Yu, The food frequency method for dietary assessment, J. Am. Diet. Assoc. 92 (1992) 681–685.

[113] NutritionQuest, Assessment & Analysis Services: Questionnaires & Screeners, NutritionQuest, 2009. Available at <http://www.nutritionquest.com/assessment/list-of-questionnaires-and-screeners>.

[114] G. Block, A.M. Hartman, C.M. Dresser, M.D. Carroll, J. Gannon, L. Gardner, A data-based approach to diet questionnaire design and testing, Am. J. Epidemiol. 124 (1986) 453–469.

[115] G. Block, M. Woods, A. Potosky, C. Clifford, Validation of a self-administered diet history questionnaire using multiple diet records, J. Clin. Epidemiol. 43 (1990) 1327–1335.

[116] S.R. Cummings, G. Block, K. McHenry, R.B. Baron, Evaluation of two food frequency methods of measuring dietary calcium intake, Am. J. Epidemiol. 126 (1987) 796–802.

[117] J. Sobell, G. Block, P. Koslowe, J. Tobin, R. Andres, Validation of a retrospective questionnaire assessing diet 10–15 years ago, Am. J. Epidemiol. 130 (1989) 173–187.

[118] G. Block, F.E. Thompson, A.M. Hartman, F.A. Larkin, K.E. Guire, Comparison of two dietary questionnaires validated against multiple dietary records collected during a 1-year period, J. Am. Diet. Assoc. 92 (1992) 686–693.

[119] J.A. Mares-Perlman, B.E. Klein, R. Klein, L.L. Ritter, M.R. Fisher, J.L. Freudenheim, A diet history questionnaire ranks nutrient intakes in middle-aged and older men and women similarly to multiple food records, J. Nutr. 123 (1993) 489–501.

[120] R.J. Coates, J.W. Eley, G. Block, E.W. Gunter, A.L. Sowell, C. Grossman, et al., An evaluation of a food frequency questionnaire for assessing dietary intake of specific carotenoids and vitamin E among low-income black women, Am. J. Epidemiol. 134 (1991) 658–671.

[121] B.J. Caan, M.L. Slattery, J. Potter, C.P. Quesenberry Jr., A.O. Coates, D.M. Schaffer, Comparison of the Block and the Willett self-administered semiquantitative food frequency questionnaires with an interviewer-administered dietary history, Am. J. Epidemiol. 148 (1998) 1137–1147.

[122] S.E. McCann, J.R. Marshall, M. Trevisan, M. Russell, P. Muti, N. Markovic, et al., Recent alcohol intake as estimated by the Health Habits and History Questionnaire, the Harvard Semiquantitative Food Frequency Questionnaire, and a more detailed alcohol intake questionnaire, Am. J. Epidemiol. 150 (1999) 334–340.

[123] A.F. Subar, F.E. Thompson, V. Kipnis, D. Midthune, P. Hurwitz, S. McNutt, et al., Comparative validation of the Block, Willett, and National Cancer Institute food frequency questionnaires: the Eating at America's Table Study, Am. J. Epidemiol. 154 (2001) 1089–1099.

[124] Fred Hutchinson Cancer Research Center, Food Frequency Questionnaires (FFQs), Fred Hutchinson Cancer Research Center, Seattle, WA, 2007. Available at: <http://sharedresources.fhcrc.org/services/food-frequency-questionnaires-ffq>.

[125] R.E. Patterson, A.R. Kristal, L.F. Tinker, R.A. Carter, M.P. Bolton, T. Agurs-Collins, Measurement characteristics of the Women's Health Initiative food frequency questionnaire, Ann. Epidemiol. 9 (1999) 178–187.

[126] Harvard School of Public Health, HSPH Nutrition Department's File Download Site: Directory Listing of /health/FFQ/files, Nutrition Department, Harvard School of Public Health, 2011. Available at <https://regepi.bwh.harvard.edu/health/FFQ/files>.

[127] E.B. Rimm, E.L. Giovannucci, M.J. Stampfer, G.A. Colditz, L.B. Litin, W.C. Willett, Reproducibility and validity of an expanded self-administered semiquantitative food frequency questionnaire among male health professionals, Am. J. Epidemiol. 135 (1992) 1114–1126.

[128] W.C. Willett, L. Sampson, M.J. Stampfer, B. Rosner, C. Bain, J. Witschi, et al., Reproducibility and validity of a semiquantitative food frequency questionnaire, Am. J. Epidemiol. 122 (1985) 51–65.

[129] W.C. Willett, R.D. Reynolds, S. Cottrell-Hoehner, L. Sampson, M.L. Browne, Validation of a semi-quantitative food frequency questionnaire: comparison with a 1-year diet record, J. Am. Diet. Assoc. 87 (1987) 43–47.

[130] S. Salvini, D.J. Hunter, L. Sampson, M.J. Stampfer, G.A. Colditz, B. Rosner, et al., Food based validation of a dietary questionnaire: the effects of week-to-week variation in food consumption, Int. J. Epidemiol. 18 (1989) 858–867.

[131] D. Feskanich, E.B. Rimm, E.L. Giovannucci, G.A. Colditz, M.J. Stampfer, L.B. Litin, et al., Reproducibility and validity of food intake measurements from a semiquantitative food frequency questionnaire, J. Am. Diet. Assoc. 93 (1993) 790–796.

[132] C.J. Suitor, J. Gardner, W.C. Willett, A comparison of food frequency and diet recall methods in studies of nutrient intake of low-income pregnant women, J. Am. Diet. Assoc. 89 (1989) 1786–1794.

[133] A.K. Wirfalt, R.W. Jeffery, P.J. Elmer, Comparison of food frequency questionnaires: the reduced Block and Willett questionnaires differ in ranking on nutrient intakes, Am. J. Epidemiol. 148 (1998) 1148–1156.

[134] National Cancer Institute, Diet History Questionnaire, Applied Research Program, National Cancer Institute, 2010. Available at: <http://riskfactor.cancer.gov/DHQ>.

[135] V. Kipnis, A.F. Subar, D. Midthune, L.S. Freedman, R. Ballard-Barbash, R.P. Troiano, et al., Structure of dietary measurement error: results of the OPEN biomarker study, Am. J. Epidemiol. 158 (2003) 14–21.

[136] A.F. Subar, F.E. Thompson, A.F. Smith, J.B. Jobe, R.G. Ziegler, N. Potischman, et al., Improving food frequency questionnaires: a qualitative approach using cognitive interviewing, J. Am. Diet. Assoc. 95 (1995) 781–788.

[137] A.F. Subar, R.G. Ziegler, F.E. Thompson, C.C. Johnson, J.L. Weissfeld, D. Reding, et al., Is shorter always better? Relative importance of questionnaire length and cognitive ease on response rates and data quality for two dietary questionnaires, Am. J. Epidemiol. 153 (2001) 404–409.

[138] A.F. Subar, D. Midthune, M. Kulldorff, C.C. Brown, F.E. Thompson, V. Kipnis, et al., Evaluation of alternative approaches to assign nutrient values to food groups in food frequency questionnaires, Am. J. Epidemiol. 152 (2000) 279–286.

[139] Arizona Cancer Center, Questionnaires, The Arizona Diet, Behavior, and Quality of Life Assessment Lab, 2012. Available at: <http://www.azcc.arizona.edu/research/shared-services/bmss/questionnaires>.

[140] C. Ritenbaugh, M. Aickin, D. Taren, N. Teufel, E. Graver, K. Woolf, et al., Use of a food frequency questionnaire to screen for dietary eligibility in a randomized cancer prevention phase III trial, Cancer Epidemiol. Biomarkers Prev. 6 (1997) 347–354.

[141] R.A. Garcia, D. Taren, N.I. Teufel, Factors associated with the reproducibility of specific food items from the Southwest Food Frequency Questionnaire, Ecol. Food Nutr. 38 (2000) 549–561.

[142] M.K. Fialkowski, M.A. McCrory, S.M. Roberts, J.K. Tracy, L.M. Grattan, C.J. Boushey, Evaluation of dietary assessment tools used to assess the diet of adults participating in the Communities Advancing the Studies of Tribal Nations Across the Lifespan cohort, J. Am. Diet. Assoc. 110 (2010) 65–73.

[143] M. Pakseresht, S. Sharma, Validation of a culturally appropriate quantitative food frequency questionnaire for Inuvialuit population in the Northwest Territories, Canada, J. Hum. Nutr. Diet. 23 (2010) 75–82.

[144] T.C. Carithers, S.A. Talegawkar, M.L. Rowser, O.R. Henry, P. M. Dubbert, M.L. Bogle, et al., Validity and calibration of food frequency questionnaires used with African-American adults in the Jackson Heart Study, J. Am. Diet. Assoc. 109 (2009) 1184–1193.

[145] A.R. Kristal, Z. Feng, R.J. Coates, A. Oberman, V. George, Associations of race/ethnicity, education, and dietary intervention with the validity and reliability of a food frequency questionnaire: the Women's Health Trial Feasibility Study in Minority Populations, Am. J. Epidemiol. 146 (1997) 856–869.

[146] G. Block, P. Wakimoto, C. Jensen, S. Mandel, R.R. Green, Validation of a food frequency questionnaire for Hispanics, Prev. Chronic. Dis. 3 (2006) A77.

[147] J.H. Hankin, C.N. Yoshizawa, L.N. Kolonel, Reproducibility of a diet history in older men in Hawaii, Nutr. Cancer 13 (1990) 129–140.

[148] J.H. Hankin, L.R. Wilkens, L.N. Kolonel, C.N. Yoshizawa, Validation of a quantitative diet history method in Hawaii, Am. J. Epidemiol. 133 (1991) 616–628.

[149] M.C. Ocke, H.B. Bueno-de-Mesquita, H.E. Goddijn, A. Jansen, M.A. Pols, W.A. van Staveren, et al., The Dutch EPIC food frequency questionnaire: I. Description of the questionnaire, and relative validity and reproducibility for food groups, Int. J. Epidemiol. 26 (1997) S37–S48.

[150] K. Katsouyanni, E.B. Rimm, C. Gnardellis, D. Trichopoulos, E. Polychronopoulos, A. Trichopoulou, Reproducibility and relative validity of an extensive semi-quantitative food frequency questionnaire using dietary records and biochemical markers among Greek schoolteachers, Int. J. Epidemiol. 26 (1997) S118–S127.

[151] S. Bohlscheid-Thomas, I. Hoting, H. Boeing, J. Wahrendorf, Reproducibility and relative validity of food group intake in a food frequency questionnaire developed for the German part of the EPIC project. European Prospective Investigation into Cancer and Nutrition, Int. J. Epidemiol. 26 (1997) S59–S70.

[152] S. Bohlscheid-Thomas, I. Hoting, H. Boeing, J. Wahrendorf, Reproducibility and relative validity of energy and macronutrient intake of a food frequency questionnaire developed for the German part of the EPIC project. European Prospective Investigation into Cancer and Nutrition, Int. J. Epidemiol. 26 (1997) S71–S81.

[153] E. Riboli, S. Elmstahl, R. Saracci, B. Gullberg, F. Lindgarde, The Malmo Food Study: validity of two dietary assessment methods for measuring nutrient intake, Int. J. Epidemiol. 26 (1997) S161–S173.

[154] P. Pisani, F. Faggiano, V. Krogh, D. Palli, P. Vineis, F. Berrino, Relative validity and reproducibility of a food frequency dietary questionnaire for use in the Italian EPIC centres, Int. J. Epidemiol. 26 (1997) S152–S160.

[155] C. Lassale, C. Guilbert, J. Keogh, J. Syrette, K. Lange, D.N. Cox, Estimating food intakes in Australia: validation of the Commonwealth Scientific and Industrial Research Organisation (CSIRO) food frequency questionnaire against weighed dietary intakes, J. Hum. Nutr. Diet. 22 (2009) 559–566.

[156] J.F. Watson, C.E. Collins, D.W. Sibbritt, M.J. Dibley, M.L. Garg, Reproducibility and comparative validity of a food frequency questionnaire for Australian children and adolescents, Int. J. Behav. Nutr. Phys. Act. 6 (2009) 62.

[157] M.C. van Dongen, M.A. Lentjes, N.E. Wijckmans, C. Dirckx, D. Lemaitre, W. Achten, et al., Validation of a food-frequency questionnaire for Flemish and Italian-native subjects in Belgium: the IMMIDIET study, Nutrition 27 (2011) 302–309.

[158] E. Kesse-Guyot, K. Castetbon, M. Touvier, S. Hercberg, P. Galan, Relative validity and reproducibility of a food frequency questionnaire designed for French adults, Ann. Nutr. Metab 57 (2010) 153–162.

[159] M. Haftenberger, T. Heuer, C. Heidemann, F. Kube, C. Krems, G.B. Mensink, Relative validation of a food frequency questionnaire for national health and nutrition monitoring, Nutr. J. 9 (2010) 36.

[160] A. Hjartaker, L.F. Andersen, E. Lund, Comparison of diet measures from a food-frequency questionnaire with measures from repeated 24-hour dietary recalls. The Norwegian Women and Cancer Study, Public Health Nutr. 10 (2007) 1094–1103.

[161] R. Takachi, J. Ishihara, M. Iwasaki, M. Hosoi, Y. Ishii, S. Sasazuki, et al., Validity of a self-administered food frequency questionnaire for middle-aged urban cancer screenees: comparison with 4-day weighed dietary records, J. Epidemiol. 21 (2011) 447–458.

[162] N. Chiba, N. Okuda, A. Okayama, T. Kadowaki, H. Ueshima, Development of a food frequency and quantity method for assessing dietary habits of Japanese individuals: comparison with results from 24-hr recall dietary survey, J. Atheroscler. Thromb. 15 (2008) 324−333.

[163] S.H. Kim, H.N. Choi, J.Y. Hwang, N. Chang, W.Y. Kim, H.W. Chung, et al., Development and evaluation of a food frequency questionnaire for Vietnamese female immigrants in Korea: the Korean Genome and Epidemiology Study (KoGES), Nutr. Res. Pract. 5 (2011) 260−265.

[164] T. Mouratidou, F.A. Ford, R.B. Fraser, Reproducibility and validity of a food frequency questionnaire in assessing dietary intakes of low-income Caucasian postpartum women living in Sheffield, United Kingdom, Matern. Child Nutr. 7 (2011) 128−139.

[165] B. Liu, H. Young, F.L. Crowe, V.S. Benson, E.A. Spencer, T.J. Key, et al., Development and evaluation of the Oxford WebQ, a low-cost, web-based method for assessment of previous 24 h dietary intakes in large-scale prospective studies, Public Health Nutr. 14 (2011) 1998−2005.

[166] F.E. Thompson, G.B. Willis, O.M. Thompson, A.L. Yaroch, The meaning of "fruits" and "vegetables," Public Health Nutr. 14 (2011) 1222−1228.

[167] A.R. Kristal, K. Glanz, Z. Feng, J.R. Hebert, C. Probart, M. Eriksen, et al., Does using a short dietary questionnaire instead of a food frequency improve response rates to a health assessment survey? J. Nutr. Educ. 26 (1994) 224−227.

[168] S. Eaker, R. Bergstrom, A. Bergstrom, H.O. Adami, O. Nyren, Response rate to mailed epidemiologic questionnaires: a population-based randomized trial of variations in design and mailing routines, Am. J. Epidemiol. 147 (1998) 74−82.

[169] M.C. Morris, G.A. Colditz, D.A. Evans, Response to a mail nutritional survey in an older bi-racial community population, Ann. Epidemiol. 8 (1998) 342−346.

[170] L. Johansson, K. Solvoll, S. Opdahl, G.E. Bjorneboe, C.A. Drevon, Response rates with different distribution methods and reward, and reproducibility of a quantitative food frequency questionnaire, Eur. J. Clin. Nutr. 51 (1997) 346−353.

[171] A. Kuskowska-Wolk, S. Holte, E.M. Ohlander, A. Bruce, L. Holmberg, H.O. Adami, et al., Effects of different designs and extension of a food frequency questionnaire on response rate, completeness of data and food frequency responses, Int. J. Epidemiol. 21 (1992) 1144−1150.

[172] F.A. Tylavsky, G.B. Sharp, Misclassification of nutrient and energy intake from use of closed-ended questions in epidemiologic research, Am. J. Epidemiol. 142 (1995) 342−352.

[173] J.A. Heady, Diets of bank clerks: development of a method of classifying the diets of individuals for use in epidemiological studies, J. R. Stat. Soc. Ser. A 124 (1961) 336−371.

[174] S. Kumanyika, G.S. Tell, L. Fried, J.K. Martel, V.M. Chinchilli, Picture-sort method for administering a food frequency questionnaire to older adults, J. Am. Diet. Assoc. 96 (1996) 137−144.

[175] S.K. Kumanyika, G.S. Tell, L. Shemanski, J. Martel, V.M. Chinchilli, Dietary assessment using a picture-sort approach, Am. J. Clin. Nutr. 65 (1997) 1123S−1129S.

[176] L.H. Eck, L.M. Klesges, R.C. Klesges, Precision and estimated accuracy of two short-term food frequency questionnaires compared with recalls and records, J. Clin. Epidemiol. 49 (1996) 1195−1200.

[177] A.F. Subar, C.M. Frey, L.C. Harlan, L. Kahle, Differences in reported food frequency by season of questionnaire administration: the 1987 National Health Interview Survey, Epidemiology 5 (1994) 226−233.

[178] Y. Tsubono, Y. Nishino, A. Fukao, S. Hisamichi, S. Tsugane, Temporal change in the reproducibility of a self-administered food frequency questionnaire, Am. J. Epidemiol. 142 (1995) 1231−1235.

[179] B. Caan, R.A. Hiatt, A.M. Owen, Mailed dietary surveys: response rates, error rates, and the effect of omitted food items on nutrient values, Epidemiology 2 (1991) 430−436.

[180] L. Holmberg, E.M. Ohlander, T. Byers, M. Zack, A. Wolk, A. Bruce, et al., A search for recall bias in a case−control study of diet and breast cancer, Int. J. Epidemiol. 25 (1996) 235−244.

[181] L.M. Hansson, M.R. Galanti, Diet-associated risks of disease and self-reported food consumption: how shall we treat partial nonresponse in a food frequency questionnaire? Nutr. Cancer 36 (2000) 1−6.

[182] C.L. Parr, A. Hjartaker, I. Scheel, E. Lund, P. Laake, M.B. Veierod, Comparing methods for handling missing values in food-frequency questionnaires and proposing k nearest neighbours imputation: effects on dietary intake in the Norwegian Women and Cancer study (NOWAC), Public Health Nutr. 11 (2008) 361−370.

[183] National Cancer Institute, Diet History Questionnaire: Web-Based DHQ, Applied Research Program, National Cancer Institute, 2010. Available at: <http://riskfactor.cancer.gov/DHQ/webquest/index.html>

[184] C. Matthys, I. Pynaert, W. De Keyzer, S. De Henauw, Validity and reproducibility of an adolescent web-based food frequency questionnaire, J. Am. Diet. Assoc. 107 (2007) 605−610.

[185] M.E. Labonte, A. Cyr, L. Baril-Gravel, M.M. Royer, B. Lamarche, Validity and reproducibility of a web-based, self-administered food frequency questionnaire, Eur. J. Clin. Nutr. 66 (2012) 166−173.

[186] A.F. Smith, Cognitive psychological issues of relevance to the validity of dietary reports, Eur. J. Clin. Nutr. 47 (1993) S6−18.

[187] S.M. Krebs-Smith, J. Heimendinger, A.F. Subar, B.H. Patterson, E. Pivonka, Estimating fruit and vegetable intake using food frequency questionnaires: a comparison of instruments, Am. J. Clin. Nutr. 59 (1994) 283s.

[188] D.J. Hunter, L. Sampson, M.J. Stampfer, G.A. Colditz, B. Rosner, W.C. Willett, Variability in portion sizes of commonly consumed foods among a population of women in the United States, Am. J. Epidemiol. 127 (1988) 1240−1249.

[189] G. Block, A.F. Subar, Estimates of nutrient intake from a food frequency questionnaire: the 1987 National Health Interview Survey, J. Am. Diet. Assoc. 92 (1992) 969−977.

[190] R.R. Briefel, K.M. Flegal, D.M. Winn, C.M. Loria, C.L. Johnson, C.T. Sempos, Assessing the nation's diet: limitations of the food frequency questionnaire, J. Am. Diet. Assoc. 92 (1992) 959−962.

[191] C.T. Sempos, Invited commentary: some limitations of semi-quantitative food frequency questionnaires, Am. J. Epidemiol. 135 (1992) 1127−1132.

[192] E.B. Rimm, E.L. Giovannucci, M.J. Stampfer, G.A. Colditz, L.B. Litin, W.C. Willett, Authors' response to "Invited commentary: some limitations of semiquantitative food frequency questionnaires," Am. J. Epidemiol. 135 (1992) 1133−1136.

[193] R.J. Carroll, L.S. Freedman, A.M. Hartman, Use of semiquantitative food frequency questionnaires to estimate the distribution of usual intake, Am. J. Epidemiol. 143 (1996) 392−404.

[194] L.H. Kushi, Gaps in epidemiologic research methods: design considerations for studies that use food-frequency questionnaires, Am. J. Clin. Nutr. 59 (1994) 180S−184S.

[195] G.H. Beaton, Approaches to analysis of dietary data: relationship between planned analyses and choice of methodology, Am. J. Clin. Nutr. 59 (1994) 253S−261S.

[196] C.T. Sempos, K. Liu, N.D. Ernst, Food and nutrient exposures: what to consider when evaluating epidemiologic evidence, Am. J. Clin. Nutr. 69 (1999) 1330S−1338S.

A. ASSESSMENT METHODS FOR RESEARCH AND PRACTICE

[197] L.S. Freedman, A. Schatzkin, Y. Wax, The impact of dietary measurement error on planning sample size required in a cohort study, Am. J. Epidemiol. 132 (1990) 1185–1195.

[198] E.J. Schaefer, J.L. Augustin, M.M. Schaefer, H. Rasmussen, J.M. Ordovas, G.E. Dallal, et al., Lack of efficacy of a food-frequency questionnaire in assessing dietary macronutrient intakes in subjects consuming diets of known composition, Am. J. Clin. Nutr. 71 (2000) 746–751.

[199] National Cancer Institute, Dietary Assessment Calibration/ Validation Register: Studies and their Associated Publications, Applied Research Program, National Cancer Institute, 2011. Available at <http://appliedresearch.cancer.gov/cgi-bin/dacv/index.pl>

[200] M.B. Livingstone, A.E. Black, Markers of the validity of reported energy intake, J. Nutr. 133 (2003) 895S–920S.

[201] S.A. Bingham, Urine nitrogen as a biomarker for the validation of dietary protein intake, J. Nutr. 133 (2003) 921S–924S.

[202] S.A. Bingham, A. Cassidy, T.J. Cole, A. Welch, S.A. Runswick, A.E. Black, et al., Validation of weighed records and other methods of dietary assessment using the 24 h urine nitrogen technique and other biological markers, Br. J. Nutr. 73 (1995) 531–550.

[203] L.T. Pijls, H. De Vries, A.J. Donker, J.T. van Eijk, Reproducibility and biomarker-based validity and responsiveness of a food frequency questionnaire to estimate protein intake, Am. J. Epidemiol. 150 (1999) 987–995.

[204] M.C. Ocke, H.B. Bueno-de-Mesquita, M.A. Pols, H.A. Smit, W. A. van Staveren, D. Kromhout, The Dutch EPIC food frequency questionnaire: II. Relative validity and reproducibility for nutrients, Int. J. Epidemiol. 26 (1997) S49–S58.

[205] S.A. Bingham, Dietary assessments in the European prospective study of diet and cancer (EPIC), Eur. J. Cancer Prev. 6 (1997) 118–124.

[206] S.A. Bingham, N.E. Day, Using biochemical markers to assess the validity of prospective dietary assessment methods and the effect of energy adjustment, Am. J. Clin. Nutr. 65 (1997) 1130S–1137S.

[207] K.M. Flegal, Evaluating epidemiologic evidence of the effects of food and nutrient exposures, Am. J. Clin. Nutr. 69 (1999) 1339S–1344S.

[208] R.C. Burack, J. Liang, The early detection of cancer in the primary-care setting: factors associated with the acceptance and completion of recommended procedures, Prev. Med. 16 (1987) 739–751.

[209] R.L. Prentice, Measurement error and results from analytic epidemiology: dietary fat and breast cancer, J. Natl. Cancer Inst. 88 (1996) 1738–1747.

[210] V. Kipnis, L.S. Freedman, C.C. Brown, A.M. Hartman, A. Schatzkin, S. Wacholder, Effect of measurement error on energy-adjustment models in nutritional epidemiology, Am. J. Epidemiol. 146 (1997) 842–855.

[211] F.B. Hu, M.J. Stampfer, E. Rimm, A. Ascherio, B.A. Rosner, D. Spiegelman, et al., Dietary fat and coronary heart disease: a comparison of approaches for adjusting for total energy intake and modeling repeated dietary measurements, Am. J. Epidemiol. 149 (1999) 531–540.

[212] R.J. Carroll, L.S. Freedman, V. Kipnis, L. Li, A new class of measurement-error models, with applications to dietary data, Can. J. Stat. 26 (1998) 467–477.

[213] L. Kohlmeier, B. Bellach, Exposure assessment error and its handling in nutritional epidemiology, Annu. Rev. Public Health 16 (1995) 43–59.

[214] R. Kaaks, E. Riboli, W. van Staveren, Calibration of dietary intake measurements in prospective cohort studies, Am. J. Epidemiol. 142 (1995) 548–556.

[215] B. Bellach, L. Kohlmeier, Energy adjustment does not control for differential recall bias in nutritional epidemiology, J. Clin. Epidemiol. 51 (1998) 393–398.

[216] V. Kipnis, R.J. Carroll, L.S. Freedman, L. Li, Implications of a new dietary measurement error model for estimation of relative risk: application to four calibration studies, Am. J. Epidemiol. 150 (1999) 642–651.

[217] S.A. Bingham, R. Luben, A. Welch, N. Wareham, K.T. Khaw, N. Day, Are imprecise methods obscuring a relation between fat and breast cancer? Lancet 362 (2003) 212–214.

[218] L.S. Freedman, N. Potischman, V. Kipnis, D. Midthune, A. Schatzkin, F.E. Thompson, et al., A comparison of two dietary instruments for evaluating the fat–breast cancer relationship, Int. J. Epidemiol. 35 (2006) 1011–1021.

[219] T.J. Key, P.N. Appleby, B.J. Cairns, R. Luben, C.C. Dahm, T. Akbaraly, et al., Dietary fat and breast cancer: comparison of results from food diaries and food-frequency questionnaires in the UK Dietary Cohort Consortium, Am. J. Clin. Nutr. 94 (2011) 1043–1052.

[220] A.R. Kristal, U. Peters, J.D. Potter, Is it time to abandon the food frequency questionnaire? Cancer Epidemiol. Biomarkers Prev. 14 (2005) 2826–2828.

[221] A.R. Kristal, J.D. Potter, Not the time to abandon the food frequency questionnaire: counterpoint, Cancer Epidemiol. Biomarkers Prev. 15 (2006) 1759–1760.

[222] R.J. Carroll, D. Midthune, A.F. Subar, M. Shumakovich, L.S. Freedman, F.E. Thompson, et al., Taking advantage of the strengths of 2 different dietary assessment instruments to improve intake estimates for nutritional epidemiology, Am. J. Epidemiol. 175 (2012) 340–347.

[223] J. Haubrock, U. Nothlings, J.L. Volatier, A. Dekkers, M. Ocke, U. Harttig, et al., Estimating usual food intake distributions by using the multiple source method in the EPIC-Potsdam Calibration Study, J. Nutr. 141 (2011) 914–920.

[224] V. Kipnis, D. Midthune, D.W. Buckman, K.W. Dodd, P.M. Guenther, S.M. Krebs-Smith, et al., Modeling data with excess zeros and measurement error: application to evaluating relationships between episodically consumed foods and health outcomes, Biometrics 65 (2009) 1003–1010.

[225] A.R. Kristal, C.H. Andrilla, T.D. Koepsell, P.H. Diehr, A. Cheadle, Dietary assessment instruments are susceptible to intervention-associated response set bias, J. Am. Diet. Assoc. 98 (1998) 40–43.

[226] M.L. Neuhouser, A.R. Kristal, D. McLerran, R.E. Patterson, J. Atkinson, Validity of short food frequency questionnaires used in cancer chemoprevention trials: results from the Prostate Cancer Prevention Trial, Cancer Epidemiol. Biomarkers Prev. 8 (1999) 721–725.

[227] National Center for Chronic Disease Prevention and Health Promotion, Behavioral Risk Factor Surveillance System (BRFSS), Centers for Disease Control and Prevention, 2012. Available at: <http://www.cdc.gov/brfss>

[228] UCLA Center for Health Policy Research, California Health Interview Survey, California Department of Health Services and the Public Health Institute, 2011. Available at: <http://www.chis.ucla.edu>

[229] F.E. Thompson, D. Midthune, A.F. Subar, T. McNeel, D. Berrigan, V. Kipnis, Dietary intake estimates in the National Health Interview Survey, 2000: methodology, results, and interpretation, J. Am. Diet. Assoc. 105 (2005) 352–363.

[230] M.L. Neuhouser, S. Lilley, A. Lund, D.B. Johnson, Development and validation of a beverage and snack questionnaire for use in evaluation of school nutrition policies, J. Am. Diet. Assoc. 109 (2009) 1587–1592.

[231] L.W. Pickle, A.M. Hartman, Indicator foods for vitamin A assessment, Nutr. Cancer 7 (1985) 3—23.

[232] T. Byers, J. Marshall, R. Fiedler, M. Zielezny, S. Graham, Assessing nutrient intake with an abbreviated dietary interview, Am. J. Epidemiol. 122 (1985) 41—50.

[233] National Cancer Institute, Register of Validated Short Dietary Assessment Instruments, Applied Research Program, National Cancer Institute, 2011. Available at: <http://riskfactor.cancer.gov/diet/shortreg>

[234] A.E. Field, G.A. Colditz, M.K. Fox, T. Byers, M. Serdula, R.J. Bosch, et al., Comparison of 4 questionnaires for assessment of fruit and vegetable intake, Am. J. Public Health 88 (1998) 1216—1218.

[235] K.W. Cullen, T. Baranowski, J. Baranowski, D. Hebert, C. de Moor, Pilot study of the validity and reliability of brief fruit, juice and vegetable screeners among inner city African-American boys and 17 to 20 year old adults, J. Am. Coll. Nutr. 18 (1999) 442—450.

[236] K. Resnicow, E. Odom, T. Wang, W.N. Dudley, D. Mitchell, R. Vaughan, et al., Validation of three food frequency questionnaires and 24-hour recalls with serum carotenoid levels in a sample of African-American adults, Am. J. Epidemiol. 152 (2000) 1072—1080.

[237] J.J. Prochaska, J.F. Sallis, Reliability and validity of a fruit and vegetable screening measure for adolescents, J. Adolesc. Health 34 (2004) 163—165.

[238] L.F. Andersen, M.B. Veierod, L. Johansson, A. Sakhi, K. Solvoll, C.A. Drevon, Evaluation of three dietary assessment methods and serum biomarkers as measures of fruit and vegetable intake, using the method of triads, Br. J. Nutr. 93 (2005) 519—527.

[239] M.K. Campbell, B. Polhamus, J.W. Mcclelland, K. Bennett, W. Kalsbeek, D. Coole, et al., Assessing fruit and vegetable consumption in a 5 a day study targeting rural blacks: the issue of portion size, J. Am. Diet. Assoc. 96 (1996) 1040—1042.

[240] T. Baranowski, M. Smith, J. Baranowski, D.T. Wang, C. Doyle, L.S. Lin, et al., Low validity of a seven-item fruit and vegetable food frequency questionnaire among third-grade students, J. Am. Diet. Assoc. 97 (1997) 66—68.

[241] M.K. Hunt, A.M. Stoddard, K. Peterson, G. Sorensen, J.R. Hebert, N. Cohen, Comparison of dietary assessment measures in the Treatwell 5 A Day worksite study, J. Am. Diet. Assoc. 98 (1998) 1021—1023.

[242] M. Serdula, R. Coates, T. Byers, A. Mokdad, S. Jewell, N. Chavez, et al., Evaluation of a brief telephone questionnaire to estimate fruit and vegetable consumption in diverse study populations, Epidemiology 4 (1993) 455—463.

[243] S.A. Smith-Warner, P.J. Elmer, L. Fosdick, T.M. Tharp, B. Randall, Reliability and comparability of three dietary assessment methods for estimating fruit and vegetable intakes, Epidemiology 8 (1997) 196—201.

[244] B. Armstrong, Diet and hormones in the epidemiology of breast and endometrial cancers, Nutr. Cancer 1 (1979) 90—95.

[245] A.R. Kristal, N.C. Vizenor, R.E. Patterson, M.L. Neuhouser, A.L. Shattuck, D. McLerran, Precision and bias of food frequency-based estimates of fruit and vegetable intakes, Cancer Epidemiol. Biomarkers Prev. 9 (2000) 939—944.

[246] F.E. Thompson, A.F. Subar, A.F. Smith, D. Midthune, K.L. Radimer, L.L. Kahle, et al., Fruit and vegetable assessment: performance of 2 new short instruments and a food frequency questionnaire, J. Am. Diet. Assoc. 102 (2002) 1764—1772.

[247] G.W. Greene, K. Resnicow, F.E. Thompson, K.E. Peterson, T.G. Hurley, J.R. Hebert, et al., Correspondence of the NCI Fruit and Vegetable Screener to repeat 24-h recalls and serum carotenoids in behavioral intervention trials, J. Nutr. 138 (2008) 200S—204S.

[248] K.E. Peterson, J.R. Hebert, T.G. Hurley, K. Resnicow, F.E. Thompson, G.W. Greene, et al., Accuracy and precision of two short screeners to assess change in fruit and vegetable consumption among diverse populations participating in health promotion intervention trials, J. Nutr. 138 (2008) 218S—225S.

[249] Centers for Disease Control and Prevention, Behavioral Risk Factor Surveillance System (BRFSS), Centers for Disease Control and Prevention, 2011. Available at: <http://www.cdc.gov/brfss>

[250] U.S. Department of Health and Human Services, Dietary Guidelines for Americans, 2010, Office of Disease Prevention and Health Promotion, U.S. Department of Health and Human Services, 2011. Available at: <http://www.health.gov/dietary-guidelines/2010.asp>

[251] G. Block, C. Clifford, M.D. Naughton, M. Henderson, M. McAdams, A brief dietary screen for high fat intake, J. Nutr. Educ. 21 (1989) 199—207.

[252] R.J. Coates, M.K. Serdula, T. Byers, A. Mokdad, S. Jewell, S.B. Leonard, et al., A brief, telephone-administered food frequency questionnaire can be useful for surveillance of dietary fat intakes, J. Nutr. 125 (1995) 1473—1483.

[253] E.H. Spencer, L.K. Elon, V.S. Hertzberg, A.D. Stein, E. Frank, Validation of a brief diet survey instrument among medical students, J. Am. Diet. Assoc. 105 (2005) 802—806.

[254] B. Caan, A. Coates, D. Schaffer, Variations in sensitivity, specificity, and predictive value of a dietary fat screener modified from Block et al, J. Am. Diet. Assoc. 95 (1995) 564—568.

[255] P. Kris-Etherton, B. Eissenstat, S. Jaax, U. Srinath, L. Scott, J. Rader, et al., Validation for MEDFICTS, a dietary assessment instrument for evaluating adherence to total and saturated fat recommendations of the National Cholesterol Education Program Step 1 and Step 2 diets, J. Am. Diet. Assoc. 101 (2001) 81—86.

[256] A.J. Taylor, H. Wong, K. Wish, J. Carrow, D. Bell, J. Bindeman, et al., Validation of the MEDFICTS dietary questionnaire: a clinical tool to assess adherence to American Heart Association dietary fat intake guidelines, Nutr. J. 2 (2003) 4.

[257] C.R. Teal, D.L. Baham, B.J. Gor, L.A. Jones, Is the MEDFICTS Rapid Dietary Fat Screener valid for premenopausal African-American women? J. Am. Diet. Assoc. 107 (2007) 773—781.

[258] A.L. Holmes, B. Sanderson, R. Maisiak, A. Brown, V. Bittner, Dietitian services are associated with improved patient outcomes and the MEDFICTS dietary assessment questionnaire is a suitable outcome measure in cardiac rehabilitation, J. Am. Diet. Assoc. 105 (2005) 1533—1540.

[259] H. Mochari, Q. Gao, L. Mosca, Validation of the MEDFICTS dietary assessment questionnaire in a diverse population, J. Am. Diet. Assoc. 108 (2008) 817—822.

[260] S. Rohrmann, G. Klein, Validation of a short questionnaire to qualitatively assess the intake of total fat, saturated, monounsaturated, polyunsaturated fatty acids, and cholesterol, J. Hum. Nutr. Diet. 16 (2003) 111—117.

[261] S. Rohrmann, G. Klein, Development and validation of a short food list to assess the intake of total fat, saturated, mono-unsaturated, polyunsaturated fatty acids and cholesterol, Eur. J. Public Health 13 (2003) 262—268.

[262] F.E. Thompson, D. Midthune, A.F. Subar, V. Kipnis, L.L. Kahle, A. Schatzkin, Development and evaluation of a short instrument to estimate usual dietary intake of percentage energy from fat, J. Am. Diet. Assoc. 107 (2007) 760—767.

[263] F.E. Thompson, D. Midthune, G.C. Williams, A.L. Yaroch, T.G. Hurley, K. Resnicow, et al., Evaluation of a short dietary assessment instrument for percentage energy from fat in an intervention study, J. Nutr. 138 (2008) 193S—199S.

[264] A.L. Yaroch, K. Resnicow, L.K. Khan, Validity and reliability of qualitative dietary fat index questionnaires: a review, J. Am. Diet. Assoc. 100 (2000) 240–244.

[265] P. van Assema, J. Brug, G. Kok, H. Brants, The reliability and validity of a Dutch questionnaire on fat consumption as a means to rank subjects according to individual fat intake, Eur. J. Cancer Prev. 1 (1992) 375–380.

[266] A.S. Ammerman, P.S. Haines, R.F. DeVellis, D.S. Strogatz, T.C. Keyserling, R.J. Simpson Jr., et al., A brief dietary assessment to guide cholesterol reduction in low-income individuals: design and validation, J. Am. Diet. Assoc. 91 (1991) 1385–1390.

[267] P.N. Hopkins, R.R. Williams, H. Kuida, B.M. Stults, S.C. Hunt, G.K. Barlow, et al., Predictive value of a short dietary questionnaire for changes in serum lipids in high-risk Utah families, Am. J. Clin. Nutr. 50 (1989) 292–300.

[268] T. Kemppainen, A. Rosendahl, O. Nuutinen, T. Ebeling, P. Pietinen, M. Uusitupa, Validation of a short dietary questionnaire and a qualitative fat index for the assessment of fat intake, Eur. J. Clin. Nutr. 47 (1993) 765–775.

[269] B.M. Retzlaff, A.A. Dowdy, C.E. Walden, V.E. Bovbjerg, R.H. Knopp, The Northwest Lipid Research Clinic Fat Intake Scale: validation and utility, Am. J. Public Health 87 (1997) 181–185.

[270] P. Little, J. Barnett, B. Margetts, A.L. Kinmonth, J. Gabbay, R. Thompson, et al., The validity of dietary assessment in general practice, J. Epidemiol. Community Health 53 (1999) 165–172.

[271] S.P. Murphy, L.L. Kaiser, M.S. Townsend, L.H. Allen, Evaluation of validity of items for a food behavior checklist, J. Am. Diet. Assoc. 101 (2001) 751–761.

[272] S. Kinlay, R.F. Heller, J.A. Halliday, A simple score and questionnaire to measure group changes in dietary fat intake, Prev. Med. 20 (1991) 378–388.

[273] S.A. Beresford, E.M. Farmer, L. Feingold, K.L. Graves, S.K. Sumner, R.M. Baker, Evaluation of a self-help dietary intervention in a primary care setting, Am. J. Public Health 82 (1992) 79–84.

[274] S.L. Connor, J.R. Gustafson, G. Sexton, N. Becker, S. Artaud-Wild, W.E. Connor, The Diet Habit Survey: a new method of dietary assessment that relates to plasma cholesterol changes, J. Am. Diet. Assoc. 92 (1992) 41–47.

[275] R.E. Glasgow, J.D. Perry, D.J. Toobert, J.F. Hollis, Brief assessments of dietary behavior in field settings, Addict. Behav. 21 (1996) 239–247.

[276] R.F. Heller, H.D. Pedoe, G. Rose, A simple method of assessing the effect of dietary advice to reduce plasma cholesterol, Prev. Med. 10 (1981) 364–370.

[277] A.R. Kristal, A.L. Shattuck, H.J. Henry, Patterns of dietary behavior associated with selecting diets low in fat: reliability and validity of a behavioral approach to dietary assessment, J. Am. Diet. Assoc. 90 (1990) 214–220.

[278] A.R. Kristal, E. White, A.L. Shattuck, S. Curry, G.L. Anderson, A. Fowler, et al., Long-term maintenance of a low-fat diet: durability of fat-related dietary habits in the Women's Health Trial, J. Am. Diet. Assoc. 92 (1992) 553–559.

[279] A.R. Kristal, S.A. Beresford, D. Lazovich, Assessing change in diet-intervention research, Am. J. Clin. Nutr. 59 (1994) 185S–189S.

[280] A.L. Yaroch, K. Resnicow, A.D. Petty, L.K. Khan, Validity and reliability of a modified qualitative dietary fat index in low-income, overweight, African American adolescent girls, J. Am. Diet. Assoc. 100 (2000) 1525–1529.

[281] P.M. Risica, G. Burkholder, K.M. Gans, T.M. Lasater, S. Acharyya, C. Davis, et al., Assessing fat-related dietary behaviors among black women: reliability and validity of a new Food Habits Questionnaire, J. Nutr. Educ. Behav. 39 (2007) 197–204.

[282] C.A. Anderson, S.K. Kumanyika, J. Shults, M.J. Kallan, K.M. Gans, P.M. Risica, Assessing change in dietary-fat behaviors in a weight-loss program for African Americans: a potential short method, J. Am. Diet. Assoc. 107 (2007) 838–842.

[283] G. Block, C. Gillespie, E.H. Rosenbaum, C. Jenson, A rapid food screener to assess fat and fruit and vegetable intake, Am. J. Prev. Med. 18 (2000) 284–288.

[284] I.M. Buzzard, C.A. Stanton, M. Figueiredo, E.A. Fries, R. Nicholson, C.J. Hogan, et al., Development and reproducibility of a brief food frequency questionnaire for assessing the fat, fiber, and fruit and vegetable intakes of rural adolescents, J. Am. Diet. Assoc. 101 (2001) 1438–1446.

[285] F.E. Thompson, D. Midthune, A.F. Subar, L.L. Kahle, A. Schatzkin, V. Kipnis, Performance of a short tool to assess dietary intakes of fruits and vegetables, percentage energy from fat and fibre, Public Health Nutr. 7 (2004) 1097–1105.

[286] A. Svilaas, E.C. Strom, T. Svilaas, A. Borgejordet, M. Thoresen, L. Ose, Reproducibility and validity of a short food questionnaire for the assessment of dietary habits, Nutr. Metab. Cardiovasc. Dis. 12 (2002) 60–70.

[287] B. Laviolle, C. Froger-Bompas, P. Guillo, A. Sevestre, C. Letellier, M. Pouchard, et al., Relative validity and reproducibility of a 14-item semi-quantitative food frequency questionnaire for cardiovascular prevention, Eur. J. Cardiovasc. Prev. Rehabil. 12 (2005) 587–595.

[288] S.L. Rifas-Shiman, W.C. Willett, R. Lobb, J. Kotch, C. Dart, M.W. Gillman, PrimeScreen, a brief dietary screening tool: reproducibility and comparability with both a longer food frequency questionnaire and biomarkers, Public Health Nutr. 4 (2001) 249–254.

[289] National Cancer Institute, Five-Factor Screener in the 2005 NHIS Cancer Control Supplement, Applied Research Program, National Cancer Institute, 2007. Available at: <http://appliedresearch.cancer.gov/surveys/nhis/5factor>

[290] National Cancer Institute, The Diet Screener in the 2005 California Health Interview Survey, Applied Research Program, National Cancer Institute, 2009. Available at: <http://appliedresearch.cancer.gov/surveys/chis/dietscreener>

[291] National Cancer Institute, Dietary Screener in the NHANES 2009–10, Applied Research Program, National Cancer Institute, 2011. Available at: <http://riskfactor.cancer.gov/studies/nhanes/dietscreen>

[292] J. Shannon, A.R. Kristal, S.J. Curry, S.A. Beresford, Application of a behavioral approach to measuring dietary change: the fat- and fiber-related diet behavior questionnaire, Cancer Epidemiol. Biomarkers Prev. 6 (1997) 355–361.

[293] D.G. Schlundt, M.K. Hargreaves, M.S. Buchowski, The Eating Behavior Patterns Questionnaire predicts dietary fat intake in African American women, J. Am. Diet. Assoc. 103 (2003) 338–345.

[294] USDA Center for Nutrition Policy and Promotion, Healthy Eating Index, U.S. Department of Agriculture, 2011. Available at: <http://www.cnpp.usda.gov/healthyeatingindex.htm>

[295] K.M. Gans, P.M. Risica, J. Wylie-Rosett, E.M. Ross, L.O. Strolla, J. McMurray, et al., Development and evaluation of the nutrition component of the Rapid Eating and Activity Assessment for Patients (REAP): a new tool for primary care providers, J. Nutr. Educ. Behav. 38 (2006) 286–292.

[296] A.R. Kristal, A.L. Shattuck, H.J. Henry, A.S. Fowler, Rapid assessment of dietary intake of fat, fiber, and saturated fat: validity of an instrument suitable for community intervention research and nutritional surveillance, Am. J. Health Promot. 4 (1990) 288–295.

[297] A.R. Kristal, B.F. Abrams, M.D. Thornquist, L. Disogra, R.T. Croyle, A.L. Shattuck, et al., Development and validation of a food use checklist for evaluation of community nutrition interventions, Am. J. Public Health 80 (1990) 1318–1322.

[298] M.L. Neuhouser, R.E. Patterson, A.R. Kristal, A.L. Eldridge, N. C. Vizenor, A brief dietary assessment instrument for assessing target foods, nutrients and eating patterns, Public Health Nutr. 4 (2001) 73–78.

[299] J. Yen, C. Zoumas-Morse, B. Pakiz, C.L. Rock, Folate intake assessment: validation of a new approach, J. Am. Diet. Assoc. 103 (2003) 991–1000.

[300] J. Haraldsdottir, I. Thorsdottir, M.D. de Almeida, L. Maes, R.C. Perez, I. Elmadfa, et al., Validity and reproducibility of a pre-coded questionnaire to assess fruit and vegetable intake in European 11- to 12-year-old schoolchildren, Ann. Nutr. Metab. 49 (2005) 221–227.

[301] C.M. Apovian, M.C. Murphy, D. Cullum-Dugan, P.H. Lin, K. M. Gilbert, G. Coffman, et al., Validation of a web-based dietary questionnaire designed for the DASH (dietary approaches to stop hypertension) diet: the DASH online questionnaire, Public Health Nutr. 13 (2010) 615–622.

[302] N.J. Birkett, J. Boulet, Validation of a food habits questionnaire: poor performance in male manual laborers, J. Am. Diet. Assoc. 95 (1995) 558–563.

[303] K. Gray-Donald, J. O'Loughlin, L. Richard, G. Paradis, Validation of a short telephone administered questionnaire to evaluate dietary interventions in low income communities in Montreal, Canada, J. Epidemiol. Community Health 51 (1997) 326–331.

[304] M.P. Spoon, P.G. Devereux, J.A. Benedict, C. Leontos, N. Constantino, D. Christy, et al., Usefulness of the food habits questionnaire in a worksite setting, J. Nutr. Educ. Behav. 34 (2002) 268–272.

[305] M.C. Nelson, L.A. Lytle, Development and evaluation of a brief screener to estimate fast-food and beverage consumption among adolescents, J. Am. Diet. Assoc. 109 (2009) 730–734.

[306] J.N. Davis, M.C. Nelson, E.E. Ventura, L.A. Lytle, M.I. Goran, A brief dietary screener: appropriate for overweight Latino adolescents? J. Am. Diet. Assoc. 109 (2009) 725–729.

[307] B.S. Burke, The dietary history as a tool in research, J. Am. Diet. Assoc. 23 (1947) 1041–1046.

[308] B.S. Burke, H.C. Stuart, A method of diet analysis: application in research and pediatric practice, J. Pediatr. 12 (1938) 493–503.

[309] A. McDonald, L. Van Horn, M. Slattery, J. Hilner, C. Bragg, B. Caan, et al., The CARDIA dietary history: development, implementation, and evaluation, J. Am. Diet. Assoc. 91 (1991) 1104–1112.

[310] M. Visser, L.C. De Groot, P. Deurenberg, W.A. van Staveren, Validation of dietary history method in a group of elderly women using measurements of total energy expenditure, Br. J. Nutr. 74 (1995) 775–785.

[311] L. Kohlmeier, M. Mendez, J. McDuffie, M. Miller, Computer-assisted self-interviewing: a multimedia approach to dietary assessment, Am. J. Clin. Nutr. 65 (1997) 1275S–1281S.

[312] J. Landig, J.G. Erhardt, J.C. Bode, C. Bode, Validation and comparison of two computerized methods of obtaining a diet history, Clin. Nutr. 17 (1998) 113–117.

[313] L. Kohlmeier, Gaps in dietary assessment methodology: meal- vs. list-based methods, Am. J. Clin. Nutr. 59 (1994) 175s–179s.

[314] W.A. van Staveren, J.O. de Boer, J. Burema, Validity and reproducibility of a dietary history method estimating the usual food intake during one month, Am. J. Clin. Nutr. 42 (1985) 554–559.

[315] M. Jain, Diet history: questionnaire and interview techniques used in some retrospective studies of cancer, J. Am. Diet. Assoc. 89 (1989) 1647–1652.

[316] S. Kune, G.A. Kune, L.F. Watson, Observations on the reliability and validity of the design and diet history method in the Melbourne Colorectal Cancer Study, Nutr. Cancer 9 (1987) 5–20.

[317] L.C. Tapsell, V. Brenninger, J. Barnard, Applying conversation analysis to foster accurate reporting in the diet history interview, J. Am. Diet. Assoc. 100 (2000) 818–824.

[318] A. Chinnock, Validation of a diet history questionnaire for use with Costa Rican adults, Public Health Nutr. 11 (2008) 65–75.

[319] E.C. van Beresteyn, M.A. van't Hof, H.J. van der Heiden-Winkeldermaat, A. ten Have-Witjes, R. Neeter, Evaluation of the usefulness of the cross-check dietary history method in longitudinal studies, J. Chronic Dis. 40 (1987) 1051–1058.

[320] B.P. Bloemberg, D. Kromhout, G.L. Obermann-De Boer, M. Van Kampen-Donker, The reproducibility of dietary intake data assessed with the cross-check dietary history method, Am. J. Epidemiol. 130 (1989) 1047–1056.

[321] G.B. Mensink, M. Haftenberger, M. Thamm, Validity of DISHES 98, a computerised dietary history interview: energy and macronutrient intake, Eur. J. Clin. Nutr. 55 (2001) 409–417.

[322] M.L. Slattery, B.J. Caan, D. Duncan, T.D. Berry, A. Coates, R. Kerber, A computerized diet history questionnaire for epidemiologic studies, J. Am. Diet. Assoc. 94 (1994) 761–766.

[323] EPIC Group of Spain, Relative validity and reproducibility of a diet history questionnaire in Spain: I. Foods, Int. J. Epidemiol. 26 (1997) S91–S99.

[324] E. Rothenberg, I. Bosaeus, B. Lernfelt, S. Landahl, B. Steen, Energy intake and expenditure: validation of a diet history by heart rate monitoring, activity diary and doubly labeled water, Eur. J. Clin. Nutr. 52 (1998) 832–838.

[325] A.E. Black, A.A. Welch, S.A. Bingham, Validation of dietary intakes measured by diet history against 24 h urinary nitrogen excretion and energy expenditure measured by the doubly-labelled water method in middle-aged women, Br. J. Nutr. 83 (2000) 341–354.

[326] J.A. Barnard, L.C. Tapsell, P.S. Davies, V.L. Brenninger, L.H. Storlien, Relationship of high energy expenditure and variation in dietary intake with reporting accuracy on 7 day food records and diet histories in a group of healthy adult volunteers, Eur. J. Clin. Nutr. 56 (2002) 358–367.

[327] L. Hagfors, K. Westerterp, L. Skoldstam, G. Johansson, Validity of reported energy expenditure and reported intake of energy, protein, sodium and potassium in rheumatoid arthritis patients in a dietary intervention study, Eur. J. Clin. Nutr. 59 (2005) 238–245.

[328] EPIC Group of Spain, Relative validity and reproducibility of a diet history questionnaire in Spain: III. Biochemical markers, Int. J. Epidemiol. 26 (1997) S110–S117.

[329] K. Murakami, S. Sasaki, Y. Takahashi, K. Uenishi, K. Yamasaki, H. Hayabuchi, et al., Misreporting of dietary energy, protein, potassium and sodium in relation to body mass index in young Japanese women, Eur. J. Clin. Nutr. 62 (2008) 111–118.

[330] M.U. Waling, C.L. Larsson, Energy intake of Swedish overweight and obese children is underestimated using a diet history interview, J. Nutr. 139 (2009) 522–527.

[331] C.L. Larsson, G.K. Johansson, Dietary intake and nutritional status of young vegans and omnivores in Sweden, Am. J. Clin. Nutr. 76 (2002) 100–106.

[332] C.L. Larsson, K.R. Westerterp, G.K. Johansson, Validity of reported energy expenditure and energy and protein intakes in Swedish adolescent vegans and omnivores, Am. J. Clin. Nutr. 75 (2002) 268–274.

[333] A. Sjoberg, F. Slinde, D. Arvidsson, L. Ellegard, E. Gramatkovski, L. Hallberg, et al., Energy intake in Swedish adolescents: validation of diet history with doubly labelled water, Eur. J. Clin. Nutr. 57 (2003) 1643–1652.

[334] U. Toft, L. Kristoffersen, S. Ladelund, A. Bysted, J. Jakobsen, C. Lau, et al., Relative validity of a food frequency questionnaire

used in the Inter99 study, Eur. J. Clin. Nutr. 62 (2008) 1038−1046.

[335] L.A. Mainvil, C.C. Horwath, J.E. McKenzie, R. Lawson, Validation of brief instruments to measure adult fruit and vegetable consumption, Appetite 56 (2011) 111−117.

[336] M. van den Heuvel, R. Horchner, A. Wijtsma, N. Bourhim, D. Willemsen, E.M. Mathus-Vliegen, Sweet eating: a definition and the development of the Dutch Sweet Eating Questionnaire, Obes. Surg. 21 (2011) 714−721.

[337] L.A. Lytle, M.Z. Nichaman, E. Obarzanek, E. Glovsky, D. Montgomery, T. Nicklas, et al., Validation of 24-hour recalls assisted by food records in third-grade children: the CATCH Collaborative Group, J. Am. Diet. Assoc. 93 (1993) 1431−1436.

[338] J.L. Weber, L. Lytle, J. Gittelsohn, L. Cunningham-Sabo, K. Heller, J.A. Anliker, et al., Validity of self-reported dietary intake at school meals by American Indian children: the Pathways Study, J. Am. Diet. Assoc. 104 (2004) 746−752.

[339] L.F. Andersen, E. Bere, N. Kolbjornsen, K.I. Klepp, Validity and reproducibility of self-reported intake of fruit and vegetable among 6th graders, Eur. J. Clin. Nutr. 58 (2004) 771−777.

[340] A. Amend, G.D. Melkus, D.A. Chyun, P. Galasso, J. Wylie-Rosett, Validation of dietary intake data in black women with type 2 diabetes, J. Am. Diet. Assoc. 107 (2007) 112−117.

[341] F. Thompson, A. Subar, N. Potischman, D. Midthune, V. Kipnis, R.P. Troiano, et al., A checklist-adjusted food frequency method for assessing dietary intake, Sixth International Conference on Dietary Assessment Methods: Complementary Advances in Diet and Physical Activity Assessment Methodologies, Diet Research Foundation, The Danish Network of Nutritional Epidemiologists, Copenhagen, Denmark, 2006.

[342] J.A. Tooze, D. Midthune, K.W. Dodd, L.S. Freedman, S.M. Krebs-Smith, A.F. Subar, et al., A new statistical method for estimating the usual intake of episodically consumed foods with application to their distribution, J. Am. Diet. Assoc. 106 (2006) 1575−1587.

[343] L.S. Freedman, D. Midthune, R.J. Carroll, N. Tasevska, A. Schatzkin, J. Mares, et al., Using regression calibration equations that combine self-reported intake and biomarker measures to obtain unbiased estimates and more powerful tests of dietary associations, Am. J. Epidemiol. 174 (2011) 1238−1245.

[344] National Center for Health Statistics, National Health and Nutrition Examination Survey, Centers for Disease Control and Prevention, 2011. Available at: <http://www.cdc.gov/nchs/nhanes/nhanes_questionnaires.htm>

[345] T. Byers, M. Serdula, S. Kuester, J. Mendlein, C. Ballew, R.S. McPherson, Dietary surveillance for states and communities, Am. J. Clin. Nutr. 65 (1997) 1210S−1214S.

[346] California Department of Public Health, California Dietary Practices Surveys (CDPS), California Department of Public Health, 2012. Available at: <http://www.cdph.ca.gov/programs/cpns/Pages/CaliforniaStatewideSurveys.aspx#1>

[347] C.M. Friedenreich, N. Slimani, E. Riboli, Measurement of past diet: review of previous and proposed methods, Epidemiol. Rev. 14 (1992) 177−196.

[348] S.S. Maruti, D. Feskanich, H.R. Rockett, G.A. Colditz, L.A. Sampson, W.C. Willett, Validation of adolescent diet recalled by adults, Epidemiology 17 (2006) 226−229.

[349] T. Eysteinsdottir, I. Gunnarsdottir, I. Thorsdottir, T. Harris, L.J. Launer, V. Gudnason, et al., Validity of retrospective diet history: assessing recall of midlife diet using food frequency questionnaire in later life, J. Nutr. Health Aging 15 (2011) 809−814.

[350] F.E. Thompson, D.E. Lamphiear, H.L. Metzner, V.M. Hawthorne, M.S. Oh, Reproducibility of reports of frequency of food use in the Tecumseh Diet Methodology Study, Am. J. Epidemiol. 125 (1987) 658−671.

[351] J.T. Dwyer, K.A. Coleman, Insights into dietary recall from a longitudinal study: accuracy over four decades, Am. J. Clin. Nutr. 65 (1997) 1153S−1158S.

[352] J.E. Chavarro, B.A. Rosner, L. Sampson, C. Willey, P. Tocco, W. C. Willett, et al., Validity of adolescent diet recall 48 years later, Am. J. Epidemiol. 170 (2009) 1563−1570.

[353] J.E. Chavarro, K.B. Michels, S. Isaq, B.A. Rosner, L. Sampson, C. Willey, et al., Validity of maternal recall of preschool diet after 43 years, Am. J. Epidemiol. 169 (2009) 1148−1157.

[354] N. Malila, M. Virtanen, P. Pietinen, J. Virtamo, D. Albanes, A. M. Hartman, et al., A comparison of prospective and retrospective assessments of diet in a study of colorectal cancer, Nutr. Cancer 32 (1998) 146−153.

[355] C.M. Friedenreich, G.R. Howe, A.B. Miller, An investigation of recall bias in the reporting of past food intake among breast cancer cases and controls, Ann. Epidemiol. 1 (1991) 439−453.

[356] C.M. Friedenreich, G.R. Howe, A.B. Miller, The effect of recall bias on the association of calorie-providing nutrients and breast cancer, Epidemiology 2 (1991) 424−429.

[357] W.C. Willett, F.B. Hu, Not the time to abandon the food frequency questionnaire: point, Cancer Epidemiol. Biomarkers Prev. 15 (2006) 1757−1758.

[358] W.C. Willett, F.B. Hu, The food frequency questionnaire, Cancer Epidemiol. Biomarkers Prev. 16 (2007) 182−183.

[359] L.S. Freedman, A. Schatzkin, A.C. Thiebaut, N. Potischman, A. F. Subar, F.E. Thompson, et al., Abandon neither the food frequency questionnaire nor the dietary fat−breast cancer hypothesis, Cancer Epidemiol. Biomarkers Prev. 16 (2007) 1321−1322.

[360] A. Schatzkin, A.F. Subar, S. Moore, Y. Park, N. Potischman, F.E. Thompson, et al., Observational epidemiologic studies of nutrition and cancer: the next generation (with better observation), Cancer Epidemiol. Biomarkers Prev. 18 (2009) 1026−1032.

[361] A.S. Kolar, R.E. Patterson, E. White, M.L. Neuhouser, L.L. Frank, J. Standley, et al., A practical method for collecting 3-day food records in a large cohort, Epidemiology 16 (2005) 579−583.

[362] M.L. Kwan, L.H. Kushi, J. Song, A.W. Timperi, A.M. Boynton, K.M. Johnson, et al., A practical method for collecting food record data in a prospective cohort study of breast cancer survivors, Am. J. Epidemiol. 172 (2010) 1315−1323.

[363] B. Rosner, W.C. Willett, D. Spiegelman, Correction of logistic regression relative risk estimates and confidence intervals for systematic within-person measurement error, Stat. Med. 8 (1989) 1051−1069.

[364] R. Kaaks, M. Plummer, E. Riboli, J. Esteve, W. van Staveren, Adjustment for bias due to errors in exposure assessments in multicenter cohort studies on diet and cancer: a calibration approach, Am. J. Clin. Nutr. 59 (1994) 245S−250S.

[365] R.J. Carroll, L.S. Freedman, V. Kipnis, Measurement error and dietary intake, Adv. Exp. Med. Biol. 445 (1998) 139−145.

[366] A.C. Thiebaut, V. Kipnis, A. Schatzkin, L.S. Freedman, The role of dietary measurement error in investigating the hypothesized link between dietary fat intake and breast cancer: a story with twists and turns, Cancer Invest 26 (2008) 68−73.

[367] L.S. Freedman, A. Schatzkin, D. Midthune, V. Kipnis, Dealing with dietary measurement error in nutritional cohort studies, J. Natl. Cancer Inst. 103 (2011) 1086−1092.

[368] C. Ritenbaugh, R.E. Patterson, R.T. Chlebowski, B. Caan, L. Fels-Tinker, B. Howard, et al., The Women's Health Initiative Dietary Modification trial: overview and baseline characteristics of participants, Ann. Epidemiol. 13 (2003) S87−S97.

[369] T. Baranowski, E. Cerin, J. Baranowski, Steps in the design, development and formative evaluation of obesity prevention-related behavior change trials, Int. J. Behav. Nutr. Phys. Act. 6 (2009) 6.

[370] T. Baranowski, D.D. Allen, L.C. Masse, M. Wilson, Does participation in an intervention affect responses on self-report questionnaires? Health Educ. Res. 21 (2006) i98—109.

[371] J.L. Forster, R.W. Jeffery, M. VanNatta, P. Pirie, Hypertension prevention trial: do 24-h food records capture usual eating behavior in a dietary change study? Am. J. Clin. Nutr. 51 (1990) 253—257.

[372] D.D. Gorder, G.E. Bartsch, J.L. Tillotson, G.A. Grandits, J. Stamler, Food group and macronutrient intakes, trial years 1—6, in the special intervention and usual care groups in the Multiple Risk Factor Intervention Trial, Am. J. Clin. Nutr. 65 (1997) 258S—271S.

[373] B. Caan, R. Ballard-Barbash, M.L. Slattery, J.L. Pinsky, F.L. Iber, D.J. Mateski, et al., Low energy reporting may increase in intervention participants enrolled in dietary intervention trials, J. Am. Diet. Assoc. 104 (2004) 357—366.

[374] G.C. Williams, T.G. Hurley, F.E. Thompson, D. Midthune, A.L. Yaroch, K. Resnicow, et al., Performance of a short percentage energy from fat tool in measuring change in dietary intervention studies, J. Nutr. 138 (2008) 212S—217S.

[375] J.O. Prochaska, C.C. DiClemente, J.C. Norcross, In search of how people change: applications to addictive behaviors, Am. Psychol. 47 (1992) 1102—1114.

[376] K. Glanz, R.E. Patterson, A.R. Kristal, C.C. DiClemente, J. Heimendinger, L. Linnan, et al., Stages of change in adopting healthy diets: fat, fiber, and correlates of nutrient intake, Health Educ. Q. 21 (1994) 499—519.

[377] J.R. Hebert, K.E. Peterson, T.G. Hurley, A.M. Stoddard, N. Cohen, A.E. Field, et al., The effect of social desirability trait on self-reported dietary measures among multi-ethnic female health center employees, Ann. Epidemiol. 11 (2001) 417—427.

[378] T.M. Miller, M.F. Abdel-Maksoud, L.A. Crane, A.C. Marcus, T.E. Byers, Effects of social approval bias on self-reported fruit and vegetable consumption: a randomized controlled trial, Nutr. J. 7 (2008) 18.

[379] L. Natarajan, M. Pu, J. Fan, R.A. Levine, R.E. Patterson, C.A. Thomson, et al., Measurement error of dietary self-report in intervention trials, Am. J. Epidemiol. 172 (2010) 819—827.

[380] A. Cheadle, B.M. Psaty, P. Diehr, T. Koepsell, E. Wagner, S. Curry, et al., Evaluating community-based nutrition programs: comparing grocery store and individual-level survey measures of program impact, Prev. Med. 24 (1995) 71—79.

[381] A. Cheadle, B.M. Psaty, S. Curry, E. Wagner, P. Diehr, T. Koepsell, et al., Can measures of the grocery store environment be used to track community-level dietary changes? Prev. Med. 22 (1993) 361—372.

[382] S.A. Smith-Warner, P.J. Elmer, T.M. Tharp, L. Fosdick, B. Randall, M. Gross, et al., Increasing vegetable and fruit intake: randomized intervention and monitoring in an at-risk population, Cancer Epidemiol. Biomarkers Prev. 9 (2000) 307—317.

[383] S. Sasaki, T. Ishikawa, R. Yanagibori, K. Amano, Responsiveness to a self-administered diet history questionnaire in a work-site dietary intervention trial for mildly hypercholesterolemic Japanese subjects: correlation between change in dietary habits and serum cholesterol levels, J. Cardiol. 33 (1999) 327—338.

[384] J.M. Samet, A.J. Alberg, Surrogate sources of dietary information, in: W. Willett (Ed.), Nutritional Epidemiology, Oxford University Press, New York, 1998.

[385] P. Emmett, Workshop 2: the use of surrogate reporters in the assessment of dietary intake, Eur. J. Clin. Nutr. 63 (2009) S78—S79.

[386] L.N. Kolonel, T. Hirohata, A.M. Nomura, Adequacy of survey data collected from substitute respondents, Am. J. Epidemiol. 106 (1977) 476—484.

[387] J. Marshall, R. Priore, B. Haughey, T. Rzepka, S. Graham, Spouse—subject interviews and the reliability of diet studies, Am. J. Epidemiol. 112 (1980) 675—683.

[388] C.G. Humble, J.M. Samet, B.E. Skipper, Comparison of self- and surrogate-reported dietary information, Am. J. Epidemiol. 119 (1984) 86—98.

[389] H.L. Metzner, D.E. Lamphiear, F.E. Thompson, M.S. Oh, V.M. Hawthorne, Comparison of surrogate and subject reports of dietary practices, smoking habits and weight among married couples in the Tecumseh Diet Methodology Study, J. Clin. Epidemiol. 42 (1989) 367—375.

[390] T.G. Hislop, A.J. Coldman, Y.Y. Zheng, V.T. Ng, T. Labo, Reliability of dietary information from surrogate respondents, Nutr. Cancer 18 (1992) 123—129.

[391] N. Herrmann, Retrospective information from questionnaires: I. Comparability of primary respondents and their next-of-kin, Am. J. Epidemiol. 121 (1985) 937—947.

[392] G.J. Petot, S.M. Debanne, T.M. Riedel, K.A. Smyth, E. Koss, A.J. Lerner, et al., Use of surrogate respondents in a case control study of dietary risk factors for Alzheimer's disease, J. Am. Diet. Assoc. 102 (2002) 848—850.

[393] J.P. Fryzek, L. Lipworth, L.B. Signorello, J.K. McLaughlin, The reliability of dietary data for self- and next-of-kin respondents, Ann. Epidemiol. 12 (2002) 278—283.

[394] J.H. Hankin, L.R. Wilkens, Development and validation of dietary assessment methods for culturally diverse populations, Am. J. Clin. Nutr. 59 (1994) 198S—200S.

[395] G.K. Lyons, S.I. Woodruff, J.I. Candelaria, J.W. Rupp, J.P. Elder, Development of a protocol to assess dietary intake among Hispanics who have low literacy skills in English, J. Am. Diet. Assoc. 96 (1996) 1276—1279.

[396] C.M. Loria, M.A. McDowell, C.L. Johnson, C.E. Woteki, Nutrient data for Mexican-American foods: are current data adequate? J. Am. Diet. Assoc. 91 (1991) 919—922.

[397] K. Levin, G.B. Willis, B.H. Forsyth, A. Norberg, M.S. Kudela, D. Stark, et al., Using cognitive interviews to evaluate the Spanish-language translation of a dietary questionnaire, Surv. Res. Methods 3 (2009) 13—25.

[398] Indian Health Service, Navajo Health and Nutrition Survey Manual, Indian Health Service, Rockville, MD, 1992.

[399] J.S. Johnson, E.D. Nobmann, E. Asay, A.P. Lanier, Developing a validated Alaska Native food frequency questionnaire for western Alaska, 2002—2006, Int. J. Circumpolar. Health 68 (2009) 99—108.

[400] M.M. Lee, F. Lee, S. Wang Ladenla, R. Miike, A semiquantitative dietary history questionnaire for Chinese Americans, Ann. Epidemiol. 4 (1994) 188—197.

[401] J.R. Hebert, P.C. Gupta, R.B. Bhonsle, P.N. Sinor, H. Mehta, F.S. Mehta, Development and testing of a quantitative food frequency questionnaire for use in Gujarat, India, Public Health Nutr. 2 (1999) 39—50.

[402] D. Taren, M. de Tobar, C. Ritenbaugh, E. Graver, R. Whitacre, M. Aickin, Evaluation of the Southwest Food Frequency Questionnaire, Ecol. Food Nutr. 38 (2000) 515—547.

[403] D. Shahar, I. Shai, H. Vardi, A. Brener-Azrad, D. Fraser, Development of a semi-quantitative Food Frequency Questionnaire (FFQ) to assess dietary intake of multiethnic populations, Eur. J. Epidemiol. 18 (2003) 855—861.

[404] A.C. Bovell-Benjamin, N. Dawkin, R.D. Pace, J.M. Shikany, Use of focus groups to understand African-Americans' dietary practices: implications for modifying a food frequency questionnaire, Prev. Med. 48 (2009) 549—554.

[405] S. Sharma, J. Cade, J. Landman, J.K. Cruickshank, Assessing the diet of the British African-Caribbean population: frequency of consumption of foods and food portion sizes, Int. J. Food Sci. Nutr. 53 (2002) 439—444.

[406] K.L. Tucker, L.A. Bianchi, J. Maras, O.I. Bermudez, Adaptation of a food frequency questionnaire to assess diets of Puerto

Rican and non-Hispanic adults, Am. J. Epidemiol. 148 (1998) 507–518.

[407] K.L. Tucker, J. Maras, C. Champagne, C. Connell, S. Goolsby, J. Weber, et al., A regional food-frequency questionnaire for the U.S. Mississippi Delta, Public Health Nutr. 8 (2005) 87–96.

[408] D.O. Stram, J.H. Hankin, L.R. Wilkens, M.C. Pike, K.R. Monroe, S. Park, et al., Calibration of the dietary questionnaire for a multiethnic cohort in Hawaii and Los Angeles, Am. J. Epidemiol. 151 (2000) 358–370.

[409] L.B. Signorello, H.M. Munro, M.S. Buchowski, D.G. Schlundt, S.S. Cohen, M.K. Hargreaves, et al., Estimating nutrient intake from a food frequency questionnaire: incorporating the elements of race and geographic region, Am. J. Epidemiol. 170 (2009) 104–111.

[410] R.J. Coates, C.P. Monteilh, Assessments of food-frequency questionnaires in minority populations, Am. J. Clin. Nutr. 65 (1997) 1108S–1115S.

[411] E.J. Mayer-Davis, M.Z. Vitolins, S.L. Carmichael, S. Hemphill, G. Tsaroucha, J. Rushing, et al., Validity and reproducibility of a food frequency interview in a multi-cultural epidemiologic study, Ann. Epidemiol. 9 (1999) 314–324.

[412] K.B. Baumgartner, F.D. Gilliland, C.S. Nicholson, R.S. McPherson, W.C. Hunt, D.R. Pathak, et al., Validity and reproducibility of a food frequency questionnaire among Hispanic and non-Hispanic white women in New Mexico, Ethn. Dis. 8 (1998) 81–92.

[413] K.W. Cullen, I. Zakeri, The youth/adolescent questionnaire has low validity and modest reliability among low-income African-American and Hispanic seventh- and eighth-grade youth, J. Am. Diet. Assoc. 104 (2004) 1415–1419.

[414] T. Baranowski, S.B. Domel, A cognitive model of children's reporting of food intake, Am. J. Clin. Nutr. 59 (1994) 212S–217S.

[415] R.S. McPherson, D.M. Hoelscher, M. Alexander, K.S. Scanlon, M.K. Serdula, Dietary assessment methods among school-aged children: validity and reliability, Prev. Med. 31 (2000) S11–S33.

[416] M.B. Livingstone, P.J. Robson, Measurement of dietary intake in children, Proc. Nutr. Soc. 59 (2000) 279–293.

[417] M.K. Serdula, M.P. Alexander, K.S. Scanlon, B.A. Bowman, What are preschool children eating? A review of dietary assessment, Annu. Rev. Nutr. 21 (2001) 475–498.

[418] H.R. Rockett, C.S. Berkey, G.A. Colditz, Evaluation of dietary assessment instruments in adolescents, Curr. Opin. Clin. Nutr. Metab. Care 6 (2003) 557–562.

[419] National Cancer Institute, NCS Dietary Assessment Literature Review, Applied Research Program, National Cancer Institute, 2009. Available at: <http://riskfactor.cancer.gov/tools/children/review>

[420] T.L. Burrows, R.J. Martin, C.E. Collins, A systematic review of the validity of dietary assessment methods in children when compared with the method of doubly labeled water, J. Am. Diet. Assoc. 110 (2010) 1501–1510.

[421] A.F. Smith, S.D. Baxter, J.W. Hardin, C.H. Guinn, J.A. Royer, Relation of children's dietary reporting accuracy to cognitive ability, Am. J. Epidemiol. 173 (2011) 103–109.

[422] S.G. Forrestal, Energy intake misreporting among children and adolescents: a literature review, Matern. Child Nutr. 7 (2011) 112–127.

[423] B.A. Dennison, P.L. Jenkins, H.L. Rockwell, Development and validation of an instrument to assess child dietary fat intake, Prev. Med. 31 (2000) 214–224.

[424] K.M. Koehler, L. Cunningham-Sabo, L.C. Lambert, R. McCalman, B.J. Skipper, S.M. Davis, Assessing food selection in a health promotion program: validation of a brief instrument for American Indian children in the southwest United States, J. Am. Diet. Assoc. 100 (2000) 205–211.

[425] L.J. Harnack, L.A. Lytle, M. Story, D.A. Galuska, K. Schmitz, D.R. Jacobs Jr., et al., Reliability and validity of a brief questionnaire to assess calcium intake of middle-school-aged children, J. Am. Diet. Assoc. 106 (2006) 1790–1795.

[426] B.G. Simons-Morton, T. Baranowski, Observation in assessment of children's dietary practices, J. Sch. Health 61 (1991) 204–207.

[427] A.F. Smith, S.D. Baxter, J.W. Hardin, J.A. Royer, C.H. Guinn, Some intrusions in dietary reports by fourth-grade children are based on specific memories: data from a validation study of the effect of interview modality, Nutr. Res. 28 (2008) 600–608.

[428] D.M. Matheson, K.A. Hanson, T.E. McDonald, T.N. Robinson, Validity of children's food portion estimates: a comparison of 2 measurement aids, Arch. Pediatr. Adolesc. Med. 156 (2002) 867–871.

[429] C. Frobisher, S.M. Maxwell, The estimation of food portion sizes: a comparison between using descriptions of portion sizes and a photographic food atlas by children and adults, J. Hum. Nutr. Diet. 16 (2003) 181–188.

[430] T. Baranowski, D. Sprague, J.H. Baranowski, J.A. Harrison, Accuracy of maternal dietary recall for preschool children, J. Am. Diet. Assoc. 91 (1991) 669–674.

[431] L.H. Eck, R.C. Klesges, C.L. Hanson, Recall of a child's intake from one meal: are parents accurate? J. Am. Diet. Assoc. 89 (1989) 784–789.

[432] E.J. Sobo, C.L. Rock, "You ate all that!?": caretaker–child interaction during children's assisted dietary recall interviews, Med. Anthropol. Q. 15 (2001) 222–244.

[433] S.D. Baxter, Cognitive processes in children's dietary recalls: insight from methodological studies, Eur. J. Clin. Nutr. 63 (2009) S19–S32.

[434] S.D. Baxter, J.W. Hardin, J.A. Royer, C.H. Guinn, A.F. Smith, Children's recalls from five dietary-reporting validation studies: intrusions in correctly reported and misreported options in school breakfast reports, Appetite 51 (2008) 489–500.

[435] S.D. Baxter, A.F. Smith, M.S. Litaker, C.H. Guinn, N.M. Shaffer, M.L. Baglio, et al., Recency affects reporting accuracy of children's dietary recalls, Ann. Epidemiol. 14 (2004) 385–390.

[436] S.D. Baxter, J.W. Hardin, C.H. Guinn, J.A. Royer, A.J. Mackelprang, A.F. Smith, Fourth-grade children's dietary recall accuracy is influenced by retention interval (target period and interview time), J. Am. Diet. Assoc. 109 (2009) 846–856.

[437] T. Baranowski, J.C. Baranowski, K.B. Watson, S. Martin, A. Beltran, N. Islam, et al., Children's accuracy of portion size estimation using digital food images: effects of interface design and size of image on computer screen, Public Health Nutr. 14 (2010) 418–425.

[438] T. Baranowski, et al., Food Intake Recording Software System, version 4 (FIRSSt4): a self-completed 24 hour dietary recall for children, J. Hum. Nutr. Diet. (2012) (e-pub (ahead of print) May 23).

[439] K.E. Storey, L.E. Forbes, S.N. Fraser, J.C. Spence, R.C. Plotnikoff, K.D. Raine, et al., Diet quality, nutrition and physical activity among adolescents: the Web-SPAN (Web-Survey of Physical Activity and Nutrition) project, Public Health Nutr. 12 (2009) 2009–2017.

[440] K.E. Storey, L.J. McCargar, Reliability and validity of Web-SPAN, a web-based method for assessing weight status, diet and physical activity in youth, J. Hum. Nutr. Diet. 25 (2012) 59–68.

[441] H.J. Moore, L.J. Ells, S.A. McLure, S. Crooks, D. Cumbor, C.D. Summerbell, et al., The development and evaluation of a novel computer program to assess previous-day dietary and physical activity behaviours in school children: the Synchronised

Nutrition and Activity Program (SNAP), Br. J. Nutr. 99 (2008) 1266–1274.

[442] C.K. Martin, R.L. Newton Jr., S.D. Anton, H.R. Allen, A. Alfonso, H. Han, et al., Measurement of children's food intake with digital photography and the effects of second servings upon food intake, Eat. Behav. 8 (2007) 148–156.

[443] E. Trolle, P. Amiano, M. Ege, E. Bower, S. Lioret, H. Brants, et al., Evaluation of 2×24-h dietary recalls combined with a food-recording booklet, against a 7-day food-record method among schoolchildren, Eur. J. Clin. Nutr. 65 (2011) S77–S83.

[444] H.R. Rockett, M. Breitenbach, A.L. Frazier, J. Witschi, A.M. Wolf, A.E. Field, et al., Validation of a youth/adolescent food frequency questionnaire, Prev. Med. 26 (1997) 808–816.

[445] D.M. Klohe, K.K. Clarke, G.C. George, T.J. Milani, H. Hanss-Nuss, J. Freeland-Graves, Relative validity and reliability of a food frequency questionnaire for a triethnic population of 1-year-old to 3-year-old children from low-income families, J. Am. Diet. Assoc. 105 (2005) 727–734.

[446] H.R. Rockett, C.S. Berkey, G.A. Colditz, Comparison of a short food frequency questionnaire with the Youth/Adolescent Questionnaire in the Growing Up Today Study, Int. J. Pediatr. Obes. 2 (2007) 31–39.

[447] R.M. Hanning, D. Royall, J.E. Toews, L. Blashill, J. Wegener, P. Driezen, Web-based Food Behaviour Questionnaire: validation with grades six to eight students, Can. J. Diet. Pract. Res. 70 (2009) 172–178.

[448] C.J. Boushey, D.A. Kerr, J. Wright, K.D. Lutes, D.S. Ebert, E.J. Delp, Use of technology in children's dietary assessment, Eur. J. Clin. Nutr. 63 (2009) S50–S57.

[449] A. Magarey, J. Watson, R.K. Golley, T. Burrows, R. Sutherland, S.A. McNaughton, et al., Assessing dietary intake in children and adolescents: considerations and recommendations for obesity research, Int. J. Pediatr. Obes. 6 (2011) 2–11.

[450] J.H. de Vries, L.C. De Groot, W.A. van Staveren, Dietary assessment in elderly people: experiences gained from studies in The Netherlands, Eur. J. Clin. Nutr. 63 (2009) S69–S74.

[451] A.J. Adamson, J. Collerton, K. Davies, E. Foster, C. Jagger, E. Stamp, et al., Nutrition in advanced age: dietary assessment in the Newcastle 85 + study, Eur. J. Clin. Nutr. 63 (2009) S6–18.

[452] E.M. Rothenberg, Experience of dietary assessment and validation from three Swedish studies in the elderly, Eur. J. Clin. Nutr. 63 (2009) S64–S68.

[453] R.L. Bailey, J.J. Gahche, C.V. Lentino, J.T. Dwyer, J.S. Engel, P.R. Thomas, et al., Dietary supplement use in the United States, 2003–2006, J. Nutr. 141 (2011) 261–266.

[454] D.C. Mitchell, H. Smiciklas-Wright, J.M. Friedmann, G. Jensen, Dietary intake assessed by the Nutrition Screening Initiative Level II Screen is a sensitive but not a specific indicator of nutrition risk in older adults, J. Am. Diet. Assoc. 102 (2002) 842–844.

[455] S. Sinnett, R. Bengle, A. Brown, A.P. Glass, M.A. Johnson, J.S. Lee, The validity of Nutrition Screening Initiative DETERMINE Checklist responses in older Georgians, J. Nutr. Elder. 29 (2010) 393–409.

[456] S. Brownie, S.P. Myers, J. Stevens, The value of the Australian nutrition screening initiative for older Australians: results from a national survey, J. Nutr. Health Aging 11 (2007) 20–25.

[457] Y. Guigoz, The Mini Nutritional Assessment (MNA) review of the literature: what does it tell us? J. Nutr. Health Aging 10 (2006) 466–485.

[458] E. Cereda, C. Pedrolli, A. Zagami, A. Vanotti, S. Piffer, A. Opizzi, et al., Nutritional screening and mortality in newly institutionalised elderly: a comparison between the Geriatric Nutritional Risk Index and the Mini Nutritional Assessment, Clin. Nutr. 30 (2011) 793–798.

[459] Y. Rolland, A. Perrin, V. Gardette, N. Filhol, B. Vellas, Screening older people at risk of malnutrition or malnourished using the Simplified Nutritional Appetite Questionnaire (SNAQ): a comparison with the Mini-Nutritional Assessment (MNA) tool, J. Am. Med. Dir. Assoc. 13 (2012) 31–34.

[460] N.J. Tomoyasu, M.J. Toth, E.T. Poehlman, Misreporting of total energy intake in older men and women, J. Am. Geriatr. Soc. 47 (1999) 710–715.

[461] P.M. Luhrmann, B.M. Herbert, M. Neuhauser-Berthold, Underreporting of energy intake in an elderly German population, Nutrition 17 (2001) 912–916.

[462] D.R. Shahar, B. Yu, D.K. Houston, S.B. Kritchevsky, A.B. Newman, D.E. Sellmeyer, et al., Misreporting of energy intake in the elderly using doubly labeled water to measure total energy expenditure and weight change, J. Am. Coll. Nutr. 29 (2010) 14–24.

[463] M.M. Chianetta, M.K. Head, Effect of prior notification on accuracy of dietary recall by the elderly, J. Am. Diet. Assoc. 92 (1992) 741–743.

[464] W.A. van Staveren, L.C. De Groot, Y.H. Blauw, R.P. van der Wielen, Assessing diets of elderly people: problems and approaches, Am. J. Clin. Nutr. 59 (1994) 221S–223S.

[465] K. Klipstein-Grobusch, J.H. den Breeijen, R.A. Goldbohm, J.M. Geleijnse, A. Hofman, D.E. Grobbee, et al., Dietary assessment in the elderly: validation of a semiquantitative food frequency questionnaire, Eur. J. Clin. Nutr. 52 (1998) 588–596.

[466] B. Shatenstein, H. Payette, S. Nadon, K. Gray-Donald, An approach for evaluating lifelong intakes of functional foods in elderly people, J. Nutr. 133 (2003) 2384–2391.

[467] M.C. Morris, C.C. Tangney, J.L. Bienias, D.A. Evans, R.S. Wilson, Validity and reproducibility of a food frequency questionnaire by cognition in an older biracial sample, Am. J. Epidemiol. 158 (2003) 1213–1217.

[468] D.A. Dillman, J.D. Smyth, L.M. Christian, Internet, Mail, and Mixed-Mode Surveys: The Tailored Design Method, Wiley, Hoboken, NJ, 2009.

[469] R.J. Voogt, W.E. Saris, Mixed mode designs: finding the balance between nonresponse bias and mode effects, J. Off. Stat. 21 (2005) 367–387.

[470] J.T. Dwyer, E.A. Krall, K.A. Coleman, The problem of memory in nutritional epidemiology research, J. Am. Diet. Assoc. 87 (1987) 1509–1512.

[471] A.F. Smith, J.B. Jobe, D.J. Mingay, Retrieval from memory of dietary information, Appl. Cogn. Psychol. 5 (1991) 269–296.

[472] C.M. Friedenreich, Improving long-term recall in epidemiologic studies, Epidemiology 5 (1994) 1–4.

[473] J.A. Satia, R.E. Patterson, V.M. Taylor, C.L. Cheney, S. Shiu-Thornton, K. Chitnarong, et al., Use of qualitative methods to study diet, acculturation, and health in Chinese-American women, J. Am. Diet. Assoc. 100 (2000) 934–940.

[474] W.S. Wolfe, E.A. Frongillo, P.A. Cassano, Evaluating brief measures of fruit and vegetable consumption frequency and variety: cognition, interpretation, and other measurement issues, J. Am. Diet. Assoc. 101 (2001) 311–318.

[475] E. Chambers, S.L. Godwin, F.A. Vecchio, Cognitive strategies for reporting portion sizes using dietary recall procedures, J. Am. Diet. Assoc. 100 (2000) 891–897.

[476] M. Johnson-Kozlow, G.E. Matt, C.L. Rock, Recall strategies used by respondents to complete a food frequency questionnaire: an exploratory study, J. Am. Diet. Assoc. 106 (2006) 430–433.

[477] G.E. Matt, C.L. Rock, M. Johnson-Kozlow, Using recall cues to improve measurement of dietary intakes with a food frequency questionnaire in an ethnically diverse population: an exploratory study, J. Am. Diet. Assoc. 106 (2006) 1209–1217.

[478] G.B. Willis, Cognitive Interviewing: A Tool for Improving Questionnaire Design, Sage, Thousand Oaks, CA, 2005.

[479] I.M. Buzzard, Y.A. Sievert, Research priorities and recommendations for dietary assessment methodology: first International Conference on Dietary Assessment Methods, Am. J. Clin. Nutr. 59 (1994) 275S–280S.

[480] T. Baranowski, R. Dworkin, J.C. Henske, D.R. Clearman, J.K. Dunn, P.R. Nader, et al., The accuracy of children's self-reports of diet: family Health Project, J. Am. Diet. Assoc. 86 (1986) 1381–1385.

[481] S.B. Domel, T. Baranowski, S.B. Leonard, H. Davis, P. Riley, J. Baranowski, Accuracy of fourth- and fifth-grade students' food records compared with school-lunch observations, Am. J. Clin. Nutr. 59 (1994) 218S–220S.

[482] S.A. Bingham, The use of 24-h urine samples and energy expenditure to validate dietary assessments, Am. J. Clin. Nutr. 59 (1994) 227S–231S.

[483] D.W. Heerstrass, M.C. Ocke, H.B. Bueno-de-Mesquita, P.H. Peeters, J.C. Seidell, Underreporting of energy, protein and potassium intake in relation to body mass index, Int. J. Epidemiol. 27 (1998) 186–193.

[484] K. Samaras, P.J. Kelly, L.V. Campbell, Dietary underreporting is prevalent in middle-aged British women and is not related to adiposity (percentage body fat), Int. J. Obes. Relat. Metab. Disord. 23 (1999) 881–888.

[485] U.A. Ajani, W.C. Willett, J.M. Seddon, Reproducibility of a food frequency questionnaire for use in ocular research: eye Disease Case–Control Study Group, Invest. Ophthalmol. Vis. Sci. 35 (1994) 2725–2733.

[486] S.D. Baxter, A.F. Smith, J.W. Hardin, M.D. Nichols, Conclusions about children's reporting accuracy for energy and macronutrients over multiple interviews depend on the analytic approach for comparing reported information to reference information, J. Am. Diet. Assoc. 107 (2007) 595–604.

[487] A.M. Hartman, G. Block, Dietary assessment methods for macronutrients, in: M.S. Micozzi, T.E. Moon (Eds), Macronutrients: Investigating Their Role in Cancer, Dekker, New York, 1992, pp. 87–124.

[488] L.S. Freedman, R.J. Carroll, Y. Wax, Estimating the relation between dietary intake obtained from a food frequency questionnaire and true average intake, Am. J. Epidemiol. 134 (1991) 310–320.

[489] F.E. Thompson, V. Kipnis, A.F. Subar, S.M. Krebs-Smith, L.L. Kahle, D. Midthune, et al., Evaluation of 2 brief instruments and a food-frequency questionnaire to estimate daily number of servings of fruit and vegetables, Am. J. Clin. Nutr. 71 (2000) 1503–1510.

[490] B. Rosner, D. Spiegelman, W.C. Willett, Correction of logistic regression relative risk estimates and confidence intervals for measurement error: the case of multiple covariates measured with error, Am. J. Epidemiol. 132 (1990) 734–745.

[491] S. Paeratakul, B.M. Popkin, I. Kohlmeier, I. Hertz-Picciotto, X. Guo, L.J. Edwards, Measurement error in dietary data: implications for the epidemiologic study of the diet–disease relationship, Eur. J. Clin. Nutr. 52 (1998) 722–727.

[492] M. Plummer, D. Clayton, Measurement error in dietary assessment: an investigation using covariance structure models: Part II, Stat. Med. 12 (1993) 937–948.

[493] M. Plummer, D. Clayton, Measurement error in dietary assessment: an investigation using covariance structure models: Part I, Stat. Med. 12 (1993) 925–935.

[494] S.J. Blumberg, J.V. Luke, M.L. Cynamon, Telephone coverage and health survey estimates: evaluating the need for concern about wireless substitution, Am. J. Public Health 96 (2006) 926–931.

[495] L.C. Lyu, J.H. Hankin, L.Q. Liu, L.R. Wilkens, J.H. Lee, M.T. Goodman, et al., Telephone vs. face-to-face interviews for quantitative food frequency assessment, J. Am. Diet. Assoc. 98 (1998) 44–48.

[496] M. Bogle, J. Stuff, L. Davis, I. Forrester, E. Strickland, P.H. Casey, et al., Validity of a telephone-administered 24-hour dietary recall in telephone and non-telephone households in the rural Lower Mississippi Delta region, J. Am. Diet. Assoc. 101 (2001) 216–222.

[497] M. Brustad, G. Skeie, T. Braaten, N. Slimani, E. Lund, Comparison of telephone vs. face-to-face interviews in the assessment of dietary intake by the 24 h recall EPIC SOFT program: the Norwegian calibration study, Eur. J. Clin. Nutr. 57 (2003) 107–113.

[498] N.J. Krantzler, B.J. Mullen, H.G. Schutz, L.E. Grivetti, C.A. Holden, H.L. Meiselman, Validity of telephoned diet recalls and records for assessment of individual food intake, Am. J. Clin. Nutr. 36 (1982) 1234–1242.

[499] S.L. Godwin, E. Chambers, L. Cleveland, Accuracy of reporting dietary intake using various portion-size aids in-person and via telephone, J. Am. Diet. Assoc. 104 (2004) 585–594.

[500] L.R. Yanek, T.F. Moy, J.V. Raqueno, D.M. Becker, Comparison of the effectiveness of a telephone 24-hour dietary recall method vs. an in-person method among urban African-American women, J. Am. Diet. Assoc. 100 (2000) 1172–1177.

[501] R. Tourangeau, L.J. Rips, K. Rasinski, The Psychology of Survey Response, Cambridge University Press, Cambridge, UK, 2000.

[502] U.S. Census Bureau, Appendix Table A: Households with a Computer and Internet Use: 1984 to 2009, U.S. Census Bureau, Current Population Survey, 2009, 2011. Available at: <http://www.census.gov/hhes/computer>.

[503] C. Matthys, I. Pynaert, M. Roe, S.J. Fairweather-Tait, A.L. Heath, S. De Henauw, Validity and reproducibility of a computerised tool for assessing the iron, calcium and vitamin C intake of Belgian women, Eur. J. Clin. Nutr. 58 (2004) 1297–1305.

[504] D.J. Toobert, L.A. Strycker, S.E. Hampson, E. Westling, S.M. Christiansen, T.G. Hurley, et al., Computerized portion-size estimation compared to multiple 24-hour dietary recalls for measurement of fat, fruit, and vegetable intake in overweight adults, J. Am. Diet. Assoc. 111 (2011) 1578–1583.

[505] T.H. Shih, X. Fan, Comparing response rates from web and mail surveys: a meta-analysis, Field Methods 20 (2008) 249–271.

[506] K.A. Balter, O. Balter, E. Fondell, Y.T. Lagerros, Web-based and mailed questionnaires: a comparison of response rates and compliance, Epidemiology 16 (2005) 577–579.

[507] S. Fricker, M. Galesic, R. Tourangeau, T. Yan, An experimental comparison of web and telephone surveys, Public Opin. Q. 69 (2005) 370–392.

[508] J.M. Beasley, A. Davis, W.T. Riley, Evaluation of a web-based, pictorial diet history questionnaire, Public Health Nutr. 12 (2009) 651–659.

[509] C.H. Thompson, M.K. Head, S.M. Rodman, Factors influencing accuracy in estimating plate waste, J. Am. Diet. Assoc. 87 (1987) 1219–1220.

[510] H.A. Guthrie, Selection and quantification of typical food portions by young adults, J. Am. Diet. Assoc. 84 (1984) 1440–1444.

[511] M. Nelson, M. Atkinson, S. Darbyshire, Food photography II: use of food photographs for estimating portion size and the nutrient content of meals, Br. J. Nutr. 76 (1996) 31–49.

[512] J.R. Hebert, P.C. Gupta, R. Bhonsle, F. Verghese, C. Ebbeling, R. Barrow, et al., Determinants of accuracy in estimating the weight and volume of commonly used foods: a cross-cultural comparison, Ecol. Food Nutr. 37 (1999) 475–502.

[513] L.R. Young, M.S. Nestle, Portion sizes in dietary assessment: issues and policy implications, Nutr. Rev. 53 (1995) 149–158.

[514] L.R. Young, M. Nestle, Variation in perceptions of a "medium" food portion: implications for dietary guidance, J. Am. Diet. Assoc. 98 (1998) 458–459.

[515] Y.S. Cypel, P.M. Guenther, G.J. Petot, Validity of portion-size measurement aids: a review, J. Am. Diet. Assoc. 97 (1997) 289–292.

[516] T. Hernandez, L. Wilder, D. Kuehn, K. Rubotzky, P.M. Veillon, S. Godwin, et al., Portion size estimation and expectation of accuracy, J. Food Compost. Anal. 19 (2006) S14–S21.

[517] E. Chambers, B. McGuire, S. Godwin, M. McDowell, F. Vecchio, Quantifying portion sizes for selected snack foods and beverages in 24-hour dietary recalls, Nutr. Res. 20 (2000) 315–326.

[518] F. Robinson, W. Morritz, P. McGuiness, A.F. Hackett, A study of the use of a photographic food atlas to estimate served and self-served portion sizes, J. Hum. Nutr. Diet. 10 (1997) 117–124.

[519] P.J. Robson, M.B. Livingstone, An evaluation of food photographs as a tool for quantifying food and nutrient intakes, Public Health Nutr. 3 (2000) 183–192.

[520] C. Vereecken, S. Dohogne, M. Covents, L. Maes, How accurate are adolescents in portion-size estimation using the computer tool Young Adolescents' Nutrition Assessment on Computer (YANA-C)? Br. J. Nutr. 103 (2010) 1844–1850.

[521] E. Foster, J.N. Matthews, J. Lloyd, L. Marshall, J.C. Mathers, M. Nelson, et al., Children's estimates of food portion size: the development and evaluation of three portion size assessment tools for use with children, Br. J. Nutr. 99 (2008) 175–184.

[522] E. Foster, M. O'Keeffe, J.N. Matthews, J.C. Mathers, M. Nelson, K.L. Barton, et al., Children's estimates of food portion size: the effect of timing of dietary interview on the accuracy of children's portion size estimates, Br. J. Nutr. 99 (2008) 185–190.

[523] M.L. Ovaskainen, M. Paturi, H. Reinivuo, M.L. Hannila, H. Sinkko, J. Lehtisalo, et al., Accuracy in the estimation of food servings against the portions in food photographs, Eur. J. Clin. Nutr. 62 (2008) 674–681.

[524] W. De Keyzer, I. Huybrechts, M. De Maeyer, M. Ocke, N. Slimani, P. van't Veer, et al., Food photographs in nutritional surveillance: errors in portion size estimation using drawings of bread and photographs of margarine and beverages consumption, Br. J. Nutr. 105 (2011) 1073–1083.

[525] T.E. Schap, B.L. Six, E.J. Delp, D.S. Ebert, D.A. Kerr, C.J. Boushey, Adolescents in the United States can identify familiar foods at the time of consumption and when prompted with an image 14 h postprandial, but poorly estimate portions, Public Health Nutr. 14 (2011) 1184–1191.

[526] M.M. Huizinga, A.J. Carlisle, K.L. Cavanaugh, D.L. Davis, R.P. Gregory, D.G. Schlundt, et al., Literacy, numeracy, and portion-size estimation skills, Am. J. Prev. Med. 36 (2009) 324–328.

[527] A.F. Smith, J.B. Jobe, D.J. Mingay, Question-induced cognitive biases in reports of dietary intake by college men and women, Health Psychol. 10 (1991) 244–251.

[528] L. Harnack, L. Steffen, D.K. Arnett, S. Gao, R.V. Luepker, Accuracy of estimation of large food portions, J. Am. Diet. Assoc. 104 (2004) 804–806.

[529] J.E. Bolland, J.A. Yuhas, T.W. Bolland, Estimation of food portion sizes: effectiveness of training, J. Am. Diet. Assoc. 88 (1988) 817–821.

[530] P.M. Howat, R. Mohan, C. Champagne, C. Monlezun, P. Wozniak, G.A. Bray, Validity and reliability of reported dietary intake data, J. Am. Diet. Assoc. 94 (1994) 169–173.

[531] J.L. Weber, A.M. Tinsley, L.B. Houtkooper, T.G. Lohman, Multimethod training increases portion-size estimation accuracy, J. Am. Diet. Assoc. 97 (1997) 176–179.

[532] D.A. Williamson, H.R. Allen, P.D. Martin, A.J. Alfonso, B. Gerald, A. Hunt, Comparison of digital photography to weighed and visual estimation of portion sizes, J. Am. Diet. Assoc. 103 (2003) 1139–1145.

[533] J.E. Bolland, J.Y. Ward, T.W. Bolland, Improved accuracy of estimating food quantities up to 4 weeks after training, J. Am. Diet. Assoc. 90 (1990) 1402–14041407.

[534] E.M. Pao, Validation of Food Intake Reporting by Men, Human Nutrition Information Service, U.S. Department of Agriculture, Hyattsville, MD, 1987 Administrative Report No. 382

[535] B.M. Posner, C. Smigelski, A. Duggal, J.L. Morgan, J. Cobb, L. A. Cupples, Validation of two-dimensional models for estimation of portion size in nutrition research, J. Am. Diet. Assoc. 92 (1992) 738–741.

[536] J. Chae, I. Woo, S. Kim, R. Maciejewski, F. Zhu, E.J. Delp, et al., Volume estimation using food specific shape templates in mobile image-based dietary assessment, Proc. SPIE 7873 (2011) 78730K.

[537] M. Sun, Q. Liu, K. Schmidt, J. Yang, N. Yao, J.D. Fernstrom, et al., Determination of food portion size by image processing, Conf. Proc. IEEE Eng. Med. Biol. Soc. 2008 (2008) 871–874.

[538] S.F. Schakel, I.M. Buzzard, S.E. Gebhardt, Procedures for estimating nutrient values for food composition databases, J. Food Compost. Anal. 10 (1997) 102–114.

[539] G.R. Beecher, R.H. Matthews, Nutrient composition of foods, in: M.L. Brown (Ed.), Present Knowledge in Nutrition, sixth ed., International Life Sciences Institute, Nutrition Foundation, Washington, DC, 1990, pp. 430–439.

[540] Interagency Board for Nutrition Monitoring and Related Research, Third Report on Nutrition Monitoring in the United States, Volume 1, U.S. Government Printing Office, Washington, DC, 1995.

[541] K.K. Stewart, What are the variances of food composition data? J. Food Compost. Anal. 10 (1997) 89.

[542] B.P. Perloff, Analysis of dietary data, Am. J. Clin. Nutr. 50 (1989) 1128–1132.

[543] U.S. Department of Agriculture, USDA Nutrient Data Laboratory, National Agricultural Library, U.S. Department of Agriculture, 2011. Available at: <http://fnic.nal.usda.gov/nal_-display/index.php?info_center=4&tax_level=2&tax_subject=279&topic_id=1387>.

[544] U.S. Department of Agriculture, USDA National Nutrient Database for Standard Reference, Release 24, Nutrient Data Laboratory home page. Agricultural Research Service, U.S. Department of Agriculture, 2012. Available at: <http://www. ars.usda.gov/main/site_main.htm?modecode=12-35-45-00>

[545] U.S. Department of Agriculture, Nutrient Data Products and Services, Agricultural Research Service, U.S. Department of Agriculture, 2011. Available at: <http://www.ars.usda.gov/services/services.htm?modecode=12-35-45-00&locpubs=yes>

[546] Food and Agricultural Organization of the United Nations, The International Network of Food Data Systems (INFOODS): International Food Composition Tables Directory, Agriculture and Consumer Protection Department, Food and Agricultural Organization of the United Nations, 2011. Available at: <http://www.fao.org/infoods/directory_en.stm>

[547] European Food Information Resource (EuroFIR), EuroFIR Home Page, European Food Information Resource, 2011. Available at: <http://eurofir.eu/home>

[548] Steering Committee of the National Nutrient Databank Conference, International Nutrient Databank Directory, National Nutrient Database Conference, 2010. Available at: <http://www.nutrientdataconf.org/indd>

[549] S.A. Smith, D.R. Campbell, P.J. Elmer, M.C. Martini, J.L. Slavin, J.D. Potter, The University of Minnesota Cancer Prevention

Research Unit vegetable and fruit classification scheme (United States), Cancer Causes Control 6 (1995) 292–302.

[550] L.E. Cleveland, D.A. Cook, S.M. Krebs-Smith, J. Friday, Method for assessing food intakes in terms of servings based on food guidance, Am. J. Clin. Nutr. 65 (1997) 1254S–1263S.

[551] USDA Center for Nutrition Policy and Promotion, USDA Food Patterns, U.S. Department of Agriculture, 2012. Available at: <http://www.cnpp.usda.gov/USDAFoodPatterns.htm>

[552] U.S. Department of Agriculture, Pyramid Servings Database for USDA Survey Codes Version 2.0, Agricultural Research Service, U.S. Department of Agriculture, 2010. Available at: <http://www.ars.usda.gov/Services/docs.htm?docid = 8634>

[553] University of Minnesota Nutrition Coordinating Center, Food and Nutrient Database, University of Minnesota, 2012. Available at: <http://www.ncc.umn.edu/products/database.html>

[554] J.K. Ahuja, L. Lemar, J.D. Goldman, A.J. Moshfegh, The impact of revising fats and oils data in the U.S. Food and Nutrient Database for Dietary Studies, J. Food Compost. Anal. 22 (2009) S63–S67.

[555] D.R. Jacobs Jr., P.J. Elmer, D. Gorder, Y. Hall, D. Moss, Comparison of nutrient calculation systems, Am. J. Epidemiol. 121 (1985) 580–592.

[556] R.D. Lee, D.C. Nieman, M. Rainwater, Comparison of eight microcomputer dietary analysis programs with the USDA Nutrient Data Base for Standard Reference, J. Am. Diet. Assoc. 95 (1995) 858–867.

[557] M.L. McCullough, N.M. Karanja, P.H. Lin, E. Obarzanek, K.M. Phillips, R.L. Laws, et al., Comparison of 4 nutrient databases with chemical composition data from the Dietary Approaches to Stop Hypertension trial: DASH Collaborative Research Group, J. Am. Diet. Assoc. 99 (1999) S45–S53.

[558] S. McNutt, T.P. Zimmerman, S.G. Hull, Development of food composition databases for food frequency questionnaires (FFQ), J. Food Compost. Anal. 21 (2008) S20–S26.

[559] A.R. Kristal, A.L. Shattuck, A.E. Williams, Current issues and concerns on the users of food composition data: food frequency questionnaires for diet intervention research, in: 17th National Nutrient Databank Conference Proceedings, June 7–10, 1992, Baltimore, MD. International Life Sciences Institute, Washington, DC, 1992, pp. 110–125.

[560] I.M. Buzzard, K.S. Price, R.A. Warren, Considerations for selecting nutrient calculation software: evaluation of the nutrient database, Am. J. Clin. Nutr. 54 (1991) 7–9.

[561] The University of Texas School of Public Health, Michael and Susan Dell Center for Healthy Living, The Food Intake Analysis System (FIAS), The University of Texas School of Public Health, 2011. Available at: <http://www.sph.uth.tmc.edu/tabDetail.aspx?id=13578&libID = 13579>

[562] K.W. Dodd, P.M. Guenther, L.S. Freedman, A.F. Subar, V. Kipnis, D. Midthune, et al., Statistical methods for estimating usual intake of nutrients and foods: a review of the theory, J. Am. Diet. Assoc. 106 (2006) 1640–1650.

[563] A.L. Carriquiry, Estimation of usual intake distributions of nutrients and foods, J. Nutr. 133 (2003) 601S–608S.

[564] P.P. Basiotis, S.O. Welsh, F.J. Cronin, J.L. Kelsay, W. Mertz, Number of days of food intake records required to estimate individual and group nutrient intakes with defined confidence, J. Nutr. 117 (1987) 1638–1641.

[565] A.M. Hartman, C.C. Brown, J. Palmgren, P. Pietinen, M. Verkasalo, D. Myer, et al., Variability in nutrient and food intakes among older middle-aged men: implications for design of epidemiologic and validation studies using food recording, Am. J. Epidemiol. 132 (1990) 999–1012.

[566] R.A. Pereira, M.C. Araujo, T.S. Lopes, E.M. Yokoo, How many 24-hour recalls or food records are required to estimate usual energy and nutrient intake? Cad. Saude Publica 26 (2010) 2101–2111.

[567] K.S. Stote, S.V. Radecki, A.J. Moshfegh, L.A. Ingwersen, D.J. Baer, The number of 24 h dietary recalls using the U.S. Department of Agriculture's automated multiple-pass method required to estimate nutrient intake in overweight and obese adults, Public Health Nutr. 14 (2011) 1736–1742.

[568] Institute of Medicine, Dietary Reference Intakes: Applications in Dietary Planning, Institute of Medicine, Food and Nutrition Board, 2003. Available at: <http://www.nap.edu/books/0309088534/html>

[569] S.M. Nusser, A.L. Carriquiry, K.W. Dodd, W.A. Fuller, A semi-parametric transformation approach to estimating usual daily intake distributions, J. Am. Stat. Assoc. 91 (1996) 1440–1449.

[570] P.M. Guenther, P.S. Kott, A.L. Carriquiry, Development of an approach for estimating usual nutrient intake distributions at the population level, J. Nutr. 127 (1997) 1106–1112.

[571] S.M. Nusser, W.A. Fuller, P.M. Guenther, Estimating usual dietary intake distributions: adjusting for measurement error and non-normality in 24-hour food intake data, in: L. Lyberg, P. Biemer, M. Collins, E. deLeeuw, C. Dippo, N. Schwartz, D. Trewin (Eds), Survey Measurement and Process Quality, Wiley, New York, 1997, pp. 689–709.

[572] W.J. de Boer, H. van der Voet, B.G. Bokkers, M.I. Bakker, P.E. Boon, Comparison of two models for the estimation of usual intake addressing zero consumption and non-normality, Food Addit. Contam Part A Chem. Anal. Control Expo. Risk Assess 26 (2009) 1433–1449.

[573] U. Harttig, J. Haubrock, S. Knuppel, H. Boeing, The MSM program: web-based statistics package for estimating usual dietary intake using the Multiple Source Method, Eur. J. Clin. Nutr. 65 (2011) S87–S91.

[574] J.A. Tooze, V. Kipnis, D.W. Buckman, R.J. Carroll, L.S. Freedman, P.M. Guenther, et al., A mixed-effects model approach for estimating the distribution of usual intake of nutrients: the NCI method, Stat. Med. 29 (2010) 2857–2868.

[575] O.W. Souverein, A.L. Dekkers, A. Geelen, J. Haubrock, J.H. de Vries, M.C. Ocke, et al., Comparing four methods to estimate usual intake distributions, Eur. J. Clin. Nutr. 65 (2011) S92–101.

[576] National Cancer Institute, Measurement ERROR Webinar Series, Applied Research Program, Division of Cancer Control and Population Sciences, National Cancer Institute, 2012. Available at: <http://riskfactor.cancer.gov/measurementerror>

2

Assessment of Dietary Supplement Use

Johanna T. Dwyer, Rebecca B. Costello

National Institutes of Health, Bethesda, Maryland

I INTRODUCTION

A Rationale

Nutritional status assessment is incomplete without assessing the intake of dietary supplements as well as food because supplements provide many essential nutrients and other bioactive substances that affect health outcomes and disease. For those suffering from health problems, specific dietary supplements may be recommended or self-prescribed. Therefore, it is essential to assess intakes of dietary supplements because Americans commonly use them today [1,2].

Dietary supplements come in a variety of product formulations, but for the purposes of discussion in this chapter, dietary supplements are defined using the legal definitions in the Dietary Supplement Health and Education Act (DSHEA), which became law in 1994. A dietary supplement is a product (other than tobacco) that is intended to supplement the diet; contains one or more dietary ingredients (including vitamins, minerals, herbs, or other botanicals, amino acids, and other substances) or their constituents; is intended to be taken by mouth as a pill, capsule, tablet, or liquid; and is labeled on the front panel as being a dietary supplement [3].

B Purposes of Dietary Supplement Intake Assessment

1 Obtain Total Intakes of Nutrients

Dietary supplements contribute substantial amounts to total intakes of some nutrients, such as calcium and vitamin D in postmenopausal women or folic acid, vitamin B_6, and vitamin B_{12} in hemodialysis patients. Failure to include these nutrient sources would lead to serious underestimation of intakes and overall diet quality. More than half of American adults use dietary supplements, and nearly half of them use multivitamin–mineral supplements. Most of the rest use single or multiple vitamin or mineral preparations that also contribute substantial nutrients to dietary intakes [2]. Therefore, it is essential to assess dietary supplement intakes among users of these products.

2 Assess Risk of Toxicities

Supplements are often very highly concentrated sources of nutrients, and especially when use of highly fortified foods is high, some individuals may have nutrient intakes that are so excessive that tolerable upper levels may be exceeded, placing the individual at risk of toxicity. Some of the bioactives in supplements can also have toxic effects, as was the case with the botanical ephedra, which was used in many weight-loss and performance-enhancing dietary supplements until banned by the Food and Drug Administration (FDA) in 2004. Also, some dietary supplements of low quality may be spiked with active drugs not declared on the label or contaminated by heavy metals, pesticides, filth, or other toxic ingredients. Noting their use on medical records may be helpful.

3 Assess Nutrient–Nutrient and Nutrient–Drug Interactions

These interactions are important to document in order to assess and plan dietary intakes and to avoid drug–supplement interactions. Supplement–nutrient and supplement–drug interactions are of particular concern. Some dietary supplements, particularly botanicals, contain many bioactive substances that may interact with other drugs or nutrients [4].

Nutrition in the Prevention and Treatment of Disease, Third Edition.
DOI: http://dx.doi.org/10.1016/B978-0-12-391884-0.00002-0

4 Clarify Associations between Dietary Supplement Intake and Health Status

It is important to clarify associations between dietary supplement use, health, and risk of various diseases and also how supplement use may change with changing patterns of disease.

5 Assess Conformity with Health Promotion and Disease Prevention Recommendations and Guidelines

The Food and Nutrition Board (FNB) of the Institute of Medicine, National Academy of Sciences, the U.S. Preventive Health Services Task Force, Healthy People 2010, the Committee on Nutrition of the American Academy of Pediatrics, and consensus statements issued on behalf of other professional societies make recommendations on the use of dietary supplements. Health screening tools may include queries to ascertain if patients are following these guidelines. For example, the FNB recommends that women in the child-bearing years who are at risk of becoming pregnant should take a dietary supplement of folic acid as well as ensure that their food intake of folate is adequate.

C Health Profiles of Dietary Supplement Users

The health profiles of dietary supplement users differ from those of non-users in some respects affecting health, which makes causative associations between supplement use and health status difficult to establish without first correcting for supplement use. These factors include physical activity, smoking status, age, income, education, and prior health status. For example, multivitamin mineral supplement users tend to have better diets and to be healthier than non-users, probably because of the differential presence of factors mentioned previously. However, generalization is hazardous. Cancer survivors often have very high levels of dietary supplement use in the hope that it will stave off a return of the malignancy [5–7]. Users of "condition-specific" supplements often suffer from specific health problems. For example, glucosamine and chondroitin or chondroitin sulfate are often used as medicines by those who are already ill or suffering from joint pain or osteoarthritis [8]. Saw palmetto is commonly used by those with prostate problems or by prostate cancer survivors [9]. There are many illnesses that consumers believe will be alleviated or cured by use of such condition-specific supplements.

D Prevalence of Dietary Supplement Use

The prevalence of dietary supplement use has increased particularly since 1994, when supplements became more widely available after the passage of DSHEA. Today, prevalence is high, with more than half of all adults using some dietary supplements. There are substantial, but somewhat lesser, numbers of children using dietary supplements. The best data are from population-based samples, such as the National Health and Nutrition Examination Survey (NHANES). On the basis of such studies, it is evident that use is particularly high in certain subgroups. For example, it is very high among elders, somewhat less but also high among young children, and lower in adolescents and adults [2,10]. Supplement use is also often positively associated with educational status, income, and, in most cases, better health status. However, those whose current health status is poor are often also heavy users of particular supplements in the hope that the products will mitigate or cure their conditions. Other studies reveal that some individuals, such as those on hemodialysis for end-stage renal disease, individuals post malabsorptive bariatric surgery, and old, frail institutionalized patients, often take special supplements.

Limited surveys of dietary supplement use have also been done for health professionals such as dietitians, but the response rates in existing surveys are too low to provide data that can be extrapolated to the profession as a whole [11].

The *Nutrition Business Journal* publishes a list of the most popular dietary supplements each year, and the latest data are summarized in Table 2.1. Although the sales data on which these lists are based do not conform precisely to the prevalence of dietary supplement use, they do give some idea of what dietary supplements Americans are buying today. The latest data in *Nutrition Business Journal 2010* show that many herbal and botanical products, including most "super fruit" products and category leaders such as echinacea and ginkgo biloba, decreased in sales compared to earlier years, whereas sales of vitamin D, probiotics, and fish/animal oils experienced double-digit increases from prior years.

The dietary supplement marketplace is constantly changing, and as it does, consumption patterns also change, so it is important to keep up with industry trends [12]. According to proprietary data collected by the Natural Marketing Institute using Harris Interactive survey data of U.S. adults (18+ years) from 2000 to 2010, "condition-specific supplements" (used for specific health issues such as memory, weight loss, and bone and joint health) more than doubled from 22% in 2000 to 48% in 2010—an 8% cumulative aggregated growth rate. Herbal supplements also showed steady growth since 2000. Use of single minerals and vitamins exhibited some minor declines, declining by approximately 1%. In addition, other supplements, such as omega-3

TABLE 2.1 Most Popular Dietary Supplements Based on 2010 Sales as Reported in *Nutrition Business Journal 2011*

Product	Consumer Sales ($ Millions)
Multivitamins	4,949
Powders/formulas	2,751
B vitamins	1,316
Calcium	1,213
Fish/animal oils	1,086
Vitamin C	966
Homeopathics	900
Glucosamine/chondroitin	744
Probiotics	626
CoQ10	480
Vitamin A/β carotene	345
Magnesium	379
Vitamin E	357
Iron	336
Drinks (for core sports)	300
Plant oils	268
Noni juice plant oils	268
Acai	277
Digestive enzymes	2,096
Mangosteen juice	193
Green tea	150
Saw palmetto	125
Echinacea	115
Garlic	109
Ginkgo biloba	90

Source: *As reported in* Nutrition Business Journal, Nutrition Business Journal Supplement Business Report, *New Hope Natural Medicines, Penton Media, Inc., San Diego, CA.*

fatty acids and probiotics, continued to drive growth in the dietary supplement category [13].

E Patterns of Dietary Supplement Use among the Ill

Nutrition professionals need to be aware that people use dietary supplements in various ways when they fall ill. They are not always forthcoming about what they are doing when discussing their health problems with their physicians or other health professionals. In part, this lack of candor may be due to the law.

DSHEA classified dietary supplements as foods, for which there are less stringent standards for quality and efficacy than would be true if they were categorized as drugs. By definition, under the law, dietary supplements are not to be used for the prevention, mitigation, or cure of disease, although in fact many people use them for these purposes [14]. Dietary supplements are inappropriate as substitutes for evidence-based medical therapies prescribed by physicians.

The vast majority of the American public turns first to prescription drugs if they are ill. A smaller proportion of the public turns first to dietary supplements or other alternative medicines for treating their illnesses, and as a result they may delay obtaining care from licensed medical practitioners. Despite the limitation of the legitimate uses of dietary supplements to health promotion under DSHEA, in fact dietary supplements are often used in ways that are different than the law intends. Caution is indicated, especially for those who are undergoing medical treatment or who are ill. Many consumers still view dietary supplements as helpful in the prevention and treatment of many conditions, including arthritis, colds and flu, osteoporosis, lack of energy, memory problems, and cancer, and hence they often self-medicate for these purposes. They also think that supplements may have a role in the prevention or treatment of depression, stress, heartburn, high cholesterol, vision, and heart and blood pressure problems.

Vitamin mineral supplements are used more commonly than herbals and botanicals and other nonvitamin, nonmineral supplements for overall health and wellness, as well as for prevention and treatment, although their efficacy in many of these regards is unproven. Many consumers use a combination of prescribed drugs, over-the-counter drugs, and dietary supplements taken simultaneously. Those who are ill run the highest risks of potential supplement–drug interactions, particularly if they are taking many medications and if they are taking medications or supplements that are especially likely to interact adversely with each other. For example, those on coumadin, a commonly used anticoagulant, may experience adverse reactions if they self-medicate with various herbal and botanical drugs that affect blood clotting [15,16].

The FDA periodically issues health advisories on dietary supplements that are posing special risk. The alerts are at http://www.fda.gov/safety/recalls/default.htm. Websites that are helpful in assessing possible interactions of dietary supplements with drugs include the National Center for Complementary and Alternative Medicine (NCCAM) website at http://www.nccam.nih.gov, the Natural Medicines database at http://www.naturaldatabase.com (subscription database), Consumer Lab at http://www.Consumerlab.com, the Natural Standard database at http://www.naturalstandard.com, and the Center for Education and Research on Therapeutics at http://www.QTdrugs.org.

NCCAM suggests that physicians and patients discuss together the use of dietary supplements to maximize benefits and minimize risks. Materials are available at the NCCAM website at http://nccam.nih.gov/health/providers.

Poor reported physical or emotional health status populations tend to be users of herbal, botanical, condition-specific, and other types of supplements. Therefore, it is important to check dietary supplement use in the ill. If patients are undergoing medical treatment and prescription drugs have been prescribed, they should be encouraged to use them as directed first and by themselves to gain the full effects of the therapy. If the patient insists on continuing dietary supplement use, possible adverse interactions with the drug regime should be investigated and the patient counseled on how to avoid potential adverse interactions. Any interactions identified should be entered into the patient's chart. If the interaction is severe or life threatening, it should be reported to the FDA at 1-800-FDA-1088 or FDA, 10903 New Hampshire Avenue, Silver Spring, MD 20993-0002.

F Motivations for Dietary Supplement Use

People have many different motivations for dietary supplement use. Motivation varies not only from person to person and by such factors as demographics (age, sex, income, education, and ethnicity) but also by attitudes such as concerns about deficiencies, readiness to engage in preventive behaviors, and health status. Motivation also varies over time within and between individuals depending on the type of product, whether it is a nutrient or non-nutrient supplement, and the definition of dietary supplement that is employed.

Motivation and use of dietary supplements are related but probably in complex ways that may differ from one individual to another. One theory is that knowledge and attitude (motivation) cause supplement use. It is also possible that people use supplements and then attitudes and knowledge (motivation) follow perhaps to rationalize or justify use. Some people apparently get into the habit and then find reasons for their behavior, often due to social influence, whereas others operate in a more deliberate manner gathering knowledge and attitudes. The implications for nutrition and other health professionals are that they must consider both ways to influence behavior when interviewing on dietary supplement use. For example, social influence may have utility in developing methods for persuading women in the

reproductive age group who might become pregnant to increase their use of folic acid.

II METHODS FOR ASSESSING DIETARY SUPPLEMENT INTAKE

A Dietary Supplement Intake (Exposure)

Most of the methods for assessing intake of dietary supplements are similar to those discussed in Chapter 1. The methods have the same strengths and limitations mentioned in that chapter. Another method applicable to supplements but not to foods is to use pill inventories, which are widely used in obtaining information about other medications. For some supplements, inferences about use can be made from blood or urine biomarkers, if available, although they provide only qualitative rather than quantitative information. The unique features of the methods for collecting dietary supplement information are detailed in Table 2.2.

B Assessing Supplement Intake in Clinical Settings

1 Inpatient Settings

Most hospitals prohibit self-medication with dietary supplements or other over-the-counter medications without the written permission of the physician, so supplement use in hospital inpatient settings is usually limited. However, prior use is of interest because some botanicals may take days or weeks to be excreted from the body. The Joint Commission, formerly known as the Joint Commission for the Accreditation of Hospitals and Healthcare Organizations, Patient Safety Goal 8 now requires documentation of any patient use of herbal remedies, vitamins, nutriceuticals, and over-the-counter drugs, and so it is important that this information be included in the patient record. Details can be found at http://www.jointcommission.org/standards_information/npsgs.aspx. The patient or a family member/caregiver should be asked to provide a list of the types and amounts of dietary supplements that the patient uses or has used in the recent past, and this information should be entered into the chart and electronic medical records as part of the dietary assessment. It is important for all health professionals who see the patient to query him or her about dietary supplement use; some patients are reluctant to tell the doctor but are willing to share their usage patterns with dietitians. It is everyone's responsibility to collect this information, and so dietitians, nurses, and pharmacists as well as physicians should be alert to these issues. When electronic medical records are developed, a question on use of dietary supplements should be included, and the

TABLE 2.2 Dietary Supplement Assessment Methods

Method	Advantages	Disadvantages	Comments
Pill inventories	Actual labels available and can be examined, doses recorded.	Patients/clients may forget or refuse to bring supplements when requested, or only produce socially acceptable/legal products. May change dietary supplement use reporting. UPC codes for dietary supplements are not unique and the formulations in a given specific UPC-coded product may change.	Technique is commonly used in studies of medication use. A variant is to ask the patient/respondent to provide drug or grocery receipts, and if these include UPC codes it may be possible to identify the supplement.
Diet records	May change eating or dietary supplement use behavior, especially if supplements have been prescribed. Provides actual record of intake going forward. Respondent has the bottle from which he or she records information and recall of items used is not necessary. May provide useful contextual information for improving adherence.	May be useful in clinical settings with willing patients to improve adherence and obtain specific details about usage patterns. However, it is extremely time-consuming for patient, usual intake may only be revealed with many days' use, and forgetting is common.	Usually, the record includes food and drink as well as dietary supplement use; can be expanded to also cover other medications when drug-supplement or food-supplement interactions are suspected.
Frequency questionnaires	Retrospective so do not affect food consumption. Lists may help to prod memory and make recall easier. May provide an estimate of usual intake. Quick to fill out. The standardized format makes it useful for large-scale studies. However, write-ins can be accommodated	Lists not usually complete and may be very nonspecific. For some condition-specific and other supplements, use is very infrequent and may not show up if the window of recall is approximately 30 days. Even semiquantitative dietary supplement intake forms are not quantitatively precise.	Frequency questionnaires for dietary supplement use range from simple checklists for categories of dietary supplements (e.g., multivitamin mineral supplements, single vitamin or mineral supplements, and others) or specific supplements to semiquantitative questionnaires that tap not only frequency but also amount used.
24 hr recalls	Retrospective so do not affect food consumption. Quantifies intake, usually easy for patient to recall. May point to problems with timing or other aspects of supplement use. Some computerized dietary assessment programs include a dietary assessment module so that both food and supplement intakes can be ascertained.	Relies on memory and some items may be forgotten or individual may not be able to provide sufficient detail about the exact supplement name, dose, etc. Many days are needed to estimate usual intake. May be useful clinically but more difficult to use in large studies in which standardization is necessary.	Individual is usually asked to provide his or her intake of dietary supplements as well as food and drink that has been consumed in the past 24 hr.
Diet histories	Food intake is not changed because method is retrospective. However, respondent may not recall usual pattern of supplement intake or may not have a usual pattern. Permits obtaining information on total diet.	Recall is involved and memory may be faulty. The amounts are usually not precise. Time-consuming for both investigator and respondent.	Individual provides the professional with information on "usual" diet.
Brief dietary supplement assessment forms	Do not change eating behavior because they are retrospective. Focus solely on dietary supplement use. Easy to fill out and inexpensive.	Only a small number of supplements or foods or both can be asked about. Often, information on dose, type of supplement, timing, etc. not provided.	Individual is asked to respond with "usual" dietary supplement intake.
Blood and urine	Does not change supplement use because it is retrospective. If the only source of the biomarker is the dietary supplement, it is possible to state with certainty that the product was consumed.	Not all micronutrients, other nutrients, or botanicals have easily identifiable biomarkers. Method is not quantifiably precise.	A blood (e.g., folic acid) or urine (e.g., creatine) biomarker is used to ascertain intake, either in conjunction with or instead of usage data on dietary supplements.

BOX 2.1

GUIDELINES FOR HEALTH PROFESSIONALS WHEN CONSIDERING
RECOMMENDATIONS FOR DIETARY SUPPLEMENTS

- Is there a shortfall in nutrient intakes from recommendations when all sources of nutrients (food, beverages, and medications such as antacids that contain nutrients and dietary supplements) are taken into account? If so, try to satisfy needs first by the use of usual foods or fortified foods, or are dietary supplements in order?
- Does the supplement contain more than 100% Daily Value and especially more than the upper level of nutrient intake recommended? If so, choose a supplement that contains lesser amounts; there is no known benefit to consuming more than the Recommended Dietary Allowance (or Adequate Intake) of a particular nutrient.
- Is the dietary supplement standardized and certified by an accredited source, such as the U.S. Phamacopoeia (USP) National Formulary (NF) showing that the USP standards for identity, purity, packaging, and labeling were followed? If so, they are labeled with the USP/NF symbol. The USP website is http://www.usp.org.
- Is the product fresh? If so, it has not exceeded its expiration date on the label.
- Does the supplement contain labeled amounts of nutrients or other constituents? Currently, there is no single source that provides verifications for label claims for nutrients and other constituents in supplements. Some useful information may be available if the product has been tested by

ConsumerLab.com and found to contain amounts of constituents claimed on the label (see www. consumerlab.com).
- Is the dietary supplement reasonable in cost and within the patient's economic means?
- Has the patient read the patient package insert and cautionary directions and dosage limits on the label? If so, the patient should be alert to adverse reactions specified and report them to his or her physician if they arise.
- Does the dietary supplement claim to prevent or cure a condition or disease? By law, dietary supplements cannot be claimed to prevent or cure disease, and so the claim is not supportable and conventional methods for doing so should be sought.
- Is the dietary supplement safe? Certain dietary supplements such as ephedra (Ma huang) have been declared unsafe by the FDA and the U.S. Department of Health and Human Services. Check the CFSAN website at FDA for updates on other products.
- Is the dietary supplement efficacious? If so, authoritative bodies such as the Food and Nutrition Board, National Academy of Sciences, the Consensus Conferences of the Agency for Healthcare Research on Quality should have indicated that such uses are safe and effective. www.ods.od.nih.gov summarizes information on many studies of safety and efficacy.

Source: Adopted and modified from Costello *et al*. [33].

---

supplements that are used should be named in the medical record.

2 Outpatient Settings

Box 2.1 provides some guidelines for health professionals when considering making recommendations on dietary supplements. During nutritional assessment, all patients should be asked about their use of dietary supplements: what supplements they use, how much they use, how often, and where they obtained them (e.g., drugstore, friends, and the Internet). Replies should be written in the medical record. Dietary supplement use should be included in diet history and in the calculation of nutrient intake. Some food frequency questionnaires and food checklists include items on the intake of the most commonly consumed dietary supplements, but these may

not include less commonly used products or supplements used only occasionally that may also be important to health. Therefore, it is wise to probe for additional supplement use and to encourage patients to write these dietary supplements on their questionnaires. If questions remain or there is need for further documentation, the patient can be asked to keep a supplement intake record that he or she can bring to the next visit. One useful way to elicit further information about dietary supplement use from ambulatory patients who report very high use but cannot remember details of what they take at home is the "brown bag" technique. The patient is asked to bring in a bag all of the dietary supplements and medications that he or she uses to the next visit. The doses and types of dietary supplements and other medications can be recorded in the chart, and their potential impact can be taken into account in dietary assessment and assessment of possible supplement—nutrient interactions. Another helpful tool is to give patients a simple diary for documenting dietary supplement use. One example is the National Institutes of Health's (NIH) brochure "Dietary Supplements: What You Need to Know." It can be downloaded and printed from the Office of Dietary Supplements' website (ods.od.nih.gov/HealthInformation/DS_WhatYouNeedToKnow.aspx). It also provides answers to some questions about dietary supplement use and medications. For patients with smart phones, an application or "App" is now available for keeping track of dietary supplements. Patients can fill this out at their leisure, and then they can share the information with health care professionals at a later time. The App can be downloaded from http://ods.od.nih.gov/about/mobile/aboutmyds.aspx.

Sources such as the "Healthcare Professional's Guide to Popular Dietary Supplements" [17] and "A Healthcare Professional's Guide to Evaluating Dietary Supplements" [18] may be helpful for obtaining estimates of ingredients and content.

C Estimating Dietary Supplement Intake

Once the patient's reported intake has been elicited, the information must be evaluated. When total nutrient intake is needed, nutrients from food, beverages, and nutrient-containing supplements must be added together to get an estimate of the individual's total dietary intake. For some, this may include capturing intakes from food bars or sports drinks that are very highly fortified.

D Assessment of Dietary Supplement Intake in Some Large-Scale National Surveys

1 National Health and Nutrition Examination Survey

NHANES is a population-based survey to assess the dietary intakes, health, and nutritional status of non-institutionalized adults and children in the United States. Approximately 5000 people are surveyed each year in five communities nationwide. In addition to food intake, information on dietary supplement use (frequency, amount, and duration) is collected from respondents during the interview in their households. The dietary supplements include vitamins, minerals, other prescription and nonprescription dietary supplements, and antacids (a major source of calcium) that have been taken in the past month. Prescription dietary supplements are also listed but in separate files. During the household interview, details on supplement use are collected. Respondents who say that they have taken dietary supplements are then asked to provide

the supplement containers. Approximately two-thirds of them do so. Supplement containers are viewed, and the interviewer records from the product label the name, strength of the ingredient (for certain vitamins and minerals), and other information. During the household interview, details on supplement use, such as how long the product has been used, how often it was taken during the past month, and how much was taken, are established [19]. Since 2007, NHANES has also collected two 24-hr recall interviews as well as interval estimates during the past 30 days.

2 National Health Interview Survey

The National Health Interview Survey (NHIS) has periodically obtained information on dietary supplement intake, especially when complementary and alternative medicine (CAM) supplements were included in the 2002 and 2007 survey years. The data products are available at the NHIS website at http://www.cdc.gov/nchs/nhis/nhis_2007_data_release_html. These data are useful in assessing use of supplements in the context of CAM use. The survey has been used in studying issues such as use of vitamin—mineral supplements among cancer survivors [20]. The latest survey is now in the field. The advantage is that the survey obtains detailed information on motivations, associations with conventional medical treatments and costs, as well as some information on dietary supplement use. Although the sampling frame is complicated, the questions asked about CAM and use of dietary supplements provide material not available in other national surveys. The disadvantage is that supplement dose information, food intake, and health indices are not included and so little can be concluded about health status other than that provided by respondent report.

3 National Cancer Institute's Diet and Health Questionnaire: A Public-Use Semiquantitative Food Frequency Questionnaire

The National Cancer Institute (NCI) has developed a semiquantitative food frequency questionnaire that is publicly available. It can be reprogrammed to add specific dietary supplements. As issued, it includes specific questions on multivitamins, herbals, antioxidant supplements, and vitamins A, C, and E during the past year and also a question on how long calcium-containing supplements or antacids have been used. There are also limited queries on approximately 10 vitamins and minerals, as well as fatty acids, and approximately 24 different herbals and botanicals that are frequently used. The questionnaire includes both foods and supplements, and it can be used for many purposes, not simply cancers. The 2006 version of the Diet and Health Questionnaire (DHQ) was validated using a checklist approach and was found to be an improvement over previous versions of the NCI questionnaire known as the 1992 NCI/Block questionnaire [21]. There have been no such validation studies with the DHQ II. However, validation findings are unlikely to be greatly modified by the minimal modifications to the food list and the updated nutrient database. The DHQ can be accessed at http://riskfactor.cancer.gov/dhq2.

4 Other Instruments for Assessing Dietary Supplement Intake in Epidemiological Studies

Many different proprietary semiquantitative questionnaires that are variations of food frequency questionnaires with additional questions on dietary supplements exist for assessing dietary supplement intakes in epidemiological studies of various large cohorts. However, the questions vary from one questionnaire to another, depending on the focus of the study. The core components of all the questionnaires are the U.S. Department of Agriculture's (USDA) Food Composition tables, combined into groups to correspond to items or recipes on the questionnaires. Data on dietary supplement composition, when available, are from manufacturers, or self-entered values are added to some of these questionnaires as well. Total intakes reported reflect intakes not only from food but also from the specific dietary supplements that were queried.

There are many examples of tools for adults that query dietary supplements as well as foods; those for children and infants are fewer in number. The questionnaires require specific food composition and dietary supplement databases to be analyzed, and these are not generally in the public domain. Adult questionnaires that query some dietary supplements include the Harvard (Willett) semiquantitative food frequency questionnaire, different versions of which have been used in a number of studies: the University of Hawaii Cancer Center's multiethnic cohort questionnaire; the Women's Health Initiative semiquantitative food frequency questionnaire; the Women's Health Study questionnaire; the National Institute of Environmental Health Sciences' Sisters Study Questionnaire; and the American Cancer Society's food frequency questionnaire. The availability of these questionnaires varies, and it depends on obtaining permission from the owners of the questionnaires and their willingness to collaborate with other investigators. Some university research groups, such as the dietary assessment groups at the University of Washington–Fred Hutchinson Cancer Center, Harvard University, and the University of Hawaii Cancer Center, will permit their questionnaires to be used, and some will analyze results for a fee.

The Fred Hutchinson Cancer Research Center at the University of Washington was the Data Coordinating Center for the Women's Health Initiative. It has developed a module based on that work and refined, for two other large NIH-sponsored clinical trials of adults, the SELECT (Selenium and Vitamin E Cancer Prevention Trial) and the VITAL (Vitamin and Lifestyle Cohort Study). It has made them available to outside groups and will process them for a fee. The VITAL study questionnaire has been further revised. The questionnaires have both nutrient supplements and herbal/botanical supplements, and they come in both male and female versions. The center's website (http://ffq.fhcrc.org) describes the services it provides to outside users.

Although use of dietary supplements is widespread, intakes from supplements, particularly by subgroups in the populations who may be heavy users, are difficult to quantify. The Supplement Reporting (SURE) study at the University of Hawaii Cancer Center developed a unique inventory method to quantify dietary supplement use. Interviewers visited participants' homes to record supplement purchase and the number of pills in each supplement bottle every 3 months over a year. The resulting inventory method markedly improves the in-depth measurement of supplement use [22]. Based on the results of the SURE study, a 1-page questionnaire for dietary supplement use (SURE-QX; Figure 2.1) has been developed and is available for use by researchers. The University of Hawaii Cancer Center food frequency questionnaire has 180 foods and 10 supplements; it is available to investigators, who can purchase it from the center and then return it for processing into nutrient intakes. The analysis provides separate variables for the intake of nutrients from food ($n = 54$) and the intake of nutrients from supplements ($n = 22$). A more extensive list of supplements is provided in the SURE-QX questionnaire described previously. The SURE-QX questionnaire has detailed questions and many defaults to permit more precise and accurate information on the dietary supplements that are used. It also includes many supplements used by Asian-Americans.

Other semiquantitative questionnaires are available from commercial services. Perhaps the best known is the Nutritionquest group, which provides the Nutritionquest or Block semiquantitative food frequency questionnaire; it can be purchased and accessed at http://www.nutritionquest.com. The basic 2005 food frequency questionnaire has approximately 110 foods and also items on multiple vitamin supplements, single vitamins and minerals, and one item on herbals. Upon request and for a fee, the Block questionnaires can be tailored for individual research purposes. The Block Nutritionquest group has also developed a

DID YOU TAKE ANY DIETARY SUPPLEMENTS DURING THE PAST YEAR, <u>AT LEAST ONCE A WEEK</u>?

① YES — If yes, did you take any of the following?　　　　② No

VITAMIN TYPE	HOW OFTEN?			FOR HOW MANY YEARS?			
	1 to 3 times a <u>week</u>	4 to 6 times a <u>week</u>	Once a <u>day</u>	1 year or <u>Less</u>	2 to 4 <u>years</u>	5 to 9 <u>years</u>	10 years or <u>more</u>
MULTIPLE VITAMINS Regular one-day-type, Centrum® or Thera-type	①	②	③	①	②	③	④
B-complex or Stress-tab type	①	②	③	①	②	③	④
SINGLE SUPPLEMENTS Vitamin C	①	②	③	①	②	③	④
Vitamin E	①	②	③	①	②	③	④
Folic acid, folate	①	②	③	①	②	③	④
Vitamin B-12	①	②	③	①	②	③	④
Vitamin B-6	①	②	③	①	②	③	④
Calcium, alone or combined with something else such as in a bone health supplement <u>OR</u> in an antacid	①	②	③	①	②	③	④
Vitamin D, alone	①	②	③	①	②	③	④
Selenium	①	②	③	①	②	③	④
Iron	①	②	③	①	②	③	④
Zinc	①	②	③	①	②	③	④
Fish oil or omega-3 fatty acids	①	②	③	①	②	③	④
Flaxseed	①	②	③	①	②	③	④
Garlic, as a pill, tablet, or capsule	①	②	③	①	②	③	④
Glucosamine, alone or combined with something else	①	②	③	①	②	③	④
Coenzyme Q-10	①	②	③	①	②	③	④
Saw Palmetto	①	②	③	①	②	③	④

IF YOU TOOK VITAMIN C OR VITAMIN E:

When you took VITAMIN C, how much did you usually take?	When you took VITAMIN E, how much did you usually take?
F 250 mg or less F 300 to 500 mg F 600 to 1000 mg F More than 1000 mg	F 200 IU or less F 250 to 400 IU F 450 to 1000 IU F More than 1000 IU

ID#._____

FIGURE 2.1　SURE-QX

brief calcium/vitamin D screener that includes 19 foods and 3 supplements as well as questions to adjust for food fortification practices. Another Block screener is the Block Folic Acid/Dietary Folate Equivalents Screener, which is based on NHANES 1999–2001 dietary recall data. It includes 21 questions and provides separate estimates of total, supplement, and food-only intakes [23]. The Block Soy Foods Screener focuses on 10 food and supplement items; it is designed to measure intakes of daidzein, genistein, coumestrol, and total isoflavones. The drawback is that the lists of dietary supplements are usually short.

E Other Instruments Used for Assessing Dietary Supplement Intake in Clinical Research Studies

Many other techniques have been used to obtain information on dietary supplement intakes. Serial random 24-hr recalls that included foods as well as supplement intakes were used successfully in the Women's Intervention Nutrition Study, a large randomized trial of diet as adjuvant therapy in women who had been treated for breast cancer [24]. In the Hemodialysis (HEMO) study of patients undergoing renal replacement therapy, food and dietary supplement intake was assessed using a 2-day diet diary assisted recall technique, in addition to medication inventories and other techniques to check on adherence to use of high-dose B vitamin supplements [25].

III DIETARY SUPPLEMENT COMPOSITION DATABASES FOR ANALYSIS OF DIETARY SUPPLEMENT INTAKE

The analysis of dietary supplement intakes ideally requires complete analytically verified tables of dietary supplement composition by chemical analyses, which still do not exist for all nutrients and even more rarely for other bioactives in supplements. Therefore, results tend to be imprecise and inaccurate, particularly for intakes of some of the botanical ingredients in dietary supplements. The situation is slowly changing, but dietary supplement databases are still incomplete with respect to both how representative they are of the universe of dietary supplements marketed and sold in the United States and how well the levels of ingredients are documented. Currently, virtually all of them rely on label claims rather than analytically verified data. For dietary supplements and many highly fortified processed foods that lack analytical data on micronutrients, intake estimates obtained from product label declarations are likely to be biased. Overages are likely, especially for vitamins because labeling regulations require that the actual nutrient content of products be equal to or greater than the declared level on the label, after taking into account processing effects and shelf life losses [26].

A Dietary Supplement Label Databases

1 NHANES Label Database

The composition of dietary supplements consumed in the NHANES is available at the National Center for Health Statistics website, although the primary purpose of the database is to store information on nutrients taken from the dietary supplement labels collected from NHANES respondents. NHANES research nutritionists obtain additional label data for the dietary supplement database by contacting manufacturers and distributors, company websites, and other Internet sources. Changes in supplement composition are tracked and entered into the database when reformulations are identified. The NHANES label database is publicly available and permits nutrition scientists to better assess total intakes of nutrients from all sources than ever before. However, it has its limitations. Only supplements that were used by respondents in the survey are provided in the database. Approximately 10,000 respondents are included in each NHANES data release. Although this may seem like a large number of respondents, for rarely used supplements, there may be few or no users who respond. Only levels of nutrients are noted, although the names of other ingredients are recorded as well. The quantitative data on nutrients that it provides rely on nutrient content declarations on the labels and are not analytically verified. Because it is a violation of the law to declare levels of a nutrient on the label as being more than what is provided, manufacturers tend to add more than the declared label value to many products. The amount added depends on the particular nutrient in question, its stability, cost, bulk, and other characteristics; there is no single "correction factor" that can be used. The supplements that are reported in NHANES during the most recent interview cycle are released every 2 years. Unfortunately, supplements change rapidly, and many of the products may not be on the market at the time the database is accessed. Default values are also included in the database because many respondents are unable to supply the exact supplement or strength that was consumed, although some information is available. Because NHANES uses a nationally representative sampling procedure, defaults developed with the NHANES data may be useful in other surveys as well, particularly if it is not possible to collect data with this level of detail. The defaults are based on the frequency of supplements reported in the latest 2-year NHANES release that is available, as well as on manufacturer information on sales. For example, default matches for adults include matching multivitamins to multivitamin minerals, as well as single ingredient formulations such as vitamin A to 8000 IU, vitamin C to 500 mg, vitamin B_6 to 100 mg, vitamin D to 400 IU, vitamin E to 400 IU, folic acid to 400 µg, calcium to 500 mg, iron to 65 mg, and zinc to 50 mg.

2 Natural Standard Database

Natural Standard is an international research collaboration that aggregates and synthesizes data on dietary supplements and other complementary and alternative therapies to provide objective and reliable information for clinicians using an evidence-based, consensus-based, and peer-reviewed procedure with reproducible grading scales. For more information, visit the website at http://www.naturalstandard.com.

The group has compiled a compendium of evidence-based reviews on herbs and dietary supplements that is available online as well as in print.

3 Natural Products Association Database

The Natural Products Association (NPA) is a trade association (formerly the National Nutritional Foods Association) that has a foundation associated with it. It operates a two-part quality assurance program that includes a third party certification program for good manufacturing practice (GMP) standards as determined by NPA based on a dialogue between suppliers and others. Those who meet the standard and pass audits can use the NPA logo. Members can also participate in the TruLabel program, which includes data on ingredients in 23,000 product labels.

4 Other Label Databases

Several other private compilations of dietary supplement label information may be purchased, such as the Natural Medicines Database (www.NaturalDatabase.com) and HealthNotes Clinical Essentials (Portland, OR; www.healthnotes.com).

B Dietary Supplement Databases with Chemical Analyses Verified

Although databases for dietary supplements are based on chemical analyses, usually the data on the label are proprietary and are disclosed only at the manufacturer's discretion. Several publicly available chemically analyzed dietary supplement databases now exist, but they contain only a few products, are not always based on representative numbers of products, and some are proprietary. The major ones are described here.

1 U.S. Department of Agriculture Dietary Supplement Ingredient Database

The Office of Dietary Supplements (ODS) at NIH collaborated with the USDA to develop an analytically substantiated dietary supplement ingredient database

(DSID) for the micronutrients and eventually for other constituents as well. Initial efforts focused on multivitamin—mineral (MVM) supplements because these are commonly consumed by Americans [26]. The database is publicly available for adult MVM and will soon be so for child MVM and later for prenatal over-the-counter MVM and omega-3 fatty acids.

2 Consumerlabs.com

ConsumerLab.com, LLC, is a provider of independent test results and information to help consumers and health care professionals evaluate dietary supplements and other health, wellness, and nutrition products. Data are published only on products that have been tested. The products are bought off the shelf in consumer outlets and chemically analyzed for various substances of interest. Consumerlabs does not publish a comprehensive database that is publicly available. However, a subscription to its reports is available for a reasonable cost at http://www.consumerlab.com.

3 NSF

NSF is an independent, not-for-profit testing organization offering product testing of dietary supplements in its NSF/American National Standards Institute. It does not simply evaluate test data submitted by manufacturers or analyze a single sample of a product and approve it; rather, NSF conducts its own product testing in its accredited laboratories. The three main components of the NSF Dietary Supplements Certification Program are verification that the contents of the supplement actually match what is printed on the label, assurance that there are no ingredients present in the supplement that are not openly disclosed on the label, and assurance that there are no unacceptable levels of contaminants present in the supplement. The major disadvantage of the values published by NSF is that they do not constitute a comprehensive database. Only products that have been certified are included in the database. Currently, approximately 540 products from 52 companies are certified on the NSF website (http://www.nsf.org/consumer).

C Computerized Dietary Assessment Programs that Include Dietary Supplements

1 University of Minnesota Dietary Supplement Module

Some computerized dietary assessment programs include dietary supplements in the interview and also have databases on their composition. For example, the University of Minnesota's Nutrient Data System has developed a dietary supplement module that can be used in conjunction with existing software to obtain information about food intake. This can be accessed at http://www.ncc.umn.edu/products/ndsr.html.

2 National Cancer Institute's Self-Administered 24-Hour Dietary Recall

The Self-Administered 24-Hour Dietary Recall (ASA24) system is a free Web-based software tool developed by the National Cancer Institute and Westat that enables automated self-administered 24-hr recalls. A new dietary supplement module, ASA24, populated from the NHANES dietary supplement data set, has been included in the current version. ASA24 consists of a Respondent application used by participants to enter recall data and a Researcher application for researchers to manage study logistics and obtain data analyses. The system allows for probing (based on USDA's automated multiple pass method), coding, and the calculation of dietary intakes using the USDA's Food and Nutrient Database for Dietary Studies. It is a highly interactive Web-based tool that uses an animated avatar to guide completion of a 24-hr dietary recall, employing more than 11,100 food images to estimate portion size. ASA24 can be used by researchers for epidemiologic, interventional, behavioral, or clinical research. Clinicians may also find it useful for dietary assessment or nutrition counseling, and educators may find it to be a useful teaching tool. Detailed information about ASA24, including information on registering a study and a demonstration of the Respondent application, is available at http://riskfactor.cancer.gov/tools/instruments/asa24.

3 Other Computerized Dietary Assessment Programs

Other computerized dietary assessment programs permit the addition of supplement information to the database even if they are not included in the food composition database, but none yet provide complete lists of the most commonly used supplements in the software package.

IV THE DIETARY SUPPLEMENT LABEL

FDA regulations require certain label information on dietary supplements, including a descriptive name of the product stating that it is a "supplement;" the name and place of business of the manufacturer, packer, or distributor; a complete list of ingredients; and the net contents of the product. The regulations are described in-depth in the FDA's Dietary Supplement Labeling Guide (accessible at http://www.fda.gov/Food/Guidance ComplianceRegulatoryInformation/GuidanceDocuments/ DietarySupplements/DietarySupplementlabelingguide/ default.htm). FDA has recently issued regulations for

GMP that touch upon such topics as verification of identity, purity, strength, and supplement composition, and these are soon to be in effect.

A Dietary Supplement Label: Ingredients

1 Differences between Food and Dietary Supplement Labels

The Supplement Facts panel on dietary supplements must list dietary ingredients that have, as well as those that do not have, recommended daily intakes (RDIs) or daily reference values (DRVs or DVs). It is optional to list the source of a dietary ingredient on the label, whereas sources of a dietary ingredient and ingredients without RDIs or DVs are not permitted on the food Nutrition Facts label. Also, the part of the plant from which a dietary ingredient is derived must be listed on the Supplement Facts panel for dietary supplements, although it cannot be listed on the food label. In contrast, the Supplement Facts panel does not permit listing of "zero" amounts of nutrients, although the Nutrition Facts panel for food requires it. The percent Daily Value (i.e., % DV or the Reference Daily Intake or Daily Reference Value) of a dietary ingredient contained in a serving of the product must be declared for all ingredients for which there are DVs except protein. Supplements for infants, children younger than 4 years, and pregnant and lactating women do not require this, however.

2 Supplement Facts Label

The panel must list the names and amounts of the dietary ingredients present in the product, the serving size, and servings per container. A serving for a dietary supplement is the maximum amount recommended for consumption at one time or, if recommendations are not given, 1 unit (e.g., tablet, capsule, packet, or teaspoon). Thus, if the label says to take one to three tablets with breakfast, the serving size is three tablets.

3 Ingredient List

Other dietary ingredients that do not have DVs are also listed in the Supplement Facts panel after the ingredients that do have them, in addition to their correct botanical (Latin) names. They are also listed by their common or usual names and must be accompanied by their weight per serving.

B Dietary Supplement Label: Claims

Box 2.2 describes the three categories of claims that can be used on dietary supplements: health claims,

---

BOX 2.2

CLAIMS THAT CAN BE USED ON DIETARY SUPPLEMENTS

Health Claims

Health claims describe a relationship between a food, food component, or dietary supplement ingredient and reducing risk of a disease or health-related condition. A "health claim" definition has two essential components: (1) a substance (whether a food, food component, or dietary ingredient) and (2) a disease or health-related condition. A statement lacking either one of these components does not meet the regulatory definition of a health claim.

FDA has oversight in determining which health claims may be used on a dietary supplement label. Its authority comes from several laws:

- NLEA Authorized Health Claims: The Nutrition Labeling and Education Act (NLEA) of 1990, the Dietary Supplement Act of 1992, and the Dietary Supplement Health and Education Act of 1994 (DSHEA) provide for health claims used on labels that characterize a relationship between a food, a food component, dietary ingredient, or dietary supplement and risk of a disease provided the claims meet certain criteria and are authorized by an FDA regulation. FDA authorizes these types of health claims based on an extensive review of the scientific literature, generally as a result of the submission of a health claim petition, using the significant scientific agreement standard to determine that the nutrient–disease relationship is well established. For an explanation of the significant scientific agreement standard, see the FDA website.
- Qualified Health Claims: FDA's 2003 *Consumer Health Information for Better Nutrition Initiative* provides for the use of qualified health claims when there is emerging evidence for a relationship between a food, food component, or dietary supplement and reduced risk of a disease or health-related condition. In this case, the evidence is not well enough established to meet the significant scientific agreement standard required for FDA to issue an authorizing regulation. Qualifying language is included as part of the claim to indicate that the evidence supporting the claim is limited. Both conventional foods and dietary supplements may use qualified health claims. FDA uses its enforcement discretion for qualified health claims after evaluating and ranking the quality and strength of the totality of the scientific evidence. Although FDA's "enforcement discretion" letters are issued to the petitioner requesting the qualified health claim, the qualified claims are available for use on any food or dietary supplement product meeting the enforcement discretion conditions specified in the letter. FDA has prepared a guide on interim procedures for qualified health claims and on the ranking of the strength of evidence supporting a qualified claim. Qualified health claim petitions that are submitted to FDA will be available for public review and comment. A listing of petitions open for public comment is at the FDA Dockets Management website. A summary of the qualified health claims authorized by FDA may be found at its website.

Nutrient Content Claims

Most nutrient content claim regulations apply only to those nutrients or dietary substances that have an established daily value and are expressed as percent Daily Value. Percentage claims for dietary supplements are another category of nutrient content claims used to describe a percentage level of a dietary ingredient for which there is no established Daily Value.

Structure–Function Claims

Statements that address a role of a specific substance in maintaining normal healthy structures or functions of the body are considered to be structure–function claims. Structure–function claims may not explicitly or implicitly link the relationship to a disease or health-related condition.

Structure–function claims on dietary supplements describe the role of a nutrient or dietary ingredient intended to affect normal structure or function in humans—for example, "calcium builds strong bones." In addition, they may characterize the means by which a nutrient or dietary ingredient acts to maintain such structure or function—for example, "fiber maintains bowel regularity" or "antioxidants maintain cell integrity"—or they may describe general well-being from consumption of a nutrient or dietary ingredient. Structure–function claims may also describe a benefit related to a nutrient deficiency disease (e.g., vitamin C and scurvy), as long as the statement also tells how widespread such a disease is in the United States. If a dietary supplement label includes such a claim, it must state in a "disclaimer" that FDA has not evaluated the claim. The disclaimer must also state that the dietary supplement product is not intended to "diagnose, treat, cure or prevent any disease" because only a drug can legally make such a claim.

nutrient content claims, and structure—function claims.

V AUTHORITATIVE INFORMATION AND RESOURCES ABOUT DIETARY SUPPLEMENTS

A Office of Dietary Supplements, National Institutes of Health

The ODS at NIH has as its mission to strengthen knowledge and understanding of dietary supplements by evaluating scientific information, stimulating and supporting research, disseminating research results, and educating the public about the efficacy and safety of dietary supplements in order to foster an enhanced quality of life and health for the U.S. population. Its website contains much useful information for health professionals and can be accessed at http://ods.od.nih.gov.

1 Computer Access to Research on Dietary Supplements

For those who wish to know about what research on dietary supplements is currently being supported by the federal government, Computer Access to Research on Dietary Supplements (CARDS) is an invaluable resource [27]. It is located at http://ods.od.nih.gov/databases/cards.html.

2 Other Resources

ODS also provides a great deal of other authoritative health information on its website. Of particular use to health professionals are dietary supplement fact sheets and the annual bibliographies of significant advances in dietary supplement research (http://ods.od.nih.gov).

B Food and Drug Administration

1 Center for Food Science and Nutrition (for Health Claims)

The FDA's Center for Food Science and Nutrition's website has a variety of materials on dietary supplements, including recent recalls, frequently asked questions, and some materials for consumers. It can be accessed at www.fda.gov/food/default.htm.

2 Center for Food Science and Nutrition's Consumer Adverse Events Reporting System and MedWatch

The Center for Food Science and Nutrition (CFSAN) has developed the Consumer Adverse Events Reporting System (CAERS), which replaces the patchwork of existing adverse event systems that were maintained previously by individual offices within CFSAN.

FDA uses the CAERS system as a monitoring tool to identify potential public health issues that may be associated with the use of a particular product already in the marketplace. Information gathered in CAERS also assists FDA in the formulation and dissemination of CFSAN's postmarketing policies and procedures. Currently, adverse event reports from the dietary supplement industry by consumers and health professionals should be submitted to MedWatch.

3 Food and Drug Administration Constituent Update

FDA produces updates for constituents that also provide other information. This information is available at http://www.fda.gov/Food/NewsEvents/ConstituentUpdates/default.htm.

C National Center for Complementary and Alternative Medicine

The NIH's NCCAM sponsors some research on dietary supplements and also provides fact sheets on a number of products, especially those that are being used for the prevention or treatment of disease. The "herbs at a glance" series contains authoritative fact sheets on a number of different herbs and botanicals, including common names, uses, potential side effects, and resources for more information. Visit http://nccam.nih.gov/health/herbsataglance.htm.

CAM on PubMed is a subset of PubMed that offers free access to more than 270,000 citations of journal articles related to complementary and alternative medicine research from the National Library of Medicine's MEDLINE database and other life science journals. Access it at http://nccam.nih.gov/research/camonpubmed.

D National Cancer Institute

The NIH's NCI operates a number of research programs that involve dietary supplements. It also occasionally produces fact sheets and papers on cancer treatment and prevention measures that include dietary supplements. The NCI's Division of Cancer Prevention and the Division of Cancer Control and Population Sciences develop and maintain a website called the Dietary Assessment Calibration and Validation Register. It is a means of keeping the international and health community aware of worldwide calibration/validation studies on dietary assessment methods. The website is accessible at http://appliedresearch.cancer.gov/cgi-bin/dacv/index.pl. It is particularly useful for researchers intending to do studies that involve nutritional assessment.

Health care providers who are treating cancer patients may wish to consult the NCI website for information on dietary supplements and other alternative and complementary therapies for cancer patients. It can be accessed at http://www.cancer.gov/cancertopics/treatment/cam.

Health professionals and patients who are seeking to enroll in clinical trials of dietary supplements or other therapies for cancers or other diseases should consult the federal government's list of registered clinical trials at http://www.clinicaltrials.gov.

E Agency for Healthcare Research and Quality (AHRQ), U.S. Department of Health and Human Services

The Agency for Healthcare Research and Quality works closely with the NIH and other federal agencies to develop systematic evidence-based reviews of the health literature on topics of public health significance. It also operates state-of-the-science and consensus conferences on these topics and publishes the deliberations. Several recent evidence-based reviews and conferences have involved dietary supplements, including MVM supplements, omega-3 fatty acids, ephedra, and ephedrine for weight loss and athletic performance; antioxidants and vitamins C, E, and CoQ10 for cardiovascular disease and cancer; B vitamins and berries for neurodegenerative diseases; and calcium and vitamin D for bone. The web address is http://www.ahrq.gov.

F National Library of Medicine

1 PubMed and MEDLINE (Public Use)

This is a world famous computerized bibliography, which includes biomedical information on dietary supplements; it is freely available to the public over the web at: www.pubmed.gov

ODS and the National Library of Medicine (NLM) partnered to create this Dietary Supplement Subset of NLM's PubMed. PubMed provides access to citations from the MEDLINE database and additional life science journals. It also includes links to many full-text articles at journal Web sites and other related Web resources.

The subset is designed to limit search results to citations from a broad spectrum of dietary supplement literature, including vitamin, mineral, phytochemical, ergogenic, botanical, and herbal supplements in human nutrition and animal models.

The PubMed Dietary Supplement Subset follows the prior International Bibliographic Information on Dietary Supplements (IBIDS) database from 1999 to 2010, which was a collaboration between the two U.S. government agencies—ODS and the U.S. Department of Agriculture's National Agricultural Library; see http://ods.od.nih.gov/Research/PubMed_Dietary_Supplement_Subset.aspx.

2 MedlinePlus (Subscription)

The National Library of Medicine sponsors a database by subscription service for specialized searches, which can be accessed at MedlinePlus: http://www.nlm.nih.gov/medlineplus/druginformation.html.

3 Bibliographies

Occasionally, the National Library of Medicine publishes bibliographies of various topics dealing with dietary supplements under its current bibliographies in medicine series.

G U.S. Department of Agriculture National Agricultural Library/Food and Nutrition Information Center

The Food and Nutrition Information Center (FNIC) compiles and disseminates authoritative bibliographies for laypeople and generalist practitioners on various topics, including dietary supplements, with partial support for these efforts from the ODS at NIH. These are available free of cost at www.nal.usda.gov/fnic. Among the recent materials available are "Dietary Supplements: General Resources for Consumers" (www.nal.usda.gov/fnic/pubs/bibs/gen/dietarysupplementsconsumers.pdf).

H Department of Defense

The U.S. Army Center for Health Promotion and Preventive Medicine website can be accessed at http://hprc-online.org/dietary-supplements. It is a resource center on various health issues for members of the armed forces as well as the general public. Some excellent materials for laypeople are available, particularly on reasonable dietary supplement use and on performance. In addition, the Human Performance Resource Center within the Uniformed Services University was established to collect, organize, and disseminate the most current information available on all aspects of human performance. Nutrition and dietary supplements are a prominent feature of this website, which can be accessed at http://humanperformanceresourcecenter.org/dietary-supplements.

I Canadian Government Resources

The Canadian government's Natural Health Product Ingredients Database includes a display of toxicity restrictions, registry numbers for the chemicals by Chemical Abstracts Service (CAS) and other registry numbers, herbals, and hyperlinks to the Canadian Natural Health Products Directorate and the Therapeutic Products Directorate monographs.

J U.S. Pharmacopoeia

The U.S. Pharmacopoeial Convention (USP) is an independent, science-based public health organization and official public standards-setting authority for all prescription and over-the-counter medicines, dietary supplements, and other health care products manufactured and sold in the United States. The standards are legally enforceable for drugs, and a dietary supplement program also exists. Quality standards are determined by a voluntary expert committee, and products that are submitted for evaluation and pass audits are listed on their website; those products that fail the evaluation are not listed. Currently, there are approximately 100 certified products. Consumer information regarding the USP certification program on dietary supplements can be found on its website as well. The data can be accessed at www.usp.org/usp-nf.

K American Dietetic Association, Also Known as the Academy of Nutrition and Dietetics

1 Position Papers and Other Materials

The American Dietetic Association (ADA), recently rechristened as the Academy of Nutrition and Dietetics in 2011, is the professional association for dietitians. It has developed a number of useful position papers, journal articles, and other materials on dietary supplements [28].

2 Evidence Library

The ADA has created an evidence analysis library that provides authoritative evaluation of the evidence on various clinical topics, including some that involve dietary supplements. Members receive access to the library as part of their dues; access to it by others is by subscription. To learn more, access the ADA website at http://www.eatright.org.

3 Practice Groups

The Complementary and Alternative Medicine Practice Group of the ADA focuses specifically on dietary supplements. It produces an excellent newsletter, and members also receive free or reduced prices on many professional resources that are useful in assessing dietary supplement intakes.

L Books

Among the useful reference books are the "Physician's Desk Reference for Nonprescription Drugs, Dietary Supplements and Herbs" [29], which covers the full spectrum of nutritional supplements, including vitamins, minerals, amino acids, probiotics, metabolites, hormones, enzymes, and cartilage products. It describes precautions, contraindications, side effects, and possible interactions with medications. The "Commission E Monographs" [30] summarizes the German Commission E monographs on various herbal medicines. "Herbs of Commerce" [31] is a comprehensive listing of more than 2000 botanicals that have current and historical uses as therapeutic agents. Botanical synonyms are included so that older botanical names that are no longer accepted can be cross-referenced. Also included are the Ayurvedic names and the Chinese names for more than 500 herbs. The book contains the Latin binomials (Linnean classification), the standardized common names, the Ayurvedic names, the Pinyin name (simplified Chinese name), and other common names. The "Encyclopedia of Dietary Supplements" [32] reviews many over-the-counter supplements carried in today's nutritional products marketplace and presents peer-reviewed, objective entries that review the most significant scientific research, including basic chemical, preclinical, and clinical studies. Other authoritative sources are also available [33,34].

VI HOW TO REPORT PROBLEMS WITH DIETARY SUPPLEMENT INTAKE

A Food and Drug Administration

The MedWatch program allows health care providers to report problems possibly caused by FDA-regulated products such as drugs, medical devices, medical foods, and dietary supplements. The identity of the patient is kept confidential. Reported adverse effects and drug interactions are also posted on the FDA Dietary Supplement Information Page of its website. If a consumer or health care provider thinks a patient has suffered a serious harmful effect or illness from a dietary supplement, it can be reported by calling FDA's MedWatch hotline at 1-800-FDA-1088 or contacting the website http://www.fda.gov/medwatch/report/hcp.htm. Consumers may also report an adverse event or illness they believe to be related to the use of a dietary supplement by calling FDA at 1-800-FDA-1088 or using the website http://www.fda.gov/medwatch/report/consumer/consumer.htm.

The FDA's Adverse Event Reporting System for dietary supplements can be completed online or by phone at 1-800 FDA-1088.

B Federal Trade Commission

The Federal Trade Commission (FTC) has authority over the advertising of dietary supplements. It can be accessed at http://www.ftc.gov/bcp/edu/microsites/whocares/supplements.shfm. It has issued advertising guidelines for the supplement industry that explain how truth in advertising applies to this industry and the kinds of claims manufacturers can and cannot make. The guidelines, titled "Dietary Supplements: An Advertising Guide for Industry," can be accessed at the FTC website. The FTC can take action against supplement manufacturers that make claims that lack "sound scientific evidence" in their advertising or that they deem false or misleading. FTC consumer protection can be accessed at www.ftc.gov/bcp/index.shtml.

C Poison Control Centers

The American Association of Poison Control Centers operates a hotline for suspected poisonings from drugs or dietary supplements at 1-800-222-1222. Its website can be accessed at http://www.aapc.org.

VII CONCLUSIONS

Best practices today include a careful assessment of dietary supplement use by consumers and patients in order to better assess their health effects. Box 2.3 provides some additional resources for those working on dietary supplement assessment. In some cases, health professionals will find it useful to encourage use of specific supplements, and in other cases they will not; in all cases, however, use should be documented.

BOX 2.3

KEY REFERENCES FOR ASSESSMENT OF USUAL INTAKES OF FOOD AND DIETARY SUPPLEMENTS

Bailey, R. L., Dodd, K. W., Goldman, J. A., Gahche, J. J., Dwyer, J. T., Moshfegh, A. J., Sempos, C. T., and Picciano, M. F. (2010). Estimation of total usual calcium and vitamin D intakes in the United States. *J. Nutr.* **140**(4), 817–822.

Carroll, R. J., Midthune, D., Subar, A. F., Shumakovich, M., Freedman, L. S., Thompson, F. E., and Kipnis, V. (2012). Taking advantage of the strengths of two different dietary assessment instruments to improve intake estimates for nutritional epidemiology. *Am. J. Epidemiol.* **175**, 340–347.

Dodd, K. W., Guenther, P. M., Freedman, L. S., Subar, A. F., Kipnis, V., Midthune, D., Tooze, J. A., and Krebs-Smith, S. M. (2006). Statistical methods for estimating usual intake of nutrients and foods: A review of the theory. *J. Am. Diet. Assoc.* **106**(10), 1640–1650.

Freedman, L. S., Kipnis, V., Schatzkin, A., Tasevska, N., and Potischman, N. (2010). Can we use biomarkers in combination with self-reports to strengthen the analysis of nutritional epidemiologic studies? *Epidemiol. Perspect. Innov.* **7**(1), 2.

Freedman, L. S., Midthune, D., Carroll, R. J., Tasevska, N., Schatzkin, A., Mares, J., Tinker, L., Potischman, N., and Kipnis, V. (2011). Using regression calibration equations that combine self-reported intake and biomarker measures to obtain unbiased estimates and more powerful tests of dietary associations. *Am. J. Epidemiol.* **174**(11), 1238–1245.

Freedman, L. S., Schatzkin, A., Midthune, D., and Kipnis, V. (2011). Dealing with dietary measurement error in nutritional cohort studies. *J. Natl. Cancer Inst.* **103**(14), 1086–1092.

Garriguet, D. (2010). Combining nutrient intake from food/beverages and vitamin/mineral supplements. *Health Rep.* **21**(4), 71–84.

Midthune, D., Schatzkin, A., Subar, A. F., Thompson, F. E., Freedman, L. S., Carroll, R. J., Shumakovich, M. A., and Kipnis, V. (2011). Validating an FFQ for intake of episodically consumed foods: Application to the National Institutes of Health-AARP Diet and Health Study. *Public Health Nutr.* **13**, 1–10.

National Cancer Institute's usual intakes website: http://riskfactor.cancer.gov/diet/usualintakes.

National Health and Nutrition Examination Survey (NHANES) dietary tutorial: http://www.cdc.gov/nchs/tutorials/Dietary/index.htm.

National Research Council (1986). "Nutrient Adequacy: Assessment Using Food Consumption Surveys." National Academies Press, Washington, DC.

Park, S. Y., Murphy, S. P., Wilkens, L. R., Yamamoto, J. F., and Kolonel, L. N. (2006). Allowing for variations in multivitamin supplement composition improves nutrient intake estimates for epidemiologic studies. *J. Nutr.* **136**(5), 1359–1364.

Source: Adapted from http://riskfactor.cancer.gov/measurementerror/sessions.

References

[1] V.L. Fulgoni, D.R. Keast, R.L. Bailey, J. Dwyer, Foods, fortificants and supplements-Where do Americans get their nutrients? J. Nutr. 141 (2011) 1805–1812.

[2] K. Radimer, B. Bindewald, J. Hughes, B. Ervin, C. Swanson, M.F. Picciano, Dietary supplement use by U.S. adults: data from the National Health and Nutrition Examination Survey, 1999–2000, Am. J. Epidemiol. 160 (2004) 339–349.

[3] Center for Food Science and Nutrition, Office of Nutritional Products, Labeling and Dietary Supplements, Guidance for Industry: A Dietary Supplement Labeling Guide, U.S. Food and Drug Administration, Washington, DC, 2005.

[4] B.B. Timbo, M.P. Ross, P.V. McCarthy, C.T.J. Lin, Dietary supplements in a national survey: prevalence of use and reports of adverse event, J. Am. Diet. Assoc. 106 (2006) 1966–1974.

[5] C.L. Rock, V.A. Newman, M.L. Neuhouser, J. Major, M.J. Carnett, Antioxidant supplement use in cancer survivors and the general population, J. Nutr. 134 (Suppl.) (1994) 3194S–3195S.

[6] C.L. Rock, V. Newman, S.W. Flatt, S. Faerber, F.A. Wright, J.P. Pierce, Nutrient intakes from foods and dietary supplements in women at risk for breast cancer recurrence, Nutr. Cancer 29 (1997) 133–139.

[7] V. Newman, C.L. Rock, S Faerber, S.W. Flatt, F.A. Wright, J.P. Pierce, Dietary supplement use by women at risk for breast cancer recurrence, J. Am. Diet. Assoc. 98 (1998) 285–292.

[8] D.T. Felson, R.C. Lawrence, M.C. Hochberg, T. McAlindon, P. Dieppe, M.A. Minor, et al., Osteoarthritis: new insights, Ann. Intern. Med. 133 (2000) 726–737.

[9] J.B. Wiygul, B.R. Evans, B.L. Peterson, et al., Supplement use among men with prostate cancer, Urology 66 (2005) 161–166.

[10] M.F. Picciano, J.T. Dwyer, K.L. Radimer, D.H. Wilson, K.D. Fisher, P.R. Thomas, et al., Dietary supplement use among infants, children, and adolescents in the United States (US): 1999–2002, Arch. Pediatr. Adolesc. Med. 161 (2007) 978–985.

[11] J.V. White, S. Pitman, J.B. Blumberg, Dietitians and multivitamin use: personal and professional practices, Nutrition Today 42 (2007) 62–68.

[12] L.G. Saldanha, The dietary supplement marketplace, Nutrition Today 42 (2007) 52–54.

[13] S. French, Personal communication, Natural Marketing Institute, Harleysville, PA, 2012, January 12.

[14] F.A. Hoffman, Regulation of dietary supplements in the United States: understanding the Dietary Supplement and Health Education Act, Clin. Obstet. Gynecol. 44 (2001) 780–788.

[15] N.C. Brazier, M.A. Levine, Drug–herb interaction among commonly used conventional medicines: a compendium for health care professionals, Am. J. Ther. 10 (2003) 163–169.

[16] R.R. Couris, Vitamins and minerals that affect hemostasis and antithrombotic therapies, Thromb. Res. 117 (2005) 25–31.

[17] American Dietetic Association/Allison Sarubin Fragakis, Healthcare Professional's Guide to Popular Dietary Supplements from the Joint Working Group on Dietary Supplements, American Dietetic Association, Chicago, 2003.

[18] ADA/APHA (2000) Special Report from the Joint Working Group on Dietary Supplements: A Healthcare Professional's Guide to Evaluating Dietary Supplements. Available at <http://www.aphanet.org>.

[19] J.T. Dwyer, M.F. Picciano, Members of the Steering Committee: National Health and Nutrition Examination Survey, Collection of food and dietary supplement intake data: What We Eat in America—NHANES, J. Nutr. 133 (2003) 575S–635S.

[20] K. McDavid, R.A. Breslow, K. Radimer, Vitamin/mineral supplementation among cancer survivors 1987 and 1992: National Health Interview Surveys, Nutr. Cancer 41 (2001) 29–32.

[21] F.E. Thompson, A.F. Subar, C.C. Brown, A.F. Smith, C.O. Sharbaugh, J.B. Jobe, et al., Cognitive research enhances accuracy of food frequency questionnaire reports: results of an experimental validation study, J. Am. Diet. Assoc. 102 (2002) 212–225.

[22] S.P. Murphy, L.R. Wilkens, K.R. Monroe, A.D. Steffen, K.M. Yonemori, Y. Morimoto, et al., Dietary supplement use within a multiethnic population as measured by a unique inventory method, J. Am. Diet. Assoc. 111 (2011) 1065–1072.

[23] A.J. Clifford, E.M. Noceti, A. Block-Jay, T. Block, G. Block, Erythrocyte folate and its response to folic acid supplementation is assay dependent in women, J. Nutr. 135 (2005) 137–143.

[24] R.T. Chlebowski, G.L. Blackburn, C.A. Thomson, D.W. Nixon, A. Shapiro, M.K. Hoy, et al., Dietary fat reduction and breast cancer outcome: interim efficacy results from the Women's Intervention Nutrition Study, J. Natl. Cancer Inst. 98 (2007) 1767–1776.

[25] Hemo Study Group (prepared by Dwyer, J.T., Cunniff, P.J., Maroni, B.J., Kopple, J.D., Burrowes, J.D., Powers, S.N., Cockram, D.B., Chumlea, W.C., Kusek, J.W., Makoff, R., Goldstein, J., Paranandi, L.), The Hemodialysis (Hemo) Pilot Study: Nutrition program and participant characteristics at baseline. J. Renal Nutr. 8 (1998) 11–20.

[26] J.T. Dwyer, J. Holden, K. Andrews, J. Roseland, C. Zhao, A. Schweitzer, et al., Measuring vitamins and minerals in dietary supplements for nutrition studies in the USA, Anal. Bioanal. Chem. 389 (2007) 37–46.

[27] C.J. Haggans, K.S. Regan, L.M. Brown, C. Wang, J. Krebs-Smith, P.M. Coates, et al., Computer access to research on dietary supplements: a database of federally funded dietary supplement research, J. Nutr. 135 (2005) 1796–1798.

[28] J. Mathieu, Sifting through the research on supplements, J. Am. Diet. Assoc. 107 (2007) 912–914.

[29] P.D.R. Thomson, PDR for Nonprescription Drugs, Dietary Supplements, and Herbs: The Definitive Guide to Over the Counter Medications, Thomson, New York, 2007.

[30] M. Blumenthal, et al., The Complete German Commission E Monographs: Therapeutic Guide to Herbal Medicines, American Botanical Council. Published by Integrative Medicine Communications, 1998.

[31] M. McGuffin, A. Leung, A.P. Tucker, Herbs of Commerce, second ed., American Herbal Products Association, Denver, CO, 2000.

[32] P.M. Coates, M.R. Blackman, G.M. Cragg, M. Levine, J. Moss, J.D. White (Eds), Encyclopedia of Dietary Supplements, Dekker, New York, 2005.

[33] R.B. Costello, M. Leser, P.M. Coates, Dietary supplements for health maintenance and risk factor reduction, Handbook of Clinical Nutrition and Aging, Humana Press, Totowa, NJ, 2005.

[34] M. McGuffin, C. Hobbs, R. Upton, A. Goldberg, Botanical Safety Handbook, CRC Press, Boca Raton, FL, 1997.

CHAPTER

3

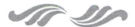

Physical and Clinical Assessment of Nutrition Status

Edward Saltzman, Kris M. Mogensen†*

*Tufts University, Boston, Massachusetts, †Brigham and Women's Hospital, Boston, Massachusetts

I INTRODUCTION

Physical assessment of nutrition status provides data, simply stated, about the size, shape, integrity, and function of the body. Physical assessment includes physical examination and anthropometric measurements, which can be combined with other components of clinical assessment (Table 3.1) to assess body weight, the presence or risk of protein-energy malnutrition (PEM), micronutrient deficiency or excess, health problems predisposing to nutritional problems, and functional status. Physical assessment alone may be used for nutrition screening, which can be defined as the use of a simple test to determine the need for further detailed assessment or intervention. For example, body mass index (BMI) and weight change are commonly used to screen for PEM. Nutrition assessment, defined as a more detailed evaluation of existing status and future nutrition risk, often includes several additional components of clinical assessment that can be synthesized to inform a plan for intervention or future rescreening [1].

The settings in which physical assessment is conducted vary considerably. Anthropometric measures are used extensively in clinical practice, population screening, and research to assess growth and prevalence of underweight or overweight and to estimate disease risk. Findings on physical examination provide evidence for morbidity related to underweight or overweight and may indicate manifestations of micronutrient deficiency or excess. Furthermore, physical assessment variables are used extensively in research to appropriately analyze data, such as the adjustment of resting energy expenditure for body weight or fat-free mass (FFM).

Clinical assessment and particularly physical assessment are commonly perceived as methods to detect malnutrition. This most often denotes PEM. As the understanding of PEM in the settings of starvation and disease has evolved, additional definitions for malnutrition have been proposed for use in clinical settings in which inflammation may play a role in compromising nutritional status. Starvation-related malnutrition occurs when there is chronic starvation without inflammation. Chronic disease-related malnutrition is present when inflammation is chronic and of a mild to moderate degree. Acute disease- or injury-related malnutrition is present when inflammation is acute and of a severe degree [2].

II COMPONENTS OF CLINICAL ASSESSMENT

The type and number of clinical assessment components, as described in Table 3.1, can be tailored to specific settings, purposes, and populations.

A Medical History and the Nutrition-Oriented Review of Systems

The medical history addresses details of the present complaint or illness, body weight change, and the past medical history. An additional nutritionally oriented review of systems (ROS) should be performed to elicit relevant factors not directly related to the present illness. The nutritionally oriented ROS should address the spectrum of behaviors and physiological functions necessary to maintain adequate nutritional status,

Nutrition in the Prevention and Treatment of Disease, Third Edition.
DOI: http://dx.doi.org/10.1016/B978-0-12-391884-0.00003-2

TABLE 3.1 Components of Clinical Assessment of Nutrition Status

Component	Examples
History	Current and past health
	Weight change
	Medications and dietary supplements
	Nutrition-oriented review of systems
	Alcohol, tobacco and illicit drug use
	Family health history
	Social history
Diet	Ability to shop and prepare food
	Appetite and taste changes
	24-Hour diet recall
	Food diaries
	Food preferences
	Food sensitivities
Anthropometrics	Weight
	Height
	Weight for height
	Skinfold thickness
	Circumferences
Physical examination	See Table 3.3
Functional assessment	Handgrip strength
	Activities of daily living
	Walking
Laboratory	Blood and urine tests
	Dual X-ray absorptiometry

including appetite and thirst, and the abilities to procure, prepare, ingest, swallow, digest, and absorb food. For example, poor dental health or use of dentures may predispose to reduced nutrient intake [3], but identification of this problem may be missed without direct questioning. Potential for abnormal nutrient losses, such as from vomiting or diarrhea, and factors that may alter protein, energy, or micronutrient requirements should be addressed.

Medications, including prescription and over-the-counter medications, vitamin and mineral supplements, and herbal preparations should be reviewed. More than 50% of the U.S. population reports use of at least one vitamin, mineral, or dietary supplement [4], but many do not consider nutritional supplements to be medications and direct questioning may be necessary to elicit this history. Medications interfere with

nutritional status by multiple mechanisms, including alterations in intake, absorption, and metabolism. Conversely, nutrition status can alter drug bioavailability and metabolism. Table 3.2 describes the mechanisms and potential effect of drug—nutrient interactions.

B Anthropometric Assessment

Anthropometric measurements quantify physical characteristics such as height, weight, weight as a function of height, circumference of body parts, and skinfold thickness. Assessment of these parameters allows comparison to population norms or to values collected over time in the same individual.

1 Height

Measurement of height is necessary to calculate BMI, body surface area, and waist-to-height ratio. When possible, height should be directly measured by a stadiometer. In infants, height, or more accurately length, is best measured by use of a length board [5]. Height begins to decline at approximately age 30 years for both men and women, and this decline accelerates with age; in one longitudinal series, between the ages of 30 and 80 years, women lost 8 cm and men lost 5 cm [6]. Height decreases as a result of vertebral bone loss as well as thinning of intervertebral disks and weight-bearing cartilage. Height may also decrease due to vertebral compression fractures in the settings of osteoporosis or trauma. Loss of vertebral mass and disk compression may induce kyphosis (curvature with backward convexity of the spine), which will further reduce measured height.

When height cannot be accurately measured, such as in acutely ill or immobilized patients, alternatives include self-reported height, estimated height, or surrogate anthropometric measures. Self-reported height is less accurate than measured height because men tend to overreport and women tend to underreport [7]. Self-reported height is more accurate, however, than estimation of height by visualization of supine patients, which has been found to overestimate height [8]. Accuracy of visual estimation of height was better for taller patients compared to shorter patients, possibly because taller patients were closer to the length of the beds in which they were lying, which provided a frame of reference for estimation [7].

Surrogate measures for height include arm span, knee height, and seated height. Use of knee height or arm span to estimate vertical height may be useful in clinical as well as research situations for individuals who cannot stand, who are debilitated, or who have experienced loss of height [6,9]. These measures correlate with vertical height but are influenced less by

TABLE 3.2 Effect of Drugs on Nutrition Status and Nutrients

Drug effect	Effect on nutrition status
Increased or decreased intake and weight gain	Weight gain or loss
Altered nutrient partitioning	Gains in fat mass
Alteration in taste or smell	Reduced interest in food consumption
Dry mouth	Dysphagia
Increased or decreased gastrointestinal motility	Food aversion or reduced intake
Nausea and vomiting	Food aversion or reduced intake
	Dehydration
	Nutrient losses
Diarrhea	Food aversion or reduced intake
	Dehydration
	Nutrient losses
Reduced nutrient bioavailability due to binding or altered transporter function	Impaired absorption of nutrients
Altered nutrient distribution	Altered tissue concentration of nutrients
Altered nutrient function	Altered conversion to active nutrient form Interference with nutrient function
Increased or decreased nutrient catabolism	Nutrient deficiency or excess
Altered excretion due to antagonism or modulation	Nutrient deficiency or excess

age-related changes in stature and impediments to the measurement of vertical height such as disability or frailty [9−12]. Surrogates of height have been used to predict both current height and previous adult maximal height. Arm span, which is the entire distance from the tip of the middle finger of one hand to the other, can be measured with arms stretched at right angles to the body by measuring tape crossing in front of the clavicles. Demi-arm span (the distance from the sternal notch to the tip of the middle finger of one hand) can also be measured and then doubled to calculate arm span. Knee height is best measured with specialized calipers and is performed either in sitting or recumbent positions, making this useful in most ambulatory and hospital settings. Prediction equations for the estimation of height from anthropometric surrogates can then be applied for specific age, gender, racial, and ethnic groups. In several trials that directly compared measured height to surrogates, disagreement between measured height and surrogates increased when the measurement was conducted in ill patients instead of healthy subjects; in these trials, compared to measured height, mean differences were 0−2 cm for self-reported height, −0.6 to4 cm for knee height, and 0−7 cm for arm span [13−16].

2 Weight

Ideally, body weight should be measured by use of calibrated beam-type or electronic scales. Alternatives are home scales, calibrated bed scales, chair scales, or wheelchair scales. To monitor changes in weight over time, the use of the same scale is recommended given variability between scales. In cases in which a person cannot be weighed or provide a self-reported weight, weight may be estimated, an inaccurate practice that does, however, improve with experience [8]. Self-reported weights are often inaccurate. Overweight women and men tend to underestimate weight, whereas lower weight men tend to overestimate [7]. In one study, use of a single self-reported weight prevented identification of weight loss in approximately one-third of patients who had lost weight [17].

Technological advances now allow automatic remote monitoring of home scales via telephone or the Internet, a method gaining popularity for management of chronic diseases such as congestive heart failure (in which rapid changes are likely due to body water) and obesity.

Involuntary loss of body weight in the setting of illness is associated with increased risk of morbidity and mortality [18−21]. In hospitalized patients with a variety of gastrointestinal, infectious, and neoplastic diseases, PEM at admission was associated with an approximately twofold risk of subsequent complications [22]. Involuntary weight loss may better predict risk for PEM-related complications in contrast to a single static measure of weight [20,23,24]. In patients with cancer who were undergoing chemotherapy, a loss of 5% or more of usual body weight was associated with impaired functional status and significantly decreased median survival compared to patients without weight loss [18]. More than 70 years ago, Studley [21] recognized that unintentional weight loss of 20% or more of usual body weight before surgery for peptic ulcer significantly increased the risk of postoperative mortality. Others have confirmed that PEM preceding surgery increases risk of postoperative complications [20,24,25]. Patients who have lost 10−20% of initial body weight over 6 months and have associated physiological defects or those who have lost 20% or more over 6 months should be considered at high risk [26,27].

In obese persons, "adjusted body weight" is used by some to estimate the metabolically active proportion of excess weight. Proposed in 1984 [28], adjustment of body weight reflects the average contribution to weight gain in obesity of 75% fat and 25% FFM: Adjusted weight = ideal body weight + [(actual weight−ideal weight) × 0.25]. There is, however, little empiric evidence to support use of this calculation despite its logical appeal [29].

Precipitous changes in weight are commonly due to alterations in body water with conditions such as congestive heart failure, cirrhosis, and renal failure or with treatments for these conditions such as diuretics.

3 Weight for Height

Weight is expressed as a function of height to facilitate comparison of individuals of varied heights. Historically, ideal body weight or desirable body weight was defined by actuarial data of weight for height with adjustment for frame size. These data have limited applicability to more current diverse populations (compared to those from which original data were obtained) and those with a longer life span [30]. Frame size can be determined by measurement of elbow or wrist breadth or of wrist circumference, which requires the use of specialized calipers or measuring tape. Percentage of ideal body weight was previously used to classify underweight and overweight, and today it is still utilized by some for these purposes or to estimate energy needs, drug dosing, or eligibility for bariatric surgery.

Body weight expressed as a function of height takes the general form weight/height^x and is called body mass index. Whereas x may be any number, Quetelet's index, or kilograms per square meter, has become synonymous with BMI. The use of BMI to assess weight for height in individuals reflects recommendations of the National Institutes of Health and World Health Organization [31].

BMI correlates with body fat for populations, but there remains considerable variation in body composition among individuals at each level of BMI. BMI may be elevated despite relatively low levels of body fat in those with edema or in bodybuilders. The relationship between BMI and body fat differs between sexes, varies among racial and ethnic groups, and also changes over the life span [32]. A single BMI classification scheme for the entire adult age range does not reflect the loss of FFM and gain in fat mass (FM) that accompany aging. Gallagher *et al.* [33] demonstrated that older (>65 years) men and women have a higher percentage of body fat compared to younger counterparts with the same BMI. Gender is also an important consideration because women have a higher percentage of body fat compared to men of the same BMI [33]. Despite these potential problems, BMI remains an easily calculated and useful method of classifying weight relative to height, especially for populations. In individuals, BMI can be used as one of several indicators of nutritional status with consideration of physical examination and other findings that may alter the expected BMI−body composition relationship.

Both low and high BMI correlate with morbidity and mortality, although there is ongoing debate regarding issues such as the magnitude of risk for those with BMI in the overweight range (25−30 kg/m^2) and how age modifies risk for morbidity and mortality [34−38]. Low levels of BMI, with underweight classified as BMI < 17.5 kg/m^2, are associated with lethargy, diminished work productivity in adults, and multiple health risks [37]. The lowest average survivable BMI, as derived from observations in starvation, famine, anorexia nervosa, or by theoretical models, has been estimated to be 12 or 13 kg/m^2 [39]. However, when weight loss is rapid or associated with illness, morbidity and mortality can occur at any level of BMI.

Obesity has deleterious effects on every organ system as well as quality of life and productivity, and the health effects of obesity are discussed in detail in this volume and elsewhere [38]. Of note, a significant proportion of weight-related co-morbidities, such as type 2 diabetes or obstructive sleep apnea, remain undiagnosed in obese persons [40,41]; this should be kept in mind when assessing obese patients.

4 Body Fat Distribution

Central distribution of body fat increases risk for type 2 diabetes, metabolic syndrome, hypertension, and coronary heart disease [42−44]. Central obesity is a predictor of risk independent of BMI. In some

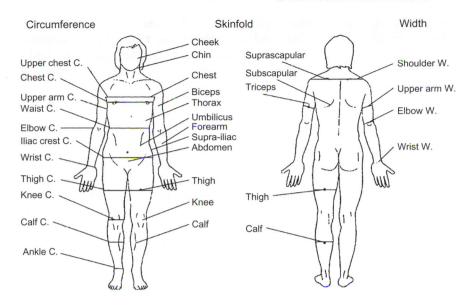

Circumference   Skinfold   Width

FIGURE 3.1 Landmarks for assessment of waist circumference. *Reprinted from The Obesity Education Initiative Expert Panel on the Identification Evaluation and Treatment of Overweight and Obesity in Adults (1998). Clinical guidelines on the identification, evaluation, and treatment of overweight and obesity in adults: The evidence report.* Obes. Res. **6** *(Suppl. 2), 51S—209S.*

investigations, when compared to BMI, central obesity has been a better predictor of disease risk [44]. Abdominal adipose depots include visceral, retroperitoneal, and subcutaneous compartments. Measures of central adiposity include a single circumference or waist-to-hip ratio. Current guidelines recommend that abdominal adiposity be assessed by waist circumference measured at the level of the top of the iliac crest [31]. Like BMI, the relationship between anthropometric measures of central obesity and disease risk varies with sex, age, and race [43]. Central obesity generally increases with increasing BMI, making the use of a single cutoff for waist circumference for the entire range of BMI problematic. The need for BMI-specific cutoffs, especially for BMI in ranges less than 30 kg/m^2, has been proposed [43].

Waist-to-height ratio (WHR) has been proposed as an alternate method to evaluate central adiposity. Like waist circumference, WHR correlates well with abdominal fat content. As with BMI, expressing waist circumference as a function of height allows comparison across varying heights. A systemic review conducted by Browning *et al.* [45] confirmed the utility of WHR as a predictor of coronary heart disease and type 2 diabetes. WHR has been found to be accurate in children and adults, men and women, and across ethnic groups. The authors suggest a cutoff of 0.5 as an indicator of risk.

5 Circumferences and Skinfold Thickness Measurements

Circumferences of the trunk or limbs reflect amounts of underlying FFM and FM. Skinfold thickness describes the amount of subcutaneous fat when the skin is pinched by specialized calipers (Figure 3.1). Combinations of circumference and skinfold thickness

measurements are utilized to predict body composition and have been validated with comparison to reference measures hydrodensitometry, dual-energy X-ray absorptiometry (DXA), or computed axial tomography [46,47]. The sites at which these measurements are conducted are illustrated in Figure 3.2. Single-site measurements may provide data regarding changes over time in the same individual but are seldom used to predict body FM or FFM.

Circumferences and skinfold thickness may be influenced by several factors, including age, sex, race, and state of hydration [48]. Prediction equations specific to the individual or population should be used when possible. Most reference data have been developed in healthy populations. Use in ill patients is problematic due to frequent body water alterations and due to uncertain effects of some disease states on body composition changes. Measurements obtained in reduced-obese persons who have lost large amounts of weight are likely influenced by redundant skin and persistent alterations in body water distribution [49].

III BODY COMPOSITION ASSESSMENT

Body composition describes and quantifies various compartments within the body. Fat content of the body is expressed as a percentage of total body mass or as absolute FM. Body composition can be assessed at the level of the body as a whole (e.g., weight or BMI); by division into FFM and FM; by division into molecules such as water, protein, and fat; or at an atomic level into elements such as carbon and potassium (Figure 3.3). Methods to assess body composition vary by the compartments being measured. Some commonly employed methods include DXA, which can divide the body into fat, fat-free, and bone compartments, and density methods such as air displacement plethysmography (ADP; using a device known as the BOD POD) and hydrostatic weighing or underwater weighing and dilution methods that measure body water. These methods utilize body density, body volume, and weight to estimate fat and fat-free compartments. Hydrostatic weighing was the traditional gold standard but has been replaced by ADP and DXA. Bioelectrical impedance (BIA) measures body water, from which FFM can be estimated. The primary use for DXA on a clinical basis is to provide a measure of bone density in order to assess osteoporosis risk, but measures of fat and FFM are not clinically available. Of the methods discussed, BIA is the least accurate for individuals, but due to its ease of use and the low expense of some devices, it has become popular in weight loss programs and health clubs.

Although excess adiposity is associated with disease in virtually every organ system, no universally agreed upon criteria for excess body fat has been accepted. The fat mass index (FMI; calculated as fat mass/$height^2$) has been proposed as a useful measure of adiposity that is independent of FFM. FMI has been validated by comparison to body composition techniques as well as BMI in NHANES [50], but its utility as a measure to predict health outcomes awaits further investigation.

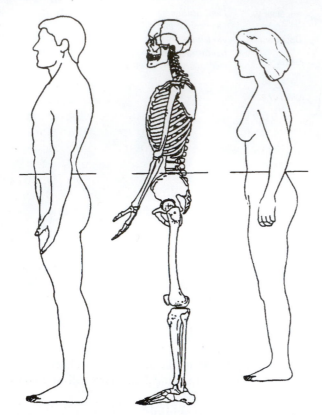

FIGURE 3.2 Body sites for measurement of circumferences, skinfold thickness, and widths. *From Wang, J., Thornton, J.C., Kolesnik, S., and Pierson, R.N., Jr. (2000). Anthropometry in body composition: An overview.* Ann. N.Y. Acad. Sci. *904, 317–326. Used with permission of Wiley-Blackwell.*

IV PHYSICAL MANIFESTATIONS OF MALNUTRITION

Physical examination may reveal manifestations of malnutrition, but there is limited sensitivity for

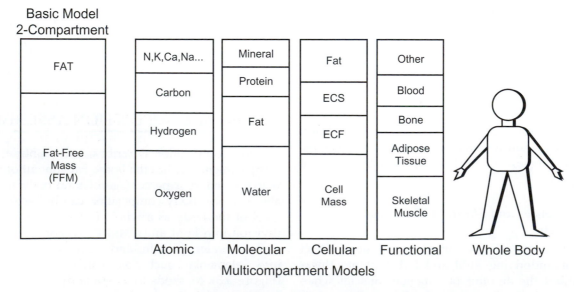

FIGURE 3.3 Models of body composition compartments. ECF, extracellular fluid; ECS, extracellular solid. *From Ellis, K.J. (2000). Human body composition:* In vivo *methods.* Physiol. Rev. *80, 649–680. Used with permission.*

micronutrient disorders because these findings may not be clearly manifest until late in the course of deficiency or excess. The specificity of physical examination is limited because deficiencies of several micronutrients may result in similar manifestations (e.g., glossitis or angular stomatitis), and micronutrient deficiencies may not occur in isolation such that physical findings may reflect multiple deficiencies. Nonetheless, physical findings that are correlated with other relevant aspects of assessment provide important data regarding the need for further investigation or treatment.

The following sections describe physical findings in organ systems or disease states. Because physical findings may be nonspecific, associated historical, anthropometric, and functional and biochemical findings are discussed. Table 3.3 summarizes selected physical findings found in nutrient deficiency or excess, some of which are depicted in Figure 3.3.

A The Head and Neck

The temporalis muscles should be visualized for evidence of wasting, a sign of PEM as well as nonnutritional diseases of muscle wasting. Hair may demonstrate alterations in color, texture, and density. PEM may result in hair that is dull or dyspigmented and easily plucked hair. Kwashiorkor may result in the Flag sign, a band of dyspigmented hair surrounded by normally colored hair that indicates a transient period of protein malnutrition. Diffuse alopecia is one of the signs of zinc deficiency, and when accompanied by rash and dysguesia, zinc deficiency should be strongly considered.

Examination of the eyes may reveal several signs of nutrient deficiency. Vitamin A deficiency is associated with reduced night vision (which may require ophthalmologic assessment to confirm) and is later manifest by Bitot's spots visible on the surface of the eye. Thiamin deficiency may result in opthalmoplegia, which classically is lateral gaze palsy.

The mouth is among the common sites that may indicate disorders of nutrition status (Figure 3.3). Cracking or ulceration of the lips (cheilosis), or cracking or ulceration at the corners of the mouth (angular stomatitis), is seen in multiple deficiencies including those of B vitamin, iron, and zinc. Angular stomatitis may also be due to poor fitting dentures, which is associated with reduced food intake.

Glossitis, or inflammation of the tongue, is associated with deficiencies of multiple vitamins, deficiencies of iron and zinc, as well as PEM. Glossitis may result in the tongue appearing swollen or "beefy," and color may be pale, red, or magenta instead of the normal pink color. Loss of papilla may result in the tongue appearing smooth or shiny (atrophic glossitis).

Pale gums may indicate anemia. Bleeding from the gums may indicate coagulopathy resulting from vitamin K deficiency or scurvy.

Cancer chemotherapy may result in pain or ulcers in the mouth and throat (mucositis), a common cause of poor intake in patients undergoing chemotherapy and in some patients undergoing radiation therapy.

Dental health directly impacts dietary intake and eating enjoyment [51,52]. Those who are edentulous or without adequate dentures are at increased risk for inadequate nutrient intake [52]. The presence of caries or periodontal disease is associated with frequent ingestion of fermentable carbohydrate or acid beverage or food.

Goiter as a result of iodine deficiency may be apparent by visualization or palpation of the thyroid. Iodine supplementation has reduced but not eliminated goiter due to iodine deficiency in endemic areas.

B Skin

The skin, like the mouth, is among the more common sites where signs of nutritional problems are observed (Figure 3.3). Tenting of the skin due to dehydration appears as a tentlike fold after pinching the skin. Alterations in skin color include pallor, which suggests anemia, and the orange-yellow hue of carotenemia, also called carotenodermia. Carotenemia is observed with high levels of intake of foods containing carotenoids, with dyslipidemia, or in conditions characterized by diminished conversion of provitamin A carotenoids to vitamin A; these condition include anorexia nervosa, hypothyroidism, liver disease, diabetes, and nephrotic syndrome [53]. Carotenemia may be distinguished from jaundice because the former does not affect the sclerae.

Dermatitis accompanies many micronutrient deficiencies as well as essential fatty acid deficiency (Table 3.3 and Figure 3.4). Classic skin manifestations include the dermatitis of sun-exposed areas in pellagra, perifollicular hyperkeratosis or petechiae of scurvy, and the erythematous perioral and perianal dermatitis of zinc deficiency.

Physical findings of anemia include pallor of the skin and mucous membranes. Populations at increased risk for nutritional anemias resulting from deficiencies of vitamin B_{12}, folate, and iron risk include alcoholics (vitamin B_{12} and folate), the elderly (vitamin B_{12}), women with menometorrhagia (iron), and vegans (iron and vitamin B_{12}). Anemias as a result of PEM and deficiencies of vitamin C, vitamin B_6, riboflavin, and copper may also occur. Copper deficiency may be induced by surgical resection or bypass of the stomach and proximal small intestine or by use of zinc supplements [54,55].

Abnormal bleeding as a result of vitamin K deficiency may be observed if deficiency is severe. Most

TABLE 3.3 Physical Signs of Nutrient Deficiency or Excess

System	Sign	Nutrient or condition
Mouth	Glossitits	Deficiencies of riboflavin, niacin, biotin, vitamin B_6, vitamin B_{12}, folate, iron, zinc
	Angular stomatitis or cheilosis	Deficiencies of riboflavin, niacin, biotin, vitamin B_6, folate, vitamin B_{12}, iron, zinc
	Gingival bleeding	Deficiencies of vitamin C or K
	Dental erosions	Bulimia nervosa
	Dental caries	Carbohydrate or acid intake
	Dental fluorosis	Discoloration or pitting of dental enamel
Eyes	Xeropthalmia	Vitamin A deficiency
	Night blindness	
	Photophobia	
	Bitot's spots	
	Corneal ulceration	
	Diplopia	Vitamin A toxicity
	Nystagmus	Thiamin deficiency
	Lateral gaze deficit	
	Optic nerve atrophy	Vitamin B_{12} deficiency
	Blindness	
	Retinitis pigmentosa	Vitamin E deficiency
	Visual deficits	
	Kayser–Fleischer ring	Copper toxicity
	Sunflower cataract	
	Xanthelasma	Dyslipidemia
Skin	Seborrheic-like dermatitis	Deficiencies of B_6, zinc
	Impaired wound healing	Deficiencies of protein vitamin C, zinc
	Erythematous or scaly rash at sun-exposed areas	Niacin deficiency
	Perifollicular petechiae	Vitamin C deficiency
	Ecchymosis (bruising)	Vitamin K deficiency
	Easy bruising	
	Dry, flaky skin	Zinc or essential fatty acid deficiency
	Depigmentation	Protein-energy malnutrition
	Yellow or orange discoloration	Carotenoid excess
	Pallor	Deficiencies of iron, vitamin B_{12}, folate
Nails	Koilonychia (spoon-shaped nails)	Iron deficiency
	Discolored or thickened nails	Selenium toxicity
Hair	Swan neck deformity	Vitamin C deficiency
	Discoloration, Flag sign	Protein-energy malnutrition
	Dullness	Biotin deficiency

(Continued)

TABLE 3.3 (*Continued*)

System	Sign	Nutrient or condition
	Easy pluckability	
	Alopecia	Zinc or biotin deficiency, vitamin A toxicity
Cardiovascular	High-output congestive heart failure	Thiamin deficiency
	Cardiomyopathy and heart failure	Selenium deficiency
Gastrointestinal	Stomatitis	Niacin deficiency
	Esophagitis	
	Proctitis	
	Hepatomegaly	Hepatic steatosis due to diabetes, obesity, Kwashiorkor, choline deficiency, carnitine deficiency
Musculoskeletal	Generalized or proximal weakness	Vitamin D deficiency
	Bone tenderness	
	Fracture	
	Weakness	PEM, hypophosphatemia, hypokalemia, hypomagnasemia, vitamin D deficiency, iron deficiency
	Muscle wasting	Protein-energy malnutrition
	Carpopedal spasm	Hypocalcemia
Neurologic and psychiatric	Peripheral neuropathy or myelopathy	Deficiencies of vitamins B_6, B_{12}, E, thiamin; toxicity of vitamin B_6
	Mental status changes	Deficiencies of thiamin, vitamins B_6, B_{12}, niacin, biotin, hypophosphatemia, hypermagnasemia
	Delirium	Deficiencies of vitamin B_{12}, thiamin, niacin
	Dementia	Deficiencies of vitamin B_{12}, thiamin, niacin

vitamin K-related bleeding is due to warfarin use, which antagonizes vitamin K action. Dietary vitamin K deficiency is observed in alcoholics and those with malabsorptive disorders or poor intake. Vitamin C deficiency may cause gingival bleeding; splinter hemorrhages of the nails; petechial hemorrhages of the skin; and larger bruises apparent on the skin, in muscles, or, in rare cases, internal organs.

Risk for decubitus ulcers and impaired wound healing is increased in deficiency states such as PEM and micronutrient deficiencies but also with obesity.

Skin lesions are not only the result of nutritional deficiencies but also may represent metabolic disorders or sensitivities to components of food. For example, hyperinsulimia may cause acanthosis nigricans, manifest as a gray discoloration around the base of the neck, the axillae, and on extensor surfaces. Dyslipidemia may result in several cutaneous lipid accumulations, such as xanthelasma, which is often found on the eyelid, and xanthoma, which can occur in multiple sites.

C Cardiovascular System

Cardiovascular abnormalities are seldom pathognomonic for specific underlying nutritional issues. Nonetheless, the contribution of nutritional issues to cardiovascular disease should be considered. For example, congestive heart failure (CHF) may be a sign of thiamin deficiency (web beriberi) or Keshan disease due to selenium deficiency in endemic areas. Wet beriberi is characterized by high-output heart failure with rapid heart rate and pulmonary and peripheral edema. Risk for thiamin deficiency may be underappreciated in CHF patients because one investigation found that one-third of patients were deficient [56]. Use of loop diuretics such as furosemide increases thiamin losses, contributing to risk of deficiency in this population [57]. Symptomatic thiamin deficiency has typically been observed in those with alcohol abuse, with very poor intake, or with carbohydrate refeeding. However, it is now recognized that patients who have undergone

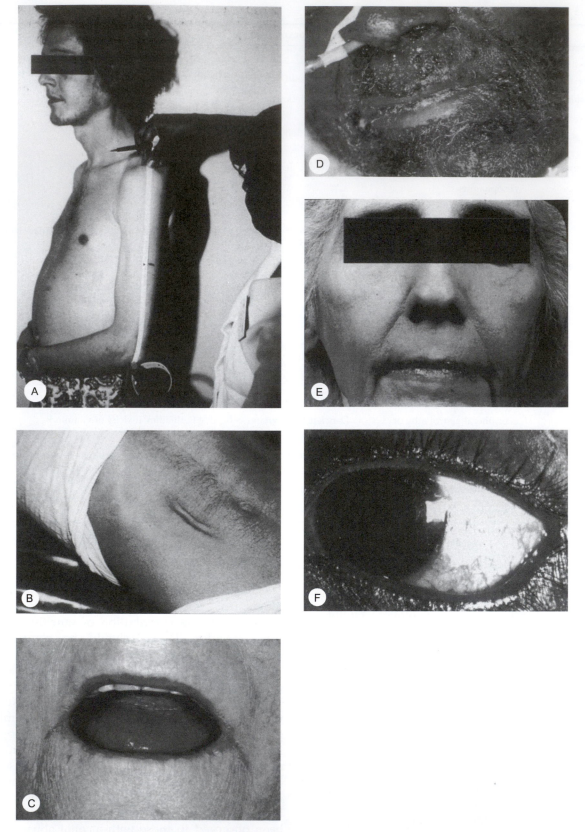

FIGURE 3.4 Physical signs associated with nutrient deficiencies. (A) Muscle wasting in severe PEM. (B) Tenting of skin in dehydration; the skin retains the tented shape after being pinched. (C) Glossitis and angular stomatitis associated with multiple B vitamin deficiencies. (D) Dermatitis associated with zinc deficiency. (E) Cheilosis, or vertical fissuring of the lips, associated with multiple B vitamin deficiencies. (F) Bitot's spot accompanying vitamin A deficiency. *Photos courtesy of Dr. Robert Russell and Dr. Joel Mason.*

bariatric surgery who experience frequent vomiting or poor intake, despite the absence of traditional risk factors, may experience symptomatic thiamin deficiency.

Cardiac cachexia may occur in patients with chronic CHF and is manifest by loss of FFM with variable loss of weight. Fat mass may remain unchanged, may decrease, or may even increase. Cachexia occurs due to inflammatory cytokines and neuroendocrine alterations that result in increased protein catabolism and decreased protein synthesis, increased resting energy expenditure, altered taste, early satiety, and diminished enjoyment of eating [58,59].

D Pulmonary System

Respiratory muscle strength may be diminished in PEM and predisposes to respiratory complications in those with chronic pulmonary disease or in acutely ill patients. Respiratory muscle strength and spirometry have been utilized as components of functional assessment for PEM.

Chronic obstructive pulmonary disease (COPD), like CHF, is associated with PEM due to several mechanisms. Food intake may be diminished by medications, cachexia, or in severe disease may be limited by shortness of breath [58,60]. Chronic treatment of COPD with corticosteroids predisposes to further loss of FFM and gains in FM with central accumulation of fat, loss of appendicular muscle, thin skin with easy bruising, glucose intolerance, and bone loss.

Acute respiratory failure may be precipitated by hypophosphatemia, which may also contribute to failure to wean from mechanical ventilation. Hypophosphatemia may accompany PEM or may occur independently due to alcohol abuse, refeeding syndrome, with correction of diabetic ketoacidosis, and with severe hypovitaminosis D.

E Gastrointestinal System

Diseases of the stomach, small intestine, colon, and liver are commonly associated with PEM and micronutrient disorders. Inflammatory bowel disease, celiac disease, resection of the intestinal tract, and short bowel syndrome may result in dehydration, PEM, and deficiencies of micronutrients and essential fatty acids. The site and extent of disease are important determinants of nutritional risk. Although active gastrointestinal disease may be associated with nutritional risk, patients with inflammatory bowel disease or celiac disease who are asymptomatic may still be at risk. Geerling *et al.* [61] found that patients with Crohn's disease in remission had persistent deficiencies in several water- and fat-soluble vitamins as well

as zinc. Patients with celiac disease are at risk for multiple deficiencies, including iron, calcium, zinc, fat-soluble vitamins, folic acid, and vitamin B_{12}. Celiac disease patients may remain at risk for metabolic bone disease even if clinically in remission [62].

Atrophic gastritis, which predisposes to vitamin B_{12} deficiency, increases in prevalence with advancing age. In one survey, more than 12% of a free-living elderly population was found to be deficient in vitamin B_{12} [63]. Drugs that reduce gastric acid secretion may also contribute by a similar mechanism, although this remains controversial. Bariatric surgery that bypasses part of the stomach, such as Roux-en-Y gastric bypass, may also lead to deficiency of vitamin B_{12} as well as deficiency of iron and copper.

End-stage liver disease or cirrhosis is frequently associated with PEM and deficiencies of fat-soluble vitamins due to poor intake, alterations in metabolism, and diminished hepatic storage. Manifestations of deficiency states may be incorrectly attributed to underlying disease, as was observed in some patients with primary sclerosing cholangitis who experienced night blindness, bone pain, or easy bleeding [64].

Chronic pancreatitis or pancreatic insufficiency (e.g., with cystic fibrosis) may lead to maldigestion of macronutrients and fat-soluble vitamins. Postprandial pain in chronic pancreatitis may further inhibit food intake.

F Musculoskeletal System

PEM may result in reductions in muscular size and strength, as well as in functional changes such as reduced work capacity or endurance. Muscle wasting as well as loss of subcutaneous fat may be observed by inspection of the temporalis muscles and the shoulder girdle and by interosseus wasting between the bones of the dorsum of the hand and the muscles of the extremities.

Generalized weakness is a common complaint. It is important to differentiate between the subjective experience of lethargy, which may be described as weakness, and actual diminished strength due to loss of skeletal muscle mass or function. The subjective experience of weakness accompanies dehydration and is an early symptom of PEM and deficiency of multiple vitamins and minerals, the most common of which is iron. Actual weakness may be observed with sarcopenia, PEM, cachexia, and disuse. Hypomagnasemia, hypokalemia, and hypovitaminosis D are among the more common micronutrient etiologies of muscle weakness [65]. Weakness due to neuropathy may also be experienced as muscle weakness.

Malnutrition in children can lead to impaired growth and bony deformities. Children with deficiencies of vitamin D or vitamin C may demonstrate bowing of long bones of the legs as well as prominence of costochondral joints (the rachitic or scorbutic rosary). Exam findings of osteomalacia in adults are subtler and may include tenderness with palpation of the sternum or long bones. A history of fractures, especially nontraumatic fractures, and bone pain should stimulate consideration of metabolic bone disease as well as calcium and vitamin D status. Persons with diseases known to influence calcium and vitamin D metabolism (e.g., those with malabsorptive disorders, chronic renal failure, and the institutionalized elderly) are at risk for metabolic bone disease, and appropriate monitoring and treatment should be undertaken. Similarly, drug–nutrient interactions that interfere with vitamin D metabolism, such as phenytoin, may increase risk of metabolic bone disease. Hypovitaminosis D and secondary hyperparathyroidism have been reported in patients who have undergone malabsorptive procedures such as gastric bypass or biliopancreatic diversion; hypocalcaemia rarely occurs after gastric bypass but has been observed after the more malabsorptive biliopancreatic diversion [66,67].

G Kidney Disease

Chronic and acute kidney disease and their treatments are associated with a host of nutritional disorders, including protein energy wasting, mineral and bone disorders, and alterations in vitamin status. Nutritional issues vary with the etiology and severity of kidney disease, whether acute or chronic, and if renal replacement therapy has been instituted. Nutrition guidelines for kidney disease are beyond the scope of this chapter but are available elsewhere [68–73].

H Neurological and Psychiatric Systems

Dementia and neurological disorders, such as stroke, Parkinson's disease, and head injury, may impair the ability to recognize, procure, and prepare food and to ingest food. The oropharyngeal phase of swallowing requires voluntary and involuntary neurologic function. A history of difficulty initiating a swallow, choking or gagging, wet cough, multiple swallowing attempts, and retained food in the mouth are signs that should stimulate evaluation for dysphagia.

Signs of bulimia may include dental erosions and parotid hyperplasia because of frequent vomiting. Nutritional problems associated with anorexia nervosa and, to a lesser extent, bulimia include PEM, electrolyte abnormalities, vitamin and mineral deficiencies, and, in the longer term, osteopenia.

Multiple psychiatric or neurological syndromes caused by nutrient deficiency (e.g., thiamin, niacin, vitamin B_6, vitamin B_{12}, vitamin E, and essential fatty acids) or excess because of supplementation or faddism have been described (Table 3.3). In the United States, common predisposing factors to deficiency syndromes are alcoholism, atrophic gastritis, malabsorptive disorders, and gastrointestinal surgery. Of particular importance is that deficiency of vitamin B_{12} may be manifest by neurological or psychiatric symptoms in the absence of anemia or macrocytosis [74]. Vitamin B_{12} deficiency may result in subtle neuropsychiatric symptoms as well as the more dramatic signs of combined systems degeneration and changes in cognition or personality. Thiamin deficiency results in deficits manifest by cognitive changes, cerebellar dysfunction, gaze palsy, sensory and motor manifestations, and eventually dementia.

The current popularity of bariatric surgery has resulted in increased prevalence and awareness of the neurological manifestations of deficiencies of thiamin, vitamin B_{12}, and copper. Kumar has comprehensively reviewed the neurological manifestations of these and other disorders [55].

V FUNCTIONAL ASSESSMENT

Functional assessment is based on the premise that PEM and other forms of malnutrition result in physiologic or functional impairment in measurable processes such as skeletal muscle or pulmonary muscle strength, mobility, and delayed-type hypersensitivity. Functional impairment may contribute to risk for malnutrition due to reduced ability to obtain, prepare, and consume food. Tools developed for functional assessment are used for both nutrition screening and assessment and vary in complexity from questionnaires about function to measurement of handgrip strength and batteries of multistage tasks requiring complex physical and cognitive processes.

A common simple functional test is handgrip strength, which is measured by handgrip dynamometry and correlates with FFM. Reductions in handgrip strength are associated with PEM and generalized muscle weakness [75–77] as well as all-cause mortality [78]. Preoperative handgrip strength has also been found to predict risk of postoperative complications [79]. Handgrip strength is useful in the serial assessment of an individual, but it can also be used for reference to age- and sex-specific norms. In malnourished patients who are provided nutrition support, an initial early increase in handgrip strength may be observed prior to significant accretion of muscle mass; this effect is likely due to repletion of intracellular energy substrates and micronutrients necessary for neuromuscular function [80]. After this initial improvement, more

TABLE 3.4 Components of Selected Multicomponent Assessment Tools

Tool	Population	Health status	Dietary intake or appetite change	Weight or BMI	Weight change	Skinfold or circumference	Physical examination	Functional status
Prognostic Nutritional Index (PNI)	Hospital							
Nutritional Risk Index (NRI)	Elderly	✓	✓		✓			
Prognostic Inflammatory and Nutritional Index (PINI)	Hospital							
Subjective Global Index (SGA)	Hospital	✓	✓		✓		✓	✓
Nutritional Risk Screening (NRS-2002)	Hospital		✓	✓	✓			
Malnutrition Universal Screening (MUST)	Hospital Community	✓	✓	✓				
Malnutrition Screening Tool (MST)	Hospital		✓		✓			
Nutrition Screening Initiative	Elderly	✓	✓	✓				✓
Mini Nutritional Assessment (MNA)	Elderly	✓	✓	✓	✓	✓		✓
Short Nutritional Assessment Questionnaire (SNAQ)	Hospital	✓	✓		✓			

gradual gains in handgrip strength occur with repletion of FFM.

VI MULTICOMPONENT ASSESSMENT TOOLS

Multicomponent tools combine elements of history, anthropometric measurements, physical examination, and biochemical assessments. Combining elements improves sensitivity and specificity in the prediction of nutrition status, need for nutrition intervention, or adverse outcomes such as hospital length of stay or mortality [81]. Depending on the purpose and setting, use of multicomponent tools may be superior to use of single parameters such as BMI, weight loss, or recent intake. Tools have been developed for specific populations, such as children, adults, and older persons, and for settings such as the community, hospitals, or nursing homes. Anthony provides an overview of six nutrition screening tools validated for use in the acute care setting [82]. Some assessment components are influenced by illness as well as by malnutrition. If these tools are used to assess risk for adverse outcomes, however, it may not be necessary to differentiate between these two influences.

Table 3.4 contrasts selected components of some multicomponent assessment tools. In studies in which tools such as those described in Table 3.4 were contrasted, none was consistently superior [83–85]. As suggested by Elia and Stratton, selection of a test should be based not only on the ability of the tool to predict the stated outcome but also on reproducibility, the setting and population, the ease of use, and the time required [81].

VII SUMMARY

Clinical assessment, including physical assessment, is integral to comprehensive nutritional assessment. Elements of physical assessment, such as BMI and weight change, are often central to nutrition screening or assessment. Physical examination findings that are interpreted in the context of other assessment components provide valuable data regarding PEM and micronutrient malnutrition status. Functional assessment and multicomponent assessment tools improve the ability to detect malnutrition, the need for intervention, and predict adverse events.

References

[1] C. Mueller, C. Compher, D.M. Ellen, A.S.P.E.N. Clinical guidelines: Nutrition screening, assessment, and intervention in adults, JPEN 35 (2011) 16–24.
[2] G.L. Jensen, J. Mirtallo, C. Compher, R. Dhaliwal, A. Forbes, R.F. Grijalba, et al., Adult starvation and disease-related malnutrition: a proposal for etiology-based diagnosis in the clinical practice setting from the international consensus guideline committee, JPEN 34 (2010) 156–159.

[3] N.R. Sahyoun, C.L. Lin, E. Krall, Nutritional status of the older adult is associated with dentition status, J. Am. Diet. Assoc. 103 (2003) 61–66.

[4] J. Gahche, R. Bailey, V. Burt, J. Hughes, E. Yetley, J. Dwyer, et al., Dietary supplement use among U.S. adults has increased since NHANES III (1988–1994), NCHS Data Brief (2011) 1–8.

[5] M.R. Corkins, J.F. Fitzgerald, S.K. Gupta, Feeding after percutaneous endoscopic gastrostomy in children: early feeding trial, J. Pediatr. Gastroenterol. Nutr. 50 (2010) 625–627.

[6] J.D. Sorkin, D.C. Muller, R. Andres, Longitudinal change in height of men and women: implications for the interpretation of the body mass index, Am. J. Epidemiol. 150 (1999) 969–977.

[7] P. Pirie, D. Jacobs, R. Jeffery, P. Hannan, Distortion in self-reported height and weight, J. Am. Diet. Assoc. 78 (1981) 601–606.

[8] T.R. Coe, M. Halkes, K. Houghton, D. Jefferson, The accuracy of visual estimation of weight and height in pre-operative surgical patients, Anaesthesia 54 (1999) 582–586.

[9] R. Roubenoff, P.W.F. Wilson, Advantage of knee height over height as an index of stature in expression of body composition in adults, Am. J. Clin. Nutr. 57 (1993) 609–613.

[10] W.C. Chumlea, S. Guo, Equations for predicting stature in white and black elderly individuals, J. Gerontol. 47 (1992) M197–M203.

[11] T. Kwok, M.N. Whitelaw, The use of armspan in nutritional assessment of the elderly, J. Am. Geriatr. Soc. 39 (1991) 494–496.

[12] C.O. Mitchell, D.A. Lipschitz, Arm length measurement as alternative to height in nutritional assessment of the elderly, JPEN 6 (1982) 226–229.

[13] M.G. Beghetto, J. Fink, V.C. Luft, E.D. De Mello, Estimates of body height in adult inpatients, Clin. Nutr. 25 (2006) 438–443.

[14] J.K. Brown, J.Y. Feng, T.R. Knapp, Is self-reported height or arm span a more accurate alternative measure of height? Clin. Nurs. Res. 11 (2002) 417–432.

[15] M. Hickson, G. Frost, A comparison of three methods for estimating height in the acutely ill elderly population, J. Hum. Nutr. Diet. 16 (2003) 13–20.

[16] J. Manonai, A. Khanacharoen, U. Theppisai, A. Chittacharoen, Relationship between height and arm span in women of different age groups, J. Obstet. Gynaecol. Res. 27 (2001) 325–327.

[17] D.B. Morgan, G.L. Hill, L. Burkinshaw, The assessment of weight loss from a single measurement of body weight: the problems and limitations, Am. J. Clin. Nutr. 33 (1980) 2101–2105.

[18] W.D. Dewys, C. Begg, P.T. Lavin, P.R. Band, J.M. Bennett, J.R. Bertino, et al., Prognostic effect of weight loss prior to chemotherapy in cancer patients, Am. J. Med. 69 (1980) 491–497.

[19] M.W. Reynolds, L. Fredman, P. Langenberg, J. Magaziner, Weight, weight change, and mortality in a random sample of older community-dwelling women, J. Am. Geriatr. Soc. 47 (1999) 1409–1414.

[20] M.H. Seltzer, B.A. Slocum, E.L. Cataldi-Bethcher, C. Fileti, N. Gerson, Instant nutritional assessment: absolute weight loss and surgical mortality, JPEN 6 (1982) 218–221.

[21] H.O. Studley, Percentage of weight loss. A basic indicator of surgical risk in patients with chronic peptic ulcer disease, JAMA 106 (1936) 458–460.

[22] T.H. Naber, A. De Bree, T.R. Schermer, J. Bakkeren, B. Bar, G. De Wild, et al., Specificity of indexes of malnutrition when applied to apparently healthy people: the effect of age, Am. J. Clin. Nutr. 65 (1997) 1721–1725.

[23] J. Fischer, M.A. Johnson, Low body weight and weight loss in the aged, J. Am. Diet. Assoc. 90 (1990) 1697–1706.

[24] J.A. Windsor, G.L. Hill, Weight loss with physiologic impairment: a basic indicator of surgical risk, Ann. Surg. 207 (1988) 290–296.

[25] D.T. Engelman, D.H. Adams, J.G. Byrne, S.F. Aranki, J.J. Collins, G.S. Couper, et al., Impact of body mass index and albumin on morbidity and mortality after cardiac surgery, J. Thorac. Cardiovasc. Surg. 118 (1999) 866–873.

[26] G.L. Hill, Body composition research: implications for the practice of clinical nutrition, JPEN 16 (1992) 197–218.

[27] J.A. Windsor, Underweight patients and the risks of major surgery, World J. Surg. 17 (1993) 165–172.

[28] J. Karkeck, Adjusted body weight for obesity, Am. Dietet. Assoc. Renal. Dietet. Practice Group Newslett. 3 (1984) 6.

[29] C. Elizabeth Weekes, Controversies in the determination of energy requirements, Proc. Nutr. Soc. 66 (2007) 367–377.

[30] N. Robinett-Weiss, M.L. Hixson, B. Keir, J. Sieberg, The metropolitan height-weight tables: perspectives for use, J. Am. Diet. Assoc. 84 (1984) 1480–1481.

[31] NHLBI Obesity Education Initiative Expert Panel on the Identification Evaluation and Treatment of Overweight and Obesity in Adults, Clinical guidelines on the identification, evaluation, and treatment of overweight and obesity in adults: the evidence report, Obes. Res. 6 (Suppl. 2) (1998) 51S–209S.

[32] A.M. Prentice, S.A. Jebb, Beyond body mass index, Obes. Rev. 2 (2001) 141–147.

[33] D. Gallagher, M. Visser, D. Sepulveda, R.N. Pierson, T. Harris, S.B. Heymsfield, How useful is body mass index for comparison of body fatness across age, sex, and ethnic groups? Am. J. Epidemiol. 143 (1996) 228–239.

[34] E.E. Calle, C. Rodriguez, K. Walker-Thurmond, M.J. Thun, Overweight, obesity, and mortality from cancer in a prospectively studied cohort of U.S. adults, N. Engl. J. Med. 348 (2003) 1625–1638.

[35] F. Landi, G. Zuccala, G. Gambassi, R.A. Incalzi, L. Manigrasso, F. Pagano, et al., Body mass index and mortality among older people living in the community, J. Am. Geriatr. Soc. 47 (1999) 1072–1076.

[36] T.L.S. Visscher, J.C. Seidell, A. Menotti, H. Blackburn, A. Nissinen, E.J.M. Feskens, et al., Underweight and overweight in relation to mortality among men aged 40–59 and 50–69, Am. J. Epidemiol. 151 (2000) 660–666.

[37] World Health Organization, Diet, nutrition, and the prevention of chronic diseases: report of a WHO study group, World Health Organ. Tech. Rep. Ser. 797 (1990) 1–204.

[38] A. Must, J. Spadano, E.H. Coakley, A.E. Field, G. Colditz, W.H. Dietz, The disease burden associated with overweight and obesity, JAMA 282 (1999) 1523–1529.

[39] C.J. Henry, Body mass index and the limits of human survival, Eur. J. Clin. Nutr. 44 (1990) 329–335.

[40] T. Young, L. Evans, L. Finn, M. Palta, Estimation of the clinically diagnosed proportion of sleep apnea syndrome middle-aged men and women, Sleep 20 (1997) 705–706.

[41] C.C. Cowie, et al., Prevalence of diabetes and impaired fasting glucose in adults—United States, 1999–2000, MMWR Morb. Mortal. Wkly. Rep. 52 (2003) 833–837.

[42] J. Despres, The insulin resistance-dyslipidemic syndrome of visceral obesity: effect on patients' risk, Obes. Res. 6 (Suppl.) (1998) 8S–17S.

[43] S. Klein, D.B. Allison, S.B. Heymsfield, D.E. Kelley, R.L. Leibel, C. Nonas, et al., Waist circumference and cardiometabolic risk: a consensus statement from Shaping America's Health: association for Weight Management and Obesity Prevention; NAASO, the Obesity Society; the American Society for Nutrition; and the American Diabetes Association, Diabetes Care 30 (2007) 1647–1652.

[44] A. Molarius, J.C. Siedell, Selection of anthropometric indicators for classification of abdominal fatness: a critical review, Int. J. Obes. 22 (1998) 719–727.

[45] L.M. Browning, S.D. Hsieh, M. Ashwell, A systematic review of waist-to-height ratio as a screening tool for the prediction of cardiovascular disease and diabetes: 0.5 could be a suitable global boundary value, Nutr. Res. Rev. 23 (2010) 247–269.

[46] A.S. Jackson, M.L. Pollock, Generalized equations for predicting body density of men, Br. J. Nutr. 40 (1978) 497–504.

[47] J.V.G.A. Durnin, M.E. Lonergan, J. Good, A. Ewan, A cross-sectional nutritional and anthropometric study, with an interval of 7 years, on 611 young adolescent schoolchildren, Br. Med. J. 32 (1974) 169–178.

[48] J. Wang, J.C. Thornton, S. Kolesnik, R.N. Pierson Jr., Anthropometry in body composition. An overview, Ann. N. Y. Acad. Sci. 904 (2000) 317–326.

[49] S.K. Das, S.B. Roberts, J.J. Kehayias, J. Wang, L.K. Hsu, S.A. Shikora, et al., Body composition assessment in extreme obesity and after massive weight loss induced by gastric bypass surgery, Am. J. Physiol. Endocrinol. Metab. 284 (2003) E1080–E1088.

[50] T.L. Kelly, K.E. Wilson, S.B. Heymsfield, Dual energy X-ray absorptiometry body composition reference values from NHANE, PLoS One 4 (2009) E7038.

[51] M. Lamy, P. Mojon, G. Kalykakis, R. Legrand, E. Butz-Jorgensen, Oral status and nutrition in the institutionalized elderly, J. Dent. 27 (1999) 443–448.

[52] A.S. Papas, C.A. Palmer, M.C. Rounds, R.M. Russell, The effects of denture status on nutrition, Spec. Care Dentist. 18 (1998) 17–25.

[53] N. Maharshak, J. Shapiro, H. Trau, Carotenoderma: a review of the current literature, Int. J. Dermatol. 42 (2003) 178–181.

[54] R. Carmel, Nutritional anemias and the elderly, Semin. Hematol. 45 (2008) 225–234.

[55] N. Kumar, Neurologic presentations of nutritional deficiencies, Neurol. Clin. 28 (2010) 107–170.

[56] S.A. Hanninen, P.B. Darling, M.J. Sole, A. Barr, M.E. Keith, The prevalence of thiamin deficiency in hospitalized patients with congestive heart failure, J. Am. Coll. Cardiol. 47 (2006) 354–361.

[57] D.A. Sica, Loop diuretic therapy, thiamine balance, and heart failure, Congest. Heart Fail 13 (2007) 244–247.

[58] W.J. Evans, J.E. Morley, J. Argiles, C. Bales, V. Baracos, D. Guttridge, et al., Cachexia: a new definition, Clin. Nutr. 27 (2008) 793–799.

[59] S. Von Haehling, W. Doehner, S.D. Anker, Nutrition, metabolism, and the complex pathophysiology of cachexia in chronic heart failure, Cardiovasc. Res. 73 (2007) 298–309.

[60] A.G. Agusti, Systemic effects of chronic obstructive pulmonary disease, Proc. Am. Thorac. Soc. 2 (2005) 367–370.

[61] B.J. Geerling, A. Badart-Smook, R.W. Stockbrugger, R.J. Brummer, Comprehensive nutritional status in patients with long-standing Crohn disease currently in remission, Am. J. Clin. Nutr. 67 (1998) 919–926.

[62] C. Cellier, C. Flobert, C. Cormier, C. Roux, J. Schmitz, Severe osteopenia in symptom-free adults with a childhood diagnosis of coeliac disease, Lancet 355 (2000) 806.

[63] J. Lindenbaum, I.H. Rosenberg, P.W. Wilson, S.P. Stabler, R.H. Allen, Prevalence of cobalamin deficiency in the Framingham elderly population, Am. J. Clin. Nutr. 60 (1994) 2–11.

[64] Y.M. Lee, M.M. Kaplan, Primary sclerosing cholangitis, N. Engl. J. Med. 332 (1995) 924–933.

[65] H.A. Bischoff-Ferrari, H.B. Staehelin, Importance of vitamin D and calcium at older age, Int. J. Vitam. Nutr. Res. 78 (2008) 286–292.

[66] C. De Prisco, S.N. Levine, Metabolic bone disease after gastric bypass surgery for obesity, Am. J. Med. Sci. 329 (2005) 57–61.

[67] N. Sinha, A. Shieh, E.M. Stein, G. Strain, A. Schulman, A. Pomp, et al., Increased PTH and 1.25(OH)(2)D levels associated with increased markers of bone turnover following bariatric surgery, Obesity 19 (2011) 2388–2393.

[68] M. Kalista-Richards, The kidney: medical nutrition therapy—Yesterday and today, Nutr. Clin. Pract. 26 (2011) 143–150.

[69] G.J. Handelman, N.W. Levin, Guidelines for vitamin supplements in chronic kidney disease patients: what is the evidence? J. Ren. Nutr. 21 (2011) 117–119.

[70] R.O. Brown, C. Compher, A.S.P.E.N. clinical guidelines: nutrition support in adult acute and chronic renal failure, JPEN 34 (2010) 366–377.

[71] N.J. Cano, M. Aparicio, G. Brunori, J.J. Carrero, B. Cianciaruso, E. Fiaccadori, et al., ESPEN guidelines on parenteral nutrition: adult renal failure, Clin. Nutr. 28 (2009) 401–414.

[72] KDOQI Work Group, KDOQI clinical practice guideline for nutrition in children with CKD: 2008 update. Executive summary, Am. J. Kidney Dis. 53 (2009) S11–S104.

[73] J.D. Kopple, National Kidney Foundation K/DOQI clinical practice guidelines for nutrition in chronic renal failure, Am. J. Kidney Dis. 37 (2001) S66–S70.

[74] J. Lindenbaum, E.B. Healton, D.G. Savage, J.C. Brust, T.J. Garrett, E.R. Podell, et al., Neuropsychiatric disorders caused by cobalamin deficiency in the absence of anemia or macrocytosis, N. Engl. J. Med. 318 (1988) 1720–1728.

[75] T. Ferdous, T. Cederholm, A. Razzaque, A. Wahlin, Z. Nahar Kabir, Nutritional status and self-reported and performance-based evaluation of physical function of elderly persons in rural Bangladesh, Scand. J. Public Health 37 (2009) 518–524.

[76] L. Valentini, L. Schaper, C. Buning, S. Hengstermann, T. Koernicke, W. Tillinger, et al., Malnutrition and impaired muscle strength in patients with Crohn's disease and ulcerative colitis in remission, Nutrition 24 (2008) 694–702.

[77] I.C. Matos, M.M. Tavares, T.F. Amaral, Handgrip strength as a hospital admission nutritional risk screening method, Eur. J. Clin. Nutr. 61 (2007) 1128–1135.

[78] T. Rantanen, S. Volpato, L. Ferrucci, E. Heikkinen, L.P. Fried, J.M. Guralnik, Handgrip strength and cause-specific and total mortality in older disabled women: exploring the mechanism, J. Am. Geriatr. Soc. 51 (2003) 636–641.

[79] V.N. Mahalakshmi, N. Ananthakrishnan, V. Kate, A. Sahai, M. Trakroo, Handgrip strength and endurance as a predictor of postoperative morbidity in surgical patients: can it serve as a simple bedside test? Int. Surg. 89 (2004) 115–121.

[80] D.M. Russell, P.J. Prendergast, P.L. Darby, P.E. Garfinkel, J. Whitwell, K.N. Jeejeebhoy, A comparison between muscle function and body composition in anorexia nervosa: the effect of refeeding, Am. J. Clin. Nutr. 38 (1983) 229–237.

[81] M. Elia, R.J. Stratton, Considerations for screening tool selection and role of predictive and concurrent validity, Curr. Opin. Clin. Nutr. Metab. Care 14 (2011) 425–433.

[82] P.S. Anthony, Nutrition screening tools for hospitalized patients, Nutr. Clin. Pract. 23 (2008) 373–382.

[83] C. Alberda, A. Graf, L. McCargar, Malnutrition: etiology, consequences, and assessment of a patient at risk, Best Pract. Res. Clin. Gastroenterol. 20 (2006) 419–439.

[84] M.R. Alvares Da Silva, T. Reverbel Da Silveira, Comparison between handgrip strength, subjective global assessment, and prognostic nutritional index in assessing malnutrition and predicting clinical outcome in cirrhotic outpatients, Nutrition 21 (2005) 113–117.

[85] M. Raslan, M.C. Gonzalez, M.C. Gonçalves Dias, M. Nascimento, M. Castro, P. Marques, et al., Comparison of nutritional risk screening tools for predicting clinical outcomes in hospitalized patients, Nutrition 26 (2010) 721–726.

4

Energy Requirement Methodology

James P. DeLany

University of Pittsburgh, Pittsburgh, Pennsylvania

I INTRODUCTION

Knowledge of energy requirements throughout the life cycle and during various physiological conditions and disease states is essential to the promotion of optimal human health. Unfortunately, available instruments for the measurement of dietary intake have demonstrated considerable misreporting [1]. Therefore, investigators have focused on measurement of energy expenditure, which can be accurately measured. Surprisingly, many of the same issues that are currently under investigation, such as gender differences, energy requirements of infants, the effect of different diets, caloric restriction, and physical activity, were first studied in the early 1900s [2–10]. The aim of this chapter is to familiarize the reader with current techniques available for the measurement of energy expenditure used to estimate energy requirements.

II COMPONENTS OF DAILY ENERGY EXPENDITURE

Total daily energy expenditure (TEE) is the sum of resting energy expenditure (REE), the thermic effect of food (TEF), and energy expended in physical activity (EEPA; Figure 4.1). The pathway of energy production from the oxidation of macronutrients in the human body is depicted in Eq. (4.1):

$$\text{Macronutrients} + O_2 \rightarrow \text{heat} + CO_2 + H_2O \qquad (4.1)$$

Examination of this equation indicates that to estimate energy expenditure, one could measure macronutrient or oxygen consumption, or the production of heat or carbon dioxide. Most energy expenditure methods in use today rely on measurement of oxygen consumption and/or carbon dioxide production.

Measurement of heat production, or direct calorimetry, is rarely used today.

A Resting Energy Expenditure

Resting metabolic rate (RMR), also called resting energy expenditure, which is the largest component of TEE (Figure 4.1), is the energy expended by a fasting individual at rest in a thermoneutral environment. The term basal metabolic rate (BMR) or basal energy expenditure (BEE), although often used to describe this component of energy expenditure, is not identical to RMR. By definition, BMR measurements are made early in the morning, in a thermoneutral environment, before the individual has engaged in any physical activity, and with no ingestion of food, tea, or coffee or inhalation of nicotine-containing tobacco smoke for at least 12 hours before the measurement. If any of the conditions for BMR are not met, the energy expenditure should be termed the resting metabolic rate. For practical reasons, BMR is rarely measured. In its place, RMR is used, which is generally higher than BMR. To estimate energy requirements, RMR is often measured or estimated based on standard equations and multiplied by a factor to estimate physical activity level.

1 Determinants of Resting Energy Expenditure

The determinants of resting energy expenditure are well-established in both adults and children. The principal factors contributing to individual variation in REE include body size and composition, gender, race, age, physical fitness, hormonal status, genetics, and environmental influences [11–17].

A BODY SIZE

Larger people have higher energy requirements than do people of smaller size because additional body

Nutrition in the Prevention and Treatment of Disease, Third Edition.
DOI: http://dx.doi.org/10.1016/B978-0-12-391884-0.00004-4

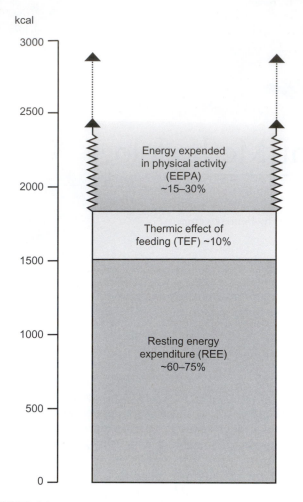

kcal

FIGURE 4.1 The components of total energy expenditure. *Source: From Poehlman, E.T., and Horton, E.S. (1988). Energy needs: Assessment and requirements in humans. In "Modern Nutrition in Health and Disease." William & Wilkins, Baltimore, MD.*

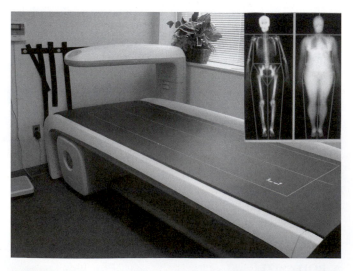

FIGURE 4.2 Dual energy x-ray absorptiometer for body composition.
See color plate.

tissue requires additional metabolic activity. Although REE is higher in larger individuals, many factors beyond body weight, such as proportion of body fat, tissue growth or repair, environment, race, and genetics, can induce major differences in metabolic rate.

B BODY COMPOSITION

The composition of the body has a major effect on REE. Fat-free mass (FFM), which serves as a surrogate for the metabolically active tissue in the body, is the primary determinant of REE [12]. Hence, most of the variation in REE between people can be accounted for by the variation in their FFM [14]. Several factors influence the amount and proportion of FFM, including age, gender, and physical fitness. FFM can be accurately measured using a number of techniques, including underwater weighing, measuring total body water using stable isotopes of deuterium or oxygen-18, and dual-energy x-ray absorptiometry (DXA). DXA is a technique that accurately estimates FFM, fat mass, and bone mineral mass. Subjects lie supine on a padded table for 6–12 minutes, during which time two very low-energy x-ray beams are passed through the body (Figure 4.2). The total x-ray dose is generally 1 mrem or less, on the order of a single day's background radiation for a whole-body composition analysis. The technique differentiates bone from soft tissue (Figure 4.2, inset) and further differentiates soft tissue between lean and fat. Svendsen *et al.* [18] discuss in detail the calculation of fat mass and lean body mass.

Because of the expense or impractical nature of research techniques for body composition, other, less accurate methods such as anthropometry and bioelectrical impedance are often used in practice to estimate body composition. However, in 1999, the National Health and Nutrition Examination Survey (NHANES) began performing DXA body composition measurements on survey subjects 8 years old or older in three mobile examination centers [19]. See Chapter 3 for a detailed description of body composition measurement techniques.

C GENDER

Gender is another factor that affects REE. The values for REE are lower in female than in male subjects, even after adjusting for differences in body composition [20,21]. Much of the differences between the sexes can be explained by differences in body composition. Females typically have more fat in proportion to muscle than males. However, females generally have metabolic rates that are 5–10% lower than those of males of the same weight and height.

D AGE

There is a well-documented age-related reduction in resting metabolic rate [22–24], with the suggested decline occurring at approximately age 40 years in men and 50 years in women [22]. This decline in REE can be partly explained by a reduction in the quantity, as well as the metabolic activity, of lean body mass [25], including changes in the relative size of organs and tissues [26]. If individuals gain weight as they age, RMR may actually increase because of gains of FFM and fat mass.

E PHYSICAL FITNESS AND ACTIVITY

Athletes generally have a higher RMR compared to nonathletic individuals [27,28]. Whether physical activity has a direct effect on RMR beyond changes in body composition is unclear [17,29,30]. Nonetheless, aerobic exercise and strength training have been shown to result in significantly higher metabolic rates in men and women as well as lean and obese individuals [29–32].

F HORMONAL STATUS

Hormonal status can impact metabolic rate, particularly in endocrine disorders affecting thyroid hormone status. Stimulation of the sympathetic nervous system, such as occurs during emotional excitement or stress, increases cellular activity by the release of epinephrine, which acts directly to promote glycogenolysis. Other hormones, such as cortisol, growth hormone, and insulin, also influence metabolic rate. Although leptin was initially considered to function as the long-sought anti-obesity hormone, it does not appear to be involved in regulating energy expenditure in humans under normal conditions except in those with a genetic deficiency [33–36]. However, recent data support a strong role for leptin signaling in energy expenditure and satiation in the weight-reduced state [37]. There appear to be no major effects of menstrual cycle on RMR in African American or Caucasian women [38–41].

G ETHNICITY AND GENETICS

Ethnic origin and genetic inheritance have been shown to affect REE. Numerous studies have reported that RMR is lower in African American adults and children compared to non-Hispanic whites even after appropriately adjusting for differences in body composition [21,39,42–48]. At least some of this difference is due to differences in the proportions of high metabolic rate tissues and organs [49]. No significant differences have been observed in RMR in other ethnic groups investigated. For example, in Pima Indians, a group believed to have a form of genetic obesity, neither RMR nor sleeping metabolic rate were found to differ from that of non-Hispanic whites after adjustment for body composition [13,50]. Mohawk Indian children were reported to have higher values of TEE than those of non-Hispanic white children, but the difference was due to higher levels of EEPA [51].

Genetic inheritance that determines body composition has a major effect on RMR, accounting for 25–50% of interindividual variability [52]. There also appears to be genetic influence beyond body composition because a significant intrafamily influence on RMR independent of FFM, age, and gender has been reported [15]. Understanding the genetic determinants of human obesity is particularly challenging because common forms of human obesity are largely polygenic. Although great strides have been made in understanding genetic determinants involved in the etiology of human obesity, the proportion of variability explained remains relatively modest [53,54]. Because currently identified genetic variants do not fully explain the heritability of obesity, other forms of variation, such as epigenetic marks, have been considered [54]. Epigenetic marks, which affect gene expression without changing the DNA sequence, have been shown to cause extreme forms of obesity such as Prader–Willi syndrome, but the epigenetic contribution to common forms of obesity is unknown.

H ENVIRONMENTAL INFLUENCES

The effects of environmental temperature on RMR are conflicting. Well-controlled studies of the acute effect of heat and cold demonstrate significant elevations in metabolic rate [55–58]. However, results from longitudinal studies of the effect of season (temperature) are conflicting, with findings of no effect, a small effect, or as much as 14% increase in metabolic rate [59–61]. High altitude has also been shown to result in increased RMR [62].

2 Adjustment of Resting Energy Expenditure for Differences in Body Size

In order to properly compare energy expenditure between individuals varying in body size or composition, it is imperative that an appropriate strategy be employed to adjust energy expenditure for these differences. Surface area was used as an early normalizing factor because heat is lost through the skin, so it was assumed that metabolic rate would be proportional to the amount of skin [63,64]. FFM is the normalizing factor used most often today, which is used as a proxy for the metabolically active tissues in the body. The use of these two factors to normalize RMR provides similar results, although higher correlations are generally observed with FFM [65].

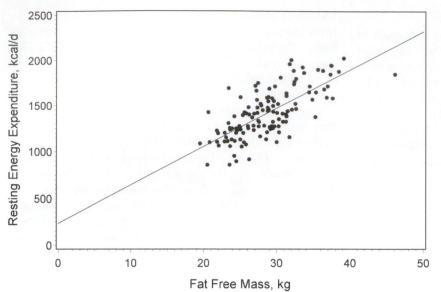

FIGURE 4.3 Resting energy expenditure versus FFM.

In the past, when examining whether there were differences in RMR between different groups differing in body weight and composition, some investigators adjusted RMR by dividing by FFM. However, although there is a very strong relationship between RMR and FFM, this relationship has a nonzero intercept, making this practice invalid [66]. As an example, in Figure 4.3, RMR is plotted against FFM for 131 lean and obese African American and Caucasian children [67]. It is fairly clear that even the most obese individuals, those with FFM >30 kg, fall on the regression line for all subjects (RMR (kcal/day) = 41.8 × FFM (kg) + 235; $r = 0.72$). It is also clear that the y-intercept is not equal to zero. When comparing a lean individual with 20 kg of FFM with an obese individual with 40 kg FFM, absolute RMR is of course higher in the obese individual (1907 kcal/day) than in the lean individual (1071 kcal/day). However, if one were to divide RMR by FFM to compare these two individuals, it would incorrectly appear that the "adjusted" RMR is 11% lower in the obese individual (53.6 vs. 47.7 kcal/kg FFM in the lean and obese individual), when in reality these two individuals fall on the same regression line and hence have similar adjusted RMR. In fact, the obese children in this study had a higher RMR when adjusted for FFM but similar RMR when adjusted for FFM and fat mass. An appropriate strategy to adjust for differences in body size is to utilize regression methods to adjust for FFM [66]. Other factors that have been included to improve energy expenditure prediction equations include age, fat mass, and sex [66,68].

3 Measuring Resting Energy Expenditure: Indirect Calorimetry

Metabolic rate has been measured using direct calorimeters [69–71] and closed-circuit indirect

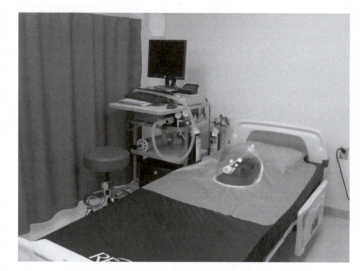

FIGURE 4.4 Indirect calorimetry system for the measurement of RMR.
See color plate.

calorimetry systems [72], but it is now generally measured with an open-flow indirect calorimetry system (Figure 4.4). Room air is drawn through a clear plastic hood covering the individual's face, and the flow and concentration of oxygen and carbon dioxide in the intake and expired air are accurately measured for calculation of RMR [73]. This technique is known as indirect calorimetry because it does not directly measure heat but, rather, measures O_2 consumption and CO_2 production, which are then used to calculate energy expenditure. The pretesting environment impacts the measurement of RMR. Food, ethanol, caffeine, nicotine, and physical activity impact RMR and should be controlled before measurements are taken

[74]. A number of commercial indirect calorimetry systems are available, with some being more reliable than others [75]. Smaller, portable indirect calorimeters are also available, allowing investigators more mobility for field measurement of metabolic rate [76—78].

4 Estimating Resting Energy Expenditure: Prediction Equations

Although numerous equations have been developed to estimate REE, the two most widely used equations are discussed here: the Harris—Benedict equations [5] and those developed by the Institute of Medicine/Food and Nutrition Board to determine dietary reference intakes (DRIs).

A HARRIS—BENEDICT EQUATIONS

The Harris—Benedict equations remain the most commonly used tool by clinicians when estimating an individual's REE. The equations are often used as a basis for prescribing energy intake for hospitalized patients and to formulate energy intake goals for weight loss. A review of the data used in the formulation of the Harris—Benedict equations in the early 1930s deduced that the methods and conclusions of Harris and Benedict appear valid but not error-free [79]. The equations in use today are shown in Table 4.1. Investigators have evaluated which equation performs best or developed new equations for specific populations [80—84]. The reader is encouraged to follow this literature as it applies to populations differing in body size, health status, race, sex, and age.

B DRI EQUATIONS

The BEE prediction equations developed for the DRIs are shown in Table 4.1. These equations were derived from observed BEE values found in the doubly labeled water (DLW) database [85]. This database was developed by searching published research that involved the use of the DLW method. The investigators associated with the identified publications were solicited to contribute to the database. Twenty investigators responded and submitted individual TEE data and ancillary data including age, gender, height, weight, BEE (both observed and estimated), and descriptors for each individual in the data set. These data were not obtained from randomly selected individuals and thus are not a representative sample of the U.S. population. However, because the measurements were obtained from men, women, and children, over a wide range of weights, heights, and ages, it is believed that the data still offer the best currently available information [85].

TABLE 4.1 Examples of Equations for Predicting Resting and Basal Energy Expenditure[a]

Harris—Benedict Equations	
Women	REE (kcal/day) = 655 + 9.56 (weight) + 1.85 (height) − 4.68 (age)
	$r^2 = 0.53$, $F = 37.8$, $P < 0.001$
Men	REE (kcal/day) = 66.5 + 13.75 (weight) + 5.0 (height) − 6.76 (age)
	$r^2 = 0.75$, $F = 135.2$, $P < 0.001$
DRI Equations	
Women	BEE (kcal/day) = 255 − (2.35 × age) + 361.6 × height + 9.39 × weight
	Residual = ±125, $R^2 = 0.39$
Men	BEE (kcal/day) = 204 − (4 × age) + 450.5 × height + 11.69 × weight
	Residual = ±149, $R^2 = 0.46$

[a]Weight is in kilograms, height is in centimeters, and age is in years.
Sources: Data from Frankenfield, D. C., Muth, E. R., and Rowe, W. A. (1998). The Harris—Benedict studies of human basal metabolism: History and limitations. J. Am. Diet. Assoc. 98, 439—445; Institute of Medicine (2005). "DRI Equations for Basal Energy Expenditure." National Academies Press, Washington, DC; and Institute of Medicine (2005). "Dietary Reference Intakes: Energy, Carbohydrate, Fiber, Fat, Fatty Acids, Cholesterol, Protein, and Amino Acids." National Academies Press, Washington, DC.

C PREDICTING REE IN DISEASE AND PHYSIOLOGICAL CONDITIONS

REE has been characterized for a variety of disease states and physiological conditions, including burns [86—88], anorexia nervosa [89,90], severe central nervous system impairment [91], cerebral palsy [92], pregnancy [93], and lactation [94]. In addition, REE has been studied in both children [81] and the elderly [95—97]. Clinicians should not assume that prediction equations, which were developed in normal, healthy people, are valid in special populations [98].

B Thermic Effect of Food

TEF, sometimes referred to as diet-induced thermogenesis, represents a small (~10%) portion of TDEE (Figure 4.1). TEF is the increase in energy expenditure that occurs after consumption of a meal. There are several protocols for measurement of TEF, but the general procedure utilizes a metabolic cart to measure metabolic rate for 3—6 hours after administration of a meal of approximately 35% of RMR, which is then compared to RMR measured either on the same day as the TEF or on a different day [21,65,99—102]. TEF is generally not measured in clinical settings but, rather, estimated as 10% of TEE.

TABLE 4.2 Examples of Activity Energy Costs

Activity	Energy cost (multiple of basal metabolism)
Lying quietly	1.0
Riding in a vehicle	1.0
Light activity while sitting	1.5
Walking (2 mph)	2.5
Watering plants	2.5
Walking the dog	3.0
Cycling leisurely and household tasks (moderate effort)	3.5
Raking the lawn	4.0
Golfing (no cart) and gardening (no lifting)	4.4
Walking (4 mph)	4.5
Dancing, ballroom (fast) or square	5.5
Dancing, aerobic or ballet	6.0
Walking (5 mph)	8.0
Jogging (10-minute miles)	10.2
Skipping rope	12.0

Source: *Reprinted with permission from the National Academies Press, Copyright 2005, National Academy of Sciences, Institute of Medicine of the National Academies (2005). "Dietary Reference Intakes for Energy, Carbohydrate, Fiber, Fat, Fatty Acids, Cholesterol, Protein, and Amino Acids." National Academies Press, Washington, DC. Adapted from Table 12-2.*

C Energy Expended in Physical Activity

EEPA is the most variable component of total energy expenditure, varying between 100 and 800 kcal/day even in the confines of a metabolic chamber [103]. EEPA includes energy expended in voluntary exercise, which includes activities of daily living (e.g., bathing, feeding, and grooming), sports and leisure, and occupational activities. EEPA also includes the energy expended in nonexercise activity thermogenesis, which is associated with fidgeting, maintenance of posture, and other physical activities of daily life [104]. Because of the alarmingly high rates of obesity in the United States, increasing EEPA through voluntary physical activity is being stressed as an effective way of achieving or maintaining a healthy weight [105].

1 Determinants of Energy Expended in Physical Activity

Differences in EEPA are due both to patterns of activity and to body size and composition. In addition, physical activity can also affect RMR in the

postexercise period by 5% or more up to 24 hours after exercise [106]. A decrease in the level of physical activity has been observed during the transition from childhood to adolescence [21,107]. A decrease in EEPA has also been observed in aging [97,108]. Cross-sectional and longitudinal studies have shown increases in body fat and decreases in muscle mass in older adults, often in the absence of differences or changes in body weight [109]. These changes in body composition are often associated with changes in physical function and metabolic risk. Fortunately, moderate intensity PA intervention has been shown to improve physical function in older adults, and free-living activity energy expenditure has been shown to be strongly associated with lower risk of mortality in healthy older adults [110,111]. Table 4.2 shows average energy costs of typical activities, with the values expressed as multiples of RMR.

2 Measuring Energy Expended in Physical Activity

Obtaining a valid and appropriate measurement of EEPA is a challenging task. Measures are classified into three general categories: objective assessment tools, including the DLW technique combined with RMR, activity monitors, and heart rate monitoring; direct observation; and subjective reports, such as physical activity questionnaires. The objective activity assessment tools are often used to validate the subjective activity measures.

A OBJECTIVE MEASURES OF EEPA

I DOUBLY LABELED WATER EEPA can be assessed by measuring TEE by DLW and subtracting measured RMR and either measured or estimated (10% of TEE) TEF. DLW has been used as a gold standard for validating other methods to measure EEPA in free-living individuals. DLW measurement of TEE is discussed in detail in Section III.

II ACTIVITY MONITORS A variety of devices (e.g., accelerometers and heart rate monitors) can provide minute-by-minute information regarding physical activity patterns. However, these devices have limitations that affect their validity for assessing EEPA [112–116]. Accelerometers are movement counters that can measure body movement and often intensity. Accelerometers cannot be used to measure the static component in exercises such as weight lifting or carrying loads. However, in normal daily life, it is assumed that the effect of static exercise on the total level of physical activity is negligible [117]. Since 1999, there has been a push to improve accelerometers because it was concluded that those available were not practical for large-scale studies due to high cost, uncertain reliability, and difficulties in interpreting data [118]. NHANES 2003–2004 began using accelerometers on survey participants ages 6 years or older who agreed to wear them, representing the largest implementation of objective physical activity monitoring [118].

Whereas accelerometry has been shown to be accurate for estimating energy expenditure during level walking, it consistently underestimates energy expenditure during other forms of activity [112,119,120]. In addition, although many devices/algorithms have been shown to perform well in a laboratory setting, they perform less well under free-living conditions. New regression models have been proposed to improve estimated energy expenditure using accelerometry [121,122]. In addition, new, multisensor devices have been developed that show promise, but they require further refinement and validation [123–128].

III HEART RATE MONITORING The use of heart rate monitoring as a proxy measure for EEPA is based on the principle that heart rate and oxygen consumption tend to be linearly related throughout a large portion of the aerobic work range. Heart rate monitors are often used to assess EEPA because the technique is relatively inexpensive and easy to use. One drawback is that the relationship between heart rate and oxygen consumption must be characterized for each subject for several exercise intensities [129]. Even when conducting individual calibration relationships and using complex modeling, heart rate monitoring can provide inaccurate estimates of energy expenditure compared to DLW and indirect calorimetry [114,130,131]. Investigators have combined heart rate monitoring and accelerometry to provide more accurate measures of EEPA [127,128].

B PHYSICAL ACTIVITY QUESTIONNAIRES

Physical activity questionnaires have been used in many studies because they are easy to administer to large numbers of people and do not intrude on people's everyday activities. Although questionnaires do not provide precise estimates of EEPA, they may be helpful in ranking groups of subjects from the least to the most active. The ranking can then be used to correlate activity levels with disease outcomes [104]. An accurate questionnaire is both reliable and valid. A reliable questionnaire consistently provides similar results in the same circumstances, whereas a valid questionnaire truly measures what it was designed to measure. The validity of a physical activity questionnaire should be determined by comparing it with an objective measure of EEPA such as the DLW method. Starling and colleagues [132] found that the Yale Physical Activity Survey estimates of EEPA compared favorably with DLW on a group basis. However, its use as a proxy measure for individual EEPA is limited. In the same study, the Minnesota Leisure Time Physical Activity Questionnaire significantly underestimated EEPA in free-living older men and women [132]. This highlights the importance of ascertaining the validity of a questionnaire before applying it in large epidemiological studies.

III TOTAL ENERGY EXPENDITURE

Measured TEE provides an estimate of energy requirements when individuals are in energy balance. If significant weight gain or loss occurs during a metabolic study, changes in body energy stores must be accounted for to assess energy intake [133].

A Measuring Total Energy Expenditure

1 Indirect Calorimetry

Metabolic chambers, also known as respiratory chambers, are utilized to study energy expenditure over periods of time from 24 hours to several days. The concepts of metabolic chambers are similar to that of metabolic carts, requiring measurement of CO_2 and O_2 concentrations and the flow rate through the chamber to calculate oxygen consumption, carbon dioxide production, respiratory quotient (RQ), and metabolic rate [103,134–137]. Metabolic chambers provide accurate measures of 24-hour and sleeping energy expenditure, as well as long-term substrate utilization. However, due to the confined environment of the chamber, they do not provide an estimate of free-living energy expenditure.

2 Doubly Labeled Water

The introduction of the DLW technique for use in humans in 1982 by Schoeller and van Santen [138] provided a scientific breakthrough in the measurement of TEE in free-living humans. The method was originally described by Lifson and McClintock in the 1950s for use in rodents [139,140]. The method is based on the principle that a dose of $^2H_2^{18}O$ mixes with total body water, and the oxygen atoms in body water are also in equilibrium with exhaled CO_2 [141]. The isotopes undergo differential elimination from the body, with ^{18}O eliminated as carbon dioxide and water and deuterium eliminated only as water. The difference between the elimination rates of oxygen and hydrogen from body water are used to calculate CO_2 flux and, hence, energy expenditure. The DLW method has been extensively validated by a number of investigators throughout the world and shown to be accurate and precise [142]. For example, very good agreement was observed between 24-hour energy expenditure using DLW (1934 ± 377 kcal/day) and metabolic chambers (1906 327 kcal/day) during caloric restriction [137].

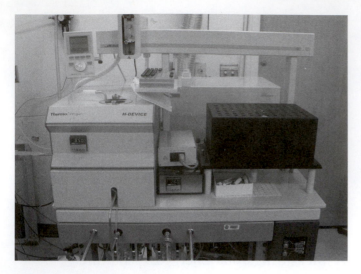

FIGURE 4.5 Mass spectrometry system used for the analysis of isotope enrichments for the DLW method.
See color plate.

TABLE 4.3 Advantages and Disadvantages of the Doubly Labeled Water Technique to Measure Total Energy Expenditure

Advantages	Disadvantages
Noninvasive, unobtrusive, and easily administered	Availability and expense of oxygen-18 (varies between $300 and $1,000 for 70-kg adult)
No reliance on participant to do anything except drink the labeled water and provide timed urine samples	Need for isotope ratio mass spectrometry for analysis of samples
Measurement performed under free-living conditions over extended time period (7–14 days)	A direct measure of CO_2 production, so need an estimate of respiratory quotient
Accurate and precise (2–8%)	Expensive for large-scale epidemiological studies
Can be used to estimate energy expended in physical activity when combined with measurement of resting metabolic rate	Does not provide information regarding time spent in activity or intensity of activities

A DLW DETAILS

The application of the DLW method can be quite flexible depending on the individuals studied, the questions being asked, and the balancing of the ideal protocol with the costs and subject burden. Baseline urine samples are collected followed by oral administration of the $^{2}H_{2}^{18}O$ dose. Initial urine samples are obtained 4–6 hours following dose administration and again at the end of the study period for measurement of final isotopic enrichment. The length of a DLW study depends on the turnover of the two isotopes, which is driven primarily by water turnover. The optimal period for studies in normal adults is 7–14 days. If measurement of energy expenditure over a longer period of time is necessary, individuals can be re-dosed with DLW [143].

The ^{18}O and deuterium isotope abundances are measured after appropriate sample preparation using a gas-inlet isotope ratio mass spectrometer (IRMS) [143]. Advancements in automated devices to prepare and introduce samples into the mass spectrometer have greatly improved the precision and throughput of the isotope analyses. For example, Figure 4.5 shows an H-Device system for injection of purified urine sample into a chromium reactor heated to 850°C for conversion to hydrogen gas before being introduced into the IRMS (just below the H-Device) for measurement of deuterium enrichment. A GasBench system (Figure 4.5, right) is used to equilibrate a cleaned urine sample with carbon dioxide gas before being introduced into a gas chromatograph to purify the CO_2 and then introduced into the IRMS for the measurement of ^{18}O enrichment. The CO_2 production rate is estimated using the measured isotope dilution spaces and elimination rates [142,144]. Energy expenditure is calculated utilizing the energy equivalent of CO_2 for a typical RQ such as 0.86 or using a calculated RQ from the macronutrient content of the diet consumed and body energy stores used during the DLW measurement period [143].

B ADVANTAGES AND DISADVANTAGES OF THE DLW TECHNIQUE

Advantages of the DLW method (Table 4.3) are that it is a true field technique for the accurate and precise (2–8%) assessment of free-living energy expenditure that requires no subject compliance, can be used to validate other techniques, and when combined with other methods can provide measures of EEPA, as described previously. The DLW method also provides an objective criterion method for validation of more subjective estimates of energy expenditure and energy intake.

Disadvantages of the DLW method include the cost and availability of the ^{18}O-labeled water, the need for expensive IRMSs and sample preparation systems, and technical difficulties with accurate measurements of isotope enrichments [145]. Another disadvantage of the DLW method is that it provides no information regarding time spent in physical activity, activity patterns, or intensity. Therefore, when conducting a DLW study, it is extremely advantageous to include other methodologies, including RMR; so that EEPA can be assessed as well as activity monitors, so that activity intensity and patterns can also be assessed.

TABLE 4.4 Doubly Labeled Water Data for Individuals with a Body Mass Index (BMI) in the Range of 18.5 to 25 kg/m^2

Age group (years)	n	Mean BMI (kg/m^2)	TEE (kcal/day)	BEE mean (kcal/day)	Mean physical activity level (TEE/BEE)
Females					
3–8	227	15.6	1487	1035	1.57
9–13	89	17.4	1907	1320	1.68
14–18	42	20.4	2302	1729	1.73
19–30	82	21.4	2436	1769	1.70
31–50	61	21.6	2404	1675	1.68
51–70	71	22.2	2066	1524	1.69
71 +	24	21.8	1564	1480	1.62
Males					
3–8	129	15.4	1441	1004	1.64
9–13	28	17.2	2079	1186	1.74
14–18	10	20.4	3116	1361	1.75
19–30	48	22.0	3081	1361	1.85
31–50	59	22.6	3021	1322	1.77
51–70	24	23.0	2469	1226	1.64
70 +	38	22.8	2238	1183	1.61

Source: Reprinted with permission from the National Academies Press, Copyright 2005, National Academy of Sciences, Institute of Medicine of the National Academies (2005). "Dietary Reference Intakes for Energy, Carbohydrate, Fiber, Fat, Fatty Acids, Cholesterol, Protein, and Amino Acids." National Academies Press, Washington, DC. From Table 5-10.

TABLE 4.5 Equations to Predict Energy Requirements in Females and Males 19 Years or Older[a]

For Females
EER = 354.1 − 6.91 × age + PA × (9.36 × weight + 726 × height)

Where PA is the physical activity coefficient:

PA = 1.00 if PAL is estimated to be ≥ 1.0 < 1.4 (sedentary)

PA = 1.12 if PAL is estimated to be ≥ 1.4 < 1.6 (low active)

PA = 1.27 if PAL is estimated to be ≥ 1.6 < 1.9 (active)

PA = 1.45 if PAL is estimated to be ≥ 1.9 < 2.5 (very active)

For Males
EER = 661.8 − 9.53 × age + PA × (15.91 × weight + 539.6 × height)

Where PA is the physical activity coefficient:

PA = 1.00 if PAL is estimated to be ≥ 1.0 < 1.4 (sedentary)

PA = 1.12 if PAL is estimated to be ≥ 1.4 < 1.6 (low active)

PA = 1.27 if PAL is estimated to be ≥ 1.6 < 1.9 (active)

PA = 1.45 if PAL is estimated to be ≥ 1.9 < 2.5 (very active)

[a]*Weight is in kilograms, height is in centimeters, and age is in years.*
Source: Institute of Medicine (2005). "Dietary Reference Intake for Energy, Carbohydrate, Fiber, Fat, Fatty Acids, Cholesterol, Protein, and Amino Acids." National Academies Press, Washington, DC.

B Estimating Total Energy Expenditure

The introduction of the DLW technique in humans has produced a large and robust database of TEE measurements in a variety of populations. A meta-analysis of 574 DLW measurements helped to establish the average and range of habitual energy expenditures in different age and sex groups [108]. Since this study, many DLW studies have been completed. The Food and Nutrition Board used data from these DLW studies to compile a worldwide TEE database [85]. Table 4.4 is a summary of data from this database. The database provides a frame of reference for energy needs in the general population and can be used to evaluate other estimates of energy expenditure. Special circumstances such as illness or enforced exertion were excluded from this database.

Because of the high cost and small numbers of laboratories with the capacity to do DLW studies, clinicians continue to rely heavily on prediction equations to estimate energy requirements. The TEE database compiled for the DRIs was used to derive equations for predicting energy expenditure requirements. These equations are provided in Table 4.5.

C Total Energy Expenditure in Special Populations

During approximately the past 20 years, there has been a proliferation of studies using DLW to examine TEE in various disease states, physiological conditions, and across the life cycle. Hence, data are now available on energy expenditure during infancy [146], childhood [21,147], adolescence [148], and in the elderly [97]. TEE during pregnancy and lactation has been well characterized in some elegant longitudinal studies [149]. In addition, TEE has been examined in adults and children with obesity [150−152]; infants and children with cystic fibrosis [153,154]; children treated for acute lymphoblastic leukemia (ALL) [155] with burns [156] and Down syndrome [157]; and adults with cerebral palsy [158], Alzheimer's disease [159], and HIV/AIDs [160]. The effects of these various conditions on energy requirements are highlighted in Table 4.6.

D Use of DLW to Estimate Energy Intake

Although knowledge of caloric intake is essential for understanding energy balance, true dietary intake is consistently underreported, regardless of the intake methodology used when compared to DLW, which can be used as an unbiased biomarker of energy intake needed to meet energy requirements [161]. For example, the large Observing Protein and Energy Nutrition Study in 484 men and women compared a food frequency questionnaire (FFQ) and the 24-hr

TABLE 4.6 Effects of Disease States and Physiological Conditions on Energy Requirements: Results from Doubly Labeled Water Studies

Disease or condition	Effect on energy requirements	Explanation
Aging	Decreased	Decreased RMR, decreased EEPA in nonagenarians
Alzheimer's disease	No change	Energy expenditure not elevated, low-energy intake predisposes to weight loss
Anorexia	Increased	To counteract increased physical activity with underweight and hypometabolism
Burns	No change	Increased resting metabolic rate counteracted by decreased physical activity
Cerebral palsy	Relative to individual	High interindividual variation in energy expended in physical activity; ambulation status an important predictor
Children treated for ALL	Decreased	Reduced physical activity
Cystic fibrosis	Increased	Mechanism unknown
HIV/AIDS	No change	Energy expenditure not elevated, reduced energy intake causes weight loss
Lactation	Increased	Energy cost of milk production partially offset by reduced physical activity
Obesity	Increased	Increased fat-free mass and fat mass, but decreased time spent in physical activity
Pregnancy	Relative to individual	No prediction of metabolic response
Spinal cord	Decreased	Lower energy expended in physical activity, resting metabolic rate, and thermic effect of food

recall (24HR) with DLW [1]. On average, men underreported energy intake by 12−14% using 24HR and 31−36% using FFQ. Women underreported energy intake by 16−20% using 24HR and by 34−38% using FFQ. Similar levels of underreporting (17−33%) have been observed in children when comparing 8-day food records with DLW, and greater underreporting has been observed in obese compared to lean children[162].

IV RECOMMENDED ENERGY INTAKES

Classically, the Recommended Dietary Allowances (RDAs) have been used as a guide to determine energy intakes for groups of normal, healthy people. The last RDA for energy, which was labeled the recommended energy intake (REI), was set in 1989. RDAs for all nutrients except energy are set at levels well above those estimated to minimize the occurrence of deficiency syndromes. For energy, this obviously is not the case because there are adverse effects to individuals who consume energy above their requirements over time resulting in weight gain. Recommendations for energy have always been set as an average of energy requirements for a population group. In the past, REIs relied heavily on data from dietary surveys that estimate energy intake. This is based on the assumption that people are in energy balance at the time of measurement and that the estimates of energy intake are valid. A large body of evidence now demonstrates that self-reported estimates of food intake do not provide accurate or unbiased estimates of people's energy intake and that underreporting of food intake is pervasive in children, teens, and adults [162−164]. Underreporting is discussed in detail in Chapter 7.

The DRIs [85] adopted an alternative approach and instead summarized data from multiple DLW studies to estimate energy requirements. There is no RDA for energy because it would be inappropriate to recommend levels that would exceed requirements of 97 or 98% of individuals. Instead, the requirement for energy for individuals of normal weight is expressed as an estimated energy requirement (EER), which reflects the energy expenditure based on the individual's sex, age, height, weight, and physical activity (see Table 4.5 for equations). For overweight individuals, these equations estimate TEE rather than the EER, which is reserved for normal-weight individuals. The equations are estimates of energy needs based on maintaining current weight and activity level and therefore were not designed to lead to weight loss in overweight individuals [85].

As the prevalence of obesity has reached epidemic proportions in the United States, people's energy expended in physical activity has become so low that it may become increasingly difficult to meet the micronutrient needs on the energy intakes required to keep people in energy balance. Hence, it will become increasingly imperative that emphasis be placed on increased energy expended in physical activity for the maintenance of optimal health.

References

[1] A.F. Subar, V. Kipnis, R.P. Troiano, D. Midthune, D.A. Schoeller, S. Bingham, et al., Using intake biomarkers to evaluate the extent of dietary misreporting in a large sample of adults: the OPEN Study, Am. J. Epidemiol. 158 (2003) 1−13.

[2] W.O. Atwater, E.B. Rosa, Description of a New Respiration Calorimeter and Experiments on the Conservation of Energy in the Human Body, U.S. Department of Agriculture, Office of Experiment Stations, Washington, DC, 1899.

[3] M. Rubner, D. Franz, Die Gesetze des Energieverbrauchsbei der Ernahrung Lepzig, 1902.

[4] W.O. Atwater, F.G. Benedict, Experiments on the Metabolism of Matter and Energy in the Human Body, 1898–1900, U.S. Department of Agriculture, Office of Experiment Stations, Washington, DC, 1902.

[5] J.A. Harris, F.G. Benedict, A Biometric Study of Basal Metabolism in Man, Carnegie Institution of Washington, Washington, DC, 1919.

[6] F.G. Benedict, L.E. Emmes, A comparison of the basal metabolism of normal men and women, Proc. Natl. Acad. Sci. USA 1 (1915) 104–105.

[7] F.G. Benedict, H. Murschhauser, Energy transformations during horizontal walking, Proc. Natl. Acad. Sci. USA 1 (1915) 597–600.

[8] F.G. Benedict, P. Roth, The basal caloric output of vegetarians as compared with that of non-vegetarians of like weight and height, Proc. Natl. Acad. Sci. USA 1 (1915) 100–101.

[9] F.G. Benedict, H.M. Smith, The influence of athletic training upon basal metabolism, Proc. Natl. Acad. Sci. USA 1 (1915) 102–103.

[10] F.G. Benedict, F.B. Talbot, The physiology of the new-born infant, Proc. Natl. Acad. Sci. USA 1 (1915) 600–602.

[11] M. Kleiber, Body size and metabolic rate, Physiol. Rev. 27 (1947) 511–541.

[12] R.L. Weinsier, Y. Schutz, D. Bracco, Reexamination of the relationship of resting metabolic rate to fat-free mass and to the metabolically active components of fat-free mass in humans, Am. J. Clin. Nutr. 55 (1992) 790–794.

[13] C. Weyer, S. Snitker, R. Rising, C. Bogardus, E. Ravussin, Determinants of energy expenditure and fuel utilization in man: effects of body composition, age, sex, ethnicity and glucose tolerance in 916 subjects, Int. J. Obes. Relat. Metab. Disord. 23 (1999) 715–722.

[14] K. Nelson, R. Weinsier, C. Long, Y. Schutz, Prediction of resting energy expenditure from fat-free mass and fat mass, Am. J. Clin. Nutr. 56 (1992) 848–856.

[15] C. Bogardus, S. Lillioja, E. Ravussin, W. Abbott, J.K. Zawadzki, A. Young, et al., Familial dependence of the resting metabolic rate, N. Engl. J. Med. 315 (1986) 96–100.

[16] N.K. Fukagawa, L.G. Bandini, W.H. Dietz, J.B. Young, Effect of age on body water and resting metabolic rate, J. Gerontol. A Biol. Sci. Med. Sci. 51 (1996) M71–M73.

[17] J.R. Speakman, C. Selman, Physical activity and resting metabolic rate, Proc. Nutrition Soc. 62 (2003) 621–634.

[18] O.L. Svendsen, J. Haarbo, C. Hassager, C. Christiansen, Accuracy of measurements of body composition by dual-energy x-ray absorptiometry in vivo, Am. J. Clin. Nutr. 57 (1993) 605–608.

[19] T.L. Kelly, K.E. Wilson, S.B. Heymsfield, Dual energy x-ray absorptiometry body composition reference values from NHANES, PLoS ONE 4 (2009) E7038.

[20] P.J. Arciero, M.I. Goran, E.T. Poehlman, Resting metabolic rate is lower in women than in men, J. Appl. Physiol. 75 (1993) 2514–2520.

[21] J.P. DeLany, G.A. Bray, D.W. Harsha, J. Volaufova, Energy expenditure in African American and white boys and girls in a 2-y follow-up of the Baton Rouge Children's Study, Am. J. Clin. Nutr. 79 (2004) 268–273.

[22] A. Keys, H.L. Taylor, F. Grande, Basal metabolism and age of adult man, Metabolism 22 (1973) 579–587.

[23] M.I. Frisard, A. Broussard, S.S. Davies, L.J. Roberts 2nd, J. Rood, L. de Jonge, et al., Aging, resting metabolic rate, and oxidative damage: results from the Louisiana Healthy Aging Study, J. Gerontol. A Biol. Sci. Med. Sci. 62 (2007) 752–759.

[24] P.M. Luhrmann, B. Edelmann-Schafer, M. Neuhauser-Berthold, Changes in resting metabolic rate in an elderly German population: cross-sectional and longitudinal data, J. Nutr. Health Aging 14 (2010) 232–236.

[25] L.S. Piers, M.J. Soares, L.M. McCormack, K. O'Dea, Is there evidence for an age-related reduction in metabolic rate? J. Appl. Physiol. 85 (1998) 2196–2204.

[26] C.J. Henry, Mechanisms of changes in basal metabolism during ageing, Eur. J. Clin. Nutr. 54 (Suppl. 3) (2000) S77–S91.

[27] E.T. Poehlman, C.L. Melby, S.F. Badylak, Resting metabolic rate and postprandial thermogenesis in highly trained and untrained males, Am. J. Clin. Nutr. 47 (1988) 793–798.

[28] C.M. Burke, R.C. Bullough, C.L. Melby, Resting metabolic rate and postprandial thermogenesis by level of aerobic fitness in young women, Eur. J. Clin. Nutr. 47 (1993) 575–585.

[29] T.J. Horton, C.A. Geissler, Effect of habitual exercise on daily energy expenditure and metabolic rate during standardized activity, Am. J. Clin. Nutr. 59 (1994) 13–19.

[30] M. Gilliat-Wimberly, M.M. Manore, K. Woolf, P.D. Swan, S.S. Carroll, Effects of habitual physical activity on the resting metabolic rates and body compositions of women aged 35 to 50 years, J. Am. Diet. Assoc. 101 (2001) 1181–1188.

[31] A. Tremblay, E. Fontaine, E.T. Poehlman, D. Mitchell, L. Perron, C. Bouchard, The effect of exercise-training on resting metabolic rate in lean and moderately obese individuals, Int. J. Obes. 10 (1986) 511–517.

[32] J.T. Lemmer, F.M. Ivey, A.S. Ryan, G.F. Martel, D.E. Hurlbut, J. E. Metter, et al., Effect of strength training on resting metabolic rate and physical activity: age and gender comparisons, Med. Sci. Sports Exerc. 33 (2001) 532–541.

[33] M. Neuhauser-Berthold, B.M. Herbert, P.M. Luhrmann, A.A. Sultemeier, W.F. Blum, J. Frey, et al., Resting metabolic rate, body composition, and serum leptin concentrations in a free-living elderly population, Eur. J. Endocrinol. 142 (2000) 486–492.

[34] S.E. Deemer, G.A. King, S. Dorgo, C.A. Vella, J.W. Tomaka, D.L. Thompson, Relationship of leptin, resting metabolic rate, and body composition in premenopausal Hispanic and non-Hispanic white women, Endocr. Res. 35 (2010) 95–105.

[35] C.J. Hukshorn, W.H. Saris, Leptin and energy expenditure, Curr. Opin. Clin. Nutr. Metab. Care 7 (2004) 629–633.

[36] J.E. Galgani, F.L. Greenway, S. Caglayan, M.L. Wong, J. Licinio, E. Ravussin, Leptin replacement prevents weight loss-induced metabolic adaptation in congenital leptin-deficient patients, J. Clin. Endocrinol. Metab. 95 (2010) 851–855.

[37] H.R. Kissileff, J.C. Thornton, M.I. Torres, K. Pavlovich, L.S. Mayer, V. Kalari, et al., Leptin reverses declines in satiation in weight-reduced obese humans, Am. J. Clin. Nutr. 95 (2012) 309–317.

[38] C.J. Henry, H.J. Lightowler, J. Marchini, Intra-individual variation in resting metabolic rate during the menstrual cycle, Br. J. Nutr. 89 (2003) 811–817.

[39] J.M. Jakicic, R.R. Wing, Differences in resting energy expenditure in African-American vs. Caucasian overweight females, Int. J. Obes. Relat. Metab. Disord. 22 (1998) 236–242.

[40] J. Weststrate, Resting metabolic rate and diet-induced thermogenesis: a methodological reappraisal, Am. J. Clin. Nutr. 58 (1993) 592–601.

[41] T.J. Horton, E.K. Miller, D. Glueck, K. Tench, No effect of menstrual cycle phase on glucose kinetics and fuel oxidation during moderate-intensity exercise, Am. J. Physiol. Endocrinol. Metab. 282 (2002) E752–E762.

[42] G.R. Hunter, R.L. Weinsier, B.E. Darnell, P.A. Zuckerman, M.I. Goran, Racial differences in energy expenditure and aerobic fitness in premenopausal women, Am. J. Clin. Nutr. 71 (2000) 500–506.

[43] R.F. Kushner, S.B. Racette, K. Neil, D.A. Schoeller, Measurement of physical activity among black and white obese women, Obes. Res. 3 (Suppl. 2) (1995) 261S—265S.

[44] T.A. Sharp, M.L. Bell, G.K. Grunwald, K.H. Schmitz, S. Sidney, C.E. Lewis, et al., Differences in resting metabolic rate between white and African-American young adults, Obes. Res. 10 (2002) 726—732.

[45] C. Weyer, S. Snitker, C. Bogardus, E. Ravussin, Energy metabolism in African Americans: potential risk factors for obesity, Am. J. Clin. Nutr. 70 (1999) 13—20.

[46] S. Blanc, D.A. Schoeller, D. Bauer, M.E. Danielson, F. Tylavsky, E.M. Simonsick, et al., Energy requirements in the eighth decade of life, Am. J. Clin. Nutr. 79 (2004) 303—310.

[47] W.H. Carpenter, T. Fonong, M.J. Toth, P.A. Ades, J. Calles-Escandon, J.D. Walston, et al., Total daily energy expenditure in free-living older African-Americans and Caucasians, Am. J. Physiol. 274 (1998) E96—E101.

[48] R.L. Weinsier, G.R. Hunter, P.A. Zuckerman, D.T. Redden, B.E. Darnell, D.E. Larson, et al., Energy expenditure and free-living physical activity in black and white women: comparison before and after weight loss, Am. J. Clin. Nutr. 71 (2000) 1138—1146.

[49] A. Jones Jr., W. Shen St, M.P. Onge, D. Gallagher, S. Heshka, Z. Wang, et al., Body-composition differences between African American and white women: relation to resting energy requirements, Am. J. Clin. Nutr. 79 (2004) 780—786.

[50] A.M. Fontvieille, J. Dwyer, E. Ravussin, Resting metabolic rate and body composition of Pima Indian and Caucasian children, Int. J. Obes. Relat. Metab. Disord. 16 (1992) 535—542.

[51] M.I. Goran, M. Kaskoun, R. Johnson, C. Martinez, B. Kelly, V. Hood, Energy expenditure and body fat distribution in Mohawk children, Pediatrics 95 (1995) 89—95.

[52] C. Bouchard, L. Perusse, O. Deriaz, J. Despres, A. Tremblay, Genetic influences on energy expenditure in humans, Crit. Rev. Food Sci. Nutr. 33 (1993) 345—350.

[53] S. Ramachandrappa, I.S. Farooqi, Genetic approaches to understanding human obesity, J. Clin. Invest. 121 (2011) 2080—2086.

[54] B.M. Herrera, S. Keildson, C.M. Lindgren, Genetics and epigenetics of obesity, Maturitas 69 (2011) 41—49.

[55] C.F. Consolazio, L.R.O. Matoush, R.A. Nelson, J.B. Torres, G.J. Isaac, Environmental temperature and energy expenditures, J. Appl. Physiol. 18 (1963) 65—68.

[56] C.F. Consolazio, R. Shapiro, J.E. Masterson, P.S.L. McKinzie, Energy requirements of men in extreme heat, J. Nutr. 73 (1961) 126—134.

[57] S. Blaza, J.S. Garrow, Thermogenic response to temperature, exercise and food stimuli in lean and obese women, studied by 24 h direct calorimetry, Br. J. Nutr. 49 (1983) 171—180.

[58] M.J. Dauncey, Influence of mild cold on 24 h energy expenditure, resting metabolism and diet-induced thermogenesis, Br. J. Nutr. 45 (1981) 257—267.

[59] O. Wilson, Basal metabolic rate in the Antarctic, Metabolism 5 (1956) 543—554.

[60] A.J. Gold, A. Zornitzer, S. Samueloff, Influence of season and heat on energy expenditure during rest and exercise, J. Appl. Physiol. 27 (1969) 9—12.

[61] M.S. Malhotra, S.S. Ramaswamy, S.N. Ray, Effect of environmental temperature on work and resting metabolism, J. Appl. Physiol. 15 (1960) 769—770.

[62] N.E. Hill, M.J. Stacey, D.R. Woods, Energy at high altitude, J. R. Army Med. Corps 157 (2011) 43—48.

[63] D. DuBois, E.F. DuBois, A formula to estimate the approximate surface area if height and weight be known, Arch. Intern. Med. 17 (1916) 863—871.

[64] W.M. Boothby, J. Berkson, H.L. Dunn, Studies of the energy of metabolism of normal individuals: a standard for basal metabolism, with a nomogram for clinical application, Am. J. Physiol. 116 (1936) 468—484.

[65] E. Ravussin, B. Burnand, Y. Schutz, E. Jequier, Twenty-four-hour energy expenditure and resting metabolic rate in obese, moderately obese, and control subjects, Am. J. Clin. Nutr. 35 (1982) 566—573.

[66] E. Ravussin, C. Bogardus, Relationship of genetics, age, and physical fitness to daily energy expenditure and fuel utilization [review], Am. J. Clin. Nutr. 49 (1989) 968—975.

[67] J.P. DeLany, G.A. Bray, D.W. Harsha, J. Volaufova, Energy expenditure in preadolescent African American and white boys and girls: The Baton Rouge Children's Study, Am. J. Clin. Nutr. 75 (2002) 705—713.

[68] L.M. Redman, L.K. Heilbronn, C.K. Martin, L. deJonge, D.A. Williamson, J.P. DeLany, et al., Metabolic and behavioral compensations in response to caloric restriction: implications for the maintenance of weight loss, PLoS ONE 4 (2009) E4377.

[69] T.H. Benzinger, C. Kitzinger, Direct calorimetry by means of the gradient principle, Rev. Sci. Instrum. 20 (1949) 849—860.

[70] J.D. Webster, G. Welsh, P. Pacy, J.S. Garrow, Description of a human direct calorimeter, with a note on the energy cost of clerical work, Br. J. Nutr. 55 (1986) 1—6.

[71] J.L. Seale, W.V. Rumpler, Synchronous direct gradient layer and indirect room calorimetry, J. Appl. Physiol. 83 (1997) 1775.

[72] F.G. Benedict, A portable respiration apparatus for clinical use, Boston Med. Surg. J. 178 (1918) 668—678.

[73] J.B. Weir, New methods for calculating metabolic rate with special reference to protein metabolism, J. Physiol. 109 (1949) 1—9.

[74] C. Compher, D. Frankenfield, N. Keim, L. Roth-Yousey, Best practice methods to apply to measurement of resting metabolic rate in adults: a systematic review, J. Am. Diet. Assoc. 106 (2006) 881—903.

[75] J.A. Cooper, A.C. Watras, M.J. O'Brien, A. Luke, J.R. Dobratz, C.P. Earthman, et al., Assessing validity and reliability of resting metabolic rate in six gas analysis systems, J. Am. Diet. Assoc. 109 (2009) 128—132.

[76] G.A. King, J.E. McLaughlin, E.T. Howley, D.R. Bassett Jr., B.E. Ainsworth, Validation of Aerosport KB1-C portable metabolic system, Int. J. Sports Med. 20 (1999) 304—308.

[77] K.E. Spears, H. Kim, K.M. Behall, J.M. Conway, Hand-held indirect calorimeter offers advantages compared with prediction equations, in a group of overweight women, to determine resting energy expenditures and estimated total energy expenditures during research screening, J. Am. Diet. Assoc. 109 (2009) 836—845.

[78] R. Duffield, B. Dawson, H.C. Pinnington, P. Wong, Accuracy and reliability of a Cosmed K4b2 portable gas analysis system, J. Sci. Med. Sport. 7 (2004) 11—22.

[79] D.C. Frankenfield, E.R. Muth, W.A. Rowe, The Harris—Benedict studies of human basal metabolism: history and limitations, J. Am. Diet. Assoc. 98 (1998) 439—445.

[80] P.M. Luhrmann, M. Neuhaeuser Berthold, Are the equations published in literature for predicting resting metabolic rate accurate for use in the elderly? J. Nutr. Health Aging 8 (2004) 144—149.

[81] J.R. McDuffie, D.C. Adler-Wailes, J. Elberg, E.N. Steinberg, E.M. Fallon, A.M. Tershakovec, et al., Prediction equations for resting energy expenditure in overweight and normal-weight black and white children, Am. J. Clin. Nutr. 80 (2004) 365—373.

[82] M.W. Vander Weg, J.M. Watson, R.C. Klesges, L.H. Eck Clemens, D.L. Slawson, B.S. McClanahan, Development and cross-validation of a prediction equation for estimating resting energy expenditure in healthy African-American and European-American women, Eur. J. Clin. Nutr. 58 (2004) 474—480.

[83] P.J. Weijs, Validity of predictive equations for resting energy expenditure in U.S. and Dutch overweight and obese class I and II adults aged 18—65 y, Am. J. Clin. Nutr. 88 (2008) 959—970.

[84] M. Skouroliakou, I. Giannopoulou, C. Kostara, M. Vasilopoulou, Comparison of predictive equations for resting metabolic rate in obese psychiatric patients taking olanzapine, Nutrition 25 (2009) 188—193.

[85] Institute of Medicine, Dietary Reference Intakes for Energy, Carbohydrate, Fiber, Fat, Fatty Acids, Cholesterol, Protein, and Amino Acids, National Academies Press, Washington, DC, 2005.

[86] M.I. Goran, L. Broemeling, D.N. Herndon, E.J. Peters, R.R. Wolfe, Estimating energy requirements in burned children: a new approach derived from measurements of resting energy expenditure, Am. J. Clin. Nutr. 54 (1991) 35—40.

[87] T. Mayes, M.M. Gottschlich, J. Khoury, G.D. Warden, Evaluation of predicted and measured energy requirements in burned children, J. Am. Diet. Assoc. 96 (1996) 24—29.

[88] D.W. Hart, S.E. Wolf, D.N. Herndon, D.L. Chinkes, S.O. Lal, M.K. Obeng, et al., Energy expenditure and caloric balance after burn: increased feeding leads to fat rather than lean mass accretion, Ann. Surg. 235 (2002) 152—161.

[89] C. Cuerda, A. Ruiz, C. Velasco, I. Breton, M. Camblor, P. Garcia-Peris, How accurate are predictive formulas calculating energy expenditure in adolescent patients with anorexia nervosa? Clin. Nutr. 26 (2007) 100—106.

[90] D.D. Krahn, C. Rock, R.E. Dechert, K.K. Nairn, S.A. Hasse, Changes in resting energy expenditure and body composition in anorexia nervosa patients during refeeding, J. Am. Diet. Assoc. 93 (1993) 434—438.

[91] L.G. Bandini, H. Puelzl-Quinn, J.A. Morelli, N.K. Fukagawa, Estimation of energy requirements in persons with severe central nervous system impairment, J. Pediatr. 126 (1995) 828—832.

[92] R.K. Johnson, M.I. Goran, M.S. Ferrara, E.T. Poehlman, Athetosis increases resting metabolic rate in adults with cerebral palsy, J. Am. Diet. Assoc. 96 (1996) 145—148.

[93] G.R. Goldberg, A.M. Prentice, W.A. Coward, H.L. Davies, P.R. Murgatroyd, C. Wensing, et al., Longitudinal assessment of energy expenditure in pregnancy by the doubly labeled water method, Am. J. Clin. Nutr. 57 (1993) 494—505.

[94] G.R. Goldberg, A.M. Prentice, W.A. Coward, H.L. Davies, P.R. Murgatroyd, M.B. Sawyer, et al., Longitudinal assessment of the components of energy balance in well-nourished lactating women, Am. J. Clin. Nutr. 54 (1991) 788—798.

[95] P.J. Arciero, M.I. Goran, A.M. Gardner, P.A. Ades, R.S. Tyzbir, E.T. Poehlman, A practical equation to predict resting metabolic rate in older females, J. Am. Geriatr. Soc. 41 (1993) 389—395.

[96] P.J. Arciero, M.I. Goran, A.W. Gardner, P.A. Ades, R.S. Tyzbir, E.T. Poehlman, A practical equation to predict resting metabolic rate in older men, Metabolism 42 (1993) 950—957.

[97] D.L. Johannsen, J.P. DeLany, M.I. Frisard, M.A. Welsch, C.K. Rowley, X. Fang, et al., Physical activity in aging: comparison among young, aged, and nonagenarian individuals, J. Appl. Physiol. 105 (2008) 495—501.

[98] J. Boullata, J. Williams, F. Cottrell, L. Hudson, C. Compher, Accurate determination of energy needs in hospitalized patients, J. Am. Diet. Assoc. 107 (2007) 393—401.

[99] K.R. Segal, A. Edano, L. Blando, F.X. Pi-Sunyer, Comparison of thermic effects of constant and relative caloric loads in lean and obese men, Am. J. Clin. Nutr. 51 (1990) 14—21.

[100] K.R. Segal, A. Edano, M.B. Tomas, Thermic effect of a meal over 3 and 6 hours in lean and obese men, Metabolism 39 (1990) 985—992.

[101] G.P. Granata, L.J. Brandon, The thermic effect of food and obesity: discrepant results and methodological variations, Nutr. Rev. 60 (2002) 223—233.

[102] G.W. Reed, J.O. Hill, Measuring the thermic effect of food, Am. J. Clin. Nutr. 63 (1996) 164—169.

[103] E. Ravussin, S. Lillioja, T.E. Anderson, L. Christin, C. Bogardus, Determinants of 24-hour energy expenditure in man: methods and results using a respiratory chamber, J. Clin. Invest. 78 (1986) 1568—1578.

[104] J.A. Levine, N.L. Eberhardt, M.D. Jensen, Role of nonexercise activity thermogenesis in resistance to fat gain in humans, Science 283 (1999) 212—214.

[105] J.E. Donnelly, S.N. Blair, J.M. Jakicic, M.M. Manore, J.W. Rankin, B.K. Smith, Appropriate physical activity intervention strategies for weight loss and prevention of weight regain for adults, Med. Sci. Sports Exerc. 41 (459—471) (2009).

[106] R. Bielinski, Y. Schutz, E. Jequier, Energy metabolism during the postexercise recovery in man, Am. J. Clin. Nutr. 42 (1985) 69—82.

[107] S.Y. Kimm, N.W. Glynn, A.M. Kriska, S.L. Fitzgerald, D.J. Aaron, S.L. Similo, et al., Longitudinal changes in physical activity in a biracial cohort during adolescence 3, Med. Sci. Sports Exerc. 32 (2000) 1445—1454.

[108] A.E. Black, W.A. Coward, T.J. Cole, A.M. Prentice, Human energy expenditure in affluent societies: an analysis of 574 doubly-labelled water measurements, Eur. J. Clin. Nutr. 50 (1996) 72—92.

[109] M.P. St.-Onge, Relationship between body composition changes and changes in physical function and metabolic risk factors in aging, Curr. Opin. Clin. Nutr. Metab. Care 8 (2005) 523—528.

[110] T.M. Manini, A.B. Newman, R. Fielding, S.N. Blair, M.G. Perri, S.D. Anton, et al., Effects of exercise on mobility in obese and nonobese older adults, Obesity 18 (2010) 1168—1175.

[111] T.M. Manini, J.E. Everhart, K.V. Patel, D.A. Schoeller, L.H. Colbert, M. Visser, et al., Daily activity energy expenditure and mortality among older adults, JAMA 296 (2006) 171—179.

[112] J.M. Jakicic, C. Winters, K. Lagally, J. Ho, R.J. Robertson, R.R. Wing, The accuracy of the TriTrac-R3D accelerometer to estimate energy expenditure, Med. Sci. Sports Exerc. 31 (1999) 747—754.

[113] E.L. Melanson, P.S. Freedson, Validity of the Computer Science and Applications, Inc. (CSA) activity monitor, Med. Sci. Sports Exerc. 27 (1995) 934—940.

[114] H.J. Montoye, Measuring Physical Activity and Energy Expenditure, Human Kinetics, Champaign, IL, 1996.

[115] G.J. Welk, S.N. Blair, K. Wood, S. Jones, R.W. Thompson, A comparative evaluation of three accelerometry-based physical activity monitors, Med. Sci. Sports Exerc. 32 (2000) S489—S497.

[116] G. Plasqui, K.R. Westerterp, Physical activity assessment with accelerometers: an evaluation against doubly labeled water, Obesity 15 (2007) 2371—2379.

[117] K.R. Westerterp, Physical activity assessment with accelerometers, Int. J. Obes. Relat. Metab. Disord. 23 (Suppl. 3) (1999) S45—S49.

[118] R.P. Troiano, D. Berrigan, K.W. Dodd, L.C. Masse, T. Tilert, M. McDowell, Physical activity in the United States measured by accelerometer, Med. Sci. Sports Exerc. 40 (2008) 181—188.

[119] D.R. Bassett, B.E. Ainsworth, A.M. Swartz, S.J. Strath, W.L. O'Brien, G.A. King, Validity of four motion sensors in measuring moderate intensity physical activity, Med. Sci. Sports Exerc. 32 (2000) S471–S480.

[120] P.C. Fehling, D.L. Smith, S.E. Warner, G.P. Dalsky, Comparison of accelerometers with oxygen consumption in older adults during exercise, Med. Sci. Sports Exerc. 31 (1999) 171–175.

[121] S.E. Crouter, K.G. Clowers, D.R. Bassett Jr., A novel method for using accelerometer data to predict energy expenditure, J. Appl. Physiol. 100 (2006) 1324–1331.

[122] D.P. Heil, Predicting activity energy expenditure using the Actical activity monitor, Res. Q. Exerc. Sport 77 (2006) 64–80.

[123] J.M. Jakicic, M. Marcus, K.I. Gallagher, C. Randall, E. Thomas, F.L. Goss, et al., Evaluation of the SenseWear Pro Armband to assess energy expenditure during exercise, Med. Sci. Sports Exerc. 36 (2004) 897–904.

[124] G.J. Welk, J.J. McClain, J.C. Eisenmann, E.E. Wickel, Field validation of the MTI Actigraph and BodyMedia armband monitor using the IDEEA monitor, Obesity 15 (2007) 918–928.

[125] D. Arvidsson, F. Slinde, L. Hulthén, Free-living energy expenditure in children using multi-sensor activity monitors, Clin. Nutr. 28 (2009) 305–312.

[126] K. Zhang, F.X. Pi-Sunyer, C.N. Boozer, Improving energy expenditure estimation for physical activity, Med. Sci. Sports Exerc. 36 (2004) 883–889.

[127] S. Brage, N. Brage, P.W. Franks, U. Ekelund, N.J. Wareham, Reliability and validity of the combined heart rate and movement sensor Actiheart, Eur. J. Clin. Nutr. 59 (2005) 561–570.

[128] S.E. Crouter, J.R. Churilla, D.R. Bassett Jr., Accuracy of the Actiheart for the assessment of energy expenditure in adults, Eur. J. Clin. Nutr. 62 (2007) 704–711.

[129] Y. Schutz, R.L. Weinsier, G.R. Hunter, Assessment of free-living physical activity in humans: an overview of currently available and proposed new measures, Obes. Res. 9 (2001) 368–379.

[130] S. Schulz, K. Westerterp, K. Bruck, Comparison of energy expenditure by the doubly labeled water technique with energy intake, heart rate, and activity recording in man, Am. J. Clin. Nutr. 49 (1989) 1146–1154.

[131] H.J. Emons, D.C. Groenenboom, K.R. Westerterp, W.H. Saris, Comparison of heart rate monitoring combined with indirect calorimetry and the doubly labelled water (2H2(18)O) method for the measurement of energy expenditure in children, Eur. J. Appl. Physiol. 65 (1992) 99–103.

[132] R.D. Starling, D.E. Matthews, P.A. Ades, E.T. Poehlman, Assessment of physical activity in older individuals: a doubly labeled water study, J. Appl. Physiol. 86 (1999) 2090–2096.

[133] S.B. Racette, S.K. Das, M. Bhapkar, E.C. Hadley, S.B. Roberts, E. Ravussin, et al., Approaches for quantifying energy intake and %calorie restriction during calorie restriction interventions in humans: the multicenter CALERIE study, Am. J. Physiol. Endocrinol. Metab. 302 (2012) E441–E448.

[134] E. Jequier, Y. Schutz, Long-term measurements of energy expenditure in humans using a respiration chamber, Am. J. Clin. Nutr. 38 (1983) 989–998.

[135] W.V. Rumpler, J.L. Seale, J.M. Conway, P.W. Moe, Repeatability of 24-h energy expenditure measurements in humans by indirect calorimetry, Am. J. Clin. Nutr. 51 (1990) 147–152.

[136] L. de Jonge, T. Nguyen, S.R. Smith, J.J. Zachwieja, H.J. Roy, G.A. Bray, Prediction of energy expenditure in a whole body indirect calorimeter at both low and high levels of physical activity, Int. J. Obes. Relat. Metab. Disord. 25 (2001) 929–934.

[137] L. de Jonge, J.P. DeLany, T. Nguyen, J. Howard, E.C. Hadley, L.M. Redman, et al., Validation study of energy expenditure and intake during calorie restriction using doubly labeled water and changes in body composition, Am. J. Clin. Nutr. 85 (2007) 73–79.

[138] D.A. Schoeller, E. van Santen, Measurement of energy expenditure in humans by doubly labeled water method, J. Appl. Physiol. 53 (1982) 955–959.

[139] N. Lifson, G.B. Gordon, R. McClintock, Measurement of total carbon dioxide production by means of D2O18, J. Appl. Physiol. 7 (1955) 704–710.

[140] R. McClintock, N. Lifson, Determination of the total carbon dioxide outputs of rats by the D2O18 method, Am. J. Physiol. 192 (1958) 76–78.

[141] N. Lifson, G.B. Gordon, M.B. Visscher, A.O. Nier, The fate of utilized molecular oxygen and the source of the oxygen of respiratory carbon dioxide, studied with the aid of heavy oxygen, J. Biol. Chem. 180 (1949) 803–811.

[142] D.A. Schoeller, Measurement of energy expenditure in free-living humans by using doubly labeled water, J. Nutr. 118 (1988) 1278–1289.

[143] J.P. DeLany, D.A. Schoeller, R.W. Hoyt, E.W. Askew, M.A. Sharp, Field use of D2 18O to measure energy expenditure of soldiers at different energy intakes, J. Appl. Physiol. 67 (1989) 1922–1929.

[144] S.B. Racette, D.A. Schoeller, A.H. Luke, K. Shay, J. Hnilicka, R.F. Kushner, Relative dilution spaces of 2H- and 18O-labeled water in humans, Am. J. Physiol. 267 (1994) E585–E590.

[145] S.B. Roberts, W. Dietz, T. Sharp, G.E. Dallal, J.O. Hill, Multiple laboratory comparison of the doubly labeled water technique, Obes. Res. 3 (Suppl. 1) (1995) 3–13.

[146] S.B. Roberts, J. Savage, W.A. Coward, B. Chew, A. Lucas, Energy expenditure and intake in infants born to lean and overweight mothers, N. Engl. J. Med. 318 (1988) 461–466.

[147] M.I. Goran, B.A. Gower, T.R. Nagy, R.K. Johnson, Developmental changes in energy expenditure and physical activity in children: evidence for a decline in physical activity in girls before puberty, Pediatrics 101 (1998) 887–891.

[148] L.E. Bratteby, B. Sandhagen, H. Fan, H. Enghardt, G. Samuelson, Total energy expenditure and physical activity as assessed by the doubly labeled water method in Swedish adolescents in whom energy intake was underestimated by 7-d diet records, Am. J. Clin. Nutr. 67 (1998) 905–911.

[149] G.R. Goldberg, A.M. Prentice, W.A. Coward, H.L. Davies, P.R. Murgatroyd, C. Wensing, et al., Longitudinal assessment of energy expenditure in pregnancy by the doubly labeled water method, Am. J. Clin. Nutr. 57 (1993) 494–505.

[150] S.W. Lichtman, K. Pisarska, E.R. Berman, M. Pestone, H. Dowling, E. Offenbacher, et al., Discrepancy between self-reported and actual caloric intake and exercise in obese subjects, N. Engl. J. Med. 327 (1992) 1893–1898.

[151] J. DeLany, G. Bray, D. Harsha, J. Volaufova, Energy expenditure and substrate oxidation predict change in body fat in children, Am. J. Clin. Nutr. 84 (2006) 862–870.

[152] B.A. Swinburn, G. Sacks, S.K. Lo, K.R. Westerterp, E.C. Rush, M. Rosenbaum, et al., Estimating the changes in energy flux that characterize the rise in obesity prevalence, Am. J. Clin. Nutr. 89 (2009) 1723–1728.

[153] P.S. Davies, J.M. Erskine, K.M. Hambidge, F.J. Accurso, Longitudinal investigation of energy expenditure in infants with cystic fibrosis, Eur. J. Clin. Nutr. 56 (2002) 940–946.

[154] R.W. Shepherd, L. Vasques-Velasquez, A. Prentice, T.L. Holt, W.A. Coward, A. Lucas, Increased energy expenditure in young children with cystic fibrosis, Lancet 331 (1988) 1300–1303.

[155] J.J. Reilly, J.C. Ventham, J.M. Ralston, M. Donaldson, B. Gibson, Reduced energy expenditure in preobese children treated for acute lymphoblastic leukemia, Pediatr. Res. 44 (1998) 557—562.

[156] M.I. Goran, E.J. Peters, D.N. Herndon, R.R. Wolfe, Total energy expenditure in burned children using the doubly labeled water technique, Am. J. Physiol. 259 (1990) E576—E585.

[157] A. Luke, N.J. Roizen, M. Sutton, D.A. Schoeller, Energy expenditure in children with Down syndrome: correcting metabolic rate for movement, J. Pediatr. 125 (1994) 829—838.

[158] R.K. Johnson, H.G. Hildreth, S.H. Contompasis, M.I. Goran, Total energy expenditure in adults with cerebral palsy as assessed by doubly labeled water, J. Am. Diet. Assoc. 97 (1997) 966—970.

[159] E.T. Poehlman, M.J. Toth, M.I. Goran, W.H. Carpenter, P. Newhouse, C.J. Rosen, Daily energy expenditure in free-living non-institutionalized Alzheimer's patients: a doubly labeled water study, Neurology 48 (1997) 997—1002.

[160] D.C. Macallan, C. Noble, C. Baldwin, S.A. Jebb, A.M. Prentice, W.A. Coward, et al., Energy expenditure and wasting in human immunodeficiency virus infection, N. Engl. J. Med. 333 (1995) 83—88.

[161] J. Trabulsi, D.A. Schoeller, Evaluation of dietary assessment instruments against doubly labeled water, a biomarker of habitual energy intake, Am. J. Physiol. Endocrinol. Metab. 281 (2001) E891—E899.

[162] C.M. Champagne, N.B. Baker, J.P. DeLany, D.W. Harsha, G.A. Bray, Assessment of energy intake underreporting by doubly labeled water and observations on reported nutrient intakes in children, J. Am. Diet. Assoc. 98 (1998) 426—433.

[163] R. Singh, B.R. Martin, Y. Hickey, D. Teegarden, W.W. Campbell, B.A. Craig, et al., Comparison of self-reported and measured metabolizable energy intake with total energy expenditure in overweight teens, Am. J. Clin. Nutr. 89 (2009) 1744—1750.

[164] R.L. Prentice, Y. Mossavar-Rahmani, Y. Huang, L. Van Horn, S. A.A. Beresford, B. Caan, et al., Evaluation and comparison of food records, recalls, and frequencies for energy and protein assessment by using recovery biomarkers, Am. J. Epidemiol. 174 (2011) 591—603.

A. ASSESSMENT METHODS FOR RESEARCH AND PRACTICE

P A R T B

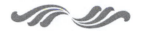

RESEARCH AND APPLIED METHODS FOR OBSERVATIONAL AND INTERVENTION STUDIES

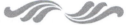

Application of Research Paradigms to Nutrition Practice

Carol J. Boushey

University of Hawaii Cancer Center, Honolulu, Hawaii

I INTRODUCTION

The importance of health-related research was eloquently stated by Professor Atkinson from the Department of Pediatrics at McMaster University while presenting the Ryley-Jeffs Memorial Lecture. In her lecture, she stated the following [1]:

> The 21st-century model of health research is founded on a broad base of multidisciplinary research that is expeditiously and effectively translated into evidence-based practice, education, policy, and advocacy. The key objective is to improve the health of populations.

Given that nutrition is involved in almost all of the metabolic processes of human life, there would be no argument that nutrition research clearly comprises an important part of health-related research. Nutrition plays critical roles in the etiology, progression, or treatment of the majority of chronic degenerative diseases contributing to the largest proportion of morbidity and mortality among the population of the United States. By virtue of the multidisciplinary role of nutrition, a field requiring knowledge in cellular and molecular biology, biochemistry, physiology, genetics, food science, and the social sciences, individuals trained in the field of nutrition are in an ideal position to discover and use health research.

To assist with the application of research to the practice of clinical and community nutrition, this chapter reviews several paradigms of research. Other chapters in this book cover specific research methods and study designs (see other chapters in Section 1). There is an emphasis on extracting information from all areas of research including the basic sciences. This chapter provides conceptual models and frameworks that can guide the practice of nutrition.

II BROAD RESEARCH AREAS

In the field of nutrition, research has been traditionally referred to as "basic" or "applied" research [2]. This dichotomous designation of nutrition research may be too simplistic. Goldstein and Brown [3] elaborated on a biomedical model that included basic science, disease-oriented research (DOR), and patient-oriented research (POR), particularly in reference to medical doctors. In the biomedical model, basic science involves the exploration of living systems at the molecular or tissue level. The DOR deliberately focuses on the pathogenesis or treatment of specific diseases, but it does not depend on patients. The POR would involve physicians treating the whole patient and observing, analyzing, and managing a patient. Recognition was made that all three areas are needed to achieve full understanding of the application of new discoveries to human health [3]. Although this model is not ideal with regard to referring to nutrition research, it does point to the difficulty of using the word "applied." In reality, this entire model is "applied" if it refers to the ultimate end point of improving the human condition. On the other hand, if "applied" refers to interaction with patients that would be only the POR. In other words, the term "applied" may not fully communicate the research activities to scientists or the public.

Nutrition in the Prevention and Treatment of Disease, Third Edition.
DOI: http://dx.doi.org/10.1016/B978-0-12-391884-0.00005-6

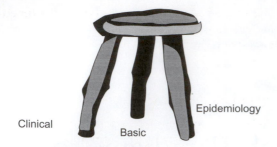

FIGURE 5.1   Research model: A three-legged stool.

One metaphor for research to consider is the three-legged stool as shown in Figure 5.1. In this model, the "legs" represent broad research areas. The "seat" represents research-based conclusions. The combined evidence from each broad research area is needed to keep the seat stable or keep the seat from falling down. An unbalanced stool would represent an incomplete picture from which to draw conclusions and recommendations. In this model, the basic research would involve examination of cellular models, biological specimens, or food components. This research is set apart in that no direct interaction occurs with human subjects. The clinical research refers to human studies that are under investigator control with regard to an intervention or treatment. The epidemiology studies would refer to observational studies using descriptive, prospective, or case—control study designs [4].

A Broad Research Areas Example

An example that demonstrates the importance of these three broad areas is the conundrum surrounding the consumption of nuts and the subsequent effect on body weight. Tree nuts and peanuts are considered to be high-fat, energy-dense foods; thus, their incorporation into a diet promoting energy balance would seem counterintuitive. However, evidence from the research areas of epidemiology, the clinical sciences, and the basic sciences suggests that the relationship between tree nuts and peanuts and weight maintenance bears reconsideration [5]. Using the broad areas represented by the three-legged stool, some examples of research regarding nuts are outlined here.

An epidemiological study design that ensures that the exposure measure (in this case, nut consumption) occurred before the outcome measure (in this case, body mass index) is the prospective cohort study [4]. Several reports from prospective analysis have been published with regard to nut consumption and body weight [6—8]. The Adventist Health Study enrolled 31,208 non-Hispanic white California Seventh-Day Adventists and collected extensive dietary data at baseline. In this cohort of adult men and women, a statistically significant negative association between the consumption of nuts and obesity as assessed by body mass index was found [6]. This was probably the earliest report indicating that those individuals with higher nut consumption were less likely to be obese compared to those individuals with lower nut consumption. Another well-known prospective analysis, the Nurses' Health Study [7], also reported a negative association between nut consumption and body mass index. Using data from the Physicians' Health Study, Albert *et al.* [8] reported no association between nut consumption and body mass index. The results from the studies noted here and from additional cross-sectional studies [9—11] have not reported a higher body mass index among frequent nut and peanut consumers compared to low consumers or nonconsumers. Collectively, these findings are compelling; however, to make a final consensus, one would want to determine if this relationship would hold under more controlled study conditions or the clinical "leg."

A quasi-experimental study was conducted with a sample of 15 healthy normal-weight adults [12]. The participants were provided additional energy as 500 kcal of peanuts to consume daily for 8 weeks on top of their usual diets. The sample size allowed the investigators to monitor the study participants closely with regard to following the protocol and collecting background dietary intake. With no compensation, the predicted weight gain was an average of 3.6 kg for the group. The measured change was only 1 kg or approximately 28% of the predicted level. These results suggest that additional energy from nuts may have less of an influence on weight than expected; however, the lack of a control group limits the conclusions that can be drawn. A study with an experimental design would be considered more useful. A prospective design using a randomized, crossover approach was completed among 20 healthy overweight adult women [13]. In this study, the women received 344 kcal of almonds daily for one 10-week period or no almonds for another 10 weeks with a 3-week washout between these two treatments. The theoretical weight gain was estimated to be 3.4 kg. However, the average weight of the participants was 70.4±9 kg at the start of the almond arm and 70.3±9 kg at the end, indicating no change. Other clinical studies have corroborated these results [5].

How might the basic science arm help with explaining these observations? Early work on this topic suggested greater energy loss from whole peanuts compared to peanut butter [14] and elevated fecal fat loss with nut consumption. As a result, a research team started to examine the nonstarch polysaccharides and phenolic compounds in the cell walls of almonds to possibly explain the epidemiological and clinical observations [15]. Using gas–liquid chromatography, high-performance liquid chromatography, and microscopy, it was observed that bioaccessibility is limited in nuts. This inefficiency stems from resistance of the parenchyma cells constituting the cell walls of nuts to microbial and enzymatic degradation. Thus, cells that are not ruptured during mastication may pass through the gastrointestinal tract without releasing the lipid they contain. Although insufficient information is available to estimate the amount of energy that may be unavailable, the findings provide an explanation for the epidemiological and clinical results.

The studies highlighted here represent only a sample of the varied research activities addressing the original observation made in 1992 from the Adventist Health Study [6]. Whereas some individuals may have been quick to change practice after reading the results of the Adventist Health Study, and other individuals may have been quick to discount the results, the lesson is that no one research area can provide a clear picture for which application to practice. Another caveat with this example is the lack of description of the contribution of results from animal models, which does not imply less importance to this research area. Admittedly, public health decisions can be made without full knowledge of biological plausibility [16]; however, practice is enhanced and more effective with a complete picture.

III EVIDENCE-BASED PRACTICE

In the 1990s, a movement within the medical profession made a concerted effort to steer away from reliance on expert opinion and start the process of informing practice decisions through a systematic examination of the scientific literature. An extensive series of manuscripts were published in *JAMA* starting with the Evidence-Based Medicine Working Group [17] and championed by two medical doctors, Gordon Guyatt and David Sackett [18]. Evidence-based medicine is a model for clinical decision making that integrates three elements: "best research evidence with clinical expertise and patient values" [19]. The research evidence includes clinically relevant research from the three areas of research discussed previously (epidemiology, clinical, and basic science). Clinical expertise recognizes that practitioners have clinical skills and past knowledge that can clarify consistent and unique patterns in patients. Each patient holds his or her own set of expectations, concerns, and preferences; thus the inclusion of patient values. These elements guide a patient's plan of care to optimize clinical outcomes and quality of life. Evidence-based medicine has broadened its scope to all health care practices to which the term "evidence-based practice" is applied.

A Steps to Achieve Evidence-Based Practice

The steps for evidence-based practice first include the recognition of a patient problem and constructing a structured clinical question [19,20]. For example, from the Evidence Analysis Library (EAL) of the American Dietetic Association, there is the question: "What gastric volume level should be reached before stopping/holding enteral nutrition?"

The second step is to efficiently and effectively search information resources to retrieve the best available evidence to answer the clinical question. This involves accessing available databases such as MEDLINE using the publicly available PubMed portal through the National Library of Medicine (www.nlm.nih.gov). Efficiently finding the best evidence may require learning about MeSH terms and appropriate filters. It would be important to use correct nomenclature. For example, prealbumin is not a precursor to albumin as implied by the name. Prealbumin is more accurately termed "transthyretin." The name selected by the Joint Commission on Biochemical Nomenclature best describes transthyretin's role as a serum transport protein for thyroxin and retinal binding protein. A PubMed search of prealbumin does not come up empty; however, a search of transthyretin generates three times the number of publications. One creates in advance some definitions of the type of study that would be most useful based on study design, patient outcomes, and exposures. Also, one decides in advance if reviews will be used.

Once applicable resources are gathered, the third step involves the critical appraisal of the evidence assembled. This step would involve assessing whether the selected report is relevant to the question and meets predetermined criteria of quality, such as study design, length of time, sample size, characteristics of sample, blinding, and use of current measures. Table 5.1 outlines the study designs of published manuscripts of original data as having an order of strongest to weakest empirical evidence when properly executed. Methods that synthesize primary research also have an order of strength of evidence. The quantitative synthesis methods, such as meta-analysis [21], are especially useful when sample sizes of individual studies tend to be small [22] or results tend to be inconsistent between studies [23]. The Agency for Healthcare and Research Quality within the U.S. Department of Health and Human Services has a number of modules for completing an evidence-based

TABLE 5.1 Study Types Listed in Order from Strongest to Weakest Evidence by Primary Research and Synthesis Research

Primary research of original data	Synthesis of primary research
EXPERIMENTAL STUDIES	**META-ANALYSIS**
Randomized controlled clinical trial	Decision analysis
Randomized crossover clinical trial	Cost–benefit analysis
Randomized controlled laboratory study	Cost-effectiveness study
OBSERVATIONAL STUDIES	**SYSTEMATIC REVIEW**
Prospective (cohort, longitudinal) study	
Case–control study	Narrative review
Ecological study	Consensus statement
Cross-sectional (prevalence) study	Consensus report
Population based	
Convenience sample	Medical opinion
Case series	
Case report	

practice review, as well as completed reports in a variety of areas (www.ahrq.gov/clinic/epcix.htm).

The fourth step is directed to gaining a full understanding of the study results through summarizing the evidence. A table outlining the results, as often used with meta-analysis, [22,23] can be useful at this stage. Various grading schemes are available for summarizing the strength of the collective evidence. Values range from 1 being good/strong to 2 being fair, 3 being limited/weak, 4 being expert opinion only, and 5 being grade not assignable. The number of studies meeting quality criteria would influence the final conclusion or recommendation.

In reality, the fifth and final step can only be made through integrating the evidence with the clinical information about the individual patient and the patient's desires and goals for care. Consideration of the best clinical care option for a patient is still the decision-making process of the health care practitioner with the patient. This can probably be best appreciated when one considers the number of options available for renal replacement therapy. The final decision is a complex process that ultimately will influence the patient's diet and the use of dietary supplements.

B Examples of Evidence-Based Practice in Nutrition

The American Dietetic Association has created an EAL that is available free to members of the association and available for a fee to others (www.adaevidencelibrary.com). Working groups have completed numerous evidence analyses and accompanying practice guidelines. This represents a rich resource for nutrition; however, the EAL does not release practitioners from actively engaging in the process. The final step still involves the application of professional judgment within the range of the patient's expressed priorities.

Other systematic reviews have been completed, and these reviews can be consulted for application to practice. The National Cholesterol Education Program has used a systematic review process to develop guidelines for cardiovascular disease [24]. Extensive systematic reviews of the influence of omega-3 fatty acids across a wide range of clinical conditions were completed [25]. For the 2010 "Dietary Guidelines," a systematic EAL review was used for the first time to develop this important policy document [26]. A number of limitations were identified regarding the published studies of omega-3 fatty acids and the "Dietary Guidelines" report. Many of the limitations were common to all health sciences research, such as poor study design, lack of information about an intervention, and nondiverse samples. However, problems unique to omega-3 fatty acids and nutrition in general were identified. When dealing with a pharmaceutical drug, there is little difference in the active substance other than dose. In contrast, omega-3 fatty acids and other nutrients may be available in different forms that vary in bioavailability or metabolic activity. Furthermore, food sources of nutrients add the complexity of variation in concentration and the possibility of other constituents in the food interfering with absorption. The circulating levels of a nutrient, which may be a biomarker of compliance, may be influenced by other metabolic factors. One of the most serious problems is the lack of attention to the baseline dietary intake or the background diet. Many studies do not even communicate that the study subjects, whether in the intervention or control groups, may have been independently consuming the nutrient of interest. Thus, the systematic compilation of evidence for nutrition will continue to present challenges not faced by other health fields.

The individual in clinical nutrition practice may question the need to be concerned with results from basic research or even research in general. A well-meaning guide for the busy clinician even suggested that just scanning an abstract and the results section of a research article would provide maximum information for the reader [27]. However, this could not be further from the truth [28]. To base practice on scientific principles, original research by necessity deserves more than a quick scan. Otherwise, a complete understanding of any results cannot be fully appreciated. The serious practitioner will make time to become familiar with each "leg" of science related to his or her area of expertise or special practice. A study of registered dietitians found that those individuals who read professional publications weekly compared to monthly had higher perceptions, attitudes, and knowledge toward evidence-based practice [29].

IV TRANSLATIONAL RESEARCH

The most recent research paradigm is "translational research." This paradigm grew from the desire to link the discoveries of molecular networks in health and disease to the patient and public benefit [30]. The challenge calls for novel interdisciplinary approaches to advance science and improve the health of the nation. The Translational Research Working Group of the National Cancer Institute reached consensus on an operational definition of translational research as "research that transforms scientific discoveries arising in the lab, clinic, or population into new clinical tools and applications that reduce cancer incidence, morbidity, and mortality." Education and practice in nutrition require knowledge and skills in the biological and social sciences [2]. As a result, nutrition is well positioned to be a player in interdisciplinary research.

Figure 5.2 depicts translational research and signifies that discovery may occur anywhere in the cycle (i.e., at the bench, clinical, or population level). As noted with the three-legged stool model, all of these areas of research interact and depend on one another. The aspect of the translational model that separates this model from the others is the additional step of developing new tools and applications for use as new chemotherapeutic drugs, new devices, nontraditional approaches [31], behavioral interventions, new screening assays, and educational training. Dissemination to health care providers, patients, and the public is considered a part of the research process. Furthermore, these new tools feed back into the discovery cycle. Should the new intervention not perform as expected, then this observation will generate new research to ensure that dissemination brings improvement to the nation's health.

The combined results from the bench, clinical, and population sciences regarding calcium and bone in youth are thoroughly covered in Chapter 44. This information is briefly summarized here to show the application of translational research in nutrition. Dietary intake data from the U.S. Department of Agriculture's "What We Eat in America, 2001–2002 NHANES" [32] showed that the average calcium intakes of adolescent girls and boys aged 9–13 years were well below the calcium recommendations set by the Institute of Medicine for girls and boys aged 9–18 years at that

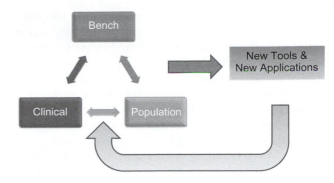

FIGURE 5.2 Translational research model.

time [33,34]. One of the major lines of evidence to establish the recommendation in this age group was calcium retention to meet peak bone mineral accretion. Furthermore, older teens tended to drink more carbonated beverages, fruit drinks, and citrus juice but less milk and noncitrus juices [35]. Because of the increase in non-calcium-rich beverages, there was a concern that the lack of calcium intake during adolescence can contribute to poor bone formation, which may potentially increase risk for osteoporosis in later life [36]. Because bone mass accrues until the peak is reached by early adulthood, maximizing peak bone mass within an individual's genetic potential requires optimal calcium intakes throughout growth. This is especially important during adolescence when the rate of calcium accretion is highest because approximately half an adult's bone mass accumulates during these few short years [37].

Clearly, the preceding information fed to the application of a targeted intervention to young girls. French and colleagues [38] developed a theoretically based intervention that incorporated behavior-changing activities into Girl Scout programs called the CAL-Girls study. The messages were directed to girls of 9–11 years old. At the end of the intensive program that was uniformly delivered, significant changes were observed for increases in dietary calcium intake; however, no significant intervention effects were observed for bone mineral content at any specific bone site. Furthermore, no gains were made in increasing weight-bearing physical activity. Therefore, the results fed back into the research cycle to initiate new research questions. Specifically, more data are needed on optimal dosages of weight-bearing physical activity and level of behavior change for consumption of calcium-rich foods needed to effect bone mass gains in early adolescent girls. Furthermore, the following question is raised: How can behavioral models be modified to better reflect positive changes in adolescents? Completely unrelated to the dosage is the concern that the methods of measuring diet and physical activity cannot adequately distinguish changes in intake or output. This type of feedback about inadequate assessment techniques has generated a number of research programs directed to improving the measurements of diet and physical activity.

The other primary target of translational research is the reduction of health disparities among subgroups. For translational linkages to occur among marginalized groups, an appreciation of the benefits of community-engaged research methods has emerged. Community-based participatory research (CBPR) refers to the formation of partnerships between community and academia to enhance the capacity to engage in discovery for translation to policy advocacy aimed at eliminating health disparities. Use of CBPR forges partnerships and breaks down the barriers between researchers and the ultimate beneficiaries. Working closely with the community and employing community members strengthens study design and implementation. The incorporation of cultural values and local knowledge creates more effective solutions to complex problems. Fialkowski and colleagues [39] outline a framework for researchers to apply CBPR drawing from historical, cultural, and current health research on Native Americans and Alaska Natives. Use of CBPR among communities in central Detroit for capacity building for public policy advocacy represents one of the more mature CBPR programs in the United States [40].

V SUMMARY

This chapter introduced several research paradigms used to assist researchers and practitioners in reaching a common goal of enhancing the health of the nation. All individuals in the field of nutrition engage with research either through the discovery process or through the learning process. The latter constitutes the synthesis of research studies to identify current best practices. With the advent of technologies, nutrition practitioners have available numerous resources to form work groups, access original published literature, and summarize evidence within the context of their working environments.

References

[1] S.A. Atkinson, A nutrition odyssey: knowledge discovery, translation, and outreach. 2006 Ryley—Jeffs Memorial Lecture, Can. J. Diet. Pract. Res. 67 (2006) 150—156.

[2] Special Committee of the Food and Nutrition Board of the Institute of Medicine, National Academy of Sciences, Opportunities in the nutritions and food sciences: research challenges and the next generation of investigators, J. Nutr. 124 (1994) 763—769.

[3] J.L. Goldstein, M.S. Brown, The clinical investigator: bewitched, bothered, and bewildered—but still beloved, J. Clin. Invest. 99 (1997) 2803—2812.

[4] C. Boushey, J. Harris, V. Bruemmer, S.L. Archer, L. Van Horn, Publishing nutrition research: a review of study design, statistical analyses, and other key elements of manuscript preparation, Part 1, J. Am. Diet. Assoc. 106 (2006) 89—96.

[5] M. St.-Onge, Dietary fats, teas, dairy, and nuts: potential functional foods for weight control? Am. J. Clin. Nutr. 81 (2005) 7—15.

[6] G.E. Fraser, J. Sabate, W.L. Beeson, T.M. Strahan, A possible protective effect of nut consumption on risk of coronary heart disease, Arch. Intern. Med. 152 (1992) 1416—1424.

[7] F.B. Hu, M.J. Stampfer, J.E. Manson, E.B. Rimm, G.A. Colditz, B. A. Rosner, et al., Frequent nut consumption and risk of coronary heart disease in women: prospective cohort study, BMJ 317 (1998) 1341—1345.

[8] C.M. Albert, J.M. Gaziano, W.C. Willett, J.E. Manson, Nut consumption and decreased risk of sudden cardiac death in the Physicians' Health Study, Arch. Intern. Med. 162 (2002) 1382—1387.

[9] J.L. Ellsworth, L.H. Kushi, A.R. Folsom, Frequent nut intake and risk of death from coronary heart disease and all causes in postmenopausal women: The Iowa Women's Health Study, Nutr. Metab. Cardiovasc. Dis. 11 (2001) 372—377.

[10] J. Sabate, Nut consumption and body weight, Am. J. Clin. Nutr. 78 (3 Suppl.) (2003) 647S—650S.

[11] A.E. Griel, B. Eissenstat, V. Juturu, G. Hsieh, P.M. Kris-Etherton, Improved diet quality with peanut consumption, J. Am. Coll. Nutr. 23 (2004) 660—668.

[12] C.M. Alper, R.D. Mattes, The effects of chronic peanut consumption on energy balance and hedonics, Int. J. Obes. 26 (2002) 1129—1137.

[13] J.H. Hollis, R.D. Mattes, Effect of chronic consumption of almonds on body weight in healthy humans, Br. J. Nutr. 98 (2007) 651—656.

[14] A.S. Levine, S.E. Silvis, Absorption of whole peanuts, peanut oil, and peanut butter, N. Engl. J. Med. 303 (1980) 917—918.

[15] P.R. Ellis, C.W.C. Kendall, Y. Ren, C. Parker, J.F. Pacy, K.W. Waldron, et al., Role of cell walls in the bioaccessibility of lipids in almond seeds, Am. J. Clin. Nutr. 80 (2004) 604—613.

[16] K.J. Rothman, Epidemiology: An Introduction, Oxford University Press, New York, 2002.

[17] Evidence-Based Medicine Working Group, Evidence-based medicine: a new approach to teaching the practice of medicine, JAMA 268 (1992) 2420—2425.

[18] A.D. Oxman, D.L. Sackett, G.H. Guyatt, Users' guides to the medical literature: i. How to get started. The Evidence-Based Medicine Working Group, JAMA 270 (1993) 2093—2095.

[19] Centre for Evidence-Based Medicine. Available at <www.cebm. net>, 2007. Accessed 08.09.07

[20] R. Hatala, S.A. Keitz, M.C. Wilson, G. Guyatt, Moving toward an integrated evidence-based medicine curriculum, J. Gen. Intern. Med. 21 (2006) 538—541.

[21] D.B. Petitti, Meta-Analysis, Decision Analysis, and Cost-Effectiveness Analysis, second ed., Oxford University Press, New York, 2000.

[22] D. Savaiano, C.J. Boushey, G.P. McCabe, Lactose intolerance symptoms assessed by meta-analysis: a grain of truth that leads to exaggeration, J. Nutr. 136 (2006) 1107—1113.

[23] C.J. Boushey, S.A.A. Beresford, G.S. Omenn, A.G. Motulsky, A quantitative assessment of plasma homocysteine as a risk factor for vascular disease: probable benefits of increasing folic acid intakes, JAMA 274 (1995) 1049−1057.

[24] L. Van Horn, N. Ernst, A summary of the science supporting the new National Cholesterol Education Program dietary recommendations: what dietitians should know, J. Am. Diet. Assoc. 101 (2001) 1148−1154.

[25] E.M. Balk, T.A. Horsley, S.J. Newberry, A.H. Lichtenstein, E.A. Yetley, H.M. Schachter, et al., A collaborative effort to apply the evidence-based review process to the field of nutrition: challenges, benefits, and lessons learned, Am. J. Clin. Nutr. 85 (2007) 1448−1456.

[26] J.M. Spahn, J.M. Lyon, J.M. Altman, D.M. Blum-Kemelor, E.V. Essery, T.V. Fungwe, et al., The systematic review methodology used to support the 2010 Dietary Guidelines Advisory Committee, J. Am. Diet. Assoc. 111 (2011) 520−523.

[27] E.A. Crist, Mapping a practice route through the journal, J. Am. Diet. Assoc. 99 (1999) 1041−1042.

[28] R.D. Mattes, C.J. Boushey, To read or not to read original research articles: it should not be a question, J. Am. Diet. Assoc. 100 (2000) 171−174.

[29] L.D. Byham-Gray, J.A. Gilbride, L.B. Dixon, F.K. Stage, Evidence-based practice: what are dietitians' perceptions, attitudes, and knowledge? J. Am. Diet. Assoc. 105 (2005) 1574−1581.

[30] E.A. Zerhouni, U.S. biomedical research: basic, translational, and clinical sciences, JAMA 294 (2005) 1352−1358.

[31] O. Szczurko, K. Cooley, J.W. Busse, D. Seely, B. Bernhardt, G.H. Guyatt, et al., Naturopathic care for chronic low back pain: a randomized trial, PLoS One 2 (2007) e919.

[32] A. Moshfegh, J. Goldman, L. Cleveland, What We Eat in America, NHANES 2001−2002: Usual Nutrient Intakes from Food Compared to Dietary Reference Intakes, U.S. Department of Agriculture, Agricultural Research Service, Washington, DC, 2005.

[33] Institute of Medicine, National Academy of Sciences, Dietary Reference Intakes for Calcium, Phosphorus, Magnesium, Vitamin D, and Fluoride, National Academies Press, Washington, DC, 1997.

[34] ARS Food Surveys Research Group, Food and Nutrient Intakes by Children 1994−96, 1998, U.S. Department of Agriculture, Agricultural Research Service, Washington, DC, 1999.

[35] L.G. Weinbery, L.A. Berner, J.E. Groves, Nutrient contributions of dairy foods in the United States: continuing survey of food intakes by individuals, 1994−1996, 1998, J. Am. Diet. Assoc. 104 (2004) 895−902.

[36] S.A. Bowman, Beverage choices of young females: changes and impact on nutrient intakes, J. Am. Diet. Assoc. 102 (2002) 1234−1239.

[37] C.M. Weaver, The growing years and prevention of osteoporosis later in life, Proc. Nutr. Soc. 59 (2000) 303−306.

[38] S.A. French, M. Storey, J.A. Fulkerson, J.H. Himes, P. Hannan, D. Neumark-Sztainer, et al., Increasing weight-bearing physical activity and calcium-rich foods to promote bone mass among 9−11 year old girls: outcome of the Cal-Girls Study, Int. J. Behav. Nutr. Phys. Act. 2 (2005) 1−11.

[39] M.K. Fialkowski, T.A. Okoror, C.J. Boushey, The relevancy of community-based methods: using diet within Native American and Alaska Native adult populations as an example, Clin. Transl. Sci. (2012) [Epub ahead of print].

[40] B.A. Israel, C.M. Coombe, R.R. Cheezum, A.J. Schulz, R.J. McGranaghan, R. Lichtenstein, et al., Community-based participatory research: a capacity-building approach for policy advocacy aimed at eliminating health disparities, Am. J. Public Health 100 (2010) 2094−2102.

Overview of Nutritional Epidemiology

Lisa Cadmus-Bertram, Ruth E. Patterson

University of California at La Jolla, San Diego, California

I INTRODUCTION

Epidemiology is the science of public health whose laboratory setting is human populations. Specifically, epidemiology is the study of the distribution and determinants of disease frequency in human populations [1]. Epidemiology addresses such questions as who gets a disease, when, and why; this information is then used to create strategies for prevention or treatment. Nutritional epidemiology is the study of how dietary factors relate to the occurrence of disease in human populations. For example, observations that persons who consumed fish at least twice a week had a lower risk of incident cardiovascular disease (CVD) and stroke as well as lower risk of sudden cardiac death than persons who ate no fish [2,3] led to widespread recommendations to include fish in the diet for CVD prevention. Similarly, population-based studies demonstrating that consumption of trans fatty acids may be associated with unfavorable blood lipid profiles have led to the decline in use of these fats by food manufacturers and outright bans by some local health departments [4–7]. Another major finding by nutritional epidemiologists that has had major public health policy implications was the observation that use of multivitamins containing folic acid during pregnancy reduced the risk of neural tube defects in the fetus. Consistent evidence from numerous epidemiologic studies led to the fortification of the U.S. food supply with folic as a primary prevention strategy in 1998 [8,9]. Thus, some of the major nutrition-related public health contributions of the past 50 years have been made possible by nutritional epidemiology.

One factor that distinguishes the discipline of nutritional epidemiology is the extraordinary challenge of accurately assessing exposure. In epidemiology, exposure is defined as participant characteristics, lifestyle behaviors, or agents (e.g., food, medications such as hormone replacement therapy, tobacco, and sun) with which a participant comes into contact that may be related to disease risk (Table 6.1) [10]. Measuring dietary intake is particularly complex for many reasons. For purposes of illustration, we can compare the assessment challenges for two common exposures: cigarette smoking and diet. Smoking is a simple (yes/no) activity, so individuals can accurately report whether or not they smoke. Because smoking is addictive, it tends to be a consistent long-term behavior. Furthermore, because smoking is a habit, most people smoke roughly the same number of cigarettes per day (i.e., one or two packs per day). In comparison, during the course of even 1 week, an individual can consume hundreds, even thousands, of distinct food items in various combinations, making it cognitively challenging for respondents to accurately report their intake. Meals can be prepared by others (e.g., in a restaurant, by a spouse, and as prepackaged food) so that the respondent may not be cognizant of preparation details such as fat or salt used in cooking or portion size. Food choices typically vary with seasons and other life activities (e.g., weekends, holidays, and vacations). In fact, the day-to-day variability in food intake can be so large that it is not possible to identify any underlying consistent dietary pattern. In addition, foods are often a surrogate for the exposure of interest (e.g., dietary fat or fiber), which means that investigators must rely on food composition databases to calculate the exposure variable. Given the problems inherent in assessing dietary intake, it is not surprising that despite some of the important contributions noted previously, it has been difficult to obtain consistent and strong evidence regarding how diet affects disease risk.

The vast majority of nutritional epidemiologic research in the past 25 years has focused on the identification

Nutrition in the Prevention and Treatment of Disease, Third Edition.
DOI: http://dx.doi.org/10.1016/B978-0-12-391884-0.00006-8

TABLE 6.1   Examples of Exposures Relevant to Nutritional Epidemiologic Studies

Exposure	Diet-related example	Other example
Agent that may cause or protect from disease	Vegetable consumption may be protective for colon cancer.	Physical activity may be protective for colon cancer.
Constitutional host factors	Genetic predisposition to nutrition-related disease.	Older adults are more predisposed to chronic disease.
Other host factors	Food preferences that determine food choices.	More educated adults may have better disease screening.
Agents that may confound the association between another agent and disease	Correlation between dietary constituents (e.g., a diet high in fruits and vegetables is usually low in fat).	Smokers are less likely to engage in physical activity.
Agents that may modify effects of other agents	Fruits and vegetables may protect against lung cancer among smokers.	Alcohol results in increased risk of lung cancer from smoking.
Agents that may determine outcome of disease	Malnutrition.	Medical treatment.

of foods and/or specific nutrients in foods that prevent or promote the occurrence of chronic diseases, such as cancer, diabetes, and CVD. Therefore, the tools and methods of nutritional epidemiology were developed to address scientific issues unique to the biology of chronic disease, including the extensive time for disease development and the multifactorial nature of these diseases. Furthermore, epidemiologic research is generally conducted in free-living humans, which establishes associations only and precludes direct tests of cause and effect. Each of these challenges is discussed here.

A Extensive Time for Disease Development

Chronic diseases develop over many years and even decades. This fact has important implications for the field of nutritional epidemiology. For example, the currently accepted model of colon cancer assumes that it is a multistep pathogenic pathway beginning with mutations (germline or somatic) leading to growth of polyps (preneoplastic growths), which become adenomas and progress to carcinoma [11]. Even after an adenoma finally develops, many years may elapse before it is clinically detected. Upon clinical detection of colon cancer, it is clear that a meal consumed that day, or the month before, could have no significant effect on the disease for two reasons. First, the critical period of

cancer initiation and promotion likely occurred many years prior to disease diagnosis. Second, the biologically relevant exposure is the long-term or usual diet, rather than any single eating occasion. Therefore, the exposure of interest in the development of cancer occurred throughout the previous 10–20 years and perhaps the previous 5 years for CVD and diabetes.

This time lag between dietary exposure and disease occurrence presents considerable difficulties in the study of diet and chronic disease. These difficulties have been addressed in two major ways. First, dietary assessment instruments for epidemiology were developed to capture information on usual, long-term dietary intake [12]. The most common is the food frequency questionnaire. Second, study designs developed in other areas of epidemiology were applied to studies of diet-disease risk: case–control and cohort studies. These designs were already being used to gather data on remote exposures (i.e., use of oral contraceptives and age at menarche) or life events (i.e., age at first pregnancy and number of full-term pregnancies), which proved to be very useful for establishing associations of various risk factors with disease risk [1]. For example, asking detailed questions about reproductive history to women with and without breast cancer has provided extremely useful and reliable data about breast cancer risk factors. Using the same approach, nutritional epidemiologists have asked people about retrospective diet in case–control studies or assessed current diet in cohort studies and followed participants over time to monitor incidence of disease. The difficulty with the latter approach is that it often takes years or decades for disease to develop, and during that time, study participants may markedly alter their usual dietary habits.

B Multifactorial Nature of Chronic Diseases

Chronic diseases such as cancer and CVD have complex etiologies that are multifactorial in nature. In addition to diet, other determinants of chronic diseases include host factors (e.g., genetic susceptibility) and other lifestyle habits (e.g., cigarette smoking, physical activity, and alcohol intake). These other factors may confound our ability to find an association of dietary intake with disease risk. For example, individuals with an interest in health may eat a low-fat diet high in fruits and vegetables and have high physical activity levels. If vegetable intake is found to be associated with reduced risk of colon cancer, it can be difficult to disentangle whether it is the high vegetable intake or the low fat intake that affects disease risk. It is also possible that diet is not related to disease risk but is merely serving as a marker for some other healthful behavior, such as physical activity or adherence to cancer screening guidelines [13].

Another illustration of the multifactorial nature of chronic disease is the complex relationship between dietary factors and a person's genetic constitution. For example, the phase II enzymes glutathione-*S*-transferases (GSTs) are upregulated by vegetables from the *Brassica* family (broccoli, Brussels sprouts, and cauliflower) such that compounds in these vegetables increase the activity of this family of enzymes [14–16]. There is also growing evidence that the health benefits of *Brassica* vegetables may vary depending on whether a person has any of the common genetic variations in these enzymes. Humans with a GSTM1 null (approximately 50% of U.S. Caucasians and 35% of African Americans) or GSTT1 null (approximately 15% of U.S. Caucasians and 25% of African Americans) have greatly reduced (heterozygote) or no (homozygote) enzyme activity [14]. Among those with the null variants, compounds in the *Brassica* vegetable, such as isothiocyanates, may be metabolized and eliminated more slowly, so they may be available for a longer period of time in target tissues and organs [17]. Several studies have found stronger associations of *Brassica* vegetables with reduced risks of lung [18], breast [19], and colon cancer [20] among persons GSTM1 and/or GSTT1 null. This example of a diet–gene interaction illustrates the complexity and multifactorial nature of diet-related chronic disease development.

C Research in Human Beings

There are several important considerations with regard to conducting research in humans. Notably, population-based nutrition research or nutritional epidemiology is often conducted among healthy persons, at least at the time of initial assessment. For studies that involve dietary interventions, federal guidelines for the protection of human subjects dictate that study participants (both healthy and diseased) cannot (knowingly) be exposed to potentially dangerous dietary regimes that restrict essential nutrients or introduce known carcinogens at high levels over long periods of time. However, short-term controlled feeding studies can reasonably test the effect of potentially harmful food constituents for the purpose of learning about nutrient metabolism and disease mechanisms in relation to food intake [21]. For example, participants can be fed charred meat containing nitrosamines to learn how humans metabolize or eliminate such potential carcinogens [22,23], or they can be fed restricted diets devoid of certain nutrients to learn about nutrient absorption, metabolism, and excretion [24,25]. Indeed, such information is critical for public health recommendations regarding nutrient requirements. These tightly controlled human feeding or intervention studies are expensive and laborious and therefore are not feasible to conduct in a large-scale manner, especially when studying general population risk. For these reasons, nutritional epidemiology is primarily an observational discipline that consists largely of (1) measuring an exposure (e.g., usual dietary intake), (2) measuring an outcome (e.g., disease occurrence), and (3) using statistical techniques to quantify the magnitude of the association between these two observations and adjust for potential confounders.

II PRINCIPLES OF EXPOSURE MEASUREMENT IN NUTRITIONAL EPIDEMIOLOGY

A variety of dietary assessment methods are used in nutritional epidemiology. The choice of instrument used depends on the hypothesis being tested, the population being studied, and cost considerations. The three primary tools are food frequency questionnaires, 24-hour dietary recalls, and food diaries or records. Here, we briefly describe these instruments and discuss the issues of error and bias associated with self-reported dietary intake.

A Food Frequency Questionnaires

Chronic disease risk develops over many years. As such, the biologically relevant exposure is usual or long-term diet, consumed many years prior to the appearance of clinical symptoms and disease diagnosis. Therefore, assessment instruments that only capture data on recent dietary intake (e.g., food records or recall) may not be as useful for studies examining chronic diseases that evolve over years or decades. For these reasons, food frequency questionnaires (FFQs) have been regarded as the dietary assessment instrument best suited for most epidemiologic applications [12]. Although the design of FFQs can vary somewhat, they typically contain the following sections: (1) adjustment questions, (2) the food checklist, and (3) summary questions.

FFQs often contain adjustment questions that assess the nutrient content of specific food items. For example, participants are asked what type of milk they usually drink and are given several options (e.g., whole, skim, and soy). Adjustment questions also permit more refined analyses of fat intake by asking about food preparation practices (e.g., removing fat from red meat) and types of added fats (e.g., use of butter vs. margarine on bread). The main section consists of a food or food group checklist, with questions on usual frequency of intake and portion size. The foods are selected to capture data on (1) major sources of energy and nutrients for most people, (2) between-person variability in food intake, and (3) major hypotheses regarding diet and disease. Frequency of consumption is typically categorized from "never or less than once per month" to "2+ per day" for foods and "6+ per day" for beverages. Portion sizes are often assessed by asking respondents to mark "small," "medium," or "large" in comparison to a given medium portion size. However, some questionnaires ask only about the frequency of intake of a "usual" portion size (e.g., 1 cup of milk). In the latter instances, respondents are asked to calculate the frequency of the amount given rather than actual serving size consumed. Summary questions ask about usual intake of fruits and vegetables because the long lists of these foods (needed to capture micronutrient intake) lead to overreporting of intake [26].

Note that development of a FFQ is a daunting, complex task requiring considerable understanding of exposure measurement in nutritional epidemiology, food composition knowledge, formatting and questionnaire design expertise, and computer programming resources [27,28]. A major limitation of FFQs are that they may be fraught with both random measurement error and bias, which limits their usefulness [29,30]. See Section V for details regarding error in FFQs.

B Measures of Short-Term Dietary Intake: Food Recalls and Records

Food records and 24-hour dietary recalls are the other common tools used in nutritional epidemiology [12]. Food records or diaries require individuals to record all foods and beverages consumed during a specified period of time, usually 3–7 days. Participants are asked to carry the record with them and to record foods as eaten in real time. Some protocols require participants to weigh and/or measure foods before eating and review the record with a registered dietitian, whereas less stringent protocols use food models or other aids to instruct respondents on estimating serving sizes and do not engage in extensive review or documentation [31]. To obtain nutrient estimates, the food consumption information from records/diaries must be entered into a specialized software program. This data-entry step is a time-consuming task and requires trained data technicians or registered dietitians. Food records are burdensome for study participants and, due to the staff time required, are expensive to administer. Therefore, for large epidemiologic studies with tens of thousands of study participants, food records are cost prohibitive.

In the foreseeable future, the use of personal digital assistants, digital cameras, mobile telephones, and other electronic devices both to record and to transmit food record data will likely alleviate some of the participant burden [32]. As with a paper-and-pencil food record, participants carry the electronic device with them during the assessment period. They are either asked to record each food and beverage as it is consumed or prompted every few hours to enter recently eaten foods. Electronic food records can produce intake estimates comparable to those from traditional food records or recalls [33]. Alternatively, mobile phones or digital cameras may be used to photograph each meal, snack, or beverage [34]. In these studies, a fiducial marker (an object of known dimensions) is often placed next to the food to provide a reference point for size. The foods are then identified and quantified either automatically by specialized software or manually by a trained technician. The participant may be asked to take both a "before" and an "after" photograph so that the amount consumed can be estimated. A third approach is the use of websites on which participants can record their intake. Because only a standard web browser is required, this can be a good strategy for individuals who already have access to a smartphone or tablet.

Electronic approaches such as these allow for more comprehensive recording than a paper-and-pencil survey and are particularly appealing for certain populations, such as school-aged children and adolescents [35]. Conversely, they may not be suitable for individuals who are unfamiliar or uncomfortable using technology. Photograph-based methods are convenient for participants but are limited by the lack of descriptive information about the foods and beverages in the photographs; even a highly trained dietician can only guess at the ingredients or preparation method used. The cost of technology-based approaches compared to paper-based recalls is variable, depending on the method used for intake quantification (automated/computerized vs. manual). Furthermore, the need to purchase, distribute, and recover the electronic devices limits the feasibility of this approach for large studies.

Twenty-four-hour dietary recalls are frequently used in population-based studies, including the National Health and Nutrition Examination (NHANES) surveys and *What We Eat in America* [36]. Data from these recalls provide snapshots of U.S. eating patterns and are used for formulations of dietary recommendations. A 24-hour dietary recall is a 20- to 30-minute interview in which the respondent is asked to recall all foods and beverages consumed during the previous 24 hours.

Ideally, the interview is conducted with real-time direct data entry into a software program for analysis. It is important that the interviewer be well trained; tone of voice, body posture (when in-person), and reactions to participant descriptions of foods consumed can influence the quality of the data.

A single recall is suitable for characterizing mean intakes of groups, such as the U.S. Department of Agriculture (USDA) survey titled *What We Eat in America* [36]. However, for individual assessment, day-to-day variability of food intake is so high that for both records and recalls, several days of data are required to characterize usual intake for an individual. Using data on variability in intake from food records completed by 194 participants in the Nurses' Health Study [12], the number of days needed to estimate the mean intakes for individuals within 10% of "true" means would be 57 days for fat, 117 days for vitamin C, and 67 days for calcium. For estimating food consumption for individuals, variability can be even greater. For example, the number of days needed to estimate foods within 10% of "true" means would be 55 days for white fish and 217 days for carrots. Unfortunately, research has shown that reported energy intake, nutrient intake, and recorded numbers of foods decrease with as few as 4 days of recording dietary intake [37]. These changes may reflect reduced accuracy and completeness of recording intake or actual changes in dietary intake to reduce the burden of recording intake. Because of the participant burden, dietary recalls or records are generally only kept for 3 or 4 days. Most protocols require that one of these days be a weekend day. Although a random selection of days would be ideal, food records are generally kept for 4 days in a row to improve response rates.

In 2009, the National Cancer Institute released a web-based 24-hour dietary recall instrument, the Automated Self-Administered 24-Hour Recall (ASA24) [38,114]. The ASA uses a modified version of the USDA's Automated Multiple-Pass Approach, which aims to improve recall quality by giving participants several opportunities at which to recall a food item. During the first step of the recall, the participant identifies foods and beverages eaten at each meal or snack. The web-based program then asks the participant whether anything was consumed during each of the gaps between meals/snacks, offering a second chance to add forgotten items. Participants are then asked about the details of each food/beverage item, such as the serving size, container type (for beverages), amount of serving consumed, and any condiments or toppings. Pictures are used to help participants select the appropriate responses. The program then asks the participant to review a list of foods and beverages that are commonly forgotten by respondents, such as water or candy. After a final review, participants are offered one additional opportunity to report items. The last item asks the participant whether the reported consumption is representative of his or her usual daily intake. Supplement information may also be collected if specified by the investigator. The ASA24 instrument is offered in English and Spanish, and efforts are underway to adapt the ASA24 for use with school-aged children.

In theory, the ASA24 offers the benefits of traditional telephone-based or in-person recalls while removing much of the expense. The ASA24 is available at no cost to researchers and is intended for self-administration by participants, eliminating the need for data entry or computation by trained dietitians. Some participant populations, however, may find it difficult to report their diet accurately using the system. This is particularly likely for individuals who are not accustomed to using a computer, are low literacy, or who eat a lot of home-prepared dishes with many ingredients. The lack of a human interviewer to answer questions and probe for clarification may exacerbate these issues. Finally, more research is needed to document its measurement characteristics. Other web-based recall approaches include the Oxford WebQ [39], DietDay [40], and the National Cancer Institute's targeted instruments (the Fruit and Vegetable Scan and Block Fat Screener) [41].

C Vitamin/Mineral Supplement Assessment

Historically, less attention has been paid to measuring vitamin/mineral supplement use compared to food intake. However, assessing vitamin/mineral supplement use is important because supplement use per se is an exposure of interest for the risk of several chronic diseases [42–46]. In addition, supplements are used by approximately half of all Americans, so they contribute a large proportion of total (diet plus supplement) micronutrient intake [27,47–49]. Epidemiologic studies typically use personal interviews or self-administered questionnaires to obtain information on three to five general classes of multiple vitamins (multivitamins with or without minerals, stress supplements, antioxidant mixtures, and other mixtures, including multivitamins with herbals), single supplements, the dose of single supplements, and sometimes frequency and/or duration of use [50].

In a validity study comparing a self-administered assessment method to label transcription among 104 supplement users, we found correlation coefficients ranging from 0.1 for iron to 0.8 for vitamin C [50]. The principal sources of error were investigator error in assigning the micronutrient composition of multiple vitamins and respondent confusion regarding the distinction between multiple vitamins and single supplements. These results suggest that commonly used epidemiologic methods of assessing supplement use may incorporate significant amounts of error in estimates of some nutrients. In a subsequent study, we found that a similar inventory reporting system captured supplement use when compared to blood, toenail, and urine biomarkers [48,51]. In a marketplace that is becoming rapidly more complex, with vitamins, minerals, and botanical compounds combined in unusual mixtures at highly variable doses, the association of dietary supplements with disease risk is becoming increasingly difficult, but important, to assess [52].

D Use of Biomarkers in Nutritional Epidemiology

Dietary biomarkers have been critical to the advancement of nutritional epidemiology and have led to huge advances in our understanding of errors in self-reported dietary intake [29,53]. Biomarkers from blood, urine, or stool specimens or toenails can provide objective estimates of dietary intake and therefore circumvent problems associated with self-reported diet such as underreporting. Two major drawbacks of biomarkers are that (1) biological specimens are expensive to collect, store, and analyze in large studies, and (2) suitable biomarkers have not been identified for all foods or nutrients. For example, there is no established biomarker for total fat or carbohydrate intake.

Dietary biomarkers fall into one of two general categories: recovery biomarkers and concentration biomarkers. Recovery biomarkers are those that have a known quantitative time-associated relationship between dietary intake and excretion or recovery in human waste (e.g., urine or feces) [54,55]. Concentration biomarkers (e.g., serum β-carotene for total fruits and vegetables) are responsive to diet and generally have a linear association with dietary intake [56,57]. However, these qualitative biomarkers are of limited usefulness in assessing overall or person-specific biases in self-report and cannot be used to estimate absolute intake in the same manner as recovery biomarkers [54,55].

Urinary nitrogen is an example of a recovery biomarker and is used to estimate protein intake. The measure is based on the following equation [58]:

Reported protein intake (g)

= (24-hour urinary nitrogen + 2) × 6.25 (g)

Like a single 24-hour recall, a single 24-hour urine collection does not reflect usual intake, but nitrogen intake has been shown to be less variable than protein intake such that only 8 days of collection are required compared to 16 days of dietary intake data to assess habitual protein intake. Although the collection of 24-hour urine is a tedious procedure, the method is readily accessible and comparatively inexpensive. In addition, other markers of dietary intake and intermediate risk markers may also be measured in the 24-hour urine that is obtained.

The "gold standard" for assessing energy intake is the use of doubly labeled water. Although this method actually measures energy expenditure (carbon dioxide output), it can be used as a measure of energy intake because energy intake and expenditure are approximately equivalent in weight-stable individuals. Doubly labeled water is water that has been "tagged" by replacing some of the hydrogen and oxygen with heavy isotopes (deuterium and oxygen-18). The participant ingests a dose of the doubly labeled water, and after a delay of a few hours, urine samples are collected to obtain a measure of the markers once they have reached equilibration with water in the body. As time continues, the deuterium will be eliminated as water and the oxygen-18 will be eliminated as water plus carbon dioxide. Thus, the rate of carbon dioxide production can be deduced by comparing the elimination of the two markers. Only one follow-up urine sample is required, and it can be collected up to a few weeks after baseline. Although it is expensive, this method has a relatively low participant burden and can accurately estimate energy intake and expenditure.

Energy expenditure can also be estimated using other methods, such as indirect calorimetry or accelerometers. In indirect calorimetry, a metabolic cart is used to measure the participant's oxygen intake and carbon dioxide output, which are then used to calculate the resting metabolic rate. A major disadvantage of this method is that it does not capture energy expended by movement or physical activity and is therefore inappropriate if free-living energy expenditure is of interest. Accelerometers are small electronic meters typically used to provide an objective measurement of physical activity. Worn on the hip during all waking hours over several days, these devices record movements during daily activity. By applying formulas to the data they collect, investigators can estimate the energy expended during the wear period. This method is practical and the cost is relatively low. It can be combined with calorimetry to estimate total energy expenditure [59].

III STUDY DESIGNS USED IN NUTRITIONAL EPIDEMIOLOGY

Epidemiologic studies can be divided into two general types: observational and experimental. The three primary observational study designs are ecologic, case–control, and cohort studies. In human studies, the main experimental study designs are intervention trials or randomized controlled trials. An overview of these study designs in relation to nutritional epidemiology is given here.

A Observational Studies

1 Ecologic and Migrant Studies

Important hypothesis-generating studies have examined the relationship of national estimates of per capita supply of foods (e.g., dietary fat) with time-lagged rates of cancer or heart disease incidence or mortality [60–63]. These analyses strongly suggest that dietary fat intake increases risk while plant foods decrease risk of these major diseases. However, there are numerous problems with country-specific measures of dietary intake. First, estimates of per capita intake from food disappearance data are extremely imprecise and include nonhuman consumption uses such as livestock feed and manufacturing use of food or food end products (e.g., corn biofuel and soybean-based inks used in newsprint). Second, it is generally not feasible to control for other differences between countries (e.g., differences in physical activity levels or smoking prevalence). Finally, it is unknown whether the individuals within the countries that are exposed to specific dietary factors are the same individuals experiencing the disease.

Migrant studies have often shown that with a single move from less developed to Westernized countries, large and significant increases occur in risk of several chronic diseases such as breast cancer [64,65]. These changes occur rapidly, often after just one generation, as immigrants become acculturated to the diet and other habits of their new country [66]. Migrant studies offer strong evidence to support a major role for lifestyle and environment exposures as disease risk factors; however, few such studies have included pertinent dietary assessment to be able to properly address these questions [66].

2 Case–Control Studies

In a case–control study, individuals are identified and studied according to a single disease outcome. Specifically, individuals who have recently been diagnosed with a disease (e.g., colon cancer) are asked about their past exposure to diet and other risk factors and often provide a blood sample. A comparable set of control individuals, usually drawn from the same population, are also enrolled in the study and are asked about their past exposures. The two groups (those with and those without the disease) are then compared for differences in dietary intake and other exposures. The major advantage of this design is that an entire study can be completed in just a few years with a smaller sample size than is needed for other study designs (it could be as small as 200 cases and controls). However, this study design can only answer questions about a single disease outcome.

In addition, these studies can introduce potentially serious biases. Two major concerns with case–control studies are recall bias and selection bias. In studies of chronic disease, investigators typically ask participants to recall behavior and other exposures (e.g., dietary intake) from the past 5–10 years, or even earlier. Bias can occur when cases recall exposure to potential risk factors differently than do controls. For example, past consumption of fatty foods might be more salient and easier to recall for individuals diagnosed with cardiovascular disease than for healthy individuals. Selection bias occurs when controls agree to join the study because of an interest in health and are therefore more likely to exhibit healthy behavior (e.g., eat healthful diets and be physically active). The higher prevalence of healthy behavior in the controls appears to be associated with reduced risk of disease when actually it is associated with willingness to participate in a research study on health. Thus, control selection is an extremely important part of study design [1,67]. Furthermore, because cases are usually recruited relatively soon after diagnosis, unless remote diet is assessed, the dietary habits reported during the previous year (or a more recent time frame) represent dietary intake in the preclinical phase of disease. Inferences from such data are not clear with respect to understanding diet–disease relationships.

Another problem with case–control studies is that biomarkers of diet (e.g., serum micronutrient concentrations) are potentially affected by the disease process and therefore may not be reliable indicators of long-term status (e.g., risk) in cases. As described in the following section, this problem is partially overcome in nested case–control studies.

3 Cohort Studies

The cohort study typically enrolls people who are free of disease, assesses baseline risk factors, and then follows the participants over time to monitor disease occurrence. The major advantage of cohort studies is that exposure to potential risk factors is assessed before the development of disease [1,67]. Therefore, exposures such as self-reported dietary intake or nutritional biomarkers from blood samples cannot be influenced by the disease process. In addition, cohort studies can examine many different exposures in relation to several different disease outcomes. A cohort study is generally a large enterprise because most diseases affect only a small proportion of a population, even if the population is followed for many years. These studies typically have sample sizes exceeding 50,000, can have a total cost in excess of $100 million, and require that the cohort be followed for 10 or more years [1,67]. Despite the cost and logistics, cohort studies have been useful in identifying diet–disease risk factors with ensuing recommendations for public health [68–73].

Because of the large size of these studies, the analysis of biologic markers (e.g., serum micronutrient concentrations) for all participants is prohibitively expensive. Therefore, cohort studies often archive (e.g., store) serum or plasma, white blood cells, toenails, DNA, or other biologic specimens for the purpose of conducting nested case–control studies in the future [74,75]. In a nested case–control study, a sample of cohort participants who developed a disease such as breast cancer (e.g., cases) are matched with other individuals in the cohort who did not develop the disease (e.g., controls). Cases and controls may be matched with respect to age, gender, and/or other important characteristics. This ensures that the sample of cases is comparable to the sample of controls with respect to potential confounding factors. Once cases and controls have been selected, biologic samples from these individuals are retrieved and analyzed to determine whether there are differences in prevalence of exposures (e.g., diet) between the two groups [76,77]. This can be an efficient and powerful study design that avoids many of the pitfalls of the classic case–control studies.

B Intervention Trials

Intervention trials prospectively examine the effect of an exposure randomly assigned by the investigators, such as a low-fat diet or a dietary supplement, on an outcome such as disease occurrence, risk factor for a disease, or a biomarker. An important consideration when designing these studies is the degree of dietary control needed. For example, depending on the hypothesis, the dietary intervention could be a controlled diet provided by the investigators, a vitamin supplement, or dietary counseling. The stringency of dietary control is determined partially by the expected size of the response (e.g., change in disease risk) and the length of the treatment period required. If the required dietary treatment period exceeds several months, a controlled feeding study is usually not logistically or financially viable.

It is also important to note that with the exception of dietary supplement intervention trials, most dietary interventions are not double-blinded. If the study compares a low-fat eating pattern to usual diet, for example, participants will know to which arm they have been randomized because they are being asked to make specific dietary changes. Furthermore, as with any intervention trial, one must account for "drop-in" and "drop-out" rates. Some study participants may find the required intervention activities too burdensome, so they may drop out or be less than 100% adherent to study activities [78,79]. Control participants, on the other hand, even if they are asked not to change their diet or take any new dietary supplements, may begin new dietary patterns that could be similar to the intervention. Both drop-in and drop-out phenomena can diminish the amount of contrast between the intervention and comparison groups, thereby attenuating any effects of the intervention.

In an intervention trial, the random assignment of participants to the control versus the intervention group means that participants with predisposing conditions or unmeasured factors that might influence the outcome are equally likely to be randomized into the intervention or the control group. Therefore, there is little or no confounding in randomized intervention studies [67]. In addition, random allocation of the exposure eliminates the potential for selection bias and recall bias. However, such trials are generally expensive and labor intensive. Therefore, randomized trials are only conducted for important public health questions where the observational data are suggestive but a controlled experiment is needed prior to issuing public health recommendations. Randomized trials are the only epidemiologic study design in which cause and effect may be concluded [1,67].

IV INTERPRETATION OF CAUSE AND EFFECT IN NUTRITIONAL EPIDEMIOLOGY

Given that nutritional epidemiology is the study of dietary intake and its association with disease risk, we must use careful scientific judgment in determining when the strength of the evidence supports a causal link between the exposure and the outcome. When assessing causality, important considerations include: (1) the main measure of association used in epidemiologic studies; (2) the major alternative explanation for an observed association in observational studies, which is confounding; and (3) methods for assessing causality in studies of associations. Other important considerations include: (1) biological plausibility, (2) temporal association, (3) the strength of the association, (4) dose–response relationship, and (5) consistency with other studies [1,67].

A Measures of Association

The most commonly used measure of association between dietary intake and disease risk is relative risk (RR). The RR estimates the magnitude of an association between the dietary exposure and disease and indicates the probability of developing the disease in the exposed group relative to those who are not exposed [1,67]. For example, an RR of 1.0 indicates that the incidence of disease in both exposed and unexposed groups is the same. An RR greater than 1.0 indicates a positive association. For example, an RR of 2.0 between dietary fat and colon cancer indicates that individuals eating a high-fat diet are twice as likely to develop colon cancer as those eating a low-fat diet. RRs less than 1.0 are typically considered protective. An RR of 0.5 for the association of vegetable intake with colon cancer risk indicates that among individuals with diets high in vegetables, the risk of colon cancer is approximately half compared to those with diets low in vegetables. Often, RRs are given for the highest category of intake (e.g., highest quartile of fat or vegetable intake) in comparison to the lowest category of intake.

Given the degree of measurement error in dietary intake estimates, RRs in nutritional epidemiology rarely exceed 3.0. RRs are typically presented with their associated confidence interval (e.g., RR 2.0, 95% confidence interval of 1.3−2.9), which provides information on the precision of the point estimate (e.g., the RR). Specifically, it is the range within which the true point estimates lie with a certain degree of assurance. Typically, 95% confidence intervals (CIs) are given, which correspond to the traditional test of statistical significance, $p < 0.05$, meaning that there is less than a 5% probability that the findings occurred by chance. A 95% CI that does not include the null value (1.0) is, by definition, statistically significant at the $p = 0.05$ level. The width of the CI also provides information about the variability in the point estimate, which is primarily a function of sample size. Therefore, the wider the CI, the more variability in the measure, the smaller the sample size, and the less confidence we can have that the observed point estimate is the true point estimate.

It is important to separate the strength of an RR from its public health relevance. For example, a large RR (e.g., RR = 5.0) might be observed between a specific food and a risk of disease. However, if consumption of that food is rare, then its overall influence on the population's total morbidity or mortality will be minimal. Conversely, an RR of 1.5 might be very important from a public health perspective if the dietary exposure is common. Once RR estimates are used to determine the strength of association, then projections of the consequence of an exposure on public health (termed population attributable risk) become important in the development of policy and allocation of resources. For example, the consistent observations from observational studies that trans fats were associated with unfavorable serum lipid profiles and cardiovascular disease led to new food labeling laws requiring that trans fats be listed among the "Nutrition Facts" [5].

B Confounding

Confounding occurs when an observed association between dietary intake and disease is actually due to another factor (e.g., physical activity) that is highly correlated with dietary intake [1,67]. Confounding is a critical concept in nutritional epidemiology because it is plausible that people who have healthful diets are likely to differ from those who did not choose healthful diets with regard to other exposures (e.g., physical activity) [12].

For example, a population-based study among 1449 adults observed that those who used vitamin/mineral supplements were more likely to be female, older, better educated, nonsmokers, regular exercisers, and to consume diets higher in fruits and vegetables and lower in fat [13]. We also found previously unreported associations of supplement use with cancer screening, use of other chemopreventive agents (e.g., aspirin), and a psychosocial factor (belief in a diet−cancer connection). These relationships could confound studies of supplement use and cancer risk in complex ways. For example, male supplement users were more likely to have had a prostate-specific antigen test, which is associated with increased diagnosis of prostate cancer [80]. Therefore, supplement use could spuriously appear to be associated with increased incidence of prostate cancer.

The observed relationship between supplement use and belief in a connection between diet and cancer is especially interesting. Health beliefs influence cancer risk through behavior such as diet and exercise. For example, in a previous prospective study, we found that belief in a connection between diet and cancer was a statistically significant predictor of changes to more healthful diets over time [81]. In cohort studies, the increasing healthfulness of supplement users' diets and other health practices over time could result in a spurious positive association between supplement use and chronic disease risk.

It is important to note that in studies in which nutrient intake is summed from foods and supplements, the intake of micronutrients in the highest exposure category is often too high to be obtained from food and reflects supplement use. Therefore, studies of nutrient intake may also be confounded by the relationship between supplement use and healthful lifestyle. In these studies, consistency of findings for the nutrient from foods and vitamin supplements separately would increase confidence that an observed association was not confounded by supplement users' healthful lifestyles.

In theory, statistical adjustment in analyses for participant characteristics and major health-related behavior controls for the effects of confounding factors are important. However, the absence of residual confounding cannot be ensured, especially if other important confounding factors are unknown, not assessed, assessed with error, or not included in the analyses.

C Evidence of Causality

Epidemiology is the study of associations, and statistical methods provide the means to conduct hypothesis testing to quantify the association. However, it is important to note that the existence of a statistically significant association does not indicate that the observed relationship is one of cause and effect. For any observed association, the following questions should be considered:

- How likely is it that the observed association is due to chance?

- Could this association be the result of poor study design, poor implementation, or inappropriate analysis?
- How well do these results meet other criteria of causality, as given in Table 6.2 [1]? Specifically, is the association weak or strong? Is there a plausible biologic mechanism? Did the exposure precede the outcome? Is there a dose–response relationship?
- How well do these results fit in the context of all available evidence on this association? Causality is supported when a number of studies, conducted at different times, using different methods, among different populations, show similar results. Note that true causality can only be inferred within the context of an experimental study, a randomized controlled trial.

In a field characterized by as much uncertainty as nutritional epidemiology, it is rare for a cause-and-effect relationship to be considered unequivocal. However, lack of complete certainty does not mean that we should ignore the information that we have or postpone action that appears needed at a given time [1,82,83]. It merely means that we exercise prudence and thoughtful consideration before acting on epidemiologic evidence.

V OBSTACLES TO FINDING ASSOCIATIONS OF DIETARY INTAKE AND DISEASE RISK

Here, we review the major obstacles to epidemiologic research, including error in exposure assessment and limitations of study designs.

A Assessing the Reliability and Validity of Measures of Dietary Intake

Reliability is generally used to refer to reproducibility, or whether an instrument will measure an exposure (e.g., nutrient intake) in the same way twice on the same respondents. Validity, which refers to the accuracy of an instrument, is a considerably higher standard. Generally, a validity study compares a practical, low-cost measurement method (e.g., an FFQ) with a more accurate but more burdensome or expensive method (e.g., food records). Reliability and validity are typically investigated by means of statistical measures of bias and precision [10].

In a reliability study, reproducibility is assessed by comparing mean intake estimates from two administrations of the instrument in the same group of respondents. If an instrument is reliable, the mean intake

TABLE 6.2 Criteria for Judging Whether Observed Associations between Diet and Disease Risk Are Causal

Criteria	
Strength of the association	The stronger the association, the less likely that it is due to the effect of an unsuspected or uncontrolled confounding variable.
Biological credibility	A known or postulated biologic mechanism supports causality. However, an association that does not appear biologically credible at one time may eventually prove to be so. Implausible associations may be the beginning of the advancement of knowledge regarding mechanisms.
Consistency	This criterion requires that the association be observed in several types of studies—for example, in more than one population and using different study methods.
Specificity	This is the degree to which one factor predicts the frequency or magnitude of a single disease.
Time sequence	The exposure of interest must precede the disease outcome by a time span consistent with known biologic mechanisms.
Dose–response	Evidence for a dose–response relationship (i.e., increased risk associated with increased exposure) is considered supportive of causality.

Source: *Adapted from Hennekens and Buring [1] and Neuhouser* et al. *[66].*

estimates should not vary substantially between the two administrations. In a validity study, bias is generally assessed by comparing the mean estimates from the instrument of interest to those from a criterion measure (e.g., a "gold standard" instrument) in the same respondents. This comparison allows us to determine whether nutrient intake estimates from the first instrument appear to be generally under- or overreported in comparison to the criterion measure [10,12]. Bias is particularly important when the objective is to measure absolute intakes for comparison to dietary recommendations or some other objective criteria. For example, bias is critical when estimating how close Americans are to meeting the dietary recommendation to eat five servings of fruits and vegetables per day.

Precision is concerned with whether an instrument accurately ranks individuals from low to high nutrient intakes, which is typically the analytic approach used to assess associations of dietary intake with risk of disease [12]. In this situation, bias in the estimate of absolute intake is not important as long as precision is good. In a validity study, precision is the correlation coefficient between nutrient intake estimates from the instrument of interest in comparison to a criterion measure. Often, dietary assessment studies also assess validity by ranking nutrient intake estimates, dividing them into categories (e.g., quartiles), and comparing these to similar categories calculated from another instrument. However, classifying a continuous exposure into a small number of categories does not reduce the effects of measurement error [10] and, therefore, this analysis does not yield additional information beyond that provided by correlation coefficients.

It is important to know that an instrument can be reliable without being accurate. That is, it can yield the same nutrient estimates two times and be wrong (e.g., biased upward or downward) both times. Alternatively, an instrument can be very reliable and consistently yield an accurate group mean (e.g., unbiased) but have poor precision such that it does not accurately rank individuals in the group from low to high in nutrient intake. Reliability is easy to measure, and nutrient correlation coefficients between two administrations of the same FFQ are generally in the range of 0.5—0.8 [12]. Estimates of reliability give an upper boundary to the accuracy of an instrument. Whereas a high reliability coefficient does not imply a high validity coefficient, a low reliability coefficient clearly means poor validity.

1 Sources of Error Associated with Self-Reported Dietary Intake

Regardless of the approach used, self-reported dietary intake is inherently subject to several sources of error (Table 6.3). Sources of random error that are common across dietary assessment methodologies include error in estimation of portion sizes, forgetting to report foods or beverages, and mistakes in reporting. Bias can occur when under- or overreporting of intake is related to some characteristic of the participants. For example, obese individuals tend to underreport their energy intake to a greater degree than normal-weight individuals [84]. Another concern is social desirability bias, which is the tendency to respond in a pleasing way. For example, participants enrolled in a program to increase fruit and vegetable intake may consciously or subconsciously overreport their intake of these foods. Susceptibility to social desirability bias varies among individuals and has been associated with differential error in the reporting of energy intake [59]. Furthermore, research indicates that dietary interventions introduce reporting bias toward the more desirable responses [85]. Finally, food records, food recalls, and FFQs are all subject to limitations in the food database and errors in the programming used to quantify nutrient intake.

2 Measurement Error Specific to FFQs

The FFQ form is a major source of error because of limitations inherent in closed-ended scannable response options, the use of a limited food list (generally approximately 100 items) to minimize respondent burden, inadequate food composition information, and the requirement that respondents mentally average intake over long periods of time.

Studies comparing FFQs with records or recalls are often called validation studies. The theory behind this type of study is that the major sources of error associated with FFQs are independent of those associated with short-term dietary recall and recording methods, which avoids spuriously high estimates of validity resulting from correlated errors. As summarized by Willett [12], errors unique to the FFQs include the restrictions imposed by a fixed list of foods, perception of portion sizes, and the cognitive challenge of assessing frequency of food consumption over a broad time frame. However, it is clear that many sources of error (e.g., underestimating portion sizes) are common to all self-report assessment instruments.

3 Measurement Error Specific to Food Records/Recalls

Unlike FFQs, food records and recalls are open-ended, do not depend on long-term memory, and allow for measurement of portion sizes. In addition to the sources of error that are common across self-reported dietary assessment methods, food records are also prone to bias that results when participants

TABLE 6.3 Sources of Error and/or Bias in Dietary Intake Estimates

Source of error	Type of error	Reason for error	FFQ	Food record	Food recall
Participant	Memory	Unable to recall food consumption. This error increases with interval of memory required.	X		X
	Frequency judgments	Respondent has cognitive difficulty accurately providing this information. May be a particular problem in low-literacy respondents.	X		
	Question comprehension	Respondent may not understand what foods are being asked about, understand the frequency categories, or be able to estimate portion sizes.	X		
	Response errors	Respondent mistakenly codes incorrect frequency or skips questions.	X		
	Portion size errors	Respondent cannot conceptualize reference portion size or his or her own portion sizes.	X	X	X
	Social desirability bias	Respondent unintentionally (or intentionally) misrepresents dietary intake in order to please investigators. For example, obese participants may underestimate intake.	X	X	X
	Fatigue/burden	Respondent alters normal food choices or omits some items to simplify record keeping.		X	
Investigator/ tool	Food list	Food list is too short or not appropriate for population being studied and therefore dietary intake data are incomplete.	X		
	Food groups	Food groups may not appropriately group foods by nutrient composition.	X		
	Portion sizes	The reference portion size may be too large or too small for a population such that it consistently over- or underestimates amounts of food consumed.	X		
	Categorization of frequencies	Loss of information by using close-ended categories (e.g., 2–4 times/week) instead of using an open-ended format.	X		
	Poor form design	Font is too small, skip patterns are not clear, or instructions are unclear.	X		
	Data collection errors	Scanning errors may occur. Data from incomplete FFQs are used in analysis.	X		
	Database	Database may have incorrect nutrient values, incomplete nutrient values, or be missing important exposures altogether (e.g., isoflavones).	X	X	X
	Programming errors	Nutrient analysis program may contain errors.	X	X	X
	Estimation	Investigator relies on estimates to quantify nutritional intake. With food records, there is no opportunity to probe participant for additional information.		X	X
Other	Seasonal variation	It may not be possible to adequately report average intake of foods where intake varies markedly over seasons.	X		
	Unusual dietary patterns	Respondents with unusual eating patterns (e.g., liquid diets) may not be able to accurately report dietary patterns.	X		
	Short time period	Short duration of reference period results in a "snapshot" that may not be representative of respondent's usual intake.		X	X
	Intervention-associated bias	Respondents in an intervention are more likely to report socially desirable responses.	X	X	X

change their eating habits during the assessment period. This may occur as the result of social desirability bias (e.g., respondent decreases intake of unhealthy foods to avoid having to report these items) or due to burden and fatigue (e.g., respondent begins eating fewer foods or more simply prepared dishes to make it easier to record intake).

Like food records, food recalls are typically open-ended. However, recalls are usually collected without advance notification. Therefore, participants cannot change what they eat retroactively and the instrument itself should not affect food intake, although misreporting due to social desirability bias is still possible. Both recalls and records are subject to coding errors because scannable forms are not typically used.

4 Comparison of Self-Reported Diet to Objective Biomarkers

Validity studies that compare self-report dietary instruments against one another are subject to certain limitations. They rely on the assumption that there will be little overlap between the sources of error and bias on the two instruments. This is unlikely to be fully true because some sources of error are common to all self-report assessments. For this reason, recent validity studies have focused on comparing self-reported diet to objective biomarkers, such as doubly labeled water. As described previously, the doubly labeled water method is a gold standard method that provides an accurate assessment of total energy expenditure (essentially equivalent to energy intake). When compared to doubly labeled water assessments, dietary recalls have been shown to underestimate energy intake by 10—20%. Food frequency questionnaires are even less accurate, underestimating energy by 25—35% [86,87]. Studies comparing energy intake estimated with an FFQ in comparison to a gold standard (doubly labeled water) have found correlations ranging from 0.1 to 0.2 [88]. These exceptionally poor correlation coefficients indicate that energy intake cannot be validly assessed using FFQs. Similarly, FFQs have been shown to underestimate protein intake by 10—15% compared to protein biomarkers measured in urine [87]. Complicating matters further, the degree of under- or overreporting is often associated with one or more participant characteristics, such as body mass index (BMI), race/ethnicity, socioeconomic status, or social desirability score [89].

5 Effects of Error in Dietary Intake Estimation and Measures of Disease Association

Error in dietary assessment can be of two types, with markedly different consequences. Random error refers to mistakes such as inadvertently marking the wrong frequency column, skipping questions, and lapses in judgment. These errors introduce noise into nutrient estimates such that our ability to find the "signal" (e.g., an association of dietary fat and breast cancer) is masked or attenuated (biased toward no association).

Systematic error refers to under- or overreporting of intake across the population (e.g., bias) as well as to person-specific sources of bias. For example, studies indicate that obese women are more likely to underestimate dietary intake than are normal-weight women [90—92]. Systematic error may result in either null associations or spurious associations. In one report, Prentice used data from FFQs collected in a low-fat

dietary intervention trial to simulate the effects of random and systematic error on an association of dietary fat and breast cancer, where the true RR was assumed to be 4.0 [93]. Assuming only random error exists in the estimate of fat intake, the projected (i.e., observed) RR for fat and breast cancer would be 1.4. Assuming both random error and systematic error exist, the projected RR would be 1.1, similar to that reported in a pooled analysis of cohort studies [94]. These results indicate that FFQs may not be adequate to detect many associations of diet with disease, even if a strong relationship exists [95,96]. In view of the error in dietary self-report, it is not surprising that results from diet—disease studies are often null or conflicting [93,97]. Because of cost or practical considerations, the use of objective biomarkers is not feasible in epidemiologic studies. One approach for large studies using self-reported diet assessment is to collect biomarker data on a subset of participants. These data can be used to calculate calibration coefficients (the degree to which specific subgroups of participants under- or overreported their intake) [87], which can then be applied to the entire study sample to produce "corrected" disease estimates.

B Limitations in Research Designs

1 Observational Studies

In studies of nutritional epidemiology, unique obstacles exist to finding clear and interpretable relationships between dietary intake and disease risk [82,97]. In roughly increasing order of importance, these obstacles include the following:

- Current or recent dietary intake may differ from intake over the time frame relevant to the development of disease, which will reduce our ability to find associations between diet and disease.
- Certain nutrient intakes within a population may not be highly variable. For example, energy from dietary fat in a population of postmenopausal women may only vary from 25 to 40%, resulting in inadequate range of disease risk to find an association with breast cancer. This situation is akin to assessing whether smoking causes cancer by studying men who smoke one pack per day in comparison to men who smoke one and a half packs per day. Minimal heterogeneity in exposures provides insufficient contrasts.
- Diet is a complex mixture of foods and nutrients, including many highly correlated compounds, making it difficult to separate the effects of any one compound from other dietary factors.
- Dietary intake may relate in a complicated manner to other risk factors such as hormonal status,

obesity, or hypertension. These relationships (some of which may be in the causal pathway) make it difficult to appropriately control for confounding factors.

- Existing dietary self-report instruments include many sources of random and systematic error, both of which obscure our ability to find associations between dietary intake and disease risk.

An important point to consider is that most of the obstacles listed previously will limit or attenuate our ability to find associations between dietary intake and disease. For example, as shown in Table 6.4, an observed association of dietary fat intake with BMI might appear too small to be clinically important. However, if we assume that significant measurement error exists in our estimate of fat intake (e.g., a correlation of 0.30 between our measure and "true" intake), then the real association would be 4.0 BMI points per 10 g of fat intake, which is considerably more important. Therefore, studies showing weak or no associations between dietary intake and disease (e.g., null results) need to be interpreted cautiously.

Observational studies are frequently referred to as hypothesis-generating studies, which set the stage for testing in a large randomized trial with disease outcomes. However, many hypotheses that were well supported by laboratory and observational epidemiologic research have proven to be null when tested in a trial:

- Experimental and epidemiological data suggested that vitamin E supplementation prevents cancer and cardiovascular events. In a trial of 7030 patients with vascular disease or diabetes mellitus, long-term vitamin E supplementation did not prevent cancer or major cardiovascular events and resulted in some increase in the risk for heart failure [98].
- β-Carotene was hypothesized to reduce tumor incidence. However, two large trials to test the effect of β-carotene supplements on lung cancer incidence in smokers found that β-carotene supplementation increased the incidence of lung cancers as well as cardiovascular and all-cause mortality [99,100].
- B vitamins were believed to lower the risk of cardiovascular disease. However, after 38 months of treatment and follow-up, supplementation with folic acid, B_{12}, and B_6 did not reduce total cardiovascular events among 3096 patients with coronary artery disease or aortic valve stenosis [101]. An analysis with long-term follow-up found that treatment with folic acid plus vitamin B_{12} was associated with increased cancer outcomes and all-cause mortality [102].
- A healthy diet was hypothesized to improve breast cancer prognosis. However, a trial of 3088 breast cancer survivors found that adoption of a diet that

TABLE 6.4 Estimates of the Observed Association[a] between Dietary Fat Intake (per 10 Grams of Fat) and BMI after Adjustment for Random Measurement Error in the Measure of Dietary Fat

Correlation coefficient[b] between the FFQ estimate and "true" fat intake	Observed increase in BMI for every 10 g of fat consumed[c]
1.00 (FFQ is a perfect measure of fat intake)	4.0
0.70 (FFQ is a good measure of fat intake)	2.8
0.50 (FFQ is a weak measure of fat intake)	2.0
0.30 (FFQ is a poor measure of fat intake)	1.2

[a]$\beta_{observed} = \beta_{true} \times validity\ coefficient$.
[b]Correlation coefficient from validity study comparing FFQ to multiple 24-hour recalls.
[c]Assume true regression coefficient from a multivariate model predicting BMI = 4.0.

was very high in vegetables, fruits, and fiber and low in fat did not reduce additional breast cancer events or mortality during a 7.3-year follow-up period [103].

- Vitamin E and selenium were thought to reduce the risk of prostate cancer. Unexpectedly, a trial of 35,533 men found that dietary supplementation with vitamin E significantly increased the risk of prostate cancer among healthy men [104,105].

Although this list of null or negative trials is in no way comprehensive, it clearly illustrates that regardless of their size or duration, observational epidemiologic studies alone may not provide reliable information on the associations of dietary intake and disease.

2 Limitations of Clinical Trials of Dietary Intake and Disease Risk

Despite the many desirable features of dietary intervention trials, unique obstacles are present in these types of studies, as summarized here.

The costs of a long-term dietary intervention trial can be formidable. For example, the National Institutes of Health-sponsored Women's Health Initiative tested whether "low-fat eating pattern" would reduce the incidence of breast cancer, colorectal cancer, and coronary heart disease among 48,837 postmenopausal women in the United States [106–108]. The dietary intervention required participants to attend monthly sessions (run by specially trained nutritionists) for the first 18 months followed by quarterly classes for the remainder of the trial—approximately 8.5 years [109]. In addition, new intervention components were added to the trial to encourage adherence. The costs of implementing this type of intervention far exceed those required for comparatively simple pill—placebo trials or observational studies.

Maintenance of dietary adherence for a sufficient period of time to be able to ascertain clinical outcomes (e.g., disease risk) can be a formidable task. On the one hand, the greater the contrast in dietary intake between the intervention and control groups, the more likely the study will be able to detect an effect on the outcome. On the other hand, it is clearly more difficult to get participants to adhere to very strict or limited regimes, which can result in such poor adherence that the trial becomes futile [110]. Monitoring of dietary adherence typically requires use of self-reported dietary instruments, with their attendant weaknesses (discussed previously).

VI FUTURE RESEARCH DIRECTIONS

As is apparent from this overview of nutritional epidemiology, the major challenge is that of addressing random, systematic, and person-specific sources of error in dietary assessment. Only when well-designed validity studies clarify these sources of error will we be able to markedly improve our ability to draw valid inferences from epidemiologic studies of diet and disease.

A promising area of research concerns diet—gene and diet—environment interactions in the etiology and pathogenesis of many chronic diseases. Despite the vigorous investigation of environmental causes of disease, it has long been recognized that not all persons exposed to the same risk factors will develop the associated disease [111,112]. For example, although it is well accepted that smoking causes lung cancer, only 10—15% of smokers will be diagnosed with the disease in their lifetime. We are beginning to understand the impact of differential genetic susceptibility in the etiology and pathogenesis of common diseases such as coronary heart disease and cancer. If only a subgroup of individuals is sensitive to certain dietary exposures, the effect will be diluted and the association will be undetectable when the entire population is the focus of study. Better understanding of these individual susceptibilities has the potential to bring considerable clarity to nutritional epidemiologic research. Another exciting area is the use of new technology to assess the influence of diet on the various "omics," such as proteomics and metabolomics [113]. These small molecules may prove to be more informative biomarkers of diet and diet—disease relationships than simple assessment of blood nutrients.

In summary, despite the challenges in nutritional epidemiology and the measurement error issues that have impeded progress in the field, nutritional epidemiology studies have made important scientific contributions that have shaped public health policy and practice. To move the field forward, we must investigate strategies to improve methods of dietary assessment and reduce measurement error. Although the complete elimination of error in dietary assessment methods is probably not a realistic objective, a better understanding of these errors (based on objective biomarkers), combined with statistical methods to address these errors, may be an attainable goal. In addition, future research on diet and disease should focus on study designs that do not rely on self-reported diet as a measure of intervention adherence or an outcome. These research approaches include use of randomized trial designs, inclusion of dietary biomarkers, and use of disease biomarkers such as insulin resistance. Ultimately, it is the combined contribution of different study types (e.g., observational, intervention, biomarker, mechanistic feeding studies, and genetic susceptibility studies) that offers the greatest potential for identification of dietary strategies for disease prevention.

References

[1] C.H. Hennekens, J.E. Buring, Epidemiology in Medicine, Little, Brown, Boston, 1987.

[2] D. Mozaffarian, J.S. Gottdiener, D.S. Siscovick, Intake of tuna or other broiled or baked fish versus fried fish and cardiac structure, function, and hemodynamics, Am. J. Cardiol. 97 (2006) 216—222.

[3] D. Mozaffarian, M.B. Katan, A. Ascherio, M. Stampfer, W.C. Willett, Trans fatty acids and cardiovascular disease [review], N. Engl. J. Med. 354 (2006) 1601—1613.

[4] W.C. Willett, Trans fatty acids and cardiovascular disease— Epidemiological data [review], Atheroscler Suppl. 7 (2006) 5—8.

[5] J. Moss, Labeling of trans fatty acid content in food, regulations and limits: the FDA view [review], Atheroscler Suppl. 7 (2006) 57—59.

[6] O. Korver, M.B. Katan, The elimination of trans fats from spreads: how science helped to turn an industry around, Nutr. Rev. 64 (2006) 275—279.

[7] S. Okie, New York to trans fats: you're out!, N. Engl. J. Med. 356 (2007) 2017—2021.

[8] M.J. Khoury, G.M. Shaw, C.A. Moore, E.J. Lammer, J. Mulinare, Does periconceptional multivitamin use reduce the risk of neural tube defects associated with other birth defects? Data from two population-based case—control studies, Am. J. Med. Genet. 61 (1996) 30—36.

[9] Anonymous, Folic acid for the prevention of neural tube defects, Am. Acad. Pediatr. 104 (1999) 325—327.

[10] B.K. Armstrong, E. White, R. Saracci, Principles of Exposure Measurement in Epidemiology, Oxford University Press, Oxford, 1992.

[11] J.D. Potter, M.L. Slattery, R.M. Bostick, S.M. Gapstur, Colon cancer: a review of the epidemiology, Epidemiol. Rev. 15 (1993) 499—545.

[12] W.C. Willett, Nutritional Epidemiology, second ed., Oxford University Press, New York, 1998.

[13] R.E. Patterson, M.L. Neuhouser, E. White, J.R. Hunt, A.R. Kristal, Cancer-related behavior of vitamin supplement users, Cancer Epidemiol. Biomarkers Prev. 7 (1998) 79−81.

[14] J.W. Lampe, C. Chen, S. Li, et al., Modulation of human glutathione S-transferases by botanically defined vegetable diets, Cancer Epidemiol. Biomarkers Prev. 9 (2000) 787−793.

[15] J.W. Lampe, S. Peterson, Brassica, biotransformation and cancer risk: genetic polymorphisms after the preventive effects of cruciferous vegetables, J. Nutr. 132 (2002) 2991−2994.

[16] J.H. Fowke, X.O. Shu, Q. Dai, et al., Urinary isothiocyanate excretion, brassica consumption, and gene polymorphisms among women living in Shanghai, China, Cancer Epidemiol. Biomarkers Prev. 12 (2003) 1536−1539.

[17] A.V. Gasper, A. Al-Janobi, J.A. Smith, et al., Glutathione S-transferase M1 polymorphism and metabolism of sulforaphane from standard and high-glucosinolate broccoli, Am. J. Clin. Nutr. 82 (2005) 1283−1291.

[18] P. Brennan, C.C. Hsu, N. Moullan, et al., Effect of cruciferous vegetables on lung cancer patients stratified by genetic status: a mendelian randomisation approach, Lancet 366 (2005) 1558−1560.

[19] J.H. Fowke, F.L. Chung, F.Q., D Jin, et al., Urinary isothiocyanate levels, brassica, and human breast cancer, Cancer Res. 63 (2003) 3980−3986.

[20] F. Turner, G. Smith, C. Sachse, et al., Vegetable, fruit and meat consumption and potential risk modifying genes in relation to colorectal cancer, Int. J. Cancer 112 (2004) 259−264.

[21] J. Lampe, Nutrition and cancer prevention: small-scale human studies for the 21st century, Cancer Epidemiol. Biomarkers Prev. 13 (2004) 1987.

[22] R. Sinha, N. Rothman, E.D. Brown, et al., Pan-fried meat containing high levels of heterocyclic aromatic amines but low levels of aromatic hydrocarbons induces cytochrome P451A2 activity in humans, Cancer Res. 54 (1994) 6154−6159.

[23] A.J. Cross, J.R. Pollock, S.A. Bingham, Haem, not protein or inorganic iron, is responsible for endogenous intestinal N-nitrosation arising from red meat, Cancer Res. 63 (2003) 1258−1260.

[24] S.R. Davis, E.P. Quinlivan, K.P. Shelnutt, et al., The methylenetetrahydrofolate reductase 677C→T polymorphism and dietary folate restriction affect plasma one-carbon metabolites and red blood cell folate concentrations and distribution in women, J. Nutr. 135 (2005) 1040−1044.

[25] S.R. Davis, E.P. Quinlivan, P.W. Stacpoole, J.F. Gregory, Plasma glutathione and cystathionine concentrations are elevated but cysteine flux is unchanged by dietary vitamin B-6 restriction in young men and women, J. Nutr. 136 (2006) 373−378.

[26] A.R. Kristal, N.C. Vizenor, R.E. Patterson, M.L. Neuhouser, A.L. Shattuck, D. McLerran, Precision and bias of food frequency-based measures of fruit and vegetable intakes, Cancer Epidemiol. Biomarkers Prev. 9 (2000) 939−944.

[27] R.E. Patterson, A.R. Kristal, R.A. Carter, L. Fels-Tinker, M.P. Bolton, T. Agurs-Collins, Measurement characteristics of the Women's Health Initiative food frequency questionnaire, Ann. Epidemiol. 9 (1999) 178−187.

[28] G. Block, A.M. Hartman, C.M. Dresser, M.D. Carroll, J. Gannon, L. Gardner, A data-based approach to diet questionnaire design and testing, Am. J. Epidemiol. 124 (1986) 453−469.

[29] A. Subar, V. Kipnis, R.P. Troiano, et al., Using intake biomarkers to evaluate the extent of dietary misreporting in a large sample of adults: The OPEN Study, Am. J. Epidemiol. 158 (2003) 1−13.

[30] V. Kipnis, D. Midthune, L.S. Freedman, et al., Empirical evidence of correlated biases in dietary assessment instruments and its implications, Am. J. Epidemiol. 153 (2001) 394−403.

[31] A.S. Kolar, R.E. Patterson, E. White, et al., A practical method for collecting 3-day food records in a large cohort, Epidemiology 16 (2005) 579−583.

[32] D.-H. Wang, M. Kogashiwa, S. Ohta, S. Kira, Validity and reliability of a dietary assessment method: the application of a digital camera with a mobile phone card attachment, J. Nutr. Sci. Vitaminol. 48 (2002) 498−504.

[33] J. Beasley, W.T. Riley, J. Jean-Mary, Accuracy of a PDA-based dietary assessment program, Nutrition 21 (2005) 672−677.

[34] B.L. Six, T.E. Schap, F.M. Zhu, et al., Evidence-based development of a mobile telephone food record, J. Am. Diet. Assoc. 110 (2010) 74−79.

[35] C.J. Boushey, D.A. Kerr, J. Wright, K.D. Lutes, D.S. Ebert, E.J. Delp, Use of technology in children's dietary assessment, Eur. J. Clin. Nutr. 63 (Suppl. 1) (2009) S50−S57.

[36] J. Dwyer, M.F. Picciano, D.J. Raiten, Collection of food and dietary supplement intake data: what We Eat in America−NHANES, J. Nutr. 133 (2003) 590−600.

[37] S. Rebro, R.E. Patterson, A.R. Kristal, C. Cheney, The effect of keeping food records on eating patterns, J. Am. Diet. Assoc. 98 (1998) 1163−1165.

[38] T.P. Zimmerman, S.G. Hull, S. McNutt, et al., Challenges in converting an interviewer-administered food probe database to self-administration in the National Cancer Institute Automated Self-Administered 24-Hour Recall (ASA24), J. Food Compost. Anal. 22 (2009) S48−S51.

[39] B. Liu, H. Young, F.L. Crowe, et al., Development and evaluation of the Oxford WebQ, a low-cost, web-based method for assessment of previous 24 h dietary intakes in large-scale prospective studies, Public Health Nutr. 14 (2011) 1998−2005.

[40] L. Arab, C.H. Tseng, A. Ang, P. Jardack, Validity of a multipass, web-based, 24-hour self-administered recall for assessment of total energy intake in blacks and whites, Am. J. Epidemiol. 174 (2011) 1256−1265.

[41] D.J. Toobert, L.A. Strycker, S.E. Hampson, et al., Computerized portion-size estimation compared to multiple 24-hour dietary recalls for measurement of fat, fruit, and vegetable intake in overweight adults, J. Am. Diet. Assoc. 111 (2011) 1578−1583.

[42] J. Satia-Abouta, A.R. Kristal, R.E. Patterson, A.J. Littman, K.L. Stratton, E. White, Dietary supplement use and medical conditions: the VITAL study, Am. J. Prev. Med. 24 (2003) 43−51.

[43] L.A. Brennan, G.M. Morris, G.R. Wasson, B.M. Hannigan, Y.A. Barnett, The effect of vitamin C or vitamin E supplementation on basal and H_2O_2-induced DNA damage in human lymphocytes, Br. J. Nutr. 84 (2000) 195−202.

[44] M.L. Neuhouser, R.E. Patterson, A. Kristal, Dietary supplements and cancer risk: epidemiological research and recommendations, in: A. Bendich, R.J. Deckelbaum (Eds), Preventive Nutrition, third ed., Humana Press, Totowa, NJ, 2005, pp. 89−121.

[45] A.R. Kristal, L.L. Stanford, J.H. Cohen, K. Wicklund, R.E. Patterson, Vitamin and mineral supplement use is associated with reduced risk of prostate cancer, Cancer Epidemiol. Biomarkers Prev. 8 (1999) 887−892.

[46] M. Leitzmann, M. Stampfer, G.A. Colditz, C.G. Willett, E. Giovannucci, Zinc supplement use and risk of prostate cancer, J. Natl. Cancer Inst. 95 (2003) 1004−1007.

[47] M.L. Neuhouser, A.R. Kristal, R.E. Patterson, P.T. Goodman, I. M. Thompson, Dietary supplement use in the Prostate Cancer Prevention Trial: implications for prevention trials, Nutr. Cancer 39 (2001) 12−18.

[48] J. Satia-Abouta, R.E. Patterson, I.B. King, et al., Reliability and validity of self-report of vitamin and mineral supplement use in the VITamins and Lifestyle Study, Am. J. Epidemiol 157 (2003) 944−954.

[49] R.B. Ervin, J.D. Wright, J.J. Kennedy-Stephenson, Use of dietary supplements in the United States, 1988–1994, Vital Health Stat. 244 (1999) 1–14.

[50] R.E. Patterson, A.R. Kristal, L. Levy, D. McLerran, E. White, Validity of methods used to assess vitamin and mineral supplement use, Am. J. Epidemiol. 148 (1998) 643–649.

[51] J.A. Satia, I.B. King, J.S. Morris, K. Stratton, E. White, Toenail and plasma levels as biomarkers of selenium exposure, Ann. Epidemiol. 16 (2006) 53–58.

[52] S. Gunther, R.E. Patterson, A.R. Kristal, K.L. Stratton, E. White, Demographic and health-related correlates of herbal and specialty supplement use, J. Am. Diet. Assoc. 104 (2004) 27–34.

[53] S.A. Bingham, Urine nitrogen as a biomarker for the validation of dietary protein intake, J. Nutr. 133 (2003) 921S–924S.

[54] R. Kaaks, Biochemical markers as additional measurements in studies of the accuracy of dietary questionnaire measurements: conceptual issues, Am. J. Clin. Nutr. 65 (1997) 1232S–1239S.

[55] V. Kipnis, A.F. Subar, D. Midthune, et al., Structure of dietary measurement error: results of the OPEN biomarker study, Am. J. Epidemiol. 158 (2003) 14–21.

[56] D.R. Campbell, M.D. Gross, M.C. Martini, G.A. Grandits, J.L. Slavin, J.D. Potter, Plasma carotenoids as biomarkers of vegetable and fruit intake, Cancer Epidemiol. Biomarkers Prev. 3 (1994) 493–500.

[57] M.L. Neuhouser, R.E. Patterson, I.B. King, N.K. Horner, J.W. Lampe, Selected nutritional biomarkers predict diet quality, Public Health Nutr. 6 (2003) 703–709.

[58] I.H.E. Rutishauser, A.E. Black, Measuring food intake, in: M. Gibney, H. Vorster, F.J. Kok (Eds), Introduction to Human Nutrition, Blackwell, Oxford, 2002, pp. 225–248.

[59] N.K. Horner, R.E. Patterson, M.L. Neuhouser, J.W. Lampe, S.A. Beresford, R.L. Prentice, Participant characteristics associated with errors in self-reported energy intake from the Women's Health Initiative food-frequency questionnaire, Am. J. Clin. Nutr. 76 (2002) 766–773.

[60] World Cancer Research Fund, Food, Nutrition and the Prevention of Cancer: A Global Perspective, American Institute for Cancer Research, Washington, DC, 1997.

[61] H. Aldercreutz, Western diet and Western diseases: some hormonal and biochemical mechanisms and associations, Scand. J. Clin. Lab. Invest. 50 (1990) 3–23.

[62] H. Yu, R.E. Harris, Y.-T. Gao, R. Gao, E.L. Wynder, Comparative epidemiology of cancers of the colon, rectum, prostate and breast in Shanghai, China versus the United States, Int. J. Epidemiol. 20 (1991) 76–81.

[63] M. Lee, S. Gomez, J. Chang, M. Wey, R. Wang, A.W. Hsing, Soy and isoflavone consumption in relation to prostate cancer risk in China, Cancer Epidemiol. Biomarkers Prev. 12 (2003) 665–668.

[64] H. Shimizu, R.K. Ross, L. Bernstein, R. Yatani, B.E. Henderson, T.M. Mack, Cancers of the prostate and breast among Japanese and white immigrants in Los Angeles County, Br. J. Cancer 63 (1991) 963–966.

[65] M.D. Pineda, E. White, A.R. Kristal, V. Taylor, Asian breast cancer survival in the U.S.: a comparison between Asian immigrants, U.S.-born Asian Americans and Caucasians, Int. J. Epidemiol. 30 (2001) 976–982.

[66] M.L. Neuhouser, B. Thompson, G.D. Coronado, C.C. Solomon, Higher fat intake and lower fruit and vegetable intakes are associated with greater acculturation among Mexicans living in Washington State, J. Am. Diet. Assoc. 104 (2004) 51–57.

[67] K.J. Rothman, Modern Epidemiology, Little, Brown, Boston, 1986.

[68] W.C. Willett, M.J. Stampfer, G.A. Colditz, B.A. Rosner, F.E. Speizer, Relation of meat, fat, and fiber intake to the risk of colon cancer in a prospective study among women, N. Engl. J. Med. 323 (1990) 1664–1672.

[69] M.F. Leitzmann, M.J. Stampfer, D.S. Michaud, et al., Dietary intake of n-3 and n-6 fatty acids and the risk of prostate cancer, Am. J. Clin. Nutr. 80 (2004) 204–216.

[70] A.J. Gonzalez, E. White, A. Kristal, A.J. Littman, Calcium intake and 10-year weight change in middle-aged adults, J. Am. Diet. Assoc. 106 (1066–1073) (2006) 1082.

[71] K. Augustsson, D.S. Michaud, E.B. Rimm, et al., A prospective study of intake of fish and marine fatty acids and prostate cancer, Cancer Epidemiol. Biomarkers Prev. 12 (2003) 64–77.

[72] R. Calle, C. Rodriguez, K. Walker-Thurmond, M. Thun, Overweight, obesity, and mortality from cancer in a prospectively studied cohort of U.S. adults, N. Engl. J. Med. 348 (2003) 1625–1638.

[73] M.L. McCullough, A.S. Robertson, C. Rodriguez, et al., Calcium, vitamin D, dairy products, and risk of colorectal cancer in the Cancer Prevention Study II Nutrition Cohort (United States), Cancer Causes Control 14 (2003) 1–12.

[74] A.R. Kristal, I.B. King, D. Albanes, et al., Centralized blood processing for the selenium and vitamin E cancer prevention trial: effects of delayed processing on carotenoids, tocopherols, insulin-like growth factor-I, insulin-like growth factor binding protein 3, steroid hormones, and lymphocyte viability, Cancer Epidemiol. Biomarkers Prev. 14 (2005) 727–730.

[75] I.B. King, J. Satia-Abouta, M.D. Thornquist, et al., Buccal cell DNA yield, quality, and collection costs: comparison of methods for large-scale studies, Cancer Epidemiol. Biomarkers Prev. 11 (2003) 1130–1133.

[76] I.B. King, A.R. Kristal, S. Schaffer, M. Thornquist, G.E. Goodman, Serum trans-fatty acids are associated with risk of prostate cancer in beta-Carotene and Retinol Efficacy Trial, Cancer Epidemiol. Biomarkers Prev. 14 (2005) 988–992.

[77] K.J. Helzlsouer, H.-Y. Huang, A.J. Alberg, et al., Association between α-tocopherol, γ-tocopherol, selenium and subsequent prostate cancer, J. Natl. Cancer Inst. 92 (2000) 2018–2023.

[78] Women's Health Initiative Study Group, Dietary adherence in the Women's Health Initiative Dietary Modification Trial, J. Am. Diet. Assoc. 104 (2004) 654–658.

[79] L. Tinker, R. Patterson, A. Kristal, D. Bowen, V. Taylor, Accuracy of two self-monitoring tools used in a low-fat intervention trial, J. Am. Diet. Assoc. 101 (2001) 1031–1040.

[80] R. Etzioni, D.F. Penson, J.M. Legler, et al., Overdiagnosis due to prostate-specific antigen screening: lessons from U.S. prostate cancer incidence trends, J. Natl. Cancer Inst. 94 (2002) 981–990.

[81] R.E. Patterson, A.R. Kristal, E. White, Do beliefs, knowledge, and perceived norms about diet and cancer predict dietary change? Am. J. Public Health 86 (1996) 1394–1400.

[82] R.L. Prentice, W.C. Willett, P. Greenwald, et al., Nutrition and physical activity and chronic disease prevention: research strategies and recommendations, J. Natl. Cancer Inst. 96 (2004) 1276–1287.

[83] M.L. Neuhouser, The long and winding road of diet and breast cancer prevention, Cancer Epidemiol. Biomarkers Prev. 15 (2006) 1755–1756.

[84] J.R. Hebert, R.E. Patterson, M. Gorfine, C.B. Ebbeling St., S.T. Jeor, R.T. Chlebowski, Differences between estimated caloric requirements and self-reported caloric intake in the Women's Health Initiative, Ann. Epidemiol. 13 (2003) 629–637.

[85] A.R. Kristal, C.H. Andrilla, T.D. Koepsell, P.H. Diehr, A. Cheadle, Dietary assessment instruments are susceptible to intervention-associated response set bias, J. Am. Diet. Assoc. 98 (1998) 40–43.

[86] J.A. Tooze, A.F. Subar, F.E. Thompson, R. Troiano, A. Schatzkin, V. Kipnis, Psychosocial predictors of energy under-reporting in a large doubly labeled water study, Am. J. Clin. Nutr. 79 (2004) 795–804.

[87] M.L. Neuhouser, L. Tinker, P.A. Shaw, et al., Use of recovery biomarkers to calibrate nutrient consumption self-reports in the Women's Health Initiative, Am. J. Epidemiol. 167 (2008) 1247–1259.

[88] V. Kipnis, A.F. Subar, D. Midthune, et al., Structure of dietary measurement error: results of the OPEN biomarker study, Am. J. Epidemiol. 158 (2003) 14–21.

[89] F.B. Scagliusi, E. Ferriolli, K. Pfrimer, et al., Characteristics of women who frequently under report their energy intake: a doubly labelled water study, Eur. J. Clin. Nutr. 63 (2009) 1192–1199.

[90] A. Black, S. Bingham, G. Johansson, W. Coward, Validation of dietary intakes of protein and energy against 24 hour urinary N and DLW energy expenditures in middle-aged women, retired men and post-obese subjects: comparisons with validation against presumed energy requirements, Eur. J. Clin. Nutr. 51 (1997) 405–413.

[91] N.K. Horner, R.E. Patterson, M.L. Neuhouser, J.W. Lampe, S.A. Beresford, R.L. Prentice, Participant characteristics associated with errors in self-reported energy intake from the Women's Health Initiative food-frequency questionnaire, Am. J. Clin. Nutr. 76 (2002) 766–773.

[92] B.L. Heitmann, L. Lissner, Dietary underreporting by obese individuals: is it specific or non-specific? Br. Med. J. 311 (1995) 986–989.

[93] R.L. Prentice, Measurement error and results from analytic epidemiology: dietary fat and breast cancer, J. Natl. Cancer Inst. 88 (1996) 1738–1747.

[94] S.A. Smith-Warner, D. Spiegelman, H.O. Adami, et al., Types of dietary fat and breast cancer: a pooled analysis of cohort studies, Int. J. Cancer 92 (2001) 767–774.

[95] S. Bingham, R. Luben, A. Welch, N. Wareham, K.T. Khaw, N. Day, Are imprecise methods obscuring a relation between fat and breast cancer? Lancet 362 (2003) 212–214.

[96] e>L.S. Freedman, N.A. Potischman, V. Kipnis et al., A comparison of two dietary instruments for evaluating the fat–breast cancer relationship. Int. J. Epidemiol.. 35 (2006) 1011–1021.

[97] R.L. Prentice, E. Sugar, C.Y. Wang, M.L. Neuhouser, R.E. Patterson, Research strategies and the use of nutrient biomarkers in studies of diet and chronic disease, Public Health Nutr. 5 (2002) 977–984.

[98] E. Lonn, J. Bosch, S. Yusuf, et al., Effects of long-term vitamin E supplementation on cardiovascular events and cancer: a randomized controlled trial, JAMA 293 (2005) 1338–1347.

[99] The Alpha-Tocopherol, Beta Carotene Cancer Prevention Study Group, The effect of vitamin E and beta carotene on the incidence of lung cancer and other cancers in male smokers, N. Engl. J. Med. 330 (1994) 1029–1035.

[100] G.S. Omenn, G.E. Goodman, M.D. Thornquist, et al., Effects of a combination of beta carotene and vitamin A on lung cancer and cardiovascular disease, N. Engl. J. Med. 334 (1996) 1150–1155.

[101] M. Ebbing, O. Bleie, P.M. Ueland, et al., Mortality and cardiovascular events in patients treated with homocysteine-lowering B vitamins after coronary angiography: a randomized controlled trial, JAMA 300 (2008) 795–804.

[102] M. Ebbing, K.H. Bonaa, O. Nygard, et al., Cancer incidence and mortality after treatment with folic acid and vitamin B_{12}, JAMA 302 (2009) 2119–2126.

[103] J.P. Pierce, L. Natarajan, B.J. Caan, et al., Influence of a diet very high in vegetables, fruit, and fiber and low in fat on prognosis following treatment for breast cancer: The Women's Healthy Eating and Living (WHEL) randomized trial, JAMA 298 (2007) 289–298.

[104] S.M. Lippman, E.A. Klein, P.J. Goodman, et al., Effect of selenium and vitamin E on risk of prostate cancer and other cancers: The Selenium and Vitamin E Cancer Prevention Trial (SELECT), JAMA 301 (2009) 39–51.

[105] E.A. Klein, I.M. Thompson Jr., C.M. Tangen, et al., Vitamin E and the risk of prostate cancer: The Selenium and Vitamin E Cancer Prevention Trial (SELECT), JAMA 306 (2011) 1549–1556.

[106] R.L. Prentice, B. Caan, R.T. Chlebowski, et al., Low-fat dietary pattern and risk of invasive breast cancer: The Women's Health Initiative Randomized Controlled Dietary Modification Trial.[see Comment], JAMA 295 (2006) 629–642.

[107] S.A. Beresford, K.C. Johnson, C. Ritenbaugh, et al., Low-fat dietary pattern and risk of colorectal cancer: The Women's Health Initiative Randomized Controlled Dietary Modification Trial, JAMA 295 (2006) 643–654.

[108] B.V. Howard, L. Van Horn, J. Hsia, et al., Low-fat dietary pattern and risk of cardiovascular disease: The Women's Health Initiative Randomized Controlled Dietary Modification Trial.[see Comment], JAMA 295 (2006) 655–666.

[109] C. Ritenbaugh, R.E. Patterson, R.T. Chlebowski, et al., The Women's Health Initiative Dietary Modification Trial: overview and baseline characteristics of participants, Ann. Epidemiol. 13 (2003) A87–A97.

[110] L.F. Tinker, M.G. Perri, R.E. Patterson, et al., The effects of physical and emotional status on adherence to a low-fat dietary pattern in the Women's Health Initiative, J. Am. Diet. Assoc. 102 (2002) 799–800.

[111] M.L. Slattery, E. Kampman, W. Samowitz, B.J. Caan, J.D. Potter, Interplay between dietary inducers of GST and the GSTM-1 genotype in colon cancer, Int. J. Cancer 87 (2000) 728–733.

[112] E.L. Goode, C.M. Ulrich, J.D. Potter, Polymorphisms in DNA repair genes and associations with cancer risk, Cancer Epidemiol. Biomarkers Prev. 11 (2002) 1513–1530.

[113] J.A. Milner, S.S. McDonald, D.E. Anderson, P. Greenwald, Molecular targets for nutrients involved with cancer prevention, Nutr. Cancer 41 (2001) 1–16.

[114] A.F. Subar, S.I. Kirkpatrick, B. Mittl, T.P. Zimmerman, F.E. Thompson, C. Bingley, G. Wallis, N.G. Islam, T. Baranowski, S. McNutt, N. Potischman, The Automated Self-Administered 24-Hour Dietary Recall (ASA24): A resource for researchers, clinicians and educators from the National Cancer Institute, Journal of the Academy of Nutrition and Diabetics, 2012.

CHAPTER

7

Analysis, Presentation, and Interpretation of Dietary Data

Deborah A. Kerr[*], *TusaRebecca E. Schap*[†], *Rachel K. Johnson*[‡]

[*]Curtin University, Perth, Western Australia, [†]Purdue University, West Lafayette, Indiana
[‡]The University of Vermont, Burlington, Vermont

I INTRODUCTION

Nutritional epidemiological studies play a critical role in relating dietary intake to risk of disease. These investigations often require the gathering of dietary intake data from various samples, which must then be translated into a usable form. This chapter focuses on research applications for the interpretation of dietary data. This includes analysis, the examination of the dietary data to determine the nutritional composition of the participants' diets; presentation, the communication of the data and results in a logical format, such as comparing the results to a standard; and interpretation, the translation of the data and results—what do the data really tell us? The type of analysis undertaken will be largely determined by the research question being addressed. The dietary assessment method chosen requires consideration of the research question as the first step. In planning the research study, dietary assessment methods may be one of the ways to assess study outcomes. It is at this planning stage that the type of analysis to be undertaken needs to be determined. In Chapter 1, the advantages and disadvantages of dietary assessment instruments were outlined in detail. The choice of method can come down to constraints of funding, research staff availability, and participant burden. With future advances in technology in dietary assessment, it may be possible to overcome some of these limitations so that more detailed methods can be undertaken without being limited by cost and participant burden.

II ANALYSIS OF DIETARY DATA

The methods most often used to obtain dietary intake information for research investigations include 24-hour dietary recalls, dietary records or diaries, and food frequency questionnaires (FFQs). The 24-hour dietary recalls and dietary records provide detailed descriptions of the types and amounts of foods and beverages consumed throughout a specified period of time, normally 1–7 days. The FFQ provides a less detailed list of selected foods and the frequency of their consumption in the past, see Chapter 1 for further description of these methods. The data received must then be analyzed to determine the total intake of nutrients or food components consumed by each subject.

A Preparation for Analysis

Prior to data analysis, the data need to be checked for missing data and data entry errors. How best to minimize measurement error should always be the researcher's primary consideration. Technology has helped a great deal with reducing data entry errors and ensuring there are no missing data (e.g., forcing a response on an electronic FFQ), but there are still areas where the researcher must make decisions on what to enter for analysis and ensure data cleaning has occurred before the analysis is undertaken.

The first step in this process is to check the returned records. All paper-based records (food records and FFQs) require thorough checking to ensure there are no

Nutrition in the Prevention and Treatment of Disease, Third Edition.
DOI: http://dx.doi.org/10.1016/B978-0-12-391884-0.00007-X

missing data. Checking of the food record on return for missing data and probing for details on food types and amounts is critical for verifying the information recorded. This step can also improve the quality of the data [1]. This requires research staff who are familiar with food composition, ethnic or regionally specific foods, and the food database system being used for analysis, as well as the format in which foods need to be entered. Popular food items may also be age-specific. For example, when working with children and adolescents, the researcher needs to be knowledgeable of the foods this age group may consume. This requires knowledge of the brand names along with the generic equivalent the food may be listed as in the food composition database [2].

Ideally, the research staff should have qualifications in nutrition and dietetics and have undergone advanced training in dietary assessment. It is recognized, however, that not all graduates may have received training in this important area of competency for dietetic professionals [3]. Ideally, record checking should be done in person with the participant so that portion size aids may be shown. Alternatively, contacting the person by telephone can also be done to verify items recorded. Although complete checking of records is ideally the best approach, there may be situations in which some details are missed or the participant is unable to provide the level of detail the researcher would like. In addition, the task of undertaking 24-hour recalls or food records can become quite tedious for participants. When the researcher probes for more details, some participants may become concerned that they have not done a good job, whereas others may become bored and lose interest in the task [4]. The researcher must to be able to balance the need for detail with the burden placed on the participant. In addition, with food records, there may be incomplete days of recording or participants may have been unwell and not eaten. For some participants, no amount of probing will result in a quality record due to a consistent lack of detail of the foods consumed. The researcher should make a decision if he or she considers the record suitable for analysis.

B Rules for Data Entry

When entering data, rules for data entry should be set up to ensure a consistent approach is applied to all records. This is particularly important when a team of researchers is entering the data. The researcher needs to be able to translate the food or drink reported to the best match in the food database. These decisions need to be recorded along with what to do about missing data so that a standardized approach is used across all records. In some situations, participants may not know the composition of the food or drink consumed. This commonly occurs with meals eaten outside the home or where they have not been involved in the food preparation. In this case, it is important to standardize the rules and decision making on what food is considered the best match for a food selected from the food database. For databases such as the Food and Nutrient Database for Dietary Studies used in the "What We Eat in America" 24-hour recalls, for most foods there is an option to select a food code "not (further) specified" (NFS or NS) when the participant is unable to provide details of the food eaten. If the quantity of food eaten is not known, then "quantity not specified" (QNS) may be chosen. These are known as defaults used for coding. Because these are based on usual consumption patterns from survey data, the use of default codes introduces more error; thus, their use should be minimized [5].

C Computer-Based Analysis

A variety of computer-based food composition databases and nutrient computation systems are available in which the foods can be entered directly by name and computation of nutrient values is automated. The food composition databases are referred to as either the reference or user database. Selection of the correct food composition database is critical because the foods in the database must be appropriate to the geographical location and the ethnicity of the population being studied. Stumbo [2] and Buzzard and colleagues [6] summarize key points for selecting dietary assessment systems; for example: (1) Does the database contain all the foods and nutrients of interest? (2) Is the database complete for nutrients of interest? (3) Do the food descriptions included in the database provide adequate specificity to accurately assess food components of interest? and (4) What quality control procedures are used to ensure the accuracy of the database? The accuracy of the data obtained from these systems will differ, depending on the following factors:

Updating of the database. New foods are constantly being introduced in the market, so the best databases are updated often to keep up with these changes. Virtually all databases use the U.S. Department of Agriculture (USDA) Nutrient Database for Standard Reference (SR) as their primary source of nutrient data. The SR contains information once published in the *Agriculture Handbook 8*, but it is no longer available in the printed form [7]. The 2011 version, Release 24 (SR24), contains data on 7906 food items and up to 146 food components [8]. This release has focused on additional foods that are major contributors of sodium to the diet and formulated foods produced by the food industry. Although the information is not complete, specific criteria have been established for evaluating foods to ensure the data are as accurate as possible [9,10]. Many databases also add information from specific food manufacturers to provide information on name-brand foods not available in the SR.

The numbers and types of food items available. This is particularly important for recalls and dietary records or for FFQs containing write-in sections in which all foods must be assigned nutrient values. In regions with ethnocultural diversity, special care must be taken when selecting databases [11,12]. Many food names can be ambiguous or spelled in a number of different ways—for example, in the United States, ketchup versus catsup versus tomato sauce in England and Australia [2]. Pennington [13] summarized a number of useful examples of food items with more than one meaning and food synonyms. Databases that contain a variety of ethnic foods will provide greater accuracy and will require less manual entry of nutrient values for foods. The researcher must have knowledge of the naming convention and the search strategy required when using food composition databases [2].

The ability to add foods or nutrients. This is most important for those investigations in areas with multiethnicity [11,14,15] or when there is a high tendency for the participants to include restaurant foods that may not be included in the database. The trend is for greater consumption of food away from home [16], especially for teenagers and young adults [17]. This has implications for the accuracy of diet assessment because it may be difficult in some situations for participants to identify the contents and amount of food they have consumed. The ability to adapt or add recipe information should also be available. For example, if a subject had homemade beef stew for lunch, the database should allow the coder to either add or delete ingredients from an existing recipe or add a new recipe to the file. The decision as to what foods to add to the database may depend on the research question and how important the composition of these foods may be to the study outcomes. There are increasing numbers of functional foods that may not appear in the database. Again, it depends on the study objectives as to how critical it is to add these foods or adjust the composition of existing foods.

The ease of data entry and analysis. Systems should be easy to use to avoid unnecessary coding errors. Entry of products by name, particularly brand names, should be available. Some databases, such as the Food Intake Analysis System [18], which is a nutrient analysis software program, offer default options. These choices provide average estimations for foods for which exact information is not known. For example, if a subject had chicken breast but was not sure of the cooking method or the serving size, the coder can choose the default option instead of making guesses. These options can help decrease differences in nutrient intake values caused by multiple coders or data entry technicians.

The nutrients available. Not every database contains all nutrients, and some contain more accurate data for particular nutrients. Systems should be evaluated for the accuracy of the nutrient values that are being studied. Analysis should include the option of choosing nutrient calculations for each food as well as summaries for an individual meal or day.

The handling of missing nutrient values. Missing values exist if the food has not been analyzed for all food components [3]. If a specific nutrient value is unknown for a particular food, the way the database handles the missing information may affect the accuracy of the nutrient information. Some systems impute values, whereas others simply use a value of zero. An imputed value is almost always a better estimation [19]. However, imputing nutrient values is a labor-intensive task and requires nutritionists with knowledge of data evaluation and imputing procedures. Therefore, caution must be taken when using databases with imputed values.

The handling of dietary supplements. In most cases, only the dietary data are entered, but this may depend on the study objectives. For example, in a calcium study, the researchers may wish to examine total calcium intake, so adding in calcium from all sources may be necessary. For single nutrients, additions can be made at the analysis stage by adding into the exported data. The assessment of dietary supplement use was presented in detail in Chapter 2.

Standardizing dietary assessment. The emergence of large multicenter trials that may span across countries has presented challenges for dietary analysis. Because food composition may differ markedly, how best to pool nutrient databases must be addressed. The European Prospective Investigation into Cancer and Nutrition (EPIC) nutrient database project is an example of how researchers have attempted to standardize nutrient databases across 10 European countries [20]. A total of 26 priority nutrients were identified by the researchers along with procedures for food matching across counties.

D Statistical Approaches to Data Checking

Statistical packages such as IBM SPSS Statistics [21] and SAS [22] are very useful for checking nutrient data for errors prior to undertaking analysis. Once the data entry has been completed, various tests should be undertaken to ensure data entry errors have not occurred. Some laboratories will perform "double entry" by two researchers of all records as a way to minimize data entry errors. Once this is complete, using the compare function in statistics, packages such as SAS can be useful to identify where data entry errors have occurred. Additional tests that should be undertaken include the use of the explore function in SPSS to check for outliers in the data. In general, results that fall well outside the mean should be further explored to determine if they are true outliers or a data entry error. It is recommended that all nutrients be checked using the explore function because some data entry errors may only show up with certain nutrients. For example, an outlier in β-carotene may have occurred if the serving size of carrots was entered incorrectly, but this may have little impact on energy (calorie) intake.

E Factors Affecting Food Composition Databases

When computing nutrient intake from food consumption data, it is assumed that the nutrient quality and content of certain foods are virtually constant and that what is consumed is available for use. However, we know that this assumption is not totally correct. There are various reasons why the actual value of a consumed nutrient may differ from the calculated value. The level of certain nutrients in foods may be affected by differences in growing and harvesting conditions (e.g., selenium [23,24]), storage, processing, and cooking (e.g., vitamin C [25]). Databases attempt to account for some of the differences by increasing the data banks to include preparation methods, cuts of meat, and specific manufacturers for processed food. For example, if chicken is entered into the database, the coder may have approximately 455 items to choose from. This large number includes name brand foods, particular pieces of chicken available (e.g., breast or thigh), and cooking methods (e.g., baked or fried, cooked with skin on or off, and skin eaten or not). Because so many choices are offered, recalls and records should be as detailed as possible to provide enough information to make an accurate selection.

The use of controlled feeding trials in a study, such as the Dietary Approaches to Stop Hypertension (DASH) trial [26], can help alleviate some of the differences between the calculated and the actual nutrient values of food. The DASH trial was a multicenter study designed to compare the effects of dietary patterns on blood pressure. The subjects were asked to consume only foods prepared by the research centers. Food procurement, production, and distribution guidelines were set and strictly adhered to at all sites to ensure that menus consistently met nutrient goals. For example, food items were given specific purchasing sizes, detailed descriptions, or defined brand names to ensure that all site recipes were of uniform composition [27]. Menu items were analyzed in a laboratory to obtain nutrient content values [28]. When possible, foods can be obtained from central suppliers to further eliminate any differences in nutritional content of foods due to regional variations in a study of this type.

The diet as a whole can also affect the availability of some nutrients. For example, phytic acid may decrease the availability of iron [29]. Computer-based analysis programs do not generally examine the overall diet and cannot determine how nutrient–nutrient interactions may affect availability. For example, iron is a mineral for which intake is not a good marker for availability. The absorption of iron is influenced by the following components: (1) the source of iron (more heme iron is absorbed than nonheme iron), (2) the iron status of the individual (decreased iron stores increase absorption), and (3) the overall composition of the meal. These components play a role in determining how much of the iron consumed is available to the body [30,31]. In turn, iron consumption can also affect the absorption of other nutrients, such as zinc. Nutrient–nutrient interactions can greatly determine how well a calculated nutrient value represents the actual available amount of a nutrient.

Other factors that should be taken into account are drug–nutrient interactions and those people who may be malnourished or suffer from malabsorption. For example, the elderly are more likely to have a decreased ability to absorb vitamin B_{12} than are younger adults. The elderly population is also at higher risk for drug–nutrient interactions because they are often prescribed many medications. Researchers must be aware of any illnesses or medications taken by subjects that could interfere with nutrient absorption.

Although food composition databases are increasingly becoming more accurate and may be closer to actual values of energy intake than laboratory analysis [28], they cannot provide exact measurements for all nutrient intakes. Furthermore, even if these values are determined to be accurate, intake does not necessarily mean the nutrient is available for use. To obtain more accurate information on nutrient status, other methods, such as external reference biomarkers (see Chapter 12) should be employed. Also, familiarity with the participants' diets is essential for more accurate calculations.

This includes, but is not limited to, factors such as dietary supplement use, medications used, the presence of diseases or illness, as well as special diets that participants may be following (e.g., vegetarian or weight loss). The decision to include or exclude individual dietary data will depend on how these factors may affect the study outcomes.

F Total Diet Analysis

There is increasing interest by researchers in examining whole foods and food groups rather than single nutrients. Researchers are interested in identifying the dietary components in food that may interact [32,33]. In addition, most countries use a food-based approach to dietary guidelines, so examining how the diet compares to dietary guidelines may be of interest to researchers. There are also non-nutrient constituents, such as phytochemicals, that may play a role in disease prevention [34]. These indexes could prove to be very useful. The usefulness of diet quality indexes appears to be their ability to quantify risk of some health outcomes [35].

In reviewing the indexes of overall diet quality, Kant [36] found that there were three major approaches to the development of indexes: (1) derived from nutrients only, (2) based on foods or food groups, and (3) based on a combination of nutrients and foods. The definition of "diet quality" differs based on the attributes chosen by the investigators of each index [36], so the index chosen will depend on the needs of the study. The indexes based on nutrients only tend to consider consumption as a percentage of one of the nutrient-based reference values of the dietary reference intakes (DRIs), such as the Recommended Dietary Allowance (RDA), as a marker for diet quality. Those based on foods and food groups examine the intake patterns of foods to identify patterns associated with adequacy [36].

Although numerous tools are available for examining overall diet quality, those most commonly applied are based on the combination of nutrients and foods. These indexes, including the Healthy Eating Index—2005 (HEI-2005) [37], the Diet Quality Index (DQI) [38,39], the Diet Quality Index—International (DQI-I) [40], and the Mediterranean Diet Score (MDS) [41—43], use the dietary guidelines [44] and food selection guides of each country to score the overall diet. With the release of the Dietary Guidelines for Americans 2010 [44] and MyPlate [45], these are likely to be incorporated into future revisions of these indexes.

Patterson et al. [39] were among the first to relate diet quality to the Dietary Guidelines for Americans.

The DQI was based on dietary recommendations from the 1989 National Academy of Sciences publication Diet and Health, in which intakes were stratified into three levels for scoring. These points were summed across eight diet variables to score the index from zero (excellent diet) to 16 (poor diet). Haines et al. [38] revised the index in 1999, now called the Dietary Quality Index—Revised (DQI-R) [38], to reflect the updated guidelines. However, no revision has been made to reflect the 2010 Dietary Guidelines for Americans.

The DQI-R incorporates both nutrients and food components to determine diet quality. It is based on 10 components, with a 100-point scale; each component is worth 10 points (Table 7.1). Components are based on total fat and saturated fat as a percentage of energy; milligrams of cholesterol consumed; recommended servings for fruit, vegetables, and grains; adequacy of calcium and iron intake; dietary diversity; and dietary moderation. The dietary diversity score was developed to show differences in intake across 23 broad food group categories, including 7 grain-based products, 7 vegetable components, 2 fruit and juice categories, and 7 animal-based products [38]. Dietary moderation scores added sugars, discretionary fat, sodium intake, and alcohol intake. The DQI-R was designed to monitor dietary changes in populations but can provide an estimate of diet quality for an individual relative to the

TABLE 7.1 Diet Quality Index—Revised

Component	Maximum score criteria[a]	Minimum score criteria[a]
Total fat (% of energy intake)	≤30%	>40%
Saturated fat (% of energy intake)	≤10%	>13%
Dietary cholesterol	≤300 mg	>400 mg
% Recommended servings of fruit per day (2—4 based on energy intake)	≥100%	<50%
% Recommended servings of vegetables/day (3—5 based on energy intake)	≥100%	<50%
% Recommended servings of bread per day (6—11 based on energy intake)	≥100%	<50%
Calcium (% adequate intake for age)	≥100%	<50%
Iron intake (% 1989 RDA for age)	≥100%	<50%
Dietary diversity score	≥6	<3
Dietary moderation score	≥7	<4

[a]Scoring range for each component is 0 (minimum) to 10 (maximum).
Source: Haines, P. S., Siega-Riz, A. M., and Popkin, B. M. (1999). The Diet Quality Index Revised: A measurement instrument for populations. Copyright © The American Dietetic Association. Reprinted by permission from Journal of the American Dietetic Association, Vol. 99: 697—704.

national guidelines and can note improvement or decline of diet quality with multiple calculations [38].

The HEI [37,46] was first developed in 1995 by the USDA Center for Nutrition Policy and Promotion to assess and monitor the dietary status of Americans [46]. It has undergone revision to reflect updated guidelines, including a revision in 2006 that is known as HEI-2005 [37], and it uses a density approach with the standards expressed as a percentage of calories or per 1000 calories (Table 7.2). Whereas the HEI resembled the DQI-R, the HEI-2005 differs in several areas. The HEI-2005 contains 12 components, not only examining the total intake of fruit, vegetables, and grains but also taking into account whole fruits and grains and specific vegetables consumed. Cholesterol intake, total fat, and food variety components were removed and replaced with "oils" and "calories from solid fat, alcohol, and added sugars."

Categorizing foods into appropriate groups, particularly combination foods, can be a problem when using these analysis techniques. Cleveland *et al.* [47] developed a method for assessing food intakes in terms of food servings. These guidelines help to overcome two major obstacles when assessing food intake with respect to the dietary guidelines—which are dealing with food mixtures and the differing units of measurement used. Because many foods are eaten as mixtures and are difficult to categorize into food groups, Cleveland *et al.* developed a recipe file that helps to break down food mixtures into ingredients so they can be assigned to their respective groups more easily. Standard serving sizes were assigned gram weights to help to overcome the units problem, allowing for the use of only one unit of measure. Approaches have also been developed for assessing whole grain servings as defined by the Food Guide Pyramid [48] or the Healthy Eating Index [49].

III PRESENTATION OF DATA

The presentation of data depends on the research questions for each study. For example, for a cross-sectional dietary assessment of an ethnic population, it may be useful to compare the data against population standards. These standards may include the DRI or comparison to a national average, such as the National Health and Nutrition Examination Surveys (NHANES). Batis *et al.* [50] demonstrate how dietary differences among ethnic populations may be presented. Researchers may also wish to evaluate menus in comparison to dietary intakes. In a study involving 40 New York child care centers, researchers compared the dietary intakes of children to the dietary recommendations and found that less than 50% of children

TABLE 7.2 Healthy Eating Index, 2005—Components and Standards for Scoring[a]

Component	Maximum points	Standard for maximum score	Standard for minimum score (0)
Total fruit (includes 100% juice)	5	≥ 0.8 cup equiv. per 1000 kcal	No fruit
Whole fruit (not juice)	5	≥ 0.4 cup equiv. per 1000 kcal	No whole fruit
Total vegetables	5	≥ 1.1 cup per 1000 kcal	No vegetables
Dark green and orange vegetables and legumes[b]	5	≥ 0.4 cup equiv. per 1000 kcal	No dark green or orange vegetables or legumes
Total grains	5	≥ 3 oz. equiv. per 1000 kcal	No grains
Whole grains	5	≥ 1.5 oz. equiv. per 1000 kcal	No whole grains
Milk[c]	10	≥ 1.3 cup equiv. per 1000 kcal	No milk
Meat and beans	10	≥ 2.5 oz. equiv. per 1000 kcal	No mean or beans
Oils[d]	10	≥ 12 g per 1000 kcal	No oil
Saturated fat	10	≤ 7% of energy	≥ 15% of energy
Sodium	10	≤ 0.7 g per 1000 kcal[e]	≥ 2.0 g per 1000 kcal
Calories from solid fat, alcohol, and added sugar	20	≤ 20% of energy[e]	≥ 50% of energy

[a]Intakes between the minimum and maximum levels are scored proportionately, except for saturated fat and sodium (see note e).
[b]Legumes counted as vegetables only after meat and beans standard is met.
[c]Includes all milk products, such as fluid milk, yogurt, and cheese.
[d]Includes nonhydrogenated vegetable oils and oils in fish, nuts, and seeds.
[e]Saturated fat and sodium get a score of 8 for intake levels that reflect the 2005 Dietary Guidelines, <10% of calories from saturated fat and 1.1 g of sodium/1000 kcal, respectively.
Source: *Reprinted from Guenther, P. M., Krebs-Smith, S. M., Reedy, J., Britten, P., Juan, W. Y., Lino, M., Carlson, A., Hiza, H. A., and Basiotis, P. P. (2006). The Healthy Eating Index—2005, CNPP-Fact Sheet No. 1. U.S. Department of Agriculture, Center for Nutritional Policy and Promotion, Alexandria, VA.*

ate at least half of the daily recommended intake for each of the five food groups [51]. When comparing data for analyses, researchers must take into account differences that may exist between survey methods,

TABLE 7.3 Uses of Dietary Reference Intakes for Healthy Individuals and Groups

Type of use	For the individual	For a group
Planning	RDA: Aim for this intake.	EAR: Use in conjunction with a measure of variability of the group's mean intake of a specific population.
	AI: Aim for this intake.	
	UL: Use as a guide to limit intake; chronic intake of higher amounts may increase risk of adverse effects.	
Assessment[a]	EAR: Use to examine the possibility of inadequacy; evaluation of true status requires clinical, biochemical, or anthropometric data.	EAR: Use in assessment of the prevalence of inadequate intakes within a group.

[a]*Requires statistically valid approximation of usual intake.*
AI, adequate intake; EAR, estimated average requirement; RDA, recommended dietary allowance; UL, tolerable upper intake level.
Source: *Reprinted with permission from the National Academies Press, Copyright 2005, National Academy of Sciences, Institute of Medicine and the National Academies (2005).* Dietary Reference Intakes for Energy, Carbohydrate, Fiber, Fat, Fatty Acids, Cholesterol, Protein, and Amino Acids. *National Academy Press, Washington, DC.*

TABLE 7.4 Overview of What We Eat in America (WWEIA)

Two days of 24-hour dietary recalls are collected using the USDA's computerized dietary data collection instrument, the Automated Multiple-Pass Method (AMPM)	Day 1: In-person interview in the mobile examination center (MEC); three-dimensional food models are available.
	Day 2: Telephone interview on a different day of the week than the MEC interview; USDA's Food Model Booklet and a limited number of three-dimensional models are provided.

Information Collected during the Interviews

For each food and beverage consumed during previous 24-hour period	Detailed description Additions to the food Amount consumed What foods were eaten in combination Time eating occasion began Name of eating occasion Food source (where obtained) Whether food was eaten at home Amounts of food energy and 60 + nutrients/food components provided by the amount of food (calculated)
For each respondent on each day	Day of the week Amount and type of water consumed, including total plain water, tap water, and plain carbonated water Source of tap water Daily intake usual, much more or much less than usual Use and type of salt at table and in preparation Whether on a special diet and type of diet Frequency of fish and shellfish consumption (children 1–5 and women 16–49 years) Daily total intakes of food energy and 60 + nutrients/food components (calculated)

questionnaire wording, data processing, and databases that could impact comparisons.

The DRIs are a set of nutrient-based reference values that include an estimated average requirement (EAR), an RDA, and an adequate intake (AI), which are defined by nutrient adequacy and may relate to the reduction of the risk of chronic disease [52]. Once the EARs have been established, they are used to set the RDAs, which should be used as a daily intake goal by healthy individuals and should be sufficient to meet the needs of 97 or 98% of all healthy people. If there is not sufficient evidence to determine an EAR, then an AI is set, once again based on groups of healthy people. A tolerable upper intake LEVEL (UL) is set when information is available as an indicator of excess for nutrients [52]. Each value has a specific goal and use [52] (Table 7.3). For example, the EAR is the estimate that is believed to meet the nutrient needs of half of the healthy people in a gender or life-stage group. When assessing nutrient intake of healthy groups, the EAR should be used instead of the RDA [52].

DRIs are set for specific subgroups based on age and gender. They are to be applied to healthy populations and may not be adequate for those who are or have been malnourished or have certain diseases or conditions that increase nutrient requirements. For individuals, the RDA and AI can serve as a goal for nutrient intake. A more complete description of the DRIs can be found in Chapter 13.

Some researchers use national survey data as a standard when presenting dietary data. What We Eat in America (WWEIA) is the dietary intake component of NHANES. This survey is a joint effort between the USDA and the U.S. Department of Health and Human Services, with data released in 2-yearly intervals. NHANES provides medical history, physical measurements, biochemical evaluation, physical signs and symptoms, and diet information from two 24-hour recalls. Table 7.4 provides an overview of the dietary information collected. Researchers may wish to compare results to the information obtained from these surveys to determine how their study sample compares to the national average. Although the data from these surveys may be applied to certain subgroups, such as specific age groups, gender, socioeconomic levels, education levels, and some ethnic groups, they cannot be used as guides for others, such as malnourished or specific disease states.

IV INTERPRETATION OF DATA

Once the dietary intake data have been checked for errors, analyzed, and compared to a standard, researchers must then examine the results to determine what the data really mean. How the data are interpreted can depend on the research questions, the dietary assessment method used and the nutrient being studied, the study type, and the accuracy of participants' responses.

A Assessment Methods

The assessment method chosen for use in a study can determine how the data collected can be interpreted. Recalls and records gather present intake data, whereas FFQs provide data based on past intake. It is known that a person's nutrient and energy intake varies not only from day to day but also from season to season. Thus, if past intake is needed, FFQs may be the better choice.

The number of days of food intake records or recalls available can also affect the interpretation of the data. If high levels of accuracy are needed for a person's nutrient intake, a greater number of days will be required than if a group average could be used. Care must be taken when determining the number of days to use in a study. For example, researchers using data from a single 24-hour recall from 832 men found that saturated fat intake was inversely associated with stroke [53]. Because of the day-to-day variability, dietary changes or recommendations for an individual should not be based on a single day's intake. Basiotis *et al.* [54] determined the number of days of food intake data needed to estimate individual intake as well as group intake for food energy and 18 nutrients. They found that for females, an average of 35 days were needed to determine a true average of energy intake for each women, whereas 3 days of food records from each subject were required to determine a group average. A minimum of 6 days of food records were needed to assess vitamin K in an elderly population [55]. However, participant burden also needs to be

considered because longer recording periods may result in lower quality records as the number of days of recording increases [56].

It is also important that data obtained from dietary assessment methods be utilized properly. The FFQ was developed to rank nutrient intakes from low to high. It was not intended to be used to determine and develop levels of nutrient intake to prevent disease. However, many researchers have chosen to use the FFQ for this purpose. For example, studies based on FFQ data have recommended levels of vitamin E intake to reduce risk for heart disease [57,58]. However, other studies have concluded that these levels may not have the effect on the development of heart disease that was previously suggested [59–61]. When choosing a method for dietary assessment, care must be taken to ensure that the data are properly interpreted.

B Data Validity

One major concern when interpreting dietary data is the accuracy of the information reported. Because most of the information gathered is self-reported, the reliability and validity of the data depend on the reporter's motivation, memory, ability to communicate, and awareness of the foods consumed. Most methods have been proven to be generally reliable; that is, they will provide the same estimate on different occasions. However, do the techniques gather true and accurate measurements, or valid measurements, of what people are really eating? In the past, assumptions were made that the information was indeed valid. The validity of the techniques was often verified by comparing the different methods to each other. This technique has been referred to as calibration [62]. For example, the results of an FFQ are compared with results obtained using a food record or repeated 24-hour recalls. The estimates by the different methods will differ for a number of reasons. FFQs rely on the participant's memory to recall foods eaten over a specified period of time. Some participants may have difficulty in remembering this level of detail. Alternatively, food records rely on participants' willingness to record in great detail all food items and beverages consumed. The burden of this task is known to lead to participants changing their intake. It is important to be aware that all self-report methods will have measurement error. This presents a major issue for data interpretation because imprecise methods may obscure the diet–disease relationship. This issue is discussed in detail by Freedman and colleagues [63]. A way to address measurement error in dietary assessment methods is by use of external recovery biomarkers [62,64]. Doubly labeled water (DLW) is the most widely used biomarker for energy intake (see

Chapter 12 for further details). Other biomarkers that have been used to validate nutrient intake include fatty acid patterns in blood to reflect fatty acid intake [65], urinary nitrogen to validate protein intake [66,67], serum carotenoids and vitamin C concentrations as markers of fruit and vegetable consumption [68], as well as urinary sucrose and fructose as a marker of total sugar intakes [69]. With the increased use of these biomarkers, particularly DLW, to determine the accuracy of dietary intake data in a variety of subjects, reporting errors will be better defined. The use of dietary biomarkers may even help to compensate for reporting errors related to some nutrients—for example, urinary sucrose and fructose as a biomarker for total sugar intakes. Misreporting of food intake—over- or underreporting—occurs with all self-report methods of dietary assessment [64].

A concerted effort is being made to develop and identify objective dietary biomarkers to aid in defining dietary exposures. Dietary biomarkers are objective biochemical indicators of dietary intake or nutritional status that accommodate the error in self-report methods and thus shed light on the diet–disease relationship [70]. Biomarkers may also be defined as a biochemical indicator of dietary intake/nutritional status, an index of nutrient metabolism, or a marker of the biological consequences of dietary intake [71]. There are three classes of nutritional biomarkers: recovery, concentration/replacement, and predictive biomarkers [71]. In order to obtain independent observations, epidemiologists have utilized concentration biomarkers assessed in biological samples as predictors of disease risk. High-density lipoprotein cholesterol and low-density lipoprotein cholesterol are examples of well-known biomarkers that are strongly associated with risk for cardiovascular disease. One of the main uses of dietary biomarkers is as a reference measurement to assess the validity and accuracy of dietary assessment methods. Recovery biomarkers are based on the concept of metabolic balance between intake and excretion over a fixed period of time [71]. Recovery biomarkers such as DLW and urinary nitrogen help to quantify errors in self-report of energy and protein intake, respectively. The concept of predictive biomarkers is relatively new. These biomarkers are sensitive, time dependent, and show a dose–response relationship with intake levels [69]. Although the correlation to intake is high, the actual recovery of the marker is quite low. Urinary fructose and sucrose concentrations represent predictive biomarkers that have been shown to significantly correlate with sugar intake and provide a useful, independent qualitative index of sugar consumption [69]. Urinary sucrose and fructose have been used in the Observing Protein and Energy Nutrition (OPEN) study to assess for error in self-reported intake of total

sugars [72]. Researchers propose that predictive biomarkers, like recovery biomarkers, may be useful for validation and calibration studies to estimate the error in self-reported dietary intakes. Predictive biomarkers may also be used independently of self-report to categorize people by their level of nutrient intake. Inherent errors (e.g., underreporting and undereating) in self-report of dietary intake may be difficult to eliminate. However, the use of dietary biomarkers will accommodate for the errors in self-report methods and thus shed light on the diet–disease relationship. For the researcher, the issue is how best to deal with implausible records as well as continuing to try to identify those participants most likely to overreport and why.

1 Overreporting

Overreporting occurs when reported intakes are higher than the measured energy expenditure levels. Overreporting has not been found to be as large of a problem with regard to reported energy intakes as underreporting, but it still has the potential to interfere with results and conclusions. This occurs particularly if the overreported foods are low in energy but high in nutrients such as many vegetables. Johansson et al. [73] found that people who overreport tend to be younger and, with lower body mass indexes, are often considered lean. The highest proportion of overreporters was found among those subjects who wanted to increase body weight. A study of the elderly population found that overreporting was higher in men [74]. Although overreporters are not common, care should be taken when obtaining data from participants who have characteristics related to risk of overreporting.

2 Underreporting

Underreporting occurs when reported intakes are lower than measured energy expenditure levels or estimated energy requirements. These reports are often so low that basal metabolic needs could not be met, and they are not biologically plausible. Depending on the age, gender, and body composition of a given sample, underreporters may comprise 2–85% of the total sample [75]. It is now understood that underreporting tends to be associated with certain groups. Prevalence of underreporting also increases as body mass index (BMI) increases. Many studies have shown that the obese underreport more often and to a greater degree—30–47%—than the lean [76–80]. Women have also been found to underreport more often than men [78,81–86]. The EPIC 24-hour recall data indicated that BMI and age were consistently related to underreporting among 35,955 men and women aged 35–74 years [86]. The researchers note, however, that the association observed may simply be due to the common

TABLE 7.5   Summary of Underreporting

Populations Most Likely to Underreport

Women [73,86]	Smokers [73,82]
Higher body mass index [73,79,80,85,86]	Lower education [79]
Low socioeconomic status, lower income [79,82,85]	Ethnicity [79]

Psychosocial Characteristics Associated with Underreporting

High scorers on restrained eating scales [88]	A history of dieting behavior [80,88]
Body dissatisfaction [85,89]	Social desirability [80,85]
Fear of negative evaluation [80]	

Foods Most Likely to Be Underreported

U.S. Survey [91]

Cake/pie	Meat, fish, poultry, egg sandwiches or mixtures
Savory snacks: chips, popcorn, pretzels	Regular soft drinks
Cheese	Fat-type spreads
White potatoes	Condiments

British Survey [92]

Cake	Breakfast cereal
Sugars	Milk
Fats	

source of variability between EI/basal metabolic rate (BMR) and its components and not to a true causal relationship between BMI, age and underreporting. Table 7.5 provides a summary of groups most likely to be underreporters. These factors are further complicated by the possibility that they are risk factors for many chronic diseases.

3 The Problem with Underreporting

A major problem with underreporting occurs when researchers begin to classify dietary intake information to determine diet and disease associations. This is often done by ranking nutrient intakes from low to high and then searching for any associations between nutrient intake and the occurrence of disease. There is a danger of misclassification of subjects if this ranking is based on false or underreported intakes. As noted previously, those who tend to be at higher risk for underreporting are also those who are at greater risk for many chronic diseases. For example, obesity is a known risk factor for coronary heart disease as well as underreporting. Because bias in measuring dietary intake has the potential of removing as well as creating associations, it can

generate misleading conclusions about the impact of diet and disease [69,70]. Underreporting is a potentially misleading problem in nutrition research. The use of biomarkers can help to validate and objectively interpret dietary intake data and, ideally, should become routine in nutritional epidemiology. However, the cost of some biomarkers such as DLW may make it impractical for routine use for researchers.

4 Reasons for Underreporting

With the aid of biomarkers for dietary intake, reporting error has been defined. Researchers continue to search for reasons why people underreport. We know that being obese is not the cause of underreporting, but it is most likely the psychological and behavioral characteristics associated with obesity that lead to underreporting [75,87]. Social desirability and self-monitoring are contributors to reporting errors [80,88]. A need for social acceptance, a desire to be liked or accepted by the interviewer, may cause the subject to underreport "sinful" foods or report "healthy" foods that were not actually consumed. A high level of body dissatisfaction—that is, if a person sees a leaner physique as being healthier or more desirable than his or her own—may cause the person to misreport foods [89]. Also, researchers found that women who scored higher on restrained eating scales, those who believe they are making a conscious effort to avoid certain foods, tend to underreport as well [75,87,88]. For some people, the act of recording dietary intake may lead to changes in eating behaviors. Thus, a person may be reporting actual, but not usual, intakes.

Another explanation for underreporting may be related more to meal size than body size. Wansink and Chandon [90] asked overweight and normal-weight adults to estimate the calories in both small and large fast-food meals. They found that both groups underestimated the number of calories in the larger meals. Therefore, greater underestimation of energy by obese individuals may be, in part, a result of their tendency to consume larger meals.

5 Foods Most Often Underreported

Underreporting does not occur for all foods and nutrients to the same degree. Foods that are perceived as unhealthy are reported less frequently and in smaller portions among low energy reporters. In a U.S. survey of 8334 adults, 1224 were found to be low energy reporters [91]. Foods that were found to be most often underreported included cakes/pies, savory snacks, cheese, white potatoes, meats, regular soft drinks, fat-type spreads, and condiments [91]. British researchers found little difference between underreporters and plausible energy reporters with regard to bread, potatoes, meat, vegetables, or fruit, but a significant

difference was seen with cakes, sugars, fat, and breakfast cereal [92]. Participants completing a 24-hour dietary recall after being observed for 24 hours in a
metabolic unit frequently did not report between-meal
eating events [93]. This may further contribute to the
most often underreported foods. Table 7.5 gives a summary of underreported foods. Some researchers have
found that underreporters tend to report lower intakes
of fat and higher intakes of protein and carbohydrates
as a percentage of total energy [93,94], whereas others
show that reports of added sugar intake are significantly lower [93]. The OPEN study used DLW to identify low energy reporters [95] and found they were
more likely to report smaller portions and female low
energy reporters reported less soft drink consumption.
No agreement has been reached as to how much, if at
all, specific macronutrients are misreported.

6 Identifying Underreporters

To help identify underreporters, researchers can
apply methods such as the Goldberg cutoff, extensively
described by Goldberg and colleagues [96] and Black
and colleagues [97,98]. The Goldberg cutoff identifies
the most obvious implausible intake values by evaluating the energy intake against estimated energy requirements. BMR can be measured using methods described
in Chapter 4, or height and weight measurements can
be used to predict BMR from a standard formula (the
Schofield equation is recommended by Goldberg et al.
[96]). A ratio of the estimated EI to measured or predicted BMR is calculated as EI/BMR. This ratio can
then be compared with a study-specific cutoff value
(see Black [97] for a practical guide to using the
Goldberg cutoff). This cutoff represents the lowest
value of EI/BMR that could reasonably reflect the
energy expenditure based on the physical activity level
if the information is available or assuming a sedentary
lifestyle if no activity information is gathered. A summary of the principles of the cutoffs can be found in
Table 7.6. Studies using the Goldberg cutoff classified
28−39% of the women and 18−27% of the men as low
energy reporters [82,91].

The Goldberg cutoff has several limitations [97]. It
has poor sensitivity for defining invalid reports at the
individual level because it identifies only the extreme
underreporters. It also does not distinguish between
varying degrees of underreporting. The major limitation is that the cutoff depends on knowledge of energy
requirements or energy expenditure. If no physical
activity information is available, the cutoff assumes a
sedentary lifestyle and will therefore underestimate the
underreporters and may lead to misclassification of
energy reporting. If researchers can gather information
on lifestyle, occupation, leisure time activities, and particularly information regarding physical activity of the

TABLE 7.6 Principles of the Goldberg Cutoff

Principle	Equations and comments
Principle 1: Validation of reported energy intake rests on the following:	Energy intake (EI) = energy expenditure (EE) − changes in body stores
Principle 2: Assumes subjects are weight stable and therefore are in energy balance:	EI = EE
Principle 3: Express energy requirements as multiples of basal metabolic rate (BMR).	EE = physical activity level (PAL) × BMR
Principle 4: Since EI = EE and EE = PAL × BMR, then the following can be assumed:	EI = PAL × BMR or EI: BMR = PAL
Principle 5: Reported energy intake expressed as:	EI$_{rep}$: BMR can be compared with expected PAL.
Principle 6: Since error exists in all the measured elements of the equation, absolute agreement cannot be expected.	
Principle 7: Confidence limits (cutoffs) of the agreement between:	EI$_{rep}$: BMR and PAL must be determined to establish if reported values within the subjects are acceptable. (For cutoff equations, see Black et al. [93].)

Source: *Data from Black, A. E. (2000). Critical evaluation of energy intake using the Goldberg cut-off for energy intake:basal metabolic rate: A practical guide to its calculation, use and limitations.* Int. J. Obes. Relat. Metab. Disord. **24**, 1119−1130.

participants, calculations can be more specific and
improve the classification of energy reporting (i.e.,
plausible, underreporting, or overreporting).

To compensate for the physical activity level limitations, McCrory et al. [99,100] proposed a method based
on the principles of the Goldberg cutoff to screen for
implausible reports by comparing reported energy
intake with predicted total energy expenditure [99,101].
Researchers offer that because total energy expenditures are predicted, not just basal metabolic rate, this
new method eliminates the potential error caused by
assigning inaccurate physical activity levels when there
is limited or no information on activity levels available
[99]. With the Goldberg method, only those participants who report ±2 standard deviation cutoffs are
considered underreporters. However, McCrory et al.
[99] suggest that in some studies, particularly those in
which relationships between habitual intakes and disease outcomes are examined, using a 1 standard deviation cutoff may help to identify those reporters who
report actual but not habitual diet. Using this method
to analyze CSFII 1994−1996 data, Huang et al. [100]
found that implausible reported energy intakes

reduced the overall validity of the sample and including misreporters could lead to inappropriate conclusions about the impact of diet on health outcomes.

7 Handling Underreporting in Dietary Data

Researchers are still not sure how to handle data sets containing large numbers of underreporters. Several approaches have been suggested, but none are ideal. One technique is to exclude anyone who is found to report implausible energy intakes. The problem with this method is that the underreporters tend to fall into specific subgroups (i.e., obese and smokers) and, as stated previously, eliminating them will alter the sample. Some investigators have analyzed their data with all the subjects and then again after the underreporters were removed [102]. Among adults from Pacific Northwest tribal nations, plausible reporters completing dietary records were found to have higher estimates of vitamins A, C, and E, magnesium, and sodium [103]. For the plausible reporters in this population, the association between reported energy intakes (from dietary records and from FFQs) and weight was significant [104]. However, when the sample was not limited to plausible reporters, the association between reported energy intakes and weight was not significant.

Other researchers have suggested adjusting nutrient intakes for energy intake using the regression of nutrient versus energy [105]. This would be feasible only if portion sizes were underestimated but the actual foods were all reported accurately. Otherwise, this method could make the reports worse [106]. As noted previously, it is most likely that foods are systematically omitted from recalls. Thus, if, for example, fat-containing foods (e.g., desserts) are often underreported, whereas vitamin A-containing foods (e.g., cantaloupe) are not, energy adjustments would provide lower than actual measures of fat intake but a higher measure of vitamin A intake. Many researchers have recognized that adjustments cannot eliminate the bias caused by selective underreporting [107].

8 Improving Dietary Assessment with Technology

Variations on the 24-hour dietary recall, food records, and FFQs have been carefully developed and improved upon throughout the years; however, the errors discussed previously still remain. Technological advances have prompted researchers to investigate the use of technology to improve diet assessment methods. Efforts to use available technology include applications for personal computers and mobile devices, as well as the development of objective biomarkers for dietary intakes [108]. Technology-based dietary assessment holds promise for engaging participants and reducing participant burden, as well as alleviating many researcher burdens (e.g., data entry and interview staff), thus improving cooperation and accuracy [108,109]. Objective biomarkers hold promise for improving associations between dietary intakes and disease outcomes in tandem with or independent of dietary assessment methods.

As technology has rapidly evolved and become more widely adopted by the general public, applications for mobile devices with integrated digital cameras have become desirable tools for use in the research community. Applications in which a participant or "user" takes images of foods and beverages consumed have become of increasing interest. Mobile applications are also viewed favorably by adolescent and adult study participants who report a preference for technology-based dietary assessment over pen-and-paper methods [4,110]. Proposed image-based dietary assessment methods can be categorized as follows: Images are reviewed by the participant/user, images are reviewed by a trained analyst, or automated systems review the images. One proposed use of digital images is to supplement a 24-hour dietary recall—in other words, an image-assisted dietary recall. Arab and Winter [111] proposed a method in which a user wears a mobile device that hangs around his or her neck for a 24-hour period. During this time, intermittent images are automatically taken. The images containing food and beverages are presented to the user to help him or her remember all foods and beverages during the 24-hour dietary recall [111]. Although the digital images of foods reviewed by the user reduce the memory-related burden, issues related to portion size estimation still exist. Applications in which images taken by a participant are reviewed by a trained analyst remove the portion size estimation burden from the user. In one example, the remote food photography method, analyst estimates range from approximately −5 to 7% of actual energy intakes [110]. Although accuracy of energy intakes would be improved with this method, there remains a burden on research staff to visually analyze the images. To further remove burden from the user as well as the researcher in an effort to improve the accuracy of dietary intakes, nutrition researchers are teaming with electrical engineers to develop an application in which the images are primarily analyzed using an automated system [112–114]. As technology continues to evolve, we can expect that image-based dietary assessment will become more mainstream as a means for ameliorating self-reporting errors currently seen in diet assessment methods.

V CONCLUSION

Dietary assessment methods provide valuable data to measure dietary exposure in nutritional epidemiology.

When undertaking dietary assessment, attention should be given to ways in which error can be minimized throughout the data gathering and analysis process. Identifying underreporters and improving dietary database validity through analytical approaches should remain in the forefront of dietary assessment until methodology improvements can be found. Improving dietary intake methodology is critical to the credibility of nutrition research, and improvements in technology may be a way forward to achieving this goal.

References

[1] M.M. Cantwell, A.E. Millen, R. Carroll, B.L. Mittl, S. Hermansen, L.A. Brinton, et al., A debriefing session with a nutritionist can improve dietary assessment using food diaries, J. Nutr. 136 (2006) 440−445.

[2] P. Stumbo, Considerations for selecting a dietary assessment system, J. Food Comp. Anal. 21 (2008) S13−S19.

[3] J.A. Pennington, P.J. Stumbo, S.P. Murphy, S.W. McNutt, A.L. Eldridge, B.J. McCabe-Sellers, et al., Food composition data: the foundation of dietetic practice and research, J. Am. Diet. Assoc. 107 (2007) 2105−2113.

[4] C.J. Boushey, D.A. Kerr, J. Wright, K.D. Lutes, D.S. Ebert, E.J. Delp, Use of technology in children's dietary assessment, Eur. J. Clin. Nutr. 63 (2009) S50−S57.

[5] U.S. Department of Agriculture, Agricultural Research Service, Beltsville Human Nutrition Research Center, Food Surveys Research Group; U.S. Department of Health and Human Services, Centers for Disease Control and Prevention, National Center for Health Statistics. "Defaults Used for Coding Foods and Amounts in What We Eat in America." Available at <http://reedir.arsnet.usda.gov/codesearchwebapp/(gjp41x2gbo4s4s45ymsivd45)/defaults.pdf>.

[6] I.M. Buzzard, K.S. Price, R.A. Warren, Considerations for selecting nutrient-calculation software: evaluation of the nutrient database, Am. J. Clin. Nutr. 54 (1991) 7−9.

[7] U.S. Department of Agriculture, Agricultural Research Service, Nutrient Data Laboratory. "About Us." Available at <http://www.ars.usda.gov/Aboutus/docs.htm?docid = 4441>(2011).

[8] U.S. Department of Agriculture, Agricultural Research Service and Nutrient Data Laboratory. "USDA National Nutrient Database for Standard Reference, Release 24." Available at <http://www.ars.usda.gov/research/publications/publications.htm?seq_no_115 = 272030>, (2011).

[9] D.B. Haytowitz, P.R. Pehrsson, J.M. Holden, The identification of key foods for food composition research, J. Food Comp. Anal. 15 (2002) 183−194.

[10] K.M. Phillips, et al., Quality-control materials in the USDA National Food and Nutrient Analysis Program, Anal. Bioanal. Chem. 384 (2006) 1341−1355.

[11] K.W. Cuthrell, S. Yuen, S. Murphy, R. Novotny, D.L. Au, Hawaii foods website: a locally based online nutrition and food-composition resource for healthcare professionals and the public, Hawaii Med. J. 69 (2010) 300−301.

[12] I.O. Akinyele, F.T. Aminu, Computerized database of ethnocultural foods commonly eaten in Nigeria, Am. J. Clin. Nutr. 65 (1997) 1331S−1335S.

[13] J.A. Pennington, Applications of food composition data: data sources and considerations for use, J. Food Comp. Anal. 21 (Suppl.) (2008) S3−S12.

[14] S. Sharma, X. Cao, J. Gittelsohn, B. Ethelbah, J. Anliker, Nutritional composition of commonly consumed traditional Apache foods in Arizona, Int. J. Food Sci. Nutr. 59 (2008) 1−10.

[15] S. Sharma, M.M. Yacavone, X. Cao, P.M. Samuda, J. Cade, K. Cruickshank, Nutritional composition of commonly consumed composite dishes for Afro-Caribbeans (mainly Jamaicans) in the United Kingdom, Int. J. Food Sci. Nutr. 60 (Suppl. 7) (2009) 140−150.

[16] J.F. Guthrie, B.H. Lin, E. Frazao, Role of food prepared away from home in the American diet, 1977−78 versus 1994−96: changes and consequences, J. Nutr. Educ. Behav. 34 (2002) 140−150.

[17] K.W. Bauer, N.I. Larson, M.C. Nelson, M. Story, D. Neumark-Sztainer, Fast food intake among adolescents: secular and longitudinal trends from 1999 to 2004, Prev. Med. 48 (2009) 284−287.

[18] University of Texas Health Science Center at Houston, School of Public Health, Food Intake Analysis System, Millennium Edition, University of Texas Health Science Center at Houston, School of Public Health, Houston, TX, 2005.

[19] I. Cowin, P. Emmett, The effect of missing data in the supplements to McCance and Widdowson's food tables on calculated nutrient intakes, Eur. J. Clin. Nutr. 53 (1999) 891−894.

[20] N. Slimani, G. Deharveng, I. Unwin, D.A. Southgate, J. Vignat, G. Skeie, et al., The EPIC Nutrient Database Project (ENDB): a first attempt to standardize nutrient databases across the 10 European countries participating in the EPIC study, Eur. J. Clin. Nutr. 61 (2007) 1037−1056.

[21] SPSS, IBM SPSS Statistics 19, SPSS, Chicago, 2010.

[22] SAS/STAT software of the SAS system, SAS Institute, Cary, NC.

[23] A.T. Diplock, Trace elements in human health with special reference to selenium, Am. J. Clin. Nutr. 45 (1987) 1313−1322.

[24] O.A. Levander, Scientific rationale for the 1989 recommended dietary allowance for selenium, J. Am. Diet. Assoc. 91 (1991) 1572−1576.

[25] R. Sinha, G. Block, P.R. Taylor, Problems with estimating vitamin C intakes, Am. J. Clin. Nutr. 57 (1993) 547−550.

[26] F.M. Sacks, L.J. Appel, T.J. Moore, E. Obarzanek, W.M. Vollmer, L.P. Svetkey, et al., A dietary approach to prevent hypertension: a review of the Dietary Approaches to Stop Hypertension (DASH) study, Clin. Cardiol. 22 (1999) III6−III10.

[27] J.F. Swain, M.M. Windhauser, K.P. Hoben, M.A. Evans, B.B. McGee, P.D. Steele, Menu design and selection for multicenter controlled feeding studies: process used in the Dietary Approaches to Stop Hypertension trial; DASH Collaborative Research Group, J. Am. Diet. Assoc. 99 (1999) S54−S59.

[28] M.L. McCullough, N.M. Karanja, P.H. Lin, E. Obarzanek, K.M. Phillips, R.L. Laws, et al., Comparison of 4 nutrient databases with chemical composition data from the Dietary Approaches to Stop Hypertension trial; DASH Collaborative Research Group, J. Am. Diet. Assoc. 99 (1999) S45−S53.

[29] M.B. Reddy, R.F. Hurrell, J.D. Cook, Estimation of nonheme-iron bioavailability from meal composition, Am. J. Clin. Nutr. 71 (2000) 937−943.

[30] S.J. Fairweather-Tait, R. Collings, Estimating the bioavailability factors needed for setting dietary reference values, Int. J. Vitam. Nutr. Res. 80 (2010) 249−256.

[31] P.A. Sharp, Intestinal iron absorption: regulation by dietary and systemic factors, Int. J. Vitam. Nutr. Res. 80 (2010) 231−242.

[32] P.M. Waijers, E.J. Feskens, M.C. Ocke, A critical review of predefined diet quality scores, Br. J. Nutr. 97 (2007) 219−231.

[33] F.B. Hu, Dietary pattern analysis: a new direction in nutritional epidemiology, Curr. Opin. Lipidol. 13 (2002) 3–9.

[34] C.M. Hasler, A.S. Bloch, C.A. Thomson, E. Enrione, C. Manning, Position of the American Dietetic Association: functional foods, J. Am. Diet. Assoc. 104 (2004) 814–826.

[35] A. Wirt, C.E. Collins, Diet quality: what is it and does it matter? Public Health Nutr. 12 (2009) 2473–2492.

[36] A.K. Kant, Indexes of overall diet quality: a review, J. Am. Diet. Assoc. 96 (1996) 785–791.

[37] P.M. Guenther, J. Reedy, S.M. Krebs-Smith, B.B. Reeve, Evaluation of the Healthy Eating Index–2005, J. Am. Diet. Assoc. 108 (2008) 1854–1864.

[38] P.S. Haines, A.M. Siega-Riz, B.M. Popkin, The Diet Quality Index revised: a measurement instrument for populations, J. Am. Diet. Assoc. 99 (1999) 697–704.

[39] R.E. Patterson, P.S. Haines, B.M. Popkin, Diet Quality Index: capturing a multidimensional behavior, J. Am. Diet. Assoc. 94 (1994) 57–64.

[40] S. Kim, P.S. Haines, A.M. Siega-Riz, B.M. Popkin, The Diet Quality Index–International (DQI-I) provides an effective tool for cross-national comparison of diet quality as illustrated by China and the United States, J. Nutr. 133 (2003) 3476–3484.

[41] A. Trichopoulou, T. Costacou, C. Bamia, D. Trichopoulos, Adherence to a Mediterranean diet and survival in a Greek population, N. Engl. J. Med. 348 (2003) 2599–2608.

[42] P. Lagiou, D. Trichopoulos, S. Sandin, A. Lagiou, L. Mucci, A. Wolk, et al., Mediterranean dietary pattern and mortality among young women: a cohort study in Sweden, Br. J. Nutr. 96 (2006) 384–392.

[43] E. Couto, P. Boffetta, P. Lagiou, P. Ferrari, G. Buckland, K. Overvad, et al., Mediterranean dietary pattern and cancer risk in the EPIC cohort, Br. J. Cancer. 104 (2011) 1493–1499.

[44] U.S. Department of Agriculture, Dietary Guidelines for Americans, U.S. Department of Agriculture, Washington, DC, 2010.

[45] U.S. Department of Agriculture. MyPlate. Available at <http://www.cnpp.usda.gov/MyPlate.htm>.

[46] E.T. Kennedy, J. Ohls, S. Carlson, K. Fleming, The Healthy Eating Index: design and applications, J. Am. Diet. Assoc. 95 (1995) 1103–1108.

[47] L.E. Cleveland, D.A. Cook, S.M. Krebs-Smith, J. Friday, Method for assessing food intakes in terms of servings based on food guidance, Am. J. Clin. Nutr. 65 (1997) 1254S–1263S.

[48] L.E. Cleveland, A.J. Moshfegh, A.M. Albertson, J.D. Goldman, Dietary intake of whole grains, J. Am. Coll. Nutr. 19 (2000) 331S–338S.

[49] C.E. O'Neil, T.A. Nicklas, M. Zanovec, S. Cho, Whole-grain consumption is associated with diet quality and nutrient intake in adults: The National Health and Nutrition Examination Survey, 1999–2004, J. Am. Diet. Assoc. 110 (2010) 1461–1468.

[50] C. Batis, L. Hernandez-Barrera, S. Barquera, J.A. Rivera, B.M. Popkin, Food acculturation drives dietary differences among Mexicans, Mexican Americans, and non-Hispanic Whites, J. Nutr. 141 (2011) 1898–1906.

[51] T. Erinosho, L.B. Dixon, C. Young, L.M. Brotman, L.L. Hayman, Nutrition practices and children's dietary intakes at 40 child-care centers in New York City, J. Am. Diet. Assoc. 111 (2011) 1391–1397.

[52] J.J. Otten, J.P. Hellwig, L.D. Meyers, DRI, Dietary Reference Intakes: The Essential Guide to Nutrient Requirements, National Academies Press, Washington, DC, 2006.

[53] M.W. Gillman, L.A. Cupples, B.E. Millen, R.C. Ellison, P.A. Wolf, Inverse association of dietary fat with development of ischemic stroke in men, JAMA 278 (1997) 2145–2150.

[54] P.P. Basiotis, S.O. Welsh, F.J. Cronin, J.L. Kelsay, W. Mertz, Number of days of food intake records required to estimate individual and group nutrient intakes with defined confidence, J. Nutr. 117 (1987) 1638–1641.

[55] N. Presse, H. Payette, B. Shatenstein, C.E. Greenwood, M.J. Kergoat, G. Ferland, A minimum of six days of diet recording is needed to assess usual vitamin K intake among older adults, J. Nutr. 141 (2011) 341–346.

[56] S.M. Rebro, R.E. Patterson, A.R. Kristal, C.L. Cheney, The effect of keeping food records on eating patterns, J. Am. Diet. Assoc. 98 (1998) 1163–1165.

[57] E.B. Rimm, M.J. Stampfer, A. Ascherio, E. Giovannucci, G.A. Colditz, W.C. Willett, Vitamin E consumption and the risk of coronary heart disease in men, N. Engl. J. Med. 328 (1993) 1450–1456.

[58] M.J. Stampfer, C.H. Hennekens, J.E. Manson, G.A. Colditz, B. Rosner, W.C. Willett, Vitamin E consumption and the risk of coronary disease in women, N. Engl. J. Med. 328 (1993) 1444–1449.

[59] S. Yusuf, G. Dagenais, J. Pogue, J. Bosch, P. Sleight, Vitamin E supplementation and cardiovascular events in high-risk patients: The Heart Outcomes Prevention Evaluation Study Investigators, N. Engl. J. Med. 342 (2000) 154–160.

[60] E. Lonn, J. Bosch, S. Yusuf, P. Sheridan, J. Pogue, J.M. Arnold, et al., Effects of long-term vitamin E supplementation on cardiovascular events and cancer: a randomized controlled trial, JAMA 293 (2005) 1338–1347.

[61] C. Chiabrando, F. Avanzini, C. Rivalta, F. Colombo, R. Fanelli, G. Palumbo, et al., Long-term vitamin E supplementation fails to reduce lipid peroxidation in people at cardiovascular risk: analysis of underlying factors, Curr. Control Trials Cardiovasc. Med. 3 (2002) 5.

[62] M.B. Livingstone, A.E. Black, Markers of the validity of reported energy intake, J. Nutr. 133 (Suppl. 3) (2003) 895S–920S.

[63] L.S. Freedman, A. Schatzkin, D. Midthune, V. Kipnis, Dealing with dietary measurement error in nutritional cohort studies, J. Natl. Cancer Inst. 103 (2011) 1086–1092.

[64] A.E. Black, A.M. Prentice, G.R. Goldberg, S.A. Jebb, et al., Measurements of total energy expenditure provide insights into the validity of dietary measurements of energy intake, J. Am. Diet. Assoc. 93 (1993) 572.

[65] L.F. Andersen, K. Solvoll, C.A. Drevon, Very-long-chain n-3 fatty acids as biomarkers for intake of fish and n-3 fatty acid concentrates, Am. J. Clin. Nutr. 64 (1996) 305–311.

[66] S.A. Bingham, J.H. Cummings, Urine nitrogen as an independent validatory measure of dietary intake: a study of nitrogen balance in individuals consuming their normal diet, Am. J. Clin. Nutr. 42 (1985) 1276–1289.

[67] S.A. Bingham, Urine nitrogen as a biomarker for the validation of dietary protein intake, J. Nutr. 133 (2003) 921S.

[68] F.R. Baldrick, J.V. Woodside, J.S. Elborn, I.S. Young, M.C. McKinley, Biomarkers of fruit and vegetable intake in human intervention studies: a systematic review, Crit. Rev. Food Sci. Nutr. 51 (2011) 795–815.

[69] N. Tasevska, S.A. Runswick, A. McTaggart, S.A. Bingham, Urinary sucrose and fructose as biomarkers for sugar consumption, Cancer Epidemiol. Biomarkers Prev. 14 (2005) 1287–1294.

[70] S.A. Bingham, Biomarkers in nutritional epidemiology, Public Health Nutr. 5 (2002) 821–827.

[71] N. Potischman, J.L. Freudenheim, Biomarkers of nutritional exposure and nutritional status: an overview, J. Nutr. 133 (Suppl. 3) (2003) 873S–874S.

[72] N. Tasevska, D. Midthune, N. Potischman, A.F. Subar, A.J. Cross, S.A. Bingham, et al., Use of the predictive sugars biomarker to evaluate self-reported total sugars intake in the Observing Protein and Energy Nutrition (OPEN) study, Cancer Epidemiol. Biomarkers Prev. 20 (2011) 490–500.

[73] L. Johansson, K. Solvoll, G.E. Bjorneboe, C.A. Drevon, Under- and overreporting of energy intake related to weight status and lifestyle in a nationwide sample, Am. J. Clin. Nutr. 68 (1998) 266−274.

[74] C. Bazelmans, C. Matthys, S. De Henauw, M. Dramaix, M. Kornitzer, G. De Backer, et al., Predictors of misreporting in an elderly population: the "Quality of Life after 65" study, Public Health Nutr. 10 (2007) 185−191.

[75] J. Maurer, D.L. Taren, P.J. Teixeira, C.A. Thomson, T.G. Lohman, S.B. Going, et al., The psychosocial and behavioral characteristics related to energy misreporting, Nutr Rev. 64 (2006) 53−66.

[76] A.M. Prentice, A.E. Black, W.A. Coward, H.L. Davies, G.R. Goldberg, P.R. Murgatroyd, et al., High levels of energy expenditure in obese women, Br. Med. J. (Clin. Res. Ed.) 292 (1986) 983−987.

[77] S.W. Lichtman, K. Pisarska, E.R. Berman, M. Pestone, H. Dowling, E. Offenbacher, et al., Discrepancy between self-reported and actual caloric intake and exercise in obese subjects, N. Engl. J. Med. 327 (1992) 1893−1898.

[78] D. Garriguet, Under-reporting of energy intake in the Canadian Community Health Survey, Health Rep. 19 (2008) 37−45.

[79] F.B. Scagliusi, E. Ferriolli, K. Pfrimer, C. Laureano, C.S. Cunha, B. Gualano, et al., Underreporting of energy intake in Brazilian women varies according to dietary assessment: a cross-sectional study using doubly labeled water, J. Am. Diet. Assoc. 108 (2008) 2031−2040.

[80] J.A. Tooze, A.F. Subar, F.E. Thompson, R. Troiano, A. Schatzkin, V. Kipnis, Psychosocial predictors of energy under-reporting in a large doubly labeled water study, Am. J. Clin. Nutr. 79 (2004) 795−804.

[81] G.M. Price, A.A. Paul, T.J. Cole, M.E. Wadsworth, Characteristics of the low-energy reporters in a longitudinal national dietary survey, Br. J. Nutr. 77 (1997) 833−851.

[82] J.A. Pryer, M. Vrijheid, R. Nichols, M. Kiggins, P. Elliott, Who are the "low energy reporters" in the dietary and nutritional survey of British adults? Int. J. Epidemiol. 26 (1997) 146−154.

[83] R.K. Johnson, R.P. Soultanakis, D.E. Matthews, Literacy and body fatness are associated with underreporting of energy intake in U.S. low-income women using the multiple-pass 24-hour recall: a doubly labeled water study, J. Am. Diet. Assoc. 98 (1998) 1136.

[84] J. Dwyer, M.F. Picciano, D.J. Raiten, Estimation of usual intakes: What We Eat in America−NHANES, J. Nutr. 133 (2003) 609S−623S.

[85] F.B. Scagliusi, E. Ferriolli, K. Pfrimer, C. Laureano, C.S. Cunha, B. Gualano, et al., Characteristics of women who frequently under report their energy intake: a doubly labelled water study, Eur. J. Clin. Nutr. 63 (2009) 1192−1199.

[86] P. Ferrari, N. Slimani, A. Ciampi, A. Trichopoulou, A. Naska, C. Lauria, et al.,). Evaluation of under- and overreporting of energy intake in the 24-hour diet recalls in the European Prospective Investigation into Cancer and Nutrition (EPIC), Public Health Nutr. 5 (2002) 1329−1345.

[87] D.L. Taren, M. Tobar, A. Hill, W. Howell, C. Shisslak, I. Bell, et al., The association of energy intake bias with psychological scores of women, Eur. J. Clin. Nutr. 53 (1999) 570−578.

[88] K.L. Rennie, M. Siervo, S.A. Jebb, Can self-reported dieting and dietary restraint identify underreporters of energy intake in dietary surveys? J. Am. Diet. Assoc. 106 (2006) 1667−1672.

[89] J.A. Novotny, W.V. Rumpler, H. Riddick, J.R. Hebert, D. Rhodes, J.T. Judd, et al., Personality characteristics as predictors of underreporting of energy intake on 24-hour dietary recall interviews, J. Am. Diet. Assoc. 103 (2003) 1146−1151.

[90] B. Wansink, P. Chandon, Meal size, not body size, explains errors in estimating the calorie content of meals, Ann. Intern. Med. 145 (2006) 326−332.

[91] S.M. Krebs-Smith, B.I. Graubard, L.L. Kahle, A.F. Subar, L.E. Cleveland, R. Ballard-Barbash, Low energy reporters vs others: a comparison of reported food intakes, Eur. J. Clin. Nutr. 54 (2000) 281−287.

[92] S.A. Bingham, A. Cassidy, T.J. Cole, A. Welch, S.A. Runswick, A.E. Black, et al., Validation of weighed records and other methods of dietary assessment using the 24 h urine nitrogen technique and other biological markers, Br. J. Nutr. 73 (1995) 531−550.

[93] S.D. Poppitt, D. Swann, A.E. Black, A.M. Prentice, Assessment of selective under-reporting of food intake by both obese and non-obese women in a metabolic facility, Int. J. Obes. Relat. Metab. Disord. 22 (1998) 303−311.

[94] S. Voss, A. Kroke, K. Klipstein-Grobusch, H. Boeing, Is macro-nutrient composition of dietary intake data affected by under-reporting? Results from the EPIC−Potsdam Study: European Prospective Investigation into Cancer and Nutrition, Eur. J. Clin. Nutr. 52 (1998) 119−126.

[95] A.E. Millen, J.A. Tooze, A.F. Subar, L.L. Kahle, A. Schatzkin, S. M. Krebs-Smith, Differences between food group reports of low-energy reporters and non-low-energy reporters on a food frequency questionnaire, J. Am. Diet. Assoc. 109 (2009) 1194−1203.

[96] G.R. Goldberg, A.E. Black, S.A. Jebb, T.J. Cole, P.R. Murgatroyd, W.A. Coward, et al., Critical evaluation of energy intake data using fundamental principles of energy physiology: 1. Derivation of cut-off limits to identify under-recording, Eur. J. Clin. Nutr. 45 (1991) 569−581.

[97] A.E. Black, Critical evaluation of energy intake using the Goldberg cut-off for energy intake:basal metabolic rate: a practical guide to its calculation, use and limitations, Int. J. Obes. Relat. Metab. Disord. 24 (2000) 1119−1130.

[98] A.E. Black, G.R. Goldberg, S.A. Jebb, M.B. Livingstone, T.J. Cole, A.M. Prentice, Critical evaluation of energy intake data using fundamental principles of energy physiology: 2. Evaluating the results of published surveys, Eur. J. Clin. Nutr. 45 (1991) 583−599.

[99] M.A. McCrory, C.L. Hajduk, S.B. Roberts, Procedures for screening out inaccurate reports of dietary energy intake, Public Health Nutr. 5 (2002) 873−882.

[100] T.T. Huang, S.B. Roberts, N.C. Howarth, M.A. McCrory, Effect of screening out implausible energy intake reports on relationships between diet and BMI, Obes. Res. 13 (2005) 1205−1217.

[101] A.G. Vinken, G.P. Bathalon, A.L. Sawaya, G.E. Dallal, K.L. Tucker, S.B. Roberts, Equations for predicting the energy requirements of healthy adults aged 18−81 y, Am. J. Clin. Nutr. 69 (1999) 920−926.

[102] K.A. Munoz, S.M. Krebs-Smith, R. Ballard-Barbash, L.E. Cleveland, Food intakes of U.S. children and adolescents compared with recommendations, Pediatrics 100 (1997) 323−329.

[103] M.K. Fialkowski, M.A. McCrory, S.M. Roberts, J.K. Tracy, L.M. Grattan, C.J. Boushey, Estimated nutrient intakes from food generally do not meet dietary reference intakes among adult members of Pacific Northwest tribal nations, J. Nutr. 140 (2010) 992−998.

[104] M.K. Fialkowski, M.A. McCrory, S.M. Roberts, J.K. Tracy, L.M. Grattan, C.J. Boushey, Evaluation of dietary assessment tools used to assess the diet of adults participating in the

Communities Advancing the Studies of Tribal Nations Across the Lifespan cohort, J. Am. Diet. Assoc. 110 (2010) 65—73.

[105] W. Willett, M.J. Stampfer, Total energy intake: implications for epidemiologic analyses, Am. J. Epidemiol. 124 (1986) 17—27.

[106] L.M. Carter, S.J. Whiting, Underreporting of energy intake, socioeconomic status, and expression of nutrient intake, Nutr. Rev. 56 (1998) 179—182.

[107] D.D. Stallone, E.J. Brunner, S.A. Bingham, M.G. Marmot, Dietary assessment in Whitehall II: the influence of reporting bias on apparent socioeconomic variation in nutrient intakes, Eur. J. Clin. Nutr. 51 (1997) 815—825.

[108] F.E. Thompson, A.F. Subar, C.M. Loria, J.L. Reedy, T. Baranowski, Need for technological innovation in dietary assessment, J. Am. Diet. Assoc. 110 (2010) 48—51.

[109] B.L. Harper, S.G. Harris, A possible approach for setting a mercury risk-based action level based on tribal fish ingestion rates, Environ. Res. 107 (2008) 60—68.

[110] C.K. Martin, H. Han, S.M. Coulon, H.R. Allen, C.M. Champagne, S. D. Anton, A novel method to remotely measure food intake of free-living individuals in real time: the remote food photography method, Br. J. Nutr. 101 (2009) 446—456.

[111] L. Arab, A. Winter, Automated camera-phone experience with the frequency of imaging necessary to capture diet, J. Am. Diet. Assoc. 110 (2010) 1238—1241.

[112] B.L. Six, T.E. Schap, F.M. Zhu, A. Mariappan, M. Bosch, E. J. Delp, et al., Evidence-based development of a mobile telephone food record, J. Am. Diet. Assoc. 110 (2010) 74—79.

[113] F. Zhu, A. Mariappan, C. Boushey, D. Kerr, K. Lutes, D. Ebert, et al., Technology-assisted dietary assessment, Proc. IS&T/SPIE Conf. Comput. Imaging VI 6814 (2008) 1—10.

[114] A. Mariappan, M. Bosch Ruiz, F. Zhu, C.J. Boushey, D.A. Kerr, D.S. Ebert, et al., Personal dietary assessment using mobile devices, Proc. IS&T/SPIE Conf. Comput. Imaging VII V7246 (2009) 72460Z.

Current Theoretical Bases for Nutrition Intervention and Their Uses

Lora E. Burke*, Rachel A. Froehlich*, Yaguang Zheng*, Karen Glanz†

*University of Pittsburgh School of Nursing, Pittsburgh, Pennsylvania
†University of Pennsylvania, Philadelphia, Pennsylvania

This chapter discusses established theories of behavior change and their use as a guide to dietary interventions targeting disease prevention and management as well as their applications in practice. Other chapters in this text provide specific recommendations regarding dietary advice for disease prevention and for nutritional management of patients. This chapter (1) introduces key concepts related to the application of theory in understanding and improving behaviors related to eating and food selection, (2) reviews behavioral issues related to healthful diets, (3) describes several theoretical models that can be helpful in planning and conducting dietary interventions, and (4) highlights important issues and constructs that cut across theories.

Dietary interventions are a central component of disease prevention and management. Health professionals' roles in dietary interventions are pivotal because of their centrality in health care and their credibility as patient educators [1–4]. The most recently published evidence-based recommendations in the United States advise including intensive behavioral dietary counseling for adults with known risk factors for chronic disease, noting that this counseling can be provided by physicians or other clinicians such as dietitians [5,6]. Although the evidence for brief, low-intensity counseling of unselected patients is not sufficient to recommend routine dietary counseling [6,7], people who report receiving advice or counseling recommending dietary change report more health-enhancing diet changes and weight loss than do those who received no such advice [8,9]. Furthermore, nonclinical community sites such as worksites, churches, schools, and community centers are becoming increasingly important as settings for nutritional information and dietary interventions, especially with the epidemic rates of obesity and diabetes among U.S. children, adolescents, and adults [10–14].

I THE IMPORTANCE OF UNDERSTANDING INFLUENCES ON DIETARY BEHAVIOR

Successful dietary interventions take many forms. Interventions to yield desirable changes in eating patterns can be best designed with an understanding of relevant theories of diet-related behavior change and the ability to use them skillfully [15]. Although earlier reports of dietary interventions did not cite a particular theory or model as the basis for the strategies they employed [16,17], the application of sound behavioral science theory in dietary interventions has become more the norm today [18]. Also, emerging evidence suggests that interventions developed with an explicit theoretical foundation are more effective than those lacking a theoretical base [19,20] and that combining multiple theories may lead to better outcomes (e.g., social cognitive theory and the transtheoretical model) [21,22].

Six theoretical models have been used often in studies targeting dietary change and thus have been demonstrated to be useful for understanding the processes of changing eating habits in clinical and community settings as well as guiding the development of dietary interventions: social cognitive theory, which includes self-efficacy and self-regulation—constructs that have

Nutrition in the Prevention and Treatment of Disease, Third Edition.
DOI: http://dx.doi.org/10.1016/B978-0-12-391884-0.00008-1

been used extensively in diet and weight loss studies; the stages of change construct from the transtheoretical model; consumer information processing, the theory of planned behavior, multiattribute utility theory, and the social ecological model [15,23,24]. This chapter describes the central elements of each theory and how the theories can be used to guide the development of interventions and provide a framework for the interpretation of outcomes.

A Multiple Determinants of Food Choice

Many social, cultural, and economic factors contribute to the development, maintenance, and change of dietary habits. No single factor or set of factors has been found to adequately account for why people eat as they do. Physiologic and psychological factors, acquired food preferences, and knowledge about foods are important individual determinants of food intake. Families, social relationships, socioeconomic status, culture, geography, and access to food are also important influences on food choices. A broad understanding of some of the key factors and models for understanding food choice can provide a foundation for well-informed clinical dietary interventions, help identify the most influential factors for a particular patient, and enable clinicians to focus on issues that are most salient for their patients.

B Multiple Levels of Influence

Common wisdom holds that nutrition interventions are most likely to be effective if they embrace an ecological perspective for health promotion [24,25]. That is, they should not only target individuals but also affect interpersonal, organizational, and environmental factors influencing diet-related behaviors [26–28]. This is most clearly illustrated when one thinks of the context of selecting and purchasing food. Consumers learn about foods through advertising and promotion via multimedia, labels on food packages, and through product information in grocery stores, cafeterias, and restaurants [29]. Their actual purchases are influenced by personal preferences, family habits, medical advice, availability, cost, packaging, placement, and intentional meal planning. The foods they consume may be further changed in the preparation process, either at home or while eating out. The process is complex and clearly determined not only by multiple factors but also by factors at multiple levels. Still, much food choice can be represented by routines and simple, internalized rules.

Traditionally, health/patient educators focus on intraindividual factors such as a person's beliefs, knowledge, and skills. Contemporary thinking suggests that thinking beyond the individual to the social milieu and environment can enhance the chance of successful health promotion and patient education [25,30]. Health providers can and should work toward understanding the various levels of influence that affect the patient's behavior and health status. This is discussed and illustrated with examples later in this chapter.

II WHAT IS THEORY?

A theory is a set of interrelated concepts, definitions, and propositions that present a systematic view of events or situations by specifying relations among variables in order to explain and predict the events or situations. The notion of generality, or broad application, is important [15]. Although various theoretical models of health behavior may reflect the same general ideas, each theory employs a unique vocabulary to articulate the specific factors considered to be important. Theories vary in the extent to which they have been conceptually developed and empirically tested.

Theory can be helpful during the various stages of planning, implementing, and evaluating interventions [15]. Theories can be used to guide the search for reasons why people are or are not consuming a healthful diet or adhering to a therapeutic dietary regimen. They can help pinpoint what you need to know before working effectively with a client, group, or patient. They also help to identify what should be monitored, measured, and/or compared in evaluating the efficacy of nutrition intervention.

III EXPLANATORY AND CHANGE THEORIES

Theories can guide the search to understand why people do or do not follow health-related or therapeutic advice, help identify what information is needed to design an effective intervention strategy, and provide insight into how to design an educational program so it is successful [15]. Thus, theories and models help explain behaviors as well as suggest how to develop more effective ways to influence and change behaviors. These types of theory often have different emphases but are quite complementary [15]. For example, understanding why someone chooses the foods he or she eats is one step toward successful dietary management, but even the best explanations are insufficient by themselves to fully guide change to improve health. Some type of change model will also be needed. All of the theories and models described here have some potential as both explanatory and change models, although they might be better for one or the other purpose.

For example, the theory of planned behavior was originally developed as an explanatory model, whereas the stages of change construct was conceived to help guide planned change efforts.

IV UNIQUE FEATURES OF DIET-RELATED BEHAVIOR TO CONSIDER WHEN USING THEORY

Diet-related behavior changes are most likely to be effective for preventing or managing disease when they are sustained over the long term and in people's natural environments, outside the clinical setting. To be effective in dietary interventions, health care providers need to understand both the principles of clinical dietary management and a variety of behavioral and educational issues [31].

There are several core issues about diet and eating-related changes that should be recognized. First, most diet-related risk factors are asymptomatic and do not present immediate or dramatic symptoms. Moreover, by the time symptoms are recognized, the changes needed are often very challenging—for example, sodium restriction in the patient with congestive heart failure. Furthermore, health-enhancing dietary changes require qualitative change, not just modification of the amount of food consumed, and eating cessation is not a viable option (as with smoking or other addictive behaviors). Finally, both the act of making changes and self-monitoring require accurate knowledge about the nutrient composition of foods or a convenient, practical reference source, as well as a commitment to make change by the individual. Thus, information acquisition and processing may be more complex for dietary change than for changes in some other health behaviors, such as smoking and exercise. As such, consumer information processing models (described later) are more important for dietary interventions than for other types of health-related behaviors. Other important issues include long-term maintenance, the format and medium for providing dietary advice, nutritional adequacy, options for initiating the change process, the ubiquitous availability of food, the ever-changing food supply, fad diets, and special populations.

A Long-Term Dietary Change

Because dietary intervention leads to meaningful improvements in health only when long-term change is achieved, both providers and patients need to "look down the road" when formulating expectations and setting goals [32]. For example, for most patients without other major risk factors or a familial disorder who follow recommended dietary changes for cholesterol reduction, significant reductions are seen within 4—6 weeks, and cholesterol reduction goals can be reached within 4—6 months [33]. Even after goals are achieved, new dietary habits must be maintained. Thus, if it takes several weeks or even months to adjust to the new dietary regimen, patience and persistence by both physician (or dietitian) and patient may be worthwhile in the long term [34,35]. Maintenance of new eating habits occurs mainly outside any clinical or therapeutic setting. Also, different skills are required to make initial changes and to maintain them over the long term, so follow-up consultations and advice should address new issues, not merely repeat or rehash old information. Reinforcement of the behavior changes that have occurred is paramount [36].

B Restrictive and Additive Recommendations: Typical Reactions

Traditionally, dietary intervention has focused on advice to restrict intake of certain foods or nutrients—for example, reducing fat and saturated fat intake, limiting calorie intake, and limiting sodium/salt. Yet the most often mentioned obstacle to achieving a healthful diet is not wanting to give up the foods we like [37]. Basic psychological principles hold that when people are faced with a restriction or loss of a choice, that choice or commodity becomes more attractive. In other words, focusing mainly on what not to eat, or on eating less of some types of foods, may evoke conscious or unconscious negativism in some people. In contrast, counseling rather than advising the individual about making behavior changes and emphasizing additive recommendations, such as increasing intake of fruits and vegetables or eating more fiber-rich foods, often appeals to people because it sanctions their doing more of something and guides them in how to do it. The challenge is to make these recommendations attractive to individuals and to ensure that they are presented in the context of an overall healthful diet.

C Implications of Counseling for Gradual Change or Very Strict Diets

A generally held view is that the chances of long-term dietary change are greater when efforts to change occur in a gradual, stepwise manner and are viewed in the context of a lifestyle change rather than a diet. This might involve setting small goals for attempting changes within specific food groups one at a time, until the total diet comes close to recommendations. A basic principle involved is that small successes (i.e., recognition of each successful behavioral change) increase confidence and motivation for each successive change. Although this is effective for many people, others become impatient or even lose their enthusiasm for changes that are minimally recognizable. An alternative is to begin with a highly restrictive diet such as a very low-calorie weight loss diet, a very low-fat diet for prevention of cardiovascular disease, or a very low-sodium diet for an individual with kidney disease. These types of programs, with very strict dietary regimens, may be useful for patients who are highly motivated (e.g., post-surgically, after a coronary incident, or newly diagnosed) or for those who have not been successful in making gradual changes. In some cases, a strict diet for an initial short period will yield visible and/or clinical changes that help motivate patients to continue adhering to a less extreme regimen; however, such diets may require careful supervision. Moreover, diets that require extreme calorie restriction for weight loss often result in a rapid weight regain after the diet is discontinued [34,35]. For these reasons, these markedly restricted diets are not recommended for most individuals.

D Special Populations

Ideally, each patient should be treated as an individual with unique circumstances and health history. Still, epidemiological research indicates that certain demographic subgroups differ in terms of both risk factors and diet. Understanding these population differences can help prepare a provider to work with various types of patients. Minority and lower socioeconomic status individuals are disproportionately affected by obesity [38] and related risk factors. Targeted interventions are needed for disadvantaged groups [39]. Age may also make a difference: Younger persons may feel invulnerable to coronary events, and older adults may be managing multiple chronic conditions and using both prescribed and over-the-counter medications that could interact with foods. These are just a few examples of how population subgroups may differ, and they serve as a reminder to be sensitive to group patterns but to avoid stereotyping in the absence of firsthand evidence about an individual.

V IMPORTANT THEORIES AND THEIR KEY CONSTRUCTS

Several available and widely used models and theories of behavior change can guide dietary interventions. This section describes the following six models and their constructs: social cognitive theory, including self-efficacy and self-regulation; stages of change from

TABLE 8.1 Statements Representing Theoretical Approaches to Understanding and Changing Dietary Behavior

Theory	Statements
Social cognitive theory	Overeating at holidays is triggered by food advertisements, store displays, and party buffets that people encounter. Work with individual to set realistic, specific, and proximal goals; for example, at holiday parties, have just one dessert.
Stages of change	If someone believes that the time is right and is "ready to change," he or she will probably be more successful with a nutrition intervention. For the person who is in a contemplative stage, provide attractive literature that is appropriate for the individual to read to possibly motivate the person to move forward.
Consumer information processing	The information on nutrition labels sometimes "overloads" consumers. Consumers who are concerned about nutrition tend to look at nutrient labels before deciding which food to buy.
Theory of planned behavior	An individual who plans to change how he or she eats and specifies what, when, how, and where the changes will happen is more likely to follow through than someone with a more general plan. Furthermore, if the person thinks that his or her spouse will be supportive, motivation will be higher.
Multiattribute utility theory	If taste and convenience are foremost in someone's mind when deciding what to eat, a nutrition intervention that zeroes in on these factors has the greatest promise of success.
Social ecological model	If healthful food is easily available and low in cost, and the company provides good cooking and food preparation facilities, then workers will be more likely to follow healthy eating patterns.

Source: *Adapted in part from McAlister et al. [15] and Rudd and Glanz [65].*

the transtheoretical model; consumer information processing; the theory of planned behavior; multiattributed utility theory; and the social ecological model [15]. The central elements of each theory and how they can be used to help formulate and guide dietary interventions are described. Table 8.1 provides illustrative statements demonstrating the application of each theory.

A Social Cognitive Theory

Social cognitive theory (SCT), the cognitive formulation of social learning theory that has been best articulated by Bandura [40,41], explains human behavior in terms of a three-way, dynamic, reciprocal model in which personal factors, environmental influences, and behavior continually interact. SCT synthesizes concepts and processes from cognitive, behavioristic, and emotional models of behavior change, so it can be readily applied to dietary interventions that target behavior change for disease prevention and management. A basic premise of SCT is that people learn not only through their own experiences but also by observing the actions of others, particularly role models who seem credible, and the results of those actions [15]. Key constructs of SCT that are relevant to dietary intervention include observational learning, self-regulation [42], reinforcement, self-control, and self-efficacy [43,44].

Principles of behavior modification, which have often been used to promote dietary change, are derived from SCT. Elements of behavioral dietary interventions based on SCT constructs of self-control, self-regulation, reinforcement, and self-efficacy include goal-setting, self-monitoring, self-evaluation, feedback, and behavioral contracting [31,45]. As discussed later, goal-setting and self-monitoring are key behavioral strategies to support behavior change [46,47].

1 Self-efficacy

Self-efficacy is a person's perception of how capable he or she is to perform a specific behavior or take action and persist in that action despite obstacles or challenges. Self-efficacy is behavior specific; for example, a person may have high self-efficacy for initiating a physical activity program but low self-efficacy for changing dietary habits [41]. Health providers can make deliberate efforts to increase patients' self-efficacy using three types of strategies: (1) setting small, incremental, and achievable goals; (2) using formalized behavioral contracting to establish goals and specify rewards; and (3) monitoring and reinforcement, including having the patient self-monitor by keeping records and providing feedback and reinforcement to the individual on the changes and progress [15,48]. Using specific, proximal goals that are achievable fosters mastery performance—the most powerful source of enhancing self-efficacy. The use of credible models to demonstrate behaviors (e.g., how to modify a recipe or cook low fat) is another important source for self-efficacy enhancement. A setting in which this is easily implemented is group sessions for cooking demonstrations. Research has provided evidence across multiple behavior domains that increased self-efficacy is associated with improved outcomes—for example, making healthy food choices, improving health-related behaviors such as glucose control in type 2 diabetes, and sustaining weight loss maintenance [48–52].

The key SCT construct of reciprocal determinism means that a person can be both an agent for change and a responder to change. Thus, changes in the environment, the examples of role models, and reinforcements can be used to promote healthier behavior. This core construct is also central to the social ecological model, which is discussed later.

2 Self-Regulation

Self-regulation, part of SCT, posits that individuals seek control over important events in their lives by self-regulating their thoughts, behaviors, and environment to achieve their defined goals [40]. According to this theory, reciprocal interactions are assumed to occur among behaviors, environment, and personal factors [41]. Kanfer [53] noted that the major self-regulative mechanism operates through three main functions: self-monitoring, self-evaluation, and self-reinforcement. The key to this process is the behavioral strategy of self-monitoring. Individuals cannot influence their motivation and actions well unless they pay deliberate attention to their own performance, as well as the conditions under which they occur and their immediate and long-term effects [54]. Thus, success in self-regulation depends in part on the fidelity, consistency, and temporal proximity of self-monitoring [55].

Studies based on self-regulation showed positive effects on dietary behavior change [56,57]. A self-regulation intervention focused on daily self-weighing and monitoring of weight with set goals for weight loss maintenance demonstrated efficacy in a clinical trial [58,59]. A behavioral weight loss trial that provided daily feedback to those using an electronic diary to self-monitor their diet showed improved self-monitoring adherence and a higher proportion losing 5% of their baseline weight compared to those who did not receive the daily feedback message [56].

B Stages of Change

Long-term dietary change for disease prevention or risk reduction involves multiple actions and adaptations over time. Some people may not be ready to attempt changes, whereas others may have already begun to change their diet and eating habits. The construct of "stage of change" is a key element of the transtheoretical model (TTM) of behavior change, and it proposes that people are at different stages of readiness to adopt healthful behaviors [51,60,61]. The notion of readiness to change, or stage of change, has been examined in dietary behavior research and found useful in explaining and predicting the adoption of dietary change [51,61].

Stages of change is a heuristic model that describes a sequence of steps in successful behavior change: precontemplation (no recognition of need for or interest in change), contemplation (thinking about changing), preparation (planning for change), action (adopting new habits), and maintenance (ongoing practice of new, healthier behavior) [51]. People do not always move through the stages of change in a linear manner. They often recycle and repeat certain stages; for example, individuals may relapse and go back to an earlier stage depending on their level of motivation and self-efficacy

The stages of change model can be used both to help understand why individuals might not be ready to undertake dietary change and to improve the success of dietary interventions [31]. Patients can be classified according to their stage of change by asking a few simple questions: Are they interested in trying to change their eating habits, thinking about changing their diet, ready to begin a new eating plan, already making dietary changes, or trying to sustain changes they have been following for some time? By knowing their current stage, clinicians can help to determine the best approach to intervening—for example, how much time to spend with the patient, whether to provide informational material for the person to consider during the contemplative stage, whether to wait until the person is more ready to attempt making changes, or whether referral for in-depth dietary counseling is warranted.

Assessing the patient's current stage of change can lead to appropriate follow-up questions about past efforts to change, obstacles and challenges, and available resources for overcoming barriers. A study that assessed readiness for change in adapting a plant-based diet found the majority of participants identified themselves to be in the precontemplation stage, recognizing fewer benefits and more barriers to adopting a plant-based diet. Reports from a few clinical trials using the stages of change theory revealed that individuals in the intervention group who were in the precontemplation or maintenance stage were more likely to achieve improved adherence to goal-setting compared to those in similar stages in the control group [62,63]. Including multiple behavior strategies such as feedback on dietary change, exercise, and management of emotional stressors improved progression through the stages of change and continued success at 1-year follow-up, suggesting that changing one behavior may lead to a second behavior change [62–64].

C Consumer Information Processing

People require information about how to choose nutritious foods in order to follow guidelines for healthy eating. A central premise of consumer information processing theory is that individuals can process only a limited amount of information at one time [65]. People tend to seek only enough information to make a satisfactory choice. They develop heuristics, or rules of thumb, to help them make choices quickly within their limited information processing capacity. The nutrition information environment is often complex and confusing; especially when programs rely heavily on print nutrition educational materials that may be written at a level higher than the audience can comprehend.

Several elements of consumer information processing theory can be applied in dietary interventions. Messages that are food focused rather than nutrient focused may be particularly helpful [66,67]. Nutrition information is most helpful when it is tailored to the comprehension level of the audience, matched to their lifestyles and experience, and is either portable or available at or near the point of food selection [67–69]. An analysis of the National Health and Nutrition Examination Survey 2005 data revealed that four out of five Americans, age 16 years or older, were aware of one of the three federal dietary guidance efforts—the Food Guide Pyramid, 5 A Day Program, and Dietary Guidelines for Americans; however, there were significant differences when comparing race and ethnic groups (non-Hispanic white Americans were more familiar), as well as among the different levels of education and income groups. These data suggest we need to make a greater effort to educate individuals from minority groups and those with lower socioeconomic status and low literacy levels about nutrition and how to read dietary information. Menu labeling, which began in California and New York City in 2008, will soon be mandated on a national level through the Patient Protection and Affordable Care Act of 2010. The objective of this initiative was to improve access to consumer information so that individuals can make informed decisions and select more healthful menu options [70,71]. The few studies that have evaluated the impact of menu labeling have found mixed results. A survey of parents, children, and adolescents of low-income minorities in New York City found no significant difference in calorie consumption before and after the implementation of menu labeling in fast-food restaurants [72]. A cross-sectional survey conducted 1 year prior to and 9 months after implementation requiring menu labeling showed no change in energy density of the meals selected [73]. A third study concluded calorie labels on restaurant menus influenced food choices and consumption; in addition, it was determined that adding the Recommended Daily Allowance to menu labels added benefit [74]. When the nutritional values of entrée options were displayed in dining facilities at the collegiate level, students were more likely to choose healthier and lower calorie menu items [75].

Knowledge about which foods to choose, and how much to consume, on a therapeutic diet, are the *sine qua non* of dietary adherence. However, knowledge of how to use nutrition information and the skills to choose or prepare healthful foods are insufficient for behavior change without motivation and support. Furthermore, patients with low literacy skills and language barriers may require more explanations and fewer printed materials, thus posing important challenges [76]. Community studies involving participants with low literacy levels and multicultural backgrounds demonstrated successful dietary changes by administering the intervention through mixed multimedia and audiovisuals [77]. Those successfully conveying education through print materials suggest using simple messages, one- or two-syllable words, large print, and, when necessary, the participant's first language [76–79].

D Theory of Planned Behavior

Often, people's food choices are influenced by how they view the actions they are considering and whether they believe important others such as family members or peers would approve or disapprove of their behavior. The theory of planned behavior (TPB), which evolved from its predecessor, the theory of reasoned action, focuses on the relationships between behavior and beliefs, attitudes, subjective norms, and intentions [80]. The concept of perceived behavioral control involves the belief about whether one can control his or her performance of a behavior [80]; that is, people may feel motivated if they believe they "can do it." A central assumption of TPB is that "behavioral intentions" are the most important determinants of behavior [81].

TPB has been applied widely to help understand and explain many types of behaviors, including eating behavior [82]. The core constructs of TPB have been found to explain fast-food consumption behaviors among middle school students whose behaviors were most influenced by subjective norms [83] and saturated fat intake among adults affected by habit strength and behavior intention [84]. The TPB has also been found to predict healthy eating such as fruit and vegetable intake [85,86] and to help explain low-fat milk consumption [87]. The TPB model was found to be more effective in predicting expectation than intention or desire for controlling weight [88]. Behavioral intentions are important and central to TPB; however, there has been some concern that they are still too far removed to be good predictors of actual behavior. The concept of *implementation intentions* involves encouraging individuals receiving an intervention to be specific about how they would change. One study found that providing implementation intention prompts led to greater weight reduction in a commercial weight loss program [89].

E Multiattribute Utility Theory

Both health professionals and marketers recognize that people seek the things they like and that give them pleasure, and that they take action to obtain these things. Identifying those concerns that are most important to a person's decision about performing a specific behavior can lead to the development of effective interventions and decision aides to promote desirable behaviors [15]. Multiattribute utility theory (MAU) is a form of value expectancy theory that aims to specify how people define and evaluate the elements of decision making about performing a specific behavior. Key elements of value expectancy theory are the valence, or importance, of a particular feature of a behavior or product and the expectancy, or subjective probability that a given consequence will occur if the behavior is performed [90].

MAU is a form of value expectancy theory with particular relevance to understanding influences on food choice and changes in eating habits. MAU posits that people evaluate decisions based on multiple attributes and somehow consciously or unconsciously weight the alternatives before deciding what actions to take. The literature on food choice has identified several key factors that appear to be important in food selection: taste, nutrition, cost, convenience, and weight control. For the general public, taste has been reported to be the most important influence on food choice, followed by cost [23]. Understanding the relative importance of various concerns to individuals can guide the design of nutrition counseling and nutrition education programs. For example, by designing and promoting a nutritious diet as tasty, an intervention might be more successful than if it is presented primarily as nutritious or inexpensive. A project that used tailored messages based on alternative food choices and the attributes among them was found to be effective for increasing dietary fiber consumption; it was based on the behavioral alternatives model, which has many similar features to MAU [91].

F Social Ecological Model

The social ecological model helps researchers understand factors affecting behavior and also provides guidance for developing successful programs through social environments. The social ecological model emphasizes multiple levels of influence (e.g., individual or intrapersonal, interpersonal, organizational, community, and public policy) and the idea that behaviors both shape and are shaped by the social environment [24,25].

The principles of the social ecological model are consistent with SCT concepts that suggest creating an environment conducive to change is important to making it easier to adopt healthy behaviors [40]. Given the widespread problems of over nutrition in developed countries, more attention is being focused on increasing the health-promoting features of communities and neighborhoods and reducing the ubiquity of high-calorie, high-fat food choices [30,92].

The social ecological model is useful to guide intervention research related to changing dietary habits because of its focus on multilevel linkages [20]. This model is often discussed in the context of the obesity epidemic [30]. Also, it has been endorsed as a foundation for diet-related behavior interventions in children considering the contextual influences on childhood obesity, and its focus on prevention is embedded in the home, school/community, and society at large [93−97]. Health promotion programs that include a focus on home and worksite environments can improve eating habits and weight management of adults [98−101]. Studies have found that social−ecological resources mediated the lifestyle intervention effects on saturated-fat consumption among postmenopausal women with type 2 diabetes [102,103]. The literature also suggests that this model can provide guidance for intervention development for pregnant women [104] and low-income African Americans to support healthy eating habits [105].

G Selecting an Appropriate Theoretical Model or Models

Effective nutrition intervention depends on marshaling the most appropriate theory and practice strategies for a given situation [106]. Different theories are best suited to different individuals and situations. For example, when attempting to overcome a patient's personal barriers to changing his diet to reduce his cholesterol level, TPB may be useful. The stages of change model may be especially useful in developing diabetes education interventions. When trying to teach low-literacy patients how to choose and prepare healthy foods, consumer information processing may be more suitable. The choice of the most fitting theory or theories should begin with identifying the problem, goal, and units of practice [15,106], not with simply selecting a theoretical framework because it is intriguing or familiar.

With regard to practical application, theories are often judged in the context of activities of fellow practitioners. To apply the criterion of usefulness to a theory, most providers are concerned with whether it is consistent with everyday observations [15,106]. In contrast, researchers usually make scientific judgments of how well a theory conforms to observable reality when empirically tested. Patient educators should review the research literature periodically to supplement their firsthand experience and that of their colleagues.

A central premise in understanding the influences on health behavior and applying them to patient education is that one can gain an understanding of a patient through an interview or written assessment and better focus on the individual's readiness, self-efficacy, knowledge level, and so on. Clearly, it is necessary to select a "short list" of factors to evaluate, and this may differ depending on clinical risk factors or a patient's history. Once there is a good understanding of that person's cognitive and/or behavioral situation, the intervention can be personalized or tailored. Tailored messages and feedback have been found to be promising strategies for encouraging healthful behavior changes in primary care, community, and home-based settings [46,107].

The challenge of successfully applying theoretical frameworks in nutrition programs involves evaluating the frameworks and their key concepts in terms of both conceptual relevance and practical value [15]. In recent years, the focus on home self-management of chronic disease such as diabetes and cardiovascular disease has increased. Nutrition professionals can assist in the development of these comprehensive approaches to patient care. The integration of multiple theories into a comprehensive model tailored for a given individual or community group requires frequent re-examination and careful analysis of the audience, resources, and treatment conditions. Psychosocial issues to consider during program development and implementation include social/cultural factors, socioeconomic status, access to community/health care resources, literacy level, personal experience, available support systems, and the individual's knowledge of the condition/management for which treatment is designed [108].

VI FINDINGS REGARDING APPLICATIONS OF THEORY TO NUTRITIONAL BEHAVIOR

In the past two decades, there has been an increase in published research applying theoretical models to the study of nutritional behavior [17,45−47,109−114]. Numerous studies have examined the determinants of eating behavior using coherent theoretical frameworks and constructs. Longitudinal studies and clinical trials testing interventions for diet-related behavior change based on SCT, stages of change, and the social ecological model are appearing increasingly more often in the literature [46]. There continues to be a need for more studies using longitudinal designs studying families and the changing food roles in families as well as the changing food environment and also studying the relationships among various eating behaviors and several nutrients or types of foods.

During the past two decades, there has been a substantial increase in research applying the stages of change model to dietary behavior [62–64,115]. Prospective intervention research examining employees' readiness to change their eating patterns has revealed "forward movement" across the stage continuum in worksite nutrition studies and has shown that changes in stage of change for healthy eating are significantly associated with dietary improvements [116].

People's initial stage of change may influence their participation in dietary interventions. Individuals who are initially in the later stages of change (preparation, action, and maintenance) tend to spend more time on complex behaviors such as dietary change [64,117–119]; they also report making more healthful food choices.

Systemic reviews of stage-based interventions have questioned the effectiveness of TTM, providing important critiques and limitations of the theory. Some argue that the theory draws arbitrary lines differentiating stages, categorizing individuals to stable coherent plans in periods of instability and mixtures of constructs, while focusing change on conscious decision making and planning, which diverts attention away from human motivation. Evidence supports limited long-term effects for smoking cessation, physical activity, and dietary change under stages of change interventions because these behaviors are more complex and require a number of specific actions to influence self-efficacy and lifestyle change [120–124].

Several large worksite nutrition programs have applied constructs from SCT [100,125,126]. A multisite study, the Working Well Trial, used an intervention rooted in SCT, consumer information processing, and the stages of change [17,127]. Several of these dietary interventions have been found to be efficacious compared to a control condition, although they have done little to test the elements of SCT that might be most associated with the observed changes.

In SCT, self-regulation-based interventions focused on improving eating habits and achieving and/or maintaining a healthy weight and lifestyle have emphasized the role of self-monitoring as a key behavior (e.g., food intake, physical activity, and weight) [128]. A systematic review of the self-monitoring literature found that there was a consistent significant association between dietary self-monitoring and weight loss [129]. Studies using personal digital assistants for self-monitoring demonstrated greater reduced energy, saturated fat intake, and weight change [130]; increased vegetable and whole-grain intake in middle-aged and older adults [131]; and reduced sodium intake in hemodialysis patients [132]. Compared to traditional methods, children and adolescents have a strong preference for capturing food images with technology, which improved cooperation and increased accuracy in reporting diet [133]. The use of new technologies for self-monitoring diet, although more expensive than traditional pen-and-paper methods, may reduce the burden of recording [134].

A widely cited report used MAU as the framework for analyzing surveys of a national sample of 2967 adults. The study examined the relative importance of taste, nutrition, cost, convenience, and weight control on personal eating choices. Taste was reported to have the most important overall influence on food choices, followed by cost. The importance of nutrition and weight control was best predicted by respondents' being within a particular health lifestyle cluster [23]. No published reports have explicitly applied MAU to design a dietary intervention, but a tailored message intervention program used the behavioral alternatives model, which has important similarities to MAU [91].

VII CONSTRUCTS AND ISSUES ACROSS THEORIES

It is important to bear in mind that the various theories that can be used for dietary interventions are not mutually exclusive. Not surprisingly, they share several constructs and common issues. It is often challenging to sort out the key issues in various models. This section focuses on important issues and constructs across models, the first of which is that successful dietary behavior change depends on a sound understanding of the patient's, or consumer's, view of the world.

A The Patient's View of the World: Perceptions, Cognitions, Emotions, and Habits

For health professionals who work with patients and provide them with advice on health and lifestyle, adherence to treatment is often disappointingly poor, even in response to relatively simple medical advice. Such poor adherence often arises because patients do not have the necessary behavioral skills to make changes to their diet. Following a heart attack, for example, patients might well understand the importance of adopting such changes to their lifestyle but be unable to make those changes. There will be other circumstances in which patients might not understand the importance of such changes and may even believe that such changes pose an additional risk to their health. In still other circumstances, patients might be experiencing depression or anxiety, such that emotional dysfunction will be a major barrier to compliance. In addition, a longitudinal study demonstrated that adherence to dietary intervention protocol declined steadily even during the intervention period as the frequency of contact declined, which suggests that it is difficult for participants to sustain the behavior changes without ongoing reinforcement [135].

Traditionally, it has been assumed that the relationship between knowledge, attitudes, and behavior is a simple and direct one. Indeed, throughout the years, many prevention and patient education programs have been based on the premise that if people understand the health consequences of a particular behavior, they will modify it accordingly. Moreover, the argument goes, if people have a negative attitude toward an existing lifestyle practice and a positive attitude toward change, they will make healthful changes. However, it is now known from research conducted during approximately the past 30 years that the relationships among knowledge, awareness of the need to change, intention to change, and an actual change in behavior are very complex.

Ideally, each patient should be treated as an individual with unique circumstances and health history. Still, epidemiological research and clinical trials indicate that certain demographic subgroups differ in terms of risk factors and health behaviors [38,136]. Understanding these population trends can help prepare a provider to work with various types of patients. For example, younger persons may feel invulnerable to coronary events, and older adults may be managing multiple chronic conditions. An active middle-aged professional may place returning to his previous level of activity above important health protective actions. These examples serve as a reminder to be sensitive to group patterns but to avoid stereotyping in the absence of firsthand evidence about an individual. Within this general context, various theories and models can guide the search for effective ways to reach and positively motivate individuals.

B Behavior Change as a Process

Sustained health behavior change involves multiple actions and adaptations over time. Some people may not be ready to attempt changes, some may be thinking about attempting change, and others may have already begun implementing behavioral modifications. One central issue that has gained wide acceptance in recent years is the simple notion that behavior change is a process, not an event. Rather, it is important to think of the change process as one that occurs in stages. It is not a question of someone deciding one day to change his or her diet and the next day becoming a low-fat eater for life. Likewise, most people will not be able to dramatically change their eating habits all at once. The idea that behavior change occurs in a number of steps is not particularly new, but it has gained wider recognition in recent years. Indeed, various multistage theories of behavior change date back more than 50 years to the work of Lewin, McGuire, Weinstein, Marlatt and Gordon, and others [15,137,138].

The notion of readiness to change, or stage of change, has been examined in health behavior research and found useful in explaining and predicting a variety of types of behaviors. Prochaska, Velicer, DiClemente, and colleagues have been leaders in beginning to formally identify the dynamics and structure of change that underlie both self-mediated and clinically facilitated health behavior change. The construct of stage of change (described previously) is a key element of their transtheoretical model of behavior change, and it proposes that people are at different stages of readiness to adopt healthful behaviors [139,140].

Although the stages of change construct cuts across various circumstances of individuals who need to change or want to change, other theories also address these processes. Here, we discuss various models to illustrate four key concerns in understanding the process of behavior change: (1) motivation versus intention, (2) intention versus action, (3) changing behavior versus maintaining behavior change, and (4) the role of biobehavioral factors.

1 Motivation Versus Intention

Behavior change is challenging for most people even if they are highly motivated to change. As previously noted, the set of relationships between knowledge, awareness of the need to change, intention to change, and an actual change in behavior are very complex. For individuals who are coping with disease and illness, and who are often having to make very significant changes to their lifestyle and other aspects of their lives, this challenge is even greater. According to the TTM, people in precontemplation are neither motivated nor planning to change, those in contemplation intend to change, and those in preparation are acting on their intentions by taking specific steps toward the action of change [140].

2 Intention Versus Action

The TTM makes a clear distinction between the stages of contemplation and preparation and overt action [139,140]. A further application of this distinction comes from the TPB [83,84], which proposes that intentions are the best predictor of behavior [80]. However, researchers are increasingly focusing attention on "implementation intentions" as being more proximal and even better predictors of behavior and behavior change [89].

3 Changing Behaviors Versus Maintaining Behavior Change

Even where there is good initial adherence to a lifestyle change program, such as changing diet or eating habits, relapse is very common. It is widely recognized that many overweight persons are able to lose weight, only to regain it within 1 or 2 years [58,141]. Thus, it has become clear to researchers and clinicians that undertaking initial behavior change and maintaining behavior change require different types of strategies. The TTM distinction between "action" and "maintenance" stages implicitly addresses this phenomenon [139,140]. Another model that is not described in detail here, Marlatt and Gordon's relapse prevention model, specifically focuses on strategies for dealing with maintenance of a recently changed behavior [137]. It involves developing self-management and coping strategies and establishing new behavior patterns that emphasize perceived control, environmental management, and improved self-efficacy. These strategies are an eclectic mix drawn from SCT [40], the TPB [80,81], and applied behavioral analysis—the forerunners of the stages of change model.

C Biobehavioral Factors

The behavioral and social theories described thus far have some important limitations, many of which are only now beginning to be understood. Notably, for some health behaviors, especially addictive or addiction-like behaviors, there are other important determinants of behavior, which may be physiological and/or metabolic. Among the best known are the addictive effects of nicotine, alcohol, and some drugs. Physiologic factors increase psychological cravings and create withdrawal syndromes that may impede even highly motivated persons from changing their behaviors (e.g., quitting smoking and not consuming alcoholic beverages). Some behavior changes, such as weight loss, also affect energy metabolism and make long-term risk factor reduction an even greater challenge than it would be if it depended on cognitive–behavioral factors alone. Research on the psychobiology of appetite offers intriguing possibilities for understanding biobehavioral models of food intake, including food addiction.

D Barriers to Actions, Pros and Cons, and Decisional Balance

According to SCT [40] a central determinant of behavior involves the interaction between individuals and their environments. Behavior and environment are said to continuously interact and influence one another, which is known as the principle of reciprocal determinism. The concept of barriers to action, or perceived barriers, can be found in several theories of health behavior, either explicitly or as an application. It is part of SCT [40] and the TPB [80]. In the TTM, there are parallel constructs labeled as the "pros" (the benefits of change) and "cons" (the costs of change) [139,140]. Taken together, these constructs are known as "decisional balance."

The idea that individuals engage in relative weighing of the pros and cons has its origins in Janis and Mann's model of decision making, published in their seminal book more than 40 years ago [142], although the idea had emerged much earlier in social psychological discourse. Lewin's idea of force field analysis [143] and other work on persuasion and decision counseling by Janis and Mann predated that important work. Indeed, this notion is basic to models of rational decision making, in which people intellectually consider the advantages and disadvantages, obstacles and facilitators, barriers and benefits, or pros and cons of engaging in a particular action.

E Control over Behavior and Health: Control Beliefs and Self-Efficacy

Sometimes, "control beliefs" and self-efficacy hold people back from achieving better health. These deterrents to positive health behavior change are common, and they can be found in several models of health behavior, including SCT, TPB, and relapse prevention. One of the most important challenges for these models—and ultimately for health professionals who apply them—is to enhance perceived behavioral control and increase self-efficacy, thereby improving patients' motivation and persistence in the face of obstacles.

VIII IMPLICATIONS AND OPPORTUNITIES

Theory and research suggest that the most effective dietary interventions are those that use multiple strategies and aim to achieve multiple goals of awareness, information transmission, skill development, and supportive environments and policies [63]. The range of dietary intervention tools and techniques is extensive and varied. Programs will differ based on their goals and objectives; the needs of clients; and the available resources, staff, and expertise. Dietary interventions can stand alone or be part of broader, multi-component, and multiple-focus health promotion and patient education programs.

What can be expected? Program design relates closely to what one can expect in terms of results. In general, minimally intensive intervention efforts such as one-time group education sessions can reach large audiences but seldom lead to behavior changes. More intensive programs typically appeal to at-risk or motivated groups; cost more to offer; and can achieve relatively greater changes in knowledge, attitudes, and eating habits [144].

Dietary interventions must be sensitive to audience and contextual factors. Food selection decisions are made for many reasons other than just nutrition: Taste, cost, convenience, and cultural factors all play significant roles [23]. Dietary change strategies must take these issues into consideration. The health promotion motto "know your audience" has a true and valuable meaning. Planning processes can consider multiple theories in a systematic way through approaches such as intervention mapping [145]. Intervention programs should be developed on the basis of the needs, behaviors, motivations, and desires of target audience [146,147].

Furthermore, change is incremental. Many people have practiced a lifetime of less than optimal diet-related behaviors. It is unreasonable to expect that significant and lasting changes will occur during the course of a program that lasts only a few months. Programs need to pull participants along the continuum of change, being sure to be just in front of those most ready to change with attractive, innovative offerings.

In population-focused programs, it appears to be of limited value to adopt a program solely oriented toward modifying individual choice (e.g., teaching and persuading individuals to choose low-fat dairy products). A more productive strategy that supports and facilitates healthy behavior changes would also include environmental change efforts, such as expanding the availability of more nutritious food choices [2,24,25,92]. When this is done, along with individual skill training, long-lasting and meaningful changes can be achieved.

Finally, when planning interventions, we need to strive to be creative. Dietary interventions should be as entertaining and engaging as the other activities with which they are competing. People will want to participate if they can have fun with the nutrition programs. Communication technologies have opened up many new channels for engaging people's interest in better nutrition. The communication of nutrition information, no matter how important it is to good health, is secondary to attracting and retaining the interest and enthusiasm of the audience.

References

[1] M.P. Fuhrman, et al., Practice paper of the American Dietetic Association: home care opportunities for food and nutrition professionals, J. Am. Diet. Assoc. 109 (6) (2009) 1092–1100.

[2] U.S. Department of Agriculture/U.S. Department of Health and Human Services (2010). Dietary guidelines for Americans 2010. Available at <http://health.gov/dietaryguidelines/dga2010/DietaryGuidelines2010.pdf>.

[3] S.M. Krebs-Smith, et al., Americans do not meet federal dietary recommendations, J. Nutr. 140 (10) (2010) 1832–1838.

[4] S. Rowe, et al., Food science challenge: translating the dietary guidelines for Americans to bring about real behavior change, J. Food Sci. 76 (1) (2011) R29–R37.

[5] A.W. Smith, et al., U.S. primary care physicians' diet-, physical activity-, and weight-related care of adult patients, Am. J. Prev. Med. 41 (1) (2011) 33–42.

[6] S. Shiffman, et al., Weight management advice: what do doctors recommend to their patients? Prev. Med. 49 (6) (2009) 482–486.

[7] K. Greiner, et al., Discussing weight with obese primary care patients: physician and patient perceptions, J. Gen. Internal Med. 23 (5) (2008) 581–587.

[8] Y.Y. Fadl, et al., Predictors of weight change in overweight patients with myocardial infarction, Am. Heart J. 154 (4) (2007) 711–717.

[9] G. Rao, et al., New and emerging weight management strategies for busy ambulatory settings: a scientific statement from the American Heart Association endorsed by the Society of Behavioral Medicine, Circulation 124 (10) (2011) 1182–1203.

[10] K.M. Flegal, et al., Prevalence and trends in obesity among U.S. adults, 1999–2008, JAMA 303 (3) (2010) 235–241.

[11] C.L. Ogden, et al., Prevalence of high body mass index in U.S. children and adolescents, 2007–2008, JAMA 303 (3) (2010) 242–249.

[12] B. Sherry, et al., Vital signs: state-specific obesity prevalence among adults—United States, 2009, Morbid. Mortal. Wkly. Rep. 59 (30) (2010) 951–955.

[13] E.M. Venditti, et al., Rationale, design and methods of the HEALTHY study behavior intervention component, Int. J. Obes. (London) 33 (Suppl. 4) (2009) S44–S51.

[14] K.M. Flegal, et al., Prevalence of obesity and trends in the distribution of body mass index among U.S. adults, 1999–2010, JAMA 307 (5) (2012) 491–497.

[15] A. McAlister, C. Perry, G. Parcel, How individuals, environments, and health behaviors interact: social cognitive theory, in: K. Glanz, B.K. Rimer, K. Viswanath (Eds), Health Behavior and Health Education: Theory, Research, and Practice, Jossey-Bass, San Francisco, 2008, pp. 169–185.

[16] K. Glanz, T. Seewald-Klein, Nutrition at the worksite: an overview, J. Nutr. Educ. 18 (1, Suppl.) (1986) S1–S12.

[17] K. Glanz, M.P. Eriksen, Individual and community models for dietary behavior change, J. Nutr. Educ. 25 (1993) 80–86.

[18] T. Baranowski, Advances in basic behavioral research will make the most important contributions to effective dietary change programs at this time, J. Am. Diet. Assoc. 106 (6) (2006) 808–811.

[19] K. Glanz, D.B. Bishop, The role of behavioral science theory in development and implementation of public health interventions, Annu. Rev. Public Health 31 (2010) 399–418.

[20] M. Story, et al., Creating healthy food and eating environments: policy and environmental approaches, Annu. Rev. Public Health 29 (2008) 253–272.

[21] R.E. Glasgow, et al., Translating what we have learned into practice: principles and hypotheses for interventions addressing multiple behaviors in primary care, Am. J. Prev. Med. 27 (2, Suppl. 1) (2004) 88–101.

[22] R.E. Glasgow, D.J. Toobert, Brief, computer-assisted diabetes dietary self-management counseling: effects on behavior, physiologic outcomes, and quality of life, Med. Care 38 (11) (2000) 1062–1073.

[23] K. Glanz, et al., Why Americans eat what they do: taste, nutrition, cost, convenience, and weight control concerns as influences on food consumption, J. Am. Diet. Assoc. 98 (10) (1998) 1118–1126.

[24] K.R. McLeroy, et al., An ecological perspective on health promotion programs, Health Educ. Q. 15 (4) (1988) 351–377.

[25] J. Sallis, N. Owen, Ecological model, in: K. Glanz, B.K. Rimer, F.M. Lewis (Eds), Health Behavior and Health Education: Theory, Research, and Practice, Jossey-Bass, San Francisco, 2002, pp. 462–484.

[26] C.K. Chow, et al., Environmental and societal influences acting on cardiovascular risk factors and disease at a population level: a review, Int. J. Epidemiol. 38 (6) (2009) 1580–1594.

[27] C.C. Nelson, et al., Allocation of household responsibilities influences change in dietary behavior, Social Sci. Med. 73 (10) (2011) 1517–1524.

[28] E. de Vet, et al., Environmental correlates of physical activity and dietary behaviours among young people: a systematic review of reviews, Obes. Rev. 12 (5) (2011) e130–e142.

[29] K. Glanz, A.M. Hewitt, J. Rudd, Consumer behavior and nutrition education: an integrative review, J. Nutr. Educ. 24 (1992) 267–277.

[30] K. Glanz, et al., Healthy nutrition environments: concepts and measures, Am. J. Health Promot. 19 (5) (2005) 330–333ii

[31] K. Glanz, Nutritional intervention: a behavioral and educational perspective, Prevention of Coronary Heart Disease, Little, Brown, Boston, 1992, pp. 231–265

[32] K. Glanz, Patient and public education for cholesterol reduction: a review of strategies and issues, Patient Educ. Couns. 12 (1988) 235–257.

[33] National Cholesterol Education Program, Third Report of the National Cholesterol Education Program (NCEP) Expert Panel on Detection, Evaluation, and Treatment of High Blood Cholesterol in Adults (Adult Treatment Panel III), National Institutes of Health, National Heart, Lung, and Blood Institute, Bethesda, MD, 2001.

[34] K.E. Hart, E.M. Warriner, Weight loss and biomedical health improvement on a very low caloric diet: the moderating role of history of weight cycling, Behav. Med. 30 (4) (2005) 161–170.

[35] R.R. Wing, et al., Year-long weight loss treatment for obese patients with type II diabetes: does inclusion of an intermittent very low calorie diet improve outcome, Am. J. Med. 9 (1994) 354–362.

[36] A.M. Coulston, C.J. Boushey, Nutrition in the Prevention and Treatment of Disease, 2nd ed., Elsevier, Boston, 2008.

[37] S.J. Morreale, N.E. Schwartz, Helping Americans eat right: developing practical and actionable public nutrition education messages based on the ADA Survey of American Dietary Habits, J. Am. Diet. Assoc. 95 (3) (1995) 305–308.

[38] Y. Wang, M.A. Beydoun, The obesity epidemic in the United States—Gender, age, socioeconomic, racial/ethnic, and geographic characteristics: a systematic review and meta-regression analysis, Epidemiol. Rev. 29 (2007) 6–28.

[39] S. Kumanyika, S. Grier, Targeting interventions for ethnic minority and low-income populations, Future Child 16 (1) (2006) 187–207.

[40] A. Bandura, Social Foundations of Thought and Action: A Social Cognitive Theory, Prentice-Hall, Englewood Cliffs, NJ, 1986.

[41] A. Bandura, Self-Efficacy: The Exercise of Control, Freeman, New York, 1997.

[42] F.H. Kanfer, A.P. Goldstein (Eds), Helping People Change: A Textbook of Methods, Pergamon, Oxford, 1975, pp. vii, 536

[43] A. Bandura, Self-Efficacy: The Exercise of Control, Freeman, New York, 1997.

[44] A. Bandura, Health promotion from the perspective of social cognitive theory, Psychol. Health 13 (1998) 623–649.

[45] K. Glanz, Behavioral research contributions and needs in cancer prevention and control: dietary change, Prev. Med. 26 (1997) S43–S55.

[46] N.T. Artinian, et al., Interventions to promote physical activity and dietary lifestyle changes for cardiovascular risk factor reduction in adults: a scientific statement from the American Heart Association, Circulation 122 (2010) 406–441.

[47] L.E. Burke, J. Wang, M.A. Sevick, Self-monitoring in weight loss: a systematic review of the literature, J. Am. Diet. Assoc. 111 (1) (2011) 92–102.

[48] M.T. Warziski, et al., Changes in self-efficacy and dietary adherence: the impact on weight loss in the PREFER study, J. Behav. Med. 31 (1) (2008) 81–92.

[49] A. Bandura, Health promotion from the perspective of social cognitive theory, Psychol. Health 13 (4) (1998) 623–649.

[50] K. Chapman-Novakofski, J. Karduck, Improvement in knowledge, social cognitive theory variables, and movement through stages of change after a community-based diabetes education program, J. Am. Diet. Assoc. 105 (10) (2005) 1613–1616.

[51] J. Di Noia, J.O. Prochaska, Dietary stages of change and decisional balance: a meta-analytic review, Am. J. Health Behav. 34 (5) (2010) 618–632.

[52] J. Di Noia, I.R. Contento, J.O. Prochaska, Computer-mediated intervention tailored on transtheoretical model stages and processes of change increases fruit and vegetable consumption among urban African-American adolescents, Am. J. Health Promotion 22 (5) (2008) 336–341.

[53] F.H. Kanfer, Self-monitoring: methodological limitations and clinical applications, J. Consult. Clin. Psychol. 35 (1970) 148–152.

[54] A. Bandura, Health promotion from the perspective of social cognitive theory, Psychol. Health 13 (1998) 623–649.

[55] A. Bandura, Social cognitive theory of self-regulation, Org. Behav. Hum. Decision Processes 50 (1991) 248–287.

[56] L. Burke, et al., The effect of electronic self-monitoring on weight loss and dietary intake: a randomized behavioral weight loss trial, Obesity 19 (2011) 338–344.

[57] L.E. Burke, et al., Self-monitoring in behavioral weight loss treatment: SMART trial short-term results, Obesity 17 (Suppl. 2) (2009) S273.

[58] R.R. Wing, et al., A self-regulation program for maintenance of weight loss, N. Engl. J. Med. 355 (15) (2006) 1563–1571.

[59] R.R. Wing, et al., STOP regain: are there negative effects of daily weighing? J. Consult. Clin. Psychol. 75 (4) (2007) 652–656.

[60] J.O. Prochaska, C.C. DiClemente, Stages and processes of self-change of smoking: toward an integrative model of change, J. Consult. Clin. Psychol. 51 (3) (1983) 390–395.

[61] J.C. Norcross, P.M. Krebs, J.O. Prochaska, Stages of change, J. Clin. Psychol. 67 (2) (2011) 143–154.

[62] S.S. Johnson, et al., Transtheoretical model-based multiple behavior intervention for weight management: effectiveness on a population basis, Prev. Med. 46 (3) (2008) 238–246.

[63] C.A. Thomson, J. Ravia, A systematic review of behavioral interventions to promote intake of fruit and vegetables, J. Am. Diet. Assoc. 111 (10) (2011) 1523–1535.

[64] G.W. Greene, et al., Change in fruit and vegetable intake over 24 months in older adults: results of the SENIOR project intervention, Gerontologist 48 (3) (2008) 378–387.

[65] J. Rudd, K. Glanz, How consumers use information for health action: consumer information processing, in: K. Glanz, F.M. Lewis, B.K. Rimer (Eds), Health Behavior and Health Education: Theory, Research, and Practice, Jossey-Bass, San Francisco, 1990, pp. 115–139.

[66] J. Barreiro-Hurlé, A. Gracia, T. de-Magistris, Does nutrition information on food products lead to healthier food choices? Food Policy 35 (3) (2010) 221–229.

[67] J.M. Mancuso, Assessment and measurement of health literacy: an integrative review of the literature, Nursing Health Sci. 11 (1) (2009) 77–89.

B. RESEARCH AND APPLIED METHODS FOR OBSERVATIONAL AND INTERVENTION STUDIES

[68] S. Campos, J. Doxey, D. Hammond, Nutrition labels on pre-packaged foods: a systematic review, Public Health Nutr. 14 (8) (2011) 1496–1506.

[69] K. Hawthorne, et al., Culturally appropriate health education for type 2 diabetes in ethnic minority groups: a systematic and narrative review of randomized controlled trials, Diabetic Med. 27 (6) (2010) 613–623.

[70] J.L. Pomeranz, K.D. Brownell, Legal and public health considerations affecting the success, reach, and impact of menu-labeling laws, Am. J. Public Health 98 (9) (2008) 1578–1583.

[71] S. Burton, et al., Attacking the obesity epidemic: the potential health benefits of providing nutrition information in restaurants, Am. J. Public Health 96 (9) (2006) 1669–1675.

[72] B. Elbel, J. Gyamfi, R. Kersh, Child and adolescent fast-food choice and the influence of calorie labeling: a natural experiment, Int. J. Obes. 35 (4) (2011) 493–500.

[73] T. Dumanovsky, et al., Changes in energy content of lunchtime purchases from fast food restaurants after introduction of calorie labelling: cross sectional customer surveys, BMJ 343 (2011) d4464.

[74] C.A. Roberto, et al., Evaluating the impact of menu labeling on food choices and intake, Am. J. Public Health 100 (2) (2010) 312–318.

[75] Y.H. Chu, et al., Improving patrons' meal selections through the use of point-of-selection nutrition labels, Am. J. Public Health 99 (11) (2009) 2001–2005.

[76] J. Zoellner, et al., Nutrition literacy status and preferred nutrition communication channels among adults in the Lower Mississippi Delta, Prev. Chronic Dis. 6 (4) (2009) A128.

[77] N.R. Kandula, et al., The relationship between health literacy and knowledge improvement after a multimedia type 2 diabetes education program, Patient Educ. Couns. 75 (3) (2009) 321–327.

[78] L.O. Strolla, Using qualitative and quantitative formative research to develop tailored nutrition intervention materials for a diverse low-income audience, Health Educ. Res. 21 (4) (2005) 465–476.

[79] C. Isarankura-Na-Ayudhya, et al., Solving the barriers to diabetes education through the use of multimedia, Nursing Health Sci. 12 (1) (2010) 58–66.

[80] D.E. Montano, D. Kasprzyk, The theory of reasoned action and the theory of planned behavior, in: K. Glanz, B.K. Rimer, F.M. Lewis (Eds), Health Behavior and Health Education: Theory, Research and Practice, Jossey-Bass, San Francisco, 2002, pp. 67–98.

[81] I. Ajzen, The theory of planned behavior, Organ. Behav. Hum. Decision Processes 50 (1991) 179–211.

[82] A.S. Anderson, et al., Take Five, a nutrition education intervention to increase fruit and vegetable intakes: impact on attitudes towards dietary change, Br. J. Nutr. 80 (2) (1998) 133–140.

[83] H.S. Seo, S.K. Lee, S. Nam, Factors influencing fast food consumption behaviors of middle-school students in Seoul: an application of theory of planned behaviors, Nutr. Res. Pract. 5 (2) (2011) 169–178.

[84] G.J. de Bruijn, et al., Saturated fat consumption and the theory of planned behaviour: exploring additive and interactive effects of habit strength, Appetite 51 (2) (2008) 318–323.

[85] L. Lautenschlager, C. Smith, Understanding gardening and dietary habits among youth garden program participants using the theory of planned behavior, Appetite 49 (1) (2007) 122–130.

[86] N. Lien, L.A. Lytle, K.A. Komro, Applying theory of planned behavior to fruit and vegetable consumption of young adolescents, Am. J. Health Promot. 16 (4) (2002) 189–197.

[87] S. Booth-Butterfield, B. Reger, The message changes belief and the rest is theory: the "1% or less" milk campaign and reasoned action, Prev. Med. 39 (3) (2004) 581–588.

[88] A. McConnon, et al., Application of the theory of planned behaviour to weight control in an overweight cohort: results from a pan-European dietary intervention trial (DiOGenes), Appetite 58 (1) (2011) 313–318.

[89] A. Luszczynska, A. Sobczyk, C. Abraham, Planning to lose weight: randomized controlled trial of an implementation intention prompt to enhance weight reduction among overweight and obese women, Health Psychol. 26 (4) (2007) 507–512.

[90] W.B. Carter, Health behavior as a rational process: theory of reasoned action and multiattribute utility theory, in: K. Glanz, F. Lewis, B. Rimer (Eds), Health Behavior and Health Education: Theory, Research and Practice, Jossey-Bass, San Francisco, 1990, pp. 63–91.

[91] D. Brinberg, M.L. Axelson, S. Price, Changing food knowledge, food choice, and dietary fiber consumption by using tailored messages, Appetite 35 (1) (2000) 35–43.

[92] K. Glanz, et al., Environmental and policy approaches to cardiovascular disease prevention through nutrition: opportunities for state and local action, Health Educ. Q. 22 (4) (1995) 512–527.

[93] M.P. Galvez, M. Pearl, I.H. Yen, Childhood obesity and the built environment, Curr. Opin. Pediatr. 22 (2) (2010) 202–207.

[94] N. Townsend, C. Foster, Developing and applying a socio-ecological model to the promotion of healthy eating in the school, Public Health Nutr. (2011) 1–8.

[95] E.G. Klein, L.A. Lytle, V. Chen, Social ecological predictors of the transition to overweight in youth: results from the Teens Eating for Energy and Nutrition at Schools (TEENS) study, J. Am. Diet. Assoc. 108 (7) (2008) 1163–1169.

[96] Y. Suarez-Balcazar, et al., Introducing systems change in the schools: the case of school luncheons and vending machines, Am. J. Community Psychol. 39 (3–4) (2007) 335–345.

[97] M. Story, M.S. Nanney, M.B. Schwartz, Schools and obesity prevention: creating school environments and policies to promote healthy eating and physical activity, Milbank Q. 87 (1) (2009) 71–100.

[98] L.H. Engbers, et al., Worksite health promotion programs with environmental changes: a systematic review, Am. J. Prev. Med. 29 (1) (2005) 61–70.

[99] A.A. Gorin, et al., Home food and exercise environments of normal-weight and overweight adults, Am. J. Health Behav. 35 (5) (2011) 618–626.

[100] L.M. Anderson, et al., The effectiveness of worksite nutrition and physical activity interventions for controlling employee overweight and obesity: a systematic review, Am. J. Prev. Med. 37 (4) (2009) 340–357.

[101] C.A. Pratt, et al., Design characteristics of worksite environmental interventions for obesity prevention, Obesity (Silver Spring) 15 (9) (2007) 2171–2180.

[102] M. Barrera, et al., Social–ecological resources as mediators of two-year diet and physical activity outcomes in type 2 diabetes patients, Health Psychol. 27 (2 Suppl.) (2008) S118–S125.

[103] M. Barrera Jr., et al., Social support and social–ecological resources as mediators of lifestyle intervention effects for type 2 diabetes, J. Health Psychol. 11 (3) (2006) 483–495.

[104] E.R. Fowles, S.L. Fowles, Healthy eating during pregnancy: determinants and supportive strategies, J. Community Health Nurs. 25 (3) (2008) 138–152.

[105] T. Robinson, Applying the socio-ecological model to improving fruit and vegetable intake among low-income African Americans, J. Community Health 33 (6) (2008) 395–406.

[106] S.M. Noar, M. Chabot, R.S. Zimmerman, Applying health behavior theory to multiple behavior change: considerations and approaches, Prev. Med. 46 (3) (2008) 275–280.

[107] H. de Vries, et al., The effectiveness of tailored feedback and action plans in an intervention addressing multiple health behaviors, Am. J. Health Promotion 22 (6) (2008) 417–425.

[108] J. Gittelsohn, S. Sharma, Physical, consumer, and social aspects of measuring the food environment among diverse low-income populations, Am. J. Prev. Med. 36 (4, Suppl.) (2009) S161–S165.

[109] L.E. Burke, et al., Improving adherence to a cholesterol-lowering diet: a behavioral intervention study, Patient Educ. Couns. 57 (1) (2005) 134–142.

[110] L.E. Burke, et al., Development and testing of the Cholesterol-Lowering Diet Self-Efficacy Scale, Eur. J. Cardiovasc. Nurs. 2 (4) (2003) 265–273.

[111] L.E. Burke, et al., Effects of a vegetarian diet and treatment preference on biochemical and dietary variables in overweight and obese adults: a randomized clinical trial, Am. J. Clin. Nutr. 86 (3) (2007) 588–596.

[112] L.E. Burke, et al., SMART trial: a randomized clinical trial of self-monitoring in behavioral weight management-design and baseline findings, Contemporary Clin. Trials 30 (6) (2009) 540–551.

[113] I. Contento, Nutrition education and implications, J. Nutr. Educ. Behav. 27 (Special Issue) (1995).

[114] C. Achterberg, C. Miller, Is one theory better than another in nutrition education? A viewpoint: more is better, J. Nutr. Educ. Behav. 36 (1) (2004) 40–42.

[115] R.C. Plotnikoff, et al., Applying the stages of change to multiple low-fat dietary behavioral contexts: an examination of stage occupation and discontinuity, Appetite 53 (3) (2009) 345–353.

[116] L.M. Anderson, et al., The effectiveness of worksite nutrition and physical activity interventions for controlling employee overweight and obesity: a systematic review, Am. J. Prev. Med. 37 (4) (2009) 340–357.

[117] E.J. Lea, D. Crawford, A. Worsley, Consumers' readiness to eat a plant-based diet, Eur. J. Clin. Nutr. 60 (3) (2006) 342–351.

[118] H. Mochari-Greenberger, M.B. Terry, L. Mosca, Does stage of change modify the effectiveness of an educational intervention to improve diet among family members of hospitalized cardiovascular disease patients? J. Am. Diet. Assoc. 110 (7) (2010) 1027–1035.

[119] M. Råberg Kjøllesdal, et al., Intention to change dietary habits, and weight loss among Norwegian–Pakistani women participating in a culturally adapted intervention, J. Immigrant Minority Health 13 (6) (2011) 1150–1158.

[120] J. Adams, M. White, Why don't stage-based activity promotion interventions work? Health Educ. Res. 20 (2) (2005) 237–243.

[121] J. Brug, et al., The transtheoretical model and stages of change: a critique: observations by five commentators on the paper by Adams, J. and White, M. (2004) Why don't stage-based activity promotion interventions work? Health Educ. Res. 20 (2) (2005) 244–258.

[122] R.P. Riemsma, et al., Systematic review of the effectiveness of stage based interventions to promote smoking cessation, Br. Med. J. 326 (7400) (2003) 1175–1177.

[123] R. West, Time for a change: putting the transtheoretical (stages of change) model to rest, Addiction 100 (8) (2005) 1036–1039.

[124] E.M. van Sluijs, M.N. van Poppel, W. van Mechelen, Stage-based lifestyle interventions in primary care: are they effective? Am. J. Prev. Med. 26 (4) (2004) 330–343.

[125] B. Sternfeld, et al., Improving diet and physical activity with ALIVE: a worksite randomized trial, Am. J. Prev. Med. 36 (6) (2009) 475–483.

[126] B. Estabrook, J. Zapka, S.C. Lemon, Evaluating the implementation of a hospital work-site obesity prevention intervention: applying the RE-AIM framework, Health Promot. Pract. 13 (2012) 190–197.

[127] D.B. Abrams, et al., Cancer control at the workplace: the Working Well Trial, Prev. Med. 23 (1) (1994) 15–27.

[128] L.E. Burke, et al., Self-monitoring dietary intake: current and future practices, J. Ren. Nutr. 15 (3) (2005) 281–290.

[129] L.E. Burke, J. Wang, M.A. Sevick, Self-monitoring in weight loss: a systematic review of the literature, J. Am. Diet. Assoc. 111 (1) (2011) 92–102.

[130] L.E. Burke, et al., The effect of electronic self-monitoring on weight loss and dietary intake: a randomized behavioral weight loss trial, Obesity (Silver Spring) 19 (2) (2011) 338–344.

[131] A.A. Atienza, et al., Using hand-held computer technologies to improve dietary intake, Am. J. Prev. Med. 34 (6) (2008) 514–518.

[132] M.A. Sevick, et al., A PDA-based dietary self-monitoring intervention to reduce sodium intake in an in-center hemodialysis patient, Patient Prefer. Adherence 2 (2008) 177–184.

[133] C.J. Boushey, et al., Use of technology in children's dietary assessment, Eur. J. Clin. Nutr. 63 (Suppl. 1) (2009) S50–S57.

[134] J.D. Long, et al., Evidence review of technology and dietary assessment, Worldviews Evid. Based Nurs. 7 (4) (2010) 191–204.

[135] S.D. Acharya, et al., Adherence to a behavioral weight loss treatment program enhances weight loss and improvements in biomarkers, Patient Prefer. Adherence 3 (2009) 151–160.

[136] J. Crandall, et al., The influence of age on the effects of lifestyle modification and metformin in prevention of diabetes, J. Gerontol. A Biol. Sci. Med. Sci. 61 (10) (2006) 1075–1081.

[137] G. Marlatt, Relapse prevention: theoretical rationale and overview of the model, in: G. Marlatt, J. Gordon (Eds), Relapse Prevention: Maintenance Strategies in the Treatment of Addictive Behaviors, Guilford, New York, 1985, pp. 3–70.

[138] N.D. Weinstein, Testing four competing theories of health-protective behavior, Health Psychol. 12 (4) (1993) 324–333.

[139] J.O. Prochaska, C.C. DiClemente, J.C. Norcross, In search of how people change: applications to addictive behaviors, Am. Psychologist 47 (9) (1992) 1102–1114.

[140] J.O. Prochaska, C. Redding, K. Evers, The transtheoretical model of behavior change, in: K. Glanz, B.K. Rimer, F.M. Lewis (Eds), Health Behavior and Health Education: Theory, Research, and Practice, Jossey-Bass, San Francisco, 2002.

[141] R.R. Wing, S. Phelan, Long-term weight loss maintenance, Am. J. Clin. Nutr. 82 (1 Suppl.) (2005) 222S–225S.

[142] I. Janis, L. Mann, Decision Making: A Psychological Analysis of Conflict, Free Press, New York, 1977.

[143] K. Lewin, A Dynamic Theory of Personality, McGraw Hill, New York, 1935.

[144] M.P. Pignone, et al., Counseling to promote a healthy diet in adults: a summary of the evidence for the U.S. Preventive Services Task Force, Am. J. Prev. Med. 24 (1) (2003) 75–92.

[145] J. Brug, A. Oenema, I. Ferreira, Theory, evidence and intervention mapping to improve behavior nutrition and physical activity interventions, Int. J. Behav. Nutr. Phys. Act. 2 (1) (2005) 2.

[146] American Dietetic Association, Position of the American Dietetic Association: nutrition education for the public, J. Am. Diet. Assoc. 96 (11) (1996) 1183–1187.

[147] S. Nitzke, J. Freeland-Graves, Position of the American Dietetic Association: total diet approach to communicating food and nutrition information, J. Am. Diet. Assoc. 107 (7) (2007) 1224–1232.

B. RESEARCH AND APPLIED METHODS FOR OBSERVATIONAL AND INTERVENTION STUDIES

C H A P T E R

9

Nutrition Intervention
Lessons from Clinical Trials

Linda G. Snetselaar

University of Iowa, Iowa City, Iowa

I INTRODUCTION

The modification of dietary patterns to prevent and optimize the management of chronic disease has been traditionally perceived as a difficult and challenging task. However, much has been learned since the 1980s about how to successfully modify eating patterns. For example, in clinical trials, several diet intervention studies focused on the prevention of cancer or cardiovascular disease have demonstrated the feasibility of reducing dietary fat intake in targeted groups. In addition, complex dietary modifications testing the effect of diet on the progression of renal disease have also been successfully achieved.

II COMMON COMPONENTS OF DIETARY INTERVENTIONS IN CLINICAL TRIALS

A Study Design

A frequently used design is the randomized control trial (RCT), in which the study begins by screening those study participants who meet the eligibility criteria. Often, very large numbers of participants are screened to arrive at the final number of participants who meet these criteria. For those who are screened into the study, each participant is randomly assigned to either dietary intervention or control, sometimes labeled the usual care group.

B Recruitment

Recruitment for an RCT can involve a variety of strategies, including newspaper advertisements, posters at pharmacies, posters in doctors' offices, booths at county and state fairs, mass mailings, and presentations to appropriate groups who may become study participants. It is wise to have a number of recruitment strategies. If one fails, others can be initiated to achieve the targeted sample size goal. Although recruiting numbers of study participants needed for optimum sample size is an important element of an RCT, recruiting participants into a study who will remain with the study for the entire dietary intervention is equally important. Carefully reviewing the required internal review board-approved study participant consent is crucial. If a potential study participant has the following responses when the study is described to him or her, he or she may not be an appropriate candidate for the study:

- Hesitant about being willing to be a part of either the control (usual care) or the intervention group and voices that only the intervention group is best for him or her
- Concerned about the time that the study intervention group will require
- Is not sure about getting supervisor-approved time off to participate in the mandatory intervention group activities
- Adamant to be a part of the study when the study has another objective that is counter to this rationale for study participation
- Concerned about being able to continue the study for the entire time it is scheduled to run
- Unsure about spouse or significant other support for study activities
- Not willing to comply with required activities explicitly stated in the consent form
- Concerned about travel time needed to participate in study

Nutrition in the Prevention and Treatment of Disease, Third Edition.
DOI: http://dx.doi.org/10.1016/B978-0-12-391884-0.00009-3

Placing a study participant in a study when these criteria exist may mean that the number of dropouts in the study increases. Losing a study participant following randomization reduces the sample size and compromises study power to show a difference between the intervention and the control group. When randomized study participants drop out of a study, this is equivalent to underrecruiting and not meeting required study sample numbers. Study participants who drop out of a study cannot be replaced.

C Intervention Design

Study interventions begin with an initial hypothesis. The following are two examples:

- This study will compare the dietary intervention and control groups using data on the number of study participants who have a change in waist circumference of 4 or 5 inches over a 2-year intervention period.
- Following a 3-year dietary intervention study, participants will have a change in hemoglobin A1c that is double that of the control group.

These hypotheses are designed to provide a comparison of the intervention and control groups. Note that each hypothesis has a numeric difference. Without this difference, the study will not show that the dietary intervention did make a difference.

The strategy for the dietary intervention should have a basis in other studies that may have had smaller numbers and short periods of intervention time compared to those of the RCT. In addition, the RCT should be backed by a pilot study to show the ability to achieve the numeric changes that the original hypothesis indicates.

A more recent study design that can benefit from the older RCT studies is the community-based participatory research study. This more community-focused study requires that community participants who will be involved in implementing the study have a voice in its design. For this study, participants will need to be involved in the beginning phases of the study design and the development of implementation strategies. Without their involvement, the study will not be truly participatory. Whereas RCTs are more structured and have many checks and balances, this more formalized method of data collection can be more difficult in a community setting. For example, absentee data collection in a school setting may be very unstructured, with different personnel collecting the data and little standardization in the recording of the reasons for a student being absent. To mimic a more structured RCT, rules and guidelines that will allow for consistent categorization of absenteeism are required. This means working with school personnel—those collecting the data and those eventually entering data—to ensure that everyone is of equal understanding with a new policy or procedure for data collection.

III CONCEPTUAL MODELS OF MOTIVATION

Interventions are developed around models to provide conceptual designs for motivation for positive directions in dietary adherence. This section discusses theories that describe models of motivation.

A Self-Regulation Theory

This theory, originally described by Kanfer, states that behavior is regulated by cycles that involve self-monitoring, comparing goal achievement with expectations, and correcting the course of action when the goal is not met [1,2]. To change dietary behavior, a person seeks to increase knowledge of the discrepancy between current status and the identified goal. Two ways to accomplish this are (1) to increase the awareness of current status (e.g., through feedback such as dietary self-monitoring) or (2) to change the goal to make it more attainable. In conflict situations, when a goal is desired and yet not seen as important enough to strive to attain, ambivalence (feeling at least two different ways about something) is a normal, key obstacle to dietary change.

B Rokeach's Value Theory

Studies in persons who have undergone sudden transformation shifts in behavior show that personality is organized around concentric layers [3]. An individual's attitudes, numbering in the thousands, represent an organizational series of steps inward. More central are our beliefs, and even more central are our core personal values. The most central is the sense of personal identity. The more central the shift, the more likely the resulting behavior change will be maintained over time.

C Health Belief Model

The health belief model attempts to explain and predict health behaviors by focusing on the attitudes and beliefs of individuals. The key variables of the health belief model are as follows [4]:

Degree of perceived risk of a disease. This variable includes perceived susceptibility of contracting a health condition associated with lack of a healthy diet and its perceived severity once the disease is contracted.

Perceived benefits of diet adherence. A second benefit is the believed effectiveness of dietary strategies designed to help reduce the threat of disease.

Perceived barriers to diet adherence. This variable includes potential negative consequences that may result from changing dietary patterns, including physical (weight gain or loss), psychological (lack of spontaneity in food selection), and financial demands (cost of new foods).

Cues to action. Events that motivate people to take action in changing their dietary habits are crucial determinants of change.

Self-efficacy. A very important variable is the belief in being able to successfully execute the dietary behavior required to produce the desired outcomes [5–7].

Other variables. Demographic, sociopsychological, and structural variables affect an individual's perceptions of dietary change and thus indirectly influence his or her ability to sustain new eating behaviors.

Motivation for change depends on the presence of a sufficient degree of perceived risk in combination with sufficient self-efficacy relative to achieving dietary change. Perceived risk without self-efficacy tends to result in defensive cognitive coping, such as denial and rationalization, rather than behavior change.

D Decisional Balance

The classic Janis and Mann decisional balance model [8] was a rational view, describing a decision as a process of weighing cognitively the pros and cons of change. Change depends on the pros of change outweighing the cons. The counselor who is adept at reflective listening skills, designed to assist the client in reviewing those ideas that result in an optimum final choice, can facilitate determining the strengths and weaknesses of a decision.

E Transtheoretical Model

This model postulates that individuals change depending on where they are in conceptual readiness to modify their behavior. Prochaska and DiClemente were the forerunners of this theory that focuses on the concept that behavioral change happens in stages of motivation as clients move to a more healthful lifestyle.

F Self-Determination Theory

The self-determination theory is based on the concept that humans have an innate tendency for personal growth. The idea behind the self-determination theory is the question of how people internalize and integrate external factors that affect their motivation to change. Eventually, they will come to self-regulate their behaviors moving toward autonomy in actions in their daily lives. The use of reflections and affirmations can be helpful in achieving this autonomy in behavior change. Motivational interviewing, although not considered a theory but rather a communications style, has been connected to this self-determination theory and uses reflections and affirmations as tools to achieve this autonomy.

G Interaction

According to Miller and Rollnick [9], motivation can be thought of not as a client trait but as an interpersonal process between nutrition counselor and participant. Rather than seeing motivational change as something the client achieves, this process is one that the nutrition counselor and the client experience in tandem.

IV THEORIES USED IN ACHIEVING DIETARY BEHAVIOR CHANGE IN CLINICAL TRIALS

The nutrition components of clinical trials require skills in long-term dietary maintenance. These skills go beyond educating participants and instead involve strategies designed to reinitiate participants who no longer comply with the recommended eating plan. The studies described here provide research data collected when the theories presented previously are initiated in a clinical trial setting.

A Women's Health Initiative

The Women's Health Initiative (WHI) [10–12] is a randomized controlled clinical trial designed to look at prevention of breast and colorectal cancer. The dietary arm of this study focused on a diet with 20% energy from fat plus five servings of fruits and vegetables and six servings of grain products per day.

To accomplish this change in dietary habits, nutritionists in the study used a variety of behavior change techniques based on the models discussed here. The stages of change model drove efforts to increase compliance in the WHI. The Prochaska–DiClemente model includes six designated stages of change: precontemplation, contemplation, determination, action, maintenance, and relapse [13]. In an effort to simplify and accommodate different levels of adherence, WHI investigators chose to use only three levels of readiness to change: ready to change, unsure, and not ready to change. The decision to simplify levels is based on work with study participants showing that strategies to modify behavior fall within these three categories.

To test the effectiveness of using motivational strategies targeted at these three levels of change, a small research study was devised. Results of that study showed a positive change in dietary behavior following its implementation [14]. In this pilot study, researchers evaluated an intensive intervention program with diet. The basis of the program was use of motivational interviewing with participants in the WHI. The goal was to meet the study nutrition goal of 20% energy from fat.

WHI dietary intervention participants ($n = 175$) from three clinical centers were randomized to intervention or control status. Those randomized to the intensive intervention program participated in three individual motivational interviewing contacts from a nutritionist, plus the usual WHI dietary intervention. Those randomized to the control group continued with the usual WHI dietary management intervention. Percentage energy from fat was estimated at intensive intervention program baseline and intensive intervention program follow-up (1 year later) using the WHI food frequency questionnaire (FFQ).

The change in percentage energy from fat between the intensive intervention program and the control group at baseline and 1-year follow-up was −1.2 percentage points from the total fat for intensive intervention program participants and +1.4 percentage points for control participants. The result was an overall difference of 2. 6 percentage points ($p < 0.001$).

Table 9.1 presents summary statistics on the intensive intervention program effects comparing baseline levels of fat consumption. The changes in fat consumed varied by intensive intervention program baseline fat intake as a percentage of energy intake. Participants having the highest intensive intervention program baseline fat intake (>30% energy) showed the largest overall change in percentage energy from fat between intensive intervention program baseline and intensive intervention program follow-up. As might be expected, the smallest change was found in participants who consumed between 25 and 30% of energy from fat at intensive intervention program baseline. These participants were closer to their goal of 20% energy from fat at baseline, allowing for less overall change.

The results of this study show that a protocol based on motivational interviewing and delivered through contacts with trained nutritionists is effective. Those subjects who participated in the intervention arm of the study further lowered their dietary fat intake to achieve study goals.

TABLE 9.1 Effect of WHI (Pilot) Intervention on FFQ Percentage Energy from Fat Stratified by Baseline Percentage Energy from Fat[a]

	n	Baseline X (SD)	Follow-up X (SD)	Difference
% Energy from fat: <20.0				
Intervention control	23	17.75 (1.8)	17.86 (3.9)	0.1
	25	17.35 (2.3)	19.70 (4.5)	2.3
Difference[b]		−0.4	1.8	2.2
% Energy from fat: =20.0 and <25.0				
Intervention control	25	22.72 (1.4)	21.68 (4.6)	−1.0
	26	23.17 (1.7)	25.29 (4.8)	2.1
Difference[b]		0.5	3.6	3.1
% Energy from fat: =25.0 and <30.0				
Intervention control	21	27.42 (1.6)	26.3 (4.6)	−1.1
	15	26.94 (1.2)	26.89 (4.6)	0.0
Difference[b]		−0.5	0.6	1.1
% Energy from fat: =30.0				
Intervention control	13	34.24 (2.5)	30.11 (6.5)	−4.1
	16	33.81 (3.1)	33.82 (5.0)	0.0
Difference[b]		−0.4	3.7	4.1

[a]Participants with missing FFQ data were excluded.
[b]p < 0.05 using paired t-test.
Source: Modified from Bowen, D., Ehret, C., Pedersen, M., Snetselaar, L., and Johnson, M. (2002). Results of an adjunct dietary intervention program in the Women's Health Initiative. J. Am. Diet. Assoc. **102**, 1631−1637.

B The Diet Intervention Study in Children

A similar protocol was used in the Diet Intervention Study in Children (DISC) [15]. DISC was a randomized, multicenter clinical trial assessing the efficacy and safety of lowering dietary fat to decrease low-density lipoprotein cholesterol in children at high risk for cardiovascular disease [16,17]. Children began this study between ages 7 and 10 years and participated in group dietary intervention programs. As they moved into adolescence (ages 13−17 years) and encountered added obstacles to dietary adherence and retention, researchers in the study designed and implemented an individual-level motivational intervention. The diet prescription in the DISC study required providing 28% energy from total fat, less than 8% energy from saturated fat, up to 9% energy from polyunsaturated fat, and less than 75 mg/day of cholesterol. The diet met

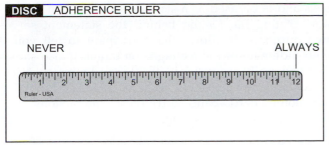

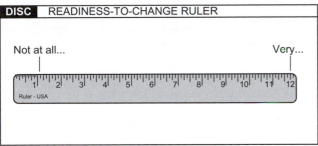

FIGURE 9.1   Assessment rulers. Source: *Data from Berg-Smith, S. M., Stevens, V. J., Brown, K. M., VanHorn, L., Gernhofer, N., Peters, E., Greenberg, R., Snetselaar, L., Ahrens, L., and Smith, K., for the Dietary Intervention Study in Children (DISC) Research Group (1999). A brief motivational intervention to improve dietary adherence in adolescents.* Health Educ. Res. *14, 399–410.*

TABLE 9.2   Changes in Total Fat Intake, Saturated Fat Intake, and Dietary Cholesterol after Two Intervention Sessions

	Mean	**SD**	*p*
Total fat intake			
Baseline	27.7	6.1	—
Follow-up	25.6	6.1	—
Change	−2.1	7.0	<0.001
Saturated fat intake			
Baseline	9.5	2.7	—
Follow-up	8.6	2.4	—
Change	−0.9	3.1	<0.001
Dietary cholesterol			
Baseline	182.9	97.6	—
Follow-up	157.3	87.6	—
Change	−25.6	92.3	<0.003

Source: *Data from Berg-Smith, S. M., Stevens, V. J., Brown, K. M., VanHorn, L., Gernhofer, N., Peters, E., Greenberg, R., Snetselaar, L., Ahrens, L., and Smith, K., for the Dietary Intervention Study in Children (DISC) Research Group (1999). A brief motivational intervention to improve dietary adherence in adolescents.* Health Educ. Res. *14, 399–410.*

the age- and sex-specific Recommended Dietary Allowance for energy, protein, and micronutrients.

Researchers used a pre- to postintervention design among a subset of the total intervention cohort ($n = 334$). The first 127 participants who appeared for regularly scheduled intervention visits after the implementation of the new intervention method were considered part of the study. These participants ranged from 13 to 17 years of age, with equal numbers of boys and girls. Nutrition interventionists asked all of the 127 participants to return in 4–8 weeks for a follow-up session. Initial sessions were conducted in person, and follow-up sessions were conducted either in person or by telephone.

Three 24-hour dietary recalls were collected within 2 weeks after the follow-up session. These dietary data were compared to three baseline 24-hour dietary recalls collected in the year preceding initial exposure to the motivational intervention method.

Self-reported data were also collected. At initial and follow-up intervention sessions, participants were shown "assessment rulers" (Figure 9.1) numbered 1–12 and asked to rate their adherence to dietary guidelines and their readiness to make new or additional dietary changes.

Results from the study show that the mean energy from total fat decreased from 27.7 to 25.6% ($p < 0.001$) (Table 9.2) and the mean energy from saturated fat decreased from 9.5 to 8.6% of the total energy intake ($p < 0.001$). In addition, dietary cholesterol decreased from 182.9 to 157.3 mg ($p < 0.003$). A comparison of males and females showed no differences in gender relative to study results. Note that for this preliminary test, no control group was randomly assigned or examined. Therefore, the researchers cannot predict if significant reductions in consumption of dietary fat and cholesterol are attributable to the intervention.

The self-reported adherence rating score and readiness to change score increased by approximately 1 point on a scale from 1 to 12 (both $p < 0.001$). To help accomplish goals, action plans were also made. The study results show that 94% of the participants made action plans and 89% successfully implemented them.

This study also examined counselor satisfaction. The results showed that nearly three-fourths of the nutrition counselors were satisfied or very satisfied with using the stages of change methods (Table 9.3).

C Motivational Intervention Method

DISC focused on the stages of change method with elements of motivational interviewing. Figure 9.2 provides a method for establishing rapport before tailoring the intervention to the readiness to change level: ready to change, unsure, and not ready to change. Figure 9.3 provides specific strategies for each level of change.

TABLE 9.3 Nutrition Counselor Satisfaction with the Motivational Intervention Method

Level of satisfaction	Percentage of the intervention sessions
Very satisfying	39
Satisfying	35
Somewhat satisfying	19
Slightly or not satisfying	7

Source: *Data from Berg-Smith, S. M., Stevens, V. J., Brown, K. M., VanHorn, L., Gernhofer, N., Peters, E., Greenberg, R., Snetselaar, L., Ahrens, L., and Smith, K., for the Dietary Intervention Study in Children (DISC) Research Group (1999). A brief motivational intervention to improve dietary adherence in adolescents. Health Educ. Res.* **14**, *399–410.*

1 First Level: Not Ready to Change

The main goal for this level of intervention is to raise awareness of the need to continue meeting goals (e.g., fat grams, carbohydrate grams, and energy intake). In addition, to achieve this goal, it is necessary to reduce resistance and barriers to meeting goals (e.g., decreasing cues to eat high-fat foods). Also, importantly, focus is placed on increasing interest in considering behavioral steps toward meeting the goals noted previously.

Throughout the initial interview, when working with a patient in this level, it is important to ask open-ended questions, listen reflectively, affirm, summarize, and elicit self-motivational statements. Figure 9.3 provides examples of questions designed to facilitate the participant's ability to make motivational statements.

A ASK OPEN-ENDED QUESTIONS

Initially for a participant at this level, it is important to ask questions that require explaining or discussing. Questions focus on requiring more than one-word answers.

The goal is to guide the participants to talk about their dietary change progress and difficulties. Figure 9.2 provides some opening questions. Other questions and statements are presented here:

"Let's discuss your experience with diet up to now. Tell me how changing your diet has been for you."
"What things would you like to discuss about your experiences with dietary change and your progress with changes? What do you like about these changes? What don't you like about these changes?"

B LISTEN REFLECTIVELY

Listening goes beyond hearing what a person has said and acknowledging those words. Crucial in responding to a patient or participant is the understanding of what is meant beyond the words. Reflective listening involves a guess at what the person feels and is phrased as a statement rather than a question. Stating the feeling behind the statement serves two purposes. It allows the participant to tell you if your judgment of the feeling is on target. It also shows that you really are trying to understand more than just words and do care about feelings also. The following are some participant–nutritionist interactions that illustrate reflective listening:

Scenario 1
  Participant: "There are times when I do a wonderful job of meeting my fat gram goal, but sometimes I don't do so well. I keep trying though."
  Nutritionist: "You seem to feel badly that you don't always meet your fat gram goal."
Scenario 2
  Participant: "I am so tired of trying to follow this diet. It seems that I have put hours into following it, and I have little to show for it. I certainly have not lost weight."
  Nutritionist: "You feel frustrated and angry about trying so hard and still getting nowhere."
Scenario 3
  Participant: "When I don't fill in a food diary, I am not sure that I am doing well or not."
  Nutritionist: "You are worried on days when you do not fill in a food diary."
Scenario 4
  Participant: "I really don't want to continue following this diet. I have other things that are more of a priority now."
  Nutritionist: "You seem hassled by these other competing desires and feel that following a new eating pattern is getting in the way."

C AFFIRM

Communicating support to participants is an excellent way of letting them know that you appreciate what they are doing. Affirmations are statements that indicate alignment and normalization of the participant's issues. Alignment means telling participants that you understand them and are with them in their difficulties. Normalization means telling the participants that they are perfectly within reason and "normal" to have such reactions and feelings. Examples of affirmations include the following:

"It is very hard to struggle with competing priorities. You've done amazingly well."
"That is an insightful idea."
"Thank you for telling me that. It must have been hard for you to tell me."
"I can see why you would have this difficulty. Many people have the same problem."

ESTABLISH RAPPORT
"How's it going?"

↓

OPENING STATEMENT

"We have ___ minutes to meet. This is what I thought we might do:

- take your height and weight measurements,
- hear how the DISC diet is going for you,
- give you some information from your last diet recall and cholesterol values, and
- talk about what, if anything, you might want to change in your eating."

"How does this sound? Is there anything else you want to do?"

↓

ASSESS CURRENT EATING BEHAVIOR AND PROGRESS

- Show Adherence Ruler.
- Ask open-ended questions to explore current eating behavior and progress.
* "Tell me more about the number you chose."
* "Why did you choose a 5, and not a 1?"
* "At what times do you follow the DISC diet, and at what times don't you?"
* "How are you feeling about the DISC diet?"
* "The last time we met, you were working on _____. How is that going?"

↓

GIVE FEEDBACK

- Show participant feedback graphs and forms.
- Compare participant results with normative data or other interpretive information.
    * "This is where you stand comapared to other teenagers."
- Elicit participant's overall response.
    * "What do you make of all this information?"
- Offer information about the meaning or significance of the results (only if participant asks or shows interest).
    * "For most teenagers who have cholesterol value around_____, they're more likely to _____."

↓

ASSESS READINESS TO CHANGE

- Introduce "change" ruler.
* "On a scale of 1–12 [1 = not at all ready; 12 = very ready], how ready are you right now to make any new changes in your life to eat foods lower in saturated fat and cholesterol?"
^ Ask participant to explain choice of number.
* "What are all the reasons you chose a ____?"

↓

TAILOR INTERVENTION APPROACH

↓

CLOSE THE COUNTER

- Summarize the session.
* "Did I get it all?"

- Support self-efficacy.
* "Again, I applaud your efforts and I know you can do it. If this plan doesn't work out, I'm sure there are other options that might work better."

- Arrange another time to meet.

FIGURE 9.2 Stages of change model. Source: *From Berg-Smith, S. M., Stevens, V. J., Brown, K. M., VanHorn, L., Gernhofer, N., Peters, E., Greenberg, R., Snetselaar, L., Ahrens, L., and Smith, K., for the Dietary Intervention Study in Children (DISC) Research Group (1999). A brief motivational intervention to improve dietary adherence in adolescents.* Health Educ. Res. **14**, 399–410.

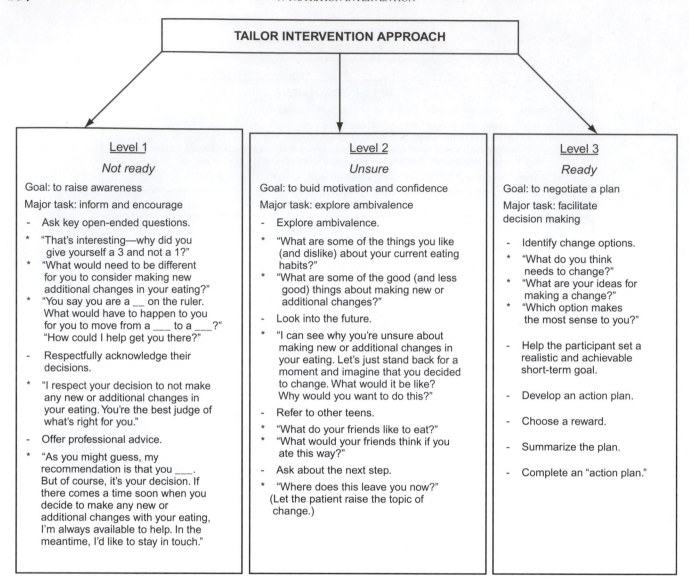

FIGURE 9.3 Stages of change components for three specific levels. Source: *Modified from Berg-Smith, S. M., Stevens, V. J., Brown, K. M., VanHorn, L., Gernhofer, N., Peters, E., Greenberg, R., Snetselaar, L., Ahrens, L., and Smith, K., for the Dietary Intervention Study in Children (DISC) Research Group (1999). A brief motivational intervention to improve dietary adherence in adolescents.* Health Educ. Res. **14**, 399–410.

D SUMMARIZE

Periodically, and at the point when you begin to elicit self-motivational statements, summarize the content of what the participant has said. Cover key points even if they involve negative feelings. You can discuss conflicting ideas that the participant has brought up by using the strategy "on the one hand, you ... and on the other hand, you.... " This reminds both of you about the issues and ensures clarity.

E ELICIT CHANGE STATEMENTS

The most important part of self-motivational statements is that they help participants realize that a problem exists, that they are concerned about the problem, that they intend to correct the problem, and that they think they can do better in the future. Figure 9.4 provides questions to elicit self-motivational statements. These statements fall into four categories: problem recognition, concern, intention to change, and optimism.

It is important to respectfully acknowledge decisions that participants make. These decisions may mean that a participant has decided not to make changes immediately (see Figure 9.3).

It is appropriate to offer professional advice but still leave the actual decision to make a change up to the participant. Figure 9.3 provides some ideas on how to approach the participant.

1. **Problem Recognition**
    What things make you think that this is a problem?
    What difficulties have you had in relation to your diet?
    In what ways do you think you or other people have been inconvenienced by your diet?
    In what ways has this been a problem for you?
    How has your diet stopped you from doing what you want to do?

2. **Concern**
    What is there about your diet that you or other people might see as reasons for concern?
    What worries you about your diet?
    How do you feel about your dietary problems?
    How much does that concern you?
    In what ways does this concern you?
    What do you think will happen if you don't make a change?

3. **Intention to Change**
    The fact that you're here indicates that at least a part of you thinks it's time to do something.
         What are the reasons you see for making a change?
    What makes you think that you need to make a change?
    If you were 100% successful and things worked out exactly as you would like, what would be
         different?
    What things make you think that you should stop following your diet? . . . And
         what about the other side? What makes you think it's time for a change?
    What are you thinking about your diet at this point?
    What would be the advantages of making a change?
    I can see that you're feeling stuck at the moment. What's going to have to change?

4. **Optimism**
    What makes you think that if you decide to make a change, you could do it?
    What encourages you that you can change if you want to?
    What do you think would work for you, if you decided to change?

FIGURE 9.4 Examples of questions designed to elicit self-motivational statements. Source: *Modified from Bowen, D., Ehret, C., Pedersen, M.,* *et al. (2002). Results of an adjunct dietary intervention program in the Women's Health Initiative.* J. Am. Diet. Assoc. *102, 1631–1637.*

Close the discussion with another summary. Concentrate on any self-motivational statements that the participant has made. End the session with the idea that both of you should think about what has been discussed and that you can revisit the issues next time.

2 Second Level: Unsure about Change

The main goal for this intervention is to tip the balance toward working to meet the goals. Four steps are important in meeting the goals: regroup, ask key questions, negotiate a plan, and conclude the work.

A REGROUP

The first step in dealing with a participant who is unsure about changing dietary habits is regrouping to focus on the transition from not being ready to deal with the problems of change to moving toward a reinitiating of behavior adjustment. This process of regrouping can serve as a reminder of what has happened in previous sessions. The following are four ways to regroup:

1. Summarize the participant's perceptions of what is going on. The summary might include self-
motivational statements that the participant has made.
2. Identify ambivalence or other conflicting issues.3. Review any self-monitoring related to dietary intake.
3. Restate intentions or plans to change or do better in the future.

B ASK KEY QUESTIONS

Ask questions that focus on the participant's statements regarding future plans to make dietary changes. The goal is to ask open-ended questions that cause the participant to think about what you have just summarized and come to the conclusion that action is necessary. The goal is for the participant to provide a statement showing the desire to change. Here are some examples of questions that facilitate positive participant statements:

"How might we work together to proceed from here?"
"Hearing my summary of how things have gone in the past, what do you want to do?"
"How might you become more involved in dietary change?"

"What are the good parts and the bad parts about continuing to change?"

"You are currently unsure of what to do. How might we work together to resolve the issue?"

C NEGOTIATE A PLAN

There are three parts to the negotiation process. The first involves setting goals; the second, considering the options; and finally, arriving at a plan:

Set goals: Past wisdom dictated that setting goals meant being specific and behavioral. "I will eat candy bars only one time per week, on Sunday." Motivational interviewing dictates that goal setting may start out broadly at first and then move to behavioral goals that are specific. To elicit broadly stated goals, the following questions might be used:

"What about your diet would you like to change?"

"How would you like things to be different from how they are now?"

Consider options: Make a list of things that might be changed to bring the participant closer to the dietary goal. Ask the participant to choose among the options. If the first one does not work, the participant has many choices as backups.

Arrive at a plan: Ask the participant to arrive at a plan. Include in the plan the specific behavioral goals with potential problems that may serve as barriers to making these changes.

D CONCLUDE THE WORK

Always end the session with an encouraging statement and a reflection on the participant's resourcefulness in identifying the plan. Follow this statement with the idea that he or she is the best expert relative to behavior change. Indicate that you will stay in touch to check on how the behavior change is going.

3 Third Level: Ready to Change

The main goal for this third intervention is to reengage the participant in meeting the dietary goals.

A REVIEW

Cover the previous discussions with the participant. Focus on the statements the participant made that show interest and a willingness to change. Use statements that show that it was the participant's idea to meet dietary goals previously set—for example, "You said that you were interested in trying again."

B ENCOURAGE CHOICES AND ACTIVITIES

Ask the participant what he or she would like to do to reengage. Encourage the participant to make his or her own choice. Collaborate and negotiate short-term, easily attained goals initially, such as "I will drink 1% milk for a week in place of 2% milk and gradually reduce to fat-free milk."

C SUMMARIZE

Review the discussion, the issues, and the difficulties on both sides. Remind the participant to keep trying and to believe in him- or herself.

D The Modification of Diet and Renal Disease Study

The Modification of Diet and Renal Disease Study (MDRD) [18] used the self-management approach to modify dietary behavior. In this population of persons diagnosed with renal disease, research nutritionists counseled participants on diets low in protein and phosphorus. Although the diets were difficult to follow, the study participants showed great motivation based on their desires to avoid renal dialysis [19]. The following strategies were used successfully in the MDRD [20]:

Single-nutrient approach to dietary behavior change: The focus in this study was on reducing protein content of the diet. With this reduction, dietary phosphorus was also reduced. When other nutrients were modified, specific food groups were identified. Even with changes in other nutrients, protein was still a primary focus.

Self-monitoring: The participant's ability to self-monitor was crucial to keeping protein intake down to goal levels. Weighing and measuring was used as a means of matching dietary change on a daily basis with the biological marker of urinary nitrogen. Further study in self-monitoring matched with the biological marker showed that problems occur in knowing how to best represent dietary intake [21]. For example, it is often difficult to closely mirror the exact amount of protein in a cut of meat if that cut is not precisely specified.

Staging changes: In the MDRD, nutritionists also staged changes in dietary protein by gradually reducing the dietary protein intake. This gradual change made day-to-day modifications easier.

Modeling: Nutritionists modeled dietary changes by offering both recipes low in protein and taste-testing sessions. Group sessions were held at which a special meal was offered with food preparation techniques modeled.

E The Diabetes Control and Complications Trial

The Diabetes Control and Complications Trial (DCCT) [22] used techniques similar to those of the MDRD study [23]:

Single-nutrient approach: Investigators focused on carbohydrate as a single nutrient, where it was matched with insulin to achieve normalized blood glucose.

Self-monitoring: Monitoring consisted of following blood glucose concentrations and dietary intakes to verify where problems might be occurring. If dietary intake was high along with blood glucose concentrations, dietary intake or insulin was modified to achieve normal blood glucose levels.

Staging changes: Changes were staged by working on specific times of day that were most problematic. If lunchtimes were most often high, we focused on dietary intake modifications to alter blood glucose levels. Also, insulin and exercise often played a role.

Modeling: Dietary modifications were facilitated by providing recipes, modeling, and going to restaurants to identify and anticipate blood glucose levels after eating a favorite lunch or other meals out of the home.

F The Brief Motivational Intervention to Reduce Body Mass Index Study

The Brief Motivational Intervention to Reduce Body Mass Index (BMI^2) study is designed to compare three groups: pediatricians without motivational interviewing training, pediatricians with motivational interviewing training, and pediatricians and registered dietitians with motivational interviewing training. The outcome for this study is children with elevated BMIs ranging from the 85th to the 97th percentile for their ages. Clinicians in this study will work with parents to try to modify their way of working with children to achieve dietary behavior change. The basis of this work is the self-determination theory, which serves as the underlying construct for the motivational interviewing communication style. This is a 2-year intervention that is currently in its first year of data collection [24].

V SUMMARY

Considerable experience in clinical trials suggests that dietary modification requires a process of making changes on an individual basis with constant negotiation with the patient or participant. Working as a team, the nutritionist and participant can achieve dietary change that alters biological markers and may reduce disease risk and optimize management.

References

[1] G. Agostinelli, J.M. Brown, W. Miller, Effects of normative feedback on consumption among heavy drinking college attendants, J. Drug Educ. 25 (1995) 31–40.

[2] J.M. Brown, W.R. Miller, Impact of motivational interviewing on participation in residential alcoholism treatment, Psychol. Addict. Behav. 7 (1993) 211–218.

[3] M. Rokeach, The Nature of Human Values, Free Press, New York, 1973.

[4] I. Rosenstock, V. Strecher, M. Becker, The health belief model and HIV risk behavior change, in: R.J. DiClemente, J.L. Peterson (Eds), Preventing AIDS: Theories and Methods of Behavioral Interventions, Plenum, New York, 1994, pp. 5–24.

[5] A. Bandura, Perceived self-efficacy in the exercise of control over AIDS infection, Primary Prevention of AIDS: Psychological Approaches, Sage, London, 1989, pp. 128–141

[6] A. Bandura, Self-efficacy: toward a unifying theory of behavioral change, Psychol. Rev. 84 (1977) 191–215.

[7] A. Bandura, Self-efficacy mechanism in physiological activation and health-promoting behavior, in: J. Madden (Ed.), Neurobiology of Learning, Emotion and Affect, Raven Press, New York, 1991, pp. 229–270.

[8] J.L. Janis, L. Mann, Decision-Making: A Psychological Analysis of Conflict, Choice and Commitment, Free Press, New York, 1977.

[9] W.R. Miller, S. Rollnick, Motivational Interviewing: Preparing People to Change Addictive Behavior, Guilford, New York, 1991.

[10] Women's Health Initiative, WHI protocol for clinical trial and observational components, Fred Hutchinson Cancer Research Center, Seattle, WA, 1994NIH Publication No. N01-WH-2-2110.

[11] R.L. Prentice, B. Caan, R.T. Chlebowski, et al., Low-fat dietary pattern and risk of invasive breast cancer: the Women's Health Initiative Randomized Controlled Dietary Modification Trial, JAMA 295 (2006) 629–642.

[12] S.A. Beresford, K.C. Johnson, C. Ritenbaugh, et al., Low-fat dietary pattern and risk of colorectal cancer: The Women's Health Initiative Randomized Controlled Dietary Modification Trial, JAMA 295 (2006) 643–654.

[13] J. Prochaska, C. DiClemente, Transtheoretical therapy: toward a more integrative model of change, Psychother. Theory Res. Prac. 19 (1982) 276–288.

[14] D. Bowen, C. Ehret, M. Pedersen, M. Johnson, Results of an adjunct dietary intervention program in the Women's Health Initiative, J. Am. Diet. Assoc. 102 (2002) 1631–1637.

[15] S.M. Berg-Smith, V.J. Stevens, K.M. Brown, L. VanHorn, N. Gernhofer, E. Peters, et al., A brief motivational intervention to improve dietary adherence in adolescents, Health Educ. Res. 14 (1999) 399–410.

[16] DISC Collaborative Research Group, Efficacy and safety of lowering dietary intake of fat and cholesterol in children with elevated low-density lipoprotein cholesterol: The Dietary Intervention Study in Children (DISC), JAMA 273 (1995) 1429–1435.

[17] DISC Collaborative Research Group, Dietary Intervention Study in Children (DISC) with elevated LDL cholesterol: design and baseline characteristics, Ann. Epidemiol 3 (1993) 393–402.

[18] S. Klahr, A.S. Levey, G.J. Beck, A.W. Caggiula, L. Hunsicker, J.W. Kusek, et al., The effects of dietary protein restriction and

blood-pressure control on the progression of chronic renal disease, N. Engl. J. Med. 330 (1994) 877—884.

[19] C. Milas, M.P. Norwalk, L. Akpele, L. Castaldo, T. Coyne, L. Doroshenko, et al., Factors associated with adherence to the dietary protein intervention in the modification of diet in renal disease, J. Am. Diet. Assoc. 95 (11) (1995) 1295—1300.

[20] L. Snetselaar, Dietary compliance issues in patients with early stage renal disease, Clin. Appl. Nutr. 2 (3) (1992) 47—52.

[21] L. Snetselaar, C.A. Chenard, L.G. Hunsicker, P.J. Stumbo, Protein calculation from food diaries underestimates biological marker, J. Nutr. 125 (1995) 2333—2340.

[22] The Diabetes Control and Complications Trial Research Group, The effect of intensive treatment of diabetes on the development and progression of long-term complications in insulin-dependent diabetes mellitus, N. Engl. J. Med. 329 (1993) 977—986.

[23] T. Greene, J. Bourgorgnie, V. Hawbe, J. Kusek, L. Snetselaar, J. Soucie, et al., Baseline characteristics in the modification of diet in renal disease study, J. Am. Soc. Nephrol. 3 (11) (1993) 1819—1834.

[24] K. Resnicow, F. McMaster, S. Woolford, E. Slora, A. Bocian, D. Harris, et al., Study design and baseline description of the BMI2 trial: reducing paediatric obesity in primary care practices, Pediatr. Obes. 7 (2011) 3—15.

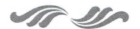

Tools and Techniques to Facilitate Nutrition Intervention

Linda M. Delahanty[*], *Joan M. Heins*[†]

[*]Massachusetts General Hospital Diabetes Center, Boston, Massachusetts
[†]Washington University School of Medicine, St. Louis, Missouri

I INTRODUCTION

To effectively facilitate nutrition interventions using medical nutrition therapy, dietitians must understand the teaching—learning process and conduct individualized assessments of learning style and motivational readiness so they can determine which tools and techniques are most appropriate to help patients make healthy changes in eating behavior.

The first section of this chapter reviews the various factors that affect the teaching—learning process, including age, literacy, culture, and learner style, and it reviews the different domains in which people learn. The next section discusses nutrition education techniques and focuses on the process that the nutrition counselor uses to assess learning needs, determine the level of education, and select the educational method and tools that match the patient's needs. The final section reviews the stages of change model and how it can be used to guide the nutrition counselor in selecting behavior change techniques that are tailored to an individual patient's level of motivational readiness. The nutrition counselor can use the behavioral counseling techniques of consciousness raising and motivational interviewing to address patients in the pre-action stages of change (precontemplation and contemplation) and use behavioral change techniques that focus on skills training such as goal setting, self-monitoring, stimulus control, problem-solving barriers, coping skills and stress management, and increasing social support for patients in the action stages (preparation, action, and maintenance). This chapter includes case scenarios demonstrating how the counselor might apply these approaches and provides examples of how to phrase the counseling dialogue.

II THE NUTRITION EDUCATION AND COUNSELING PROCESS

The potential effect of nutrition interventions and medical nutrition therapy to improve health outcomes from cardiovascular, cancer, diabetes, obesity, gastrointestinal, and other health conditions is clearly described in other chapters in this text. However, the process of implementing medical nutrition therapy is not as straightforward and is based on thorough assessment of each client's lifestyle, capabilities, and motivation to change.

At a glance, one might perceive the nutrition education and counseling process to be routine, where nutrition information and recommended food choices are discussed as they pertain to particular health concerns of a client. For a patient with a high cholesterol level, teach the National Cholesterol Education Program's (NCEP) multifaceted therapeutic lifestyle changes (TLC) approach; for high blood pressure, teach weight loss and Dietary Approaches to Stop Hypertension (DASH) diet; and for type 2 diabetes, teach weight loss, exercise, and carbohydrate counting. If only changing eating behavior was that straightforward! The truth is that each person who is referred for nutrition counseling presents with varying levels of knowledge and motivation for changing eating habits. Today's nutrition counselor must draw on knowledge from the biomedical and behavioral sciences to define the nutrition prescription and design an intervention that will truly impact eating.

The traditional model for delivery of nutrition interventions has been individual consultations in health care settings. This paradigm is changing. Increased focus on chronic disease prevention has resulted in an enhanced need for nutrition education at a time when economic constraints in health care have led to a decline in traditional hospital-based nutrition counseling services. Thus, dietitians are providing counseling services in shopping centers, offering cholesterol education classes in health clubs, and communicating with clients via telephone and the Internet. Although individualized counseling will continue as an important component of clinical nutrition, the use of alternative methods, such as group sessions or guided self-study, has been shown to be both efficient and effective. Regardless of the setting, nutrition counseling has a common goal: to help people make healthy changes in eating behaviors. This chapter discusses tools and techniques for applying education and behavior change theories in the practice of medical nutrition therapy.

III THE TEACHING/LEARNING PROCESS

Knowledge is not sufficient but is essential for behavior change [1]. To be effective, nutrition counselors need to understand the elements that influence learning and the different domains in which people learn.

A Factors Influencing Learning

Learning is influenced by many factors, including age, literacy, culture, and individual learner style.

1 Age

Much of our understanding of the differences in the way adults and children learn comes from the work of Knowles [2], who identified concepts of *need to know*, *performance centered*, and *experiential learning* as important to the adult learner. These concepts have been expanded by the research of others who describe self-directed learning [3] and critical thinking techniques [4] as elements that enhance adult learning. A common theme that emerges across learning theories and studies of adult learning is the importance of active involvement of the individual in the learning process [5].

2 Literacy

The term "literacy" includes not only the ability to read and write but also the ability to process information. With the wide use of printed materials to support nutrition education, client literacy and the reading level of teaching materials are important issues. Assessing level of formal education is easy, but unfortunately it is not always an accurate indicator of literacy. Tests such as ABLE [6], WRAT [7], and the Cloze procedure [8] can be used to evaluate an individual's literacy level. These tests, however, take time to administer and can be embarrassing to the client. Their best use may be to assess reading levels in targeted groups before developing educational materials rather than for individual assessment in clinical practice. The steps for evaluating nutrition education materials are relatively simple, and dietitians can use them when information on the reading level of material is not provided. Methods such as the SMOG readability formula [9], Gunning's FOG Index [10], Flesch Reading Ease and Flesch–Kincaid Grade Level [11], and the Fry Readability Graph [12] are described in the reading and health education literature [13–15]. These formulas use the number of words, the number of syllables, and similar criteria to assign a grade or reading level. They can be scored by hand or with computer programs. The Flesch Reading Ease and Flesch–Kincaid Grade Level are available on Microsoft Office Word versions 2003 and 2007 [16]. One of the difficulties of using readability formulas in clinical nutrition is that core words such as "calories," "carbohydrate," "vitamins," "minerals," and "cholesterol" contain three or more syllables and consequently raise the reading level of materials. These words may be sufficiently common, however, so that people with reading abilities lower than the assigned grade level can process and comprehend the materials based on their familiarity with the words as well as the organization of the written text [17]. Recognition that poor health outcomes are not related exclusively to reading levels has led to an emerging field of health literacy. Health literacy is defined as "the degree to which individuals have the capacity to obtain, process, and understand basic health information and services needed to make appropriate health decisions" [18]. A simple technique such as giving a client a nutrition tool to read and then asking what the information means to him or her can identify important limitations in the individual's health literacy. The U.S. Department of Health and Human Services website for health literacy (http://www.hrsa.gov/healthliteracy) provides basic information and practical tips for health professionals to use in communicating with patients as well as links to additional resources.

3 Culture

Ethnicity and culture influence the way people learn. Addressing cultural difference is not simply translating educational materials into the primary language of the client. Fundamentals of values, health beliefs, and communication styles also vary by culture. The changing demographics of the American population have resulted in an increased need for nutrition education materials appropriate for a wide range of cultures. In response to this need, the Diabetes Care and Education practice group of the American Dietetic Association developed the *Ethnic and Regional Food Practice* series [19]. Written for health professionals, this series was revised into a book titled *Cultural Food Practices*, which details information on 15 different cultures. Each chapter discusses traditions and beliefs influencing health behaviors, traditional meal patterns and holiday foods, current food practices, and communication and learning preferences. The book comes with a CD with 20 reproducible, culturally specific client education handouts including four Spanish translations [20]. Other sources for ethnically appropriate teaching materials include government printing agencies, volunteer health organizations, ethnic special interest groups, and vendors of health education materials. Even when specific guidelines are not available, an appreciation that food and health hold different meanings to people of different cultures can aid dietitians in counseling individuals from diverse ethnic backgrounds. Dietitians can use a model for multicultural nutrition counseling competencies, developed by Harris-Davis and Haughton, as a basis for self-evaluation and selection of opportunities to enhance their skills [21].

4 Learner Style

"Learner style" is a phrase that has been used to describe the way people cognitively process information [22] and the interaction of the individual with the learning environment [23]. Drawing from the work of Carl Jung, Osterman identified four types of learners: feelers, thinkers, sensors, and intuitors [24]. Table 10.1 summarizes key characteristics that differentiate these styles. Teaching strategies can be selected to match the learning style or characteristic of the individual. When working with groups, an education session can be constructed to include components that will appeal to all learning styles [24]. Walker, in her review of adult learner characteristics [23], contrasts different environmental methods of learning, such as group versus individual, computer versus print versus video, didactic versus emotional appeal in messages, and directed learning versus self-directed approaches. A number of studies have examined the effectiveness of different methods for delivering education and counseling for health behavior change. Findings show that group settings are both clinically and cost-effective and an efficient use of clinicians' time [25−28]. A comparison of group versus self-directed education for blood cholesterol reduction found that the self-directed approach was a viable alternative to group diet instruction [29]. Studies of telephone, e-mail, and Internet counseling show these approaches can change health behaviors in diverse patient populations [30−32]. These findings support use of alternatives to individual counseling sessions to match client learning styles and provide efficient methods for dietitians to use to extend nutrition services to more people.

B Domains of Learning

Learning includes knowledge, attitude, and skill. The education literature describes these areas of learning as domains: cognitive (knowledge), affective (attitude), and psychomotor (skill) [33,34]. Within each domain there is a range or level of learning that can be achieved.

The cognitive domain concentrates on knowledge outcome and includes six hierarchical levels: knowledge, comprehension, application, analysis, synthesis, and evaluation. The affective domain encompasses an individual's feelings or attitudes associated with a particular topic. The affective domain progresses through five levels from receiving to responding, valuing, organizing, and characterizing within a value or a value complex. The psychomotor domain looks at skill development including perception set (prepared for learning), guided response (performance), mechanism (response more habitual), complex overt response

TABLE 10.1 Learning Styles

	Feelers	Thinkers	Sensors	Intuitors
Looks for:	Meaning, clarity	Facts and information	Practical application	Alternatives
Learns by:	Listening and sharing	Thinking through ideas	Problem solving	Trial and error
Best format:	Discussion	Lecture	Demonstration	Self-discovery
Favorite question:	Why?	What?	How?	If?

Source: *Adapted from Osterman, D. N. (1984). The feedback lecture: Matching teaching and learning styles.* J. Am. Diet. Assoc. *84, 1221−1222.*

(response is effective and routine), and adaptation (response continues in new situations).

Detailed classification systems or taxonomies have been developed that include action verbs to define levels of learning [35,36]. The taxonomies are used to set learning objectives. Objectives can be written for any domain and for any level within that domain, depending on the desired outcome of the counseling session. A learning plan can be developed for an individual that systematically advances him or her from a low level to a high level of competence.

Application of the taxonomies of learning to nutrition counseling offers a framework for integrating learning and behavior change theories. Learning objectives are written in language that clearly identifies who will do what, when, where, and how. *Who* is the client, *what* is the information, *how* is the measurable behavior, and *when* and *where* define the situation. For example, a behavioral objective for a patient with hyperlipidemia, targeted at the application level of the cognitive domain, could be as follows: At the end of the counseling session (*when*), the client (*who*) will be able to identify (*how*) low-fat entrée options (*what*) from sample menus (*where*).

The value of setting behavioral objectives for nutrition interventions is well supported in the literature. A review by Contento and colleagues [5] found that programs that were more behaviorally focused were more effective. This extensive review identified education and behavior change strategies that were successful in changing eating habits. Educational strategies of self-evaluation or self-assessment and active participation worked well for individual or group interventions. Effective behavioral strategies included the use of a systematic behavior change process, tailoring the intervention to the specific needs of the individual, involvement of others to provide social support, and an empowerment approach that enhances personal control.

In summary, for nutrition counseling to be successful, learning principles suggest that as much attention must be given to selecting the most effective way to communicate the diet to the individual as is given to assessing what would be the most effective diet for the individual. Health professionals often have strong grounding in the biological sciences but less exposure to the behavioral sciences. For this reason, the comfort level for determining the appropriate nutrient intake is greater than for evaluating learner needs and setting behavioral objectives. The current demand in all areas of health care to measure effectiveness in terms of patient outcomes requires clinicians to look beyond the diagnosis and intervention phases of care and evaluate the ultimate results. Nutrition interventions that do not show measurable improvement in patient status are not effective.

The argument that treatment failure is due to patient noncompliance does not negate the lack of effect. Dietitians and other health care providers must be adept at combining nutrition, learning, and behavior change principles in the process of nutrition education.

IV NUTRITION EDUCATION TECHNIQUES

Length of time since diagnosis, acuity of disease condition, complexity of the nutrition intervention, preferred client learning style, and readiness to change behaviors are factors to consider in developing a client's education plan. The counselor needs to assess learning needs, decide on the level of education, select an optimal method, and choose appropriate nutrition education tools.

A Assessing Learning Needs

Assessment of learning needs should be an integral part of nutrition counseling. Table 10.2 provides a basic list of variables that should be assessed. Additional items are added to gather information pertinent to the individual and the clinical condition. The amount of

TABLE 10.2 Nutrition Educational Assessment

Demographic	Clinical
Age	Medical history
Gender	Medication
Occupation	Height/weight
Education	Food allergies/intolerances
Social	**Health habits**
Family status	Eating patterns
Living environment	Physical activity
Social network	Smoking status
Cultural factors	Alcohol intake
Religious practices	Health practices
Health beliefs	Use of health services
Learner characteristics	
Previous health education	
Expectations for current education	
Preferred learning methods	
Learning style	
Health literacy	
Readiness for change	

time spent in assessment can limit time spent in counseling. Some studies report up to 55% of a counseling session devoted to the assessment phase [37]. However, time spent on a comprehensive assessment is regained by the effectiveness of a nutrition counseling session that has been tailored to the individual's needs. A variety of approaches can be used to reduce time spent on assessment. Before the counseling session, data can be collected from medical records, and patients can be asked to submit information. Questionnaires can be sent and received by mail, via fax, through the Internet, or completed by the client in the waiting room before the visit. If advanced data collection has not been successful, the counselor may ask about this information in the counseling session. Although clients may not recount a comprehensive description of their referring physician's intent, their perception of what the interaction should achieve provides a basis for assessing learning needs and willingness to make behavior changes.

B Levels of Education

Nutrition education should be planned as a continuum of learning that starts with fundamental guidelines and then incrementally adds more complex information as basic applications are mastered. The terms "initial/survival," "practical," and "continuing" have been used to differentiate three levels of education [37]. The wide availability of topic-specific reproducible handouts provides dietitians with the opportunity to tailor the information to address specific learning needs.

1 Initial/Survival Level

The first level focuses on essential information that the client needs to make important fundamental adjustments in health behaviors. Ideally, initial education will occur soon after diagnosis. The extent of information included at the survival level differs by disease condition and learner characteristics. A person with diabetes treated with insulin needs enough information to understand the association between food, activity, and insulin so that he or she can select appropriate meals to avoid hyper- and hypoglycemia. For the patient with congestive heart failure with frequent hospital admissions, the survival information would focus on the sodium content of foods and avoidance of fluid retention. Education needs to be simple; the dietitian serves as a teacher by providing concrete guidelines on what the patient should or should not do.

2 Practical Level

The practical level of education can occur as follow-up to initial counseling or as a new encounter,

with the patient having had initial instruction some time before. Information should expand on the fundamentals learned for survival by applying them to a variety of situations. New topics can be introduced as well. Clients often will identify "need to know" information they have found important to learn, such as how to eat in restaurants, modify recipes, or interpret food labels. At this level, the dietitian serves as a counselor by providing guidelines for patients to use in making decisions.

3 Continuing Education

Once a client has mastered the basic skills and can apply them successfully in his or her life, continuing education can be used to reinforce learning, update information, and achieve higher levels of knowledge. In-depth knowledge of the relationship between nutrition and the disease process, nutrition principles, food preparation, and eating behaviors can enable patients to "take charge" of their disease management. The dietitian at this level serves as a consultant, helping the client synthesize and personalize information.

C Educational Methods

In addition to the content of the educational intervention, the process or method offers different techniques to make nutrition education more effective. In-person individual or group sessions have been the most common formats used for nutrition counseling. Technical advances now provide an array of opportunities for distance counseling thru Internet sites [38] and mobile applications [39]. Although decisions on the method for nutrition counseling may be made by feasibility criteria (i.e., availability, time, and money), the client's learning preference should be considered as well. Using Osterman's classification of learning styles (Table 10.1), *feelers* would like group sessions that have discussion opportunities, whereas *thinkers* could be frustrated by this method because they "just want the facts." *Sensors* would respond to either method as long as an application exercise is included. A combination of individual and group sessions offers practical advantages. Information presented during group sessions can be tailored to the individual in a one-on-one discussion either in-person or by telephone, e-mail, or an online forum. In the highly successful Diabetes Prevention Program (DPP), a standardized lifestyle curriculum was delivered in individual sessions [40]. The Look AHEAD trial that followed adapted the DPP curriculum to group sessions supplemented with individual counseling [41]. The DPP curriculum has also been adapted for delivery in group sessions, community settings, and pilot tested with the YMCA [42]. In 2010, the Centers for Disease Control and Prevention initiated a standardized program to introduce community-based DPPs using the YMCA model [43]. Interactive, online, Internet programs, some of which are based on the DPP curriculum, are appearing. Many use dietitians as facilitators or consultants. Some have negotiated reimbursement of program fees from health insurers.

Another method for nutrition education is the use of self-study materials. Self-study modules offer advantages in terms of convenience, pace of learning, active involvement of the individual, and economics. Two classic examples are the Shape Up America program [44], now available online [45], and the Learn Program [46]. The American Dietetic Association introduced "Real Solutions: Weight Loss Workbook" in 2004 [47]. Self-study modules generally include self-assessment exercises, information on the health topic, steps for identifying behaviors to modify and guidelines for making changes, methods for monitoring, and tips on sustaining the new behaviors. A variety of self-study programs are now available on CD-ROM, applications for mobile devices, and on the Internet. The U.S. Department of Agriculture's (USDA) My Plate is available in a self-help module via the Internet at http://www.choosemyplate.gov. A Food and Drug Administration-approved mobile application for diabetes management was tested in primary care settings and resulted in a 1.9% decline in glycated hemoglobin [39]. Dietitians can incorporate self-study tools in their practice to help clients make daily lifestyle decisions.

Caban and colleagues [48] developed a model for using patient assessment to guide selection of education methods for weight management (Figure 10.1). They use a comprehensive set of physical and psychological indicators to classify individuals by risk status, and then they select interventions with an intensity that matches individual needs. People who are in stable clinical condition and highly motivated with few behaviors to change are classified as low risk and candidates for self-directed learning methods. Those with clinical conditions targeted for improvement and who are less motivated with several behaviors to change require more structure and support. Group interaction, periodic monitoring, and structured activities are appropriate for this type of client. The high-risk individual, who has multiple health problems, little motivation, and requires a great deal of support, will need individualized care. Dietitians can use this model to determine the best type of program for individual clients.

D Nutrition Educational Tools

Nutrition counseling does not suffer from a lack of tools. Information on nutrition education materials can be found in the catalogs of publishing houses, volunteer health and professional organizations, government agencies, reviews published in professional journals, and by professional networking. Education materials are also available from companies manufacturing health products (e.g., pharmaceutical companies) and associations that promote a food or food group (e.g., the National Dairy Council). Although there may not be a teaching tool that matches all aspects of a patient's learning profile, the availability of electronic educational materials allows dietitians to manage a large number of tools that can be quickly accessed and printed during a nutrition counseling session.

1 Meal Planning Tools

Several formats for nutrition education tools have been applied in multiple areas of clinical nutrition.

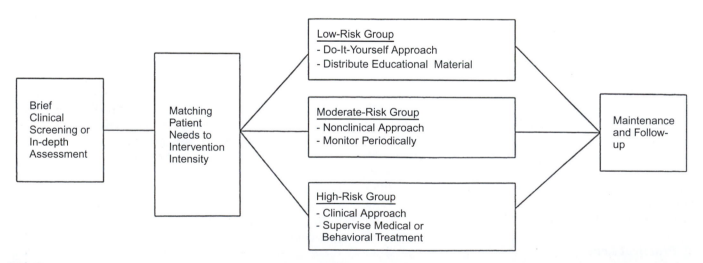

FIGURE 10.1 Model for individualizing treatment approaches. Source: *Adapted with permission from Caban, A., Johnson, P., Marseille, D., and Wylie-Rosett, J. (1999). Tailoring a lifestyle change approach and resources to the patient. Diab. Spectrum 12, 33—38.*

These include guidelines, menu approaches, counting methods, and exchange systems.

Guidelines such as the USDA My Plate are tools that provide basic information to help people make healthy food choices. They may include some information on servings and food preparation but not the specificity of nutrient information that can be found with other methods. Guidelines work well for initial education if precision in nutrient intake is not required. They may contain sufficient information for some people to be able to make eating behavior changes that reduce health risks and improve clinical indicators.

Menus are a tool to give clients specific direction on what to eat, including food type, preparation method, and serving size. For survival education, several days of menus can be written using familiar foods that ensure appropriate nutrition. Menu planning tools generally rely on input from the patient so that food likes and dislikes can be taken into consideration. Menu planning can be combined with other instructional formats and used at the practical and ongoing education levels as well. Computer programs are available that plan menus, taking into account the nutrient prescription and individual food preferences.

Counting methods are popular for diverse nutrition interventions. Calorie counting is a standard approach for weight management. Fat gram counting is utilized in teaching materials for cholesterol reduction, cancer prevention, and weight management. Carbohydrate counting, initially considered a technique for intensive insulin therapy, is now being used with all types of diabetes for initial as well as continuing education.

Exchange approaches focus on food groups versus individual foods to teach nutrition principles. The *Exchange Lists for Meal Planning* [49] has been used for decades to instruct patients with diabetes. The system provides a tool for teaching patients how to select a diet that meets a macronutrient prescription. The exchange lists concept has been adapted for weight management education and is sometimes applied to nutrient information provided with recipes and manufactured food products.

The plate model, recently introduced by the USDA as My Plate, has origins in Sweden. It was first described in a 1970 magazine and then incorporated into a book titled *Food for People with Diabetes and Heart Disease: Good Food for Everyone*. In 1993, five members of the Idaho Diabetes Care and Education practice group adapted it to the "Idaho Plate Method" [50]. When used in the Diabetes Atherosclerosis Intervention Study, it was found to be as effective as the more quantitative exchange lists [51]. The method uses a visual tool of a plate divided into sections: Different divisions of the plate space exist, but the common theme is limiting meat and starches and increasing fruit and vegetable consumption. The plate model has been widely adapted for diverse nutrition education topics and offers a simple method for encouraging portion control as well as healthy food choices.

Different versions of meal planning tools can be found to match many idiosyncratic learner characteristics. Simplified versions appropriate for initial education or for low-literacy clients and versions that have been translated into Spanish are the most common. Computer programs allow the provider to tailor materials to patient characteristics and to change content when it becomes obsolete.

2 Skills Training

Meal planning tools, even those carefully selected and matched to individual learner characteristics, are not sufficient for nutrition education. People may learn what they need to do but lack the "skill" or ability to translate knowledge into practice. Teaching an individual how to read a nutrition label provides the knowledge necessary to interpret the information. Applying that knowledge to decisions made at the point of purchase or in meal preparation requires skill. Comparing nutrition labels on two products requires analytical skills if the products have different serving sizes. After using the nutrition label to select a product, additional skills are required to integrate the selected food into the total diet. Tools are available in print, on video, on CD-ROM, from the Internet, and as two- and three-dimensional models for teaching clients a wide range of nutrition skills.

Some clients, however, cannot or choose not to master certain skills. Meal planning is a prime example. No matter how well educated and trained, there are some people who find meal planning a real barrier to following their diet. "Just tell me what to eat" is their common complaint. Preprinted menus offer a solution in some cases. The American Diabetes Association introduced the first of their *Month of Meals* publications in 1989 and quickly added several more editions in response to the demand [52]. The *Month of Meals* series has been consolidated into one volume, *The American Diabetes Association Month of Meals Diabetes Meal Planner* [53]. The association also offers *The Ultimate Diabetes Meal Planner* with weekly plans for three meals and snacks at five calorie levels [54]. Books offering low-fat and/or low-calorie menus are abundant as well.

Menus, however, do not meet the needs of people who lack the skills and interest to prepare meals. The Cardiovascular Risk Reduction Dietary Intervention Trial addressed the difficulty many people have in translating complex dietary recommendations into meals. The trial compared a nutritionally complete prepared meals program with (1) a diet prescribed to meet the same nutrient levels established for the prepared meals and (2) usual-care dietary therapy [55,56]. The prepared meals program resulted in significantly greater weight loss and reduction in blood pressure than the other two interventions, and it also resulted in improvement in lipid and glucose levels compared with the usual-care therapy.

This "need" for more specific information that will help people choose healthy meals is not limited to clinical nutrition. The food industry, recognizing that each generation of Americans spends less time cooking, has responded with carry-out and order-in meals from restaurants and deli, salad bar, and complete "meals to go" in supermarkets. Chef-prepared meals for home delivery can be ordered online from a long list of vendors, and meal prep franchises are flourishing. Today's nutrition counselor must be just as adept at helping clients develop the skills to select healthy prepared meals as teaching the fundamentals of reducing dietary fat intake.

To change eating habits, nutrition counseling needs to include more than well-selected education techniques. A review has found that many studies based on dissemination of information and teaching skills were not effective in changing eating behavior [5]. Even studies supposedly following the knowledge, attitude, behavior communications model were not successful if the behavioral components were simply skills training (e.g., label reading and food preparation). Only in studies in which participants were self-selected and already motivated were they able to show changes in eating patterns with an intervention that did not have a true behavior change technique. Unfortunately, a diagnosis of a disease or health risk does not automatically result in a motivated patient; therefore, nutrition counselors need to include behavior change techniques in their practice.

V BEHAVIOR CHANGE TECHNIQUES

Theories for behavior change are extensive, and some offer techniques that are practical for use in nutrition counseling. Some techniques, such as self-monitoring, behavioral contracting, and goal setting, are patient focused. They allow the individual to "personalize" the nutrition intervention, to be an active participant in the process, and to receive feedback on progress made toward identified goals. Counselors typically implement other techniques such as motivational interviewing, consciousness raising, and assessing readiness for change. The stages of change transtheoretical model [57] offers dietitians a systematic framework for applying behavior change techniques to nutrition education and counseling. Although the model can be used with all education methods, the following section describes its application in nutrition counseling sessions.

A Stages of Change

The stages of change model was described by Prochaska and colleagues. It postulates that both cessation of high-risk behaviors and the acquisition of healthy behaviors involve progression through five stages of change: precontemplation, contemplation, preparation, action, and maintenance (Table 10.3) [57]. The precontemplation stage is characterized by having no intention of changing the behavior in question in the foreseeable future. People in this stage tend to be unaware that they have a problem and are resistant to efforts to modify the behavior in question. Contemplation is characterized by awareness that the particular behavior is a problem and serious consideration about resolving the problem but having no commitment to take action in the near future. The preparation stage is the stage of decision making. The person has made a commitment to take action within the next 30 days and is already making small behavioral changes. In the action stage, clients make notable overt efforts to change. Maintenance involves working to stabilize the particular behavior change and avoid relapse for the next 6 months. People do not simply progress through the stages in a straight line; they may recycle by relapsing and repeating stage progressions, and they can enter or exit at any point [58,59]. This transtheoretical model has been shown to generalize across a broad range of problem behaviors (including diet, exercise, and weight control) and populations [58].

Integral to the stages of change model is a "standard" or goal for the behavior that has been proven to produce results. For example, the goal of the NCEP TLC diet for a dietary saturated fat intake of less than 7% of energy and less than 200 mg cholesterol per day was established based on research showing associated reduction in serum low-density lipoprotein cholesterol concentration. Stages of change techniques help individuals evaluate current behaviors against a defined standard and then assess their readiness to change. The objective is to help patients achieve the standard for the behavior; however, incremental goals are often required. Fortunately, many nutrition interventions in clinical nutrition show benefits associated with stepwise progression to the goal.

If dietitians use the stages of change model as a basic technique for approaching nutrition counseling sessions, it often requires a modification in their teaching and counseling style [60]. The focus of attention shifts from establishing an agenda to merely educate the individual and shifts toward an approach that assesses the status of the individual as a basis for tailoring the counseling session. For example, instructing a client with hypercholesterolemia who is clearly in the precontemplation stage on an NCEP TLC diet will be less effective than discussing the risks associated with high cholesterol levels and the

TABLE 10.3 Stages of Change

Stage	Definition	Client characteristics	Expressions client may say
Precontemplation	Person is not interested in making changes within the next 6 months.	May be unaware a problem exists.	It's not my problem.
		Sees no reason or need to change.	I can't change.
		Not interested in talking about the situation or behavior.	Leave me alone.
			Quit nagging me.
Contemplation	Person is thinking about making changes within the next 6 months.	Has limited knowledge about the problem.	I'll change when the time is better—someday.
		Is weighing risks/benefits of changing a behavior.	Why should I? I don't understand.
		Is waiting for the "magic moment" to start.	I know I should, but _____.
		Is wishing problem behavior would solve itself.	It takes too much effort.
Preparation	Person is planning to make changes within the next 30 days or has tried making some small changes but is not consistent with new behavior yet.	Is motivated and ready to learn.	I am ready to _____.
		Knows what to do but not sure how to start.	I want to _____.
		May have tried small changes, but now ready to try more.	How can I start?
			Where can I go to learn _____?
Action	Person has changed a behavior within the past 6 months and is becoming more consistent with it.	Efforts to change are more visible to others and are more consistent.	I can _____.
		Believes change is possible.	It's getting easier for me to _____.
		Started making changes in his or her environment to support the changed behavior.	I'm doing it, but sometimes _____.
			I was amazed to learn that _____.
Maintenance	Person has maintained a new behavior longer than 6 months.	Is maintaining the new behavior—the change has become a part of his or her daily routine.	I just do it now.
		Is trying to avoid slipping back into old habits.	It's not a problem for me to _____.
		Is confident about ability to maintain change.	I feel good about _____.
			I don't have to think about it much anymore.

Source: Reprinted with permission from HealthPartners, Inc., Bloomington, MN. © 2000. All other rights reserved. For more information, contact HealthPartners, Center for Health Promotion.

B. RESEARCH AND APPLIED METHODS FOR OBSERVATIONAL AND INTERVENTION STUDIES

benefits of reducing the saturated fat content of the diet. Although the counselor may feel an obligation to impart specific information, mismatching stages and interventions could break rapport and may lead the client to avoid further follow-up sessions.

B Effective Use of Stages of Change Technique in Nutrition Counseling

Nutrition assessments are typically done at the initial counseling session. It is important for dietitians to use the stages of change model in each session to assess attitudes toward nutrition and health, readiness to learn, and willingness to change. Assessment of these attitudes requires proficient use of open-ended questions and listening skills.

Open-ended questions begin with "what," "how," "why," and "could." The first clue about a client's stage of change is in the response to opening questions such as "How can I help you?" "What are your goals for our meeting today?" Attentive listening is an important tool to assess the client's responses to these questions. Attentive listening involves not only allowing sufficient silence to hear the client's verbal response but also paying attention to facial expression, voice tone, and body language as the person is speaking. The nutrition counselor can use the listening technique of paraphrasing to determine if he or she has accurately understood the content of the client's statements or the listening technique of reflection to find out if he or she understands the emotional feeling that the client is trying to convey [61]. It is the combination of open-ended questioning and proficient listening skills that builds rapport.

As the counselor collects assessment information in the first part of the counseling session, there are repeated opportunities to evaluate a client's stage of change through the use of open-ended questions and effective listening skills.

C Consciousness Raising: A Technique for Precontemplators

1 A Case of Precontemplation

Dietitian: "How can I help you?" "What are your goals for today's session?"
Client: "I don't know. The doctor sent me." "I feel fine." "I already have so many problems, so why bother?" (arms crossed, sitting back in the chair, stiff body posture, voice tone may display resignation, anger, upset, or denial concerning necessity for changing habits or coming to see the dietitian)
Dietitian: "Did your doctor say why he wanted you to come?" "What did your doctor tell you about

your _____ (e.g., cholesterol levels/diabetes control/blood pressure)?"

Patients in the precontemplation stage tend to focus more on the difficulties or disadvantages of changing eating behavior—the diet restriction, the inconvenience, or the expense of making healthy food choices or keeping food records. They tend to put much less emphasis on the benefits of changing eating behavior. Patients can be in the precontemplation stage for various reasons, including lack of knowledge, lack of skills, lack of resources, distorted health beliefs, or competing priorities [62]. The counselor needs to explore and assess the reasons particular to each client before proceeding further with the session.

A QUESTIONS TO ASSESS KNOWLEDGE, SKILLS, RESOURCES, HEALTH BELIEFS, AND COMPETING PRIORITIES

- "What did your doctor tell you about your _____ (e.g., cholesterol level/diabetes control/blood pressure)?"
- "What did your doctor tell you about your laboratory results?"
- "Do you know what the goals are for _____ (cholesterol levels/hemoglobin A1c levels/blood glucose levels)?"
- "What are your personal goals?"
- "What do you know about how your diet affects your _____ (e.g., cholesterol level/hemoglobin A1c/ blood glucose patterns)?"
- "What do you think is most important when reading a nutrition label if you have _____ (e.g., diabetes/high cholesterol)?"
- "Do you have a blood glucose meter?"
- "Do you test your blood glucose levels at home?"
- "How often and what times of day?"
- "What do you think that you would need to do to improve your _____ (e.g., cholesterol levels/ hemoglobin A1c levels/blood glucose levels/activity level)?"
- "Are there any factors that you feel make it difficult for you to focus on improving your _____ (e.g., cholesterol levels/hemoglobin A1c levels/blood glucose levels/ activity level)?"

2 Consciousness Raising

Consciousness raising is an important strategy for dietitians to use if a client presents to a session in the precontemplation stage [59]. The following steps can be used to facilitate consciousness raising (Table 10.4):

- Discuss the medical problem or condition of concern.
- Review lab results related to the condition versus target/normal values for the test results.

TABLE 10.4 Stage-Matched Counseling Techniques

Stage	Counseling strategies	Do's/don'ts that motivate/hinder change
Precontemplation	Raise self-awareness of their behavior.	Don't be judgmental.
	Raise awareness of health concern and implications.	Don't rush them into action.
	Show how their behavior may affect others around them.	Don't ignore their emotional reaction to idea of change.
	Encourage them to express their feelings.	Do listen and acknowledge their feelings.
		Do help them understand effects of their behavior.
		Do help them become aware a problem exists.
Contemplation	Identify and discuss their concerns, beliefs, and perceived barriers toward their behavior.	Don't ignore the potential impact the change may have on their family.
	Show how benefits of change outweigh the risks of not changing.	Don't nag or preach to them demanding they change.
	Clarify any ambivalence felt toward changing.	Don't provide "how to" information.
	Provide or suggest resources for learning more about the solution.	Do listen to their concerns.
		Do help them identify benefits they'll receive if they decide to change a behavior.
		Do provide "facts" answering the "why" questions they have.
Preparation	Help them develop a plan of action.	Don't recommend general behavior change—be specific.
	Teach specific "how to" skills.	Don't refer to small changes as "not good enough."
	Help build their self-confidence so they can form a new behavior.	Don't create new barriers for them to overcome.
	Help them access an educational program and obtain resources needed for change.	Do provide specific ideas on how to change.
		Do remind them that "change" is hard work.
		Do help them realize that "any change" is better than "no change."
Action	Reinforce their decision to change.	Don't nag or preach.
	Provide emotional support to continue behavior change they've started.	Don't make assumptions that they're not having lapses.
	Explain the difference between lapse and relapse.	Don't overpraise so that they only report successful outcomes.
	Help them evaluate their progress, and teach additional skills, as needed.	Do explore their feelings about changes they've made.
		Do celebrate "milestones," big and small.
		Do compliment positive behavior changes you observe.
Maintenance	Offer ideas or ways to maintain change.	Don't assume that initial action means permanent change.
	Help them build a supportive environment around them to maintain the change.	Don't be discouraged or disappointed when lapses happen.
	Continue teaching relapse prevention techniques.	Don't underestimate environmental barriers.
	Help validate rationale for change.	Do remind them of their overall progress (from the start).
	Do review benefits they've received from changing their behavior.	Do ask open-ended questions about how they are coping with change and how they feel about their changed behavior.

Source: *Reprinted with permission from HealthPartners, Inc., Bloomington, MN. © 2000. All other rights reserved. For more information, contact Health Partners, Center for Health Promotion.*

B. RESEARCH AND APPLIED METHODS FOR OBSERVATIONAL AND INTERVENTION STUDIES

- Review the relationship of diet, exercise, and other self-care habits to the medical condition and personal lab data.
- Use visual aids (e.g., test tubes of fat and 1- or 5-lb fat models), audiovisuals, and personalized profile sheets to enhance the message.
- Elicit feedback from the client regarding this information.

As the interaction between the counselor and the patient proceeds, the counselor can watch for changes in body language (leaning forward, changing voice tone, and arms uncrossing) and in level of interaction (asking more questions). Once this information-sharing process is complete, the counselor has provided the client with the information necessary to make an informed choice about changing eating behavior. The clients who are in the precontemplation stage because of lack of knowledge or skills may move toward contemplation or preparation stages once these issues are addressed. On the other hand, some clients may be fully informed about their medical condition, lab data, and the impact of eating, activity, and self-care habits on their health and still do not view changing eating habits as a priority. These clients are less likely to progress to contemplation or preparation within one session. In these cases, it is important to avoid judgment and show understanding by acknowledging their feelings and choices. For example, a client may feel too depressed to consider change at the time of the session, and a competing priority may be to seek counseling and treatment for depression first. The counselor's responsibility is to provide information and then reassess the client's stage of change. It is the client's responsibility to make an informed choice.

D Motivational Interviewing: A Technique for Contemplators

1 A Case of Contemplation

Dietitian: "How can I help you?" "What would you like to accomplish at our meeting today?"
Patient: "I'm not sure. I know what to do. I just need motivation." "I know that I should (e.g., lose weight/eat less fat), but _____."

Patients in the contemplation stage view the advantages and disadvantages of changing eating, exercise, or self-care habits as about equal, with the disadvantages slightly greater than the advantages. They may focus on the short-term costs of changing eating behaviors (e.g., limiting food choices, adjusting food purchases when shopping or menu selections when eating out, and investing time in keeping food records or nutrition appointments) and pay less attention to the long-term health benefits [62]. Clients

can be in the contemplation stage because of limited knowledge about the problem, wishing that someone else would fix the problem or that the problem would solve itself, competing priorities, or low self-efficacy regarding ability to change eating habits.

If limited knowledge is the problem, then the counselor can use the technique of consciousness raising to provide information, clarify any misconceptions, and respond to specific questions. The counselor also needs to evaluate each client's self-efficacy for changing eating behavior because perceived self-efficacy influences the acquisition of new behaviors and the inhibition of existing behaviors. It also affects people's choices of behavioral settings, the amount of effort they will expend on a task, and the length of time they will persist in the face of obstacles. Finally, self-efficacy affects people's emotional reactions and thought patterns [63].

For clients to move from the contemplation stage toward the preparation stage of change, they must believe that the advantages of changing their eating behavior outweigh the disadvantages. The counselor can help reduce or minimize barriers to change by assisting the client with practical problem solving (some barriers may be related to access to treatment and resources and other barriers will be more attitudinal, such as fear of change or the results of change). It is also helpful to identify the client's positive incentives for continuing with current behaviors (i.e., the payoff for staying the same) and use strategies to decrease the perceived desirability of the behavior (e.g., increase awareness of the negative consequences of the behavior using facts and audiovisuals) [62].

Motivational interviewing (MI) is a client-centered technique designed to build commitment and reach a decision to change [64]. It focuses on increasing the client's intrinsic motivation to change and self-confidence in ability to do so. Results from several studies support the use of MI to improve glycemic control and enhance weight loss, particularly for those who are struggling with weight loss or have hit a weight loss plateau. The increased weight loss with MI appears to be mediated by enhanced treatment engagement and program adherence [65].

MI involves an interview process that elicits "change talk" or personally relevant reasons that support movement in the direction of healthful behavior change. "Change talk" may express a concern, recognition of a problem, optimism about change, or an intention to change [65].

The goal of MI is to increase the frequency, range, and strength of client "change talk" and to minimize "staying the same" talk. Although motivational interviewing acknowledges that ambivalence is normal and exists among most people considering a behavior change, it does not seek to pull for or emphasize the reasons to stay the same (the disadvantages). This is because people who talk more about reasons not to change, do not change, whereas, those who express more "change talk" have a greater likelihood of making targeted behavior changes [66]. When clients hear themselves articulate why they want to change, it has a motivating effect.

Thus, rather than actively eliciting the advantages and disadvantages of behavior change, MI focuses on (1) asking strategic open-ended questions and (2) responding by spending a short time recognizing and acknowledging a client's reasons for staying the same but spending the most time emphasizing personalized reasons for change. Dietitians can use the all EARS approach to increase the proportion of "change talk" that a client offers [65].

2 The EARS Approach

E: Elaboration: Ask for more detail about the personal reasons for change (advantages of behavior change).

A: Affirmation: Comment positively on the client's "change talk" statements.

R: Reflection: Use reflective statements to further strengthen client "change talk."

S: Strategic summary: Collect a bouquet of all the "change talk," put it together, and give it back to the client.

When all of the personal reasons are grouped together and reflected back to the client in a succinct summary, it can be powerfully motivating [65].

Dietitian: "What makes you want to _____ (reduce fat intake, lose weight, lower blood sugars) right now?

Client: "I'd really like to be on less medications and I know if I lose weight and increase my activity, then I might be able to reduce or get off of some of these medications." I've had a hard time focusing because of other family stresses. I tend to eat when I am worried but I am trying to walk to help my stress."

Dietitian: "What concerns you about being on more medications?" (E)

Client: "The more medications that I take, the less healthy I feel. All of these medications have side effects."

Dietitian: "So for you, a major benefit of losing weight and increasing your activity is to reduce the amount of medications that you take and to feel healthier as well." (R)

Client: "Yes that is right!"

Dietitian: "The fact that you've started walking to relieve stress instead of eating for stress is a very positive step that you have made toward your goal." (A)

Client: "Yes, I want to keep that up. I noticed that my energy level is better after I walk."

Dietitian: "You seem pleased that you have been able to fit walking into your schedule and that it is a constructive way to deal with your stress. It also seems to energize you." (R)

Client: "Yes I really want to try to do more."

Dietitian: "That sounds good. What are you ready to work on?" (E)

Client: "I would like to start using frozen proportioned meals for dinner 4 timers per week." This will save me some time and help me eat less at dinner."

Dietitian: "That sounds like a really good idea because it will save you time, help you lose weight and get closer to your goal of being on less medication." "Out of 100% confidence, how confident are you that you will be able to eat frozen dinners 4 days per week?" (A)

Client: "80% confident. I can do it."

Dietitian: So, you definitely would like to be on less medication and you believe that losing weight and increasing your activity level is the key. It is clear that the walking that you have been doing energizes you and helps manage your stress. You feel that the next step is to use frozen dinners 4 times per week and that this is doable and will help you lose weight." (S)

Client: "I definitely feel I can do this. I can pick up the frozen dinners on the way home."

Each client's motivation to change is influenced by two components: importance and confidence [67]. Assessing importance and confidence is a technique that dietitians can use to help decide what steps to take with patients who are in the contemplation stage of change.

3 Importance and Confidence Technique[1]

A INTRODUCE THE DISCUSSION

"I'm not really sure how you feel about _____ (e.g., reducing your fat intake/losing weight/ exercising more). Can you help me by answering two simple questions and then we can see where to go from there?"

B ASSESS IMPORTANCE AND CONFIDENCE

"How do you feel *right now* about _____ (fat/ losing weight/exercising more)? On a scale from 0 to 10, with 0 meaning 'not important at all' and 10 meaning 'very important,' how *important* is it to you

---

[1]This section is reprinted with permission of Allan Zuckoff, M. A., University of Pittsburgh Medical Center; adapted from S. Rollnick, P. Mason, and C. Butler (1999). "Health Behavior Change: A Guide for Practitioners." Churchill Livingstone, London.

personally to _____ (eat less fat/lose weight/
exercise more)?"

"If you decided *right now* to _____ (eat less fat/
lose weight/exercise more), how *confident* do you
feel that you would succeed? If 0 is 'not confident at
all' and 10 is 'very confident,' what number would
you give yourself?"

Summarize the answers:

C SELECTING THE FOCUS

- If importance is low (<3), focus on importance first.
- If both are the same, focus on importance first.
- If one number is distinctly lower than the other, focus on the lower number first.
- If both are very low (<3), explore feelings about participating further in the session.

D EXPLORING IMPORTANCE

"This is _____ (very/pretty/somewhat/a little bit) important to you. What made you choose _____ and not 1 or 2?"

- Reflect reasons given (self-motivational statements).
- Ask for elaboration. ("What makes that important to you?" "Tell me more about that.")
- Ask for more reasons. ("What else makes it [very/pretty/somewhat/a little] important?")
- Summarize. ("So what makes this [very/pretty/somewhat/a little] important right now is. ..." "What would have to happen for you to move up to a _____ [score plus 3 or 4]?" "What stops you from being at a _____ [score plus 3 or 4]?")
- Reflect, ask for elaboration, ask "What else?"
- Summarize. ("So what makes this [very/pretty/somewhat/a little] important is.. ..." "It would become more important to you if. ..." "What has kept it from being more important is.. ..")

E EXPLORING CONFIDENCE

"You feel (very/pretty/somewhat/a little) confident that you could do this if you tried. What made you choose _____ and not 1 or 2?"

- Reflect reasons given (self-motivational statements).
- Ask for elaboration. ("Tell me more about that.")
- Ask for more reasons. ("What else makes you feel [very/pretty/somewhat/a little] confident?")
- Summarize ("So what makes you [very/pretty/somewhat/a little] confident right now is.. ...") "What would help you move up to a _____ [score plus 3 or 4]?" "What stops you from being at a _____ [score plus 3 or 4]?")

- Reflect, ask for elaboration, ask "What else?"
- Summarize. ("So what makes you [very /pretty/somewhat/a little] confident is...." "You would feel more confident if...." "What has kept you from feeling more confident is....")

The following types of questions can be used in the motivational interviewing process to reinforce confidence/self-efficacy. These types of questions are referred to as *competency-focused interviewing* [61].

F QUESTIONS THAT ARE COMPETENCY FOCUSED AND SUCCESS ORIENTED

- "What do you know about _____ (e.g., diabetes, high cholesterol)?"
- "What kind of changes have you made in your diet so far?"
- "How have you fit exercise into your schedule in the past?"
- "What is the most important thing that you were able to learn?"
- "What do you think you would do differently this time to enable you to _____ (lose weight/lower your cholesterol/improve your blood glucose levels?)"
- "How do you think you would feel when you reach your goal?"
- "What do you see as the next step?"

4 FRAMES Strategy

Miller and Rollnick [62] suggested that the following specific motivational techniques can be combined to achieve an effective motivational interviewing strategy (FRAMES):

Feedback: Clearly discuss the client's current health situation and risks and explain results of objective tests; share observations based on food records and weight trends. Clarify goals by comparing feedback on the patient's current situation to some standard, and set goals toward that standard that are realistic and attainable.

Responsibility: Emphasize that it is the client's responsibility to change.

Advice: Clearly identify the problem or risk area, explain why change is important, and advocate specific change.

Menu: Offer the client a menu of alternative strategies for changing eating habits. Offering each client a range of options allows the individual to select strategies that match his or her particular situation and enhance the sense of perceived personal choice.

Empathy: Show warmth, respect, support, caring, concern, understanding, commitment, and active interest through attentive listening skills.

Self-efficacy: Reinforce the client's self-efficacy via competency-based questions and statements. Research has shown that the counselor's belief in the client's ability to change can be a significant determinant of outcome [62].

The dietitian's responsibility in counseling patients in the contemplation stage is to help the client reduce the barriers to making changes, focus more on the benefits, recognize and elicit "change talk," simplify the "to do" steps, and enhance self-efficacy. Once the dietitian has completed this process, it is the client's responsibility and choice to make a decision about changing eating habits.

E Goal Setting: A Technique for the Preparation Stage

1 A Case of Preparation

Dietitian: "How can I help you?" "What are your goals for today's session?"

Patient: "I want to _____ (improve my blood glucose control/lower my cholesterol level/lose weight)."

Patients in the preparation stage feel that the advantages of changing their eating habits outweigh the disadvantages. They may have already tried making small changes, but they are looking for more specific guidance and support.

Their ambivalence may not have disappeared. However, they show more interest in change by making self-motivational statements and by asking more questions about change and experimenting with small changes [62]. The dietitian's responsibility is to strengthen the client's commitment to change and to assist the client in making realistic plans to modify his or her lifestyle and eating habits. It is the client's responsibility to participate in goal setting by considering the options and selecting a strategy that provides sufficient direction to prevent floundering but not so many goals that it undermines self-efficacy and success.

It is important for the dietitian to accentuate and reinforce behaviors that the client is doing right and then set goals from there. Goals that are specific, realistic, positive, short term, and measurable are best. It is also important to help the client anticipate obstacles to success and problem-solve strategies to deal with those barriers (Figure 10.2). Finally, the counselor can ask questions to be sure that the client has set reasonable achievable goals. If clients are not at least 80% confident in their ability to achieve their goals, it is important to help them reset their goals to a level at which they feel they can be successful.

2 Goal Setting

For clients to move toward the action stage, they must resolve their ambivalence and establish a firm commitment to a plan of action. The counselor can use the FRAMES technique to guide the client toward a specific action plan. In addition, the counselor can ask questions and make statements that imply competency and build self-efficacy.

A QUESTIONS TO FACILITATE GOAL SETTING

- "What do you think you would like to do?"
- "What would you say is the first step that you need to take?"
- "What other changes would you like to make?"
- "What options would you consider trying?"
- "What obstacles can you anticipate that might interfere with your ability to accomplish your goals?"
- "How do you think you will handle these obstacles?"
- "How confident are you that you will be able to accomplish your goals?"

Patient: "I'd like to start to increase my activity to improve my blood sugars."

Dietitian: "That's great! It's good that you have so many options for exercise—a treadmill, outdoor walking, an exercise bike. You've also already got a great start on increasing your activity by walking with your co-worker at lunch two times per week for 20 minutes each time. If you could increase your activity toward 150 minutes per week, that is a good target. What would you say would be a reasonable next step to increase your activity?"

Patient: "I'd like to try to walk four times per week for 20 minutes at lunch."

Dietitian: "Are there any problems or roadblocks that you can anticipate that would get in the way of accomplishing this goal?"

Patient: "If it rains, we might not go out."

Dietitian: "How will you handle that situation?"

Patient: "I'll either suggest that we walk indoors, or I'll make a plan to walk on my own on the weekend."

Dietitian: "Are there any other barriers or obstacles that you can anticipate?"

Patient: "No, not right now."

Dietitian: "Out of 100% confidence, how confident are you that you can do 80 minutes of activity in the next week?"

Patient: "I'm 80% confident."

Dietitian: "Good, because if you were less than 80% confident, that would mean that we should consider changing the goal so that you feel that the likelihood of success is fairly high."

WEEKLY GOALS

NUTRITION /BEHAVIOR   1._____
                            2._____

EXERCISE   1._____
                            2._____

The following roadblocks could interfere with my ability to achieve these goals.
Therefore, I have devised these coping strategies.

_____

Roadblock #1:

Plan:

_____

Roadblock #2:

Plan:

_____

Roadblock #3:

Plan:

_____

Evaluation

How did it go? _____

What did you learn? _____

Would you do anything differently next time? _____

FIGURE 10.2   Weekly goals form.

F Self-Management Skills Training: Techniques for Action

1 A Case of Action

Dietitian: "How can I help you?" "What would you like to accomplish in our meeting today?"
Patient: "I'm doing well with my food choices and exercise during the week, but on weekends it can be harder if I go out to eat."

Patients in the action stage have started making changes in their environment to support changes in eating habits. They need positive reinforcement for making behavioral changes and assistance strengthening self-management skills. The counselor's responsibility is to provide continued praise and support for positive behavioral changes and offer ongoing information and advice

to enhance self-management skills. The client's responsibility is to actively participate in the session by sharing feelings about changes that he or she has made and discussing questions and concerns about maintaining the behavior changes.

2 Self-Management Skills Training

The core techniques that dietitians can combine to help clients in the action stage to strengthen self-management skills are concrete nutrition information and advice, self-monitoring, stimulus control, and exercise [1].

Concrete nutrition information and advice: Dietitians' expertise in translating nutrition recommendations into food choices that are meaningful and satisfying is key in supporting clients in the action stage. In particular, dietitians can assist patients in trying new recipe ideas/modifying favorite recipes, finding healthier food choices, and suggesting new and interesting food combinations at meals and snacks. In this way, dietitians can help patients learn that dietary change can occur without disrupting family food patterns or personal enjoyment of food. *Self-monitoring:* Dietitians can encourage clients to use self-monitoring as a tool to enhance behavior change. When clients keep track of their eating habits by recording the amounts and types of food eaten, they become more aware of how their food choices affect their health outcomes (e.g., weight, cholesterol, and blood sugar). Patients who are overweight or have hypercholesterolemia may focus on food records that track their weight, fat gram, or energy intake, whereas patients with diabetes may focus on self-monitoring food, carbohydrate intake, activity, and blood sugar patterns and then use the data to learn a problem-solving approach for understanding food-activity–blood sugar relationships.

Stimulus control: Dietitians can discuss with patients how to set up their environment for success. If patients remove problem foods from their environment and follow a shopping list that includes only healthy food choices, then they can create an environment conducive to successful dietary change. Clients can also learn strategies to reduce the temptations for undesired foods by minimizing exposure to these food items at parties or buffets.

Exercise: Increasing exercise is a positive lifestyle change that can improve high-density lipoprotein cholesterol, blood glucose control, blood pressure, weight loss and weight maintenance, self-esteem, and motivation. Increasing physical activity can therefore enhance the impact of dietary change on health outcomes and may also strengthen the self-esteem, self-efficacy, and motivation necessary to maintain diet behavior change.

G Problem-Solving Skills and Coping Strategies: Techniques for Maintenance

1 A Case of Maintenance

Dietitian: "How can I help you?" "What are your goals for today's session?"

Patient: "I feel good about the way that I'm eating now. It has become more of a habit to _____ (eat less fat/exercise more/count carbohydrates)."

Patients in the maintenance stage have been actively working on changing eating habits for at least 6 months. Although the changes in eating habits may have become part of a patient's routine, there is still a risk of lapse or relapse. The dietitian's responsibility is to help clients plan ahead for high-risk situations and develop the problem-solving and coping skills necessary to avoid relapsing. The client's responsibility is to share any feelings or concerns related to the changes that he or she has made, discuss the particular situations that challenge his or her ability to continue with eating behavior change, and actively participate in the problem-solving process.

2 Problem-Solving Skills and Coping Strategies

Some examples of high-risk situations that can lead to lapse or relapse of eating behavior change are eating out, stress and other emotions (feeling anxious or depressed), hunger, and vacations. If clients do not develop coping strategies to deal with high-risk situations, then they are likely to interpret an experience of overeating as a failure. This can diminish self-efficacy and undermine long-term success. Alternatively, if clients can respond to high-risk situations with effective problem-solving and coping strategies, then the experience of managing the situation improves self-efficacy and increases the likelihood of sustaining behavior change [1].

When patients can identify barriers to achieving their goals and anticipate high-risk situations, then the nutrition counselor can teach them the following steps to the problem-solving approach:

1. Describe the problem or barrier in detail.
2. Brainstorm options to address it.
3. Pick an option to try.
4. Make a positive action plan or goal (see Figure 10.2).
5. Anticipate and plan to handle roadblocks.
6. Identify ways to increase the likelihood of success.
7. Try the plan and see how it goes.

When the nutrition counselor models the problem-solving approach with the client and the client practices this skill successfully, then self-efficacy improves [68].

The best way to help clients prevent relapse is to focus on both cognitive and behavioral techniques to appropriately respond to lapses. The behavioral steps to help clients include the following: (1) anticipate and identify high-risk situations, (2) facilitate a problem-solving approach to determine possible solutions, (3) select a coping strategy, and (4) evaluate the effectiveness of the plan. The cognitive techniques that are important in preventing relapse are directed at how clients think and feel in response to a relapse. Cognitive restructuring techniques include the following: (1) listen to self-talk associated with a lapse and evaluate if thoughts are logical, reasonable, or helpful; (2) counter any negative self-talk with positive statements; and (3) stay focused on the progress so far and the advantages of making changes in eating behavior [46].

In the process of discussing lapses in high-risk situations, it is important for dietitians to remind clients that lapses are normal and to ask open-ended questions about how clients feel regarding changes they have made in eating habits and respond to them with empathy and not judgment [62].

A QUESTIONS TO FACILITATE DISCUSSION OF HIGH-RISK SITUATIONS

- "How are you feeling about the changes that you have made in your eating habits so far?"
- "Are there any situations that make it more challenging for you to sustain your _____ (activity level/reduced fat intake/weight loss)?"
- "What strategies have you tried so far to deal with the situation?"
- "How did they work?"
- "Are there any other ideas that you might try?"
- "Would you like to hear about some strategies that have worked for other people in the same situation?"
- "If we take a moment to review the various options that we have discussed, are there any that you would like to try?"
- "Which ones?" (See Figure 10.2.)

The problem-solving skills and coping strategies that are important for working with clients in the maintenance stage often incorporate the techniques used to help move the client forward through the stages of change. Note that patients can recycle by relapsing and repeating stage progressions, and they can exit and reenter at any point. In fact, many new clients that dietitians see are relapsers who are coming to reenter and recycle through the eating behavior change process. In these cases, there are some important questions that the counselor can ask to assess each client's experience.

B QUESTIONS TO ASSESS PRIOR EXPERIENCE OF RELAPSERS

- "What were your three most important reasons for _____ (losing weight/eating less fat/exercising more)?"
- "How long did you sustain the behavior change?" "Who supported you at that time?" "How did you handle temptations?"
- "What coping strategies did you use?"
- "What was going on in your life and how were you feeling when you started slipping?"
- "What did you learn from that experience?"

In summary, the stages of change model is a useful technique for approaching nutrition counseling sessions. At first glance, however, adding a new component to counseling sessions may appear difficult when allocation of time is already an issue [37]. Fisher uses a three-phase model to show that stages of change techniques can be applied in sessions as brief as 15 minutes (Figure 10.3). The model expedites identification of the behavior, clarification of patient's readiness to change, and selection of stage-appropriate tools and techniques. The time the dietitian allocates to tailor counseling to information that the patient is receptive to learning will result in a more productive session.

H Social Support

Social support influences all stages of behavior change. A number of studies have shown the benefit of

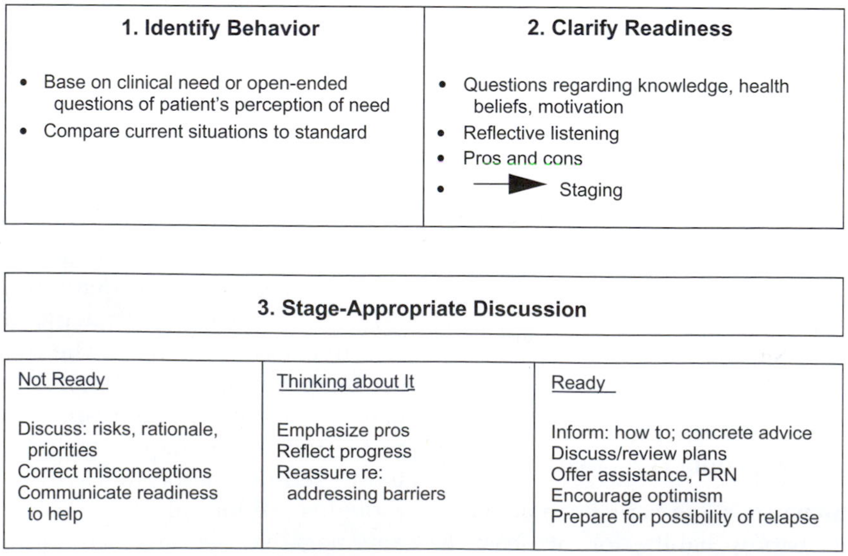

1. Identify Behavior	2. Clarify Readiness
• Base on clinical need or open-ended questions of patient's perception of need • Compare current situations to standard	• Questions regarding knowledge, health beliefs, motivation • Reflective listening • Pros and cons • ——► Staging

3. Stage-Appropriate Discussion

Not Ready	Thinking about It	Ready
Discuss: risks, rationale, priorities Correct misconceptions Communicate readiness to help	Emphasize pros Reflect progress Reassure re: addressing barriers	Inform: how to; concrete advice Discuss/review plans Offer assistance, PRN Encourage optimism Prepare for possibility of relapse

FIGURE 10.3 Three-phase model within 15-minute encounter. Source: *Adapted with verbal permission from E. B. Fisher, Jr.*

support from family, friends, co-workers, and clinicians [1,5,69]. Dietitians can use social support to reinforce behavior change by including resources for support in their counseling practice.

Social support is complex. The specific action, the recipient's perception, as well as the individuals integration into a social network are variables mentioned in describing the concept of social support. Studies examining the role of social support in diabetes management have found that nondirective types of support (suggests, willing to help but does not take over) were mentioned more often than directive types of support (tells, assumes responsibility) [69,70]. Studies of staff support conducted with patients with acute as well as chronic illnesses indicate that stage or phase of the patient's clinical condition may influence the type of staff support that is most helpful [71]. Patients newly diagnosed or in an acute phase of their illness appear to appreciate directive support (gives me great solutions), whereas those in stable conditions value nondirective support (gives me suggestions but lets me make up my own mind). Applying type of social support to stages of change techniques, nondirective support is most appropriate for the precontemplation, contemplation, and maintenance phases, whereas directive support would be appropriate for problem solving in the preparation and action stages.

The unique role of social support from peers has been demonstrated in a number of community-based studies. The Chronic Disease Self-Management Program developed out of a research grant received by Stanford University's Division of Family and Community Medicine. Workshops are held in community settings, and participants with different chronic health problems attended together. Stanford provides a 6-week curriculum and leader training with a specification that one or both leaders be a non-health professional with a chronic condition [72]. The Robert Wood Johnson Diabetes Initiative focused on improving self-management supports for adults with diabetes in real-world clinic and community settings. Lay health workers, called Promotoras in Hispanic communities, were found to be an important component of successful interventions. The Diabetes Initiative website (http://diabetesnpo.im.wustl.edu/index.html) provides a wealth of resources, including information on training lay health workers. The Centers for Disease Control and Prevention's National Diabetes Prevention Program (described previously) trains YMCA employees to deliver the program. Peers for Progress, a program of the American Academy of Family Physicians Foundation, was introduced in 2008 with the mission "to accelerate the availability of best practices in peer support around the world." The website (http://www.peersforprogress.org) has a variety of resources, including a Twitter networking link.

Social support through online networks is an emerging resource for clients and for health professionals. Individuals with chronic conditions can receive emotional support as well as practical information on how to handle day-to-day challenges of disease self-management. For dietitians, it offers an opportunity to stay abreast of current issues, gain a sense of patient struggles, and establish the dietetics profession as the preferred nutrition source for consumers. A variety of online communities are available on the American Dietetic Association website (http://www.eatright.org), and it provides a resource for nutrition counselors to use to refer clients to lay online communities.

VI CONCLUSION

The challenge in facilitating nutrition interventions is to prevent or treat disease by changing people's eating habits. Research on nutrition education is extensive but not conclusive. Although a definitive model has not been identified, a variety of strategies has shown success and can be incorporated into nutrition education programs. There is consensus on two elements: (1) Education needs to be tailored to the individual's learning needs, and (2) both education and behavior change techniques are necessary. Understanding factors that influence the learning and behavior change processes enables better selection of educational tools and techniques to make counseling more effective. The stages of change model is a useful technique for tailoring education to the individual and applying behavior change strategies.

References

[1] K.D. Brownell, L.R. Cohen, Adherence to dietary regimens 2: components of effective interventions, Behav. Med. 20 (1995) 155−164.

[2] M. Knowles, The Adult Learner: A Neglected Species, Gulf Publishing, Houston, TX, 1990.

[3] A. Tough, How adults learn and change, Diabetes Educator 11 (1985) 12−25.

[4] S.D. Brookfield, Developing Critical Thinkers: Challenging Adults to Explore Alternative Ways of Thinking and Acting, Jossey-Bass, San Francisco, 1987.

[5] I. Contento, Y.I. Bronner, D.M. Paige, S.M. Gross, L. Bisignani, L.A. Lytle, et al., The effectiveness of nutrition education and implications for nutrition education policy, programs, and research: a review of research, J. Nutr. Educ. 27 (1995) 355−364.

[6] B. Karlsen, E.F. Gardner, Adult Basic Learning Examination Norms Booklet, Harcourt Brace, San Antonio, TX, 1986.

[7] G.S. Wilkinson, Wide Range Achievement Test Administration Manual, Wide Range, Wilmington, DE, 1993.

[8] S.C. Taylor, Cloze procedure: a new test for measuring readability, Journalism Q 10 (1953) 425−433.

[9] G.H. McLaughlin, SMOG grading: a new readability formula, J. Reading 12 (1969) 639−646.

[10] R. Gunning, The Technique of Clear Writing, McGraw-Hill, New York, 1952.

[11] R. Flesch, How to Write Plain English, (see Chapter 2). Harper & Row, New York, 1979.

[12] E.B. Fry, Fry's readability graph: clarifications, validity, and extension to level 17, J. Reading 21 (1977) 242–252.

[13] R.D. Powers, W.A. Summer, B.E. Kearl, A recalculation of four readability formulas, J. Educ. Psychol. 48 (1958) 99–105.

[14] J. Vaughn Jr., Interpreting readability assessments, J. Reading 19 (1976) 635–639.

[15] J. Pitchert, P. Elam, Readability formulas may mislead you, Patient Educ. Couns. 7 (1985) 181–191.

[16] Microsoft Office Support. Test your document's readability. Available at <http://office.microsoft.com/en-us/word-help/test-your-document-s-readability-HP010148506.aspx> (accessed 26.08.11).

[17] S.V.J. Nitzke, Overview of reading and literacy research and applications in nutrition education, J. Nutr. Educ. 24 (1992) 261–265.

[18] U.S. Department of Health and Human Services. Healthy People 2010: Understanding and Improving Health. Available at <http://www.healthypeople.gov/Document/pdf/uih/2010uih.pdf>, 2000 (accessed 24.04.07).

[19] American Dietetic Association. Ethnic and Regional Food Practices: A Series (1989–2002). American Dietetic Association, Chicago.

[20] Diabetes Care and Education DPG, in: C.M. Goody, L. Drago (Eds.), Cultural Food Practices, American Dietetic Association, Chicago, 2010.

[21] E. Harris-Davis, B. Haughton, Model for multicultural nutrition counseling competencies, J. Am Diet. Assoc. 100 (2000) 1178–1185.

[22] C. Achterberg, Factors that influence learner readiness, J. Am. Diet. Assoc. 88 (1988) 1426–1429.

[23] E. Walker, Characteristics of the adult learner, Diabetes Educator 25 (1999) 16–24.

[24] D.N. Osterman, The feedback lecture: matching teaching and learning styles, J. Am. Diet. Assoc. 84 (1984) 1221–1222.

[25] S.L. Norris, M.M. Engelgau, K.M. Narayan, Effective of self-management training in type 2 diabetes: a systematic review of randomized controlled trials, Diabetes Care 24 (2001) 561–587.

[26] T. Deakin, C.E. McShane, J.E. Cade, R.D.R. Williams, Group based training for self-management strategies in people with type 2 diabetes mellitus, Cochrane LIBR (4) (2006) (CD003417).

[27] G.S. Goldfield, L.H. Epstein, C.K. Kilanowski, R.A. Paluch, B. Kogut-Bossler, Cost-effectiveness of group and mixed family-based treatment for childhood obesity, Int. J. Obes. 25 (2001) 1843–1849.

[28] A. Murphy, A. Guilar, D. Donat, Nutrition education for women with newly diagnosed gestational diabetes mellitus: small-group vs. individual counseling, Can. J. Diabetes 28 (2004) 1–5.

[29] J.M. Johnston, G.R. Jansen, J. Anderson, P. Kendell, Comparison of group diet instruction to a self-directed education program for cholesterol reduction, J. Nutr. Educ. 26 (1994) 140–145.

[30] D.F. Tate, E.H. Jackvony, R.R. Wing, Effects of Internet counseling on weight loss in adults at risk for type 2 diabetes: a randomized trial, JAMA 289 (2003) 1833–1836.

[31] D.A. Williamson, P. Martin, M. Davis, A. White, R. Newton, H. Walden, et al., Efficacy of an Internet-based behavioral weight loss program for overweight adolescent African-American girls, Eating Weight Disord. 10 (2005) 193–203.

[32] D.F. Tate, E.H. Jackvony, R.R. Wing, A randomized trial comparing human e-mail counseling, computer-automated tailored counseling, and no counseling in an Internet weight loss program, Arch. Intern. Med. 166 (2006) 1620–1625.

[33] R.F. Mager, Preparing Instructional Objectives, Fearon, Belmont, CA, 1975.

[34] C. Houston, D. Haire-Joshu, Application of health behavior models, in: D. Haire-Joshu (Ed.), Management of Diabetes Mellitus: Perspectives Across the Lifespan, Mosby-Year Book, St. Louis, MO, 1995.

[35] B.S. Bloom, A Taxonomy of Educational Objectives. Handbook 1: Cognitive Domain, McKay, New York, 1956.

[36] A. Harrow, A Taxonomy of the Psychomotor Domain, McKay, New York, 1971.

[37] J.W. Pichert, Teaching strategies for effective nutrition counseling, in: M.A. Powers (Ed.), Handbook of Diabetes Nutritional Counseling, Aspen, Rockville, MD, 1987.

[38] R.A. Krukowski., D.S. West., J. Harvey-Berino, Recent advances in Internet-delivered, evidence-based weight control programs for adults, J. Diabetes Sci. Technol. 3 (1) (2009) 184–189.

[39] C.C. Quinn, M.D. Shardell, M.L. Terrin, E.A. Barr, S.H. Ballew, A.L. Gruber-Baldini, Cluster-randomized trial of a mobile phone personalized behavioral intervention for blood glucose control, Diabetes Care 34 (2011) 1934–1942.

[40] Diabetes Prevention Program. Lifestyle Balance: DPP Lifestyle Change Program Manual of Operations. Available at http://www.bsc.gwu.edu/dpp/lifestyle/DPP_duringcore.pdf, 1996 (accessed 22.09.11).

[41] L.M. Delahanty, D.M. Nathan, Implications of the Diabetes Prevention Program (DPP) and Look AHEAD clinical trials for lifestyle interventions, J. Am. Diet. Assoc. 108 (4 Suppl. 1) (2008) S66–S72.

[42] R.T. Ackermann, E.A. Finch, E. Brizendine, et al., Translating the diabetes prevention program into the community: the DEPLOY pilot study, Am. J. Prev. Med. 35 (2008) 357–363.

[43] Centers for Disease Control and Prevention. National Diabetes Prevention Program. Available at <http://www.cdc.gov/diabetes/projects/prevention_program.htm>, 2011 (accessed 21.09.11).

[44] W. Glass, On Your Way to Fitness, Shape Up America, Bethesda, MD, 1996.

[45] Shape Up America. On Your Way to Fitness, 1996. Available at <http://www.shapeup.org/publications/on.your.way.to.fitness/index.html> (accessed 24.04.07).

[46] K.D. Brownell, The Learn Program for Weight Control, American Health Publishing, Dallas, TX, 2004.

[47] T. Piechota, Real Solutions: Weight Loss Workbook, American Dietetic Association, Chicago, 2004.

[48] A. Caban, P. Johnson, D. Marseille, J. Wylie-Rosett, Tailoring a lifestyle change approach and resources to the patient, Diab. Spectrum 12 (1999) 33–38.

[49] American Dietetic Association/American Diabetes Association, Exchange Lists for Meal Planning, American Dietetic Association/American Diabetes Association, Chicago/Alexandria, VA, 2002.

[50] Idaho Plate Method. Available at <http://www.platemethod.com/about.html>. (accessed 07. 09.11).

[51] K.M. Camelon, K. Hadell, P.T. Jamsen, K.J. Ketonen, H.M. Kohtamaki, S. Makimatilla, et al., The plate model: a visual method of teaching meal planning, J. Am. Diet. Assoc. 98 (1998) 1155–1162.

[52] Month of Meals series. (1989–1994). American Diabetes Association, Alexandria, VA.

[53] American Diabetes Association, The American Diabetes Association Month of Meals Diabetes Meal Planner, American Diabetes Association, Alexandria, VA, 2010.

[54] J.F. Higgins, D. Groetzinger, The Ultimate Diabetes Meal Planner, American Diabetes Association, Alexandria, VA, 2009.

[55] J.A. Metz, P.M. Kris-Etherton, C.D. Morris, V.A. Mustad, J.S. Stern, S. Oparil, et al., Dietary compliance and cardiovascular risk reduction with a prepared meal plan compared to a self-selected diet, Am. J. Clin. Nutr. 66 (1997) 373–385.

[56] R.B. Haynes, P. Kris-Etherton, D.A. McCarron, S. Oparil, A. Chait, L.M. Resnick, et al., Nutritionally complete prepared meal

plan to reduce cardiovascular risk factors: a randomized clinical trial, J. Am. Diet. Assoc. 99 (1999) 1077–1083.

[57] J.O. Prochaska, C.C. DiClementi, Stages and processes of self-change in smoking: toward an integrative model of change, J. Consult. Clin. Psychol. 51 (1983) 390–395.

[58] J.O. Prochaska, W.F. Velicier, J.S. Rossi, M.G. Goldstein, B.H. Marcus, W. Rakowski, et al., Stages of change and decisional balance for 12 problem behaviors, Health Psychol. 13 (1994) 39–46.

[59] J.O. Prochaska, C.C. DiClementi, J.C. Norcross, In search of how people change: applications to addictive behaviors, Diab. Spectrum 6 (1993) 25–33.

[60] E. Gehling, The next step: changing us or changing them? Diab. Care Educ. Newsflash 20 (1999) 31–33.

[61] M.J. Powers, Counseling skills for improved behavior change, in: M.A. Powers (Ed.), Handbook of Diabetes Nutritional Counseling, Aspen, Gaithersburg, MD, 1996.

[62] W.R. Miller, S. Rollnick, Motivational Interviewing: Preparing People for Change, second ed., Guilford, New York, 2002.

[63] V.J. Strecher, B. McEvoy Devellis, M.H. Becker, I.M. Rosenstock, The role of self-efficacy in achieving health behavior change, Health Educ. Q. 13 (1986) 73–91.

[64] V. DiLillo, N.J. Siegfried, West D. Smith, Incorporating motivational interviewing into behavioral obesity treatment, Cogn. Behav. Pract. 10 (2003) 120–130.

[65] V. DiLillo, D. Smith West, Incorporating motivational interviewing into counseling for lifestyle change among overweight individuals with type 2 diabetes, Diab. Spectrum 24 (2) (2011) 80–84.

[66] T.B. Moyers, T. Martin, J. Houck, P. Christopher, J. Tonigan, From in-session behaviors to drinking outcomes: a causal chain for motivational interviewing, J. Consult. Clin. Psychol. 77 (2009) 113–124.

[67] S. Rollnick, P. Mason, C. Butler, Health Behavior Change: A Guide for Practitioners, Churchill Livingstone, London, 1999.

[68] T.J. D'Zurilla, A.C. Nezu, Social problem solving skills in adults, in: P.C. Kendall (Ed.), Advances in Cognitive-Behavioral Research and Therapy, Academic Press, New York, 1982, pp. 201–274.

[69] E.B. Fisher Jr., A.M. La Greca, C. Arfken, N. Schneiderman, Directive and nondirective support in diabetes management, Int. J. Behav. Med. 4 (1997) 131–144.

[70] K. Davis, J. Heins, E.B. Fisher Jr., Types of social support deemed important by participants in the DCCT, Diabetes 46 (Suppl. 1) (1997) 89A.

[71] M.S. Walker, D.M. Zona, E.B. Fisher, Depressive symptoms after lung cancer surgery: their relation to coping style and social support, Psychooncology 15 (2006) 684–693.

[72] Stanford School of Medicine. Chronic Disease Self-Management Program. Available at <http://patienteducation.stanford.edu/programs/cdsmp.html> (accessed 13.09.11).

11

Evaluation of Nutrition Interventions

Alan R. Kristal[*], *Nicholas J. Ollberding*[†]

[*]Fred Hutchinson Cancer Research Center, Seattle, Washington [†]University of Chicago, Chicago, Illinois

I INTRODUCTION

Nutrition interventions include a broad array of programs and activities with many different goals. Interventions may be designed for treatment of acute or chronic disease, prevention of specific diseases, or simply improvement of nutritional status. Interventions can focus on changing an individual's dietary behavior, both directly and indirectly, or they can target the composition, manufacture, and availability of food. Research in dietary intervention can be either behavioral, to test whether a dietary intervention program can promote dietary change, or clinical/epidemiological, to test whether dietary change can affect a disease end point or disease risk. Nutrition intervention programs can be delivered as services to individual clients, groups, or entire communities. The evaluation needs of each nutrition intervention program will differ, based on the program content, design, and goals.

The optimal way to evaluate a nutrition intervention is to complete a hypothesis-driven, randomized trial. This means that an *a priori* hypothesis should be used to evaluate whether or not the intervention was effective, an experimental design created, and careful attention paid to factors that contribute to the overall validity of a scientific experiment, such as protocol development, measurement, and statistical analysis. Although expertise from many scientific disciplines is required to complete such a trial, it is important for nutritional scientists to understand the methodological issues that underlie the design of a valid intervention evaluation.

This chapter provides a general overview of quantitative evaluation, with an emphasis on those aspects likely to be the responsibility of a nutritional scientist. The focus is on quantitative outcomes and, in particular, on whether or not an intervention is effective in achieving change in dietary behavior.

II OVERVIEW: TYPES OF NUTRITION INTERVENTION PROGRAM EVALUATIONS

A well-designed and clearly articulated evaluation plan is a key aspect of a successful nutrition intervention program. An evaluation plan requires an intervention program to have clearly defined and realistic objectives. An evaluation plan can also give timely feedback at each stage of program implementation, allowing modifications to improve program effectiveness. The three types of evaluations that are most suitable for nutrition intervention programs are (1) formative evaluation, focusing on program design; (2) process evaluation, emphasizing program implementation, quality assurance, and participant reaction; and (3) outcome evaluation, measuring the achievement of program objectives.

A Formative Evaluation

One challenge for nutrition intervention programs is matching the content of the interventions to the interests and needs of the intended audience. Nutrition information is inherently complex, and it must balance between being scientifically correct and still comprehensible and useful to the intended audience. Intervention activities should also be reasonable for the context in which they are delivered. At the stage of formative evaluation, a nutritionist assesses whether or not materials and programs are appropriately

Nutrition in the Prevention and Treatment of Disease, Third Edition.
DOI: http://dx.doi.org/10.1016/B978-0-12-391884-0.00011-1

intensive, scientifically coherent, convenient, and otherwise consistent with their intended uses.

B Process Evaluation

Once in place, it is important to know if the intervention program is reaching its audience and how it is being received. There is a tendency for persons who are already interested in nutrition and motivated to change to participate in intervention trials. Thus, if an intervention is to be generalizable, it is important to ensure that program components successfully reach men, younger persons, racial and ethnic minorities, and other groups less likely to be drawn to programs in nutrition. This is also the stage at which to evaluate whether the program is being implemented as intended and whether the audiences' reactions to the program are favorable or changes are needed to have a broader impact.

C Outcome Evaluation

Ultimately, the effectiveness of a nutrition intervention will be judged based on its ability to achieve program objectives. The authors judge the specification and collection of outcome measures, and their correct analysis, to be essential to any nutrition intervention evaluation.

III OUTCOMES OR END POINTS USED TO ASSESS INTERVENTION EFFECTIVENESS

The most obvious intervention outcomes or end points are based on changes in nutrient intake, but for comprehensive evaluations of dietary interventions, this is too limited. Often, indirect measures of intervention effectiveness—for example, changes in supermarket sales or implementation of a worksite catering policy—can serve as meaningful outcomes. In addition, to understand how an intervention did or did not work, it is necessary to measure intermediate or mediating factors for dietary change, such as beliefs, attitudes, or nutritional knowledge [1].

Before discussing outcomes in detail, two overarching points need to be emphasized. First, the most important consideration for selecting outcomes is that they must have clear interpretations that relate directly to the intervention you are evaluating. Examples of poor evaluation outcomes include "compliance with the USDA MyPlate recommendations," "dietary adequacy," or "compliance with the Dietary Reference Intakes." These types of outcomes are not useful as

evaluation end points because they are too multidimensional, cannot be precisely defined, or their interpretations are too subjective. Second, if you will not measure dietary change per se, then the outcomes you select should have a known and reasonably strong relationship to dietary behavior. For example, increased nutrition knowledge or awareness of relationships between diet and disease are not sufficient in themselves as intervention end points because they have low or no predictive value for dietary behavior change. Experience suggests that it is best to carefully formulate and define intervention outcomes as a part of the overall intervention design. This results in a more focused intervention program and yields evaluation data that are optimally informative.

A Types of Outcomes or End Points Used to Assess Intervention Effectiveness

Outcomes can be classified most broadly into four types: (1) physiological or biological measures, (2) behavioral measures based on self-report, (3) diet-related psychosocial measures, and (4) environmental or surrogate measures of dietary behavior.

Biological or physiological measures are objective indicators of dietary change. For well-funded and relatively small clinical intervention trials, measures based on serological concentration of nutrients or metabolic changes associated with dietary change are optimal approaches to evaluation. The strength of biological measures is that they are objective and unbiased. Their weaknesses are that they do not exist for many outcomes of interest (e.g., reduced percentage of energy from fat in the diet) and they are rarely sufficiently sensitive to detect the relatively modest dietary changes one can expect from low-intensity health-promotion interventions. It can also be procedurally difficult and prohibitively expensive to add biological measures to large, health-promotion intervention trials.

Self-reported dietary behavior is the most often used basis for intervention evaluation. There are two conceptually distinct types of measures based on self-reported diet. The most common measures are the intakes of specific nutrients in an individual's diet, such as percentage of energy from fat or milligrams of β-carotene, or measures of food use, such as servings per day of fruits and vegetables. One can also characterize dietary habits—for example, removing the skin before eating chicken or using low-fat instead of regular salad dressings. The primary weakness of all self-reported behavioral outcomes is that persons exposed to an intervention may bias their reports of behavior to exaggerate true behavior change [2,3]. The strengths of self-reported behavioral outcomes are that they are easy to interpret and often reflect an intervention's specified goals.

Psychosocial outcomes consist of theoretical constructs that relate to diet or dietary change. These include nutrition knowledge, attitudes, and beliefs about diet and intentions and self-efficacy to change diet. These constructs are best interpreted in the context of structured theoretical models of behavior change. For example, an intervention based on the precede/proceed model [4] would assess changes in predisposing, enabling, and reinforcing factors for dietary change. The primary weakness of psychosocial outcomes is that they do not measure dietary change; rather, they measure factors that relate, often quite weakly, to dietary behavior. Their strength is that they are often the actual target or focus of the intervention. For example, an intervention designed to increase awareness of the benefits of eating more fruits and vegetables could be evaluated by measuring changes in perceived benefits. Psychosocial measures are best considered as mediating factors for dietary change—that is, factors that explain how an intervention ultimately results in changed behavior [5–8]. Collecting information on psychosocial factors can yield valuable insights into how to improve the design and content of dietary interventions [9] and thus should be given high priority in research designs.

Environmental measures assess characteristics of communities, organizations, or the physical environment that in some way reflect dietary behavior or dietary change. Measures some researchers have used are the percentage of supermarket shelf space used for healthful versions of staple foods (e.g., low-fat milk or whole-grain breads) and the percentage of foods in vending machines that are low in fat. The weakness of these measures is that there is relatively little research to support their validity as measures of dietary change, and the available evidence suggests that associations between change in environmental measures and individual dietary behavior are modest. However, the strengths of these measures are that they are objective and unbiased, and they are frequently inexpensive to collect.

Selection from among these various types of intervention outcomes is based on many criteria. However, the primary criterion is that they should be meaningful measures of the desired intervention outcome. This requires judgment and thoughtful consideration of both the goals of the intervention and the goals of the evaluation. The following examples illustrate the diversity of options available for evaluating different types of interventions. For an intensive, clinical intervention with a goal of lowering fat intake from 35 to 20% of energy, outcomes could include self-reported diet and measured body weight. For a worksite-based intervention to increase the availability of healthful foods to workers during the workday, outcomes could include foods offered at cafeterias and in vending machines. For a worksite-based intervention designed to test different approaches to promoting healthy dietary patterns, outcomes could include self-reported diet as well as mediating psychosocial factors such as knowledge of fat in foods and stage of change to adopt a low-fat diet. For a public health campaign to increase the use of lower fat milk products, outcomes could include supermarket sales data and random digit dial surveys to assess consumption of low-fat milk.

IV DESIGN OF NUTRITION INTERVENTION EVALUATIONS

Evaluation design encompasses the protocols for participant recruitment, measuring intervention delivery and outcomes, and analyzing and presenting results. Choices made during the development of an evaluation design are primarily guided by two considerations: (1) the content, type, or design of the nutrition intervention and (2) the purpose of the evaluation.

By type of intervention, the broadest distinctions are between clinical interventions and public health interventions. Clinical interventions target high-risk individuals and generally consist of intensive, multiple individual or group sessions that address both dietary behavior (nutrition education) and psychological support for maintaining dietary change. In contrast, public health interventions target large groups of individuals, usually not limited to persons at high risk, and generally consist of a broad range of low-intensity and low-cost components such as media messages and self-help materials. Some interventions fall between these two extremes (e.g., worksite-based health-promotion programs may offer a series of intensive nutrition education classes), and some interventions may fall outside of this classification altogether (e.g., the decision to fortify cereal-grain products with folic acid). For purposes of evaluation, the two most important distinctions between clinical and public health interventions are the timing and amount of expected change: Intensive clinical interventions produce rapid and dramatic change, whereas public health interventions yield slow change over long periods of time.

For the purposes of the evaluation, a broad distinction is made between research that contributes to scientific knowledge and documentation that serves the needs of practitioners and administrators. Comprehensive scientific evaluations are generally beyond the financial means of any but the most well-funded research trials because the costs of evaluation generally far exceed those for intervention design and delivery. Practitioners and administrators must assume that the interventions being delivered are at least somewhat effective. As a result, evaluation is focused on evidence that the program is reaching the intended target population and is benefiting those who participate.

A Design Components of Nutrition Intervention Evaluations

Five components characterize the design of an intervention evaluation:

1. A representative sample of persons who would be likely program participants or targets of an intervention.
2. One or more measures of the evaluation outcome at preintervention.
3. One or more comparison groups, most often a control group not receiving an intervention.
4. Randomized assignment to treatment (intervention or control) groups.
5. One or more measures of the evaluation outcome at postintervention.

The most robust research evaluations include all of these design characteristics. However, not all of these components need be present to have a scientifically valid design. The only necessary characteristics are that there be postintervention outcome measures and a comparison group. Intervention evaluations not based on a randomized trial can be either quasi-experimental, in which treatment is assigned in a manner other than randomization, or observational, in which epidemiological methods are used to statistically model differences between those receiving and those not receiving an intervention. Because of their complexity, nutritionists should consult with appropriate experts before choosing such design alternatives.

Administrative evaluation of program effectiveness should strive to incorporate as many of these evaluation components as feasible. In practice, however, an administrative evaluation may simply consist of documenting the number of persons receiving the intervention and measuring changes among those exposed. One improvement in this design would be to calculate participation rates based, for example, on the number of persons offered the intervention or the number eligible. This would give administrators insight into the acceptability and penetration of the intervention into eligible populations. Another improvement would be to document the level of exposure to or participation in the intervention and to correlate the level of exposure to changes in outcome. This type of dose–response analysis can suggest whether more intensive intervention would be cost-effective.

1 Representative Sample

Evaluation of a representative sample means that evaluation participants include persons from demographic and socioeconomic groups who would be targets for the intervention. Representativeness in dietary interventions is often difficult because participation in nutrition interventions tends to be higher among women and older people [10]. However, representativeness is not always important or even desirable. If the purpose of the evaluation is to test whether an intervention can work at all (e.g., in the best of all possible circumstances), it will be preferable to recruit only highly motivated volunteers using highly selective enrollment criteria. It may even be appropriate to require participants to complete a prerandomization run-in activity, such as completing a 4-day food record, to eliminate participants not likely to complete the trial [11]. Alternatively, if an evaluation is designed to examine how an intervention will work as it is to be delivered in practice, then participants are best recruited from representative samples from defined populations in an attempt to achieve as high a recruitment rate as possible [12].

2 Preintervention Measures

Measures before intervention are desirable for two reasons. First, even in randomized experiments, there might be differences in baseline measures across treatment groups. Second, pre- and postintervention measures allow evaluators to calculate change from baseline. Basing evaluation on differences in change between treatment groups rather than simply on differences in outcome measures postintervention almost always yields superior statistical power. If possible, preintervention assessments should be completed before treatment group assignment so that neither the evaluation staff nor the participant can be biased by knowing which intervention they will receive.

3 Comparison Group

The choice of comparison group(s) depends on the goal of the intervention. The most common design is to compare outcomes in a group receiving an intervention to one not receiving an intervention. Options include comparisons between a new and a standard intervention or between groups receiving different levels of the same intervention. It is rarely satisfactory to have no comparison group because it is not possible to determine whether any observed changes can be attributed to the intervention or to other factors outside of an investigator's control or not directly associated with the intervention.

4 Randomized Assignment to Treatment Groups

Randomization is the best way to ensure comparability between treatment groups, but it is not always possible. In this case, it may be feasible to devise an unbiased approach to assign individuals to contrasting treatments, for example, based on health care practitioner, day of the week, or hospital clinic. One entirely unacceptable design is to offer an intervention and compare results in self-selected participants to those refusing to participate. Participation in a nutrition intervention is strongly associated with characteristics that *a priori* predict dietary change, such as sex, age, and interest in nutrition and health. With this approach, comparisons between participants and nonparticipants are so strongly biased that they should be excluded from consideration for any type of evaluation design. Examination of change among participants alone would be a better design because no inferences can be made beyond documentation that change occurred in those who received the intervention.

5 Postintervention Assessments

It is optimal to complete two postintervention measures, one after the intervention is complete and one delayed by at least several months. The first measure assesses the immediate impact of the intervention, whereas the latter gives insight into whether effects are durable and whether there is continued change over time. Basing an evaluation on an early measure alone can be misleading: Some interventions may have no long-term effect because behavior change is not sustained. Some interventions may yield continual, gradual change over time, in which case only a long-term assessment will demonstrate intervention effectiveness.

B Analysis of Intervention Effects

Statistical analysis of nutrition interventions can pose many challenges. Some of these statistical issues are described here, and nontechnical recommendations for the most commonly used designs and statistical models are given.

1 Level of Measurement and Units of Analysis

There are many choices for how outcomes are assessed and analyzed. Unit of measurement describes whether the outcomes are assessed on individual participants (e.g., self-reported diet) or on a group-level or environmental characteristic (e.g., supermarket sales or availability of fresh fruit in worksite cafeterias). Unit of analysis describes whether analyses of outcomes are based on individual observations (e.g., individual changes in fat intake), on aggregated measures of individual observations (e.g., percentage of population drinking low-fat milk in the previous day), or on group-level or environmental outcomes. For clinical interventions and for public health interventions in which outcome assessments are based on measurements of individuals, the units of measurement and analysis are almost always at the individual level. For some public health interventions, especially those that target large groups or communities, there are many options for combinations of unit of measurement and unit of analysis. The most common is to aggregate measures on a sample of individuals and interpret these as measures of the community [13]. One can also measure outcomes at the community level, such as availability of healthful foods in supermarkets and restaurants, existence of nutrition programs in the community, or media coverage of nutrition-related information. It is of utmost importance to match the evaluation design, particularly the randomization scheme, to the unit of analysis. In grouped randomized designs, for example, a trial randomizing worksites or schools to different intervention treatments, the analysis must be based on the unit of randomization, not the individuals participating in the intervention. Unlike individually randomized designs, the sample size for analysis of grouped randomized designs is a function of both the number of groups and the number of participants in each group. Consider an intervention trial that is evaluating whether a school nutrition unit can affect students' lunch choices. If 12 schools with 2000 students were each randomized such that 6 implemented the curriculum and 6 did not, the number of experimental units is 12, not 24,000. Readers will find an excellent and nontechnical overview of these issues in reviews by Koepsell [14,15].

2 Calculating the Simple Intervention Effect

The best and most comprehensible measure of intervention effectiveness is the difference between the change in intervention group participants minus the change in control (or alternative treatment) group participants. This measure can be considered the intervention effect. As an example, in an intervention with a goal to decrease the percentage of energy from fat, the intervention effect is defined as:

$$[Fat(\%en)_b - Fat(\%en)_f]_I - [Fat(\%en)_b - Fat(\%en)_F]_C$$

where fat(%en) is the percentage of energy from dietary fat; subscripts b and f refer to baseline and follow-up, respectively; and subscripts I and C refer to intervention and control groups, respectively. The statistical test of whether or not the intervention effect is different from zero is based on the standard error of the intervention effect, which is defined as:

$$\sqrt{\frac{\text{var}[\text{fat}(\%\text{en})_b - \text{fat}(\%\text{en})_f]_I}{n_I} + \frac{\text{var}[\text{fat}(\%\text{en})_b - \text{fat}(\%\text{en})_f]_C}{n_C}}$$

where n_I is the sample size in the intervention group, and n_c is the sample size in the control group.

Most measures of dietary intake and serum nutrient concentrations have log-normal or other non-normal distributions; however, changes in these measures are characteristically normally distributed. It is therefore rarely necessary to transform measures before analysis, and for simplicity of interpretation it should be avoided.

3 Calculating Intervention Effects Adjusted for Sociodemographic and Confounding Factors

The intervention effect is best estimated after adjustment for characteristics that are associated with dietary behavior. This is because (1) randomization may not have resulted in these characteristics being evenly divided between treatment groups, and (2) there may be increased statistical power to detect a statistically significant intervention effect if variance associated with these factors is controlled for in the analyses. Here are two approaches to calculating adjusted intervention effects, which differ depending on the scale of measurement of the outcome variable. Most outcome measures are either continuous (e.g., percentage of energy from fat) or ordered categories (e.g., motivation to change measured on a scale of 1 to 10), and thus multiple linear regression can be used to calculate adjusted intervention effects. For a simple, two-treatment randomized design, the best approach is to build a regression model as follows: The dependent variable is calculated as the change from baseline to follow-up in the outcome measure; the covariates are the baseline value of the outcome measure plus the characteristics and diet-related measures you wish to control for in the analysis; the independent variable representing treatment group is an indicator variable coded 0 = control and 1 = treatment. In this model, the regression coefficient for the treatment indicator variable is the adjusted treatment effect, and the standard error of this regression coefficient is used to test the statistical significance of the adjusted intervention effect. Table 11.1 gives an example of how this approach is used for the primary analysis of a two-group randomized trial of a dietary intervention.

If an outcome measure is categorical—for example, whether or not a participant lost 10 pounds or more—it is then appropriate to use logistic regression models. For a simple, two-treatment design, the following model would be appropriate: The dependent variable

TABLE 11.1 Example of Statistical Analyses Used to Report Outcome of a Dietary Intervention to Reduce Fat and Increase Fruit and Vegetable Intakes

	n	Baseline	Change at 3 months	Change at 12 months
Fat-related diet habits[a]				
Intervention ($x \pm SD$)	601	2.29 ± 0.49	−0.09 ± 0.37	−0.09 ± 0.38
Control ($x \pm SD$)	604	2.30 ± 0.49	−0.01 ± 0.36	−0.00 ± 0.40
Intervention effect ($x \pm SE$)		Unadjusted	−0.08 ± 0.02	−0.09 ± 0.02
		Adjusted[β]	−0.09 ± 0.02	−0.10 ± 0.02
		p value	<0.0001	<0.0001
Fruit and vegetables (servings/day)				
Intervention ($x \pm SD$)	601	3.62 ± 1.49	0.41 ± 1.88	0.47 ± 1.83
Control ($x \pm SD$)	604	3.47 ± 1.41	0.08 ± 1.63	0.14 ± 1.80
Intervention effect ($x \pm SE$)		Unadjusted	0.33 ± 0.09	0.33 ± 0.10
		Adjusted[β]	0.39 ± 0.10	0.46 ± 0.10
		p value	<0.0001	<0.0001

[a]Score from 21-item scale, scored from 1.0 (low fat) to 4.0 (high fat).
[β]Adjusted for baseline value, age, sex, race, body mass index, and income.
Source: From Kristal, A., Curry, S., Shattuck, A., Feng, Z., and Li, S. (2000). A randomized trial of a tailored, self-help dietary intervention: The Puget Sound Eating Patterns Study. Prev. Med. **31**, 380−389.

is an indicator variable, coded 0 or 1, representing whether or not the outcome is absent or present; the covariates are variables you wish to control in the analysis; and the independent variable representing treatment group is an indicator variable coded 0 = control and 1 = treatment. The exponentiated regression coefficient of the treatment group indicator variable (e'^3) is the relative odds of the outcome comparing the control to treatment group. The standard error of the regression coefficient is used to determine whether the relative odds are statistically different from 1.0. Multiple categorical outcomes, such as movement through stages of dietary change, pose considerable statistical challenges [16,17]. Consultation with a biostatistician is important in modeling these types of outcomes, and some approach to simplifying the analysis may prove to yield more interpretable and useful results.

C Statistical Power

A final aspect of an evaluation design is to choose an appropriate sample size. This requires making a judgment on what size intervention effect is worth detecting. Even a trivially small intervention effect can be found statistically significant given a large enough sample size, and a clinically meaningful intervention effect may not reach statistical significance if the sample size is too small. For clinical interventions, it is reasonable to choose an effect size that is meaningful for an individual. For a public health intervention, the effect size will be much smaller and needs only be meaningful in terms of changes in population distributions of the outcome measure. When choosing minimum effect sizes, it is worthwhile to review what other interventions have achieved. The general recommendation is to never set a minimum detectable intervention effect larger than 1.5 times that observed in other interventions unless there is strong reason to believe that the new intervention being evaluated is far superior.

V MEASUREMENT ISSUES WHEN ASSESSING DIETARY CHANGE AND OTHER INTERVENTION OUTCOMES

Once outcomes are well-defined and an evaluation design is established, one must select, modify, or develop measures. The two standard characteristics of dietary assessment methods, validity and reliability, are described in detail elsewhere in this text (see Chapter 1). Here, the discussion extends to cover measures of psychosocial factors and aspects of measurement that are relevant to measuring dietary change, as well as practical considerations that have important implications for trial design and feasibility. Section VI describes how these measurement issues influence selection from among alternative measures of intervention outcomes.

A Validity

Simply stated, validity is the extent to which your assessment tool measures what you want it to measure. Validity is not necessarily an intrinsic aspect of a particular tool or assessment instrument because validity can vary as a function of method of administration, participants, or time. There are many types of validity, each with implications for intervention evaluation. Content validity is the extent to which you have sampled the domain of what you are trying to measure. For example, if your intervention goal were to lower total fat intake, high content validity would mean that you have measured all foods with meaningful amounts of fat. A limited but nevertheless important part of content validity is commonly referred to as face validity. Face validity is a judgment made by experts about whether or not a completed questionnaire measures what it is supposed to measure [18]. Construct validity is primarily a consideration for psychosocial measures. In this context, high construct validity means that the items used to form a scale are a good measure of some meaningful, underlying, or latent construct. An example is a scale that measures enabling factors for dietary change, consisting of six items on barriers, norms, and social support [19]. Criterion validity considers how well one measure correlates with another measure of the same construct. A type of criterion validity most important for nutrition intervention evaluations is predictive validity, which is based on whether a measure made at one time point predicts change at a later point in time. For example, based on the theory of reasoned action [20], one would validate a measure of intention to eat more fruits and vegetables by examining how well it predicts increased intake.

B Reliability

Two types of reliability are important for evaluating intervention trials. Test—retest reliability measures agreement between multiple assessments. In practice, this means that a measure taken on one day would be strongly correlated with a measure taken on another day. Although no measures have perfect reliability, measures of daily nutrient intake or specific dietary behavior have particularly low reliability because of the variability in the amounts and types of foods people eat from day to day. This type of variability, termed intraindividual or within-persons variability, makes even a perfect assessment of a single day's diet not informative for evaluating whether or not a person has changed his or her usual diet as a response to an intervention.

A second and entirely different type of reliability, which is relevant primarily to measures of psychosocial factors, is internal consistency reliability. Most psychosocial factors cannot be assessed directly (e.g., social support for eating low-fat foods), and they are generally measured using a set of items that taken together characterize the construct (e.g., "How much support do you get from your co-workers to select healthy foods from the cafeteria at lunch?"). The statistic called Cronbach's alpha, which ranges from 0 to 1, is a measure of how well the mean of scale items measures an underlying construct. High internal consistency reliability is a function of two factors—the average correlation among items in the scale and the number of items in the scale. Most scientists suggest a minimum of 0.7 for internal consistency; however, this ignores the practical problem that in applied evaluations it is not feasible to use lengthy scales. When scales are restricted to three or four items, a Cronbach's alpha of 0.50 is satisfactory.

C Intervention-Associated Recall Bias

Bias is a measure of the extent to which an instrument under- or overestimates what it is attempting to measure. Ample evidence indicates that person-specific biases exist in self-reports of diet; for example, overweight persons tend to systematically underestimate energy intake [21]. If person-specific biases are constant, they will have little impact on evaluation because analyses will be based on differences between measures assessed at baseline and follow-up. However, two unique sources of bias are introduced whenever evaluation of a dietary intervention is based on self-reported behavior. First, repeated monitoring results in changed responses to assessment instruments. For example, the number of different foods reported on a 4-day diet record decreases from day 1 to day 4, suggesting that study participants simplify their diets [22]. There is also some evidence that the quality of dietary intake data improves with repeated assessments, and this may differ by intervention treatment group [22]. Second, although well-designed dietary intervention trials randomize participants to intervention and control groups, the delivery of the behavioral intervention cannot be blinded as in conventional placebo-controlled trials [23]. Thus, if intervention group participants report eating diets that match the goals of the intervention program rather than what they actually ate, there will be a bias toward overestimating intervention effectiveness. This bias can be substantial [2,3,24], and it appears to be larger in women than in men [25–27]. The potential for this type of bias, known as social desirability or demand bias, warrants consideration in the design and in the analysis of dietary intervention studies.

D Responsiveness

A measure related specifically to measuring change is termed "responsiveness." Conceptually, responsiveness is a measure of whether an instrument captures information on intervention-related dietary patterns [28]. In intensive clinical interventions, in which a successful intervention results in large changes in foods consumed and food-preparation techniques, a sensitive instrument will capture information both on the most common foods and dietary practices of the sample at baseline and on new practices adopted because of the intervention. In public health interventions, in which there are only modest changes in dietary behavior, a sensitive measure will detect very small changes in behavior targeted by the intervention. Statistically, responsiveness is the ratio of the intervention effect divided by the standard deviation of the intervention effect. Responsiveness is thus a function of several aspects of a measure: (1) how well an instrument measures the intervention outcome both pre- and post-intervention, (2) the magnitude of the intervention effect, and (3) the variance in the dietary or other measure used as the intervention outcome.

E Participant Burden

If outcome assessments are too long or complicated, require biological samples, or must be repeated many times, high participant burden results. High participant burden can significantly compromise an evaluation. During recruitment, participation rates will be poor and participants will be less representative of the intervention target population. Once entered into the study, long or repeated follow-up assessments will contribute to high dropout rates. Once recruited and assigned to a treatment group, all participants should be included in the evaluation whether or not they complete the intervention or subsequent follow-up assessments (intent-to-treat analysis). Thus, high dropout rates (>25%) make an evaluation suspect.

F Instrument Complexity

Accurate assessment of nutrient intake requires complex instrumentation, regardless of whether instruments are interviewer- or self-administered. Some diet-related psychosocial factors may also require many questions with complicated skip patterns. It is important to remember that nutrition knowledge and literacy may be poor in some populations. Intervention participants may have difficulty answering detailed questions about food preparation or serving sizes, or they may not be able to understand complex questions about attitudes and beliefs [29].

Complexity of analysis is an issue that is often overlooked. Before using an evaluation instrument, understand how it will be analyzed, evaluate the underlying nutrient database and associated software, and make sure that these analyses produce the variables you wish to measure. Dietary records, food frequency questionnaires, or scales to measure diet-related psychosocial factors are not useful unless there are means to transform data from these instruments into interpretable measures of the evaluation outcomes. Similarly, although it is simple to collect blood for serological outcomes, an analysis of many diet-related serological measures is possible only in specialized research laboratories. These laboratories are primarily in academic research centers, and they are rarely capable of or interested in processing the large numbers of samples required for evaluating a dietary intervention.

G Costs

Randomized trials are expensive, and the costs of evaluating a nutrition intervention are often far greater than the costs of intervention delivery. A large proportion of evaluation cost can be attributed to outcome assessments, especially if they are based on dietary records or recalls or on serological measures of micronutrient concentrations. Not surprisingly, the high cost of dietary assessments strongly motivates the use of alternative measures.

VI DIETARY ASSESSMENT INSTRUMENTS AND THEIR APPLICABILITY FOR INTERVENTION EVALUATION

Most research on dietary assessment is motivated by the needs of nutritional epidemiologists and is focused on how to best understand relationships between diet and health outcomes or on surveillance of population-level nutritional status. Dietary intervention studies have tended to use dietary assessment methods developed for other purposes, with the hope that they will serve the current intended purpose. However, as described previously in this chapter, evaluating dietary interventions and measuring dietary change have many special nuances. Here, the available tools for measuring intervention effectiveness are reviewed with a focus on the characteristics most relevant for outcome evaluation.

A Anthropometric and Biochemical Measures

Many anthropometric and biochemical measures correlate with nutrient intake, but relatively few of these are useful or appropriate for the evaluation of interventions to change dietary behavior (Table 11.2). The exceptions will be interventions that are designed to increase intake of a specific micronutrient—for example, the fortification of cereal-grain products in the United States with folic acid or the fortification of sugar with vitamin A in Guatemala [30].

The most useful anthropometric measure is change in body weight, which can either be the goal of the nutritional intervention or a marker of decreased energy intake relative to expenditure or fat intakes. Given the lack of objective markers of dietary fat reduction, this relationship with weight deserves more comment. Randomized trials of fat reduction show intervention effects for weight of approximately 3 kg associated with a 10-percentage point decrease in the percentage energy from fat [11,31] and of approximately 0.25 kg with decreases of 1 percentage point [12]. Weight loss associated with fat reduction is likely

TABLE 11.2 Anthropometric and Biochemical Measures Suitable for Intervention Evaluation

Measure	Intervention(s)	Comments/references
Weight	Energy or possibly fat	[11,31]
Serum carotenoids	Fruits and vegetables	Fasting blood samples are optimal. Control for serum cholesterol, body mass index, and smoking are necessary. Confounded by β-carotene supplements. [33–35,37]
Urinary isoflavonoids	Soy products	Spot sample may be adequate. Hidden sources of soy (e.g., processed meats) may confound measure. [102,103]
Red cell or phospholipid	Fish	Confounded by fish oil supplements.
Fatty acid	Fat modification	[104–106]
Plasma/urinary isothiocyanates	Cruciferous vegetables	[107,108]
Serum cholesterol	Fat modification	[109,110]

due to incomplete substitution of nonfat sources of energy in a fat-restricted diet [32].

Biochemical measures are useful for assessing changes in foods containing unique constituents that can be measured easily in blood or urine. The most often used measure is change in total serum carotenoids, which reflects usual intakes of carotenoid-containing fruits and vegetables [33–36]; however, total carotenoids minus lycopene is a superior measure [37] because of the low correlation of serum lycopene with other serum carotenoids. Biochemical measures are also useful to assess metabolic changes that result from dietary change. Lipids, such as low-density lipoprotein and serum cholesterol, can be used as a measure of polyunsaturated and decreased saturated fatty acid intake in some target groups [38,39]. Because biochemical measures are expensive and typically require invasive collection procedures, they are impractical to use as primary outcome measures in public health interventions. An alternative is to collect biochemical measures on a small subsample of volunteers and use these data as secondary outcomes to confirm results based on dietary self-report and to incorporate less invasive biochemical measures when possible [40].

B Self-Reported Dietary Behavior

Table 11.3 gives an overview of measures used to collect data on self-reported diet. Selection from among these many choices requires balancing the costs and participant burden of "gold standard" measures such as multiple 24-hour dietary recalls with the practical benefits of using short, self-administered questionnaires that assess specific dietary patterns.

The primary distinctions among types of instruments are based on whether diet is measured as foods actually consumed, foods "usually" consumed, or patterns of food consumption. Note that there is an inherent hierarchy across these types of instruments: One can measure dietary patterns based on any dietary assessment instrument or foods usually consumed based on foods actually consumed. Measuring nutrients from foods actually consumed is a gold standard for intervention evaluation because any changes in foods, portion sizes, and preparation techniques can be captured.

However, because many days of foods must be assessed to characterize an individual's usual diet, any measure based on actual foods consumed will be expensive and have high participant burden. The benefit of assessing nutrients from foods usually consumed is that only a single measure is needed at each time point, but it is not possible to capture details on all foods and their preparation methods in precise detail. The benefits of assessing dietary patterns alone are that it is a less burdensome task and is often a more direct measure of whether new dietary behaviors were adopted. The limitation is that changes in dietary patterns cannot be directly interpreted as changes in nutrient intake and are thus less well accepted in the nutritional science community.

1 Nutrients from Foods Actually Consumed

The best approach to measuring nutrients from foods actually consumed is unannounced (unscheduled), interviewer-administered 24-hour dietary recalls. Unannounced recalls are administered by telephone, which in practice is facilitated by collecting information at the beginning of an evaluation on convenient days, places, and times to call. Participants can be given serving size booklets so that they can refer to specific pictures when reporting amounts of foods consumed. The protocol or script used for collecting 24-hour recalls can also be modified to focus on assessing the intervention outcomes (e.g., for an intervention to decrease saturated fat, type of margarine will be important) and deemphasize details that are uninformative (e.g., for a fruit and vegetable intervention, probes for added salt are not relevant). Finally, it is important to consider the limitations to the accuracy of 24-hour recalls because respondents often do not know answers to questions about food composition, preparation, or portion size.

High costs (between $35 and $55 per day) and participant burden are serious drawbacks to any study whose goal is to evaluate intervention effectiveness using interviewer-administered dietary recalls. This is especially true when the evaluation is at the individual level and therefore many days of intake must be captured for each participant. The development of an automated, self-administered 24-hour recall (ASA24) may substantially reduce the cost associated with collecting multiple unannounced 24-hour recalls [41]; however, limitations of the use of such technology include computer and high-speed Internet access, as well as some degree of basic and computer literacy. In addition, the development of dietary data recorders (DDRs), as shown in Figure 11.1, may improve the ability to measure foods actually consumed by integrating video and audio/text recordings with user-provided information on food preparation and purchasing decisions. These data, used in conjunction with a standard nutrient database and specialized operating software, will provide researchers with digital food records collected in real time and enable objective estimates of portion size while reducing participant burden and cost.

For randomized designs, it may be sufficient to calculate intervention effects based on one pre- and one postintervention recall per participant. This measure of the intervention effect will be unbiased, but there are problems because of the low reliability of a single day's measure of nutrient intake. Most important, because the group-level intervention effect will have high variance, there will be low statistical power to detect differences across treatment groups. Furthermore, it is statistically inappropriate to adjust this measure of the intervention effect for individuals' characteristics or other diet-related factors [42]. Intervention effects calculated from a single 24-hour recall can be used in much the same way as biochemical measures; as a secondary outcome, are used to corroborate a more practical but less valid measure of nutrient intake.

TABLE 11.3 Measures of Self-Reported Diet Suitable for Intervention Evaluation

Nutrients from foods consumed
24-Hour dietary recalls
Nutrients from "usual diet"
Food frequency questionnaires
Dietary patterns
Diet behavior questionnaires
Short food frequency questionnaires
"Focused" 24-hour dietary recalls

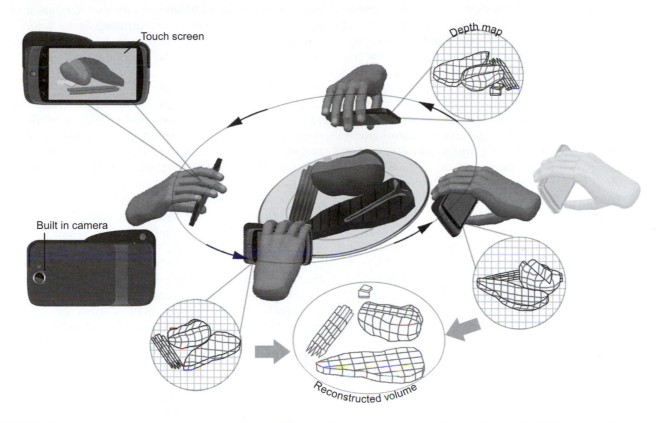

FIGURE 11.1   Volume estimation concept map for DDR. As the phone is rotated around the food items, the DDR system collects a short video, which is enough to ascertain multiple video angles for depth image generation and volume calculation. Through a series of automated queries, users can also provide additional information pertaining to the preparation, location, or time of consumption. See color plate.

Other methods of capturing foods actually consumed, including food records and scheduled 24-hour recalls, are inappropriate for intervention evaluation. This is because both record keeping and anticipating a dietary recall can substantially change dietary behavior [2]. Although unannounced 24-hour recalls may be subject to intervention-associated bias through differential recall of foods consumed, food records or announced recalls are much more likely to be biased because of their effects on food choice. For example, three multipass 24-hour recalls were used at baseline, 6, and 12 months to generate Diet Quality Index scores [43,44] using the Diet Quality Index—Revised (DQI-R) [45] among female cancer survivors (>65 years of age) participating in an intervention to improve diet quality. Investigators reported significant improvements among the intervention group at 6 months but not at 12 months. These results could be due to the reasons mentioned previously or a diminishing effect of the intervention over time. The true reason explaining these results may have been elucidated had an appropriate biomarker been available for use (see Chapter 12).

2 Nutrients from Foods Usually Consumed

Since the mid-1980s, food frequency questionnaires (FFQs) have become a standard measure in nutritional epidemiology. They have also become quite common for intervention evaluations because they can be self-administered, processed using mark-sense technology, and cost less than $15 per administration.

Two characteristics of any FFQ detract from their use for measuring dietary change. First, whereas FFQs are convenient for investigators, they are burdensome to participants because they require time, high literacy, and knowledge about food. Second, the cognitive processes required to complete an FFQ might make them highly subject to intervention-associated bias. Respondents must construct answers to FFQ items using knowledge about their characteristic diet because memory about actual eating and drinking episodes erodes after only a few days [46]. Thus, not knowing the true answer to most questions, it is likely that perceptions of behavior deemed desirable because of the intervention would bias FFQ responses [27]. Nevertheless, practical considerations often require using FFQs. For these evaluations, it is necessary to incorporate methods to minimize response burden and increase response rates, such as limiting total questionnaire length and giving incentives. In addition, the use of a computerized FFQ that allows for complex skip patterns and the logical flow of questions may reduce response burden.

Standard FFQs developed for epidemiological studies are not necessarily good for intervention evaluation. An intervention-focused FFQ must usually collect detailed information on food choices that reflect the intervention goals. This may require any of the following: (1) regrouping foods into categories relevant to the intervention (e.g., grouping soups into "creamed," "vegetable," "bean," and "broth" to capture fat, carotenoids, and fiber), (2) assessing relatively fine distinctions between similar foods (e.g., nonfat versus regular mayonnaise, refried versus baked beans, or plain lettuce salads versus mixed salads with carrots and tomatoes), (3) assessing preparation methods (e.g., chicken with or without skin and shellfish boiled or fried), and (4) collecting information on portion sizes. It is also important to examine the nutrient database and computer algorithms underlying analysis of the FFQ. Several approaches are available for assigning nutrient values to FFQ items [47,48], and some may not produce a nutrient database that reflects substantial differences in relevant nutrients between foods targeted by the intervention. There are also different approaches in how FFQ analysis software incorporates information about types of foods (e.g., type of milk) or preparations (e.g., chicken with or without skin) when computing nutrients. It may be necessary to modify these algorithms to better reflect changes targeted by an intervention. Unfortunately, developing a new FFQ is time-consuming and complex, and most evaluations must choose wisely from among those available based on how well they capture the dietary behavior of interest. Some commercially available FFQ software packages do allow minor modifications that can be helpful in developing FFQs for intervention trials [49], and some FFQs are available that were developed specifically for evaluating interventions [23,47,50].

3 Dietary Patterns

The many practical and scientific benefits to using short, simple instruments to measure dietary patterns targeted by an intervention were described previously in this chapter. A modest amount of research has been done in this area, and it has yielded four approaches to short dietary assessment: (1) short FFQs; (2) prediction equations, based on regression models; (3) diet-habits questionnaires; and (4) focused 24-hour recalls. These approaches differ substantially in their underlying statistical assumptions and their use of behavioral theory related to dietary behavior change. Understanding these differences can help nutritionists to select and modify available instruments or to develop instruments suited to the intervention under evaluation.

A SHORT FOOD FREQUENCY QUESTIONNAIRES

These instruments typically contain between 10 and 15 FFQ items and are designed to assess intake of a specific nutrient or frequency of eating a specific group of foods. Examples in the literature include instruments for fat [51], calcium [52], and fruits and vegetables [53–56]. For intervention evaluation, a short FFQ should be based on knowledge of dietary patterns in the sample receiving the intervention [57,58] and the behavioral targets of the intervention. There is modest evidence that an approach based solely on statistical criteria can be valid in epidemiological studies [48], but this approach lacks face validity when evaluating an intervention. Short FFQs are appropriate for intervention evaluation only if a small number of foods are being targeted by the intervention or if the outcome is a nutrient that is concentrated in very few foods. Thus, short FFQs are best for nutrients such as calcium [59] or for food groups such as fruits and vegetables, and they are suspect for nutrients such as fat or sodium that are spread throughout the food supply.

B PREDICTION EQUATIONS

Many nutritional scientists have proposed using regression models to predict nutrient intake from a short set of questions. These models are built typically on data from FFQs, in which the frequencies of eating specific foods are entered into a stepwise linear regression model predicting the nutrient of interest. A relatively small number of foods will predict a large amount of variance in most nutrients [60], and on the surface this appears to be a useful way to simplify dietary assessment. However, these models have poor face validity because these prediction equations assign coefficients (weights) to food items that often have little to do with the nutrient of interest [61]. The models also have poor criterion validity because models developed from one sample typically do not predict nutrient intake in a different, independent sample [62,63].

A related approach is based on using factor analysis to identify patterns of association among foods on an FFQ. These patterns are given descriptive names (e.g., "junk food" or "plain home cooking") based on the interpretation of the foods in the factor, and these factors are treated as meaningful measures of an underlying dietary pattern. These patterns lack both face validity and criterion validity and are not reproducible between samples. One of the reasons both regression and factor analysis do not yield useful measures is that they are based on correlations among FFQ items in a specific sample. There is little consistency in the correlations among FFQ items across time or across samples and even less consistency if a dietary intervention changes dietary patterns. Measures based on regression models or factor analysis are entirely inappropriate for intervention evaluation.

C DIET-HABITS QUESTIONNAIRES

Diet-habits questionnaires are unique because they have been developed specifically to measure intervention outcomes. These questionnaires typically contain between 15 and 30 questions, with response options that are qualitative (e.g., rarely/never to usually/always) or ordered frequency categories. The most robust of these measures is based on theoretical or at least explicit models of dietary behavior change [64,65], and their development is facilitated by an understanding of nutrition, psychometric theory, and cognitive psychology, as well as skill in item construction and questionnaire design. There is ample evidence that these measures can be valid measures of dietary change [64−72], and they tend to have higher responsiveness than alternatives such as short FFQs, full FFQs, or repeated 24-hour recalls [10,12,28,73,74].

Diet behavior questionnaires are well suited to evaluations of public health interventions because of their low participant burden and high sensitivity to change, and they are less well suited for clinical interventions requiring a measure of changes in nutrient intake. Before beginning an evaluation, it is important to pilot these measures in the target population to make sure that the questionnaire format language and diet patterns being measured are appropriate. Nutritionists should take the liberty of modifying existing questionnaires to better suit their target population, as long as the basic structure and content of the instrument remains intact.

D FOCUSED 24-HOUR RECALLS

A focused recall uses techniques similar to those used to collect standard 24-hour recalls, but it collects only information related to the evaluation outcome. For example, if the intervention goal is to increase servings of fruits and vegetables, then the only information captured during the interview is about fruits and vegetables. The amount of detail collected can also vary. A focused recall could collect details about the type and serving size of all targeted foods, or an interviewer could simply read a list of foods and ask respondents whether or not they ate them in the previous day[75]. Focused recalls are far simpler to administer and analyze than standard 24-hour recalls, but they share the characteristic of low bias because of their reliance on episodic rather than general memory [46]. Similar to a 24-hour recall, only repeated assessments can be used to characterize behavior of an individual,

but a single measure is fine for characterizing a group. For example, one could contrast the percentages of participants in the intervention and control groups who drank skim milk or ate french fried potatoes on the previous day. More complex focused recalls have been developed to measure carotenoid intake [76], and more research on developing these measures is warranted. Nutritionists should consider developing instruments based on this approach when the 24-hour recalls are the desired evaluation tool but cannot be used because of costs or participant burden.

4 Diet-Related Psychosocial Factors

Table 11.4 gives an overview of psychosocial factors that can be used to assess intervention outcomes. Comprehensive behavioral models are built from many constructs [77], but in the context of an intervention evaluation it is generally both feasible and necessary to measure only those constructs that are central to the model. Thus, for each of the behavioral models used to design nutrition interventions, those psychosocial factors that are key to their evaluation are selected.

Little research exists on the validity and responsiveness of diet-related psychosocial measures. Measures developed and validated for one behavioral domain— for example, for smoking cessation—are often adapted for dietary intervention research without consideration of their face or construct validity. For some diet-related psychosocial constructs, measurement is simple and little validation is necessary. For example, one could measure intention to change diet with a single item such as "In the next 6 months, how likely is it that you will change your diet to eat less fat?" Alternatively, measuring a construct such as stage of dietary change can be complex and requires considerable developmental research. When adopting psychosocial measures

TABLE 11.4 Diet-Related Psychosocial Factors Suitable for Intervention Evaluation

Theoretical model	Key constructs	References
Utilization of health services	Predisposing (knowledge, attitudes, beliefs) Enabling (barriers, norms) Reinforcing (social support)	[82,111,112]
The theory of reasoned action	Intention	[112−114]
Health belief model	Perceived benefits, susceptibility, and severity	[112,115,116]
Social learning theory	Self-efficacy	[117]
Transtheoretical model	Stages of change	[80,118−120]

from other behavioral domains, it is important to remember that dietary behavior is unique. First, dietary behavior is not a single behavior but a composite of many behaviors consisting of food choice, preparation, and frequency of consumption. Psychosocial factors related to one aspect of dietary behavior may differ from those relating to another. Second, dietary behavior is not discrete, such as smoking; rather, it occurs on a continuum in which any discrete definition of desirable dietary behavior is necessarily arbitrary (e.g., <30% energy from fat). Thus, diet-related psychosocial factors related to a discrete criterion, such as eating five or more servings a day of fruits and vegetables, may not capture the intent of an intervention to simply increase servings regardless of baseline intake.

One of the most popular approaches to organizing dietary intervention programs is based on using the "stage of change" construct from the transtheoretical model [78]. Interventions are designed to move participants from pre-action stages of dietary change (precontemplation, contemplation, and decision) into action and then maintenance. There is increasing evidence that interventions can move people through stages of dietary change [79], and that movement through stages of change is associated with dietary behavior change [16,17]. However, much controversy surrounds the conceptualization of stages of change when applied to dietary behavior and thus little agreement exists in the literature on how it should be assessed [79–81].

A second popular approach for organizing nutrition interventions is precede/proceed, which is not a behavioral model but, rather, a planning model for intervention development and delivery. Practical measures of the main constructs from this model—predisposing, enabling, and reinforcing factors—have been developed and validated [19,82]. One study demonstrated that change in these factors, in addition to stage of dietary change, explained up to 55% of the intervention effect in a large randomized trial [17].

C Environmental and Surrogate Measures of Diet

Table 11.5 gives an overview of environmental indicators and other surrogate measures that can be used to assess outcomes of dietary interventions. With the exception of household food inventories, these measures are only useful to evaluate intervention outcomes at the group or community level, and thus they are best suited to evaluate environmental-level interventions.

Household food inventories consist of asking a set of questions about whether or not specific foods are

TABLE 11.5 Surrogate and Environmental Measures Suitable for Intervention Evaluation

Measure	References
Individual or household level	[84,87]
Household food (pantry) inventory	
Group or community level	
Cafeteria plate observation	[121]
Cafeteria sales	[94,95]
Vending machine sales	[93]
Supermarket sales	[89]
Supermarket environment	

currently available in the household. Characteristically, the list consists of 10–15 foods that relate to the intervention. Examples of foods that could be included are types of staple foods (e.g., regular versus low-fat mayonnaise) or the types of foods available for snacks (potato chips, fresh fruit, or baby carrots). There are no studies that formally evaluate household inventories as intervention outcome measures, but there is evidence that study participants can recall foods in their households accurately [83] and that the types of foods correlate with individually assessed nutrient intake [84,85]. Because of the simplicity of this approach, further efforts to evaluate these measures are well motivated.

Monitoring food sales can be used as a direct measure of an intervention effect, but it is extraordinarily challenging [86–89]. Relating changes in supermarket sales to nutrition interventions is difficult, and most interventions attempting this approach have failed. Reasons are many, including the complexity of the food supply, the large number of food items that are sold in typical supermarkets, business confidentiality of sales data, and poor match between the data needs for business and the needs of nutrition researchers. Careful planning, pilot studies, and ongoing contact between researchers and persons responsible for data collection are necessary to make supermarket sales data useful for outcome evaluation. Monitoring sales in food services such as worksite and school cafeterias or vending machines is much simpler and has been used successfully to evaluate interventions [90–95]. One good approach is to devise a simple scheme for unobtrusively observing and recording food choices as customers move through a cafeteria line [96].

Changes in the food environment, such as supermarket signage or distribution of supermarket shelf space, are also potential surrogate measures of intervention outcomes. A series of studies has shown that it is possible to reliably measure supermarket environments, that measures of shelf space correlate with community-level measures of diet, and that changes in supermarket shelf space correlate weakly with changes in community-level diet [97–101]. It is possible that changes in supermarket signage or foods offered in restaurants could reflect an effective community-level intervention, as businesses adjust to demands from consumers for information about and access to healthier foods. These are not likely to be sensitive measures because the supermarket environment is saturated with signage, and restaurant menus are difficult to evaluate objectively.

VII CONCLUSION

Evaluations of nutrition interventions can be both scientifically and operationally challenging. Nutritionists can and should take the lead in conceptualizing and interpreting the evaluation of a nutrition intervention, but they should also seek collaborations or consultations with scientists in other disciplines to ensure that methods are optimal. When planning an evaluation, make sure that the time line allows you to test, pilot, and, if necessary, refine measures and procedures, even if you are using previously developed instruments and methods. Know that your measures will have sufficient responsiveness to detect an intervention effect. Make sure that your measures assess the behaviors targeted by the intervention and that the effect sizes you expect are reasonable. These steps are often expensive and slow, but the ultimate result of using appropriate evaluation methods is that you will obtain clearly interpretable and valid results.

References

[1] T. Baranowski, Advances in basic behavioral research will make the most important contributions to effective dietary change programs at this time, J. Am. Diet. Assoc. 106 (2006) 808–811.

[2] B. Caan, R. Ballard-Barbash, M.L. Slattery, J.L. Pinsky, F.L. Iber, D.J. Mateski, et al., Low energy reporting may increase in intervention participants enrolled in dietary intervention trials, J. Am. Diet. Assoc. 104 (2004) 357–366.

[3] T. Baranowski, D.D. Allen, L.C. Masse, M. Wilson, Does participation in an intervention affect responses on self-reported questionnaires? Health Educ. Res. 21 (2006) i98–i109.

[4] A. Bandura, Social Foundations of Thought and Action: A Social Cognitive Theory, Prentice-Hall, Englewood Cliffs, NJ, 1986.

[5] D.P. MacKinnon, J.H. Dwyer, Estimating mediated effect in prevention studies, Eval. Rev. 17 (1993) 144–148.

[6] W.B. Hansen, R.B. McNeal, The law of maximum expected potential effect: constraints placed on program effectiveness by mediator relationships, Health Educ. Res. 11 (1996) 501–507.

[7] T. Baranowski, L.S. Lin, D.W. Wetter, K. Resnicow, M.D. Hearn, Theory as mediating variables: why aren't community interventions working as desired? Ann. Epidemiol. 7 (1997) S89–S95.

[8] C. Framson, A.R. Kristal, J.M. Schenk, A.J. Littman, S. Zeliadt, D. Benitez, Development and validation of the mindful eating questionnaire, J. Am. Diet. Assoc. 109 (8) (2009) 1439–1444.

[9] K. Glanz, A. Steffen, Development and reliability testing for measures of psychosocial constructs associated with adolescent girls' calcium intake, J. Am. Diet. Assoc. 108 (5) (2008) 857–861.

[10] S.A. Beresford, S.J. Curry, A.R. Kristal, D. Lazovich, Z. Feng, E.H. Wagner, A dietary intervention in primary care practice: the eating patterns study, Am. J. Public Health 87 (1997) 610–616.

[11] A.R. Kristal, A.L. Shattuck, D.J. Bowen, R.W. Sponzo, D.W. Nixon, Feasibility of using volunteer research staff to deliver and evaluate a low-fat dietary intervention: the American Cancer Society Breast Cancer Dietary Intervention project, Cancer Epidemiol. Biomarkers Prev. 6 (1997) 459–467.

[12] A.R. Kristal, S.J. Curry, A.L. Shattuck, Z. Feng, S. Li, A randomized trial of a tailored, self-help dietary intervention: The Puget Sound Eating Patterns Study, Prev. Med. 31 (2000) 380–389.

[13] S.A. French, M. Story, J.A. Fulkerson, J.H. Himes, P. Hannan, D. Neumark-Sztainer, et al., Increasing weight-bearing physical activity and calcium-rich foods to promote bone mass gains among 9–11 year old girls: outcomes of the Cal-Girls study, Int. J. Behav. Nutr. Phys. Act. 2 (2005) 1–11.

[14] T.D. Koepsell, P.H. Diehr, A. Cheadle, A. Kristal, Invited commentary: symposium at community intervention trials, Am. J. Epidemiol. 142 (1995) 594–599.

[15] T.D. Koepsell, E.H. Wagner, A.C. Cheadle, D.L. Patrick, D.C. Martin, P.H. Diehr, et al., Selected methodological issues in evaluating community-based health promotion and disease prevention programs, Annu. Rev. Nutr. 13 (1992) 31–57.

[16] K. Glanz, R.E. Patterson, A.R. Kristal, Z. Feng, L. Linnan, J. Heimendinger, et al., Impact of worksite health promotion on stages of dietary change: The Working Well trial, Health Educ. Behav. 25 (1998) 448–463.

[17] A.R. Kristal, K. Glanz, B.C. Tilley, S. Li, Mediating factors in dietary change: understanding the impact of a worksite nutrition intervention, Health Educ. Behav. 27 (2000) 112–125.

[18] J.C. Nunally, I.H. Bernstein, Psychometric Theory, McGraw-Hill, New York, 1994.

[19] K. Glanz, A.R. Kristal, G. Sorensen, R. Palombo, J. Heimendinger, C. Probart, Development and validation of measures of psychosocial factors influencing fat- and fiber-related dietary behavior, Prev. Med. 22 (1993) 373–387.

[20] I. Ajzen, M. Fishbein, Understanding Attitudes and Predicting Social Behavior, Prentice Hall, Englewood Cliffs, NJ, 1980.

[21] R.K. Johnson, R.P. Soultanakis, D.E. Matthews, Literacy and body fatness are associated with underreporting of energy intake in U.S. low-income women using the multiple-pass 24-hour recall: a doubly labeled water study, J. Am. Diet. Assoc. 98 (1998) 1136–1140.

[22] S.M. Rebro, R.E. Patterson, A.R. Kristal, C.L. Cheney, The effect of keeping food records on eating patterns, J. Am. Diet. Assoc. 98 (1998) 1163–1165.

[23] A.R. Kristal, Z. Feng, R.J. Coates, A. Oberman, V. George, Associations of race, ethnicity, education and dietary intervention on validity and reliability of a food frequency questionnaire in the Women's Health Initiative Feasibility Study in Minority Populations, Am. J. Epidemiol. 146 (1997) 856–869.

[24] J. Forster, R. Jeffrey, M. Van Natta, P. Pirie, Hypertension prevention trial: do 24-h food records capture usual eating behavior in a dietary change study? Am. J. Clin. Nutr. 51 (1990) 253–257.

[25] J.R. Hebert, L. Clemow, L. Pbert, J. Ockene, Social desirability bias in dietary self-report may compromise the validity of dietary intake measures, Int. J. Epidemiol. 24 (1995) 389–398.

[26] J.R. Herbert, Y. Ma, L. Clemow, I.S. Ockene, G. Saperia, E.J. Stanek, et al., Gender differences in social desirability and social approval bias in dietary self-report, Am. J. Epidemiol. 146 (1997) 1046–1055.

[27] A.R. Kristal, C.H.A. Andrilla, T.D. Koepsell, P.H. Diehr, A. Cheadle, Dietary assessment instruments are susceptible to intervention-associated response set bias, J. Am. Diet. Assoc. 98 (1998) 40–43.

[28] A.R. Kristal, S.A.A. Beresford, D. Lazovich, Assessing change in diet-intervention research, Am. J. Clin. Nutr. 59 (Suppl.) (1994) 185S–189S.

[29] S. Weinrich, M. Boyde, B. Pow, Tool adaptation for socioeconomically disadvantaged populations, in: M. Stromburd, S. Olson (Eds.), Instruments for Clinical Health Care Research, Jones & Bartlett, Norwalk, CT, 1997, pp. 20–29.

[30] G. Arroyave, L.A. Mejia, J. Aguilar, The effect of vitamin A fortification of sugar on the serum vitamin A levels of preschool Guatemalan children, Am. J. Clin. Nutr. 34 (1981) 41–49.

[31] L. Sheppard, A.R. Kristal, L.H. Kushi, Weight loss in women participating in randomized low-fat diets, Am. J. Clin. Nutr. 54 (1991) 821–828.

[32] J.O. Hill, J.C. Peters, Environmental contributions to the obesity epidemic, Science 280 (1998) 1371–1375.

[33] A. Drewnowski, C.L. Rock, S.A. Henderson, A.B. Shore, C. Fischler, P. Galan, et al., Serum beta-carotene and vitamin C as biomarkers of vegetable and fruit intakes in a community-based sample of French adults, Arch. Intern. Med. 65 (1997) 1796–1802.

[34] C.L. Rock, S.W. Flatt, F.A. Wright, S. Faerber, V. Newman, J.P. Pierce, Responsiveness of carotenoids to a high vegetable diet intervention designed to prevent breast cancer recurrence, Cancer Epidemiol. Biomarkers Prev. 6 (1997) 617–623.

[35] C.L. Rock, M.D. Thornquist, A.R. Kristal, R.E. Patterson, D.A. Cooper, M.L. Newhouser, et al., Demographic, dietary and lifestyle factors differentially explain variability in serum carotenoids and fat soluble vitamins: baseline results from the Olestra Post-Marketing Surveillance Study, J. Nutr. 129 (1999) 855–864.

[36] S.P. Murphy, L.L. Kaiser, M.S. Townsend, L.H. Allen, Evaluation of validity of items for a food behavior checklist, J. Am. Diet. Assoc. 101 (2001) 761.

[37] D.R. Campbell, M.D. Gross, M.C. Martini, G.A. Grandits, J.L. Slavin, J.D. Potter, Plasma carotenoids as biomarkers of vegetable and fruit intake, Cancer Epidemiol. Biomarkers Prev. 3 (1994) 493–500.

[38] M.J. Mazier, P.J. Jones, Dietary fat saturation, but not the feeding state, modulates rates of cholesterol esterification in normolipidemic men, Metabolism 48 (1999) 1210–1215.

[39] A.L. Holmes, B. Sanderson, R. Maisiak, A. Brown, V. Bittner, Dietitian services are associated with improved patient outcomes and the MEDFICTS dietary assessment questionnaire is a suitable outcome measure in cardiac rehabilitation, J. Am. Diet. Assoc. 105 (2005) 1533–1540.

[40] S.T. Mayne, B. Cartmel, S. Scarmo, H. Lin, D.J. Leffell, E. Welch, et al., Noninvasive assessment of dermal carotenoids as a biomarker of fruit and vegetable intake, Am. J. Clin. Nutr. 92 (4) (2010) 794–800.

[41] National Cancer Institute, ASA24: Automated Self-Administered 24-Hour Recall, Version 1. National Cancer Institute, Bethesda, MD, 2011. Available at http://riskfactor.cancer.gov/tools/instruments/asa24

[42] K. Lui, Measurement error and its impact on partial correlation and multiple regression analysis, Am. J. Epidemiol. 127 (1988) 864–874.

[43] P.S. Haines, A.M. Siega-Riz, B.M. Popkin, The Diet Quality Index Revised: a measurement instrument for populations, J. Am. Diet. Assoc. 99 (1999) 697–704.

[44] R.E. Patterson, P.S. Haines, B.M. Popkin, Diet Quality Index: capturing a multidimensional behavior, J. Am. Diet. Assoc. 94 (1994) 57–64.

[45] D.C. Snyder, R. Sloane, P.S. Haines, P. Miller, E.C. Clipp, M.C. Morey, et al., The Diet Quality Index-Revised: a tool to promote and evaluate dietary change among older cancer survivors enrolled in a home-based intervention trial, J. Am. Diet. Assoc. 107 (2007) 1519–1529.

[46] A.F. Smith, J.B. Jobe, D.J. Mingay, Retrieval from memory of dietary information, Appl. Cogn. Psychol. 5 (1991) 269–296.

[47] A.R. Kristal, A.L. Shattuck, A.E. Williams, Food frequency questionnaires for diet intervention research, in:17th National Nutrient Databank Conference, International Life Sciences Institute, Baltimore, MD, 1992, pp. 110–125.

[48] G. Block, A.M. Hartman, C.M. Dresser, M.D. Carroll, J. Gannon, L. Gardner, A data-based approach to diet questionnaire design and testing, Am. J. Epidemiol. 124 (4) (1986) 53–469.

[49] G. Block, L.M. Coyle, A.M. Hartman, S.M. Scoppa, Revision of dietary analysis software for the Health Habits and History Questionnaire, Am. J. Epidemiol. 139 (1994) 1190–1196.

[50] R.E. Patterson, A.R. Kristal, R.A. Carter, L. Fels-Tinker, M.P. Bolton, T. Agurs-Collins, Measurement characteristics of the Women's Health Initiative food frequency questionnaire, Ann. Epidemiol. 9 (1999) 178–187.

[51] G. Block, C. Clifford, M.P. Naughton, M. Henderson, M. McAdams, A brief dietary screen for high fat intake, J. Nutr. Educ. 21 (1989) 199–207.

[52] S.R. Cummings, G. Block, K. McHenry, R.B. Baron, Evaluation of two food frequency methods of measuring dietary calcium intake, Am. J. Epidemiol. 126 (1987) 796–802.

[53] M. Serdula, R. Coates, T. Byers, A. Mokdad, S. Jewell, N. Chavez, et al., Evaluation of a brief telephone questionnaire to estimate fruit and vegetable consumption in diverse study populations, Epidemiology 4 (1993) 455–463.

[54] A.E. Field, G.A. Colditz, M.K. Fox, T. Byers, M. Serdula, R.J. Bosch, et al., Comparison of 4 questionnaires for assessment of fruit and vegetable intake, Am. J. Public Health 88 (1998) 1216–1218.

[55] M.K. Hunt, A.M. Stoddard, K. Peterson, G. Sorensen, J.R. Herbert, N. Cohen, Comparison of dietary assessment measures in the Treatwell 5 A Day worksite study, J. Am. Diet. Assoc. 98 (1998) 1021–1023.

[56] A.R. Kristal, N.C. Vizenor, R.E. Patterson, M.L. Neuhouser, A.L. Shattuck, Validity of food frequency based measures of fruit and vegetable intakes, Cancer Epidemiol. Biomarkers Prev. 9 (2000) 939–944.

[57] G. Block, C.M. Dresser, A.M. Hartman, M.D. Carroll, Nutrient sources in the American diet: quantitative data from the NHANES II survey. II. Macronutrients and fats, Am. J. Epidemiol. 122 (1985) 27–38.

[58] G. Block, C.M. Dresser, A.M. Hartman, M.D. Carroll, Nutrient sources in the American diet: Quantitative data from the NHANES II survey. I. Vitamins and minerals, Am. J. Epidemiol. 122 (1985) 13–26.

[59] J.K. Jensen, D. Gustafson, C.J. Boushey, G. Auld, M.A. Bock, C.M. Bruhn, et al., Development of a food frequency questionnaire to measure calcium intake of Asian, Hispanic, and White youth, J. Am. Diet. Assoc. 104 (2004) 762–769.

[60] T. Byers, J. Marshall, R. Fielder, M. Zielezny, S. Graham, Assessing nutrient intake with an abbreviated dietary interview, Am. J. Epidemiol. 122 (1985) 41–50.

[61] G.E. Gray, A. Paganini-Hill, R.K. Ross, B.E. Henderson, Assessment of three brief methods of estimation of vitamin A and C intakes for a prospective study of cancer: comparison with dietary history, Am. J. Epidemiol. 119 (1984) 581–590.

B. RESEARCH AND APPLIED METHODS FOR OBSERVATIONAL AND INTERVENTION STUDIES

[62] J.H. Hankin, H.B. Messinger, R.A. Stallones, A short dietary method for epidemiological studies: IV. Evaluation of questionnaire, Am. J. Epidemiol. 91 (1968) 562–567.

[63] J.H. Hankin, V. Rawlings, A. Nomura, Assessment of a short dietary method for a prospective study on cancer, Am. J. Clin. Nutr. 31 (1978) 355–359.

[64] A.R. Kristal, A.L. Shattuck, H.J. Henry, Patterns of dietary behavior associated with selecting diets low in fat: reliability and validity of a behavioral approach to dietary assessment, J. Am. Diet. Assoc. 90 (1990) 214–220.

[65] J. Shannon, A.R. Kristal, S.J. Curry, S.A. Beresford, Application of a behavioral approach to measuring dietary change: the fat- and fiber-related diet behavior questionnaire, Cancer Epidemiol. Biomarkers Prev. 6 (1997) 355–361.

[66] S.L. Conner, J.R. Gustafson, G. Sexton, N. Becker, S. Artaud-Wild, W.E. Conner, The Diet Habit Survey: a new method of dietary assessment that relates to plasma cholesterol changes, J. Am. Diet. Assoc. 92 (1992) 41–47.

[67] K. Gans, S. Sundaram, J. McPhillips, M. Hixson, L. Linnan, R. Carleson, Rate your plate: an eating pattern assessment and educational tool that relates to plasma cholesterol changes, J. Nutr. Educ. 25 (1993) 29–36.

[68] J.R. Peters, E.S. Quiter, M.L. Brekke, J. Admire, M.J. Brekke, R.M. Mullins, et al., The eating pattern assessment tool: a simple instrument for assessing dietary fat and cholesterol intake, J. Am. Diet. Assoc. 94 (1994) 1008–1013.

[69] A.R. Kristal, E. White, A.L. Shattuck, S. Curry, G.L. Anderson, A. Fowler, et al., Long-term maintenance of a low-fat diet: durability of fat-related dietary habits in the Women's Health Trial, J. Am. Diet. Assoc. 92 (1992) 553–559.

[70] A.R. Kristal, A.L. Shattuck, R.E. Patterson, Differences in fat related dietary patterns between black, Hispanic, and white women: results from the Women's Health Trial Feasibility Study in minority populations, Public Health Nutr. 2 (1999) 273–276.

[71] S. Kinlay, R.F. Heller, J.A. Halliday, A simple score and questionnaire to measure group changes in dietary fat intake, Prev. Med. 20 (1991) 378–388.

[72] T.J. Hartman, P.R. McCarthy, J.H. Himes, Use of eating-pattern messages to evaluate changes in eating behaviors in a worksite cholesterol education program, J. Am. Diet. Assoc. 93 (1993) 1119–1123.

[73] T.J. Hartman, P.R. McCarthy, R.J. Park, E. Schuster, L. Kushi, Results of a community-based low-literacy nutrition education program, J. Community Health 22 (1997) 325–341.

[74] R.E. Glasgow, J.D. Perry, D.J. Toobert, J.F. Hollins, Brief assessments of dietary behavior in field settings, Addict. Behav. 21 (1996) 239–247.

[75] A.R. Kristal, B.F. Abrams, M.D. Thornquist, L. DiSorga, R.T. Croyle, A.L. Shattuck, et al., Development and validation of a food use checklist for evaluation of community nutrition interventions, Am. J. Public Health 80 (1990) 1318–1322.

[76] M.L. Neuhouser, R.E. Patterson, A.R. Kristal, A.L. Eldridge, N.C. Vizenor, A brief dietary assessment instrument for assessing target foods, nutrients and eating patterns, Public Health Nutr. 4 (2000) 73–78.

[77] K. Glanz, F.M. Lewis, B.K. Rimer, Health Behavior and Health Education Theory, Research, and Practice, Jossey-Bass, San Francisco, 1997.

[78] J.O. Prochaska, W.F. Velicer, The transtheoretical model of health behavior change, Am. J. Health Promot. 12 (1997) 38–48.

[79] A.R. Kristal, K. Glanz, S.J. Curry, R.E. Patterson, How can stages of change be best used in dietary interventions? J. Am. Diet. Assoc. 99 (1999) 679–684.

[80] R. Povey, M. Conner, P. Sparks, R. James, R. Shepherd, A critical examination of the application of the transtheoretical model's stages of change to dietary behaviours, Health Educ. Res. 14 (1999) 641–651.

[81] G.W. Greene, S.R. Rossi, J.S. Rossi, W.F. Velicer, J.L. Fava, J.O. Prochaska, Dietary applications of the stages of change model, J. Am. Diet. Assoc. 99 (1999) 673–678.

[82] K. Glanz, A.R. Kristal, B.C. Tilley, K. Hirst, Psychosocial correlates of healthful diets among male autoworkers, Cancer Epidemiol. Biomarkers Prev. 7 (1998) 119–126.

[83] S.J. Crocket, J.D. Potter, M.S. Wright, A. Bacheller, Validation of a self-reported shelf inventory to measure food purchases behavior, J. Am. Diet. Assoc. 92 (1992) 694–697.

[84] J.A. Satia, R.E. Patterson, A. Kristal, M. Pineda, T.G. Hislop, A household food inventory for North American Chinese, Public Health Nutr. 2 (2001) 241–247.

[85] R.E. Patterson, A.R. Kristal, J. Shannon, J.R. Hunt, E. White, Using a brief household inventory as an environmental indicator of individual dietary practices, Am. J. Public Health 87 (1997) 272–275.

[86] R. Shucker, A. Levy, J. Tenny, O. Mathews, Nutrition self-labeling and consumer purchase behavior, J. Nutr. 24 (1992) 553–559.

[87] B.H. Patterson, L.G. Kessler, Y. Wax, A. Bernstein, L. Light, D.N. Midthune, et al., Evaluation of a supermarket intervention, Eval. Res. 16 (2002) 464–490.

[88] A.R. Kristal, L. Goldenhar, J. Muldoon, R.F. Morton, A randomized trial of a supermarket intervention to increase consumption of fruits and vegetables, Am. J. Health Promot. 11 (1997) 422–425.

[89] J. Odenkirchen, B. Portnoy, J. Blair, A. Rodgers, L. Light, J. Tenny, In-store monitoring of a supermarket nutrition intervention, Fam. Community Health 14 (1992) 1–9.

[90] C.S. Wilbur, S.M. Zifferblatt, J.L. Pinsky, S. Zifferblatt, Healthy vending: a cooperative pilot research program to stimulate good health in the marketplace, Prev. Med. 10 (1981) 85–89.

[91] M.F. Schmitz, J.E. Fielding, Point-of-choice nutrition labeling: evaluation in a worksite cafeteria, J. Nutr. Educ. 19 (1986) 85–92.

[92] P.M. Cincirpini, Changing food selections in a public cafeteria, Behav. Modif. 8 (1984) 520–539.

[93] S.M. Hoerr, V.A. Louden, Can nutrition information increase sales of healthful vended snacks? J. Sch. Health 63 (1993) 386–390.

[94] R.W. Jeffery, S.A. French, C. Raether, J.E. Baxter, An environmental intervention to increase fruit and salad purchases in a cafeteria, Prev. Med. 23 (1994) 788–792.

[95] C.C. Perlmutter, D.D. Canter, M.B. Gregoire, Profitability and acceptability of fat- and sodium-modified hot entrees in a worksite cafeteria, J. Am. Diet. Assoc. 97 (1997) 391–395.

[96] J. Mayer, T. Brown, J. Heins, D. Bishop, A multi-component intervention for modifying food selection in a worksite cafeteria, J. Nutr. Educ. 6 (1987) 277–280.

[97] A. Cheadle, B. Psaty, E. Wagner, P. Diehr, T. Koepsell, S. Curry, et al., Evaluating community-based nutrition programs: assessing reliability of a survey of grocery store product displays, Am. J. Public Health 80 (1990) 709–711.

[98] A. Cheadle, B.M. Psaty, S. Curry, E. Wagner, P. Diehr, T. Koepsell, et al., Community-level comparisons between the grocery store environment and individual dietary practices, Prev. Med. 20 (1991) 250–261.

[99] A. Cheadle, E. Wagner, T. Koepsell, A. Kristal, D. Patrick, Environmental indicators: a tool for evaluating community-based health-promotion programs, Am. J. Prev. Med. 9 (1992) 78–84.

[100] A. Cheadle, B.M. Psaty, S. Curry, E. Wagner, P. Diehr, T. Koepsell, et al., Can measures of the grocery story environment be used to track community-level dietary changes? Prev. Med. 22 (1993) 361–372.

[101] A. Cheadle, B. Psaty, P. Diehr, T. Koepsell, E. Wagner, S. Curry, et al., Evaluating community-based nutrition programs: comparing grocery store and individual-level survey measures of program impact, Prev. Med. 24 (1995) 71–79.

[102] S.C. Karr, J.W. Lampe, A.M. Hutchins, J.L. Slavin, Urinary isoflavonoid excretion in humans is dose-dependent at low to moderate levels of soy protein consumption, Am. J. Clin. Nutr. 66 (1997) 46–51.

[103] A. Seow, C.C. Shi, A.A. Franke, J.H. Hankin, H.P. Lee, M.C. Yu, Isoflavonoid levels in spot urine are associated with frequency of dietary soy intake in a population-based sample of middle-aged and older Chinese in Singapore, Cancer Epidemiol. Biomarkers Prev. 7 (1998) 135–140.

[104] J.L. Stanford, I. King, A.R. Kristal, Long-term storage of red blood cells and correlations between red cell and dietary fatty acids: results from a pilot study, Nutr. Cancer 16 (1991) 183–188.

[105] J. Agren, O. Hanninen, A. Julkunen, L. Fogelholm, H. Vidgred, U. Schwab, et al., Fish diet, fish oil and docosahexaenoic acid rich oil lower fasting and postprandial plasma lipid levels, Eur. J. Clin. Nutr. 50 (1996) 765–771.

[106] M.L. Burr, A.M. Fehily, J.F. Gilbert, S. Rogers, R.M. Holliday, P.M. Sweetnam, et al., Effects of changes in fat, fish, and fibre intakes on death and myocardial reinfarction: Diet and Reinfarction Trial (DART), Lancet 2 (1989) 757–761.

[107] F. Chung, D. Jiao, S. Getahun, M. Yu, A urinary biomarker for uptake of dietary isothiocyanates in humans, Cancer Epidemiol. Biomarkers Prev. 7 (1998) 103–108.

[108] A. Seow, C. Shi, F. Chung, D. Jioa, J. Hankin, H. Lee, et al., Urinary total isothiocyanate (ITC) in a population-based sample of middle-aged and older Chinese in Singapore: relationship with dietary total ITC and glutathione S-transferase MI/TI/PI genotypes, Cancer Epidemiol. Biomarkers Prev. 7 (1998) 775–781.

[109] J. McDougall, K. Litzau, E. Haver, V. Saunders, G. Spiller, Rapid reduction of serum cholesterol and blood pressure by a twelve-day, very low fat, strictly vegetarian diet, J. Am. Coll. Nutr. 14 (1995) 491–496.

[110] W.H. Howell, D.J. McNamara, M.A. Tosca, B.T. Smith, J.A. Gaines, Plasma lipid and lipoprotein responses to dietary fat and cholesterol: a meta-analysis, Am. J. Clin. Nutr. 65 (1997) 1747–1764.

[111] L.W. Green, M.W. Kreuter, Health Promotion Planning: An Educational and Environmental Approach, Mayfield, Mountain View, CA, 1991.

[112] G. Paradis, J. O'Loughlin, M. Elliot, P. Masson, L. Renaud, G. Sacks-Silver, et al., Coeur en sante St.-Henri: a heart health promotion programme in a low income, low education neighborhood in Montreal, Canada: theoretical model and early field experience, J. Epidemiol. Community Health 49 (1995) 503–512.

[113] N.J. Richardson, R. Shepherd, N.A. Elliman, Current attitudes and future influences on meat consumption in the U.K, Appetite 21 (1993) 41–51.

[114] J.L. Brewer, A.J. Blake, S.A. Rankin, L.W. Douglass, Theory of reasoned action predicts milk consumption in women, J. Am. Diet. Assoc. 99 (1999) 33–44.

[115] A.S. Kloeblen, S.S. Batish, Understanding the intention to permanently follow a high folate diet among a sample of low-income pregnant women according to the health belief model, Health Educ. Res. 14 (1999) 327–388.

[116] R.B. Schafer, P.M. Keith, E. Schafer, Predicting fat in diets of marital partners using the health belief model, J. Behav. Med. 18 (1995) 419–433.

[117] A. Ling, C. Howarth, Self-efficacy and consumption of fruit and vegetables: validation of a summated scale, Am. J. Health Promot. 13 (1999) 290–298.

[118] K. Glanz, R.E. Patterson, A.R. Kristal, C.C. DiClemente, J. Heimendinger, L. Linnan, et al., Stages of change in adopting healthy diets: fat, fiber, and correlates of nutrient intake, Health Educ. Q. 21 (1994) 499–519.

[119] M.K. Campbell, M. Symons, W. Demark-Wahnefried, B. Polhamus, J.M. Bernhardt, J.W. McClelland, et al., Stages of change and psychosocial correlates of fruit and vegetable consumption among rural African-American church members, Am. J. Health Promot. 12 (1998) 185–191.

[120] S. Nitzke, G. Auld, J. McNulty, M. Bock, C. Bruhn, K. Gabel, et al., Stages of change for reducing fat and increasing fiber among dietitians and adults with diet-related chronic disease, J. Am. Diet. Assoc. 99 (1999) 728–731.

[121] K. Graves, B. Shannon, Using visual plate waste measurement to assess school lunch behavior, J. Am. Diet. Assoc. 83 (1983) 163–165.

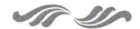

Biomarkers and Their Use in Nutrition Intervention

*Amanda J. Cross**, *Johanna W. Lampe*[†], *Cheryl L. Rock*[‡]

[*]**National Cancer Institute, National Institutes of Health, Department of Health and Human Services, Rockville, Maryland** [†]**Fred Hutchinson Cancer Research Center, Seattle, Washington** [‡]**University of California at San Diego, La Jolla, California**

I INTRODUCTION

A biomarker or biological indicator is a characteristic that is measured and evaluated as a marker of normal biological processes, pathogenic processes, or responses to an intervention. In theory, almost any measurement that reflects a change in a biochemical process, structure, or function can be used as a biomarker. In addition, an exogenous compound that, as a result of ingestion, inhalation, or absorption, can be measured in tissues or body fluids can also be considered a biomarker.

Biomarkers can be classified broadly into markers of exposure, effect, and susceptibility and have numerous applications in nutrition. They can be used to assess dietary intakes (exposure), biochemical or physiological responses to a dietary behavior or nutrition intervention (effect), a clinical endpoint or disease outcome (surrogate endpoint biomarker), and predisposition to a disease or response to treatment (genetic susceptibility).

Although clinicians have used certain biological markers, such as serum cholesterol and glucose, for generations, the use of biomarkers has taken on new importance with the dramatic advances in various fields of biology and desire for objective measures in large-scale, population-based, descriptive and intervention nutrition research. Exquisitely sensitive laboratory techniques can detect subtle alterations in molecular processes that reflect events known or believed to occur along the continuum between health and disease.

This chapter presents the basic concepts and key issues related to the various uses of biomarkers in nutrition intervention research; it is not intended to be a comprehensive review. Identification and use of biomarkers is continuously evolving with the growing understanding of biological processes and the improved sensitivity of laboratory assays. Consequently, our examples of existing biomarkers are snapshots of the greater scheme of biomarker development and application.

II BIOMARKERS OF DIETARY INTAKE OR EXPOSURE

Biomarkers are used to monitor dietary exposure and for nutritional assessment for several reasons. One reason is to provide biochemical data on nutritional status by generating objective evidence that enables the evaluation of dietary adequacy or ranking of individuals on exposure to particular nutrients or dietary constituents. Biochemical or biological measurements may also be collected to characterize objectively a dietary pattern, such as fruit and vegetable consumption; to validate dietary assessment instruments or self-reported dietary data; or to monitor compliance to a dietary intervention. Another purpose for obtaining these biological measures is to establish the biological link between the nutritional factor and a physiological or biochemical process—often a hallmark of nutrition intervention studies—when the concentration of the micronutrient or dietary constituent is measured in a peripheral tissue.

Biomarkers of dietary intake can be classified as either recovery biomarkers, which are considered the best, or concentration biomarkers. Recovery biomarkers reflect

Nutrition in the Prevention and Treatment of Disease, Third Edition.
DOI: http://dx.doi.org/10.1016/B978-0-12-391884-0.00012-3

absolute intake over a defined period of time; an example is nitrogen in 24-hour urine collections as a recovery biomarker of dietary protein intake [1]. Concentration biomarkers, on the other hand, are correlated with intake but cannot be used to calculate an absolute level of intake; an example of a concentration biomarker is plasma vitamin E [2].

A Biomarkers of Energy Intake

To date, few biological measures are available that objectively monitor overall energy intake, and those that are available are cumbersome in free-living populations or expensive. Under steady-state conditions, indirect calorimetry provides an estimate of energy expenditure and some insight about intake. Indirect calorimetry estimates the rate of oxidation or energy expenditure from the rate of oxygen consumption (VO_2) and the rate of carbon dioxide production (VCO_2). This technique is relatively inexpensive and portable, although some participant cooperation is required. These traits make the technique attractive primarily for clinical applications [3].

Energy expenditure can also be measured using a doubly labeled water technique [4], as discussed in detail in Chapter 4, which is an example of a recovery biomarker in which energy intake is indirectly ascertained by measuring energy expenditure. This method uses nonradioactive isotopes of hydrogen (^{2}H) and oxygen (^{18}O) to measure free-living total energy expenditure by monitoring urinary isotope excretion. Energy expenditures determined by room calorimetry, indirect calorimetry, and doubly labeled water measures are not significantly different within the calorimeter environment; however, in free-living individuals, doubly labeled water-derived energy expenditures are found to be 13−15% higher than those for other methods [5]. The doubly labeled water method has the distinct advantage of allowing the study participants to go about their usual activities, with energy expenditure calculated after a study period of 7−14 days. Unfortunately, the ^{18}O isotope required to conduct doubly labeled water studies is expensive and is often in short supply. Although doubly labeled water methodology is suited to nutrition research aimed at quantifying total energy expenditure for specific groups, the cost for large samples limits broad use.

B Biomarkers of Nutrient Intake

Biochemical measures of nutrients can be a valuable component of nutritional assessment and monitoring. Overall, the usefulness of biochemical indicators of nutritional status or exposure is based on knowledge of the physiological and other determinants of the measure. For several micronutrients, the concentration of the nutrient in the circulating body pool (i.e., serum) appears to be a reasonably accurate reflection of overall status for the nutrient. In contrast, the amount of some micronutrients in the circulating pool may be homeostatically regulated when the storage pool is adequate, or may be unrelated to intake, and thus has little relationship with total body reserves or overall status. Figure 12.1 illustrates the relation between various compartments or body pools that may be sampled in the measurement of biological indicators.

Knowledge of the influencing nondietary factors is particularly important for accurate interpretation of the nutrient concentration in tissues. For example, tocopherols and carotenoids are transported in the circulation nonspecifically by the cholesterol-rich lipoproteins [6,7], so higher concentrations of these lipoproteins are predictive of higher concentrations of the associated micronutrients in the circulation, independent of dietary intake or total body pool. Smoking and alcohol consumption need to be considered in the interpretation of serum and other tissue concentrations of several micronutrients, particularly compounds that may be subject to oxidation (e.g., vitamin C, tocopherols, carotenoids, folate). Knowledge of the relationship between the indicator and the risk of nutrient depletion, in addition to the responsiveness of the indicator to interventions or change, is also necessary [8]. For some nutrients, a specific sensitive exposure marker of diet simply has not yet been identified.

Table 12.1 lists examples of biochemical measures of nutrients that may serve as useful biomarkers in nutritional assessment or monitoring of dietary intake; all of these are examples of concentration biomarkers and may not be proportionately related to intake because their levels are the result of other influencing factors. For more details, the reader is referred to in-depth reviews addressing the use of biomarkers for assessing nutrient exposure [9−12].

C Biomarkers of Other Dietary Exposures

Numerous dietary constituents, particularly of plant origin, although not recognized as essential for life, have demonstrated biological activity and are thought to play an important role in the prevention of chronic disease [13,14]. These phytochemicals are absorbed to various degrees, often metabolized in the intestinal epithelium and liver, and excreted; thus, the metabolites can be monitored in serum or plasma or urine.

Some classes of compounds such as flavonoids are found in many plant foods, whereas others such as isoflavones are limited to select sources (Table 12.2). The isoflavones daidzein and genistein are highly

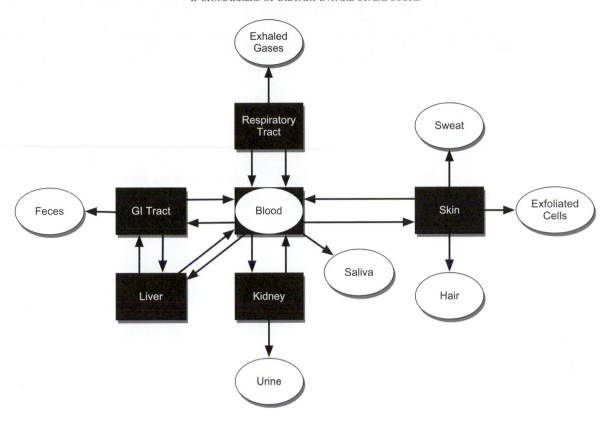

FIGURE 12.1 The relation between body compartments and biological specimens that can be assayed for dietary biomarkers.

concentrated in soybeans and soy products [15,16]. Urinary isoflavone excretion is associated strongly and directly with soy protein intake under controlled dietary conditions [17]. In intervention studies of soy foods or isoflavone supplementation, urinary isoflavonoid excretion and serum or plasma isoflavone concentrations are useful markers of study compliance [18,19]. However, because the plasma half-lives of the isoflavones genistein and daidzein are short (6—8 hours) [20], the timing of soy consumption in relation to urine or blood sampling may under- or overestimate isoflavone exposure. Metabolism of isoflavones is also linked to the health of colonic bacterial populations, and therefore the effects of diet and drugs on the colonic environment may influence plasma and urinary levels.

Dietary exposure to flavonoids and other polyphenols can be monitored by measuring parent compounds and metabolites in urine or plasma [21,22]. Several compounds in cruciferous vegetables, such as sulforaphane and other isothiocyanates, have been of interest because of their potential chemopreventive effects. Concentrations of these compounds and their metabolic derivatives can be measured in plasma and urine by liquid chromatography—mass spectrometry (LC-MS) [23]. In addition, dithiocarbamates (conversion products of isothiocyanates and their metabolites) can be quantified

readily in urine, following extraction and measurement by high-performance liquid chromatography (HPLC). Both of these approaches provide a way to monitor cruciferous-vegetable exposure during an intervention [24].

Biomarkers also exist for monitoring exposure to less desirable food constituents, such as mycotoxins (e.g., aflatoxin) in mold-contaminated grain products and pyrolysis products that result from cooking meat at high temperatures (e.g., heterocyclic amines). Because of the nature of these compounds, exposure to potentially carcinogenic compounds can be determined by measuring the presence of adducts—the result of covalent binding of the chemicals to proteins or to nucleic acids in DNA. The rationale for using measurements of carcinogen—DNA adducts is based on the assumption that DNA adducts formed *in vivo* are responsible for genetic alterations in genes critical for carcinogenesis and that protein adducts formed through the same processes reflect the formation of DNA adducts [25]. Because adducts represent an integration of exposure and interindividual variability in carcinogen metabolism and DNA repair, they may provide a more relevant measure of exposure (i.e., a biologically effective dose [25]). Some adducts are specific for dietary exposure; aflatoxin—albumin adducts result from ingestion of aflatoxin. Other adducts, such as benzo[*a*]pyrene—DNA

TABLE 12.1   Biomarkers of Nutrient Intake[a]

Nutrient	Biomarkers of dietary exposure	Possible functional markers
Dietary fiber, nonstarch polysaccharides	Fecal hemicellulose	Fecal weight
		Fecal short-chain fatty acids
	Urinary or plasma lignans	
	Urinary or plasma alkylresorcinols (whole grains)	
Thiamin		Erythrocyte transketolase activation
Biotin	Urinary 3-hydroxy-isovalerate with a loading dose of leucine	Erythrocyte pyruvate carboxylase activity
Riboflavin	Plasma FAD	EGRAC
	Erythrocyte FAD	
Niacin	Erythrocyte NAD	Erythrocyte nicotinate-nucleotide: pyrophosphate phosphoribosyltransferase activity (not very responsive)
	Urinary metabolites of niacin	
Vitamin B_6	Plasma pyridoxal 5-phosphate	Erythrocyte aspartate or alanine aminotransferase
	Urinary 4-pyridoxic acid	
Folate	Plasma folate	Plasma homocysteine
	Erythrocyte folate	
Vitamin B_{12}	Plasma B_{12}	
Vitamin C	Plasma vitamin C	Urinary deoxypyridinoline:total collagen cross-links
	Erythrocyte, lymphocyte, or platelet vitamin C	Urinary carnitine
Vitamin A	Plasma retinol:retinol-binding protein	
Vitamin E	α-and/or γ-tocopherol in serum or plasma, erythrocytes, lymphocytes, lipoproteins, adipose tissue, or buccal mucosal cells	LDL oxidation
		Breath pentane and ethane
		Platelet adhesion and aggregation
Vitamin D	Serum 25-hydroxyvitamin D	
Vitamin K	Plasma vitamin K	Plasma prothrombin concentrations
Phosphorus	Serum inorganic phosphate	
Magnesium	Erythrocyte or lymphocyte magnesium	
Calcium	Calcium retention	Bone mass
		Serum osteocalcin
		Serum levels of skeletal alkaline phosphatase
		Urinary and serum measures of collagen turnover
Iron		Serum ferritin[b]
		Transferrin saturation
		Erythrocyte protoporphyrin

(Continued)

TABLE 12.1 (*Continued*)

Nutrient	Biomarkers of dietary exposure	Possible functional markers
		Mean corpuscular volume
		Serum transferrin receptor
		Hemoglobin or packed cell volume
Copper	Platelet copper	Erythrocyte SOD
		Platelet cytochrome c oxidase activity
		Serum peptidylglycine α-aminating monooxygenase activity
		Plasma diamine oxidase
Zinc		Erythrocyte metallothionein
		Erythrocyte SOD
		Monocyte metallothionein mRNA
		Serum thymulin activity
		Plasma 5-nucleotidase activity
Manganese	Serum manganese	Lymphocyte Mn-SOD activity
		Blood arginase activity
Molybdenum		Urinary levels of sulfate, uric acid, sulfite, hypoxanthine, xanthine, and other sulfur-containing compounds
Iodine	Urinary or plasma iodine	Plasma TSH, T$_4$, and T$_3$ (total and free)
Selenium	Plasma or whole-blood selenium	Plasma GSH peroxidase activities
	Hair or toenail selenium	Erythrocyte GSH peroxidase activities
		Blood cell selenoperoxidase activities

[a]*Direct measures of dietary exposure and nutrient-specific functional markers. This table includes both established markers and additional markers that show promise.*
[b]*In approximate order of increasing severity of iron shortage [104].*
EGRAC, FAD-dependent erythrocyte glutathione reductase activation coefficient; FAD, flavin adenine dinucleotide; GSH, glutathione; LDL, low-density lipoprotein; NAD, nicotinamide adenine dinucleotide; SOD, superoxide dismutase; T$_3$, triiodothyronine; T$_4$, thyroxine; TSH, thyroid-stimulating hormone.

adducts, are nonspecific because benzo[*a*]pyrene comes from a variety of sources besides diet, including air pollution, tobacco, and occupational exposures. Adducts can be used to monitor exposure within individuals. They can also serve as early markers of the efficacy of interventions designed to prevent exposure to genotoxic agents or to modify the metabolism of procarcinogens once exposure has occurred. An example of this latter use is an intervention to reduce aflatoxin−DNA adducts using a broccoli sprout supplement [26].

D Biomarkers as General Dietary Indicators

Although biomarkers of energy intake, specific nutrients, and other dietary variables can themselves be useful indicators of general diet, there are additional broad biomarkers to consider. Monitoring changes in patterns in response to dietary interventions presents additional challenges. The goal in this case is to monitor the intake of certain types of foods or food groups rather than specific nutrients; therefore, these dietary indicators should ideally be distributed within certain types of foods.

Plasma carotenoids provide a good example of the use of biomarkers as a dietary indicator when the goal is to assess and monitor dietary patterns. Vegetables and fruits contribute the vast majority of carotenoids in the diet, and plasma carotenoid concentrations have been shown to be useful biomarkers of vegetable and fruit intakes in cross-sectional descriptive studies, controlled feeding studies, and clinical trials [27−30]. The consistency of this relationship across diverse groups and involving various concurrent dietary manipulations (with differences in amounts of dietary factors that could alter carotenoid

TABLE 12.2   Phytochemical Content of Plant Food Families and Select Plant Foods[a]

Plant foods	Flavonoids	Isoflavones	Lignans	Carotenoids	Organosulfides	Isothiocyanates	Terpenes	Phytates
Cruciferae[b]	✓			✓	✓	✓	✓	
Rutaceae[c]	✓			✓			✓	
Alliaceae[d]	✓			✓	✓		✓	
Solanaceae[e]	✓			✓			✓	
Umbelliferae[f]	✓			✓			✓	
Curcurbitaceae[g]	✓			✓			✓	
Cereals	✓		✓				✓	✓
Soybeans	✓	✓		✓			✓	✓
Flaxseed	✓		✓					
Measurable in biological samples	Urine Blood Stool	Urine Blood Stool	Blood	Blood	Blood Breath	Urine Blood	Blood Stool	Urine Blood

[a]Some phytochemicals are present in most plant foods; others are restricted to particular botanical families or even particular plant species.
[b]Cabbage family.
[c]Citrus family.
[d]Onion family.
[e]Tomato family.
[f]Carrot family
[g]Squash family.

Source: *Adapted from Caragay, A. B. (1992). Cancer-preventive foods and ingredients. Food Technol.* **46**, *65–68; and Fahey, J. W., Clevidence, B. A., and Russell, R. M. (1999). Methods for assessing the biological effects of specific plant components. Nutr. Rev.* **57**, *S34–S40.*

bioavailability) is notable, although considerable inter-individual variation in the degree of response is typically observed. Also, nondietary factors that are among the determinants of plasma carotenoid concentrations (e.g., body mass and plasma cholesterol concentration) will influence the absolute concentration that is observed in response to dietary intake, so these characteristics must be used as adjustment factors.

Although vitamin C also is provided predominantly by fruits and vegetables in the diet, this measure is much less useful as a biomarker of this dietary pattern because the relationship between vitamin C intake and plasma concentration is linear only up to a certain threshold [31]. The use of vitamin C supplements (which is common in the U.S. population) often increases the intake level beyond the range in which linearity between intake and plasma concentration occurs and thus obscures the relationship between food choices and tissue concentrations.

Lignans are a group of compounds present in high-fiber foods, particularly cereals and fruits and vegetables [32]. These compounds are not found in animal products and, similar to carotenoids, may be useful markers of a plant-based diet [33]. Lignans provide an example of how using dietary constituents as biomarkers requires an understanding of the metabolism of the compounds. Lignans in plant foods are altered by intestinal microbiota so that the specific compounds, enterodiol and enterolactone, monitored in plasma or urine are actually bacterial metabolites. Because of this bacterial conversion, lignan concentrations in urine or plasma in response to a similar dietary dose vary significantly among individuals. In addition, nondietary factors (e.g., use of oral antibiotics) reduce enterolactone and enterodiol production [34].

Although whole grain foods are a source of fiber, they have independently been inversely associated with some chronic diseases, such as cardiovascular disease [35], type 2 diabetes [36], and some cancers [37,38]. It is difficult to accurately assess intake of whole grains from standard dietary questionnaires; therefore, a biomarker of intake is essential. Plasma concentrations and urinary excretion of alkylresorcinols and alkylresorcinol metabolites have been identified as a good indicator of whole grains intake, specifically [39,40].

In contrast to fiber, red and processed meats have been positively associated with stroke, cardiovascular disease, diabetes, and cancer [41–43]; these associations were identified using self-reported dietary assessment methods known to result in measurement error. Two controlled feeding studies were used to investigate potential biomarkers of meat intake by analyzing known breakdown products, including creatinine, creatine, carnitine, taurine, 1-methylhistidine, and 3-methylhistidine. It was reported that urinary levels of 1-methyhistidine and 3-methylhistidine dose-dependently reflected red meat intake [44]; however, this needs to be investigated in free-living individuals, in whom diet is not tightly controlled, to determine whether they can be successfully used in an epidemiologic setting as potential biomarkers of meat intake.

Investigating specific fatty acids can reveal important dietary patterns. The fatty acid composition of membrane phospholipids is in part determined by the omega-6 and omega-3 fatty acid composition of the diet. Thus, the fatty acid pattern of serum phospholipids or plasma aliquots has been used as a biomarker of compliance with omega-3 fatty acid supplementation in clinical trials [45,46]. Although enzyme selectivity and other physiological factors are also important determinants of the fatty acid composition of phospholipids, a diet high in omega-3 polyunsaturated fats will result in increased amounts of eicosapentaenoic and docosahexaenoic acids in circulating tissue pools. Specific fatty acids can also be associated with certain types of foods. Pentadecanoic acid (15:0) and heptadecanoic acid (17:0) are fatty acids produced by bacteria in the rumen of ruminant animals. These fatty acids, with uneven numbers of carbon atoms, are not synthesized by humans; therefore, their presence in human biological samples can indicate dietary exposure to milk fat. Proportions of 15:0 and 17:0 in adipose tissue and concentrations of 15:0 in serum have been found to correlate with milk fat intake in men and women [47,48].

III FUNCTIONAL BIOMARKERS AND MARKERS OF BIOLOGICAL EFFECTS

If a nutrient or dietary constituent has an identified impact on physiological, biochemical, or genetic factors, measuring markers of those effects can be extremely useful. Such indices can be classified as those that are measures of discrete functions of a nutritional factor and those that are measures of more general functions or activities [49]. A discrete functional index often relates to the first limiting biochemical system—for example, a particular enzymatic pathway [50]. These markers can be used to identify the dosage or concentration of a nutritional factor necessary to achieve a clinically meaningful response or to define optimum nutrient status (Table 12.1). Unfortunately, for many nutritional factors, the first limiting biochemical system is unknown or not readily measured or accessible in humans. A general functional index is less specific but may be more directly linked to the pathogenesis of disease or ill health. Often, a panel of markers, rather than one specific measure, provides a better picture. Examples of general functional indices or markers are oxidative stress, immune function, bone health, and cell turnover—processes that have been shown to play roles in the risk of various diseases.

For a functional index to be an effective nutritional biomarker for intervention studies related to disease risk, a cause-and-effect relationship must be established (1) between nutritional status and the functional index, (2) between the functional index and ill health, and (3) between nutrient status and ill health. Such an undertaking is a daunting and time-consuming task, but it is especially important if a functional biomarker is going to be used as a proxy, or surrogate, for a clinical end point or disease outcome. A clinical end point is a characteristic or variable that measures how a patient feels, functions, or survives. A surrogate end point biomarker is an index whose modulation has been shown to indicate the progression or reversal of the disease process; it is a biomarker that is intended to substitute for a clinical end point. In an intervention trial, the use of surrogate end point biomarkers (rather than the frank diagnosis of disease) requires substantially less time and fewer resources in the evaluation of efforts aimed toward reducing risk for chronic diseases such as cancer, cardiovascular disease, and osteoporosis [51].

To date, few markers have been established as true surrogate end point biomarkers (i.e., they can accurately substitute for a clinical end point [52]). The evidence supporting the linkage of a biomarker to a clinical end point may be derived from epidemiological studies, clinical trials, *in vitro* analyses, animal models, and simulated biological systems. Many biomarkers have been proposed as potential surrogate end points, but relatively few are likely to achieve this status because of the complexity of disease mechanisms and the limited capability of a single biomarker to reflect the collective impact of multiple therapeutic effects on ultimate outcome.

A Biomarkers of Enzyme Function

Understanding how diet influences enzyme systems is important in developing strategies for disease prevention and treatment. For example, dietary modulation of enzymes involved in carcinogen metabolism may be important in reducing cancer risk, and a dietary intervention that reduces expression of rate-limiting enzymes in cholesterol synthesis may alter cardiovascular disease risk. Enzymes that require micronutrients as cofactors are also used as biomarkers of nutritional status (Table 12.1).

Components of the diet have the capacity to modulate protein synthesis and function. An ideal discrete functional marker would be one that reflects the direct effect of a dietary constituent—for example, mRNA amount when the dietary factor regulates gene expression or level of enzyme activity when the factor acts as a competitive inhibitor of the enzyme (Figure 12.2). Unfortunately, monitoring at these levels in the pathway in an intact human is not always feasible. Often, we rely primarily on a downstream marker, whose measurement may be influenced by subsequent or parallel pathways and may give a diluted signal.

Often, the enzymes of interest are located primarily in tissues that are not readily accessible (e.g., liver, intestine, and lung). One approach to meeting this challenge is to measure the enzymes in more accessible tissue; for example, enzymes that are present in high levels in the liver can often be measured in plasma or serum as a result of normal hepatocyte turnover. Enzyme activity of glutathione S-transferase (GST), a biotransformation enzyme important in carcinogen detoxification, can be measured spectrophotometrically in serum [53] or concentrations of the enzyme can be determined in serum by immunoassay [54]. Serum concentration of the GST isoenzyme GST-α has been shown to increase when cruciferous vegetables are added to the diet [55]. A limitation of using serum measures of a hepatic enzyme is that the assumption is made that liver function is normal. Thus, including other measures of liver function in the data collection is important to verify that no underlying hepatic disease is resulting in spurious GST values. In addition, some enzymes are present in isoforms in various tissues. GST-μ, another GST isoenzyme, is present in lymphocytes as well as in liver; therefore, for this isoenzyme, GST activity or protein concentration can be measured in cells extracted from blood samples [54].

Another approach to monitor enzyme activity *in vivo* is to use a drug probe. Many of the same xenobiotic metabolizing enzymes that metabolize carcinogens also metabolize and are modulated by commonly used drugs. The metabolites of these drugs can be monitored in serum, plasma, or urine and used to determine enzyme activities. For example, measuring caffeine metabolites in urine samples collected 4 hours after consumption of a defined caffeine dose allows determination of cytochrome P4501A2, N-acetyltransferase, and xanthine oxidase activities [55], and urinary concentrations of the glucuronide and sulfate conjugates of acetaminophen (paracetamol) are used to measure UDP-glucuronosyltransferase and sulfotransferase activities [56]. Drugs can be administered as probes during a nutrition intervention to determine the degree of change in enzyme activity in response to diet and to examine gene—diet interactions [57—59].

Measurement of arachidonic acid metabolism, which involves measuring the concentration of prostaglandins or leukotrienes (metabolic products) or enzymes in the eicosanoid metabolic pathway (i.e., cyclooxygenase), provides another example. Altered arachidonic acid metabolism is among the biochemical activities of nonsteroidal anti-inflammatory agents and may also be influenced by antioxidant micronutrients such as vitamin E [60], and quantitative changes in these products or enzymes in tissues serve as biomarkers of this activity [61]. A reasonable amount of biological evidence suggests some role for this enzymatic pathway in colon carcinogenesis [62], but the overall relationship with the disease process is still under investigation.

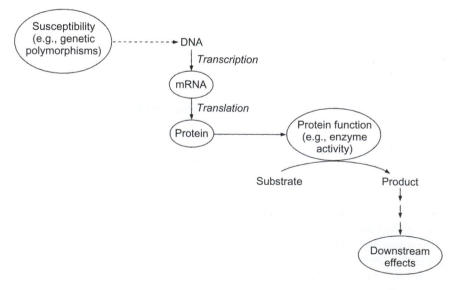

FIGURE 12.2 Direct functional markers of dietary exposure.

Similarly, endogenous compounds can serve as probes to monitor enzyme activity. Serum concentrations of the amino acid homocysteine, compared to serum and red blood cell folate concentration, are a more sensitive systemic measure of cellular folate depletion [63,64]. Serum concentrations of homocysteine increase with folate inadequacy because the remethylation of homocysteine requires N-5-methyltetrahydrofolate as a cosubstrate [65], which therefore provides a functional marker for folate status. Nonetheless, because homocysteine is at the intersection of two metabolic pathways, remethylation and transsulfuration, deficiencies in other nutrients in these pathways—namely vitamin B_{12}, vitamin B_6, and possibly riboflavin—can contribute to elevated serum homocysteine concentrations [63].

B Biomarkers of Oxidative Stress

Oxidative stress has been suggested to play a role in the pathophysiological disease process in cancer, atherosclerotic cardiovascular disease, and many other acute and chronic conditions [66], although the specific relationship with the disease process remains to be established in most instances. Cellular damage caused by reactive oxygen species, which are generated from cellular respiration, co-oxidation during metabolism, and the activity of phagocytic cells of the immune system, is controlled by antioxidant defense mechanisms that involve several micronutrients. Oxidative stress describes the condition of oxidative damage resulting when the balance between free radical generation and antioxidant defenses is unfavorable. Direct measurement of active oxygen and related species in biological samples is challenging, mainly because these compounds have short half-lives. Thus, the oxidative stress biomarkers used in human studies are typically adducts or end products that reflect reactions that have occurred between free radicals and compounds such as lipids, proteins, carbohydrates, DNA, and other molecules that are potential targets [67].

One frequently described assay used as an oxidative stress biomarker is the thiobarbituric acid reactive substances (TBARS) assay. The TBARS assay basically quantifies a product of malondialdehyde, which presumably reflects lipid hydroperoxides in the sample. Direct measurement of malondialdehyde in biological samples using HPLC has also been examined as an alternative approach, and plasma malondialdehyde concentrations have been reported to respond to alterations in antioxidant nutrient status, albeit not consistently [67].

Measurement of breath pentane is another biomarker of oxidative stress that has been utilized in human studies [68]. The approach basically involves collecting exhaled air for the measurement of the products of peroxidation of unsaturated fatty acids, a portion of which are volatile and released in the breath, using gas chromatography methods. However, the specific measurement methodologies vary a great deal and are not always reliable, and standardization of the procedure and knowledge of various influencing factors are needed to improve the usefulness of this approach [67].

Another biomarker of oxidative stress is urinary 8-hydroxydeoxyguanosine (8OHdG), which can be measured by several different methods with high sensitivity [69]. The 8-hydroxylation of the guanine base is a frequent type of oxidative DNA damage, and 8OHdG is subsequently excreted without further metabolism in the urine after repair *in vivo* by exonucleases. In previous studies, certain demographic factors and physiological characteristics such as gender and body mass [70] have been observed to influence urinary 8OHdG concentration, so these factors may need to be considered in interpretation. Urinary 8OHdG is increased in association with conditions known to be characterized by increased oxidative stress, such as smoking, whole-body irradiation, and cytotoxic chemotherapy [69–71]. Urinary 8OHdG (unadjusted or adjusted for urinary creatinine) has also been observed to decline in response to a high vegetable and fruit diet intervention in human subjects [72], which is particularly interesting because this type of diet has been suggested to promote reduced oxidative stress [13,72,73].

Prostaglandin-like compounds produced by nonenzymatic free radical-catalyzed peroxidation of arachidonic acid, termed F_2 isoprostanes, are currently of great interest as useful biomarkers of oxidative damage [74]. Specific gas chromatography—mass spectrometry (GC-MS) assays for the measurement of some of these compounds, such as iPF2a-III (also called 8-iso-$PGPF_2$) and iPF$_2$-VI, have been developed and used to quantify the compounds in urine and blood samples. These markers have been shown to be less variable than 8OHdG [75]. Elevated levels have been observed in plasma and urine samples from subjects under a wide variety of conditions of enhanced oxidative stress [76], and the measure can be altered in dietary intervention studies designed to reduce oxidative damage [77].

Another approach to measuring DNA oxidative damage that has been evaluated for use in human nutrition intervention research is the measurement of 5-hydroxymethyluracil levels in DNA in blood. 5-Hydroxymethyluracil is produced when DNA is exposed to oxidants, is relatively stable compared to other oxidation products, and can be quantified with GC-MS [78,79]. At the same time, its high intraindividual variation reduces its utility as a biomarker [80].

Oxidative damage to low-density lipoprotein (LDL) has been specifically linked to atherogenesis, and in an application of this biological activity, measurement of LDL oxidation *ex vivo* has been used in clinical studies as a biomarker of oxidative stress [81]. Basically, this process involves isolating the LDL fraction from a blood sample, exposing this fraction to oxidants such as Cu^{2+}, and measuring the time lag before oxidation. Also, various specific methodologies are used across laboratories, and the lack of standardization in the approaches in use constrains the ability to make comparisons across studies.

Several other approaches to measuring biomarkers of oxidative stress have been proposed and are under study, and the reader is referred to a review of this topic [67]. Because of their inherent variability and uncertain responsiveness to dietary manipulations, clinical researchers often employ a panel of potential measures of oxidative stress rather than relying on a single indicator [72].

C Biomarkers of Immune Function

The human immune system is a complex and highly interactive network of cells and their products that has a central role in protecting against various external disease-promoting factors and perhaps against malignant cells. Many of the components of the immune system can serve as biomarkers and are monitored *in vivo* or *ex vivo* [82,83]. Because of the complexity of the system, the selection of assays should be closely aligned with the research question being asked. Furthermore, multiple parameters need to be measured; one single biomarker is inadequate to monitor immune function.

Cell-mediated immune variables include the absolute amounts or ratios of various white blood cell (WBC) types (e.g., total counts, WBC differentials, T cell subsets) and measures of T cell function (e.g., lymphocyte proliferation, cytokine release from mitogen-stimulated cultures, cytotoxic capacities, and delayed-type hypersensitivity). Both number and activity of natural killer cells (one of the cell types that play an important role in immune surveillance) are used as biomarkers in nutrition intervention trials [84,85]. Cytokines (e.g., the interleukins) are soluble factors released by immune cells, which control and direct the function of other immune effectors. Some of these have been used as markers of immune response in randomized trials of vitamin supplementation [85,86].

An *in vivo* functional test, the delayed-type hypersensitivity (DTH) skin test, is widely used to monitor the immune system in humans, including in studies of dietary modulation of immune function [87]. It measures the capacity of an individual's immune system to mount a response to antigenic stimulation. The DTH test typically involves the simultaneous intradermal application of one or several DTH antigens. These antigens elicit an immunological reaction involving the release of lymphokines by antigen-sensitized T cells. These compounds, in turn, activate macrophages, which release inflammatory mediators, resulting in measurable skin induration.

D Biomarkers of Bone Health

Bone mass measurements and biomarkers of bone turnover are used as functional indices of bone health and, to a certain extent, can also be used as markers of the adequacy of calcium intake. Measures of bone mass include bone mineral content (i.e., the amount of mineral at a particular skeletal site, such as the femoral neck, lumbar spine, or total body) and bone mineral density (BMD; i.e., bone mineral content divided by the area of the scanned region). Both are strong predictors of fracture risk [88−90]. Controlled calcium intervention trials that measure change in BMD provide evidence for the intake requirement for calcium [91] (see Chapters 44 and 45 for more details).

Biochemical markers of bone turnover predict bone mass changes and fracture risk and respond to dietary calcium intake [91]; thus, they provide some promise for a biochemical indicator of calcium status. Unlike BMD, they reflect more subtle changes in bone metabolism. Bone turnover is the cyclical process by which the skeleton undergoes renewal by a coupled, but time-separated, sequence of bone resorption and bone formation [92]. Markers of bone turnover rely on the measurement in serum or urine of enzymes or matrix proteins synthesized by osteoblasts or osteoclasts that spill over into body fluids, or of osteoclast-generated degradation products of the bone matrix [91]. Currently, serum levels of skeletal alkaline phosphatase and osteocalcin are used as markers of bone formation, and products of collagen degradation measured in urine are used to measure bone resorption. These markers exhibit substantial short-term and long-term fluctuations related to time of day, phase of menstrual cycle, and season of the year, as well as other factors that alter bone remodeling (e.g., exercise) [93].

E Biomarkers of Cell Turnover

Cellular markers of proliferation, differentiation, and apoptosis (i.e., programmed cell death) can be useful as biomarkers in research focused on nutritional factors and cancer, although the measured effect is a general indicator of an altered cell growth regulation effect. Use of such markers is severely restricted by the difficulty accessing the tissue of interest. Consequently, research in this area has been limited primarily to tissue available via endoscopic or fine-needle biopsy procedures (e.g., gastrointestinal tract, breast, and prostate).

As a general rule, increased proliferation of undifferentiated cells defines one aspect or characteristic of carcinogenesis, and in colon cancer, this relationship has been well-established. For example, cell proliferation occurs at the base of the colonic crypts, and as cells migrate from the crypts to the luminal surface, they become increasingly differentiated and mature and lose their proliferative capabilities [94]. The shift in which the proliferative zone extends to the surface so that cells on the luminal surface retain proliferative capabilities and are immature and underdifferentiated may be considered a field defect that sets the stage for current and future neoplastic changes [94–96]. Early work in this area relied on the incorporation of tritiated thymidine or bromodeoxyuridine into the DNA of dividing cells during incubation of a biopsy specimen. These methods required that the tissue be freshly obtained, so the cells were viable and replicating. Often, label incorporation was incomplete. Now, with increased sensitivity in immunohistochemical techniques, proteins present in proliferating cells (e.g., proliferating cell nuclear antigen [PCNA] and Ki67) are used more widely to quantify proliferative activity in tissue specimens. Labeling indices involving tritiated thymidine and PCNA have been used to quantify the proliferative activity in colonic mucosal samples from human subjects [97] and have been used successfully as end points in several nutrition intervention studies to prevent colon cancer [98]. These indices are being further refined by staining for proteins present during apoptosis (e.g., Bax and Bcl-2) and in differentiated cells in order to provide a more complete picture of cell dynamics.

Adoption of aberrant crypt foci (early morphological changes in colonic epithelium that are considered potential precursors of adenomatous polyps) as biomarkers in humans is an example of how improvements in technology have led to the adoption of a biomarker that until recently could only be used in animal studies. Development of magnifying endoscopes with improved resolution now allows investigators to monitor aberrant crypt foci in colon tissue samples from healthy humans [99].

IV BIOMARKERS OF GENETIC SUSCEPTIBILITY

The health of individuals and the population in general is the result of interaction between genetic and environmental factors. For the great majority of human diseases, purely genetic or purely environmental etiologies are insufficient to explain individual variability in occurrence, prognosis, or outcome [100]. This is especially the case with chronic diseases, such as heart disease and cancer. Genetically determined susceptibility factors alter disease frequency or treatment response through variations in the DNA coding sequences of genes. As a result, genetically susceptible individuals produce proteins that are structurally different from those of individuals who are not at increased risk of disease, or they produce them in greater or lesser amounts.

By genetic standards, traits with a frequency of between 1/100 and 1/10,000 in a population are considered uncommon, and rare traits are those with a frequency of less than 1/10,000 [101]. Typically, these are low-prevalence and high-penetrance genes (e.g., genes associated with familial cancers). Common genetic traits are those in which the least common allele is present in at least 1% of the population [101]. Traits with this characteristic are known as genetic polymorphisms. They include the high-prevalence, low-penetrance genes—"susceptibility genes"—thought to contribute to disease risk.

In cases in which specific genetic mutations or variations may indicate disease risk or progression or may be modified by nutritional factors, genetic markers can also be useful biomarkers. Various molecular techniques have been developed to help characterize genetic abnormalities or differences. Genetic factors are important to consider in nutrition research for several reasons. One reason is that it is increasingly evident that genetic polymorphisms may contribute substantially to differences in the response to environmental and dietary exposures [102]. For example, genetic variations in the expression of the xenobiotic metabolizing enzymes may mediate the potentially mutagenic effect of heterocyclic amines (obtained from meat cooked at high temperature) [103] (see also Chapter 34). Also, results from laboratory animal studies suggest that dietary modifications can promote alterations in genetic factors [104] so that measuring genetic abnormalities may be considered an approach to demonstrating a biological link between dietary factors and disease risk.

Some polymorphic traits may only be important in the presence of a particular dietary exposure. For example, carrying the 5,10-methylenetetrahydrofolate reductase (MTHFR) thermal-labile variant has been shown to be a risk factor for colorectal adenomatous polyps, but only in the context of low folate, vitamin B_{12}, and vitamin B_6 intake [105].

Given that a goal of nutrition research and interventions is the prevention and treatment of disease, genetic markers may aid in this effort by identifying population subgroups at high risk of disease in the presence of particular dietary exposures. Genetic susceptibility markers may also strengthen our understanding of disease by focusing attention on possible pathways of disease causation and progression. There is considerable heterogeneity in disease risk within populations; thus, markers of susceptibility may also help to clarify associations between dietary exposures and diseases within population subgroups [106].

V METABOLOMICS FOR BIOMARKER DISCOVERY

Metabolomics involves the quantitative and qualitative study of a large number (e.g., 400−800) of small molecules (typically less than 850 Da) in biological fluids, including serum or plasma and urine. Metabolomic profiles can be measured by using GC-MS, LC-MS, or nuclear magnetic resonance spectroscopy. This metabolic phenotyping integrates exposure and functional biomarkers, and it allows the investigation of biomarkers of exposures as well as disease processes. The advantage for nutritional studies is the ability to investigate an array of dietary variables rather than single exposures; furthermore, an individual's metabolic profile reflects environmental and genetic factors as well as gut microbiota, all of which play an important role in diet and metabolism.

In controlled feeding studies, metabolomics has identified metabolic signatures for consumption of diets varying in composition of fats [107], proteins [108], and phytochemicals [109,110], as well as black versus green tea [111]. Additional focused and comprehensive efforts are underway to identify metabolites related to diet, physical activity, energy balance, and disease end points [112−115]. Although preliminary data suggest that only 20% of metabolites are affected when samples are nonfasting [116,117], more studies are required to investigate the sources of variation in metabolic profiles between biological fluids, as well as inter- and intraindividual variation.

VI CRITERIA FOR SELECTING AND USING BIOMARKERS

When a candidate biomarker is identified, certain basic considerations need to be addressed before it can be adopted for use in research or in a clinical setting [118]. These considerations relate to the reliability of the laboratory assay, the biological relevance of the marker, and the characteristics of the marker within a population. Whether or not a particular established marker is used also depends on the purpose the marker will serve.

Development of a biomarker usually builds on scientific knowledge from various types of laboratory studies, including tissue culture and animal studies. In the laboratory, an initial priority is to determine a marker's reliability or reproducibility. Assay performance can be evaluated using coefficients of variation (CV%; $[SD/mean] \times 100$) to estimate within- and between-batch precision; these are measures of analytical, laboratory performance and do not reflect intra- or interindividual variation. The within-batch precision is determined by dividing single samples into multiple aliquots and analyzing them together. Between-batch precision is determined by analyzing multiple aliquots on separate days. It is difficult to generalize about acceptable numerical values for the laboratory CV% because the degree of error acceptable depends on the use of the biomarker data. For epidemiological studies, if the goal is to establish a stable estimate of the group mean, an acceptable CV% may depend on the number of samples available, the mean concentration of the biomarker, and between-individual variation [119]. Techniques of quality control [120,121] and statistical methodologies for managing quality control data [122] have been established and are used in clinical laboratories.

Biomarkers should be relatively easy to measure and require relatively noninvasive techniques of tissue sampling. This requires that the biological relevance or validity—that is, the relationship between biomarkers in tissues readily available for human monitoring (e.g., peripheral blood) to those in target tissue (e.g., lung and liver) and the relationship between the biomarker and the disease or exposure being studied—of the measure be established. One example is the use of serum ferritin as a marker of body iron stores. Serum ferritin was validated as a measure of iron stores against bone marrow examination for stainable iron, the criterion—but very invasive—method for measuring iron stores [123]. As a result, serum ferritin has been adopted as a simple, quantitative biomarker of iron stores in otherwise healthy individuals.

If a particular biomarker is to be used as a measure of dietary exposure, it must be evaluated with respect to its sensitivity to that intake. Several approaches, both observational and interventional, can be used to define the relationship between long-term dietary intake and biological levels. Investigators can rely on geographical differences in exposure: Tissue samples from areas of known nutrient deficiency of a specific nutrient can be compared with samples from average and high-exposure areas. This approach has the advantage that it can reflect the long-term intake of a settled group of individuals; however, identifying and controlling confounding factors is a major challenge [119]. Another observational approach is to establish within individuals the relation between a dietary exposure and the biochemical marker. Participants for such a study can be selected randomly or can be selected specifically to maximize the range of intakes. Rigorous testing of the relationship between intake of the dietary factor and a biomarker under controlled dietary conditions is also valuable to establish dose—response relations; however, these trials are usually limited to weeks or months, and if they involve extensive changes to usual diet, blinding of participants may not be feasible.

Depending on the biomarker, significant variability can be seen in a biomarker. Sources of variation can be internal (e.g., age, sex, genetics, body build, and biological rhythm) or environmental (e.g., diet, season, time of day, immobilization, exercise, and drugs). These can contribute to both within- and interindividual variation. Additional external sources of variation, beyond laboratory accuracy and precision, can include an individual's posture during sample collection and sample handling and storage; protocols should be established to minimize these latter sources of variability.

Selection of a biomarker is dependent in part on its use. A biological indicator that is going to be used as a measure of a dietary exposure in an epidemiological study needs to be a valid representation of long-term intake [119]. Repeated sampling and measurement of a biomarker over time can provide some estimate of the within-individual variability and, therefore, the likelihood that the biomarker is a stable estimate of long-term intake. If repeated measures of a biochemical indicator vary substantially over time in the same individuals, then a single measure will not accurately reflect true, long-term intake [119]. This lack of consistency may occur because diet has changed over the sampling interval or because the measure is overly sensitive to short-term influences, such as recent intake. When using dietary constituents or their metabolites as biomarkers, an understanding of the metabolism and pharmacokinetics of the compound and the frequency of exposure will help to establish the utility of the measure as a biomarker of long-term intake.

A nutrition intervention study may require a biomarker that is a short-term measure of response to treatment. A biomarker that is to serve as a short-term measure of response needs to change within the time frame of the intervention. For example, serum folate provides a measure of recent folic acid exposure; however, erythrocyte concentrations are dependent on the life span of the cells and therefore will not reflect short-term changes in dietary folate. Serum folate concentrations decline within 3 weeks after the initiation of a low-folate diet, whereas erythrocyte folate concentration remains in the normal range for at least 17 weeks [124].

Additional practical considerations in the use of established biomarkers include the ability to conveniently access the body compartment for measurement, the procedures necessary to collect and process the sample, the burden to study participants or patients, and the resources for laboratory analysis. For example, multiday collections of feces or urine can be a major burden for many individuals. In addition, they can result in incomplete collections, which also compromise the final results. An accurate quantification of vitamin C or folate in a circulating body pool requires processing steps that must be conducted immediately after blood collection to preserve the sample appropriately and prevent degradation that would otherwise make the resulting measurement inaccurate. These extra steps can add time and effort to the labor of blood processing. Furthermore, the complexity of an assay method can vary from the ability to analyze hundreds of samples a day at a cost of a few dollars per sample to a labor-intensive, week-long process that costs hundreds of dollars per sample.

The ability to measure particular biomarkers is also often linked to technological challenges and existing capabilities. For example, HPLC (developed in the 1970s) and improved separation and detection technologies that are currently emerging facilitate the quantification of many micronutrients and other dietary constituents that are present in very low concentrations in biological samples. Similarly, immunoassays allow for quantitation of phytochemicals, proteins, and so on in small volumes of serum or plasma, whereas previous methods required substantial quantities of sample. The development of microarray technology has provided the ability to analyze the expression profiles for thousands of genes in parallel [125,126]. This technique will rapidly advance knowledge regarding the mechanisms by which nutrition and diet affect disease risk; however, its application in intact humans will still be limited by access to the tissue of interest and the capacity to detect small but relevant changes in gene expression in response to diet.

A summary of the ideal characteristics of a biomarker, the assay involved, as well as study-specific questions is given in Table 12.3. Many of the prerequisites of a potential biomarker depend on the research question and study design.

VII SUMMARY

The use of biomarkers in humans is an integral component of nutrition intervention research. Biochemical measurements of dietary constituents in blood or other tissues can provide a useful assessment of the intake of certain dietary factors. However, for some nutrients, functional markers, or direct functional indices,

TABLE 12.3   Criteria for Selecting Biomarkers

Qualities of a good biomarker:

Sensitive

Specific

Biologic relevance to target tissue

Found in accessible biospecimen—not invasive

Easy to measure

Applicable to many populations.

Qualities of a good biomarker assay:

Reliable

Reproducible

Sensitive.

Identify sources of variability in the biomarker:

Interindividual variation (e.g., age, sex, genetics, diet, lifestyle, season, time of day, drugs).

Intraindividual variation.

The effect of sample handling and storage; for example, is the biomarker stable during long-term storage?

Identify the type of biomarker needed:

Is the biomarker applicable to the setting? For example, cohort studies usually have biospecimens from only one time point—Is a single measure representative and sufficient?

Is the assay applicable to the setting? For example, the assay would need to have relatively high throughput for cohort studies, whereas for small intervention studies this would be less important.

Does the study require a short-term or a long-term biomarker?

Does the biomarker reflect a dose—response?

Do the biospecimens need to be collected after fasting or should they be nonfasting?

persistence; and assessing the contribution of genetic and acquired susceptibility factors to interindividual variability.

References

[1] S.A. Bingham, Urine nitrogen as an independent validatory measure of protein intake, Br. J. Nutr. 77 (1) (1997) 144—148.

[2] P. Galan, S. Briancon, A. Favier, S. Bertrais, P. Preziosi, H. Faure, et al., Antioxidant status and risk of cancer in the Su.Vi.Max study: is the effect of supplementation dependent on baseline levels? Br. J. Nutr. 94 (1) (2005) 125—132.

[3] S.A. McClave, H.L. Snider, Use of indirect calorimetry in clinical nutrition, Nutr. Clin. Pract. 7 (1992) 207—221.

[4] J.R. Speakman, The history and theory of the doubly labeled water technique, Am. J. Clin. Nutr. 68 (Suppl) (1998) 932S—938S.

[5] J. Seale, Energy expenditure measurements in relation to energy requirements, Am. J. Clin. Nutr. 62 (Suppl) (1995) 1042S—1046S.

[6] B.A. Clevidence, J.G. Bieri, Association of carotenoids with human plasma lipoproteins, Methods Enzymol. 214 (1993) 33—46.

[7] J.E. Romanchik, D.W. Morel, E.H. Harrison, Distribution of carotenoids and a-tocopherol among lipoproteins do not change when human plasma is incubated in vitro, J. Nutr. 125 (1995) 2610—2617.

[8] J.P. Habicht, D.L. Pelletier, The importance of context in choosing nutritional indicators, J. Nutr. 120 (Suppl) (1990) 1519—1524.

[9] M.E. Shils, J.A. Olson, M. Shike, A.C. Ross (Eds), Modern Nutrition in Health and Disease, ninth ed., Williams & Wilkins, Philadelphia, 1999.

[10] E.E. Ziegler, L.J. Filer (Eds), Present Knowledge in Nutrition, seventh ed., ILSI Press, Washington, DC, 1996.

[11] F.A.N. Board, Dietary Reference Intakes for Thiamin, Riboflavin, Niacin, Vitamin B_6, Folate, Vitamin B_{12}, Pantothenic Acid, Biotin, and Choline, National Academy Press, Washington, DC, 1998.

[12] R. Kaaks, E. Riboli, R. Sinha, Biochemical markers of dietary intake, in: P. Toniolo, P. Boffetta, D.E.G. Shuker, N. Rothman, B. Hulka, N. Pearce (Eds), Application of Biomarkers in Cancer Epidemiology, International Agency for Research on Cancer, Lyon, France, 1997, pp. 103—126.

[13] International Agency for Research on Cancer (IARC), Fruit and Vegetables: IARC Handbook of Cancer Prevention, vol. 8, IARC, Lyon, France, 2003.

[14] L.J. Ignarro, M.L. Balestrieri, C. Napoli, Nutrition, physical activity, and cardiovascular disease: An update, Cardiovasc. Res. 73 (2007) 326—340.

[15] L. Coward, N. Barnes, K.D.R. Setchell, S. Barnes, Genistein, daidzein and their β-glycoside conjugates: antitumor isoflavones in soybean foods from American and Asian diets, J. Agric. Food Chem. 41 (1993) 1961—1967.

[16] A.A. Franke, L.J. Custer, C.M. Cerna, K. Narala, Quantitation of phytoestrogens in legumes by HPLC, J. Agric. Food Chem. 42 (1994) 1905—1913.

[17] S.C. Karr, J.W. Lampe, A.M. Hutchins, J.L. Slavin, Urinary isoflavonoid excretion in humans is dose-dependent at low to moderate levels of soy protein consumption, Am. J. Clin. Nutr. 66 (1997) 46—51.

[18] G. Maskarinec, A.A. Franke, A.E. Williams, S. Hebshi, C. Oshiro, S. Murphy, et al., Effects of a 2-year randomized soy intervention on sex hormone levels in premenopausal women, Cancer Epidemiol. Biomarkers Prev. 13 (2004) 1736—1744.

[19] H. Marini, L. Minutoli, F. Polito, A. Bitto, D. Altavilla, M. Atteritano, et al., Effects of the phytoestrogen genistein on bone metabolism in

provide a better estimate of the significance of the true status for a nutrient. More general functional indices and indicators of biological activity relating to processes associated with disease risk are important for establishing the relationships between diet and disease prevention and response to treatment.

The development of biomarkers continues at a rapid pace. New types of markers are being proposed constantly, and analytical techniques for existing markers are improved. This advancement requires establishing the accuracy, reliability, and interpretability of the biomarkers; obtaining data on marker distributions within different age and sex groupings in normal populations; determining the extent of intraindividual variation in markers with respect to tissue localization and osteopenic postmenopausal women: a randomized trial, Ann. Intern. Med. 146 (2007) 839–847.

[20] S. Watanabe, M. Yamaguchi, T. Sobue, T. Takahashi, T. Miura, Y. Arai, et al., Pharmacokinetics of soybean isoflavones in plasma, urine and feces of men after ingestion of 60 g baked soybean powder (kinako), J. Nutr. 128 (1998) 1710–1715.

[21] M.D. Gross, M. Pfeiffer, M. Martini, D. Campbell, J. Slavin, J. Potter, The quantitation of metabolites of quercetin flavonols in human urine, Cancer Epidemiol. Biomarkers Prev. 5 (1996) 711–720.

[22] M. Noroozi, J. Burns, A. Crozier, I.E. Kelly, M.E.J. Lean, Prediction of dietary flavonol consumption from fasting plasma concentration or urinary excretion, Eur. J. Clin. Nutr. 54 (2000) 143–149.

[23] A.V. Gasper, A. Al-Janobi, J.A. Smith, J.R. Bacon, P. Fortun, C. Atherton, et al., Glutathione S-transferase M1 polymorphism and metabolism of sulforaphine from standard and high-glucosinolate broccoli, Am. J. Clin. Nutr. 82 (2005) 1283–1291.

[24] T.A. Shapiro, J.W. Fahey, A.T. Dinkova-Kostova, W.D. Holtzclaw, K.K. Stephenson, K.L. Wade, et al., Safety, tolerance, and metabolism of broccoli sprout glucosinolates and isothiocyanates: a clinical phase I study, Nutr. Cancer 55 (2006) 53–62.

[25] C.P. Wild, P. Pisani, Carcinogen–DNA and carcinogen–protein adducts in molecular epidemiology, in: P. Toniolo, P. Boffetta, D.E.G. Shuker, N. Rothman, B. Hulka, N. Pearce (Eds), Application of Biomarkers in Cancer Epidemiology, International Agency for Research on Cancer, Lyon, France, 1997, pp. 143–158.

[26] T.W. Kensler, J.G. Chen, P.A. Egner, J.W. Fahey, L.P. Jacobson, K.K. Stephenson, et al., Effects of glucosinolate-rich broccoli sprouts on urinary levels of aflatoxin-DNA adducts and phenanthrene tetraols in a randomized clinical trial in He Zuo township, Qidong, People's Republic of China, Cancer Epidemiol. Biomarkers Prev. 14 (2005) 2605–2613.

[27] M.C. Martini, D.R. Campbell, M.D. Gross, G.A. Grandits, J.D. Potter, J.L. Slavin, Plasma carotenoids as biomarkers of vegetable intake: the Minnesota CPRU feeding studies, Cancer Epidemiol. Biomarkers Prev. 4 (1995) 491–496.

[28] D.R. Campbell, M.D. Gross, M.C. Martini, G.A. Grandits, J.L. Slavin, J.D. Potter, Plasma carotenoids as biomarkers of vegetable and fruit intake, Cancer Epidemiol. Biomarkers Prev. 3 (1994) 493–500.

[29] C.L. Rock, S.W. Flatt, F.A. Wright, S. Faerber, V. Newman, S. Kealey, et al., Responsiveness of carotenoids to a high vegetable diet intervention designed to prevent breast cancer recurrence, Cancer Epidemiol. Biomarkers Prev. 6 (1997) 617–623.

[30] L. Le Marchand, J.H. Hankin, F.S. Carter, C. Essling, D. Luffey, A.A. Franke, et al., A pilot study on the use of plasma carotenoids and ascorbic acid as markers of compliance to a high fruit and vegetable diet intervention, Cancer Epidemiol. Biomarkers Prev. 3 (1994) 245–251.

[31] J. Blanchard, T.N. Toxer, M. Rowland, Pharmacokinetic perspectives on megadoses of ascorbic acid, Am. J. Clin. Nutr. 66 (1997) 1165–1171.

[32] I.E.J. Milder, I.C.W. Arts, B. van de Putte, D.P. Venema, P.C.H. Hollman, Lignan contents of Dutch plant foods: a database including lariciresinol, pinoresinol, secoisolariciresinol and matairesinol, Br. J. Nutr. 93 (2005) 393–402.

[33] L.M. Kirkman, J.W. Lampe, D.R. Campbell, M.C. Martini, J.L. Slavin, Urinary lignan and isoflavonoid excretion in men and women consuming vegetable and soy diets, Nutr. Cancer 24 (1995) 1–12.

[34] A. Kilkkinen, P. Pietinen, T. Klaukka, J. Virtamo, P. Korhonen, H. Adlercreutz, Use of oral antimicrobials decreases serum enterolactone concentrations, Am. J. Epidemiol. 155 (2002) 472–477.

[35] M.K. Jensen, P. Koh-Banerjee, F.B. Hu, M. Franz, L. Sampson, M. Gronbaek, et al., Intakes of whole grains, bran, and germ and the risk of coronary heart disease in men, Am. J. Clin. Nutr. 80 (6) (2004) 1492–1499.

[36] J.S. de Munter, F.B. Hu, D. Spiegelman, M. Franz, R.M. van Dam, Whole grain, bran, and germ intake and risk of type 2 diabetes: a prospective cohort study and systematic review, PLoS Med. 4 (8) (2007) e261.

[37] A. Schatzkin, Y. Park, M.F. Leitzmann, A.R. Hollenbeck, A.J. Cross, Prospective study of dietary fiber, whole grain foods, and small intestinal cancer, Gastroenterology 135 (4) (2008) 1163–1167.

[38] A. Schatzkin, T. Mouw, Y. Park, A.F. Subar, V. Kipnis, A. Hollenbeck, et al., Dietary fiber and whole-grain consumption in relation to colorectal cancer in the Nih-Aarp Diet and Health Study, Am. J. Clin. Nutr. 85 (5) (2007) 1353–1360.

[39] R. Landberg, A. Kamal-Eldin, A. Andersson, B. Vessby, P. Aman, Alkylresorcinols as biomarkers of whole-grain wheat and rye intake: plasma concentration and intake estimated from dietary records, Am. J. Clin. Nutr. 87 (4) (2008) 832–838.

[40] L.A. Guyman, H. Adlercreutz, A. Koskela, L. Li, S.A. Beresford, J.W. Lampe, Urinary 3-(3,5-dihydroxyphenyl)-1-propanoic acid, an alkylresorcinol metabolite, is a potential biomarker of whole-grain intake in a U.S. population, J. Nutr. 138 (10) (2008) 1957–1962.

[41] S.C. Larsson, J. Virtamo, A. Wolk, Red meat consumption and risk of stroke in Swedish men, Am. J. Clin. Nutr. 94 (2) (2011) 417–421.

[42] R. Micha, S.K. Wallace, D. Mozaffarian, Red and processed meat consumption and risk of incident coronary heart disease, stroke, and diabetes mellitus: a systematic review and meta-analysis, Circulation 121 (21) (2010) 2271–2283.

[43] World Cancer Research Fund/American Institute for Cancer Research (WCRF/AICR), Food, Nutrition, Physical Activity, and the Prevention of Cancer: A Global Perspective, WCRF/AICR, Washington, DC, 2007.

[44] A.J. Cross, J.M. Major, R. Sinha, Urinary biomarkers of meat consumption, Cancer Epidemiol. Biomarkers Prev. 20 (6) (2011) 1107–1111.

[45] S.N. Meydani, S. Endres, M.M. Woods, B.R. Goldin, C. Soo, A. Morrill-Labrode, et al., Oral (n-3) fatty acid supplementation suppresses cytokine production and lymphocyte proliferation: comparison between young and older women, J. Nutr. 121 (1991) 547–555.

[46] E. Soyland, J. Funk, G. Rajka, M. Sandberg, P. Thune, L. Rustad, et al., Effect of dietary supplementation with very-long-chain n-3 fatty acids in patients with psoriasis, N. Engl. J. Med. 328 (1993) 1812–1816.

[47] A. Wolk, B. Vessby, H. Ljung, P. Barrefors, Evaluation of a biologic marker for dairy fat intake, Am. J. Clin. Nutr. 68 (1998) 291–295.

[48] A.E.M. Smedman, I.B. Gustafsson, L.G.T. Berglund, B.O.H. Vessby, Pentadecanoic acid in serum as a marker for intake of milk fat: relations between intake of milk fat and metabolic risk factors, Am. J. Clin. Nutr. 69 (1999) 22–29.

[49] J.R. Turnlund, Future directions for establishing mineral/trace element requirements, J. Nutr. 124 (1994) 1765S–1770S.

[50] J.J. Strain, Optimal nutrition: an overview, Proc. Nutr. Soc. 58 (1999) 395–396.

[51] G.J. Kelloff, C.C. Sigman, K.M. Johnson, C.W. Boone, P. Greenwald, J.A. Crowell, et al., Perspectives on surrogate end points in the development of drugs that reduce the risk of cancer, Cancer Epidemiol. Biomarkers Prev. 9 (2000) 127–137.

[52] T.R. Fleming, D.L. DeMets, Surrogate end points in clinical trials: are we being misled? Ann. Int. Med. 125 (1996) 605–613.

[53] W.H. Habig, M.J. Pabst, W.B. Jakoby, Glutathione S-transferases: the first enzymatic step in mercapturic acid formation, J. Biol. Chem. 249 (1974) 7130–7139.

[54] J.J.P. Bogaards, H. Verhagen, M.I. Willems, G. van Poppel, P.J. van Bladeren, Consumption of Brussels sprouts results in elevated a-class glutathione S-transferase levels in human blood plasma, Carcinogenesis 15 (1994) 1073−1075.

[55] A.D.M. Kashuba, J.S. Bertino, G.L. Kearns, J.S. Leeder, A.W. James, R. Gotschall, et al., Quantitation of three-month intraindividual variability and influence of sex and menstrual cycle phase on CYP1A2, N-acetyltransferase-2, and xanthine oxidase activity determined with caffeine phenotyping, Clin. Pharmacol. Ther. 63 (1998) 540−551.

[56] E.J. Pantuck, C.B. Pantuck, K.E. Anderson, L.W. Wattenberg, A.H. Conney, A. Kappas, Effect of Brussels sprouts and cabbage on drug conjugation, Clin. Pharmacol. Ther. 35 (1984) 161−169.

[57] R. Sinha, N. Rothman, E.D. Brown, S.D. Mark, R.N. Hoover, N.E. Caprasо, et al., Pan-fried meat containing high levels of heterocyclic aromatic amines but low levels of polycyclic aromatic hydrocarbons induces cytochrome P4501A2 activity in humans, Cancer Res. 54 (1994) 6154−6159.

[58] M.A. Kall, O. Vang, J. Clausen, Effects of dietary broccoli on human drug metabolising activity, Cancer Lett. 114 (1997) 169−170.

[59] J.W. Lampe, C. Chen, S. Li, J. Prunty, M.T. Grate, D.E. Meehan, et al., Modulation of human glutathione S-transferases by botanically defined vegetable diets, Cancer Epidemiol. Biomarkers Prev. 9 (2000) 787−793.

[60] K. Lauritsen, L.S. Laursen, K. Bukhave, J. Rask-Madsen, Does vitamin E supplementation modulate in vivo arachidonate metabolism in human inflammation?, Pharmacol. Toxicol. 61 (1987) 246−249.

[61] M.T. Ruffin, K. Krishnan, C.L. Rock, D. Normolle, M.A. Vaerten, M. Peters-Golden, et al., Suppression of human colorectal mucosal prostaglandins: determining the lowest effective aspirin dose, J. Natl. Cancer Inst. 89 (1997) 1152−1160.

[62] K. Krishnan, M.T. Ruffin, D.E. Brenner, Clinical models of chemoprevention for colon cancer, Hematol. Oncol. Clin. North Am. 12 (1998) 1079−1113.

[63] J. Selhub, J.W. Miller, The pathogenesis of homocysteinemia: interruption of the coordinate regulation by S-adenosylmethionine of the remethylation and transsulfuration of homocysteine, Am. J. Clin. Nutr. 55 (1992) 131−138.

[64] Y.I. Kim, K. Fawaz, T. Knox, Y.M. Lee, R. Norton, S. Arora, et al., Colonic mucosal concentrations of folate correlate well with blood measurements of folate status in persons with colorectal polyps, Am. J. Clin. Nutr. 68 (1998) 866−872.

[65] S.P. Stabler, P.D. Marcell, E.R. Podell, R.H. Allen, D.G. Savage, J. Lindenbaum, Elevation of total homocysteine in the serum of patients with cobalamin or folate deficiency detected by capillary gas chromatography−mass spectrometry, J. Clin. Invest. 81 (1988) 466−474.

[66] C.L. Rock, R.A. Jacob, P.A. Bowen, Update on the biological characteristics of the antioxidant micronutrients: vitamin C, vitamin E, and the carotenoids, J. Am. Diet. Assoc. 96 (1996) 693−702.

[67] S.T. Mayne, Antioxidant nutrients and chronic disease: use of biomarkers of exposure and oxidative stress status in epidemiologic research, J. Nutr. 133 (Suppl. 3) (2003) 933S−940S.

[68] M. Lemoyne, A.V. Gossum, R. Kurian, M. Ostro, J. Azler, K.N. Jeejeebhoy, Breath pentane analysis as an index of lipid peroxidation: a functional test of vitamin E status, Am. J. Clin. Nutr. 46 (1987) 267−272.

[69] S. Mei, Q. Yao, C. Wu, G. Xu, Determination of urinary 8-hydroxy-2'-deoxyguanosine by two approaches—capillary electrophoresis and GC/MS: an assay for in vivo oxidative DNA damage in cancer patients, J. Chromatogr. B Analyt. Technol. Biomed. Life Sci. 827 (2005) 83−87.

[70] S. Loft, K. Vistisen, M. Ewertz, A. Tjonneland, K. Overvad, H.E. Poulsen, Oxidative DNA damage estimated by 8-hydroxydeoxyguanosine excretion in humans: influence of smoking, gender and body mass index, Carcinogenesis 13 (1992) 2241−2247.

[71] C. Tagesson, M. Kallberg, C. Klintenberg, H. Starkhammar, Determination of urinary 8-hydroxydeoxyguanosine by automated coupled-column high performance liquid chromatography: a powerful technique for assaying in vivo oxidative DNA damage in cancer patients, Eur. J. Cancer 31A (1995) 934−940.

[72] H.J. Thompson, J. Heimendinger, A. Haegele, S.M. Sedlacek, C. Gillette, C. O'Neill, et al., Effect of increased vegetable and fruit consumption on markers of oxidative cellular damage, Carcinogenesis 20 (1999) 2261−2266.

[73] G. Johansson, A. Holmen, L. Persson, R. Hogstedt, C. Wassen, L. Ottova, et al., The effect of a shift from a mixed diet to a lactovegetarian diet on human urinary and fecal mutagenic activity, Carcinogenesis 13 (1992) 153−157.

[74] J.L. Witztum, To E or not to E—How do we tell? Circulation 98 (1998) 2785−2787.

[75] J.D. Morrow, T.M. Harris, L.J. Roberts, Noncyclooxygenase oxidative formation of a series of novel prostaglandins: analytical ramifications for measurement of eicosanoids, Anal. Biochem. 184 (1990) 1−10.

[76] J.D. Morrow, L.J. Roberts, The isoprostanes: unique bioactive products of lipid peroxidation, Prog. Lipid Res. 36 (1997) 1−21.

[77] M. Atteritano, H. Marini, L. Minutoli, F. Polito, A. Bitto, D. Altavilla, et al., Effects of the phytoestrogen genistein on some predictors of cardiovascular risk in osteopenic, postmenopausal women: a 2-year randomized, double-blind, placebo-controlled study, J. Clin. Endocrinol. Metab. 92 (2007) 3068−3075.

[78] Z. Djuric, M.H. Lu, S.M. Lewis, D.A. Luongo, X.W. Chen, L.K. Heilbrun, et al., Oxidative DNA damage levels in rats fed low-fat, high-fat, or calorie-restricted diets, Toxicol. Appl. Pharmacol. 115 (1992) 156−160.

[79] Z. Djuric, L.K. Heilbrun, B.A. Reading, A. Boomer, F.A. Valeriote, S. Martino, Effects of a low-fat diet on levels of oxidative damage to DNA in human peripheral nucleated blood cells, J. Natl. Cancer Inst. 83 (1991) 766−769.

[80] I. Kato, J. Ren, L.K. Heilbrun, Z. Djuric, Intra- and inter-individual variability in measurements of biomarkers for oxidative damage in vivo: nutrition and breast health study, Biomarkers 11 (2006) 143−152.

[81] L. Mosca, M. Rubenfire, C. Mandel, C. Rock, T. Tarshis, A. Tsai, et al., Antioxidant nutrient supple mentation reduces the susceptibility of low density lipoprotein to oxidation in patients with coronary artery disease, J. Am. Coll. Cardiol. 30 (1997) 392−399.

[82] C.J. Field, Use of T cell function to determine the effect of physiologically active food components, Am. J. Clin. Nutr. 71 (6 Suppl.) (2000) 1720S−1750S.

[83] B. Lourd, L. Mazari, Nutrition and immunity in the elderly, Proc. Nutr. Soc. 58 (1999) 685−695.

[84] T. Murata, H. Tamai, T.M.M. Morinobu, H. Takenaka, K. Hayashi, M. Mino, Effect of long-term administration of β-carotene on lymphocyte subsets in humans, Am. J. Clin. Nutr. 60 (1994) 597−602.

[85] M.S. Santos, S.N. Meydani, L. Leka, D. Wu, N. Fotouhi, M. Meydani, et al., Natural killer cell activity in elderly men is enhanced by β-carotene supplementation, Am. J. Clin. Nutr. 64 (1996) 772−777.

[86] K.-C.G. Jeng, C.-S. Yang, W.-Y. Siu, Y.-S. Tsai, W.J. Liao, J.-S. Kuo, Supplementation of vitamins C and E enhances cytokine production by peripheral blood mononuclear cells in healthy adults, Am. J. Clin. Nutr. 64 (1996) 960−965.

[87] J.D. Bogden, A. Bendich, F.W. Kemp, K.S. Bruening, J.H. Skurnick, T. Denny, et al., Daily micronutrient supplements enhance delayed-hypersensitivity skin test responses in older people, Am. J. Clin. Nutr. 60 (1994) 437−447.

B. RESEARCH AND APPLIED METHODS FOR OBSERVATIONAL AND INTERVENTION STUDIES

[88] D.M. Black, S.R. Cummings, H.K. Genant, M.C. Nevitt, L. Palermo, W. Browner, Axial and appendicular bone density predict fractures in older women, J. Bone Miner. Res. 7 (1992) 633–638.

[89] S.R. Cummings, D.M. Black, M.C. Nevitt, W. Browner, J. Cauley, K. Ensrud, et al., Bone density at various sites for prediction of hip fracture: the Study of Osteoporotic Fractures Research Group, Lancet 341 (1993) 72–75.

[90] L.J.I. Melton, E.J. Atkinson, W.M. O'Fallon, H.W. Wahner, B.L. Riggs, Long-term fracture pre diction by bone mineral assessed at different skeletal sites, J. Bone Miner. Res. 8 (1993) 1227–1233.

[91] K.D. Cashman, A. Flynn, Optimal nutrition: calcium, magnesium and phosphorus, Proc. Nutr. Soc. 58 (1999) 477–487.

[92] J.A. Kanis, Calcium requirements for optimal skeletal health in women, Calcified Tissue Int. 49 (1991) S33–S41.

[93] N.B. Watts, Clinical utility of biochemical markers of bone remodeling, Clin. Chem. 45 (1999) 1359–1368.

[94] C.R. Boland, The biology of colorectal cancer, Cancer 71 (Suppl.) (1993) 4181–4186.

[95] J.G. Einspahr, D.S. Alberts, S.M. Gapstur, R.M. Bostick, S.S. Emerson, E.W. Gerner, Surrogate end-point biomarkers as measures of colon cancer risk and their use in cancer chemoprevention trials, Cancer Epidemiol. Biomarkers Prev. 6 (1997) 37–48.

[96] M. Lipkin, H. Newmark, Effect of added dietary calcium on colonic epithelial-cell proliferation in subjects at high risk for familial colonic cancer, N. Engl. J. Med. 313 (1985) 1381–1384.

[97] R.M. Bostick, L. Fosdick, T.J. Lillemoe, P. Overn, J.R. Wood, P. Grambsch, et al., Methodological findings and considerations in measuring colorectal epithelial cell proliferation in humans, Cancer Epidemiol. Biomarkers Prev. 6 (1997) 931–942.

[98] P.A. Vargas, D.S. Alberts, Primary prevention of colorectal cancer through dietary modification, Cancer 70 (1992) 1229–1235.

[99] T. Takayama, S. Katsuki, Y. Takahashi, M. Ohi, S. Nojiri, S. Sakamaki, et al., Aberrant crypt foci of the colon as precursors of adenoma and cancer, N Engl. J. Med. 339 (1998) 1277–1284.

[100] S. Garte, C. Zocchetti, E. Taioli, Gene- environment interactions in the application of biomarkers of cancer susceptibility in epidemiology, in: P. Toniolo, P. Boffetta, D.E.G. Shuker, N. Rothman, B. Hulka, N. Pearce (Eds), Application of Biomarkers in Cancer Epidemiology, International Agency for Research on Cancer, Lyon, France, 1997, pp. 251–264.

[101] R.F. Murray, Tests of so-called susceptibility, J. Occup. Med. 28 (1986) 1103–1107.

[102] C. Lai, P.G. Shields, The role of interindividual variation in human carcinogenesis, J. Nutr. 129 (Suppl.) (1999) 552S–555S.

[103] U. Peters, R. Sinha, D.A. Bell, N. Rothman, D.J. Grant, M.A. Watson, et al., Urinary mutagenesis and fried red meat intake: influence of cooking temperature, phenotype, and genotype of metabolizing enzymes in a controlled feeding study, Environ. Mol. Mutagen. 43 (2004) 53–74.

[104] Y.I. Kim, I.P. Pogribney, A.G. Basnakian, J.W. Miller, J. Selhub, S.J. James, et al., Folate deficiency in rats induces DNA strand breaks and hypomethylation within the p53 tumor suppressor gene, Am. J. Clin. Nutr. 65 (1997) 46–52.

[105] C.M. Ulrich, E. Kampman, J. Bigler, S.M. Schwartz, C. Chen, R. Bostick, et al., Colorectal adenomas and the C677T MTHFR polymorphism: evidence for gene–environment interaction?, Cancer Epidemiol. Biomarkers Prev. 8 (1999) 659–668.

[106] M.F. Vine, L.T. McFarland, Markers of susceptibility, in: B.S. Hulka, T.C. Wilcosky, J.D. Griffith (Eds), Biological Markers in Epidemiology, Oxford University Press, New York, 1990, pp. 196–213.

[107] A.D. Watson, Thematic review series: systems biology approaches to metabolic and cardiovascular disorders.

[108] C. Stella, B. Beckwith-Hall, O. Cloarec, E. Holmes, J.C. Lindon, J. Powell, et al., Susceptibility of human metabolic phenotypes to dietary modulation, J. Proteome Res. 5 (10) (2006) 2780–2788.

[109] F.A. van Dorsten, C.H. Grun, E.J. van Velzen, D.M. Jacobs, R. Draijer, J.P. van Duynhoven, The metabolic fate of red wine and grape juice polyphenols in humans assessed by metabolomics, Mol. Nutr. Food Res. 54 (2010) 897–908.

[110] M.C. Walsh, L. Brennan, E. Pujos-Guillot, J.L. Sebedio, A. Scalbert, A. Fagan, et al., Influence of acute phytochemical intake on human urinary metabolomic profiles, Am. J. Clin. Nutr. 86 (6) (2007) 1687–1693.

[111] E.J. van Velzen, J.A. Westerhuis, J.P. van Duynhoven, F.A. van Dorsten, C.H. Grun, D.M. Jacobs, et al., Phenotyping tea consumers by nutrikinetic analysis of polyphenolic end-metabolites, J. Proteome Res. 8 (7) (2009) 3317–3330.

[112] C.B. Newgard, J. An, J.R. Bain, M.J. Muehlbauer, R.D. Stevens, L.F. Lien, et al., A branched-chain amino acid-related metabolic signature that differentiates obese and lean humans and contributes to insulin resistance, Cell Metab. 9 (4) (2009) 311–326.

[113] M.E. Dumas, E.C. Maibaum, C. Teague, H. Ueshima, B. Zhou, J.C. Lindon, et al., Assessment of analytical reproducibility of 1H NMR spectroscopy based metabonomics for large-scale epidemiological research: the Intermap Study, Anal. Chem. 78 (7) (2006) 2199–2208.

[114] J.F. Fearnside, M.E. Dumas, A.R. Rothwell, S.P. Wilder, O. Cloarec, A. Toye, et al., Phylometabonomic patterns of adaptation to high fat diet feeding in inbred mice, PLoS ONE 3 (2) (2008) e1668.

[115] E. Holmes, R.L. Loo, J. Stamler, M. Bictash, I.K. Yap, Q. Chan, et al., Human metabolic phenotype diversity and its association with diet and blood pressure, Nature 453 (7193) (2008) 396–400.

[116] O. Shaham, R. Wei, T.J. Wang, C. Ricciardi, G.D. Lewis, R.S. Vasan, et al., Metabolic profiling of the human response to a glucose challenge reveals distinct axes of insulin sensitivity, Mol. Syst. Biol. 4 (2008) 214.

[117] X. Zhao, A. Peter, J. Fritsche, M. Elcnerova, A. Fritsche, H.U. Haring, et al., Changes of the plasma metabolome during an oral glucose tolerance test: is there more than glucose to look at, Am. J. Physiol. Endocrinol. Metab. 296 (2) (2009) E384–E393.

[118] H.M. Blanck, B.A. Bowman, G.R. Cooper, G.L. Myers, D.T. Miller, Laboratory issues: use of nutritional biomarkers, J. Nutr. 133 (Suppl. 3) (2003) 888S–894S.

[119] D. Hunter, Biochemical indicators of dietary intake, in: W. Willett (Ed.), Nutritional Epidemiology, second ed., Oxford University Press, New York, 1998, pp. 174–243.

[120] T.P. Whitehead, Quality Control in Clinical Chemistry, Wiley, New York, 1977.

[121] A. Aitio, P. Apostoli, Quality assurance in biomarker measurement, Toxicol. Lett. 77 (1995) 195–204.

[122] J.O. Westgard, P.L. Barry, M.R. Hunt, T. Groth, A multi-rule Shewhart chart for quality control in clinical chemistry, Clin. Chem. 27 (1981) 493–501.

[123] D.A. Lipschitz, J.D. Cook, C.A. Finch, A clinical evaluation of serum ferritin, N. Engl. J. Med. 290 (1974) 1213–1216.

[124] V. Herbert, Recommended dietary intakes (RDI) of folate in humans, Am. J. Clin. Nutr. 45 (1987) 661–670.

[125] E. Trujillo, C. Davis, J. Milner, Nutrigenomics, proteomics, metabolomics, and the practice of dietetics, J. Am. Diet. Assoc. 106 (2006) 403–413.

[126] M.D. Niculescu, K.A. da Costa, L.M. Fischer, S.H. Zeisel, Lymphocyte gene expression in subjects fed a low-choline diet differs between those who develop organ dysfunction and those who do not, Am. J. Clin. Nutr. 86 (2007) 230–239.

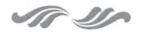

NUTRITION FOR HEALTH MAINTAINENCE, PREVENTION, AND DISEASE-SPECIFIC TREATMENT

PART A

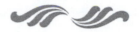

FOOD AND NUTRITION INTAKE
FOR HEALTH

Nutrition Guidelines to Maintain Health

Carol West Suitor*, Suzanne P. Murphy†

*Nutrition Consultant, Winooski, Vermont †University of Hawaii Cancer Center, Honolulu, Hawaii

I INTRODUCTION

Nutrition guidelines for Americans fall into two broad categories: those that focus primarily on nutrient intakes and those that are primarily oriented to food choices. In addition, because healthy food and nutrient intakes are closely linked to healthy activity levels, physical activity guidance is often included with dietary guidance.

The Food and Nutrition Board of the National Academies has periodically released recommendations for nutrient intakes by Americans. Beginning in 1997, its nutrient recommendations took the form of Dietary Reference Intakes (DRIs) [1−7]. DRI is an umbrella term for four types of nutrient recommendations:

- Estimated average requirement (EAR)
- Recommended Dietary Allowance (RDA)
- Adequate intake (AI)
- Tolerable upper intake level (UL)

The EAR, RDA, and AI all relate to nutrient adequacy, and the UL relates to safety. DRIs have been set for energy, 14 vitamins, 15 minerals (with ULs for an additional 3), and 7 macronutrients. A summary of all the DRI values is given in the Appendix. Prior to 1997, nutrient recommendations were limited to RDAs and Safe and Adequate Daily Dietary Intakes [8].

The U.S. Department of Agriculture (USDA) and the U.S. Department of Health and Human Services (HHS) have jointly issued the Dietary Guidelines for Americans every 5 years since 1980. The *Dietary Guidelines* are to be used to develop educational materials and to assist policymakers to design and implement federal food, nutrition education, and information programs. The policy document *Dietary Guidelines for Americans 2010* was released in 2011 [9]. In 2008, HHS developed *Physical Activity Guidelines for Americans* [10]. A summary of those guidelines is included in the 2010 *Dietary Guidelines* policy document [9]. Advice to increase physical activity now frequently accompanies dietary guidance because health professionals recognize that maintenance of a healthy body size and sustained cardiopulmonary fitness can be achieved only through an active lifestyle coupled with healthy dietary choices.

USDA plays a key role in developing educational materials to support the implementation of the *Dietary Guidelines*. USDA developed MyPlate and many other materials that may be found at the website http://www.choosemyplate.gov. The site provides tools to be used by professionals in nutrition education efforts and to help the public make healthy food choices. The Food and Drug Administration (FDA) is responsible for regulations governing the Nutrition Facts panel [11] and the Supplement Facts label [12], both of which are required by law. These regulations provide consumers with nutrition information at the point of purchase and are intended to help consumers meet the *Dietary Guidelines*.

II GUIDELINES FOR NUTRIENT INTAKES

A Overview

The DRIs offer guidance on the level of nutrient intake that will promote health, reduce the risk of chronic disease, and reduce risk associated with excessive nutrient intake. The Food and Nutrition Board sought substantial input from nutrition professionals [13] as it developed the process for setting the DRIs, and it incorporated several new concepts into the process:

- An increased focus on the reduction of chronic disease.

Nutrition in the Prevention and Treatment of Disease, Third Edition.
DOI: http://dx.doi.org/10.1016/B978-0-12-391884-0.00013-5

- Determination of the EAR, which would be the intake that would be adequate for approximately 50% of a healthy population.
- Calculation of the RDA from the EAR, by adding two standard deviations of the requirement distribution. The RDA is thus the level of intake that would be adequate for 97.5% of the population.
- Use of the AI when the scientific database is not sufficient to set an EAR (and its associated RDA).
- Determination of the UL, which represents the upper level of intake that poses a low risk of adverse effects. Usual intakes above this level are not recommended.

The first DRI reports were issued for six sets of nutrients: bone-related nutrients (calcium, phosphorus, magnesium, vitamin D, and fluoride) [1], B vitamins (e.g., thiamin, riboflavin, niacin, vitamin B_6, vitamin B_{12}, folate, and choline) [2], antioxidant nutrients (e.g., vitamin C, vitamin E, and selenium) [3], micronutrients (vitamins A and K, iron, zinc, copper, iodine, molybdenum, and several other minerals) [4], macronutrients (e.g., energy, protein, fat, carbohydrates, and dietary fiber) [5], and electrolytes (e.g., potassium, sodium, and chloride) [6]. In 2010, the Institute of Medicine (IOM) released a DRI report that updates the recommendations for calcium and vitamin D [7]. The Appendix includes updated values from this report.

To address appropriate ways to use the DRIs, IOM released two reports—one on assessing nutrient intakes [14] and the other on planning nutrient intakes [15]. A summary report on the DRIs is available [16] and provides a concise reference to the DRI values and appropriate uses, but it does not encompass the recent changes in the DRIs for calcium and vitamin D.

B Dietary Reference Intakes for Nutrient Adequacy

The RDA (or the AI if an RDA is not available) is the appropriate target for guidance to consumers on healthy nutrient intakes. Because an individual's actual requirement is almost never known, the goal is to reduce to a very low level the risk that an intake is inadequate. By definition, usual intake at the level of the RDA or AI has a low risk of inadequacy (2 or 3% for the RDA). The appropriate target for vitamin D intake for a woman 31–50 years of age, for example, is the RDA of 600 IU (15 μg)/day [7]. Her target for potassium would be the AI of 4.7 g/day [6].

To reflect current information on bioavailability, the RDAs for two nutrients are expressed in forms that are unfamiliar to many consumers and clients: Folate is in micrograms of dietary folate equivalents (DFE) rather than total micrograms of folate, and vitamin E is in milligrams of α-tocopherol rather than in milligrams of α-tocopherol equivalents. The new DFE unit reflects the higher availability of fortification and supplemental forms of folate compared with naturally occurring folate in foods. Thus, the use of DFEs tends to increase estimates of an individual's intakes of this nutrient. The newer vitamin E unit reflects the lower bioavailability of forms of tocopherol other than the RRR and 2R stereoisomeric forms of α-tocopherol. The less available forms include β-tocopherol and γ-tocopherol, which are not transported well from the liver. Furthermore, the all-racemic α-tocopherol form that is commonly used for fortification and in dietary supplements has a lower activity than does α-tocopherol. Therefore, intakes measured in the older units (α-tocopherol equivalents) will overestimate intakes of the active forms of the vitamin.

Recent changes in the DRIs for calcium and vitamin D merit special attention. In 1997, AIs had been set for calcium and vitamin D because the data were judged insufficient to set EARs and RDAs. The new reference values for these two nutrients are based on an exhaustive review of a much larger amount of information, including studies of higher quality than were available by 1997 [1]. The 2010 report [7] provides EARs and RDAs for both nutrients. Compared with the original DRI values, the RDAs for calcium are the same as the previous AIs for nearly all the age–gender groups. The exceptions apply to children ages 1–3 and 4–8 years, for whom the 2010 RDAs for calcium are 200 mg lower than the 1997 AIs. The changes in the DRIs for vitamin D are much more extensive. In particular, the 2010 RDAs for vitamin D are higher than the 1997 AIs for all the age–gender groups. They are 1.5 times higher for persons ages 1–70 years, 1.33 times higher for persons ages 71 or older, and 3 times higher for pregnant and lactating females. For infants ages 0–11 months, the 2010 AIs are twice as high as the 1997 AIs. For both the nutrients, the availability of EARs for all age groups above infants makes it possible to better assess the extent to which inadequate dietary intake may be a problem for groups of people.

C Dietary Reference Intake for Safety: The Tolerable Upper Intake Level

The UL indicates a level of nutrient intake that should not be exceeded. A UL should never be considered a target intake; the RDA and AI are the appropriate targets. Health professionals may guide consumers in using the UL to ensure that nutrient intakes are not too high. The Appendix shows the ULs that have been set for 8 vitamins and 16 minerals.

In the most recent DRI report [7], the UL for calcium of 2500 mg/day was not changed for children younger than 9 years or for adults ages 19–50 years, but it was increased to 3000 mg/day for older children through age 18 years and decreased to 2000 mg/day for adults ages 51 years or older. Intakes that exceed the UL are most likely to occur through the consumption of many calcium-fortified foods or calcium supplements or a combination. Intakes above the UL for calcium carry an increased risk of kidney stone formation, especially in adults. The recent DRI report also includes changes in the ULs for vitamin D—all of which are higher. They now range from 2500 IU (63 µg) for children ages 1–3 years to 3000 IU (75 µg) for children ages 4–9 years and 4000 IU (100 µg) for older children and adults of all ages.

The DRIs specify different forms for the RDA and the UL for four nutrients: magnesium, niacin, folate, and vitamin E. The UL for magnesium for adults is 350 mg/day, but this value applies to pharmacological forms only. (Magnesium salts can cause osmotic diarrhea.) For niacin and folate, the ULs apply to forms used in fortification or supplements only. For vitamin E, the UL applies to all forms of α-tocopherol.

ULs are not available for all nutrients, not because intake at any level in considered safe but, rather, because there was not sufficient scientific data to set a UL. In some circumstances (controlled trials, feeding studies, or therapeutic prescriptions), intakes above the UL may be appropriate if medical supervision is provided.

D How Current Nutrient Intakes Compare to the DRIs

To evaluate the intakes of groups of people, the recommended method [14] involves evaluating intakes from large dietary intake surveys and estimating the percentage of the population whose usual intake is below the EAR. That percentage is an accurate estimate of the prevalence of inadequate intakes for most nutrients. When nutrient requirements are skewed, however, as is the case with iron requirements for menstruating women, a somewhat modified approach is used [17]. For nutrients with an AI rather than an EAR, it is not possible to quantify the prevalence of inadequacy, but mean intakes above the AI indicate that a low prevalence of inadequacy is likely. The National Health and Nutrition Examination Survey (NHANES), which is conducted continuously by the USDA and the HHS, is a widely used source of dietary intake data for the assessment of adequate and excessive intakes. Many authors acknowledge the challenges of evaluating the nutrient intakes of either individuals or groups [18–20].

1 Adequacy

Table 13.1 shows the recommended intakes (RDAs or AIs) for selected nutrients by gender; using NHANES data, it also shows the estimated mean intake of each nutrient from food and the estimated prevalence of dietary inadequacy as the percentage of the population with intakes below the EAR. Comparable estimates using more recent data were not available, with the partial exception of calcium and vitamin D. Estimates obtained using NHANES 2003–2006 data indicate that median calcium intake by male adults ranged from 728 to 942 mg/day, and median calcium intake by female adults ranged from 589 to 686 mg/day. For both genders, median calcium intakes decreased with age and with median energy intake [21]. With regard to vitamin D, the IOM [7] examined data on serum values of 25-hydroxyvitamin D as an additional way to assess adequacy. The committee stated that some of the cut points for serum values used in identifying vitamin D deficiency appear to be excessively high. The IOM concluded that consensus cutoff points for vitamin D deficiency and excess are needed for public health and clinical care.

Comparing mean intake with the RDA, as could be done using Table 13.1, may give a misleading picture of the extent of inadequacy. For example, the estimated mean intake of vitamin C by women exceeded the RDA, but 32% of women were found to have intakes below the EAR. For fiber and potassium, which have AIs rather than EARs, the prevalence of inadequacy would be assumed to be low if the mean intake were above the AI. In these two cases, however, the mean intake is far below the AI, and thus the prevalence of inadequacy is unknown. According to the 2010 Dietary Guidelines Advisory Committee [22], fewer than 4% of Americans had fiber intakes above the AI, and fewer than 3% had potassium intakes above the AI.

The prevalence of dietary inadequacy is 10% or less for vitamin B_{12} and iron for both men and women and for vitamin B_6 and folate for men (see Table 13.1). The estimate for vitamin B_{12}, however, does not take into consideration the reduced absorption of naturally occurring vitamin B_{12} that occurs among many individuals beginning at approximately age 51 years. Although the estimated prevalence of inadequacy is especially high for vitamin E (89% for men and 97% for women), clinical deficiencies of vitamin E are rare [3].

Low intakes of calcium and vitamin D are of special concern because of their association with reduced skeletal health, and low intakes of potassium and fiber are of concern because of their association with chronic conditions. Thus, given the relatively high prevalence of inadequacy for these and several other nutrients (vitamins A, C, and E and magnesium), it appears that nutrient intakes need to be improved.

TABLE 13.1 How Adequate Are the Dietary Nutrient Intakes of American Adults? Selected Nutrients for Men and Women 19 Years of Age or Older

Nutrient	Gender	Recommended intake[a]	Reported intake[b]	Prevalence of dietary inadequacy (%)[b,c]
Vitamin A (RAE/day)	Men	900	656	57
	Women	700	564	48
Vitamin C (mg/day)[d]	Men	90	105	36
	Women	75	84	32
Vitamin D (IU/day)	Men	600–800	200–216[e]	ND[f]
	Women	15–20	140–176[e]	ND[g]
Vitamin E (mg α-tocopherol/day)	Men	15	8.2	89
	Women	15	6.3	97
Dietary fiber (g/day)	Men	30–38	18.0	Unknown
	Women	21–25	14.3	Unknown
Vitamin B$_6$ (mg/day)	Men	1.3–1.7	2.23	7
	Women	1.3–1.5	1.53	28
Folate (μg DFE/day)	Men	400	636	6
	Women	400	483	16
Vitamin B$_{12}$ (μg/day)[h]	Men	2.4	6.45	<3
	Women	2.4	4.33	7–9
Iron (mg/day)	Men	8	18.0	<3
	Women	8–18	13.1	10
Zinc (mg/day)	Men	11	14.2	11
	Women	8	9.7	17
Calcium (mg/day)	Men	1000–1200	984	ND[i]
	Women	1000–1200	735	ND[j]
Magnesium (mg/day)	Men	400–420	322	64
	Women	310–320	240	67
Potassium (mg/day)	Men	4700	3141	Unknown
	Women	4700	2267	Unknown

[a]Adequate intake (AI) or Recommended Dietary Allowance (RDA) as shown in the Appendix excluding values for pregnant and lactating women.

[b]From What We Eat in America, NHANES, 2001–2002 [23]; mean intake from food only. Mean intakes would increase if supplements were included.

[c]The percentage of intakes below the estimated average requirement (EAR) [14]. All intake data were adjusted for day-to-day variation in intakes before examining the proportion below the EAR.

[d]Vitamin C recommendations are for nonsmokers; they are 35 mg/day higher for smokers. The prevalences of vitamin C inadequacy are for nonsmokers. Corresponding prevalences for smokers are 69% for men and 76% for women.

[e]Range of means for adults presented in Table H-3a of the recent DRI Dietary Reference Intakes Calcium and Vitamin D [7]; data from NHANES 2005–2006.

[f]Based on NHANES 2005–2006 data, food sources only [7], more than 75% of men had vitamin D intakes below the EAR.

[g]Based on NHANES 2005–2006 data, food sources only [7], more than 95% of women had vitamin D intakes below the EAR except for the women ages 31–50 years, whose vitamin D intakes were higher.

[h]Prevalence for participants 19–50 years of age. Prevalence was not calculated for participants age 50 or older because 10–30% of older adults may not absorb vitamin B$_{12}$ in foods, so this age group should take a supplement or consume foods that are fortified with vitamin B$_{12}$.

[i]Based on NHANES 2003–2006 data, food sources only [7], fewer than 25% of men ages 19–50 years had calcium intakes below the EAR, but more than 50% of older men did.

[j]Based on NHANES 2003–2006 data, food sources only [7], more than 50% of women had calcium intakes below the EAR.

DFE, Dietary folate equivalents; ND, not determined; RAE, retinol activity equivalents.

2 Risk of Excessive Intake

Because ULs have been set for many nutrients, it is possible to examine the prevalence of intakes at risk of being excessive. As shown in Table 13.2, which covers intakes from food, the prevalence of intakes that exceed the UL tends to be low for adults for all nutrients except sodium. In particular, sodium intakes are above the UL for 94% of men and 74% of women. Sodium

TABLE 13.2   What Is the Prevalence of Intakes from Food That Are above the Tolerable Upper Intake Level?[a]

Nutrient	Prevalence for children, 1—18 years	Prevalence for adults, 19 years or older
Retinol	1—3 years: 12%	<3%
	Other ages: <3%	
Folic acid	1—3 years: 5%	<3%
	4—8 years: 4%	
	Other ages: <3%	
Vitamin B$_6$	<3%	<3%
Vitamin C	<3%	<3%
Calcium	<3%	<3%
Phosphorus	<3%	<3%
Iron	<3%	<3%
Zinc	1—3 years: 69%	<3%
	4—8 years: 22%	
	Other ages: <3%	
Copper	1—3 years: 15%	<3%
	Other ages: <3%	
Selenium	1—3 years: 8%	<3%
	Other ages: <3%	
Sodium	1—3 years: 83%	Men: 94%
	4—8 years: 94%	Women: 74%
	9—18 years: 74—97%	

[a]Intake from food only. Prevalence of intakes above the UL would increase if supplements were included.
Source: What We Eat in America, NHANES 2001—2002 [23].

intakes are also above the UL for all ages of children and adolescents. These findings are of concern because high sodium intake is linked with hypertension [6]. Although few adults have intakes that exceed the UL for other nutrients, high intakes of some nutrients may be of concern for children. For example, high zinc intakes are a concern up to 8 years, as are retinol, copper, and selenium intakes for children 1—3 years of age. Because many of the ULs are extrapolated from data for adults, it is possible that they are unnecessarily low for some nutrients.

An important consideration when evaluating intakes is whether all sources of a nutrient are measured and included in total intake. In particular, many Americans take dietary supplements, and the contribution of supplements to intakes should be considered before evaluating the adequacy of an individual diet or the prevalence of inadequacy for a group of individuals. Although NHANES 2001—2002 collected and quantified nutrient intakes from supplements, the sources of the data in Tables 13.1 and 13.2 [7,24] do not reflect intakes from supplements. Therefore, the mean intakes reported in these tables for many of these nutrients are lower than they would have been with supplements included. In addition, the percentage of the population with intakes below the EAR is probably an overestimate of the true prevalence of dietary inadequacy, and the prevalence of intakes above the UL may be underestimated.

III GUIDELINES FOR HEALTHY FOOD CHOICES: DIETARY GUIDELINES FOR AMERICANS

A Overview

By law, the secretaries of USDA and HHS are required to jointly issue *Dietary Guidelines for Americans* every 5 years. *Dietary Guidelines for Americans, 2010* [9], the policy document, is the most recent edition. One of the major ways in which the 2010 *Dietary Guidelines* differs from earlier editions is that it addresses an American public of whom the majority are overweight or obese. It is intended for Americans age 2 years or older even if they are at increased risk of chronic diseases such as cardiovascular disease, hypertension, type 2 diabetes mellitus, and osteoporosis. Following the guidelines may help Americans "attain and maintain a healthy weight, reduce the risk of chronic disease, and promote overall health" [9, p. 5].

To provide the scientific basis for the *Dietary Guidelines*, the 2010 Dietary Guidelines Advisory Committee conducted an evidence-based review of diet and health [22]. The committee's process led to the development of two overarching concepts:

1. Maintain calorie balance over time to achieve and sustain a healthy weight.
2. Focus on consuming nutrient-dense foods and beverages.

The policy document [9] gives a relatively lengthy explanation of the term *nutrient dense*. Key elements of the term include the following:

- "The term 'nutrient dense' indicates that the nutrients and other beneficial substances in a food have not been 'diluted' by the addition of calories from added solid fats, added sugars, or added refined starches, or by the solid fats naturally present in the food."

- "All vegetables, fruits, whole grains, seafood, eggs, beans and peas, unsalted nuts and seeds, fat-free and low-fat milk and milk products, and lean meats and poultry—when prepared without adding solid fats or sugars—are nutrient-dense foods." [9, p. 5]

Dietary Guidelines focuses more on the forms of food than on the actual density of specific vitamins,

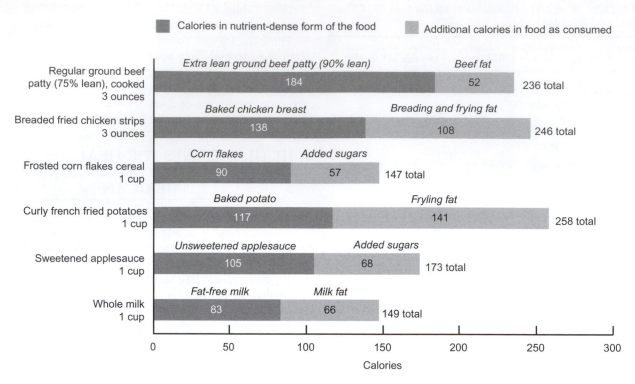

FIGURE 13.1   Examples of the calories in food choices that are not in nutrient-dense forms and the calories in nutrient-dense forms of these foods. Based on data from the U.S. Department of Agriculture, Agricultural Research Service, Food and Nutrient Database for Dietary Studies 4.1 (http://www.ars.usda.gov/Services/docs.htm?docid=20511) and the National Nutrient Database for Standard Reference, Release 23 (http://www.nal.usda.gov/fnic/foodcomp/search). Source: *USDA/HHS [9], Figure 5-2, p. 47.* See color plate.

minerals, or protein in the food. By the previous definition, both iceberg and romaine lettuce are nutrient-dense foods even though the content of several nutrients is considerably higher in the romaine, whether expressed per unit weight or per kilocalorie. Figure 13.1 provides examples of the calories in food choices that are in nutrient-dense forms and the additional calories in forms of the food as commonly consumed.

The *Dietary Guidelines* are linked to the DRIs in that the guidelines and materials that support them are designed to help people meet the DRIs—primarily through consuming foods rather than supplements. Key recommendations taken from the 2010 *Dietary Guidelines* appear in Box 13.1.

The 2010 *Dietary Guidelines* include the following key recommendations for specific population groups:

- Women capable of becoming pregnant: (1) Choose foods that supply heme iron, additional iron sources, and enhancers of iron absorption; and (2) consume 400 μg/day of synthetic folic acid from fortified foods and/or supplements.
- Pregnant women: (1) Consume 8–12 oz. of a variety of seafood per week, (2) limit the intake of fish that are high in methylmercury content, and (3) take an

iron supplement as recommended by one's health care provider. The first two recommendations for pregnant women also apply to breast-feeding women.
- Individuals ages 50 years and older: Consume foods fortified with vitamin B_{12} or a vitamin B_{12} supplement.

B New Aspects of Key Recommendations

This section provides information about some of the new aspects of the key recommendations in *Dietary Guidelines for Americans* [9].

1 Balancing Calories to Manage Weight

Dietary Guidelines covers the epidemic of overweight and obesity, the meaning of the terms overweight and obese, the obesogenic environment, current dietary intake, calorie balance, and weight management (including guidelines for physical activity). As can be seen in Box 13.1, the *Dietary Guidelines* takes an integrated approach to healthy eating that incorporates a number of aspects of weight management. Thus, the following discussion is limited to calorie needs, sources of calories, and physical activity guidelines.

BOX 13.1

DIETARY GUIDELINES FOR AMERICANS 2010 KEY RECOMMENDATIONS

Balancing Calories to Manage Weight

- Prevent and/or reduce overweight and obesity through improved eating and physical activity behaviors.
- Control total calorie intake to manage body weight. For people who are overweight or obese, this will mean consuming fewer calories from foods and beverages.
- Increase physical activity and reduce time spent in sedentary behaviors.
- Maintain appropriate calorie balance during each stage of life—childhood, adolescence, adulthood, pregnancy and breast-feeding, and older age.

Foods and Food Components to Reduce

- Reduce daily sodium intake to less than 2300 milligrams (mg) and further reduce intake to 1500 mg among persons who are 51 and older and those of any age who are African American or have hypertension, diabetes, or chronic kidney disease. The 1500 mg recommendation applies to about half of the U.S. population, including children, and the majority of adults.
- Consume less than 10 percent of calories from saturated fatty acids by replacing them with monounsaturated and polyunsaturated fatty acids.
- Consume less than 300 mg per day of dietary cholesterol.
- Keep trans fatty acid consumption as low as possible by limiting foods that contain synthetic sources of trans fats, such as partially hydrogenated oils, and by limiting other solid fats.
- Reduce the intake of calories from solid fats and added sugars.
- Limit the consumption of foods that contain refined grains, especially refined grain foods that contain solid fats, added sugars, and sodium.
- If alcohol is consumed, it should be consumed in moderation—up to one drink per day for women and two drinks per day for men—and only by adults of legal drinking age.

Foods and Nutrients to Increase

Individuals should meet the following recommendations as part of a healthy eating pattern while staying within their calorie needs.

- Increase vegetable and fruit intake.
- Eat a variety of vegetables, especially dark-green and red and orange vegetables and beans and peas.
- Consume at least half of all grains as whole grains. Increase whole-grain intake by replacing refined grains with whole grains.
- Increase intake of fat-free or low-fat milk and milk products, such as milk, yogurt, cheese, or fortified soy beverages.
- Choose a variety of protein foods, which include seafood, lean meat and poultry, eggs, beans and peas, soy products, and unsalted nuts and seeds.
- Increase the amount and variety of seafood consumed by choosing seafood in place of some meat and poultry.
- Replace protein foods that are higher in solid fats with choices that are lower in solid fats and calories and/or are sources of oils.
- Use oils to replace solid fats where possible.
- Choose foods that provide more potassium, dietary fiber, calcium, and vitamin D, which are nutrients of concern in American diets. These foods include vegetables, fruits, whole grains, and milk and milk products.

Building Healthy Eating Patterns

- Select an eating pattern that meets nutrient needs over time at an appropriate calorie level.
- Account for all foods and beverages consumed and assess how they fit within a total healthy eating pattern.
- Follow food safety recommendations when preparing and eating foods to reduce the risk of foodborne illnesses.

Source: *U.S. Department of Agriculture/U.S. Department of Health and Human Services* [9].

a CALORIE NEEDS

Table 13.3 gives an estimate of individual calorie needs. The calorie range for each age/sex group is based on physical activity level, from sedentary to active.

b SOURCES OF CALORIES

The policy document includes a table that lists the top 25 sources of calories among all Americans ages 2 years or older and by two age groups. Table 13.4 provides an excerpt that highlights the five top sources of calories

TABLE 13.3 Estimated Calorie Needs per Day by Age, Gender, and Physical Activity Level[a]

Gender	Age (years)	Physical activity level (kcal)		
		Sedentary[b]	Moderately Active[c]	Active[d]
Child	2–3	1000–1200[e]	1000–1400[e]	1000–1400[e]
Female[f]	4–8	1200–1400	1400–1600	1400–1800
	9–13	1400–1600	1600–2000	1800–2200
	14–18	1800	2000	2400
	19–30	1800–2000	2000–2200	2400
	31–50	1800	2000	2200
	51+	1600	1800	2000–2200
Male	4–8	1200–1400	1400–1600	1600–2000
	9–13	1600–2000	1800–2200	2000–2600
	14–18	2000–2400	2400–2800	2800–3200
	19–30	2400–2600	2600–2800	3000
	31–50	2200–2400	2400–2600	2800–3000
	51+	2000–2200	2200–2400	2400–2800

[a]Based on estimated energy requirement (EER) equations, using reference heights (average) and reference weights (healthy) for each age/gender group. For children and adolescents, reference height and weight vary. For adults, the reference man is 5 feet 10 inches tall and weighs 154 pounds. The reference woman is 5 feet 4 inches tall and weighs 126 pounds. EER equations are from [5].
[b]Sedentary means a lifestyle that includes only the light physical activity associated with typical day-to-day life.
[c]Moderately active means a lifestyle that includes physical activity equivalent to walking approximately 1.5–3 miles per day at 3 or 4 miles per hour, in addition to the light physical activity associated with typical day-to-day life.
[d]Active means a lifestyle that includes physical activity equivalent to walking more than 3 miles per day at 3 or 4 miles per hour, in addition to the light physical activity associated with typical day-to-day life.
[e]The calorie ranges shown are to accommodate the needs of different ages within the group. For children and adolescents, more calories are needed at older ages. For adults, fewer calories are needed at older ages.
[f]Estimates for females do not include women who are pregnant or breast-feeding.
Source: U.S. Department of Agriculture/U.S. Department of Health and Human Services [9], Table 2-3, p. 14.

consumed by children ages 2–18 years and adults ages 19 years or older. The calorie values in parentheses are daily means. Considerable day-to-day variation would be expected.

Clearly, the top five calorie sources are similar for adults and children. The major differences are that pizza appears in the top five for the younger age group, whereas alcoholic beverages appear in the top five for adults. Each food category includes commonly eaten foods that are high in solid fats or added sugars, high in refined grain rather than whole grain, or low in essential nutrients—or that have two or more of these characteristics. In Figure 13.1, for example, one can see that nearly half the calories in the very popular breaded fried chicken strips come from the breading and the frying fat. For many Americans, balancing calories is likely to require

TABLE 13.4 Top Five Sources of Calories among Americans, by Age Group, 2005–2006

Rank	Food category (mean kcal/day)	
	Ages 2–18 years (mean total daily calories = 2027)	Ages 19+ years (mean total daily calories = 2199)
1	Grain-based desserts (138 kcal)[a]	Grain-based desserts (138 kcal)[a]
2	Pizza (136 kcal)	Yeast breads (134 kcal)
3	Soda/energy/sports drinks (118 kcal)	Chicken and chicken mixed dishes (123 kcal)[b]
4	Yeast breads (114 kcal)	Soda/energy/sports drinks (112 kcal)
5	Chicken and chicken mixed dishes (113 kcal)[b]	Alcoholic beverages (106 kcal)

[a]Includes cake, cookies, pie, cobbler, sweet rolls, pastries, and donuts.
[b]Includes fried or baked chicken parts and chicken strips/patties, chicken stir-fries, chicken casseroles, chicken sandwiches, chicken salads, stewed chicken, and other chicken mixed dishes.
Source: Excerpt from USDA/HHS [9]; 2011 data from NHANES 2005–2006, as analyzed by the National Cancer Institute.

lower intake of commonly consumed foods that are low in nutrient density.

c PHYSICAL ACTIVITY GUIDELINES

Beginning in 2000, increasing concerns about both fitness levels and the obesity rates among Americans led to a dietary guideline that focused specifically on physical activity. *Dietary Guidelines for Americans, 2010* supports the *2008 Physical Activity Guidelines for Americans* [10] developed by HHS. According to the Physical Activity Guidelines Advisory Committee [25],

> Very strong scientific evidence based on a wide range of well-conducted studies shows that physically active people have higher levels of health-related fitness, a lower risk profile for developing a number of disabling medical conditions, and lower rates of various chronic diseases than do people who are inactive. [25, p. A-2]

Among the health benefits for adults are lower rates of all-cause mortality, coronary heart disease, high blood pressure, stroke, type 2 diabetes, metabolic syndrome, colon cancer, breast cancer, and depression. For children, "well-documented health benefits include reduced body fatness, more favorable cardiovascular and metabolic disease risk profiles, enhanced bone health, and reduced symptoms of anxiety and depression" [25, p. A-2–3].

An active lifestyle can promote a healthy diet by increasing energy requirements. With a larger energy budget, individuals can spare calories for additional foods that contain added sugars or fats, for example, without displacing foods from the healthy foundation

---

BOX 13.2

SELECTED POINTS MADE IN 2008 PHYSICAL ACTIVITY GUIDELINES

Children and adolescents: Do 60 minutes or more of physical activity daily.

- Have most of it be of moderate or vigorous intensity.
- At least 3 days/week, include
  - vigorous intensity exercise
  - muscle-strengthening exercise
  - bone-strengthening exercise

Adults: Avoid inactivity, and, for substantial health benefits, do at least 150 minutes of moderate-intensity or 75 minutes of vigorous-intensity aerobic physical activity over the week, performed in episodes of at least 10 minutes.

- For more extensive health benefits, do at least 300 minutes of moderate-intensity or 150 minutes of vigorous-intensity aerobic physical activity over the week.

- Do moderate-intensity or high-intensity muscle-strengthening activities that involve all the major muscle groups on 2 or more days per week.

Older adults: Follow the guidelines for adults if physically able.

- Be as active physically as your condition allows.
- Do exercises for balance if at risk of falling.
- Determine your level of effort relative to your level of fitness.
- If applicable, find out whether and how your condition affects your ability to do physical activity safely.

Source: *Excerpted and adapted from the U.S. Department of Health and Human Services* [10].

---

of their diets. When people can eat more food without gaining weight, they may experience greater enjoyment from eating.

Box 13.2 summarizes the key physical activity guidelines that are specified for children and adolescents, adults, and older adults. To reduce risks posed by physical activity, the 2008 guidelines also address safety, covering topics such as tailoring the physical activity to one's current fitness level and health goals, increasing physical activity gradually, using appropriate gear, following rules, choosing safe environments, and (if applicable because of a chronic condition) consulting with a health care provider about appropriate types and amounts of physical activity. In addition, the 2008 guidelines include recommendations for women during and after pregnancy, adults with disabilities, and people with chronic medical conditions.

Cross-sectional self-reported data on physical activity levels show that a majority of Americans do not meet physical activity recommendations. Such data have been collected through the Behavior Risk Factor Surveillance System (BRFSS; http://www.cdc.gov/brfss), the Youth Risk Behavior Surveillance System (YRBSS; NHANES (http://www.cdc.gov/nchs/nhanes.htm)), and the National Health Interview Survey (http://www.cdc.gov/nchs/nhis.htm). Using a criterion of participation in moderate-intensity activities for at least 30 minutes per day at least 5 days per week or vigorous-intensity activities for at least 10 minutes per day at least 3 days per

week or both, approximately 45–50% of all U.S. adults meet the physical activity recommendation. Compared with females, more males meet the recommendation, and the percentage of adults meeting the recommendation decreases substantially with age (e.g., data from BRFSS indicate a decrease from 60.5% for males ages 18–24 years to 43.1% for males age 65 years or older). In 2006, only 19% of adults reported participation in strength and endurance activities [10]. Similarly, data on the activity levels of youth indicate that much improvement is needed. YRBSS data for 2005 show fewer than 36% of high school students met current physical activity recommendations. For youth, the criterion is moderate to vigorous physical activity (causing an increase in heart rate and hard breathing at least some of the time) for at least 60 minutes per day on 5 or more days per week [10].

Recent publications provide further support for the *2008 Physical Activity Guidelines*. For example, the IOM report, *Early Childhood Obesity Prevention Policies* [26], includes four goals and recommendations directed to improving the physical activity levels of young children, and the American College of Sports Medicine (ACSM) released a new position stand called "Quantity and Quality of Exercise for Developing and Maintaining Cardiorespiratory, Musculoskeletal, and Neuromotor Fitness in Apparently Healthy Adults" [27]. The ACSM position additionally calls for both reducing the total time spent in sedentary activities and including frequent,

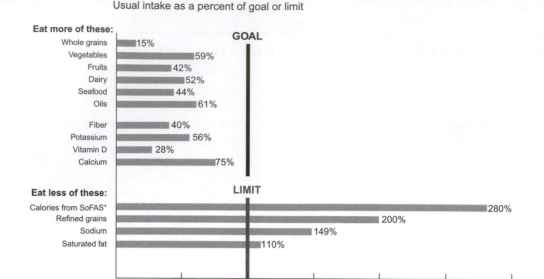

FIGURE 13.2   A comparison of typical American diets to selected recommended intake levels (goals) or limits. Bars show average intakes for all individuals (ages 1 or 2 years or older, depending on the data source) as a percentage of the recommended intake level or limit. Recommended intakes for food groups and limits for refined grains and solid fats and added sugars are based on amounts in the USDA 2000-calorie food pattern. Recommended intakes for fiber, potassium, vitamin D, and calcium are based on the highest adequate intake or Recommended Dietary Allowance for ages 14−70 years. Limits for sodium are based on the tolerable upper intake level and for saturated fat on 10% of calories. The protein foods group is not shown here because, on average, intake is close to recommended levels. *SoFAS, solid fats and added sugars. Based on data from the U.S. Department of Agriculture, Agricultural Research Service, and the U.S. Department of Health and Human Services, Centers for Disease Control and Prevention. What We Eat in America, NHANES 2001−2004 or 2005−2006. *Source: USDA/HHS [9], Figure 5-1, p. 46.* See color plate.

short bouts of standing and physical activity between periods of sedentary activity—even for physically active adults.

2 What to Reduce and What to Increase

Information about the dietary intakes of Americans provides a partial basis for the two key recommendations regarding dietary components to reduce and those to increase. Figure 13.2 illustrates how typical U.S. diets compare to recommended intake levels of selected food groups, food components, and nutrients.

a FOODS AND FOOD COMPONENTS TO REDUCE

This key recommendation addresses the consumption of sodium, saturated fat, dietary cholesterol, trans fatty acids, calories from solid fats and added sugars, refined grains, and alcohol. Each of these foods or food components is consumed in excessive amounts by a substantial percentage of the U.S. population, each may contribute to the risk of certain chronic diseases, and several of them contribute to the risk of overweight and obesity. Solid fats are listed in addition to saturated fat and trans fatty acids because of their abundant presence in U.S. diets and because they may make substantial contributions to excess calorie intake [9]. The four foods and food components that are highlighted in Figure 13.2 as items to be reduced are calories from solid fats and added sugars, refined grains, sodium, and saturated fat.

The *Dietary Guidelines* policy document places sodium first on the list of foods and food components to reduce and states that daily sodium intake should be lower than 1500 mg/day for approximately half of the population (African Americans; people with hypertension, diabetes, or chronic kidney disease; and all those age 51 years or older). For the rest of the U.S. population, the recommended sodium intake is less than 2300 mg/day. This is an especially challenging recommendation for individuals to meet because sodium is widely used by food manufacturers. Just prior to the release of the *Dietary Guidelines*, the IOM recommended a comprehensive set of strategies to reduce sodium intake [28].

Dietary Guidelines also gives special attention to reducing the intake of calories from solid fats and added sugars (SoFAS). As shown in Figure 13.2, intake of SoFAS far exceeds the recommended limit. On average, they contribute approximately 35% of the calories consumed by Americans each day without contributing essential nutrients. Curbing one's intake of SoFAS makes it easier to achieve nutrient adequacy without excessive calories.

b FOODS AND NUTRIENTS TO INCREASE

The food groups or subgroups to be increased are whole grains, vegetables, fruits, dairy, seafood, and oils high in unsaturated fatty acids. As can be seen in Figure 13.2, average intake of each of these food groups and subgroups by Americans is well below the goal that was set to promote health. Meeting the goals for the consumption of these types of foods is associated with improved nutrient intake and reduced risk of several chronic diseases. For example,

- High vegetable and fruit intake is associated with reduced risk of cardiovascular disease, and intake of specific vegetables and fruits may reduce the risk of some types of cancer.
- The consumption of whole grains may reduce the risk of cardiovascular disease, and it is associated with a lower body weight. More limited evidence suggests that whole grain intake is associated with reduced risk of type 2 diabetes.

The four nutrients to increase (vitamin D, calcium, potassium, and dietary fiber; Figure 13.2) are the only nutrients that the 2010 Dietary Guidelines Advisory Committee identified to be of public health concern for both adults and children [22]. The committee stated, "These four shortfall nutrients are clearly linked to indicators of nutrient inadequacy or disease prevalence and require special consideration in developing dietary guidance to meet recommended food intakes" [22, p. D2−25]. For other nutrients reported to be underconsumed, biochemical or clinical evidence did not support their identification as nutrients of public health concern. The *Dietary Guidelines* policy document, however, states that the first reason for recommending increased intake of fruits and vegetables is that they are major contributors of a number of underconsumed nutrients (folate, magnesium, potassium, dietary fiber, and vitamins A, C, and K).

The types of evidence used to support the identification of the four underconsumed nutrients as of public health concern included the following [22]:

- Vitamin D: Low wintertime serum 25-hydroxyvitamin D concentrations.
- Calcium: Data on the high prevalence of osteoporosis, osteopenia, and low bone mass.
- Potassium: Data on the high prevalence of U.S. adults who have prehypertension or hypertension,

and evidence that higher potassium consumption reduces both systolic and diastolic blood pressure.
- Dietary fiber: The role of dietary fiber in reducing the risk of coronary heart disease, the leading cause of death in the United States, and the possibility that fiber contributes to satiety and may thereby aid weight control.

With regard to vitamin D, the 2010 Dietary Guidelines Advisory Committee also referred to concurrent work by the IOM to reassess the DRIs for vitamin D. The DRI report on calcium and vitamin D, which was released in late 2010 [7], included evidence that vitamin D intakes of most Americans are below the new EARs but stated, "the estimated intake data for vitamin D cannot stand alone as a basis for broad public health action." A partial reason for this statement is that available data on serum 25-hydroxy D concentrations suggest that requirements are being met. Exposure to the sun may account for at least some of this discrepancy.

3 Building Healthy Eating Patterns

To achieve a healthy eating pattern, the *Dietary Guidelines* highlights four principles [9]:

1. Focus on nutrient-dense foods.
2. Remember that beverages count.
3. Follow food safety principles (often abbreviated as clean, separate, cook, and chill).
4. Consider the role of supplements and fortified foods.

Several templates for healthy eating are offered: the USDA Food Patterns, adaptation of those food patterns for vegetarians and vegans, and the DASH Eating Plan. The key recommendations for food group intake, however, do not specify amounts to consume. Table 13.5 provides a comparison of the average daily amounts of foods from different food groups recommended by two of those eating plans and the usual intake by adults in the United States as reported for the years 2001−2004.

The daily averages shown in Table 13.5 are useful for assessing intakes but not for providing practical guidance regarding how to plan menus for a day. See Section IV.A for more guidance on menu planning. Examination of Table 13.5 shows why key recommendations in the *Dietary Guidelines* include statements to increase total intake of fruits and vegetables, the variety of vegetables, and the proportion of whole grains and to decrease intake of solid fats and added sugars. Clearly, Americans' average intake of these foods or ingredients deviates substantially from the recommended amounts.

TABLE 13.5 Eating Pattern Comparison: USDA and DASH Food Patterns and Usual Adult Intake—At or Adjusted to *Daily* Averages across All Ages of Adults and Both Sexes

Food groups and subgroups (measure)	USDA food pattern	DASH pattern	Usual adult intake
Vegetables: total (c)	2.5	2.1	1.6
Dark green (c)	0.2	ND	0.1
Dried beans and peas (c)	0.2	See protein foods	0.1
Red and orange (c)	0.8	ND	0.4
Other (c)	0.6	ND	0.5
Starchy (c)	0.7	ND	0.5
Fruits and juices (c)	2.0	2.5	1.0
Grains: total (oz.)	6.0	7.3	6.4
Whole grains (oz.)	>3.0	3.9	0.6
Milk and milk products (dairy products) (c)	3.0	2.6	1.5
Protein foods:	5.5	5.8	5.1
Meat (oz.)	1.8	1.4	2.5
Poultry (oz.)	1.5	1.7	1.2
Eggs (oz.)	.4	ND	0.4
Fish/seafood (oz.)	1.2	1.4	0.5
Dried peas and beans (oz.)	See vegetables	0.4 (0.1 c)	See vegetables
Nuts, seeds, and soy products (oz.)	0.6	0.9	0.5
Oils (g)	27	25	18
Solid fats (g)	16	ND	43
Added sugars (g)	32	12	79
Alcohol (g)	ND	ND	9.9

c, cup; ND, not determined.

Source: *Adapted from U.S. Department of Agriculture/U.S. Department of Health and Human Services [9], Table 5-1, p. 51.*

4 Helping Americans Make Healthy Choices

One new aspect of the *Dietary Guidelines* policy document is the section that calls for environmental improvements that will promote physical activity and healthy eating. Health care professionals are among the many influential sectors that are called upon to become involved in systematic and coordinated efforts to effect such improvements. The 2010 *Dietary Guidelines'* call to action encompasses three principles [9, p. 57]:

1. Ensure that all Americans have access to nutritious foods and opportunities for physical activity

2. Facilitate individual behavior change through environmental strategies

3. Set the stage for lifelong healthy eating, physical activity, and weight management behaviors

Similarly, five key documents—*Healthy People 2010* [29] and IOM reports that address the prevention of childhood obesity [26,30] and food deserts [31] and the reduction of sodium intake [28]—emphasize the necessity for environmental improvements to promote the health and nutrition of Americans.

IV SELECTED GOVERNMENT RESOURCES TO PROMOTE NUTRITIONAL HEALTH

A MyPlate and Related Nutrition Education Materials

Dietary Guidelines for Americans, 2010 [9] was written for policymakers and a broad spectrum of health professionals, not for consumers. USDA has taken the lead in developing consumer messages and a new food icon based on the content of the policy document, as described in its *Executive Summary of Formative Research* [32]. To do so, USDA used an iterative consumer research approach that included (1) interviews with federal nutrition education staff, (2) an analysis of media coverage of the 2005 guidelines, (3) a review of six communication programs intended to influence consumers, and (4) a literature review. Then USDA conducted a series of focus groups that asked consumers to assess messages and submessages in terms of their effectiveness in helping to make healthier food choices. USDA acknowledged that some thought MyPyramid—the logo that was developed after the release of the 2005 *Dietary Guidelines*—was too complicated, whereas others thought it was too simplistic [32]. USDA also considered a recommendation of the White House Childhood Obesity Task Force, namely "Recommendation 2.1. The Federal government, working with local communities, should disseminate information about the 2010 *Dietary Guidelines for Americans* through simple, easily actionable messages for consumers and a next generation Food Pyramid" [33]. USDA concluded that a comprehensive, layered approach should be used to communicate the 2010 guidelines—an approach that uses a new logo in place of MyPyramid and provides practical tips, resources, and tools to help follow the guidelines in a way that fits individual consumers and their lifestyles.

MyPlate is the communication tool (food logo) that was designed to help Americans make better food choices and to remind them to eat healthfully [34]

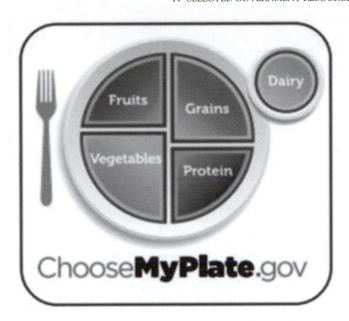

FIGURE 13.3 MyPlate. *Source: U.S. Department of Agriculture (http://www.cnpp.usda.gov/Publications/MyPlate/ MyPlateGraphicsStandards.pdf).*

(Figure 13.3). MyPlate emphasizes the key message: Make half your plate fruits and vegetables.

Compared to MyPyramid, MyPlate presents less information but uses a more understandable format [34]. Consumers can go to http://www.choosemyplate.gov and click on the segments of the MyPlate icon to learn what foods are in each food group, amounts to consume (expressed in cups or ounces), what counts as a cup or an ounce, benefits of consuming foods from the food group, and various tips. One can also find recipes, look up a food, get a personalized eating plan based on the 2010 *Dietary Guidelines*, get healthy eating tips and weight loss information, plan a healthy menu, review frequently asked questions and answers, and link with physical activity guidance. The website has a section for professionals (http://www.choosemyplate.gov/information-healthcare-professionals.html) that covers such topics as "Getting Started with MyPlate," "MyPlate Community Tool Kit," "A Brief History of USDA Food Guides," the communications message calendar for *Dietary Guidelines*, "Executive Summary of Formative Research," "Sample Menus at 2000 Calorie Level," "Food Group Recipes," "Daily Food Plans," and "MyPlateGraphic Standards." Box 13.3 provides an example of the kind of daily food plan that can be accessed for an adult. Notably, the plan gives target levels for the weekly consumption of different types of vegetables and of seafood.

Among the new materials for consumers is the *Dietary Guidelines* consumer brochure, which is a 4-page publication called "Let's Eat for the Health of It" [35]. This publication highlights four tips for healthy eating that are designed to help consumers focus on the most important aspects of the *Dietary Guidelines*:

1. Build a healthy plate.
2. Cut back on foods high in solid fats, added sugars, and salt.
3. Eat the right amount of calories for you.
4. Be physically active your way.

To date, 14 TipSheets have been developed [36] in conjunction with USDA. Topics include "10 Tips to a Great Plate" (Box 13.4), the five food groups shown in the MyPlate icon, healthy meal planning, vegetarian eating, shopping, strategies that address children, and salt and sodium.

B Food and Supplement Nutrition Labeling

Information on packaged foods can assist consumers to follow the *Dietary Guidelines*. Three parts of the packaging may be helpful: the Nutrition Facts panel, the ingredient listing, and, possibly, front-of-package information. The labeling of supplements is similar to that of foods but requires the listing of non-nutritive components.

1 Nutrition Facts and Supplement Facts Panels

a NUTRITION FACTS PANEL

The Nutrition Labeling and Education Act (NLEA) of 1990 requires a Nutrition Facts panel on most packaged food products [37] to help consumers follow the *Dietary Guidelines*. Nutrition information on unpackaged fruits and vegetables must be posted in the produce department of grocery stores. The FDA provides useful information about food labeling for consumers, professionals, and manufacturers at the FDA website [38,39]. The nutrient content of a food is shown as a percentage of a Daily Value (DV) [38]; DVs have not been updated in more than 20 years.

Accurate interpretation of the Nutrition Facts panel requires close attention to the listed portion size, which does not always correspond to the size used in the educational materials that support MyPlate. The serving sizes on the food label, which are specified by the NLEA, are intended to reflect the usual portion sizes that a consumer might typically select, whereas the portions specified in educational materials are used in planning meals for persons of different ages and activity levels.

Consumers can readily scan the %DVs on food labels to determine if a food item is a high or low source of specific food components and, if the serving size is the same, to compare two or more products. For example, the consumer may want to choose the food

BOX 13.3

RECOMMENDED DAILY FOOD PLAN FOR AN ADULT WHO NEEDS 2000 KCAL/DAY

My Daily Food Plan

Based on the information you provided, this is your daily recommended amount for each food group.

GRAINS 6 ounces	VEGETABLES 2½ cups	FRUITS 2 cups	DAIRY 3 cups	PROTEIN FOODS 5½ ounces
Make half your grains whole	**Vary your veggies**	**Focus on fruits**	**Get your calcium-rich foods**	**Go lean with protein**
Aim for at least **3 ounces** of whole grains a day	Aim for these amounts **each week:** **Dark green veggies** = 1½ cups **Red & orange veggies** = 5½ cups **Beans & peas** = 1½ cups **Starchy veggies** = 5 cups **Other veggies** = 4 cups	Eat a variety of fruit Choose whole or cut-up fruits more often than fruit juice	Drink fat-free or low-fat (1%) milk, for the same amount of calcium and other nutrients as whole milk, but less fat and Calories Select fat-free or low-fat yogurt and cheese, or try calcium-fortified soy products	Twice a week, make seafood the protein on your plate Vary your protein routine—choose beans, peas, nuts, and seeds more often Keep meat and poultry portions small and lean

Find your balance between food and physical activity
Be physically active for at least **150 minutes** each week

Know your limits on fats, sugars, and sodium
Your allowance for oils is **6 teaspoons** a day
Limit Calories from solid fats and added sugars to **260 Calories** a day
Reduce sodium intake to less than **2300 mg** a day

This Calorie level is only an estimate of your needs. Monitor your body weight to see if you need to adjust your Calorie intake.

Note: This box shows the plan for a 2000-calorie diet as presented at http://www.choosemyplate.gov, which produces plans based on age, gender, height, weight, and activity level—in this case, a 25 year-old woman, 130 lb, 5 ft. 5 in., less than 30 min of moderate to vigorous physical activity daily). Note that daily totals are provided and that some additional specifications apply to amounts from the food groups and food components on a daily or weekly basis.

Source: *Adapted from the U.S. Department of Agriculture (http://www.choosemyplate.gov/myplate/index.aspx).*

BOX 13.4

DIETARY GUIDELINES TIPSHEET NO. 1

1. Balance calories.
2. Enjoy your food but eat less.
3. Avoid oversized portions.
4. Foods to eat more often (vegetables, fruit, whole grains, fat-free or 1% milk, and dairy products).
5. Make half your plate fruits and vegetables.
6. Switch to fat-free or low-fat (1%) milk.
7. Make half your grains whole grains.
8. Foods to eat less often (foods high in solid fats, added sugars, and salt).
9. Compare sodium in foods.
10. Drink water instead of sugary drinks.

Source: *Adapted from the U.S. Department of Agriculture (http://fcs. tamu.edu/food_and_nutrition/family-nutrition/myplate-tip-sheets.pdf).*

---

that is lowest in sodium or highest in dietary fiber. Although listing of the potassium content of foods is currently optional, increasingly manufacturers are including it on the Nutrition Facts panel.

b SUPPLEMENT FACTS PANEL

A Supplement Facts label is required for most dietary supplements [12]. The format of this label is similar to that for the Nutrition Facts label on foods, but it also allows for more flexibility in reporting non-nutrient components. For example, the label on a ginseng supplement would indicate the number of milligrams of ginseng in the supplement, but it would not include a %DV for ginseng.

2 Ingredient Listing

All ingredients in a food must be listed on the label, in descending order by weight. Currently, the ingredient listing is suggested for use in identifying foods that have a high content of whole grains. For example, if the only grain ingredient in bread is whole wheat flour, it is sure to be a whole grain product. If the first ingredient is wheat flour, however, and the only other grain ingredient is whole wheat or rye flour, one knows that the product is higher in refined grain than in whole grain. The ingredient listing also helps identify foods that contain added solid fats and sugars.

3 Front-of-Package Labeling

At the request of Congress and the FDA, IOM conducted a two-part study to examine front-of-package nutrition systems and symbols and the scientific basis of underlying nutrient criteria, consider the strengths and limitations of the approaches, identify the systems and symbols that are most effective with consumers, address ways to maximize their use, and consider the potential benefits of a single front-of-label food guidance system that would be regulated by the FDA. The final report recommends the development, testing, and implementation of a single front-of-package symbol system to be used for all foods and beverages [40]. The symbol would display calories in common household measure sizes and 0–3 nutritional points for saturated and trans fats, sodium, and added sugars.

V CONCLUSION

Together, DRIs and *Dietary Guidelines for Americans* provide a strong basis for dietary guidance to promote the health of Americans. A broad array of new resource materials is now available to assist professionals in working with clients. Improvements in the labeling of food packages may be on the horizon. Key recommendations presented in the *Dietary Guidelines* can form the basis for consistent messages related to diet and physical activity. Evidence on the dietary intake, weight status, and health of Americans makes it clear that improvements are needed. The burden falls on nutrition educators and behavioral scientists to provide approaches that will inspire the public to change their food practices and activity levels in a positive direction and to be proactive in initiating environmental changes that will facilitate healthy behaviors. The rewards are many, both at the individual level (in improved well-being and reduced rates of chronic disease and disability) and at the societal level (in reduced medical care costs and lost productivity). One estimate suggests that 15.2% of all deaths in the United States in 2000 (350,000 deaths) were due to poor diet and activity patterns [41]. Health professionals have a crucial role in promoting healthful diet and activity patterns by the American public. Successful and practical intervention programs are greatly needed.

References

[1] Institute of Medicine, Dietary Reference Intakes for Calcium, Phosphorus, Magnesium, Vitamin D, and Fluoride, National Academy Press, Washington, DC, 1997.

[2] Institute of Medicine, Dietary Reference Intakes for Thiamin, Riboflavin, Niacin, Vitamin B_6, Folate, Vitamin B_{12}, Pantothenic Acid, Biotin, and Choline, National Academy Press, Washington, DC, 1998.

[3] Institute of Medicine, Dietary Reference Intakes for Vitamin C, Vitamin E, Selenium, and Carotenoids, National Academy Press, Washington, DC, 2000.

[4] Institute of Medicine, Dietary Reference Intakes for Vitamin A, Vitamin K, Arsenic, Boron, Chromium, Copper, Iodine, Iron, Manganese, Molybdenum, Nickel, Silicon, Vanadium, and Zinc, National Academy Press, Washington, DC, 2001.

[5] Institute of Medicine, Dietary Reference Intakes for Energy, Carbohydrate, Fiber, Fat, Fatty Acids, Cholesterol, Protein, and Amino Acids, National Academy Press, Washington, DC, 2002/2005.

[6] Institute of Medicine, Dietary Reference Intakes for Water, Potassium, Sodium, Chloride, and Sulfate, National Academies Press, Washington, DC, 2005.

[7] Institute of Medicine, DRI Dietary Reference Intakes for Calcium and Vitamin D, National Academies Press, Washington, DC, 2010.

[8] National Research Council, Food and Nutrition Board, Recommended Dietary Allowances, National Academy Press, Washington, DC, 1989.

[9] U.S. Department of Agriculture/U.S. Department of Health and Human Services, Dietary Guidelines for Americans, 2010, seventh ed., U.S. Government Printing Office, Washington, DC, 2010. Available at <http://health.gov/dietaryguidelines/dga2010/DietaryGuidelines2010.pdf> (accessed 14.07.11).

[10] U.S. Department of Health and Human Services. 2008 Physical Activity Guidelines for Americans, Publication No. U0036. Available at <http://www.health.gov/paguidelines/pdf/paguide.pdf>, 2008 (accessed 17.07.11).

[11] U.S. Food and Drug Administration. Labeling & Nutrition. Available at <http://www.fda.gov/food/labelingnutrition/default.htm>, 2011 (accessed 11.07.11).

[12] U.S. Food and Drug Administration. Overview of Dietary Supplements. Available at <http://www.fda.gov/food/dietarysupplements/consumerinformation/ucm110417.htm>, 2009 (accessed 11.07.11).

[13] Institute of Medicine, How Should the Recommended Dietary Allowances Be Revised? National Academy Press, Washington, DC, 1994.

[14] Institute of Medicine, Dietary Reference Intakes: Applications in Dietary Assessment, National Academy Press, Washington, DC, 2000.

[15] Institute of Medicine, Dietary Reference Intakes: Applications in Dietary Planning, National Academies Press, Washington, DC, 2003.

[16] Institute of Medicine, Dietary Reference Intakes: The Essential Guide to Nutrient Requirements, National Academies Press, Washington, DC, 2006.

[17] National Research Council, Food and Nutrition Board, Nutrient Adequacy: Assessment Using Food Consumption Surveys, National Academy Press, Washington, DC, 1986.

[18] A.F. Subar, V. Kipnis, R.P. Troiano, D. Midthune, D.A. Schoeller, S. Bingham, et al., Using intake biomarkers to evaluate the extent of dietary misreporting in a large sample of adults: The OPEN study, Am. J. Epidemiol. 158 (1) (2003) 1–13.

[19] K. Poslusna, J. Ruprich, J.H. de Vries, M. Jakubikova, P. van't Veer, Misreporting of energy and micronutrient intake estimated by food records and 24 hour recalls, control and adjustment methods in practice, Br. J. Nutr. 101 (Suppl. 2) (2009) S73–S85.

[20] T.L. Burrows, R.J. Martin, C.E. Collins, A systematic review of the validity of dietary assessment methods in children when compared with the method of doubly labeled water, J. Am. Diet. Assoc. 110 (10) (2010) 1501–1510.

[21] K.M. Mangano, S.J. Walsh, K.L. Insogna, A.M. Kenny, J.E. Kerstetter, Calcium intake in the United States from dietary and supplemental sources across adult age groups: new estimates from the National Health and Nutrition Examination Survey 2003–2006, J. Am. Diet. Assoc. 111 (2011) 687–695.

[22] Dietary Guidelines Advisory Committee, Report of the Dietary Guidelines Advisory Committee on the Dietary Guidelines for Americans, 2010, to the Secretary of Agriculture and the Secretary of Health and Human Services, U.S. Department of Agriculture, Agricultural Research Service, Washington, DC, 2010. Available at <http://www.cnpp.usda.gov/dgas2010-dga-creport.htm>, (accessed 09.07.11).

[23] Food Surveys Research Group, U.S. Department of Agriculture. What We Eat in America, NHANES 2001–2002: Usual Nutrient Intakes from Food Compared to Dietary Reference Intakes. Available at <http://www.ars.usda.gov/SP2UserFiles/Place/12355000/pdf/0102/usualintaketables2001-02.pdf>, 2005 (accessed 15.04.07).

[24] Food Surveys Research Group, U.S. Department of Agriculture. What We Eat in America, NHANES 2007–2008: Nutrient Intakes from Food and Dietary Supplements. Available at <http://www.ars.usda.gov/Services/docs.htm?docid=18349>, 2011 (accessed 30.08.11).

[25] Physical Activity Guidelines Advisory Committee. in: Physical Activity Guidelines Advisory Committee Report, U.S. Department of Health and Human Services. Washington, DC, 2008. Available at <http://www.health.gov/PAGuidelines/Report/pdf/CommitteeReport.pdf> (accessed 07.07.11).

[26] Institute of Medicine, Early Childhood Obesity Prevention Policies, National Academies Press, Washington, DC, 2011.

[27] C.E. Garber, B. Blissmer, M.R. Deschenes, B.A. Franklin, M.J. Lamonte, I.-M. Lee, et al., Quantity and quality of exercise for developing and maintaining cardiorespiratory, musculoskeletal, and neuromotor fitness in apparently healthy adults: guidance for prescribing exercise, Med. Sci. Sports Exercise. 43 (7) (2011) 1334–1359.

[28] Institute of Medicine, Strategies to Reduce Sodium Intake in the United States, National Academies Press, Washington, DC, 2010.

[29] U.S. Department of Health and Human Services. Healthy People 2020. Available at <http://www.healthypeople.gov/2020/topicsobjectives2020/objectiveslist.aspx?topicId=29>, 2010 (accessed 12.07.11).

[30] Institute of Medicine, Local Government Actions to Prevent Childhood Obesity, National Academies Press, Washington, DC, 2009.

[31] P. Tarnapol, P.T. Whitacre, J. Mulligan, The Public Health Effects of Food Deserts: Workshop Summary, National Academies Press, Washington, DC, 2009.

[32] Center for Nutrition Policy and Promotion, U.S. Department of Agriculture. Development of 2010 Dietary Guidelines for Americans, Consumer Messages and New Food Icon, Executive Summary of Formative Research. Available at <http://www.choosemyplate.gov/downloads/MyPlate/ExecutiveSummaryOfFormativeResearch.pdf>, 2011 (accessed 01.07.11).

[33] White House Task Force on Childhood Obesity. White House Task Force on Childhood Obesity Report to the President: Solving the Problem of Childhood Obesity within a Generation, p. 26. Available at <http://www.letsmove.gov/white-house-task-force-childhood-obesity-report-president>, 2010 (accessed 03.09.11).

[34] U.S. Department of Agriculture. <http://www.choosemyplate.gov> (accessed 01.07.11).

[35] U.S. Department of Agriculture. Let's eat for the health of it. *Home and Garden Bulletin* No. 252-CP. Available at <http://www.choosemyplate.gov/food-groups/downloads/MyPlate/DG2010Brochure.pdf>, 2011 (accessed 26.06.11).

[36] Center for Nutrition Policy and Promotion, U.S. Department of Agriculture. 10 Tips Nutrition Education Series. Available at <http://fcs.tamu.edu/food_and_nutrition/family-nutrition/myplate-tip-sheets.pdf>, 2011 (accessed 30.06.11).

[37] U.S. Food and Drug Administration. Nutritional Labeling and Education Act (NLEA) Requirements (8/94−2/95). Available at <http://www.fda.gov/ICECI/Inspections/InspectionGuides/ucm074948.htm?utm_campaign=Google2&utm_source=fdaSearch&utm_medium=website&utm_term=nlea&utm_content=1>.

[38] U.S. Food and Drug Administration/U.S. Department of Health and Human Services/U.S. Department of Agriculture. Eating Healthier and Feeling Better Using the Nutrition Facts Label. Available at <http://www.fda.gov/Food/ResourcesForYou/Consumers/ucm266853.htm>, 2006, August (accessed 01.09.11).

[39] U.S. Food and Drug Administration. Food Facts from the U.S. Food and Drug Administration: A Key to Choosing Healthful Foods: Using the Nutrition Facts Food Label. Available at <http://www.fda.gov/downloads/Food/ResourcesForYou/Consumers/UCM079504.pdf>, 2007 (accessed 01.09.11).

[40] Institute of Medicine, Front-of Package Nutrition Rating Systems and Symbols: Promoting Healthier Choices, National Academies Press, Washington, DC, 2011.

[41] A.H. Mokdad, J.S. Marks, D.F. Stroup, J.L. Gerberding, Actual causes of death in the United States, 2000, JAMA 291 (10) (2004) 1238−1245 [Erratum in *JAMA* 2005; 293(3), 293−294].

A. FOOD AND NUTRITION INTAKE FOR HEALTH

Nutrition, Health Policy, and the Problem of Proof

Robert P. Heaney*, Sarah Roller†

*Creighton University, Omaha, Nebraska
†Kelley Drye & Warren LLP, Washington, DC

I BACKGROUND CONSIDERATIONS

In the early days of molecular biology, there was a dictum that went "one gene, one protein," expressing first, the insight that the blueprints for proteins were encoded in the genome, and, second, the speculation that because each protein was unique, it had a unique genetic blueprint. The latter belief had to be abandoned quickly when it became apparent that there were a great many more proteins than there were genes. Rather than a setback, the resulting revisions in the blueprint model greatly enriched the science of cell biology. Nutrition today faces a similar need to reformulate the basic approach to its own science.

Although less explicitly articulated than the one-gene–one-protein principle, nutrition implicitly holds to a "one-nutrient–one-disease" conceptual model. As commonly taught, *the* disease of thiamin deficiency is beriberi; *the* disease of niacin deficiency is pellagra; *the* disease of vitamin D deficiency is rickets (or osteomalacia in adults); and so on. Although there is no expressed objection by nutritional scientists to recognizing multiple systemic consequences of nutrient inadequacy, the hold of the one-nutrient–one-disease model continues to dominate both nutritional policy and the regulation of health claims. Specifically, it has been the organizing principle not only for nutrition scientists but also for food and nutrition policymakers.

The public health triumphs of the model could rightly be celebrated during the early days of nutrition policy, as mandatory food fortification, under the then novel food regulations, proved to be efficacious for the treatment and prevention of classical nutrient deficiency diseases. With time, however, the inadequacies of the conceptual model have been exposed by the peculiar outcomes it yields in the face of contemporary nutrition problems, which suggest that the model too often functions today to frustrate rather than serve public health needs. As just one example, we cite the reluctance, in the case of vitamin D, to label as "deficiency" the osteoporosis, fracture risk, propensity to falls, immune defects, hypertension, and cancer risk that accompany low vitamin D status. Clinical scientists generally call all this morbidity "vitamin D insufficiency." It cannot be "deficiency," so the thinking goes, because such patients do not have rickets or osteomalacia.

A Scientific Limits and Policy Issues

Nutrient–disease relationships are increasingly subjected to modes of evaluation and regulation that were borrowed from the medical model and were designed for the evaluation of drug efficacy. The one-nutrient–one-disease conceptual model casts nutrients, like drugs, in an essentially acute, therapeutic relationship with a predefined disease end point (i.e., "vitamin C is to scurvy as lipid-lowering drug is to serum cholesterol"). Not surprisingly, the model has offered little resistance to those who have repurposed the tools designed by evidence-based medicine to evaluate drug efficacy in creating "evidence-based review" methods for selecting, grading, ranking, and gauging the "strength" of the evidence showing

Nutrition in the Prevention and Treatment of Disease, Third Edition.
DOI: http://dx.doi.org/10.1016/B978-0-12-391884-0.00014-7

that nutrition is effective in addressing one public health need or another. Unfortunately, the codification[1] of such methods for nutrition policy and food regulatory purposes has further obscured the fundamental differences between the nutrients delivered by foods and the active ingredients delivered by drugs, and it has compounded the problem by devaluing the kinds of scientific evidence [1] that have the capability to expose the truth and chart a more effective course for achieving public health nutrition goals (see Section II).

The structural limitations of nutrition policies premised on the one-nutrient—one-disease model can be illustrated through a stepwise examination of the standards that define and govern what are termed "structure—function claims," "disease claims," and "health claims" under the Federal Food, Drug, and Cosmetic Act (FDCA).

1 Structure—Function Claims

To a significant degree, the extent to which the health benefits of a food product can be conveyed through product marketing claims depends on whether the benefit can be directly attributed to the nutritional value of the particular food. Although FDCA standards generally classify and regulate products that are "intended to affect the structure or any function of the body" as "drugs," in adopting these standards in 1938, the Congress apparently recognized that these "drug" standards should not be applied to foods because foods, by their very nature and purpose, affect body structures and functions of the body.[2] This is reflected in the "carveout" that excludes from this particular "drug" standard those products that qualify as "food."[3] It is this carve-out that allows "structure—function" claims to be made for a food or essential nutrient

---

[1]See U.S. Food and Drug Administration (FDA), "Guidance for Industry: Evidence-Based Review System for the Scientific Evaluation of Health Claims—Final" (January 2009), which states, "Evaluating the Totality of Scientific Evidence. Under the approach set out in this guidance, at this point, FDA intends to evaluate the results of the studies from which scientific conclusions can be drawn and rate the strength of the total body of publicly available evidence. The agency plans to conduct this evaluation by considering the study type (e.g., intervention, prospective cohort, case—control, cross-sectional) methodological quality rating previously assigned, number of the various types of studies and sample sizes, relevance of the body of scientific evidence to the U.S. population or target subgroup, whether study results supporting the proposed claim have been replicated, and the overall consistency of the total body of evidence…. In general, intervention studies provide the strongest evidence for the claimed effect, regardless of existing observational studies on the same relationship. Intervention studies are designed to avoid selection bias and avoid findings that are due to chance or other confounders of disease. Although the evaluation of substance—disease relationships often involves both intervention and observational studies, observational studies generally cannot be used to rule out the findings from more reliable intervention studies. One intervention study would not be sufficient to rule out consistent findings of observational studies. However, when several randomized, controlled intervention studies are consistent in showing or not showing a substance—disease relationship, they trump the findings of any number of observational studies. This is because intervention studies are designed and controlled to test whether there is evidence of a cause-and-effect relationship between the substance and the reduced risk of a disease, whereas observational studies are only able to identify possible associations. There are numerous examples—such as vitamin E and CVD and beta-carotene and lung cancer—where associations identified in observational studies have been publicized. However, when randomized, controlled intervention studies were later conducted to test these possible associations, the intervention studies found no evidence to support the relationships" (references omitted). See also USDA Evidence Library, which states, "What is a NEL systematic review? A NEL evidence-based systematic review is a state-of-the-art method for evaluating scientific evidence to answer a precise question or series of questions" and defining the "NEL systematic review process" to include recruiting a multidisciplinary team, formulating systematic review questions, identifying and selecting relevant studies to review, conducting literature review for each question, extracting evidence and critically appraising each study, synthesizing the evidence, and developing and grading conclusion statements (http://www.nel.gov; accessed September 29, 2011).

[2]See 21 U.S.C. § 321(g)(1)(C) (defining "drug" to mean "articles (other than food) intended to affect the structure or any function of the body of man or other animals."); see also 21 U.S.C. § 321(f) (defining "food" to mean "(1) articles used for food or drink for man or other animals, (2) chewing gum, and (3) articles used for components of any such article."); *Nutrilab, Inc. v. Schweiker* 713 F. 2d 335 (1983); FDA Food Labeling Guide at H3 and H4 (stating that "structure—function … claims describe the effect that a substance has on the structure or function of the body and do not make reference to a disease…." "Calcium builds strong bones;" and characterizing more general health benefit claims to be "dietary guidance" claims (e.g., "Carrots are good for your health" or "Calcium is good for you.")). See also 21 U.S.C. § 343(r)(6); 21 C.F.R. § 101.93 (authorizing certain structure—function claims for dietary supplements).

[3]21 U.S.C. §§ 321(f) and 321(g)(1)(C). Note that the "food" carve-out applies to articles that qualify as "food" under 21 U.S.C. § 321(f) but *not* those that qualify as "food" exclusively under 21 U.S.C.§ 321(ff), such as herbal and botanical ingredients of dietary supplement products, for which structure—function claims are governed by 21 U.S.C. § 343(r)(6) *but not* 21 U.S.C. § 321(g)(1)(C) and its "food" carve-out.

without triggering "drug" regulation or other pre-market clearance requirements.[4] For example, such structure–function claims as "calcium helps build strong bones" can be employed to market calcium-rich foods provided that the claims are conveyed in a manner that is factually accurate and supported by appropriate scientific evidence. In addition, as a matter of regulatory policy, the U.S. Food and Drug Administration (FDA) requires substantiation to establish that the health benefits claimed are conferred through a "nutritive" mechanism of action.[5] As a result, well-substantiated structure–function claims that describe calcium benefits for body functions and parts beyond the skeletal system would nonetheless be prohibited by the FDA policy unless the benefit could be attributed to the nutritive value of calcium.

2 Disease Claims

At the same time, the "nutritive value" test operates to constrain the scope of permissible structure–function claims. The breadth of FDA's definition of prohibited "disease" claims[6] sweeps virtually all foods for which disease-related benefit claims can be made into the same regulatory class as therapeutic drugs. For example, FDCA standards require products that are represented "for use in the diagnosis, cure, mitigation, treatment, or prevention of disease" to be regulated as "drugs,"[7] and they prohibit "drug" products from being marketed except in compliance with the applicable FDA monograph.[8] In brief, FDA regulatory policies will apply this "drug" standard—that is, regulating food products as "drugs"—whenever marketing claims suggest that the product may have disease-related benefits.[9] Because compliance with FDA's requirements for approval of new drug applications (and related standards) is not feasible for most food products,[10] the ultimate effect of the FDA policy is to ban all express and implied disease-related claims for foods, except for those that are specifically authorized by FDA as "health claims." Relatively few health claims have been authorized by FDA since the FDCA health claim provisions were adopted in 1990. As a result of the unduly burdensome premarket clearance procedures and the restrictive FDA requirements governing the language of authorized health claims, such claims typically have little marketing value and are not widely

---

[4]This does not mean that all "structure–function" claims are permissible for food or nutrients. FDCA sections 403(a) and 201(n) require structure–function claims, like other claims, to be conveyed in a manner that is accurate and substantiated by appropriate scientific evidence. 21 U.S.C. §§ 321(n) and 343(a). Similar requirements also apply to structure–function claims that appear in product labeling and/or advertising and other marketing communications under the Federal Trade Commission Act and state food and drug and consumer protection statutes. See, e.g., Fairchild-Dzanis, M., Roller, S., et al., "Can We Say That? A Practical Guide to Substantiating Claims for Foods and Consumer Health Products," Food Drug Law Institute Monograph Volume 2, Number 3 (2011) (http://www.fdli.org).

[5]See, e.g., 62 Fed. Reg. 49859, 49860 (September 23, 1997) (explaining that the scope of permissible structure–function claims for foods regulated by FDA is confined to those that are attributable to the nutritive value of the food or food substance to which the claim refers, as follows: "The claim that cranberry juice cocktail prevents the recurrence of urinary tract infections is a claim that brings the product within the 'drug' definition whether it appears on a conventional food or on a dietary supplement because it is a claim that the product will prevent disease." However, a claim that cranberry products help to maintain urinary tract health may be permissible on both cranberry products in conventional food form and dietary supplement form if it is truthful, not misleading, and derives from the nutritional value of cranberries. If the effect derives from the nutritive value of cranberries, the claim would describe an effect of a food on the structure or function of the body and thus fall under one exception to the definition for the term "drug" found in [21 U.S.C. § 321(g)(1)(C)]).

[6]See 21 U.S.C. § 321(g)(1)(B) and 21 C.F.R. § 101.93(g) (distinguishing structure–function claims from prohibited "disease claims").

[7]21 U.S.C. § 321(g)(1)(B).

[8]See FDLI Monograph Section III.D. See, e.g., Fairchild-Dzanis, M., Roller, S., et al., "Can We Say That? A Practical Guide to Substantiating Claims for Foods and Consumer Health Products," Food Drug Law Institute Monograph Volume 2, Number 3 (2011) Section III.D. (www.fdli.org).

[9]See Roller, S., and Pippins R., "Marketing Nutrition and Health Benefits of Food and Beverage Products: Enforcement, Litigation & Liability Issues," 65 Food and Drug Law Journal 447 (2010) (analyzing FDA warning letters alleging that breakfast cereal, walnuts, and other food products are "drugs" as a result of marketing claims).

[10]Dietary supplements are "foods" for most FDCA regulatory purposes. See 21 U.S.C. 321(ff). There are a few FDA-approved "drugs" that are used for dietary supplement purposes. These include more concentrated dosage forms of essential nutrients (e.g., vitamin D) and fish oils (e.g., EPA/DHA supplement).

used to market foods that qualify for the health claim.[11]

3 Health Claims

Under FDCA standards, claims that characterize any relationship between a food and a "disease" or "health-related condition" (e.g., blood pressure and serum cholesterol) qualify as "health claims" and must be authorized by FDA.[12] FDA has interpreted the FDCA standards expansively. Health claims are evaluated on a claim-by-claim basis through premarket clearance procedures rather than requiring health claims to be constructed in alignment with more general consumer protection law principles such as those the Federal Trade Commission relies on to regulate marketing claims for consumer products.[13] In addition, the FDA premarket clearance procedures generally require the submission of a petition reviewing a large body of substantiating scientific evidence, which FDA evaluates using evidence-based review methods that give greatest weight to evidence from randomized controlled trials (RCTs) in determining whether the claim will be authorized and, if so, how the model claim language will be stated (see Section II).[14,15]

Another way in which the FDA policy disadvantages claims concerning nutrient–disease relationships is found in the way FDA defines "disease." FDA regulations define "disease" to encompass any type of "damage" to an organ, part, structure, or system of the body such that it does not function properly … or a state of health leading to such dysfunctioning."[16] The FDA regulations go on to exclude from the "disease" definition "diseases resulting from essential nutrient deficiencies (e.g., scurvy, pellagra)."[17] The effect of this exclusion is to place all disease claims relating to an "essential nutrient deficiency disease" on the same legal footing as a structure–function claim concerning the same nutrient. Although this much of the FDA regulatory standard is justified from a nutrition policy standpoint, the substantial difficulty comes from the way that FDA construes "essential nutrient deficiency disease," which is constrained by the one-nutrient–one-disease conceptual model, as reflected by the following statement of rationale from the FDA rulemaking record:

> The relationships between nutrients and classical deficiency diseases are well-established. Moreover, such diseases are of little public health significance in this country. Under such circumstances, FDA believes that it would not be appropriate to subject such relationships to the health claims regime…. [A] claim about the benefits of vitamin D in preventing vitamin D deficiency, for example, would be misleading where the claim does not explain that few individuals in the United States are at risk of such a deficiency.[18]

---

[11]See Government Accountability Office, "Food Labeling: FDA Needs to Reassess Its Approach to Protecting Consumers from False or Misleading Claims" at 12–13 (GAO-11-102) (January 2011) (stating, "FDA data and other research indicate that companies' interest in qualified health claims has slowed…. FDA's and industry's initial expectation of a flood of petitions for qualified health claims on food was never realized…. In addition, research by FDA and others shows that companies are making minimal use of qualified health claims. In 2010 … only 0.4% of [food labels] had qualified health claims"; and reporting that 4.3% of food labels had "significant scientific agreement claims" of the type which are covered by FDA regulations at 21 C.F.R. Part 101, Subpart E). See also Roller, S., Voorhees, T., and Lunkenheimer, A., "Obesity, Food Marketing and Consumer Litigation: Threat or Opportunity?" (discussing research studies conducted by the Federal Trade Commission (FTC) examining the relationship between FDA food labeling regulations and healthy food marketing practices and reporting a sharp decline in comparative nutrition claims and health claims in the marketplace, including in advertising for "good foods," after FDA regulations governing health claims and other nutrition-related claims were implemented).

[12]21 U.S.C. § 343(r).

[13]See 15 C.F.R. Part 260 (FTC, "Guides for the Use of Environmental Marketing Claims"); see also 75 *Fed. Reg.* 63552 (October 15, 2010) (proposing amendments to 15 C.F.R. Part 260). Compare 21 C.F.R. § 101.72 (regulating health claims relating to calcium, vitamin D, and osteoporosis).

[14]See Food and Drug Administration (FDA), "Guidance for Industry: Evidence-Based Review System for the Scientific Evaluation of Health Claims—Final" (January 2009).

[15]See 21 C.F.R. § 101.70; see also 21 U.S.C. § 343(r) (authorizing expedited clearance for health claims that are substantiated by certain statements of authoritative government bodies and related requirements through premarket notification procedures).

[16]21 C.F.R. § 101.14(a)(5).

[17]Id.

[18]58 *Fed. Reg.* 2478, 2481–2482 (January 6, 1993) (explaining that the FDA regulation excluding claims concerning essential nutrient diseases from regulation as "health claims" is supported by the relevant legislative history, and stating, "[t]here is no indication that [the Congress] intended [the health claim requirements] to cover classical deficiency diseases (diseases resulting directly from a deficiency of a vitamin, essential mineral, or other essential nutrient)…. Under such circumstances, FDA believes that it would not be appropriate to subject such relationships to the health claims regime. Claims about such classical nutrient deficiency diseases are adequately regulated under the provisions of [21 U.S.C. 343(a)] and thus must be truthful and not misleading").

With the benefit of hindsight and experience, current health claim policies seem more likely to frustrate than advance public health interests, particularly with respect to essential nutrient–disease relationships. The sharp decline in the incidence of neural tube defects that has occurred during the past 15 years as a result of folic acid fortification (Figure 14.1) demonstrates the ongoing public health importance of adequate nutrient intakes and the disease burdens associated with inadequate intakes.[19,20] Had FDA adopted a sufficiently generous interpretation of "essential nutrient deficiency disease" to encompass neural tube defects resulting from inadequate folate/folic acid intake, there would have been no need to subject such claims to the restrictions that are imposed under FDA health claim regulations,[21] and, in all likelihood, food marketers would have created more inspiring ways to convey the health message than those that were designed through rulemaking procedures.[22]

Despite the peculiar outcomes for public health, in the case of osteoporosis, the FDA policy has relied on a strained distinction between "essential nutrient deficiency diseases" and "chronic disease,"[23] with essential nutrient–osteoporosis relationships being classified as a chronic disease that is "affected" by diet, together with saturated fat–heart disease, sodium–hypertension, and other relationships between the avoidance of a dietary substance and health benefits. Had FDA instead construed "essential nutrient deficiency disease" broadly enough to encompass osteoporosis and its relationship to intakes of calcium and vitamin D, food marketers would have had greater freedom to convey the benefits of both of these nutrients for osteoporosis prevention, and for a much longer time.

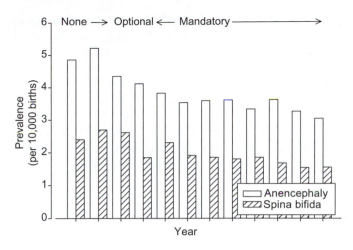

FIGURE 14.1 Neural tube defect prevalence from 1995 to 2006 in the 27 U.S. states with surveillance systems for the birth defect. Folate fortification of cereal grain products became optional in 1996 and mandatory by 1999. Since then, there has been a reduction of nearly 40% in these devastating defects, at an estimated annual savings of more than $50 million per year in first year medical costs alone. *Source: Centers for Disease Control and Prevention (cdc.gov/ncbddd/folicacid/data.html). Copyright Robert P. Heaney, 2011. Used with permission.*

For many years, the FDA health claim regulations permitted only calcium–osteoporosis health claims, and only later in response to a health claim petition did the agency expand the scope, authorizing health claims to permit vitamin D to be mentioned in addition to calcium. In the meantime, the scientific evidence suggests that the FDA regulation required food marketers to employ a misleading health calcium–osteoporosis claim because it compelled nondisclosure of the additional vitamin

---

[19]21 C.F.R. § 172.345 (authorizing the addition of folic acid to certain foods including breakfast cereal, enriched bread products, meal replacements (i.e., 400µg/serving or less), and corn grits (1.0 mg/pound).

[20]http://www.cdc.gov/ncbddd/folicacid/data.html.

[21]21 C.F.R. §§ 101.14 and 101.79.

[22]21 C.F.R. § 0101.79(d) (authorizing the following model claims: "(1) *Examples 1 and 2.* Model health claims appropriate for foods containing 100% or less of the DV for folate per serving or per unit (general population). The examples contain only the required elements: (i) Healthful diets with adequate folate may reduce a woman's risk of having a child with a brain or spinal cord birth defect. (ii) Adequate folate in healthful diets may reduce a woman's risk of having a child with a brain or spinal cord birth defect. (2) *Example 3.* Model health claim appropriate for foods containing 100% or less of the DV for folate per serving or per unit. The example contains all required elements plus optional information: Women who consume healthful diets with adequate folate throughout their childbearing years may reduce their risk of having a child with a birth defect of the brain or spinal cord. Sources of folate include fruits, vegetables, whole grain products, fortified cereals, and dietary supplements. (3) *Example 4.* Model health claim appropriate for foods intended for use by the general population and containing more than 100% of the DV of folate per serving or per unit: Women who consume healthful diets with adequate folate may reduce their risk of having a child with birth defects of the brain or spinal cord. Folate intake should not exceed 250% of the DV (1000 µg)"); see also 61 *Fed. Reg.* 8779 (March 5, 1996) and 65 *Fed. Reg.* 58918 (October 3, 2000).

[23]21 C.F.R. § 101.72 (regulating health claims pertaining to diets adequate in calcium and vitamin D and the reduced risk of osteoporosis); see also 21 C.F.R. 101.79 (regulating claims pertaining to diets adequate in folate and a woman's reduced risk of having a child with a brain or spinal cord birth defect as health claims).

D—osteoporosis relationship.[24] In addition, any reference to vitamin D in the health claim on a voluntary basis would have run the risk of triggering "drug" regulation for the product in question, as illustrated by the FDA enforcement record.[25]

Another questionable result of the FDA policy is the fact that the only disease-related benefits that can be represented for calcium and vitamin D in food marketing claims without triggering "drug" status relate to the classical essential nutrient deficiency disease, rickets,[26] or osteoporosis.[27] In addition, if a food were lawfully marketed with an osteoporosis health claim but added to it additional information conveying the benefits of the calcium and/or vitamin D with respect to other diseases or conditions (e.g., fracture risk and propensity to falls), such claims would trigger drug regulation for the food in question.

A further difficulty of the FDA health claims policy concerns the methods that are employed to evaluate the scientific evidence supporting beneficial nutrient—disease relationships and the standards of proof that must be satisfied (see Section II). For instance, the starting assumptions are the same regardless of whether the health claim being evaluated concerns health benefits that result from avoiding a risk-increasing substance in food (e.g., saturated fat) or adding a substance that is not an essential nutrient (e.g., plant sterol/stanol esters), or whether the benefits result from simply ensuring that intakes of essential nutrients are adequate.[28]

The same positivist standard of proof must be satisfied to prove that intake of the substance at the level in question is beneficial. There is no presumption of benefit that is factored into the evaluation of a health claims concerning essential nutrients. This approach to evaluating cause-and-effect relationships in the diet/health context is made worse by the prejudicial weighting system that places greatest importance on results from RCTs. This method departs radically from the well-established principles for evaluating environmental hazards and disease [1]. In this regard, the evaluation of benefits that result from correcting the inadequate intakes of essential nutrients are comparable to those that result from reducing exposure to an environmental hazard, such as reducing lead in drinking water, because when it comes to levels of dietary exposure to essential nutrients, by definition, "inadequate" levels present a health hazard. From there, the only real scientific question to be answered to serve public health needs is how much hazard, at what intake level will it occur, and in whom.

Although research into the workings of nutrients in ways that are distinct from the those involved in "classical" nutrient deficiency diseases is ongoing, and even flourishing, the opportunities to translate all that is already known and can foreseeably be known about nutrition—disease relationships into nutrition and food regulatory policies that are effective in alleviating the heavy burdens of noncommunicable disease are at one and the same time obscured and hobbled by the one-nutrient—one-disease model. The obstacles are further compounded by the evidence-based review methods that are being used with increasing frequency to evaluate whether adequate nutrition is important enough to warrant strategies such as nutrition education programs, food fortification, and other public health measures. Unfortunately, the prevailing conceptual model and evidence-based review methods are instruments that are too unreliable to ensure that the resulting nutrition policies can chart the best course for alleviating noncommunicable disease burdens.

B Nutritional Relationships between Chronic Undernutrition and Systemic Disease

These important regulatory issues aside, there is a fundamental need to reformulate the very scientific framework for nutrition—that is, how we think about the topic. We need to develop alternatives to the one-nutrient—one-disease model not just for more intelligent regulation but also for purposes of characterizing the manifestations of disease that result from chronic, suboptimal intake of essential nutrients.

Several years ago, an alternative conceptual framework was proposed, one that explicitly recognized two main classes of mechanisms of nutrient action and

---

[24]See 73 *Fed. Reg.* 56486 (September 29, 2008) (amending 21 C.F.R. § 101.72 to include vitamin D in the osteoporosis health claim, in addition to calcium); see also 21 U.S.C. 321(n) (providing that nondisclosure of material factual information is misleading and causes a food to be unlawful).

[25]See Roller, S., and Pippins, R., "Marketing Nutrition and Health Benefits of Food and Beverage Products: Enforcement, Litigation & Liability Issues," 65 *Food and Drug Law Journal* 447 (2010).

[26]21 C.F.R. § 101.14(a)(5).

[27]21 C.F.R. § 101.72 (authorizing the following model claims: "Adequate calcium and vitamin D throughout life, as part of a well-balanced diet, may reduce the risk of osteoporosis"; "Adequate calcium and vitamin D as part of a healthful diet, along with physical activity, may reduce the risk of osteoporosis later in life").

[28]See generally, 21 C.F.R. Part 101, Subpart E.

that made explicit provision for a spectrum of latency periods for disease expression. Examples of its application to three nutrients—calcium, vitamin D, and folate—were given [2]. This model is set forth diagrammatically in Figures 14.2 and 14.3. (Figure 14.2 is applicable to all nutrients, whereas Figure 14.3 exemplifies the model for one nutrient, vitamin D.) The model is arbitrary in that it makes an artificial distinction between so-called "index" and "non-index" mechanisms and diseases. Doing so simply pays homage to the diseases classically associated with each nutrient (their "index" diseases) and to the mechanisms elucidated for their pathogenesis. These "index" diseases are the "one disease" of the one-nutrient–one-disease model. The expanded model is artificial in that it gives special place to the disorder first associated with the nutrient, which, as it turns out, may not always be the most important expression of deficiency. Moreover, it lumps all of the other disorders into a catch-all category of "non-index" diseases, most of which are excluded by the FDA (as just detailed) from its "essential nutrient deficiency disease category." Nevertheless, the value of the expanded model is that it forces attention to the multiplicity of effects, and it gives explicit

recognition to long latency disorders, in contrast to the short latency that is characteristic of all the index diseases.

With vitamin D, for example, it is now clear that non-index processes certainly account for the great majority of the nutrient's actions in the body, literally dwarfing its effects on bone and the calcium economy (which, at the same time, remain real and important in their own right).

Behind this revised conceptualization lies the fact that all cells and tissues need essentially all nutrients. They all need energy; they all need raw materials and building blocks; and they all need co-factors, catalysts, and minerals. When an organism's diet is deficient in any given nutrient, all cells and tissues are to some extent functionally impaired. In the early days of nutritional science, we recognized only the most rapidly developing disorders involving only the most vulnerable tissues or systems. We can do better today.

There are two important considerations that flow from this broader understanding: (1) Nutrient deficiency states, even when one defect is more prominent than others, tend to be pluriform; and (2) although their public health impact may be large, measurable effects of nutrients in isolated, single tissues or systems are often small (see Section II.C). The problems created by these features can be exemplified by two observations relating specifically to calcium.

Many papers describing trials of calcium conclude somewhat as follows: "Although the reduction in blood pressure [or fracture or obesity or colon cancer or premenstrual syndrome] was statistically significant, the effect was too small to warrant recommending a change in calcium intake for the general population" [3,4]. Such a conclusion is usually incorrect because it ignores the public health impact of even small changes (see Section II.C) and also because it ignores all the other real, but sometimes equally small, measurable effects involving other body systems and diseases.

The problem is further exemplified by a study analyzing diet quality in women using a diet score based on nine essential nutrients that exhibit low covariance in foods [5]. Diets poor in calcium were typically poor in five of the nine selected nutrients, whereas diets adequate in calcium were adequate in at least eight of the nine. In other words, calcium deficiency is rarely the only problem with a given diet.

Both of these features have implications (1) for nutritional policy because manifestly multiple system effects have to be factored into the decision process and (2) for nutritional interventions because mononutrient supplementation or fortification will be an inadequate response to what is commonly a polynutrient problem.

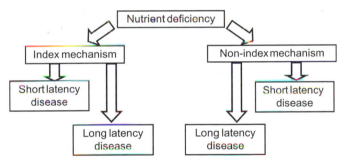

FIGURE 14.2 Scheme setting forth broad classes of latencies and mechanisms by which deficiency of a given nutrient produces disease or dysfunction. Source: *Copyright Robert P. Heaney, 2007. Used with permission.*

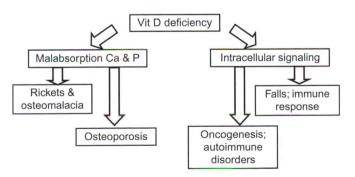

FIGURE 14.3 The scheme of Figure 14.2, made specific for vitamin D. Source: *Copyright Robert P. Heaney, 2007. Used with permission.*

II THE MATTER OF PROOF

Both current clinical science and regulatory policy are eagerly pursuing an approach to certainty described as "evidence-based," despite frequently overlooked shortcomings in this approach both as practiced [5,7] and as discussed previously (see Section I.A). Evidence-based medicine (EBM), even before it got that name, had typically been applied to evaluation of procedural or pharmacological interventions in individual patients, such as "Does radical mastectomy for breast cancer produce better outcomes than lumpectomy?" or "Do beta blockers improve survival after myocardial infarction?" Such questions tend to be discrete and narrowly defined, and indeed every attempt is made to make them so. EBM attempts to rank the studies addressing such questions according to study design (or type), assigning greatest weight to the RCT and then cohort studies, case—control studies, case reports, and, finally, little or no weight to expert opinion.[29]

Despite its many problems [6,7], this approach is generally held to be the best way to evaluate new medical treatments. Unfortunately, because nutrition has no corresponding approach of its own, EBM and its criteria, developed for medical treatments, are today being applied to nutritional questions and to issues of nutritional policy [8]. We say "unfortunately" because the drug model is poorly suited to the nutrient context. Table 14.1 summarizes several of the principal inherent differences between the two, which we explore in more detail next.

A Contrast Groups

It is relatively easy to measure drug effects because drugs are added to a drug-free state. In addition, drugs are not normally present in the body except when administered by a physician or investigator, and when introduced, their concentration is not homeostatically regulated. Nutrients, by contrast, can essentially never have a nutrient-free state, either in the diet or in the body. Even when deficient, they are always still present in both, and often their serum concentration is tightly regulated (e.g., calcium and magnesium), which is why that concentration is often a poor index of nutrient status.

TABLE 14.1 Structural Differences between Drugs and Nutrients Related to Tests of Efficacy

Characteristic	Drug	Nutrient
Contrast groups	Drug-free	Regular diet (or low)
	Drug-added	Augmented diet
Scope of action	Largely single system	Usually multisystem
Effect size	Measurably large	Measurably small, system-by-system
Response characteristic	Linear	Threshold
Adjuvants	Minimize co-therapy	Optimize total nutrition

B Scope

It is easy to measure drug effects for yet another reason: Those effects are narrow in scope. The primary outcome variable for an antihypertensive is blood pressure. However, the primary outcome variable for any given nutrient is not easy to define adequately because it will usually be multiple. Despite a vast literature of nutrient efficacy studies with unitary end points, the fact is that nutrients should almost never be evaluated using single-system outcomes. They require some sort of global index, which nutrition today lacks.

C Effect Size

It is easy to observe drug effects for another reason: They are, by design, measurably large in size. An antihypertensive agent that lowers blood pressure by 4 mm Hg in patients with hypertension would not be considered useful and would not be tested. Instead, agents would be designed to lower blood pressure by perhaps 40 mm Hg. Such drugs could be tested satisfactorily and economically in sample sizes of less than 50 patients. By contrast, a nutrient that lowers blood pressure at a population level by 4 mm Hg would have a profound effect on public health, but it would require sample sizes in excess of 1000 healthy individuals simply to demonstrate that it had any effect at all.

It is important to stress that the apparent smallness of nutrient effects does not mean that they are thereby unimportant. Figure 14.4 makes this point

---

[29]DHHS, FDA, Interim Evidence Based Ranking System for Scientific Data (July 10, 2003) weighting studies by design type in descending order from Type One to Type Four:
Type One: Randomized, controlled intervention trials;
Type Two: Prospective observational cohort studies;
Type Three: Nonrandomized intervention trials with concurrent or historical controls; case—control studies; and
Type Four: Cross-sectional studies; analyses of secondary disease end points in intervention trials; case series.

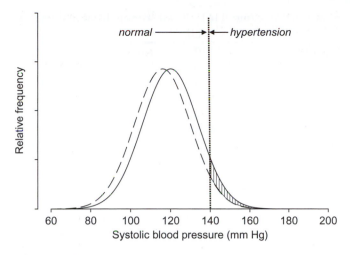

FIGURE 14.4 Typical frequency distribution for systolic blood pressure in perimenopausal women (with mean 120 mm Hg and SD 14 mm Hg) (the solid line). Approximately 8% of this population has a value above 140 mm Hg and hence would be considered hypertensive. Shifting the distribution downwards (i.e., to the left) by just 4 mm Hg (the dashed curve) lowers the proportion above 140 mm Hg to approximately 4.3%, or a reduction of nearly 50%. The shaded zone is the graphic representation of the difference in population proportions that are hypertensive, which is produced by the lowering of the distribution of blood pressure values. Source: *Copyright Robert P. Heaney, 2007. Used with permission.*

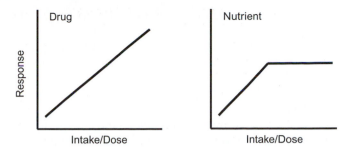

FIGURE 14.5 Response curves typical of drugs (left) and nutrients (right). The drug response tends to be monotonic so that higher doses produce larger effects across the range of plausible doses, whereas for nutrients, there is usually a response threshold or plateau, above which the benefit of the nutrient is constant, irrespective of intake. Source: *Copyright Robert P. Heaney, 2007. Used with permission.*

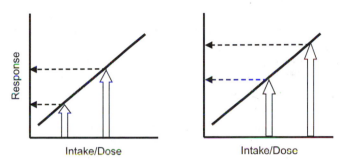

FIGURE 14.6 For drugs, the response can be detected along much or all of the response range. Left, low dose; right, high dose. Source: *Copyright Robert P. Heaney, 2007. Used with permission.*

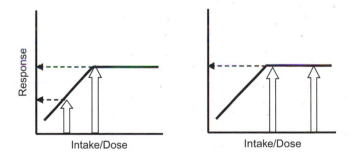

FIGURE 14.7 For nutrients, response occurs only if one or both of the contrasting intakes is below the response threshold (left). If both are at or above the threshold (right), no difference in response occurs. Source: *Copyright Robert P. Heaney, 2007. Used with permission.*

graphically for a typical distribution of systolic blood pressure values in adult women. A downward shift of the distribution by just 4 mm Hg reduces the fraction of the population above 140 mm Hg (i.e., the cutoff for the diagnosis, hypertension) by nearly 50%—a profoundly important public health benefit from a change that, in individuals, may seem trivially small. Further examples of large cumulative impacts of small changes are seen in the fact that negative calcium balance of just 30 mg/day translates to 1% bone loss/year or 30% in 30 years—that is, a skeletal deterioration from normal status to osteoporosis. Weight gain presents a similar contrast. Energy imbalance of as little as 70 kcal/day (less than one-half can of a typical carbonated beverage) leads to a weight gain of 70 lbs in just 10 years; that is, it accounts for a transition from normal weight to obesity. Such small changes underlie many of the long latency disorders, but they are effectively imperceptible when viewed up close.

D Response Characteristic

Drug effects are usually linear across a broad range of doses, whereas nutrient effects typically exhibit a sigmoid response (Figure 14.5). The drug response is monotonic; that is, it is directionally the same (and hence is detectable) everywhere along the plausible intake range (Figure 14.6). By contrast, a perceptible nutrient effect occurs only if at least one of the contrasted intakes is below the response threshold (Figure 14.7). If both groups have intakes above the threshold, no difference in response to the two intakes will occur or should be expected.

E Adjuvants

An additional and very important difference between the two investigative challenges lies in the role of helper agents in enabling or obscuring the proper effects of an intervention. When testing drugs, co-therapies are usually excluded so as to allow clearer definition of precisely what the particular drug is doing. However, in evaluating individual nutrients, not only must intakes of other nutrients continue but also ensuring adequacy of their intakes can become critically important if the test nutrient is to exert a measurable effect. Calcium, vitamin D, and protein provide useful examples of this interdependency.

It can easily be shown that practicable calcium intakes will not produce useful quantities of absorbed calcium in the absence of vitamin D and, conversely, that inadequate calcium intake will not permit adequate absorption even in the presence of full vitamin D repletion [9]. If, as is generally recognized, the effect of either calcium or vitamin D is considered to be increased calcium delivery into the body, it follows that one needs both nutrients to obtain (and observe) the effect of either. Using a drug model would typically require studying each nutrient alone, as some of the published meta-analyses of calcium and vitamin D have mistakenly done [10–12].

Taking the example a step further, studies have shown that simply getting more calcium into the body is not enough to ensure protection of bone. The effect of calcium on bone mass turns out to be dependent on protein intake. Dawson-Hughes and Harris [13] showed that the improvement in bone density by supplementation with calcium and vitamin D was confined to individuals in the highest tertile of protein intakes. Also, in the Omaha Nun database in midlife women, the positive association of calcium intake with skeletal calcium retention was confined to women with protein intakes above the median for the group [14]. The results from these two studies are entirely concordant, and they ought not be surprising because protein makes up nearly 50% of the volume of bone, and bone remodeling requires a continuing supply of fresh dietary protein if bone replacement is to keep pace with bone removal. Finally, data suggest that magnesium may also be crucial inasmuch as vitamin D deficiency seems to be associated with subclinical magnesium deficiency [15]. In brief, as already noted, diets are seldom deficient in just one nutrient, and tests of the efficacy of single nutrients may fail, as many have done [16], if all other intake shortfalls are not corrected as well.

Efforts can be made to overcome or compensate for many of these structural problems, once recognized. However, contextual issues are more difficult to deal with. Table 14.2 lists three important contextual differences between drugs and nutrients in the testing of efficacy, each of which is discussed briefly next.

F Profits and Patents

With drugs, the cost of establishing efficacy (estimated at approximately $1 billion for an average drug today) will be recovered from the "profits" derived from drug sales throughout the years for which patent protection prevents unfair competition. Neither recourse is usually available for foods or nutrients. Profit margins are low, and patent protection is limited or nonexistent. Thus, the food industry is effectively precluded from funding the sorts of EBM-recommended testing needed to show population-level benefits.

G Ethics

Because of the difference in response characteristic between drugs and nutrients, a valid RCT for a nutrient requires that the control group be placed on an inadequate intake. With new drugs, one can always summon equipoise. One does not know, in advance, whether the agent being tested will confer any net benefit, and it is not, in fact, a deprivation to be "deprived" of a drug that is ineffective. However, that posture is never possible for nutrients. All nutrients are, ultimately, essential, and to test the putative benefit of any single nutrient requires, in effect, that our trial measure what happens to someone who clearly does not get enough. Once that necessity is recognized, it is immediately apparent why there is an ethical problem because to

TABLE 14.2 Contextual Differences between Drugs and Nutrients Related to Tests of Efficacy

Characteristic	Drug	Nutrient
Profit margin (access to funds for testing)	Large	Small
Patent protection	Usually available	Usually not available
Ethics	Placebo controls often acceptable	Placebo controls usually unacceptable when outcome involves serious disease

show a benefit, the investigators must harm the control group [17]. Such a trial becomes even more clearly indefensible when the outcome concerned is a serious health problem such as hip fracture or preeclampsia.[30]

III APPROACHES

The validity of the foregoing analysis must be judged on its own merits, not on the feasibility or attractiveness of any solutions the authors may propose. Nevertheless, suggesting alternative approaches seems appropriate, if only to illustrate how the problem of establishing efficacy for nutrients might be handled or to evoke other and perhaps better suggestions. For purposes of this chapter, we confine ourselves to two distinct strategies and, within them, three approaches that together attempt to address most of the problems of the drug model listed in Tables 14.1 and 14.2. The two strategies are (1) defining "normal" for nutrients on physiological rather than empirical grounds and (2) developing empirical approaches better suited to nutrients than the RCT.

A Defining "Normal"

"Normal" for nutrition and nutrients can be operationally defined as the intake (or nutrient status) above which further increases in intake (or status) produce no further benefit. In other words, "normal" status exists when the function of the body system(s) concerned is/are not limited by nutrient availability.

The empirical approach attempts to locate that intake by RCTs of intakes approaching or exceeding that critical value. Although straightforward in concept, this general strategy can only work very crudely because the approach to normal is asymptotic; that is, the closer one gets to normal, the smaller will be the change produced and thus more difficult to find. In fact, it leads to a "Catch-22" situation. Either a significant improvement in function is not found (because, for example, the study was not adequately powered) or, if found, it will necessarily be small, and hence likely to be dismissed as unimportant.

An alternate strategy is to define "normal" in physiological terms. Five such model referents can be suggested:

- The negative feedback control loop model.
- The plateau model.
- The primitive intake model.
- The mutational model.
- A homeostasis model.

These have been discussed at greater length elsewhere [19]. Here, it may be useful to describe each, if only very briefly. The negative feedback model is the one currently used in clinical endocrinology to define "normal" for hormone replacement therapy. It is the intake that minimizes the control loop stimulus (e.g., TSH in thyroid hormone replacement). In the plateau model, "normal" is the intake that gets a function up onto its response plateau, and in nutrition it is is exemplified by iron intake as it relates to blood hemoglobin concentration. The primitive intake model (when that intake can reasonably be ascertained) is the exposure that prevailed during the evolution of human physiology. It presumes, reasonably we believe, that it is the intake for which human physiology is fine-tuned. The mutational model recognizes that certain micronutrients are autologously synthesized in mammals closely related to *Homo sapiens*, and when the environment provided ample quantities of such substances, that synthetic capacity was often lost through mutation. "Normal" in this context would be the amount synthesized by closely related animals just prior to mutational loss of that ability during primate (or hominid) evolution. Finally, the homeostatic model is based on the recognition that "normal" involves an ability to respond to perturbations and to return the organism to a certain resting state. A familiar example would be the glucose tolerance test used to assess insulin sensitivity and responsiveness.

These models would not be universally applicable. Nor are they all clearly distinct from one another. Nor is it obvious that a useable model could be found for every nutrient. Nevertheless, some are effectively in use today, and that use could profitably be expanded.

B Alternative Empirical Strategies

1 A Global Index

Because nutrients affect many systems and organs, it seems desirable to test nutrient effects in a way that

---

[30]The CPEP trial (Calcium in Preeclampsia Prevention) is a case in point [18]. Calcium supplementation in this trial did not significantly reduce preeclampsia incidence, in contrast to results from previous RCTs. However, there was no low calcium contrast group in CPEP. The control group received a calcium intake averaging above the current recommendations for pregnancy. It would not, in fact, have been ethically permissible to design the trial with a low calcium intake group because for the trial to be successful, there would have had to have been an excess of well over 20 cases of preeclampsia in the control group, relative to the intervention group.

captures that multiplicity. Such an approach calls for a global index that aggregates the multiple, sometimes small, yet measurable changes produced in as many systems. Unfortunately, no such index exists for nutrients. There have been recent and promising attempts to define food quality in a positive way—that is, by what a food contains rather than by what it does not have (or has less of) [20,21]. An analogous approach might be taken to health promotion by individual nutrients. Although it is unlikely that a single index could be developed for all nutrients, the components of the index for a specific nutrient would logically be made up of those functions or outcomes clinically linked to the nutrient concerned. An illustration of the value of capturing multiple end points is provided in Figure 14.8, showing important health benefits for vitamin D in four distinct systems [22]. Although in this example, each benefit had been established individually, the required sample sizes and costs were large. Manifestly, an aggregate outcome measure that incorporated all four end points would both more fairly and more accurately represent the health benefit of vitamin D and could have rendered detection of benefit less difficult and less costly.

Also, with respect to vitamin D, Cannell [23] has proposed recognition of a "vitamin D deficiency syndrome" consisting of low serum 25(OH)D levels together with some combination of osteoporosis, osteomalacia, poor calcium absorption, heart disease, hypertension, autoimmune disease, certain cancers, depression, and chronic pain, or any of the other disorders that have been plausibly linked to low vitamin D

status. This approach explicitly recognizes the number of ways that vitamin D functions and, therefore, the ways deficiency may manifest itself. The features of this syndrome definition could simply be inverted, thus characterizing the benefit of improved vitamin D status. A global index could be fabricated, constructing it so that high values would be indicative of greater benefit and low values of less benefit (or increased risk of frank disease). A certain number of points might be given for every incremental lowering in systolic blood pressure, a certain number of points for every incremental improvement in calcium absorption, a certain number of points for every incremental lowering in frequency of falls, a certain number of points for every incremental reduction in prevalence of key cancers (e.g., breast, colon, prostate, lung, and marrow—lymphoma), and a certain number of points for insulin responsiveness (expressed, for example, in response to a standard glucose challenge).

This example is intended solely to illustrate the type of approach that might be taken, and not to suggest specific components or the values attached to them. Issues that would need to be resolved would be the relative importance of the various end points to the individual concerned, to the public health, or to the health care budget of the nation. Such relative importance would be expressed in the index by the weights (number of points) given to each component of the index. However the score may be confected, and however its various components may be weighted, the score itself would be the primary outcome variable of an appropriately designed clinical investigation, explicitly comparing the aggregate of system effects in individuals having better vitamin D status with those with poorer status.

Comparable scores could surely be developed for other nutrients. For example, the components of a calcium score would include blood pressure, colon cancer risk, bone remodeling rate, bone mass, fracture risk, kidney stone risk, and body composition. Much work would have to be done in order to elicit a sufficient consensus in the scientific community to make the use of such indices persuasive, but lacking that effort, the field has no good way to assess the multiplicity of system effects that is characteristic of nutrients. Such indices for vitamin D and calcium seem a good place to start because their components represent already established end points. Thus, in their case, experimentation with the index will be a test of the concept, not a test of the nutrient—that is, how well the index works in identifying a health benefit, not how well vitamin D or calcium work. Interestingly, global indices can easily be constructed to incorporate negative effects (if any) of a nutrient, thereby facilitating straightforward quantification of net benefit.

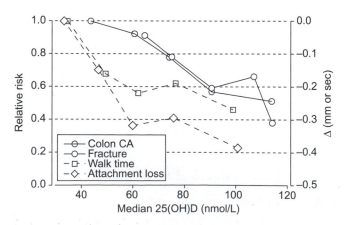

FIGURE 14.8 Health status improvement in several clinical studies of four health outcomes (periodontal disease, neuromuscular function, fractures, and colon cancer), plotted as a function of median achieved vitamin D status in the various studies assembled in this analysis, as assessed by serum 25(OH)D concentration. The solid lines are for relative risk of colon cancer and fracture (left-hand axis) and the dashed lines for reductions in walk time in the elderly and tooth attachment loss in periodontal disease (right-hand axis). Source: Redrawn from Bischoff-Ferrari et al. [22]. Used with permission.

C An Alternative to the Randomized Controlled Trial

Before describing a design that might solve some of the problems implicit in Tables 14.1 and 14.2, it is useful to review the major design types, with particular emphasis on their propensity to bias—that is, what makes them, structurally, more or less persuasive.

By way of background, it is useful to recall one inescapable fact of clinical research: Individuals respond differently to any given nutritional state, disease context, or treatment intervention. These differences are based in countless genetic variations in receptor binding, enzyme efficiency, gene promotion, and all of the other signaling and response mechanisms of cells and tissues of the body. In addition, individuals bring different life experiences, different comorbidities, differing nutritional status, differing motivations, and differing abilities to adhere to or sustain a given therapeutic intervention.

The result is that when one envisions an investigation of a nutrient or drug intervention in a given sample of the population, one knows in advance that some will do better than others. Some will have got better or worse by themselves, irrespective of the intervention. In brief, some will show improvement or worsening of a particular physiological function for reasons unrelated to the intervention being tested. The problem lies in the fact that we cannot tell who these persons are in advance, nor do we know who will actually get better or worse until we have done the investigation. Then the challenge is to determine whether it was the intervention that was responsible for a measured difference between treated groups or some of the other myriad factors that vary among the subjects—factors that may, by chance, have been disproportionately represented in the contrast groups of the investigation.

1 The Randomized, Controlled Trial

As already noted, the preferred approach to this issue is the RCT. Its strength lies in the fact that in randomly allocating the members of the sample to one intervention or the other, we actually randomly allocate the unrecognizable "improvers" and "worseners" to the treatment and control groups. From centuries of experience with the laws of probability, we are able to estimate the likelihood that a substantial disproportion of the improvers were by chance allocated to the active agent and, correspondingly, a substantial fraction of the worseners to the control group. When we make a probability statement about the results, such as "$P < 0.05$" or "$P < 0.01$," we are simply saying that the

chances are less than 1 in 20 or less than 1 in 100 that the difference we observed between the two treatment groups was due to this luck-of-the-draw disproportion in responders rather than to the effect of the intervention we are studying.

Although the RCT permits strong causal inference, the problems enumerated in Tables 14.1 and 14.2 and in the foregoing discussion make the RCT unsuitable (or even unacceptable) for much research involving nutrients. In addition, the RCT has serious generalizability problems, too often ignored [24].

Nevertheless, an RCT is favored by EBM because it allows us to quantify our chances of being wrong when we impute causality to the intervention. It is sobering to bear in mind that we can never truly prove causality; all we can do is state our chances of being wrong when we make that imputation. There is always the possibility that we will have been unlucky, that we had chosen that one time in 100 when pure random chance "put" an excess of the improvers in the treatment group and an excess of the worseners in the control group.[31]

2 Observational Studies

By contrast, all other investigational designs (generally termed "observational" studies) have to contend with the fact that the assignment of one group of individuals to a given intervention, and another to no treatment at all (or to low or high intakes of the nutrient being investigated), will not be due to random chance but to other factors not under the control of the investigator—factors that may be related to the measured outcome. With all such designs, although one can assess the chances that a given difference is greater than might have been expected from random chance, one has no way of knowing whether that difference was due to the intervention or to other, unrelated factors that influenced who received the intervention and who did not, simply because those factors were not distributed randomly to the contrast groups.

3 Investigative Interference

An additional and crucial feature of a properly designed RCT is the double-blind. This is important because the placebo effect is a powerful one, and individuals in a trial, knowing that they are receiving a potentially efficacious treatment for a serious health problem, respond differently than do individuals outside the investigative context. This difference in response is known technically as "interference" of the investigation in the outcome. In any concurrent investigation, whether an RCT or a concurrent cohort

---

[31]Moreover, given the multiplicity of randomized controlled trials that are reported every week in the literature, one can be certain that some of them will have fallen victim to that chance.

study, the placebo effect will always be present and may be responsible for a substantial portion of the response. The purpose of the blind in an RCT is to equalize that interference; that is, both the placebo and the treatment group experience a real placebo response, and any difference in outcome will therefore likely be due to the intervention. However, with a concurrent cohort study (often termed a "prospective" design), we must contend not only with the influence of other, unrecognized factors but also with unbalanced interference. Because both the study participants and the investigative staff are aware of who is a member of the active and the placebo arms of the study, there is unequal interference.

Two observational designs avoid this unequal interference problem: the case–control study and the non-concurrent cohort study. In the former, the contrast groups are assembled from individuals who have and have not actually developed the outcome under study, and then their exposure to the factor being tested is determined after the fact. In the latter, the exposure is also determined after the fact, but the study is basically prospective, inasmuch as one assembles the contrast groups by exposure, not outcomes, using various previously recorded databases or personal recall. In both cases, the investigation occurs after the outcome has developed, and hence no interference of the investigation in the outcome is possible.

The weakness of case–control studies lies in their tendency to "admission rate bias" [25], a problem that can be avoided only by either obtaining one's samples from the population, using random sampling methods, or by total sampling of the outcomes concerned. (Then, with either approach, admission into the study is not influenced by factors related to the outcome.) However, such stratagems are rarely possible and even more rarely implemented. Hence, case–control studies, as commonly reported, rank low on EBM's scale of persuasiveness.

4 The Non-Concurrent Cohort Design

Like its concurrent cousin, the non-concurrent cohort study assembles its contrast groups on the basis of exposure to the intervention (or in the case of nutrients, to high or low intakes of the nutrient concerned). However, it does so after the fact. An example would be a study of the effects of smoking. Contrast groups can be accurately assembled many years after onset of smoking.

Non-concurrent cohort studies circumvent some of the problems of the RCT and, when feasible, may well be the preferred nonexperimental design, and perhaps the only one reasonably suited to the study of nutrients. Non-concurrent cohort designs sidestep the ethical problem because the low intake group is self-

determined, and the exposure (or lack thereof) is not under investigative control. We may deplore the inadequate intake, but we neither cause it nor tolerate it.

The principal problem with a non-concurrent cohort study lies not in its design per se but in its execution. This is because it is not always easy to establish with any certainty, after the fact, to which contrast group an individual might have belonged. How can we be certain that one group has had a high intake of vitamin B_6 for the past 10 years and a contrasting group had a low intake? (There are exceptions. For example, individuals with lactose intolerance, because they avoid most dairy products, have lifelong, low calcium intakes and thus constitute a ready-made low intake contrast group for a non-concurrent cohort study of calcium benefits.)

In addition, there are now many large databases and specimen banks, both in Europe and in North America, that do permit such kinds of assessment. One example is the demonstration by Munger et al. [26] of an association between low vitamin D status and risk of development of multiple sclerosis (MS). That study was possible because the U.S. military has a huge repository of frozen serum samples, which could be analyzed, in this case for 25(OH)D, in order to ascertain vitamin D status prior to the development of MS. This study, as executed, used a case–control design (rather than a non-concurrent cohort design), but that was purely for reasons of cost. (Because MS is a rare disorder, starting with the cases greatly reduced the required investigative and analytical work.) However, there would have been no theoretical barrier to ascertaining 25(OH)D concentrations in all of the millions of frozen specimens or some reasonable sample thereof and thus constructing the study as a non-concurrent design. Just 2 years earlier, Munger et al. [25] had done precisely that for the Nurses' Health Study (however, using recorded vitamin D intakes rather than serum 25(OH)D to define the exposure cohorts) and had found a similar apparent protection of vitamin D with respect to risk of MS. In both cases, it was possible to estimate the actual vitamin D status prior to development of MS. However, because that status was unknown to both the participants and the investigators until after development of the outcome, no interference could have occurred. That leaves only the possibility of some extraneous, but unrelated, factor being responsible for allocation of the improvers and worseners to the two contrast groups. In many cases, this problem can be mitigated.

There will never be a method of estimating the chance that the observed effect was caused by unrelated factors as foolproof as random allocation, but that does not mean that one cannot take steps to reduce disproportions in the distribution of these other factors or to match the contrast groups for them. For example, regarding the issue of postmenopausal estrogen use in coronary artery disease risk, in addition to taking estrogen use as a determinant of the contrast groups, hindsight instructs us that we could have matched the groups for other markers of health-promoting behaviors such as smoking, alcohol use, regular dental visits, weekly exercise, body mass index, family history, co-therapy with a progestogen, and undoubtedly many others. In other words, in assembling the contrast groups that constitute the two cohorts of a non-concurrent cohort study, one needs to use not only exposure to the agent being tested but also all other factors that we know, at the time of the investigation, may be associated with the outcome of interest. Manifestly, this is not easy, and it will not always be possible. However, where possible, such an approach, particularly when combined with a global index, offers the best possible chance of skirting both the ethical problem of RCTs and the inferential weakness often faced by observational studies of the efficacy of nutrients.

Many reports from observational studies attempt to evaluate the impact of these factors by "adjusting" for various confounders. In reports from such studies, the method of adjustment is almost never stated and the reader (and often the investigator as well) does not know the basis for the adjustment. Rather than adjusting, it would seem to be far preferable to match the contrast groups for the confounding factors in advance of the analysis.

IV CONCLUSION

This chapter has attempted to address an issue that is both a challenge and an opportunity for nutritional science at the beginning of its second century as a scientific discipline. It is a challenge in that the drug model, widely used as a basis for claims of efficacy, is ill-suited for the task of establishing nutrient effects but is increasingly being applied to nutrients, particularly for the framing of nutritional policy. It is an opportunity in that it gives nutrition a chance to break out of its implicit one-nutrient–one-disease mold and to focus more explicitly on total body health, not as a sop to a romanticized "holistic" approach to science but simply because total body health is precisely the proper object of nutrition per se.

For nutrition to live up to its promise of reducing the substantial burden of diet-related morbidity and mortality, both the conceptualization of nutrition and the systems for evaluating relevant scientific evidence will need to be reframed to characterize more fully and accurately the human relationship of dependency on the food environment which nutrition, ultimately, endeavors to understand. Given the ecological nature

and evolutionary origins of this relationship, this reframing will need to consider features of historic food environments that have shaped the evolution of human nutritional needs, as well as those of contemporary food environments that are shaping current food consumption patterns and nutritional inadequacies. These, in turn, will have to be integrated into a system of evaluation that places clinical, observational, and other research findings into an appropriate environmental health context, both to expose those disease relationships with greater biological plausibility and significance and to minimize the risk of overlooking subtler relationships of substantial importance to public health. Ultimately, a reformulated approach for evaluating a more diverse range of relevant scientific evidence will be necessary if the nutritional relationships to disease that have greatest importance for improving both personal and public health are to be recognized and woven into the fabric of nutrition policy.

This chapter is little more than a first step. Although the investigational design that avoids most of the problems presented by randomized trials—that is, the non-concurrent cohort study—would seem to offer promise, much more thought and testing need to be done to better define the probably nutrient-specific confounding factors that ought to be factored into assembling the intake cohorts needed to discern total body effects of nutrients. Even more important, nutrition needs to define "normal" on physiological grounds rather than basing that definition solely on empirical grounds. In addition, better tools, such as global effect indices, need to be developed and tested. Unfortunately, the EBM juggernaut is rapidly rolling downhill and threatens to crush public health nutrition with its reductionist methods. Hence, the challenge is both real and urgent.

References

[1] A.B. Hill, The environment and disease: association or causation? Proc. R. Soc. Med. 58 (1965) 295–300.
[2] R.P. Heaney, Long-latency deficiency disease: insights from calcium and vitamin D, Am. J. Clin. Nutr. 78 (2003) 912–919.
[3] L.E. Griffith, G.H. Guyatt, R.J. Cook, H.C. Bucher, D.J. Cook, The influence of dietary and nondietary calcium supplementation on blood pressure: an updated meta-analysis of randomized controlled trials, Am. J. Hypertens. 12 (1999) 84–92.
[4] P.S. Allender, J.A. Cutler, D. Follmann, F.P. Cappuccio, J. Pryer, P. Elliott, Dietary calcium and blood pressure: a meta-analysis of randomized clinical trials, Ann. Intern. Med. 124 (1996) 825–831.
[5] M.J. Barger-Lux, R.P. Heaney, P.T. Packard, J.M. Lappe, R.R. Recker, Nutritional correlates of low calcium intake, Clinics Appl. Nutr. 2 (1992) 39–44.
[6] F.J. Service, Idle thoughts from an addled mind, Endocr. Prac. 8 (2002) 135–136.

[7] R.P. Heaney, Evidence-based medicine and common sense: practical and ethical issues in clinical trials for osteoporosis, Future Rheumatol. 2 (2007) 104–110.

[8] S.T. Roller, T. Voorhees Jr., A.K. Lunkenheimer, Obesity, food marketing and consumer litigation: threat or opportunity? Food Drug Law J. 61 (2006) 419–444.

[9] R.P. Heaney, Vitamin D: Role in the Calcium Economy, in: D. Feldman, F.H. Glorieux, J.W. Pike (Eds), Vitamin D, second ed., Academic Press, San Diego, 2005, pp. 773–787.

[10] B. Shea, G. Wells, A. Cranney, N. Zytaruk, V. Robinson, L. Griffith, et al., VII: meta-analysis of calcium supplementation for the prevention of postmenopausal osteoporosis, Endocr. Rev. 23 (2002) 552–559.

[11] E. Papadimitropoulos, G. Wells, B. Shea, W. Gillespie, B. Weaver, N. Zytaruk, et al., VIII: meta-analysis of the efficacy of vitamin D treatment in preventing osteoporosis in postmenopausal women, Endocr. Rev. 23 (2002) 560–569.

[12] A. Cranney, G. Guyatt, L. Griffith, G. Wells, P. Tugwell, C. Rosen, IX: summary of meta-analyses of therapies for postmenopausal osteoporosis, Endocr. Rev. 23 (2002) 570–578.

[13] B. Dawson-Hughes, S.S. Harris, Calcium intake influences the association of protein intake with rates of bone loss in elderly men and women., Am. J. Clin. Nutr. 75 (2002) 773–779.

[14] R.P. Heaney, Effects of protein on the calcium economy, in: P. Burckhardt, B. Dawson-Hughes, R.P. Heaney (Eds), Nutritional Aspects of Osteoporosis, Elsevier, Amsterdam, 2007, pp. 191–197.

[15] O. Sahota, M.K. Mundey, P. San, I.M. Godber, D.J. Hosking, Vitamin D insufficiency and the blunted PTH response in established osteoporosis: the role of magnesium deficiency, Osteoporos. Int. 17 (2006) 1013–1021.

[16] G.S. Omenn, G.E. Goodman, M.D. Thornquist, J. Balmes, M.R. Cullen, A. Glass, et al., Effects of a combination of beta carotene and vitamin A on lung cancer and cardiovascular disease, N. Engl. J. Med. 334 (1996) 1150–1155.

[17] R.J. Levine, Placebo controls in clinical trials of new therapies for osteoporosis, J. Bone Miner. Res. 18 (2003) 1154–1159.

[18] R.J. Levine, J.C. Hauth, L.B. Curet, B.M. Sibai, P.M. Catalano, C.D. Morris, et al., Trial of calcium to prevent preeclampsia, N. Engl. J. Med. 337 (1997) 69–76.

[19] R.P. Heaney, The nutrient problem, Nutr. Rev. 70 (2012) 165–169.

[20] A. Drewnowski, Concept of a nutritious food: toward a nutrient density score, Am. J. Clin. Nutr. 82 (2005) 721–732.

[21] R.P. Heaney, K. Rafferty, Assessing nutritional quality, Am. J. Clin. Nutr. 83 (2006) 722–723.

[22] H.A. Bischoff-Ferrari, E. Giovannucci, W.C. Willett, T. Dietrich, B. Dawson-Hughes, Estimation of optimal serum concentrations of 25-hydroxyvitamin D for multiple health outcomes, Am. J. Clin. Nutr. 84 (2006) 18–28.

[23] Vitamin D Council. "Vitamin D Deficiency: A Global Epidemic." Available at <http://www.vitamindcouncil.com/vdds.shtml> (accessed 23.03.07).

[24] A.R. Feinstein, Epidemiologic analyses of causation: the unlearned scientific lessons of randomized trials, J. Clin. Epidemiol. 42 (1989) 481–489.

[25] K.L. Munger, S.M. Zhang, E. O'Reilly, M.A. Hernan, M.J. Olek, W.C. Willett, et al., Vitamin D intake and incidence of multiple sclerosis, Neurology 62 (2004) 60–65.

[26] K.L. Munger, L.I. Levin, B.W. Hollis, N.S. Howard, A. Ascherio, Serum 25-hydroxyvitamin D levels and risk of multiple sclerosis, JAMA 296 (2006) 2832–2838.

15

Choline and Brain Development

Mihai D. Niculescu

University of North Carolina at Chapel Hill, Chapel Hill, North Carolina

I INTRODUCTION

An increasing amount of evidence supports the hypothesis that chronic illness in adult life has, in part, its origins before birth due to various environmental exposures [1]. In such cases, prevention rather than treatment becomes the active principle in establishing long-term public health policies that will enable an overall improvement in the health status of the general population [2]. Various nutrient deficiencies (omega-3/6 fatty acids, iron, protein/amino acids, energy restriction, folate, choline, etc.), occurring during pregnancy or perinatally, have been associated with defects in brain development that range from impaired physiological functions such as decreased visual acuity to severe birth defects [3−9]. Moreover, such early alterations in brain development have been associated, in many cases, with long-term functional alterations of brain functions, within adulthood and the aging period [10−12].

The importance of adequate nutrition during brain development has been repeatedly reinforced by many studies. A growing body of evidence indicates that the relationship between various nutrients and the development of the nervous system is complex and not necessarily confined to one specific period of gestation, but there is no doubt that specific nutrients play essential roles in neural development [10,13,14]. This chapter discusses the role that choline and its metabolite betaine have in brain development and also the subsequent implications in the physiology of memory and brain aging.

II CHOLINE METABOLISM AND BIOCHEMISTRY

A Intestinal Absorption

Dietary free choline or choline-containing esters (e.g., phosphatidylcholine) are first hydrolized in the intestine. The free choline is oxidized, in part, by the gut bacteria to betaine (Figure 15.1) or further metabolized to methyl-amines [15], whereas the choline-containing esters are hydrolyzed by enzymes from the pancreatic secretions and from intestinal mucosal cells, such as phospholipases A_1, A_2, and B [16]. The remaining free choline is absorbed by the enterocytes via carrier-mediated transport [17,18], whereas betaine is absorbed most probably via active Na^+ or Cl^--coupled, and also via passive Na^+-independent transport systems (reviewed in [19]), at a faster rate than choline [17,18]. The bioavailability of choline-containing compounds is different in infants than in adults, probably as a consequence of differences in both the physiology of their digestive system [16] and the choline content of the milk [20].

B Transport and Tissue Uptake

Once absorbed into enterocytes, choline is transported to the liver via the portal circulation mainly as phosphatidylcholine [21], or it is incorporated into chylomicrons and released into the systemic circulation via the lymphatic system [22,23]. Choline accumulates in all tissues [24] by diffusion and mediated transport (reviewed in [25,26]) using three distinct uptake systems: low-affinity facilitated diffusion, high-affinity Na^+-dependent transport, and an Na^+-independent transport with intermediate affinity [25,26]. Based on the affinity for choline, three types of transporters have been identified: cation transporters (OCTs) with low affinity, choline-transporter-like (CTLs) with intermediate affinity, and choline transporters (CHTs) with high affinity [25,26]. In addition, phosphatidylcholine (PC) is trafficked via the ATP-binding cassette transporters (especially ABCA1 and ABCG1) [27−29]. In liver, choline uptake is also dependent on the remodeling of HDL-PC by secretory phospholipase A_2 [30]. Choline

Nutrition in the Prevention and Treatment of Disease, Third Edition.
DOI: http://dx.doi.org/10.1016/B978-0-12-391884-0.00015-9

is transported across the blood—brain barrier by the CHT high-affinity system, represented by the solute carrier family 5 (choline transporter), member 7 (SLC5A7, known also as CHT or CHT1) [31—34]. Within the brain cells, this system depends partially on the integrity of endosomal apparatus [35], and it supplies choline for acetylcholine synthesis in presynaptic neurons [36]. Preliminary studies suggested that the CHT system could be enhanced by treatment with cytidine-5′-diphosphocholine (CDP-choline), specifically within cognitive areas such as the frontal cortex [37]. The CDP-choline pathway is the main source of endogenous phosphatidylcholine synthesis in brain, and it contributes to axon formation, growth, and branching of primary sympathetic neurons [38]. Preliminary studies suggested that CHT trafficking to cell membrane (and the consequent increase in choline uptake) may be under the transient control of protein kinase C activation [39].

Choline is excreted in the primary urine by glomerular filtration, but only 2% of the filtered choline is found in the final urine because of the intense reabsorption present mainly in the proximal tubules [40], operated by an organic cation transport system [41].

C Metabolism

Figure 15.2 presents a general overview of choline metabolism. Of special importance is the accumulation of choline by liver, kidney, brain, mammary gland, and placenta [24,25,42]. Choline is involved in three major pathways: acetylcholine synthesis, methyl donation via its oxidation to betaine, and phosphatidylcholine synthesis. The latter two have a special importance in brain development [43,44]. Phosphatidylcholine synthesis occurs by two independent pathways (Figure 15.2). Choline is phosphorylated by choline kinase and converted subsequently to CDP-choline. In combination with diacylglycerol, CDP-choline forms phosphatidylcholine (reaction catalyzed by diacylglycerol cholinephosphotransferase). In an alternate pathway, choline is synthesized *de novo* by the methylation of phosphatidylethanolamine (PtdEtn) to phosphatidylcholine in a reaction catalyzed by phosphatidylethanolamine-*N*-methyltransferase (Pemt,EC 2.1.1.17) using *S*-adenosylmethionine as methyl donor [45,46]. Although most active in liver, this pathway is also

FIGURE 15.1   Molecular structure of choline and betaine.

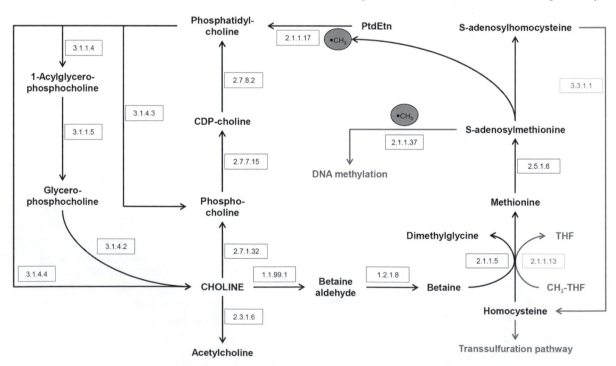

FIGURE 15.2   Choline metabolism. Enzymes are represented by EC numbers (1.1.99.1, choline dehydrogenase; 1.2.1.8, betaine-aldehyde dehydrogenase; 2.1.1.5, betaine-homocysteine *S*-methyltransferase; 2.1.1.13, methionine synthase; 2.1.1.17, phosphatidylethanolamine *N*-methyltransferase; 2.1.1.37, DNA (cytosine-5-)-methyltransferase; 2.3.1.6, choline *O*-acetyltransferase; 2.5.1.6, methionine adenosyltransferase; 2.7.1.32, choline kinase; 2.7.7.15, choline-phosphate cytidylyltransferase; 2.7.8.2, diacylglycerol cholinephosphotransferase; 3.1.1.4, phospholipase A2; 3.1.1.5, lysophospholipase; 3.1.4.2, glycerophosphocholine phosphodiesterase; 3.1.4.3, phospholipase C; 3.1.4.4, phospholipase D; 3.3.1.1, adenosylhomocysteinase). PtdEtn, phosphatidylethanolamine; THF, tetrahydrofolate.

active in other tissues, such as fetal brain and mammary gland [47–49]. In brain, choline regulates the Na^+, K^+-ATPase activity, although its mechanism of action is not yet completely understood [50].

Choline is also involved in the one-carbon metabolism via its irreversible oxidation to betaine [51], which methylates homocysteine to form methionine, thus contributing to the *S*-adenosylmethionine synthesis and linking choline with folate metabolism (Figure 15.2). Note that choline and folate metabolisms interact dynamically. Relative to brain, folate-deficient intakes or *Mthfr* heterozygosity enhanced the conversion of choline to betaine in order to sustain the homeostasis of methyl groups available for homocysteine methylation [52]. When rats were exposed to a folate-deficient diet for 10 weeks, choline levels decreased in liver, lung, kidneys, and heart [53]. Surprisingly, choline levels were moderately elevated in the cortex and striatum [53].

During pregnancy, choline is transported across the placenta by active mechanisms, against a concentration gradient [54]. The fetus is exposed to a high concentration of choline, and plasma choline concentration progressively declines after the first weeks of life [55]. In human newborns, plasma-free choline can reach concentrations of approximately 70 μM [56], whereas in adults, plasma-free choline is much lower (7–20 μM) [56,57]. The majority of choline in blood circulates as phosphatidylcholine (1–2.5 mM) [56,57].

III CHOLINE IN FOODS AND DIETARY REQUIREMENTS

A Dietary Sources

Most of the foods we eat contain various amounts of free choline, choline esters, and betaine [48]. In 2004, the U.S. Department of Agriculture (USDA) released its first database on choline content in common foods (http://www.nal.usda.gov/fnic/foodcomp/Data/Choline/Choln02.pdf). In most foods, free choline and phosphatidylcholine are the most abundant compounds. The foods most abundant in choline are of animal origin, especially eggs and liver, but some vegetables also have significant amounts of free choline and phosphatidylcholine (Brussels sprouts, cauliflower, nuts, etc.). Cereals and many baked products contain high amounts of betaine as well.

In human breast milk, free choline and all main choline esters are abundant, with total choline levels between 0.6 and 2 mM [58]. Manufacturers of infant formulas have modified the content of choline compounds to levels similar to those of human breast milk [20,58].

B Dietary Requirements

Although choline was not initially considered an essential nutrient because of its endogenous *de novo* synthesis from phosphatidylethanolamine [59], human studies during the past two decades have demonstrated that dietary choline is required (reviewed in [60]). In 1998, the U.S. Institute of Medicine (Food and Nutrition Board) established for the first time adequate intake (AI) and tolerable upper intake limit (UL) values for choline based on limited human studies [61] (Table 15.1). These values remained unchanged after the 2010 revision of the Dietary Reference Intakes by the USDA. UL values range from 1000 mg/day in children to 3500 mg/day in adults [61]. However, for some age categories for which adequate data were missing, AI values have been set by extrapolating from adult values (for ages 1–18 years) and for infants (for ages 7–12 months) [61]. Although a previous controlled study indicated that choline intakes may be adequate [62], a later epidemiological study using participants from the Framingham Offspring Study indicated that the mean intake for total choline (energy adjusted) is below the AI values, with a mean intake of 313 mg/day; moreover, there was an inverse association between choline intake and plasma total homocysteine concentration in subjects with low folate intakes [63]. This study strengthened previous similar findings in pregnant women, where a significant percentage of individuals had lower choline intakes than the recommended AI values [64,65]. The realization that choline intakes in the general U.S. population may not

TABLE 15.1 Adequate Intakes for Choline

Group	Age	Adequate intake (mg/day)
Infants and children	0–6 months	125
	7–12 months	150
	1–3 years	200
	4–8 years	250
	9–13 years	375
Boys	14–18 years	550
Girls	14–18 years	400
Pregnant women	All ages	450
Lactating women	All ages	550
Other men		550
Other women		425

Source: *Adapted from Institute of Medicine and National Academy of Sciences USA (1998). Choline. In "Dietary Reference Intakes for Folate, Thiamin, Riboflavin, Niacin, Vitamin B₁₂, Pantothenic Acid, Biotin, and Choline," pp. 390–422. National Academy Press, Washington, DC.*

be adequate has been refined by studies indicating that high-frequency genetic variations within genes involved in choline and folate metabolism can significantly alter the threshold for dietary requirements, thus raising the issue of individual-specific AIs for choline, rather than the general recommendations that are in place today (Table 15.1) [60,66–69]. Age- and gender-specific differences have also been reported for choline concentrations in plasma and human brain, indicating that the definition of dietary choline intakes should also take into consideration the physiological variations associated with gender and age [70,71].

C Interactions with Other Nutrients and Environment-Related Chemicals

Several animal studies have indicated that choline metabolism can be modulated by interaction with other nutrients and vitamins or by chemicals present in foods, water, food packaging, or food containers.

Dietary choline supplementation has proved beneficial against physical, neurological, and behavioral alterations induced by alcohol exposure. When pregnant rats were subjected to both alcohol and choline supplementation, behavioral measures in the offspring were improved compared to those of a group exposed only to alcohol, indicating that early choline supplementation could reduce the severity of fetal alcohol outcomes [72]. Within the same model, alterations induced by alcohol exposure in working memory were mitigated by choline supplementation [73]. Rats exposed postnatally to alcohol, and later choline supplemented, had significant reductions in the severity of trace eyeblink deficits induced by alcohol exposure [74].

The exposure to nicotine has been reported to adversely affect choline metabolism and brain development, although not all reported results are convergent. Gestational exposure of rats to nicotine decreased the choline uptake in the brains from offspring, due to lower binding to the high-affinity transporter, whereas changes in the acetylcholine esterase and choline acetyltransferase levels were variable and brain-area specific [75]. When young mice were exposed to cigarette smoke (containing a high and a low nicotine dose), those exposed to high nicotine smoke had increased choline uptake in the hippocampus and cerebral cortex compared to those exposed to low nicotine smoke or controls [76].

In rats, choline supplementation reversed the long-term alterations in learning and memory induced by Pb^{2+} exposure, which associated with higher gene and protein expression for the N-methyl-D-aspartate (NMDA) receptor subunit 1 (NR1), compared to the group exposed only to Pb_{2+} [77].

Mice fed a choline-deficient diet registered increased non-heme iron in the liver. The assessment of protein and mRNA expression of genes involved in iron metabolism and transport suggested that dietary choline deficiency may be associated with enhanced iron intake and reduced hepatic iron efflux [78].

Choline availability is enhanced by supplementation with vitamins B_6 and B_{12}, which are involved in folate and homocysteine metabolism (Figure 15.2) [79]. However, it is not clear whether these interactions have consequences for brain development.

Choline metabolism is also altered by the presence of other chemicals that, although not nutrients, can be found in packaging materials, drinking water, cosmetics, or other plastics used for foods. Examples are bisphenol A, diethanolamine, and arsenic [80–85].

D Consequences of Dietary Choline Deficiency in Humans

Studies performed in animals and humans have categorized the effects induced by dietary choline deficiency into three groups: (1) changes in acetylcholine synthesis and release in brain, (2) organ dysfunction/metabolic changes in adults eating a low-choline diet for a relatively short time, and (3) birth defects (abnormal neural tube closure and cleft palate) in newborns from mothers eating diets lower in choline content, as well as effects of choline on neural-related cell proliferation and survival in rodents.

Historically, the first reports on the effects induced by changing dietary choline focused on acetylcholine release in human brain and the consequences this had on memory, small motor movements, and the release of other neurotransmitters such as 7-aminobutyric acid (reviewed in [86]). In this context, the effectiveness of choline supplementation in improving the acetylcholine release was, for most of the studies, limited to individuals with neurological disorders such as tardive dyskinesia and Alzheimer's disease [87]. Using rodent models, dietary choline has been shown to modulate the density of the benzodiazepine receptors and the function of the GABAergic receptors in the cortex [86], but whether these findings can be applied to healthy humans remains unclear.

Human dietary requirements for choline have been studied in subjects fed low-choline diets under controlled conditions; they developed reversible fatty liver as well as liver and muscle damage [88,89]. These clinical outcomes were associated with increased apoptosis in lymphocytes [90]. Premenopausal women were less likely to develop organ dysfunction when fed a low-choline diet than were men or postmenopausal women, most likely because estrogen contributes to the activation of the gene that regulates the endogenous synthesis of choline (phosphatidylethanolamine *N*-methyltransferase gene (*PEMT*)) [91]. Interestingly, the risk of developing such clinical signs was associated with the presence of several polymorphisms within genes involved in folate and choline metabolism, such as the *PEMT* gene, the choline dehydrogenase gene (*CHDH*), and the 5,10-methylenetetrahydrofolate dehydrogenase (*MTHFD1*) gene, suggesting that dietary choline requirements may differ with genotype, gender, and estrogen status [68,92].

The third category of effects relates to critical periods when choline is needed for fetal and infant development, for which most studies have focused on neural and brain development.

IV CHOLINE AND NEURAL DEVELOPMENT

Dietary choline is essential in at least two distinct stages of brain development: neurulation (formation and closure of the neural tube) and a later stage (late pregnancy and potentially the neonatal period) during the maturation of hippocampus and other brain areas. Although the mechanisms responsible for these outcomes have been partially elucidated in animal models, confirmation in human studies is available only for early pregnancy.

A Choline Availability in Early Pregnancy

When gestation day 9 mouse embryos were exposed *in vitro* to either an inhibitor of choline uptake (2-dimethylaminoethanol; DMAE) or an inhibitor of phosphatidylcholine synthesis (1-*O*-octadecyl-2-*O*-methyl-rac-glycero-3-phosphocholine; ET-18-OCH3), they developed craniofacial hypoplasia and open neural tube defects in the forebrain, midbrain, and hindbrain regions [93]—alterations that are similar to those induced by folate deficiency [94]. Increased cell death was associated especially with the inhibition of phosphatidylcholine synthesis [93]. A subsequent study using the same mouse embryo model revealed that the mechanisms responsible for these outcomes were related to alterations in choline metabolism pathways [95], stressing the importance of dietary choline. These two animal studies were enhanced by data from human epidemiological studies describing similar outcomes in newborns from mothers who ate diets low in choline during pregnancy. In these studies, Shaw *et al.* reported that maternal dietary choline and betaine intakes during pregnancy inversely correlated with the risk of having a baby with neural tube defects and

orofacial clefts [64,65]. Women in the lowest quartile of total choline intake during the periconceptional period (290.41 mg/day) and eating diets low in folate content had a fourfold higher risk of having a baby with neural tube defects (spina bifida and anencephaly) than the women in the highest quartile for choline intake and with a low folate diet [65]. A similar relationship was also found between maternal choline intake and the increased risk of cleft lip with cleft palate [64]. However, a recent study by the same group failed to replicate these findings [96]. It is not clear whether this discrepancy was due to differences in study design or differences in the recruited populations [96]. Another study performed by the same team found a surprising association between higher intakes of choline and increased risk for metopic synostosis [97].

Independent of the maternal choline intake, the presence in infants of single nucleotide polymorphisms of two genes involved in choline metabolism—choline kinase A (*CHKA*) and CTP: phosphocholine cytidylyltransferase 1 (*PCYT1A*)—increased the risk of spina bifida in infants, regardless of the maternal choline intake [98]. Together, these data suggest that the risk for neural tube defects may be related to the maternal dietary choline and folate intakes and to the presence in the offspring of genetic polymorphisms in genes related to the metabolism of these two nutrients.

B Choline Availability in Late Pregnancy

During later gestation, rat and mouse models have been used to explore the role of choline in fetal brain development.

1 Choline Deficiency Inhibits Cell Proliferation

Rats and mice fed a low-choline diet in late pregnancy (gestational days 12—17 in mice and days 12 to 18 or 20 in rats) had reduced neural precursor cell proliferation and increased apoptosis in fetal hippocampus and cortex [99—101]. Similar outcomes were reported when pregnant mice were fed a low-folate diet [102], again suggesting the potential synergistic mechanisms of action between folate and choline. These alterations were confirmed in cell culture studies using primary neurons, pheochromocytoma cells, and human neuroblastoma cells. Dividing neuron-like cells (PC 12) exposed to a choline-deficient medium had decreased cell division and increased apoptosis and had diminished concentrations of phosphatidylcholine in their membranes [99,103]. The induced apoptosis is caspase 3-dependent in both cell culture and fetal brain models [101,103]. These changes were associated with important alterations of proteins involved in cell signaling, neuronal differentiation, and the regulation of cell cycle progression. Choline deficiency altered the expression of structural and signaling proteins such as TGF-β_1, vimentin, and MAP1 in the rat hippocampus [104]. Decreased cell proliferation was also associated with increased expression of neuronal and glial differentiation markers vimentin, TOAD-64 (dihydropyriminidase-like 2; Dpysl2), and calretinin [100,104,105]. Moreover, choline deficiency altered the protein expression of netrin and DCC, two proteins required for axonal growth and guidance in the developing nervous system [106]. These data suggested that choline deficiency induces a net trend toward the differentiation of neural progenitors and a subsequent reduction of the pool of the available precursor cells. Some differences persist for the lifetime of the offspring of treated mothers; prenatal choline supplementation decreased calretinin protein levels in the adult (24-month) mouse hippocampus [105].

A study revealed that the alterations in cell proliferations induced by fetal choline deficiency are not confined to neural cells. Angiogenesis in mouse fetal hippocampus was inhibited by choline deficiency (gestational day 17) due to decreased proliferation of endothelial cells [107]. The reduction was associated with increased expression of genes involved in angiogenic signaling (Vegfc and Angpt2) [107].

Regarding the link between choline and folate metabolisms (discussed previously), limited studies indicated that choline supplementation could partially offset the deleterious effects of folate deficiency on fetal brain development. Whereas folate deficiency during late pregnancy (gestational days 11–17) presented less cell proliferation and increased apoptosis within septum, hippocampus, striatum, and the anterior and midposterior neocortex, the concomitant exposure to a folate-deficient, choline-supplemented diet partially mitigated these outcomes in some of the brain areas but not all [108].

The mechanisms associating choline deficiency with decreased cell proliferation are, in part, related to the overexpression of cyclin-dependent kinase inhibitors p27Kip1 [109], p15Ink4b [109,110], and Cdkn3 [110,111], indicating that choline deficiency inhibits cell proliferation by inducing G_1 arrest because of the inhibition of the interaction between cyclin-dependent kinases and cyclins. Moreover, in human neuroblastoma cells (IMR-32), choline deficiency decreased the phosphorylation of the retinoblastoma protein (p110, Rb) [111]. This interaction model between p27Kip1 and p15Ink4b cyclin-dependent kinase inhibitors, TGF-β, and the Rb proteins fits the previously described model of cell cycle regulation (reviewed in [112]), in which the net outcome is cell cycle arrest in the G_1 phase of the cell cycle. These findings were reinforced by a study using mouse hippocampal and cortical progenitor cells exposed to choline deficiency for 48 hours. Using oligonucleotide arrays, the authors reported extensive changes in more than 1000 genes, of which 331 were related to cell division, apoptosis, neuronal and glial differentiation, methyl metabolism, and calcium-binding protein ontology classes [113], where, again, the net result was toward reduced cell proliferation, increased apoptosis, and increased neuronal and glial differentiation.

2 Choline Deficiency Alters Gene Expression via Epigenetic Mechanisms

Epigenetic mechanisms consist of chemical changes of the chromatin (DNA and histones) that do not alter the DNA sequence and that establish meiotically and mitotically stable, heritable patters of gene expression [114,115]. These mechanisms consist of DNA methylation and hydroxymethylation, histone modifications, along with the modulation of epigenetic marks by noncoding RNA species [14,115,116].

a EPIGENETIC MECHANISMS REGULATE GENE EXPRESSION

DNA methylation is represented by the substitution of hydrogen with methyl groups to DNA (reviewed in [117]). In mammalians, the majority of DNA methylation occurs at carbon 5 of the cytosine ring (5-methylcytosine; 5mC) only when the cytosine is followed by a guanine nucleotide (CpG site), but methyl groups can be also added to other nucleotides [117]. This process is catalyzed by DNA methyltransferases (DNMTs). During the S-phase of cell cycle progression, the DNA methylation status of the parental DNA strand is duplicated on the newly synthesized DNA by maintenance DNA methyltransferase DNMT1 [118]. However, DNA methylation can also occur at previously unmethylated CpG sites (de novo DNA methylation), catalyzed by de novo DNA methyltransferases DNMT3a and 3b, and with participation of DNMT2 and 3L [118].

When DNA methylation occurs within promoter regions, it usually associates with gene underexpression and chromatin compaction [51], but instances have been described in which promoter hypermethylation prevented the binding of inhibitory factors, thus allowing for promoter activation and gene overexpression [119]. The establishment of cell type-specific DNA methylation patterns contributes decisively to shaping the cellular phenotypes of differentiated cells [118].

Within the concept of epigenetic regulation of gene expression, an important feature is genomic imprinting, allowing genes to be expressed in a parent-of-origin manner (imprinted genes), this process being the molecular basis for mono-allelic expression [120]. During early embryogenesis, most of the parental DNA methylation patterns are erased by active and passive demethylation mechanisms (with the exception of some imprinted regions), whereas new DNA methylation patterns are established by *de novo* methylation. The establishment of new epigenetic patterns continues during fetal morphogenesis and in the early postnatal period [121].

The epigenetics of DNA also includes the hydroxylation of methyl groups attached to cytosine, as an intermediary step in active DNA demethylation, with important functional consequences on gene activation [122]. This groundbreaking discovery provided the first plausible mechanism for the previously observed active DNA demethylation [116].

Chromatin modifications occur at the flexible tail regions of histones. These modifications include, but are not limited to, methylation, acetylation, phosphorylation, ubiquitination, and ADP ribosylation [123]. In concert with DNA methylation, histone modifications allow for the reversible switch between chromatin relaxation and compaction and also the establishment of the degree of access that transcription factors have to promoter regions [118,123]. Examples are methylation of histone H3 at its lysine 9 and 27 residues (K9 and K27), allowing for chromatin compaction and inhibition of gene expression, and trimethylation of H3K4 that induces transcriptional activation and promoter activation [123].

MicroRNAs (miRNAs) are noncoding RNA species, up to 25 nucleotides in length, that contribute to gene expression regulation through RNA interference [124]. Their epigenetic role consists of the modulation of expression for several genes involved in the epigenetic machinery, which are responsible for DNA and histone modifications (e.g., *DNMT3a/b*, *HDAC1/4*, and *MeCP2*) [124]. Some genes encoding miRNA species can also be epigenetically regulated because their gene expression is highly dependent on their promoter methylation (reviewed in [124]).

b DNA METHYLATION, FETAL DEVELOPMENT, AND CELL DIFFERENTIATION

DNA methylation is very important during embryogenesis and late fetal development. Although the original DNA methylation pattern is germline specific (sperm DNA is hypermethylated compared to oocyte DNA), almost immediately after fertilization (within one or two cell divisions) there is a dramatic erasure of methylation, which continues until blastocyst implantation [121]. Following implantation, mouse embryonic stem cells are subjected to *de novo* methylation catalyzed by *Dnmt3a* and *Dnmt3b* genes (*de novo* methylases), with the exception of certain tissue-specific genes that remain unmethylated [121]. Once established, the new methylation pattern is conserved during cell replication (catalyzed by Dnmt1 in the S phase

of cell division [125]). These methylation patterns can be changed as cells differentiate (cell differentiation is associated with a genome-wide DNA hypomethylation followed by remethylation [117]) and can be altered by dietary intake of methyl donors (discussed next).

c DNA METHYLATION AND NEURAL DEVELOPMENT

Neural development is influenced by DNA methylation. Overall levels of methylation decrease as neuronal differentiation proceeds [126] and the treatment of neural precursor cells with demethylating agents induces them to differentiate into cholinergic and adrenergic neurons [127]. These methylation patterns are cell type-specific: Whereas mature neurons express DNA methyltransferases, these genes have much lower levels of expression in oligodendrocytes and astrocytes in the white matter [128]. The expression of DNA methyltransferases has a different importance, based on the differentiation stage of the cell: Deletion of Dnmt1 in postmitotic neurons does not affect overall levels of DNA methylation, whereas the same deletion in neural progenitors markedly decreases methylation levels and causes severe defects in neurogenesis [129]. Astrocyte differentiation is also dependent on the methylation status of glial fibrillary acidic protein (*Gfap*) promoter at the binding site of STAT3 transcription factor. This promoter site becomes hypomethylated before differentiation, and its methylation prevents gene activation by STAT3 and astrocyte differentiation in fetal brain [130].

d CHOLINE DEFICIENCY ALTERS EPIGENETIC STATUS IN FETAL BRAIN

Although the relationship between nutrition and epigenetics has been firmly established [131], less is known about the epigenetic mechanisms involved in nutritionally triggered alterations in fetal brain development. However, available data allow us to identify an important role for choline in DNA methylation during brain development (reviewed in [132]). Maternal choline deficiency decreased the global DNA methylation in the neuroepithelial layer of the fetal hippocampus [110], whereas opposite effects were reported in the fetal brains from Pemt$^{-/-}$ mice, which also had increased *S*-adenosylmethionine levels [133]. Interestingly, Pemt$^{-/-}$ mice also had altered methylation of the lysine 4 and 9 residues within histone 3, suggesting that alterations in choline availability to the fetal brain may be crucial for both DNA and histone methylation [133]. Along with decreased global methylation, changes in gene-specific methylation were reported, where the promoter of cyclin-dependent kinase 3 (*Cdkn3*) was hypomethylated by choline deficiency in the progenitor layer of the hippocampus and in human neuroblastoma cells [110,111]. These alterations were associated with increased protein expression of this cyclin-dependent kinase inhibitor [110], and this model is consistent with previous findings regarding the epigenetic regulation of cyclin-dependent kinase inhibitors and their roles in cell proliferation [134]. Choline deficiency also induced DNA hypermethylation of the calbindin 1 promoter on the mouse fetal hippocampus, which associated with region-specific hypomethylation of monomethyl-lysine 9 of histone 3 (H3K9me1) and dimethyl-lysine of histone 3 (H3K9me2) in the hippocampus [119].

The epigenetic roles of choline are not confined to neural cells. Within the fetal hippocampus, the reduction in angiogenesis induced by choline deficiency also involved the DNA hypomethylation of CpG islands within the *Vegfc* and *Angpt2* promoters, two genes that are implicated in angiogenic signaling [107].

Because dietary choline is important in the maintenance of the *S*-adenosylmethionine pool (the methyl donor for DNA methylation), along with folate and methionine (Figure 15.2), it is attractive to hypothesize that choline, by influencing the epigenetic status of the developing brain, could thereby induce permanent epigenetic changes associated with alterations of brain function at later ages [14]. Figure 15.3 summarizes the hypothesized role that choline may play in the regulation of early brain development.

V LONG-LASTING CONSEQUENCES OF PRENATAL CHOLINE AVAILABILITY

A Molecular and Functional Changes

The changes induced by dietary choline in fetal brain have long-lasting effects that alter the neuronal function throughout the adult life. When pregnant rats were choline supplemented during late gestation, basal and receptor-stimulated phospholipase D activity was upregulated in the hippocampus of the offspring during postnatal development [135]. Acetylcholine metabolism and choline uptake mechanisms were also permanently altered in the adult brain. Choline acetyltransferase (ChAT) and acetylcholinesterase (AChE) activities were increased in the adult hippocampus of rats exposed to choline deficiency while *in utero*, and choline incorporation into acetylcholine was more dependent on high-affinity choline uptake mechanisms, compared to controls or to rats that were choline supplemented while *in utero* [136]. The increase in AChE activity was later found to be due to increased AChE protein synthesis [137], strongly suggesting that gene expression or post-transcriptional regulation was permanently altered by choline deficiency. This hypothesis was confirmed later in a study showing that the gene expression of the choline transporter Cht

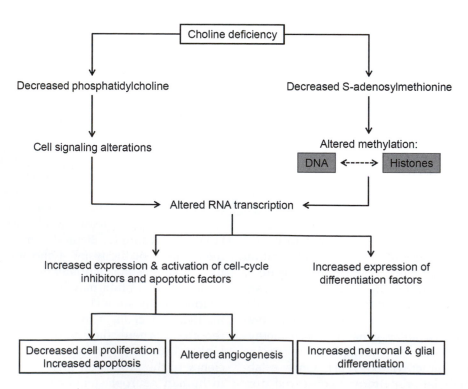

FIGURE 15.3   Choline deficiency alters brain development.

was increased in the adult hippocampus from rats exposed to prenatal choline deficiency, and that this correlated with an increased number of neurons that were CHT immunoreactive [138]. In addition, many other changes in gene expression were described to occur in the adult hippocampus and cortex, initiated by prenatal choline manipulation [139].

Cell signaling is also influenced by prenatal choline availability. In juvenile rats, the phosphorylation and activation of hippocampal mitogen-activated protein kinase and cAMP response element binding protein in response to glutamate, NMDA stimulation, or depolarizing concentrations of K^+ were increased by choline supplementation and reduced by choline deficiency while *in utero* [140]. Choline supplementation while *in utero* also increased the levels of nerve growth factor (NGF) in the adult rat hippocampus and cortex [141], suggesting that prenatal choline availability has an important role in promoting neurogenesis in the adult hippocampus, which is mediated by the nootropic action of NGF [142]. Opposite changes were reported for choline deficiency while *in utero* in other areas of the forebrain, such as medial septal nucleus, nucleus of the diagonal band, and the nucleus basalis of Meynert [143].

Although confirmation in humans is needed, these findings provided evidence that prenatal choline availability initiates a pattern of permanent metabolic alterations (metabolic imprinting) that, once established, plays an important role in later life [144].

B Choline Deficiency Induces Cognitive and Memory Deficits

The functional and molecular changes previously described are, at least in part, responsible for behavioral and memory changes initiated by prenatal variation in the availability of choline to developing brain (reviewed in [43]). Prenatal choline supplementation protects against the neurotoxicity induced by the administration of the NMDA receptor antagonist dizocilpine (MK-801) to female adolescent rats [145,146]. When status epilepticus was induced in adult rats using kainic acid, rats receiving supplemental choline between gestational day 11 and postnatal day 7 performed better in the water maze tests than did the deficient and control groups, whereas the hippocampal ChAT activity was 18% lower in the choline-deficient animals compared with the other two groups [147]. However, prenatal choline-deficient rats were not more susceptible to seizure induction by kainic acid than the group receiving adequate choline during fetal development [148].

Maternal dietary choline availability during late pregnancy was associated with long-lasting changes in the hippocampal function of the adult offspring. Choline supplementation during this period enhanced visuospatial and auditory memory in the adult rats throughout their life span [149–153]. It also enhanced a property of the hippocampus, long-term potentiation [154–156]. The offspring from mothers fed a choline-deficient diet manifested opposite outcomes [150,154].

In men, the choline concentration in the anterior cingulated cortex correlated with age, and higher total choline values were positively correlated with faster performance on the Stroop Interference task [157]. Postmortem assessment of choline levels in the brains of men with Alzheimer's disease indicated lower levels of plasmalogen choline in the prefrontal cortex than in controls, but it was unclear whether there was a mechanistic association between choline levels and disease because other components within phospholipids were also altered (i.e., docosahexaenoic acid; DHA) [158].

VI IMPLICATIONS FOR HUMAN BRAIN DEVELOPMENT

It is difficult to extrapolate to humans the findings reported using animal models. However, data are available to support the hypothesis that similar mechanisms are involved in humans. Because of ethical constraints, no studies are available in children or pregnant mothers to validate the rodent model. Because pregnant women are at risk of becoming choline deficient [60,159–161], and possibly having increased risk of giving birth to infants with neural tube defects [65], the recommendation that pregnant women should attempt to consume diets adequate in choline content seems reasonable. In addition, because half of the population has gene polymorphisms that affect choline and folate metabolisms [68,92], it is likely that different individuals may have different dietary requirements for choline and may need to pay special attention to choline intake not only during pregnancy but also during all other life stages.

Acknowledgment

The author acknowledges and thanks A.R. Niculescu for his contribution to the artwork included in this chapter.

References

[1] P.D. Gluckman, M.A. Hanson, F.M. Low, The role of developmental plasticity and epigenetics in human health, Birth Defects Res. C Embryo Today 93 (2011) 12–18.

[2] M.D. Niculescu, Epigenetic transgenerational inheritance: should obesity-prevention policies be reconsidered? Synesis 2 (2011) G18–G26.

[3] N. Gordon, Nutrition and cognitive function, Brain Dev. 19 (1997) 165−170.

[4] P. Guesry, The role of nutrition in brain development, Prev. Med. 27 (1998) 189−194.

[5] M.P. Mattson, Gene−diet interactions in brain aging and neurodegenerative disorders, Ann. Intern. Med. 139 (2003) 441−444.

[6] M.P. Mattson, T.B. Shea, Folate and homocysteine metabolism in neural plasticity and neurodegenerative disorders, Trends Neurosci. 26 (2003) 137−146.

[7] S.M. Innis, Dietary lipids in early development: relevance to obesity, immune and inflammatory disorders, Curr. Opin. Endocrinol. Diabetes Obes. 14 (2007) 359−364.

[8] S.M. Innis, Omega-3 fatty acids and neural development to 2 years of age: do we know enough for dietary recommendations? J. Pediatr. Gastroenterol. Nutr. 48 (Suppl. 1) (2009) S16−S24.

[9] M.K. Georgieff, Nutrition and the developing brain: nutrient priorities and measurement, Am. J. Clin. Nutr. 85 (2007) 614S−620S.

[10] D. Benton, Neurodevelopment and neurodegeneration: are there critical stages for nutritional intervention? Nutr. Rev. 68 (2010) S6−S10.

[11] J.T. Brenna, Animal studies of the functional consequences of suboptimal polyunsaturated fatty acid status during pregnancy, lactation and early post-natal life, Maternal Child Nutr. 7 (2011) 59−79.

[12] M.F. Laus, L.D. Vales, T.M. Costa, S.S. Almeida, Early postnatal protein-calorie malnutrition and cognition: a review of human and animal studies, Int. J. Environ. Res. Public Health 8 (2011) 590−612.

[13] I.C.G. Weaver, Shaping adult phenotypes through early life environments, Birth Defects Res. C Embryo Today Rev. 87 (2009) 314−326.

[14] M.D. Niculescu, D.S. Lupu, Nutritional influence on epigenetics and effects on longevity, Curr. Opin. Clin. Nutr. Metab. Care 14 (2011) 35−40.

[15] S.H. Zeisel, J.S. Wishnok, J.K. Blusztajn, Formation of methylamines from ingested choline and lecithin, J. Pharmacol. Exp. Ther. 225 (1983) 320−324.

[16] P.J.H. Jones, S. Kubow, Lipids, sterols, and their metabolites, in: M.E. Shils, M. Shike, A.C. Ross, B. Caballero, R.J. Cousins (Eds), Modern Nutrition in Health and Disease, Lippincott Williams & Wilkins, Philadelphia, 2006, pp. 92−122.

[17] H. Kettunen, S. Peuranen, K. Tiihonen, M. Saarinen, Intestinal uptake of betaine in vitro and the distribution of methyl groups from betaine, choline, and methionine in the body of broiler chicks, Comp. Biochem. Physiol. A Mol. Integr. Physiol. 128 (2001) 269−278.

[18] U. Schwab, A. Torronen, E. Meririnne, M. Saarinen, G. Alfthan, A. Aro, M. Uusitupa, Orally administered betaine has an acute and dose-dependent effect on serum betaine and plasma homocysteine concentrations in healthy humans, J. Nutr. 136 (2006) 34−38.

[19] S.A. Craig, Betaine in human nutrition, Am. J. Clin. Nutr. 80 (2004) 539−549.

[20] M.Q. Holmes-McNary, W.L. Cheng, M.H. Mar, S. Fussell, S.H. Zeisel, Choline and choline esters in human and rat milk and in infant formulas, Am. J. Clin. Nutr. 64 (1996) 572−576.

[21] L. Savendahl, M.H. Mar, L.E. Underwood, S.H. Zeisel, Prolonged fasting in humans results in diminished plasma choline concentrations but does not cause liver dysfunction, Am. J. Clin. Nutr. 66 (1997) 622−625.

[22] C. Schlierf, W.H. Falor, P.D. Wood, Y.L. Lee, L.W. Kinsell, Composition of human chyle chylomicrons following single fat feedings, Am. J. Clin. Nutr. 22 (1969) 79−86.

[23] L.Y. Yang, A. Kuksis, J.J. Myher, Similarities in surface lipids of chylomicrons from glyceryl and alkyl ester feeding: major components, Lipids 26 (1991) 806−818.

[24] S.H. Zeisel, J.K. Blusztajn, Choline and human nutrition, Annu. Rev. Nutr. 14 (1994) 269−296.

[25] P.R. Lockman, D.D. Allen, The transport of choline, Drug Dev. Ind. Pharm. 28 (2002) 749−771.

[26] V. Michel, Z. Yuan, S. Ramsubir, M. Bakovic, Choline transport for phospholipid synthesis, Exp. Biol. Med. (Maywood) 231 (2006) 490−504.

[27] A. Kobayashi, Y. Takanezawa, T. Hirata, Y. Shimizu, K. Misasa, N. Kioka, H. Arai, K. Ueda, M. Matsuo, Efflux of sphingomyelin, cholesterol, and phosphatidylcholine by ABCG1, J. Lipid Res. 47 (2006) 1791−1802.

[28] G. Schmitz, T. Langmann, Structure, function and regulation of the ABC1 gene product, Curr. Opin. Lipidol. 12 (2001) 129−140.

[29] G. Schmitz, T. Langmann, S. Heimerl, Role of ABCG1 and other ABCG family members in lipid metabolism, J. Lipid Res. 42 (2001) 1513−1520.

[30] J.C. Robichaud, J.N. van der Veen, Z. Yao, B. Trigatti, D.E. Vance, Hepatic uptake and metabolism of phosphatidylcholine associated with high density lipoproteins, Biochim. Biophys. Acta 1790 (2009) 538−551.

[31] D.D. Allen, P.R. Lockman, The blood−brain barrier choline transporter as a brain drug delivery vector, Life Sci. 73 (2003) 1609−1615.

[32] D.D. Allen, P.R. Lockman, K.E. Roder, L.P. Dwoskin, P.A. Crooks, Active transport of high-affinity choline and nicotine analogs into the central nervous system by the blood−brain barrier choline transporter, J. Pharmacol. Exp. Ther. 304 (2003) 1268−1274.

[33] P.R. Lockman, J.H. McAfee, W.J. Geldenhuys, D.D. Allen, Cation transport specificity at the blood−brain barrier, Neurochem. Res. 29 (2004) 2245−2250.

[34] W.J. Geldenhuys, D.D. Allen, P.R. Lockman, 3-D-QSAR and docking studies on the neuronal choline transporter, Bioorg. Med. Chem. Lett. 20 (2010) 4870−4877.

[35] M.T. Ivy, R.F. Newkirk, Y. Wang, J.G. Townsel, A novel choline cotransporter sequestration compartment in cholinergic neurons revealed by selective endosomal ablation, J. Neurochem. 112 (2010) 1295−1304.

[36] D. Lund, A.M. Ruggiero, S.M. Ferguson, J. Wright, B.A. English, P.A. Reisz, S.M. Whitaker, A.C. Peltier, R.D. Blakely, Motor neuron-specific overexpression of the presynaptic choline transporter: impact on motor endurance and evoked muscle activity, Neuroscience 171 (2010) 1041−1053.

[37] S.K. Tayebati, D. Tomassoni, A. Di Stefano, P. Sozio, L.S. Cerasa, F. Amenta, Effect of choline-containing phospholipids on brain cholinergic transporters in the rat, J. Neurol. Sci. 302 (2011) 49−57.

[38] J. Strakova, L. Demizieux, R.B. Campenot, D.E. Vance, J.E. Vance, Involvement of CTP: phosphocholine cytidylyltransferase-beta2 in axonal phosphatidylcholine synthesis and branching of neurons, Biochim. Biophys. Acta. 1811 (2011) 617−625.

[39] S.A. Black, F.M. Ribeiro, S.S. Ferguson, R.J. Rylett, Rapid, transient effects of the protein kinase C activator phorbol 12-myristate 13-acetate on activity and trafficking of the rat high-affinity choline transporter, Neuroscience 167 (2010) 765−773.

[40] M. Acara, F. Roch-Ramel, B. Rennick, Bidirectional renal tubular transport of free choline: a micropuncture study, Am. J. Physiol. 236 (1979) F112−F118.

[41] F. Pietruck, M. Horbelt, T. Feldkamp, K. Engeln, S. Herget-Rosenthal, T. Philipp, A. Kribben, Digital fluorescence imaging of organic cation transport in freshly isolated rat proximal tubules, Drug Metab. Dispos. 34 (2006) 339−342.

[42] S.H. Zeisel, K.A. da Costa, Choline: an essential nutrient for public health, Nutr. Rev. 67 (2009) 615—623.

[43] S.H. Zeisel, The fetal origins of memory: the role of dietary choline in optimal brain development, J. Pediatr. 149 (2006) S131—S136.

[44] S.H. Zeisel, M.D. Niculescu, Perinatal choline influences brain structure and function, Nutr. Rev. 64 (2006) 197—203.

[45] J.K. Blusztajn, S.H. Zeisel, R.J. Wurtman, Synthesis of lecithin (phosphatidylcholine) from phosphatidylethanolamine in bovine brain, Brain Res. 179 (1979) 319—327.

[46] T. Kaneshiro, J.H. Law, Phosphatidylcholine synthesis in Agrobacterium tumefaciens: I. Purification and properties of a phosphatidylethanolamine N-methyltransferase, J. Biol. Chem. 239 (1964) 1705—1713.

[47] J.K. Blusztajn, S.H. Zeisel, R.J. Wurtman, Developmental changes in the activity of phosphatidylethanolamine N-methyltransferases in rat brain, Biochem. J. 232 (1985) 505—511.

[48] J.E. Vance, S.J. Stone, J.R. Faust, Abnormalities in mitochondria-associated membranes and phospholipid biosynthetic enzymes in the mnd/mnd mouse model of neuronal ceroid lipofuscinosis, Biochim. Biophys. Acta 1344 (1997) 286—299.

[49] E.K. Yang, J.K. Blusztajn, E.A. Pomfret, S.H. Zeisel, Rat and human mammary tissue can synthesize choline moiety via the methylation of phosphatidylethanolamine, Biochem. J. 256 (1988) 821—828.

[50] C. Liapi, A. Kyriakaki, A. Zarros, P. Galanopoulou, H. Al-Humadi, I. Dontas, K. Voumvourakis, S. Tsakiris, Choline-deprivation alters crucial brain enzyme activities in a rat model of diabetic encephalopathy, Metab. Brain Dis. 25 (2010) 269—276.

[51] M.D. Niculescu, S.H. Zeisel, Diet, methyl donors and DNA methylation: Interactions between dietary folate, methionine and choline, J. Nutr. 132 (2002) 2333S—2335S.

[52] T.W. Chew, X. Jiang, J. Yan, W. Wang, A.L. Lusa, B.J. Carrier, A.A. West, O.V. Malysheva, J.T. Brenna, J.F. Gregory III, M.A. Caudill, Folate intake, MTHFR genotype, and sex modulate choline metabolism in mice, J. Nutr. 141 (2011) 1475—1481.

[53] N.A. Crivello, J.K. Blusztajn, J.A. Joseph, B. Shukitt-Hale, D.E. Smith, Short-term nutritional folate deficiency in rats has a greater effect on choline and acetylcholine metabolism in the peripheral nervous system than in the brain, and this effect escalates with age, Nutr. Res. 30 (2010) 722—730.

[54] J.H. Sweiry, K.R. Page, C.G. Dacke, D.R. Abramovich, D.L. Yudilevich, Evidence of saturable uptake mechanisms at maternal and fetal sides of the perfused human placenta by rapid paired-tracer dilution: studies with calcium and choline, J. Dev. Physiol. 8 (1986) 435—445.

[55] K.E. McMahon, P.M. Farrell, Measurement of free choline concentrations in maternal and neonatal blood by micropyrolysis gas chromatography, Clin. Chim. Acta 149 (1985) 1—12.

[56] A.L. Buchman, M. Sohel, A. Moukarzel, D. Bryant, R. Schanler, M. Awal, P. Burns, K. Dorman, M. Belfort, D.J. Jenden, D. Killip, M. Roch, Plasma choline in normal newborns, infants, toddlers, and in very-low-birth-weight neonates requiring total parenteral nutrition, Nutrition 17 (2001) 18—21.

[57] S.H. Zeisel, Choline: an essential nutrient for humans, Nutrition 16 (2000) 669—671.

[58] Y.O. Ilcol, R. Ozbek, E. Hamurtekin, I.H. Ulus, Choline status in newborns, infants, children, breast-feeding women, breast-fed infants and human breast milk, J. Nutr. Biochem. 16 (2005) 489—499.

[59] J. Bremer, D.M. Greenberg, Biosynthesis of choline in vitro, Biochim. Biophys. Acta 37 (1960) 173—175.

[60] S.H. Zeisel, Nutritional genomics: defining the dietary requirement and effects of choline, J. Nutr. 141 (2011) 531—534.

[61] Institute of Medicine and National Academy of Sciences USA, Choline, Dietary Reference Intakes for Folate, Thiamin, Riboflavin, Niacin, Vitamin B$_{12}$, Panthothenic Acid, Biotin, and Choline, National Academy Press, Washington, DC, 1998, pp. 390—422

[62] L.M. Fischer, J.A. Scearce, M.H. Mar, J.R. Patel, R.T. Blanchard, B.A. Macintosh, M.G. Busby, S.H. Zeisel, Ad libitum choline intake in healthy individuals meets or exceeds the proposed adequate intake level, J. Nutr. 135 (2005) 826—829.

[63] E. Cho, S.H. Zeisel, P. Jacques, J. Selhub, L. Dougherty, G.A. Colditz, W.C. Willett, Dietary choline and betaine assessed by food-frequency questionnaire in relation to plasma total homocysteine concentration in the Framingham Offspring Study, Am. J. Clin. Nutr. 83 (2006) 905—911.

[64] G.M. Shaw, S.L. Carmichael, C. Laurent, S.A. Rasmussen, Maternal nutrient intakes and risk of orofacial clefts, Epidemiology 17 (2006) 285—291.

[65] G.M. Shaw, S.L. Carmichael, W. Yang, S. Selvin, D.M. Schaffer, Periconceptional dietary intake of choline and betaine and neural tube defects in offspring, Am. J. Epidemiol. 160 (2004) 102—109.

[66] L.M. Fischer, K.A. da Costa, L. Kwock, J. Galanko, S.H. Zeisel, Dietary choline requirements of women: effects of estrogen and genetic variation, Am. J. Clin. Nutr. 92 (2010) 1113—1119.

[67] L.M. Fischer, K.A. da Costa, J. Galanko, W. Sha, B. Stephenson, J. Vick, S.H. Zeisel, Choline intake and genetic polymorphisms influence choline metabolite concentrations in human breast milk and plasma, Am. J. Clin. Nutr. 92 (2010) 336—346.

[68] K.A. da Costa, O.G. Kozyreva, J. Song, J.A. Galanko, L.M. Fischer, S.H. Zeisel, Common genetic polymorphisms affect the human requirement for the nutrient choline, FASEB J. 20 (2006) 1336—1344.

[69] M.A. Caudill, Pre- and postnatal health: evidence of increased choline needs, J. Am. Diet. Assoc. 110 (2010) 1198—1206.

[70] L.M. Fischer, K.A. daCosta, L. Kwock, P.W. Stewart, T.S. Lu, S.P. Stabler, R.H. Allen, S.H. Zeisel, Sex and menopausal status influence human dietary requirements for the nutrient choline, Am. J. Clin. Nutr. 85 (2007) 1275—1285.

[71] C.S. Chen, Y.T. Kuo, H.Y. Tsai, C.W. Li, C.C. Lee, C.F. Yen, H.F. Lin, C.H. Ko, S.H. Juo, Y.C. Yeh, G.C. Liu, Brain biochemical correlates of the plasma homocysteine level: a proton magnetic resonance spectroscopy study in the elderly subjects, Am. J. Geriatr. Psychiatry 19 (2011) 618—626.

[72] J.D. Thomas, E.J. Abou, H.D. Dominguez, Prenatal choline supplementation mitigates the adverse effects of prenatal alcohol exposure on development in rats, Neurotoxicol. Teratol. 31 (2009) 303—311.

[73] J.D. Thomas, N.M. Idrus, B.R. Monk, H.D. Dominguez, Prenatal choline supplementation mitigates behavioral alterations associated with prenatal alcohol exposure in rats, Birth Defects Res. A Clin. Mol. Teratol. 88 (2010) 827—837.

[74] J.D. Thomas, T.D. Tran, Choline supplementation mitigates trace, but not delay, eyeblink conditioning deficits in rats exposed to alcohol during development, Hippocampus 22 (2011) 619—630.

[75] A.L. Nunes-Freitas, A. Ribeiro-Carvalho, C.S. Lima, A.C. Dutra-Tavares, A.C. Manhaes, P.C. Lisboa, E. Oliveira, E. Gaspar de Moura, C.C. Filgueiras, Y. Abreu-Villaca, Nicotine exposure during the third trimester equivalent of human gestation: time course of effects on the central cholinergic system of rats, Toxicol. Sci. 123 (2011) 144—154.

[76] Y. Abreu-Villaca, C.C. Filgueiras, M. Guthierrez, A.H. Medeiros, M.A. Mattos, S. Pereira Mdos, A.C. Manhaes, R.C. Kubrusly, Exposure to tobacco smoke containing either high or low levels of nicotine during adolescence: differential effects on choline uptake in the cerebral cortex and hippocampus, Nicotine Tob. Res. 12 (2010) 776—780.

[77] G. Fan, C. Feng, F. Wu, W. Ye, F. Lin, C. Wang, J. Yan, G. Zhu, Y. Xiao, Y. Bi, Methionine choline reverses lead-induced cognitive and N-methyl-D-aspartate receptor subunit 1 deficits, Toxicology 272 (2010) 23—31.

[78] H. Tsuchiya, T. Sakabe, Y. Akechi, R. Ikeda, R. Nishio, K. Terabayashi, Y. Matsumi, Y. Hoshikawa, A. Kurimasa, G. Shiota, A close association of abnormal iron metabolism with steatosis in the mice fed a choline-deficient diet, Biol. Pharm. Bull. 33 (2010) 1101–1104.

[79] N. van Wijk, C.J. Watkins, M. Bohlke, T.J. Maher, R.J. Hageman, P.J. Kamphuis, L.M. Broersen, R.J. Wurtman, Plasma choline concentration varies with different dietary levels of vitamins B_6, B_{12} and folic acid in rats maintained on choline-adequate diets, Br. J. Nutr. (2011) 1–5.

[80] M. Vahter, E. Marafante, Effects of low dietary intake of methionine, choline or proteins on the biotransformation of arsenite in the rabbit, Toxicol. Lett. 37 (1987) 41–46.

[81] G. Song, Y. Cui, Z.J. Han, H.F. Xia, X. Ma, Effects of choline on sodium arsenite-induced neural tube defects in chick embryos, Food Chem. Toxicol. (2011) (Epub ahead of print).

[82] C.N. Craciunescu, M.D. Niculescu, Z. Guo, A.R. Johnson, L. Fischer, S.H. Zeisel, Dose response effects of dermally applied diethanolamine on neurogenesis in fetal mouse hippocampus and potential exposure of humans, Toxicol. Sci. 107 (2009) 220–226.

[83] C.N. Craciunescu, R. Wu, S.H. Zeisel, Diethanolamine alters neurogenesis and induces apoptosis in fetal mouse hippocampus, FASEB J. 20 (2006) 1635–1640.

[84] M.D. Niculescu, R. Wu, Z. Guo, K.A. da Costa, S.H. Zeisel, Diethanolamine alters proliferation and choline metabolism in mouse neural precursor cells, Toxicol. Sci. 96 (2007) 321–326.

[85] D.C. Dolinoy, D. Huang, R.L. Jirtle, Maternal nutrient supplementation counteracts bisphenol A-induced DNA hypomethylation in early development, Proc. Natl. Acad. Sci. USA 104 (2007) 13056–13061.

[86] L.G. Miller, Dietary choline alteration: implications for gamma-aminobutyric acid and other neurotransmitter receptors, Biochem. Pharmacol. 40 (1990) 1179–1182.

[87] R.J. Wurtman, J.H. Growdon, Dietary enhancement of CNS neurotransmitters, Hosp. Pract. 13 (1978) 71–77.

[88] K.A. da Costa, M. Badea, L.M. Fischer, S.H. Zeisel, Elevated serum creatine phosphokinase in choline-deficient humans: mechanistic studies in C2C12 mouse myoblasts, Am. J. Clin. Nutr. 80 (2004) 163–170.

[89] K.A. da Costa, C.E. Gaffney, L.M. Fischer, S.H. Zeisel, Choline deficiency in mice and humans is associated with increased plasma homocysteine concentration after a methionine load, Am. J. Clin. Nutr. 81 (2005) 440–444.

[90] K.A. da Costa, M.D. Niculescu, C.N. Craciunescu, L.M. Fischer, S.H. Zeisel, Choline deficiency increases lymphocyte apoptosis and DNA damage in humans, Am. J. Clin. Nutr. 84 (2006) 88–94.

[91] M. Resseguie, J. Song, M.D. Niculescu, K.A. da Costa, T.A. Randall, S.H. Zeisel, Phosphatidylethanolamine N-methyltransferase (PEMT) gene expression is induced by estrogen in human and mouse primary hepatocytes, FASEB J. 21 (2007) 2622–2632.

[92] M. Kohlmeier, K.A. da Costa, L.M. Fischer, S.H. Zeisel, Genetic variation of folate-mediated one-carbon transfer pathway predicts susceptibility to choline deficiency in humans, Proc. Natl. Acad. Sci. USA 102 (2005) 16025–16030.

[93] M.C. Fisher, S.H. Zeisel, M.H. Mar, T.W. Sadler, Inhibitors of choline uptake and metabolism cause developmental abnormalities in neurulating mouse embryos, Teratology 64 (2001) 114–122.

[94] A.C. Antony, In utero physiology: role of folic acid in nutrient delivery and fetal development, Am. J. Clin. Nutr. 85 (2007) 598S–603S.

[95] M.C. Fisher, S.H. Zeisel, M.H. Mar, T.W. Sadler, Perturbations in choline metabolism cause neural tube defects in mouse embryos in vitro, FASEB J. 16 (2002) 619–621.

[96] S.L. Carmichael, W. Yang, G.M. Shaw, Periconceptional nutrient intakes and risks of neural tube defects in California, Birth Defects Res. A Clin. Mol. Teratol. 88 (2010) 670–678.

[97] S.L. Carmichael, S.A. Rasmussen, E.J. Lammer, C. Ma, G.M. Shaw, Craniosynostosis and nutrient intake during pregnancy, Birth Defects Res. A Clin. Mol. Teratol. 88 (2010) 1032–1039.

[98] J.O. Enaw, H. Zhu, W. Yang, W. Lu, G.M. Shaw, E.J. Lammer, R.H. Finnell, CHKA and PCYT1A gene polymorphisms, choline intake and spina bifida risk in a California population, BMC Med. 4 (2006) 36.

[99] M.Q. Holmes-McNary, R. Loy, M.H. Mar, C.D. Albright, S.H. Zeisel, Apoptosis is induced by choline deficiency in fetal brain and in PC12 cells, Brain Res. Dev. Brain Res. 101 (1997) 9–16.

[100] C.D. Albright, C.B. Friedrich, E.C. Brown, M.H. Mar, S.H. Zeisel, Maternal dietary choline availability alters mitosis, apoptosis and the localization of TOAD-64 protein in the developing fetal rat septum, Brain Res. Dev. Brain Res. 115 (1999) 123–129.

[101] C.N. Craciunescu, C.D. Albright, M.H. Mar, J. Song, S.H. Zeisel, Choline availability during embryonic development alters progenitor cell mitosis in developing mouse hippocampus, J. Nutr. 133 (2003) 3614–3618.

[102] C.N. Craciunescu, E.C. Brown, M.H. Mar, C.D. Albright, M.R. Nadeau, S.H. Zeisel, Folic acid deficiency during late gestation decreases progenitor cell proliferation and increases apoptosis in fetal mouse brain, J. Nutr. 134 (2004) 162–166.

[103] C.L. Yen, M.H. Mar, S.H. Zeisel, Choline deficiency-induced apoptosis in PC12 cells is associated with diminished membrane phosphatidylcholine and sphingomyelin, accumulation of ceramide and diacylglycerol, and activation of a caspase, FASEB J. 13 (1999) 135–142.

[104] C.D. Albright, A.Y. Tsai, M.H. Mar, S.H. Zeisel, Choline availability modulates the expression of TGFbeta1 and cytoskeletal proteins in the hippocampus of developing rat brain, Neurochem. Res. 23 (1998) 751–758.

[105] C.D. Albright, D.F. Siwek, C.N. Craciunescu, M.H. Mar, N.W. Kowall, C.L. Williams, S.H. Zeisel, Choline availability during embryonic development alters the localization of calretinin in developing and aging mouse hippocampus, Nutr. Neurosci. 6 (2003) 129–134.

[106] C.D. Albright, M.H. Mar, C.N. Craciunescu, J. Song, S.H. Zeisel, Maternal dietary choline availability alters the balance of netrin-1 and DCC neuronal migration proteins in fetal mouse brain hippocampus, Brain Res. Dev. Brain Res. 159 (2005) 149–154.

[107] M.G. Mehedint, C.N. Craciunescu, S.H. Zeisel, Maternal dietary choline deficiency alters angiogenesis in fetal mouse hippocampus, Proc. Natl. Acad. Sci. USA 107 (2010) 12834–12839.

[108] C.N. Craciunescu, A.R. Johnson, S.H. Zeisel, Dietary choline reverses some, but not all, effects of folate deficiency on neurogenesis and apoptosis in fetal mouse brain, J. Nutr. 140 (2010) 1162–1166.

[109] C.D. Albright, M.H. Mar, C.B. Friedrich, E.C. Brown, S.H. Zeisel, Maternal choline availability alters the localization of p15Ink4B and p27Kip1 cyclin-dependent kinase inhibitors in the developing fetal rat brain hippocampus, Dev. Neurosci. 23 (2001) 100–106.

[110] M.D. Niculescu, C.N. Craciunescu, S.H. Zeisel, Dietary choline deficiency alters global and gene-specific DNA methylation in the developing hippocampus of mouse fetal brains, FASEB J. 20 (2006) 43–49.

[111] M.D. Niculescu, Y. Yamamuro, S.H. Zeisel, Choline availability modulates human neuroblastoma cell proliferation and alters the methylation of the promoter region of the cyclin-dependent kinase inhibitor 3 gene, J. Neurochem. 89 (2004) 1252–1259.

[112] M.J. Ravitz, C.E. Wenner, Cyclin-dependent kinase regulation during G1 phase and cell cycle regulation by TGF-beta, Adv. Cancer Res. 71 (1997) 165–207.

[113] M.D. Niculescu, C.N. Craciunescu, S.H. Zeisel, Gene expression profiling of choline-deprived neural precursor cells isolated from mouse brain, Brain Res. Mol. Brain Res. 134 (2005) 309–322.

[114] S. Gravina, J. Vijg, Epigenetic factors in aging and longevity, Pflugers Arch. 459 (2010) 247–258.

[115] M.K. Skinner, Role of epigenetics in developmental biology and transgenerational inheritance, Birth Defects Res. C Embryo Today 93 (2011) 51–55.

[116] F. Mohr, K. Dohner, C. Buske, V.P. Rawat, TET genes: new players in DNA demethylation and important determinants for stemness, Exp. Hematol. 39 (2011) 272–281.

[117] N.V. Cucu, DNA methylation, in: M.D. Niculescu, P. Haggarty (Eds), Nutrition in Epigenetics, Wiley, Ames, IA, 2011, pp. 15–46.

[118] C. Bonifer, P.N. Cockerill, Chromatin mechanisms regulating gene expression in health and disease, Adv. Exp. Med. Biol. 711 (2011) 12–25.

[119] M.G. Mehedint, M.D. Niculescu, C.N. Craciunescu, S.H. Zeisel, Choline deficiency alters global histone methylation and epigenetic marking at the Re1 site of the calbindin 1 gene, FASEB J. 24 (2010) 184–195.

[120] A.C. Ferguson-Smith, Genomic imprinting: the emergence of an epigenetic paradigm, Nat. Rev. Genet. 12 (2011) 565–575.

[121] N.J. Kaminen-Ahola, A.I. Ahola, E. Whitelaw, Epigenetic inheritance: Both mitotic and meiotic, in: M.D. Niculescu, P. Haggarty (Eds), Nutrition in Epigenetics, Wiley, Ames, IA, 2011, pp. 87–103.

[122] M. Tahiliani, K.P. Koh, Y. Shen, W.A. Pastor, H. Bandukwala, Y. Brudno, S. Agarwal, L.M. Iyer, D.R. Liu, L. Aravind, A. Rao, Conversion of 5-methylcytosine to 5-hydroxymethylcytosine in mammalian DNA by MLL partner TET1, Science 324 (2009) 930–935.

[123] S.B. Hake, Chromatin modifications, in: M.D. Niculescu, P. Haggarty (Eds), Nutrition in Epigenetics, Wiley, Ames, IA, 2011, pp. 47–71.

[124] F. Sato, S. Tsuchiya, S.J. Meltzer, K. Shimizu, MicroRNAs and epigenetics, FEBS J. 278 (2011) 1598–1609.

[125] J. Cerny, P.J. Quesenberry, Chromatin remodeling and stem cell theory of relativity, J. Cell Physiol. 201 (2004) 1–16.

[126] J.F. Costello, DNA methylation in brain development and gliomagenesis, Front. Biosci. 8 (2003) s175–s184.

[127] M.P. Mattson, Methylation and acetylation in nervous system development and neurodegenerative disorders, Ageing Res. Rev. 2 (2003) 329–342.

[128] K. Goto, M. Numata, J.I. Komura, T. Ono, T.H. Bestor, H. Kondo, Expression of DNA methyltransferase gene in mature and immature neurons as well as proliferating cells in mice, Differentiation 56 (1994) 39–44.

[129] G. Fan, C. Beard, R.Z. Chen, G. Csankovszki, Y. Sun, M. Siniaia, D. Biniszkiewicz, B. Bates, P.P. Lee, R. Kuhn, A. Trumpp, C. Poon, C.B. Wilson, R. Jaenisch, DNA hypomethylation perturbs the function and survival of CNS neurons in postnatal animals, J. Neurosci. 21 (2001) 788–797.

[130] T. Takizawa, K. Nakashima, M. Namihira, W. Ochiai, A. Uemura, M. Yanagisawa, N. Fujita, M. Nakao, T. Taga, DNA methylation is a critical cell-intrinsic determinant of astrocyte differentiation in the fetal brain, Dev. Cell 1 (2001) 749–758.

[131] J.A. McKay, J.C. Mathers, Diet induced epigenetic changes and their implications for health, Acta Physiol. (Oxford) 202 (2011) 103–118.

[132] S.H. Zeisel, Choline: clinical nutrigenetic/nutrigenomic approaches for identification of functions and dietary requirements, World Rev. Nutr. Diet. 101 (2010) 73–83.

[133] X. Zhu, M.H. Mar, J. Song, S.H. Zeisel, Deletion of the Pemt gene increases progenitor cell mitosis, DNA and protein methylation and decreases calretinin expression in embryonic day 17 mouse hippocampus, Brain Res. Dev. Brain Res. 149 (2004) 121–129.

[134] K. Fukai, O. Yokosuka, F. Imazeki, M. Tada, R. Mikata, M. Miyazaki, T. Ochiai, H. Saisho, Methylation status of p14ARF, p15INK4b, and p16INK4a genes in human hepatocellular carcinoma, Liver Int. 25 (2005) 1209–1216.

[135] T. Holler, J.M. Cermak, J.K. Blusztajn, Dietary choline supplementation in pregnant rats increases hippocampal phospholipase D activity of the offspring, FASEB J. 10 (1996) 1653–1659.

[136] J.M. Cermak, T. Holler, D.A. Jackson, J.K. Blusztajn, Prenatal availability of choline modifies development of the hippocampal cholinergic system, FASEB J. 12 (1998) 349–357.

[137] J.M. Cermak, J.K. Blusztajn, W.H. Meck, C.L. Williams, C.M. Fitzgerald, D.L. Rosene, R. Loy, Prenatal availability of choline alters the development of acetylcholinesterase in the rat hippocampus, Dev. Neurosci. 21 (1999) 94–104.

[138] T.J. Mellott, N.W. Kowall, I. Lopez-Coviella, J.K. Blusztajn, Prenatal choline deficiency increases choline transporter expression in the septum and hippocampus during postnatal development and in adulthood in rats, Brain Res. 1151 (2007) 1–11.

[139] T.J. Mellott, M.T. Follettie, V. Diesl, A.A. Hill, I. Lopez-Coviella, J.K. Blusztajn, Prenatal choline availability modulates hippocampal and cerebral cortical gene expression, FASEB J. 21 (2007) 1311–1323.

[140] T.J. Mellott, C.L. Williams, W.H. Meck, J.K. Blusztajn, Prenatal choline supplementation advances hippocampal development and enhances MAPK and CREB activation, FASEB J. 18 (2004) 545–547.

[141] N.J. Sandstrom, R. Loy, C.L. Williams, Prenatal choline supplementation increases NGF levels in the hippocampus and frontal cortex of young and adult rats, Brain Res. 947 (2002) 9–16.

[142] H. Frielingsdorf, D.R. Simpson, L.J. Thal, D.P. Pizzo, Nerve growth factor promotes survival of new neurons in the adult hippocampus, Neurobiol. Dis. 26 (2007) 47–55.

[143] C. McKeon-O'Malley, D. Siwek, J.A. Lamoureux, C.L. Williams, N.W. Kowall, Prenatal choline deficiency decreases the cross-sectional area of cholinergic neurons in the medial septal nucleus, Brain Res. 977 (2003) 278–283.

[144] W.H. Meck, C.L. Williams, Metabolic imprinting of choline by its availability during gestation: implications for memory and attentional processing across the lifespan, Neurosci. Biobehav. Rev. 27 (2003) 385–399.

[145] S.X. Guo-Ross, S. Clark, D.A. Montoya, K.H. Jones, J. Obernier, A.K. Shetty, A.M. White, J.K. Blusztajn, W.A. Wilson, H.S. Swartzwelder, Prenatal choline supplementation protects against postnatal neurotoxicity, J. Neurosci. 22 (2002) RC195.

[146] S.X. Guo-Ross, K.H. Jones, A.K. Shetty, W.A. Wilson, H.S. Swartzwelder, Prenatal dietary choline availability alters postnatal neurotoxic vulnerability in the adult rat, Neurosci. Lett. 341 (2003) 161–163.

[147] G.L. Holmes, Y. Yang, Z. Liu, J.M. Cermak, M.R. Sarkisian, C.E. Stafstrom, J.C. Neill, J.K. Blusztajn, Seizure-induced memory impairment is reduced by choline supplementation before or after status epilepticus, Epilepsy Res. 48 (2002) 3–13.

[148] S.J. Wong-Goodrich, C.M. Tognoni, T.J. Mellott, M.J. Glenn, J.K. Blusztajn, C.L. Williams, Prenatal choline deficiency does not enhance hippocampal vulnerability after kainic

acid-induced seizures in adulthood, Brain Res. 1413 (2011) 84−97.

[149] W.H. Meck, C.L. Williams, Perinatal choline supplementation increases the threshold for chunking in spatial memory, Neuroreport 8 (1997) 3053−3059.

[150] W.H. Meck, C.L. Williams, Simultaneous temporal processing is sensitive to prenatal choline availability in mature and aged rats, Neuroreport 8 (1997) 3045−3051.

[151] W.H. Meck, C.L. Williams, Characterization of the facilitative effects of perinatal choline supplementation on timing and temporal memory, Neuroreport 8 (1997) 2831−2835.

[152] W.H. Meck, C.L. Williams, Choline supplementation during prenatal development reduces proactive interference in spatial memory, Brain Res. Dev. Brain Res. 118 (1999) 51−59.

[153] C.L. Williams, W.H. Meck, D.D. Heyer, R. Loy, Hypertrophy of basal forebrain neurons and enhanced visuospatial memory in perinatally choline-supplemented rats, Brain Res. 794 (1998) 225−238.

[154] J.P. Jones, W. Meck, C.L. Williams, W.A. Wilson, H.S. Swartzwelder, Choline availability to the developing rat fetus alters adult hippocampal long-term potentiation, Brain Res Dev Brain Res. 118 (1999) 159−167.

[155] D.A. Montoya, A.M. White, C.L. Williams, J.K. Blusztajn, W.H. Meck, H.S. Swartzwelder, Prenatal choline exposure alters hippocampal responsiveness to cholinergic stimulation in adulthood, Brain Res. Dev. Brain Res. 123 (2000) 25−32.

[156] G. Pyapali, D. Turner, C. Williams, W. Meck, H.S. Swartzwelder, Prenatal choline supplementation decreases the threshold for induction of long-term potentiation in young adult rats, J. Neurophysiol. 79 (1998) 1790−1796.

[157] C.C. Cloak, D. Alicata, L. Chang, B. Andrews-Shigaki, T. Ernst, Age and sex effects levels of choline compounds in the anterior cingulate cortex of adolescent methamphetamine users, Drug Alcohol Depend. 119 (2011) 207−215.

[158] M. Igarashi, K. Ma, F. Gao, H.W. Kim, S.I. Rapoport, J.S. Rao, Disturbed choline plasmalogen and phospholipid fatty acid concentrations in Alzheimer's disease prefrontal cortex, J. Alzheimer's Dis. 24 (2011) 507−517.

[159] S.H. Zeisel, Is maternal diet supplementation beneficial? Optimal development of infant depends on mother's diet, Am. J. Clin. Nutr. 89 (2009) 685S−687S.

[160] S.H. Zeisel, Importance of methyl donors during reproduction, Am. J. Clin. Nutr. 89 (2009) 673S−677S.

[161] S.H. Zeisel, H.C. Freake, D.E. Bauman, D.M. Bier, D.G. Burrin, J.B. German, S. Klein, G.S. Marquis, J.A. Milner, G.H. Pelto, K.M. Rasmussen, The nutritional phenotype in the age of metabolomics, J. Nutr. 135 (2005) 1613−1616.

CHAPTER

16

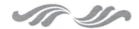

Nutritional Recommendations for Athletes

Sara C. Campbell

Rutgers, The State University of New Jersey,
New Brunswick, New Jersey

I INTRODUCTION

Successful performance in sport is a result of many different factors. Arguably one of the most important factors is genetic predisposition; however, meeting optimal energy requirements is also critical for performance. Athletes who make poor food choices may prevent themselves from achieving their optimal potential. There is a strong evidence base that has established a role for optimal dietary strategies to enhance performance [1]. This begins with the recognition that when performing regular exercise, hard physical labor, or exercise training, utilization of carbohydrate (CHO), fat, and protein to make energy increases. As a result, the requirements of macro- and micronutrients increase.

The relationship between nutrition and physical performance has fascinated people for a long time. It has become clear that different types of exercise and different sports have different energy and nutrient requirements, and therefore food intake must be adjusted accordingly. It has been clearly shown that certain nutritional strategies can enhance performance, improve recovery, and result in more profound training adaptations. However, the diets of athletes are often reported as nutritionally inadequate [2]. The knowledge an athlete possess on proper nutrition, which is typically greater than that of the general public, is still lacking and mostly based on coach-driven advice and may be influenced by financial constraints [3]. The role of the sports nutritionist becomes increasingly critical to correct dietary inadequacies and promote health by creating a positive impact on the optimal performance of the athlete [4]. Nutrition strategies should be aimed at modulating training-induced adaptations, most important in muscle. This chapter reviews the nutritional demands of exercise in relation to the physiological demands and examines strategies to fuel exercise performance.

II ENERGY REQUIREMENTS FOR ATHLETES

Adequate energy requirement is a delicate balance between the amount of food intake required to maintain total daily energy expenditure (TDEE) and body weight [5]. TDEE is the sum of resting metabolic rate (RMR; 60–75%), diet-induced thermogenesis (DIT; 10%), and thermic effect of exercise (TEE; 15–30%). During exercise, the energy expenditure increases several-fold mostly as a result of skeletal muscle contraction. Therefore, depending on how much exercise an individual performs, TEE is by far the most variable component of TDEE. Thermic effect of exercise includes all energy expended above the RMR and DIT. In addition, it is influenced by lifestyle activities, the nature of exercise performed, gender, and prior nutritional status. TEE can contribute from virtually nothing to more than 80% of energy expenditure. In highly trained, very active individuals, the TEE can amount to up to 8000 kcal per day. In sedentary people, the thermic effect of exercise may be as low as 100 kcal per day. Energy expenditure during physical activity ranges from 5 kcal/min for very light activities to up to 25 kcal/min for very high-intensity exercise (Table 16.1).

Because of the variable nature of TEE, it is imperative that athletes understand how much energy they use to perform their sport, which will be indicative of energy intake required to maintain this performance. Energy restriction in athletes has deleterious side effects because in most situations, substrate (carbohydrates, fats, and proteins) availability can become critical for

Nutrition in the Prevention and Treatment of Disease, Third Edition.
DOI: http://dx.doi.org/10.1016/B978-0-12-391884-0.00016-0

TABLE 16.1   Rough Estimation of Energy Expenditure in a Variety of Sports[a]

Activity level	kJ/min	kcal/min	Examples
Resting	4	1	Sleeping, watching TV
Very light activities	12–20	3–5	Sitting and standing activities, driving, cooking, card playing, desk work, typing
Light activities	20–28	5–7	Walking (slowly), baseball, bowling, horseback riding, cycling (very slowly), gymnastics, golf
Moderate activities	28–36	7–9	Jogging, cycling (at a moderate pace), basketball, badminton, soccer, tennis, volleyball, brisk walking, swimming (at an easy pace)
Strenuous activities	36–52	9–13	Running (10–13 km/h), cross-country skiing, boxing, cycling (30–35 km/h), swimming, judo
Very strenuous activities	>52	>13	Running (>14 km/h), cycling (>35 km/h)

[a]*Energy expenditure depends on body mass, the intensity, and the duration of rest periods.*
Source: *McArdle, W. D., Katch, F. I., and Katch, V. L. (2006). Exercise Physiology: Energy, Nutrition and Human Performance, 5th ed. Lippincott, Williams & Wilkins, Philadelphia.*

the continuation of exercise. These substrates and their availability for energy production during exercise must be obtained through nutrition. In endurance athletes, for example, carbohydrate depletion is one of the most common causes of fatigue. Therefore, adequate carbohydrate intake is essential to prevent early fatigue as a result of carbohydrate depletion.

A Energy Balance

Energy balance represents the difference between energy intake and energy expenditure. When the energy intake exceeds the energy expenditure, there is a positive energy balance, which results in weight gain. When the energy intake is below the energy expenditure, there is a negative energy balance and weight loss results. Over the long term, energy balance is maintained in weight-stable individuals, even though on a day-to-day basis this balance may sometimes be positive and sometimes negative. Although life is not always that simple, basic manipulation of the energy balance equation will yield weight loss or gain. For example, if someone wishes to lose weight, it is important to increase the energy expenditure relative to the energy intake or decrease energy intake below daily energy expenditure. The opposite would be true if an individual is trying to achieve weight gain.

B Energy Balance in Different Activities

Some physical activities require higher energy outputs than others, as shown in Table 16.1. Tennis, for example, has relatively low energy expenditure if played recreationally. However, during a match the exercise can be intense, and energy expenditure during that short burst of exercise can be very high. However,

because this is typically followed by a longer period of relatively low intensity (walking) or even standing, the average energy expenditure for this activity is relatively low. On the other hand, in continuous sports such as cycling and running, in which there is usually no recovery during the activity, energy expenditures can be relatively high.

Physically active individuals need to be aware of the energy input necessary to maintain weight and performance. The simplest way to do this is to calculate resting daily energy expenditure (RDEE): RDEE (kcal) = 370 + 21.6 (fat-free mass, kg). In order to calculate fat-free mass (FFM), two simple steps must be followed. First, determine your weight in kilograms. This can be done by taking your body weight in pounds and dividing it by 2.2; for example, if you weigh 220 pounds, your weight in kilograms is 220/2.2 = 100 kg. Second, calculate FFM in kilograms. Take your weight in kilograms and multiply it by [1 − your body fat percentage]. For example, if you weigh 100 kg and your body fat percentage is 12%, then your FFM = 100 kg × (1 − 0.12) = 88 kg. These simple calculations allow individuals to understand exactly what their energy requirements are so that they can match energy intake with expenditure. As stated previously, inadequate energy intake relative to energy expenditure can compromise performance and will negate the benefits of training. This is because limiting nutrient intake can result in loss of lean tissue mass that results in the loss of strength and endurance as well as compromising the immune, endocrine, and musculoskeletal systems.

Energy expenditure varies by type, frequency, intensity, and duration of the activity. The energy systems (Table 16.2) used during exercise will dictate expenditure. These energy systems are the immediate energy system (i.e., the ATP-PC system, phosphagen system, and power system), short-term energy system (i.e.,

TABLE 16.2 Energy Systems and Energy Use

Energy system	Rate[a]	Capacity[b]
ATP-creatine phosphate	1.6–6.0	24
Anaerobic glycolysis	1.0–1.5	240
Aerobic		
Carbohydrate	0.5	3000
Fat	0.24	Unlimited

[a] *μmol/g muscle/sec (power).*
[b] *μmol/g muscle (energy supply).*

TABLE 16.3 Sources of Energy for Exercise

Source	Storage form	Total body calories (kcal)	Distance covered
ATP	Tissues	1	17.5 yards
Creatine phosphate	Tissues	4	70 yards
Carbohydrate	Serum glucose	20	350 yards
	Liver glycogen	400	4 miles
	Muscle glycogen	1500	15 miles
Fat	Serum fatty acids	7	123 yards
	Serum triglyceride	75	0.75 mile
	Muscle triglyceride	2500	25 miles
	Adipose tissue	80,000	800 miles
Protein	Muscle	30,000	300 miles

anaerobic energy system, glycolytic system, and lactic acid system), and long-term energy system (i.e., aerobic energy system). The immediate energy system uses adenosine triphosphate (ATP) and phosphocreatine (PCr) to supply muscles with energy to do work, and exercises of this nature typically last only approximately 6–10 seconds so they are short, powerful, and high-intensity activities. Examples include the golf swing, tennis serve, and 40-yard dash. The short-term energy system is the anaerobic system, meaning that it does not require oxygen to produce energy. This system's primary substrate is carbohydrate in the forms of glycogen and glucose, which is broken down via glycolysis. A result of no oxygen being used for ATP production in this system is the overaccumulation of hydrogen ions in the muscle, thus lowering the pH (more acidic environment) and leading to a cessation in exercise due to the disruption of the glycolytic enzymes. This system can provide energy for approximately 60 seconds to 3 minutes, and some examples of exercises include a 440-m run or 100-m swim. Finally, the long-term energy system will provide fuel for exercise lasting longer than 3 minutes. This fuel is provided by muscle and liver glycogen; intramuscular, blood, and adipose tissue triglycerides; and a small amount of amino acids. This system requires oxygen for ATP production, and as it becomes available, oxidative pathways are used, which can produce large amounts of ATP for exercise events such as marathons, endurance cycling, and swimming. Because each energy system is supplied by various macronutrients, it is imperative that athletes eat a well-balanced diet that meets the recommendations. A summary of the macronutrients that are used to make ATP for muscular contraction is provided in Table 16.3.

1 What is the Role of Body Composition?

Body weight and body composition are two factors that govern an athlete's decisions in food choices. Body weight may be an important influence on speed, endurance, and power, whereas body composition may influence strength, agility, and appearance. For example, a lean (more muscle than fat) appearance may be important for speed. In many sports in which body composition or body weight is believed to be important (gymnastics, dancing, body building, and weight category sports such as wrestling, judo, and boxing), athletes often try to maintain a negative energy balance in order to lose weight [6]. It is known that the energy intakes in these sports can be very low [7,8] and that this can be a detriment to performance.

At the other extreme are endurance or ultraendurance sports, such as marathons, triathlons, and cross-country skiing, in which extremely high energy expenditures are known to occur that must be matched by appropriate calorie intake. Optimum performance in these sports depends on the individual maintaining energy balance on a day-to-day basis.

Females generally have lower energy intakes than males and often have lower intakes than would be necessary for being physically active [8,9]. For females, energy intake ranged from 5.1 MJ (1600 kcal) to 10.2 MJ (3200 kcal). For males, energy intake ranged from 12.1 MJ (2900 kcal) to 24.7 MJ (10,500 kcal). These differences in energy intake may be related to body size and weight, body composition, and the training volume. Team sport athletes have a moderate energy intake, whereas some of the endurance sports have been characterized by very high energy intakes. In fact, energy intakes in excess of 12.6 MJ (3000 kcal) for females and 16.7 MJ (4000 kcal) for males were reported only in endurance sports.

In summary, an individualize assessment of the athlete's body composition is warranted to determine an optimal competitive body weight and relative fatness, with the goal to optimize the athlete's health and performance. In addition, particular attention should be paid to female athletes, who are frequently known to underconsume calories, and sports in which weight is of particular importance for competition.

2 How Do Athletes Assess Energy Cost of Activity?

As mentioned previously, one can use the RDEE equation to calculate resting energy requirements; however, there is also a need to understand how much energy is being used during exercise. There are several ways to accomplish this, including both direct and indirect means of measurement. To directly measure energy cost, one would use a human calorimeter. Although use of a human calorimeter is the most accurate way to assess energy cost, few facilities have one of these and it is not the most convenient or practical means of measurement. As such, indirect calorimetry has become the standard of measurement for this purpose. These measurements can be obtained by placing the subject on a metabolic cart, which can measure the amount of oxygen consumed and carbon dioxide produced. These values can then be used to calculate the respiratory quotient (RQ). Each macronutrient has its own RQ value. It is important to note that the RQ for protein is approximated at 0.80; however, an equation for protein is typically more convoluted and mostly unavailable compared to those for fats and carbohydrates. This is because proteins are not simply oxidized to carbon dioxide and water during energy metabolism. During metabolism, the protein is deaminated and the nitrogen and sulfur are excreted. The resulting keto fragments are then oxidized. All of this complicates things; however, the actual contribution of protein to energy metabolism is very low. For example, see the following equations:

$$\text{Respiratory quotient (RQ)} = \frac{CO_2 \text{ produced}}{CO_2 \text{ consumed}}$$

Examples of macronutrient RQ calculations
  CHO RQ calculation

$C_6H_{12}O_6 + 6O_2 = 6CO_2 + 6H_2O + 38 \text{ ATP (CHO)}$
$RQ = 6CO_2/6O_2 = 1.0 = 5.05 \text{ kcal/lO}_2$

  Fat RQ calculation

$C_{16}H_{32}O_2 + 23O_2 = 16CO_2 + 16H_2O + 129 \text{ ATP (fat)}$
$RQ = 16CO_2/23O_2 = 0.7 = 4.68 \text{ kcal/lO}_2$

Additional indirect means of measurement include doubly labeled water (deuterium), heart rate monitors,

accelerometers, or activity tracking by keeping daily activity logs. During activity tracking, each activity is given a metabolic equivalent (MET) that corresponds to how many times resting level the activity corresponds to. For example, an activity that is 6 METs would be six times resting metabolism. A full list of activities and their MET values are found in the "Compendium of Physical Activities" [10].

III MACRONUTRIENT RECOMMENDATIONS FOR ATHLETES

The previous sections provided a summary emphasizing the importance of proper nutrition with the understanding that this nutrition is what ultimately provides one with the substrate necessary to make ATP for muscular contraction (i.e., work). The remaining sections of this chapter summarize the pertinent literature related to appropriate recommendations for macro- and micronutrient intake.

A Carbohydrate

Carbohydrate fuel plays a major role in the performance of many types of exercise and sport. The depletion of body carbohydrate stores is a cause of fatigue or performance impairments during exercise, particularly during prolonged (>90 minutes) sessions of submaximal or intermittent high-intensity activity (Figure 16.1). Unfortunately, total body carbohydrate stores are limited and are often substantially less than the fuel requirements of the training and

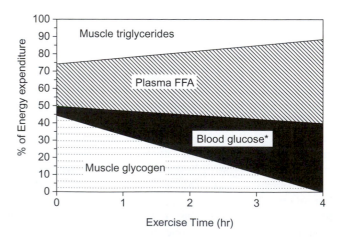

FIGURE 16.1 Percentage of energy derived from the four major substrates during prolonged exercise at 65–75% VO$_{2max}$. The asterisk designates the importance of blood glucose contributing as a source of carbohydrate energy for muscle as exercise is prolonged. Source: *Reproduced with permission from Coyle, E. F. (1995). Substrate utilization during exercise in active people. Am. J. Clin. Nutr. 61(Suppl.), S968–S979.*

competition sessions undertaken by athletes. Maximizing glycogen stores in both liver and muscle prior to the exercise bout is essential for optimal performance. Studies have shown that after exercise, muscle glycogen stores can be returned to normal resting levels (350–500 mmol/kg dry weight muscle) with 24–36 hours of rest and an adequate carbohydrate intake (6–10 g/kg body weight per day) [1,11,12]. Therefore, strategies for athletes include consuming carbohydrate before, during, and in the recovery period between prolonged exercise bouts.

1 Pre-Exercise Carbohydrate Intake

Feeding prior to exercise should take into account the timing of the meal prior to exercise, the intensity of the exercise that will be performed, and the type of carbohydrate ingested—that is, the glycemic index of the food and whether it is a solid or liquid. Glycemic index is assessed by how rapidly blood glucose levels rise after a fixed amount of ingested CHO. The glycemic index of some foods can be found in Table 16.4.

Studies examining pre-exercise feedings have focused on various times prior to the bout and types of CHO given. Early research [13] examined feeding glucola (glucose solution), milk, or water 30 minutes prior to exercise at 80% maximal oxygen uptake (VO$_2$ max). Results of this study showed that glucola participants could not exercise for as long because of the stimulated insulin response to the skeletal muscle glucose uptake. This early study raised some issues about potentially restricting CHO consumption prior to competition so that exercise hypoglycemia could be avoided. Later findings, however, do not fully support this early study. Although research has consistently found clear metabolic differences in response to the timing of pre-exercise carbohydrate ingestion within the hour before exercise, the performance effects have been somewhat equivocal. With the exception of the Foster study [13], research has either found no performance effects [14–21] or a performance improvement [22–24]. Based on current research, it appears that there is little evidence to suggest benefits from avoiding carbohydrate intake in the hour before exercise. If one is concerned that he or she might be susceptible to hypoglycemia during exercise, carbohydrate

can be ingested just prior to exercise (in the last 5 minutes), or foods that have a low glycemic index can be consumed. This can be done to minimize the risks of hypoglycemia because as exercise begins and the glucose transporter-4 (GLUT-4) is stimulated to translocate to the cell membrane, it will be responsible for bringing in glucose to the cell for energy metabolism. To support this idea, Thomas et al. [25] fed participants glucose, potato, lentils, or water 60 minutes prior to exercise at 75% VO$_2$ max. Results showed that blood glucose and insulin response was higher in the glucose and potato groups compared to the lentil group. Finally, a large body of work has shown that the intake of a substantial amount of carbohydrate (~200–300 g) 3 or 4 hours before exercise enhances various measures of exercise performance compared to performance undertaken after an overnight fast [26–28].

The form of carbohydrates ingested—solid versus liquid—before exercise has also been examined for its potential effects on metabolism and performance. It is known and accepted that ingestion of solid foods significantly slows gastric emptying, digestion, and absorption rates compared with liquid foods [29]. This will have an impact on blood glucose concentration, and because this can be a concern for athletes, is has been suggested that consuming solid food may provide a slower release of glucose to the blood for maintenance of levels during exercise [30]. Interestingly, data from studies comparing ingestion of solid versus liquid carbohydrate [31] and solid versus gel carbohydrate [32] found no significant differences in blood glucose concentrations between groups. Furthermore, additional research has found no differences in carbohydrate oxidation rates between solid versus liquid [33] or liquid versus gel [34] carbohydrate consumed during exercise. Performance studies have found no significant differences following pre-exercise ingestion of solid versus liquid [32] or solid versus gel [31,32] carbohydrates. It appears that the form of carbohydrate consumed does not play a significant role in performance or metabolism, and it is therefore suggested that whatever the athlete's preference is to consume can be supported.

Finally, the amount of carbohydrate consumed prior to exercise does not appear to play a major role in performance or changes in blood glucose concentrations. Ultimately, the concerns that should be addressed by athletes prior to competition should be: (1) to ensure that optimal levels of liver and muscle glycogen are attained to sustain performance, and (2) if the individual is concerned that he or she might be a hypoglycemic responder during exercise, to consume low glycemic index foods prior to exercise, consume carbohydrate right before exercise, or avoid carbohydrate completely for at least 60 minutes prior to exercise bouts.

TABLE 16.4 Glycemic Index (GI) of Select Foods

High GI (>85)	Medium GI (60–85)	Low GI (<60)
Glucose	Banana	Fructose
Sucrose	Oatmeal	Apple
Bread	Pasta	Lentils
Potatoes	Rice	Milk
Sports drinks	Corn	Yogurt

2 Carbohydrate Feedings during Exercise and Post-Exercise

Numerous studies have documented that consumption of carbohydrates (glucose or glucose polymers) during exercise improves endurance performance in events lasting 60 minutes or longer [31,35,36]. Feeding for bouts lasting less than 60 minutes has produced mixed results [37,38] unless the intensity is high, in which case it appears to be beneficial [39]. The mechanisms appear to be the maintenance of blood glucose levels and the additional carbohydrate to maintain muscular contraction. In the literature, most of the results that support these notions have been obtained using tracer techniques and naturally enriched ^{13}C glucose. What does this body of literature tell us? It suggests that carbohydrate is being oxidized at a rate of approximately $1-1.1$ g/min. This will be influenced by several factors, including: (1) The rate of gastric emptying, which is known to decrease as the concentration of carbohydrate increases and the rate of administration increases. (2) The decreases in absorption that are seen with exogenous levels of carbohydrate administration of $1.2-1.7$ g/min; and (3) The liver, which can potentially release up to 1 g/min of exogenous carbohydrate to the bloodstream.

Carbohydrate restoration post-exercise is imperative for athletes, especially for those who train multiple times in one day or on successive days so that performance during these sessions can be at the highest level. Optimizing glycogenesis, the making of glycogen for storage, can be achieved by consuming $6-10$ g/kg per body weight per day [40]. This is equivalent to roughly 65% carbohydrate diet when a 70-kg person is consuming 3000 calories (Figure 16.2). Glycogen synthase (GS-1) is the enzyme responsible for reforming glycogen, and it is aided by GLUT-4 (glucose transporter mentioned

previously). When muscle is inactive, GLUT-4 remains in the center of the muscle cell; however, when we are exercising, it is translocated to the cell membrane, allowing glucose to enter the cell, and this starts glycogenesis. Upon cessation of exercise, GLUT-4 does not immediately return to the center of the cell. It is by this premise that high glycemic index carbohydrate foods and drinks may be more favorable for glycogen storage than some low glycemic index food choices [40] because glycogen storage may occur at a slightly faster rate during the first few hours after exercise [12]. Again, this is especially true for athletes who have limited time between workouts. For athletes who have extended time periods of inactivity, it is not as critical to consume carbohydrate immediately; however, these athletes still need to meet the goals for total carbohydrate intake throughout the day.

In summary, the recommendations for carbohydrates for after exercise are:

1. Feed approximately $100-150$ g of carbohydrate within the first hour post-exercise.
2. Over a 24-hour period, feed $6-8$ g/kg/body weight for females and $8-10$ g/kg/body weight for males.
3. High glycemic index foods provide the best glycogen replacement to increase the insulin response and glucose transport into the cell for glycogenesis.
4. Beverages containing $70-90$ g carbohydrate ($4-6$% CHO) can be used immediately post-exercise and consumed at a rate of 1.2 g CHO/kg/hr.

3 Carbohydrate Loading (Supercompensation)

Carbohydrate loading is a special practice that aims to maximize or "supercompensate" muscle glycogen stores up to twice the normal resting level (e.g., $\sim 500-900$ mmol/kg dry weight). The first protocol was devised in the late 1960s by Scandinavian exercise

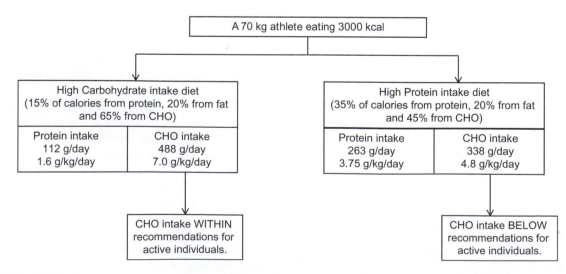

FIGURE 16.2 Carbohydrate consumption and meeting daily needs.

physiologists who found, using the muscle biopsy technique, that the size of pre-exercise muscle glycogen stores affected submaximal exercise capacity [41–43]. Several days of a low-carbohydrate diet resulted in depleted muscle glycogen stores and reduced endurance capacity compared with a mixed diet. However, high carbohydrate intake for several days caused a "supercompensation" of muscle glycogen stores and prolonged the cycling time to exhaustion. These pioneering studies produced the "classical" 7-day model of carbohydrate loading. This model consists of a 3- or 4-day "depletion" phase of hard training and low carbohydrate intake, followed by a 3- or 4-day "loading" phase of high carbohydrate intake and exercise taper (i.e., decreased amounts of training) [44]. Early field studies of prolonged running events showed that carbohydrate loading enhanced performance not by allowing the athlete to run faster but, rather, by prolonging the time that the athlete could maintain the race pace.

Further studies undertaken on trained subjects have produced a "modified" carbohydrate loading strategy [45]. The muscle of well-trained athletes has been found to be able to supercompensate its glycogen stores without a prior depletion or "glycogen stripping" phase. For well-trained athletes at least, carbohydrate loading may be seen as an extension of "fuelling up"—involving rest/taper and high carbohydrate intake over 3 or 4 days. The modified carbohydrate loading protocol offers a more practical strategy for competition preparation by avoiding the fatigue and complexity of the extreme diet and training protocols associated with the previous depletion phase. Typically, carbohydrate loading postpones fatigue and extends the duration of steady-state exercise by approximately 20% and improves performance over a set distance or workload by 2 or 3% [46–48].

B Fat

Fat represents the primary substrate for aerobic exercise; however; athletes typically avoid fat as a part of their diet. As mentioned previously, this is especially true for athletes for whom body weight and/or composition is an important part of the sport. It would be remiss not to discuss, even briefly, fat and its importance in energy metabolism during exercise because it is the primary substrate used at rest and during low- and moderate-intensity exercise (Figure 16.3). In addition, exercise training substantially enhances fat oxidation and utilization (Figure 16.4) by increasing enzyme concentration in the major metabolic pathways associated with fat oxidation; muscles also become more densely populated with capillaries to facilitate greater blood flow and oxygen extraction, and mitochondrial volume is increased (major site for fat oxidative pathways).

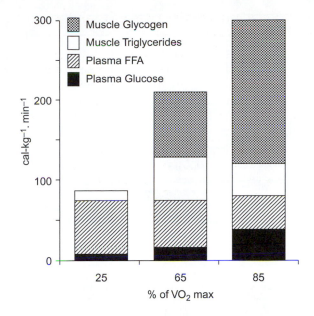

FIGURE 16.3 Contribution of the four major substrates during low (25%), moderate (65%), and high (85%) intensity exercise. During low and moderate intensity, IMTG and plasma free fatty acids provide the substrate for ATP production, whereas at high intensity muscle glycogen is the major contributor. *Source: Reproduced with permission from Romijn, J. A., Coyle, E. F., Sidossis, L. S., Gastaldelli, A., Horowitz, J. F., Endert, E., and Wolf, R. R. (1993). Regulation of endogenous fat and carbohydrate metabolism in relation to exercise intensity and duration. Am. J. Physiol.* **265**, *E380–E391.*

Research in this area has focused on gender differences, which seem to support women having a greater reliance on fat oxidation compared to men. Several studies specifically showed that women increased the amount of intramuscular triglycerides (IMTG) stored in the muscle and had a significant decrease in IMTG post-exercise compared to men [33,34,49]. These men and women were matched for VO_2 ml/kg FFM/min and training volume, and the women were tested during the same menstrual phase to control for the influence of sex hormones. These studies suggest that athletes, especially female athletes, should consume enough fat in the diet to adequately replenish what they use during their training sessions. It has been shown that women who consume low-fat diets and who perform endurance events can have depleted IMTG levels 2 days after these events. This will compromise performance [50–53], and as such it is recommended that for females who perform this type of exercise, energy intake from fat can be as high as 30% of daily caloric intake. Furthermore, low-fat diets also compromise the intake of the important fat-soluble vitamins A, D, E, and K as well as the essential fatty acids (α-linolenic acid and linoleic acid) [54].

There are no specific recommendations for fat intake for athletes as there are for carbohydrate and protein

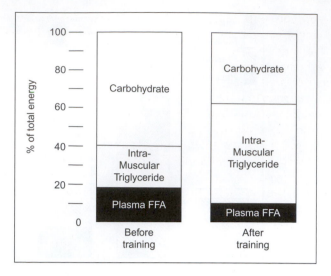

FIGURE 16.4 Changes in substrate use after training. The asterisk denotes a significant increase in using IMTG for ATP production with a significant decrease in carbohydrate use. Source: *Reproduced with permission from Hurley, B. F., Nemeth, P. M., Martin, W. H., 3rd, Hagberg, J. M., Dalsky, G. P., and Holloszy, J. O. (1986). Muscle triglyceride utilization during exercise: Effect of training.* J. Appl. Physiol. **60**, 562–567.

(discussed next) other than not to restrict levels that would be detrimental to health by limiting important vitamin and essential fatty acid intake. It is important to remind the athlete that fat oxidation is the primary way to produce ATP during aerobic exercise, and IMTG stores need to be replaced like the glycogen stores. Athletes should be advised to take in healthy fats such as mono- and polyunsaturated fatty acids. These are healthier and examples include consuming foods such as nuts, using olive oil for cooking, and consuming "fatty" fish, which contain the essential fatty acids.

C Protein

There is still considerable debate about how much dietary protein is required for optimal athletic performance. This is most likely because muscle contains a large proportion of the total protein in a human body (∼40%). Muscle also accounts for 30–50% of all protein turnover in the body. In muscle, the majority of amino acids are incorporated into tissue proteins, with a small pool of free amino acids. This pool undergoes turnover, receiving free amino acids from the breakdown of protein and contributing amino acids for protein synthesis. Protein break in skeletal muscle serves two main purposes: (1) To provide essential amino acids when individual amino acids are converted to acetyl CoA or tricarboxylic acid cycle intermediates. (2) In addition it provides individual amino acids that can be used elsewhere in the body for the synthesis of neurotransmitters, hormones, glucose, and proteins. If protein

degradation rates are greater than the rates of synthesis, there will be a reduction of protein content; conversely, muscle protein content can only increase if the rate of synthesis exceeds that of degradation.

Exercise (especially endurance exercise) results in increased oxidation of the branched-chain amino acids, which are essential amino acids and cannot be synthesized within the body. Therefore, increased oxidation would imply that the dietary protein requirements are increased. Some studies in which the nitrogen balance technique was used showed that the dietary protein requirements for athletes involved in prolonged endurance training were higher than those for sedentary individuals. Whether requirements are really higher remains somewhat controversial (for review, see [55,56]).

It has been estimated that protein may contribute up to approximately 15% to energy expenditure in resting conditions. During exercise, this relative contribution is likely to decrease because energy expenditure is increased and most of this energy is provided by carbohydrate and fat. During very prolonged exercise when carbohydrate availability becomes limited, the contribution of protein to energy expenditure may amount to approximately 5% of the total energy expenditure. Thus, although protein oxidation is increased during endurance exercise, the relative contribution of protein to energy expenditure remains small. Protein requirements may increase somewhat, but this increased need may be met easily by a moderate protein intake. The research groups that advocate an increased protein intake for endurance athletes usually recommend a daily intake of 1.2–1.8 g/kg body mass. This is approximately twice the level of protein intake that is recommended for sedentary populations.

There are reports of increased protein breakdown after resistance exercise. The suggested increased dietary protein requirements with resistance training are related to increased muscle bulk (hypertrophy) rather than increased oxidation of amino acids. Muscle protein breakdown increases after resistance training, but to a smaller degree than muscle protein synthesis. The elevations in protein degradation and synthesis are transient. Protein breakdown and synthesis after exercise are elevated at 3 and 24 hours after exercise but return to baseline levels after 48 hours. These results seem to apply to resistance exercise and high-intensity dynamic exercise.

There is controversy regarding whether strength athletes really need to eat large amounts of protein. Nitrogen balance studies conducted on such athletes have been criticized because they generally have been of short duration and a steady-state situation may not be established [56]. The recommendation for protein intakes for strength athletes is therefore generally 1.4–2.0 g/kg, depending on body mass, per day.

Again, this seems to be met easily with a normal diet, and no extra attention to protein intake is needed. Protein supplements are often used but are not necessary to meet the recommended protein intake. There is also no evidence that supplements would be more effective than normal foods.

In conclusion, it is very important to understand the difference between complete and incomplete proteins when planning meals. Complete proteins contain all of the essential amino acids (those that the body cannot produce), including the branch-chain amino acids. Food sources include meats, fish, poultry, eggs, and dairy. Incomplete proteins are those that do not contain all of the essential amino acids and are typically plant-based sources such as legumes and grains. Animal protein sources (complete proteins) have a high digestibility, whereas the plant sources do not. This is not to suggest that athletes cannot be vegetarian; however, it does suggest that these athletes need to pay particular attention to their protein intake and ensure that they are eating complimentary proteins. This means they must eat a variety of plant-based protein sources to ensure that they get all of the essential amino acids required each day.

IV MICRONUTRIENT REQUIREMENTS FOR ATHLETES

A Vitamins

Vitamins are essential organic compounds that serve to regulate metabolic processes, energy synthesis, and neurological processes and to prevent cell degradation and/or death. Vitamins can be either water or fat soluble. Fat-soluble vitamins are A, D, E, and K (as previously mentioned), and examples of water-soluble vitamins are C and the B vitamins. The body can store fat-soluble vitamins and therefore consumption of these in excess can result in toxicity. In contrast, water-soluble vitamins cannot be stored by the body, with a few exceptions such as vitamin B_6, so they are excreted in the urine when consumed in excess. Research has suggested that some vitamins may possess some health benefits (e.g., vitamins C and E, niacin, and folic acid); few of these have been shown to enhance performance in athletes when sufficient intake is present.

Studies have reported that active individuals tend to be deficient in certain B vitamins including B_6, thiamin, and riboflavin [57,58]. The B vitamins are an important group because they act as coenzymes in metabolism. This means that they can help donate or accept methyl group items, especially in substrate metabolism. For example, the active form of thiamin, thiamin pyrophosphate, can help to remove carbon dioxide and

hydrogen ions from pyruvate to help create acetyl CoA. Acetyl CoA is the molecule required to enter the Kreb's cycle and initiate oxidative metabolism. As a result, deficiency in the B vitamins can be detrimental to energy metabolism. In addition, vitamin B_{12} and folate deficiencies manifest themselves as either pernicious or megaloblastic anemia, respectively. This is a serious concern as well because improper red blood cell function will adversely affect the oxygen carrying ability of the body, which will limit performance. Finally, for vegetarian athletes, vitamin B_{12} should be carefully monitored because the best sources of B vitamins are found in meat products; as such, supplementation of B_{12} in vegetarian athletes is essential.

Other vitamins, such as A, C, and E, are known antioxidants. This means they have the ability to scavenge free radicals and decrease oxidative stress. This may be of particular interest to athletes because theoretically it may help athletes to tolerate heavy training loads and potentially accelerate recovery. However, the literature on antioxidant supplementation is convoluted and in some cases inconclusive. What is known is that athletes do have enhanced antioxidant status and enzymes as a result of exercise training [59]. In addition, it has been suggested that supplying antioxidants to athletes may actually negate the natural antioxidant health-promoting effects of exercise [60]. As such, caution should be exercised with regard to the efficacy on intake and the purpose for supplementation.

Finally, vitamin D is important to ensure proper intake (Recommended Daily Allowance (RDA) 600 IU/day for males and females ages 19—50 years)). Its partnership with calcium and their role in bone health are well-established [61]. Although this vitamin is typically not a concern with regard to deficiency, it can be in sports in which body composition is an issue. This has previously been mentioned and it is likely because these athletes tend to underconsume fat, which will be reflected in the status of the fat-soluble vitamins and essential fatty acid intake. As a result, it is recommended that these types of athletes would benefit from supplementation of vitamin D.

In summary, athletes who consume a balanced diet with appropriate calorie intake will meet their vitamin requirements and there is no need to for additional supplementation. However, as mentioned previously, athletes do tend to have some dietary inadequacies and as such a multivitamin is sometimes recommended to ensure all vitamin requirements are met.

B Minerals

Minerals are essential inorganic compounds that help with tissue structure and metabolic processes such as components of enzymes and hormones and regulators of metabolic and neural control. As is the case with vitamins, some minerals that have been found to be deficient in athletes—for example, iron (RDA 8 mg/day for males and 18 mg/day for females age 19—50 years) and calcium (RDA 1000 mg/day for males and females age 19—50 years). Lacking these minerals will negatively impact performance. Conversely, supplementing these minerals can improve performance.

Exercise is an outstanding form of weight-bearing activity; however, many athletes still have low bone density, especially female distance runners. The more common problem with this group of athletes, however, is menstrual disturbances that disrupt hormonal status and predispose women to the female athlete triad (disordered eating, low bone density, and menstrual dysfunction). In these athletes, calcium supplementation may be increased to 1200—1500 mg/day, and this has been shown to help maintain bone mass.

Iron is a common mineral found to be deficient especially in early training periods. This is reflected by reductions in both hematocrit (percentage of red blood cells) and hemoglobin (oxygen-carrying component of the red blood cell). This can be due to several factors, including changes in plasma volume that dilute hemoglobin, exertional hemolysis, and dietary practices that include low iron intake, low iron bioavailability, and increased iron excretion. Heme iron, such as that found in meats, fish, and poultry, is better absorbed and bioavailable compared to non-heme iron, which is found in grains, vegetables, and legumes. Factors that enhance iron absorption include vitamin C, peptides from fish/meat/chicken, alcohol, and food acids, whereas factors that inhibit absorption include phytates, polyphenols, calcium, and peptides from plant sources such as soy protein. The absorption of both heme and non-heme iron is increased as an adaptive response in people who are iron deficient or have increased iron requirements. Prevention and treatment of iron deficiency may include iron supplementation, with a recommended therapeutic dose of 100 mg/day of elemental iron for 2 or 3 months. However, the management plan should include dietary counseling to increase the intake of bioavailable iron and appropriate strategies to reduce any unwarranted iron loss.

In addition, zinc and magnesium are two other minerals that are important for energy production. Zinc plays a role in growth, building, and repair of muscle tissue; energy production; and immune function. Survey data suggest that Americans have zinc levels below the recommended intake [62—64] and that female athletes are at a particular risk for deficiency [64]. Zinc levels can be difficult to measure; however, deficiency has serious consequences, including decreases in cardiorespiratory function, muscle strength, and endurance. Vegetarian athletes are again at a particular risk for zinc deficiency. The RDA for zinc is currently 11 mg/day for males and 8 mg/day for females. There is no reason to consume more than 40 mg/day because this is the upper limit for toxicity [62]; however, intake at 25 mg/day has been shown to minimize exercise-induced changes in immune function [65—68]. Magnesium plays a role in cellular metabolism; membrane stability; and neuromuscular, immune, and hormonal status. Magnesium deficiency impairs performance due to inefficient oxygen use, and in sports in which weight is an issue; deficiency has been reported [69,70]. The RDA for magnesium is 420 mg/day for males and 320 mg/day for females.

V FLUID REQUIREMENTS FOR ATHLETES

Water represents approximately 50—60% of total body weight and functions as a transport medium, lubricant, solvent, and thermal regulator (Figure 16.5). The body is constantly exchanging fluids between the interstitial fluid (fluid between tissues) and intracellular fluid (fluid within the cells) compartments to maintain both hydrostatic and osmotic pressures. The maintenance of these fluid compartments occurs through osmotic forces that are regulated by properly working sodium—potassium pumps. Sodium controls the extracellular fluid (fluid outside the cell) volume, regulates osmolality, helps with acid—base balance, and maintains resting cell membrane potential. Potassium controls the intracellular fluid volume, and it also regulates osmolality, acid—base balance, and cell membrane potential. The body has active mechanisms in place for monitoring sodium levels, ensuring that they are always in acceptable ranges. No such mechanism exists for potassium; potassium simply relies on ion exchange pumps for maintenance.

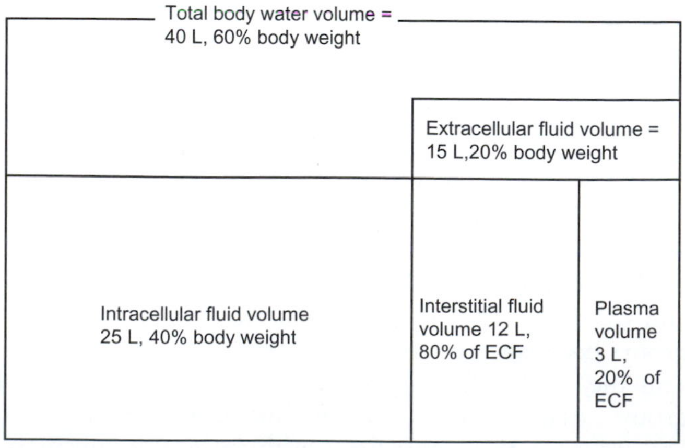

Total body water volume = 40 L, 60% body weight		
Intracellular fluid volume 25 L, 40% body weight	Extracellular fluid volume = 15 L, 20% body weight	
	Interstitial fluid volume 12 L, 80% of ECF	Plasma volume 3 L, 20% of ECF

FIGURE 16.5　Body water distribution.

When we sweat during exercise, we lose fluid from the interstitial fluid compartment and this will disrupt balance, calling on our electrolytes to help correct the disruption. The issue is that when we sweat, we also lose electrolytes, so the replenishing of the fluid and electrolytes before, during, and after exercise sessions is of utmost importance. Regulation of fluid balance is dictated by our thirst mechanism (the sensation of feeling thirsty is not perceived until a person has lost at least 2% of body mass), monitoring of the extracellular fluid volume, and blood pressure. To maintain fluid balance, water intake may vary from 1 liter to approximately 12 liters per day. However, during exercise and especially during exercise in hot conditions, sweat rates (and thus water losses) may increase dramatically and dehydration may occur (i.e., the body is in negative fluid balance). Depending on the sport, sweat rates can range from 0.3 to 2.4 l/hr [71], with the average sodium concentration in sweat approximately 1 g/l [1].

A Dehydration and Performance

The literature is clear that dehydration will negatively impact performance (Figure 16.6). Dehydration can cause several physiological disturbances, all of which negatively impact performance (Figure 16.7). Several studies have shown that mild dehydration, equivalent to the loss of only 2% body weight, is sufficient to significantly impair exercise performance [71,72]. In addition, it is often reported that greater losses result in greater reductions in performance. Even very low-intensity exercise (i.e., walking) is affected by dehydration. The capacity to perform high-intensity exercise that results in exhaustion within only a few minutes has been shown to be reduced by as much as 45% by prior dehydration (2.5% of body weight) [73]. Although there is little opportunity for sweat loss during such short-duration, high-intensity events, athletes who travel to compete in hot climates are likely to experience acute dehydration, which can persist for several days and can be of sufficient magnitude to have a detrimental effect on performance in competition. Although dehydration has detrimental effects especially on performance in hot conditions, such effects can also be observed in cool conditions. Both decreases in maximal aerobic power (VO_2 max) and decreases in endurance capacity have been reported with dehydration in temperate conditions [74], although not all studies have found such an effect [75,76].

B Dehydration and Heat Illness

Dehydration also puts the athlete at increased risk for heat illness. Heat illness can be assessed by calculating

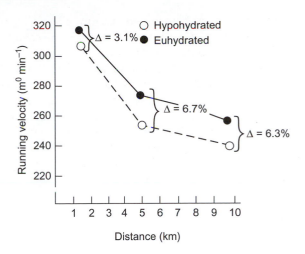

FIGURE 16.6 Effects of dehydration on running velocity over distance covered. Results clearly show that velocity is significantly different at all three distances. Source: *Reproduced with permission from Sawka, M. N., Francesconi, R. P., Young, A. J., and Pandolf, K. B. (1984). Influence of hydration level and body fluids on exercise performance in the heat.* J. Am. Med. Assoc. **252**, 1165–1169.

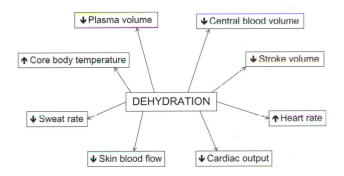

FIGURE 16.7 Physiological side effects of dehydration.

wet bulb globe temperature (WBGT) index = 0.7 T_{wb} + 0.2 T_g + 0.1 T_a, where T_{wb} is the wet-bulb temperature, T_g is the globe temperature, and T_a is the ambient or dry bulb temperature. Risks based on this formula are as follows: very high risk; WBGT > 28°C (82°F)—race should be postponed, rescheduled, or canceled. High risk; WBGT 23–28°C (73–82°F)—runners should be aware that heat illnesses may occur, particularly in susceptible persons. Moderate risk; WBGT 18–23°C (65–73°F)—remind runners that heat and humidity will increase during the race if early in the day. Low risk; WBGT < 18°C (<65°F)—does not guarantee heat illness will not occur (Figure 16.8). Early symptoms of heat injury are excessive sweating, headache, nausea, dizziness, a reduced consciousness, and impaired mental function. When core body temperature rises to more than 40°C, heat stroke may develop; heat stroke is characterized by hot dry skin, confusion, and loss of consciousness.

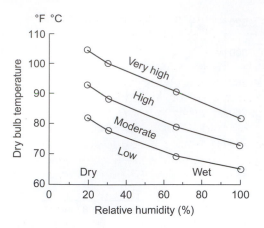

FIGURE 16.8 Temperature, relative humidity, and risk for heat illness. Source: *Reproduced with permission from Armstrong, L. E., and Maresh, C. M. (1996). Fluid replacement during exercise and recovery from exercise. In "Body Fluid Balance: Exercise and Sport" (E. R. Burkirk and S. M. Puhl, Eds.), pp. 259–281. CRC Press, Boca Raton, FL.*

C Hyponatremia

Hyponatremia or low sodium level is defined by dilution of serum sodium from normal levels of 135–145 to less than 130 mEq/l. Causes of hyponatremia include sodium loss, water retention, or both due to excessive sweating, vomiting, diarrhea, or excessive use of diuretics. The most common symptoms, if water intake is excessive and hyponatremia develops slowly, are mental confusion, giddiness, and coma. Muscle twitching, irritability, and convulsions occur if the development is rapid.

Hyponatremia appears to be most common among slow runners in marathon and ultramarathon races and probably arises because of the loss of sodium in sweat coupled with very high intakes of water. This means that there can be a danger of misdiagnosis of this condition when it occurs in individuals participating in endurance races. The usual treatment for dehydration is administration of fluid intravenously and orally. If this treatment were to be given to a hyponatremic individual, the consequences could be fatal.

D Fluid Intake before, during, and after Exercise

The American College of Sports Medicine's (ACSM) position stand [71] on exercise and fluid replacement provides a comprehensive review of the research and recommendations for hydration before, during, and after exercise. ACSM has also published position stands on exercising in environmental conditions [77,78]. This section summarizes the position stand on fluid replacement and serves as a guide that athletes should follow.

1 Before Exercise

Athletes should start drinking at least 4 hours prior to exercise approximately 5–7 ml/kg body weight of water or sport beverage. This allows for adequate time to optimize hydration status and excrete any excess fluids in the urine prior to competition when it would not be timely to do so. Overhydrating (hyperhydration) with excess water or glycerol solutions will substantially expand intra- and extracellular fluid volumes and will increase the risk of voiding during the competition. In addition, it confers no clear performance benefit.

2 During Exercise

As mentioned previously, decreases that are 2% or more of body weight initiate the thirst response and are typically indicative of dehydration, which is detrimental to performance. Fluid intake during exercise should be aimed at preventing this from occurring. Although this seems easy in theory, this is highly dependent on the athlete due to body size, sweat rate, and the exercise being performed. In addition, fluid balance during exercise may not occur because sweat rates may be greater than gastric emptying rates that limit fluid absorption and ultimately fluid ingestion rate by the athlete. To help, gastric emptying rates can be maximized when the stomach is full, and absorption rates can be maximized when the carbohydrate concentration in the beverage is approximately 6–8%. Athletes should start drinking fluids right away during exercise and at regular intervals to replace water loss. Athletes should ingest fluids cooler than the ambient temperature (15–22°C). Carbohydrate–electrolyte drinks are beneficial for exercises that last longer than 1 hour; these help replace electrolytes and maintain blood glucose levels. The sodium level in fluids when exercise lasts longer than 1 hour should be approximately 0.5–0.7 g/l.

3 After Exercise

Because most athletes will not consume enough liquids during exercise, post-exercise hydration is critical. If the athlete has adequate time between exercise sessions, then intake of normal meals and beverage should replenish hydration status. Rapid and complete recovery from exercise can be accomplished by drinking at least 16–24 oz. (450–675 ml) of fluid for every pound of body weight lost during the exercise bout. This can easily be tracked by simply weighing oneself before and after exercise and then hydrate accordingly. Another easy way to determine hydration status is to observe the color of the urine (Figure 16.9).

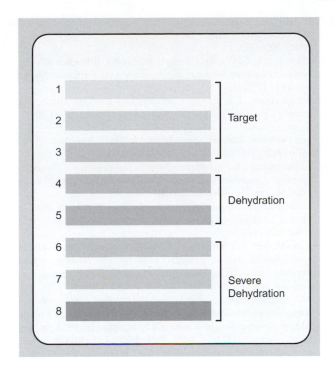

FIGURE 16.9 Urine color hydration chart. Scientific validation for this chart can be found in the *International Journal of Sport Nutrition*, Volume 4, 1994, pp. 265–279 and Volume 8, 1998, pp. 345–355. See color plate.

VI SUMMARY AND CONCLUSIONS

The basic difference between athletes and the general population is that athletes typically need more fluids to recover sweat and electrolyte loss during physical activity and greater food intake to maintain energy balance demands that are associated with exercise. Much of this energy can be in the form of carbohydrate, but neglecting protein or fat could be detrimental to performance. Although there are general rules for how to govern these increased energy demands, each individual is different and the concept of one diet fits all is obsolete. However, the types of foods recommended can be standard in that good carbohydrates in the forms of grains, fruits, vegetables, and breads should be encouraged along with fats that are high in mono- and polyunsaturated fatty acids such as nuts, olive oil, and "fatty" fish and proteins that are lean and complete (e.g., that contain all of the essential amino acids) such as meat, poultry, and fish. Requirements for these macronutrients may vary between strength-trained and aerobic-trained athletes and also may vary between genders. Special attention is warranted for sports that place a strong emphasis on body composition and weight to ensure that these athletes are consuming enough calories. Furthermore, vegetarian athletes need to be mindful of ensuring that

they are consuming complimentary proteins to obtain all of the essential amino acids recommended as well as vitamin B_{12}, which is typically found only in animal products. In addition, female athletes, especially in body composition and weight-dependent sports, need to be counseled on the importance of maintaining adequate calorie intake for both macro- and micronutrients to avoid disturbances such as those seen in the female athlete triad. Consuming adequate nutrients is essential for an athlete to achieve optimal performance. The guidelines put forth in this chapter provide a thorough overview of the evidence-based nutritional recommendations to help athletes understand energy requirements allowing for both energy balance and peak performance.

References

[1] American College of Sports Medicine; American Dietetic Association; Dietitians of Canada, Joint position statement: nutrition and athletic performance. American College of Sports Medicine, American Dietetic Association, and Dietitians of Canada, Med. Sci. Sports Exerc. 41 (3) (2009) 709–731.

[2] L.M. Burke, G.R. Cox, N.K. Cummings, B. Desbrow, Guidelines for carbohydrate intake: do athletes achieve them? Sports Med. 31 (4) (2001) 267–299.

[3] C. Zinn, G. Schofield, C. Wall, Evaluation of sports nutrition knowledge of New Zealand premier club rugby coaches, Int. J. Sports Nutr. Exer. Metab. 16 (2) (2006) 214–225.

[4] S. Heaney, H. O'Connor, S. Michael, J. Gifford, G. Naughton, Nutrition knowledge in athletes: a systematic review, Int. J. Sports Nutr. Exer. Metab. 21 (2011) 248–261.

[5] W.W. Campbell, R.A. Geik, Nutritional requirements for the older athlete, Nutrition 20 (2004) 603–608.

[6] A.B. Loucks, Energy balance and body composition in sports and exercise, J. Sports Sci. 22 (2004) 1–14.

[7] A.M.J. Erp van-Baart, W.H.M. Saris, R.A. Binkhorst, J.A. Vos, J.W.H. Elvers, Nationwide survey on nutritional habits in elite athletes: Part II. Mineral and vitamin intake, Int. J. Sports Med. 10 (1989) S11–S16.

[8] M. Dahlstrom, E. Jansson, E. Nordevang, L. Kaijser, Discrepancy between estimated energy intake and requirement in female dancers, Clin. Physiol. 10 (1990) 11–25.

[9] P. Ziegler, R. Sharp, V. Hughes, W. Evans, C.S. Khoo, Nutritional status of teenage female competitive figure skaters, J. Am. Diet. Assoc. 102 (3) (2002) 374–379.

[10] B.E. Ainsworth, W.L. Haskell, S.D. Herrmann, N. Meckes, D.R. Bassett Jr., C. Tudor-Locke, et al., Compendium of physical activities: a second update of codes and MET values, Med. Sci. Sports Exerc. 43 (8) (2011) 1575–1581.

[11] J.L. Ivy, M.C. Lee, J.T. Brozinick Jr., M.J. Reed, Muscle glycogen storage after different amounts of carbohydrate ingestion, J. Appl. Physiol. 65 (5) (1988) 2018–2023.

[12] J.L. Ivy, A.L. Katz, C.L. Cutler, W.M. Sherman, E.F. Coyle, Muscle glycogen synthesis after exercise: effect of time of carbohydrate ingestion, J. Appl. Physiol. 64 (4) (1988) 1480–1485.

[13] C. Foster, D.L. Costill, W.J. Fink, Effects of preexercise feedings on endurance performance, Med. Sci. Sports 11 (1979) 1–5.

[14] A.E. Jeukendrup, N.P. Craig, J.A. Hawley, The bioenergetics of world class cycling, J. Sci. Med. Sport 3 (2000) 414–433.

[15] F. Brouns, W.H.M. Saris, J. Stroecken, E. Beckers, R. Thijssen, N.J. Rehrer, et al., Eating, drinking, and cycling: a controlled

Tour de France simulation study, Part I, Int. J. Sports Med. 10 (1989) S32–S40.

[16] A.M. Sjodin, A.B. Andersson, J.M. Hogberg, K.R. Westerterp, Energy balance in cross-country skiers: a study using doubly labeled water, Med. Sci. Sports Exerc. 26 (1994) 720–724.

[17] G.P. Rontoyannis, T. Skoulis, K.N. Pavlou, Energy balance in ultramarathon running, Am. J. Clin. Nutr. 49 (1989) 976–979.

[18] K.A. Beals, N.L. Meyer, Female athlete triad update, Clin. Sports Med. 26 (2007) 69–89.

[19] K. Birch, Female athlete triad, Br. Med. J. 330 (2005) 244–246.

[20] A.B. Loucks, Introduction to menstrual disturbances in athletes, Med. Sci. Sports Exerc. 35 (2003) 1551–1552.

[21] L. Nybo, CNS fatigue and prolonged exercise: effect of glucose supplementation, Med. Sci. Sports Exerc. 35 (2003) 589–594.

[22] T.D. Noakes, Physiological models to understand exercise fatigue and the adaptations that predict or enhance athletic performance, Scand. J. Med. Sci. Sports 10 (2000) 123–145.

[23] J. Bergstrom, E. Hultman, A study of glycogen metabolism during exercise in man, Scand. J. Clin. Invest. 19 (1967) 218–228.

[24] J. Bergstrom, L. Hermansen, E. Hultman, B. Saltin, Diet, muscle glycogen and physical performance, Acta Physiol. Scand. 71 (1967) 140–150.

[25] D.E. Thomas, J.R. Brotherhood, J.C. Brand, Carbohydrate feeding before exercise: effect of glycemic index, Int. J. Sports Med. 12 (2) (1991) 180–186.

[26] W.M. Sherman, G. Brodowicz, D.A. Wright, W.K. Allen, J. Simonsen, A. Dernbach, Effects of 4 h pre-exercise carbohydrate feedings on cycling performance, Med. Sci. Sports Exerc. 21 (1989) 598–604.

[27] D.A. Wright, W.M. Sherman, A.R. Dernbach, Carbohydrate feedings before, during, or in combination improve cycling endurance performance, J. Appl. Physiol. 71 (1991) 1082–1088.

[28] E.J. Schabort, A.N. Bosch, S.M. Weltan, T.D. Noakes, The effect of a preexercise meal on time to fatigue during prolonged cycling exercise, Med. Sci. Sports Exerc. 31 (1999) 464–471.

[29] R.L. Jentjens, A.E. Jeukendrup, Prevalence of hypoglycemia following pre-exercise carbohydrate ingestion is not accompanied by higher insulin sensitivity, Int. J. Sport Nutr. Exerc. Metab. 12 (2002) 398–413.

[30] O.K. Tsintzas, C. Williams, L. Boobis, P. Greenhaff, Carbohydrate ingestion and glycogen utilisation in different muscle fibre types in man, J. Physiol. 489 (1995) 243–250.

[31] D.P. Leijssen, W.H. Saris, A.E. Jeukendrup, A.J. Wagenmakers, Oxidation of exogenous [13C] galactose and [13C] glucose during exercise, J. Appl. Physiol. 79 (1995) 720–725.

[32] X. Shi, R.W. Summers, H.P. Schedl, S.W. Flanagan, R. Chang, C.V. Gisolfi, Effects of carbohydrate type and concentration and solution osmolality on water absorption, Med. Sci. Sports Exerc. 27 (1995) 1607–1615.

[33] C. Roepstorff, C.H. Steffensen, M. Madsen, B. Stallknecht, I.L. Kanstrup, E.A. Richter, et al., Gender differences in substrate utilization during submaximal exercise in endurance-trained subjects, Am. J. Physiol. Endocrinol. Metab. 282 (2) (2002) E435–E447.

[34] C.H. Steffensen, C. Roepstorff, M. Madsen, B. Kiens, Myocellular triacylglycerol breakdown in females but not in males during exercise, Am. J. Physiol. Endocrinol. Metab. 282 (3) (2002) E634–E642.

[35] R.L. Jentjens, M.C. Venables, A.E. Jeukendrup, Oxidation of exogenous glucose, sucrose and maltose during prolonged cycling exercise, J. Appl. Physiol. 96 (4) (2004) 1285–1291.

[36] J.L. Ivy, W. Miller, V. Dover, L.G. Goodyear, W.M. Sherman, S. Farrel, et al., Endurance improved by ingestion of a glucose polymer supplement, Med. Sci. Sports Exerc. 15 (1983) 466–471.

[37] P. Felig, A. Cherif, A. Minagawa, J. Wahren, Hypoglycemia during prolonged exercise in normal men, N. Engl. J. Med. 306 (1982) 895–900.

[38] J.L. Ivy, D.L. Costili, W.J. Fink, R.W. Lower, Influence of caffeine and carbohydrate feedings on endurance performance, Med. Sci. Sports 11 (1979) 6–11.

[39] A.R. Coggan, E.F. Coyle, Carbohydrate feedings during high-intensity exercise, J. Appl. Physiol. 65 (4) (1988) 1703–1709.

[40] R. Jentjens, A. Jeukendrup, Determinants of post-exercise glycogen synthesis during short-term recovery, Sports Med. 33 (2003) 117–144.

[41] J. Bergstrom, E. Hultman, Muscle glycogen synthesis after exercise: an enhancing factor localized to the muscle cells in man, Nature 210 (1966) 309–310.

[42] E. Hultman, J. Bergström, Muscle glycogen synthesis in relation to diet studied in normal subjects, Acta Med. Scand. 182 (1) (1967) 109–117.

[43] J. Bergström, E. Hultman, A.E. Roch-Norlund, Muscle glycogen synthetase in normal subjects: basal values, effect of glycogen depletion by exercise and of a carbohydrate-rich diet following exercise, Scand. J. Clin. Lab. Invest. 29 (2) (1972) 231–236.

[44] W. Sherman, Carbohydrates, muscle glycogen, and muscle glycogen supercompensation, in: M.H. Williams (Ed.), Ergogenic Aids in Sports, Human Kinetics, Champaign, IL, 1983, pp. 1–25.

[45] W.M. Sherman, D.L. Costill, W.J. Fink, J.M. Miller, Effect of exercise–diet manipulation on muscle glycogen and its subsequent utilisation during performance, Int. J. Sports Med. 2 (1981) 114–118.

[46] J.A. Hawley, E.J. Schabort, T.D. Noakes, S.C. Dennis, Carbohydrate loading and exercise performance, Sports Med. 24 (1997) 1–10.

[47] E.F. Coyle, A.R. Coggan, M.K. Hemmert, J.L. Ivy, Muscle glycogen utilization during prolonged strenuous exercise when fed carbohydrate, J. Appl. Physiol. 61 (1986) 165–172.

[48] J.A. Hawley, E.J. Schabort, T.D. Noakes, S.C. Dennis, Carbohydrate loading and exercise performance, Sports Med. 24 (1997) 1–10.

[49] M.A. Tarnopolsky, Gender differences in substrate metabolism during endurance exercise, Can. J. Appl. Physiol. 25 (4) (2000) 312–327.

[50] D.R. Larson-Meyer, B.R. Newcomer, G.R. Hunter, Influence of endurance running and recovery diet on intramyocellular lipid content in women: a ^{1}H NMR study, Am. J. Physiol. Endocrinol. Metab. 282 (1) (2002) E95–E106.

[51] D.E. Larson-Meyer, O.N. Borkhsenious, J.C. Gullett, R.R. Russell, M.C. Devries, S.R. Smith, et al., Effect of dietary fat on serum and intramyocellular lipids and running performance, Med. Sci. Sports Exerc. 40 (5) (2008) 892–902.

[52] K.A. Beals, M.M. Manore, Nutritional status of female athletes with subclinical eating disorders, J. Am. Diet. Assoc. 98 (4) (1998) 419–425.

[53] D.M. Muoio, J.J. Leddy, P.J. Horvath, A.B. Awad, D.R. Pendergast, Effect of dietary fat on metabolic adjustments to maximal VO_2 and endurance in runners, Med. Sci. Sports Exerc. 26 (1) (1994) 81–88.

[54] M.M. Manore, Dietary recommendations and athletic menstrual dysfunction, Sports Med. 32 (14) (2002) 887–901.

[55] S.M. Phillips, Dietary protein for athletes: from requirements to metabolic advantage, Appl. Physiol. Nutr. Metab. 31 (2006) 647–654.

[56] K.D. Tipton, O.C. Witard, Protein requirements and recommendations for athletes: relevance of ivory tower arguments for practical recommendations, Clin. Sports Med. 26 (2007) 17–36.

[57] M. Fogelholm, Micronutrient status in females during a 24-week fitness-type exercise program, Ann. Nutr. Metab. 36 (4) (1992) 209–218.

[58] L. Rokitzki, A.N. Sagredos, F. Reuss, D. Cufi, J. Keul, Assessment of vitamin B_6 status of strength and speedpower athletes, J. Am. Coll. Nutr. 13 (1) (1994) 87–94.

[59] S.K. Powers, M.J. Jackson, Exercise-induced oxidative stress: cellular mechanisms and impact on muscle force production, Physiol. Rev. 88 (2008) 1243–1276.

[60] M. Ristow, K. Zarse, A. Oberbach, N. Klöting, M. Birringer, M. Kiehntopf, et al., Antioxidants prevent health-promoting effects of physical exercise in humans, Proc. Natl. Acad. Sci. USA 106 (21) (2009) 8665–8670.

[61] A.C. Ross, J.E. Manson, S.A. Abrams, J.F. Aloia, P.M. Brannon, S. K. Clinton, et al., The 2011 Dietary Reference Intakes for Calcium and Vitamin D: what dietetics practitioners need to know, J. Am. Diet. Assoc. 111 (4) (2011) 524–527.

[62] Institute of Medicine, Dietary Reference Intakes for Vitamin A, Vitamin K, Arsenic, Boron, Chromium, Copper, Iodine, Iron, Manganese, Molybdenum, Nickel, Silicon, Vanadium, and Zinc, National Academies Press, Washington, DC, 2001.

[63] E. Haymes, Iron, in: J. Driskell, I. Wolinsky (Eds), Sports Nutrition. Vitamins and Trace Elements, CRC Press/Taylor & Francis, New York, 2006, pp. 203–216.

[64] A. Micheletti, R. Rossi, S. Rufini, Zinc status in athletes: relation to diet and exercise, Sports Med. 31 (2001) 577–582.

[65] D.C. Nieman, Nutrition, exercise, and immune system function, Clin. Sports Med. 18 (3) (1999) 537–548.

[66] M. Gleeson, N.C. Bishop, Elite athlete immunology: importance of nutrition, Int. J. Sports Med. 21 (Suppl. 1) (2000) S44–S50.

[67] R.S. Gibson, A.L. Heath, E.L. Ferguson, Risk of suboptimal iron and zinc nutriture among adolescent girls in Australia and New Zealand: causes, consequences, and solutions, Asia Pac. J. Clin. Nutr. 11 (Suppl. 3) (2002) S543–S552.

[68] A. Singh, M.L. Failla, P.A. Deuster, Exercise-induced changes in immune function: effects of zinc supplementation, J. Appl. Physiol. 76 (6) (1994) 2298–2303.

[69] C.H. Bohl, S.L. Volpe, Magnesium and exercise, Crit. Rev. Food Sci. Nutr. 42 (6) (2002) 533–563.

[70] H.C. Lukaski, Magnesium, zinc, and chromium nutrition and athletic performance, Can. J. Appl. Physiol. 26 (Suppl.) (2001) S13–S22.

[71] M.N. Sawka, L.M. Burke, E.R. Eichner, R.J. Maughan, S.J. Montain, N.S. Stachenfeld, American College of Sports Medicine position stand: exercise and fluid replacement, Med. Sci. Sports Exerc. 39 (2007) 377–390.

[72] S.N. Cheuvront, R. Carter III, M.N. Sawka, Fluid balance and endurance exercise performance, Curr. Sports Med. Rep. 2 (2003) 202–208.

[73] R.M. Walsh, T.D. Noakes, J.A. Hawley, S.C. Dennis, Impaired high-intensity cycling performance time at low levels of dehydration, Int. J. Sports Med. 15 (1994) 392–398.

[74] G.K. McConell, C.M. Burge, S.L. Skinner, M. Hargreaves, Influence of ingested fluid volume on physiological responses during prolonged exercise, Acta Physiol. Scand. 160 (1997) 149–156.

[75] T.A. Robinson, J.A. Hawley, G.S. Palmer, G.R. Wilson, D.A. Gray, T.D. Noakes, et al., Water ingestion does not improve 1-H cycling performance in moderate ambient temperatures, Eur. J. Appl. Physiol. Occup. Physiol. 71 (1995) 153–160.

[76] R.J. Maughan, C.E. Fenn, J.B. Leiper, Effects of fluid, electrolyte and substrate ingestion on endurance capacity, Eur. J. Appl. Physiol. Occup. Physiol. 58 (1989) 481–486.

[77] L.E. Armstrong, D.J. Casa, M. Millard-Stafford, D.S. Moran, S.W. Pyne, W.O. Roberts, American College of Sports Medicine position stand: exertional heat illness during training and competition, Med. Sci. Sports Exerc. 39 (2007) 556–572.

[78] J.W. Castellani, A.J. Young, M.B. Ducharme, G.G. Giesbrecht, E. Glickman, R.E. Sallis, American College of Sports Medicine position stand: prevention of cold injuries during exercise, Med. Sci. Sports Exerc. 38 (2006) 2012–2029.

A. FOOD AND NUTRITION INTAKE FOR HEALTH

C H A P T E R

17

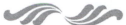

Nutrition for Children with Special Health Care Needs

Anne Bradford Harris[*], *Marion Taylor Baer*[†], *Cristine M. Trahms*[‡], *Beth Ogata*[‡]

[*]University of Wisconsin—Madison, Madison, Wisconsin [†]University of California at Los Angeles, Los Angeles, California [‡]University of Washington, Seattle, Washington

I INTRODUCTION

According to data available from the National Survey of Children with Special Health Care Needs, 10.2 million children in the United States (13.9%) have special conditions that increase their need for health care services and educational supports beyond those of children without special needs [1,2]. Children with special health care needs include those with specific diagnoses related to developmental disabilities such as genetic disorders (e.g., trisomy 21 (Down syndrome) and phenylketonuria (PKU), cognitive and behavioral challenges (e.g., autism and intellectual disabilities), and neuromotor impairments (e.g., cerebral palsy and spina bifida). Children who are born prematurely or with a low birth weight are considered to be at high risk for developing a special health care need. There are also children with common chronic health concerns (e.g., asthma, diabetes, and obesity) who can be included in the broader definition of children with special health care needs, but the focus of this chapter is on children with functional conditions related to prematurity or a known developmental disability.

As many as 40–60% of children with special health care needs are at risk for one or more problems with nutritional status, ranging from slow growth and poor feeding to more severe gastrointestinal problems and metabolic disorders [3,4]. Table 17.1 provides a list of special health care needs, including the sequelae of prematurity, the more common genetic disorders, and other developmental disabilities, and the associated functional problems with nutrition. Because of the increasing prevalence of children with special health care needs,

the essential role that nutrition therapy plays in treating several conditions, and the high risk of developing comorbid nutrition problems (e.g., underweight and overweight), nutrition professionals will encounter children with special health care needs in their practices and should be able to anticipate their most commonly seen nutrition problems [5,6].

Intrauterine nutrition insults occurring prenatally can predispose children to developmental disabilities and poor growth, as well as to problems with obesity and chronic illnesses later in life. Children with special health care needs receive services in multiple settings, including prenatal public health nutrition programs such as WIC (the Special Supplemental Nutrition Program for Women, Infants and Children; http://www.fns.usda.gov/wic), schools, and primary and tertiary care practices. To ensure that those at high risk for nutrition problems are identified and referred for appropriate services, nutrition screening is an important part of care in all of these settings [7]. Evidence is mounting establishing the cost-effectiveness of appropriate nutrition interventions, especially preventive interventions, for high-risk populations of mothers and children [3,8,9]. Mothers who receive adequate nutrition during pregnancy have better birth outcomes, and children who have their nutritional risks identified and receive appropriate interventions demonstrate better growth, health, and developmental outcomes than those who do not.

This chapter describes nutritional risk for mothers during pregnancy that affects their offspring and for infants and children identified with a special health care need, with the intent to prevent disability through good nutrition, to provide secondary prevention of

Nutrition in the Prevention and Treatment of Disease, Third Edition.
DOI: http://dx.doi.org/10.1016/B978-0-12-391884-0.00017-2

TABLE 17.1   A Comparison of Specific Developmental Conditions with Types of Nutrition Risks

Disorder	Growth			Diet		Medical		
	Underweight	Overweight	Short stature	Low energy needs	High energy needs	Feeding issues/ special diet	Constipation	Chronic medications
Autism	X	X				X		X
Prematurity with bronchopulmonary dysplasia	X		X		X	X		X
Cerebral palsy	X	X	X	X	X	X	X	X
Down syndrome		X	X	X		X		
Inborn errors of metabolism						X		X
Prader–Willi syndrome		X	X	X				
Spina bifida	X	X	X	X		X	X	X

further disability in specific conditions with known nutrition issues, and to preserve and promote function in order to enable the child with special health care needs to reach his or her potential in terms of growth and development.

Section II addresses primary and secondary prevention of developmental problems by examining the evidence that nutrition, and specific nutrients, during fetal development and infancy affects developmental outcomes and subsequent special needs for children.

Section III outlines the functional approach to identifying nutritional needs—how growth, diet, and medical issues are assessed, including issues specific to children with special health care needs in each of these areas.

Section IV covers selected pediatric conditions in more depth—inborn errors of metabolism, Prader–Willi syndrome, feeding problems, and autism spectrum disorders—including a description of the diagnosis, assessment of nutritional status, and ongoing intervention, where there is evidence for nutrition interventions.

II THE ROLE OF NUTRITION IN PREVENTING DEVELOPMENTAL PROBLEMS

An adequate supply of nutrients, both macro and micro, may be the most important environmental factor in determining the optimal growth and development of the fetus. Low birth weight (LBW), resulting from preterm birth or intrauterine growth retardation, has long been established as a major risk factor for developmental disabilities (discussed next), but, relatively recently, maternal nutritional status is being considered to be more important than previously

recognized. This includes epidemiological and experimental studies (beyond the scope of this chapter), which have suggested that early nutrition plays a key role in the later development of obesity and its associated chronic diseases—the theory that early "nutrition programming" determines the set point of energy balance in the fetus [10]. The following brief review of research findings illustrates that associations between nutrition and pregnancy outcome in terms of disability, as well as chronic illness, are becoming more apparent.

A Low Birth Weight and Preterm Birth

Risk of preterm birth (before 37 weeks of gestation), LBW ($<2500\,g$), or being small for gestational age (SGA) increases by approximately 50% with short interpregnancy intervals (<18 months) and less than 2 years postmenarche in young adult U.S. women compared to those who are older or who have an interpregnancy interval of 18–23 months; this cannot be entirely explained by social or behavioral factors [11]. Evidence is accumulating that if the pregnant woman is still growing herself, or has not had sufficient time since her last pregnancy to replace depleted stores, the physiological changes that normally favor improved nutrient utilization during gestation may not be adequate to meet the needs of both mother and fetus. In such cases, it appears that nutrients are partitioned between the mother and the fetus depending on the initial nutritional status of the mother [11]. In one study, the incidence of preterm birth was lowered in women given a diet of fish, oils, low-fat meats and dairy, whole grains, fruits, vegetables, and legumes compared to women who continued their usual diet. Although the study goal was to lower cholesterol in the mothers, it is likely that this diet also improved their nutritional status [12]. Other studies have shown that zinc [13], folate [14], and iron [15] deficiencies all increase the risk of preterm birth and LBW. In addition, low serum selenium early in pregnancy has been shown to predict lower birth weight [16].

A large study of women in the Danish National Birth Cohort ($\sim$36,000 subjects) indicates that periconceptional use of multivitamins, particularly regular use, is associated with a lowered risk of infants being born SGA [17]. This study also showed that the association between pre- and post-multivitamin use and preterm birth varied according to prepregnancy weight; women whose body mass index (BMI) was less than 25 had significantly less risk of either preterm labor or delivery, whereas the same was not true for overweight women [17]. In a report that was part of the "Generation R" study—a large (> 6000 women) but prospective study in The Netherlands—Timmermans and colleagues [18] showed that periconceptional folic acid supplementation (starting prior to conception or up to the eighth week of pregnancy) was associated with decreased risk of preterm birth and LBW, whereas preconception use also reduced the risk for birth of an infant SGA.

B Other Risks

In addition to the risk of developmental disabilities subsequent to preterm delivery or LBW, intellectual disability (ID) in children has long been linked to known maternal nutrition-related conditions such as iodine deficiency. ID of unknown cause, including autism spectrum disorders (ASD), has been found to be higher in children of mothers with diabetes, epilepsy (possibly due to drug–nutrient interactions), and anemia [19]. This large population-based study in Western Australia used linked databases of children born between 1983 and 1992. It was studied in 2002 to identify 2865 children with ID of unknown cause (grouped into mild to moderate, $n = 2462$; severe to profound, $n = 212$; and ASD with ID, $n = 181$) and 236,964 children without ID. Mothers with anemia ($n = 1101$) were five times more likely (odds ratio (OR) = 5.26) to have a child with severe ID (IQ <35 to 40), even after socioeconomic variables were introduced into the stepwise logistic regression model (OR = 4.93).

In a large population-based study of children in Hungary with ($n = 781$) and without ($n = 22,843$) Down syndrome, the investigators found a protective effect for maternal iron supplementation (150–300 mg/day of ferrous sulfate) during the first month of gestation [20]. Note that iron and folate, two nutrients related to LBW, are both depleted in pregnancy and must be replaced [11].

The toxic effects of mercury on the developing fetus are well-known [21], and the U.S. Department of Health and Human Services has recommended limiting seafood consumption by pregnant women because of its high mercury content. However, a large study (11,875 women) in the United Kingdom [22] indicated that restricting seafood intake to 340 g/day resulted in adverse neurodevelopmental outcomes in children, whereas higher intakes had no ill effects. The assumption is that this is due to a deficiency of omega-3 fatty acids because few women took fish oil supplements. These fatty acids have been shown to have positive effects on neurodevelopment [23,24], as have other nutrients found in fish, such as choline, zinc, and copper [25]. Although protective effects of other dietary components were not considered in the Australian study, there is evidence that selenium plays a protective role by reducing the bioavailability of mercury [26].

C Spina Bifida and Other Birth Defects

The recognition of a relationship between nutrition and the etiology of certain developmental disabilities has been most fully realized in the case of spina bifida and other neural tube defects (NTDs). Although the link between diet and NTDs was suspected as early as the 1960s [27,28] and demonstrated repeatedly in studies that implicated vitamins and minerals in general [28], and gradually focused on folate in particular [29], there was no public health campaign in the United States to increase folate intake until the mid-1990s after the publication of the Medical Research Council's definitive study [30]. Then, rather than directing efforts toward increasing women's intake of folate-containing foods, the emphasis was on folate supplementation for pregnant women followed by the passage of the mandatory fortification of cereal grain products that went into effect in January 1998. Since then, the Centers for Disease Control and Prevention (CDC) has reported a 36% decrease in the prevalence of NTDs, comparing data from 1995–1996 (10.8/10,000 population) with those from 2006 (6.9/10,000 population) [31]. In an earlier report [32], the CDC estimated an approximate decrease of 26% in the reported prevalence of NTDs, comparing data from 1995–1996 with those from 1999–2000, the year following the mandate [32]. The report from the Center on Birth Defects and Developmental Disabilities (CBDDD) noted that the decrease is less than predicted from research trials [33], which led to the Healthy People 2010 goal of a 50% reduction. The Healthy People 2020 goal, MCH 28-1, is a more modest 10% improvement in the incidence of spina bifida using a baseline of 34.2 live births or fetal deaths/100,000 live births (2005–2006 data from the National Birth Defects Prevention Network, CDC, and CBDDD) and a target of 30.8/100,000 live births [34]. It is worth noting that the incidence of spina bifida births is not equally spread among racial groups. The rate is higher among Hispanic groups (36.7) than whites (34.4), and it is much lower among non-Hispanic blacks (28.4), despite this group having the lowest blood folate levels both before and after fortification.

The CDC recommends increased folic acid intake (supplements or fortified breakfast cereals) and charges health care professionals to recommend these to women of child-bearing age [32]. There is no mention of the desirability of improving the general diet of these women, although the editor acknowledges that there may be other causes of NTDs besides folate insufficiency, and this may explain the slow reduction in incidence past the initial period of fortification. A group of investigators in The Netherlands reported significantly lower dietary intakes of iron, magnesium, niacin, fiber, plant protein, and polysaccharides in mothers of infants with spina bifida ($n = 106$) compared to controls ($n = 181$), independent of periconceptional folic acid use [35]. They also found increased risk related to dietary intake of mono- and disaccharides, which they suggest supports the importance of optimal carbohydrate intake during neural tube formation. In addition, it has been suggested that choline is another nutrient that, along with folate and B_{12}, may increase the risk of NTDs when inadequate in the diet due to its important role in the methionine cycle, which is crucial to brain development [36]. The dietary recommendations for choline were set for the first time in 1998 [37].

Our current understanding of the role of folate in the pathogenesis of NTDs awaited the unraveling of the mystery of the human genome and the development of the field of epigenetics. The research on DNA, RNA, and human chromosomes tells us that the genome, or the inheritable information held in the chromosomes, is not immutable but may be affected by epigenetic markers that interact with other components of the genome. Nutrigenomics, also referred to as nutritional genomics, introduces a molecular approach that integrates genomics, nutrition, and health [38,39]. The science focuses on the differential influences that nutrients have on the regulation of gene expression by way of nuclear receptors that regulate processes such as embryonic development and cell differentiation and proliferation [40]. It is thought that in the case of folate, because of its role in the methylation of DNA, a deficiency occurring during the periconceptional period can lead to epigenetic alterations in the DNA of the embryo and to NTDs in the fetus of those women who are genetically susceptible and/or whose need for folate is elevated. Interestingly, the gene that encodes the enzyme methylenetetrahydrofolate reductase (MTHFR), important in the methylation cycle, has a polymorphism that is common in Mexico (32%) but has a very low frequency among African Americans, paralleling the racial demographics of the prevalence of spina bifida alluded to previously [39]. It is certain

that nutrigenomics holds future promise in improving maternal and child health.

Another food-related factor that has been implicated in the high incidence of NTDs among Mexican Americans is fumonisins, a class of mycotoxins produced by mold, which interferes with folate metabolism. In response to an "outbreak" of NTDs along the Texas—Mexico border in 1990—1991, an epidemiological study linked it to high levels of fumonisins in the corn used to make tortillas, and other corn products, which form a large part of the diet of this population [41]. Other risk factors, such as folate intake (dietary plus multivitamin), were not confounders. In fact, B_{12} levels have been shown to be a more important predictor of risk in this population than folate levels [42], and low maternal B_{12} status has been shown to be an independent risk factor in a folic acid-fortified population in Canada [43].

Although orofacial clefts (cleft lip or palate or both) are not considered a developmental disability per se, there is evidence of an association between their occurrence and maternal nutrition as well as a rationale for the potential contribution of several nutrients (folate, niacin, thiamine, B_6, B_{12}, riboflavin, zinc, amino acids, and carbohydrates) to their etiology. In a large multistate case—control study using 1997—2000 data from the National Birth Defects Prevention Study, Shaw and colleagues [44], via phone interviews and food frequency questionnaires, found an association between iron and riboflavin intakes and a reduction in risk. Other studies point to the contribution of vitamins B_1 and B_6 and niacin [45].

D Fetal Alcohol Syndrome

Fetal alcohol syndrome (FAS) or, as proposed by the American Academy of Pediatrics, alcohol-related neurodevelopmental disorder and alcohol-related birth defects, is defined by pre- and postnatal growth disturbances, dysmorphic facial features, and intellectual disability; behavioral abnormalities are common, as are motor problems, facial anomalies, and cardiac defects [46]. FAS represents an example of a developmental disability in which prenatal nutrition likely plays a major role in the etiology. This is due to (1) the dietary energy provided by alcohol (7.1 kcal/g or 29.7 kJ), which replaces foods containing essential micronutrients, thereby putting the mother and fetus at risk for nutrient deficiencies, and (2) the interference of alcohol with the metabolism of all fat- and water-soluble vitamins, especially folate, and zinc [47]. These nutrients are key to fetal development because of their involvement in multiple systems: enzyme, gene transcription, and transport. Folate insufficiency, mentioned previously in the etiology of spina bifida and cleft lip and palate, has also been implicated in the etiology of limb and heart abnormalities and Down syndrome [48]. Severe zinc deficiency has been linked to intrauterine growth retardation and teratogenesis; mild to moderate deficiency has been associated with congenital malformations, LBW, and preterm delivery [49]. Because of the wide array of nutrients that have been implicated in promoting optimal birth outcomes, it would seem of utmost importance that clinicians and public health professionals urge women of childbearing age to eat a well-balanced diet rather than relying primarily on vitamin and mineral supplements or population-based fortification of foods or food ingredients, as has been suggested by some [50].

E Newborn Screening for Metabolic Disorders

Population-based newborn screening (NBS) for metabolic disorders has been established as a preventive public health measure available to all neonates. If infants with specific metabolic, endocrine, and other disorders are identified by NBS in the first few days of life, the diagnostic process can be completed and treatment started before physical and neurological damage occurs. Many of the disorders screened by NBS programs are autosomal recessive. This means that each parent carries the affected gene, and the risk of having an affected infant is one in four for each pregnancy. Thus, affected infants identified by NBS usually do not have a positive family history of the disorder.

Successful NBS of infants depends on reliable, valid, and timely laboratory results. Many states have established a central NBS laboratory, which supports a rigid quality control process. The initial NBS report provides a presumptive positive result that must be confirmed by mandatory laboratory confirmation of the diagnosis.

The American Academy of Pediatrics [51] recommends that an NBS blood sample be collected before the infant is discharged from the hospital nursery. If the blood sample is collected before the infant is 24 hours of age, it is essential that a second screening sample be obtained. NBS programs require a small sample of dried blood, which is submitted on filter paper. This type of sample is easily transported to the central laboratory, and many tests can be completed on a single blood sample. Tandem mass spectrometry technology has increased the number of disorders that can be effectively screened [52].

An effective NBS program involves timely community-based collection of initial blood samples, laboratory confirmation, education of primary care providers and families, as well as specific disorder follow-up, management, and evaluation components [53]. Each

TABLE 17.2 Generally Accepted Criteria for Newborn Screening for a Specific Disorder

Symptoms are usually absent in newborns.

Disease results in developmental impairment, serious illness, or death.

Sensitive, specific laboratory tests are available on a mass population basis.

Disease occurs frequently enough to warrant screening.

Successful treatment procedures are available.

Benefits of screening justify the cost.

Follow-up and treatment programs are available.

Source: *Adapted from Kaye, C. I., and the Committee on Genetics (2006). Newborn screening fact sheets.* Pediatrics 118, 934–963.

state has developed individual legislative NBS mandates. However, the March of Dimes [54], the American Academy of Pediatrics [52], and the American Society of Human Genetics [55] have developed recommendations and guidelines for expanded NBS, which, it is hoped, will be universally adopted. The general criteria for inclusion of a disorder in an NBS panel are shown in Table 17.2. Resources for up-to-date information on expanded NBS programs are shown in Table 17.3.

Expanded NBS programs provide the opportunity for earlier presumptive positive identification. Recent laboratory and clinical developments provide an increased specificity in diagnosis and treatment modalities. Thus, the long-term outcome for persons with inborn errors of metabolism is brighter than in the past. The contrast between outcomes without early treatment and expected outcomes with early identification and treatment are shown in Table 17.4 and discussed further in Section IV.

III THE FUNCTIONAL APPROACH TO NUTRITION ASSESSMENT FOR CHILDREN WITH SPECIAL NEEDS

There are five functional areas to be assessed when measuring a child's nutritional status: growth, dietary intake, elimination patterns, medical status and medications, and feeding behaviors and skills [56]. For children with special health care needs, these five areas may all contain specific and relevant information that relates to nutritional status. Special needs vary widely, from conditions that may only mildly affect nutritional status, such as ID, to those with severe and chronic nutritional implications, such as some neuromotor or metabolic disorders. However, these five functional areas can provide a framework for the nutritional assessment regardless of the type of special health care need.

TABLE 17.3 Newborn Screening Informational Resources

Resource	Description	URL
American College of Human Genetics (ACMG) model ACT sheets and screening algorithms	ACTion (ACT) sheets and algorithms developed by experts of the ACMG involved in newborn screening for endocrine, hematological, genetic, and metabolic diseases. The material describes the interrelationships between the conditions screened in newborn screening laboratories and the markers (analytes) used for screening. For each marker(s), there is (1) an ACT sheet that describes the short-term actions a health professional should follow in communicating with the family and determining the appropriate steps in the follow-up of the infant who has screened positive and (2) an algorithm that presents an overview of the basic steps involved in determining the final diagnosis in the infant.	http://www.acmg.net/resources/policies/ACT/condition-analyte-links.htm
The National Newborn Screening and Genetics Resource Center (NNSGRC)	Provides information and resources in the area of newborn screening and genetics to benefit health professionals, the public health community, consumers, and government officials; describes the newborn screening program in each state.	http://genes-r-us.uthscsa.edu
March of Dimes (MOD)	MOD recommends that all infants in all states receive newborn screening for 29 disorders for which effective treatment is available. The 29 disorders can be grouped into five categories: (1) amino acid metabolism disorders, (2) organic acid metabolism disorders, (3) fatty acid oxidation disorders, (4) the hemoglobinopathies, and (5) others; the basic description and treatment for each disorder are provided.	http://www.marchofdimes.com/professionals/14332_15455.asp
Kaye, C. I., and the Committee on Genetics (2006). Newborn screening fact sheets. *Pediatrics* 118, 934–963.	Fact sheets from the American Academy of Pediatrics that describe each disorder, frequency, treatment, and outcome.	http://genes-r-us.uthscsa.edu/NBS_%20Fact%20Sheets.pdf

Levels of nutrition assessment can be categorized from screening (level 1) to more comprehensive but still generalized (level 2) and specialized assessment as part of an interdisciplinary team (level 3) [7]. All three levels of nutrition screening and assessment should cover the five functional areas, but the amount and type of information gathered are different depending on the purpose of the interaction and the training of the health care provider. The purpose of screening is to identify children at risk for nutrition problems, to refer children with more severe problems to the next level of care, and to provide anticipatory guidance and educational materials to children and their families regarding the prevention of nutrition problems [7]. Although screening can be completed with information from the caregiver working with health care providers from other disciplines [57], more in-depth nutrition assessment and intervention usually require a registered dietitian (RD), often in conjunction with a specialized interdisciplinary team. For many children with special health care needs, their nutritional status will be assessed, monitored, and intervention provided on an ongoing basis by a pediatric RD (preferably master's prepared) who has been trained in a particular area, such as pulmonary disease, metabolic disorders, or feeding skill development. These dietitians, working with the health care team, utilize their specialized skills to optimize a child's nutritional status in the context of the child's developmental level and medical conditions, as well as the other therapies being provided.

A Measuring Growth

Growth information is used in nutrition assessment to compare an individual child's growth to that of his or her peers and to evaluate the growth pattern over time. For the information to be valuable, anthropometric measurements must be accurate, the data must be plotted correctly, and the appropriate reference data should be used for comparison [58,59]. At a minimum, weight, height (or length for children who cannot stand independently), and head circumference (especially for children up to 3 years of age) should be measured. Ideally, some form of body composition measurement is also used, with the simplest and most well referenced being skinfold measurements obtained with calipers, which have been shown to be helpful in determining differences in body composition in children with developmental disabilities [60].

To determine growth rate in children, weight and height for age can be plotted on the CDC growth

TABLE 17.4 Selected Metabolic Disorders That Require Medical Nutrition Therapy (MNT)

Disorder	Pathway affected	Outcome without treatment	Outcome with early identification and treatment	MNT	Supplements/ medications	Biochemical parameters monitored
Disorders of amino acid metabolism						
Phenylketonuria (PKU)	Phenylalanine hydroxylase	Mental retardation (IQ < 40)	Normal IQ (requires lifelong treatment)	Low phenylalanine, supplemented tyrosine	Potentially, BH4 for some patients	Plasma phenylalanine, tyrosine
Maple syrup urine disease (MSUD)	Branched-chain ketoacid dehydrogenase complex	Encephalopathy → death	Variable; may be cognitively compromised	Low leucine, isoleucine, valine	L-Carnitine	Plasma leucine, isoleucine, valine, alloisoleucine
Glutaric acidemia, type 1	Glutaryl-CoA dehydrogenase	Impaired movement, dystonia, vomiting, seizures, coma	No long-term data	Low lysine, tryptophan	L-Carnitine; riboflavin	Electrolytes, blood glucose, plasma amino acids
Homocystinuria (HCY)	Cystathionine β-synthase	Cardiac problems, organ damage, psychiatric disturbances, death	Variable; may be physically and cognitively compromised	Low methionine, supplement cysteine	Folate, betaine	Plasma methionine, total and free homocysteine
Isovaleric acidemia	Isovaleryl-CoA dehydrogenase	Metabolic acidosis → coma → death	Variable; may be cognitively compromised	Low leucine	L-Carnitine, glycine	Plasma amino acids (isovaleryl carnitine), urine organic acids (isovaleryl glycine)
Tyrosinemia, type 1	Fumarylacetoacetate hydrolase	Liver failure → death	Prevention of neurologic crisis, renal and hepatic failure, rickets	Low tyrosine, phenylalanine	Orfadin (nitisionine)	Plasma tyrosine, phenylalanine, methionine, succinate, alpha-fetoprotein
Disorders of carbohydrate metabolism						
Hereditary fructose intolerance (HFI)	Fructose-1-phosphate aldolase B	Hypoglycemia, liver cancer → death	Typical growth, development	Restrict fructose, sucrose		Liver function enzymes
Galactosemia	Galactose-1-phosphate uridyl transferase	Sepsis → severe delays, death	Often learning disabilities	Restrict galactose, use soy formula		Galactose-1-phosphate
Glycogen storage disease, type 1a	Glucose-6-phosphatase	Glycogen stored in liver, severe hypoglycemia, liver cancer → death	Normalization of glucose levels, moderation in liver size, decreased risk of liver cancer	Low lactose, fructose, sucrose; low-fat, high complex carbohydrate	Raw cornstarch, iron and calcium supplements	Cholesterol, triglycerides, uric acid, liver function (AST, ALT, GGT), blood glucose levels
Disorders of fatty acid oxidation						
Long-chain acyl-CoA dehydrogenase deficiency (LCAD)	Long-chain acyl-CoA dehydrogenase	Cardiomyopathy, hepatomegaly, encephalopathy, hypotonia	Variable	Low-fat, low long-chain fatty acids, avoid fasting	L-Carnitine, medium-chain triglycerides, thiamine, DHA, glycine	Plasma acylcarnitines, CK, uric acid, liver function studies, CBC, iron status
Medium-chain acyl-CoA dehydrogenase deficiency (MCAD)	Medium-chain acyl-CoA dehydrogenase	Encephalopathy, hepatomegaly, disability due to severe episodes	No sequelae if no episodes of severe hypoglycemia	Moderate fat, low medium-chain fatty acids, avoid fasting	L-Carnitine	If well, plasma carnitine; if ill, electrolytes, blood glucose

(Continued)

A. FOOD AND NUTRITION INTAKE FOR HEALTH

TABLE 17.4   *(Continued)*

Disorder	Pathway affected	Outcome without treatment	Outcome with early identification and treatment	MNT	Supplements/ medications	Biochemical parameters monitored
Disorders of organic acid metabolism						
Methylmalonic aciduria (MMA)	Methylmalonyl-CoA mutase or cobalamin co-factor synthesis	Metabolic acidosis coma → death	Variable; may be cognitively compromised	Low protein, isoleucine, methionine, threonine, valine	L-Carnitine, sodium benzoate,[a] bicitra	Methylmalonic acid, electrolytes, kidney function (BUN, creatinine), carnitine
Propionic academia (PA)	Propionyl-CoA carboxylase	Metabolic acidosis coma → death	Variable; may be cognitively compromised	Low protein, isoleucine, methionine, threonine, valine, long-chain unsaturated fatty acids	L-Carnitine, sodium benzoate, biotin, bicitra	Urine organic acids, plasma electrolytes, L-carnitine, kidney function
Disorders of urea cycle metabolism						
Ornithine transcarbamylase deficiency (OTC)	Ornithine transcarbamylase	Hyperammonemia → severe delays or death	Variable; may be cognitively compromised	Low protein, supplement essential amino acids, increased energy	L-Carnitine, sodium benzoate, sodium phenylbutyrate,[a] L-arginine	Plasma amino acids, ammonia, electrolytes, L-carnitine, citrulline, arginine
Citrullinemia (CIT)	Argininosuccinate synthetase		Variable; may be cognitively compromised	Low protein, supplement essential amino acids, increased energy	L-Carnitine, sodium benzoate, sodium phenylbutyrate, L-citrulline	Plasma amino acids, ammonia, electrolytes, L-carnitine, citrulline, arginine
Carbamyl phosphate synthetase deficiency (CPS)	Carbamyl phosphate synthetase	Hyperammonemia → severe delays or death	Variable; may be cognitively compromised	Low protein, supplement essential amino acids, increased energy	L-Carnitine, sodium benzoate, sodium phenylbutyrate, L-arginine	Plasma amino acids, ammonia, electrolytes, L-carnitine, citrulline, arginine
Argininosuccinic aciduria (ASA)	Argininosuccinate lyase	Hyperammonemia → severe delays or death	Variable; may be cognitively compromised	Low protein, supplement essential amino acids, increased energy	L-carnitine, sodium benzoate, sodium phenylbutyrate	Plasma amino acids, ammonia, electrolytes, L-carnitine, arginine

[a]*Sodium benzoate and sodium phenylbutyrate are chemicals administered to enhance waste ammonia excretion; other compounds producing the same effect are also used.*

charts [61]. The CDC charts provide a useful reference to monitor weight in relation to stature, including BMI for children older than 2 years. In most cases, BMI-for-age charts are not available for special conditions and have not been validated for use with children with special health care needs whose body composition often differs from that of typically developing children. Triceps and subscapular skinfolds along with arm circumference measurements can further define the growth and body composition data for the child. All of these anthropometric data used together can give a general picture of the nutritional status of the child, whether the child is underweight or overfat, and how linear growth is progressing. In children with neuromotor disorders that make measuring length difficult (e.g. spasticity and contractures), other types of anthropometric measurements have been developed (e. g., knee height or segmental measurements) with which to estimate stature and linear growth [62], although their clinical usefulness depends on the knowledge and skill of the clinicians obtaining the measurements.

Although the CDC growth charts, which are based on the growth of large numbers of healthy children, can be used to plot growth, some physical conditions affect growth potential. There are specialized charts that may be considered for use with children affected by these conditions. The rationale for using specialized growth charts is clear for genetic disorders where there is evidence that linear growth potential is different. However, the development and use of growth charts for nongenetic conditions, such as cerebral palsy, is complicated by the fact that the underlying cause of the disorder does not change the genetic growth potential. The online training module, "Children with Special Health Care Needs," is available for a full discussion of these charts (HRSA Growth Charts Training website at depts.washington.edu/growth). Although specialized growth charts may serve as useful references, they have significant limitations. Generally, they are developed from relatively small, homogeneous samples of children with unknown nutritional status, and data used to develop the charts may have been obtained using inconsistent measuring techniques. One recommendation is to plot the growth patterns of children on both the specialized charts, when appropriate, and the CDC growth charts [59]. This will allow comparisons of growth to the general population of children and to the references for children identified with a similar condition. Assessing serial growth measurements and using disorder-specific growth charts available for some genetic disorders (e.g., Down syndrome and Prader–Willi syndrome) will help differentiate between normal growth and alterations in growth rate resulting from poor nutrition. To interpret the growth data and understand the causes for unusual growth patterns, further information is needed.

B Assessing Dietary Intake

Analysis of a child's dietary pattern can predict and prevent nutrient deficiencies and, as with anthropometric data, requires accurate information to be useful. Data collection techniques may range from screening based on food groups and frequency of consumption to conducting a 24-hour recall and computer-assisted analysis of food records kept for 3 or more days. The assessment method should depend on the type and accuracy of information needed. Nutrient adequacy is usually compared to the daily recommended intakes (DRIs) for a child's age and size, unless there are known high-risk nutrients [59]. For some conditions, there are known issues of marginal micronutrient status, such as vitamin D status with chronic use of some anticonvulsant medications [63] and for several nutrients when low food intake is a chronic problem (e.g., for some children with cerebral palsy) [64,65]. Dietary analysis will reveal if there are any specific nutrients or groups of nutrients of concern. In addition, energy intake must be assessed and compared to estimated needs for each

child. If anthropometric measurement data provide evidence that the child is overweight or underweight (indicating chronic or current inappropriate energy intake) or has altered lean or adipose tissue patterns, this information should be considered along with the dietary assessment in determining the child's energy needs. For children with short stature or who are overweight or underweight, it is best to calculate energy intake recommendations based on current height (kcal/cm) rather than weight (kcal/kg).

Information relating to other functional areas—elimination patterns, the use of medications (and nutrition supplements), and feeding skills and behaviors—can be included as part of the dietary assessment. When conducting a 24-hour dietary recall or analyzing a food record, information is gathered about: (1) food textures; (2) feeding frequency, methods, and caregiver and child behaviors and interactions; and (3) type, amount, and timing of supplement and medication use. Along with the nutrient analysis, dietary assessment should include checking for possible drug–nutrient interactions. Also, fluid intake and output, and the frequency and texture of bowel movements are assessed to determine if chronic constipation or diarrhea are present, which can compromise feeding behaviors and nutritional status. Children with special needs may have significant feeding skill delays, or feeding patterns that fit their developmental level rather than their chronological age, which will alter the type, texture, and quantity of foods they are able to consume. This may pose a challenge to meeting the nutrient and energy needs of the child in the volume of food consumed. Food preferences and refusals, which may be related to past or current medical conditions, need to be taken into account when designing dietary interventions. Often, working with a team that includes the parent/caregiver, a feeding therapist, and a nurse or physician can aid in determining the most appropriate type and texture of foods to use to facilitate the child's optimal feeding skill development, as well as his or her nutritional intake (see Section IV).

C Considering Medical Conditions

Medical conditions can have an impact on nutritional status in a number of ways (shown in Table 17.1). Some conditions (e.g., Prader–Willi syndrome) actually alter a child's energy and other nutrient needs, whereas other conditions interfere with adequate nutrient intake or utilization (e.g., feeding problems in some types of cerebral palsy). Examples of conditions that increase energy demands are cardiac and pulmonary complications of prematurity and cerebral palsy in which there are significant hypertonia/spasticity or athetoid movements. Other chronic illnesses associated with high energy needs are HIV/AIDS, cystic fibrosis, and mitochondrial disorders. Some genetic disorders are associated with lowered metabolic rates resulting in decreased energy needs (e.g., Down syndrome and Prader–Willi syndrome). Conditions associated with reduced or low muscle mass (as in muscular dystrophies) also result in decreased energy needs. In genetic disorders in which short stature occurs, overall food, nutrient, and energy needs may be lower than those of age peers throughout adolescence and adulthood. If a child has reduced activity levels because of immobility, energy demands will also be lower.

With a few exceptions, such as copper deficiency in Wilson's disease and some metabolic disorders, most medical conditions do not have a primary effect on an individual's micronutrient needs [58]. There is not enough evidence to suggest that nutrients associated with energy metabolism be adjusted even with very high or low energy intakes. Therefore, the DRIs are still the most appropriate guideline for nutrient requirements for children with special needs. In the self-study curriculum "Nutrition for Children with Special Health Care Needs" (available online at www.pacificwestmch.org), the following questions are suggested to assess whether and how a medical condition will affect nutritional status:

1. Does the condition (or medication used to treat the condition) have an effect on the child's nutrient needs?
2. Does the condition change the types of foods the child can eat?
3. Does the condition alter the amount of food that the child can reasonably be expected to consume?
4. Does the condition affect the amount of time the child can spend at the table (eating)? Does this make a smaller intake likely?
5. Does the medication or therapy schedule interfere with scheduled meal or snack times?

Consideration of these issues and the impact on overall nutrient intake and nutritional status should be the final component of the nutrition assessment for children with special needs.

IV EVIDENCE-BASED INTERVENTIONS FOR SELECTED CONDITIONS

A Inborn Errors of Metabolism

Inborn errors of metabolism (IEM) are the classic example of the secondary prevention of disability through nutrition therapy. The basic concepts, principles, and strategies of treatment of selected disorders of protein, carbohydrate, and fat metabolism are presented here. A complete discussion of diagnosis and management of the array of metabolic disorders

TABLE 17.5 Components of Medical Nutrition Therapy for Metabolic Disorders

Identify precise modifications required for treatment of the disorder.

Provide nutritional surveillance to ensure that medical nutrition therapy is adequate.

Provide a mechanism for follow-up of child for symptoms of nutritional deficiency or toxicity.

Provide emotional and educational support for child and family.

can be found elsewhere [66,67]. Table 17.5 outlines the essential components of medical nutrition therapy (MNT) for treatment of metabolic disorders. Although the clinical and biochemical presentation of each metabolic disorder is unique and the disorders present a range from mild to life-threatening illness, metabolic disorders can be thought of as a group in which the absence or inactivity of a specific enzyme or co-factor causes the buildup of the substrate and deficiency of the product. The goal of treatment for IEM is to strive for correction of the biochemical abnormality. The outcome of treatment for these disorders is variable and depends on early diagnosis and intensive and continuous intervention. MNT is the primary mode of treating metabolic disorders.

1 Principles of Medical Nutrition Therapy

The two major principles of MNT for IEM are (1) to mitigate the effects of the altered enzyme by modifying components of dietary intake to adjust the environment at the cellular level and (2) to provide protein, energy, and nutrients to support growth and development.

For many disorders, the treatment is determined by the identification of the missing or inactive enzyme. In an effort to modify the detrimental effect of the decreased or absent enzyme activity, the paradigm of "working around" the enzyme is used. In many cases, decreasing the substrate available for the reaction and supplementing the product to promote "normal" blood levels prevents or decreases the deleterious effects of the disorder. For example, in the treatment of PKU, phenylalanine (substrate) is restricted because of the absence or inactivity of phenylalanine hydroxylase (enzyme), and tyrosine (product) is supplemented. In some disorders, the absent or inactive enzyme is further down the amino acid degradation pathway and may affect the metabolism of two or more amino acids—for example, leucine, isoleucine, and valine in maple syrup urine disease (MSUD).

The affected amino acids in most disorders of amino acid metabolism are "essential"—that is, they cannot be synthesized by the body and therefore must be provided in the diet. These critical essential amino acids (EAAs) must be provided at a level that promotes growth and development but is restricted enough to prevent toxic buildup of amino acid(s) that cannot be metabolized.

In some disorders, the additional step of enhancing enzyme activity by supplying its co-factor can be helpful. An example of this is providing pharmacological doses of biotin in biotinidase deficiency [68] or providing vitamin B_6, on which cystathionine β-synthase is dependent, in some forms of homocystinuria [69]. Drug trials with a synthetic co-factor (tetrahydrobiopterin) have shown promise in providing a drug therapy that aids in the management of PKU based on this principle [70,71].

In metabolic disorders of carbohydrate metabolism, such as galactosemia, the nutrient of concern (galactose) is not essential. Therefore, the goal of effective MNT is to eliminate as much of the exogenous component as possible from the diet. There is no established requirement for galactose because it is produced endogenously [72]. Other sources of nourishment need to be provided to compensate for the omitted foods and their nutrients.

Disorders of fatty acid metabolism require a source of energy other than fat because fat cannot be metabolized to meet energy needs. Fatty acids of specific carbon lengths are often minimized or eliminated, depending on whether or not the fatty acid is essential for growth and development. For example, in long-chain acyl-CoA dehydrogenase deficiency or very long-chain acyl-CoA dehydrogenase deficiency, shorter chain fats can be metabolized and are often supplemented; for example, medium-chain triglycerides are provided as MCT oil [66]. However, in medium-chain acyl-CoA dehydrogenase deficiency, sources of medium-chain fat should be modestly restricted. Other essential components of treatment are (1) supplementation of L-carnitine, an amino acid that functions in the transport of fatty acid acyl-CoA esters during mitochondrial β-oxidation, and (2) avoidance of fasting because of the accumulation of partially oxidized metabolites associated with impaired energy production [73].

2 Providing Medical Nutrition Therapy

The general principles of protein and energy management that support general nourishment as well as the issues of biochemical control specific to the disorder must be addressed [74,75]. The infant or child needs to be provided with adequate amino acids, total protein, nitrogen, and energy to support growth. Energy needs may be increased when L-amino acids provide the protein equivalent, and maintaining an adequate energy intake is essential in preventing catabolism. It must also be noted that suppression of destructive metabolites can produce striking biochemical and clinical improvement.

3 Providing Adequate Nourishment

For some disorders, total protein is not restricted, but the composition of the protein may be adjusted. For example, treatment of PKU requires the restriction of phenylalanine intake but not total protein. This is accomplished by using a specially designed semisynthetic medical formula. Infants and children with IEM must obtain most of their protein from specialized metabolic formulas. Natural foods seldom provide more than 25% (often 10%) of the protein requirements of infants and children with amino acid, organic acid, or urea cycle disorders.

Protein in the specialized formulas is provided as individual L-amino acids (excluding those amino acids that are contraindicated for each condition). L-Amino acids are more readily oxidized than intact protein; thus, the requirement for protein when L-amino acids are the protein source is greater than usual. Adequate protein and energy are required to maintain an anabolic state. If adequate formula is not prescribed or consumed, a catabolic state will develop, causing both high plasma amino acids levels and clinical problems. Advances in food technology, combined with clinical nutrition research, have produced a naturally occurring protein moiety called glycomacropeptide, refined from whey, which is very low in phenylalanine and has been shown to improve protein retention, phenylalanine utilization, and to reduce hunger when substituted for some of the amino acid formula in the diets of people with PKU [76,77].

The urea cycle disorders require the restriction of overall protein intake because excess nitrogen from any source can be neurotoxic. However, it is also imperative to provide enough protein and energy to support growth. The formulas for the treatment of urea cycle disorders have a high concentration of amino acids to ensure ready incorporation into protein. Most children with these disorders also require medications to enhance the excretion of excess nitrogen through secondary pathways other than the urea cycle. For infants and children with urea cycle disorders, catabolism from excess protein, weight loss, illness, or infection is a danger. Hyperammonemia can occur rapidly (in several hours) and be life-threatening. The total amount of protein tolerated by the individual child depends on residual enzyme activity, age, and growth rate.

4 Supplying Restricted Amino Acids

Small amounts of the restricted EAAs specific to each disorder are required for growth and development. These EAAs are provided to the infant by including small amounts of proprietary infant formula in the metabolic formula mixture. As the child grows and matures, adding small amounts of cow or soy milk or fruits, vegetables, and grains can provide these essential amino acids.

5 Breast-Feeding

Some infants with metabolic disorders are able to maintain low and stable plasma amino acid levels with a combination of breast milk and metabolic formula feedings. Many infants are too metabolically fragile to maintain appropriate plasma levels with breast-feeding; for example, some infants with PKU are able to tolerate partial breast-feeding and maintain low plasma phenylalanine levels. Breast-feeding is overtly contraindicated for infants with some disorders, such as galactosemia.

6 Feeding

Poor appetite is not uncommon for children with IEM, especially urea cycle disorders, MSUD, and the organic acidemias. Reasons for poor appetite and poor feeding may be organic, behavioral, or both. Many children with IEM who have had acute episodes may also have a history of vomiting, which may lead to feeding avoidance.

7 Growth

Poor growth is often a reflection of several factors: (1) Infants who have endured a severe neonatal illness may require an extended time of appropriate nourishment before they catch up in growth, (2) frequent febrile illness may interfere with achieving expected physical growth, or (3) poor metabolic control or an inadequate protein or energy intake may interfere with growth. Many children with IEM who have little or no enzyme activity are medically fragile, and it is difficult to maintain metabolic balance and support typical growth patterns.

8 Monitoring for Children with Metabolic Disorders

The frequency of monitoring biochemical parameters depends on the age and health status of the child. Maintaining metabolic balance for children with IEM requires frequent and intensive monitoring of biochemical parameters specific to the disorder as well as those that reflect general nutritional status. The goal of treatment for all disorders is to achieve biochemical levels at or near the normal range. Laboratory parameters that are frequently monitored include plasma amino acids, urine organic acids, hematological status, protein status, electrolytes, blood lipids, and ammonia levels. A general plan to guide biochemical assessment is shown in Table 17.4.

9 Specialized Metabolic Team

As a group, children with IEM comprise a small percentage of the pediatric population, and even the most common of these disorders is rare in the general population. However, the health care needs of these children are specific and urgent. The American Academy of Pediatrics has recommended that a team experienced in management supervise the therapy of these children [51]. Effective treatment generally requires the expertise of a geneticist, dietitian, nurse, genetic counselor, psychologist, and neurologist. The complex nutritional and medical management of these children cannot occur effectively without the follow-up and support of the community teams. Communication among the team at the tertiary center, the community, and the family is crucial for supporting the best possible medical, nutritional, and intellectual outcome for these children.

B Prader—Willi Syndrome

Prader—Willi syndrome (PWS) is caused by a microdeletion on paternally inherited genes on chromosome 15. PWS is associated with early failure to thrive, hypotonia, abnormal body composition, hypogonadism, short stature, and behavioral and learning issues [78]. Hyperphagia, which usually begins toward the end of the first year and is thought to be due to a hypothalamic abnormality, is accompanied by a lack of satiety. Thus, delay in identification and treatment of PWS can lead to the onset of gross obesity after infancy.

Abnormal food-seeking behavior is characteristic of PWS and includes hoarding and foraging for food as well as eating items generally considered to be inedible, such as garbage, pet food, or uncooked frozen food. Infants and children with PWS demonstrate a low metabolic rate and thus decreased energy needs. An intake as low as 1000—1200 kcal/day is often required to maintain a stable weight in older children [78]. Strict and consistent behavioral limits and the establishment of regular routines are helpful behavioral management strategies for food intake and behavioral concerns for children with PWS [79].

Controlled trials have shown that children with PWS benefit from growth hormone therapy from infancy through childhood and into adulthood [80,81]. However, growth hormone treatment does not "cure" the underlying causes of short stature in PWS, and it may not completely reverse short stature, relative hypotonia, and adiposity characteristic of PWS [82]. New standardized growth curves based on white children with PWS from birth to 36 months of age not treated with growth hormone have been generated [83]. These charts can be used to monitor growth patterns and assess nutritional status for similar infants and children with PWS both treated and not treated with growth hormone.

C Dietary Interventions for Children with Feeding Problems

With increased survival rates of premature and medically fragile infants, there is an increased population of children who are at risk for, or who demonstrate, feeding difficulties with multifactorial origins, depending on the degree of prematurity or LBW. For example, in premature infants, gastroesophageal reflux, a physiological and developmental consequence of prematurity, may occur three to five times per hour [84]. Poor coordination of the suck—swallow and suck—respiration is often predictive of feeding abnormalities [85]. Nutritional status and feeding development are of primary concern in the neonatal intensive care unit (NICU). Feeding skill development and transitions from parenteral to enteral nutrition in the medically fragile newborn are facilitated by an interdisciplinary team of health care providers, which includes the parents. Breast-feeding, or the feeding of breast milk, is encouraged as much as is possible for the newborn and his or her mother as an important means of nourishment, developing attachment, and for feeding skills to develop at the appropriate gestational age. Fortified human milk is often indicated in preterm infants to support optimal growth and bone mineralization [86]. Many infants are discharged from the NICU only after achieving at least a portion of their nutritional intake through oral routes, although the use of nasogastric, orogastric, and gastrostomy tube feedings has increased. However, to prevent later feeding problems, it is best to minimize the use of tube feedings or to encourage developmentally appropriate oral feedings as soon as the child is medically stable and physically able. Early introduction of feedings, as early as 33 weeks' gestational age, has been shown to accelerate the rate at which preterm infants are able to attain full oral feedings [87].

Among children with developmental delays and special health care needs, especially those born prematurely, the estimated incidence of feeding disorders ranges from 33 to 80%, depending on the definitions of feeding disorders [88—90]. Problems with feeding occur when: the components of normal feeding development are missing or delayed, there are significant behavioral refusals due to multiple etiologies, there are medical interventions and medications that interfere with appetite and regulation, or there are physiological problems related to the medical condition or disability (Table 17.6). An extensive discussion of the physiological and behavioral contributors to feeding problems is included in a special issue of *Developmental Disabilities Research Reviews* devoted to this topic [91]. Whereas inpatient behavioral therapy has been shown to be effective for children with feeding interaction problems [90], children with persistent physical challenges resulting in swallowing and other difficulties often require supplemental or total tube feedings for long periods of time and may never become independent oral feeders. Utilizing a sophisticated statistical method (latent class analysis) of chart review data from 286 children referred to a feeding team, Berlin and colleagues [92] demonstrated that children fed by gastrostomy tube had both more behavioral feeding problems and higher weights across all categories sharing common medical, developmental, and behavioral conditions. This group concluded that the presence of multiple, co-morbid conditions confers general, rather than specific, risk for feeding problems.

TABLE 17.6 Feeding Problems in Children with Special Health Care Needs

Feeding difficulty	Frequent causes	Associated conditions
Delayed or slow development	Hypertonia	Developmental delay
Posturing or seating difficulties	Hypotonia	Cerebral palsy
Persistence of primitive reflexes	Hypersensitivity	Cleft lip and cleft palate
Craniofacial anatomic problems	Developmental immaturity (prematurity)	Down syndrome (trisomy 21)
Uncoordinated sucking, chewing, swallowing	Gastroesophageal reflux	Prader—Willi syndrome
Behavioral refusals	Unpleasant intrusions into the oral cavity	Rett syndrome
Decreased appetite	Unpleasant feeding experiences (past or present)	Muscular dystrophy
	Constipation	Williams syndrome
	Increased secretions	Myelomeningocele with accompanying Arnold—Chiari malformation
	Decreased gastric motility	Autism
	Medications	Chronic respiratory diseases (cystic fibrosis, BPD, RDS)

An interdisciplinary team that can determine which factors are interacting as causes of the feeding difficulties is helpful in determining and coordinating appropriate interventions [89,91]. The challenge for the nutritionist on the interdisciplinary feeding team is to assess nutritional status and dietary intake and to determine how best the child can meet his or her nutritional needs using the most developmentally appropriate feeding methods and forms of foods whenever possible [56,59]. Use of dietary supplements, including nutritionally complete formulas, either orally or through a tube, is sometimes necessary to supply the necessary energy, protein, and other nutrients needed. It is often best to use the child's size and developmental stage (e.g., pubertal and prepubertal) to estimate nutrient needs rather than the child's chronological age. When estimating energy needs for children with feeding problems who are smaller, shorter, or heavier than their same-aged peers, it is recommended to use the child's height or length, rather than weight or ideal body weight or age, to determine the estimated energy needs.

Nutrition interventions for children with ASD are discussed in the next section, but it should be mentioned here that although children with ASD often have feeding challenges, the diet often meets or exceeds the RDA for protein, carbohydrates, and fat [93,94]. However, rigid mealtime patterns or limited food repertoires are common feeding issues for children with ASD [93,95,96]. For example, the child with ASD may insist on only white foods or demand a particular plate. The child may have a preference for only salty or only sweet foods or only foods of a certain texture. These behaviors may make family meals difficult, and severe food jags can lead to nutrient deficiency. If entire food groups are missing, or if there is excessive intake of a particular nutrient, a vitamin/mineral supplement may be appropriate. Pica (the eating of "nonfood" items) may also be more common than in the general population [93], and nutrition education and intervention may need to address this behavior. Therapies to expand food choices vary and can be difficult to implement. Families can be encouraged to offer new items with preferred foods [97] and to offer them repeatedly, possibly over a period of months. Interdisciplinary intervention is usually necessary, including a behavior specialist, or an occupational or speech therapist where texture or oral issues are also present.

Identifying the need for nutrition intervention early in a child's life—and providing ongoing and coordinated services between inpatient, early intervention, and school- and community-based services—is ideal but often challenging based on the complexity of the health care system and lack of nutritionist services available in many settings [6,98]. A practical and detailed description of feeding problems, developmental conditions leading to feeding problems, and suggested feeding and nutrition assessment strategies is included in the self-study curriculum referred to earlier, "Nutrition for Children with Special Health Care Needs," Module 3: Feeding Skills (available at www.pacificwestmch.org) [58].

D Autism Spectrum Disorders

1 Definition and Etiology

ASD is a group of disorders that includes pervasive developmental disorder not otherwise specified (PDD-NOS), Asperger syndrome, and autism. All diagnostic instruments rely on behavioral criteria outlined by the *Diagnostic and Statistical Manual of Mental Disorders*, fourth edition (*DSM-IV*), which include stereotyped behaviors, interactions, and activities, as well as limited social and communication abilities [99]. The *DSM-V* diagnostic criteria (under development) may also include unusual sensory processing because this is common in children with autism [100,101]. Intellectual abilities can range from typical to profound ID, but the majority of children with ASD display challenging behaviors, including distractibility, lack of focus/decreased attention span, and hyperactivity [102]. Although the reasons are not clear, the prevalence of ASD appears to be increasing in the United States; surveillance data from the CDC indicate that 1 out of 110 U.S. children has a potential diagnosis of ASD [103], and for boys, the estimated prevalence is even higher at 1 in 80 [104]. However, the National Survey of Children's Health, a large ($N = 78,037$) survey of children ages 3–17 years based on parent report, places the prevalence even higher at 1 in 91 children, or 1 in 58 boys [105]. This survey showed that non-Hispanic black and multiracial children were at lower risk of having an ASD than were white children.

The etiology of ASD is unknown, although it is likely that both genetic and environmental factors, possibly including nutrition, are involved. For example, it has been speculated that the steep rise in the prevalence of autism, which parallels the rise in the use of folic acid supplements and the fortification of foods implemented in 1998 to prevent neural tube defects, may be linked [106]. Children with autism and their mothers, compared to typically developing children and their mothers, have a decreased methylation capacity [107]. Rogers hypothesizes that MTHFR, the enzyme needed to activate folate as a methyl donor and that is subject to a gene variant (polymorphism) seen frequently in individuals with autism, may be key. Researchers at the University of California at Davis Mind Institute reported that mothers of children with autism in the Childhood Autism Risks from Genetics and Environment (CHARGE) study were less likely than the case-controlled mothers of typically developing children to have taken prenatal (not "ordinary") vitamins during the 3 months before and the first month of pregnancy [108]. This study also examined interaction effects between seven gene variants involved in the folate and transmethylation pathways, and it found significant interactions between prenatal vitamins and MTHFR and catechol-*O*-methyl transferase, further suggesting the involvement of an epigenetic (gene–environment) mechanism, probably involving the methyl donors folate and vitamin B_{12}. Evidence for the role of dysfunctional folate and/or methionine metabolism in autism was reviewed by Main and colleagues [109]. Although their findings did not conclusively implicate alterations in these metabolic pathways, largely due to methodological issues such as subject heterogeneity, inclusion of multiple polymorphisms, and lack of sufficient power in the studies reviewed, the indications underline the need for further research into maternal nutrition as an important environmental factor involved in epigenetic phenomena potentially involved in the etiology of autism.

Co-morbidities often seen in the ASD population, which may affect feeding or nutritional status, include fragile X syndrome, seizure disorder, oppositional disorder, and immune system dysregulation [94,110]. Currently, there is active research focused on gastrointestinal, nutrition, and feeding issues in children with ASD. Each is briefly discussed next.

2 Gastrointestinal Issues

Although the current diagnostic criteria for ASD do not include gastrointestinal (GI) symptoms, multiple reports since the 1970s describe chronic GI dysfunctions/symptoms of some sort in 30–80% of children with ASD [111], including diarrhea, constipation, abdominal bloating, discomfort, irritability, GI reflux, and vomiting [95]. Other studies have reported pathological findings in the GI tract of children with ASD, including increased intestinal permeability and compromised gut microflora [93,112]. Campbell and colleagues [113] showed that a variant in the promoter of the gene encoding the MET receptor tyrosine kinase is associated with ASD. This was the first study to demonstrate a possible genetic cause for the association between autism and GI disease, although as far back as 1961, Asperger suggested a link between autism and celiac disease [114].

The theories in the case of GI symptoms and ASD relate to possible food sensitivities and/or allergies, altered immune responses, and altered intestinal microflora. For example, there may be undigested opioid-like peptides from the proteins gluten and casein that cross the intestinal wall ("leaky gut") and the blood–brain barrier, where they stimulate opioid receptors, resulting in disturbances in brain neurotransmission causing, or increasing, behavioral symptoms [94,115]. Although some earlier studies reported increased urinary peptides in some children with ASD, a case–control study found no differences between those with ASD and typically developing controls [116]. Another theory holds that harmful gut flora, possibly resulting from overuse of antibiotics, may secrete neurological toxins and contribute to the intestinal permeability or "leaky gut." This is based on studies of stool samples that have shown an excess of pathogenic bacteria in some children with ASD. A survey of 600 primary care physicians indicated that 19% recommended probiotics for children with ASD; 59% supported families who wanted to use them [117]. An alternate theory is that children with ASD have an increased incidence of GI disorders such as gluten intolerance [93] because of autoimmune responses [118], as histopathologies of children with ASD have shown an irregular immune response [119]. This is the rationale for some regimens to include di- or trimethylglycine as methyl donors to enhance the immune response as well as neurotransmitters. Based on evidence that methylation pathways may be altered, compromising antioxidant/detoxification capacity (single-nucleotide polymorphisms have been identified in children with ASD and their families [107]), methyl donors vitamin B_{12} and folic acid/glutathione are recommended by some.

Finally, some nutrient deficiencies, or relative deficiencies, have been implicated in the etiology of some of the behavioral symptoms of autism. Vitamin B_6 is an example because of the role it plays in neurotransmission and based on evidence that there is a lack of an enzyme needed to convert it to its active form. Omega-3 fatty acids, essential for brain development, have been found to be low in the plasma of some children with ASD; oral supplementation has been reportedly used by 25% of families of children with ASD [120]. Improvements in behavior following a well-designed pilot trial have been reported [121].

Highly publicized case studies often lead families to choose an alternative diet for their child. Inflammation of the GI tract resulting from exposure to irritants is uncomfortable or even painful. Because of a limited ability to communicate, the child with ASD may not be able to make known his or her discomfort, which may worsen behavioral symptoms. Because most studies use parent or caregiver report of behavior changes in children after implementing the diet, a significant potential confounder is the parental placebo effect because parents seeking to find any treatment for their child may be susceptible to suggestion. Also, most studies have not been of a prospective, randomized, blinded design [122]; for example, they begin with a population of children with ASD who already have GI issues [123]. This makes it difficult to generalize findings to the entire ASD population. It remains unclear whether the gluten-/casein-free diet is a valid treatment for ASD or simply a treatment for co-morbid gluten/casein sensitivity in a subgroup of these children. Worse, the recommendations for alternative diets may be influenced by profit or ideology (some physicians sell the products they recommend).

In an effort to sort through the conflicting reports, a consensus report sponsored by the Autism Forum, a group of 28 participants in seven working groups (including nutrition) representing 10 disciplines and multiple organizations identified, graded, and evaluated publications related to GI issues and autism and found a general absence of high-quality research data, which precludes evidence-based recommendations at this time [124]. They developed and published 23 consensus statements, including the following:

- GI disturbances in ASD, likely highly prevalent, are incompletely understood and may be difficult to evaluate because of problems communicating discomfort/pain.
- Children with ASD and GI symptoms may have more problem behaviors than others with ASD; these may be a sign that a GI evaluation is warranted. (Consensus statements (CS) 1–3, 6, and 7)
- GI disturbance specific to ASD has not been established; evidence for abnormal GI permeability in ASD is limited, and the studies are methodologically challenged. (CS 4 and 5)
- ASD caregivers and health care providers need to know how to recognize signs and symptoms of GI disorders and other nutritional problems. (CS 8 and 9)
- Evaluation by a nutritionist recommended; anthropometry should be monitored; those with limited diets or taking supplements should be evaluated. (CS 9, 10, and 16)
- Additional studies are needed before recommending specific diets for ASD; data do not support the use of a casein-free or gluten-free diet (or both) as primary treatment. (CS 11 and 12)
- Detailed history to identify potential associations between GI and/or behavioral symptoms and allergies; involvement of specialists (GI, nutrition, and feeding therapists) can be beneficial. (CS 13–17)
- Direct relationship between immune dysfunction and ASD is not yet proven, but it warrants further investigation. (CS 17 and 18)
- Well-defined phenotypes and genotypes will enhance further clinical investigations. (CS 20–23)

At this time, therefore, there are no recommended diet therapies for ASD.

3 Nutrition Issues

The growth patterns of children with ASD are thought to be normal. However, studies have shown an increased rate of head growth in children with ASD [125]. Others have shown an increased rate of linear growth, weight gain, and body mass index [126]. Anthropometric data for this population should still consist of length, weight, weight/length, and head circumference. When the child is found to have a large head size, this should be considered when making weight/height comparisons because they could be deceptively increased. In children with ASD, it is not unusual to see a very low or very high BMI as a result of feeding issues.

The fact that the etiology of ASD is not well understood makes the diagnosis difficult for many families to accept, and they may try multiple interventions to improve their child's symptomatology, including dietary regimens. Complementary therapies are very popular; dramatic testimonials abound, and there is an active promotion of alternative and diet therapies at autism conferences attended by parents. Many books have been written, and websites touting alternative therapies are common. Levy and colleagues found that 30% of children with ASD had had dietary interventions by the time of diagnosis [127,128]; another study reported that 41% of respondents claimed that their children had benefited from dietary and nutritional treatments [129]. In a survey by the Interactive Autism Network, 54% of respondents reported using supplements, and 30% reported using dietary interventions (S.L. Hyman, personal communication, 2009). Given the lack of scientific evidence, the question is why do parents choose dietary therapies? Answers include: (1) frustration with the limitations of current therapies coupled with hope for a cure or at least an improvement in behavior, (2) comfort in knowing parents have done everything possible for their child, and (3) wanting to have some control over the treatment. Some parents prefer "harmless" treatments over drugs. Finally, parents may give the therapy credit for changes that would have occurred anyway. The greater the efforts, the more biased they may be toward seeing them "pay off."

Potential nutrition problems with the casein-free, gluten-free diet—an example of a popular diet—include risks associated with the avoidance of casein such as insufficiency of vitamin D and calcium [130]. Hediger and colleagues found decreased cortical bone in males with ASD [131]. Milk is often a major source of protein for children as well. The elimination of gluten leads to a risk of inadequate sources for B vitamins in the diet. Vitamin/mineral supplementation for these children may not be appropriate, sufficient, or safe (not regulated). For example, children's multivitamins typically lack enough calcium and vitamin D to make up for the lack of milk in the diet; the popular chewable children's "gummy" brand formulations lack iron.

"Diet and Nutrition in Children with Autism Spectrum Disorders: An Autism Treatment Network Collaborative Study" is a national research project (four sites throughout the country) that is studying the nutritional intake, including supplements and dietary modifications, of approximately 450 children with ASD. The purpose is to describe the nutritional status of these children, their associated medical and behavioral symptoms, and investigate any relationships among dietary intake, feeding behaviors, and food preferences of the children and their families [132].

The role of the dietitian/nutritionist who works with families of children with autism is to ensure adequate growth and development and to support the family who wants to try an alternative diet. Parents need to understand what is currently known about the efficacy of the diet (based on current evidence) and if there are any potential deficiencies; the more restrictive the diet, the greater the risk. It is important to help families clearly understand the difficulties that may arise in attempting to follow a special diet, especially when a child eats outside of the home on a daily basis (e.g., at school or with other caregivers). At school, eating separately or different foods may further isolate the child from his or her peers. The diet can be more costly than a traditional diet. If the child is a "picky eater" or has feeding problems, these may be complicating factors when introducing a restrictive diet. Because of an increased incidence of a limited food repertoire and resultant limited nutrient intake, children with ASD are at particular risk for anemia. Similarly, an increased prevalence of pica may suggest the need to measure hemoglobin and lead levels to rule out lead toxicity [93].

Currently, there are no drugs used specifically to treat ASD, but drug–nutrient interactions should be assessed if children are prescribed drugs to treat co-morbidities such as seizures or psychiatric symptoms. The most common drugs used in this population that have significant drug–nutrient interactions have been reviewed by Geraghty and colleagues [111]. They include those used for ADHD (Concerta and Strattera), which may cause a decrease in appetite and also nausea, vomiting, constipation, and diarrhea in the case of Strattera. Another category of commonly used medications are anticonvulsants (Depakote and Keppra); Depakote may also decrease appetite with associated nausea, vomiting, and diarrhea and also decrease serum vitamin D and calcium. The antipsychotic drugs (Zyprexa and Risperdal), on the other hand, may increase appetite and cause weight gain, at least in the case of Zyprexa. The use of secretin as an experimental therapy in the ASD population is currently being investigated and may have GI side effects [93]. An extensive review of the drugs used to treat symptoms associated with ASD is provided by Wink *et al.* [133].

4 Feeding Issues

Some behaviors seen with ASD, especially those related to sensory processing, which include taste, smell, and oral sensitivities [100], can lead to feeding or eating disorders. Despite the fact that sensory processing difficulties are not yet recognized as a core deficit in children with ASD, one study reported that these children showed differences in 92% of the sensory processing behaviors measured compared to typically developing children [134]. In fact, in a study in which children with autism were compared to other children with or without developmental delays, children with autism were more abnormal in responses to taste and smell than any of the other groups, and the differences were not related to either developmental level or IQ [101].

These sensory issues may be responsible for the high prevalence of problem eating behaviors seen in children with autism [135], which have been estimated to range between 46 and 89% [136]. These behaviors may include selective food refusals such as textures, colors, and food groups [137]. Schreck and Williams [95] reported that restrictive food acceptance was common in children with ASD across all food groups except carbohydrates. Other selective behaviors affecting feeding may relate to the GI issues referred to previously, fear of new foods, or obsessive mealtime rituals such as the need for sameness. The child with ASD may also have difficulties with changes in the environment [95], which may lead to problems with school mealtimes where a loud and boisterous cafeteria may be overwhelming such that a child with ASD may have difficulty eating lunch with a group of peers.

V CONCLUSION

In this review, we provided examples of nutrition issues related to the role of nutrition in the primary (maternal nutrition) and secondary (MNT for IEM) prevention of developmental disabilities and in the secondary prevention of nutrition-related disorders that are commonly seen in children with special health care needs. Emphasis was given to several important concepts. First is the growing evidence regarding the contributory role of nutrition on the life course trajectory, through epigenetic and nutrigenomic relationships as yet not fully understood, in the etiology of preterm birth, low birth weight, and some birth defects, as well as the essential role of nutrition in early postnatal development. Because of the growing numbers of nutrients shown to be involved in normal development, the importance of whole foods versus supplements is also becoming apparent. The second major point, which follows from the first, is that early nutrition intervention is crucial to the individual child's attaining his or her highest potential and optimizing human development throughout the life course. Third, we presented a functional approach to assessment, early detection, and treatment of nutrition problems in children with special health care needs, stressing the point that although diagnoses may differ, the nutrition issues are often similar. Finally, although we did not cover the importance of training dietetics professionals in this area or the need to improve families' access to nutrition services for children with special needs, we refer the reader to the latest position paper of the American Dietetic Association for an excellent review of the legislative history and a presentation of the challenges that remain for the profession [6].

References

[1] M. McPherson, P. Arango, H. Fox, C. Lauver, M. McManus, P.W. Newacheck, et al., A new definition of children with special health care needs, Pediatrics 102 (1998) 137–140.

[2] U.S. Department of Health and Human Services, Health Resources and Services Administration, Maternal and Child Health Bureau, The National Survey of Children with Special Health Care Needs Chartbook 2005–2006, U.S. Department of Health and Human Services, Rockville, MD, 2007.

[3] B. Lucas, M. Nardella, Cost Considerations: The Benefits of Nutrition Services for a Case Series of Children with Special Health Care Needs in Washington State, Washington State Department of Health, Olympia, WA, 1998.

[4] P.B. Sullivan, B. Lambert, M. Rose, M. Ford-Adams, A. Johnson, P. Griffiths, Prevalence and severity of feeding problems in children with neurological impairment: Oxford feeding study, Dev. Med. Child Neurol. 42 (2000) 674–680.

[5] B.B. Strickland, P. van Dyck, M.D. Kogan, C. Lauver, S.J. Blumberg, C.D. Bethell, et al., Assessing and ensuring a comprehensive system of services for children with special health care needs: a public health approach, Am. J. Public Health 101 (2011) 224–231.

[6] American Dietetic Association, Position of the American Dietetic Association: providing nutrition services for people with developmental disabilities and special health care needs, J. Am. Diet. Assoc. 110 (2010) 296–307.

[7] M.T. Baer, A. Harris, Pediatric nutrition assessment: identifying children at risk, J. Am. Diet. Assoc. 97 (Suppl. 2) (1997) S107–S115.

[8] MP Bitler, J. Currie, Does WIC work? The effects of WIC on pregnancy and birth outcomes, J. Policy Anal. Manage. 24 (1) (2005) 73–91.

[9] T. Joyce, A. Racine, C. Yunzal-Butler, Reassessing the WIC effect: evidence from the Pregnancy Nutrition Surveillance System, J. Policy Anal. Manage. 272 (2) (2008) 277–303.

[10] D.J. Barker, C. Osmond, T.J. Forsén, E. Kajantie, J.G. Eriksson, Trajectories of growth among children who have coronary events as adults, N. Engl. J. Med. 353 (17) (2005) 1802–1809.

[11] J.C. King, The risk of maternal nutritional depletion and poor outcomes increases in early or closely spaced pregnancies, J. Nutr. 133 (2003) 1732S–1736S.

[12] J. Khoury, T. Henriksen, B. Christophersen, S. Tonstad, Effect of a cholesterol-lowering diet on maternal, cord and neonatal lipids, and pregnancy outcome: a randomized clinical trial, Am. J. Obstet. Gynecol. 193 (4) (2005) 1292–1301.

[13] T.O. Scholl, M.L. Hediger, J.I. Schall, R.L. Fischer, C.S. Khoo, Low zinc intake during pregnancy: its association with preterm and very preterm delivery, Am. J. Epidemiol. 137 (1993) 1115–1124.

[14] T.O. Scholl, M.L. Hediger, J.I. Schall, C.S. Khoo, R.L. Fischer, Dietary and serum folate: their influence on the outcome of pregnancy, Am. J. Clin. Nutr. 63 (1996) 520–525.

[15] T.O. Scholl, High third trimester ferritin concentration: association with very preterm delivery, infection, and maternal nutritional status, Obstet. Gynecol. 92 (1998) 161–166.

[16] J.D. Bogden, F.W. Kemp, X. Chen, A. Stagnaro-Green, T.P. Stein, T.O. Scholl, Low-normal serum selenium early in human pregnancy predicts lower birth weight, Nutr. Res. 29 (10) (2006) 497–502.

[17] J.M. Catov, L. Bodnar, J. Olsen, S. Olsen, E.A. Nohr, Periconceptional multivitamin use and risk of preterm or small-for-gestational-age births in the Danish National Birth Cohort, Am. J. Clin. Nutr. 94 (2011) 906–912.

[18] S. Timmermans, V. Jaddoe, A. Hofman, R.P. Steegers-Theunissen, E.A. Steegers, Periconception folic acid supplementation, fetal growth and the risks of low birth weight and preterm birth: the Generation R Study, Br. J. Nutr. 102 (2009) 777–985.

[19] H. Leonard, N. de Keirk, J. Bourke, C. Bower, Maternal health in pregnancy and intellectual disability in the offspring: a population-based study, Ann. Epidemiol 16 (6) (2006) 446–454.

[20] A.E. Czeizel, E. Puho, Maternal use of nutritional supplements during the first month of pregnancy and decreased risk of Down's syndrome: case–control study, Int. J. Appl. Basic Nutr. Sci. 21 (2005) 698–704.

[21] W. Jedrychowski, J. Jankowski, E. Flak, A. Skarupa, E. Mroz, E. Sochack-Tatara, et al., Effects of prenatal exposure to mercury on cognitive and psychomotor function in one-year-old infants: epidemiologic cohort study in Poland, Ann. Epidemiol. 16 (6) (2006) 439–447.

[22] J.R. Hibbeln, J.M. Davis, C. Steer, P. Emmett, I. Rogers, C. Williams, et al., Maternal seafood consumption in pregnancy and neurodevelopmental outcomes in childhood (ALSPAC study): an observational cohort study, Lancet 369 (2007) 578–585.

[23] J. Colombo, K.N. Dannass, D.J. Shaddy, S. Kundurthi, J.M. Maidranz, C.J. Anderson, et al., Maternal DHA and the development of attention in infancy and toddlerhood, Child Dev. 75 (2004) 1254–1267.

[24] R. Willatts, J.S. Forsyth, M.K. DiModugno, S. Varma, M. Colvin, Effect of long-chain polyunsaturated fatty acids in infant formula on infant cognitive function, Lipids 33 (1998) 973–980.

[25] J.J. Strain, M.P. Bonham, E.M. Duffy, J.M.W. Wallace, P.J. Robson, T.W. Clarkson, et al., Nutrition and neurodevelopment: the search for candidate nutrients in the Seychelles Child Development Nutrition Study, Seychelles Med. Dent. J. 7 (1) (2004) 77.

[26] L.J. Raymond, N.V.C. Ralston, Mercury: selenium interactions and health implications, Seychelles Med. Dent. J. 7 (1) (2004) 72–77.

[27] J. Fedrick, Anencephalus: variation with maternal age, parity, social class and region in England, Wales and Scotland, Ann. Hum. Genet. 34 (1970) 31–38.

[28] R.W. Smithells, S. Sheppard, C.J. Schorah, Vitamin deficiencies and neural tube defects, Arch. Dis. Child 51 (1976) 944–950.

[29] K.M. Laurence, N. James, M.H. Miller, G.B. Tennant, H. Campbell, Double blind randomized controlled trial of folate treatment before conception to prevent recurrence of neural tube defects, Fr. Med. J. 282 (1981) 1509–1511.

[30] Medical Research Council Vitamin Study Research Group, The epidemiology of neural tube defects: a review of the Medical Research Council Vitamin Study, Lancet 336 (1991) 131—137.

[31] Centers for Disease Control and Prevention, Grand rounds: additional opportunities to prevent neural tube defects with folic acid fortification, MMWR 59 (31) (2010) 980—984.

[32] Centers for Disease Control and Prevention, Spina bifida and anencephaly before and after folic acid mandate—United States, 1995—1996 and 1999—2000, MMWR 53 (17) (2004) 362—365.

[33] Centers for Disease Control and Prevention, Recommendations for the use of folic acid to reduce the number of cases of spina bifida and other neural tube defects, MMWR 41 (1992) RR-14.

[34] "Healthy People 2020 Objectives". Available at <http://www.healthypeople.gov/2020/topicsobjectives2020/objectiveslist.aspx?topicId = 26>, 2011 (Accessed 12.10.2011).

[35] P.M.W. Groenen, I.A.L.M. van Rooij, P.G.M. Peer, M.C. Ocke, G.A. Zielhuis, R.P.M. Steegers-Theunissen, Low maternal dietary intakes of iron, magnesium, and niacin are associated with spina bifida in the offspring, J. Nutr. 134 (2004) 1516—1522.

[36] M. Caudill, Pre- and postnatal health: evidence of increased choline needs, J. Am. Diet. Assoc. 110 (2010) 1198—1206.

[37] Institute of Medicine, Dietary Reference Intakes for Thiamin, Riboflavin, Niacin, Vitamin B_6, Folate, Vitamin B_{12}, Pantothenic Acid, Biotin and Choline, National Academies Press, Washington, DC, 1998.

[38] P. Gillies, Nutrigenomics: the rubicon of molecular nutrition, J. Am. Diet. Assoc. 103 (2003) S50—S55.

[39] S. Barnes, Nutritional genomics, polyphenols, diets, and their impact on dietetics, J. Am. Diet. Assoc. 108 (2008) 1888—1895.

[40] L Afman, M. Muller, Nutrigenomics: from molecular nutrition to prevention of disease, J. Am. Diet. Assoc. 106 (2006) 569—576.

[41] S.A. Missmer, L. Suarez, M. Felkner, D. Wang, A.H. Merrill Jr., K.J. Rothman, et al., Exposure to fumonisins and the occurrence of neural tube defects along the Texas—Mexico border, Environ. Health Perspect. 114 (2) (2006) 237—241.

[42] L. Suarez, K. Hendricks, S.P. Cooper, A.M. Sweeney, R.J. Hardy, R.D. Larsen, Maternal serum B-12 levels and risk for neural tube defects in a Texas—Mexico border population, Ann. Epidemiol. 13 (2003) 81—88.

[43] J.G. Ray, P.R. Wyatt, M.D. Thompson, M.J. Vermeulen, C. Meier, P.-Y. Wong, et al., Vitamin B-12 and the risk of neural tube defects in a folic-acid fortified population, Epidemiology 18 (3) (2007) 362—366.

[44] G.M. Shaw, S.L. Carmichael, C. Laurent, S.A. Rasmussen, Maternal nutrient intakes and risk of orofacial clefts, Epidemiology 17 (2006) 285—291.

[45] I.P.C. Krapels, I.A.L.M. van Rooij, M.C. Ocke, B.A. van Cleef, A.M.M. Duijpers-Jagtman, R.P.M. Steegers-Theunissen, Maternal dietary B vitamin intake, other than folate, and the association with orofacial cleft in the offspring, Eur. J. Nutr. 43 (2004) 7—14.

[46] American Academy of Pediatrics, Fetal alcohol syndrome and alcohol-related neurodevelopmental disorders: policy statement, Pediatrics 196 (2) (2000) 359—361.

[47] P.M. Suter, Alcohol: Its role in health and nutrition, in: B.A. Bowman, R.M. Russell (Eds), Present Knowledge in Nutrition, ILSI Press, Washington, DC, 2001.

[48] L.B. Bailey, S. Moyers, J.F. Gregory, Folate, in: B.A. Bowman, R.M. Russell (Eds), Present Knowledge in Nutrition, ILSI Press, Washington, DC, 2001.

[49] M.J. Dibley, Zinc, in: B.A. Bowman, R.M. Russell (Eds), Present Knowledge in Nutrition, ILSI Press, Washington, DC, 2001.

[50] G.P. Oakley, When will we eliminate folic acid-preventable spina bifida? Epidemiology 1 (3) (2007) 367—368.

[51] C.I. Kaye, Committee on Genetics, Newborn screening fact sheets, Pediatrics 118 (2006) 934—963.

[52] L.E. Cipriano, C.A. Rupar, G.S. Zaric, The cost-effectiveness of expanding newborn screening for up to 21 inherited metabolic disorders using tandem mass spectrometry: results from a decision-analytic model, Value Health 10 (2007) 83—97.

[53] M.S. Watson, M.Y. Mann, M.A. Lloye-Puryear, P. Rinaldo, R.R. Howell, American College of Medical Genetics Newborn Screening Expert Group, Pediatrics 117 (2006) S296—S307.

[54] March of Dimes (2007). Available at <www.marchofdimes.com/pnhec/298_834.asp>.

[55] American Society of Human Genetics. Available at <www.acmg.net/resources/policies/ACT/condition-analyte-links.htm>, 2007 (Accessed 2.08.07).

[56] B.L. Lucas, S.A. Feucht, L. Grieger (Eds), Pediatric Nutrition Practice Group and Dietetics in Developmental and Psychiatric Disorders, American Dietetic Association, Chicago, 2004.

[57] J.A. Randall Simpson, H. Keller, L.A. Rysdale, J.E. Beyers, Nutrition Screening Tool for Every Preschooler (NutriSTEP): validation and test—retest reliability of a parent-administered questionnaire assessing nutrition risk of preschoolers, Eur. J. Clin. Nutr. 62 (6) (2008) 770—780.

[58] Pacific West MCH Distance Learning Network (2005). Self-study modules: "Nutrition for Children with Special Health Care Needs," Module 3: Feeding Skills; and group-study modules: "Nutrition for Children with Special Health Care Needs." Available at <www.pacificwestmch.org>.

[59] Y. Yang, B.L. Lucas, S.A. Feucht (Eds), Nutrition Interventions for Children with Special Health Care Needs, third ed., Washington State Department of Health, Tumwater, WA, 2010 (DOH Publication No. 961-158).

[60] T. Bellou, Skinfold measurements enhance nutrition assessments and care planning for children with developmental delays and disabilities, Infant Child Adolescent Nutr. 3 (3) (2011) 158—170.

[61] National Center for Health Statistics (2000). "CDC Clinical Growth Charts." Available at <www.cdc.gov/growthcharts>.

[62] R.D. Stevenson, Use of segmental measures to estimate stature in children with cerebral palsy, Arch. Pediatr. Adolesc. Med. 149 (6) (1995) 658—662.

[63] M.T. Baer, B. Kozlowski, E.M. Blyler, C.M. Trahms, M.L. Taylor, M.P. Hogan, Vitamin D, calcium, and bone status in children with developmental delay in relation to anticonvulsant use and ambulatory status, Am. J. Clin. Nutr. 65 (4) (1997) 1042—1051.

[64] E. Hillesund, J. Skranes, K.U. Trygg, T. Bohmer, Micronutrient status in children with cerebral palsy, Acta Pediatr. 96 (2007) 1195—1198.

[65] N. Schoendorfer, R. Boyd, P.S.W. Davies, Micronutrient adequacy and morbidity: paucity of information in children with cerebral palsy, Nutr. Rev. 68 (12) (2010) 739—748.

[66] C.R. Scriver, A.L. Beaud, W.S. Sly, D. Valle (Eds), The Metabolic and Molecular Basis of Inherited Disease, McGraw Hill, New York, 1995.

[67] McKusick-Nathans Institute for Genetic Medicine. "Online Mendelian Inheritance in Man." Available at <www.ncbi.nlm.nih.gov/omim>, 2000 (Accessed 25.07.07).

[68] B. Wolf, Biotinidase deficiency, GeneReviews (2007).

[69] J.D. Picker, H.L. Levy, Homocystinuria caused by cystathionine β-synthase deficiency, GeneReviews (2007).

[70] B.K. Burton, D. Adams, D.K. Grange, J.I. Malone, E. Jurecki, H. Bausell, et al., Tetrahydrobiopterin therapy for phenylketonuria in infants and young children, J. Pediatr. 158 (2011) 410—415.

[71] F.K. Trefz, B. Burton, N. Longo, M.M.P. Casanova, D.J. Gruskin, A. Dorenbaum, et al., Efficacy of sapropterin dihydrochloride in increasing phenylalanine tolerance in children with phenylketonuria: a phase III, randomized, double-blind, placebo-controlled study, J. Pediatr. 154 (2009) 700—707.

[72] A.M. Bosch, Classical galactosemia revisited, J. Inherit. Metab. Dis. 29 (2006) 516—525.

[73] D. Matern, P Rinaldo, Medium chain acyl-coenzyme a dehydrogenase deficiency, GeneReviews (2007).

[74] P.B. Acosta, S. Yanicelli, Nutrition support of inherited disorders of amino acid metabolism: Part 1, Top. Clin. Nutr. 9 (1993) 65—82.

[75] P.B. Acosta, S. Yanicelli, Nutrition support of inherited disorders of amino acid metabolism: Part 2, Top. Clin. Nutr. 9 (1993) 48—72.

[76] E.L. MacLeod, M. Clayton, S.C. van Calcar, D.M. Ney, Breakfast with glycomacropeptide compared with amino acids suppresses plasma ghrelin levels in individuals with phenylketonuria, Mol. Genet. Metab. 100 (4) (2010) 303—308.

[77] S.C. van Calcar, E. MacLeod, S.T. Gleason, M.R. Etzel, M.K. Clayton, J.A. Wolff, et al., Improved nutritional management of phenylketonuria by using a diet containing glycomacropeptide compared with amino acids, Am. J. Clin. Nutr. 89 (2009) 1068—1077.

[78] C. Chen, J. Visootsak, S. Dills, J.M. Graham, Prader—Willi syndrome: an update and review for the primary pediatrician, Clin. Pediatr. 46 (2007) 580—591.

[79] F. Benarroch, H.J. Hirsch, L. Genstil, M.A. Landau, V. Gross-Tsur, Prader—Willi syndrome: medical prevention and behavioral challenges, Child Adolesc. Psych. Clin. North Am. 16 (2007) 695—708.

[80] D.A. Festen, R. de Lind van Wijngaarden, M. van Eekelen, B.J. Otten, J.M. Wit, H.J. Duivenvoorden, et al., Randomized controlled GH trial: effects on anthropometry, body composition and body proportions in a large group of children with Prader—Willi syndrome, Clin. Endocrinol. (Oxford) 69 (3) (2008) 443—451.

[81] M.A. Angulo, M. Castro-Magana, M. Lamerson, R. Arguello, S. Accacha, A. Khan, Final adult height in children with Prader—Willi syndrome with and without human growth hormone treatment, Am. J. Med. Genet. 143A (2007) 1456—1461.

[82] P.F. Collett-Solberg, Update in growth hormone therapy of children, J. Clin. Endocrinol. Metab. 96 (3) (2011) 573—579.

[83] M.G. Butler, J. Sturich, J. Lee, S.E. Myers, B.Y. Whitman, J.A. Gold, et al., Growth standards of infants with Prader—Willi syndrome, Pediatrics 127 (2011) 687—695.

[84] C.F. Poets, Gastroesophageal reflux: a critical review of its role in preterm infants, Pediatrics 113 (2004) E128—E132.

[85] I.H. Gewolb, F.L. Vice, Abnormalities in the coordination of respiration and swallow in preterm infants with bronchopulmonary dysplasia, Dev. Med. Child Neurol. 48 (7) (2006) 595—599.

[86] H. Heiman, R.J. Schanler, Enteral nutrition for premature infants: the role of human milk, Sem. Fetal Neonatal Med. 1291 (2007) 26—34.

[87] C. Simpson, R. Schanler, C. Lau, Early introduction of oral feeding in preterm infants, Pediatrics 110 (3) (2002) 517—522.

[88] T. Linsheid, K. Budd, L. Rasnake, Pediatric feeding problems, in: E.M. Roberts (Ed.), Handbook of Pediatric Psychology, Guilford, New York, 2003, pp. 481—498.

[89] R. Manikam, J. Perman, Pediatric feeding disorders, J. Clin. Gastroenterol. 30 (2000) 34—36.

[90] G. Schadler, H. Suss-Burghart, A.M. Toschke, H. von Voss, R. von Kries, Feeding disorders in ex-prematures: causes—response to therapy—long term outcome, Eur. J. Pediatr. 166 (2007) 803—808.

[91] M.C. Petersen, B.T. Rogers, Introduction: feeding and swallowing and developmental disabilities, Dev. Disabil. Res. Rev. 14 (2008) 75—76.

[92] K.S. Berlin, D. Lobato, B. Pinkos, C.S. Cerezo, N.S. LeLeiko, Patterns of medical and developmental comorbidities among children presenting with feeding problems: a latent class analysis, J. Dev. Behav. Pediatr. 32 (2011) 41—47.

[93] C.A. Erickson, K.A. Stigler, M.R. Corkins, D.J. Posey, J.F. Fitzgerald, J. McDougle, Gastrointestinal factors in autistic disorder: a critical review, J. Autism Dev. Disord. 35 (2005) 713—727.

[94] S.E. Levy, M.C. Souders, R.F. Ittenbach, E. Giarelli, A.E. Mulberg, J.A. Pinto-Martin, Relationship of dietary intake to gastrointestinal symptoms in children with autistic spectrum disorders, Biol. Psychiatry 61 (2007) 492—497.

[95] K.A. Schreck, K. Williams, Food preferences and factors influencing food selectivity for children with autism spectrum disorders, Res. Dev. Disabil. 27 (2006) 353—363.

[96] K.A. Schreck, K. Williams, A.F. Smith, A comparison of eating behaviors between children with and without autism, J. Autism Dev. Disord. 34 (2004) 433—438.

[97] W.H. Ahearn, Using simultaneous presentation to increase vegetable consumption in a mildly selective child with autism, J. Appl. Behav. Anal. 26 (2003) 361—365.

[98] C. Baranoski, T. Grutza, G.L. Hagen, J. Humphrey, C. Kedzierski, K. Schrock, Nutrition practice in the early intervention system: Illinois. ICAN, Infant Child Adolescent Nutr. 3 (3) (2011) 133—139.

[99] American Psychiatric Association, Diagnostic and Statistical Manual of Mental Disorders, fourth ed., American Psychiatric Association, Washington, DC, 1994.

[100] A.D. Lane, R. Young, A.E.Z. Baker, M.T. Angley, Sensory processing subtypes in autism: association with adaptive behavior, J. Autism Dev. Disord. 40 (2010) 112—122.

[101] S.J. Rogers, S. Hepburn, E. Wehner, Parent reports of sensory symptoms in toddlers with autism and those with other developmental disorders, J. Autism Dev. Disord. 33 (6) (2003) 631—642.

[102] L. Lecavalier, Behavioral and emotional problems in young people with pervasive developmental disorders: relative prevalence, effects of subject characteristics, and empirical classification, J. Autism Dev. Disord. 36 (8) (2006) 1101—1114.

[103] B.M. Kuehn, CDC: autism spectrum disorders common, JAMA 297 (9) (2007) 940.

[104] Anonymous, Announcement: Autism Awareness Month—April 2011, MMWR 60 (2011) 379.

[105] M.D. Kogan, S. Blumberg, L.A. Schieve, C.A. Boyle, J.M. Perrin, R.M. Ghandour, et al., Prevalence of patient-reported autism spectrum disorder among children in the U.S., 2007, Pediatrics 124 (5) (2007) 1395—1403.

[106] E. Rogers, Has enhanced folate status during pregnancy altered natural selection and possibly autism prevalence? A closer look at a possible link, Medical Hypotheses 71 (2008) 406—410.

[107] S.J. James, P. Cutler, S. Melnyk, S. Jernigan, L. Janak, D.W. Gaylor, et al., Metabolic biomarkers of increased oxidative stress and impaired methylation capacity in children with autism, Am. J. Clin. Nutr. 80 (2004) 1611—1617.

[108] R.J. Schmidt, R. Hansen, J. Hartiala, H. Allayee, L.C. Schmidt, D.J. Tancredi, et al., Prenatal vitamins, one-carbon metabolism gene variants, and risk for autism, Epidemiology 22 (4) (2011) 476—485.

[109] A.E. Main, M. Angley, P. Thosmas, C.E. O'Doherty, M. Fenech, Folate and methionine metabolism in autism: a systematic review, Am. J. Clin. Nutr. 91 (2010) 1598—1620.

[110] C.J. Newschaffer, D. Fallin, N.L. Lee, Heritable and nonheritable risk factors for autism spectrum disorders, Epidemiol. Rev. 24 (2002) 137—153.

[111] M.E. Geraghty, G. DePasquale, A.E. Lane, Nutritional intake and therapies in autism: a spectrum of what we know: Part 1, Infant Child Adolescent Nutr. 2 (2010) 62—69.

[112] D. Horvath, J. Perman, Autism and gastrointestinal symptoms, Curr. Gastroenterol. Rep. 4 (2002) 231—258.

[113] D.B. Campbell, T. Buie, H. Winter, M. Bauman, J.S. Sutcliffe, J.M. Perrin, et al., Distinct genetic risk based on association of MET in families with co-occurring autism and gastrointestinal conditions, Pediatrics 123 (3) (2009) 1018—1024.

[114] H. Asperger, Psychopathology of children with celiac disease, Ann. Paediatr. 197 (1961) 346–351.

[115] G.W. Christison, K. Ivany, Elimination dies in autism spectrum disorders: any wheat amidst the chaff? J. Dev. Behav. Pediatr. 27 (2 Suppl.) (2006) S162–S171.

[116] H. Cass, P. Gringras, J. March, I. McKendrick, A.E. O'Hare, L. Owen, et al., Absence of urinary opioid peptides in children with autism, Arch. Dis. Child 93 (2008) 745–750.

[117] A.E. Golnik, M. Ireland, Complementary alternative medicine for children with autism: a physician survey, J. Autism Dev. Disord. 39 (2009) 996–1005.

[118] H. Jyonouchi, L. Geng, A. Ruby, C. Reddy, B. Zimmerman-Bier, Evaluation of an association between gastrointestinal symptoms and cytokine production against common dietary proteins in children with autism spectrum disorders, J. Pediatr. 146 (2005) 605–610.

[119] H. Jyonouchi, L. Geng, A. Ruby, B. Zimmerman-Bier, Dysregulation innate immune responses in young children with autism spectrum disorders: their relationship to gastrointestinal symptoms and dietary intervention, Neuropsychobiology 51 (2005) 77–85.

[120] M.E. Geraghty, J. Bates-Wall, K. Ratliff-Schaub, A.E. Lane, Nutrition interventions and therapies in autism: a spectrum of what we know: Part 2, Infant Child Adolescent Nutr. 2 (2010) 120–133.

[121] G.P. Amminger, G. Berger, M.R. Schafer, C. Klier, M.H. Friedrich, M. Feucht, Omega-3 fatty acid supplementation in children with autism: a double-blind randomized placebo controlled pilot study, Biol. Psychiatry 61 (2007) 551–553.

[122] H.H. Wong, R.G. Smith, Patterns of complementary and alternative medical therapy use in children diagnosed with autism spectrum disorders, J. Autism Dev. Disord. 36 (2006) 902–909.

[123] J.H. Elder, M. Shankar, J. Shuster, D. Theriaque, S. Burns, L. Sherrill, The gluten-free, casein-free diet in autism: results of a preliminary double blind clinical trial, J. Autism Dev. Disord. 36 (2006) 413–420.

[124] T. Buie, D. Campbell, G.J. Fuchs III, G.T. Furuta, J. Levy, J. Vandewater, et al., Evaluation, diagnosis, and treatment of gastrointestinal disorders in individuals with ASD: a consensus report, Pediatrics 125 (2010) S1–S18.

[125] C. Dissanayake, Q.M. Bui, R. Huggins, D.Z. Loesch, Growth in stature and head circumference in high-functioning autism and asperger disorder during the first 3 years of life, Dev. Psychopathol. 18 (2006) 381–393.

[126] J.L. Mills, M.L. Hediger, C.A. Molloy, G.P. Chrousos, P. Manning-Courtney, K.F. Yu, et al., Elevated levels of growth-related hormones in autism and autism spectrum disorder, Clin. Endocrinol. 67 (2007) 230–237.

[127] S.E. Levy, D. Mandell, S. Merhar, R.F. Ittenbach, J.A. Pinto-Martin, Use of complementary and alternative medicine among children recently diagnosed with autistic spectrum disorder, J. Dev. Behav. Pediatr. 24 (6) (2003) 418–423.

[128] S.E. Levy, S. Hyman, Complementary and alternative medicine treatments for children with autism spectrum disorders, Child Adolesc. Psychiatr. Clin. North Am. 17 (4) (2008) 803–820.

[129] E. Hanson, L. Kalish, E. Bunce, C. Curtis, S. McDaniel, J. Ware, et al., Use of complementary and alternative medicine among children diagnosed with autism spectrum disorder, J. Autism Dev. Disord. 37 (4) (2007) 628–636.

[130] A.C. Herndon, C. DiGuiseppi, S.L. Johnson, J. Leiferman, A. Reynolds, Does nutritional intake differ between children with autism spectrum disorders and children with typical development? J. Autism Dev. Disord. 39 (2) (2009) 212–222.

[131] M.L. Hediger, L. England, C.A. Molloy, K.F. Yu, P. Manning-Courtney, J.L. Mills, Reduced bone cortical thickness in boys with autism or autism spectrum disorder, J. Autism Dev. Disord. 38 (2008) 848–856.

[132] Autism Intervention Research Network on Physical Health (2010). AIR-Perspectives.

[133] L.K. Wink, M. Plawecki, C.A. Erickson, K.A. Stigler, C.J. McDougle, Emerging drugs for the treatment of symptoms associated with autism spectrum disorders, Expert Opin. Emerge. Drugs 15 (3) (2010) 481–494.

[134] S.D. Tomchek, W. Dunn, Sensory processing in children with and without autism: a comparative study using the short sensory profile, Am. J. Occup. Ther. 1 (2) (2007) 190–200.

[135] C.T. Lukens, T. Linscheid, Development and validation of an inventory to assess mealtime behavior problems in children with autism, J. Autism Dev. Disord. 38 (2008) 342–352.

[136] J.R. Ledford, D. Gast, D. Luscre, K.M. Ayres, Observational and incidental learning by children with autism during small group instruction, J. Autism Dev. Disord. 38 (1) (2008) 86–103.

[137] L.G. Bandini, S. Anderson, C. Curtin, S.A. Cermak, W.E. Evans, R. Scampini, et al., Food selectivity and sensory issues in children with autism spectrum disorders, J. Peds. 157 (2) (2010) 259–264.

DIETARY BIOACTIVE COMPOUNDS
FOR HEALTH

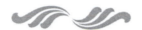
Antioxidants in Health and Disease

Harold E. Seifried*, Susan M. Pilch†

*National Cancer Institute, Rockville, Maryland, †National Institutes of Health Library, Bethesda, Maryland

I INTRODUCTION

Antioxidants are a loosely characterized group of compounds that are defined by their general ability to decrease or delay oxidation. Dietary antioxidants are recognized to have the ability to inhibit the formation of both reactive oxygen species (ROS) and reactive nitrogen species (RNS), which can adversely affect normal cellular processes and physiological functions [1–3]. Under normal conditions, the balance between production and elimination of free radicals is maintained by enzymes (e.g., glutathione peroxidases, catalase and superoxide dismutases, thioredoxin reductase, and heme oxygenase) and a host of nonenzymatic components (some metals, glutathione, thiols, certain vitamins, and phytochemicals such as isoflavones, flavonoids, and polyphenols), which can be influenced by eating behaviors [1–3]. Table 18.1 includes a number of these antioxidants with their respective structures and properties.

The range of chemical classes within the antioxidant domain is unprecedented and is part of the reason why the grouping of compounds by their ability to interact with reactive species (ROS and RNS) can lead to oversimplification and generalization. Hence, descriptors such as "conundrum" and "double-edged sword" are often used to characterize the relationship between antioxidants and health. Part of the controversy stems from the innate properties of ROS because this class of compounds can influence both disease prevention and disease promotion. Although the generation of ROS had been viewed as primarily, or solely, detrimental to health, advances in research have shown ROS can have crucial roles in normal physiological processes, including functioning as growth factors, influencing immunocompetence, and initiating apoptosis in damaged cells.

Despite these beneficial functions of ROS, abnormal production or nonhomeostatic regulation of ROS is positively linked to the development of common diseases and associated conditions, including cancer and cardiovascular disease (CVD), as well as a number of neurological and metabolic diseases. As a result, antioxidants have been deemed promising for the prevention and possibly treatment of several of these diseases. Some of this optimism is based on the frequently observed case–control association between diets high in fruits and vegetables (and presumably antioxidant exposures) and decreased disease risk. Although there is evidence that antioxidants may offer health benefits in populations that are at increased risk because of environmental or medical conditions, there are many inconsistencies in the literature. Some of this inconsistency stems from different study end points (i.e., mortality, cancer, or CVD occurrence and individual study results versus meta-analysis of several "related" studies) and study design (prospective versus retrospective, the use of food frequency data versus controlled dietary or purified agent clinical trials, healthy population epidemiological versus disease intervention studies, and so on). The effect of the vehicle that contains the antioxidant also introduced variability because the bioavailability in a food matrix can be quite different from that in a pure compound and synergistic interactions are likely within the whole food because there are several antioxidants present in most food groups. Because evidence does exist that several antioxidants at "normal" exposure levels can regulate signal transduction and, thus, regulate proliferation and the immune response, both normal physiological processes and mechanisms other than their antioxidant properties may be functioning. Overall, the physiological or pharmacological importance of antioxidants as regulators of radicals as a possible means for promoting health continues to receive widespread scientific attention and debate in the literature (http://www.dukehealth.org/health_library/health_articles/the_andioxidant_controversy).

Nutrition in the Prevention and Treatment of Disease, Third Edition.
DOI: http://dx.doi.org/10.1016/B978-0-12-391884-0.00018-4

TABLE 18.1 Some Antioxidants and Their Biological Activity

Antioxidant	structure	Detected or effective level	Cancer activity	CVD activity	Hormonal response	Deficiency symptoms
Carotenoids: β-Carotene		5–50 µg/dL	Induces connexin–differentiation, immune function	Food sources lower CVD	No	Only vitamin A—xeroderma, night vision
Curcumin		>2 µmol/l at 8 g/day	Anti-inflammatory; increases apoptosis, interferes with chemotherapeutics and cell signaling; interferes with Phase I enzymes, stimulates Phase II	??	No	No
Flavonoids: Genistein		1–10 µmol/l	Modulates cell signaling, inhibits angiogenesis, increases apoptosis, much dat from cell studies	Food sources lower CVD, minimal lowering	Some are estrogenic, some anti, some both (dose related)	No
Glutathione			Substrate of GSH glutathione peroxidase reduction of H_2O_2 and lipid hydroperoxides and substrate for Phase II carcinogen metabolism	??	No	??
Oleanic acid			Inhibits proliferation angiogenesis, metastasis; induces apoptosis and cell differentiation; anti-inflammatory	Antiatherosclerotic, hypolioidemic	No	No
Reseratrol		Mostly in cell culture	Inhibits proliferation angiogenesis, induces apoptosis and cell cycle arrest in cancer cells in culture	Inhibits platelet aggregation cell adhesion in culture	Both estrogen (E2) agonist without E2 and antagonist with E2	No

	Structure	Level	Effect	CVD		Deficiency
Selenium	Se	45–80 µg/1 40–100 µg/d	Increases glutathione peroxidase, stimulates immunity	Weakly cardio-protective	No	Muscle wasting, cardiomyopathy
Vitamin C		Saturated blood levels at 400 mg per dau ~70 µmol/1	Reduces lung, breast, oral, upper GI, gastric, colorectal CA with oral C; IV doses increase survival	Mixed results on CVD reduction, more + than −, lowers blood pressure, coronary artery dilation	No	Scurvy, impaired collagen synthesis
Vitamin D			Induces differentiation, lowers proliferation	Lowers blood pressure	No	Rickets, seizures, osteomalacia
Vitamin E		20 µmol/1	Affects cell signaling, boosts immunity, inflammation; minimal CA effect	Platelet aggregation, lower MI, carotid atherosclerosis	No	27 to 40 + % of population below 20 µmol/1

B. DIETARY BIOACTIVE COMPOUNDS FOR HEALTH

A Antioxidant Usage and Measures of Oxidative Stress

Attention of the public and the scientific literature to the purported health benefits of antioxidants [4–7] has paralleled the increased use of antioxidant supplements by the U.S. adult population. Data from the National Health and Nutrition Examination Surveys (NHANES), first conducted in 1971, indicated an overall prevalence of dietary supplement usage of 23% in NHANES I; prevalence rates increased to 35% in NHANES II and 40% in NHANES III, with women's usage approximately 12% higher than that of men [8,9]. However, the total male intake was somewhat higher than that of females of all ages [10]. Based on 1999–2000 NHANES III data, approximately 33% take multivitamins and more than 12% use vitamin E or C supplements [6]. The increased interest in the effects of vitamins in general and specifically the class of "antioxidants" as protecting agents was sparked by a series of articles beginning in the 1970s. In the decades since, an expanded knowledge base in the nutritional sciences about the potential molecular targets and interactions that may account for the health benefits of antioxidants has surfaced from a wide range of preclinical, clinical, and population studies [7,11].

The major cellular targets of ROS include membrane lipids, proteins, nucleic acids, and carbohydrates. Several biomarkers for oxidative damage and antioxidant defense have been introduced as potential indicators of alterations in normal homeostatic mechanisms. Basically, oxidative stress biomarkers can be separated into those that (1) reflect modified molecules caused by ROS and (2) reflect shifts in biological measures of low-molecular-weight compounds or the induction of enzymes (Table 18.2). The ability to monitor these biomarkers at multiple time points in blood, urine, ductal lavage, and so on allows for repeated measurement and greater sensitivity in detecting and understanding stress status, which is not always possible for multiple reasons, including ethical and patient compliance concerns with more invasive procedures. Unfortunately, it is not simple to link these biomarkers to a specific clinical outcome. However, the field is expanding and maturing. The uncertainty about normal and abnormal values, appropriate target tissues, and the unsubstantiated relationship of a change in a biomarker to a specific phenotypic response also raises significant concerns about many of these measures. Eventually, an "oxidative stress profile" that incorporates changes in multiple biomarkers could be useful in establishing who may benefit or who may potentially be placed at risk by the exaggerated use of antioxidants through foods or dietary supplements.

Two main types of methods have been used to evaluate the antioxidant properties of foods; these assays are based on hydrogen atom transfer (HAT) reactions or on electron transfer (ET). Most HAT-based assays use a competitive reaction scheme in which antioxidant and substrate compete for thermally generated peroxyl radicals through the decomposition of azo compounds. These assays include inhibition of induced low-density lipoprotein auto-oxidation, oxygen radical absorbance capacity, total radical trapping antioxidant parameter, and crocin bleaching assays. The ET-based assays measure the capacity of an antioxidant in the reduction of an oxidant and corresponding change in color when reduced. ET-based assays include the total phenols assay by Folin–Ciocalteu reagent, Trolox equivalence antioxidant capacity, ferric ion reducing antioxidant power, "total antioxidant potential" assay using a Cu(II) complex as an oxidant, and DPPH, the oxygen radical absorbance capacity [12,13]. Although each of the methods has value for a relative comparison across a variety of food items, it remains unclear whether the measures truly reflect their physiological value after consumption because they do not measure true biomarkers of physiological activity. In addition, the lack of detailed information about multiple exposures and with variable durations makes the interpretation of existing studies with sometimes subtle changes in fluids and cells in humans extremely challenging. The merits of these analyses may also be questioned because possible postprandial or diurnal variations

TABLE 18.2 Some Biomarkers of Oxidative Damage

Total antioxidant potential	Total radical trapping antioxidant
Lipid peroxidation	Malondialdehyde-lysine, 4-hydroxy-2-nonenallysine, acrolein-lysine, F2-isoprostane, thiobarbituric acid reactive substances
DNA oxidation	8-Hydroxy-2'-deoxyguanosine
Glyco-oxidation	Carboxymethyl-lysine, pentosidine, argpyrimidine, methylglyoxal
Nitro-oxidation	Nitrotyrosine, nitrite to nitrate
Protein oxidation	o,o'-Dityrosine, *ortho*-tyrosine, bilirubin oxidative metabolites, oxidized glutathione
Enzyme activities	Superoxide dismutase, catalase, glutathione peroxidase, glutathione reductase, glutathione-*S*-transferase, thioredoxin reductase, heme oxygenase
Protein concentrations	Albumin, ferritin, transferrin, lactoferrin, ceruloplasmin, thioredoxin
Concentrations of low-molecular-weight molecules	Bilirubin, tocopherols, carotenoids, ubiquinol/ubiquinone, ascorbate, glutathione, cysteine, urate, selenium

that are not directly related to the intake of dietary antioxidants per se are not considered. Finally, plasma antioxidant capacity may be significantly affected by non-antioxidant dietary constituents, which influence uptake, tissue mobilization, or metabolism of endogenous or exogenous antioxidants [2,11,12,14,15].

The beneficial health effects of fruits and vegetables have been attributed, at least in part, to their antioxidant content. Significant and generally transient increases in plasma total antioxidant capacity are frequently observed following the human consumption of flavonoid-rich foods [14]. That these flavonoids or possibly other bioactive food components function by modifying oxidative stress has been challenged by observations that typical intakes only result in minimal shifts in circulating biomarkers in plasma, and that extensive metabolism of the agents likely diminishes their *in vivo* antioxidant capacity. Lotito and Frei [14] concluded that the large increase in plasma total antioxidant capacity observed after the consumption of flavonoid-rich foods is not caused by the flavonoids per se but is likely the consequence of increased uric acid levels. However, work on the metabolism of the glycoside or aglycone forms of the flavonoids has shown that metabolic products, including products of intestinal and hepatic metabolism, can have very different properties than the parent compounds, calling into question the extrapolation of observed *in vitro* anti-inflammatory and antioxidant effects to the *in vivo* situation [15].

The possible usefulness of antioxidants in disease prevention, particularly for cardiovascular diseases and cancer, stems from a number of epidemiological findings and a number of follow-up intervention studies. However, a substantive compendium of negative cardiovascular and cancer effects of antioxidant use, especially relating to dietary supplements, has also emerged, as will be discussed subsequently. A resulting concern is the potentially deleterious effects of antioxidant supplements on normal ROS levels because precise modulation of ROS levels is needed to allow normal cell function or to promote apoptotic cell death of aged, precancerous, or transformed cells [16]. Conflicting findings on risks and benefits have led to the careful reviews of antioxidant efficacy, such as evidence reports from the Agency for Healthcare Research and Quality (AHRQ) on vitamin C, vitamin E, and coenzyme Q10 [17,18]. These AHRQ reports included broad, systematic searches of the literature. The report on prevention and treatment of cardiovascular disease [17] concluded that the evidence did not support a positive benefit of vitamin E supplementation for cardiovascular events; neither did it support significant potential for harm. Conclusions about vitamin C and coenzyme Q were mixed. The review of the cancer literature [18] did not support the hypothesis that

supplements of vitamins C or E or coenzyme Q10 generally help prevent or treat cancer. Isolated findings of benefit require confirmation. Taylor and Greenwald [19] reviewed a number of completed nutritional cancer prevention trials, helping to fill out the background picture on this question.

This collection of potential positive and negative antioxidant effects on ROS deserves further examination because of the molecular evidence for the multiple roles of ROS in development and progression of cancer, CVD, and other diseases [2,11]. This increased attention is timely because there have been studies [2] that link some nutritional antioxidants with increased mortality from cancer and CVD, as well as some clinical studies that do not support the cancer prevention efficacy of some antioxidants. A review [20] indicated there are a number of European antioxidant and cancer clinical and epidemiological studies under way, so the subject will continue to be closely scrutinized and debated as new information becomes available.

B Reactive Oxygen Species and Normal Physiology

ROS typically arise as by-products of cellular metabolism and ionizing radiation, usually reflected in the formation of the following four species: superoxide anion (O_2^-), hydrogen peroxide (H_2O_2), hydroxyl radical (OH•), and singlet oxygen ($^1O_2$). Although H_2O_2 and $^1O_2$ are not free radicals per se, these species often initiate and promote oxidation by their ability to react directly with electron-rich organic species. The reactivity of O_2^- or H_2O_2 with other molecules is not appreciable, but the presence of trace amounts of transition metals fosters their conversion to OH via the Fenton or Haber–Weiss reactions. ROS formation is a natural consequence of aerobic metabolism and is integral for maintaining tissue oxygen homeostasis [21].

Oxygen homeostasis—the balance between constitutive oxidants and antioxidants—is maintained through a natural series of reduction–oxidation (redox) reactions involving the transfer of electrons between two chemical species: compounds that lose electrons (oxidized) and those that gain electrons (reduced). When oxygen homeostasis is not maintained, the cellular environment becomes oxidatively stressed. Approximately 1–3% of oxygen consumed by the body is converted into ROS [22]. Three of the major ROS—superoxide radical O_2^-, hydrogen peroxide, and hydroxyl radical OH•—are normal metabolic by-products that are generated continuously by the mitochondria in growing cells [21,23,24]. Other significant intracellular sources of ROS include microsomal cytochrome P450 enzymes, flavoprotein oxidases, and peroxisomal enzymes involved in fatty acid metabolism [21]. The potentially damaging oxidative stress can be caused by excess ROS, which are kept in check by endogenous cellular antioxidant mechanisms. Oxidative stress-related enzymes include superoxide dismutases for eliminating the superoxide radical, as well as catalase and glutathione peroxidases for removing hydrogen peroxide and organic peroxides [21,23]. Polymorphisms have been observed in these enzymes, which can affect an individual's capacity to respond to changes in ROS; this is discussed in more detail later.

Transient fluctuations of ROS levels can influence activity of signal transduction pathways leading to cell proliferation or to apoptosis or necrosis, depending on the dosage and duration of ROS changes and also on cell type. Typically, low levels of ROS can be mitogenic, whereas medium (normal homeostatic) levels lead to temporary or permanent growth arrest (replicative senescence), and elevated levels usually result in cell death either by apoptosis or by necrosis [24–26]. Although necrosis and apoptosis may be viewed as negative events in terms of cell loss, these processes also have positive roles in the downregulation of immune responses [3] and the elimination of transformed cells ("tumor suppression" via apoptosis).

C Reactive Oxygen Species in Disease Conditions

Imbalanced ROS homeostasis has been linked to increased risk of several diseases such as cancer, CVD, atherosclerosis, diabetes, and neurodegenerative conditions including Alzheimer's disease. Understanding the molecular effects of ROS on these different disease processes should assist in unraveling the varied and sometimes contradictory evidence about these diseases and assist in evaluating the importance and safety of antioxidants.

1 Cancer

Cancer is a number of somewhat distinct diseases that can be characterized on the basis of uncontrolled cellular growth resulting from a series of altered sets of genetic and epigenetic manifestations. Hanahan and Weinberg [27] indicated the "hallmark capabilities" necessary for tumorigenesis: (1) self-sufficiency in growth signals, (2) insensitivity to antigrowth signals, (3) evasion of apoptosis, (4) limitless potential for replication, (5) sustained angiogenesis, and (6) tissue invasion and metastasis. Excessive ROS and RNS are involved in all these processes and thus contribute to cancer progression either positively by promoting cell division or negatively by stimulating apoptosis and slowing the growth. Belief in the protective effects of antioxidant supplements has led to their widespread use by cancer patients [28].

The expanded use of nutritional aides is not limited to the United States because many other countries are reporting increased use of various alternative and complementary approaches and strategies [29]. A greater understanding of both the negative and the positive consequences of ROS and antioxidants in the etiology and progression of carcinogenesis is crucial to making clear advances in cancer prevention and treatment. Currently, the two faces (benefit/risk) of ROS/RNS in malignant diseases make it difficult to present a true, clear, and concise message to consumers.

2 Cardiovascular Disease

CVD, encompassing atherosclerosis and its associated vascular disorders, is the leading cause of mortality in developed countries [30,31]. In addition, other vascular insults such as those associated with cigarette smoking, diabetes mellitus, hypertension, and hyperlipidemia can trigger an inflammatory response in blood vessels. Chronic low-grade inflammation is generally accepted to accompany atherogenesis [32,33]. This inflammatory state, which has been linked in part to ROS mediation, can result in damage to smooth muscle and vascular endothelial cells. This in turn leads to a dysfunctional endothelium characterized by pathological alterations in the endothelial cell's anticoagulant, anti-inflammatory, and vascular-relaxation properties, which can promote the recruitment of monocytes, macrophages, growth factors, and cellular hypertrophy. All of these factors can contribute to atherosclerotic plaque formation. In summary, increased ROS activity helps drive many of these processes involved in the development of CVD if left unchecked.

II ANTIOXIDANTS IN DISEASE ETIOLOGY, PREVENTION, AND TREATMENT

Several studies have reported that diets high in fruits and vegetables can be associated with a markedly decreased risk of CVD and cancer. This has been frequently attributed to high levels of antioxidants present in these foods. Other studies, however, do not provide clear and unequivocal support for this assumption. For example, data from historical food frequency questionnaires collected during the cohort Nurses' Health and Health Professionals Follow-Up Studies indicated that cancer incidence was not influenced by increased fruit or vegetable consumption; however, modest reductions in CVD were detected (Table 18.3) [34]. Similarly, studies of dietary supplements and individual antioxidants are not consistent; observed effects have ranged from benefit to possible harm [35,36]. A number of factors may contribute to these contradictory findings, including participant

TABLE 18.3 Human Intervention Studies on Antioxidants

Study and publication date	Study details, size, and duration	Intervention details	Study results
Linxian Study, China (1993) [41]	29,584 men (5 years)	βC (15 mg), vitamin E (30 mg), and selenium (50 μg), daily	Protective effects: cancer, −13%; mortality, −9%
ATBC study, Finland (1994) [51,53,54,61−65,83]	29,133 male smokers (5−8 years) with up to 19-year follow-up	βC (20 mg)±vitamin E (50 mg) daily	Lung cancer: +18% but mortality mixed
			Prostate cancer: −32%
			Colorectal cancer: −22%
			No decrease CVD or angina
			Slight excess hemorrhagic stroke and βC-related mortality (+7%), but decreased with vitamin E
CARET study, United States (1996) [36,52,55]	18,314 male smokers or asbestos exposed (4 years + 6-year follow-up)	βC (30 mg)±vitamin A (25,000 IU) daily	Lung cancer, +28%; mortality, +17% baseline levels after 10 years
CHAOS, United Kingdom (1996) [87]	2,002 atherosclerosis patients, ∼80% males (510 days)	535 or 263 mg vitamin E daily	Decreased nonfatal myocardial infarction (MI) (77%)
PHS study, United States (1996) [42,44,96]	22,071 physicians (12 years) (11% smokers, 39% former smokers)	50 mg βC every other day	No significant overall effect on cancer or CVD; decreased prostate cancer −32%
NPC Trial, United States (1996) [70−72]	1,312 men and women with dermal basal or squamous cell carcinoma (4.5 years + 16.4-year follow-up)	200 μg selenium daily	No effect on skin cancer; lung, −46%; colorectal, −58%; prostate, −63%; mortality, −50%
WHS study, United States (1999) [43,76,85]	39,876 females 45+ year-old health professionals (2.1 years +10-year follow-up) (13% smokers)	50 mg βC or vitamin E (400 mg) every other day±aspirin	No βC effect on cancer rates nor on CVD; CVD death decreased 24% with vitamin E; no change cancer, MI, or stroke; high fruit and vegetable intake associated with lower MI
GISSI, Italy (1999) [99]	11,324 MI survivors, ∼85% male (3−5 years)	Vitamin E (300 mg)±PUFA (1 g) daily	No effect of vitamin E on CVD; PUFA effects protective; cardiovascular deaths, −30%; mortality, −20%
Antioxidant Supplementation in Atherosclerosis Prevention (ASAP), Finland (2002) [93]	520 high-cholesterol male and female (postmenopausal) smokers and nonsmokers (6 years)	Vitamin C (250 mg) and 91 mg α-tocopherol, twice daily	Carotid atherosclerosis −25% combined, −30% in men; decreased plaque size in >50%
Intravascular Ultrasonography (IVUS), United States (2002) [94]	40 cardiac transplant patients (1 year)	Vitamin C (500 mg) and vitamin E (263 mg) twice daily	Decreased atherosclerotic plaque size
British Heart Protection Study, United Kingdom (2002) [95]	20,536 increased risk of MI; 15,454 males, 5,082 females (5 years)	Vitamin C (250 mg) vitamin E (600 mg) and 20 mg βC	No effect on cancer, stroke, or dementia
SU.VI.MAX, France (2003) [66−69]	12,741 men (aged 45−60 years) and women (aged 35−60 years) (7.1 years)	βC (6 mg), vitamin E (30 mg), vitamin C (120 mg) + Zn (20 mg) and selenium (100 μg) daily dosing	Protective in men: prostate cancer, ∼ −58%; all cancer, −31%; mortality, −37%; no supplement effect in women but lower CVD with high fruits and vegetables
HOPE & HOPE-TOO, Canada, United States, Europe, South America (2005) [100,101]	1138 men and women (older than 55 years) with left ventricular dysfunction or diabetes (4 years + follow-up to 7 years)	Vitamin E (400 mg) daily	No significant effect on cancer incidence or mortality; no significant effect on CVD events but heart failure +13%

(Continued)

TABLE 18.3   *(Continued)*

Study and publication date	Study details, size, and duration	Intervention details	Study results
E3N Prospective Cohort Study, France (2006) [58]	59,910 women—selected 700 with smoking-related cancers (7.4 years)	βC intake divided into quartiles from diet reports	Nonsmokers 20 to 60 + % reduction lung cancer; smokers 1.5–2 × increase
SELECT, United States (2008) [50]	35,533 men (5.46 years) PSA <4 ng/ml and normal digital exam (aged 50 or 55 years) (5.5 years)	Se 200 μg/day as selenomethionine, racemic vitamin E 400 (IU)/day	No significant effect on prostate cancer or diabetes for combination; nonsignificant increase in prostate with vitamin E
PHS II study, United States (2008) [49]	14,641 male physicians (50 years or older) + 8-year follow-up	Vitamin C (500 mg daily), vitamin E 400 (IU) every other day	No significant effect on lung, colorectal, prostate, or total cancer; vitamin E-associated hemorrhagic stroke
Women's Antioxidant Cardiovascular Study (WASC), United States (2009) [48]	7627 cancer-free women (40 years or older) (9.4 years)	Vitamin C (500 mg daily) and vitamin E 600 (IU) + βC (50 mg) every other day	No significant effect on total cancer incidence or cancer mortality

baseline health and ROS levels, exposure to environmental carcinogens, and genetic differences in ROS metabolism [37]. Some argue that higher doses of some antioxidants have a pro-oxidant effect [2], and there is a high probability that pharmacokinetics including absorption, distribution, metabolism, and excretion of a simple ingested supplement is quite different from the complex matrix in fruits and vegetables, which contains many different types of antioxidants as well as other macro- and micronutrients and other phytochemicals.

Because many examples of J- and U-shaped dose–response curves have been reported among vitamins, other nutrients, and food additives, a critical question for cancer patients should be the following: What is the potential interaction of ROS and antioxidants with chemotherapy and radiation therapy? The interaction occurs sometimes in a positive manner, enhancing the efficacy of the treatment, but also sometimes negatively, interfering with the agent or treatment. Similarly, individual antioxidants can inhibit or stimulate tumor cell growth or survival depending on the tumor, the antioxidant, and the oxidative status; this means that there is no simple answer regarding the overall effectiveness of antioxidants, and each must be considered on a case-by-case basis. The following sections provide the results of some major clinical and epidemiological trials on the antioxidant effects on cancer and observed side effects, particularly on CVD, focusing on the antioxidants selenium, vitamin E, vitamin C, and β-carotene, all of which are readily available in the marketplace as dietary supplements. Key study findings and some experimental details are presented Table 18.3.

A Antioxidants and Cancer

The potential benefits of the dietary antioxidants selenium, vitamin E, vitamin C, and β-carotene in numerous observational and clinical trials have been examined for several years [7,38]. Since the 1990s, however, evidence has emerged indicating that some antioxidants, in certain individuals, perhaps at untoward high doses or in the presence of specific conditions or cancer treatments, may modulate normal protective benefits, whereas others may bring about deleterious effects, such as interfering with the efficacy of cancer drug treatment or increasing an individual's risk for cancer or heart disease [39,40].

1 Antioxidant Supplementation and Cancer Prevention

On initial examination of Table 18.3, large-scale trials do not consistently demonstrate a definite benefit of antioxidant supplements in healthy individuals. However, closer examination suggests that in individuals with initially low background antioxidant status, supplementation to achieve a normal range may bring about some health benefit [41]. In some cases, however, high-dose supplementation may lead to potentially harmfully elevated blood levels, especially in oxidatively stressed individuals such as smokers who consume large amounts of β-carotene.

a β-CAROTENE

A major issue in assessing antioxidant efficacy is whether any antioxidant interventions, especially at elevated doses above the normal nutritional level, result in a dose-dependent benefit to individuals at risk from disease. For example, two large-scale, randomized intervention trials evaluated the effect of β-carotene supplementation over 12 years on the primary prevention of cancer and CVD in male physicians (Physicians Health Study (PHS)) [42] and over 2 years in female health professionals (Women's Health Study (WHS)) [43]. The dose administered was

50 µg β-carotene every other day. Upon initial evaluation, no evidence of either stimulation or inhibition of either disease was noted when placebo and treated groups were compared. However, subgroup analyses of the PHS data later found that men with the lowest quartile for plasma β-carotene at initial baseline had a lower risk for total cancer, particularly prostate cancer, when β-carotene supplement users were compared with placebo [44]. The average blood levels achieved during the PHS study were 120 µg/dl [45], whereas normal serum β-carotene is in the 5 to 50 µg/dl range [1]. An effect on smokers was not observable in these two studies, possibly because only 11% of the physicians and 13% of the women were smokers; therefore, the study was not adequately powered to examine this aspect. There is no reason to suspect that these individuals were nutritionally compromised, so the results may not be universally applicable to the general population. Additional β-carotene findings were derived from nested cohort subsets of randomized clinical trials of β-carotene. These studies found no evidence that β-carotene supplementation prevented recurrence of basal or squamous carcinomas of the skin (50 µg/day) in the United States [46] or of colorectal adenomas (20 mg/day) in Australia [47].

Similarly, several randomized trials in high-risk populations have reported reduced disease risk using antioxidants, at least in baseline deficient populations when subsets of the populations are examined. The NCI trials, conducted in Linxian, China, with a population at high risk for esophageal cancer, noted a significant benefit for those receiving a β-carotene/vitamin E/selenium combination: a 13% decrease in the cancer mortality rate, a 21% decrease in stomach cancer mortality, a 4% decrease in esophageal cancer mortality, a 10% decrease in deaths from strokes, and a 9% decrease in deaths from all causes [41]. However, the generalizability of these findings from Linxian may not be universally appropriate because individuals in this study appear to have limited intakes of several micronutrients. Thus, these trial findings may not be applicable to well-nourished populations. Indeed, several studies did not show stimulatory or inhibitory effects on total cancers or the target organs in U.S. populations [48−50] (Table 18.3).

2 Effects in Smokers

When smokers were selected as the target population, very different views surfaced about the health consequences of β-carotene supplements. Two highly publicized trials provided evidence for potentially adverse effects of antioxidants, particularly in smokers and in individuals exposed to certain environmental hazards, such as asbestos. These two independent, randomized, clinical trials—the 5- to 8-year ATBC (Alpha-Tocopherol Beta-Carotene) [51] and the 4-year CARET (Beta-Carotene and Retinol Efficacy Trial) [52]—reported adverse effects of 20- and 30-mg β-carotene daily supplementation on lung cancer risk in these high-risk populations. The ATBC studied effects primarily in smokers, whereas the PHS included more than half who were nonsmokers [42]. Similar to the PHS study results for β-carotene, the ATBC study data demonstrated a reduction (32%) in prostate cancer incidence in the α-tocopherol (vitamin E) supplemented group [53] and 22% fewer cases of colorectal cancer [54] upon reanalysis. Although lung cancer incidence was elevated in both ATBC and CARET smokers with β-carotene, after a 12-year follow-up of CARET participants, a significant decrease in lung cancer incidence in the placebo arm was observed that was linked to fruit and vegetable intake when the lowest versus highest quintiles were compared [55]. An earlier case−control study of lung cancer in nonsmokers conducted in New York concluded that dietary β-carotene, raw fruits and vegetables, and vitamin E supplements reduced the risk of lung cancer in nonsmoking men and women [56]. A subsequent evaluation of the Nurses' Health Study from Harvard implicated carrots but not β-carotene, further adding to the confusion [57]. Interestingly, in the French Etude Epidemiologique de Femmes de la Mutuelle Generale de l'Education Nationale (E3N) prospective investigation, the nonsmoking women showed a dose-dependent lowering of lung cancer risk when intakes were considered. The largest reduction was observed in women taking β-carotene supplements, but smokers showed the commonly observed increased risk [58]. Research has implicated β-carotene cleavage products as likely factors in the increased cancer activity of high β-carotene doses, exacerbated by smoking-induced alterations in β-carotene metabolism [45,59,60].

3 Follow-Up Examinations of Existing Studies

Follow-up examinations of a subset of the ATBC cohort have reported a marked association between elevated serum levels of α-tocopherol and reduced prostate cancer risk in a 6-year prospective study with 100 prostate cancer patients and 200 controls [61]; however, a separate post-intervention study reported that the excess risk for lung cancer and the beneficial effect for prostate cancer were no longer significantly different from controls [62]. In addition, with the exception of a slight carotene protective effect on early stage laryngeal cancer, other upper aerodigestive cancers were not affected [63], although a dose−responsive decrease in mortality with increasing vitamin E serum levels was noted [64]. Interestingly, evaluation of dietary records in the ATBC study indicated that consumption of fruits and vegetables was associated with a lower lung cancer risk, as were the levels of dietary lycopene and other carotenoids, as well as actual serum levels of β-carotene and retinol, when the highest and lowest baseline quintiles were compared [65]. A 6-year follow-up of the CARET cohort reported that the increased risk was no longer significant for either lung cancer or cardiovascular disease, but subgroup analysis suggests excess risk in heretofore unreported susceptible groups (females and former smokers), a difference from the ATBC study that may be due to the higher β-carotene dose in CARET [36] or perhaps the presence of vitamin E (α-tocopherol). The return to normal risk levels in the smokers suggests that subtle changes were introduced such that this group may have actually achieved protection from prior treatment. Thus, it is conceivable that the increased risk observed in the ATBC study may have reflected an increase in those with a preexisting precancerous lesion or tumor but protection in those without. This hypothesis would also explain the lack of increased cancer in the Women's Antioxidant Cardiovascular Study, in which cancer-free women were given vitamins C and E plus 50 mg β-carotene [48]. Thus, the question of benefits or merits of β-carotene in smokers remains controversial because it may depend on the presence or absence of precancerous lesions.

Further follow-up and reexamination of subgroup analysis may also help explain these unexpected results. For example, the French study, SUppléments en VItamines et Minéraux AntioXydants (Antioxidant Vitamin and Mineral Supplements (SU.VI.MAX)), examined the effects of supplementation with vitamins C and E (120 and 30 mg, respectively), 6 mg β-carotene, 100 μg selenium, and 20 mg zinc on the health of approximately 13,000 men (45–60 years) and women (35–60 years) [66–69]. In men only, antioxidant supplementation reduced the risk of developing all types of cancers by 31%. This effect was most pronounced in men with low baseline levels of β-carotene who had the greatest increased risk of developing cancer. An evaluation of the study data showed that there was a nonsignificant reduction in prostate cancer rate associated with the supplementation in all men, but there was a significant difference between men with normal baseline prostate-specific antigen (PSA) and those with elevated PSA. Among men with normal PSA, there was a statistically significant reduction in the prostate cancer rate among those receiving the supplements. Surprisingly, the supplementation was associated with an increased incidence of prostate cancer, with borderline statistical significance in men with elevated PSA at baseline [69]. The average β-carotene blood levels both at the beginning of the study ($\sim$39 μg/dl in women and $\sim$25 μg/dl in men) and at the end ($\sim$90 μg/dl for women and $\sim$50 μg/dl for men) were below those

seen in the PHS, whereas no such change was observed for serum levels of vitamins E or C, selenium, or zinc.

a SELENIUM

Dietary selenium is another potentially important antioxidant and potential chemopreventive agent because of its importance in the functionality of glutathione peroxidase. Strong evidence linking selenium supplementation and decreased cancer risk comes from the secondary analysis of the Nutritional Prevention of Cancer (NPC) trial, a study designed for patients with a history of basal or squamous cell carcinomas [70]. Although no benefit was observed for skin cancer, the primary end point of the study, secondary end point analyses showed significant reductions in relative risk for total cancer mortality (50%), total cancer incidence (37%), as well as incidences of lung (46%), colorectal (58%), and prostate (63%) cancer for patients who received selenium supplements. Further reanalysis of the NPC data confirmed a 49% reduction in prostate cancer incidence in men receiving selenium supplements compared to controls, although follow-up suggests the benefits may be decreasing with time [71]. Another reanalysis that included 3 additional years of follow-up data found a nonsignificant decrease in lung cancer risk for all patients who received selenium supplements; however, the analysis suggested a significant risk reduction following supplementation among those with the lowest baseline plasma selenium [72]. A separate study by Li et al. [73] also indicated that a reduction in prostate cancer incidence occurred following selenium supplementation. The authors of these various studies differ in their conclusions concerning whether selenium prevents initiation of carcinogenesis or inhibits tumor progression; nevertheless, the benefit of selenium for prostate cancer prevention is fairly consistent. A wealth of preclinical studies support the anticancer properties of selenium. Much of the evidence concerning selenium's anticancer/antitumor properties suggests mechanisms of action other than those associated with its antioxidant properties [74]. A clinical trial of selenium as selenomethionine in combination with vitamin E, however, failed to show a significant effect on prostate cancer or diabetes, but selenium alone gave a nonsignificant increase in diabetes and selenium a similar effect on the prostate in a very large cohort of relatively healthy U.S. men [50].

4 Antioxidant Combinations

More broadly, a meta-analysis of antioxidant supplementation in patients at elevated risk of gastrointestinal cancers revealed no protective effect for vitamins A, C, and E on esophageal, gastric, colorectal, pancreatic, and liver cancers. However, selenium supplementation was noted as possibly a cancer deterrent. The authors have noted that the findings may not be easily extrapolated to the effects of fruits and vegetables, which are rich sources of only some of these antioxidants [35]. Likewise, the applicability of these findings to healthy individuals is unclear. The follow-up examination of fruit and vegetable use and breast cancer risk within the European Prospective Investigation into Cancer and Nutrition (EPIC) study indicated that fruits and vegetables had no effect on cancer when the highest versus the lowest quintiles were compared [75]. These findings add to the confusion in light of other studies that suggest fruits and vegetables have benefits, particularly when associated with their antioxidant content [55,56,58]. The WHS, however, saw a reduction in myocardial infarction [76]. These inconsistencies may reflect the variation in the intake of individual fruits and vegetables, their interactions with environmental insults, or the genetic background of the consumer.

Completion of the human genome sequence and the advent of DNA microarrays using cDNAs enhanced the detection and identification of hundreds of differentially expressed genes in response to antioxidants including flavonoids, selenium, zinc, and several vitamins [77]. The phenolic antioxidant resveratrol found in berries and grapes has been reported to inhibit the growth formation of prostate tumor cells by acting on the regulatory genes such as p53 while activating a cascade of genes involved in cell cycle and apoptosis, including p300, Apaf-1, cdk inhibitor p21, p57 (KIP2), p53-induced Pig 7, Pig 8, Pig 10, cyclin D, and DNA fragmentation factor 45, although some findings were not confirmed by reverse transcriptase—polymerase chain reaction [78]. Likewise, the expression of a host of genes is influenced by selenium supplementation [79].

B Antioxidants and Cardiovascular Disease

Despite the general acceptance of antioxidants' safety and potential efficacy [38], meta-analysis of clinically based studies of vitamin E supplementation showing increased mortality above a 400-mg dose [80], compared to a protective effect of fruit and vegetable consumption in EPIC [75] and a meta-analysis of fruit and vegetable cohort studies [81], provides mixed evidence. A study by Kushi *et al.* in 1996 examined the role of dietary antioxidants in randomly chosen members of the prospective Iowa Women's Health Study [82]. A dose-dependent inverse relationship between vitamin E consumption and coronary heart disease mortality was detected. The strongest inverse association was observed among the approximately 22,000 women who did not consume vitamin supplements compared to those who did [82]. The meta-analysis of high-dose vitamin E supplementation by Miller *et al.* [80], however, suggested

a positive association of all-cause mortality when supplementation was above 400 IU/day. Despite a number of issues with the choice of studies to be included and excluded in the meta-analysis, as well as the failure to consider a dose—response relationship in the physiological range, Wright's earlier analysis of continuous serum α-tocopherol values in the ATBC study indicated a dose-dependent reduction in mortality because of chronic disease with increasing concentrations up to approximately 13 or 14 mg/l (30—33 mmol/l), after which no further benefit was noted. Those with the higher baseline blood levels showed decreased mortality [64]. The use of superphysiological exposures with questionable health benefits, especially for those at the highest status, raises serious concerns about the wisdom of megadoses of vitamin E supplements. A meta-analysis of more than 60 clinical trials that focused on antioxidant use (including vitamin E) reached similar conclusions about slightly increased mortality but again may have introduced some biases in the evaluation [83]. Another study, the Canadian Heart Outcomes Prevention Evaluation (HOPE)—a randomized controlled prospective investigation of vitamin E supplementation (400 IU/day) in approximately 4700 patients with diabetes and other cardiovascular risk factors—linked supplementation with an increased risk of heart failure but no protection from cancer in the 2.6-year follow-up portion of the study; no differences in cardiovascular effects were noted during the first 4.6 years [84].

Research evidence from large-scale trials also indicated no clear benefit of antioxidant supplements in healthy individuals when considered *in toto*. Upon closer examination, supplementing individuals with low background levels to a normal range may be beneficial, but high-dose supplementation leading to markedly elevated blood levels may be harmful, especially in oxidatively stressed individuals, such as smokers in the case of β-carotene or in unhealthy or older patients in the case of vitamin E.

1 Targets of Antioxidant-Related Disease Protection

Vitamin E, vitamin C, and β-carotene intake, whether by supplementation or as components of foods, has been extensively studied for their potential to reduce CVD or conditions related to the sequelae of CVD and other vascular diseases. A number of older studies suggest that vitamin E, alone or in combination with other antioxidants, may be protective against atherosclerosis in at-risk populations. In the WHS, there was a significant (24%) reduction in cardiovascular deaths [85] in the vitamin E group. However, other studies question the overall benefits [51,86—88]. In addition to a potential role in minimizing oxidative DNA damage and lipid peroxidation, vitamin E may modify several other functions, some of which specifically protect against processes known to contribute to atherosclerosis, including inhibiting protein kinase C activity and smooth muscle cell proliferation, inhibiting cell adhesion and platelet aggregation, counteracting inflammation, and enhancing bioavailability of nitric oxide to improve endothelium-dependent vasodilator function [89—91]. Vitamin E may also improve insulin-mediated glucose uptake, thus possibly decreasing risk for type 2 diabetes, a condition that also contributes to atherosclerosis [92].

2 Clinical Trial Interventions for CVD Amelioration

Antioxidants have been tested for the ability to ameliorate development of CVD in some at-risk populations. The Antioxidant Supplementation in Atherosclerosis Prevention (ASAP) study, a 6-year randomized trial, supplemented 520 hypercholesterolemic men and postmenopausal women (45—69 years old) with vitamin C and vitamin E [93]. A significant decrease (26%) in the progression of carotid atherosclerosis was observed in men, although no significant effect was seen in women. In the Harvard Intravascular Ultrasonography (IVUS) study, a combination of vitamin C and vitamin E was given to 40 (35 males) cardiac transplant patients. Cardiac transplantation leads to oxidative stress, which may contribute to atherosclerosis; supplementation of patients with these vitamins slowed progress of coronary atherosclerosis [94].

Two large studies have reported preliminary results. The British Heart Protection Study, a multicenter, randomized, double-blind, placebo-controlled trial with a 2×2 factorial design, enrolled 20,536 patients aged 55—75 years who were at an increased 5-year risk of myocardial infarction [95]. Participants received antioxidant vitamins (combination of 600 IU vitamin E, 250 mg vitamin C, and 20 mg β-carotene) and simvastatin or each separately. No adverse or beneficial effect on vascular or nonvascular morbidity or mortality could be attributed to supplementation with vitamins. The American PHS II enrolled 15,000 physicians aged 55 years or older in a randomized, double-blind, placebo-controlled trial to test β-carotene, vitamin E (400 IU synthetic on alternate days), vitamin C (500 mg/day), and multivitamin (Recommended Dietary Allowance (RDA) of most vitamins and minerals) in a $2 \times 2 \times 2 \times 2$ factorial design [96]. This study was completed in September 2007 [49]. The effects of supplementation on the prevention of total and prostate cancer, CVD, and age-related eye diseases (cataracts and macular degeneration) have been examined. No effects on cancer were observed. Preliminary analysis reported no significant effect of any of the vitamins on cardiovascular outcomes, but a greater number of hemorrhagic strokes were observed in

the vitamin E versus placebo group; the effects of multivitamin use are still being evaluated [49]. The WHS tested the ability of aspirin, vitamin E, and β-carotene to prevent cancer and CVD [43,85]. Analysis of β-carotene supplementation showed no effect of β-carotene on risk of CVD. In the vitamin E group, there was a significant (24%) reduction in cardiovascular deaths [85]. Despite the lack of evidence for an effect of the combined discrete nutrients on CVD, high fruit and vegetable intake was associated with lower risk for myocardial infarction in the WHS study [76].

As seen in the WHS, dietary habits may sometimes be linked to decreased CVD risk, despite a lack of effectiveness for individual supplements. Similarly, Mennen et al. [97] found that a diet rich in flavonoids reduced cardiovascular disease risk in a subset of women participating in the SU.VI.MAX study [66—69]. Dietary intakes were estimated using six 24-hour dietary records collected during the course of 1 year. In women, flavonoid-rich food consumption was associated with decreased systolic blood pressure and a decreased risk for CVD; this relationship was not observed in men. The lack of an effect in men could be attributed to the men's higher risk for CVD; inconsistencies in dietary reporting and measuring of flavonoid consumption could also contribute to this discrepancy. However, this study found that after 7.5 years of follow-up, no protective effect against ischemic heart disease attributable to antioxidant supplementation could be discerned in either men or women [97].

Four large, randomized clinical trials specifically tested the ability of vitamin E supplementation to slow the progression of CVD in individuals at increased risk for CVD death (reviewed by Salonen [98]). The ATBC trial, originally designed to test cancer prevention abilities of vitamins C and E and β-carotene, tested supplementation with 50 mg α-tocopherol acetate daily for 5—8 years [51]. In this study of male smokers, α-tocopherol supplementation was associated with a modest trend toward decreased incidence of angina pectoris but no decrease in CVD mortality. β-Carotene supplementation had no preventive effect and was associated with a slight increase in the occurrence of angina [86]. An apparent excess of hemorrhagic stroke in the treatment group complicated this study. The Cambridge Heart Antioxidant Study (CHAOS) tested RRR-α-tocopherol from "natural sources" in 2002 participants with clinical evidence of CVD [87]. Trial analysis identified a 77% decrease in nonfatal myocardial infarction but also a nonsignificant increase in early deaths from CVD and total mortality, although no increase in risk of hemorrhagic stroke was observed. Interpretation of this study was complicated by unbalanced randomization, incomplete follow-up, and a midstudy change in vitamin E dose (800 IU per day to 400 IU per day) [88]. The Italian Gruppo Italiano per lo Studio della Supravvivenza nell Infarto Miocardio (GISSI) study supplemented 11,324 participants with previous myocardial infarction with 300 mg all-racemic α-tocopherol daily, with or without 1 g polyunsaturated fatty acids (PUFAs) [99]. No effect was observed in the group receiving both supplements, but a significant 20% decrease in cardiovascular death was observed in the group receiving only PUFAs [99]. In the HOPE study, 2545 women and 6996 men at high risk for CVD received either 400 IU per day "natural source" vitamin E or ramipril; this study found no effect of supplementation on any parameters related to CVD [100,101]. As noted previously, however, the follow-up study suggests an increase in CVD after an additional 2.6 years [84]. The Women's Health Initiative examined multivitamin use in more than 160,000 women during an 8-year clinical trial follow-up period with nearly 8 years of observational follow-up. More than 40% used multivitamins, and this was not linked to increases in several common cancers, CVD, myocardial infarction, stroke, and overall mortality [102].

ROS can influence the inflammatory process. Because inflammation is thought to be a significant cause of damage to blood vessels, contributing to CVD, it may be a target for treatment with antioxidants. Vascular smooth muscle cell accumulation and hypertrophy, and nitric oxide regulation of endothelial vasorelaxation and vasodilation, are processes that may also be therapeutically modulated by antioxidants. Although individual supplements have not proven to be strongly effective, diets high in fruit and vegetables, and their attendant antioxidant and phytochemical combinations, generally have been shown to be somewhat protective [81]. Of course, diets high in fruits and vegetables may indirectly reduce the risk of CVD by promoting healthy body weight, decreasing the risk of developing conditions contributing to CVD such as hyperlipidemia and type 2 diabetes.

Studies with defined populations have generally failed to demonstrate marked prevention potential for cancer or heart disease, but animal studies suggest benefits should occur. There are a number of possible explanations for this inconsistency. Foremost among these is that significant nutrient–nutrient interactions are likely occurring along with the importance of environmental insults as determinants of the overall response. Some of the case–control studies may actually be selecting participants with a general interest in the pursuit of a healthy lifestyle. It is known that volunteers for observational antioxidant studies tend to have better diets, exercise more, use less alcohol, and come from higher socioeconomic backgrounds, all of which all may contribute to a decreased baseline risk for CVD and other disease conditions [103].

In addition, supplement users tend to have healthy lifestyles and diets favorable for disease prevention [103].

C Polymorphism: An Additional Risk Factor in Cancer

Evidence is increasing that genetic polymorphisms can influence the response to an arsenal of agents used in the battle against cancer, including both drugs and dietary components. However, these investigations are often conflicting because the development of cancer is not a simple process but, rather, involves multiple cellular events, many of which are likely influenced by genetic polymorphisms at the site of the target or by how the agent is modified through absorption, metabolism, or excretion.

Although ROS are integral to many cellular and biomolecular processes associated with acute coronary syndromes, metabolism, and early stages of cancer, the relationship to specific genetic polymorphisms has not been overly compelling and remains controversial. It may be that current eating behaviors prevent the easy identification of diet–gene–health interactions in this disease condition. However, mechanistically, the linkage with free radical-related gene polymorphisms is logical and deserves additional attention as a potential subtle long-term regulator of both cancer and heart disease risk. Little attention has been given to genes associated with oxidative stress and heart disease; the primary focus has been on cholesterol homeostasis and control [104]. However, two papers have focused on ROS and antioxidant vitamins. The overall view is that ROS are strongly linked with atherosclerosis, hypertension, and congestive heart failure, but a demonstrated efficacy of antioxidants has proved elusive [105,106].

A number of scientists have been exploring the effects of genetic polymorphisms on oxidative stress or the ability of antioxidants to influence the cancer process. Several examples concerning the possible utility of using specific polymorphisms as predictors of cancer risk have surfaced. For example, the manganese superoxide dismutase (MnSOD) protein is involved in decreasing the levels of superoxide anion generated during normal biochemical processes. A polymorphism that changes an alanine residue to valine in position 9 or valine to alanine in position 16 in the protein has been suspected to be a risk factor in prostate and breast carcinogenesis and has been found with higher frequency in individuals with prostate cancer [107–109] and, in some studies, with increased severity of the disease and earlier onset [109,110]. Likewise, breast cancer risk was observed to be slightly increased (odds ratio 1.3) in women with Ala/Ala genotype compared to those with Val/Val genotype [111].

Interestingly, patients carrying the Val allele may have a higher prevalence of cardiomyopathy [112]. However, these early findings need to be further investigated because a number of clinical and meta-analysis studies [108–110,113–120] examining the link of these mutations to both cancers are inconsistent, with some having failed to verify an association and others supporting it (Table 18.4). Some studies have shown the association to be primarily in those with low antioxidant consumption [108,118,121].

The catalase (CAT) gene polymorphism at 262C→T may also have a role in breast cancer development. This antioxidant enzyme neutralizes hydrogen peroxide and is known to be induced by oxidative challenges. A 262C→T polymorphism in the promoter region of CAT is associated with risk of several conditions related to oxidative stress. Interestingly, the CC genotype relationship with breast cancer reduction was only observed among Caucasians and not in African Americans [122]. CAT polymorphism at codon 262 does not appear to be related to diabetes and the risk of heart disease [123]. The reason for the disconnect among genetic polymorphisms (CAT and MnSOD), oxidative damage, and risk of cancer and heart disease warrants additional attention but may be due to an enhanced response to antioxidants in the CC genotype [121].

Still another gene involved in antioxidant activity and cancer risk is glutathione peroxidase 1 (GPX-1) [100]. Although codon 198 can lead to leucine or proline, it was determined that the leucine-containing allele was more frequently associated with breast cancer than was the proline-containing allele [124]; however, there are inconsistencies in the literature [125,126]. Combinations of gene polymorphism may offer additional insights into risk. Cox et al. [127] observed an increased breast cancer relative risk (OR = 1.87) in individuals with the MnSOD Ala16Ala genotype and the Leu198Leu genotype of GPX-1, whereas neither surfaced as risk modifiers when considered independently.

Environmental factors may also dictate the importance of genetic polymorphisms in determining cancer risk. For example, the T allele in the GPX-1 gene at position 198 is considered to be protective in smokers. In a study of smokers with 432 lung cancer cases and 366 controls, those possessing the variant T allele were significantly less likely to develop lung cancer than individuals without it [128]. Likewise, patients with alcohol-induced cirrhosis who had the genotype consistent with low MnSOD activity and also with high GPX-1 activity had much lower levels of potentially toxic levels of iron. In individuals with both polymorphisms, none developed hepatocellular carcinoma, as opposed to other polymorphism combinations, for which 16–32% of the individuals developed liver cancer [129]. In addition, consumption of a number of food items may influence the relationship between individual polymorphisms and health. Both aldehyde dehydrogenase-2 (ALDH2) and X-ray repair cross-complementing 1 (XRCC1) genes have been identified as having a role in the response to dietary selenium. The glutamic acid 487 lysine polymorphism in the ALDH2 gene and the arginine 399 glutamine polymorphism in the XRCC1 gene are both associated with an increased risk of esophageal cancer in individuals consuming a low-selenium diet. In addition, this risk becomes even more pronounced in individuals who smoke or consume alcohol [130]. This may reflect the individual pharmacokinetics in handling supplemental selenium. Likewise, the protective effect of the catalase CC genotype was even more pronounced among women who used dietary supplements, as well as those with high fruit and vegetable intakes [131]. In another study, an inverse association between fruit and vegetable consumption and breast cancer risk was observed among women with the wild-type genotype for codon 84 of their O^6-methylguanine-DNA methyltransferase (MGMT) gene [132]. In this group, the observed OR was 0.8, whereas for individuals with other polymorphisms, the effects of a varied intake were not statistically significant. The association between fruit and vegetable consumption and reduced breast cancer risk was also seen

TABLE 18.4 Meta-Analyses of Prostate and Breast Cancer Risk with SOD Mutations

Mutation	Organ	No. of studies	Cases	Controls	Results	Reference
Ala-9Val	Prostate	5	889	1841	Nonsignificant increase	[119]
Ala-9Val	Prostate	9	1660	2594	Positive	[108]
Ala-9Val	Breast	13	4278	5057	Nonsignificant increase	[108]
Ala-16Val	Prostate	4	2379	4066	Nonsignificant increase	[119]
Ala-16Val	Prostate	32	26,022	32,426	Negative	[120]
Ala-16Val	Prostate	12	3574	5388	Positive	[117]
Ala-16Val	Breast	17	9710	11,041	Negative	[113]

in individuals with a variant allele for codon 143 in their MGMT gene. In one study, the intake of α- and β-carotene as modifiers of skin cancer was found to relate to MnSOD V16A polymorphism, such that an inverse association of intake was limited to the Val carriers, whereas no association was observed among women with the AA genotype [133].

D Antioxidants: Prevention Versus Treatment in Clinical Applications

As has been indicated, antioxidants can have both beneficial and deleterious effects on disease. In the case of cardiovascular disease in general and atherosclerosis in particular, the effects of antioxidants would be expected to be primarily beneficial because lipid oxidation and inflammation are important factors in the sequelae involving atherosclerotic plaque development. The overall consensus is that dietary antioxidant interventions seem to have a minor effect on improving atherosclerosis prevention [134]. However, reviews on the relationships of the statin drugs with free radical generation and inflammation provide evidence that statin drugs have a strong protective effect over and above their more well-known cholesterol-lowering activity [135]. Some of these protective effects, however, may be due to increased expression of antioxidant enzymes such as catalases and a suppression of pro-oxidant enzyme systems that reduce the production of the free radicals superoxide and peroxynitrite [136,137].

Antioxidant and ROS effects on the cancer process are in part dependent on the status and behaviors of the consumer as well as the stage of development and type of cancer involved. The ability to predict and distinguish between the positive and negative effects of antioxidants is especially crucial in those receiving cancer treatments.

Many cancer patients take vitamin supplements for protection and health promotion. A survey of patients at a comprehensive cancer center found that 60% of patients used vitamins and the majority combined them with conventional therapy [138]. Similarly, among a Massachusetts cohort of women with early stage breast cancer, 60% used megavitamin therapy along with surgery, chemotherapy, and/or radiation therapy [139]. Given the large numbers of cancer patients taking antioxidant vitamins, with or without the knowledge of their oncologists, greater understanding of the actions of antioxidants within the cancer disease and treatment milieu is crucial. Consumer awareness of the issues between antioxidants and cancer appears to be increasing but is far behind other health-related dietary practices [140].

Radiotherapy, as well as many chemotherapeutic agents, eliminates cancer cells by inducing apoptosis via generation of ROS. Thus, it was feared that antioxidants, especially in megadoses, may decrease ROS production and thus decrease the benefits of these treatments. Nevertheless, a number of in vitro and some clinical studies have shown that antioxidant treatment during standard cancer therapy does not always interfere with these therapies. The use of high-dose levels of antioxidants appears to be critical to achieve a beneficial outcome when antioxidants are used with more conventional treatments. In several reported studies, low doses of antioxidants stimulated the growth of human cancer cells in culture, and a single low dose of antioxidant before radiation therapy protected cells against radiation damage, suggesting that low doses of antioxidants might have detrimental effects on cancer treatment [141,142]. High-dose levels have been defined in humans as up to 10 g vitamin C/day, up to 1000 IU vitamin E/day, and up to 60 μg β-carotene/day; in tissue culture, high levels have been considered up to 200 μg vitamin C/ml, up to 20 μg vitamin E/ml, and up to 15 μg β-carotene/ml [143]. Low-dose levels have been defined in humans as approximately the RDA values and in tissue culture as up to 50 μg vitamin C/ml, up to 5 μg vitamin E/ml, and up to 1 μg β-carotene/ml [141].

Although antioxidants may cause some inhibition of ROS production caused by chemo- or radiation therapy, at high levels the antioxidant can directly inhibit tumor growth and can appear to stimulate the drug effects. Prasad et al. [143] described the ability of the α-tocopherol succinate form of vitamin E to enhance the cytotoxic effects of adriamycin in human prostate cancer, glioma, and HeLa cells; enhance cisplatin, tamoxifen, and decarbazine in human melanoma and parotid acinar carcinoma cells; and promote doxorubicin to inhibit murine leukemia cell lines.

The subject of antioxidants during cancer care has been reviewed [144], but data from large-scale trials with antioxidants are not available. Interestingly, some smaller studies provide limited evidence that antioxidant supplementation can increase the efficacy of standard chemotherapies in humans. In 18 nonrandomized patients with small cell lung cancer, supplementation with multiple antioxidants along with chemotherapy or radiation therapy resulted in increased survival times. Retinoic acid and interferon enhanced the effect of radiation on locally advanced cervical adenoma, again improving survival times [145]. Two patients with advanced epithelial ovarian carcinoma (stage IIIC) received antioxidant therapy (1200 IU vitamin E, 300 mg coenzyme Q10, 9000 mg vitamin C, 25 mg mixed carotenoids, and 10,000 IU vitamin A) before conventional chemotherapy and 60 g ascorbic acid twice weekly at the end of therapy. Both women had normal CA-125 levels and remained disease-free more than 3 years after initial diagnosis [146]. In an open trial in patients with small cell lung cancer, patients who received individualized daily supplements of trace elements, fatty acids, and vitamins (including 15,000–40,000 IU vitamin A, 10,000–20,000 IU β-carotene, 300–800 IU vitamin E, 2–5 g vitamin C, and 1600–3400 μg selenium) had a greater 2-year survival rate than historical controls (33 versus <15%) [147,148]. Furthermore, an analysis of 385 breast cancer patients asked to recall antioxidant supplement use showed that users of supplements were less likely to have a breast cancer recurrence or breast cancer-related death than nonusers [149]. In contrast, an analysis of outcomes for 90 women with unilateral nonmetastatic breast cancer who received megadoses of vitamins and minerals (β-carotene, vitamin C, niacin, selenium, coenzyme Q10, and zinc) showed no improvement in survival compared to matched controls (the 5-year survival rate was 72% for cases and 81% for controls) [150]. Although definitive conclusions cannot be drawn from this limited number of studies, improvement in survival of patients receiving antioxidants in addition to chemotherapy has been observed. The use of antioxidant vitamins in conjunction with standard therapy warrants additional attention [151].

III OVERALL CONCLUSION AND DISCUSSION

ROS are a potential double-edged sword in disease promotion and prevention. Whereas the generation of ROS once was viewed as detrimental to the overall health of the organism, advances in research have shown that ROS play crucial roles in normal physiological processes, including response to growth factors, the immune response, and apoptotic elimination of damaged cells. Notwithstanding these beneficial functions, aberrant production or regulation of ROS activity has been demonstrated to contribute to the development of some prevalent diseases and conditions, including cancer and CVD. Antioxidant supplementation has historically been viewed as a promising therapy for prevention and treatment of these diseases, especially given the tantalizing but sometimes conflicting links observed between diets high in fruits and vegetables (and presumably antioxidants) and decreased risks for cancer and CVD. Trials of individual antioxidants, however, have rarely shown strongly beneficial effects. In most healthy individuals, endogenous antioxidant defenses may be sufficient, and extra supplementation may have little effect on disease susceptibility. In some populations, particularly those with underlying illness or compromised nutritional

status, dietary or other supplementation may be helpful. A better understanding of the impact of supplementation on disease risk may also be furthered by increased knowledge of individual genetic polymorphisms related to the metabolism and detoxification of ROS and antioxidants, as well as interactions of metabolic intermediates. A more critical issue is the interaction of antioxidants and orthodox cancer therapy.

Advances in tools used to determine oxidative status may allow for the estimating of an individual antioxidant profile. Whether supplements have positive or negative effects may depend on an individual's baseline antioxidant and ROS levels. Antioxidant supplementation in those with low baseline ROS could be detrimental because it may impair normal immune function and prevent ROS-mediated apoptotic elimination of precancerous or cancerous cells. Similarly, better measurements of ROS status may help to predict the potential for antioxidants in individuals exposed to specific environmental toxins, including but not limited to cigarette smoke, which may influence the magnitude and direction of the response.

Current measures of antioxidant status in an individual vary greatly among different research settings, making comparison of results problematic. The establishment of "gold standard" biomarkers of oxidative stress and establishment of guidelines to accurately and precisely determine levels of a given marker in normal, healthy individuals should help to resolve the uncertainties in the literature. Better measurements may also help to determine why a diet high in fruits and vegetables is often more beneficial than specific antioxidant supplements. Additional research focusing on critical events that contribute to disease progression will help in defining the most efficient times for intervention with antioxidant supplementation.

Future research must focus on defining molecular mechanisms that engender oxidative stress, transforming healthy conditions to diseased states, and identifying timelines for effective interventions with antioxidants as either preventive or therapeutic agents. Although much of the current literature about antioxidants, including administration of pharmacological or dietary amounts, focuses on enhancing ROS elimination and inhibiting ROS generation, many other cellular processes are likely involved. An improved understanding of these cellular processes and how they relate to measures of oxidative stress will provide important clues about those who will benefit most or be placed at risk from antioxidant usage, whether provided as foods or supplements. The identification of the reliable and sensitive biomarkers of antioxidant exposures, of their biological effects or consequences, and of susceptibility factors including genetic and environmental modifiers will have far-reaching implications for the monitoring and treatment of oxidative stress related to health and disease conditions.

References

[1] Panel on Dietary Antioxidants and Related Compounds, A Report by the Panel on Dietary Antioxidants and Related Compounds: Dietary Reference Intakes for Vitamin C, Vitamin E, Selenium, and Carotenoids, Food and Nutrition Board, Institute of Medicine, Washington, DC, 2000.

[2] B. Halliwell, Oxidative stress and cancer: have we moved forward? Biochem. J. 401 (2007) 1–11.

[3] H.E. Seifried, D.E. Anderson, J.A. Milner, P. Greenwald, Reactive oxygen species and dietary antioxidants: double-edged swords? in: H. Panglossi (Ed.), New Developments in Antioxidant Research, Nova Science, Hauppauge, NY, 2006, pp. 1–25.

[4] U.S. Surgeon General, Healthy People: The Surgeon General's Report on Health Promotion and Disease Prevention, U.S. Public Health Service, Washington, DC, 1979 (see Chapter 11).

[5] American Institute for Cancer Research/World Cancer Research Fund, Food, Nutrition and the Prevention of Cancer: A Global Perspective, American Institute for Cancer Research, Washington, DC, 1997.

[6] K. Radimer, B. Bindewald, J. Hughes, B. Ervin, C. Swanson, M.F. Picciano, Dietary supplement use by U.S. adults: data from the National Health and Nutrition Examination Survey, 1999–2000, Am. J. Epidemiol. 160 (2004) 339–349.

[7] V. Mishra, Oxidative stress and role of antioxidant supplementation in critical illness, Clin. Lab. 53 (2007) 199–209.

[8] J. Gahche, R. Bailey, V. Burt, J. Hughes, E. Yetley, J. Dwyer, et al., Dietary supplement use among U.S. adults has increased since NHANES III (1988–1994), NCHS Data Brief (2011) 1–8.

[9] U.S. Department of Health and Human Services/Centers for Disease Control and Prevention/National Center for Health Statistics, Health, United States, 2010: with Special Feature on Death and Dying, National Center for Health Statistics, Hyattsville, MD, 2011 (p. 322, Table 96).

[10] R.B. Ervin, J.D. Wright, C.Y. Wang, J. Kennedy-Stephenson, Dietary intake of selected vitamins for the United States population: 1999–2000, Adv. Data (2004) 1–4.

[11] H.E. Seifried, D.E. Anderson, E.I. Fisher, J.A. Milner, A review of the interaction among dietary antioxidants and reactive oxygen species, J. Nutr. Biochem. 18 (2007) 567–579.

[12] R.L. Prior, X. Wu, K. Schaich, Standardized methods for the determination of antioxidant capacity and phenolics in foods and dietary supplements, J. Agric. Food Chem. 53 (2005) 4290–4302.

[13] D. Huang, B. Ou, R.L. Prior, The chemistry behind antioxidant capacity assays, J. Agric. Food Chem. 53 (2005) 1841–1856.

[14] S.B. Lotito, B. Frei, Consumption of flavonoid-rich foods and increased plasma antioxidant capacity in humans: cause, consequence, or epiphenomenon? Free Radic. Biol. Med. 41 (2006) 1727–1746.

[15] S.B. Lotito, W.J. Zhang, C.S. Yang, A. Crozier, B. Frei, Metabolic conversion of dietary flavonoids alters their anti-inflammatory and antioxidant properties, Free Radic. Biol. Med 51 (2011) 454–463.

[16] J.L. Martindale, N.J. Holbrook, Cellular response to oxidative stress: signaling for suicide and survival, J. Cell Physiol. 192 (2002) 1–15.

[17] P. Shekelle, S.C. Morton, M. Hardy, Effect of supplemental antioxidants vitamin C, vitamin E, and coenzyme Q10 for the prevention and treatment of cardiovascular disease, Evidence Report/Technology Assessment, Agency for Healthcare Research and Quality, Rockville, MD, 2003.

[18] I. Coulter, M. Hardy, P. Shekelle, S.C. Morton, Effect of the supplemental use of antioxidants vitamin C, vitamin E, and coenzyme Q10 for the prevention and treatment of cancer, Evidence Report/Technology Assessment, Agency for Healthcare Research and Quality, Rockville, MD, 2003 (No. 75).

[19] P.R. Taylor, P. Greenwald, Nutritional interventions in cancer prevention, J. Clin. Oncol. 23 (2005) 333–345.

[20] M. Goodman, R.M. Bostick, O. Kucuk, D.P. Jones, Clinical trials of antioxidants as cancer prevention agents: past, present, and future, Free Radic. Biol. Med. 51 (2011) 1068–1084.

[21] L. Castro, B.A. Freeman, Reactive oxygen species in human health and disease, Nutrition 17 (161) (2001) 163–165.

[22] R.S. Sohal, R. Weindruch, Oxidative stress, caloric restriction, and aging, Science 273 (1996) 59–63.

[23] J.M. McCord, The evolution of free radicals and oxidative stress, Am. J. Med. 108 (2000) 652–659.

[24] W. Lopaczynski, S.H. Zeisel, Antioxidants, programmed cell death, and cancer, Nutr. Res. 21 (2001) 295–307.

[25] T. Finkel, N.J. Holbrook, Oxidants, oxidative stress and the biology of ageing, Nature 408 (2000) 239–247.

[26] N.J. Holbrook, S. Ikeyama, Age-related decline in cellular response to oxidative stress: links to growth factor signaling pathways with common defects, Biochem. Pharmacol. 64 (2002) 999–1005.

[27] D. Hanahan, R.A. Weinberg, The hallmarks of cancer, Cell 100 (2000) 57–70.

[28] G.K. Dy, L. Bekele, L.J. Hanson, A. Furth, S. Mandrekar, J.A. Sloan, et al., Complementary and alternative medicine use by patients enrolled onto phase I clinical trials, J. Clin. Oncol. 22 (2004) 4810–4815.

[29] R. Gerson-Cwilich, A. Serrano-Olvera, A. Villalobos-Prieto, Complementary and alternative medicine (CAM) in Mexican patients with cancer, Clin. Transl. Oncol. 8 (2006) 200–207.

[30] H. Itabe, Oxidized low-density lipoproteins: what is understood and what remains to be clarified, Biol. Pharm. Bull. 26 (2003) 1–9.

[31] C. Duval, A.V. Cantero, N. Auge, L. Mabile, J.C. Thiers, A. Negre-Salvayre, et al., Proliferation and wound healing of vascular cells trigger the generation of extracellular reactive oxygen species and LDL oxidation, Free Radic. Biol. Med. 35 (2003) 1589–1598.

[32] W. Droge, Free radicals in the physiological control of cell function, Physiol. Rev. 82 (2002) 47–95.

[33] G.W. Sullivan, I.J. Sarembock, J. Linden, The role of inflammation in vascular diseases, J. Leukoc. Biol. 67 (2000) 591–602.

[34] H.C. Hung, K.J. Joshipura, R. Jiang, F.B. Hu, D. Hunter, S.A. Smith-Warner, et al., Fruit and vegetable intake and risk of major chronic disease, J. Natl. Cancer Inst. 96 (2004) 1577–1584.

[35] G. Bjelakovic, D. Nikolova, R.G. Simonetti, C. Gluud, Antioxidant supplements for prevention of gastrointestinal cancers: a systematic review and meta-analysis, Lancet 364 (2004) 1219–1228.

[36] G.E. Goodman, M.D. Thornquist, J. Balmes, M.R. Cullen, F.L. Meyskens Jr., G.S. Omenn, et al., The Beta-Carotene and Retinol Efficacy Trial: incidence of lung cancer and cardiovascular disease mortality during 6-year follow-up after stopping beta-carotene and retinol supplements, J. Natl. Cancer Inst. 96 (2004) 1743–1750.

[37] R.I. Salganik, The benefits and hazards of antioxidants: controlling apoptosis and other protective mechanisms in cancer patients and the human population, J. Am. Coll. Nutr. 20 (2001) 464S–475S.

[38] U.S. Food and Drug Administration Office of Special Nutritionals, Conference on Antioxidant Vitamins and Cancer and Cardiovascular Disease, U.S. Food and Drug Administration, Washington, DC, 1993.

[39] H.E. Seifried, S.S. McDonald, D.E. Anderson, P. Greenwald, J.A. Milner, The antioxidant conundrum in cancer, Cancer Res. 63 (2003) 4295—4298.

[40] H.E. Seifried, D.E. Anderson, B.C. Sorkin, R.B. Costello, Free radicals: the pros and cons of antioxidants: executive summary report, J. Nutr. 134 (2004) 3143S—3163S.

[41] W.J. Blot, J.Y. Li, P.R. Taylor, W. Guo, S. Dawsey, G.Q. Wang, et al., Nutrition intervention trials in Linxian, China: supplementation with specific vitamin/mineral combinations, cancer incidence, and disease-specific mortality in the general population, J. Natl. Cancer Inst. 85 (1993) 1483—1492.

[42] C.H. Hennekens, J.E. Buring, J.E. Manson, M. Stampfer, B. Rosner, N.R. Cook, et al., Lack of effect of long-term supplementation with beta carotene on the incidence of malignant neoplasms and cardiovascular disease, N. Engl. J. Med. 334 (1996) 1145—1149.

[43] I.M. Lee, N.R. Cook, J.E. Manson, J.E. Buring, C.H. Hennekens, Beta-carotene supplementation and incidence of cancer and cardiovascular disease: The Women's Health Study, J. Natl. Cancer Inst. 91 (1999) 2102—2106.

[44] N.R. Cook, M.J. Stampfer, J. Ma, J.E. Manson, F.M. Sacks, J.E. Buring, et al., Beta-carotene supplementation for patients with low baseline levels and decreased risks of total and prostate carcinoma, Cancer 86 (1999) 1783—1792.

[45] R.M. Russell, The enigma of beta-carotene in carcinogenesis: what can be learned from animal studies, J. Nutr. 134 (2004) 262S—268S.

[46] E.R. Greenberg, J.A. Baron, T.A. Stukel, M.M. Stevens, J.S. Mandel, S.K. Spencer, et al., A clinical trial of beta carotene to prevent basal-cell and squamous-cell cancers of the skin: The Skin Cancer Prevention Study Group, N. Engl. J. Med. 323 (1990) 789—795.

[47] R. MacLennan, F. Macrae, C. Bain, D. Battistutta, P. Chapuis, H. Gratten, et al., Randomized trial of intake of fat, fiber, and beta carotene to prevent colorectal adenomas, J. Natl. Cancer Inst. 87 (1995) 1760—1766.

[48] J. Lin, N.R. Cook, C. Albert, E. Zaharris, J.M. Gaziano, M. Van Denburgh, et al., Vitamins C and E and beta carotene supplementation and cancer risk: a randomized controlled trial, J. Natl. Cancer Inst. 101 (2009) 14—23.

[49] J.M. Gaziano, R.J. Glynn, W.G. Christen, T. Kurth, C. Belanger, J. MacFadyen, et al., Vitamins E and C in the prevention of prostate and total cancer in men: The Physicians' Health Study II randomized controlled trial, JAMA 301 (2009) 52—62.

[50] S.M. Lippman, E.A. Klein, P.J. Goodman, M.S. Lucia, I.M. Thompson, L.G. Ford, et al., Effect of selenium and vitamin E on risk of prostate cancer and other cancers: The Selenium and Vitamin E Cancer Prevention Trial (SELECT), JAMA 301 (2009) 39—51.

[51] D. Albanes, O.P. Heinonen, J.K. Huttunen, P.R. Taylor, J. Virtamo, B.K. Edwards, et al., Effects of alpha-tocopherol and beta-carotene supplements on cancer incidence in the Alpha-Tocopherol Beta-Carotene Cancer Prevention Study, Am. J. Clin. Nutr. 62 (1995) 1427S—1430S.

[52] G.S. Omenn, G.E. Goodman, M.D. Thornquist, J. Balmes, M.R. Cullen, A. Glass, et al., Risk factors for lung cancer and for intervention effects in CARET, the Beta-Carotene and Retinol Efficacy Trial, J. Natl. Cancer Inst. 88 (1996) 1550—1559.

[53] O.P. Heinonen, D. Albanes, J. Virtamo, P.R. Taylor, J.K. Huttunen, A.M. Hartman, et al., Prostate cancer and supplementation with alpha-tocopherol and beta-carotene: incidence and mortality in a controlled trial, J. Natl. Cancer Inst. 90 (1998) 440—446.

[54] D. Albanes, N. Malila, P.R. Taylor, J.K. Huttunen, J. Virtamo, B.K. Edwards, et al., Effects of supplemental alpha-tocopherol and beta-carotene on colorectal cancer: results from a controlled trial (Finland), Cancer Causes Control 11 (2000) 197—205.

[55] M.L. Neuhouser, R.E. Patterson, M.D. Thornquist, G.S. Omenn, I.B. King, G.E. Goodman, Fruits and vegetables are associated with lower lung cancer risk only in the placebo arm of the Beta-Carotene and Retinol Efficacy Trial (CARET), Cancer Epidemiol. Biomarkers Prev. 12 (2003) 350—358.

[56] S.T. Mayne, D.T. Janerich, P. Greenwald, S. Chorost, C. Tucci, M.B. Zaman, et al., Dietary beta carotene and lung cancer risk in U.S. nonsmokers, J. Natl. Cancer Inst. 86 (1994) 33—38.

[57] F.E. Speizer, G.A. Colditz, D.J. Hunter, B. Rosner, C. Hennekens, Prospective study of smoking, antioxidant intake, and lung cancer in middle-aged women (USA), Cancer Causes Control 10 (1999) 475—482.

[58] M. Touvier, E. Kesse, F. Clavel-Chapelon, M.C. Boutron-Ruault, Dual association of beta-carotene with risk of tobacco-related cancers in a cohort of French women, J. Natl. Cancer Inst. 97 (2005) 1338—1344.

[59] C. Liu, R.M. Russell, X.D. Wang, Alpha-tocopherol and ascorbic acid decrease the production of beta-apo-carotenals and increase the formation of retinoids from beta-carotene in the lung tissues of cigarette smoke-exposed ferrets in vitro, J. Nutr. 134 (2004) 426—430.

[60] A.J. Alija, N. Bresgen, O. Sommerburg, C.D. Langhans, W. Siems, P.M. Eckl, Beta-carotene breakdown products enhance genotoxic effects of oxidative stress in primary rat hepatocytes, Carcinogenesis 27 (2006) 1128—1133.

[61] S.J. Weinstein, M.E. Wright, P. Pietinen, I. King, C. Tan, P.R. Taylor, et al., Serum alpha-tocopherol and gamma-tocopherol in relation to prostate cancer risk in a prospective study, J. Natl. Cancer Inst. 97 (2005) 396—399.

[62] J. Virtamo, P. Pietinen, J.K. Huttunen, P. Korhonen, N. Malila, M.J. Virtanen, et al., Incidence of cancer and mortality following alpha-tocopherol and beta-carotene supplementation: a postintervention follow-up, JAMA 290 (2003) 476—485.

[63] M.E. Wright, J. Virtamo, A.M. Hartman, P. Pietinen, B.K. Edwards, P.R. Taylor, et al., Effects of alpha-tocopherol and beta-carotene supplementation on upper aerodigestive tract cancers in a large, randomized controlled trial, Cancer 109 (2007) 891—898.

[64] M.E. Wright, K.A. Lawson, S.J. Weinstein, P. Pietinen, P.R. Taylor, J. Virtamo, et al., Higher baseline serum concentrations of vitamin E are associated with lower total and cause-specific mortality in the Alpha-Tocopherol, Beta-Carotene Cancer Prevention Study, Am. J. Clin. Nutr. 84 (2006) 1200—1207.

[65] C.N. Holick, D.S. Michaud, R. Stolzenberg-Solomon, S.T. Mayne, P. Pietinen, P.R. Taylor, et al., Dietary carotenoids, serum beta-carotene, and retinol and risk of lung cancer in the alpha-tocopherol, beta-carotene cohort study, Am. J. Epidemiol. 156 (2002) 536—547.

[66] S. Hercberg, P. Preziosi, P. Galan, H. Faure, J. Arnaud, N. Duport, et al., "The SU.VI.MAX Study": a primary prevention trial using nutritional doses of antioxidant vitamins and minerals in cardiovascular diseases and cancers. SUpplementation on VItamines et Mineraux AntioXydants, Food Chem. Toxicol. 37 (1999) 925—930.

[67] S. Hercberg, P. Galan, P. Preziosi, M. Malvy, S. Briancon, H.M. Ait, et al., The SU.VI.MAX trial on antioxidants, IARC Sci. Publ. 156 (2002) 451—455.

[68] S. Hercberg, P. Galan, P. Preziosi, S. Bertrais, L. Mennen, D. Malvy, et al., The SU.VI.MAX Study: a randomized, placebo-controlled trial of the health effects of antioxidant vitamins and minerals, Arch. Intern. Med. 164 (2004) 2335—2342.

[69] F. Meyer, P. Galan, P. Douville, I. Bairati, P. Kegle, S. Bertrais, et al., Antioxidant vitamin and mineral supplementation and

prostate cancer prevention in the SU.VI.MAX trial, Int. J. Cancer 116 (2005) 182–186.

[70] L.C. Clark, G.F. Combs Jr., B.W. Turnbull, E.H. Slate, D.K. Chalker, J. Chow, et al., Effects of selenium supplementation for cancer prevention in patients with carcinoma of the skin: a randomized controlled trial. Nutritional Prevention of Cancer Study Group, JAMA 276 (1996) 1957–1963.

[71] A.J. Duffield-Lillico, B.L. Dalkin, M.E. Reid, B.W. Turnbull, E.H. Slate, E.T. Jacobs, et al., Selenium supplementation, baseline plasma selenium status and incidence of prostate cancer: an analysis of the complete treatment period of the Nutritional Prevention of Cancer Trial, BJU Int. 91 (2003) 608–612.

[72] M.E. Reid, A.J. Duffield-Lillico, L. Garland, B.W. Turnbull, L.C. Clark, J.R. Marshall, Selenium supplementation and lung cancer incidence: an update of the Nutritional Prevention of Cancer Trial, Cancer Epidemiol. Biomarkers Prev. 11 (2002) 1285–1291.

[73] H. Li, M.J. Stampfer, E.L. Giovannucci, J.S. Morris, W.C. Willett, J.M. Gaziano, et al., A prospective study of plasma selenium levels and prostate cancer risk, J. Natl. Cancer Inst. 96 (2004) 696–703.

[74] T.W. Fan, R.M. Higashi, A.N. Lane, Integrating metabolomics and transcriptomics for probing SE anticancer mechanisms, Drug Metab. Rev. 38 (2006) 707–732.

[75] C.H. van Gils, P.H. Peeters, H.B. Bueno-de-Mesquita, H.C. Boshuizen, P.H. Lahmann, F. Clavel-Chapelon, et al., Consumption of vegetables and fruits and risk of breast cancer, JAMA 293 (2005) 183–193.

[76] S. Liu, J.E. Manson, I.M. Lee, S.R. Cole, C.H. Hennekens, W.C. Willett, et al., Fruit and vegetable intake and risk of cardiovascular disease: The Women's Health Study, Am. J. Clin. Nutr. 72 (2000) 922–928.

[77] B.A. Narayanan, Chemopreventive agents alters global gene expression pattern: predicting their mode of action and targets, Curr. Cancer Drug Targets 6 (2006) 711–727.

[78] B.A. Narayanan, N.K. Narayanan, G.G. Re, D.W. Nixon, Differential expression of genes induced by resveratrol in LNCaP cells: P53-mediated molecular targets, Int. J. Cancer 104 (2003) 204–212.

[79] A.C. Goulet, G. Watts, J.L. Lord, M.A. Nelson, Profiling of selenomethionine responsive genes in colon cancer by microarray analysis, Cancer Biol. Ther. 6 (2007) 494–503.

[80] E.R. Miller III, R. Pastor-Barriuso, D. Dalal, R.A. Riemersma, L.J. Appel, E. Guallar, Meta-analysis: high-dosage vitamin E supplementation may increase all-cause mortality, Ann. Intern. Med. 142 (2005) 37–46.

[81] L. Dauchet, P. Amouyel, S. Hercberg, J. Dallongeville, Fruit and vegetable consumption and risk of coronary heart disease: a meta-analysis of cohort studies, J. Nutr. 136 (2006) 2588–2593.

[82] L.H. Kushi, A.R. Folsom, R.J. Prineas, P.J. Mink, Y. Wu, R.M. Bostick, Dietary antioxidant vitamins and death from coronary heart disease in postmenopausal women, N. Engl. J. Med. 334 (1996) 1156–1162.

[83] G. Bjelakovic, D. Nikolova, L.L. Gluud, R.G. Simonetti, C. Gluud, Mortality in randomized trials of antioxidant supplements for primary and secondary prevention: systematic review and meta-analysis, JAMA 297 (2007) 842–857.

[84] E. Lonn, J. Bosch, S. Yusuf, P. Sheridan, J. Pogue, J.M. Arnold, et al., Effects of long-term vitamin E supplementation on cardiovascular events and cancer: a randomized controlled trial, JAMA 293 (2005) 1338–1347.

[85] I.M. Lee, N.R. Cook, J.M. Gaziano, D. Gordon, P.M. Ridker, J.E. Manson, et al., Vitamin E in the primary prevention of cardiovascular disease and cancer: The Women's Health Study: a randomized controlled trial, JAMA 294 (2005) 56–65.

[86] J.M. Rapola, J. Virtamo, J.K. Haukka, O.P. Heinonen, D. Albanes, P.R. Taylor, et al., Effect of vitamin E and beta carotene on the incidence of angina pectoris: a randomized, double-blind, controlled trial, JAMA 275 (1996) 693–698.

[87] N.G. Stephens, A. Parsons, P.M. Schofield, F. Kelly, K. Cheeseman, M.J. Mitchinson, Randomised controlled trial of vitamin E in patients with coronary disease: Cambridge Heart Antioxidant Study (CHAOS), Lancet 347 (1996) 781–786.

[88] C.D. Morris, S. Carson, Routine vitamin supplementation to prevent cardiovascular disease: a summary of the evidence for the U.S. Preventive Services Task Force, Ann. Intern. Med. 139 (2003) 56–70.

[89] A. Azzi, I. Breyer, M. Feher, M. Pastori, R. Ricciarelli, S. Spycher, et al., Specific cellular responses to alpha-tocopherol, J. Nutr. 130 (2000) 1649–1652.

[90] A. Azzi, R. Gysin, P. Kempna, R. Ricciarelli, L. Villacorta, T. Visarius, et al., The role of alpha-tocopherol in preventing disease: from epidemiology to molecular events, Mol. Aspects Med. 24 (2003) 325–336.

[91] L. Sung, M.L. Greenberg, G. Koren, G.A. Tomlinson, A. Tong, D. Malkin, et al., Vitamin E: the evidence for multiple roles in cancer, Nutr. Cancer 46 (2003) 1–14.

[92] C. Gokkusu, S. Palanduz, E. Ademoglu, S. Tamer, Oxidant and antioxidant systems in niddm patients: influence of vitamin E supplementation, Endocr. Res. 27 (2001) 377–386.

[93] R.M. Salonen, K. Nyyssonen, J. Kaikkonen, E. Porkkala-Sarataho, S. Voutilainen, T.H. Rissanen, et al., Six-year effect of combined vitamin C and E supplementation on atherosclerotic progression: The Antioxidant Supplementation in Atherosclerosis Prevention (ASAP) study, Circulation 107 (2003) 947–953.

[94] J.C. Fang, S. Kinlay, J. Beltrame, H. Hikiti, M. Wainstein, D. Behrendt, et al., Effect of vitamins C and E on progression of transplant-associated arteriosclerosis: a randomised trial, Lancet 359 (2002) 1108–1113.

[95] Heart Protection Study Collaborative Group, MRC/BHF Heart Protection Study of antioxidant vitamin supplementation in 20,536 high-risk individuals: a randomised placebo-controlled trial, Lancet 360 (2002) 23–33.

[96] W.G. Christen, J.M. Gaziano, C.H. Hennekens, Design of Physicians' Health Study II—A randomized trial of beta-carotene, vitamins E and C, and multivitamins, in prevention of cancer, cardiovascular disease, and eye disease, and review of results of completed trials, Ann. Epidemiol. 10 (2000) 125–134.

[97] L.I. Mennen, D. Sapinho, A. de Bree, N. Arnault, S. Bertrais, P. Galan, et al., Consumption of foods rich in flavonoids is related to a decreased cardiovascular risk in apparently healthy French women, J. Nutr. 134 (2004) 923–926.

[98] J.T. Salonen, Clinical trials testing cardiovascular benefits of antioxidant supplementation, Free Radic. Res. 36 (2002) 1299–1306.

[99] Gruppo Italiano per lo Studio della Sopravvivenza nell'Infarto miocardico, Dietary supplementation with n-3 polyunsaturated fatty acids and vitamin E after myocardial infarction: results of the GISSI-Prevenzione trial. Gruppo Italiano per lo Studio della Sopravvivenza nell'Infarto miocardico, Lancet 354 (1999) 447–455.

[100] S. Yusuf, P. Sleight, J. Pogue, J. Bosch, R. Davies, G. Dagenais, Effects of an angiotensin-converting-enzyme inhibitor, ramipril, on cardiovascular events in high-risk patients: The Heart Outcomes Prevention Evaluation Study Investigators, N. Engl. J. Med. 342 (2000) 145–153.

[101] G.R. Dagenais, S. Yusuf, M.G. Bourassa, Q. Yi, J. Bosch, E.M. Lonn, et al., Effects of ramipril on coronary events in high-risk

persons: results of the Heart Outcomes Prevention Evaluation Study, Circulation 104 (2001) 522−526.

[102] M.L. Neuhouser, S. Wassertheil-Smoller, C. Thomson, A. Aragaki, G.L. Anderson, J.E. Manson, et al., Multivitamin use and risk of cancer and cardiovascular disease in the Women's Health Initiative cohorts, Arch. Intern. Med. 169 (2009) 294−304.

[103] R.A. Harrison, D. Holt, D.J. Pattison, P.J. Elton, Are those in need taking dietary supplements? A survey of 21,923 adults, Br. J. Nutr. 91 (2004) 617−623.

[104] J.M. Ordovas, Identification of a functional polymorphism at the adipose fatty acid binding protein gene (FABP4) and demonstration of its association with cardiovascular disease: a path to follow, Nutr. Rev. 65 (2007) 130−134.

[105] K. Sugamura, J.F. Keaney Jr., Reactive oxygen species in cardiovascular disease, Free Radic. Biol. Med. 51 (2011) 978−992.

[106] J.M. Núñez-Córdoba, M.A. Martínez-González, Antioxidant vitamins and cardiovascular disease, Curr. Top. Med. Chem. 11 (2011) 1861−1869.

[107] H.A. Ergen, F. Narter, O. Timirci, T. Isbir, Effects of manganese superoxide dismutase Ala-9Val polymorphism on prostate cancer: a case−control study, Anticancer Res. 27 (2007) 1227−1230.

[108] S. Wang, F. Wang, X. Shi, J. Dai, Y. Peng, X. Guo, et al., Association between manganese superoxide dismutase (MnSOD) Val-9Ala polymorphism and cancer risk: a meta-analysis, Eur. J. Cancer 45 (2009) 2874−2881.

[109] C. Kucukgergin, O. Sanli, T. Tefik, M. Aydin, F. Ozcan, S. Seckin, Increased risk of advanced prostate cancer associated with MnSOD Ala-9-Val gene polymorphism, Mol. Biol. Rep. 39 (2011) 193−198.

[110] Z. Arsova-Sarafinovska, N. Matevska, D. Petrovski, S. Banev, S. Dzikova, V. Georgiev, et al., Manganese superoxide dismutase (MnSOD) genetic polymorphism is associated with risk of early-onset prostate cancer, Cell Biochem. Funct. 26 (2008) 771−777.

[111] Q. Cai, X.O. Shu, W. Wen, J.R. Cheng, Q. Dai, Y.T. Gao, et al., Genetic polymorphism in the manganese superoxide dismutase gene, antioxidant intake, and breast cancer risk: results from the Shanghai Breast Cancer Study, Breast Cancer Res. 6 (2004) R647−R655.

[112] L. Valenti, D. Conte, A. Piperno, P. Dongiovanni, A.L. Fracanzani, M. Fraquelli, et al., The mitochondrial superoxide dismutase A16V polymorphism in the cardiomyopathy associated with hereditary haemochromatosis, J. Med. Genet. 41 (2004) 946−950.

[113] X. Ma, C. Chen, H. Xiong, J. Fan, Y. Li, H. Lin, et al., No association between SOD2 Val16Ala polymorphism and breast cancer susceptibility: a meta-analysis based on 9,710 cases and 11,041 controls, Breast Cancer Res. Treat. 122 (2010) 509−514.

[114] N. Eras-Erdogan, E. Akbas, H. Senli, S. Kul, T. Colak, Relationship between polymorphism in the manganese superoxide dismutase gene and breast cancer, Mutat. Res. 680 (2009) 7−11.

[115] N.A. Kocabas, S. Sardas, S. Cholerton, A.K. Daly, A.H. Elhan, A.E. Karakaya, Genetic polymorphism of manganese superoxide dismutase (MnSOD) and breast cancer susceptibility, Cell Biochem. Funct. 23 (2005) 73−76.

[116] A. Bag, N. Bag, Target sequence polymorphism of human manganese superoxide dismutase gene and its association with cancer risk: a review, Cancer Epidemiol. Biomarkers Prev. 17 (2008) 3298−3305.

[117] C. Mao, L.X. Qiu, P. Zhan, K. Xue, H. Ding, F.B. Du, et al., MnSOD Val16Ala polymorphism and prostate cancer susceptibility: a meta-analysis involving 8962 subjects, J. Cancer Res. Clin. Oncol. 136 (2010) 975−979.

[118] B. Mikhak, D.J. Hunter, D. Spiegelman, E.A. Platz, K. Wu, J.W. Erdman Jr., et al., Manganese superoxide dismutase (MnSOD) gene polymorphism, interactions with carotenoid levels and prostate cancer risk, Carcinogenesis 29 (2008) 2335−2340.

[119] L. Liwei, L. Chunyu, H. Ruifa, Association between manganese superoxide dismutase gene polymorphism and risk of prostate cancer: a meta-analysis, Urology 74 (2009) 884−888.

[120] L.X. Qiu, L. Yao, C. Mao, B. Chen, P. Zhan, H. Yuan, et al., Lack of association between MnSOD Val16Ala polymorphism and breast cancer risk: a meta-analysis involving 58,448 subjects, Breast Cancer Res. Treat. 123 (2010) 543−547.

[121] Y. Li, C.B. Ambrosone, M.J. McCullough, J. Ahn, V.L. Stevens, M.J. Thun, et al., Oxidative stress-related genotypes, fruit and vegetable consumption and breast cancer risk, Carcinogenesis 30 (2009) 777−784.

[122] J. Ahn, S. Nowell, S.E. McCann, J. Yu, L. Carter, N.P. Lang, et al., Associations between catalase phenotype and genotype: modification by epidemiologic factors, Cancer Epidemiol. Biomarkers Prev. 15 (2006) 1217−1222.

[123] O. Ukkola, P.H. Erkkila, M.J. Savolainen, Y.A. Kesaniemi, Lack of association between polymorphisms of catalase, copper-zinc superoxide dismutase (SOD), extracellular SOD and endothelial nitric oxide synthase genes and macroangiopathy in patients with type 2 diabetes mellitus, J. Intern. Med. 249 (2001) 451−459.

[124] Y.J. Hu, A.M. Diamond, Role of glutathione peroxidase 1 in breast cancer: loss of heterozygosity and allelic differences in the response to selenium, Cancer Res. 63 (2003) 3347−3351.

[125] J. Ahn, M.D. Gammon, R.M. Santella, M.M. Gaudet, J.A. Britton, S.L. Teitelbaum, et al., No association between glutathione peroxidase Pro198Leu polymorphism and breast cancer risk, Cancer Epidemiol. Biomarkers Prev. 14 (2005) 2459−2461.

[126] J. Hu, G.W. Zhou, N. Wang, Y.J. Wang, GPX1 Pro198Leu polymorphism and breast cancer risk: a meta-analysis, Breast Cancer Res. Treat. 124 (2010) 425−431.

[127] D.G. Cox, R.M. Tamimi, D.J. Hunter, Gene × gene interaction between MnSOD and GPX-1 and breast cancer risk: a nested case−control study, BMC Cancer 6 (2006) 217.

[128] O. Raaschou-Nielsen, M. Sorensen, R.D. Hansen, K. Frederiksen, A. Tjonneland, K. Overvad, et al., GPX1 Pro198Leu polymorphism, interactions with smoking and alcohol consumption, and risk for lung cancer, Cancer Lett. 247 (2007) 293−300.

[129] A. Sutton, P. Nahon, D. Pessayre, P. Rufat, A. Poire, M. Ziol, et al., Genetic polymorphisms in antioxidant enzymes modulate hepatic iron accumulation and hepatocellular carcinoma development in patients with alcohol-induced cirrhosis, Cancer Res. 66 (2006) 2844−2852.

[130] L. Cai, N.C. You, H. Lu, L.N. Mu, Q.Y. Lu, S.Z. Yu, et al., Dietary selenium intake, aldehyde dehydrogenase-2 and X-ray repair cross-complementing 1 genetic polymorphisms, and the risk of esophageal squamous cell carcinoma, Cancer 106 (2006) 2345−2354.

[131] J. Ahn, M.D. Gammon, R.M. Santella, M.M. Gaudet, J.A. Britton, S.L. Teitelbaum, et al., Associations between breast cancer risk and the catalase genotype, fruit and vegetable consumption, and supplement use, Am. J. Epidemiol. 162 (2005) 943−952.

[132] J. Shen, M.B. Terry, M.D. Gammon, M.M. Gaudet, S.L. Teitelbaum, S.M. Eng, et al., MGMT genotype modulates the associations between cigarette smoking, dietary antioxidants and breast cancer risk, Carcinogenesis 26 (2005) 2131−2137.

[133] J. Han, G.A. Colditz, D.J. Hunter, Manganese superoxide dismutase polymorphism and risk of skin cancer (United States), Cancer Causes Control 18 (2007) 79—89.

[134] G.M. Puddu, E. Cravero, G. Arnone, A. Muscari, P. Puddu, Molecular aspects of atherogenesis: new insights and unsolved questions, J. Biomed. Sci. 12 (2005) 839—853.

[135] L.L. Stoll, M.L. McCormick, G.M. Denning, N.L. Weintraub, Antioxidant effects of statins, Drugs Today (Barcelona) 40 (2004) 975—990.

[136] S.V. Drinitsina, D.A. Zateishchikov, Antioxidant properties of statins, Kardiologiia 45 (2005) 65—72.

[137] T.J. Guzik, D.G. Harrison, Vascular NADPH oxidases as drug targets for novel antioxidant strategies, Drug Discov. Today 11 (2006) 524—533.

[138] M.A. Richardson, T. Sanders, J.L. Palmer, A. Greisinger, S.E. Singletary, Complementary/alternative medicine use in a comprehensive cancer center and the implications for oncology, J. Clin. Oncol. 18 (2000) 2505—2514.

[139] H.J. Burstein, S. Gelber, E. Guadagnoli, J.C. Weeks, Use of alternative medicine by women with early-stage breast cancer, N. Engl. J. Med. 340 (1999) 1733—1739.

[140] C. Toner, Consumer perspectives about antioxidants, J. Nutr. 134 (2004) 3192S—3193S.

[141] K.N. Prasad, W.C. Cole, B. Kumar, K. Che Prasad, Pros and cons of antioxidant use during radiation therapy, Cancer Treat. Rev. 28 (2002) 79—91.

[142] K.N. Prasad, Rationale for using high-dose multiple dietary antioxidants as an adjunct to radiation therapy and chemotherapy, J. Nutr. 134 (2004) 3182S—3183S.

[143] K.N. Prasad, B. Kumar, X.D. Yan, A.J. Hanson, W.C. Cole, Alpha-tocopheryl succinate, the most effective form of vitamin E for adjuvant cancer treatment: a review, J. Am. Coll. Nutr. 22 (2003) 108—117.

[144] K.N. Prasad, Antioxidants in cancer care: when and how to use them as an adjunct to standard and experimental therapies, Expert Rev. Anticancer Ther. 3 (2003) 903—915.

[145] K.N. Prasad, W.C. Cole, B. Kumar, K.C. Prasad, Scientific rationale for using high-dose multiple micronutrients as an adjunct to standard and experimental cancer therapies, J. Am. Coll. Nutr. 20 (450S—463S) (2001) 473S—475S.

[146] J.A. Drisko, J. Chapman, V.J. Hunter, The use of antioxidants with first-line chemotherapy in two cases of ovarian cancer, J. Am. Coll. Nutr. 22 (2003) 118—123.

[147] D.W. Lamson, M.S. Brignall, Antioxidants in cancer therapy; Their actions and interactions with oncologic therapies, Altern. Med. Rev. 4 (1999) 304—329.

[148] K. Jaakkola, P. Lahteenmaki, J. Laakso, E. Harju, H. Tykka, K. Mahlberg, Treatment with antioxidant and other nutrients in combination with chemotherapy and irradiation in patients with small-cell lung cancer, Anticancer Res. 12 (1992) 599—606.

[149] A.T. Fleischauer, N. Simonsen, L. Arab, Antioxidant supplements and risk of breast cancer recurrence and breast cancer-related mortality among postmenopausal women, Nutr. Cancer 46 (2003) 15—22.

[150] M.L. Lesperance, I.A. Olivotto, N. Forde, Y. Zhao, C. Speers, H. Foster, et al., Mega-dose vitamins and minerals in the treatment of non-metastatic breast cancer: an historical cohort study, Breast Cancer Res. Treat. 76 (2002) 137—143.

[151] K.A. Conklin, Dietary antioxidants during cancer chemotherapy: impact on chemotherapeutic effectiveness and development of side effects, Nutr. Cancer 37 (2000) 1—18.

19

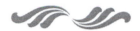

Diet and Supplements in the Prevention and Treatment of Eye Diseases

Julie A. Mares*, Amy E. Millen†, Kristin J. Meyers*

*University of Wisconsin−Madison, Madison, Wisconsin, †University at Buffalo, The State University of New York, Buffalo, New York

I INTRODUCTION

A Nutrition and Common Age-Related Eye Diseases

The deterioration of human vision advances with age. More than 80% of blindness worldwide occurs in people older than age 50 years. This chapter addresses the influence of diet on the most common causes of vision loss in middle-aged and older people: age-related cataract, age-related macular degeneration, and diabetic retinopathy.

Significant advances in the understanding of how nutrition may influence eye diseases of the aging population have been made since the 1980s. The aging public's awareness of the decline in vision with age, and of the possibility that nutrition may influence this decline, has driven the marketing of nutritional supplements which are sometimes costly and of uncertain benefit. In this chapter, we consider the existing evidence for the benefits of certain diets and supplements in slowing age-related visual problems associated with cataracts, macular degeneration, and diabetic retinopathy (summarized in Tables 19.1−19.3).

B Nutrition and Other Aspects of Vision

The reader is referred to other texts and reviews that describe the role of nutrition in other aspects of vision that are briefly summarized in the following paragraphs. The role of vitamin A in preventing night blindness and xerophthalmia, which remain common problems in developing countries, has been widely discussed [1]. Food shortages, as occurred in Cuba in 1991−1994 and among the allied prisoners of World War II, or chronic alcohol use can result in a condition broadly referred to as nutritional amblyopia, which results in blurred vision and reduced visual acuity [2]. This may be the result of poor intake and absorption of B vitamins or antioxidants, alcohol and tobacco toxicity, or a combination of these factors.

Nutrition may be important to some patients with hereditary visual disorders. One such condition is retinitis pigmentosa, an autosomal dominant condition resulting in progressive visual loss. It begins with the loss of night vision in childhood or adolescence. This is followed by the loss of peripheral vision because of the degeneration of rods and, finally, the loss of central vision because of the degeneration of cones [3]. Vitamin A supplements have improved some aspects of retina function in patients with retinitis pigmentosa [4]. In addition, preliminary research suggests potential benefit of lutein [5] and omega-3 fats [6] in slowing rates of retina degeneration and of visual decline in retinitis pigmentosa patients. However, the benefits of vitamin A, lutein, and omega-3 supplements are not conclusive, and adequate intakes through dietary means may pose less risk over the long term [7].

Nutrition may also be important to the development of the visual system in newborns. Some studies, but not all, have observed better visual development in infants who were breast-fed, as opposed to those who were bottle fed. This has led to a search for the nutritional differences between breast milk and infant formulas that may explain better vision in breast-fed infants. In two studies, breast-feeding was associated

Nutrition in the Prevention and Treatment of Disease, Third Edition.
DOI: http://dx.doi.org/10.1016/B978-0-12-391884-0.00019-6

TABLE 19.1   Summary of Evidence Relating Nutritional Exposures to Cataract

Nutritional exposure	Strength of evidence	Comments
Healthy diet patterns	**Benefit of following micronutrient-rich diet patterns is likely:**	Two studies suggest that the benefit of healthy diets on lowering risk of nuclear cataract is stronger than the benefit of high intake of single nutrients.
		Many studies in animals and humans support the benefit of numerous specific micronutrients and phytochemicals.
Carbohydrate	**Possible increased risk associated with high levels of specific or overall refined carbohydrates:**	Results in population studies might reflect an influence of diabetes on cataract rather than carbohydrates specifically.
	Animal studies suggest several mechanisms.	
	Population studies are limited in number and conflicting.	
Antioxidants	**Benefit of food antioxidants is likely:** Animal studies prove that oxidative stress leads to lens opacities and that antioxidants lower indicators of oxidative stress and/or damage.	In population studies, diets rich in specific antioxidant nutrients are likely to be markers for diets rich in plant foods (fruits, vegetables, and whole grains), which contribute a wide range of nutritive and non-nutritive antioxidants.
	Population studies in many samples indicate lower risk of cataract with higher intake or blood levels of various antioxidants (vitamins C and E or lutein and zeaxanthin); data are most consistent for diets rich in lutein and zeaxanthin.	Clinical trials do not generally support benefit of one or two specific antioxidant nutrients or a combination of high-dose antioxidants.
Lead	**Exposure possibly increases risk:**	
	Evidence is limited to one study. This risk factor and the influence of other heavy metals require further research.	
Multivitamin supplements	**Benefit is unlikely. Harm is possible**	Protective associations in population studies may reflect better diets or other healthy lifestyles in multivitamin supplement users. Data from clinical trials suggest benefit for nuclear cataract but harm for posterior subcapsular cataract and no overall lowering of risk of cataract extractions.
High-dose antioxidants	**Benefit is unlikely. Harm is possible.**	

with better visual acuity at age 3.5 [8] and 4–6 years [9]. Breast milk contains high levels of the long-chain fatty acid, docosahexaenoic acid (DHA), which rapidly accumulates in retinal photoreceptor membranes neonatally. DHA supplementation has been reported in some, but not all, studies to improve visual functions in some preterm and term infants (reviewed in [10]). Some suggest that improvements may only be transient. One study reported that DHA supplementation for 6 months postnatally did not improve vision in later childhood [9]. This suggests the possibility that other components of breast milk missing from infant formulas, such as carotenoids, may be responsible for better vision in breast-fed infants (discussed in the next section).

Overall nutritional intake in infancy, childhood, and adolescence might influence chronic age-related eye diseases that develop in later life. Evidence suggests that childhood diet influences the risk of cardiovascular disease later in life [11], but the influence on age-related eye diseases, which are the focus of this chapter, has not been investigated.

C Lutein and Zeaxanthin and Eye Health throughout the Life Span

There is evidence that the eye may uniquely require two oxygenated carotenoids, lutein and zeaxanthin, for quality vision throughout life, as well as to limit degeneration of the retina and lens of the eye, which contributes to age-related macular degeneration and cataracts in later life. Thus, although these carotenoids are not yet considered essential for life, growth, and reproduction (the criteria that historically defined essential nutrients), they may be uniquely important to the eye and essential for optimal vision in both the young and aging. Overall, the evidence is limited, but it is suggestive and actively under investigation. Here, an overview of these carotenoids is given and their

TABLE 19.2 Summary of Evidence Relating Diet to Age-Related Macular Degeneration (AMD)

Nutritional exposure	Strength of evidence	Comments
Healthy diet patterns	**Benefit of following micronutrient-rich diet patterns is likely:**	Two studies suggest that scores on overall healthy diet patterns lower risk. One study suggests risk lowering is particularly marked when combined with physical activity and not smoking. Many studies in animals and humans support the benefit of numerous specific micronutrients and phytochemicals.
Lutein and zeaxanthin	**Benefit in slowing AMD and/or improving vision is possible:**	Diets rich in lutein and zeaxanthin may reflect the overall benefit of high intakes of many micronutrient-rich foods.
	Supplementation in animal studies reduces light damage to retina.	The benefit of lutein and zeaxanthin supplements in slowing or preventing AMD is currently being studied in clinical trials.
	The biological plausibility that lutein and zeaxanthin could lower risk by protection against oxidative stress and/or reduction of damage due to light exposure is strong, but impact in humans has not been proven.	The ability to accumulate lutein and zeaxanthin (and therefore the potential benefit) varies across people.
	In population studies, diets high in foods that contain lutein and zeaxanthin are consistently related to lower risk for advanced AMD but inconsistently related to lower risk for earlier stages.	
	Several small and short-term clinical trials provide preliminary evidence to suggest that lutein and zeaxanthin supplementation may improve vision in people with AMD. Benefit in slowing advanced AMD is being tested in a large clinical trial (AREDS2).	
Zinc	**Benefit in slowing progression is proven:**	The long-term benefits and risks of high-dose zinc supplementation are unknown (and are being further studied).
	High-dose zinc supplements slowed the progression of intermediate to advanced AMD in a large, multicenter, placebo-controlled clinical trial over 6 years. In combination with antioxidant supplements, this supplement also reduced moderate visual acuity loss.	The safest dose with benefit is unknown.
	Benefit of adequate zinc intake from foods in slowing development of AMD is likely:	
	Zinc deficiency impairs retinal function in animals and humans.	
	Diets high in zinc have been related to lower AMD in some, but not all, epidemiological studies but may reflect other aspects of consuming foods rich in zinc (milk, beans, meats, and shellfish).	
Dietary fat	**High intake of total fat is likely to encourage development of AMD:**	Higher risk for AMD among people with diets high in fat might reflect lower overall nutrient density of high-fat diets or other aspects of lifestyle associated with the intake of high-fat diets.
	Overall fat intake is associated with lower prevalence or progression of AMD in most population studies (although not always statistically significant).	
	Benefit of foods rich in long-chain omega-3 fatty acids is likely:	Diets high in long-chain omega-3 fats or fish may be related to lower AMD risk due to unmeasured and controlled for aspects of diet (intake of vitamin D and/or selenium) or lifestyle. Benefits should be considered in conjunction with the possibility that fish and some fish oils may contain mercury or other contaminants.
	High intake of long-chain omega-3 fatty acids or fish is associated with lower risk for AMD in 8 of 9 study samples.	
		The benefit of fish oil supplements is unknown and being tested.

(Continued)

TABLE 19.2   (*Continued*)

Nutritional exposure	Strength of evidence	Comments
Vitamin D	**Benefit of good vitamin D status (from moderate sunlight, foods, and/or supplements) is possible but only recently studied:** Animal and cell studies suggest anti-inflammatory properties of vitamin D. Lower risk for AMD was observed in three population studies but not one other.	Higher blood levels of vitamin D may be related to other aspects of diet or lifestyle that could protect against AMD.
Glycemic index	**Diets with low glycemic index score might reduce risk of developing AMD:**	A low glycemic index score is likely to be a marker for a plant-food and nutrient-rich diet that might protect against AMD.
Multivitamin supplements	**Benefit is unknown:** The use of multivitamin supplements has not been associated with lower risk for AMD in population studies (except in Americans who did not report drinking milk daily).	The impact of multivitamins on the onset or worsening of AMD has not been tested in clinical trials.
Antioxidants	**Benefits of a specific combination antioxidant supplement in slowing progression have been demonstrated in one large study sample (AREDS) and suggested by the results of several smaller studies:**	Caveats regarding AREDS-tested supplements: —There is no evidence that high-dose antioxidants lower the onset of AMD among people with early signs of the disease or who merely have a family history of AMD. —The longer term risks and benefits are unknown. —Whether lower doses or different combinations of nutrients may have more benefit or lower long-term risk is unknown (and is being studied). Trials of one or two high-dose antioxidants have not shown benefit.

possible role in vision throughout life is described. In Sections II–IV, the evidence that suggests their importance in slowing age-related cataract, macular degeneration, and diabetic retinopathy is discussed.

Lutein and zeaxanthin are the most abundant carotenoids in the eye, and they are selectively concentrated into the macula [12–14] but also into other ocular tissues, such as the lens, to the exclusion of other carotenoids commonly found in human diets, blood, and tissues such as lycopene and intact β-carotene [12,15]. Monkeys deprived of plant foods do not have these carotenoids in their eyes [16], demonstrating that obtaining them from the diet is essential. In humans, their concentration in the macular area of the retina is highly variable. It is also low in autopsy samples of newborn infants and higher in samples from older infants and children up to 4 years of age [13]. This suggests that they might accumulate in early life from diet in humans.

Breast milk appears to be selectively enriched in lutein and zeaxanthin over other carotenoids [17–19], particularly 1–3 months postpartum [20]. This, along with the evidence for specific binding protein for these carotenoids in the retina, suggests the existence of selective mechanisms to provide lutein and zeaxanthin

in the first few months of life. This time period corresponds to the period of time in which the retinal is developing and specifically in the area where these carotenoids accumulate most markedly, the macula. The macula is the area of the retina with the highest density of cones and is responsible for seeing directly ahead and for seeing fine detail sharply. At birth, the macula is not yet formed. This process happens largely in the first year but to some extent during the first 3 or 4 years of life. (For a review and description of fatty acids in visual development, see [21].)

Carotenoids that accumulate in the macula may influence vision in several ways, as described previously [22,23]. The yellow patch on the retina that they comprise, referred to as macular pigment, absorbs short-wavelength (∼480 nm) light in the blue range of the spectrum. Evidence (summarized later) is accumulating to suggest that this might: (1) Influence the morphological development of this region, (2) influence vision function, and (3) protect against age-related damage contributing to age-related macular degeneration in later life.

In monkeys, depletion of lutein and zeaxanthin in early life results in morphological changes such as

TABLE 19.3 Summary of Evidence Relating Diet to Diabetic Retinopathy (DR)

Nutritional exposure	Strength of evidence	Comments
Dietary fat, fiber, and sodium	**High-fiber diets and diets low or moderate in total or saturated fat and sodium may be related to the development or progression of DR:** Some observational studies support lower risk of DR among people whose diets are high in fiber and low in fat and sodium. Such a diet may be beneficial by helping maintain blood glucose control and by lowering blood lipids and hypertension.	High-fiber diets that are low or moderate in fat are also likely to be rich in other micronutrients, which may explain benefit in studies to date. Existing studies are limited by their cross-sectional designs, short-term assessment of dietary intake, small sample sizes, and lack of adjustment for confounding factors. No conclusions can be made thus far regarding intake of fiber, fat, and sodium and risk of DR development or progression.
Antioxidants	**Benefit of foods rich in antioxidants is likely but inadequately studied:** Data from animal studies strongly support a protective effect of antioxidant intake and protection against development of DR. Five observational studies have investigated the association between antioxidants, in the serum or diet, and risk of prevalent DR. These studies do not conclusively support a protective effect of antioxidants on DR. Some studies suggest that antioxidant exposure could be potentially detrimental; however, this may be explained by study bias. One observation study suggested that long-term intake of antioxidant supplements or multivitamins may protect against prevalent DR.	Population studies are limited in number and cross-sectional design, and results may be biased by changes in diet and supplementation practices upon development of diabetic complications. Long-term, observational prospective studies are needed.
Other potential dietary factors	**The benefit of consuming diets rich in many nutrients is suggested:** Potential roles of magnesium, B vitamins, and vitamin D in DR development are suggested by emerging evidence. New studies also suggest that genetic differences in enzymes involved in the metabolism of these nutrients may modify associations between diet and DR relationships. Certain dietary patterns may lower risk for the onset or worsening of DR. Existing data from observational studies suggest that plant-based diets, or diets that comply with the American Diabetes Association dietary recommendations, may be protective.	Long-term, prospective studies are needed to investigate the putative role of newly implicated nutrients, as well as overall dietary patterns, in protection against the development of DR.

a lower density of the single cells that metabolically support the photoreceptors (retinal pigment epithelium) [24]. In addition, preterm infants supplemented with lutein had greater sensitivity responses of rod photoreceptors [25]. However, the extent to which this creates lasting visual advantages or prevents lifelong vision problems is unknown. Vision throughout life might also be modified by the degree to which lutein and zeaxanthin have accumulated *in utero* and by the intake of foods containing these carotenoids in later infancy and childhood.

It has long been proposed and recently demonstrated that these carotenoids enhance vision function. Supplementation has resulted in improvements in the ability to see under conditions of glare, to recover vision after a bright light is flashed [26], and to detect items in the natural world at a distance or under low light conditions [27]. Lutein supplementation slowed vision loss in adults with retinitis pigmentosa who were also taking vitamin A [5]. Although promising, the practical significance of these measurable influences on vision functions in daily life remains unclear.

Finally, the density of lutein and zeaxanthin in the lens and retina may influence eye diseases that occur in later life [23]. It has been reasoned that infant eyes are particularly vulnerable to oxidative damage in early life, which may have consequences decades later [23]. Because of the redundancy of the visual system, it may be difficult to observe the impact of early life nutrition on vision function in later life in small samples of people.

Given the possibility that lutein and zeaxanthin might be important for visual system development and function, it seems prudent to provide infants with nutrition early in life such as can be provided by breast-feeding from mothers with adequate intake of these carotenoids. The need for these carotenoids might be particularly high in premature infants, who do not have the benefit of optimally accumulating carotenoids *in utero* and are limited in ability to obtain them after birth.

Food sources of lutein and zeaxanthin include a wide variety of fruits and vegetables, seeds, and eggs [28]. They are particularly concentrated in green leafy vegetables, but corn products and eggs may comprise significant sources for some people, such as American Hispanics.

Trends in food consumption and obesity in the past two decades may also be contributing to the poor status for these carotenoids and, ultimately, eye health. The average daily intake of lutein and zeaxanthin in Americans in 2003 was estimated to be approximately 0.4–0.6 mg from 1 to 30 years of age and 1 mg among Americans older than age 31 years and into old age [28]. In adult populations, this is lower than estimated averages in 1988–1994 of 1.5 or 1.6 mg/day in The Third National Health and Nutrition Examination Survey [29]. This may reflect a reduction in vegetable intake observed in U.S. adults between these two time periods [30]. Increasing obesity in the United States is likely another factor contributing to reductions in carotenoid status because obesity is associated with lower levels of lutein and zeaxanthin in serum and macular pigment [31] even after accounting for dietary intake [32].

II CATARACT

Cataract is the leading cause of blindness worldwide, accounting for almost half of all blindness globally [33]. The visual burden of cataract is largest in developing countries, where the relatively simple surgical excision of cataract is less available. However, the economic burden of cataract in developed countries is also high. In the United States, an estimated 17% of Americans older than 40 years have cataract in either eyes, and 5% have had cataracts extracted [34]. Cataract surgery accounted for more than 12% of the total Medicare budget the last time this was evaluated in 1992 [35]. Even though cataract surgery has become less expensive, the occurrence of cataract will dramatically increase in the next 20 years as the aging U.S. population increases [34]. The large increase in cataract surgical procedures predicted for the U.S. population is expected to have a substantial effect on health care spending and, potentially, on the fiscal stability of the Medicare system [36]. Nutrition appears to be a primary means to substantially reduce the burden of age-related cataract; it has been estimated that if preventive

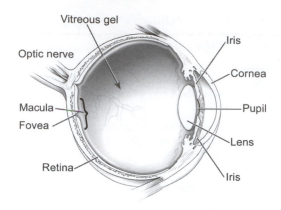

FIGURE 19.1 Anatomical features of the human eye. *Source: Courtesy of the National Eye Institute, National Institutes of Health.*

measures could delay cataract by only 10 years, the visual and surgical burden would be reduced by half [37].

Cataracts develop as opaque regions in the lens of the eye (Figure 19.1) as a result of either acute metabolic insults or, slowly, the gradual accumulation of damage with age. The lens must remain clear in order to collect light and focus it on the retina. However, lens opacities scatter light, blurring vision. When light transmission is blocked substantially enough to reduce visual acuity, a cataract exists; if opacities become severe, blindness can occur.

Cataracts generally occur in three regions of the lens: (1) the nucleus, or center, of the lens (nuclear cataract); (2) the region just under the lens capsule that separates the lens from the vitreous humor (posterior subcapsular cataracts (PSC)), and (3) the fiber layer between the outside edges of the lens and the nucleus (cortical cataract). Cataracts sometimes occur exclusively in one or the other of these regions; however, sometimes opacities occur in multiple regions, particularly as cataracts become more severe, and along with the advancement of age.

Nuclear cataracts may reflect cumulative insults that have occurred since early childhood. This is because nuclear lens fibers do not have mitochondria, nuclei, or other cytoplasmic organelles and thus lack the capacity to repair damage over one's lifetime. Nuclear cataracts are the most common type of cataract in whites [38–40], whereas cortical cataracts are most common in blacks [40,41]. Least frequently, cataracts develop in the PSC region of the lens; however, when they do, they often necessitate lens extraction [42] because opacities in this region often severely limit vision.

A Causes

The pathogenesis of cataract is known to involve the accumulated stresses resulting from inability of the eye to sufficiently defend against, or repair, the damage caused by physiological and environmental stressors that arise from such things as the photochemical formation of free radicals and osmotic imbalances. Smoking is the most common modifiable risk factor for cataract in population studies [43–51]. Exposure to smoke from combustion of wood or other biofuels may similarly increase cataract risk [52]. Other probable risk factors include exposure to ultraviolet (UV)-B light (particularly in the cortical region of the lens) [53–55], myopia [56], and diabetes (especially for cortical cataract and sometimes nuclear cataract and PSC) [51,57–60]. Risk is sometimes, but not always, higher among people who have a higher body mass index [61–63], use alcoholic beverages heavily [64–66], and have elevated markers of systemic and local inflammation [67,68] or arthritis [51]. Several aspects of diet could modify these risk factors or independently influence the risk of cataracts.

Animal studies have indicated that cataract can be induced by high-galactose diets, experimental diabetes, nutrient deficiencies (riboflavin, calcium, zinc, and selenium), or nutrient excesses (selenium) (reviewed previously [69,70]). In humans, nutritional influences on the development of cataract are also suggested by the high prevalence of cataract in developing countries [33], although this may also reflect the higher concentration of sunlight to which people living near the equator are exposed, high exposure to wood smoke or other biofuels used in cooking [52], or the increased prevalence of diarrheal diseases. In samples of people from a few developing countries, a higher occurrence of cataract has been reported among those with low intakes of protein-containing foods [71], fruits and vegetables [72], or other selected nutrients [73].

In the absence of extreme metabolic insults or deficiencies, lens opacities develop slowly over many years, beginning in the second decade in life and progressing more rapidly in middle and older age. A gradual influence of nutrition on the development of cataract over adult life is suspected and is supported by studies in the Emory mouse, a mouse strain that develops cataracts in adulthood. In these mice, calorie restriction, which is generally associated with reduced oxidative stress and improved glucoregulation [74], slows the development of lens opacities [75]. Since the 1980s, a body of evidence has accumulated to indicate lower rates of cataracts among populations of people who eat micronutrient-rich diets or take multivitamins (summarized in Table 19.1). These findings, discussed later, support the idea that nutritional status over adult life influences the development of cataract with age. However, most epidemiological studies of relationships of diet to cataract have been conducted in relatively well-nourished and older populations in developed countries and over short time periods. Therefore, these studies may underestimate the role of diet in the development of cataracts over time and accompanied by conditions of extreme limitations of food intake.

B Healthy Diet Patterns

Broadly healthy diets or vegetarian diets have been associated with lower risk of cataract extraction or nuclear cataract in three separate studies [76–78]. Experimental studies in animals and people and epidemiological studies in populations (discussed later) suggest specific food components may be responsible. The risk lowering associated with healthy diets in epidemiological studies [76,77] is approximately twofold and not explained by single nutrients [77], suggesting additional unknown food components that may lower risk and/or that food components work jointly to lower risk.

C Carbohydrates

In experimental animals, sugar cataracts are easily developed by feeding monosaccharide-rich diets or agents that promote diabetes (reviewed in [70]), which itself is a risk factor for cataract. In humans, these effects are demonstrated in individuals with galactosemia, a rare, autosomal recessive disorder leading to an inability to break down dietary galactose, as found in milk. One of the clinical consequences of galactosemia is cataracts, which can present in untreated infants [79]. Galactosemia is largely detected in infants via state-mandated newborn screening and treated with a galactose-free diet. However, treated individuals are still at higher risk of developing cataract throughout life [80,81], and milk intake in the broader population of adults has yet to be studied in association with age-related cataract.

Sugars do not require insulin to enter the lens. When the metabolic pathways to utilize them are overwhelmed, sugar alcohols are formed by aldose reductase, accumulate in the lens, and can cause osmotic cataracts. Moreover, prolonged exposure to monosaccharides can lead to nonenzymatic glycosylation and the accumulation of advanced glycation end products in the lens [82], or cataracts [83]. In people with diabetes, poor glycemic control has been associated with higher lens density [84]. The prediabetic state has also been associated with cataract [85]. In animals, the development of diabetes- or galactosemia-induced cataract has been reduced by intake of specific plant extracts [86] or a wide variety of nutrients and phytochemicals, including vitamins C and E [87], soy isoflavones [88], caffeine [89], resveratrol [90], cumin [91], and curcumin (in tumeric) [92].

However, the overall impact of blood glucose, specifically on cataract risk, is uncertain. Based on epidemiological studies, dietary carbohydrate has been associated with higher risk for cataract, particularly in the cortical region of the lens and less consistently in the nuclear area [93]. However, it remains to be determined if this reflects an effect of carbohydrate, per se, or a prediabetic state [94]. In addition, high dietary carbohydrate intake in developed countries may reflect an abundance of foods that are nutrient poor.

D Antioxidants

It is well-known that oxidative stress increases lens damage. Relationships of antioxidant nutrients to cataract development in animals, and to the occurrence of cataract in populations, have been extensively reviewed [52,69,70,87,95,96]. Deficiencies of riboflavin, selenium, and zinc—co-factors for enzymes that play important roles in oxidative defense—cause cataracts in some species [70]. Deficiencies of vitamins C or E and major water and lipid-soluble antioxidants, respectively, have not been reported to cause cataracts independently, but they do protect against oxidative damage in a variety of animal and cell systems. Vitamin C is abundant in human lenses, and its levels in the lens reflect those in the diet [97]. Lipid-soluble antioxidants in lenses include vitamin E and the carotenoids lutein and zeaxanthin [15], which have both been demonstrated to protect against UV light-induced peroxidation in lens cells [98].

In several population studies, blood levels of antioxidants or diets rich in one or more antioxidants (vitamins C and E or lutein and zeaxanthin) are often related to lower prevalence or incidence of cataracts or cataract extractions [99–109]. However, protective associations are not observed in other studies [105,110]. In a large prospective study of approximately 25,000 Swedish women, taking vitamin C supplements was associated with an increased risk of cataract extraction over 10 years [111]. One explanation for these conflicting pieces of evidence is that both deficiencies and excess of antioxidants could be harmful. In the lens, vitamin C can enhance oxidative stress [112] and contribute to glycation of lens proteins [113,114]. Moreover, there is evidence that oxidation of vitamin C can enhance photosensitivity, which could further promote cataracts [115].

In order to attempt to account for the joint influence of antioxidants, some researchers have noted lower rates of cataract among persons with a combination of high levels of antioxidants in diet or serum [17,99,106] (and in people with plant-rich diets, which would also be high in nutritive and non-nutritive antioxidants

discussed previously). Clinical trials of high doses of only one or two antioxidant nutrients for up to 12 years have not been generally effective in slowing cataract [116–119]. In one clinical trial, the rate of progression of lens opacities was lower among 81 persons who took three antioxidant nutrients (18 mg of β-carotene, 750 mg of vitamin C, and 600 IU of vitamin E) for 3 years compared to 77 people who did not take these supplements. However, in a large (4629 subjects) double-masked, placebo-controlled trial—the Age-Related Eye Disease Study (AREDS)—a similar formulation of high-dose antioxidants (containing 15 mg β-carotene, 500 mg vitamin C, and 400 IU vitamin E) taken for an average of 6.3 years did not influence progression of age-related lens opacities. A study of multiple antioxidants over 5 years in a South Indian population also found no evidence of benefit [120].

The potential importance of the xanthophyll carotenoids lutein and zeaxanthin, which are also antioxidants, to lens health was not recognized when population studies and clinical trials of antioxidants were conducted during the past two decades. However, there is mounting evidence that their intake may explain, in part, the lower cataract risk associated with people who eat diets rich in vegetables (discussed later). Diets and resulting serum rich in lutein and zeaxanthin are consistently related to lower incidence or prevalence of nuclear cataract or cataract extraction in longitudinal studies [99–104]. However, foods rich in these carotenoids, such as green vegetables and dark green leafy vegetables, are rich in many antioxidants and micronutrients so that the consistency of this association may simply reflect antioxidant-rich diets in general.

Some evidence for specific beneficial roles of lutein in the lens exists, even though the levels of lutein in the human lens are generally much lower than those in the macula of the eye. Experimental evidence indicates that lutein supplementation to cultured human lens epithelial cells results in lower oxidative damage due to UV light [98] and supplementation to diabetic rats slows cataract progression [121].

Supplements containing lutein and zeaxanthin have only been common since approximately 1995. There are no studies that report the influence of supplementation on cataract development. As with other antioxidants, there is theoretically the potential for a pro-oxidant effect in very high doses, but this has not been studied.

Thus, the overall body of evidence from animal and population studies suggests that antioxidant components of the diet may contribute to protection against cataract development. However, there is little evidence that short-term supplementation with one or a few antioxidants is likely to have an important impact on cataracts, which develop over many years and are influenced by a wide variety of dietary, health, and lifestyle factors. Moreover, adverse incidences affecting cataract development are possible when supplements are taken in high doses.

E Heavy Metals

Research on the benefits of antioxidants has not considered the potential larger importance that antioxidant protection might have under conditions of high oxidative stress. One such stress is the exposure to heavy metals. There is emerging evidence that the exposure of the lens to heavy metals that accompany air, soil, or water pollution and/or smoking, such as lead, cadmium [122], and mercury [123], can promote cataract development. It is thought that mechanisms for toxicity of heavy metals may be by depleting cellular glutathione and/or by heavy metals displacing zinc and copper on enzymes involved in protection against free radicals, causing oxidative stress [124]. Most epidemiological studies have not examined the joint effect of low intake of antioxidant-rich foods and heavy metal exposure. However, it is possible that the antioxidant protection afforded by foods or supplements is of greater importance in people at elevated risk, such as those exposed to heavy metals. Consistent with this idea, in a sample of fish-eating people living in an area of the Amazon with among the highest levels of mercury exposure in the world, the joint existence of poor plasma selenium and high blood mercury was associated with a dramatically higher (16 fold) prevalence of age-related cataract. In one clinical trial, β-carotene was protective against cataract only in smokers, who could have been expected to have higher exposure to heavy metals [117]. Thus, a benefit of food antioxidants may be greater in high-risk individuals such as smokers or people who are exposed to industrial pollutants.

F Dietary Supplements

Numerous studies have evaluated the relationships of dietary supplement use with the occurrence of cataract and are the subject of several reviews [125−128]. A protective effect of multivitamin use on nuclear cataract is indicated by three clinical trials [24,129,130]. However, evidence does not support a benefit on cortical opacities in studies up to 9 years, and the risk of cataracts in the posterior subcapsular region of the lens was increased twofold [24]. Therefore, no overall benefit on risk of cataract extraction has been observed in clinical trials.

The body of evidence does not support a benefit of high-dose antioxidant supplements, as previously discussed. Possible risk is suggested by evidence that use of vitamin C supplements was associated with increased risk of cataract extraction in a large prospective study of Swedish women [111].

III AGE-RELATED MACULAR DEGENERATION

A Overview

Age-related macular degeneration (AMD) is a result of deterioration of the part of the retina, the macula (see Figure 19.1), that is responsible for central vision and reading fine detail. It is the leading cause of blindness in developed countries and the third leading cause worldwide [33]. In the United States, by age 65 years, approximately 8% of people have an intermediate form of AMD that has a high risk of progressing to advanced AMD [131], and 2% of Americans older than 80 years have advanced AMD [131]. There is no cure for this condition, and medical and surgical treatments are limited to people with one type of advanced AMD (wet AMD) and are of limited long-term effectiveness. Because of the steep increase in AMD with age, prevention is likely to have a large impact on the social and economic burden of this condition.

The early stages of AMD are signaled by yellowish white deposits, or drusen (Figure 19.2), which can vary in size and area; more extensive drusen development is predictive of greater eventual progression to advanced stages. In intermediate stages, there are sometimes areas of hyper - or hypopigmentation (retinal pigment abnormalities) in the retina pigment epithelial (RPE) cells, a single layer of cells that support the rods and cones (photoreceptors), caused by disturbances in the distribution of melanin pigments. Extensive drusen and retinal pigment abnormalities are thought to signal the existence of pathological processes associated with a distressed central retina. These changes are theorized to compromise the ability of nutrients and oxygen to flow from the choroidal blood supply, through Bruch's membrane, to the RPE cells and the photoreceptors they support. Drusen may also reflect the existence of inflammatory processes that contribute to degradation of this area.

When deterioration proceeds to the extent that the RPE cells and the photoreceptors they support die, advanced AMD occurs. This type of advanced AMD is sometimes referred to as "dry" AMD. If growth of new blood vessels occurs, then the advanced AMD is referred to as "wet" AMD. Bleeding or leaking of these vessels can also cause acute limits in vision. Advanced AMD of both types interferes with vision in the center of the visual field (such as that needed to view a person's face straight on) and the ability to read fine detail needed, for example, to read newspapers.

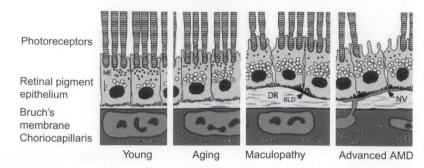

FIGURE 19.2 Changes to layers of retina in the macular region during aging, and progression of age-related macular degeneration (AMD) in early and advanced stages. With age, there is an accumulation of lipofuscin (LF), a decline in melanin (ME) in the retinal pigment epithelium, and a thickening and lipid enrichment of Bruch's membrane. Basal laminar deposits (BLD) are seen in early maculopathy but may also reflect aging. Drusen (DR) accumulation also characterizes early maculopathy. In intermediate AMD, drusen becomes more extensive, and there are areas of the retinal pigment epithelium that are hypopigmented or hyperpigmented (because of melanin clumping). In more advanced AMD, there is atrophy of the photoreceptors and there may be neovascularization (NV)—the growth of new blood vessels and narrowing of the choriocapillaris. *Source: Courtesy of Francois Delori, Schepens Eye Research Institute/Harvard Medical School, Boston, Massachusetts.*

B Causes

AMD appears to develop as a result of a complex interplay of multiple dietary, environmental, and genetic factors that influence oxidative stress [132], inflammation [133–135], and light damage [136]. Smoking is the most commonly reported risk factor [137] for AMD in epidemiological studies. Although it is commonly thought that damage by light, especially in the blue range, promotes AMD, epidemiological studies have not consistently observed higher rates of AMD among people with high levels of sunlight exposure. This might be due to the difficulty in assessing the amount, type, and timing of sun exposure. Some studies indicate high risk for AMD among people with cardiovascular disease [138,139] or its risk factors [140]. Aspects of diet that may explain these risk factors or be independently related are discussed later.

After smoking, the most consistent, strong risk factor for AMD is family history [141]. People with AMD more commonly have certain variants within genes related to complement activation in the inflammatory response. Although multiple complement related genes have been associated with AMD risk, the complement factor H (*CFH*) and age-related maculopathy susceptibility-2 (*ARMS2*) genes carry the greatest amount of risk. A variant within *CFH* (rs1061170), referred to as the Y402H variant because it results in a change in amino acid 402, explains more than half of the population risk of AMD and is associated with 2.5–6.0 times greater AMD risk than individuals without the risk variant [142]. A variant with independent but similarly strong effects is the A69S variant (rs10490924) within *ARMS2* [143]. The genetic predisposition to AMD may involve a propensity for inflammation or exacerbation of an inflammatory response [135]. Some studies find a high prevalence of AMD among people with elevated C-reactive protein

[144,145], an indicator of systemic inflammation, or among people with inflammatory diseases, such as gout [146], or who have used anti-inflammatory medicines, which may signal the presence of inflammatory disease [147]. The evidence that diet and supplements may prevent or slow progression of AMD is discussed here and summarized in Table 19.2.

C Healthy Diets

A wide body of evidence from a variety of study types supports the idea that food choices influence the development and progression of AMD. The body of evidence has been recently enhanced with results of studies that directly indicate that diets which are healthy in many ways (as indicated by high scores on healthy diet indices or two or more joint aspects of healthy diets) are related to lower prevalence of early [148,149] and advanced AMD [149,150] and lower incidence of early AMD [16] and progression to advanced AMD [151], particularly among people with the common high-risk Y402H variant in the complement factor H gene [152]. The reduction in the chance of having AMD may be particularly large (3-fold lower) when jointly accompanied by moderate to high levels of physical activity and avoidance of smoking [148]. Having high levels of body fat, which likely reflects a combination of genetic factors, diet, and physical activity, has been associated with a 12-fold higher risk for incidence of early or advanced AMD in people with two high-risk alleles for *CFH* Y402H [153]. Together with smoking, obesity has been observed to increase risk for progression of AMD 19-fold among people who have two copies of the risk allele at each of the *CFH* and *ARMS2* loci and 8-fold among people who have one copy of two common risk alleles [154]. Collectively, healthy diets, physical activity, not smoking, and genetic factors may contribute jointly to the lowering of oxidative stress, inflammation, and blood pressure and improving blood lipids, all of which are thought to be pathogenic mechanisms that promote AMD.

The following section describes evidence for a role of specific foods or nutrients. However, the level of risk reduction that might be achieved is likely highest when many beneficial aspects of diet are optimized, in the context of healthy diets, as discussed previously. The epidemiological evidence discussed here was gathered largely from the results of studies that do not adequately take into consideration the fact that high levels of one nutrient might reflect and be a marker for high levels of many other nutrients, or that the observed result might be modified by other aspects of diet. In the future, it might be possible to gain a better understanding of optimizing specific aspects of diet by combining data from several large epidemiological studies and examining relationships with specific foods or nutrients within groups of people who have similar overall diet quality. Combining data will also allow for investigators to power studies suitably to examine aspects of diet jointly with level of genetic risk and levels of physical activity. Thus, the reader must consider the evidence for specific nutrients with the caveat that the available evidence does not adequately isolate nutrients in a way that a benefit from supplements containing the nutrients can be generally inferred.

D Antioxidants

Oxidative damage to proteins, lipids, and DNA by free radicals within the photoreceptor outer segments or RPE can be the result of photo-oxidation of lipids from light exposure; it can also be the by-product of metabolic events, such as oxidative metabolism or enzyme reactions that use oxygen (e.g., xanthine oxidase). The retina is particularly susceptible to oxidative stress because of free radicals that result from light exposure, high rates of oxidative metabolism, and a high concentration of lipids with double bonds that are vulnerable to attack by free radicals. Free radicals that propagate oxidative damage may also be produced directly as a mechanism for biological defense, as is the case when white blood cells respond immunologically to pathogens with an oxidant boost.

The retina is generally rich in antioxidants and antioxidant enzymes that quench reactive oxygen species, including vitamins C and E [155], carotenoids [12,13], and zinc [156], a co-factor for superoxide dismutase. Eighty percent or more of carotenoids in the retina are lutein and zeaxanthin (discussed later). Lycopene, an efficient quencher of singlet oxygen, is also found in the RPE/choroidal area [12]. Although other carotenoids are not commonly found in human eye tissues, it is possible that they may have systemic effects on oxidative damage, which could modify processes that promote AMD (e.g., cardiovascular disease) or spare carotenoids that accumulate in the retina. In studies with experimental animals, deficiencies of vitamins E and C, carotenoids, or nutrients such as zinc, which are components in enzymes that protect against oxidative stress, result in pathological changes to the retina (as previously reviewed [132,157−159]).

Results of clinical trials of antioxidant supplements have been varied. Single or dual high-dose antioxidant supplements have not been associated with lower risk or progression of AMD [160,161]. This is consistent with evidence that oxidant defense is carried out by a highly complex system of mechanisms, in which antioxidant effects of several different individual antioxidant molecules have been found to be synergistic [162−164]. Differently, in the AREDS study—a 6.2-year randomized, placebo-controlled clinical trial [165]—high doses of a combination of antioxidants (500 mg of vitamin C, 400 IU of vitamin E, 15 mg of β-carotene, and 80 mg of zinc along with 2 mg of copper) slowed the progression of AMD from intermediate to more advanced stages by 28%. There is also evidence that this treatment reduces the age-related oxidation of cysteine in the blood, which supports the possibility that the benefit is due to an improvement in oxidative stress [166]. A small short-term study of men with atrophic AMD, who received antioxidant supplements along with lutein, reported improved visual function [167]. Men randomized to the control group did not report improved vision.

Although these studies suggest that a combination of dietary antioxidants may be important in slowing the progression of AMD, questions remain regarding the optimal dose and combination of nutrients in supplements, their long-term benefit and safety, and whether other aspects of diet are equally or more important. There is no evidence that people who have early AMD or who are at risk for AMD because of a family history will benefit from high-dose antioxidant supplements. Moreover, results of a large meta-analysis suggest that vitamin A, β-carotene, and vitamin E may increase mortality [168].

Epidemiological studies also generally support the idea that the intake of foods that are rich in antioxidants is associated with lower risk for AMD. Although the level of individual antioxidants in foods is usually much lower than levels provided by current high-dose antioxidant supplements, foods provide a more varied array of antioxidants than do supplements, and the impact of decades of consuming dietary antioxidants on AMD may be substantial and has not been adequately studied. In epidemiological studies, when associations with antioxidant nutrients are considered one at a time, low levels of one or more antioxidants in the blood or diet have often, but not always, been related to higher prevalence or incidence of certain age-related changes in the macula. Dietary nutrients related to lower occurrence of AMD include vitamin E [16,169,170] or one or more carotenoids (reviewed in [171] and subsequently reported in [172–175]) or zinc [16,170,176].

In the Rotterdam Eye Study [16], a 35% lower risk of incident AMD was observed among the 10% of participants who were consuming antioxidant-rich diets (i.e., diets with above the median intake of all four antioxidants in AREDS supplements) compared with those consuming above median intake for only one antioxidant. In this sample, high dietary intake of antioxidants particularly lowered the risk of developing AMD associated with high genetic risk [152].

Although the level of antioxidant vitamins in foods is usually lower than that in high-dose antioxidant supplements, the numbers of different known and unknown antioxidants in foods are likely to exceed those in supplements. Foods high in antioxidants, such as vegetables, might lower oxidative stress to a greater degree than supplements. In a randomized, crossover trial, eating two or more cups of brassica vegetables (e.g.,broccoli) lowered a urinary marker of oxidative stress, whereas moderate levels of supplementation with antioxidants in multivitamins did not [177]. A number of the polyphenolic flavonoids have been documented to have antioxidant or anti-inflammatory activity or increase ocular blood flow (reviewed in [178]). The polyphenol resveratrol, found in foods such as grapes, peanuts, wine, raisins, and some berries, acts as an antioxidant and anti-inflammatory agent under some conditions and was found to inhibit damage to human retinal pigment epithelial cells in culture resulting from exposure to substances found in cigarette smoke (as did lutein) [179]. However, the evidence regarding the effectiveness of these in limiting AMD-related pathology is limited and conflicting. The impact of decades of consuming dietary nutrient and non-nutrient antioxidants on AMD may be substantial [180] but has not been adequately studied to date.

E Lutein and Zeaxanthin

Lutein and its structural isomer zeaxanthin, which are obtained from certain fruits and vegetables (discussed previously), are selectively concentrated in the retina and are thought to protect against damage due to light and oxidative stress that would otherwise promote AMD. They may also lower AMD risk by lowering inflammation in the retina resulting from light damage (discussed later) or by lowering inflammation in other areas of the body [25,181] which may indirectly protect against AMD.

The highest density of these carotenoids is found in the inner retina, in the Henle fiber and inner plexiform layers [182], where they comprise a yellow pigment referred to as macular pigment. At these locations, they are likely to function as an optical filter that absorbs short-wavelength visible (blue) light [183]. This might protect against AMD or simply enhance vision (as discussed previously). They are also present in the lipid-rich photoreceptor outer segments, where they are likely to act as antioxidants in specific membrane domains which are rich in unsaturated lipids that are vulnerable to oxidation [184].

The macular pigment density reduces approximately 2-fold between the central macula, where the zeaxanthin isomer predominates, and the periphery of the fovea, where the lutein isomer predominates [13]. The total concentration reduces 100-fold from the center of the cone-dominated fovea to the rod-dominated peripheral retina [185].

One mechanism by which the absorption of blue light by macular pigment could protect against the development and progression of AMD is by blocking light-induced formation of a toxic di-retinal conjugate, A2E. Drusen deposits, characteristic of early AMD, which may be promoted by inflammatory processes [134], contain lipofuscin, the principal component of which is the toxic compound A2E, which forms as a consequence of light-related vitamin A cycling in the retina. A2E accumulates in the RPE during phagocytosis of the rods and cones, and it is taken up by the lysosomes. In excess, A2E has a variety of potential toxic effects, including sensitivity to blue light damage [186]. When a critical intracellular level of this compound is reached, cell damage to DNA occurs, induced by blue light irradiation [187]. Because macular pigment can absorb 40–90% of incident blue light [183], it can reduce A2E toxicity.

There is evidence in animals that lutein and zeaxanthin protect areas of the retina influenced by AMD in humans. Animal models that are best for studying the impact of macular pigment on AMD or related photoreceptor health are species that accumulate these carotenoids in their ocular tissues, including primates and some birds. Primates fed diets deficient in these xanthophyll carotenoids [159,188] suffer a loss of RPE cells and increased photoreceptor cell death [189]. Subsequent supplementation with lutein protected the fovea of the retina against blue light damage [128]. Retinal zeaxanthin has also been demonstrated to prevent light-induced photoreceptor death in quail [190]. Dietary lutein supplementation has been reported to inhibit inflammatory and angiogenic molecules related to neovascularization in mice and to inhibit inflammatory and angiogenic processes in human retinal cell cultures [191].

The evidence for protection in humans derives mostly from epidemiological studies, which consistently indicate lower rates of advanced stages of AMD in people with higher dietary levels of these carotenoids [17,29,192–194]. Associations between the intake or serum levels of lutein and zeaxanthin and earlier stages of AMD are inconsistent [16,17,29,170,175,192]. However, results from the Carotenoids in Age-Related Eye Disease Study indicate that a protective association between dietary lutein and AMD is observed after excluding people who have made marked dietary changes and women younger than 75 years of age, in whom the association is less likely to be influenced by survivor bias [195].

The relationships between dietary lutein and zeaxanthin and AMD may also depend on a person's ability to absorb and accumulate carotenoids from the diet or supplements. This appears to vary among individuals. Between 20 and 50% of subjects in previous investigations had low serum or retinal response to oral supplementation with these carotenoids [196–198]. In general, blood responses to oral carotenoids vary among individuals as well [199,200]. The influences on the ability to absorb carotenoids by the intestinal tract and the eye are largely unknown. Having high levels of body fat, diabetes [31,32], or certain genetic variants [201–203] is related to lower macular density. These may influence the ability to absorb and accumulate lutein and zeaxanthin in the eye or may increase the turnover of carotenoids in the eye due to inflammation and oxidative stress.

Synergistic relationships between dietary lutein and genetic predisposition for AMD are possible and may explain some inconsistency in the relationships of dietary lutein with AMD. The presence of the common genetic risk variant in the *CFH* gene (Y402H), which increases risk for AMD, was less predictive of AMD in people whose diets were rich in lutein and zeaxanthin [152].

The strong biological plausibility that the macular pigment protects against degeneration is supported by the observation of lower levels of lutein and zeaxanthin in autopsy specimens of donor eyes with AMD compared with donor eyes in people without AMD [185]. However, to date, relationships of AMD to macular pigment density, measured noninvasively in living persons, have not been detected in cross-sectional studies [204–208]. This may be due, in part, to bias as a result of recent lutein supplement use in people who have been diagnosed with or have a family history of macular degeneration or due to survivor bias common in epidemiological studies of older people. Significant [204] or marginally significant [208] trends for a protective association have been observed when such people are excluded from analyses. A trend in the direction of protection of macular pigment on AMD progression was observed in the only longitudinal study [209], but it was not statistically significant nor well powered (only 27 people developed AMD over 10 years). For this reason, larger longitudinal studies are needed to evaluate the magnitude of protection that higher macular pigment density may have on lowering risk for AMD.

Even if higher macular pigment density is found to be related to lower risk for developing or worsening macular pigment in future studies, it remains to be determined whether this is due to the dietary intake of lutein and zeaxanthin, or the many other components in fruits and vegetables, or the healthy lifestyles of people with lutein-rich diets that may slow the development of AMD. Women who had a combination of healthy lifestyles (fruit- and vegetable-rich diet, not smoking, and high levels of physical activity) had higher macular pigment density than women who did not, despite having only slightly greater intake of lutein and zeaxanthin [148]. This suggests that these may be other means of enhancing macular pigment.

The benefits and risks of taking lutein and zeaxanthin supplements have been studied in only a limited number of small clinical trials. Visual acuity improved slightly in the fewer than 30 subjects who received exclusively lutein supplements for 1 year [167] and in those receiving lutein and zeaxanthin in combination with other antioxidants [210]. In another trial, data suggest that lutein or zeaxanthin supplementation may improve visual performance at low illumination [27]. However, in a different small trial, supplementation did not improve contrast sensitivity over 9 months [211]. Larger and longer term trials are needed to more conclusively address potential benefits (and risks) of supplementation with lutein and zeaxanthin. Results of a large multicenter trial of these carotenoids (and omega-3 fatty acids) on the progression of advanced AMD (AREDS 2) are expected in 2013 [212].

Despite the possibility that vegetables, particularly green vegetables and dark leafy greens, may lower the risk for AMD (and cataract, as discussed previously), some older people limit their intake because these contain high levels of vitamin K, which could interfere with warfarin that has been prescribed to prevent blood clotting. A sudden increase in vitamin K intake from these foods can reduce the effectiveness of the drug. However, patients can be advised to consult with the physician who manages their warfarin dose to adjust it to the highest daily green vegetable intake that the patient can consistently eat.

F Zinc and Other Metals

Zinc may be particularly important to the retina because concentrations of zinc in the retina exceed those elsewhere in the body, with the exception of the prostate [156]. Deficiency of zinc in both animals and people impairs retinal functioning, as previously reviewed [157]. There is evidence for numerous mechanisms (catalytic, regulatory, and structural [213]) by which zinc could influence retinal integrity. Zinc catalyzes enzymatic reactions and is a co-factor of more than 100 enzymes, some of which are involved in oxidant defense. Zinc depletion in RPE cells has reduced levels of catalase, glutathione peroxidase, and metallothionein and has reduced the ability to phagocytize photoreceptor outer segments [214]. Zinc performs structural roles; it facilitates protein folding to produce biologically active molecules (zinc fingers). Zinc is also involved in immune responses [215,216]. Both zinc deficiency and excesses impair immunity [216]. Zinc binds to and inhibits the activity of factor H protein in the complement system and has been proposed to contribute to deposit formation and inflammation associated with early AMD [217]. Zinc depletion may also trigger apoptosis of RPE cells or increase the vulnerability of RPE cells to photic injury [218]. However, zinc supplementation can also enhance stress-induced effects in RPE cells [219]. Both lower and higher [220] levels of zinc in the choroid and retinal pigment epithelium were observed in autopsy specimens from patients with AMD compared to those without the condition [221].

The longer term benefit of zinc on risk for AMD is suggested by the results of several [16,17,170,176] but not all [222,223] observational studies involving at least 500 participants [17]. The use of high-dose zinc supplements (80 mg as zinc oxide, along with 2 mg of cupric oxide) for 6 years with or without antioxidants was associated with modestly lower progression from intermediate to advanced AMD in AREDS [224]. One smaller zinc supplementation trial had previously reported a benefit of zinc supplementation on vision loss in patients with AMD [225], whereas another did not [226]. No serious safety issues with zinc supplementation were identified in the 6-year AREDS study (aside from more frequent hospitalization for genitourinary problems in men and more frequent anemia, unsupported by differences in hematocrit), and zinc supplementation was related to lower mortality in this sample [227]. However, the longer term benefits and risks of zinc supplementation at the high levels tested in AREDS are unknown. Furthermore, the benefit associated with zinc may be dependent on genetics. One study reported a protection against early AMD only in individuals with high dietary zinc intake who also carried either of the high-risk AMD variants from *CFH* or *ARMS2* [152]. However, subsequent analysis of the AREDS trial reported that the benefit of high-dose zinc, in lowering the risk of progressing from intermediate

to advanced AMD, were only effective in those without the high-risk CFH [228]. Joint influences of genes and zinc status in relation to AMD risk remain understudied.

That a protective association of zinc on AMD is observed in most, but not all, observational studies and clinical trials may reflect the possibility that protection is limited to individuals who are exposed to high levels of heavy metals through cigarette smoke or other environmental contaminants. Such high-risk individuals may comprise different proportions of the study samples in observational studies and trials. Two metals that have been suggested to place persons at high risk for age-related macular degeneration are cadmium and lead [229]. These divalent cations often compete for the same binding sites as copper and zinc and have the capacity to displace these essential metals [230]. Relationships between these common and toxic metals and AMD have not been directly studied in epidemiological studies.

Cadmium, a naturally occurring metal that is increasing in the environment as a by-product of industrial activities, smoking, and fertilizers, is a potent inflammatory agent and increases oxidative stress [231]. Cadmium levels in the retinal tissues were approximately double in smokers compared to non-smokers [232] and may explain, in part, the higher risk of AMD in smokers. Higher urinary cadmium levels were found in smokers who had AMD compared to smokers who did not have AMD [233]. Lead is also a naturally occurring metal that accumulates in body tissues with age as a function of smoking, drinking water, and other types of environmental contamination. Like cadmium, it can lead to the production of inflammatory cytokines and oxidative stress. Lead in the neural retina has been associated with the presence of AMD [229].

In summary, the benefit of diets with adequate levels of zinc from foods (dairy, meat, or beans) or from supplements may depend on exposure to toxic metals that compete with zinc. The benefit may also depend on genetic risk for enhanced inflammation and/or oxidative stress. These interactions have not been well studied in humans. Very large studies are needed to do this.

G Dietary Fat

There are at least three broad mechanisms by which dietary fats might either enhance or slow AMD. First, because of the high caloric density of fats, eating high-fat foods can displace other nutrient-dense foods that may have otherwise protected against AMD. Second, eating high-fat and low nutrient density foods may contribute to high body mass, which is reported to be a risk factor for AMD [234–236]. Third, fatty acids have numerous biological effects as components of biological membranes and regulators of biochemical pathways. Some dietary fats increase risk for atherosclerosis, which is related to AMD risk in some studies [138,139] and in a mouse model of atherogenesis [237]. Certain fatty acids can also have direct human physiological effects on the retina by modulating oxidative stress or by the inflammatory response, which can promote AMD pathogenesis (discussed later).

In mouse models of atherosclerosis, feeding high-fat diets resulted in the accumulation of lipid-like droplets in the retina and degenerative changes in RPE cells and Bruch's membrane [238–241]. In epidemiological studies, high dietary fat levels have been generally associated with increased risk for early and late AMD [234–236,242–245], even though these associations have not always been statistically significant. Some exceptions to this trend include prevalence or short-term incidence studies with low power to evaluate associations with either early AMD [246] or advanced AMD [242–244].

However, there is inconsistency across studies in the type of fat that was most related to AMD. AMD was more strongly related to a high intake of saturated fats in some studies [236,243–245,247] and to a high intake of polyunsaturated fatty acids [223] or monounsaturated fatty acids in other studies [234,236,247]. A high intake of monounsaturated fatty acids, nuts, or olive oil was associated with a lower risk in other studies [223,248,249]. The intake of trans-fatty acids, provided in diets by margarines and other processed foods, was related to higher risk for AMD in three studies [234,236,248]. Because fat intake often changes, particularly in relation to the common diagnosis for cardiovascular diseases, which can be related to AMD, these relationships are difficult to interpret.

In addition, there is limited knowledge about the combined effects of other risk factors that might influence the observed associations. For example, chronic light exposure reduces the loss of DHA from photoreceptors in rats [250]. This suggests that light exposure may modify the impact of dietary fats on AMD. The protective association of nuts on the incidence of early AMD was greater in people without other risk factors (smoking, low dietary carotenoids, and low ratio of total to high-density lipoprotein cholesterol in one study) [249]. Omega-3 fatty acid intake in one study [152] and weekly fish intake in another [251] reduced the AMD risk in patients with common high-risk genetic variants. However, joint effects are highly inconsistent across single studies. Larger pooled studies are needed to evaluate such joint effects in human epidemiological studies. Moreover, there is limited ability in such studies to adjust for the numerous other protective aspects of diet that accompany a more moderate, compared to high, intake of fat.

In contrast, lower risk for early or late AMD among people with higher intake of fish, fatty fish, or long-chain omega-3 polyunsaturated fatty acids (LC omega-3 PUFAs) is reported in most published observational studies [236,245–249,252–254]. Two studies found no such associations [223,243]. Curiously, however, the rates of intermediate and advanced AMD (characterized by pigmentary abnormalities and geography atrophy) in a sample of older adults from Iceland are markedly higher than rates in three other populations of European ancestry [254], despite having the highest per capita fish intake among Europeans and the fact that 56% report the use cod liver oil, a rich source of LC omega-3 fatty acids.

The protective influence of omega-3 fatty acids could be somewhat dependent on the omega-6 content of the diet. A higher ratio of omega-3 to -6 fatty acids could increase formation of anti-inflammatory eicosanoids from omega-3 fatty acids because the omega-6 fatty acids compete for the desaturase enzyme that creates them [256] or replace the omega-6 content of membranes. A high ratio of omega-6 to omega-3 fatty acids also upregulates genes involved in lipid trafficking in the neuroretina [257]. In three studies, the risk reduction associated with a high intake of LC omega-3 PUFAs was stronger among subjects who had low intake of omega-6 PUFAs [234,236,247].

LC omega-3 PUFAs, such as DHA or eicosapentaenoic acid (EPA), may be particularly important to the health of the retina. The pathogenesis of AMD may be influenced by atherosclerosis or involve parallel processes [140]. There is a large body of evidence to suggest that EPA and DHA lower cardiovascular disease mortality by several mechanisms: by an improvement of blood lipids by lowering blood triglycerides; decreasing inflammation, blood pressure, and platelet aggregation; and improving vascular reactivity [258]. These may influence AMD pathogenesis directly or indirectly. DHA is the most abundant LC omega-3 PUFA in rod outer segment membranes [259,260] at a concentration that exceeds levels found elsewhere in the body (reviewed in [261]). Its presence in membranes affects their biophysical properties and may influence membrane-bound enzymes, receptors, and transport. This is important in visual transduction [262], but it may also influence the pathogenesis of AMD. LC omega-3 PUFAs may protect against AMD by direct influence on retinal cell survival [263]. DHA has also been demonstrated to protect RPE cells from oxidative stress [263,264]. Deficiency of omega-3 fatty acids in nonhuman primates increases sensitivity to blue light damage [128].

DHA may also lower risk for AMD through its anti-inflammatory properties [256]. Numerous cell culture studies provide clues for possible mechanisms by which LC omega-3 PUFAs could enhance the integrity of vascular and basement membranes and prevent neo-vascularization (reviewed in [265]). The benefit of supplementing with 1 g per day of LC omega-3 PUFAs is unknown and is currently being tested in a large clinical trial (AREDS 2).

H Vitamin D

Data are emerging to suggest that vitamin D might also play a role in protection against AMD by virtue of vitamin D's anti-inflammatory and anti-angiogenic properties. Vitamin D is a fat-soluble vitamin that can be obtained from food, supplements, or synthesis in the skin on exposure to sunlight. Vitamin D is hydroxylated in the liver to form 25-hydroxyvitamin D (25(OH)D), the preferred biomarker to assess vitamin D status. 25(OH)D can be further hydroxylated in the kidneys and other tissues to form 1,25-dihydroxyvitamin D (1,25(OH)2D), the active hormone that interacts with the vitamin D receptor to influence gene transcription.

The vitamin D receptor (VDR) has been found on human retinal cells, indicating that it may have a role in eye health [266,267]. Localized inflammation is thought to be involved in the etiology of AMD [268]. This is supported by the high prevalence of *CFH* polymorphisms among people with AMD [142] and the observation of immunocompetent proteins entrapped in drusen [133].

Vitamin D is thought to suppress localized inflammatory responses. The VDR is found on cells of the immune system [269−271], and vitamin D has been shown to alter the proliferation and differentiation of immune cells, decrease immunoglobin production [272−276], and promote a Th1 over a Th2 cell response [269−271,276]. Vitamin D may also prevent later development of neovascular AMD due to its anti-angiogenic properties. Endothelial cells express the VDR [277], and studies in cell culture [278,279] and animal models of retinal disease [280,281] show that vitamin D has anti-angiogenic properties.

Blood concentrations of 25(OH)D generally reflect intake of vitamin D from foods, supplements, as well as endogenous production of vitamin D that occurs upon exposure of skin to ultraviolet B radiation in sunlight [282]. Two studies have observed decreased odds of prevalent, early AMD among persons with high compared to low blood concentrations of 25(OH)D [283,284], and one study observed no association between 25(OH)D and any AMD [285]. Consistent evidence from epidemiological studies in other samples and persons with different levels of healthy diets and lifestyles, in studies using prospective designs and in studies with larger numbers of people with advanced AMD are needed to better evaluate the possibility that better vitamin D status protects against AMD.

Food sources for vitamin D include naturally occurring sources such as fatty fish, fish liver oil, shiitake mushrooms, and egg yolk and also fortified food sources such as milk, orange juice, breakfast cereals, and margarine [282,286]. Observations of a protective effect of blood measures of vitamin D on AMD are supported by the observation that high compared to low intake of milk [283] and vitamin D from food and supplements combined [284] has been associated with a decreased odds of early AMD. In a study of male monozygotic twins with discordant AMD, vitamin D intake from foods was associated with a lower grade of AMD [287]. However, in a separate case—control study, no statistically significant association was observed between dietary vitamin D intake and neovascular AMD [288]. Interestingly, previously reported dietary associations between AMD and fish, omega-3 fatty acids (found in fish), and zinc (for which milk is an important source) might reflect, in part, a protective effect from vitamin D.

Data from studies investigating associations between AMD and food and supplement sources of vitamin D should be examined with caution, however, because total intake of vitamin D from foods and supplements may not reflect an individual's true vitamin D status [289]; vitamin D can also be obtained from sunlight exposure. Studies of vitamin D and AMD are also difficult to assess because they may also be confounded by the potentially detrimental effects of sun exposure. Sun exposure is needed to endogenously synthesize vitamin D. However, sun exposure may also increase risk for AMD (reviewed in [290]). The avoidance of excessive sunlight to minimize risk for skin cancers, cataract, and AMD might jeopardize systemic vitamin D status in older people, leading to potentially increased risk of AMD if adequate vitamin D status is shown to be protective. Collectively, the existing data suggest that vitamin D might be another nutrient that protects the aging retina. If confirmed, vitamin D status could have an impact on risk for AMD, given that portions of the U.S. population are at risk for poor vitamin D status [291,292].

I Glycemic Index

The glycemic index of foods was recently introduced as another possible aspect of diet that could influence the development of AMD [293]. Although advanced glycation end products have been found in drusen, it is not yet known whether they are a cause or consequence of degenerative changes. Degeneration of the retinal vasculature is a well-known complication of diabetes mellitus; however, the presence of diabetes has sometimes, but not always, been related to AMD in epidemiological studies. The biological plausibility that elevation in blood sugar promotes AMD, particularly in the absence of diabetes, remains untested. Nevertheless, diets with a low glycemic index often include few refined grains and sugars and plenty of fruits, vegetables, whole grains, legumes, and milk, which have numerous ingredients that could protect against AMD. Thus, high glycemic index diets, like high-fat diets, may be related to higher rates of AMD, in part or in whole, because they are poorer in a wide variety of protective nutrients and other diet components.

J Botanical Supplements

The use of herbal supplements has increased in the United States. Several botanical supplements, such as those containing ginkgo biloba and bilberry, have been promoted to benefit the health of the retina. However, no scientific studies support their benefit except for one very small (20 persons) study of ginkgo biloba in patients with AMD, in which improvement in visual acuity was indicated in a preliminary report (previously reviewed [294]).

IV DIABETIC RETINOPATHY

A Overview

Diabetic retinopathy (DR) is a complication of diabetes, type 1 or type 2, that is considered to be the result of damage to the microvasculature of the retina. It is the leading cause of new cases of blindness in working-aged U.S. adults (20–74 years) [295]. Approximately 12.3% of Americans ages 20 years or older have diabetes, and this is estimated to increase to 14.0% by 2030 [296]. Diabetes is especially burdensome in minority populations, such as African Americans, Mexican Americans [297], and Native Americans [298], in whom the prevalence and incidence are higher than the national averages. The burden of associated complications like DR will likely also increase in the coming years.

Previous work has described the natural history of the disease (reviewed in [299,300]). In brief, preclinical stages of DR include changes in retinal blood flow. Nonproliferative DR consists of the formation of clinical lesions (microaneurysms and intraretinal hemorrhages), the appearance of retinal exudates (lipid deposits from leaky blood vessels) and cotton wool spots (resulting from localized ischemia), and the appearance of venous bleeding and loops. Blindness can result at theses stages if macular edema occurs. In the later proliferative stage (PDR), new vessels and fibrous tissue can originate from the optic disc or elsewhere in the retina. Problems arise if the vessels grow through the inner limiting membrane into the vitreous humor of the eye, which is constantly contracting and condensing. Often, this movement can lead to vessel tear, hemorrhage, and blindness.

The only effective medical treatment is laser photocoagulation [299] to cauterize leaking, newly developed blood vessels that have grown as a result of DR. Photocoagulation does not necessarily prevent vision loss in all individuals, and it involves investing time in treatment that may cause discomfort.

B Causes

Randomized controlled trials have demonstrated that maintenance of tight blood glucose control via intensive insulin therapy is associated with lower incidence and progression of DR in individuals with types 1 and 2 diabetes [301–304]. Even so, intensive insulin therapy did not prevent the occurrence of DR in all individuals and was often associated with increased bouts of hypoglycemia [301,302]. Other risk factors for DR are duration of diabetes [305], hypertension [306], and elevated blood lipids [304]. Although such strong risk factors have been identified, they have been estimated to account for a small percentage (~10%) of the risk of DR incidence or progression [307]. There is still a need to continue to investigate possible preventive measures for DR incidence and progression.

Nutrition may significantly influence risk of DR, and its role has been relatively unexplored (summarized in Table 19.3). Various types of diets may contribute to risk for DR (1) by contributing to the maintenance of tight blood glucose control, (2) by lowering blood pressure or serum lipid levels, or (3) via mechanisms independent of such factors. However, few large epidemiologic studies have investigated the overall impact of differing diets and supplementation on the risk for DR. Medical nutrition therapy for patients with diabetes could be targeted at preventing DR or its progression and may be less costly than current treatment. Next, a few areas of promising research in nutrition and diabetic retinopathy are highlighted.

C Dietary Fat, Fiber, and Sodium

Some of the original investigations of the associations between dietary intake and DR were conducted in the 1980s and involved small intervention studies of linoleic acid, an omega-6 PUFA, among individuals with type 2 diabetes [308,309]. These studies suggested that intake of diets enriched with linoleic acid decreased the development and progression of DR, especially among those with poor glycemic control. The authors hypothesized that linoleic acid enrichment of cell membranes would increase the sensitivity of the insulin receptor and thus improve blood glucose control [308]. However, these earlier intervention studies' effects could have been due to linoleic acid consumption displacing consumption of other more harmful fatty acids, such as saturated fat.

Since then, published studies have suggested that high calorie and fat (% kcal) intake may increase risk for DR. Data from one ecological study showed a greater prevalence of DR in persons with type 1 diabetes in European regions with higher, compared to lower, mean intakes of cholesterol, total fat, and saturated fat (% kcal) [310]. Results of the Diabetes Control and Complications Trial (DCCT) of 1041 patients with type 1 diabetes showed positive correlations between DR progression and the intake of total, saturated, and monosaturated fat (% kcal) and cholesterol and a negative correlation between DR progression and intake of carbohydrates (% kcal) [311]. A prospective study of 649 African Americans with type 1 diabetes [312] investigated associations between DR progression and usual intake of total calories, protein, fat (total, saturated, oleic, and linoleic), cholesterol, and sodium. Total kilocalories along with age, glycosylated hemoglobin (Ghb), and hypertension were found to be significant predictors of vision threatening DR and severe hard exudates, whereas sodium, age, Ghb, and hypertension were found to be significant predictors of macula edema progression. The authors suggest that increasing kilocalories increases hyperglycemia and dyslipidemia and thus oxidative stress, a proposed etiologic mechanism for DR [313], and that high sodium intake increases hypertension, a known risk factor for DR. On the other hand, two cross-sectional studies [314,315] observed no statistically significant differences in total calories, total fat consumption (% kcal) [314,315], or saturated fat consumption (% kcal) [314] between persons with and without prevalent DR.

Diets rich in fiber, especially soluble fiber, have been shown to improve glycemic control and insulin sensitivity [316] and thus likely reduce risk for DR. The DCCT observed that intake of dietary fiber (% kcal) was inversely correlated with the progression of DR [311]. One [314] of three [315,317] earlier conducted studies observed a higher intake of fiber in persons without compared to those with DR. A population-based, cross-sectional study of 1261 individuals with type 2 diabetes observed 41 and 24% increased odds, respectively, of overall and sight-threatening DR among persons with a low compared to a high consumption of fiber-rich foods with adjustment for confounding factors [318]. However, the total quantity or type of fiber in the diet from consumed foods was not determined.

More research is needed to assess the effects of long-term calorie, dietary fat, and fiber intake with respect to the incidence and progression of DR. The published studies of calories, dietary fat, and fiber have a number of limitations: cross-sectional designs [314,315,318]; dietary assessment methods, which do not accurately assess long-term dietary intake [314]; lack of adjustment for confounding factors [311,314,315]; and small sample sizes [314].

D Diet Patterns

A few published studies suggest that dietary patterns, including those high in fiber and low in fat (and most likely rich in certain micronutrients), may be beneficial in protecting against DR. Results of a small case—control study of people with type 2 diabetes, conducted in India, indicated that diets high in energy, animal proteins, and fats were more common among persons with proliferative DR than controls [319]. Controls tended to eat more pulses and vegetables, sources of dietary fiber. The DCCT reported that conventionally treated participants who followed the American Diabetes Association's dietary recommendations with respect to fat and total calorie intake were less likely to experience DR progression [311]. In addition, a 20-year follow-up of a 6-year lifestyle intervention study of 542 individuals with impaired glucose tolerance in Da Qing, China, showed lower incidence of severe DR in the group receiving combined diet and exercise intervention compared to the control group [320]. The dietary intervention group was targeted to increase vegetable intake and lower alcohol and sugar intake. The authors suggest these results are explained by a reduction in incidence of diabetes among individuals in the intervention group. No other published studies have investigated relationships of dietary patterns to risk of DR.

E Antioxidants

Hyperglycemia is thought to increase oxidative stress through a number of proposed mechanisms, including damage to DNA, lipids, proteins, and carbohydrates as well as functional alterations of a number of other metabolic pathways that promote oxidative stress (reviewed in detail elsewhere [313,321]). Increased oxidative stress is hypothesized to promote diabetic vascular complications such as DR [313,321]. The retina is especially susceptible to damage from reactive oxygen species due to the PUFA-rich endothelial cells of the retinal microvasculature [313,322].

Furthermore, some studies have shown that individuals with diabetes compared to individuals without diabetes have lower blood levels of antioxidants [323,324], as well as lower carotenoids in the retina [31], perhaps as a result of increased oxidative stress. Antioxidant intake has been proposed to help alleviate the observed increased state of oxidative stress in individuals with diabetes and help to prevent the development of microvascular complications such as DR. Supplementation of streptozotocin-induced diabetic rats for 12 months with micronutrients in the AREDS trial resulted in less degeneration of the retinal microvasculature (indicating early signs of DR) than in nonsupplemented animals [325]. However, numerous studies investigating associations between antioxidant micronutrients biomarkers (primarily vitamins C and E) and diabetic retinopathy in small patient samples have yielded conflicting results [326].

There is currently insufficient data from epidemiological studies to conclude that diets or supplements high in antioxidants prevent or slow DR [327–329]. One study observed no relationship between levels of vitamin C or E in the diet (assessed 6 years earlier) and prevalent DR [329]. In a second cross-sectional population-based study, vitamin C in the serum was unrelated to the prevalence of DR, but serum vitamin E concentrations were positively associated with increased odds of DR [328]. This relationship was attenuated when current supplement users were removed from the analysis. In a different cross-sectional study, the severity of prevalent DR was higher in subjects who had high intakes of vitamin C and in subjects who did not use insulin and had high intakes of vitamin E [327]. Data from a clinical trial of vitamin E supplementation did not show differences in the history of DR laser therapy between supplementation and placebo arms [330]. However, DR was not the primary end point for the trial. In addition, three cross-sectional studies investigating associations between carotenoids and DR suggest that intake [327,331,332] or blood levels [327,331,332] of carotenoids (more so non-provitamin A (PVA) compared to PVA carotenoids [327,331,332]) are inversely associated with the odds of DR.

Associations of prevalent DR to short-term diet and blood nutrient levels in cross-sectional studies may be biased by the recent use of popular antioxidant supplements, particularly in people who may be experiencing more severe symptoms of diabetes. Also, long-term use of antioxidant supplements may protect against DR. In one study, participants who reported as using multivitamins, vitamin C, or vitamin E supplements 3 or more years before DR was assessed had lower odds of DR [329]. To date, no published studies of clinical trials have examined the effect of antioxidant therapy with the primary outcome of DR. Moreover, there are no prospective cohort studies of the influence of a wider range of dietary antioxidants on the onset or worsening of DR. Given the strong evidence for protection by antioxidants in animal studies, and the suggestion of the benefit of long-term antioxidant use in one large observational study, additional studies are needed to better assess these relationships.

F Vitamin D

Vitamin D has anti-inflammatory and anti-angiogenic properties, as previously discussed, which may also help prevent DR development and progression. The etiology of DR is hypothesized to involve hyperglycemia-induced chronic low-grade inflammation [333], and advanced DR involves angiogenesis. Three studies have investigated associations between vitamin D status and DR [334–336] with conflicting results. Aksoy et al. [334], in a study of 66 participants with diabetes, observed lower serum 1,25 (OH)2D, but not 25(OH)D concentrations, in participants with more severe DR compared to those with less severe or no DR. One cross-sectional study of 581 outpatients with type 2 diabetes observed lower 25(OH)D concentrations in patients with prevalent PDR compared to no DR [335]. Results from a 26-year prospective study of 220 patients with type 1 diabetes observed no associations between serum 25(OH)D concentrations of incident background or PDR in adjusted analyses [336]. Other studies have suggested associations between different polymorphisms of the vitamin D receptor and risk of DR [337–339], whereas others have not [340,341].

Additional work in larger epidemiologic studies is needed that can account for pertinent confounding variables as well as provide adequate cases to investigate associations between vitamin D status and PDR. Furthermore, work in minority populations with the greatest burden of diabetes and the greatest risk for vitamin D deficiency (e.g., African Americans) [291] should be conducted.

G Other Dietary Factors

Hypomagnesemia is common in persons with diabetes, and it is hypothesized to be associated with decreased glycemic control and insulin sensitivity [342,343]. Inconsistent evidence exists from small studies on the relationship between blood measures of magnesium and the presence, severity, or progression of DR (reviewed in [326]). These observations have yet to be investigated in large prospective epidemiological studies.

Deficiencies in B vitamins (B_{12}, B_6, and folate) can lead to hyperhomocysteinemia. Hyperhomocysteinemia is thought to increase risk for cardiovascular disease via a number of proposed mechanisms, including increased oxidative stress [344]. Hyperhomocysteinemia has been shown to be associated with DR in some small studies, and previous work has related polymorphisms in the methylenetetrahydrofolate reductase gene (MTHFR), responsible for homocysteine metabolism, to risk of DR (reviewed in [345]). No epidemiologic studies focusing on folate intake in relation to DR have been published.

Alcohol consumption in relation to DR has been studied in a number of observational studies [346–350]. Only one study found that moderate alcohol consumption was associated with reduced odds of DR [348]. Other studies found no relationship.

H Summary

Prospective observational research is needed in population studies of individuals with diabetes to determine whether the protective effects of antioxidant intake, observed in experimental animals and small, hospital-based studies, can be generalized to people over the long term. Limited data exist on the role of vitamin D in DR. A strong biological rational exists to suggest vitamin D may influence prevalent DR. Additional research is needed to evaluate the importance of overall dietary patterns, rich in different nutrients, on the prevalence and progression of DR in the general population. Given the broad aspects of diet that could protect against DR, such data will particularly assist in making public health recommendations and individual dietary recommendations.

V OVERALL SUMMARY

Scientific evidence suggests that food matters in the maintenance of eye health, as with other parts of the body. That is, there is mounting evidence to support the notion that specific food components exert effects that are likely to promote or delay the development of the most common and costly causes of vision loss: age-related cataract and macular degeneration and diabetic retinopathy. Research on nutrition's effects on the specific development and progression of the three conditions has taken place largely since the 1980s. Therefore, less evidence has accumulated for these than for other common chronic diseases. Nevertheless, these conditions each share common pathogenic mechanisms (oxidative stress, inflammation, hypertension, hyperglycemia, and angiogenesis) with other chronic diseases of aging that are known to be influenced by diet (hypertension, stroke, heart disease, diabetes, and cancer).

Evidence to support the idea that broadly healthy diet patterns lower risk for these common causes of vision loss is limited to a few studies. However, research has shown that dietary patterns such as those high in plant foods [351], low in refined carbohydrates, and low or moderate in fat (e.g., the DASH diet or the Mediterranean diet pattern), are related to reduced occurrence of many chronic diseases of aging [352–355]. Therefore, such nutrient-rich diet patterns are also likely to provide benefit in slowing the development of age-related cataract, AMD, and DR. Although research on diet in relation to other less common eye conditions, such as glaucoma, is minimal, it is likely that healthy diets lower risk for these understudied conditions, as well, because of the shared pathogenic mechanisms and evidence for the impact of food on them.

One pathogenic mechanism for degeneration of eye health that differs from most other chronic diseases (except those in skin) is the damage caused by overexposure to sunlight. In this respect, the need for the carotenoids lutein and zeaxanthin, which absorb light, may be uniquely important in maintaining eye health. These carotenoids may also be important in filtering light in ways that optimize the ability to see, particularly in certain circumstances. Research in this area is new and emerging.

We are only beginning to understand how food works jointly with other aspects of healthy lifestyles and genetics to modify risk for eye diseases. It is likely that food and nutrition, in conjunction with other aspects of healthy lifestyles such as physical activity and avoiding smoking, may have an even larger impact on limiting these causes of vision loss than results of human studies reflect. This is suggested by an observational study of AMD [148]. There is evidence that these healthy lifestyles minimize many processes that might otherwise promote oxidative stress, inflammation, hyperglycemia, and hypertension. Therefore, the effects of food may compound these benefits.

There is evidence that genetic variation can also influence propensity for these deleterious processes. Therefore, it is possible that healthy diets and lifestyles matter more (or less) in people genetically prone to these processes. Research on these possibilities is suggestive but limited.

Despite the evidence that food matters, evidence that dietary supplements of single or a combination of select nutrients slow age-related cataract, macular degeneration, or diabetic retinopathy is limited to slowing the development of late stages of AMD in people who already have this condition. In most cases, nutrient-dense foods provide a larger array of potentially protective substances than do supplements. Increasing evidence suggests a larger impact of foods than supplements in preventing age-related eye disease. One possible exception of vitamin D, which is sometimes difficult to obtain from natural food sources. This may be most important in extreme Northern and Southern Hemispheres, which provide inadequate ultraviolet light in winter to permit the synthesis of this vitamin in skin. The most sustainable way to ensure nutritional health of individuals that promotes eye health over the long term may be to foster the ability to grow nutritious food locally-and get physical activity and sun exposure in moderation.

References

[1] K.P. West Jr., D. McLaren, The epidemiology of vitamin A deficiency disorders (VADD), in: G.J. Johnson, D.C. Minassian, R.A. Weale, S.K. West (Eds), The Epidemiology of Eye Disease, second ed., Arnold, London, 2003, pp. 240–260.

[2] R. Semba, Handbook of Nutrition and Ophthalmology, Human Press, Totowa, NJ, 2007.

[3] D.T. Hartong, E.L. Berson, T.P. Dryja, Retinitis pigmentosa, Lancet 368 (9549) (2006) 1795–1809.

[4] E.L. Berson, B. Rosner, M.A. Sandberg, K.C. Hayes, B.W. Nicholson, C. Weigel-DiFranco, et al., A randomized trial of vitamin A and vitamin E supplementation for retinitis pigmentosa, Arch. Ophthalmol. 111 (6) (1993) 761–772.

[5] E.L. Berson, B. Rosner, M.A. Sandberg, C. Weigel-DiFranco, R.J. Brockhurst, K.C. Hayes, et al., Clinical trial of lutein in patients with retinitis pigmentosa receiving vitamin A, Arch. Ophthalmol. 128 (4) (2010) 403–411.

[6] W.G. Hodge, H.M. Schachter, D. Barnes, Y. Pan, E.C. Lowcock, L. Zhang, et al., Efficacy of [omega]-3 fatty acids in preventing age-related macular degeneration: a systematic review, Ophthalmology 113 (7) (2006) 1165–1173.

[7] R.W. Massof, G.A. Fishman, How strong is the evidence that nutritional supplements slow the progression of retinitis pigmentosa? Arch. Ophthalmol. 128 (4) (2010) 493–495.

[8] C. Williams, E.E. Birch, P.M. Emmett, K. Northstone, Stereoacuity at age 3.5 y in children born full-term is associated with prenatal and postnatal dietary factors: a report from a population-based cohort study, Am. J. Clin. Nutr. 73 (2) (2001) 316–322.

[9] A. Singhal, R. Morley, T.J. Cole, K. Kennedy, P. Sonksen, E. Isaacs, et al., Infant nutrition and stereoacuity at age 4–6 y, Am. J. Clin. Nutr. 85 (1) (2007) 152–159.

[10] M. Fleith, M.T. Clandinin, Dietary PUFA for preterm and term infants: review of clinical studies, Crit. Rev. Food Sci. Nutr. 45 (3) (2005) 205–229.

[11] A.R. Ness, M. Maynard, S. Frankel, G.D. Smith, C. Frobisher, S.D. Leary, et al., Diet in childhood and adult cardiovascular and all-cause mortality: The Boyd Orr cohort, Heart 91 (7) (2005) 894–898.

[12] P.S. Bernstein, F. Khachik, L.S. Carvalho, G.J. Muir, D.Y. Zhao, N.B. Katz, Identification and quantitation of carotenoids and their metabolites in the tissues of the human eye, Exp. Eye Res. 72 (3) (2001) 215–223.

[13] R.A. Bone, J.T. Landrum, L. Fernandez, S.L. Tarsis, Analysis of the macular pigment by HPLC: retinal distribution and age study, Invest. Ophthalmol. Vis. Sci. 29 (6) (1988) 843–849.

[14] B. Li, P. Vachali, J.M. Frederick, P.S. Bernstein, Identification of StARD3 as a lutein-binding protein in the macula of the primate retina, Biochemistry 50 (13) (2011) 2541–2549.

[15] K.J. Yeum, F.M. Shang, W.M. Schalch, R.M. Russell, A. Taylor, Fat-soluble nutrient concentrations in different layers of human cataractous lens, Curr. Eye Res. 19 (6) (1999) 502–505.

[16] R. van Leeuwen, S. Boekhoorn, J.R. Vingerling, J.C. Witteman, C.C. Klaver, A. Hofman, et al., Dietary intake of antioxidants and risk of age-related macular degeneration, JAMA 294 (24) (2005) 3101–3107.

[17] J.S.L. Tan, J.J. Wang, V. Flood, E. Rochtchina, W. Smith, P. Mitchell, Dietary antioxidants and the long-term incidence of age-related macular degeneration: The Blue Mountains Eye Study, Ophthalmology 115 (2) (2008) 334–341.

[18] F.J. Schweigert, K. Bathe, F. Chen, U. Buscher, J.W. Dudenhausen, Effect of the stage of lactation in humans on carotenoid levels in milk, blood plasma and plasma lipoprotein fractions, Eur. J. Nutr. 43 (1) (2004) 39–44.

[19] C. Macias, F.J. Schweigert, Changes in the concentration of carotenoids, vitamin A, alpha-tocopherol and total lipids in human milk throughout early lactation, Ann. Nutr. Metab. 45 (2) (2001) 82–85.

[20] G. Lietz, G. Mulokozi, J.C.K. Henry, A.M. Tomkins, Xanthophyll and hydrocarbon carotenoid patterns differ in plasma and breast milk of women supplemented with red palm oil during pregnancy and lactation, J. Nutr. 136 (7) (2006) 1821–1827.

[21] R. Semba, Fatty acids and visual development, Handbook of Nutrition and Ophthalmology, Human Press, Totawa, NJ, 2007.

[22] J.P. Zimmer, B.R. Hammond Jr., Possible influences of lutein and zeaxanthin on the developing retina, Clin. Ophthalmol. 1 (1) (2007) 25–35.

[23] B.R. Hammond Jr., Possible role for dietary lutein and zeaxanthin in visual development, Nutr. Rev. 66 (12) (2008) 695–702.

[24] G. Maraini, R.D. Sperduto, F. Ferris, T.E. Clemons, F. Rosmini, L. Ferrigno, A randomized, double-masked, placebo-controlled clinical trial of multivitamin supplementation for age-related lens opacities: Clinical Trial of Nutritional Supplements and Age-Related Cataract Report No. 3, Ophthalmology 115 (4) (2008) 599–607.

[25] L.P. Rubin, G.M. Chan, B.M. Barrett-Reis, A.B. Fulton, R.M. Hansen, T.L. Ashmeade, et al., Effect of carotenoid supplementation on plasma carotenoids, inflammation and visual development in preterm infants, J. Perinatol. (2011) [Epub ahead of print]

[26] J.M. Stringham, B.R. Hammond, Macular pigment and visual performance under glare conditions, Optom. Vis. Sci. 85 (2) (2008) 82–88.

[27] J. Kvansakul, M. Rodriguez-Carmona, D.F. Edgar, F.M. Barker, W. Kopcke, W. Schalch, et al., Supplementation with the carotenoids lutein or zeaxanthin improves human visual performance, Ophthalmic Physiol. Opt. 26 (4) (2006) 362–371.

[28] E.J. Johnson, J.E. Maras, H.M. Rasmussen, K.L. Tucker, Intake of lutein and zeaxanthin differ with age, sex, and ethnicity, J. Am. Diet. Assoc. 110 (9) (2010) 1357–1362.

[29] J.A. Mares-Perlman, A.I. Fisher, R. Klein, M. Palta, G. Block, A.E. Millen, et al., Lutein and zeaxanthin in the diet and serum and their relation to age-related maculopathy in the third National Health and Nutrition Examination Survey, Am. J. Epidemiol. 153 (5) (2001) 424–432.

[30] S.S. Casagrande, Y. Wang, C. Anderson, T.L. Gary, Have Americans increased their fruit and vegetable intake? The trends between 1988 and 2002, Am. J. Prev. Med. 32 (4) (2007) 257–263.

[31] J.A. Mares, T.L. LaRowe, D.M. Snodderly, S.M. Moeller, M.J. Gruber, M.L. Klein, et al., Predictors of optical density of lutein and zeaxanthin in retinas of older women in the Carotenoids in Age-Related Eye Disease Study, an ancillary study of the Women's Health Initiative, Am. J. Clin. Nutr. 84 (5) (2006) 1107–1122.

[32] S.M. Moeller, R. Voland, G.E. Sarto, V.L. Gobel, S.L. Streicher, J.A. Mares, Women's Health Initiative diet intervention did not increase macular pigment optical density in an ancillary study of a subsample of the Women's Health Initiative, J. Nutr. 139 (9) (2009) 1692–1699.

[33] S. Resnikoff, D. Pascolini, D. Etya'ale, I. Kocur, R. Pararajasegaram, G.P. Pokharel, et al., Global data on visual impairment in the year 2002, Bull. World Health Organization 82 (11) (2004) 844–851.

[34] N. Congdon, J.R. Vingerling, B.E. Klein, S. West, D.S. Friedman, J. Kempen, et al., Prevalence of cataract and pseudophakia/aphakia among adults in the United States, Arch. Ophthalmol. 122 (4) (2004) 487–494.

[35] E.P. Steinberg, J.C. Javitt, P.D. Sharkey, A. Zuckerman, M.W. Legro, G.F. Anderson, et al., The content and cost of cataract surgery, Arch. Ophthalmol. 111 (8) (1993) 1041–1049.

[36] L.B. Ellwein, C.J. Urato, Use of eye care and associated charges among the Medicare population: 1991–1998, Arch. Ophthalmol. 120 (6) (2002) 804–811.

[37] C. Kupfer, Bowman lecture. The conquest of cataract: a global challenge, Trans. Ophthalmol. Soc. UK 104 (Pt. 1) (1985) 1–10.

[38] B.E. Klein, R. Klein, K.L. Linton, Prevalence of age-related lens opacities in a population: The Beaver Dam Eye Study, Ophthalmology 99 (4) (1992) 546–552.

[39] B.E. Klein, R. Klein, K.E. Lee, Incidence of age-related cataract over a 10-year interval: The Beaver Dam Eye Study, Ophthalmology 109 (11) (2002) 2052–2057.

[40] S.K. West, B. Munoz, O.D. Schein, D.D. Duncan, G.S. Rubin, Racial differences in lens opacities: The Salisbury Eye Evaluation (SEE) project, Am. J. Epidemiol. 148 (11) (1998) 1033–1039.

[41] M.C. Leske, S.Y. Wu, A.M. Connell, L. Hyman, A.P. Schachat, Lens opacities, demographic factors and nutritional supplements in the Barbados Eye Study, Int. J. Epidemiol. 26 (6) (1997) 1314–1322.

[42] B.E. Klein, R. Klein, S.E. Moss, Incident cataract surgery: The Beaver Dam Eye Study, Ophthalmology 104 (4) (1997) 573–580.

[43] B.E. Klein, R. Klein, K.E. Lee, Cardiovascular disease, selected cardiovascular disease risk factors, and age-related cataracts: The Beaver Dam Eye Study, Am. J. Ophthalmol. 123 (3) (1997) 338–346.

[44] B.E. Klein, R. Klein, K.E. Lee, S.M. Meuer, Socioeconomic and lifestyle factors and the 10-year incidence of age-related cataracts, Am. J. Ophthalmol. 136 (3) (2003) 506–512.

[45] W.G. Christen, R.J. Glynn, J.E. Manson, U.A. Ajani, J.E. Buring, A prospective study of cigarette smoking and risk of age-related macular degeneration in men, JAMA 276 (14) (1996) 1147–1151.

[46] J.M. Weintraub, W.C. Willett, B. Rosner, G.A. Colditz, J.M. Seddon, S.E. Hankinson, Smoking cessation and risk of cataract extraction among U.S. women and men, Am. J. Epidemiol. 155 (1) (2002) 72–79.

[47] S. West, B. Munoz, O.D. Schein, S. Vitale, M. Maguire, H.R. Taylor, et al., Cigarette smoking and risk for progression of nuclear opacities, Arch. Ophthalmol. 113 (11) (1995) 1377–1380.

[48] Age-Related Eye Disease Study Research Group, Risk factors associated with age-related nuclear and cortical cataract: a case-control study in the Age-Related Eye Disease Study, AREDS Report No. 5, Ophthalmology 108 (8) (2001) 1400–1408.

[49] W. Smith, P. Mitchell, S.R. Leeder, Smoking and age-related maculopathy: The Blue Mountains Eye Study, Arch. Ophthalmol. 114 (12) (1996) 1518–1523.

[50] S.Y. Tsai, W.M. Hsu, C.Y. Cheng, J.H. Liu, P. Chou, Epidemiologic study of age-related cataracts among an elderly Chinese population in Shih-Pai, Taiwan, Ophthalmology 110 (6) (2003) 1089–1095.

[51] B.N. Mukesh, A. Le, P.N. Dimitrov, S. Ahmed, H.R. Taylor, C.A. McCarty, Development of cataract and associated risk factors: The Visual Impairment Project, Arch. Ophthalmol. 124 (1) (2006) 79–85.

[52] A.E. Fletcher, Free radicals, antioxidants and eye diseases: evidence from epidemiological studies on cataract and age-related macular degeneration, Ophthalmic Res. 44 (3) (2010) 191–198.

[53] S.K. West, D.D. Duncan, B. Munoz, G.S. Rubin, L.P. Fried, K. Bandeen-Roche, et al., Sunlight exposure and risk of lens opacities in a population-based study: The Salisbury Eye Evaluation Project, JAMA 280 (8) (1998) 714–718.

[54] H.R. Taylor, S.K. West, F.S. Rosenthal, B. Munoz, H.S. Newland, H. Abbey, et al., Effect of ultraviolet radiation on cataract formation, N. Engl. J. Med. 319 (22) (1988) 1429–1433.

[55] C.A. McCarty, H.R. Taylor, A review of the epidemiologic evidence linking ultraviolet radiation and cataracts, Dev. Ophthalmol. 35 (2002) 21–31.

[56] C.A. McCarty, Cataract in the 21st century: lessons from previous epidemiological research, Clin. Exp. Optom. 85 (2) (2002) 91–96.

[57] N.G. Rowe, P.G. Mitchell, R.G. Cumming, J.J. Wans, Diabetes, fasting blood glucose and age-related cataract: The Blue Mountains Eye Study, Ophthalmic Epidemiol. 7 (2) (2000) 103–114.

[58] M.C. Leske, S.Y. Wu, A. Hennis, A.M. Connell, L. Hyman, A. Schachat, Diabetes, hypertension, and central obesity as cataract risk factors in a black population: The Barbados Eye Study, Ophthalmology 106 (1) (1999) 35–41.

[59] C.A. McCarty, B.N. Mukesh, C.L. Fu, H.R. Taylor, The epidemiology of cataract in Australia, Am. J. Ophthalmol. 128 (4) (1999) 446–465.

[60] B.E. Klein, R. Klein, Q. Wang, S.E. Moss, Older-onset diabetes and lens opacities: The Beaver Dam Eye Study, Ophthalmic Epidemiol. 2 (1) (1995) 49–55.

[61] L.E. Caulfield, S.K. West, Y. Barron, J. Cid-Ruzafa, Anthropometric status and cataract: The Salisbury Eye Evaluation project, Am. J. Clin. Nutr. 69 (2) (1999) 237–242.

[62] R.J. Glynn, W.G. Christen, J.E. Manson, J. Bernheimer, C.H. Hennekens, Body mass index: an independent predictor of cataract, Arch. Ophthalmol. 113 (9) (1995) 1131–1137.

[63] R. Hiller, M.J. Podgor, R.D. Sperduto, L. Nowroozi, P.W. Wilson, R.B. D'Agostino, et al., A longitudinal study of body mass index and lens opacities: The Framingham Studies, Ophthalmology 105 (7) (1998) 1244–1250.

[64] M.S. Morris, P.F. Jacques, S.E. Hankinson, L.T. Chylack Jr., W.C. Willett, A. Taylor, Moderate alcoholic beverage intake and early nuclear and cortical lens opacities, Ophthalmic Epidemiol. 11 (1) (2004) 53–65.

[65] B.E. Klein, R.E. Klein, K.E. Lee, Incident cataract after a five-year interval and lifestyle factors: The Beaver Dam Eye Study, Ophthalmic Epidemiol. 6 (4) (1999) 247–255.

[66] R.G. Cumming, P. Mitchell, Alcohol, smoking, and cataracts: The Blue Mountains Eye Study, Arch. Ophthalmol. 115 (10) (1997) 1296–1303.

[67] B.E. Klein, R. Klein, K.E. Lee, M.D. Knudtson, M.Y. Tsai, Markers of inflammation, vascular endothelial dysfunction, and age-related cataract, Am. J. Ophthalmol. 141 (1) (2006) 116–122.

[68] B.E. Klein, R. Klein, K.E. Lee, L.M. Grady, Statin use and incident nuclear cataract, JAMA 295 (23) (2006) 2752–2758.

[69] G.E. Bunce, J. Kinoshita, J. Horwitz, Nutritional factors in cataract, Annu. Rev. Nutr. 10 (1990) 233–254.

[70] G.E. Bunce, Animal studies on cataract, in: A. Taylor (Ed.), Nutritional and Environmental Influences on the Eye, CRC Press, Boca Raton, FL, 1999, pp. 105–115.

[71] A. Chatterjee, R.C. Milton, S. Thyle, Prevalence and aetiology of cataract in Punjab, Br. J. Ophthalmol. 66 (1) (1982) 35–42.

[72] E.O. Ojofeitimi, D.A. Adelekan, A. Adeoye, T.G. Ogungbe, A.O. Imoru, E.C. Oduah, Dietary and lifestyle patterns in the aetiology of cataracts in Nigerian patients, Nutr. Health 13 (2) (1999) 61–68.

[73] M. Mohan, R.D. Sperduto, S.K. Angra, R.C. Milton, R.L. Mathur, B.A. Underwood, et al., India–U.S. case–control study of age-related cataracts: India–U.S. Case–Control Study Group, Arch. Ophthalmol. 107 (5) (1989) 670–676.

[74] L. Fontana, S. Klein, Aging, adiposity, and calorie restriction, JAMA 297 (9) (2007) 986–994.

[75] A. Taylor, R.D. Lipman, J. Jahngen-Hodge, V. Palmer, D. Smith, N. Padhye, et al., Dietary calorie restriction in the Emory mouse: effects on lifespan, eye lens cataract prevalence and progression, levels of ascorbate, glutathione, glucose, and glycohemoglobin, tail collagen breaktime, DNA and RNA oxidation, skin integrity, fecundity, and cancer, Mech. Aging Dev. 79 (1) (1995) 33–57.

[76] S.M. Moeller, A. Taylor, K.L. Tucker, M.L. McCullough, L.T. Chylack Jr., S.E. Hankinson, et al., Overall adherence to the dietary guidelines for Americans is associated with reduced prevalence of early age-related nuclear lens opacities in women, J. Nutr. 134 (7) (2004) 1812–1819.

[77] J.A. Mares, R. Voland, R. Adler, L. Tinker, A.E. Millen, S.M. Moeller, et al., Healthy diets and the subsequent prevalence of nuclear cataract in women, Arch. Ophthalmol. 128 (6) (2010) 738–749.

[78] P.N. Appleby, N.E. Allen, T.J. Key, Diet, vegetarianism, and cataract risk, Am. J. Clin. Nutr. 93 (5) (2011) 1128–1135.

[79] A.M. Bosch, Classical galactosaemia revisited, J. Inherit. Metab. Dis. 29 (4) (2006) 516–525.

[80] S.E. Waisbren, N.L. Potter, C.M. Gordon, R.C. Green, P. Greenstein, C.S. Gubbels, et al., The adult galactosemic phenotype, J. Inherit. Metab. Dis. 35 (2012) 279–286.

[81] S. Illsinger, N. Janzen, U. Meyer, Y.S. Shin, J. Sander, T. Lucke, et al., Early cataract formation due to galactokinase deficiency: impact of newborn screening, Arch. Med. Res. 42 (2011) 608–612.

[82] M.A. van Boekel, H.J. Hoenders, Glycation of crystallins in lenses from aging and diabetic individuals, FEBS Lett. 314 (1) (1992) 1–4.

[83] S. Swamy-Mruthinti, S.M. Shaw, H.R. Zhao, K. Green, E.C. Abraham, Evidence of a glycemic threshold for the development of cataracts in diabetic rats, Curr. Eye Res. 18 (6) (1999) 423–429.

[84] A. Di Benedetto, P. Aragona, G. Romano, G. Romeo, E. Di Cesare, R. Spinella, et al., Age and metabolic control influence lens opacity in type I, insulin-dependent diabetic patients, J. Diabetes Complications 13 (3) (1999) 159–162.

[85] C. Costagliola, R. Dell'Omo, F. Prisco, D. Iafusco, F. Landolfo, F. Parmeggiani, Bilateral isolated acute cataracts in three newly diagnosed insulin dependent diabetes mellitus young patients, Diab. Res. Clin. Pract. 76 (2) (2007) 313–315.

[86] R.N. Gacche, N.A. Dhole, Aldose reductase inhibitory, anticataract and antioxidant potential of selected medicinal plants from the Marathwada region, India, Nat. Prod. Res. 25 (7) (2011) 760–763.

[87] P. Jacques, Nutritional antioxidants and prevention of age-related eye disease, in: H. Garewal (Ed.), Antioxidants and Disease Prevention, CRC Press, Boca Raton, FL, 1997, pp. 149–177.

[88] M.P. Lu, R. Wang, X. Song, R. Chibbar, X. Wang, L. Wu, et al., Dietary soy isoflavones increase insulin secretion and prevent the development of diabetic cataracts in streptozotocin-induced diabetic rats, Nutr. Res. 28 (7) (2008) 464–471.

[89] S.D. Varma, S. Kovtun, K. Hegde, Effectiveness of topical caffeine in cataract prevention: studies with galactose cataract, Mol. Vis. 16 (2010) 2626–2633.

[90] K.J. Pearson, J.A. Baur, K.N. Lewis, L. Peshkin, N.L. Price, N. Labinskyy, et al., Resveratrol delays age-related deterioration and mimics transcriptional aspects of dietary restriction without extending life span, Cell Metab. 8 (2) (2008) 157–168.

[91] P.A. Kumar, P.Y. Reddy, P.N. Srinivas, G.B. Reddy, Delay of diabetic cataract in rats by the antiglycating potential of cumin through modulation of alpha-crystallin chaperone activity, J. Nutr. Biochem. 20 (7) (2009) 553–562.

[92] R. Manikandan, R. Thiagarajan, S. Beulaja, G. Sudhandiran, M. Arumugam, Effect of curcumin on selenite-induced cataractogenesis in Wistar rat pups, Curr. Eye Res. 35 (2) (2010) 122–129.

[93] C.J. Chiu, L. Robman, C.A. McCarty, B.N. Mukesh, A. Hodge, H.R. Taylor, et al., Dietary carbohydrate in relation to cortical and nuclear lens opacities in the Melbourne Visual Impairment project, Invest. Ophthalmol. Vis. Sci. 51 (6) (2010) 2897–2905.

[94] C. Costagliola, L. Lobefalo, P.E. Gallenga, Role of higher dietary carbohydrate intake in cataract development, Invest. Ophthalmol. Vis. Sci. 52 (6) (2011) 3593.

[95] W.G. Christen, Antioxidant vitamins and age-related eye disease, Proc. Assoc. Am. Phys. 111 (1) (1999) 16–21.

[96] C.J. Chiu, A. Taylor, Nutritional antioxidants and age-related cataract and maculopathy, Exp. Eye Res. 84 (2) (2007) 229–245.

[97] A. Taylor, P.F. Jacques, T. Nowell, G. Perrone, J. Blumberg, G. Handelman, et al., Vitamin C in human and guinea pig aqueous, lens and plasma in relation to intake, Curr. Eye Res. 16 (9) (1997) 857–864.

[98] C. Chitchumroonchokchai, J.A. Bomser, J.E. Glamm, M.L. Failla, Xanthophylls and alpha-tocopherol decrease UVB-induced lipid peroxidation and stress signaling in human lens epithelial cells, J. Nutr. 134 (12) (2004) 3225–3232.

[99] J.A. Mares-Perlman, W.E. Brady, B.E. Klein, R. Klein, G.J. Haus, M. Palta, et al., Diet and nuclear lens opacities, Am. J. Epidemiol. 141 (4) (1995) 322–334.

[100] B.J. Lyle, J.A. Mares-Perlman, B.E. Klein, R. Klein, J.L. Greger, Antioxidant intake and risk of incident age-related nuclear cataracts in the Beaver Dam Eye Study, Am. J. Epidemiol. 149 (9) (1999) 801–809.

[101] L. Chasan-Taber, W.C. Willett, J.M. Seddon, M.J. Stampfer, B. Rosner, G.A. Colditz, et al., A prospective study of carotenoid and vitamin A intakes and risk of cataract extraction in U.S. women, Am. J. Clin. Nutr. 70 (4) (1999) 509–516.

[102] L. Brown, E.B. Rimm, J.M. Seddon, E.L. Giovannucci, L. Chasan-Taber, D. Spiegelman, et al., A prospective study of carotenoid intake and risk of cataract extraction in U.S. men [see Comment], Am. J. Clin. Nutr. 70 (4) (1999) 517–524.

[103] P.F. Jacques, L.T. Chylack Jr., S.E. Hankinson, P.M. Khu, G. Rogers, J. Friend, et al., Long-term nutrient intake and early age-related nuclear lens opacities, Arch. Ophthalmol. 119 (7) (2001) 1009–1019.

[104] H.T.V. Vu, L. Robman, A. Hodge, C.A. McCarty, H.R. Taylor, Lutein and zeaxanthin and the risk of cataract: The Melbourne Visual Impairment Project, Invest. Ophthalmol. Vis. Sci. 47 (9) (2006) 3783–3786.

[105] L. Ferrigno, R. Aldigeri, F. Rosmini, R.D. Sperduto, G. Maraini, Associations between plasma levels of vitamins and cataract in the Italian–American Clinical Trial of Nutritional Supplements and Age-Related Cataract (CTNS): CTNS Report 2, Ophthalmic Epidemiol. 12 (2) (2005) 71–80.

[106] P.F. Jacques, L.T. Chylack Jr., R.B. McGandy, S.C. Hartz, Antioxidant status in persons with and without senile cataract, Arch. Ophthalmol. 106 (3) (1988) 337–340.

[107] M. Dherani, G.V. Murthy, S.K. Gupta, I.S. Young, G. Maraini, M. Camparini, et al., Blood levels of vitamin C, carotenoids and retinol are inversely associated with cataract in a North Indian population, Invest. Ophthalmol. Vis. Sci. 49 (8) (2008) 3328–3335.

[108] M. Yoshida, Y. Takashima, M. Inoue, M. Iwasaki, T. Otani, S. Sasaki, et al., Prospective study showing that dietary vitamin C reduced the risk of age-related cataracts in a middle-aged Japanese population, Eur. J. Nutr. 46 (2) (2007) 118–124.

[109] R.D. Ravindran, P. Vashist, S.K. Gupta, I.S. Young, G. Maraini, M. Camparini, et al., Inverse association of vitamin C with cataract in older people in India, Ophthalmology 118 (10) (2011) 1958–1965.

[110] J.A. Mares-Perlman, W.E. Brady, B.E. Klein, R. Klein, M. Palta, P. Bowen, et al., Serum carotenoids and tocopherols and

severity of nuclear and cortical opacities, Invest. Ophthalmol. Vis. Sci. 36 (2) (1995) 276−288.

[111] S. Rautiainen, B.E. Lindblad, R. Morgenstern, A. Wolk, Vitamin C supplements and the risk of age-related cataract: a population-based prospective cohort study in women, Am. J. Clin. Nutr. 91 (2) (2010) 487−493.

[112] M. Linetsky, H.L. James, B.J. Ortwerth, Spontaneous generation of superoxide anion by human lens proteins and by calf lens proteins ascorbylated *in vitro*, Exp. Eye Res. 69 (2) (1999) 239−248.

[113] M. Linetsky, E. Shipova, R. Cheng, B.J. Ortwerth, Glycation by ascorbic acid oxidation products leads to the aggregation of lens proteins, Biochim. Biophys. Acta 1782 (1) (2008) 22−34.

[114] X. Fan, L.W. Reneker, M.E. Obrenovich, C. Strauch, R. Cheng, S.M. Jarvis, et al., Vitamin C mediates chemical aging of lens crystallins by the Maillard reaction in a humanized mouse model, Proc. Natl. Acad. Sci. USA 103 (45) (2006) 16912−16917.

[115] F. Avila, B. Friguet, E. Silva, Simultaneous chemical and photochemical protein crosslinking induced by irradiation of eye lens proteins in the presence of ascorbate: the photosensitizing role of an UVA-visible-absorbing decomposition product of vitamin C, Photochem. Photobiol. Sci. 9 (10) (2010) 1351−1358.

[116] M.C. Mathew, A.M. Ervin, J. Tao, R.M. Davis, Antioxidant vitamin supplementation for preventing and slowing the progress of age-related cataract, Cochrane Database Syst. Rev. 6 (CD004567) (2012).

[117] W.G. Christen, J.E. Manson, R.J. Glynn, J.M. Gaziano, R.D. Sperduto, J.E. Buring, et al., A randomized trial of beta carotene and age-related cataract in U.S. physicians, Arch. Ophthalmol. 121 (3) (2003) 372−378.

[118] J.J. McNeil, L. Robman, G. Tikellis, M.I. Sinclair, C.A. McCarty, H.R. Taylor, Vitamin E supplementation and cataract: randomized controlled trial, Ophthalmology 111 (1) (2004) 75−84.

[119] W. Christen, R. Glynn, R. Sperduto, E. Chew, J. Buring, Age-related cataract in a randomized trial of beta-carotene in women, Ophthalmic Epidemiol. 11 (5) (2004) 401−412.

[120] D.C. Gritz, M. Srinivasan, S.D. Smith, U. Kim, T.M. Lietman, J.H. Wilkins, et al., The antioxidants in prevention of cataracts study: effects of antioxidant supplements on cataract progression in South India, Br. J. Ophthalmol. 90 (7) (2006) 847−851.

[121] E. Arnal, M. Miranda, I. Almansa, M. Muriach, J.M. Barcia, F.J. Romero, et al., Lutein prevents cataract development and progression in diabetic rats, Graefes Arch. Clin. Exp. Ophthalmol. 247 (1) (2009) 115−120.

[122] N.M. Kalariya, B. Nair, D.K. Kalariya, N.K. Wills, F.J. van Kuijk, Cadmium-induced induction of cell death in human lens epithelial cells: implications to smoking associated cataractogenesis, Toxicol. Lett. 198 (1) (2010) 56−62.

[123] M. Lemire, M. Fillion, B. Frenette, A. Mayer, A. Philibert, C.J. Passos, et al., Selenium and mercury in the Brazilian Amazon: opposing influences on age-related cataracts, Environ. Health Perspect. 118 (11) (2010) 1584−1589.

[124] M. Valko, H. Morris, M.T. Cronin, Metals, toxicity and oxidative stress, Curr. Med. Chem. 12 (10) (2005) 1161−1208.

[125] J.M. Seddon, Multivitamin−multimineral supplements and eye disease: age-related macular degeneration and cataract, Am. J. Clin. Nutr. 85 (1) (2007) 304S−307S.

[126] J.A. Mares, High-dose antioxidant supplementation and cataract risk, Nutr. Rev. 62 (1) (2004) 28−32.

[127] J.A. Mares, T.L. La Rowe, B.A. Blodi, Doctor, what vitamins should I take for my eyes? Arch. Ophthalmol. 122 (4) (2004) 628−635.

[128] F.M. Barker II, D.M. Snodderly, E.J. Johnson, W. Schalch, W. Koepcke, J. Gerss, et al., Nutritional manipulation of

primate retinas, V: effects of lutein, zeaxanthin, and n-3 fatty acids on retinal sensitivity to blue-light-induced damage, Invest. Ophthalmol. Vis. Sci. 52 (7) (2011) 3934−3942.

[129] R.C. Milton, R.D. Sperduto, T.E. Clemons, F.L. Ferris III, Centrum use and progression of age-related cataract in the Age-Related Eye Disease Study: a propensity score approach, AREDS Report No. 21, Ophthalmology 113 (8) (2006) 1264−1270.

[130] R.D. Sperduto, T.S. Hu, R.C. Milton, J.L. Zhao, D.F. Everett, Q.F. Cheng, et al., The Linxian cataract studies: Two nutrition intervention trials, Arch. Ophthalmol. 111 (9) (1993) 1246−1253.

[131] D.S. Friedman, B.J. O'Colmain, B. Munoz, S.C. Tomany, C. McCarty, P.T. de Jong, et al., Prevalence of age-related macular degeneration in the United States, Arch. Ophthalmol. 122 (4) (2004) 564−572.

[132] S. Beatty, H. Koh, M. Phil, D. Henson, M. Boulton, The role of oxidative stress in the pathogenesis of age-related macular degeneration, Surv. Ophthalmol. 45 (2) (2000) 115−134.

[133] D.H. Anderson, R.F. Mullins, G.S. Hageman, L.V. Johnson, A role for local inflammation in the formation of drusen in the aging eye, Am. J. Ophthalmol. 134 (3) (2002) 411−431.

[134] G. Hagemen, P. Luthert, N. Victor-Chong, L. Johnson, D. Anderson, R. Mullins, An integrated hypothesis that considers drusen as biomarkers of immune-medicated processes at the RPE−Brunch's membrane interface in aging and age-related macular degeneration, Prog. Retin. Eye Res. 20 (2001) 705−732.

[135] G.S. Hageman, D.H. Anderson, L.V. Johnson, L.S. Hancox, A.J. Taiber, L.I. Hardisty, et al., A common haplotype in the complement regulatory gene factor H (HF1/CFH) predisposes individuals to age-related macular degeneration, Proc. Natl. Acad. Sci. USA 102 (20) (2005) 7227−7232.

[136] H. Shaban, C. Richter, A2E and blue light in the retina: the paradigm of age-related macular degeneration, Biol. Chem 383 (3−4) (2002) 537−545.

[137] R. Klein, B.E.K. Klein, Smoke gets in your eyes too, JAMA 276 (14) (1996) 1179−1180.

[138] R. van Leeuwen, M.K. Ikram, J.R. Vingerling, J.C. Witteman, A. Hofman, P.T. de Jong, Blood pressure, atherosclerosis, and the incidence of age-related maculopathy: The Rotterdam Study, Invest. Ophthalmol. Vis. Sci. 44 (9) (2003) 3771−3777.

[139] J.R. Vingerling, I. Dielemans, A. Hofman, M. Bots, Age-related macular degeneration is associated with atherosclerosis, Am. J. Epidemiol. 142 (4) (1995) 404−409.

[140] K.K. Snow, J.M. Seddon, Do age-related macular degeneration and cardiovascular disease share common antecedents? Ophthalmic Epidemiol. 6 (2) (1999) 125−143.

[141] U. Chakravarthy, T.Y. Wong, A. Fletcher, E. Piault, C. Evans, G. Zlateva, et al., Clinical risk factors for age-related macular degeneration: a systematic review and meta-analysis, BMC Ophthalmol. 10 (2010) 31.

[142] A. Thakkinstian, P. Han, M. McEvoy, W. Smith, J. Hoh, K. Magnusson, et al., Systematic review and meta-analysis of the association between complement factor H Y402H polymorphisms and age-related macular degeneration, Hum. Mol. Genet. 15 (18) (2006) 2784−2790.

[143] Y. Tong, J. Liao, Y. Zhang, J. Zhou, H. Zhang, M. Mao, LOC387715/HTRA1 gene polymorphisms and susceptibility to age-related macular degeneration: a HuGE review and meta-analysis, Mol. Vis. 16 (2010) 1958−1981.

[144] J.M. Seddon, G. Gensler, R.C. Milton, M.L. Klein, N. Rifai, Association between C-reactive protein and age-related macular degeneration.[see Comments], JAMA 291 (6) (2004) 704−710.

[145] J.M. Seddon, S. George, B. Rosner, N. Rifai, Progression of age-related macular degeneration: prospective assessment of C-reactive protein, interleukin 6, and other cardiovascular biomarkers, Arch. Ophthalmol. 123 (6) (2005) 774–782.

[146] R. Klein, B.E. Klein, S.C. Tomany, K.J. Cruickshanks, Association of emphysema, gout, and inflammatory markers with long-term incidence of age-related maculopathy, Arch. Ophthalmol. 121 (5) (2003) 674–678.

[147] T.E. Clemons, R.C. Milton, R. Klein, J.M. Seddon, F.L. Ferris III, Risk factors for the incidence of advanced age-related macular degeneration in the Age-Related Eye Disease Study (AREDS), AREDS Report No. 19, Ophthalmology 112 (4) (2005) 533–539.

[148] J.A. Mares, R.P. Voland, S.A. Sondel, A.E. Millen, T. Larowe, S.M. Moeller, et al., Healthy lifestyles related to subsequent prevalence of age-related macular degeneration, Arch. Ophthalmol. 129 (4) (2011) 470–480.

[149] C.J. Chiu, R.C. Milton, R. Klein, G. Gensler, A. Taylor, Dietary compound score and risk of age-related macular degeneration in the Age-Related Eye Disease Study, Ophthalmology 116 (5) (2009) 939–946.

[150] M.P. Montgomery, F. Kamel, M.A. Pericak-Vance, J.L. Haines, E.A. Postel, A. Agarwal, et al., Overall diet quality and age-related macular degeneration, Ophthalmic Epidemiol. 17 (1) (2010) 58–65.

[151] C.J. Chiu, R. Klein, R.C. Milton, G. Gensler, A. Taylor, Does eating particular diets alter the risk of age-related macular degeneration in users of the Age-Related Eye Disease Study supplements? Br. J. Ophthalmol. 93 (9) (2009) 1241–1246.

[152] L. Ho, R. van Leeuwen, J.C. Witteman, C.M. van Duijn, A.G. Uitterlinden, A. Hofman, et al., Reducing the genetic risk of age-related macular degeneration with dietary antioxidants, zinc, and omega-3 fatty acids: The Rotterdam study, Arch. Ophthalmol. 129 (6) (2011) 758–766.

[153] D.A. Schaumberg, S.E. Hankinson, Q. Guo, E. Rimm, D.J. Hunter, A prospective study of 2 major age-related macular degeneration susceptibility alleles and interactions with modifiable risk factors, Arch. Ophthalmol. 125 (1) (2007) 55–62.

[154] J.M. Seddon, P.J. Francis, S. George, D.W. Schultz, B. Rosner, M.L. Klein, Association of CFH Y402H and LOC387715 A69S with progression of age-related macular degeneration, JAMA 297 (16) (2007) 1793–1800.

[155] J.C. Nielsen, M.I. Naash, R.E. Anderson, The regional distribution of vitamins E and C in mature and premature human retinas, Invest. Ophthalmol. Vis. Sci. 29 (1) (1988) 22–26.

[156] Z.A. Karcioglu, Zinc in the eye, Surv. Ophthalmol. 27 (2) (1982) 114–122.

[157] J. Mares, R. Klein, Diet and age-related macular degeneration, in: A. Taylor (Ed.), Nutritional and Environmental Influences on the Eye, CRC Press, Boca Raton, FL, 1999, pp. 181–214.

[158] G.J. Handelman, E.A. Dratz, The role of antioxidants in the retina and retinal pigment epithelium and the nature of prooxidant damage, Adv. Free Radic. Biol. Med. 2 (1986) 1–89.

[159] M.R. Malinow, L. Feeney-Burns, L.H. Peterson, M.L. Klein, M. Neuringer, Diet-related macular anomalies in monkeys, Invest. Ophthalmol. Vis. Sci. 19 (8) (1980) 857–863.

[160] J.M. Teikari, L. Laatikainen, J. Virtamo, J. Haukka, M. Rautalahti, K. Liesto, et al., Six-year supplementation with alpha-tocopherol and beta-carotene and age-related maculopathy, Acta Ophthalmol. Scand. 76 (2) (1998) 224–229.

[161] H.R. Taylor, G. Tikellis, L.D. Robman, C.A. McCarty, J.J. McNeil, Vitamin E supplementation and macular degeneration: randomised controlled trial, BMJ 325 (7354) (2002) 11.

[162] W. Stahl, A. Junghans, B. de Boer, E.S. Driomina, K. Briviba, H. Sies, Carotenoid mixtures protect multilamellar liposomes against oxidative damage: synergistic effects of lycopene and lutein, FEBS Lett. 427 (2) (1998) 305–308.

[163] M. Wrona, W. Korytowski, M. Rozanowska, T. Sarna, T.G. Truscott, Cooperation of antioxidants in protection against photosensitized oxidation, Free Radic. Biol. Med. 35 (10) (2003) 1319–1329.

[164] M. Wrona, M. Rozanowska, T. Sarna, Zeaxanthin in combination with ascorbic acid or alpha-tocopherol protects ARPE-19 cells against photosensitized peroxidation of lipids, Free Radic. Biol. Med. 36 (9) (2004) 1094–1101.

[165] Age-Related Eye Disease Study Research Group, A randomized, placebo-controlled, clinical trial of high-dose supplementation with vitamins C and E and beta carotene for age-related cataract and vision loss: AREDS Report No. 9, Arch. Ophthalmol. 119 (10) (2001) 1439–1452.

[166] S.E. Moriarty-Craige, J. Adkison, M. Lynn, G. Gensler, S. Bressler, D.P. Jones, et al., Antioxidant supplements prevent oxidation of cysteine/cystine redox in patients with age-related macular degeneration, Am. J. Ophthalmol. 140 (6) (2005) 1020–1026.

[167] S. Richer, W. Stiles, L. Statkute, J. Pulido, J. Frankowski, D. Rudy, et al., Double-masked, placebo-controlled, randomized trial of lutein and antioxidant supplementation in the intervention of atrophic age-related macular degeneration: The Veterans LAST study (Lutein Antioxidant Supplementation Trial), Optometry 75 (4) (2004) 216–230.

[168] G. Bjelakovic, D. Nikolova, L.L. Gluud, R.G. Simonetti, C. Gluud, Antioxidant supplements for prevention of mortality in healthy participants and patients with various diseases, Cochrane Database Syst. Rev. (2012) 3 (CD007176).

[169] S. West, S. Vitale, J. Hallfrisch, B. Munoz, D. Muller, S. Bressler, et al., Are antioxidants or supplements protective for age-related macular degeneration? Arch. Ophthalmol. 112 (2) (1994) 222–227.

[170] G.M. VandenLangenberg, J.A. Mares-Perlman, R. Klein, B.E. Klein, W.E. Brady, M. Palta, Associations between antioxidant and zinc intake and the 5-year incidence of early age-related maculopathy in the Beaver Dam Eye Study, Am. J. Epidemiol. 148 (2) (1998) 204–214.

[171] J. Mares, Carotenoids and eye disease: epidemiologic evidence, in: N.I. Krinsky, S. Mayne (Eds), Carotenoids in Health and Disease, Dekker, New York, 2003.

[172] C. Delcourt, I. Carriere, M. Delage, P. Barberger-Gateau, W. Schalch, the POLA Study Group, Plasma lutein and zeaxanthin and other carotenoids as modifiable risk factors for age-related maculopathy and cataract: The POLA study, Invest. Ophthalmol. Vis. Sci. 47 (6) (2006) 2329–2335.

[173] N. Cardinault, J.-H. Abalain, B. Sairafi, C. Coudray, P. Grolier, M. Rambeau, et al., Lycopene but not lutein nor zeaxanthin decreases in serum and lipoproteins in age-related macular degeneration patients, Clin. Chim. Acta 357 (1) (2005) 34–42.

[174] C.R. Gale, N.F. Hall, D.I. Phillips, C.N. Martyn, Lutein and zeaxanthin status and risk of age-related macular degeneration, Invest. Ophthalmol. Vis. Sci. 44 (6) (2003) 2461–2465.

[175] S.M. Moeller, N. Parekh, L. Tinker, C. Ritenbaugh, B. Blodi, R.B. Wallace, et al., Associations between intermediate age-related macular degeneration and lutein and zeaxanthin in the Carotenoids in Age-Related Eye Disease Study (CAREDS): ancillary study of the Women's Health Initiative, Arch. Ophthalmol. 124 (8) (2006) 1151–1162.

[176] J.A. Mares-Perlman, R. Klein, B.E. Klein, J.L. Greger, W.E. Brady, M. Palta, et al., Association of zinc and antioxidant nutrients with age-related maculopathy, Arch. Ophthalmol. 114 (8) (1996) 991–997.

[177] J.H. Fowke, J.D. Morrow, S. Motley, R.M. Bostick, R.M. Ness, Brassica vegetable consumption reduces urinary F2-isoprostane

levels independent of micronutrient intake, Carcinogenesis 27 (2006) 2096–2102.

[178] S. Majumdar, R. Srirangam, Potential of the bioflavonoids in the prevention/treatment of ocular disorders, J. Pharm. Pharmacol. 62 (8) (2010) 951–965.

[179] S.J. Sheu, N.C. Liu, J.L. Chen, Resveratrol protects human retinal pigment epithelial cells from acrolein-induced damage, J. Ocul. Pharmacol. Ther. 26 (3) (2010) 231–236.

[180] J.A. Mares, Potential value of antioxidant-rich foods in slowing age-related macular degeneration, Arch. Ophthalmol. 124 (9) (2006) 1339–1340.

[181] J.E. Kim, J.O. Leite, R. DeOgburn, J.A. Smyth, R.M. Clark, M.L. Fernandez, A lutein-enriched diet prevents cholesterol accumulation and decreases oxidized LDL and inflammatory cytokines in the aorta of guinea pigs, J. Nutr. 141 (8) (2011) 1458–1463.

[182] D.M. Snodderly, P.K. Brown, F.C. Delori, J.D. Auran, The macular pigment: I. Absorbance spectra, localization, and discrimination from other yellow pigments in primate retinas, Invest. Ophthalmol. Vis. Sci. 25 (6) (1984) 660–673.

[183] A. Junghans, H. Sies, W. Stahl, Macular pigments lutein and zeaxanthin as blue light filters studied in liposomes, Arch. Biochem. Biophys. 391 (2) (2001) 160–164.

[184] W.K. Subczynski, A. Wisniewska, J. Widomska, Location of macular xanthophylls in the most vulnerable regions of photoreceptor outer-segment membranes, Arch. Biochem. Biophys. 504 (1) (2010) 61–66.

[185] R.A. Bone, J.T. Landrum, S.T. Mayne, C.M. Gomez, S.E. Tibor, E.E. Twaroska, Macular pigment in donor eyes with and without AMD: a case–control study, Invest. Ophthalmol. Vis. Sci. 42 (1) (2001) 235–240.

[186] J.R. Sparrow, K. Nakanishi, C.A. Parish, The lipofuscin fluorophore A2E mediates blue light-induced damage to retinal pigmented epithelial cells, Invest. Ophthalmol. Vis. Sci. 41 (7) (2000) 1981–1989.

[187] J.R. Sparrow, H.R. Vollmer-Snarr, J. Zhou, Y.P. Jang, S. Jockusch, Y. Itagaki, et al., A2E-epoxides damage DNA in retinal pigment epithelial cells: Vitamin E and other antioxidants inhibit A2E-epoxide formation, J. Biol. Chem. 278 (20) (2003) 18207–18213.

[188] I.Y. Leung, M.M. Sandstrom, C.L. Zucker, M. Neuringer, D.M. Snodderly, Nutritional manipulation of primate retinas: II. Effects of age, n-3 fatty acids, lutein, and zeaxanthin on retinal pigment epithelium, Invest. Ophthalmol. Vis. Sci. 45 (2004) 3244–3256.

[189] L. Feeney-Burns, M. Neuringer, C.L. Gao, Macular pathology in monkeys fed semipurified diets, Prog. Clin. Biol. Res. 314 (1989) 601–622.

[190] L.R. Thomson, Y. Toyoda, A. Langner, et al., Elevated retinal zeaxanthin and prevention of light-induced photoreceptor cell death in quail, Investigative Ophthalmology & Visual Science 43 (11) (2002) 3538–3549.

[191] K. Izumi-Nagai, N. Nagai, K. Ohgami, S. Satofuka, Y. Ozawa, K. Tsubota, et al., Macular pigment lutein is antiinflammatory in preventing choroidal neovascularization, Arterioscler. Thromb. Vasc. Biol. 27 (12) (2007) 2555–2562.

[192] E. Cho, S.E. Hankinson, B. Rosner, W.C. Willett, G.A. Colditz, Prospective study of lutein/zeaxanthin intake and risk of age-related macular degeneration, Am. J. Clin. Nutr. 87 (6) (2008) 1837–1843.

[193] J. Seddon, et al., Dietary carotenoids, vitamins A, C, and E, and advanced age related macular degeneration, JAMA 272 (1994) 1413–1420.

[194] J.P. SanGiovanni, E.Y. Chew, T.E. Clemons, F.L. Ferris III, G. Gensler, A.S. Lindblad, et al., The relationship of dietary carotenoid and vitamin A, E, and C intake with age-related macular degeneration in a case–control study: AREDS Report No. 22, Arch. Ophthalmol. 125 (9) (2007) 1225–1232.

[195] S.M. Moeller, N.R. Mehta, L.F. Tinker, C. Ritenbaugh, B.A. Blodi, R.B. Wallace, et al., Associations between intermediate age-related macular degeneration and lutein and zeaxanthin in the Carotenoids in Age-Related Eye Disease Study (CAREDS), an ancillary study of the Women's Health Initiative, Arch. Ophthalmol. 124 (2006) 1–24.

[196] B.R. Hammond Jr., E.J. Johnson, R.M. Russell, N.I. Krinsky, K.J. Yeum, R.B. Edwards, et al., Dietary modification of human macular pigment density, Invest. Ophthalmol. Vis. Sci. 38 (9) (1997) 1795–1801.

[197] R.A. Bone, J.T. Landrum, L.H. Guerra, C.A. Ruiz, Lutein and zeaxanthin dietary supplements raise macular pigment density and serum concentrations of these carotenoids in humans, J. Nutr. 133 (4) (2003) 992–998.

[198] T.S. Aleman, J.L. Duncan, M.L. Bieber, E. de Castro, D.A. Marks, L.M. Gardner, et al., Macular pigment and lutein supplementation in retinitis pigmentosa and Usher syndrome, Invest. Ophthalmol. Vis. Sci. 42 (8) (2001) 1873–1881.

[199] P.E. Bowen, V. Garg, M. Stacewicz-Sapuntzakis, L. Yelton, R.S. Schreiner, Variability of serum carotenoids in response to controlled diets containing six servings of fruits and vegetables per day, Ann. N. Y. Acad. Sci. 691 (1993) 241–243.

[200] P.E. Bowen, S.M. Herbst-Espinosa, E.A. Hussain, M. Stacewicz-Sapuntzakis, Esterification does not impair lutein bioavailability in humans, J. Nutr. 132 (12) (2002) 3668–3673.

[201] E. Loane, J.M. Nolan, G.J. McKay, S. Beatty, The association between macular pigment optical density and CFH, ARMS2, C2/BF, and C3 genotype, Exp. Eye Res. 93 (2011) 592–598.

[202] P. Borel, F.S. de Edelenyi, S. Vincent-Baudry, C. Malezet-Desmoulin, A. Margotat, B. Lyan, et al., Genetic variants in BCMO1 and CD36 are associated with plasma lutein concentrations and macular pigment optical density in humans, Ann. Med. 43 (1) (2011) 47–59.

[203] E. Loane, G.J. McKay, J.M. Nolan, S. Beatty, Apolipoprotein E genotype is associated with macular pigment optical density, Invest. Ophthalmol. Vis. Sci. 51 (5) (2010) 2636–2643.

[204] P.S. Bernstein, D.Y. Zhao, S.W. Wintch, I.V. Ermakov, R.W. McClane, W. Gellermann, Resonance Raman measurement of macular carotenoids in normal subjects and in age-related macular degeneration patients, Ophthalmology 109 (10) (2002) 1780–1787.

[205] M. Dietzel, M. Zeimer, B. Heimes, B. Claes, D. Pauleikhoff, H.W. Hense,). Determinants of macular pigment optical density and its relation to age-related maculopathy: results from the Muenster Aging and Retina Study (MARS), Invest. Ophthalmol. Vis. Sci. 52 (6) (2011) 3452–3457.

[206] A. Obana, T. Hiramitsu, Y. Gohto, A. Ohira, S. Mizuno, T. Hirano, et al., Macular carotenoid levels of normal subjects and age-related maculopathy patients in a Japanese population, Ophthalmology 115 (1) (2008) 147–157.

[207] T.T. Berendschot, J.J. Willemse-Assink, M. Bastiaanse, P.T. de Jong, D. van Norren, Macular pigment and melanin in age-related maculopathy in a general population, Invest. Ophthalmol. Vis. Sci. 43 (6) (2002) 1928–1932.

[208] T.L. LaRowe, J.A. Mares, D.M. Snodderly, M.L. Klein, B.R. Wooten, R. Chappell, Macular pigment density and age-related maculopathy in the Carotenoids in Age-Related Eye Disease Study, an ancillary study of the Women's Health Initiative, Ophthalmology 115 (5) (2008) 876–883.

[209] M.J. Kanis, T.T. Berendschot, D. van Norren, Influence of macular pigment and melanin on incident early AMD in a white

population, Graefes Arch. Clin. Exp. Ophthalmol. 245 (6) (2007) 767–773.

[210] F.E. Cangemi, TOZAL Study: an open case–control study of an oral antioxidant and omega-3 supplement for dry AMD, BMC Ophthalmol. 7 (2007) 3.

[211] H.E. Bartlett, F. Eperjesi, Effect of lutein and antioxidant dietary supplementation on contrast sensitivity in age-related macular disease: a randomized controlled trial, Eur. J. Clin. Nutr. 61 (2007) 1121–1127.

[212] H. Coleman, E. Chew, Nutritional supplementation in age-related macular degeneration, Curr. Opin. Ophthalmol. 18 (3) (2007) 220–223.

[213] Food and Nutrition Board, Institute of Medicine, Dietary Reference Intakes for Vitamin C, Vitamin E, Selenium, and Carotenoids, National Academy Press, Washington, DC, 2000.

[214] D.J. Tate Jr., M.V. Miceli, D.A. Newsome, Zinc protects against oxidative damage in cultured human retinal pigment epithelial cells, Free Radic. Biol. Med. 26 (5–6) (1999) 704–713.

[215] E. Mocchegiani, M. Muzzioli, R. Giacconi, Zinc, metallothioneins, immune responses, survival and ageing, Biogerontology 1 (2) (2000) 133–143.

[216] A.H. Shankar, A.S. Prasad, Zinc and immune function: the biological basis of altered resistance to infection, Am. J. Clin. Nutr. 68 (2 Suppl.) (1998) 447S–463S.

[217] R. Nan, I. Farabella, F.F. Schumacher, A. Miller, J. Gor, A.C. Martin, et al., Zinc binding to the Tyr402 and His402 allotypes of complement factor H: possible implications for age-related macular degeneration, J. Mol. Biol. 408 (4) (2011) 714–735.

[218] H.J. Hyun, J.H. Sohn, D.W. Ha, Y.H. Ahn, J.-Y. Koh, Y.H. Yoon, Depletion of intracellular zinc and copper with TPEN results in apoptosis of cultured human retinal pigment epithelial cells, Invest. Ophthalmol. Vis. Sci. 42 (2) (2001) 460–465.

[219] J.P.M. Wood, N.N. Osborne, Zinc and energy requirements in induction of oxidative stress to retinal pigmented epithelial cells, Neurochem. Res. 28 (10) (2003) 1525–1533.

[220] N.K. Wills, N. Kalariya, V.M. Sadagopa Ramanujam, J.R. Lewis, S. Haji Abdollahi, A. Husain, et al., Human retinal cadmium accumulation as a factor in the etiology of age-related macular degeneration, Exp. Eye Res. 89 (1) (2009) 79–87.

[221] J.C. Erie, J.A. Good, J.A. Butz, J.S. Pulido, Reduced zinc and copper in the retinal pigment epithelium and choroid in age-related macular degeneration, Am. J. Ophthalmol. 147 (2) (2009) 276–282.

[222] E. Cho, M.J. Stampfer, J.M. Seddon, S. Hung, D. Spiegelman, E.B. Rimm, et al., Prospective study of zinc intake and the risk of age-related macular degeneration, Ann. Epidemiol. 11 (5) (2001) 328–336.

[223] N. Parekh, R.P. Voland, S.M. Moeller, B.A. Blodi, C. Ritenbaugh, R.J. Chappell, et al., Association between dietary fat intake and age-related macular degeneration in the Carotenoids in Age-Related Eye Disease Study (CAREDS): an ancillary study of the Women's Health Initiative, Arch. Ophthalmol. 127 (11) (2009) 1483–1493.

[224] Age-Related Eye Disease Study Research Group, A randomized, placebo-controlled, clinical trial of high-dose supplementation with vitamins C and E and beta carotene for age-related cataract and vision loss: AREDS Report No. 9, Arch. Ophthalmol 119 (10) (2001) 1439–1452.

[225] D.A. Newsome, M. Swartz, N.C. Leone, R.C. Elston, E. Miller, Oral zinc in macular degeneration.[see Comments], Arch. Ophthalmol. 106 (2) (1988) 192–198.

[226] M. Stur, M. Tittl, A. Reitner, V. Meisinger, Oral zinc and the second eye in age-related macular degeneration, Invest. Ophthalmol. Vis. Sci. 37 (7) (1996) 1225–1235.

[227] T.E. Clemons, N. Kurinij, R.D. Sperduto, Associations of mortality with ocular disorders and an intervention of high-dose antioxidants and zinc in the Age-Related Eye Disease Study: AREDS Report No. 13, Arch. Ophthalmol. 122 (5) (2004) 716–726.

[228] M.L. Klein, P.J. Francis, B. Rosner, R. Reynolds, S.C. Hamon, D.W. Schultz, et al., CFH and LOC387715/ARMS2 genotypes and treatment with antioxidants and zinc for age-related macular degeneration, Ophthalmology 115 (6) (2008) 1019–1025.

[229] J.C. Erie, J.A. Good, J.A. Butz, Excess lead in the neural retina in age-related macular degeneration, Am. J. Ophthalmol. 148 (6) (2009) 890–894.

[230] T. Sarna, J.S. Hyde, H.M. Swartz, Ion-exchange in melanin: an electron spin resonance study with lanthanide probes, Science 192 (4244) (1976) 1132–1134.

[231] M. Bhattacharyya, A. Wilson, S.S. Rajan, M. Jonah, Biochemical pathways in cadmium toxicity, in: R.Z. Zalups, J. Koropatnick (Eds), Molecular Biology and Toxicology of Metals, Taylor & Francis, New York, 2000, pp. 276–299.

[232] J.C. Erie, J.A. Butz, J.A. Good, E.A. Erie, M.F. Burritt, J.D. Cameron, Heavy metal concentrations in human eyes, Am. J. Ophthalmol. 139 (5) (2005) 888–893.

[233] J.C. Erie, J.A. Good, J.A. Butz, D.O. Hodge, J.S. Pulido, Urinary cadmium and age-related macular degeneration, Am. J. Ophthalmol. 144 (3) (2007) 414–418.

[234] J.M. Seddon, B. Rosner, R.D. Sperduto, L. Yannuzzi, J.A. Haller, N. P. Blair, et al., Dietary fat and risk for advanced age-related macular degeneration, Arch. Ophthalmol. 119 (8) (2001) 1191–1199.

[235] D.A. Schaumberg, W.G. Christen, S.E. Hankinson, R.J. Glynn, Body mass index and the incidence of visually significant age-related maculopathy in men, Arch. Ophthalmol. 119 (9) (2001) 1259–1265.

[236] J.M. Seddon, J. Cote, B. Rosner, Progression of age related macular degeneration: association with dietary fat, transunsaturated fat, nuts, and fish intake, Arch. Ophthalmol. 121 (12) (2003) 1728–1737.

[237] A.C. Provost, L. Vede, K. Bigot, N. Keller, A. Tailleux, J.P. Jais, et al., Morphologic and electroretinographic phenotype of SR-BI knockout mice after a long-term atherogenic diet, Invest. Ophthalmol. Vis. Sci. 50 (8) (2009) 3931–3942.

[238] M.V. Miceli, D.A. Newsome, D.J. Tate Jr., T.G. Sarphie, Pathologic changes in the retinal pigment epithelium and Bruch's membrane of fat-fed atherogenic mice, Curr. Eye Res. 20 (1) (2000) 8–16.

[239] M. Kliffen, E. Lutgens, M.J. Daemen, E.D. de Muinck, C.M. Mooy, P.T. de Jong, The APO(*)E3-Leiden mouse as an animal model for basal laminar deposit, Br. J. Ophthalmol. 84 (12) (2000) 1415–1419.

[240] D.G. Espinosa-Heidmann, J. Sall, E.P. Hernandez, S.W. Cousins, Basal laminar deposit formation in APO B100 transgenic mice: complex interactions between dietary fat, blue light, and vitamin E, Invest. Ophthalmol. Vis. Sci. 45 (1) (2004) 260–266.

[241] S. Dithmar, N.A. Sharara, C.A. Curcio, N.A. Le, Y. Zhang, S. Brown, et al., Murine high-fat diet and laser photochemical model of basal deposits in Bruch membrane, Arch. Ophthalmol. 119 (11) (2001) 1643–1649.

[242] R.A. Heuberger, J.A. Mares-Perlman, R. Klein, B.E. Klein, A.E. Millen, M. Palta, Relationship of dietary fat to age-related maculopathy in the Third National Health and Nutrition Examination Survey, Arch. Ophthalmol. 119 (12) (2001) 1833–1838.

[243] J.A. Mares-Perlman, W.E. Brady, R. Klein, G.M. VandenLangenberg, B.E. Klein, M. Palta, Dietary fat and age-related maculopathy, Arch. Ophthalmol. 113 (6) (1995) 743–748.

[244] W. Smith, P. Mitchell, S.R. Leeder, Dietary fat and fish intake and age-related maculopathy, Arch. Ophthalmol. 118 (3) (2000) 401–404.

[245] E. Cho, S. Hung, W.C. Willett, D. Spiegelman, E.B. Rimm, J.M. Seddon, et al., Prospective study of dietary fat and the risk of age-related macular degeneration, Am. J. Clin. Nutr. 73 (2) (2001) 209–218.

[246] B. Chua, V. Flood., E. Rochtchina, J.J. Wang, W. Smith, P. Mitchell, Dietary fatty acids and the 5-year incidence of age-related maculopathy, Arch. Ophthalmol. 124 (7) (2006) 981–986.

[247] Age-Related Eye Disease Study Research Group, The relationship of dietary lipid intake and age-related macular degeneration in a case–control study: AREDS Report No. 20, Arch. Ophthalmol 125 (5) (2007) 671–679.

[248] E.W. Chong, L.D. Robman, J.A. Simpson, A.M. Hodge, K.Z. Aung, T.K. Dolphin, et al., Fat consumption and its association with age-related macular degeneration, Arch. Ophthalmol. 127 (5) (2009) 674–680.

[249] J.S. Tan, J.J. Wang, V. Flood, P. Mitchell, Dietary fatty acids and the 10-year incidence of age-related macular degeneration: The Blue Mountains Eye Study, Arch. Ophthalmol. 127 (5) (2009) 656–665.

[250] F. Li, W. Cao, R.E. Anderson, Protection of photoreceptor cells in adult rats from light-induced degeneration by adaptation to bright cyclic light, Exp. Eye Res. 73 (4) (2001) 569–577.

[251] J.J. Wang, E. Rochtchina, W. Smith, R. Klein, B.E. Klein, T. Joshi, et al., Combined effects of complement factor H genotypes, fish consumption, and inflammatory markers on long-term risk for age-related macular degeneration in a cohort, Am. J. Epidemiol. 169 (5) (2009) 633–641.

[252] J.M. Seddon, S. George, B. Rosner, Cigarette smoking, fish consumption, omega-3 fatty acid intake, and associations with age-related macular degeneration: The U.S. Twin Study of Age-Related Macular Degeneration, Arch. Ophthalmol. 124 (7) (2006) 995–1001.

[253] J.P. SanGiovanni, E.Y. Chew, E. Agron, et al., The relationship of dietary omega-3 long-chain polyunsaturated fatty acid intake with incident age-related macular degeneration: AREDS report No. 23, Arch. Ophthalmol. 126 (9) (2008) 1274–1279.

[254] A. Arnarsson, T. Sverrisson, E. Stefansson, H. Sigurdsson, H. Sasaki, K. Sasaki, et al., Risk factors for five-year incident age-related macular degeneration: The Reykjavik Eye Study, Am. J. Ophthalmol. 142 (3) (2006) 419–428.

[255] F. Jonasson, A. Arnarsson, T. Peto, H. Sasaki, K. Sasaki, A.C. Bird, 5-Year incidence of age-related maculopathy in the Reykjavik Eye Study, Ophthalmology 112 (1) (2005) 132–138.

[256] S.C. Larsson, M. Kumlin, M. Ingelman-Sundberg, A. Wolk, Dietary long-chain n-3 fatty acids for the prevention of cancer: a review of potential mechanisms, Am. J. Clin. Nutr. 79 (6) (2004) 935–945.

[257] E. Simon, B. Bardet, S. Gregoire, N. Acar, A.M. Bron, C.P. Creuzot-Garcher, et al., Decreasing dietary linoleic acid promotes long chain omega-3 fatty acid incorporation into rat retina and modifies gene expression, Exp. Eye Res. 93 (2011) 628–635.

[258] J.L. Breslow, n-3 Fatty acids and cardiovascular disease, Am. J. Clin. Nutr. 83 (6) (2006) S1477–S1482.

[259] N.G. Bazan, B.L. Scott, Dietary omega-3 fatty acids and accumulation of docosahexaenoic acid in rod photoreceptor cells of the retina and at synapses, Ups. J. Med. Sci. (1990) 97–107.

[260] S.J. Fliesler, R.E. Anderson, Chemistry and metabolism of lipids in the vertebrate retina, Prog. Lipid Res. 22 (2) (1983) 79–131.

[261] L.M. Arterburn, E.B. Hall, H. Oken, Distribution, interconversion, and dose response of n-3 fatty acids in humans, Am. J. Clin. Nutr. 83 (6) (2006) S1467–S1476.

[262] B.J. Litman, S.L. Niu, A. Polozova, D.C. Mitchell, The role of docosahexaenoic acid containing phospholipids in modulating G protein-coupled signaling pathways: visual transduction, J. Mol. Neurosci. 16 (2–3) (2001) 237–242.

[263] N.P. Rotstein, L.E. Politi, O.L. German, R. Girotti, Protective effect of docosahexaenoic acid on oxidative stress-induced apoptosis of retina photoreceptors, Invest. Ophthalmol. Vis. Sci. 44 (5) (2003) 2252–2259.

[264] P.K. Mukherjee, V.L. Marcheselli, C.N. Serhan, N.G. Bazan, Neuroprotectin D1: a docosahexaenoic acid-derived docosatriene protects human retinal pigment epithelial cells from oxidative stress, Proc. Natl. Acad. Sci. USA 101 (22) (2004) 8491–8496.

[265] J.P. SanGiovanni, E.Y. Chew, The role of omega-3 long-chain polyunsaturated fatty acids in health and disease of the retina, Prog. Retinal Eye Res. 24 (1) (2005) 87–138.

[266] J.A. Johnson, J.P. Grande, P.C. Roche, R.J. Campbell, R. Kumar, Immuno-localization of the calcitriol receptor, calbindin-D28k and the plasma membrane calcium pump in the human eye, Curr. Eye Res. 14 (2) (1995) 101–108.

[267] D. Choi, B. Appukuttan, S.J. Binek, S.R. Planck, J.T. Stout, J.T. Rosenbaum, et al., Prediction of cis-regulatory elements controlling genes differentially expressed by retinal and choroidal vascular endothelial cells, J. Ocul. Biol. Dis. Infor. 1 (1) (2008) 37–45.

[268] F.C. Barouch, J.W. Miller, The role of inflammation and infection in age-related macular degeneration, Int. Ophthalmol. Clin. 47 (2) (2007) 185–197.

[269] D.L. Kamen, V. Tangpricha, Vitamin D and molecular actions on the immune system: modulation of innate and autoimmunity, J. Mol. Med. (Berlin) 88 (5) (2010) 441–450.

[270] J.R. Mora, M. Iwata, U.H. von Andrian, Vitamin effects on the immune system: Vitamins A and D take centre stage, Nature Rev. 8 (9) (2008) 685–698.

[271] D.D. Bikle, Vitamin D and immune function: understanding common pathways, Curr. Osteoporosis Rep. 7 (2) (2009) 58–63.

[272] W.F. Rigby, T. Stacy, M.W. Fanger, Inhibition of T lymphocyte mitogenesis by 1,25-dihydroxyvitamin D3 (calcitriol), J. Clin. Invest. 74 (4) (1984) 1451–1455.

[273] S. Chen, G.P. Sims, X.X. Chen, Y.Y. Gu, S. Chen, P.E. Lipsky, Modulatory effects of 1,25-dihydroxyvitamin D3 on human B cell differentiation, J. Immunol. 179 (3) (2007) 1634–1647.

[274] J.M. Lemire, J.S. Adams, R. Sakai, S.C. Jordan, 1 Alpha,25-dihydroxyvitamin D3 suppresses proliferation and immunoglobulin production by normal human peripheral blood mononuclear cells, J. Clin. Invest. 74 (2) (1984) 657–661.

[275] G. Penna, L. Adorini, 1 Alpha,25-dihydroxyvitamin D3 inhibits differentiation, maturation, activation, and survival of dendritic cells leading to impaired alloreactive T cell activation, J. Immunol. 164 (5) (2000) 2405–2411.

[276] C. Daniel, N.A. Sartory, N. Zahn, H.H. Radeke, J.M. Stein, Immune modulatory treatment of trinitrobenzene sulfonic acid colitis with calcitriol is associated with a change of a T helper (Th) 1/Th17 to a Th2 and regulatory T cell profile, J. Pharmacol. Exp. Ther. 324 (1) (2008) 23–33.

[277] I. Chung, W.D. Yu, A.R. Karpf, G. Flynn, R.J. Bernardi, R.A. Modzelewski, et al., Anti-proliferative effects of calcitriol on endothelial cells derived from two different microenvironments, J. Steroid Biochem. Mol. Biol. 103 (3–5) (2007) 768–770.

[278] D.J. Mantell, P.E. Owens, N.J. Bundred, E.B. Mawer, A.E. Canfield, 1 Alpha,25-dihydroxyvitamin D(3) inhibits angiogenesis in vitro and in vivo, Circ. Res. 87 (3) (2000) 214–220.

[279] I. Chung, G. Han, M. Seshadri, B.M. Gillard, W.D. Yu, B.A. Foster, et al., Role of vitamin D receptor in the antiproliferative effects of calcitriol in tumor-derived endothelial cells and tumor angiogenesis in vivo, Cancer Res. 69 (3) (2009) 967–975.

[280] D.M. Albert, R.W. Nickells, D.M. Gamm, M.L. Zimbric, C.L. Schlamp, M.J. Lindstrom, et al., Vitamin D analogs, a new treatment for retinoblastoma: the first Ellsworth Lecture, Ophthalmic Genet. 23 (3) (2002) 137–156.

[281] D.M. Albert, E.A. Scheef, S. Wang, F. Mehraein, S.R. Darjatmoko, C.M. Sorenson, et al., Calcitriol is a potent inhibitor of retinal neovascularization, Invest. Ophthalmol. Vis. Sci. 48 (5) (2007) 2327–2334.

[282] M.F. Holick, Vitamin D deficiency, N. Engl. J. Med. 357 (3) (2007) 266–281.

[283] N. Parekh, R.J. Chappell, A.E. Millen, D.M. Albert, J.A. Mares, Association between vitamin D and age-related macular degeneration in the Third National Health and Nutrition Examination Survey, 1988 through 1994, Arch. Ophthalmol. 125 (5) (2007) 661–669.

[284] A.E. Millen, R. Voland, S.A. Sondel, N. Parekh, R.L. Horst, R.B. Wallace, et al., Vitamin D status and early age-related macular degeneration in postmenopausal women, Arch. Ophthalmol. 129 (4) (2011) 481–489.

[285] S. Golan, V. Shalev, G. Treister, G. Chodick, A. Loewenstein, Reconsidering the connection between vitamin D levels and age-related macular degeneration, Eye (London) 25 (9) (2011) 1122–1129.

[286] S.C. Manolagas, D.M. Provvedini, E.J. Murray, C.D. Tsoukas, L.J. Deftos, The antiproliferative effect of calcitriol on human peripheral blood mononuclear cells, J. Clin. Endocrinol. Metab. 63 (2) (1986) 394–400.

[287] J.M. Seddon, R. Reynolds, H.R. Shah, B. Rosner, Smoking, dietary betaine, methionine, and vitamin D in monozygotic twins with discordant macular degeneration: epigenetic implications, Ophthalmology 118 (2011) 1386–1394.

[288] C. Augood, U. Chakravarthy, I. Young, J. Vioque, P.T. de Jong, G. Bentham, et al., Oily fish consumption, dietary docosahexaenoic acid and eicosapentaenoic acid intakes, and associations with neovascular age-related macular degeneration, Am. J. Clin. Nutr. 88 (2) (2008) 398–406.

[289] A.E. Millen, J. Wactawski-Wende, M. Pettinger, M.L. Melamed, F.A. Tylavsky, S. Liu, et al., Predictors of serum 25-hydroxyvitamin D concentrations among postmenopausal women: The Women's Health Initiative Calcium plus Vitamin D clinical trial, Am. J. Clin. Nutr. 91 (5) (2010) 1324–1335.

[290] E.S. West, O.D. Schein, Sunlight and age-related macular degeneration, Int. Ophthalmol. Clin. 45 (1) (2005) 41–47.

[291] A.A. Ginde, M.C. Liu, C.A. Camargo Jr., Demographic differences and trends of vitamin D insufficiency in the U.S. population, 1988–2004, Arch. Internal Med. 169 (6) (2009) 626–632.

[292] A.C. Looker, C.M. Pfeiffer, D.A. Lacher, R.L. Schleicher, M.F. Picciano, E.A. Yetley, Serum 25-hydroxyvitamin D status of the U.S. population: 1988–1994 compared with 2000–2004, Am. J. Clin. Nutr. 88 (6) (2008) 1519–1527.

[293] C.J. Chiu, L.D. Hubbard, J. Armstrong, G. Rogers, P.F. Jacques, L.T. Chylack Jr., et al., Dietary glycemic index and carbohydrate in relation to early age-related macular degeneration, Am. J. Clin. Nutr. 83 (4) (2006) 880–886.

[294] A.L. West, G.A. Oren, S.E. Moroi, Evidence for the use of nutritional supplements and herbal medicines in common eye diseases, Am. J. Ophthalmol. 141 (1) (2006) 157–166.

[295] C. Mathieu, M. Waer, K. Casteels, J. Laureys, R. Bouillon, Prevention of type I diabetes in NOD mice by nonhypercalcemic doses of a new structural analog of 1,25-dihydroxyvitamin D3, KH1060, Endocrinology 136 (3) (1995) 866–872.

[296] J.E. Shaw, R.A. Sicree, P.Z. Zimmet, Global estimates of the prevalence of diabetes for 2010 and 2030, Diabetes Res. Clin. Pract. 87 (1) (2010) 4–14.

[297] C.C. Cowie, K.F. Rust, D.D. Byrd-Holt, E.W. Gregg, E.S. Ford, L.S. Geiss, et al., Prevalence of diabetes and high risk for diabetes using A1C criteria in the U.S. population in 1988–2006, Diabetes Care 33 (3) (2010) 562–568.

[298] W.C. Knowler, D.J. Pettitt, M.F. Saad, P.H. Bennett, Diabetes mellitus in the Pima Indians: incidence, risk factors and pathogenesis, Diabetes Metab. Rev. 6 (1) (1990) 1–27.

[299] M. Porta, A. Allione, Current approaches and perspectives in the medical treatment of diabetic retinopathy, Pharmacol. Ther. 103 (2) (2004) 167–177.

[300] L.P. Aiello, T.W. Gardner, G.L. King, G. Blankenship, J.D. Cavallerano, F.L. Ferris III, et al., Diabetic retinopathy, Diabetes Care 21 (1) (1998) 143–156.

[301] The Diabetes Control and Complications Trial Research Group, The effect of intensive treatment of diabetes on the development and progression of long-term complications in insulin-dependent diabetes mellitus, N. Engl. J. Med. 329 (14) (1993) 977–986.

[302] UK Prospective Diabetes Study (UKPDS) Group, Intensive blood-glucose control with sulphonylureas or insulin compared with conventional treatment and risk of complications in patients with type 2 diabetes (UKPDS 33), Lancet 352 (9131) (1998) 837–853.

[303] M. Shichiri, H. Kishikawa, Y. Ohkubo, N. Wake, Long-term results of the Kumamoto Study on optimal diabetes control in type 2 diabetic patients, Diabetes Care 23 (Suppl. 2) (2000) B21–B29.

[304] E.Y. Chew, W.T. Ambrosius, M.D. Davis, R.P. Danis, S. Gangaputra, C.M. Greven, et al., Effects of medical therapies on retinopathy progression in type 2 diabetes, N. Engl. J. Med. 363 (3) (2011) 233–244.

[305] R. Klein, B.E. Klein, S.E. Moss, M.D. Davis, D.L. DeMets, The Wisconsin Epidemiologic Study of Diabetic Retinopathy: III. Prevalence and risk of diabetic retinopathy when age at diagnosis is 30 or more years, Arch. Ophthalmol. 102 (4) (1984) 527–532.

[306] D.R. Matthews, I.M. Stratton, S.J. Aldington, R.R. Holman, E.M. Kohner, Risks of progression of retinopathy and vision loss related to tight blood pressure control in type 2 diabetes mellitus: UKPDS 69, Arch. Ophthalmol. 122 (11) (2004) 1631–1640.

[307] B.E. Klein, M.D. Knudtson, M.Y. Tsai, R. Klein, The relation of markers of inflammation and endothelial dysfunction to the prevalence and progression of diabetic retinopathy: Wisconsin Epidemiologic Study of Diabetic Retinopathy, Arch. Ophthalmol. 127 (9) (2009) 1175–1182.

[308] A.J. Houtsmuller, J. van Hal-Ferwerda, K.J. Zahn, H.E. Henkes, Influence of different diets on the progression of diabetic retinopathy, Prog. Food Nutr. Sci. 4 (5) (1980) 41–46.

[309] J. Howard-Williams, P. Patel, R. Jelfs, R.D. Carter, P. Awdry, A. Bron, et al., Polyunsaturated fatty acids and diabetic retinopathy, Br. J. Ophthalmol. 69 (1) (1985) 15–18.

[310] M. Toeller, A.E. Buyken, G. Heitkamp, G. Berg, W.A. Scherbaum, Prevalence of chronic complications, metabolic control and nutritional intake in type 1 diabetes: comparison between different European regions: EURODIAB Complications Study group, Horm. Metab. Res. 31 (12) (1999) 680–685.

[311] D.K. Cundiff, C.R. Nigg, Diet and diabetic retinopathy: insights from the Diabetes Control and Complications Trial (DCCT), MedGenMed 7 (1) (2005) 3.

[312] M.S. Roy, M.N. Janal, High caloric and sodium intakes as risk factors for progression of retinopathy in type 1 diabetes mellitus, Arch. Ophthalmol. 128 (1) (2011) 33–39.

[313] R.A. Kowluru, P.S. Chan, Oxidative stress and diabetic retinopathy, Exp. Diabetes Res. 2007 (2007) 43603.

[314] M.S. Roy, G. Stables, B. Collier, A. Roy, E. Bou, Nutritional factors in diabetics with and without retinopathy, Am. J. Clin. Nutr. 50 (4) (1989) 728–730.

[315] R.B. Paisey, G. Arredondo, A. Villalobos, O. Lozano, L. Guevara, S. Kelly, Association of differing dietary, metabolic, and clinical risk factors with microvascular complications of diabetes: a prevalence study of 503 Mexican type II diabetic subjects, Diabetes Care 7(5), 428–433.

[316] J.W. Anderson, P. Baird, R.H. Davis Jr., S. Ferreri, M. Knudtson, A. Koraym, et al., Health benefits of dietary fiber, Nutr. Rev. 67 (4) (2009) 188–205.

[317] M.S. Roy, R. Klein, B.J. O'Colmain, B.E. Klein, S.E. Moss, J.H. Kempen, The prevalence of diabetic retinopathy among adult type 1 diabetic persons in the United States, Arch. Ophthalmol. 122 (4) (2004) 546–551.

[318] S. Ganesan, R. Raman, V. Kulothungan, T. Sharma, Influence of dietary fibre intake on diabetes and diabetic retinopathy: Sankara Nethralaya Diabetic Retinopathy Epidemiology and Molecular Genetic Study (SN-DREAM, Report 26), Clin. Exp. Ophthalmol. 40 (2012) 288–294.

[319] B. Raheja, K. Modi, J. Barua, S. Jain, V. Shahani, G. Koppikar, Proliferative diabetic retinopathy in NIDDM and Indian diet, J. Med. Assoc. Thailand 70 (Suppl. 2) (1987) 139–143.

[320] Q. Gong, E.W. Gregg, J. Wang, Y. An, P. Zhang, W. Yang, et al., Long-term effects of a randomised trial of a 6-year lifestyle intervention in impaired glucose tolerance on diabetes-related microvascular complications: The China Da Qing Diabetes Prevention Outcome Study, Diabetologia 54 (2) (2011) 300–307.

[321] D. Giugliano, A. Ceriello, G. Paolisso, Oxidative stress and diabetic vascular complications, Diabetes Care 19 (3) (1996) 257–267.

[322] D.M. van Reyk, M.C. Gillies, M.J. Davies, The retina: oxidative stress and diabetes, Redox Rep. 8 (4) (2003) 187–192.

[323] S.R. Maxwell, H. Thomason, D. Sandler, C. Leguen, M.A. Baxter, G.H. Thorpe, et al., Antioxidant status in patients with uncomplicated insulin-dependent and non-insulin-dependent diabetes mellitus, Eur. J. Clin. Invest. 27 (6) (1997) 484–490.

[324] J. Nourooz-Zadeh, A. Rahimi, J. Tajaddini-Sarmadi, H. Tritschler, P. Rosen, B. Halliwell, et al., Relationships between plasma measures of oxidative stress and metabolic control in NIDDM, Diabetologia 40 (6) (1997) 647–653.

[325] R.A. Kowluru, M. Kanwar, P.S. Chan, J.P. Zhang, Inhibition of retinopathy and retinal metabolic abnormalities in diabetic rats with AREDS-based micronutrients, Arch. Ophthalmol. 126 (9) (2008) 1266–1272.

[326] C.T. Lee, E.L. Gayton, J.W. Beulens, D.W. Flanagan, A.I. Adler, Micronutrients and diabetic retinopathy: a systematic review, Ophthalmology 117 (1) (2010) 71–78.

[327] E.J. Mayer-Davis, R.A. Bell, B.A. Reboussin, J. Rushing, J.A. Marshall, R.F. Hamman, Antioxidant nutrient intake and diabetic retinopathy: The San Luis Valley Diabetes Study, Ophthalmology 105 (12) (1998) 2264–2270.

[328] A.E. Millen, M. Gruber, R. Klein, B.E. Klein, M. Palta, J.A. Mares, Relations of serum ascorbic acid and alpha-tocopherol to diabetic retinopathy in the Third National Health and Nutrition Examination Survey, Am. J. Epidemiol. 158 (3) (2003) 225–233.

[329] A.E. Millen, R. Klein, A.R. Folsom, J. Stevens, M. Palta, J.A. Mares, Relation between intake of vitamins C and E and risk of diabetic retinopathy in the Atherosclerosis Risk in Communities Study, Am. J. Clin. Nutr. 79 (5) (2004) 865–873.

[330] E. Lonn, S. Yusuf, B. Hoogwerf, J. Pogue, Q. Yi, B. Zinman, et al., Effects of vitamin E on cardiovascular and microvascular outcomes in high-risk patients with diabetes: Results of the HOPE study and MICRO-HOPE substudy, Diabetes Care 25 (11) (2002) 1919–1927.

[331] L. Brazionis, K. Rowley, C. Itsiopoulos, K. O'Dea, Plasma carotenoids and diabetic retinopathy, Br. J. Nutr. 101 (2) (2009) 270–277.

[332] Z.Z. Li, X.Z. Lu, C.C. Ma, L. Chen, Serum lycopene levels in patients with diabetic retinopathy, Eur J Ophthalmol. 20 (4) (2010) 719–723.

[333] T.S. Kern, Contributions of inflammatory processes to the development of the early stages of diabetic retinopathy, Exp. Diabetes Res. 2007 (2007) 95103.

[334] H. Aksoy, F. Akcay, N. Kurtul, O. Baykal, B. Avci, Serum 1,25 dihydroxy vitamin D (1,25(OH)2D), 25 hydroxy vitamin D (25 (OH)D) and parathormone levels in diabetic retinopathy, Clin. Biochem. 33 (1) (2000) 47–51.

[335] A. Suzuki, M. Kotake, Y. Ono, T. Kato, N. Oda, N. Hayakawa, et al., Hypovitaminosis D in type 2 diabetes mellitus: association with microvascular complications and type of treatment, Endocr. J. 53 (4) (2006) 503–510.

[336] C. Joergensen, P. Hovind, A. Schmedes, H.H. Parving, P. Rossing, Vitamin D levels, microvascular complications, and mortality in type 1 diabetes, Diabetes Care 34 (5) (2011) 1081–1085.

[337] M.J. Taverna, A. Sola, C. Guyot-Argenton, N. Pacher, F. Bruzzo, G. Slama, et al., Taq I polymorphism of the vitamin D receptor and risk of severe diabetic retinopathy, Diabetologia 45 (3) (2002) 436–442.

[338] M.J. Taverna, J.L. Selam, G. Slama, Association between a protein polymorphism in the start codon of the vitamin D receptor gene and severe diabetic retinopathy in C-peptide-negative type 1 diabetes, J. Clin. Endocrinol. Metab. 90 (8) (2005) 4803–4808.

[339] K. Bucan, M. Ivanisevic, T. Zemunik, V. Boraska, V. Skrabic, Z. Vatavuk, et al., Retinopathy and nephropathy in type 1 diabetic patients—Association with polymorphysms of vitamin D-receptor, TNF, Neuro-D and IL-1 receptor 1 genes, Coll. Antropol. 33 (Suppl. 2) (2009) 99–105.

[340] E. Capoluongo, D. Pitocco, P. Concolino, C. Santonocito, E. Di Stasio, G. d'Onofrio, et al., Slight association between type 1 diabetes and "ff" VDR FokI genotype in patients from the Italian Lazio Region: lack of association with diabetes complications, Clin. Biochem. 39 (9) (2006) 888–892.

[341] K. Cyganek, B. Mirkiewicz-Sieradzka, M.T. Malecki, P. Wolkow, J. Skupien, J. Bobrek, et al., Clinical risk factors and the role of VDR gene polymorphisms in diabetic retinopathy in Polish type 2 diabetes patients, Acta Diabetol. 43 (4) (2006) 114–119.

[342] C.H. Sales, L.F. Pedrosa, Magnesium and diabetes mellitus: their relation, Clin. Nutr. 25 (4) (2006) 554–562.

[343] M. Barbagallo, L.J. Dominguez, Magnesium metabolism in type 2 diabetes mellitus, metabolic syndrome and insulin resistance, Arch. Biochem. Biophys. 458 (1) (2007) 40–47.

[344] W. Herrmann, M. Herrmann, R. Obeid, Hyperhomocysteinaemia: a critical review of old and new aspects, Curr. Drug Metab. 8 (1) (2007) 17–31.

[345] M. Maeda, Y. Fujio, J. Azuma, MTHFR gene polymorphism and diabetic retinopathy, Curr. Diabetes Rev. 2 (4) (2006) 467–476.

[346] C.C. Lee, R.P. Stolk, A.I. Adler, A. Patel, J. Chalmers, B. Neal, et al., Association between alcohol consumption and diabetic retinopathy and visual acuity-the AdRem Study, Diabetes Med. 27 (10) (2010) 1130–1137.

[347] S.E. Moss, R. Klein, B.E. Klein, Alcohol consumption and the prevalence of diabetic retinopathy, Ophthalmology 99 (6) (1992) 926–932.

B. DIETARY BIOACTIVE COMPOUNDS FOR HEALTH

[348] J.W. Beulens, J.S. Kruidhof, D.E. Grobbee, N. Chaturvedi, J.H. Fuller, S.S. Soedamah-Muthu, Alcohol consumption and risk of microvascular complications in type 1 diabetes patients: The EURODIAB Prospective Complications Study, Diabetologia 51 (9) (2008) 1631–1638.

[349] G. Giuffre, G. Lodato, G. Dardanoni, Prevalence and risk factors of diabetic retinopathy in adult and elderly subjects: The Casteldaccia Eye Study, Graefes Arch. Clin. Exp. Ophthalmol. 242 (7) (2004) 535–540.

[350] L. Xu, Q.S. You, J.B. Jonas, Prevalence of alcohol consumption and risk of ocular diseases in a general population: The Beijing Eye Study, Ophthalmology 116 (10) (2009) 1872–1879.

[351] F.B. Hu, Plant-based foods and prevention of cardiovascular disease: an overview, Am. J. Clin. Nutr. 78 (3) (2003) 544S–551S.

[352] M.L. McCullough, D. Feskanich, M.J. Stampfer, E.L. Giovannucci, E.B. Rimm, F.B. Hu, et al., Diet quality and major chronic disease risk in men and women: moving toward improved dietary guidance, Am. J. Clin. Nutr. 76 (6) (2002) 1261–1271.

[353] K. Hoffmann, B.-C. Zyriax, H. Boeing, E. Windler, A dietary pattern derived to explain biomarker variation is strongly associated with the risk of coronary artery disease, Am. J. Clin. Nutr. 80 (3) (2004) 633–640.

[354] L.J. Appel, T.J. Moore, E. Obarzanek, W.M. Vollmer, L.P. Svetkey, F.M. Sacks, et al., A clinical trial of the effects of dietary patterns on blood pressure: DASH Collaborative Research Group, N. Engl. J. Med. 336 (16) (1997) 1117–1124.

[355] K.L. Tucker, H. Chen, M.T. Hannan, L.A. Cupples, P.W. Wilson, D. Felson, et al., Bone mineral density and dietary patterns in older adults: The Framingham Osteoporosis Study, Am. J. Clin. Nutr. 76 (1) (2002) 245–252.

Nutrients and Food Constituents in Cognitive Decline and Neurodegenerative Disease

James A. Joseph[*], *Gemma Casadesus*[†], *Mark A. Smith*[†], *George Perry*[‡], *Barbara Shukitt-Hale*[*]

[*]USDA, HNRCA at Tufts University, Boston, Massachusetts [†]Case Western Reserve University, Cleveland, Ohio [‡]University of Texas at San Antonio, San Antonio, Texas

I INTRODUCTION

According to Wikipedia, "Pollyanna tells the story of Pollyanna Whittier, a young girl who goes to live with her wealthy Aunt Polly after her father's death. Pollyanna's philosophy of life centers around what she calls 'The Glad Game': She always tries to find something to be glad about in every situation." Given the increasing proportion of aged individuals in the United States and other countries, with all of their attendant ills, if there was ever a time when a "Pollyanna" is needed, it is now. The purpose of this review is to provide some additional "Pollyannas" in the form of polyphenols contained in berries, Concord grape juice, curcumin, and other natural products such as tea catechins, and the polyunsaturated fatty acids contained in such commodities as fish oils and nuts that may act as harbingers of good news for healthy aging. Note, however, that because there have already been multiple reviews of vitamins E and C (e.g., [1,2]) and such supplements as ginkgo biloba (e.g., [3]), these topics will not be covered here.

As is well-known, with aging there is an increase in the number of multiple co-occurring chronic conditions, including cognitive decline and dementia. Because the proportion of the population in the United States and other nations that are aged continues to increase, cognitive and motor deficits are growing rapidly. Cognitive impairment and dementia are major causes of disability in our nation, and their financial impact and long-term care costs are enormous.

The major cause of dementia is Alzheimer's disease (AD). Aging clearly results in declines in brain size, weight, and function [4–6]. However, to date, the cellular and morphological substrates underlying these changes remain poorly characterized. Although dogma suggests that aging is associated with a significant loss of neurons in the brain, careful studies have uncovered only modest, if any, change in cell number and size in a variety of brain regions with aging, including the neocortex and hippocampus [7–10]. A lack of evident morphological changes associated with neurodegeneration in the entorhinal cortex with aging further supports the concept that there are fundamental differences between the types of changes that occur in normal "healthy" aging and the pathological changes that occur in age-related neurodegenerative processes, such as AD.

Among the clear functional changes that occur in the brain with aging are declines in various aspects of cognition and memory. In particular, short-term memory [11], memory acquisition and early retrieval [5], working memory [12], recognition memory [13,14], reasoning [15], and processing speed [16,17] are affected with aging. In fact, a great deal of research has shown, in both humans and animal models, the occurrence of numerous neuronal and behavioral deficits during aging in the absence of neurodegenerative disease. These changes may include decrements in receptor sensitivity, most notably adrenergic [18], dopaminergic [19,20], muscarinic [21,22], and opioid [23]. These decrements, and those involving neuronal

Nutrition in the Prevention and Treatment of Disease, Third Edition.
DOI: http://dx.doi.org/10.1016/B978-0-12-391884-0.00020-2

signaling [24] and decreases in neurogenesis [25], can be expressed, ultimately, as alterations in both motor [26,27] and cognitive behaviors [28]. The alterations in motor function may include decreases in balance, muscle strength, and coordination [26], whereas cognitive deficits are seen primarily with respect to spatial learning and memory [29,30]. Indeed, these characterizations have been supported by a great deal of research both in animals [28–30] and in humans [31]. Age-related deficits in motor performance are thought to be the result of alterations either in the striatal dopamine (DA) system (as the striatum shows marked structural and functional changes with age in Parkinson's disease [PD]) or in the cerebellum, which also shows age-related alterations [32,33].

Memory alterations appear to occur primarily in secondary memory systems and are reflected in the storage of newly acquired information [22,34]. It is thought that the hippocampus mediates allocentric spatial navigation (i.e., place learning), and that the prefrontal cortex is critical to acquiring the rules that govern performance in particular tasks (i.e., procedural knowledge), whereas the dorsomedial striatum mediates egocentric spatial orientation (i.e., response and cue learning) [35–38]. More important, data from a variety of experiments suggest that the contributing factors to the behavioral decrements seen in aging involve oxidative stress (OS) [39] and inflammation (INF) [40,41]. This review discusses some of the nutritional interventions in aging and their putative utility in neurodegenerative disease.

II GENDER DIFFERENCES IN DEMENTIA

Epidemiological observations and evidence of gender-related differences in cognition and behavior suggest that there may be important genetic or biological factors related to gender that are operating in the pathogenesis of neurological disease, particularly in AD. Clinicians who diagnose and treat patients with AD recognize that there is heterogeneity in its cognitive and behavioral manifestations. Research suggests that gender may be an important modifying factor in AD development and expression. One of the most intriguing aspects concerning the epidemiology of AD is that the prevalence rate in women is roughly twice that in men, and this skewed sex ratio is specific for AD but not for other dementias. Age is the most important risk factor associated with dementia. Males tend to have shorter life spans than females, and even though the life-span gap narrows as men live longer, still at the age of 75 and older, there are significantly more women than men with AD.

Long-term effects of the metabolic and hormonal differences between men and women may play a relevant role on the observed age-associated cognitive impairment and behavioral changes. Some studies have considered metabolic differences in cerebral glucose between men and women as an important factor in cognitive decline. These studies have only shown a decreased parietal activity in early onset dementia of AD, independent of a gender effect [42]. Another aspect regarding differences in prevalence of AD among men and women focuses on the roles of estrogen and testosterone in disease pathogenesis, and there are a number of lines of evidence suggesting that estrogen deficiency, following menopause, may contribute to the etiology of AD in women [43,44]. The decreased incidence [45] and a delay in the onset [46] of AD among women on hormone replacement therapy following menopause [47] has also contributed to a belief that these agents may play a relevant role in brain function and cognitive decline associated with aging [48]. However, a decline in estrogen or testosterone does not explain why males with Down's syndrome are at significantly higher risk of developing AD-type changes and at an earlier age than their female counterparts [49]. Indeed, the concentration of estrogen and testosterone in both sexes is similar in patients with Down's syndrome compared to those in the general population. Studies have also cast doubt on estrogen replacement therapy as being protective against AD [50–53].

There are a number of other hormones involved in the hypothalamic–pituitary–gonadal axis that regulate reproductive function and, importantly, receptors for these other hormones are expressed in many nonreproductive tissues including the brain. Supporting evidence indicates that other hormones of the hypothalamic–pituitary–gonadal axis may be playing a central role in the pathogenesis of AD [54].

Several studies of gender differences in cognition have pointed to greater language deficits in women with AD compared with men [55,56]. However, other studies have reported the absence of gender-related language differences or other measures of cognition, including memory and perception, in AD [57,58]. Although the most prominent change noted in patients with AD is decreased cognition, behavioral disturbances also frequently occur. Interestingly, although several reports have suggested that increased behavioral disturbance in AD is related to dementia severity across gender, qualitative differences between men and women in the manifestation of the disturbances have also been reported. Female patients with AD exhibit tendencies to be more reclusive and emotionally labile. In comparison, men with AD show more psychomotor and vegetative changes and aggressive behaviors [59]. Male patients exhibit greater problems than female patients in wandering, abusiveness, and social impropriety, particularly in the more advanced stages of the disorder. In addition, male patients with AD have increased physical, verbal, and sexual aggression than women [60−63]. Depression, on the other hand, does appear to be more prevalent in female than in male patients with AD [63]. Thus, several observations suggest that there may be important genetic factors related to gender that are operative in the pathogenesis of AD. However, it remains controversial whether men and women differ in the incidence of AD and whether there are clearly recognizable sex disparities operating in the cognitive and behavioral changes among those afflicted.

III OXIDATIVE STRESS IN AGING

Oxidative stress results from the shift toward reactive oxygen species (ROS) production in the equilibrium between ROS generation and the antioxidant defense system [64]. In the brain, this is particularly important because studies have found indications of increased OS in brain aging, including reductions in redox active iron [65,66], as well as increases in Bcl-2 [67] and membrane lipid peroxidation [68]. Studies have also shown that there are significant increases in cellular hydrogen peroxide [69]. In addition, there is significant lipofuscin accumulation [65] along with alterations in membrane lipids [70]. Studies have also suggested the involvement of lipid rafts with oxidative stress sensitivity [71]. Importantly, the consequences of these increases in oxidative stress at several levels may result in reduced calcium homeostasis, alterations in cellular signaling cascades, and changes in gene expression [72−77], which combine to contribute to the increased vulnerability to OS seen in the aging population [78,79] and which is elevated in neurodegenerative diseases, such as AD [80−82] and PD [83,84].

Oxidative stress vulnerability in aging may also be the result of microvasculature changes and increases in oxidized proteins and lipids [85], as well as alterations in (1) membrane microenvironment and structure [86,87], (2) calcium buffering ability, and (3) the vulnerability of neurotransmitter receptors to OS (discussed later). Additional "vulnerability factors" include critical declines in endogenous antioxidant protection, involving alterations in the ratio of oxidized to total glutathione [88] and reduced glutamine synthetase [89]. Taken together, these findings indicate that there are increases in OS in aging, that the central nervous system (CNS) may be particularly vulnerable to these increases (for review, see [87,90]), and that the efficacy of antioxidants may be reduced in aging.

Calcium buffering has been shown to be significantly reduced in senescence [91−93]. The consequences of such long-lasting increases in cytosolic calcium may involve cell death induced by several mechanisms (e.g., xanthine oxidase activation [94]), with subsequent pro-oxidant generation and loss of functional capacity of the cell.

However, it is important to note that OS may only be a partial contributor to neuronal and behavioral changes in senescence. For example, OS may contribute to these age-related diseases by inducing the expression of proinflammatory cytokines through activation of the oxidative stress-sensitive nuclear factor kappa B (NF-κB) [95,96]. NF-κB in turn upregulates the inflammatory response leading to a further increase in ROS [97], which results in a continuous increase in oxidative stress and inflammation and thus vulnerability to further stressors.

A Oxidative Stress in Alzheimer's Disease

Various reports have shown increased reactive carbonyls in association with AD [98]. These changes have been identified in senile plaques [99,100], neurofibrillary tangles (NFT) [100,101], and the primary component of the latter, tau protein [101,102]. The significance of these findings was initially questioned by suggestions that the lesions of AD, such as those that occur in vessel walls [103,104], accumulate damage through low protein turnover [105]. What was missing from this criticism was not the accumulative nature of carbonyl modification but, rather, that the products first identified, advanced glycation end products (AGE), are "active modifications," by which we mean they are the result of metal-catalyzed redox chemistry and are continuing sites of redox chemistry [106]. Also, we have demonstrated that the lesions not only are sites of AGE accumulation but also continuing sites of glycation because the initial Amadori product is closely associated with NFT [107].

Early reports of oxidative modifications were followed in close succession by the identification in NFT of reactive carbonyls [108,109] and protein adducts of the lipid per oxidation product, hydroxynonenal [110,111]. What was remarkable in using these different markers resulting either from carbonyl adduction or, in the case of reactive carbonyls, from direct protein oxidation is that whereas highly stable modifications involving cross-linked proteins are predominantly associated with the lesions, metastable modifications are more commonly associated with the neuronal cytoplasm. Specifically, populations of neurons involved in AD, and not others, show this change, suggesting that the most active site of oxidative damage is the neuronal cytoplasm.

Studies analyzing certain physical properties of the oxidized proteins forming cross-linking compounds, specifically those properties that make these biological molecules refractory to light, have shown the presence of modified proteins in the brain of AD patients [112]. In addition, oxidation of the modified proteins not only renders the modified protein more resistant to degradation but also appears to competitively inhibit the proteosome [112]. These changes may underlie the accumulation of ubiquitin conjugates observed in the neurons in AD [113]. Protein nitration is a non-cross-link-related oxidative modification of protein resulting from either peroxynitrite attack or peroxidative nitration. In investigating the distribution of nitrotyrosine in AD, we found that the major site of nitrotyrosine was in the cytoplasm of non-NFT-containing neurons [114] and that neurons containing NFT actually showed lower levels of nitrotyrosine than did similar neurons lacking NFT. These relationships were confirmed when we examined RNA, a cellular component with a relatively rapid turnover rate. A major oxidation product of RNA, 8-hydroxyguanosine (8OHG), has a distribution similar to nitrotyrosine, except that it is absent from NFT and reduced in the surrounding cytoplasm [115], even though NFT contain associated RNA [116]. The concurrence of RNA and protein damage suggests that the major site of oxidative damage in AD is localized predominantly in the neuronal cytoplasm.

B Source of Reactive Oxygen Species

Both location and type of damage are important to understand the source of oxidative damage. First, the location of damage, which involves every category of biomacromolecules, appears to be restricted to neurons. Classically, nitrotyrosine is considered the product of peroxynitrite attack of tyrosine, and 8OHG is considered the product of −OH attack of guanosine. However, the separation is not simple; nitrotyrosine can be formed from peroxidative nitration by nitrite and H_2O_2 and peroxynitrite is produced by the reaction of nitric oxide (NO^-) with superoxide (O_2^-). In the case of peroxidative nitration, treating tissue sections with nitrite and H_2O_2 yields increased nitrotyrosine of the same distribution found during the disease in AD, but not control, cases [117]. An issue with peroxynitrite is diffusibility, being the result of the fusion of NO and O_2^-; it can diffuse several cell diameters from its source to attack vulnerable target proteins [118]. In AD, one of the most striking findings is the restriction of damage to the cell bodies of vulnerable neurons. Although amyloid-β deposits and NFT contain redox-active iron, like oxidative damage, the most conspicuous changes in iron are within the cytoplasm of vulnerable neurons [119,120].

Significantly, cytoplasmic redox-active iron is barely detectable in controls. Redox-active iron is the critical element for Fenton chemistry generation of −OH from H_2O_2. Ultrastructural localization of iron shows it is diffusely associated with the cytoplasm, primarily in the endoplasmic reticulum but also in granules identified as lipofuscin as well as their associated vacuoles.

Lipofuscin is thought to represent the terminal phase of autophagic lysosomes that involve iron-rich mitochondria [121]. Therefore, the increased redox-active iron in such lysosomes in AD lends credence to the notion of mitochondrial abnormalities in AD. Mitochondrial DNA, as well as the protein cytochrome oxidase-I, is increased severalfold in vulnerable neurons in AD. Ultrastructural examination showed, although both markers were in mitochondria, that in AD the increased levels were in the cytoplasm and, in the case of mDNA, in vacuoles associated with lipofuscin, the same sites that showed increased redox-active iron. The majority of iron is in the endoplasmic reticulum, suggesting that the role for mitochondria is probably not to directly supply −OH but instead to supply its precursors, H_2O_2 and redox-active metals. Although the proposed mechanism is distinct from nonmetal-catalyzed peroxynitrite formation, it does not discount an important role for NO. Neurons in AD show activation of NO synthetase as well as its modulator, dimethylargininase [122]. Nitric oxide has strong antioxidant activity (see the next section) as well as inhibitor activity for cytochromes. The latter could play a role in the hypometabolism consistently found in AD [123] as well as the altered mitochondrial dynamics noted here.

C Relationship to Lesions

In AD, the putative source of the ROS was supposed to be the lesions. Amyloid-β by itself was proposed to generate ROS [124]. This mechanism has fallen into question for both chemical and biological issues [125]. Nevertheless, amyloid-β, in some circumstances, can bind iron and promote catalytic redox cycling, yielding reactive oxygen [126]. *In vivo* oxidative damage is inversely correlated to amyloid-β load, indicating that rather than being a source of the reactive oxygen, amyloid-β may be a modulator that can either increase or decrease reactive oxygen production [86,127,128]. Furthermore, the relative paucity of short-lived oxidative changes surrounding amyloid-β deposits [115], rather than those that accumulate in long-lived proteins [100], also puts into question the idea that reactive oxygen resulting from inflammation is an important mechanism for oxidative damage. In fact, although the notion of inflammation in AD is well established [129], this appears to be a secondary response to the underlying pathological changes.

IV INFLAMMATION

As mentioned previously, evidence also suggests that in addition to oxidative stress, CNS inflammatory events may have an important role in affecting neuronal and behavioral deficits in aging [130]. It has been shown that activated glial cells increase in the normal aging brain, which exhibits greater immunoreactivity in markers for both microglia and astrocytes [131–133]. In addition, increased glial fibrillary acid protein expression is observed by middle age [131], and in the elderly this increase even occurs in the absence of a defined stimulus [134]. Glial cells mediate the endogenous immune system within the microenvironment in the CNS [135], and their activation is the hallmark of inflammation in the brain [136]. Activated microglia produce inflammatory molecules such as cytokines, growth factors, and complement proteins [134,137,138]. These proinflammatory mediators in turn activate other cells to produce additional signaling molecules that further activate microglia in a positive feedback loop to perpetuate and amplify the inflammatory signaling cascade [139]. Activated microglia produce proinflammatory cytokines such as interleukin-1 (IL-1), IL-6, and tumor necrosis factor-α (TNF-α) [140,141].

Increases in TNF-α have also been reported as a function of age [142], as well as associated inhibition of glia [143]. Similarly, research in both aged mice and humans has found increases in TNF-α, IL-6 [142–145], and C-reactive protein [146]. All of these changes appear to be accompanied by upregulations in downstream indicators of inflammation (e.g., complement C1q) in microarray studies [147].

In addition, studies indicate that the expression of cyclooxygenase-2 (COX-2) appears to be associated with amyloid-β deposition in the hippocampus [148,149], and inflammatory prostaglandins (PG) such as PGE show increases in the hippocampus, as well as other areas in aging [150]. Because the PG synthesis pathway appears to be a major source of ROS in brain [151] and in other organ systems, these findings indicate that inflammation may be accompanied by and even generate its "evil twin," OS, in producing the deleterious effects of aging. Thus, such factors as cytokines, cyclooxygenases, prostaglandins, and others may act as extracellular signals in generating additional ROS that are associated with decrements in neuronal function or glial neuronal interactions [152–156] and ultimately the deficits in behavior that have been observed in aging.

If this is the case, it should be possible to induce behavioral (cognitive and motor) deficits similar to those seen in aging using procedures that induce oxidative or inflammatory stressors. Indeed, these changes have been induced in several experiments. Rodent studies have suggested that young animals exposed to OS show similar neuronal and behavioral changes to those seen in aged animals. The results have shown that young animals irradiated with particles of high energy and charge show behavioral deficits paralleling those observed in aging [157–159]. High energy and charged particles (specifically 600 MeV or 1 GeV ^{56}Fe) also disrupt the functioning of the dopamine-mediated behaviors, such as motor behavior [160], spatial learning and memory behavior [161], and amphetamine-induced conditioned taste aversion [162].

Inflammatory mediators have been shown to produce similar deficits in behavior [41]. For example, the administration of lipopolysaccharide (LPS) intrahippocampally was found to upregulate inflammatory mediators, inducing degeneration of hippocampal pyramidal neurons, and produced decrements in working memory [40,163,164]. Similarly, the chronic ventricular infusion of LPS into young rats produces many of the same alterations in behavior that have been reported in AD. These changes are accompanied by inflammatory, neurochemical, and neuropathological alterations [40,41,163,165].

Thus, these studies and those reviewed previously suggest that one method to forestall or perhaps even reverse the behavioral declines that have been observed in aging might be to increase endogenous antioxidant/anti-inflammatory protection.

V AGE–ALZHEIMER'S DISEASE PARALLELS

As discussed previously, there are increases in oxidative and inflammatory stressors as a function of age that appear to be involved in the decrements seen in both cognitive and motor behaviors. If this is the case, then it might be postulated that neurodegenerative diseases, which are age dependent, would be superimposed upon an environment already vulnerable to these insults. Indeed, OS plays a major role in the cascade of effects associated with AD (e.g., damage to DNA, protein oxidation, lipid peroxidation [90], and abnormal sequestration of metals [166–168]) that may be independent of amyloid-β deposition. Thus, the free radical perturbations would have an even greater effect in an aged organism because, as noted in the previous sections, there is increased vulnerability to OS and inflammatory insults in senescence. These inflammatory mediators are prominent in the AD brain, and they have also been observed in lower concentrations in nondemented brains from aged individuals. As noted in the previous section, multiple endogenous sources including microglia, astrocytes, and brain endothelial cells can produce these inflammatory mediators in AD [169–172]. Glial cells play important roles in supporting survival of neurons [173–176] and are extraordinarily sensitive to changes in the brain microenvironment. Brain astrocytes (reactive astrocytes) in particular show reactive gliosis to several forms of CNS lesions [177,178]. In addition, gliosis, which can lead to brain damage by several mechanisms [179], is a feature common to virtually every neurodegenerative disease (e.g., multiple sclerosis, AD, tumor, HIV encephalitis, and prion disease) [180–184].

VI POLYPHENOL SUPPLEMENTATION AND REDUCTIONS OF OXIDATIVE STRESS AND INFLAMMATION

There have been numerous studies in which antioxidants have been examined with respect to reducing the deleterious effects of brain aging, with mixed results. However, our research suggests that the combinations of antioxidant/anti-inflammatory polyphenolics found in fruits and vegetables may show efficacy in aging. Plants, including food plants (fruits and vegetables), synthesize a vast array of chemical compounds that are not involved in their primary metabolism. These "secondary metabolites" instead serve a variety of ecological functions, ultimately to enhance the plant's survivability. Interestingly, these compounds also may be responsible for the multitude of beneficial effects of fruits and vegetables on an array of health-related bioactivities; two of the most important may be their antioxidant and anti-inflammatory properties. Because OS appears to be involved in the signaling and behavioral losses seen in senescence, an important question is whether increasing antioxidant or anti-inflammatory intake would forestall or prevent these changes, and the literature is replete with studies (e.g., vitamins E and C [185]) in which a large variety of dietary agents have been employed to alter behavioral and neuronal deficits with aging. Instead, because recent studies have indicated that they have been shown to have considerable efficacy in reducing the deleterious effects of neuronal aging, this chapter focuses more on the antioxidant/anti-inflammatory potential of green tea catechins, curcumin, and berry fruits.

A Green Tea Catechins

Catechins are derived from a number of sources, including green tea, red wine, apples, grapes, and dark chocolate [186]. The most extensively studied have been those from green tea. (−) Epigallocatechin-3-gallate (EGCG) is the primary compound in green tea

that is thought to provide the numerous beneficial effects that have been shown in many studies to provide a number of health benefits ranging from cancer treatment to cardiovascular function. Youdim, Mandel, and colleagues have provided several extensive reviews of the properties and molecular mechanisms involved in the health benefits of EGCG [187]. Thus, an extensive review is not provided here except as these effects relate to neuroprotection, where it appears that the strongest evidence suggests that the primary beneficial properties of EGCG may be its antioxidant, anti-inflammatory, and metal chelating abilities. In addition, these catechins appear to enhance prosurvival genes and, as described later for blueberries, act to enhance neuroprotection and reduce stress signaling. This multiplicity of effects appears to provide a significant protection against oxidative and inflammatory stressors. By far the bulk of the data concerning neuroprotection have been provided by studies showing reduced ischemic-induced neuronal degeneration in various models of cerebral artery occlusion [188–194]. Green tea catechins have also been found to provide significant neuroprotection against N-methyl-4-phenyl-1,2,3,6-tetrahydropyridine (MPTP)-induced neurotoxicity in mice in several experiments (e.g., see [188]). Significant protection has also been seen in numerous *in vitro* experiments in several cell models (as reviewed in [194,195]). Clearly, there appear to be numerous beneficial properties of green tea catechins on several oxidative stress- or inflammatory-mediated conditions. However, the possible benefits in a human population and the amounts of green tea necessary to produce beneficial effects remain to be determined.

B Curcumin

One of the most exciting polyphenolic-containing dietary products that has emerged in the neuroscience literature in recent years is curcumin. Largely as a result of the groundbreaking work of Dr. Greg Cole and colleagues [196], this spice, which has been used to treat illnesses for hundreds of years, has been shown to possess some putative important beneficial effects for neuroprotection and possible treatment in AD. In a manner similar to that seen with respect to the green tea catechins discussed previously and the berries discussed in the next section, curcumin, which is derived from *Curcuma longa* Linn (aka turmeric), appears to have potent anti-inflammatory/antioxidant properties. Moreover, it has also been shown to have potent anticancer effects (for review, see [196]). However, of interest here is curcumin's putative effect on AD. Curcumin supplementation prevented extensive damage following transient forebrain ischemia in

CA1 neurons in the rat [197], suggesting that it may have important neuroprotective properties. In addition, *in vitro* studies have demonstrated that curcumin reduces inflammatory activity of microglial cells [198,199]. Several studies in AD transgenic mice also showed that curcumin downregulated amyloid expression and reduced inflammatory markers [200–202]. Data in humans are still forthcoming, but from the animal and cell experiments, it appears that curcumin may be important in altering the course of plaque deposition and expression of AD.

C Berry Fruits

In our first study, we utilized fruits and vegetables identified as being high in antioxidant activity via the oxygen radical absorbance capacity assay [203–205] and showed that long-term (from age 6 to 15 months in F344 rats) feeding with a supplemented American Institute of Nutrition (AIN)-93 diet (strawberry extract or spinach extract [1 or 2% of the diet] or vitamin E [500 IUD]) retarded age-related decrements in cognitive or neuronal function. Results indicated that the supplemented diets could prevent the onset of age-related deficits in several indices (e.g., cognitive behavior and Morris water maze performance) [206].

In a subsequent experiment [91], we found that dietary supplementation (for 8 weeks) with spinach, strawberry, or blueberry (BB) extracts in an AIN-93 diet was effective in reversing age-related deficits in neuronal and behavioral (cognitive) function in aged (19 months) F344 rats. However, only the BB-supplemented group exhibited improved performance on tests of motor function. Specifically, the BB-supplemented group displayed improved performance on two motor tests that rely on balance and coordination, rod walking, and the accelerating rotarod, whereas none of the other supplemented groups differed from control on these tasks [91]. The rodents in all diet groups, but not the control group, showed improved working memory (short-term memory) performance in the Morris water maze, demonstrated as one-trial learning following the 10-minute retention interval [91]. We also observed significant increases in several indices of neuronal signaling (e.g., muscarinic receptor [MAChR] sensitivity) and found that the BB diet reversed age-related "dysregulation" in Ca^{45} buffering capacity. Examinations of ROS in the brain tissue obtained from animals in the various diet groups indicated that the striata obtained from all of the supplemented groups exhibited significantly lower ROS levels (by assaying DCF; 2′,7′-dichlorofluorescein diacetate) than the controls. A subsequent study using a BB-supplemented NIH-31 diet replicated the previous findings [207]. However, it was clear from these supplementation studies [91,207] that the significant effects of BBs on both motor and cognitive behavior were due to a multiplicity of actions, in addition to those involving antioxidant and anti-inflammatory activity. We have also shown that BB-supplemented senescent animals show increased neurogenesis [208].

With respect to AD, we have shown that BB-supplemented (from age 1 to 12 months) mice transgenic for amyloid precursor protein and presenilin-1 mutations (which show the formation of numerous plaques in the brain, similar to those seen in AD) do not show behavioral deficits in Y-maze performance as seen by those given a control diet [209]. The supplemented mice also showed enhancements in several signaling molecules associated with cognitive function (e.g., extracellular signal-regulated kinase activity). These findings suggest that it is possible to delay or prevent cognitive dysfunction despite the pathological changes in this mouse model and further suggest that the inclusion in the diet of fruits high in antioxidant activity may help prevent the deleterious effects of this disease later in life (Figure 20.1).

D Polyunsaturated Fatty Acids

The major source of omega-3 (eicosapentaenoic acid [EPA]) and omega-6 (docosahexaenoic acid [DHA]) fatty acids is fish oil. Numerous studies have suggested that dietary supplementation with EPA and DHA has a host of beneficial effects in many of the diseases that increase as a function of aging, such as heart disease [210–212], hypertriglyceridemia [213], cancer [214,215], and neurodegenerative disease [216,217]. Studies suggest, for example, that aging mice, which have reduced levels of brain polyunsaturated fatty acids, appear to show alterations in neuronal membranes, such that the mice show memory loss, learning disabilities, cognitive alterations, and even decrements in visual acuity, which can be reduced by supplementing the mice with DHA containing fish oil or DHA [218]. Similar findings have also been seen in the rat [219]. It also appears that AD patients exhibit lower amounts of DHA in plasma [220] and brain [221]. Epidemiologically, it appears that increased DHA or dietary fatty fish intake reduce the risk of AD [222]. Importantly, however, the mechanisms involved in the putative beneficial effects of DHA in these models are not well understood. Florent and colleagues [223] showed that protection against amyloid-β involved activation of ERK1/2 survival pathways. They showed that cortical neurons pretreated with DHA showed less cell death and reduced apoptosis, caspase activity, and arachidonic acid activity. The study by Florent and colleagues [223] supports previous studies in a variety of cell types showing DHA protective effects [224]. In addition to its effects on ERK protective signaling, DHA has also been shown to be the derivative of the docosanoid neuroprotectin D1 (NPD1) that was shown to provide protection against oxidative stress in retinal cells [225]. It also appears that DHA alters membrane lipid rafts to induce phosphatidylserine accumulation in cell membranes, to impinge on additional points in the cell survival pathways (e.g., Akt and Raf-1 [226,227]). Thus, it appears that the protective effects of polyunsaturated fatty acids, much as the fruit polyphenols, may involve enhancing protective signaling pathways.

Results from several studies have indicated that the regular consumption of foods containing omega-3 fatty acid including soybean oil, fish oil, and nuts may lower mortality from cardiovascular disease [228–235]. Importantly, evidence also indicates that tree nuts such as walnuts may be beneficial in cardiovascular disease for their effects on serum lipids (reviewed in [236]). Although studies of nuts are not nearly as extensive as studies on the effects of fish oil, and few studies have focused on the brain effects of tree nuts such as walnuts, one could surmise based on the cardiovascular findings that there may be secondary or primary benefits on neuronal function. Moreover, because tree nuts such as walnuts also contain flavonoids similar to those found in fruits and vegetables, additional benefits might occur from synergistic interactions with the nut-derived fatty acids. Preliminary research from our lab, for example, has shown that senescent rats maintained on a diet containing walnuts showed enhanced performance in both cognitive and motor behaviors relative to the animals maintained on the control diets (unpublished results).

E Putative Signaling Mechanisms Involved in Polyphenol Regulation of Oxidative Stress and Inflammation

There are multiple sources of OS in the cell that result from food metabolism, ionizing radiation, smoking, and so on. There are also mitochondrial sources of ROS that emerge from the energy metabolism of the cell. Importantly, ROS are also generated from inflammatory processes. Subsequently, a great deal of research has shown that there is a cascade of stress signals that are generated from ROS. For example, ROS are believed to play an important role in the pathophysiology of neurodegenerative diseases such as AD or PD, involving the production of inflammatory mediators [237,238].

One of the first steps in the production of these mediators is the generation of the protein kinase C (PKC) family. Of particular importance is the generation of the protein kinase Cγ (PKCγ) isoform, one of the major forms that is found in memory control brain areas such as the hippocampus. Of the different isoforms of PKC present in the brain, the γ subtype is the most abundant representative in the rat hippocampus [239,240]. The PKC pathway is part of a major signal transduction system in inflammation [241] and is activated by several inflammatory agents, including the tumor-promoting phorbol ester PMA (phorbol 12-myristate 13-acetate). The exact mechanism of the involvement of PKC in the stress pathway remains to be determined, but it has been suggested that ROS-induced PKCγ may target lipid rafts [242]. Importantly, PKC isoforms

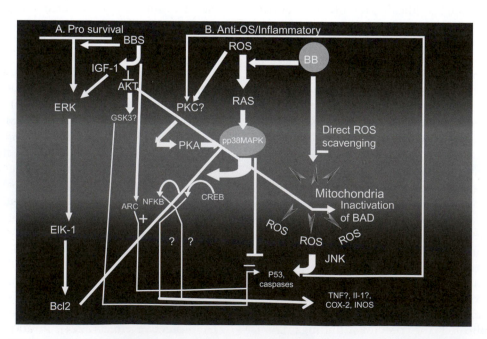

FIGURE 20.1   Possible direct and indirect effects of blueberry supplementation (BBS) that reduce stress signaling and increase survival.

have been associated with the LPS-generated increased production of NO and inducible NO synthase (iNOS) [243]. Moreover, Hall and colleagues [244] found that the induction of PKC from microglial cells via amyloid-β (Aβ)25−35 induced COX-2 expression.

In this respect, microglial cells are a major source of inflammation increasing the production of cytokines and NO, among other compounds, that can induce cell death and decrements in neuronal activity [134,245]. It has been shown that p38 MAPK is intimately involved with microglia activation, the stress response [246], and c-Jun N-terminal kinase (JNK) [247]. Importantly, activation of neuronal p38 MAPK and JNK has been shown to directly disrupt long-term potentiation (LTP), and inhibition of microglial activation was found to prevent LTP disruption [248−251].

An integral part of the stress pathway is the activation of NF-κB. It is present in the cytoplasm in an inhibitory form and attached to an inhibitory protein, IκB, where it is tightly controlled [252]. During stimulation with the uncoupling of IκB, NF-κB translocates to the nucleus and mediates the transcription of many "inflammatory" genes (e.g., COX-2, TNF-α, IL-1β, and iNOS) to further promulgate inflammatory signals and neuronal degeneration [253]. NF-κB usually acts in concert with cyclic AMP response element binding protein (CREB), and research has shown that acute mild hypoxia upregulates CREB at serine 133 (for reviews, see [254,255]). It has also been shown that CREB is activated by hydrogen per oxide in Jurkat T lymphocytes [256] and by cadmium in mouse neuronal cells [257], as well as during stroke [258].

Thus, this brief discussion shows that inflammatory and oxidative stressors can elicit a cascade of signals that result ultimately in the generation of additional stressors, loss of cell function, and, in the case of neurodegenerative disease, reductions in the protective capacity of the organism in senescence. However, it appears from our findings and those of others that polyphenols similar to those contained in berry fruits such as blueberries can activate protective pathways to reduce the deleterious effects of inflammation and oxidative stress. In addition, previous research has shown that under OS or inflammatory conditions, polyphenols similar to those contained in blueberries, tea, red wine, or ginkgo biloba altered signaling in ERK activity (e.g., see [259,260]), as well as PKC [261,262] and CREB [263] in several models described next).

1 BV2 Mouse Microglial Cells

As mentioned previously, accumulating evidence indicates that inflammation in the CNS increases during normal aging and age-related neurodegenerative diseases augment neuroinflammation. Neuroinflammation is largely mediated through the activation of microglial cells. Microglial activation has been attributed to enhanced signal transduction leading to the induction of inflammatory enzymes such as iNOS and COX-2, as well as cytokines such as IL-1β and TNF-α. In an earlier study, we showed that blueberries were effective in attenuating the production of these inflammatory mediators in LPS-activated murine BV2 microglia [264]. To extend these findings, we also examined a purified extract of blueberries (post-C18) and showed a suppression in the LPS-induced increases in iNOS, p38 MAPK, and NF-κB in the BV2 mouse microglial cells.

2 Muscarinic-Transfected Receptors

We and others have shown that there are increases in vulnerability to OS in aging that include striatal MAChR sensitivity to hydrogen peroxide application [265]. Given their importance in a variety of functions including memory [266], amyloid precursor protein (APP) processing [267], and vascular functioning [268], OS and age-sensitive deficits in MAChR may result in the cognitive, behavioral, and neuronal aberrations observed in aging that are exacerbated in AD and vascular dementia. In this regard, findings have indicated that COS-7 cells transfected with one of the five MAChRs and exposed to DA [259] showed differences in OS sensitivity expressed as a function of Ca^{2+} buffering (i.e., the ability to extrude or sequester Ca^{2+} following oxotremorine-induced depolarization). The loss of calcium buffering in these experiments is similar to that reported in many studies with respect to aging [269,270], and such losses can have a profound effect on the functioning and viability of the cell [271−273], further increasing OS [274] and leading ultimately to decrements in motor and memory function in senescent rats [30,275]. It is also important to note that there are significant differences in the rates of aging among various brain regions, with areas such as the hippocampus [275,276], cerebellum [277,278], and striatum [265,279] showing profound alterations with aging in such factors as morphology, electrophysiology, and receptor sensitivity. However, we showed [280] that COS-7 cells transfected with M1 muscarinic receptors (which show increased vulnerability to DA-induced OS) are protected from these changes if pretreated with blueberry extract. Additional analyses suggested that mechanistically the protective effects of blueberries may be derived from their ability to reduce stress signaling. These analyses revealed that blueberry treatment decreased both CREB- and PKCγ-induced signaling increases induced by DA, while increasing protective MAPK signals.

3 Primary Hippocampal Cells

In a subsequent experiment, we showed that deficits in Ca^{2+} buffering induced by DA or Aβ42 in primary hippocampal neuronal cells were antagonized by blueberry extract. The results indicated that Aβ-induced increases in *p*-MAPK were suppressed by blueberries while blueberries further enhanced DA-induced increases in *p*-MAPK. However, blueberries antagonized both DA- and Aβ42-induced increases in PKCγ, *p*-CREB, *p*-p38 MAPK, *p*-JNK, and IGF-1. Previous studies have shown that OS/INF stressors such as Aβ can increase transcription factors (e.g., *p*-CREB) associated with OS/INF and possibly decrease Ca^{2+} homeostasis, but it appears that the beneficial effects of blueberry polyphenols may involve reductions in stress signaling.

VII CONCLUSION

From the previous discussion, it should be clear that there are a number of sources of oxidative stress and inflammation and that these insults are superimposed on an increasingly vulnerable environment in aging. Moreover, in genetic aberrations in conditions such as AD or PD, this vulnerability increases even further. Because this is the case, it is critical that methods be explored to reduce this vulnerability. In this review, we have tried to show that one method of accomplishing this may be through diets containing polyphenols and polyunsaturated fatty acids. An abundance of epidemiological data indicate that diets rich in these compounds, which have antioxidant and anti-inflammatory activities, may play a pivotal role in maintaining human health [281–283]. As data on the brain levels of specific polyphenol forms and their metabolites become available, associations and specific mechanism can be explored in detail.

Therefore, it is important for the diets to contain fruits and vegetables, and this appears to be especially true in fostering healthy aging and possibly in preventing the onset of AD. We have reviewed studies that have shown reversals in age-related cognitive and motor behaviors with fruit or vegetable supplementation [91] and have increased signaling and prevented cognitive decline in APP/PSI mice [209]. In the case of AD, there is an inverse correlation between the intake of wine flavonoids [284] or fruit and vegetable intake [285] and the development of dementia. Thus, these studies, as well as those reviewed previously, suggest a positive role for dietary polyphenols and polyunsaturated fatty acids in both the prevention and the delay of the deleterious effects of aging and AD. Finally, note that studies in cell models indicate that green tea extracts may also be of some benefit in reducing the neurotoxicity associated with PD [286–288]. Given these considerations, it is evident that polyphenols and polyunsaturated fatty acids that have antioxidant and anti-inflammatory properties may be critical elements in a diet to maintain motor and cognitive health throughout the life span and should increase the likelihood of achieving successful aging.

Acknowledgments

The authors thank Dr. Donna Bielinski and Vivian Cheng for their help in the preparation and editing of this chapter.

References

[1] A. Martin, D. Janigian, B. Shukitt-Hale, R.L Prior, J.A. Joseph, Effect of vitamin E intake on levels of vitamins E and C in the central nervous system and peripheral tissues: implications for health recommendations, Brain Res. 845 (1999) 50–59.

[2] A. Martin, A. Cherubini, C. Andres-Lacueva, M. Paniagua, J.A. Joseph, Effects of fruits and vegetables on levels of vitamins E and C in the brain and their association with cognitive performance, J. Nutr. Health Aging 6 (2002) 392–404.

[3] Y. Christen, Ginkgo biloba and neurodegenerative disorders, Front. Biosci. 9 (2004) 3091–3104.

[4] R. Cabeza, C.L. Grady, L. Nyberg, et al., Age- related differences in neural activity during memory encoding and retrieval: a positron emission tomography study, J. Neurosci. 17 (1997) 391–400.

[5] S.A. Small, Y. Stern, M. Tang, R. Mayeux, Selective decline in memory function among healthy elderly, Neurology 52 (1999) 1392–1396.

[6] D.G. Murphy, C. DeCarli, M.B. Schapiro, et al., Age-related differences in volumes of subcortical nuclei, brain matter, and cerebrospinal fluid in healthy men as measured with magnetic resonance imaging, Arch. Neurol. 49 (1992) 839–845.

[7] J.H. Morrison, P.R. Hof, Life and death of neurons in the aging brain, Science 278 (1997) 412–419.

[8] M.J. West, Regionally specific loss of neurons in the aging human hippocampus, Neurobiol. Aging 14 (1993) 287–293.

[9] M.J. Ball, M.J. West, Aging in the human brain: a clarion call to stay the course, Neurobiol. Aging 19 (1998) 1.

[10] A. Peters, J.H. Morrison, D.L. Rosene, B.T. Hyman, Feature article: are neurons lost from the primate cerebral cortex during normal aging? Cereb. Cortex 8 (1998) 295–300.

[11] R.T. Bartus, D. Fleming, H.R. Johnson, Aging in the rhesus monkey: debilitating effects on short-term memory, J. *Gerontol.* 33 (1978) 858–871.

[12] C.L. Grady, A.R. McIntosh, F. Bookstein, et al., Age-related changes in regional cerebral blood flow during working memory for faces, Neuroimage 8 (1998) 409–425.

[13] M.B. Moss, R.J. Killiany, Z.C. Lai, et al., Recognition memory span in rhesus monkeys of advanced age, Neurobiol. Aging 18 (1997) 13–19.

[14] P.R. Rapp, D.G. Amaral, Recognition memory deficits in a subpopulation of aged monkeys resemble the effects of medial temporal lobe damage, Neurobiol. Aging 12 (1991) 481–486.

[15] A.S. Gilinsky, B.B. Judd, Working memory and bias in reasoning across the life span, Psychol. Aging 9 (1994) 356–371.

[16] R. Kail, T.A. Salthouse, Processing speed as a mental capacity, Acta Psychol. (Amst.) (1994) 199–225.

[17] T.W. Robbins, M. James, A.M. Owen, et al., Cambridge Neuropsychological Test Automated Battery (CANTAB): a factor analytic study of a large sample of normal elderly volunteers, Dementia 5 (1994) 266–281.

[18] N. Gould, K. Chadman, PC. Bickford, Antioxidant protection of cerebellar beta-adrenergic receptor function in aged F344 rats, Neurosci. Lett. 250 (1998) 165–168.

[19] J.A. Joseph, R.E. Berger, B.T. Engel, G.S. Roth, Age-related changes in the nigrostriatum: a behavioral and biochemical analysis, J. Gerontol. 33 (1978) 643–649.

[20] C. Cepeda, C.S. Colwell, I.N. Itri, et al., Dopaminergic modulation of NMDA-induced whole cell currents in neostriatal neurons in slices: contribution of calcium conductances, J. Neurophysiol. 79 (1998) 82–94.

[21] T. Egashira, Effects of breeding conditions on neurochemical cholinergic and monoaminergic markers in aged rat brain, Nippon Ronen Igakkai Zasshi 37 (2000) 233–238.

[22] J.A. Joseph, The putative role of free radicals in the loss of neuronal functioning in senescence, Integr. Physiol. Behav. Sci. 27 (1992) 216–227.

[23] J. Kornhuber, K. Schoppmeyer, C. Bendig, P. Riederer, Characterization of [3H]pentazocine binding sites in postmortem human frontal cortex, Neural. Transm. 103 (1996) 45–53.

[24] R.L. Galli, B. Shukitt-Hale, K.A. Youdim, J.A. Joseph, Fruit polyphenolics and brain aging: nutritional interventions targeting age-related neuronal and behavioral deficits, Ann. N. Y. Acad. Sci. 959 (2002) 128–132.

[25] H.G. Kuhn, H. Dickinson-Anson, F.H. Gage, Neurogenesis in the dentate gyrus of the adult rat: age-related decrease of neuronal progenitor proliferation, J. Neurosci. 16 (1996) 2027–2033.

[26] J.A. Joseph, R.T. Bartus, D. Clody, et al., Psychomotor performance in the senescent rodent: reduction of deficits via striatal dopamine receptor up-regulation, Neurobiol. Aging 4 (1983) 313–319.

[27] A. Kluger, J.G. Gianutsos, J. Golomb, et al., Motor/psychomotor dysfunction in normal aging, mild cognitive decline, and early Alzheimer's disease: diagnostic and differential diagnostic features, Int. Psychogeriatr. 9 (Suppl) (1997) 307–321.

[28] R.T. Bartus, Drugs to treat age-related neurodegenerative problems: the final frontier of medical science? J. Am. Geriatr. Soc. 38 (1990) 680–695.

[29] D.K. Ingram, E.L. Spangler, S. Iijima, et al., New pharmacological strategies for cognitive enhancement using a rat model of age-related memory impairment, Ann. N. Y. Acad. Sci. 717 (1994) 16–32.

[30] B. Shukitt-Hale, G. Mouzakis, J.A. Joseph, Psychomotor and spatial memory performance in aging male Fischer 344 rats, Exp. Gerontol. 33 (1998) 615–624.

[31] J.L. Muir, Acetylcholine, aging, and Alzheimer's disease, Pharmacol. Biochem. Behav. 56 (1997) 687–696.

[32] P. Bickford, C. Heron, D.A. Young, Impaired acquisition of novel locomotor tasks in aged and norepinephrine-depleted F344 rats, Neurobiol. Aging 13 (1992) 475–481.

[33] P. Bickford, Motor leaning deficits in aged rats are correlated with loss of cerebellar noradrenergic function, Brain Res. 620 (1993) 133–138.

[34] R.T. Bartus, R.L. Dean, B. Beer, Neuropeptide effects on memory in aged monkeys, Neurobiol. Aging 3 (1982) 61–68.

[35] B.D. Devan, E.H. Goad, H.L. Petri, Dissociation of hippocampal and striatal contributions to spatial navigation in the water maze, Neurobiol. Learn. Mem. 66 (1996) 305–323.

[36] R.J. McDonald, N.M. White, Parallel information processing in the water maze: evidence for independent memory systems involving dorsal striatum and hippocampus, Behav. Neural. Biol. 61 (1994) 260–270.

[37] M.G. Oliveira, O.F. Bueno, A.C. Pomarico, E.B. Gugliano, Strategies used by hippocampal- and caudate putamen-lesioned rats in a learning task, Neurobiol. Learn. Mem. 68 (1997) 32–41.

[38] D.R. Zyzak, T. Otto, H. Eichenbaum, M. Gallagher, Cognitive decline associated with normal aging in rats: a neuropsychological approach, Learn. Mem. 2 (1995) 1–16.

[39] B. Shukitt-Hale, D.E. Smith, M. Meydani, J.A. Ioseph, The effects of dietary antioxidants on psychomotor performance in aged mice, Exp. Gerontol. 34 (1999) 797–808.

[40] B. Hauss-Wegrzyniak, L.B. Willard, P. Del Soldato, et al., Peripheral administration of novel anti-inflammatories can attenuate the effects of chronic inflammation within the CNS, Brain Res. 815 (1999) 36–43.

[41] B. Hauss-Wegrzyniak, M.G. Vannucchi, G.L. Wenk, Behavioral and ultrastructural changes induced by chronic neuroinflammation in young rats, Brain Res. 859 (2000) 157–166.

[42] G.W. Small, D.E. Kuhl, W.H. Riege, et al., Cerebral glucose metabolic patterns in Alzheimer's disease: effect of gender and age at dementia onset, Arch. Gen. Psychiatry 46 (1989) 527–532.

[43] A.F. Jorm, A.E. Korten, A.S. Henderson, The prevalence of dementia: a quantitative integration of the literature, Acta Psychiatr. Scand. 76 (1987) 465–479.

[44] G. McGonigal, B. Thomas, C. McQuade, et al., Epidemiology of Alzheimer's presenile dementia in Scotland, 1974–88, BMJ 306 (1993) 680–683.

[45] V.W. Henderson, A. Paganini-Hill, C.K. Emanuel, et al., Estrogen replacement therapy in older women: comparisons between Alzheimer's disease cases and nondemented control subjects, Arch. Neurol. 51 (1994) 896–900.

[46] M.X. Tang, D. Jacobs, Y. Stem, et al., Effect of oestrogen during menopause on risk and age at onset of Alzheimer's disease, Lancet 348 (1996) 429–432.

[47] C. Kawas, S. Resnick, A. Morrison, et al., A prospective study of estrogen replacement therapy and the risk of developing Alzheimer's disease: the Baltimore Longitudinal Study of Aging, Neurology 48 (1997) 1517–1521.

[48] F.C. Stam, J.M. Wigboldus, A.W. Smeulders, Age incidence of senile brain amyloidosis, Pathol. Res. Pract. 181 (1986) 558–562.

[49] N. Schupf, D. Kapell, B. Nightingale, et al., Earlier onset of Alzheimer's disease in men with Down syndrome, Neurology 50 (1998) 991–995.

[50] R.A. Mulnard, Estrogen as a treatment for Alzheimer's disease, JAMA 284 (2000) 307–308.

[51] R.A. Mulnard, C.W. Cotmau, C. Kawas, et al., Estrogen replacement therapy for treatment of mild to moderate Alzheimer disease: a randomized controlled trial. Alzheimer's disease cooperative study, JAMA 283 (2000) 1007–1015.

[52] P.N. Wang, S.Q. Liao, R.S. Liu, et al., Effects of estrogen on cognition, mood, and cerebral blood flow in AD: a controlled study, Neurology 54 (2000) 2061–2066.

[53] S. Seshadri, G.L. Zornberg, L.E. Derby, et al., Postmenopausal estrogen replacement therapy and the risk of Alzheimer disease, Arch. Neurol. 58 (2001) 435–440.

[54] A.R. Genazzani, M. Gastaldi, B. Bidzinska, et al., The brain as a target organ of gonadal steroids, Psychoneuroendocrinology 17 (1992) 385–390.

[55] D.N. Ripich, S.A. Petrill, P.J. Whitehouse, E.W. Ziol, Gender differences in language of AD patients: a longitudinal study, Neurology 45 (1995) 299–302.

[56] J.G. Buckwalter, E. Sobel, M.E. Dunn, et al., Gender differences on a brief measure of cognitive functioning in Alzheimer's disease, Arch. Neurol. 50 (1993) 757–760.

[57] L.E. Hebert, R.S. Wilson, D.W. Gilley, et al., Decline of language among women and men with Alzheimer's disease, J. Gerontol. B Psychol. Sci. Soc. 55 (2000) P354–P360.

[58] K.A. Bayles, T. Azuma, R.F. Cruz, et al., Gender differences in language of Alzheimer disease patients revisited, Alzheimer Dis. Assoc. Disord. 13 (1999) 138–146.

[59] B.R. Ott, C.A. Tate, N.M. Gordon, W.E. Heindel, Gender differences in the behavioral manifestations of Alzheimer's disease, J. Am. Geriatr. Soc. 44 (1996) 583–587.

[60] D.A. Drachman, J.M. Swearer, B.F. O'Donnell, et al., The Caretaker Obstreperous-Behavior Rating Assessment (COBRA) scale, J. Am. Geriatr. Soc. 40 (1992) 463–470.

[61] C.G. Lyketsos, C. Steele, E. Galik, et al., Physical aggression in dementia patients and its relationship to depression, Am. J. Psychiatry 156 (1999) 66–71.

[62] C.G. Lyketsos, L.S. Chen, J.C. Authony, Cognitive decline in adulthood: an 11.5-year follow-up of the Baltimore Epidemiologic Catchment Area Study, Am. J. Psychiatry 156 (1999) 58–65.

[63] D Cohen, C. Eisdorfer, P. Gorelick, Sex differences in the psychiatric manifestations of Alzheimer's disease, J. Am. Geriatr. Soc. 41 (1993) 229–232.

[64] B. Halliwell, J.M. Gutteridge, Oxygen radicals and the nervous system, Trends Neurosci. 8 (1985) 22–26.

[65] E.P. Gilissen, R.E. Jacobs, J.M. Allman, Magnetic resonance microscopy of iron in the basal forebrain cholinergic structures of the aged mouse lemur, J. Neurol. Sci. 168 (1999) 21–27.

[66] J. Savory, J.K. Rao, Y. Huang, P.R. Letada, M.M. Herman, Age-related hippocampal changes in Bcl-2:Baxratio, oxidative stress, redox-active iron and apoptosis associated with aluminum-induced neurodegeneration: increased susceptibility with aging, Neurotoxicology 20 (1999) 805–817.

[67] R. Sadoul, Bcl-2 family members in the development and degenerative pathologies of the nervous system, Cell Death Differ. 5 (1998) 805–815.

[68] B.P. Yu, Cellular defenses against damage from reactive oxygen species (published erratum appears in *Physiol. Rev.* 1995 Jan., **75** (1): preceding 1) Physiol. Rev. 74 (1994) 139–162.

[69] M. Cavazzoni, S. Barogi, A. Baracca, G. Parenti Castelli, G. Lenaz, The effect of aging and an oxidative stress on peroxide levels and the mitochondrial membrane potential in isolated rat hepatocytes, FEBS Lett. 449 (1999) 53–56.

[70] N.A. Denisova, S.A. Erat, J.F. Kelly, G.S. Roth, Differential effect of aging on cholesterol modulation of carbachol-stimulated low-K(m) GTPase in striatal synaptosomes, Exp. Gerontol. 33 (1998) 249–265.

[71] H.M. Shen, Y. Lin, S. Choksi, J. Tran, T. Jin, L. Chang, et al., Essential roles of receptor-interacting protein and TRAF2 in oxidative stress-induced cell death, Mol. Cell Biol. 24 (2004) 5914–5922.

[72] L. Annunziato, A. Pannaccione, M. Cataldi, A. Secondo, P. Castaldo, G. Di Renzo, et al., Modulation of ion channels by reactive oxygen and nitrogen species: a pathophysiological role in brain aging? Neurobiol. Aging 23 (2002) 819–834.

[73] T.P. Dalton, H.G. Shertzer, A. Puga, Regulation of gene expression by reactive oxygen, Annu. Rev. Pharmacol. Toxicol. 39 (1999) 67–101.

[74] K.J. Davies, Oxidative stress, antioxidant defenses, and damage removal, repair, and replacement systems, IUBMB Life 50 (2000) 279–289.

[75] K.A. Hughes, R.M. Reynolds, Evolutionary and mechanistic theories of aging, Annu. Rev. Entomol. 50 (2005) 421–445.

[76] R. Perez-Campo, M. Lopez-Torres, S. Cadenas, C. Rojas, G. Barja, The rate of free radical production as a determinant of the rate of aging: evidence from the comparative approach, J. Comp. Physiol. B 168 (1998) 149–158.

[77] P. Waring, Redox active calcium ion channels and cell death, Arch. Biochem. Biophys. 434 (2005) 33–42.

[78] B. Halliwell, Role of free radicals in the neurodegenerative diseases: therapeutic implications for antioxidant treatment, Drugs Aging 18 (2001) 685–716.

[79] A.C. Rego, C.R. Oliveira, Mitochondrial dysfunction and reactive oxygen species in excitotoxicity and apoptosis: implications for the pathogenesis of neurodegenerative diseases, Neurochem. Res. 28 (2003) 1563–1574.

[80] M.A. Lovell, W.D. Ehmann, S.M. Butler, W.R. Markesbery, Elevated thiobarbituric acid-reactive substances and antioxidant enzyme activity in the brain in Alzheimer's disease, Neurology 45 (1995) 1594–1601.

[81] D.L. Marcus, C. Thomas, C. Rodriguez, K. Simberkoff, J.S. Tsai, J.A. Strafaci, et al., Increased peroxidation and reduced antioxidant enzyme activity in Alzheimer's disease, Exp. Neurol. 150 (1998) 40–44.

[82] C.D. Smith, J.M. Carney, P.E. Starke-Reed, C.N. Oliver, E.R. Stadtman, R.A. Floyd, et al., Excess brain protein oxidation and enzyme dysfunction in normal aging and in Alzheimer disease, Proc. Natl. Acad. Sci. USA 88 (1991) 10540–10543.

[83] D.T. Dexter, A.E. Holley, W.D. Flitter, T.F. Slater, F.R. Wells, S.E. Daniel, et al., Increased levels of lipid hydroperoxides in the parkinsonian substantia nigra: an HPLC and ESR study, Mov. Disord. 9 (1994) 92–97.

[84] J.P. Spencer, P. Jenner, S.E. Daniel, A.J. Lees, D.C. Marsden, B. Halliwell, Conjugates of catecholamines with cysteine and GSH in Parkinson's disease: possible mechanisms of formation involving reactive oxygen species, J. Neurochem. 71 (1998) 2112–2222.

[85] R.A. Floyd, K. Hensley, Oxidative stress in brain aging: implications for therapeutics of neurodegenerative diseases, Neurobiol. Aging 23 (2002) 795–807.

[86] J. Joseph, B. Shukitt-Hale, N.A. Denisova, A. Martin, G. Perry, M.A. Smith, Copernicus revisited: amyloid beta in Alzheimer's disease, Neurobiol. Aging 22 (2001) 131–146.

[87] J.A. Joseph, N. Denisova, D. Fisher, B. Shukitt-Hale, P. Bickford, R. Prior, et al., Membrane and receptor modifications of oxidative stress vulnerability in aging: nutritional considerations, Ann. N. Y. Acad. Sci. 854 (1998) 268–276.

[88] C.W. Olanow, An introduction to the free radical hypothesis in Parkinson's disease, Ann. Neurol. 32 (Suppl.) (1992) S2–S9.

[89] J.M. Carney, C.D. Smith, A.M. Carney, D.A. Butterfield, Aging- and oxygen-induced modifications in brain biochemistry and behavior, Ann. N. Y. Acad. Sci. 738 (1994) 44–53.

[90] J.A. Joseph, N. Denisova, D. Fisher, P. Bickford, R. Prior, G. Cao, Age-related neurodegeneration and oxidative stress: putative nutritional intervention, Neurol. Clin. 16 (1998) 747–755.

[91] J.A. Joseph, B. Shukitt-Hale, N.A. Denisova, D. Bielinski, A. Martin, J.J. McEwen, et al., Reversals of age-related declines in neuronal signal transduction, cognitive, and motor behavioral deficits with blueberry, spinach, or strawberry dietary supplementation, J. Neurosci. 19 (1999) 8114–8121.

[92] P.W. Landfield, J.C. Eldridge, The glucocorticoid hypothesis of age-related hippocampal neurodegeneration: role of dysregulated intraneuronal Ca2þ, Ann. N. Y. Acad. Sci. 746 (1994) 308–321.

[93] E.C. Toescu, A. Verkhratsky, Ca2þ and mitochondria as substrates for deficits in synaptic plasticity in normal brain ageing, J. Cell Mol. Med. 8 (2004) 181–190.

[94] Y. Cheng, P. Wixom, M.R. James-Kracke, A.Y. Sun, Effects of extracellular ATP on Fe2þ-induced cytotoxicity in PC-12 cells, J. Neurochem. 66 (1994) 895–902.

[95] N. Durany, G. Munch, T. Michel, P. Riederer, Investigations on oxidative stress and therapeutical implications in dementia, Eur. Arch. Psychiatry Clin. Neurosci. 249 (Suppl. 3) (1999) 68–73.

[96] G. Munch, R. Schinzel, C. Loske, A. Wong, N. Durany, J.J. Li, et al., Alzheimer's disease—Synergistic effects of glucose deficit, oxidative stress and advanced glycation endproducts, J. Neural. Transm. 105 (1998) 439–461.

[97] N. Lane, A unifying view of ageing and disease: the double-agent theory, J. Theor. Biol. 225 (2003) 531–540.

[98] C.D. Smith, J.M. Carney, T. Tatsumo, et al., Protein oxidation in aging brain, Ann. N. Y. Acad. Sci. 663 (1992) 110–119.

[99] M.P. Vitek, K. Bhattacharya, J.M. Glendening, et al., Advanced glycation end products contribute to amyloidosis in Alzheimer disease, Proc. Natl. Acad. Sci. USA 91 (1994) 4766–4770.

[100] M.A. Smith, S. Taneda, P.I. Richey, et al., Advanced Maillard reaction end products are associated with Alzheimer disease pathology, Proc. Natl. Acad. Sci. USA 91 (1994) 5710–5714.

[101] S.D. Yan, X. Chen, A.M. Schmidt, et al., Glycated tau protein in Alzheimer disease: a mechanism for induction of oxidant stress, Proc. Natl. Acad. Sci. USA 91 (1994) 7787–7791.

[102] M.D. Ledesma, P. Bonay, C. Colaco, J. Avila, Analysis of microtubule associated protein tau glycation in paired helical filaments, J. Biol. Chem. 269 (1994) 21614–21619.

[103] R.G. Salomon, G. Subbanagounder, J. O'Neil, et al., Levuglandin E2-protein adducts in human plasma and vasculature, Chem. Res. Toxicol. 10 (1997) 536–545.

[104] L.M. Sayre, G. Perry, M.A. Smith, In situ methods for detection and localization of markers of oxidative stress: application in neurodegenerative disorders, Methods Enzymol. 309 (1999) 133–152.

[105] M.P. Mattson, J.W. Carney, D.A. Butterfield, A tombstone in Alzheimer's? Nature 373 (1995) 481.

[106] M.A. Smith, L.M. Sayre, M.P. Vitek, et al., Early AGEing and Alzheimer's, Nature 374 (1995) 316.

[107] R.J. Castellani, P.I. Harris, L.M. Sayre, et al., Active glycation in neurofibrillary pathology of Alzheimer disease: N(epsilon)-(carboxymethyl) lysine and hexitol-lysine, Free Radic. Biol. Med. 31 (2001) 175–180.

[108] M.A. Smith, G. Perry, P.I. Richey, et al., Oxidative damage in Alzheimer's, Nature 382 (1996) 120–121.

[109] M.A. Smith, L.M. Sayre, V.E. Anderson, et al., Cytochemical demonstration of oxidative damage in Alzheimer disease by immunochemical enhancement of the carbonyl reaction with 2,4-dinitrophenylhydrazine, J. Histochem. Cytochem. 46 (1998) 731–735.

[110] T.J. Montine, V. Amarnath, M.E. Martin, et al., E-4-hydroxy-2-nonenal is cytotoxic and cross-links cytoskeletal proteins in P19 neuroglial cultures, Am. J. Pathol. 148 (1996) 8993.

[111] L.M. Sayre, D.A. Zelasko, P.I. Harris, et al., 4-Hydroxynoueual-derived advanced lipid peroxidation end products are increased in Alzheimer's disease, J. Neurochem. 68 (1997) 2092–2097.

[112] B. Friguet, E.R. Stadtman, L.I. Szweda, Modification of glucose-6-phosphate dehydrogenase by 4-hydroxy-2-nonenal: formation of cross-linked protein that inhibits the multicatalytic protease, J. Biol. Chem. 269 (1994) 21639–21643.

[113] H. Mori, J. Kondo, Y. Ihara, Ubiquitin is a component of paired helical filaments in Alzheimer's disease, Science 235 (1987) 1641–1644.

[114] M.A. Smith, P.I. Richey Harris, L.M Sayre, et al., Widespread peroxynitrite-mediated damage in Alzheimer's disease, J. Neurosci. 17 (1997) 2653–2657.

[115] A. Nunomura, G. Perry, M.A Pappolla, et al., RNA oxidation is a prominent feature of vulnerable neurons in Alzheimer's disease, J. Neurosci. 19 (1999) 1959–1964.

[116] S.D. Ginsberg, P.B. Crino, V.M. Lee, et al., Sequestration of RNA in Alzheimer's disease neurofibrillary tangles and senile plaques, Ann. Neurol. 41 (1997) 200–209.

[117] A. Nunomura, G. Perry, G. Aliev, et al., Oxidative damage is the earliest event in Alzheimer disease, J. Neuropathol. Exp. Neurol. 60 (2001) 759–767.

[118] J.B. Sampson, Y. Ye, H. Rosen, J.S. Beckman, Myeloperoxidase and horseradish peroxidase catalyze tyrosine nitration in proteins from nitrite and hydrogen peroxide, Arch. Bioehem. Biophys. 356 (1998) 207–213.

[119] M.A. Smith, P.I. Harris, L.M. Sayre, G. Pelty, Iron accumulation in Alzheimer disease is a source of redox-generated free radicals, Proc. Natl. Acad. Sci. USA 94 (1997) 9866–9868.

[120] L.M. Sayre, G. Perry, P.I. Hatris, et al., In situ oxidative catalysis by neurofibrillary tangles and senile plaques in Alzheimer's disease: a central role for bound transition metals, J. Neurochem. 74 (2000) 270–279.

[121] U.T. Brunk, C.B. Jones, R.S. Sohal, A novel hypothesis of lipofuscinogenesis and cellular aging based on interactions between oxidative stress and autophagocytosis, Mutat. Res. 275 (1992) 395–403.

[122] M.A. Smith, M. Vasak, M. Knipp, et al., Dimethylargininase, a nitric oxide regulatory protein, in Alzheimer disease, Free Radic. Biol. Med. 25 (1998) 898–902.

[123] G.W. Small, J.C. Mazziotta, M.T. Collins, et al., Apolipoprotein E type 4 allele and cerebral glucose metabolism in relatives at risk for familial Alzheimer disease, JAMA 273 (1995) 942–947.

[124] K. Hensley, J.M. Carney, M.P. Mattson, et al., A model for beta-amyloid aggregation and neurotoxicity based on free radical generation by the peptide: relevance to Alzheimer disease, Proc. Natl. Acad. Sci. USA 91 (1994) 3270–3274.

[125] L.M. Sayre, M.G. Zagorski, W.K. Surewicz, et al., Mechanisms of neurotoxicity associated with amyloid beta deposition and the role of free radicals in the pathogenesis of Alzheimer's disease: a critical appraisal, Chem. Res. Toxicol. 10 (1997) 518–526.

[126] C.A. Rottkamp, A.K. Raina, X. Zhu, et al., Redox-active iron mediates amyloid-beta toxicity, Free Radic. Biol. Med. 30 (2001) 447–450.

[127] G. Perry, A. Nunomura, A.K. Raina, M.A. Smith, Amyloid-beta junkies, Lancet 355 (2000) 757.

[128] M.A. Smith, J.A. Joseph, G. Peny, Arson: tracking the culprit in Alzheimer's disease, Ann. N. Y. Acad. Sci. 924 (2000) 35–38.

[129] W.J. Lukiw, N.G. Bazan, Neuroinflammatory signaling upregulation in Alzheimer's disease, Neurochem. Res. 25 (2000) 1173–1184.

[130] A.M. Bodles, S.W. Barger, Cytokines and the aging brain: what we don't know might help us, Trends Neurosci. 27 (2004) 621–626.

[131] I. Rozovsky, C.E. Finch, T.E. Morgan, Age-related activation of microglia and astrocytes, Neurobiol. Aging 19 (1998) 97–103.

[132] J.G. Sheng, R.E. Mrak, W.S. Griffin, Enlarged and phagocytic, but not primed, interleukin-1 alpha-immunoreactive microglia increase with age in normal human brain, Acta Neuropathol. (Berlin) 95 (1998) 229–234.

[133] J.A. Sloane, W. Hollander, M.B. Moss, D.L. Rosene, C.R. Abraham, Increased microglial activation and protein nitration in white matter of the aging monkey, Neurobiol. Aging 20 (1999) 395–405.

[134] P.L. McGeer, E.G. McGeer, The inflammatory response system of brain: implications for therapy of Alzheimer and other neurodegenerative diseases, Brain Res. Rev. 21 (2) (1995) 195–218.

[135] G.W. Kreutzberg, Microglia: a sensor for pathological events in the CNS, Trends Neurosci. 19 (1996) 312–318.

[136] C.F. Orr, D.B. Rowe, G.M. Halliday, An inflammatory review of Parkinson's disease, Prog. Neurobiol. 68 (2002) 325–340.

[137] S. Chen, R.C. Frederickson, K.R. Brunden, Neuroglial-mediated immunoinflammatory responses in Alzheimer's disease: complement activation and therapeutic approaches, Neurobiol. Aging 17 (1996) 781–787.

[138] V. Darley-Usmar, H. Wiseman, B. Halliwell, Nitric oxide and oxygen radicals: a question of balance, FEBS Lett. 369 (1995) 131–135.

[139] R.A. Floyd, Neuroinflammatory processes are important in neurodegenerative diseases: an hypothesis to explain the increased formation of reactive oxygen and nitrogen species as major factors involved in neurodegenerative disease development, Free Radic. Biol. Med. 26 (1999) 1346–1355.

[140] J.D. Luterman, V. Haroutunian, S. Yemul, L. Ho, D. Purohit, P.S. Aisen, et al., Cytokine gene expression as a function of the clinical progression of Alzheimer disease dementia, Arch. Neurol. 57 (2000) 1153–1160.

[141] E. Tarkowski, A.M. Liljeroth, L. Minthon, A. Tarkowski, A. Wallin, K. Blennow, Cerebral pattern of pro- and anti-inflammatory cytokines in dementias, Brain Res. Bull. 61 (2003) 255–260.

[142] H.N. Chang, S.R. Wang, S.C. Chiang, W.J. Teng, M.L. Chen, J.J. Tsai, et al., The relationship of aging to endotoxin shock and to production of TNF-α, J. Gerontol. 51 (1996) M220–M222.

[143] R.C. Chang, W. Chen, P. Hudson, B. Wilson, D.S. Han, J.S. Hong, Neurons reduce glial responses to lipopolysaccharide (LPS) and prevent injury of microglial cells from over-activation by LPS, J. Neurochem. 76 (2001) 1042–1049.

[144] C.C. Spaulding, R.L. Walford, R.B. Effros, Calorie restriction inhibits the age-related dysregulation of the cytokines TNF-alpha and IL-6 in C3B10RF1 mice, Mech. Ageing Dev. 93 (1997) 87–94.

[145] S. Volpato, J.M. Guralnik, L. Ferrucci, J. Balfour, P. Chaves, L.P. Fried, et al., Cardiovascular disease, interleukin-6, and risk of mortality in older women: the Women's Health and Aging Study, Circulation 103 (2001) 947–953.

[146] I. Kushner, C-reactive protein elevation can be caused by conditions other than inflammation and may reflect biologic aging, Cleveland Clin. J. Med. 68 (2001) 535–537.

[147] R. Weindruch, T. Kayo, C.K. Lee, T.A. Prolla, Microarray profiling of gene expression in aging and its alteration by caloric restriction in mice, J. Nutr. 131 (2001) 918S–923S.

[148] L. Ho, C. Pieroni, D. Winger, D.P. Purohit, P.S. Aisen, G.M. Pasinetti, Regional distribution of cyclooxygenase-2 in the hippocampal formation in Alzheimer's disease, J. Neurosci. Res. 57 (1999) 295–303.

[149] J.J. Hoozemans, M.K. Bruckner, A.J. Rozemuller, R. Veerhuis, P. Eikelenboom, T. Arendt, Cyclin D1 and cyclin E are co-localized with cyclooxygenase 2 (COX-2) in pyramidal neurons in Alzheimer disease temporal cortex, J. Neuropathol. Exp. Neurol. 61 (2002) 678–688.

[150] P. Casolini, A. Catalani, A.R. Zuena, L. Angelucci, Inhibition of COX-2 reduces the age-dependent increase of hippocampal inflammatory markers, corticosterone secretion, and behavioral impairments in the rat, J. Neurosci. Res. 68 (2002) 337–343.

[151] B.S. Baek, J.W. Kim, J.H. Lee, H.J. Kwon, N.D. Kim, H.S. Kang, et al., Age-related increase of brain cyclooxygenase activity and dietary modulation of oxidative status, J. Gerontol. A Biol. Sci. Med. Sci. 56 (2001) B426–B431.

[152] S. Rosenman, P. Shrikant, L. Dubb, E. Benveniste, R. Ransohoff, Cytokine-induced expression of vascular cell adhesion molecule-1 (VCAM-1) by astrocytes and astrocytoma cell lines, J. Immunol. 154 (1995) 1888–1899.

[153] H. Schipper, Astrocytes, brain aging, and neurodegeneration, Neurobiol. Aging 17 (1996) 467–480.

[154] B. Steffen, G. Breier, E. Butcher, M. Schulz, B. Engelhardt, ICAM-1, VCAM-1, and MAdCAM-1 are expressed on choroid plexus epithelium but not endothelium and mediate binding of lymphocytes in vitro, Am. J. Pathol. 148 (1996) 1819–1838.

[155] N. Stella, A. Estelles, J. Siciliano, M. Tence, S. Desagher, D. Piomelli, et al., Interleukin-1 enhances the ATP-evoked release of arachidonic acid from mouse astrocytes, J. Neurosci. 17 (9) (1997) 2939–2946.

[156] M.N. Woodroofe, Cytokine production in the central nervous system, Neurology 45 (Suppl. 6) (1995) S6–S10.

[157] J.A. Joseph, S. Erat, B.M. Rabin, CNS effects of heavy particle irradiation in space: behavioral implications, Adv. Space Res. 22 (1998) 209–216.

[158] J.A. Joseph, B. Shukitt-Hale, J. McEwen, B.M. Rabin, CNS-induced deficits of heavy particle irradiation in space: the aging connection, Adv. Space Res. 25 (2000) 2057–2064.

[159] B. Shukitt-Hale, G. Casadesus, J.J. McEwen, B.M. Rabin, J.A. Joseph, Spatial learning and memory deficits induced by exposure to iron-56-particle radiation, Radiat. Res. 154 (2000) 28–33.

[160] J.A. Joseph, W.A. Hunt, B.M. Rabin, T.K. Dalton, Possible "accelerated striatal aging" induced by 56Fe heavy-particle irradiation: implications for manned space flights, Radiat. Res. 130 (1992) 88–93.

[161] B.M. Rabin, J.A. Joseph, S. Erat, Effects of exposure to different types of radiation on behaviors mediated by peripheral or central systems, Adv. Space Res. 22 (1998) 217–225.

[162] P.C. Bickford, B. Shukitt-Hale, J.A. Joseph, Effects of aging on cerebellar noradrenergic function and motor learning: nutritional interventions, Mech. Ageing Dev. 111 (1999) 141–154.

[163] B. Hauss-Wegrzyniak, P. Dobrzanski, J.D. Stoehr, G.L. Wenk, Chronic neuroinflammation in rats reproduces components of the neurobiology of Alzheimer's disease, Brain Res. 780 (1998) 294–303.

[164] K. Yamada, Y. Komori, T. Tanaka, K. Senzaki, T. Nikai, H. Sugihara, et al., Brain dysfunction associated with an induction of nitric oxide synthase following an intracerebral injection of lipopolysaccharide in rats, Neuroscience 88 (1999) 281–294.

[165] B. Hauss-Wegrzyniak, P. Vraniak, G.L. Wenk, The effects of a novel NSAID on chronic neuroinflammation are age dependent, Neurobiol. Aging 20 (1999) 305–313.

[166] Y. Christen, Oxidative stress and Alzheimer disease, Am. J. Clin. Nutr. 71 (2000) 621S–629S.

[167] W.R. Markesbery, J.M. Carney, Oxidative alterations in Alzheimer's disease, Brain Pathol. 9 (1999) 133–146.

[168] D. Ham, H.M. Schipper, Heme oxygenase-I induction and mitochondrial iron sequestration in astroglia exposed to amyloid peptides, Cell Mol. Biol. (Noisy-le-grand) 46 (2000) 587–596.

[169] U. Agrimi, G. Di Guardo, Amyloid, amyloid inducers, cytokines and heavy metals in scrapie and other human and animal subacute spongiform encephalopathies: some hypotheses, Med. Hypotheses 40 (1993) 113–116.

[170] D. Paris, K.P. Townsend, D.F. Obregon, et al., Pro-inflammatory effect of freshly solubilized beta-amyloid peptides in the brain, Prostaglandins Other Lipid Mediat. 70 (2002) 1–12.

[171] L Meda, P. Baron, G. Scarlato, Glial activation in Alzheimer's disease: the role of Aβ and its associated proteins, Neurobiol. Aging 22 (2001) 885–893.

[172] E. McGeer, P. McGeer, The importance of inflammatory mechanisms in Alzheimer disease, Exp. Gerontol. 33 (1998) 371–378.

[173] M. Yoshida, H. Saito, H. Katsuki, Neurotrophic effects of conditioned media of astrocytes isolated from different brain regions on hippocampal and cortical neurons, Experientia 51 (1995) 133–136.

[174] S. Wiese, F. Metzger, B. Holtmann, M. Sendtner, Mechanical and excitotoxic lesion of motoneurons: effects of neurotrophins and ciliary neurotrophic factor on survival and regeneration, Acta Neurochir. Suppl. (Wien) 73 (1999) 31–39.

[175] G. Paratcha, F. Ledda, L. Baars, et al., Released GFR alpha 1 potentiates downstream signaling, neuronal survival, and

differentiation via a novel mechanism of recruitment of c-Ret to lipid rafts, Neuron 29 (2001) 171–184.

[176] W.P. Rakowicz, C.S. Staples, J. Milbrandt, et al., Glial cell line-derived neurotrophic factor promotes the survival of early postnatal spinal motor neurons in the lateral and medial motor columns in slice culture, J. Neurosci. 22 (2002) 3953–3962.

[177] D. Garcia-Ovejero, S. Veiga, L.M. Garcia-Segura, L.L. Doncarlos, Glial expression of estrogen and androgen receptors after rat brain injury, J. Camp. Neurol. 450 (2002) 256–271.

[178] S.K. Malhotra, T.K. Shnitka, J. Elbrink, Reactive astrocytes: a review, Cytobios 61 (1990) 133–160.

[179] J. McGraw, G.W. Hiebert, J.D. Steeves, Modulating astrogliosis after neurotrauma, J. Neurosci. Res. 63 (2001) 109–115.

[180] D.R. Brown, Microglia and prion disease, Microsc. Res. Tech. 54 (2001) 71–80.

[181] Y. Persidsky, J. Limoges, J. Rasmussen, et al., Reduction in glial immunity and neuropathology by a PAF antagonist and an MMP and TNFα inhibitor in SCID mice with HIV-I encephalitis, J. Neuroimmunol. 114 (2001) 57–68.

[182] F.P. Gendron, J.T. Neary, P.M. Theiss, et al., Mechanisms of P2X7 receptor-mediated ERKl/2 phosphorylation in human astrocytoma cells, Am. J. Physiol. Cell. Physiol. 284 (2003) C571–C581.

[183] M.C. Irizarry, B.T. Hyman, Alzheimer disease therapeutics, J. Neuropathol. Exp. Neural. 60 (2001) 923–928.

[184] K. Kobayashi, M. Hayashi, H. Nakano, et al., Apoptosis of astrocytes with enhanced lysosomal activity and oligodendrocytes in white matter lesions in Alzheimer's disease, Neuropathol. Appl. Neurobiol. 28 (2002) 238–251.

[185] A. Martin, R. Prior, B. Shukitt-Hale, G. Cao, J.A. Joseph, Effect of fruits, vegetables, or vitamin E-rich diet on vitamins E and C distribution in peripheral and brain tissues: implications for brain function, J. Gerontol. A Biol. Sci. Med. Sci. 55 (2000) B144–B151.

[186] B.A. Sutherland, R.M. Rahman, I. Appleton, Mechanisms of action of green tea catechins, with a focus on ischemia-induced neurodegeneration, J. Nutr. Biochem. 17 (2006) 291–306.

[187] S.A. Mandel, Y. Avramovich-Tirosh, L. Reznichenko, H. Zheng, O. Weinreb, T. Amit, et al., Multi functional activities of green tea catechins in neuroprotection: modulation of cell survival genes, iron-dependent oxidative stress and PKC signaling pathway, Neurosignals 14 (2005) 46–60.

[188] F. Dajas, F. Rivera, F. Blasina, F. Arredondo, C. Echeverry, L. Lafon, et al., Cell culture protection and in vivo neuroprotective capacity of flavonoids, Neurotox. Res. 5 (2003) 425–432.

[189] F. Rivera, J. Urbanavicius, E. Gervaz, A. Morquio, F. Dajas, Some aspects of the in vivo neuroprotective capacity of flavonoids: bioavailability and structure–activity relationship, Neurotox. Res. 6 (2004) 543–553.

[190] J.T. Hong, S.R. Ryu, H.J. Kim, J.K. Lee, S.H. Lee, D.B. Kim, et al., Neuroprotective effect of green tea extract in experimental ischemia–reperfusion brain injury, Brain Res. Bull. 53 (2000) 743–749.

[191] Y.B. Choi, Y.I. Kim, K.S. Lee, B.S. Kim, D.J. Kim, Protective effect of epigallocatechin gallate on brain damage after transient middle cerebral artery occlusion in rats, Brain Res. 1019 (2004) 47–54.

[192] Y. Matsuoka, H. Hasegawa, S. Okuda, T. Muraki, T. Uruno, K. Kubota, Ameliorative effects of tea catechins on active oxygen-related nerve cell injuries, J. Pharmacol. Exp. Ther. 274 (1995) 602–608.

[193] M. Suzuki, M. Tabuchi, M. Ikeda, K. Umegaki, T. Tomita, Protective effects of green tea catechins on cerebral ischemic damage, Med. Sci. Monit. 10 (2004) BR166–BR174.

[194] B.A. Sutherland, O.M. Shaw, A.N. Clarkson, D.N. Jackson, I.A. Sammut, I. Appleton, Neuroprotective effects of (−)-epigallocatechin gallate following hypoxia–ischemia-induced brain damage: novel mechanisms of action, FASEB J 19 (2005) 258–260.

[195] Y. Levites, O. Weinreb, G. Maor, M.B.H. Youdim, S. Mandel, Green tea polyphenol (−)-epigallocatechin-3-gallate prevents N-methyl-4-phenyl-1,2,3,6-tetrahydropyridine-induced dopaminergic neurodegeneration, J. Neurochem. 78 (2001) 1073–1082.

[196] J.M. Ringman, S.A. Frautschy, G.M. Cole, D.L. Masterman, J.L. Cummings, A potential role of the curry spice curcumin in Alzheimer's disease, Curr. Alzheimer Res. 2 (2005) 131–136.

[197] F.A. Al-Omar, M.N. Nagi, M.M. Abdulgadir, K.S. Al Joni, A.A. Al-Majed, Immediate and delayed treatments with curcumin prevents forebrain ischemia induced neuronal damage and oxidative insult in the rat hippocampus, Neurochem. Res. 31 (2006) 611–618.

[198] H.Y. Kim, E.J. Park, E.H. Joe, I Jou, Curcumin suppresses Janus kinase-STAT inflammatory signaling through activation of Src homology 2 domain containing tyrosine phosphatase 2 in brain microglia, J. Immunol. 171 (2003) 6072–6079.

[199] K.K. Jung, H.S. Lee, J.Y. Cho, W.C. Shin, M.H. Rhee, T.G. Kim, et al., Inhibitory effect of curcumin on nitric oxide production from lipopolysaccharide-activated primary microglia, Life Sci. 79 (2006) 2022–2031.

[200] M. Garcia-Alloza, L.A. Borrelli, A. Rozkalne, B.T. Hyman, B.J. Bacskai, Curcumin labels amyloid pathology in vivo, disrupts existing plaques, and partially restores distorted neurites in an Alzheimer mouse model, J. Neurochem. 102 (2007) 1095–1104.

[201] F. Yang, G.P. Lim, A.N. Begum, O.J. Ubeda, M.R. Simmons, S.S. Ambegaokar, et al., Curcumin inhibits formation of amyloid beta oligomers and fibrils, binds plaques, and reduces amyloid in vivo, J. Biol. Chem. 280 (2005) 5892–5901.

[202] P.R. Holt, S. Katz, R. Kirshoff, Curcumin therapy in inflammatory bowel disease: a pilot study, Dig. Dis. Sci. 50 (2005) 2191–2193.

[203] G. Cao, M. Giovanoni, R.L. Prior, Antioxidant capacity in different tissues of young and old rats, Proc. Soc. Exp. Biol. Med. 211 (1996) 359–365.

[204] R.L. Prior, G. Cao, Antioxidant capacity and polyphenolic components of teas: implications for altering in vivo antioxidant status, Proc. Soc. Exp. Biol. Med. 220 (1999) 255–261.

[205] S.Y. Wang, H.S. Lin, Antioxidant activity in fruits and leaves of blackberry, raspberry, and strawberry varies with cultivar and developmental stage, J. Agric. Food Chem. 48 (2000) 140–146.

[206] J.A. Joseph, B. Shukitt-Hale, N.A. Denisova, R.L. Prior, G. Cao, A. Martin, et al., Long-term dietary strawberry, spinach, or vitamin E supplementation retards the onset of age-related neuronal signal-transduction and cognitive behavioral deficits, J. Neurosci. 18 (1998) 8047–8055.

[207] K.A. Youdim, B. Shukitt-Hale, S. MacKinnon, et al., Polyphenolics enhance red blood cell resistance to oxidative stress: in vitro and in vivo, Biochim. Biophys. Acta 1523 (2000) 117–122.

[208] G. Casadesus, H. Stellwagen, A. Szprengiel, et al., Modulation of hippocampal neurogenesis and cognitive performance in the aged rat: the blueberry effect, Soc. Neurosci. Abs. 28 (2002) 294.

[209] G.E. Billman, J.X. Kang, A. Leaf, Prevention of sudden cardiac death by dietary pure omega-3 polyunsaturated fatty acids in dogs, Circulation 99 (1999) 2452–2457.

[210] J.A. Joseph, G. Arendash, M. Gordon, D. Diamond, B. Shukitt-Hale, D. Morgan, Blueberry supplementation enhances signaling and prevents behavioral deficits in an Alzheimer disease model, Nutr. Neurosci. 6 (2003) 153–162.

[211] F. Grimminger, H. Grimm, D. Fuhrer, C. Papavassilis, G. Lindemann, C. Blecher, et al., Omega-3 lipid infusion in a heart allotransplant model: shift in fatty acid and lipid mediator profiles and prolongation of transplant survival, Circulation 93 (1996) 365–371.

[212] F. Biscione, C. Pignalberi, A. Totteri, F. Messina, G. Altamura, Cardiovascular effects of omega-3 free fatty acids, Curr. Vasc. Pharmacol. 5 (2007) 163–172.

[213] R.C. Oh, J.B. Lanier, Management of hypertriglyceridemia, Am. Fam. Physician 75 (2007) 1365–1371.

[214] R.S. Chapkin, L.A. Davidson, L. Ly, B.R. Weeks, J.R. Lupton, D.N. McMurray, Immunomodulatory effects of (n-3) fatty acids: putative link to inflammation and colon cancer, J. Nutr. 137 (2007) 200S–204S.

[215] A.P. Simopoulos, Evolutionary aspects of diet, the omega-6/omega-3 ratio and genetic variation: nutritional implications for chronic diseases, Biomed. Pharmacother. 60 (2006) 502–507.

[216] G.M. Cole, S.A. Frautschy, Docosahexaenoic acid protects from amyloid and dendritic pathology in an Alzheimer's disease mouse model, Nutr. Health 18 (2006) 249–259.

[217] G.M. Cole, G.P. Lim, F. Yang, B. Teter, A. Begum, Q. Ma, et al., Prevention of Alzheimer's disease: omega-3 fatty acid and phenolic antioxidant interventions, Neurobiol. Aging 26 (Suppl. 1) (2005) 133–136.

[218] S. Yehuda, S Rabinovitz, R.L. Carasso, D.I. Mostofsky, The role of polyunsaturated fatty acids in restoring the aging neuronal membrane, Neurobiol. Aging 23 (2002) 843–853.

[219] A. Ikemoto, M. Ohishi, Y. Sato, N Hata, Y. Misawa, Y. Fujii, et al., Reversibility of n-3 fatty acid deficiency-induced alterations of learning behavior in the rat: level of n-6 fatty acids as another critical factor, J. Lipid Res. 42 (2001) 1655–1663.

[220] J.A. Conquer, M.C. Tierney, J. Zecevic, W.J. Bettger, R.H. Fisher, Fatty acid analysis of blood plasma of patients with Alzheimer's disease, other types of dementia, and cognitive impairment, Lipids 35 (2000) 1305–1312.

[221] M. Soderberg, C. Edlund, K. Kristensson, G. Dallner, Fatty acid composition of brain phospholipids in aging and in Alzheimer's disease, Lipids 26 (1991) 421–425.

[222] S. Kalmijn, M.P. van Boxtel, M. Ocke, W.M. Verschuren, D. Kromhout, L.J. Launer, Dietary intake of fatty acids and fish in relation to cognitive performance at middle age, Neurology 62 (2004) 275–280.

[223] S. Florent, C. Malaplate-Armand, I. Youssef, B. Kriem, V. Koziel, M.C. Escanye, et al., Docosahexaenoic acid prevents neuronal apoptosis induced by soluble amyloid-beta oligomers, J. Neurochem. 96 (2006) 385–395.

[224] W. Stillwell, S.R. Wassall, Docosahexaenoic acid: membrane properties of a unique fatty acid, Chem. Phys. Lipids 126 (2003) 1–27.

[225] N.G. Bazan, The onset of brain injury and neurodegeneration triggers the synthesis of docosanoid neuroprotective signaling, Cell Mol. Neurobiol. 26 (2006) 901–913.

[226] M. Akbar, H.Y. Kim, Protective effects of docosahexaenoic acid in staurosporine-induced apoptosis: involvement of phosphatidylinositol-3 kinase pathway, J. Neurochem 82 (2002) 655–665.

[227] M. Akbar, F. Calderon, Z. Wen, H.Y. Kim, Docosahexaenoic acid: a positive modulator of Akt signaling in neuronal survival, Proc. Natl. Acad. Sci. USA 102 (2005) 10858–10863.

[228] A.T. Erkkila, S. Lehto, K. Pyorala, M.I. Uusitupa, n-3 Fatty acids and 5-y risks of death and cardiovascular disease events in patients with coronary artery disease, Am. J. Clin. Nutr. 78 (2003) 65–71.

[229] K. He, Y. Song, M.L. Daviglus, K. Liu, L. Van Horn, A.R. Dyer, et al., Accumulated evidence on fish consumption and coronary heart disease mortality: a meta-analysis of cohort studies, Circulation 109 (2004) 2705–2711.

[230] F.B. Hu, L. Bronner, W.C. Willett, M.J. Stampfer, K.M. Rexrode, C.M. Albert, et al., Fish and omega-3 fatty acid intake and risk of coronary heart disease in women, JAMA 287 (2002) 1815–1821.

[231] K. He, Y. Song, M.L. Daviglus, K. Liu, L. Van Horn, A.R. Dyer, et al., Fish consumption and incidence of stroke: a meta-analysis of cohort studies, Stroke 35 (2004) 1538–1542.

[232] M. de Lorgeril, P. Salen, J.L. Martin, I. Monjaud, J. Delaye, N. Mamelle, Mediterranean diet, traditional risk factors, and the rate of cardiovascular complications after myocardial infarction: final report of the Lyon Diet Heart Study, Circulation 99 (1999) 779–785.

[233] H.C. Bucher, P. Hengstler, C. Schindler, G. Meier, N-3 polyunsaturated fatty acids in coronary heart disease: a meta-analysis of randomized controlled trials, Am. J. Med. 112 (2002) 298–304.

[234] M.L. Burr, Fish food, fish oil and cardiovascular disease, Clin. Exp. Hypertens. A 14 (1992) 181–192.

[235] T.A. Dolecek, G. Granditis,). Dietary polyunsaturated fatty acids and mortality in the Multiple Risk Factor Intervention Trial (MRFIT), World Rev. Nutr. Diet. 66 (1991) 205–216.

[236] E.B. Feldman, The scientific evidence for a beneficial health relationship between walnuts and coronary heart disease, J. Nutr. 132 (2002) 1062S–1101S.

[237] Y. Akiyama-Oda, Y. Hotta, S. Tsukita, H. Oda, Mechanism of glia–neuron cell-fate switch in the Drosophila thoracic neuroblast 6-4 lineage, Development 127 (2000) 3513–3522.

[238] K.J. Barnham, C.L. Masters, A.I. Bush, Neurodegenerative diseases and oxidative stress, Nat. Rev. Drug Discov. 3 (2004) 205–214.

[239] F.L. Huang, Y. Yoshida, H. Nakabayashi, W.S. Young 3rd, K.P. Huang, Immunocytochemical localization of protein kinase C isozymes in rat brain, J. Neurosci. 8 (1988) 4734–4744.

[240] N. Saito, A. Kose, A. Ito, K. Hosoda, M. Mori, M. Hirata, et al., Immunocytochemical localization of beta II subspecies of protein kinase C in rat brain, Proc. Natl. Acad. Sci. USA 86 (1989) 3409–3413.

[241] M. Spitaler, D.A. Cantrell, Protein kinase C and beyond, Nat. Immunol. 5 (2004) 785–790.

[242] D. Lin, D.J. Takemoto, Oxidative activation of protein kinase C gamma through the C1 domain: effects on gap junctions, J. Biol. Chem. 280 (2005) 13682–13693.

[243] T. Salonen, O. Sareila, U. Jalonen, H. Kankaanranta, R. Tuominen, E. Moilanen, Inhibition of classical PKC isoenzymes downregulates STAT1 activation and iNOS expression in LPS-treated murine J774 macrophages, Br. J. Pharmacol. 147 (2006) 790–799.

[244] A.J. Hall, M. Tripp, T. Howell, G. Darland, J.S. Bland, J.G. Babish, Gastric mucosal cell model for estimating relative gastrointestinal toxicity of non-steroidal anti-inflammatory drugs, Prostaglandins Leukot. Essent. Fatty Acids 75 (2006) 9–17.

[245] E.G. McGeer, P.L. McGeer, Inflammatory processes in Alzheimer's disease, Prog. Neuropsychopharmacol. Biol. Psychiatry 27 (2003) 741–749.

[246] X. Zhu, A.K. Raina, H.G. Lee, G. Casadesus, M.A. Smith, G. Perry, Oxidative stress signalling in Alzheimer's disease, Brain Res. 1000 (2004) 32–39.

[247] K. Hensley, R.A. Floyd, N.Y. Zheng, R. Nael, K.A. Robinson, X. Nguyen, et al., p38 kinase is activated in the Alzheimer's disease brain, J. Neurochem. 72 (1999) 2053–2058.

[248] J. Yrjanheikki, R. Keinanen, M. Pellikka, T. Hokfelt, J. Koistinaho, Tetracyclines inhibit microglial activation and are neuroprotective in global brain ischemia, Proc. Natl. Acad. Sci. USA 95 (1998) 15769–15774.

[249] T. Tikka, B.L. Fiebich, G. Goldsteins, R. Keinanen, J. Koistinaho, Minocycline, a tetracycline derivative, is neuroprotective against excitotoxicity by inhibiting activation and proliferation of microglia, J. Neurosci. 21 (2001) 2580–2588.

[250] S. Zhu, I.G. Stavrovskaya, M. Drozda, B.Y. Kim, V. Ona, M. Li, et al., Minocycline inhibits cytochrome c release and delays progression of amyotrophic lateral sclerosis in mice, Nature 417 (2002) 74–78.

[251] X.X. Dong, Z.J. Hui, W.X. Xiang, Z.F. Rong, S. Jian, C.J. Zhu, Ginkgo biloba extract reduces endothelial progenitor-cell senescence through augmentation of telomerase activity, J. Cardiovasc. Pharmacol. 49 (2007) 111–115.

[252] Y. Yamamoto, R.B. Gaynor, IκB kinases: key regulators of the NF-κB pathway, Trends Biochem. Sci. 29 (2004) 72–79.

[253] A.A. Farooqui, L.A. Horrocks, T. Farooqui, Modulation of inflammation in brain: a matter of fat, J. Neurochem. 101 (2007) 577–599.

[254] D. Beitner-Johnson, D.E. Millhorn, Hypoxia induces phosphorylation of the cyclic AMP response element-binding protein by a novel signaling mechanism, J. Biol. Chem. 273 (1998) 19834–19839.

[255] E.P. Cummins, C.T. Taylor, Hypoxia-responsive transcription factors, Pflugers Arch. 450 (2005) 363–371.

[256] O.G. Rodriguez-Mora, C.J. Howe, M.M. Lahair, J.A. McCubrey, R.A. Franklin, Inhibition of CREB transcriptional activity in human T lymphocytes by oxidative stress, Free Radic. Biol. Med. 38 (2005) 1653–1661.

[257] P. Rockwell, J. Martinez, L. Papa, E. Gomes, Redox regulates COX-2 upregulation and cell death in the neuronal response to cadmium, Cell Signal 16 (2004) 343–353.

[258] V. Gerzanich, S. Ivanova, J.M. Simard, Early pathophysiological changes in cerebral vessels predisposing to stroke, Clin. Hemorheol. Microcirc. 29 (2003) 291–294.

[259] J.A. Joseph, D.R. Fisher, J. Strain, Muscarinic receptor subtype determines vulnerability to oxidative stress in COS-7 cells, Free Radic. Biol. Med. 32 (2002) 153–161.

[260] J.A. Joseph, D.R. Fisher, D. Bielinski, Blueberry extract alters oxidative stress-mediated signaling in COS-7 cells transfected with selectively vulnerable muscarinic receptor subtypes, J. Alzheimer's Dis. 9 (2006) 35–42.

[261] L.M. He, L.Y. Chen, X.L. Lou, A.L. Qu, Z. Zhou, T. Xu, Evaluation of beta-amyloid peptide 25–35 on calcium homeostasis in cultured rat dorsal root ganglion neurons, Brain Res. 939 (2002) 65–75.

[262] G.E. Stutzmann, I. Smith, A. Caccamo, S. Oddo, F.M. Laferla, I. Parker, Enhanced ryanodine receptor recruitment contributes to Ca^{2+} disruptions in young, adult, and aged Alzheimer's disease mice, J. Neurosci. 26 (2006) 5180–5189.

[263] C. O'Neill, R.F. Cowburn, W.L. Bonkale, T.G. Ohm, J. Fastbom, M. Carmody, et al., Dysfunctional intracellular calcium homeostasis: a central cause of neurodegeneration in Alzheimer's disease, Biochem. Soc. Symp. (2001) 177–194.

[264] F.C. Lau, D.F. Bielinski, J.A. Joseph, Inhibitory effects of blueberry extract on the production of inflammatory mediators in lipopolysaccharide-activated BV2 microglia, J. Neurosci. Res. 85 (2007) 1010–1017.

[265] J.A. Joseph, R. Villalobos-Molina, N. Denisova, S. Erat, R. Cutler, J.G. Strain, Age differences in sensitivity to H$_2$O$_2$- or

[266] R.T. Bartus, R.L. Dean, B. Beer, A.S. Lippa, The cholinergic hypothesis of geriatric memory dysfunction, Science 217 (1982) 408–417.

[267] S. Rossner, U. Ueberham, R. Schliebs, J.R. Perez-Polo, V. Bigl, The regulation of amyloid precursor protein metabolism by cholinergic mechanisms and neurotrophin receptor signaling, Prog. Neurobiol. 56 (1998) 541–569.

[268] A. Elhusseiny, Z. Cohen, A. Olivier, D.B. Stanimirovic, E. Hamel, Functional acetylcholine muscarinic receptor subtypes in human brain microcirculation: identification and cellular localization, J. Cereb. Blood Flow Metab. 19 (1999) 794–802.

[269] E.C. Toescu, A. Verkhratsky, Parameters of calcium homeostasis in normal neuronal ageing, J. Anat. 197 (2000) 563–569.

[270] J.P. Herman, K.C. Chen, R. Booze, P.W. Landfield, Upregulation of alpha1D Ca^{2+} channel subunit mRNA expression in the hippocampus of aged 344 rats, Neurobiol. Aging 19 (1998) 581–587.

[271] D.R. Lynch, T.M. Dawson, Secondary mechanisms in neuronal trauma, Curr. Opin. Neurobiol. 7 (1994) 510–516.

[272] R.C. Vannucci, R.M. Brucklacher, S.J. Vannucci, Intracellular calcium accumulation during the evolution of hypoxic–ischemic brain damage in the immature rat, Brain Res. Dev. 126 (2001) 117–120.

[273] M.P. Mattson, Emerging apoptosis in neurodegenerative disorders, Mol. Cell Biol. 1 (2000) 120–129.

[274] P. DeSarno, S.A. Shestopal, T.D. King, A. Zmijewska, L. Songand, R.S. Jope, Muscarinic receptor activation protects cells from apoptotic effects of DNA damage, oxidative stress and mitochondrial inhibition, J. Biol. Chem. 278 (2003) 11086–11093.

[275] A. Huidobro, P. Blanco, M Villalba, P. Gomez-Puertas, A. Villa, R. Pereira, et al., Age-related changes in calcium homeostatic mechanisms in synaptosomes in relation with working memory deficiency, Neurobiol. Aging 14 (1993) 479–486.

[276] C. Nyakas, B.J. Oosterink, J. Keijser, K. Felszeghy, G.I. de Jong, J. Korf, et al., Selective decline of 5-HT1A receptor binding sites in rat cortex, hippocampus and cholinergic basal forebrain nuclei during aging, J. Chem. Neuroanat. 13 (1997) 53–61.

[277] J.L. Kaufmann, P.C. Bickford, G. Taglialatela, Oxidative stress dependent upregulation of Bcl-2 expression in the central nervous system of aged Fisher 344 rats, J. Neurochem. 76 (2001) 1099–1108.

[278] H. Hartmann, K. Velbinger, A. Eckert, W.E. Muller, Region-specific downregulation of free intracellular calcium in the aged rat brain, Neurobiol. Aging 17 (1996) 557–563.

[279] V. Kaasinen, H. Vilkman, J. Hietala, K. Nagren, H. Helenius, H. Olsson, et al., Age-related dopamine D2/D3 receptor loss in extrastriatal regions of the human brain, Neurobiol. Aging 21 (2000) 683–688.

[280] J.A. Joseph, D.R. Fisher, A.N. Carey, A. Neuman, D.F. Bielinski, Dopamine-induced stress signaling in COS-7 cells transfected with selectively vulnerable muscarinic receptor subtypes is partially mediated via the i3 loop and antagonized by blueberry extract, J. Alzheimer's Dis. 10 (2006) 423–437.

[281] J. Miquel, Nutrition and ageing, Public Health Nutr. 4 (2001) 1385–1388.

[282] P.M. Kris-Etherton, C.L. Keen, Evidence that the antioxidant flavonoids in tea and cocoa are beneficial for cardiovascular health, Curr. Opin. Lipidol. 13 (2002) 41–49.

[283] P.M. Kris-Etherton, K.D. Hecker, A. Bonanome, et al., Bioactive compounds in foods: their role in the prevention of

cardiovascular disease and cancer, Am. J. Med. I13 (Suppl. 9B) (2002) 71S–88S.

[284] D. Commenges, V. Scotet, S. Renaud, H. Jacqmin-Gadda, P. Barberger-Gateau, J.F. Dartigues, Intake of flavonoids and risk of dementia, Eur. J. Epidemiol. 16 (2000) 357–363.

[285] W.B. Grant, A. Campbell, R.F. Itzhaki, J. Savory, The significance of environmental factors in the etiology of Alzheimer's disease, J. Alzheimer's Dis. 4 (2002) 179–189.

[286] Y. Levites, T. Amit, M.B. Youdim, S. Mandel, Involvement of protein kinase C activation and cell survival/cell cycle genes in green tea polyphenolepigallocatechin 3-gallate neuroprotective action, J. Biol. Chem. 277 (2002) 30574–30580.

[287] Y. Levites, O. Weinreb, G. Maor, et al., Green tea polyphenol (−)-epigallocatechin-3-gallate prevents N-methyl-4-phenyl-1,2,3,6-tetrahydropyridine induced dopaminergic neurodegeneration, J. Neurochem. 78 (2001) 1073–1082.

[288] Y. Levites, M.B. Youdim, G. Maor, S. Mandel, Attenuation of 6-hydroxydopamine (6-OHDA)-induced nuclear factor-κB (NF-κB) activation and cell death by tea extracts in neuronal cultures, Biochem. Pharmacol. 63 (2002) 21–29.

Phytochemicals in the Prevention and Treatment of Obesity and Its Related Cancers

Kee-Hong Kim[*], *Gyo-Nam Kim*[*], *Ki Won Lee*[†]

[*]Purdue University, West Lafayette, Indiana, [†]Seoul National University, Seoul, Republic of Korea

I INTRODUCTION

The prevalence of obesity is a significant global health problem. Obesity is the result of excess body fat due to an imbalance between energy intake and energy expenditure. Energy balance is influenced by numerous environmental factors (e.g., metabolic rate, exercise, and culture) and genetic factors (e.g., monogenic syndromes and susceptibility genes) (Figure 21.1). Indeed, the excessive body fat accumulation in adipose tissue is a consequence of impaired energy expenditure, such as reduced physical activity, basal metabolism, and thermogenesis [1]. On the other hand, an increase in food intake by consuming foods with more simple sugars, less fiber, and/or elevated fat content impacts on positive energy balance, resulting in an expansion of adipocyte size and weight and an increased number of new adipocytes. In addition, complex interactions among these variables contribute to individual differences not only in adipose mass gain but also in the response to interventions and/or treatments of obesity. Brain and peripheral tissues such as adipose tissue, liver, and intestine play an important role in regulating systemic energy balance and therefore the development of obesity. Among these tissues, adipose tissue is known to play both causative and consequential roles in obesity. Although adipose tissue is traditionally known as an energy reservoir, storing lipids during periods of energy excess and positive energy balance, generation of new fat cells and metabolic and endocrine changes in adipose tissue also contribute to metabolic dysfunction of other peripheral tissues and dysregulation of central signals

of energy balance. This suggests that the generation of new adipose tissue and its metabolic and endocrine function could be preventive and/or therapeutic targets of obesity.

Despite many reported beneficial effects of dietary phytochemicals on health, less attention has been drawn to modulation of obesity and its associated diseases by phytochemicals. Thus, this chapter focuses on understanding the cellular processes involved in the generation and function of adipose tissue and obesity-related cancers. Furthermore, the current understanding of regulation of obesity by dietary phytochemicals found in fruits, vegetables, and edible plants (e.g., spices) is discussed.

II ROLE OF ADIPOSE TISSUE IN OBESITY

A Development of Adipose Tissue

Adipose tissue develops as a result of both hypertrophy (i.e., cell size increase) and hyperplasia (i.e., cell number increase) of mature adipocytes and preadipocytes, respectively. Adipocyte hypertrophy plays an important role in regulating cells' lipid storage and secretion of adipose-specific hormones/factors that contribute to systemic energy balance, inflammation, and energy homeostasis. On the other hand, adipocyte hyperplasia, termed adipogenesis, is known to contribute to the generation of new adipocytes during childhood and adolescence, as well as adipocyte turnover in adults [2]. This makes adipogenesis an effective cellular process for prevention of the generation of adipose tissue and, therefore, the development of obesity.

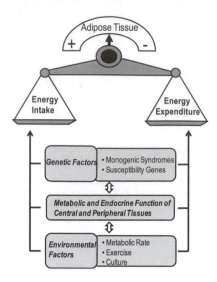

FIGURE 21.1   Factors influencing energy balance.

Mesodermal pluripotent stem cell-driven preadipocytes undergo adipogenesis when cells are exposed to appropriate hormonal and nutritional signals. Adipogenesis consists of four distinct steps: (1) early growth arrest of confluent preadipocytes, (2) mitotic clonal expansion (MCE), (3) transcription of adipogenic transcription factors, and (4) terminal cell differentiation [3]. Growth arrest of preadipocytes in the early phase of adipogenesis is coordinately regulated by transcriptional control of genes involved in the cell cycle by adipogenic transcription factors CCAAT/enhancer binding protein α (C/EBPα) and peroxisome proliferator-activated receptor γ (PPARγ) [3]. Upon exposure to mitogenic and adipogenic signals, the growth-arrested preadipocytes undergo at least one round of cell cycle with DNA replication and cell division. Although MCE appears to be required for promoting adipogenesis of most established preadipocyte cell lines *in vitro*, it is reported to not be necessary for adipogenesis of other cells such as primary human preadipocytes [3]. Nevertheless, inhibition of MCE by cell cycle inhibitors [4] and modulation of genes encoding cell cycle components [5,6] have been shown to impair adipogenesis. In addition, phosphorylational activation of the adipogenic insulin signaling pathway such as insulin receptor, insulin receptor substrate-1 and -2, phosphoinositide 3-kinase, and protein kinase B/Akt in the early phase of adipogenesis also participates in the promotion of adipogenesis. Cell cycle regulators such as cyclin D, Rb, and E2Fs [7] appear to link between MCE and the transcriptional events in the early phase of adipogenesis. Concomitant with the MCE process, the DNA binding ability of C/EBPβ, an early adipogenic transcription factor, and its transcriptional activity are acquired. This occurs through sequential phosphorylation of C/EBPβ by a cell cycle regulator cdk2/cyclin A,

mitogen-activated protein kinase (MAPK), and glycogen synthase kinase-3β during MCE [8]. Phosphorylated C/EBPβ subsequently induces its target adipogenic transcription factors C/EBPα and PPARγ.

Whereas C/EBPβ-induced expression of C/EBPα is required for promotion of adipogenesis and formation of white adipose tissue, PPARγ is reported to reverse the defective function of C/EBPβ and C/EBPα in adipogenesis [7], suggesting that PPARγ is the central regulator of adipogenesis. PPARγ forms a heterodimer with retinoid X receptor, and this heterodimeric complex binds to the PPAR response element located in the promoter regions of many genes involved in fat storage and adipokine production. Several agonists such as 15-deoxy-$\Delta^{12,14}$-prostaglandin J_2 and thiazolidinediones are also known to promote transactivation of PPARγ.

During the terminal phase of adipogenesis, genes encoding enzymes in lipid metabolism, such as glycerol-3-phosphate acyltransferase (GPAT), glycerol-3-phosphate dehydrogenase, glyceraldehyde-3-phosphate dehydrogenase, fatty acid synthase (FAS), acetyl coenzyme A (CoA) carboxylase (ACC), and stearoyl-CoA desaturase (SCD), are activated. Levels of genes involved in fatty acid update and transport and lipid droplet formation, including an adipose-specific fatty acid binding protein (aP2), a fatty acid transporter (FAT/CD36), and perilipin, are also increased. In addition, mature adipocytes produce adipocyte-specific hormones such as leptin, adiponectin, resistin, adipsin, and plasminogen activator inhibitor-1, as well as a number of inflammatory cytokines such as tumor necrosis factor-α (TNF-α), interleukin-6 (IL-6), IL-1α, and monocyte chemotactic protein-1. These adipocyte-secreted factors are known to modulate peripheral and systemic energy balance.

Molecular and dietary regulation of adipogenesis is suggested to prevent body weight gain and the development of obesity. However, inhibition of adipogenesis alone could possibly result in adipocyte hypertrophy and/or redirection of body fat to other non-adipose tissues, which increases the risk of the development of obesity-related diseases. Thus, additional approaches to improve whole-body energy expenditure possibly through activation of thermogenesis and/or fatty acid oxidation should be accompanied by the blockage of adipogenesis.

B Role of Adipose Tissue in Energy Metabolism

Adipose tissue is traditionally viewed as a storage organ of lipids. During approximately the past decade, adipose tissue has been further revealed as an endocrine tissue secreting a number of hormones and factors that modulate systemic glucose and lipid homeostasis. *De novo* lipogenesis plays a key role in adipocyte hypertrophy as well as hepatic lipid synthesis. The substrates for *de novo* lipogenesis are fatty acid esters and CoA. Transport of mitochondrial citrate to cytosol by tricarboxylate transporter initiates the generation of acetyl-CoA and malonyl-CoA by ATP-citrate synthase and ACC, respectively, followed by subsequent synthesis of fatty acids, mostly palmitate, by FAS. The most abundant saturated and unsaturated fatty acids found in adipocytes are stearate and oleate, respectively. A single *cis* double bond at the Δ^9 of oleate is introduced by SCD-1. Conversely, mice deficient in ACC [9] or SCD-1 [10] were found to be resistant to adiposity. Similarly, administration of an inhibitor of FAS such as a fungal-derived cerulenin and synthetic C75 promoted long-term weight reduction in obese animals [11,12], suggesting that FAS is an effective target protein for the control of *de novo* lipogenesis.

Triglycerides are synthesized by esterification of glycerol with three molecules of fatty acids. Thus, glycerol 3-phosphoate, a glycolytic metabolite, and fatty acyl-CoAs are the key substrates for triglyceride synthesis. Fatty acids used for triglyceride synthesis are mainly derived from *de novo* lipogenesis, hydrolysis of triglycerides in the cell, or fatty acids transported from circulation. The first step of esterification of a fatty acyl-CoA to glycerol 3-phosphate is catalyzed by GPAT, and this is followed by subsequent esterification of two fatty acyl-CoAs catalyzed by endoplasmic reticulum (ER) resident enzymes, such as GPAT, *sn*-1-acylglycerol-3-phosphate acyltransferase (AGPAT), phosphatidic acid phosphatase, and diacylglycerol acyltransferase (DGAT). The newly synthesized triglycerides in the ER are then coated by several lipid droplet envelope binding proteins, such as perilipin and adipose differentiation-related protein, which are required for the formation of triglyceride-enriched lipid droplets and an effective mobilization of lipid droplets under energy-demanding conditions. In support of the importance of these enzymes in triglyceride metabolism, genetic deletion of a gene encoding one of these enzymes in mice [13−16] and humans [17−19] with mutation of one of these genes have been shown to lower adiposity and/or energy balance. However, total inhibition of enzyme activities by genetic deletion of their corresponding genes is associated with side effects such as insulin resistance, skin barrier abnormalities, and/or neonatal lethality [20]. This could be avoided if a selective and moderate inhibition of the function of enzymes involved in triglyceride synthesis could be achieved. In this regard, identification of natural phytochemicals that significantly, but not completely, inhibit activities of enzymes involved in triglyceride synthesis would effectively modulate the development of obesity [21].

Adipokines secreted from differentiated adipocytes regulate energy metabolism in peripheral tissues and brain in a paracrine and endocrine manner. Among the many adipokines, evidence suggests the important function of leptin and adiponectin in modulation of lipid metabolism both in adipose tissue and in nonadipose tissues such as liver and muscle. Leptin is a 16-kDa peptide that belongs to the cytokine class 1 superfamily. Leptin is encoded by *Lep* in mice and *LEP* in humans. Leptin exerts its biological functions by binding to its receptor encoded by *Lepr* in mice and *LEPR* in humans. Circulating leptin is correlated with body mass index (BMI), and defects in leptin and leptin receptor genes trigger the development of obesity and diabetes in both humans and animals [22,23]. The activated leptin−leptin receptor signaling pathway in peripheral tissues and in hypothalamus influences lipid metabolism and food intake, respectively. Leptin is known to induce the mobilization of triglycerides in lipid droplets (i.e., lipolysis) by activation of AMP-activated protein kinase (AMPK) and its dependent fatty acid oxidation in skeletal muscle [24]. On the other hand, leptin is suggested to inhibit triglyceride synthesis and increase lipolysis in adipocytes through activation of leptin signaling pathway and suppression of genes involved in lipogenesis [25]. Although leptin appears to directly regulate the function of AMPK and its related triglyceride turnover, it also indirectly modulates lipid metabolism through interference of insulin-induced lipogenesis and insulin-inhibited fatty acid oxidation, suggesting that leptin functions as a counterregulatory hormone to insulin.

Adiponectin is a 244-amino acid hormone mainly secreted from adipose tissue. Studies have further identified the expression of adiponectin mRNA in the liver and muscle tissues [26,27]. A number of animal studies indicate that adiponectin promotes fatty acid oxidation and suppresses gluconeogenesis in the liver, thereby promoting energy expenditure and protecting animals from high diet-induced obesity and insulin resistance [28,29]. Conversely, obesity is associated with a low level of circulating adiponectin. Adiponectin-induced resistance to obesity and improvement of insulin sensitivity occur through interaction between adiponectin and the two receptors—a muscle-specific ADIPOR1 and a liver-specific ADIPOR2 [30]. The adiponectin−ADIPOR axis also appears to have direct and indirect effects on protection from obesity-related diseases such as atherosclerosis, cardiovascular diseases, and nonalcoholic steatohepatitis. These health benefit effects of adiponectin are exerted largely through allosteric activation of AMPK activity and transcription of genes involved in fatty acid oxidation, such as PPARα and PPARγ. Adiponectin expression and secretion is modulated by various nutritional and inflammatory cues. For instance, fasting−refeeding [31], long-term caloric restriction [32], insulin treatment [33], and PPARγ agonists [34] induce adiponectin production, whereas inflammatory cytokines (e.g., TNF-α and IL-6) [35,36] and glucocorticoid [35] suppress adiponectin production.

C Function of Adipose Tissue in Energy Balance

Adipose tissue mass is closely associated with food intake regulation. As an endocrine organ, adipose tissue transmits a signal to the brain for central control of energy balance. Much attention has been given to the effect of an adipose-specific hormone leptin on central food intake. The interaction between leptin and its receptor expressed in hypothalamus is known to coordinately regulate central food intake signaling such as the proopiomelanocortin (POMC)-dependent anorexic pathway and the neuropeptide Y (NPY)/ agouti-related protein (AgRP)-dependent hyperphagic pathway. Leptin-induced cleavage of POMC and its subsequent activation of α-melanocyte-stimulating hormone (α-MSH) and melanocortin receptor contribute to a decrease in food intake. On the other hand, reduction of circulating leptin level triggers the release of hyperphagic hormones NPY and AgRP in hypothalamus. AgRP released under the leptin deficiency in turn inhibits the anorexic function of α-MSH, resulting in stimulation of food intake [37,38]. Analogous to leptin, the level of plasma insulin, which is directly correlated with adipocyte hypertrophy, also modulates central food intake through the interaction of plasma insulin with insulin receptor expressed in the hypothalamus for controlling anorexic and hyperphagic pathways [38,39]. Collectively, when adipose mass is reduced, low levels of circulating leptin and insulin are known to stimulate food intake and reduce energy expenditure. In contrast, increased levels of these hormones in circulation result in suppression of food intake and increased energy expenditure.

AMPK, a whole-body energy sensor protein, not only controls peripheral energy homeostasis but also integrates nutritional and hormonal signals in the brain to control central food intake and energy balance. Leptin-induced dephosphorylation and inactivation of the hypothalamic AMPK has been shown to inhibit food intake. AMPK also plays an important role in hypothalamic *de novo* lipogenesis and its impact on food intake. AMPK activation in the hypothalamus under insulin deficiency, for example, results in inhibition of ACC activity with a reduced level of malonyl-CoA, which in turn modulates the function of hypothalamic neurons and increases food intake. On the other hand, inhibition of AMPK activity in the hypothalamus by central administration of glucose [40], metabolic intermediate citrate [41], or α-lipoic acid [42] resulted in suppression of food intake. Moreover, inhibition of *de novo* lipogenic enzyme FAS activity by C75 [43] in the hypothalamus resulted in accumulation of malonyl-CoA with inhibition of food intake.

Central regulation of energy balance is also attributed by endocrine function of some intestinal hormones. Intestinal hormones such as cholecystokinin [44], peptide YY [45], and glucagon-like peptide-1 [46] are major representatives of endocrine—gut—brain communications that sense the size and frequency of meals in the intestine. Thus, elevated levels of the release of these hormones from the intestine are known to lower food intake, appetite, and weight gain through interaction with their specific receptors in the brain. Interestingly, some dietary compounds in coffee, such as chlorogenic acid and caffeine [47], and isoflavones [48] are known to modulate the release of intestinal hormones and lower satiety.

III OBESITY-RELATED CANCERS

Obesity is a global health crisis. Nearly 300 million adults are obese worldwide, and approximately two-thirds of U.S. adults are overweight or obese [49]. Obesity has been implicated in a number of chronic diseases, including diabetes and cardiovascular diseases [50]. As one of the life-threatening diseases, cancer has a high mortality rate. Increased cancer incidence has been observed in developing countries as well as in developed countries, including the United States. Risk factors for developing cancer include tobacco smoke (including secondhand smoke); exposure to sun, air pollution, or other toxic chemicals; infections; alcohol intake; and family history. Obesity is a critical risk factor for developing specific types of cancers. A cohort study estimated that 15—20% of deaths from all cancers in the United States are attributable to overweight and obesity [51]. Epidemiological studies have also suggested that greater BMI is associated with increased incidence and/or death from a few forms of cancer, including colon, breast, esophageal, and endometrial cancers [52]. Studies of the associations between obesity and the mortality from cancers often yield inconsistent results, and the mechanisms by which obesity mediates tumorformation and progression are not been clearly understood.

The World Cancer Research Fund found that obesity is associated with greater risk of colorectal, breast (postmenopausal), endometrial, esophageal, and probably other types of cancers [53]. In obesity, adipose tissue dysfunction is a key contributor to the development hyperinsulinemia and insulin resistance. Insulin stimulates the production of insulin-like growth factor (IGF)-1 in adipose tissue, where it plays an important role in cancer development by inducing cell proliferation and inhibiting apoptosis [54]. Binding IGF-1 to its receptor (IGF-1R) activates multiple signaling cascades, including phosphatidylinositol 3-kinase (PI3K)-Akt and Ras/Raf/MAPK, which in turn lead to cellular growth, proliferation, differentiation, and motility [54].

Another mechanism associated with adiposity and carcinogenesis is the bioavailability of sex steroids [55]. Particularly, estrogen is mainly synthesized from adipose tissue, and its circulating level is directly associated with BMI in postmenopausal women [56]. Increased circulating levels and bioactivity of IGF-1 can decrease hepatic synthesis and circulating levels of sex hormone-binding globulin (SHBG), which has a high affinity to testosterone and estradiol [57]. Indeed, in both men and women, decreased SHBG levels due to higher adiposity lead to increased concentrations of free estradiol and testosterone [57]. After binding their receptors, estrogen and testosterone can diffuse into the target cells and subsequently promote cell proliferation and inhibit apoptosis [55].

A Colorectal Cancer

Colorectal cancer is the third leading cause of cancer in the world. It is estimated that nearly 9.7% (1.23 million) of all commonly diagnosed cancers worldwide are attributed to colon [58]. An epidemiological study suggested that obesity is associated with an increased risk of colorectal cancer [59]. A prospective cohort study found direct associations between obesity measures such as waist circumference, waist:hip ratio, body weight, and BMI and the risk for colorectal cancer in men [60]. Another clinical study performed in Japan found that colorectal cancer is significantly correlated with the accumulation of visceral fat but not subcutaneous fat [61]. This study suggests that visceral adipose tissue accumulation is likely to be a stronger predictor for colorectal cancer development [61].

Although the mechanisms by which greater adiposity regulates colorectal cancer development are not clearly understood, increased circulating levels of leptin may be associated with obesity and colon cancer. A cohort study indicated that people with high leptin levels had an approximately 30-fold higher risk of colon cancer [62]. Increased levels of leptin receptors have been found in colon tumors, polyps, and adjacent mucosa, as well as human colon cancer cells [63]. Obese mice also had greater body and epididymal fat mass and increased levels of serum leptin and leptin receptor. An experimental study showed that obese mice fed a high-fat diet were more susceptible to carcinogen-induced colon tumorigenesis than were mice fed a normal diet [64]. This study suggests that obesity induced by a high-fat diet stimulates colon tumor formation, which is likely mediated by increased levels of circulating leptin and its binding to the leptin receptor. Supporting this notion, leptin is suggested to

stimulate cell proliferation via activation of nuclear factor-κB (NF-κB) and extracellular signal-regulated kinase (ERK)1/2-mediated pathways in colonic epithelial cells [63,65]. Leptin is also known to induce angiogenesis [66], which results in tumor growth, invasion, and metastasis [67].

B Breast Cancer

Breast cancer is the second most common cancer in the world, and it is the leading cause of cancer-related mortality in U.S. women [68]. In particular, obesity increases the risk of breast cancer among postmenopausal women partially due to obesity-mediated upregulation of serum-free estradiol [69]. Whereas estrogen is produced mainly in the ovaries in premenopausal women, it is alternatively produced from adipose tissue in postmenopausal women [70]. Hence, the positive association between obesity and the risk of breast cancer among postmenopausal women is likely attributable to greater estrogen production from adipose tissue.

The mechanisms underlying the link between obesity and breast cancer risk are not fully understood. However, the potential mechanisms may involve obesity-mediated alterations in the levels of growth factors (i.e., IGF-1), subsequently modified sex hormones, and elevated levels of inflammatory cytokines and adipokines. Obesity is associated with increased levels of insulin and IGF-1, leading to the downregulation of circulating SHBG, which in turn increases bioavailability of free estradiol [57]. This increased amount of estradiol is considered to be a strong risk factor for the development of postmenopausal breast cancer [70].

Patients with breast cancer exhibit increased concentrations of plasma inflammatory cytokines, such as TNF-α and IL-1β, -6, and -8, compared to their age-matched controls [71]. Conversely, elevated level of inflammation may also contribute to the increased risk of breast cancer. Indeed, obesity is considered to be a low-grade systemic inflammation. Obesity-induced production of inflammatory cytokine TNF-α causes insulin resistance through activation of the I-κ B kinase (IKK) complex, which in turn induces phosphorylation of serine residues of insulin resistance substrate [72]. In addition, the proinflammatory cytokine IL-6 activates Janus kinase (JAK)/signal transducer and activator of transcription (STAT)-3 signaling pathways, which induce cancer cell proliferation [73].

Lastly, the positive relations between obesity and breast cancer development can be explained by obesity-mediated reductions in plasma levels of adipokines [74]. Among breast cancer patients, postmenopausal women exhibited significantly decreased serum adiponectin levels compared to premenopausal women [75].

An *in vitro* study demonstrated that adiponectin suppresses cell proliferation and promotes cell growth arrest and apoptosis in MDA-MB-231 breast cancer cells [76]. The mechanism by which adiponectin prevents cancer progression is the ADIPOR1 and R2-medicated activation of AMPK. Epidemiological studies have found a lower cancer incidence in patients with type 2 diabetes after treatment with a metformin, an AMPK activator [77], indicating a key role of AMPK in cancer prevention.

C Endometrial Cancer

Endometrial cancer has the highest incidence in Western countries [78]. Case—control and cohort studies strongly suggested a positive association between overweight and/or obesity and endometrial cancers risk [51,79].

As with breast cancer, obesity-associated induction of circulating estrogen and reduction of SHBG level is likely to contribute to the development of endometrial cancer [80]. In addition, studies have also found a close relation between obesity-caused induction of leptin and the risk of endometrial cancer [81]. Leptin has been shown to stimulate proliferation of human endometrial cancer cells through functional activation of cyclooxygenase-2 (COX-2), which is mediated via JAK2/STAT3, MAPK/ERK, and PI3K/AKT signaling pathways [82]. This finding emphasizes the importance of leptin and leptin-mediated activation of COX-2 in obesity-triggered endometrial cancer development.

D Esophageal Cancer

In addition to alcohol and tobacco use, obesity is a critical risk factor for esophageal disorders: esophageal cancer, Barrett esophagus, and gastroesophageal reflux disease (GERD) [78], as supported by a meta-analysis that included 12 case—control studies and 2 cohort studies [83]. Among these disorders, esophageal cancer and GERD are reported to be positively correlated with obesity indices such as BMI and body fat distribution (i.e., abdominal body fat). Mechanisms underlying the relationship between esophageal cancer risk and obesity are not fully understood, but leptin is also suggested to play an important role in the development of esophageal cancer. Leptin promotes proliferation and mobility of human esophageal cancer cells [54], likely through the activation of ERK and epidermal growth factor receptor (EGFR) [84]. In addition, both esophageal cancer and GERD are associated with systemic inflammation [85,86]. Because obesity is associated with a state of low-grade inflammation, obesity-induced systemic inflammation and elevated levels of

secreted proinflammatory cytokines may promote the development of these esophageal disorders.

E Other Obesity-Related Cancers

Several studies have examined the potential relationship between obesity and the risk of cancers such as bladder, prostate, and pancreatic cancers. However, the findings have yielded inconstant results. A case—control study found a positive association between greater adiposity and the risk of bladder cancer [87]. However, a prospective cohort study of approximately 500,000 men and women revealed a positive but modest correlation between adiposity and bladder cancer risk [88]. Although more than 40 studies, including various prospective and case—control studies, were conducted to examine the relationship between obesity and prostate cancer risk, the results were conflicting [89]. Several studies have suggested that increased BMI is likely associated with an approximately twofold greater risk of pancreatic cancer in both men and women [90], but a meta-analysis using case—control and cohort studies did not find a relationship between BMI and pancreatic cancer risk [91]. Thus, whether obesity plays a role in the development and progression of bladder, prostate, and pancreatic cancers remains inconclusive.

IV PHYTOCHEMICALS IN OBESITY AND ITS RELATED CANCERS

Currently, surgery, chemotherapy, and radiation treatment are widely used to decrease mortality rates and improve survival rates from cancers. However, these treatments are associated with several side effects, and cancer patients treated with these strategies often cannot be completely cured. It is reported that appropriate dietary modification contributes to an approximately one-third decrease in death rates for all cancers in the United States [92,93]. Natural bioactive compounds have been demonstrated to regulate a wide range of cellular and signaling processes in a variety of cancer cell types [94]. Fruits, vegetables, and edible plants (e.g., spices) are good sources of vitamins, minerals, and fibers for basic nutrition. In addition, they are excellent sources of micronutrients and natural bioactive phytochemicals such as polyphenols, phenolics, and alkaloids, which provide significant health benefits. During the past several decades, a great deal of research has revealed that dietary phytochemicals modulate inflammatory, oxidative, and cell proliferative processes that substantially contribute to the initiation of many human diseases such as carcinogenesis.

Consumption of food containing natural phytochemicals is believed to promote health by protecting or delaying against the development of various chronic diseases. Indeed, a number of epidemiological studies support the hypothesis that phytochemicals in fruits, vegetables, and plants reduce the risk of various forms of cancer [95–100]. Whereas many natural phytochemicals have been identified to be chemopreventive, efforts to identify anti-obese phytochemicals and their mode of actions have recently been emerging. Therefore, natural phytochemicals, which have both anti-obese and chemopreventive properties, could be promising dietary approaches for the prevention of the development of obesity and its related cancer progression. The dietary phytochemicals reported to exhibit potential anti-obese and chemopreventive properties are summarized in Table 21.1 and discussed next.

A Curcumin

Curcumin (diferuloylmethane) is a yellow pigment derived from turmeric, a powdered rhizome of *Curcuma longa Linn* (Table 21.1). Curcumin's protective activities against various diseases, such as diabetes, obesity, and cancers, have been intensively studied during the past several decades. Accumulating evidence suggests that curcumin exhibits antioxidant, anti-inflammatory, anticarcinogenic, and cardioprotective properties [101], which are attributed to modulation of multiple targets in the cells and development of various diseases [94].

Curcumin has been reported to improve the profile of plasma lipid metabolites in obese animals. Curcuminoids (commercial-grade curcumin (73.4 %) mixed with demethoxycurcumin (16.1 %) and bisdemethoxycurcumin (10.5 %)) lower the liver triglyceride and cholesterol levels and plasma triglycerides and very low-density lipoprotein (VLDL) fraction in animals fed a high-fat diet [102]. In diabetic mice, curcumin significantly suppressed body weight gain and blood glucose and insulin levels [103] largely through lowering hepatic lipid metabolism. The direct effect of curcumin intake on obesity has been addressed By Weisberg *et al.* [104], who examined the therapeutic effect of curcumin on obese and diabetic animals. Oral administration of 3% dietary curcumin to obese and diabetic mice for 6 weeks exhibited lower body fat gain and reversed obesity-induced glucose and insulin tolerance. Curcumin treatment also reduced lipid accumulation and inflammation in the liver and macrophage infiltration of adipose tissue. On the other hand, curcumin appears to prevent the development of obesity. A long-term feeding study showed that mice with a high-fat diet supplemented with a low dose of curcumin (i.e., 500 mg/kg diet) for at least 12 weeks showed a reduction of body weight gain, adiposity, and

angiogenesis in adipose tissue without any effects on food intake behavior [105]. This was associated with activation of AMPK, transcriptional suppression of genes involved in lipogenesis and angiogenesis in adipose tissue, and an increase in fatty acid oxidation. In addition, curcumin was demonstrated to have an anti-adipogenic property both *in vitro* [106–109] and *in vivo* [105] through suppression of C/EBPα and PPARγ gene expression, mitotic clonal expansion, activation of Wnt/β-catenin signaling, AMPK activity, and apoptosis of preadipocytes in the early phase of adipogenesis.

Although the molecular mechanisms underlying curcumin's anticancer activities are not completely understood, several mechanisms underlying the chemopreventive function of curcumin have been proposed. Upon activation of cancer cells by free radicals, inflammatory mediators, carcinogens, or ultraviolet light, the transcription factor NF-κB senses these signals and induces expression of several genes involved in cell survival, transformation, proliferation, and metastasis [110]. Curcumin suppresses NF-κB activation by inhibiting the DNA binding ability of NF-κB, and reducing the activation of IKK complex, which in turn lead to the inhibition of inhibitory factor I-κ B (IκB) phosphorylation and subsequent translocation of NF-κB into the nucleus [111]. Curcumin-inhibited NF-κB activation results in suppression of transcriptions of NF-κB-regulated genes involved in cancer cell proliferation, such as COX-2, TNF-α, cyclin D1, adhesion molecules, and metalloproteinases [112], thereby inducing apoptosis. Curcumin has also been reported to promote cell cycle arrest in the G1/S phase in human colon carcinoma cells [113] by downregulating NF-κB-dependent cyclin D1 expression [112]. Curcumin also inhibits activity of transcription factor activating protein-1 (AP-1). AP-1 regulates expression of several genes involved in apoptosis, cell proliferation, and progression. Importantly, AP-1 promotes tumor metastasis by repressing tumor-suppressor genes, including p53, p21, and p16 [110]. Curcumin suppresses AP-1 activation in prostate cancer cell lines such as LNCaP, PC-3, and DU1145 [110]. Inhibition of AP-1 transcriptional activity may be attributed to curcumin-mediated inhibition of c-Jun N-terminal kinase (JNK) phosphorylation [114] that otherwise leads to cell proliferation and tumorigenesis.

Although curcumin is safe even at doses of 2 g/day in humans, poor bioavailability of curcumin limits its therapeutic and/or preventive use in human diseases. This includes poor absorption of curcumin in intestine, rapid metabolism and clearance in various tissues, and rapid clearance in the physiological system. Developments of liposome, micelle, and phospholipid complex [115–118] with curcumin have long been studied and are promising approaches to improve bioavailability of curcumin. In addition, recently developed nanoparticle-based delivery of curcumin [119] and conjugation of curcumin with polyethylene glycol [106] could improve the

TABLE 21.1   Summary of Molecular Targets and End Point Modulation of Potential Anti-Obese and Chemopreventive Phytochemicals

Name	Structure	Molecular targets and end point modulation	References
Curcumin		Lowered plasma triglycerides and VLDL levels, and liver triglycerides and cholesterol levels	[102]
		Lowered body weight gain, blood glucose and insulin levels	[103]
		Lowered body fat gain	[104]
		Reversed obesity-induced glucose and insulin tolerance	[105]
		Reduced lipid accumulation and inflammation	[105,109]
		Reduced body weight gain, adiposity, angiogenesis	[106−109]
		Activation of AMPK in adipose tissue	[110−112]
		Inhibited adipogenesis	[113]
		Reduced NF-κB activity and cell proliferation	[110,112]
		Induction of apoptosis of cancer cells	
		Inhibition of AP-1 activity	
Resveratrol		Decreased PPARγ expression	[112]
		Induced glucose uptake	[122]
		Reduced *de novo* lipogenesis	[123,124]
		Induction of apoptosis	[125,126]
		Increased insulin sensitivity, AMPK function, PGC-1α expression	[127]
		Improved mitochondria function	[128,130]
		Reduced adiposity	[130]
		Suppressed leptin	
		Reduced EGFR, IGF1-R	
		Induced apoptosis and p53 signaling pathway	
EGCG		Decreased fat mass	[134,135]
		Reduced levels of serum lipid metabolites and/or body fat	[137−140]
		Increased thermogenesis and energy expenditure	[142−144]
		Inhibited gene expression and/or activity of lipogenic enzymes	[143,148]
		Activated AMPK	[143−148]
		Inhibited adipogenesis and adipocyte function	[152]
		Reduced the levels of IGF-1, IGFBP-3	[154,155]
		Suppressed TNF-α expression and NF-κB activity	[155,156]
		Induced apoptosis	
		Promoted cell cycle arrest	
Soy phytoestrogens	Genistein	Lowered BMI	[162]
		Improved insulin sensitivity and blood HDL level	[163,164]

(Continued)

B. DIETARY BIOACTIVE COMPOUNDS FOR HEALTH

TABLE 21.1 (*Continued*)

Name	Structure	Molecular targets and end point modulation	References
Daidzein		Reduced body and fat weight gain	[165]
		Suppressed *de novo* lipogenesis	[143]
		Stimulated lipolysis	[165—167]
		Inhibited adipogenesis	[167,168]
		Activated apoptosis and AMPK	[169]
		Inhibited apoptosis	[175]
		Inhibited hepatic triglyceride content and fatty acid synthesis	[176]
		Reduced sex steroid receptor protein expression	[177,178]
		Suppressed NF-κB activity	
		Inhibited ER-α, ER-β, and AR gene expression	
		Suppressed protein tyrosine kinase activity	
		Inhibited TGF-β1-mediated cell growth	

bioavailability of curcumin, but the efficacy and safety of these complexes should be investigated.

B Resveratrol

Resveratrol (Table 21.1), a phenolic compound found in diverse plants, has received much scientific interest throughout the years. It is a naturally occurring stilbenoid found in grapes, berries, peanuts, and sugarcane. As known from the "French paradox," resveratrol has a therapeutic potential against chronic diseases. Its numerous health benefits include hypolipidemic, chemopreventive, anti-inflammatory, and antioxidant activities by largely targeting Sirtuin 1 (Sirt1) [120].

Resveratrol modulates adipose development and function via regulation of various cellular processes. As a dietary activator of Sirt1, resveratrol decreases lipid accumulation and promotes free fatty acid release from adipocytes through Sirt1-dependent repression of PPARγ function [121]. Resveratrol also inhibits adipogenesis of human adipocytes in a Sirt1-dependent manner through stimulation of basal and insulin-induced glucose uptake with a reduced level of *de novo* lipogenesis *in vitro* [122]. In addition, Sirt1-independent function of resveratrol in fat cells has been proposed in which resveratrol regulates the number of differentiated human adipocytes through induction of apoptosis [123]. Indeed, resveratrol has been shown to be an effective proapoptotic agent both in preadipocytes [124] and in adipocytes, by which it controls, at least in part, the function and number of adipocytes. Nevertheless, mice administrated a high-fat diet supplemented with resveratrol at 0.04% (w/w) of diet for

50 weeks [125] or at 0.4% (w/w) for 8 weeks [126] displayed enhanced insulin sensitivity, AMPK function, PPARγ coactivator-1α (PGC-1α) expression, and improvement of mitochondria function as well as reduced adiposity, suggesting a protective function of resveratrol against diet-induced obesity and its related metabolic disorders. However, more studies are needed to improve bioavailability of resveratrol in circulation and target metabolic tissues and also to prove its health benefits in humans.

Although data are still insufficient to reach a conclusion, the protective actions of resveratrol against cancer development are likely attributable to the suppression of leptin secretion [127]. Leptin acts as an important protein linking obesity and cancer [62]. Indeed, a high-fat diet increases circulating levels of serum leptin, and leptin treatment has been shown to increase colonic cell proliferation in mice [64] and human colon cancer cells [63]. Given that resveratrol is known to suppress adipogenesis, resveratrol-mediated suppression of leptin secretion in adipose tissue likely contributes to prevent cancer development.

In addition, growth factor receptors are known to play an important role in the development and progression of colon cancer [128] via stimulating cell growth, angiogenesis, and metastasis. Evidence suggests that resveratrol-suppressed growth factor receptors, including EGFR and IGF-1R, also appear to mediate its chemopreventive function. In fact, an animal experiment with Wistar rats demonstrated that resveratrol administration for 30 weeks significantly attenuated colonic tumor incidence [129]. Resveratrol has been shown to suppress IGF-1-induced cell proliferation and induce apoptosis in human colon cancer cells by inhibiting IGF-1R/Wnt function and activating p53 signaling pathways [130].

C Tea Catechins

Consumption of teas, including green, black, white, and oolong, is commonly associated with a number of positive impacts on human health. The beneficial effect of consuming tea on body weight management appears to be largely through the modulation of whole-body energy balance. Long-term consumption of catechins, which are natural phenolic antioxidants found in teas, is associated with reduction in body weight and body fat in humans [131,132]. Catechins largely consist of epicatechin, epicatechin gallate, epigallocatechin, and epigallocatechin gallate (EGCG). In particular, EGCG is the most abundant polyphenol found in green tea (Table 21.1), and it is most effective in preventing the development of various diseases, including obesity and type 2 diabetes [133]. EGCG decreased subcutaneous fat mass by an average of 55% and abdominal fat by an average of 28% in lean rats after 1 week of intraperitoneal injection of a dose of 70−92 mg EGCG/kg body weight [134]. A 4-day EGCG treatment also induced a 20% body fat loss in obese rats [135]. Although the anti-obesity function of EGCG in humans is inconclusive, a number of human epidemiological studies suggest a possible benefit of EGCG and tea consumption in weight loss [96,98]. Consumption of high levels of green tea (more than 10 cups/day) [136], habitual tea consumption (more than 10 years) [137], and consumption of a bottle of oolong tea containing 690 mg catechins/day for 12 weeks [138] in different human populations resulted in lower levels of serum lipid metabolites and/or body fat, as well as greater thermogenesis and energy expenditure [139,140]. Note that other nonphytochemicals in the tea, such as caffeine, are also suggested to contribute, at least in part, to the health benefit of tea consumption [141]. Despite the important health benefit of EGCG, the detailed mechanism of its action in regulating body weight and adipose mass is relatively unclear. In general, EGCG and other catechins are known to inhibit gene expression and/or activity of lipogenic enzymes such as FAS, SCD-1, and glucose-6-phosphate dehydrogenase, thereby reducing fatty acid and triglyceride synthesis in adipose tissue and the liver [142−144] partly through activation of AMPK [143] and/or inhibition of adipogenesis of adipocytes. EGCG also displays a direct inhibitory effect on adipogenesis via regulation of multiple cellular processes and the transcriptional program in adipogenesis. In addition to its anti-adipogenic property, EGCG has been reported to exhibit anti-mitogenic [145] and/or proapoptotic [146] effect and to act as a transcriptional suppressor [147] and/or AMPK activator [148] during adipogenesis.

Numerous studies have suggested that EGCG may be effective in preventing cancer development [149]. A meta-analysis showed a positive association between increased green tea consumption and a significant reduction of breast cancer risk [150]. An *in vivo* study using rats fed a high-fat diet supplemented with black tea found decreased tumor numbers, size, and multiplicity after the administration of a chemical carcinogen [151].

The chemopreventive mechanisms of catechins found in green and/or black tea have been proposed in a number of studies. Catechins appear to inhibit the function of growth factor receptors and their downstream mediators and NF-κB activation. Catechins also induce cancer cell apoptosis and cell cycle arrest. Oral administration of green tea polyphenol mixture to the transgenic adenocarcinoma of the mouse prostate (TRAMP) mouse model has been shown to inhibit the development and progression of prostate tumor by reducing the levels of IGF-1 and IGF-binding protein (IGFBP)-3 and its downstream signaling pathways in dorsolateral prostate [152]. The role of TNF-α is important in carcinogenesis because it acts as a growth factor for most of the tumor cells [153]. However, EGCG has been shown to suppress TNF-α expression [154] through inhibition of NF-κB activity [155]. On the other hand, EGCG induces apoptosis by stabilizing p53 in human prostate carcinoma LNCaP cells [156]. Likewise, promotion of cell cycle arrest through alteration of cell cycle regulatory protein expression by EGCG may be another molecular mechanism by which EGCG blocks carcinogenesis [155].

Anti-obesity activities of EGCG have been well-defined. As discussed previously, green tea, particularly EGCG, has been suggested to decrease body mass and exert hypolipidemic activity. The potential mechanisms by which green tea regulates body weight and adiposity may be attributed to an increase in energy expenditure and fat oxidation, and a decrease in intestinal lipid absorption [157]. Although it is not clear whether EGCG-lowered body weight and adiposity directly contribute to the prevention of the development of obesity-related cancers, based on the aforementioned studies, it is plausible to hypothesize that EGCG-mediated reductions in body and adipose tissue mass may contribute to the decreased risk of the development of various cancers. Hence, more studies are needed to address this hypothesis and to elucidate whether EGCG could be an ideal candidate to protect against both obesity and its related cancers.

D Soy Phytoestrogens

Dietary phytoestrogens are known to benefit human health [158]. Due to the fact that phytoestrogens have chemical structures similar to that of estradiol, it is suggested that phytoestrogens are able to modulate cellular estrogenic processes through binding to the estrogen receptors in various cell types. Indeed, these phytoestrogens are largely known to have protective function against menopausal disorders, cardiovascular disease, cancer, and osteoporosis [159—161]. The major bioactive isoflavones in the dietary phytoestrogens are genistein and daidzein (Table 21.1). These are largely found in soybean and soybean products, and they are tightly conjugated with soy proteins. In approximately the past decade, a number of studies of humans and animals have provided evidence of a potential anti-obesity function of soy proteins and soy isoflavones such as daidzein and genistein. Consumption of soy isoflavones was associated with lower BMI, improved insulin sensitivity, and blood high-density lipoprotein (HDL) level in postmenopausal women of normal weight [162]. Moreover, soy protein isolate and its hydrolysate effectively reduced weight gain by lowering adipose tissue mass in genetically obese mice [163] and obese rats fed a high-fat diet [164]. Although the mechanisms underlying the anti-obese function of phytoestrogens are largely unclear, the phytoestrogens appear to modulate systemic energy balance by targeting energy metabolism of a variety of cell types, including adipocytes and hepatocytes. Genistein is shown to suppress *de novo* lipogenesis and stimulate lipolysis in isolated adipocytes [165]. Moreover, genistein is known to inhibit adipogenesis by suppressing C/EBPβ activity [166] and by activation of AMPK [148] and apoptosis [167] in differentiating preadipocytes. Contrary to genistein's anti-adipogenic effect, daidzein, an analog of genistein, is reported to have proadipogenic property with improved PPARγ-mediated transcriptional activity and insulin-stimulated glucose uptake [168]. Genistein has also been reported to inhibit hepatic triglyceride content and fatty acid synthesis in the liver and adipose tissue [169]. Collectively, these phytoestrogens seem to have favorable actions on energy metabolism that could partly explain their protective and/or therapeutic effect on obesity and its related glucose disorders.

Epidemiological studies suggest that increased consumption of phytoestrogens may contribute to a decrease in the rates of recurrence and mortality of breast and prostate cancers [170,171]. A cross-sectional study of 100 women who had been treated for breast cancer and were in remission reported that two-third of the patients consumed some type of soy food with average daily intake of 11.6 mg genistein and 7.4 mg daidzein [172]. Among many other soy isoflavones, genistein has been studied extensively due to its abundance in soy foods and its protective activities against hormone-dependent cancers [173]. Indeed, many animal studies suggest an anticancer property of genistein

in prostate cancer. Dietary supplementation with genistein decreased the percentage of TRAMP mice that developed adenocarcinomas of the prostate [174]. Consistent with this finding, supplementation with genistein and daidzein resulted in inhibition of chemical-induced prostate carcinomas in F344 rats [175]. Soy isoflavones are known to be converted to equol and 5-hydroxyl-equol by intestinal bacteria, which exhibit biological function that exceeds those of their precursors. Thus, soy isoflavone's anti-obesity and anticancer properties are suggested to result from equol-modulated estrogen- and androgen-dependent cellular conditions.

Although the mechanisms by which genistein protects against obesity-related cancer development are not fully elucidated, downregulation of sex steroid receptor protein expression, suppression of NF-κB activation, and inhibition of tyrosine kinase in cancer cells by genistein and daidzein have been proposed. Because of the structural similarity to the endogenous hormone 17β-estradiol, the potential chemopreventive function of genistein and daidzein is likely to be through modulation of ER function and its related signaling pathways, and this could be mediated by the soy isoflavone metabolite equol. In support, dietary genistein downregulates mRNA expressions of ER-α and -β as well as androgen receptor (AR) in the dorsolateral prostate of Sprague—Dawley rats [176]. This study suggests that dietary genistein may protect against prostate cancer due to its high affinity with sex steroid hormone receptor. These phytoestrogens also play an inhibitory role in the binding between NF-κB and DNA and in the protein tyrosine kinase (PTK) activity observed in prostate and breast cells [177]. In addition, genistein is suggested to target various cellular pathways such as transforming growth factor-β1 (TGF-β1) and its downstream pathways [178]. Collectively, the anticarcinogenic actions of genistein and daidzein are likely mediated through modulation of the functions of NF-κB and PTK and also TGF-β1-dependent signaling cascades mostly in prostate and breast cancer cells, which otherwise are known to stimulate cancer cell proliferation.

V CONCLUSION

During the past several decades, there has been a substantial increase in our understanding of the molecular basis of the development of obesity and obesity-related cancers. The identification of specific molecular targets that contribute to the incidence of these diseases provides the ability to screen new anti-obesity and/or chemopreventive dietary components. This chapter summarized the potential use of some food components in the dietary prevention of obesity and its related cancers. Given the poor bioavailability of most of the aforementioned dietary components in physiological condition, further research should focus on developing new methods to enhance the efficacy and stability of these in circulation and/or target tissues. In addition, detailed preclinical studies and human studies should be performed.

References

[1] P.G. Kopelman, Obesity as a medical problem, Nature 404 (2000) 635–643.

[2] K.L. Spalding, E. Arner, P.O. Westermark, S. Bernard, B.A. Buchholz, O. Bergmann, et al., Dynamics of fat cell turnover in humans, Nature 453 (2008) 783–787.

[3] F.M. Gregoire, C.M. Smas, H.S. Sul, Understanding adipocyte differentiation, Physiol. Rev. 78 (1998) 783–809.

[4] Q.Q. Tang, T.C. Otto, M.D. Lane, Mitotic clonal expansion: a synchronous process required for adipogenesis, Proc. Natl. Acad. Sci. USA 100 (2003) 44–49.

[5] P.L. Chen, D.J. Riley, Y. Chen, W.H. Lee, Retinoblastoma protein positively regulates terminal adipocyte differentiation through direct interaction with C/EBPs, Genes Dev. 10 (1996) 2794–2804.

[6] M. Classon, B.K. Kennedy, R. Mulloy, E. Harlow, Opposing roles of pRB and p107 in adipocyte differentiation, Proc. Natl. Acad. Sci. USA 97 (2000) 10826–10831.

[7] S.R. Farmer, Transcriptional control of adipocyte formation, Cell Metab. 4 (2006) 263–273.

[8] X. Li, J.W. Kim, M. Gronborg, H. Urlaub, M.D. Lane, Q.Q. Tang, Role of cdk2 in the sequential phosphorylation/activation of C/EBPbeta during adipocyte differentiation, Proc. Natl. Acad. Sci. USA 104 (2007) 11597–11602.

[9] L. Abu-Elheiga, W. Oh, P. Kordari, S.J. Wakil, Acetyl-CoA carboxylase 2 mutant mice are protected against obesity and diabetes induced by high-fat/high-carbohydrate diets, Proc. Natl. Acad. Sci. USA 100 (2003) 10207–10212.

[10] J.M. Ntambi, M. Miyazaki, J.P. Stoehr, H. Lan, C.M. Kendziorski, B.S. Yandell, et al., Loss of stearoyl-CoA desaturase-1 function protects mice against adiposity, Proc. Natl. Acad. Sci. USA 99 (2002) 11482–11486.

[11] S.H. Cha, Z. Hu, M.D. Lane, Long-term effects of a fatty acid synthase inhibitor on obese mice: food intake, hypothalamic neuropeptides, and UCP3, Biochem. Biophys. Res. Commun. 317 (2004) 301–308.

[12] T.M. Loftus, D.E. Jaworsky, G.L. Frehywot, C.A. Townsend, G.V. Ronnett, M.D. Lane, et al., Reduced food intake and body weight in mice treated with fatty acid synthase inhibitors, Science 288 (2000) 2379–2381.

[13] L.E. Hammond, S. Neschen, A.J. Romanelli, G.W. Cline, O.R. Ilkayeva, G.I. Shulman, et al., Mitochondrial glycerol-3-phosphate acyltransferase-1 is essential in liver for the metabolism of excess acyl-CoAs, J. Biol. Chem. 280 (2005) 25629–25636.

[14] L. Vergnes, A.P. Beigneux, R. Davis, S.M. Watkins, S.G. Young, K. Reue, Agpat6 deficiency causes subdermal lipodystrophy and resistance to obesity, J. Lipid Res. 47 (2006) 745–754.

[15] K. Reue, P. Xu, X.P. Wang, B.G. Slavin, Adipose tissue deficiency, glucose intolerance, and increased atherosclerosis result from mutation in the mouse fatty liver dystrophy (fld) gene, J. Lipid Res. 41 (2000) 1067–1076.

[16] S.J. Smith, S. Cases, D.R. Jensen, H.C. Chen, E. Sande, B. Tow, et al., Obesity resistance and multiple mechanisms of triglyceride synthesis in mice lacking DGAT, Nat. Genet. 25 (2000) 87–90.

[17] A.K. Agarwal, A. Garg, Congenital generalized lipodystrophy: significance of triglyceride biosynthetic pathways, Trends Endocrinol. Metab. 14 (2003) 214–221.

[18] E.H. Ludwig, R.W. Mahley, E. Palaoglu, S. Ozbayrakci, M.E. Balestra, I.B. Borecki, et al., DGAT1 promoter polymorphism associated with alterations in body mass index, high density lipoprotein levels and blood pressure in Turkish women, Clin. Genet. 62 (2002) 68–73.

[19] M. Peterfy, J. Phan, P. Xu, K. Reue, Lipodystrophy in the fld mouse results from mutation of a new gene encoding a nuclear protein, lipin, Nat. Genet. 27 (2001) 121–124.

[20] S.J. Stone, H.M. Myers, S.M. Watkins, B.E. Brown, K.R. Feingold, P.M. Elias, et al., Lipopenia and skin barrier abnormalities in DGAT2-deficient mice, J. Biol. Chem. 279 (2004) 11767–11776.

[21] Y. Shi, P. Burn, Lipid metabolic enzymes: emerging drug targets for the treatment of obesity, Nat. Rev. Drug Discov. 3 (2004) 695–710.

[22] J.L. Halaas, K.S. Gajiwala, M. Maffei, S.L. Cohen, B.T. Chait, D. Rabinowitz, et al., Weight-reducing effects of the plasma protein encoded by the obese gene, Science 269 (1995) 543–546.

[23] F. Lonnqvist, P. Arner, L. Nordfors, M. Schalling, Overexpression of the obese (ob) gene in adipose tissue of human obese subjects, Nat. Med. 1 (1995) 950–953.

[24] Y. Minokoshi, Y.B. Kim, O.D. Peroni, L.G. Fryer, C. Muller, D. Carling, et al., Leptin stimulates fatty-acid oxidation by activating AMP-activated protein kinase, Nature 415 (2002) 339–343.

[25] C.A. Siegrist-Kaiser, V. Pauli, C.E. Juge-Aubry, O. Boss, A. Pernin, W.W. Chin, et al., Direct effects of leptin on brown and white adipose tissue, J. Clin. Invest. 100 (1997) 2858–2864.

[26] S. Kaser, A. Moschen, A. Cayon, A. Kaser, J. Crespo, F. Pons-Romero, et al., Adiponectin and its receptors in non-alcoholic steatohepatitis, Gut 54 (2005) 117–121.

[27] W.J. Freeman, Neurodynamic models of brain in psychiatry, Neuropsychopharmacology 28 (Suppl. 1) (2003) S54–S63.

[28] T. Yamauchi, J. Kamon, H. Waki, Y. Terauchi, N. Kubota, K. Hara, et al., The fat-derived hormone adiponectin reverses insulin resistance associated with both lipoatrophy and obesity, Nat. Med. 7 (2001) 941–946.

[29] T.P. Combs, A.H. Berg, S. Obici, P.E. Scherer, L. Rossetti, Endogenous glucose production is inhibited by the adipose-derived protein Acrp30, J. Clin. Invest. 108 (2001) 1875–1881.

[30] T. Yamauchi, Y. Nio, T. Maki, M. Kobayashi, T. Takazawa, M. Iwabu, et al., Targeted disruption of AdipoR1 and AdipoR2 causes abrogation of adiponectin binding and metabolic actions, Nat. Med. 13 (2007) 332–339.

[31] Y. Zhang, M. Matheny, S. Zolotukhin, N. Tumer, P.J. Scarpace, Regulation of adiponectin and leptin gene expression in white and brown adipose tissues: influence of beta3-adrenergic agonists, retinoic acid, leptin and fasting, Biochim. Biophys. Acta 1584 (2002) 115–122.

[32] T.P. Combs, A.H. Berg, M.W. Rajala, S. Klebanov, P. Iyengar, J.C. Jimenez-Chillaron, et al., Sexual differentiation, pregnancy, calorie restriction, and aging affect the adipocyte-specific secretory protein adiponectin, Diabetes 52 (2003) 268–276.

[33] J.S. Bogan, H.F. Lodish, Two compartments for insulin-stimulated exocytosis in 3T3-L1 adipocytes defined by endogenous ACRP30 and GLUT4, J. Cell Biol. 146 (1999) 609–620.

[34] T.P. Combs, J.A. Wagner, J. Berger, T. Doebber, W.J. Wang, B.B. Zhang, et al., Induction of adipocyte complement-related protein of 30 kilodaltons by PPARgamma agonists: a potential mechanism of insulin sensitization, Endocrinology 143 (2002) 998–1007.

[35] M. Fasshauer, J. Klein, S. Neumann, M. Eszlinger, R. Paschke, Hormonal regulation of adiponectin gene expression in 3T3-L1 adipocytes, Biochem. Biophys. Res. Commun. 290 (2002) 1084–1089.

[36] M. Fasshauer, S. Kralisch, M. Klier, U. Lossner, M. Bluher, J. Klein, et al., Adiponectin gene expression and secretion is inhibited by interleukin-6 in 3T3-L1 adipocytes, Biochem. Biophys. Res. Commun. 301 (2003) 1045–1050.

[37] L.A. Tartaglia, M. Dembski, X. Weng, N. Deng, J. Culpepper, R. Devos, et al., Identification and expression cloning of a leptin receptor, OB-R, Cell 83 (1995) 1263–1271.

[38] M.W. Schwartz, S.C. Woods, D. Porte Jr., R.J. Seeley, D.G. Baskin, Central nervous system control of food intake, Nature 404 (2000) 661–671.

[39] S.P. Grossman, The role of glucose, insulin and glucagon in the regulation of food intake and body weight, Neurosci. Biobehav. Rev. 10 (1986) 295–315.

[40] Y. Minokoshi, T. Alquier, N. Furukawa, Y.B. Kim, A. Lee, B. Xue, et al., AMP-kinase regulates food intake by responding to hormonal and nutrient signals in the hypothalamus, Nature 428 (2004) 569–574.

[41] G.R. Stoppa, M. Cesquini, E.A. Roman, P.O. Prada, A.S. Torsoni, T. Romanatto, et al., Intracerebroventricular injection of citrate inhibits hypothalamic AMPK and modulates feeding behavior and peripheral insulin signaling, J. Endocrinol. 198 (2008) 157–168.

[42] M.S. Kim, J.Y. Park, C. Namkoong, P.G. Jang, J.W. Ryu, H.S. Song, et al., Anti-obesity effects of alpha-lipoic acid mediated by suppression of hypothalamic AMP-activated protein kinase, Nat. Med. 10 (2004) 727–733.

[43] T. Shimokawa, M.V. Kumar, M.D. Lane, Effect of a fatty acid synthase inhibitor on food intake and expression of hypothalamic neuropeptides, Proc. Natl. Acad. Sci. USA 99 (2002) 66–71.

[44] T.H. Moran, Cholecystokinin and satiety: current perspectives, Nutrition 16 (2000) 858–865.

[45] D. Larhammar, Structural diversity of receptors for neuropeptide Y, peptide YY and pancreatic polypeptide, Regul. Pept. 65 (1996) 165–174.

[46] J.J. Holst, On the physiology of GIP and GLP-1, Horm. Metab. Res. 36 (2004) 747–754.

[47] K.L. Johnston, M.N. Clifford, L.M. Morgan, Coffee acutely modifies gastrointestinal hormone secretion and glucose tolerance in humans: Glycemic effects of chlorogenic acid and caffeine, Am. J. Clin. Nutr. 78 (2003) 728–733.

[48] Y. Zhang, X. Na, L. Li, X. Zhao, H. Cui, Isoflavone reduces body weight by decreasing food intake in ovariectomized rats, Ann. Nutr. Metab. 54 (2009) 163–170.

[49] K.M. Flegal, M.D. Carroll, C.L. Ogden, L.R. Curtin, Prevalence and trends in obesity among U.S. adults, 1999–2008, JAMA 303 (2010) 235–241.

[50] R.I. Meijer, E.H. Serne, Y.M. Smulders, V.W. van Hinsbergh, J.S. Yudkin, E.C. Eringa, Perivascular adipose tissue and its role in type 2 diabetes and cardiovascular disease, Curr. Diab. Rep. 11 (2011) 211–217.

[51] E.E. Calle, C. Rodriguez, K. Walker-Thurmond, M.J. Thun, Overweight, obesity, and mortality from cancer in a prospectively studied cohort of U.S. adults, N. Engl. J. Med. 348 (2003) 1625–1638.

[52] A.G. Renehan, M. Tyson, M. Egger, R.F. Heller, M. Zwahlen, Body-mass index and incidence of cancer: a systematic review and meta-analysis of prospective observational studies, Lancet 371 (2008) 569–578.

[53] W.C.R. Fund, Food, Nutrition, Physical Activity and the Prevention of Cancer: A Global Perspective, American Institute for Cancer Research, Washington, DC, 2007.

[54] S. Yakar, D. Leroith, P. Brodt, The role of the growth hormone/insulin-like growth factor axis in tumor growth and progression: lessons from animal models, Cytokine Growth Factor Rev. 16 (2005) 407–420.

[55] E.E. Calle, R. Kaaks, Overweight, obesity and cancer: epidemiological evidence and proposed mechanisms, Nat. Rev. Cancer 4 (2004) 579–591.

[56] T.J. Key, P.N. Appleby, G.K. Reeves, A. Roddam, J.F. Dorgan, C. Longcope, et al., Body mass index, serum sex hormones, and breast cancer risk in postmenopausal women, J. Natl. Cancer Inst. 95 (2003) 1218–1226.

[57] M. Pugeat, J.C. Crave, M. Elmidani, M.H. Nicolas, M. Garoscio-Cholet, H. Lejeune, et al., Pathophysiology of sex hormone binding globulin (SHBG): relation to insulin, J. Steroid Biochem. Mol. Biol. 40 (1991) 841–849.

[58] J. Ferlay, H.R. Shin, F. Bray, D. Forman, C. Mathers, D.M. Parkin, Estimates of worldwide burden of cancer in 2008: GLOBOCAN 2008, Int. J. Cancer 127 (2010) 2893–2917.

[59] E.M. Siegel, C.M. Ulrich, E.M. Poole, R.S. Holmes, P.B. Jacobsen, D. Shibata, The effects of obesity and obesity-related conditions on colorectal cancer prognosis, Cancer Control 17 (2010) 52–57.

[60] E. Giovannucci, A. Ascherio, E.B. Rimm, G.A. Colditz, M.J. Stampfer, W.C. Willett, Physical activity, obesity, and risk for colon cancer and adenoma in men, Ann. Intern. Med. 122 (1995) 327–334.

[61] S. Yamamoto, T. Nakagawa, Y. Matsushita, S. Kusano, T. Hayashi, M. Irokawa, et al., Visceral fat area and markers of insulin resistance in relation to colorectal neoplasia, Diabetes Care 33 (2010) 184–189.

[62] P. Stattin, A. Lukanova, C. Biessy, S. Soderberg, R. Palmqvist, R. Kaaks, et al., Obesity and colon cancer: does leptin provide a link? Int. J. Cancer 109 (2004) 149–152.

[63] J.C. Hardwick, G.R. Van Den Brink, G.J. Offerhaus, S.J. Van Deventer, M.P. Peppelenbosch, Leptin is a growth factor for colonic epithelial cells, Gastroenterology 121 (2001) 79–90.

[64] S.Y. Park, J.S. Kim, Y.R. Seo, M.K. Sung, Effects of diet-induced obesity on colitis-associated colon tumor formation in A/J mice, Int. J. Obes. (London) 36 (2011) 273–280.

[65] P. Rouet-Benzineb, T. Aparicio, S. Guilmeau, C. Pouzet, V. Descatoire, M. Buyse, et al., Leptin counteracts sodium butyrate-induced apoptosis in human colon cancer HT-29 cells via NF-kappaB signaling, J. Biol. Chem. 279 (2004) 16495–16502.

[66] M.R. Sierra-Honigmann, A.K. Nath, C. Murakami, G. Garcia-Cardena, A. Papapetropoulos, W.C. Sessa, et al., Biological action of leptin as an angiogenic factor, Science 281 (1998) 1683–1686.

[67] S.B. Fox, G. Gasparini, A.L. Harris, Angiogenesis: pathological, prognostic, and growth-factor pathways and their link to trial design and anticancer drugs, Lancet Oncol. 2 (2001) 278–289.

[68] J.E. Kim, J.Y. Kim, K.W. Lee, H.J. Lee, Cancer chemopreventive effects of lactic acid bacteria, J. Microbiol. Biotechnol. 17 (2007) 1227–1235.

[69] P.H. Lahmann, K. Hoffmann, N. Allen, C.H. van Gils, K.T. Khaw, B. Tehard, et al., Body size and breast cancer risk: findings from the European Prospective Investigation into Cancer and Nutrition (EPIC), Int. J. Cancer 111 (2004) 762–771.

[70] M.K. Sung, J.Y. Yeon, S.Y. Park, J.H. Park, M.S. Choi, Obesity-induced metabolic stresses in breast and colon cancer, Ann. N. Y. Acad. Sci. 1229 (2011) 61–68.

[71] J.Y. Yeon, Y.J. Suh, S.W. Kim, H.W. Baik, C.J. Sung, H.S. Kim, et al., Evaluation of dietary factors in relation to the biomarkers of oxidative stress and inflammation in breast cancer risk, Nutrition 27 (2011) 912–918.

[72] I. Nieto-Vazquez, S. Fernandez-Veledo, D.K. Kramer, R. Vila-Bedmar, L. Garcia-Guerra, M. Lorenzo, Insulin resistance associated to obesity: the link TNF-alpha, Arch. Physiol. Biochem. 114 (2008) 183–194.

[73] D.R. Hodge, E.M. Hurt, W.L. Farrar, The role of IL-6 and STAT3 in inflammation and cancer, Eur. J. Cancer 41 (2005) 2502–2512.

[74] A. Schaffler, J. Scholmerich, C. Buechler, Mechanisms of disease: Adipokines and breast cancer—Endocrine and paracrine mechanisms that connect adiposity and breast cancer, Nat. Clin. Pract. Endocrinol. Metab. 3 (2007) 345–354.

[75] C. Mantzoros, E. Petridou, N. Dessypris, C. Chavelas, M. Dalamaga, D.M. Alexe, et al., Adiponectin and breast cancer risk, J. Clin. Endocrinol. Metab. 89 (2004) 1102–1107.

[76] J.H. Kang, Y.Y. Lee, B.Y. Yu, B.S. Yang, K.H. Cho, D.K. Yoon, et al., Adiponectin induces growth arrest and apoptosis of MDA-MB-231 breast cancer cell, Arch. Pharm. Res. 28 (2005) 1263–1269.

[77] Z. Luo, M. Zang, W. Guo, AMPK as a metabolic tumor suppressor: control of metabolism and cell growth, Future Oncol. 6 (2010) 457–470.

[78] T.J. Key, A. Schatzkin, W.C. Willett, N.E. Allen, E.A. Spencer, R.C. Travis, Diet, nutrition and the prevention of cancer, Public Health Nutr. 7 (2004) 187–200.

[79] R. Kaaks, A. Lukanova, M.S. Kurzer, Obesity, endogenous hormones, and endometrial cancer risk: a synthetic review, Cancer Epidemiol. Biomarkers Prev. 11 (2002) 1531–1543.

[80] Iu, S. Maleta, Effect of ampicillin, oxacillin, benzylpenicillin and phenoxymethylpenicillin on the outcome of acute radiation sickness in albino mice, Antibiotiki 13 (1968) 727–728.

[81] E. Petridou, M. Belechri, N. Dessypris, P. Koukoulomatis, E. Diakomanolis, E. Spanos, et al., Leptin and body mass index in relation to endometrial cancer risk, Ann. Nutr. Metab. 46 (2002) 147–151.

[82] J. Gao, J. Tian, J. Lv, F. Shi, F. Kong, H. Shi, et al., Leptin induces functional activation of cyclooxygenase-2 through JAK2/STAT3, MAPK/ERK, and PI3K/AKT pathways in human endometrial cancer cells, Cancer Sci. 100 (2009) 389–395.

[83] A. Kubo, D.A. Corley, Body mass index and adenocarcinomas of the esophagus or gastric cardia: a systematic review and meta-analysis, Cancer Epidemiol. Biomarkers Prev. 15 (2006) 872–878.

[84] J.M. Howard, G.P. Pidgeon, J.V. Reynolds, Leptin and gastrointestinal malignancies, Obes. Rev. 11 (2010) 863–874.

[85] M.M. Abdel-Latif, S. Duggan, J.V. Reynolds, D. Kelleher, Inflammation and esophageal carcinogenesis, Curr. Opin. Pharmacol. 9 (2009) 396–404.

[86] A. Kandulski, P. Malfertheiner, Gastroesophageal reflux disease: from reflux episodes to mucosal inflammation, Nat. Rev. Gastroenterol. Hepatol. 9 (2011) 15–22.

[87] S.Y. Pan, K.C. Johnson, A.M. Ugnat, S.W. Wen, Y. Mao, Association of obesity and cancer risk in Canada, Am. J. Epidemiol. 159 (2004) 259–268.

[88] C. Koebnick, D. Michaud, S.C. Moore, Y. Park, A. Hollenbeck, R. Ballard-Barbash, et al., Body mass index, physical activity, and bladder cancer in a large prospective study, Cancer Epidemiol. Biomarkers Prev. 17 (2008) 1214–1221.

[89] A.W. Hsing, L.C. Sakoda, S. Chua Jr., Obesity, metabolic syndrome, and prostate cancer, Am. J. Clin. Nutr. 86 (2007) s843–s857.

[90] E.E. Calle, M.J. Thun, Obesity and cancer, Oncogene 23 (2004) 6365–6378.

[91] A. Berrington de Gonzalez, S. Sweetland, E. Spencer, A meta-analysis of obesity and the risk of pancreatic cancer, Br. J. Cancer 89 (2003) 519–523.

[92] S. Shukla, S. Gupta, Dietary agents in the chemoprevention of prostate cancer, Nutr. Cancer 53 (2005) 18–32.

[93] Y.A. Vano, M.J. Rodrigues, S.M. Schneider, Epidemiological link between eating habits and cancer: the example of colorectal cancer, Bull. Cancer 96 (2009) 647–658.

[94] K.W. Lee, A.M. Bode, Z. Dong, Molecular targets of phytochemicals for cancer prevention, Nat. Rev. Cancer 11 (2011) 211–218.

[95] J.K. Campbell, K. Canene-Adams, B.L. Lindshield, T.W. Boileau, S.K. Clinton, J.W. Erdman Jr., Tomato phytochemicals and prostate cancer risk, J. Nutr. 134 (2004) 3486S–3492S.

[96] L.M. Butler, A.H. Wu, Green and black tea in relation to gynecologic cancers, Mol. Nutr. Food Res. 55 (2011) 931–940.

[97] X. Zhang, X.O. Shu, Y.B. Xiang, G. Yang, H. Li, J. Gao, et al., Cruciferous vegetable consumption is associated with a reduced risk of total and cardiovascular disease mortality, Am. J. Clin. Nutr. 94 (2011) 240–246.

[98] J.M. Yuan, Green tea and prevention of esophageal and lung cancers, Mol. Nutr. Food Res. 55 (2011) 886–904.

[99] Z.C. Nelson, R.M. Ray, C. Wu, H. Stalsberg, P. Porter, J.W. Lampe, et al., Fruit and vegetable intakes are associated with lower risk of breast fibroadenomas in Chinese women, J. Nutr. 140 (2010) 1294–1301.

[100] X.O. Shu, Y. Zheng, H. Cai, K. Gu, Z. Chen, W. Zheng, et al., Soy food intake and breast cancer survival, JAMA 302 (2009) 2437–2443.

[101] A. Goel, B.B. Aggarwal, Curcumin, the golden spice from Indian saffron, is a chemosensitizer and radiosensitizer for tumors and chemoprotector and radioprotector for normal organs, Nutr. Cancer 62 (2010) 919–930.

[102] A. Asai, T. Miyazawa, Dietary curcuminoids prevent high-fat diet-induced lipid accumulation in rat liver and epididymal adipose tissue, J. Nutr. 131 (2001) 2932–2935.

[103] K.I. Seo, M.S. Choi, U.J. Jung, H.J. Kim, J. Yeo, S.M. Jeon, et al., Effect of curcumin supplementation on blood glucose, plasma insulin, and glucose homeostasis related enzyme activities in diabetic db/db mice, Mol. Nutr. Food Res. 52 (2008) 995–1004.

[104] S.P. Weisberg, R. Leibel, D.V. Tortoriello, Dietary curcumin significantly improves obesity-associated inflammation and diabetes in mouse models of diabesity, Endocrinology 149 (2008) 3549–3558.

[105] A. Ejaz, D. Wu, P. Kwan, M. Meydani, Curcumin inhibits adipogenesis in 3T3-L1 adipocytes and angiogenesis and obesity in C57/BL mice, J. Nutr. 139 (2009) 919–925.

[106] C.Y. Kim, N. Bordenave, M.G. Ferruzzi, A. Safavy, K.H. Kim, Modification of curcumin with polyethylene glycol enhances the delivery of curcumin in preadipocytes and its antiadipogenic property, J. Agric. Food Chem. 59 (2011) 1012–1019.

[107] J. Ahn, H. Lee, S. Kim, T. Ha, Curcumin-induced suppression of adipogenic differentiation is accompanied by activation of Wnt/beta-catenin signaling, Am. J. Physiol. Cell. Physiol. 298 (2010) C1510–C1516.

[108] J. Zhao, X.B. Sun, F. Ye, W.X. Tian, Suppression of fatty acid synthase, differentiation and lipid accumulation in adipocytes by curcumin, Mol. Cell. Biochem. 351 (2011) 19–28.

[109] Y.K. Lee, W.S. Lee, J.T. Hwang, D.Y. Kwon, Y.J. Surh, O.J. Park, Curcumin exerts antidifferentiation effect through AMPKalpha-PPAR-gamma in 3T3-L1 adipocytes and antiproliferatory effect through AMPKalpha-COX-2 in cancer cells, J. Agric. Food Chem. 57 (2009) 305–310.

[110] B.B. Aggarwal, S. Shishodia, Molecular targets of dietary agents for prevention and therapy of cancer, Biochem. Pharmacol. 71 (2006) 1397–1421.

[111] C. Jobin, C.A. Bradham, M.P. Russo, B. Juma, A.S. Narula, D.A. Brenner, et al., Curcumin blocks cytokine-mediated NF-kappa B activation and proinflammatory gene expression by inhibiting inhibitory factor I-kappa B kinase activity, J. Immunol. 163 (1999) 3474–3483.

[112] S. Shishodia, G. Sethi, B.B. Aggarwal, Curcumin: getting back to the roots, Ann. N. Y. Acad. Sci. 1056 (2005) 206–217.

[113] H. Chen, Z.S. Zhang, Y.L. Zhang, D.Y. Zhou, Curcumin inhibits cell proliferation by interfering with the cell cycle and inducing apoptosis in colon carcinoma cells, Anticancer Res. 19 (1999) 3675–3680.

[114] Y. Xia, C. Makris, B. Su, E. Li, J. Yang, G.R. Nemerow, et al., MEK kinase 1 is critically required for c-Jun N-terminal kinase activation by proinflammatory stimuli and growth factor-induced cell migration, Proc. Natl. Acad. Sci. USA 97 (2000) 5243–5248.

[115] L. Li, B. Ahmed, K. Mehta, R. Kurzrock, Liposomal curcumin with and without oxaliplatin: effects on cell growth, apoptosis, and angiogenesis in colorectal cancer, Mol. Cancer Ther. 6 (2007) 1276–1282.

[116] D. Suresh, K. Srinivasan, Studies on the *in vitro* absorption of spice principles—Curcumin, capsaicin and piperine in rat intestines, Food Chem. Toxicol. 45 (2007) 1437—1442.

[117] Z. Ma, A. Shayeganpour, D.R. Brocks, A. Lavasanifar, J. Samuel, High-performance liquid chromatography analysis of curcumin in rat plasma: application to pharmacokinetics of polymeric micellar formulation of curcumin, Biomed. Chromatogr. 21 (2007) 546—552.

[118] A. Liu, H. Lou, L. Zhao, P. Fan, Validated LC/MS/MS assay for curcumin and tetrahydrocurcumin in rat plasma and application to pharmacokinetic study of phospholipid complex of curcumin, J. Pharm. Biomed. Anal. 40 (2006) 720—727.

[119] S. Bisht, G. Feldmann, S. Soni, R. Ravi, C. Karikar, A. Maitra, Polymeric nanoparticle-encapsulated curcumin ("nanocurcumin"): a novel strategy for human cancer therapy, J. Nanobiotechnol. 5 (2007) 3.

[120] S. Chung, H. Yao, S. Caito, J.W. Hwang, G. Arunachalam, I. Rahman, Regulation of SIRT1 in cellular functions: role of polyphenols, Arch. Biochem. Biophys. 501 (2010) 79—90.

[121] F. Picard, M. Kurtev, N. Chung, A. Topark-Ngarm, T. Senawong, R. Machado De Oliveira, et al., Sirt1 promotes fat mobilization in white adipocytes by repressing PPAR-gamma, Nature 429 (2004) 771—776.

[122] P. Fischer-Posovszky, V. Kukulus, D. Tews, T. Unterkircher, K.M. Debatin, S. Fulda, et al., Resveratrol regulates human adipocyte number and function in a Sirt1-dependent manner, Am. J. Clin. Nutr. 92 (2010) 5—15.

[123] I. Mader, M. Wabitsch, K.M. Debatin, P. Fischer-Posovszky, S. Fulda, Identification of a novel proapoptotic function of resveratrol in fat cells: SIRT1-independent sensitization to TRAIL-induced apoptosis, FASEB J. 24 (2010) 1997—2009.

[124] S. Rayalam, J.Y. Yang, S. Ambati, M.A. Della-Fera, C.A. Baile, Resveratrol induces apoptosis and inhibits adipogenesis in 3T3-L1 adipocytes, Phytother. Res. 22 (2008) 1367—1371.

[125] J.A. Baur, K.J. Pearson, N.L. Price, H.A. Jamieson, C. Lerin, A. Kalra, et al., Resveratrol improves health and survival of mice on a high-calorie diet, Nature 444 (2006) 337—342.

[126] M. Lagouge, C. Argmann, Z. Gerhart-Hines, H. Meziane, C. Lerin, F. Daussin, et al., Resveratrol improves mitochondrial function and protects against metabolic disease by activating SIRT1 and PGC-1alpha, Cell 127 (2006) 1109—1122.

[127] K. Szkudelska, L. Nogowski, T. Szkudelski, The inhibitory effect of resveratrol on leptin secretion from rat adipocytes, Eur. J. Clin. Invest. 39 (2009) 899—905.

[128] A.P. Majumdar, S. Banerjee, J. Nautiyal, B.B. Patel, V. Patel, J. Du, et al., Curcumin synergizes with resveratrol to inhibit colon cancer, Nutr. Cancer 61 (2009) 544—553.

[129] M. Sengottuvelan, N. Nalini, Dietary supplementation of resveratrol suppresses colonic tumour incidence in 1,2-dimethylhydrazine-treated rats by modulating biotransforming enzymes and aberrant crypt foci development, Br. J. Nutr. 96 (2006) 145—153.

[130] J. Vanamala, L. Reddivari, S. Radhakrishnan, C. Tarver, Resveratrol suppresses IGF-1 induced human colon cancer cell proliferation and elevates apoptosis via suppression of IGF-1R/Wnt and activation of p53 signaling pathways, BMC Cancer 10 (2010) 238.

[131] K. Diepvens, K.R. Westerterp, M.S. Westerterp-Plantenga, Obesity and thermogenesis related to the consumption of caffeine, ephedrine, capsaicin, and green tea, Am. J. Physiol. Regul. Integr. Comp. Physiol. 292 (2007) R77—R85.

[132] R. Hursel, M.S. Westerterp-Plantenga, Thermogenic ingredients and body weight regulation, Int. J. Obes. 34 (2010) 659—669.

[133] F. Thielecke, M. Boschmann, The potential role of green tea catechins in the prevention of the metabolic syndrome: a review, Phytochemistry 70 (2009) 11—24.

[134] Y.H. Kao, R.A. Hiipakka, S. Liao, Modulation of endocrine systems and food intake by green tea epigallocatechin gallate, Endocrinology 141 (2000) 980—987.

[135] Y.H. Kao, R.A. Hiipakka, S. Liao, Modulation of obesity by a green tea catechin, Am. J. Clin. Nutr. 72 (2000) 1232—1234.

[136] K. Imai, K. Nakachi, Cross sectional study of effects of drinking green tea on cardiovascular and liver diseases, BMJ 310 (1995) 693—696.

[137] C.H. Wu, F.H. Lu, C.S. Chang, T.C. Chang, R.H. Wang, C.J. Chang, Relationship among habitual tea consumption, percent body fat, and body fat distribution, Obes. Res. 11 (2003) 1088—1095.

[138] T. Nagao, Y. Komine, S. Soga, S. Meguro, T. Hase, Y. Tanaka, et al., Ingestion of a tea rich in catechins leads to a reduction in body fat and malondialdehyde-modified LDL in men, Am. J. Clin. Nutr. 81 (2005) 122—129.

[139] S. Berube-Parent, C. Pelletier, J. Dore, A. Tremblay, Effects of encapsulated green tea and Guarana extracts containing a mixture of epigallocatechin-3-gallate and caffeine on 24 h energy expenditure and fat oxidation in men, Br. J. Nutr. 94 (2005) 432—436.

[140] M. Boschmann, F. Thielecke, The effects of epigallocatechin-3-gallate on thermogenesis and fat oxidation in obese men: a pilot study, J. Am. Coll. Nutr. 26 (2007) 389S—395S.

[141] A.G. Dulloo, C. Duret, D. Rohrer, L. Girardier, N. Mensi, M. Fathi, et al., Efficacy of a green tea extract rich in catechin polyphenols and caffeine in increasing 24-h energy expenditure and fat oxidation in humans, Am. J. Clin. Nutr. 70 (1999) 1040—1045.

[142] M. Friedrich, K.J. Petzke, D. Raederstorff, S. Wolfram, S. Klaus, Acute effects of epigallocatechin gallate from green tea on oxidation and tissue incorporation of dietary lipids in mice fed a high-fat diet, Int. J. Obes. (London) (2011) (Epub ahead of print)

[143] C.H. Huang, S.J. Tsai, Y.J. Wang, M.H. Pan, J.Y. Kao, T.D. Way, EGCG inhibits protein synthesis, lipogenesis, and cell cycle progression through activation of AMPK in p53 positive and negative human hepatoma cells, Mol. Nutr. Food Res. 53 (2009) 1156—1165.

[144] S.Y. Cho, P.J. Park, H.J. Shin, Y.K. Kim, D.W. Shin, E.S. Shin, et al., (−)-Catechin suppresses expression of Kruppel-like factor 7 and increases expression and secretion of adiponectin protein in 3T3-L1 cells, Am. J. Physiol. Endocrinol. Metab. 292 (2007) E1166—E1172.

[145] P.F. Hung, B.T. Wu, H.C. Chen, Y.H. Chen, C.L. Chen, M.H. Wu, et al., Antimitogenic effect of green tea (−)-epigallocatechin gallate on 3T3-L1 preadipocytes depends on the ERK and Cdk2 pathways, Am. J. Physiol. Cell. Physiol. 288 (2005) C1094—C1108.

[146] J. Lin, M.A. Della-Fera, C.A. Baile, Green tea polyphenol epigallocatechin gallate inhibits adipogenesis and induces apoptosis in 3T3-L1 adipocytes, Obes. Res. 13 (2005) 982—990.

[147] H.S. Moon, C.S. Chung, H.G. Lee, T.G. Kim, Y.J. Choi, C.S. Cho, Inhibitory effect of (−)-epigallocatechin-3-gallate on lipid accumulation of 3T3-L1 cells, Obesity (Silver Spring) 15 (2007) 2571—2582.

[148] J.T. Hwang, I.J. Park, J.I. Shin, Y.K. Lee, S.K. Lee, H.W. Baik, et al., Genistein, EGCG, and capsaicin inhibit adipocyte differentiation process via activating AMP-activated protein kinase, Biochem. Biophys. Res. Commun. 338 (2005) 694—699.

[149] D. Chen, S.B. Wan, H. Yang, J. Yuan, T.H. Chan, Q.P. Dou, EGCG, green tea polyphenols and their synthetic analogs and prodrugs for human cancer prevention and treatment, Adv. Clin. Chem. 53 (2011) 155—177.

[150] C.L. Sun, J.M. Yuan, W.P. Koh, M.C. Yu, Green tea, black tea and breast cancer risk: a meta-analysis of epidemiological studies, Carcinogenesis 27 (2006) 1310—1315.

[151] A.E. Rogers, L.J. Hafer, Y.S. Iskander, S. Yang, Black tea and mammary gland carcinogenesis by 7,12-dimethylbenz[*a*]

anthracene in rats fed control or high fat diets, Carcinogenesis 19 (1998) 1269–1273.

[152] V.M. Adhami, I.A. Siddiqui, N. Ahmad, S. Gupta, H. Mukhtar, Oral consumption of green tea polyphenols inhibits insulin-like growth factor-I-induced signaling in an autochthonous mouse model of prostate cancer, Cancer Res 64 (2004) 8715–8722.

[153] B.J. Sugarman, B.B. Aggarwal, P.E. Hass, I.S. Figari, M.A. Palladino Jr., H.M. Shepard, Recombinant human tumor necrosis factor-alpha: effects on proliferation of normal and transformed cells *in vitro*, Science 230 (1985) 943–945.

[154] H. Fujiki, M. Suganuma, S. Okabe, E. Sueoka, K. Suga, K. Imai, et al., Mechanistic findings of green tea as cancer preventive for humans, Proc. Soc. Exp. Biol. Med. 220 (1999) 225–228.

[155] S. Shankar, Q. Chen, R.K. Srivastava, Inhibition of PI3K/AKT and MEK/ERK pathways act synergistically to enhance antiangiogenic effects of EGCG through activation of FOXO transcription factor, J. Mol. Signal 3 (2008) 7.

[156] K. Hastak, S. Gupta, N. Ahmad, M.K. Agarwal, M.L. Agarwal, H. Mukhtar, Role of p53 and NF-kappaB in epigallocatechin-3-gallate-induced apoptosis of LNCaP cells, Oncogene 22 (2003) 4851–4859.

[157] H.J. Park, R.S. Bruno, Hepatoprotective activities of green tea in nonalcoholic fatty liver disease, Agro Food Industry Hi-Tech 21 (2010) 37–40.

[158] S.J. Bhathena, M.T. Velasquez, Beneficial role of dietary phytoestrogens in obesity and diabetes, Am. J. Clin. Nutr. 76 (2002) 1191–1201.

[159] H. Adlercreutz, W. Mazur, Phyto-oestrogens and Western diseases, Ann. Med. 29 (1997) 95–120.

[160] K.D. Setchell, Phytoestrogens: the biochemistry, physiology, and implications for human health of soy isoflavones, Am. J. Clin. Nutr. 68 (1998) 1333S–1346S.

[161] L.W. Lissin, J.P. Cooke, Phytoestrogens and cardiovascular health, J. Am. Coll. Cardiol. 35 (2000) 1403–1410.

[162] D. Goodman-Gruen, D. Kritz-Silverstein, Usual dietary isoflavone intake is associated with cardiovascular disease risk factors in postmenopausal women, J. Nutr. 131 (2001) 1202–1206.

[163] T. Aoyama, K. Fukui, T. Nakamori, Y. Hashimoto, T. Yamamoto, K. Takamatsu, et al., Effect of soy and milk whey protein isolates and their hydrolysates on weight reduction in genetically obese mice, Biosci. Biotechnol. Biochem. 64 (2000) 2594–2600.

[164] T. Aoyama, K. Fukui, K. Takamatsu, Y. Hashimoto, T. Yamamoto, Soy protein isolate and its hydrolysate reduce body fat of dietary obese rats and genetically obese mice (yellow KK), Nutrition 16 (2000) 349–354.

[165] H.K. Kim, C. Nelson-Dooley, M.A. Della-Fera, J.Y. Yang, W. Zhang, J. Duan, et al., Genistein decreases food intake, body weight, and fat pad weight and causes adipose tissue apoptosis in ovariectomized female mice, J. Nutr. 136 (2006) 409–414.

[166] A.W. Harmon, Y.M. Patel, J.B. Harp, Genistein inhibits CCAAT/enhancer-binding protein beta (C/EBPbeta) activity and 3T3-L1 adipogenesis by increasing C/EBP homologous protein expression, Biochem. J. 367 (2002) 203–208.

[167] S. Rayalam, M.A. Della-Fera, J.Y. Yang, H.J. Park, S. Ambati, C.A. Baile, Resveratrol potentiates genistein's antiadipogenic and proapoptotic effects in 3T3-L1 adipocytes, J. Nutr. 137 (2007) 2668–2673.

[168] K.W. Cho, O.H. Lee, W.J. Banz, N. Moustaid-Moussa, N.F. Shay, Y.C. Kim, Daidzein and the daidzein metabolite, equol, enhance adipocyte differentiation and PPARgamma transcriptional activity, J. Nutr. Biochem. 21 (2009) 841–847.

[169] L. Nogowski, P. Mackowiak, K. Kandulska, T. Szkudelski, K.W. Nowak, Genistein-induced changes in lipid metabolism of ovariectomized rats, Ann. Nutr. Metab. 42 (1998) 360–366.

[170] A.H. Wu, R.G. Ziegler, P.L. Horn-Ross, A.M. Nomura, D.W. West, L.N. Kolonel, et al., Tofu and risk of breast cancer in Asian-Americans, Cancer Epidemiol. Biomarkers Prev. 5 (1996) 901–906.

[171] N. Kurahashi, M. Iwasaki, S. Sasazuki, T. Otani, M. Inoue, S. Tsugane, Soy product and isoflavone consumption in relation to prostate cancer in Japanese men, Cancer Epidemiol. Biomarkers Prev. 16 (2007) 538–545.

[172] M.K. Virk-Baker, T.R. Nagy, S. Barnes, Role of phytoestrogens in cancer therapy, Planta Med. 76 (2010) 1132–1142.

[173] P.J. Magee, I.R. Rowland, Phyto-oestrogens, their mechanism of action: current evidence for a role in breast and prostate cancer, Br. J. Nutr. 91 (2004) 513–531.

[174] R. Mentor-Marcel, C.A. Lamartiniere, I.E. Eltoum, N.M. Greenberg, A. Elgavish, Genistein in the diet reduces the incidence of poorly differentiated prostatic adenocarcinoma in transgenic mice (TRAMP), Cancer Res. 61 (2001) 6777–6782.

[175] K. Kato, S. Takahashi, L. Cui, T. Toda, S. Suzuki, M. Futakuchi, et al., Suppressive effects of dietary genistin and daidzin on rat prostate carcinogenesis, Jpn. J. Cancer Res. 91 (2000) 786–791.

[176] W.A. Fritz, J. Wang, I.E. Eltoum, C.A. Lamartiniere, Dietary genistein down-regulates androgen and estrogen receptor expression in the rat prostate, Mol. Cell. Endocrinol. 186 (2002) 89–99.

[177] T. Akiyama, J. Ishida, S. Nakagawa, H. Ogawara, S. Watanabe, N. Itoh, et al., Genistein, a specific inhibitor of tyrosine-specific protein kinases, J. Biol. Chem. 262 (1987) 5592–5595.

[178] H. Kim, T.G. Peterson, S. Barnes, Mechanisms of action of the soy isoflavone genistein: emerging role for its effects via transforming growth factor beta signaling pathways, Am. J. Clin. Nutr. 68 (1998) 1418S–1425S.

CHAPTER

22

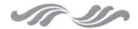

Bioavailability and Metabolism of Bioactive Compounds from Foods

Andrew P. Neilson*, Mario G. Ferruzzi†

*Virginia Polytechnic Institute and State University, Blacksburg, Virginia
†Purdue University, West Lafayette, Indiana

I INTRODUCTION

A Dietary Phytochemicals

Plants produce a wide variety of compounds that can exert biological activities in humans and animals. Bioactive components present in edible plants are of particular interest for the prevention of disease because their widespread use with minimal toxicity has the potential to impact human health on the population level. The majority of plant bioactive compounds are secondary (2°) metabolites, as opposed to primary (1°) metabolites. Whereas 1° metabolites are compounds central to required biochemical processes of cells (e.g., amino acid, energy, and nucleic acid metabolism), 2° metabolites are not absolutely required for the survival of the organism. Rather, 2° metabolites are specialized compounds that confer added survival and competitive advantages to the plant. More generally, plant 2° metabolites are referred to as natural products as well as phytochemicals (although "phytochemical" technically refers to any plant metabolite).

Major classes of plant phytochemicals include the phenolics/polyphenols, alkaloids, and terpenoids. Minor classes include polyacetylenes, polyenes, miscellaneous pigments, cyanogenic glucosides, glucosinolates, and nonprotein amino acids. Refer to Table 22.1 for the chemical properties of the major classes. The majority of the dietary bioactives associated with disease prevention are either phenolics or terpenoids, and those classes are discussed further.

Dietary phytochemicals are typically divided into two distinct classes based on their structure, solubility, and physiological absorption properties: water-soluble and lipid-soluble. In terms of relevance to diet and disease, the principal water-soluble dietary phytochemicals include the phenolics and polyphenols. The principal lipid-soluble compounds include the carotenoids, tocochromanols (vitamin E derivatives), and curcuminoids. Although curcuminoids are technically phenolics, their hydrophobic nature and digestive properties make them more lipophilic and hence they are grouped with the lipid-soluble compounds for the purposes of this chapter.

Dietary phytochemicals have a variety of roles in nutrition and health. Some (e.g., certain carotenoids, through provitamin A activity, and tocochromanols, with vitamin E activity) are essential nutrients required for development, maintenance, and health. These nutrients may also exert supplemental non-nutrient benefits, such as reduced risk of chronic diseases including cancer. The majority of dietary phytochemicals are not essential nutrients, and as such, they are classified as xenobiotics—chemicals found in an organism but that are not normally produced by the organism (metabolites from the organism's own biochemical pathways) and are not expected to be present in the organism or used for normal metabolic function. The term xenobiotic does not imply harmful or beneficial biological activity but, rather, denotes that the compound is regarded as a foreign substance by the body and is metabolized and excreted as such. This may include pharmaceuticals, pollutants, and natural products such as phytochemicals. A growing body of research in the fields of medicine, biochemistry, nutrition, and epidemiology has provided evidence to support the role of both dietary nutrients and xenobiotic phytochemicals in the prevention of disease (Table 22.2) [1–17].

Nutrition in the Prevention and Treatment of Disease, Third Edition.
DOI: http://dx.doi.org/10.1016/B978-0-12-391884-0.00022-6

TABLE 22.1   Properties of Plant Natural Products

	Natural product class		
	Terpenoids	**Alkaloids**	**Phenolics**
Biosynthetic precursor			
	Isoprene	Amino acids	Phenylalanine, tyrosine
Chemical nature	Hydrocarbon	Nitrogen-containing	Phenol ring(s)
Characterized compounds	>25,000	>12,000	>8000
Example			
	(−)-Limonene	Morphine	Coniferyl alcohol

TABLE 22.2   Reported Roles of Dietary Phytochemicals in Basic Health and Disease Prevention

Solubility	Class	Functions as essential nutrients	Putative functions in prevention of disease
Water-soluble	Phenolic acids	None	Inflammation, cancer, vascular function and cardiovascular disease, general antioxidant activity
	Flavonoids	None	Inflammation, cancer, vascular function and cardiovascular disease, metabolic syndrome (obesity, diabetes, low-grade inflammation), neuroprotection, general antioxidant activity, modulation of colon microflora and immune stimulation
Lipid-soluble	Carotenoids	Eye health and vision, cell growth and differentiation, cell signaling, reproduction, immune function	Cancer, cardiovascular disease, osteoporosis, skin health, general antioxidant activity
	Tocochromanols	Antioxidant activity, membrane function, immune function	Cardiovascular disease, neuroprotection, general antioxidant activity
	Curcuminoids	None	Inflammation, cancer, neuroprotection, skin health, general antioxidant activity

B Definition of Bioavailability

The bioavailability of dietary phytochemicals is used as a measurement of their exposure to body fluids and tissues, as a means to assess their potential for beneficial and/or harmful activity. A standardized definition of bioavailability for pharmaceutical agents is defined in the United States as follows:

> The rate and extent to which the active ingredient or active moiety is absorbed from a drug product and becomes available at the site of action. For drug products that are not intended to be absorbed into the bloodstream, bioavailability may be assessed by measurements intended to reflect the rate and extent to which the active ingredient or active moiety becomes available at the site of action (21 CFR 320.1).

This definition can be modified to apply to functional compounds, including phytochemicals, from the diet (foods, dietary supplements, etc.) as follows: Bioavailability is defined as the rate and extent to which the active ingredient or active moiety is absorbed from the ingested matrix and becomes available at the site of action.

Essentially, this definition results from the two factors governing the activity of any compound *in vivo*: (1) The active compound must be present at the site of action to impart its biological activity, and (2) the concentration and the length of exposure of the active compound at the site of action determine the magnitude of the activity.

Interest in the biological activities and the resultant health-promoting and/or health-protecting functions of plant foods and their constituent compounds has resulted in numerous research endeavors to elucidate the factors that impact the bioavailability of dietary phytochemicals. The aim of this research is primarily to identify food factors (macro- and microcomposition, physical form, phytochemical concentration, etc.) and *in vivo* biological factors (digestion, absorption, metabolism, distribution, and excretion processes) that limit bioavailability. Such knowledge is then used to improve the bioavailability of dietary phytochemicals and, by extension, their activities at the tissue of interest.

Note that the definition of bioavailability specifically refers to the availability of one specific compound/moiety or a few compounds/moieties of interest at their known or desired site of action. This definition is more easily applicable in its purest intended sense to pharmaceuticals than to dietary phytochemicals originating from complex food matrices. Pharmaceuticals are composed of one or a few known compounds with rigorously established activity, and they are designed to exert a specific function in a specific tissue in a specific "intent to treat" population (age, gender, disease state, etc.), with a specific indication of an existing or likely disease (an indication is a symptom or cause that suggests the proper and efficacious treatment of disease). Foods and dietary supplements generally do not meet these criteria, greatly complicating the utility of bioavailability as a means to optimize the efficacy of dietary compounds in several ways.

First, with the exception of a few essential nutrient deficiencies, the exact mechanisms linking diet to the prevention or amelioration of diseases have not been definitively established. Dietary phytochemicals, other dietary components (fiber, toxins, pesticides, etc.), genetic factors modulating disease susceptibility, environmental factors, age, gender, and lifestyle all contribute to the interaction between diet and disease risk.

Second, many foods and dietary supplements typically contain hundreds, if not thousands, of phytochemicals with diverse and largely unknown biological activities. It is probable that the observed biological activities of foods and supplements are due to the combined effects of numerous phytochemicals rather than a single compound or small group of compounds. This is a potential obstacle for bioavailability research because it is both desirable and practical to measure only a small percentage of the compounds ingested. Typically, bioavailability studies select the phytochemicals to be measured based on three main criteria: (1) predominance of the compound(s) in the dietary source to be studied, (2) epidemiological or other evidence suggesting a link between consumption of the phytochemical(s) or foods rich in the phytochemical(s) with the biological outcome of interest, or (3) *in vitro* studies or *in vivo* studies suggesting that the phytochemical(s) provides the desired biological outcome when administered in purified or semipurified form.

Third, the observed biological effect of a phytochemical is not necessarily due to the native form found in foods. This is due to a variety of metabolic processes that occur during and postabsorption and are discussed further later. These metabolic systems break down native dietary phytochemicals into simpler compounds (the gut microflora, pre-absorption) and alter their functional groups (phase I and II detoxification systems, post-absorption). Therefore, these metabolites may, in fact, be the active compounds that are responsible for some or all of the observed biological activities. However, many studies measure the bioavailability of the native phytochemicals for several reasons: (1) Most phytochemicals can be converted into many metabolites (in some cases, dozens), which exponentially increases the number of compounds to measure; (2) in many cases, the profile of metabolites arising from a single phytochemical is unknown or incomplete; (3) the activities of the native compound are better characterized both *in vivo* and *in vitro*; and (4) the native compound serves as a marker for all of its metabolites (albeit an imperfect one).

Finally, the actual disease-modulating activity of a particular dietary compound may occur throughout different known and unknown sites in the body. Furthermore, the actual site where the compound exerts its activity need not be the site of the desired effect. For example, stimulation of sensory, neurological, endocrine, and immune function by the active compound at one site may result in a significant biological response at another distant site where the active compound either is not present or is present but does not produce the observed effect locally. Therefore, selection of the site at which bioavailability is to be determined is critical for accurately assessing phytochemical delivery with relevance to the specific biological outcomes. Typically, bioavailability studies measure the concentration of the phytochemicals (s) of interest in one of several blood fractions (plasma, serum, lipoprotein fraction, or whole blood). This has several advantages: (1) It provides a measure of general systemic availability and distribution, (2) it is readily accessible in a healthy clinical study population and does not require highly invasive collection procedures, and (3) data from blood bioavailability are believed in some cases to be representative of a wide variety of tissues. Blood bioavailability, however, does present the disadvantage of not being specific to the desired organ or tissue of interest (unless blood or the circulatory system is in fact the site of interest) and may not be representative of chronic dietary exposure for rapidly cleared compounds. Tissues for which venous blood from an extremity is less than ideal for assessing bioavailability include the brain (due to the high selectivity of the blood−brain barrier), the kidneys (urine may be a better marker), adipose tissues (in which lipid-soluble compounds may accumulate over chronic exposure), and the intestines (due to flow of absorbed dietary components from the intestines to the liver prior to systemic circulation). These limitations should be taken into consideration when planning and interpreting bioavailability studies.

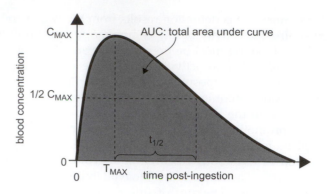

FIGURE 22.1 **Pharmacokinetic parameters used to assess systemic bioavailability of dietary bioactive compounds.** AUC, area under the concentration × time curve; C_{max}, the maximal concentration obtained in the blood; T_{max}, the time at which the maximal blood concentration occurs; $t_{1/2}$, the elimination half-life, which is the time required for 50% clearance from the blood.

C Measurement of Bioavailability

The bioavailability of dietary phytochemicals is commonly assessed through characterization of their acute absorption, also termed pharmacokinetic (PK) behavior, following ingestion. PK refers to the kinetics (i.e., data with respect to time) of appearance of the phytochemical in and subsequence clearance from circulation, typically measured in plasma or serum blood fractions. Typically, PK data are obtained by measuring the blood concentration following an acute dose at several time points, starting with baseline (time of ingestion, where the concentration is essentially zero), and continuing until the compound has been cleared from the blood (the concentration returns to zero). This approach of studying PK from baseline to complete clearance is more accurate and less subject to bias than collecting data at a single time point or a few time points following a single or chronic dosing. PK parameters may then be calculated from the concentration−time data based on several distinct mathematical models. Bioavailability can also be assessed by quantifying delivery to a specific target tissue, as opposed to blood, as a function of time.

PK calculations and comparisons are of interest as a means to quantify the availability of selected compounds of interest for delivery to target tissues and subsequent bioactivity. Although kinetic calculations and parameters can be complex, typically four main PK parameters are observed in the phytochemical bioavailability literature: C_{max}, T_{max}, AUC, and $t_{1/2}$ (Figure 22.1). C_{max} refers to the maximal concentration obtained in the blood fraction of interest in the specified experimental period. The magnitude of C_{max} indicates the maximal concentration to which tissues may be exposed, and higher C_{max} values

are commonly desirable for improved delivery to tissues with additional endothelial barriers such as brain. T_{max} refers to the time at which the maximal concentration was obtained in the blood fraction of interest in the specified experimental period. Smaller T_{max} values indicate more rapid absorption and appearance in the blood. AUC, or area under the curve, represents the calculated area (in units of concentration × time) under the concentration (y-axis) versus time (x-axis) pharmacokinetic curve. AUC is typically used as the best measure of bioavailability (total systemic exposure) because it reflects both concentration and time parameters and accounts for the entire shape of the PK curve. The elimination half-life, $t_{1/2}$, is a calculated parameter reflecting the time required for 50% clearance (excretion and/or degradation) from the blood fraction of interest in the specified experimental period. Smaller $t_{1/2}$ values indicate rapid clearance from the blood, which may limit exposure and efficacy. These parameters are therefore commonly used to quantify the bioavailability and clearance of selected compounds of interest from circulation.

II BIOAVAILABILITY OF WATER-SOLUBLE COMPOUNDS

A Polyphenols

Polyphenols are a large, structurally diverse group of organic compounds that contain multiple phenol functional groups (a hydroxyl group bonded to an aromatic ring) [18]. Thousands of polyphenolic compounds are distributed in fruits, vegetables, and common beverages such as tea and coffee. Constituent compounds comprise several broad structural classes that each have closely related subclasses of compounds with differing oxidation states and/or substitution patterns [18]. Polyphenolic compounds are divided into four principal structural classes: phenolic acids, stilbenes, lignans, and flavonoids [18]. This section focuses on the phenolic acids and flavonoids.

1 Phenolic Acids

The phenolic acids are the simplest polyphenols in terms of chemical structure. Phenolic acids are carboxylic acids derived from either benzoic or cinnamic acid skeletons (Figure 22.2). Predominant dietary phenolic acids and their dietary sources are listed in Table 22.3 [18–21].

2 Flavonoids

Flavonoids are composed of two phenyl rings linked by a propane bridge to form an oxygenated heterocyclic ring with a benzo-γ-pyrone structure, resulting in the characteristic 15-carbon (C6—C3—C6) flavan skeleton with three rings (Figure 22.3) [19,22–25]. The A and B rings are benzenes, and the C ring is the central pyran heterocycle. The flavonoids are further divided into subclasses based on the oxidation state, substitution pattern, and functional group composition of the C ring as well as the nature of the B—C ring linkage [18,19,24,25]. The six major classes of flavonoids are the anthocyanins, flavonols, flavan-3-ols, flavanones, flavones, and isoflavones (Figure 22.4) [18,19,22,23]. Predominant plant-derived flavonoids and their key dietary sources are listed in Table 22.1 [18–21].

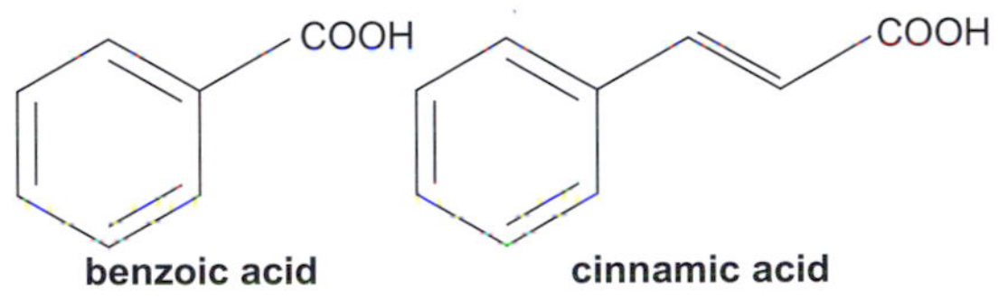

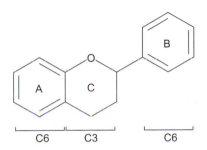

FIGURE 22.2 Structures of benzoic acid and cinnamic acid, the backbones of phenolic acids.

FIGURE 22.3 The C_6—C_3—C_6 three-ring flavan skeleton characteristic of flavonoids.

TABLE 22.3 Major Dietary Sources of Water-Soluble and Lipid-Soluble Phytochemicals

Class	Subclass	Representative compounds	Food sources
Phenolic acids	Benzoic acids	Gallic acid, protochatechuic acid, hydroxybenzoic acids	Tea, berries
	Cinnamic acids	Chlorogenic acid, coumaric acids, caffeic acids, ferulic acids	Coffee, berries, cherries, apples, cereal grains
Flavonoids	Anthocyanins	Cyanidin, delphinidin, malvidin, pelargondidin, petunidin, peonidin	Grapes, berries
	Flavonols	Kaempferol, myrecitin, quercitin	Apples, onions, leeks, broccoli, tomato
	Flavan-3-ols	Catechins, procyanidins	Tea, grapes, chocolate, apples, berries
	Flavanones	Hesperitin, naringenin, eriodictyol	Citrus and citrus products
	Flavones	Apigenin, luteolin	Green leafy herbs and spices, peppers
	Isoflavones	Daidzein, genestein, glycetin	Soybeans, legumes
Carotenoids	Xanthophylls	Lutein, zeaxanthin, β-cryptoxanthin	Green leafy vegetables, other green vegetables
	Carotenes	α-Carotene, β-carotene, lycopene	Tomatoes, red vegetables, yellow/orange vegetables
Tocochromanols	Tocopherols, tocotrienols	α-, β-, γ-, and δ-tocopherols and tocotrienols	nuts, seeds, plant oils, green leafy vegetables, cereal grains
Curcuminoids		Curcumin, desmethoxycurcumin, bis-desmethoxycurcumin	Turmeric, mustard

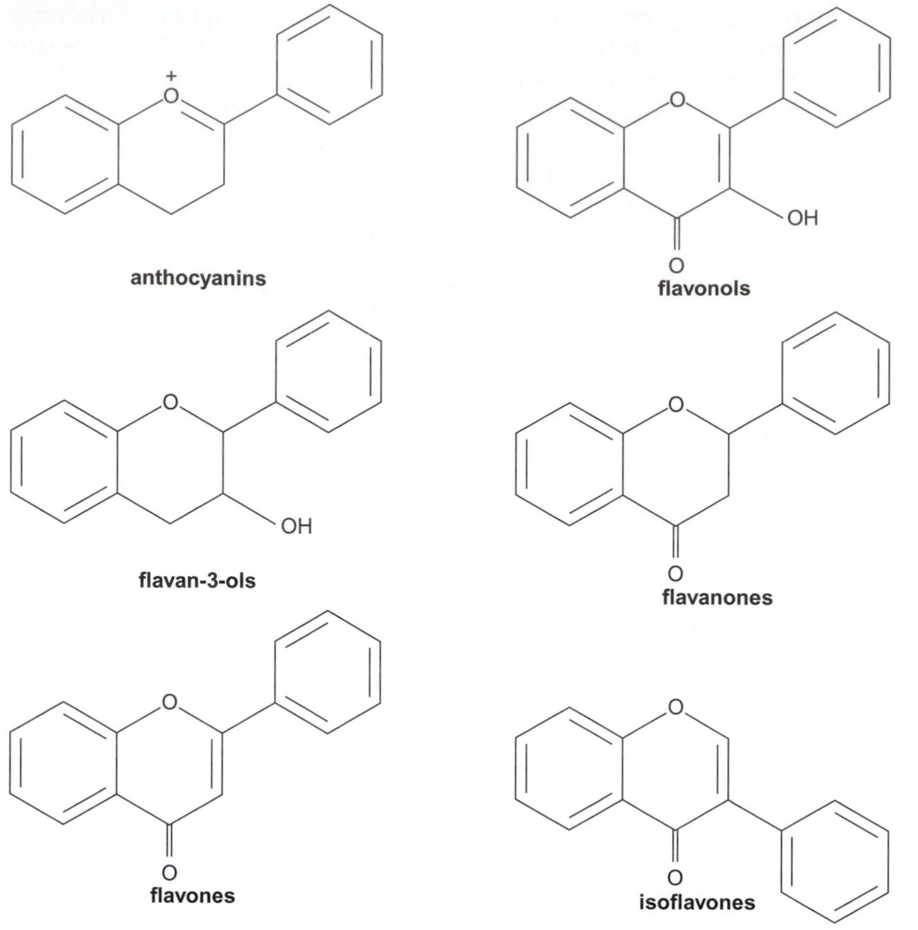

FIGURE 22.4   Basic structural features of the six major subclasses of flavonoids.

B Bioavailability of Polyphenols

1 Absorption

Polyphenols ingested from foods and beverages technically remain outside of the body until they have been absorbed through the membrane of epithelial (surface) cells lining the gastrointestinal tract. The majority of intact polyphenol absorption occurs in the small intestine, with subsequent absorption in the lower intestine of colonic metabolites. In order for dietary polyphenols to be absorbed in the small intestine, they must first be made bioaccessible. Bioaccessibility is defined as presentation of the compound to the luminal (apical) surface of intestinal epithelial cells (enterocytes) on the intestinal wall. The bioaccessible fraction (or percentage bioaccessibility) is the fraction of the consumed dose of any phytochemical that is extracted from a food during normal digestion and made accessible and available for absorption by enterocytes.

Several factors determine the bioaccessibility of polyphenols. First, in order to be absorbable, polyphenols must be released from molecular interactions with other food components as well as bulk-phase physical interactions with the food matrix. During digestion, polyphenols are released from the food matrix by mechanical action such as chewing and grinding in the oral cavity. Further digestive release continues in the stomach and small intestine due to the action of gastric acid as well as a variety of gastric and intestinal enzymes that hydrolyze lipids, proteins, and carbohydrates.

Second, the stability of these species in the gastrointestinal tract will greatly affect the concentration reaching the surface of the intestinal epithelia [26]. Saliva, gastric juice, and intestinal secretions contain a wide array of enzymes designed to degrade food components (pepsin, trypsin, esterases, lipases, amylases, etc.) as well as wide pH variations, which will affect the amount of the ingested dose that remains intact during digestion.

Third, polyphenols must be soluble in the bulk aqueous phase of the gastrointestinal milieu in order to facilitate the final step—diffusion across the unstirred water layer that protects the enterocyte surface [27]. Only the fraction of the ingested dose that meets these criteria of stability, release, solubility, and diffusion

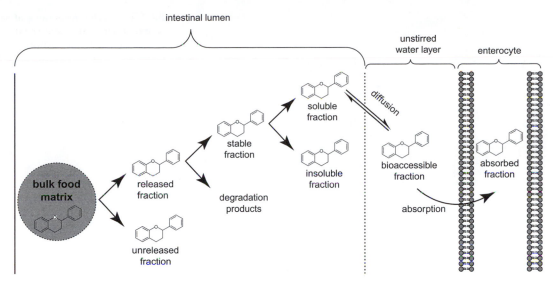

FIGURE 22.5 Digestive and absorptive processes involved in the bioaccessibility of polyphenols.

will be available for absorption (i.e., bioaccessible) (Figure 22.5). The sum of digestive release, stability, solubility, and diffusion processes determines the extent to which a particular dietary polyphenol is bioaccessible. The fractional bioaccessibility can vary greatly, depending on the compound, the nature of the food matrix (macronutrient composition, physical form, etc.), and meal composition [28].

The portion of the ingested polyphenol dose that reaches the surface of the small intestine is available for absorption into the enterocytes. Polyphenols must pass through enterocytes in order to access the bloodstream for systemic distribution. Although the identification of specific transport systems for polyphenols remains an active area of research, it is generally believed that absorption of polyphenols into enterocytes does occur through the action of monocarboxylic acid (MCT) transporter, as well as by passive diffusion [29–31]. Polyphenols appear to compete for MCT transport [32]. Passive diffusion appears to contribute significantly to the absorption of some flavonoids because the lipophilicity (log P) appears to highly correlate with intestinal permeability [29]. Passive diffusion can contribute significantly to the absorption of flavonoids with high log P values (isoflavones and flavanones), but it contributes little to the absorption of other flavonoids, particularly those that are highly hydroxylated and have lower log P values (flavan-3-ols, amongst others).

Less than 100% of the dose absorbed by the enterocytes is subsequently transported into the bloodstream. Enterocytes act as the body's first barrier against foreign compounds (xenobiotics) through the action of efflux transporters. These transporters limit cellular accumulation of xenobiotic compounds, and subsequent systemic distribution, by actively removing them from the cell and returning them to the lumen or by transporting them to interstitial space or into the bloodstream. The efflux of polyphenols by enterocytes appears to be facilitated by members of the ATP-binding cassette (ABC) superfamily of transmembrane transporters, specifically P-glycoprotein (Pgp) and the multidrug resistant protein (MRP) 1 and MRP2 [33,34]. This active efflux of xenobiotics has been termed phase III metabolism. Pgp and MRP2 are apical (luminal) transporters that reduce the net absorption of the xenobiotics by effluxing them back into the intestinal lumen rather than into the bloodstream [30]. MRP1 is a basolateral transporter (expressed on the bloodstream side) by which accumulated polyphenols are introduced into the circulation via the mesenteric veins on the serosal side of the intestinal epithelia. From the mesenteric veins, these compounds enter the portal vein and are circulated into the liver.

2 Metabolism and Excretion

Like xenobiotic compounds, polyphenols are substrates for the body's detoxification system. This system is designed to reduce the potential toxicity of foreign compounds by metabolizing them to compounds that are more readily excreted or have reduced biological activity. This detoxification system consists of three primary activities, called phase I, phase II, and phase III metabolism. Phase I metabolism is performed by members of the cytochrome p450 (CYP) superfamily of enzymes and typically involves hydroxylation. The addition of a hydroxyl group is a functionalization step that renders xenobiotics more reactive for subsequent metabolism, such as in phase II.

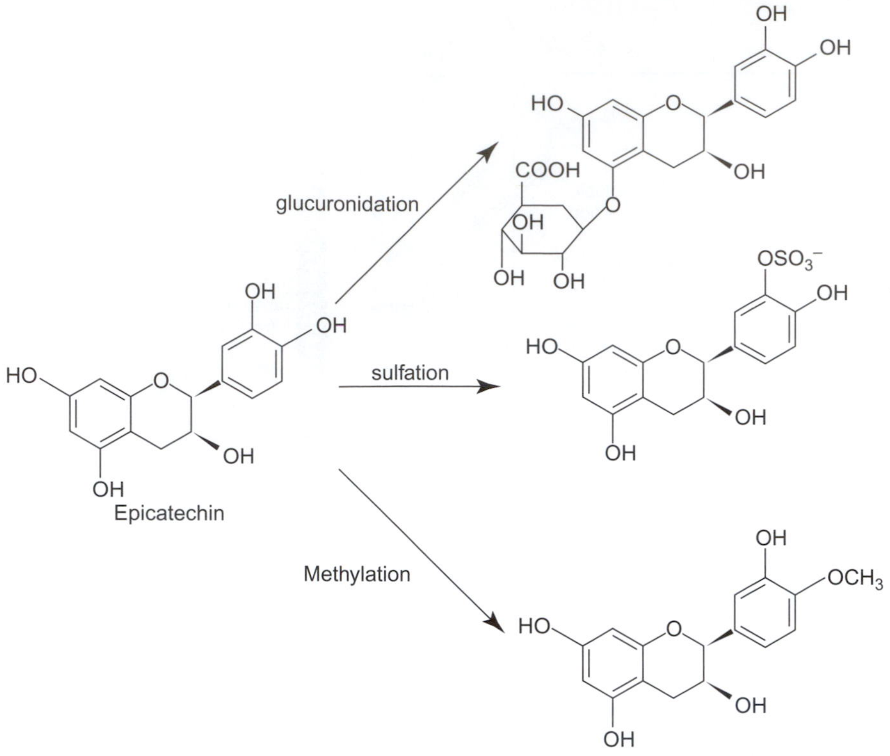

FIGURE 22.6 Structures of selected phase II metabolites of a representative flavonoid compound [(−)-epicatechin]. Conjugation may occur at a variety of positions on the molecule. Polyphenols may also undergo multiple phase II modifications on the same molecule.

Phase II metabolism typically involves conjugation reactions whereby a hydroxyl group on the xenobiotic is modified by addition of a sulfate, glucuronic acid, or methyl group. Glucuronidation is carried out by uridine diphosphate glucuronyl-transferase (UDPGT), sulfation is carried out by sulfotransferase (SULT) or phenol sulfotransferase (PST), and O-methylation is carried out by catechol O-methyl transferase (COMT) [33,35−37]. These reactions can typically occur at any phenol group on the molecule. The products of these reactions can also be substrates for further phase II metabolism, resulting in the generation of multiply conjugated and/or methylated products. These reactions decrease the potential toxicity of xenobiotics and facilitate their excretion into bile and/or urine by the liver and kidneys, respectively [35]. Structures of predominant phase II metabolites of a representative flavonoid are shown in Figure 22.6.

Finally, phase III metabolism involves the efflux of both native xenobiotics and their phase I/II metabolites from the enterocyte as a means to lower their intracellular concentration. Due to their hydroxylation, polyphenols are not typically substrates for phase I activation by most CYP phase-I detoxification enzymes [35,38]. Polyphenol readily undergo phase II conjugation in a variety of tissues, particularly the intestinal epithelium, liver, and kidneys.

Polyphenols absorbed from the intestinal lumen by enterocytes are subjected to phase II detoxification reactions in the cell interior, which may be the predominant site of phase II metabolism of these compounds in the body. The phase II conjugates formed in the enterocytes appear to be efficiently effluxed into the interstitial space and bloodstream by MRP1 and into the gut lumen by MRP2, but they do not appear to be effectively transported by Pgp [33,34,39,40]. Like the native compounds, phase II conjugates effluxed into the bloodstream enter the mesenteric veins and are circulated into the liver by the portal vein prior to systemic circulation.

From intestinal tissues, both native compounds and phase II metabolites secreted into the bloodstream are passed to the liver through the portal vein. The liver is another site of extensive xenobiotic metabolism, including phase II metabolism. Studies have indicated that the activity of COMT is highest in the liver [33,37,41,42]. The liver also possesses strong glucuronidation and sulfation activity from UDPGT and SULT, respectively [33]. The metabolism of dietary xenobiotics in the liver is termed "first-pass" metabolism because this is where absorbed compounds are first exposed to metabolism prior to entering general circulation.

Circulating forms of polyphenols are largely extracted from the bloodstream by the kidneys and subsequently excreted in the urine [43]. Glucuronide and sulfate conjugates appear to be more readily excreted into the urine than the native forms [44,45]. In addition to urinary elimination, data from rat as well as human studies suggest that native polyphenols and their O-methylated forms

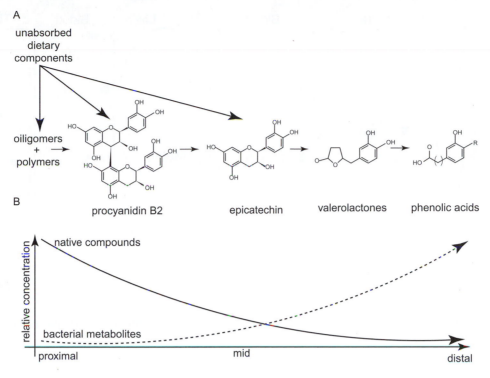

FIGURE 22.7 (A) Highly schematic representation of the colonic metabolism of unabsorbed dietary flavonoids. (B) Representation of the concentration gradients of native flavonoids and their bacterial metabolites that are likely generated along the length of the colon during progressive bacterial metabolism.

are secreted from the liver into bile, either by first-pass or subsequent metabolism, and are subsequently recovered in feces [46–48].

The majority of studies indicate that the total small intestinal absorption of dietary polyphenols is relatively poor, typically accounting for 0.3–43% of the total amount ingested depending on the compound, with most values at the extreme lower end of this range [49]. Therefore, the majority of the ingested dose passes through the small intestine unabsorbed and reaches the colon. The colon harbors a complex bacterial community composed of more than 500 species, mainly anaerobes of the *Firmicutes* and *Bacteroides* groups [50,51]. These bacteria reside in both the lumen and the epithelium/mucosa of the colon. The bacterial load of the colon is extremely high, with roughly 10^9–10^{12} cells/g luminal contents, and bacteria can comprise up to 60% of fecal matter by weight [52]. Colonic bacteria essentially possess the metabolic potential of an organ and perform numerous functions critical to the health of the host, including competition versus invasive pathogens, salvage of unabsorbed energy, stimulation of immune function, and control of colonocyte differentiation and proliferation [52–54]. The varied metabolic capacity of colonic bacteria results in extensive fermentation of unabsorbed material. Studies have consistently demonstrated that the

colonic bacteria of animals and humans metabolize polyphenols to a variety of simpler metabolites. Similar to the native compounds, these metabolites may be absorbed into the bloodstream, subjected to xenobiotics metabolism, and excreted. Microbial metabolites may account for many of the reported bioactivities of dietary polyphenols *in vivo*.

The contribution of colonic fermentation products to overall bioavailability of polyphenols is illustrated well by the flavan-3-ols. Both monomeric flavan-3-ols (catechins) and their oligomeric/polymeric forms (procyanidins) have modest net small intestinal absorption. Typical reports indicate systemic bioavailability of intact flavan-3-ols is generally poor (<25%), with most studies reporting from 0.1 to 10% of the ingested amount for C, EC, EGC, and EGCG and their phase II conjugated metabolites [20,41,55–59] and much less for procyanidins (0.3–4%) [60–64]. These data suggest instead that a large portion of the ingested dose of these compounds is not absorbed in the small intestine but, rather, reaches the colon and its associated microflora as native compounds or as phase II metabolites that have been generated and effluxed by enterocytes [20,41,65,66].

Polyphenol glycosides found in many foods and polyphenol conjugates, produced by phase I/II metabolism and apical efflux by enterocytes, are hydrolyzed

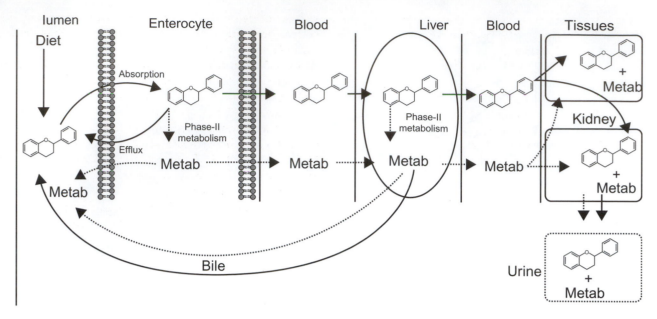

FIGURE 22.8 **Schematic of processes that affect the systemic bioavailability and metabolism of dietary polyphenols.** Dotted lines indicate metabolism/metabolites.

to generate native polyphenols [67,68]. The native polyphenols are extensively degraded by a variety of depolymerization, hydrolysis, ring cleavage, dehydroxylation, and chain-shortening reactions to generate a wide array of 1,3-diphenylpropanes, γ-valerolactones, benzoic acids, phenylacetic acids, phenylpropionic acids, and other aromatic compounds [41,61,67−88] (Figure 22.7A). The bacterial degradation of flavan-3-ols is extensive, with estimates of up to 100% for catechins and procyanidins (PCs). Therefore, gradients of native PCs and their microbial metabolites are likely established along the length of the colon [61]. The proximal colon is likely exposed to higher levels of native PCs, whereas the distal colon is exposed to higher levels of metabolites (Figure 22.7B). However, there are few data regarding distinct profiles present in the lumen and mucosa of the proximal, mid, and distal colon.

These colonic metabolites are readily absorbed from the colon and have greater systemic bioavailability than native catechins or PCs [81,82]. These absorbed metabolites may account for many of the observed effects of dietary polyphenols. Native polyphenols and their bacterial metabolites appear to exert distinct activities, with distinct efficacies, on pathways and outcomes critical to a variety of diseases, such as cancer and inflammation [80,89−93]. Therefore, the bacterial metabolism of flavan-3-ols in the colon may represent a major contributing factor to their bioavailability, systemic distribution, and bioactivity. However, these metabolites may be generated from a variety of

sources, including amino acids. Therefore, the role of these colonic metabolites in the health-protective activities of phytochemicals remains to be fully elucidated.

A schematic of the bioavailability of polyphenols is shown in Figure 22.8.

III LIPID-SOLUBLE COMPOUNDS

A Classes of Lipid-Soluble Phytochemicals

As described previously, three main classes of lipid-soluble phytochemicals predominate in commonly consumed fruits, vegetables, and spices: carotenoids, tocochromanols, and curcuminoids. The carotenoids are bright yellow and orange plant pigments characterized by their 40-carbon structures derived from the 5-carbon precursor molecule isoprene. As such, carotenoids are long-chain hydrocarbons with highly conjugated double-bond systems and bilateral or near bilateral symmetry around a central bond [10,94,95]. Carotenoids are further classified based on the presence or absence of end cyclization (e.g., straight-chain carotenoid lycopene vs. cyclized α- and β-carotenes) and the presence or absence of oxygen (the strict hydrocarbons such as lycopene and β-carotene are called carotenes, whereas the oxygenated carotenoids such as lutein and zeaxanthin are called xanthophylls) [10,94,95]. Representative carotenoid structures are shown in Figure 22.9.

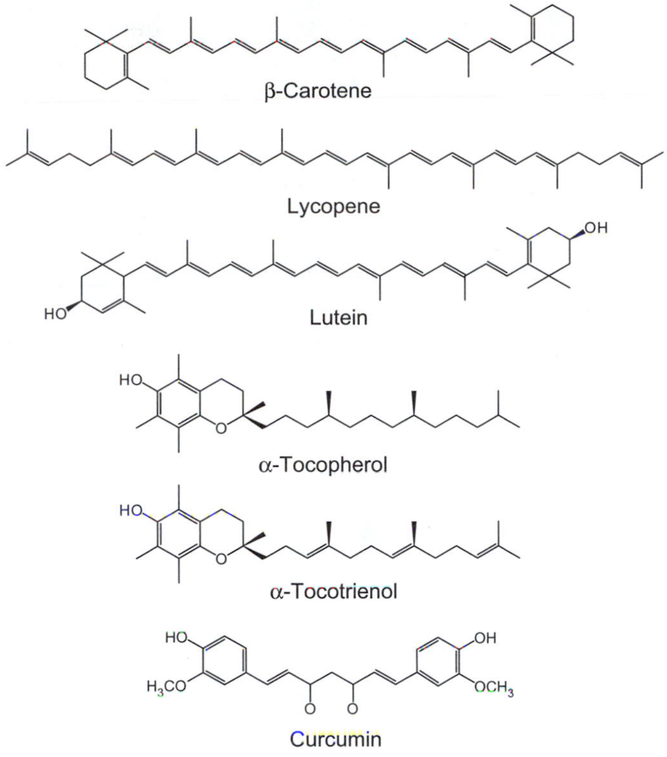

FIGURE 22.9 Structures of lipophilic phytochemicals from various classes: carotene carotenoids (β-carotene and lycopene), a xanthophyll carotenoid (lutein), a tocopherol tocochromanol (α-tocopherol), a tocotrienol tocochromanol, (α-tocotrienol), and a curcuminoid (curcumin).

The tocochromanols, or vitamin E compounds, are isoprenoids similar to the carotenoids. Tocochromanols are amphipathic molecules, with a polar chromane ring head and a nonpolar 16-carbon phytyl tail [96—99]. Tocochromanols have varying methylation patterns in the chromane group, designated as the α-, β-, γ-, and δ-tocochromanols. The tocochromanol are composed of two distinct classes—the tocopherols and the toco-trienols—each with the α-, β-, γ-, and δ-tocochroma-nols. Tocopherols have a saturated phytyl tail, whereas tocotrienols have three double bonds in the phytyl tail. Therefore, tocopherols have three chiral centers and can exist as eight stereoisomers (naturally occurring α-tocopherol is in the all-*R* configuration, whereas synthetic α-tocopherol is all-racemic, or an equal mixture of all eight stereoisomers). Due to the phytyl unsatura-tion, the tocotrienols have only one chiral center and two stereoisomers (naturally occurring tocotrienols have the *R* configuration at carbon 2 and *trans* double bonds at carbons 3′ and 7′). The structures of represen-tative tocochromanols are shown in Figure 22.9.

The curcuminoids are classified as diarylheptanoids (two aryl rings linked by a seven-carbon chain). The curcuminoids have varying functional group substitutions on the aryl rings (hydroxy, methoxy, and sulfate and sugar groups), and the aryl rings may be symmetrical or different. Curcuminoids may also have distinct seven-carbon chain patterns (unsaturation, oxo groups, enone groups, 1,3-diols, 1,3-diketones, and cyclization), with all double bonds in the *trans* configuration. The main curcuminoids in the diet are curcumin, demethoxycurcumin, and bisdemethoxycur-cumin, which have the 1,3-diketone chain and differ by the number of aryl rings having a methoxy group (both, one, and neither, respectively). The structure of curcumin is shown in Figure 22.9. Although curcumi-noids are not isoprenoids, they are classified as lipid-soluble phytochemicals due to their poor solubility in water and their digestive properties.

B Bioavailability of Lipid-Soluble Phytochemicals

As with the water-soluble compounds, only the bioaccessible fraction of any lipid-soluble phyto-chemical that is ingested will be available in the small intestine for subsequent absorption. However, factors governing the bioaccessibility of lipid-soluble phyto-chemicals are dependent on their hydrophobicity and thus poor solubility in the aqueous milieu of the gastrointestinal tract lumen. Solubilization in the gut lumen requires co-consumed lipid in the form of tria-cylglycerols, which, once digested, facilitate formation of bile salt lipid micelles (Figure 22.10).

1 Bioavailability and Metabolism of Carotenoids

Due to the requirement for humans and animals to obtain vitamin A from dietary sources in the form of pro-vitamin A carotenoids from plants (as well as retinyl esters from animals, which are not discussed here), carotenoid bioavailability has been extensively studied [100].

Digestive release and bioaccessibility represent signif-icant obstacles to carotenoid bioavailability. First, the carotenoids must be released from physical entrapment in the bulk food matrix in order to become bioaccessible [100,101]. For plant tissues, this involves disruption of the plant cell walls and organelles containing the carote-noids [102]. Thus, food processing such as heating and mechanical breakdown can significantly increase carot-enoid bioavailability simply by increasing the amount able to be released from the food matrix during the nor-mal digestive process [102]. Following digestive release in the stomach and upper small intestine, the hydropho-bic components aggregate to form crude lipid emulsion droplets in the gastric chyme, which progressively become smaller as mechanical disruption continues [101]. The carotenoids are then partitioned into mixed

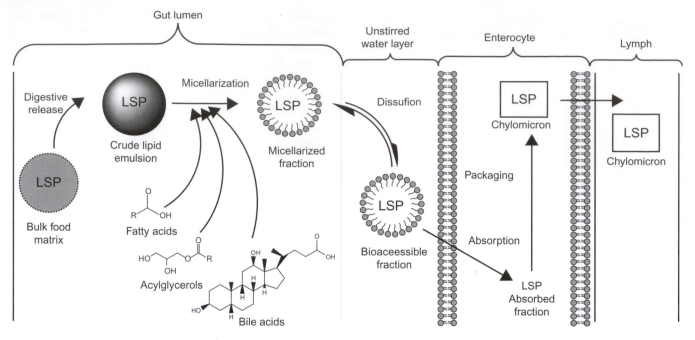

FIGURE 22.10   Schematic of processes impacting systemic bioavailability and metabolism of dietary lipophilic compounds.

micelles in the small intestine. Mixed micelles are heterogeneous aggregates with hydrophilic exteriors and hydrophobic interiors, composed of bile salts, fatty acids, mono- and diacylglycerols, cholesterol, carotenoids, tocochromanols, etc. [95,101,103]. The formation of micelles allows carotenoids to be soluble in the hydrophobic interior while the micelle crosses the unstirred water layer at the intestinal epithelial surface. Carotenoids that escape micellarization are not typically bioaccessible and remain unabsorbed [100–103]. Due to their relative polarity, xanthophylls (oxygenated carotenoids) are more readily micellarized than apolar carotenes, and they are hence more bioaccessible [100].

Co-consumption of dietary fat has consistently been shown to improve the absorption of carotenoids [104–110]. Fat stimulates secretion of bile salts and lipases during digestion, and it also provides essential components for the formation of mixed micelles (phospholipids, acylglycerols, and fatty acids). Fat also assists in extracting carotenoids from the food matrix into the crude lipid emulsion during digestion. Co-ingestion of 3–5 g fat is thought to provide optimal carotenoid absorption from a meal, and long-chain dietary fatty acids enhance absorption more than do short- and medium-chain fatty acids [95,101,103]. However, the threshold value of co-consumed lipid required for efficient carotenoid absorption is still the subject of several investigations.

Upon diffusing across the unstirred water layer, mixed micelles come into contact with the intestinal epithelium, where the micelles are disrupted and the carotenoids are released onto the epithelial surface and then absorbed into the enterocytes by both passive and facilitated diffusion processes. Transporters participating in facilitated diffusion include SR-B1, CD36, and NPC1L1 [100,101]. Once inside the enterocytes, carotenoids are transported to the Golgi apparatus with the assistance of fatty acid binding protein, where they are incorporated into chylomicron particles along with other lipid-soluble compounds and fatty acids and apoprotein B-48 [100]. These chylomicrons are then secreted into the lymphatic system for transport through the thoracic duct and subclavian vein to the liver [101]. During transport, chylomicrons are disrupted by the action of lipoprotein lipase in the vascular compartment, and the resulting chylomicron remnants are taken up by the liver [102]. In the liver, carotenoids are repackaged into very low-density lipoproteins (VLDLs) for systemic export. VLDLs are subsequently converted into low-density lipoproteins (LDLs) and then high-density lipoproteins (HDLs) [100]. The apolar carotenes are believed to reside at the interior of these lipoproteins, whereas the more polar xanthophylls reside on the exterior [100,102]. During the conversion of VLDL to LDL and HDL, LDL becomes enriched in carotenes, whereas HDL becomes enriched in xanthophylls [100].

The subsequent metabolism of both pro-vitamin A carotenoids to retinol as well as the conversion of other carotenoids (lycopene, etc.) is the subject of intensive investigation beyond the scope of this chapter [101]. Although carotenoids are generally not metabolized by the classic phase I, and II xenobiotic detoxification pathways, new information on generation of apo-carotenoids through cleavage of intact species will likely yield insight into the disease-preventative activities of these plant pigments.

2 Bioavailability and Metabolism of Tocochromanols

The processes governing the bioavailability of tocochromanols appear to be very similar to those for carotenoids [111,112]. Tocochromanols must be released from the bulk food matrix, micellarized, and presented onto the enterocyte surface for absorption, and dietary fat also plays a crucial role in this process [111–116]. The absorption of tocochromanols occurs through both passive and facilitated diffusion, with the potential involvement of SR-BI [112,113,117]. In the enterocytes, tocochromanols are assembled into chylomicrons with the assistance of microsomal triglyceride transport protein and secreted into the lymph [112,117]. In addition, some fraction may be exported directly into portal circulation via HDL [112,113,117]. The liver absorbs chylomicron remnants, and tocochromanols are then repacked into VLDL for systemic distribution [99,113]. The majority of circulating tocochromanols reside in LDL and HDL, from which they are quickly deposited into tissues with the assistance of lipoprotein lipase [113]. In cells, tocochromanols are incorporated into cell membranes as antioxidants, and they are not generally metabolized by the xenobiotic detoxification systems.

3 Bioavailability and Metabolism of Curcuminoids

Less is known regarding the bioavailability of the curcuminoids compared to the carotenoids and tocochromanols. Due to their observed pleiotropic effects *in vitro* via a wide assortment of molecular targets and mechanisms, there is great interest in their potential preventive and therapeutic activities, including: antimicrobial, antioxidant, anti-inflammatory, anticarcinogenic, antithrombotic, neuroprotective, antirheumatic, and hypoglycemic activities [16,17,118–120].

Curcuminoids are hydrophobic polyphenols, with poor solubility in water, limited solubility in methanol, and good solubility in ethanol, dimethyl sulfoxide, acetone, and chloroform [17,18,121]. This hydrophobicity leads to poor solubilization and limited diffusion across the unstirred water layer, resulting in extremely low gut absorption and bioavailability relative to those of other polyphenols and also the lipid-soluble phytochemicals. The majority of an oral curcumin dose is not absorbed but is excreted intact in feces (which also indicates limited metabolism by colonic microbiota) [17,118,119]. In many cases, native curcumin and its metabolites are present at levels near or below the analytical limit of detection (typically high-performance liquid chromatography analysis with ultraviolet, electrochemical, or mass spectrometric detection) in human blood fractions or urine following oral ingestion of gram quantities of curcuminoids [17,118]. Therefore, the gastrointestinal tract is the major site exposed to native curcumin. The small fraction of curcumin that is absorbed is then rapidly biotransformed by reduction reactions (to tetrahydro- and hexahydrocurcumin derivatives), as well as conjugated to sulfates and glucuronides, in the intestinal mucosa, liver, and kidneys [118,121–123]. The low levels of curcumin detected in blood and urine are almost exclusively conjugates of curcumin or reduced curcumin derivatives, and the half-lives of these compounds are exceedingly short due to rapid clearance [118,121–123].

Poor absorption, extensive biotransformation, and rapid elimination pose a major hurdle in exploiting the bioactivities of orally administered curcuminoids [16,17,118,121–123]. Studies of curcumin pharmacokinetics and pharmacodynamics typically of necessity involve doses of gram/kilogram quantities and gram quantities to animals and humans, respectively, which are much higher than doses typically employed for other phytochemicals [118,124]. Although curcumin is generally thought to be safe at high doses for short-term use, and it has "generally recognized as safe" (GRAS) status in the United States, concerns have arisen over its long-term safety [17,118,121,123,124]. This is of particular importance for long-term use of curcumin as a preventive agent in healthy populations, in which toxicity is less acceptable than in therapeutic uses for existing disease.

Several delivery strategies have been developed to improve the bioavailability and efficacy of curcuminoids *in vivo*, including (1) co-administration with adjuvants to inhibit metabolism; (2) formulation of nanoparticles targeting delivery of curcumin to specific regions of the gastrointestinal tract; (3) incorporation of curcumin into micelles, phospholipid complexes, and liposomes to improve diffusion across the unstirred water layer, (4) development of synthetic curcumin analogues with improved solubility, (5) heat-assisted solubilization, (6) synthesis of curcumin prodrugs that yield curcumin upon hydrolysis, and (7) formulation of curcumin metal chelation complexes to improve solubility [16,17,118,121,123–126]. Particularly noteworthy is the use of the adjuvant piperine, which is an alkaloid from black pepper. Co-administration of milligram quantities of piperine with curcumin has been shown to increase the bioavailability of curcumin by up to 2000% [16,118,123,124]. Piperine acts by inhibiting phase II biotransformation and clearance of curcumin, thus increasing the persistence of native curcumin in circulation [16,118,123,124]. Piperine may also increase gut permeability [127,128]. Concern has arisen regarding this adjuvant because reduced biotransformation of other drugs may result in toxicity due to abnormal accumulation [124].

Curcumin poses a particular challenge for correlating bioavailability to efficacy because: (1) Curcumin appears to exert some efficacy even when no native or conjugated curcumin is detectable in blood, and (2) curcumin exerts activities distant from the gastrointestinal tract, even though this is the primary site of delivery and accumulation. Therefore, the effective dose, active moiety, and mechanisms of action of curcumin remain to be fully characterized *in vivo* [17,119].

IV SUMMARY

Numerous bioactive phytochemicals are found in commonly consumed plant foods, including fruits, vegetables, beverages, and spices. Their widespread presence in the diet and apparent low toxicity suggest that phytochemicals have the potential to impact human health and disease risk on the population level. Considering this potential benefit, interest in factors affecting their bioavailability from common dietary sources has grown. When considering bioavailability, dietary phytochemicals can be divided into two distinct classes: water-soluble (phenolics and polyphenols) and lipid-soluble (carotenoids, tocochromanols, and curcuminoids). Significant effort has been placed on the identification of food factors (macro- and microcomposition, physical form, phytochemical concentration, etc.) and *in vivo* biological factors (digestion, absorption, metabolism, distribution, and excretion processes) that impact bioavailability in humans and experimental animal models. Such knowledge is critical to improve the bioavailability of health-promoting phytochemicals and to better understand the mechanisms by which they exert their biological activities at target tissues.

References

[1] L. Hooper, P.A. Kroon, E.B. Rimm, J.S. Cohn, I. Harvey, K.A. Le Cornu, et al., Flavonoids, flavonoid-rich foods, and cardiovascular risk: a meta-analysis of randomized controlled trials, Am. J. Clin. Nutr. 88 (2008) 38–50.

[2] E. Herrera, R. Jiménez, O.I. Aruoma, S. Hercberg, I. Sánchez-García, C. Fraga, Aspects of antioxidant foods and supplements in health and disease, Nutr. Rev. 67 (2009) S140–S144.

[3] S. Prasad, K. Phromnoi, V.R. Yadav, M.M. Chaturvedi, B.B. Aggarwal, Targeting inflammatory pathways by flavonoids for prevention and treatment of cancer, Planta Med. 76 (2010) 1044–1063.

[4] A. Kale, S. Gawande, S. Kotwal, Cancer phytotherapeutics: role for flavonoids at the cellular level, Phytother. Res. 22 (2008) 567–577.

[5] G. Davì, F. Santilli, C. Patrono, Nutraceuticals in diabetes and metabolic syndrome, Cardiovasc. Ther. 28 (2010) 216–226.

[6] M.G. Traber, B. Frei, J.S. Beckman, Vitamin E revisited: do new data validate benefits for chronic disease prevention? Curr. Opin. Lipidol. 19 (2008) 30–38.

[7] J.A. Vita, Polyphenols and cardiovascular disease: effects on endothelial and platelet function, Am. J. Clin. Nutr. 81 (2005) 292S–297S.

[8] D. Grassi, G. Desideri, G. Croce, S. Tiberti, A. Aggio, C. Ferri, Flavonoids, vascular function and cardiovascular protection, Curr. Pharm. Design 15 (2009) 1072–1084.

[9] S.C. Thomasset, D.P. Berry, G. Garcea, T. Marczylo, W.P. Steward, A.J. Gescher, Dietary polyphenolic phytochemicals—Promising cancer chemopreventive agents in humans? A review of their clinical properties, Int. J. Cancer 120 (2007) 451–458.

[10] A.V. Rao, Carotenoids and human health, Pharmacol. Res. 55 (2007) 207–216.

[11] G. Riccioni, Carotenoids and cardiovascular disease, Curr. Atheroscler. Rep 11 (2009) 434–439.

[12] C.L. Rock, Carotenoids and cancer, in: G. Britton, H. Pfander, S. Liaaen-Jensen (Eds.), Carotenoids, Vol. 5, Birkhauser, Basel, 2009, pp. 269–286.

[13] F. Galli, A. Azzi, Present trends in vitamin E research, Biofactors 36 (2010) 33–42.

[14] J.M. Tucker, D.M. Townsend, Alpha-tocopherol: roles in prevention and therapy of human disease, Biomed. Pharmacother. 59 (2005) 380–387.

[15] R. Thangapazham, A. Sharma, R. Maheshwari, Multiple molecular targets in cancer chemoprevention by curcumin, AAPS J 8 (2006) E443–E449.

[16] P. Anand, C. Sundaram, S. Jhurani, A.B. Kunnumakkara, B.B. Aggarwal, Curcumin and cancer: an "old-age" disease with an "age-old" solution, Cancer Lett. 267 (2008) 133–164.

[17] H. Hatcher, R. Planalp, J. Cho, F. Torti, S. Torti, Curcumin: from ancient medicine to current clinical trials, Cell. Mol. Life Sci. 65 (2008) 1631–1652.

[18] C. Manach, A. Scalbert, C. Morand, C. Remesy, L. Jimenez, Polyphenols: food sources and bioavailability, Am. J. Clin. Nutr. 79 (2004) 727–747.

[19] G.R. Beecher, Overview of dietary flavonoids: Nomenclature, occurrence and intake, J. Nutr. 133 (2003) 3248S–3254S.

[20] A. Scalbert, G. Williamson, Dietary intake and bioavailability of polyphenols, J. Nutr. 130 (2000) 2073S–2085S.

[21] L. Bravo, Polyphenols: Chemistry, dietary sources, metabolism, and nutritional significance, Nutr. Rev. 56 (1998) 317–333.

[22] K.E. Heim, A.R. Tagliaferro, D.J. Bobilya, Flavonoid antioxidants: Chemistry, metabolism and structure—activity relationships, J. Nutr. Biochem. 13 (2002) 572–584.

[23] T. Iwashina, The structure and distribution of the flavonoids in plants, J. Plant Res 113 (2000) 287–299.

[24] P.G. Pietta, Flavonoids as antioxidants, J. Nat. Prod. 63 (2000) 1035–1042.

[25] L.H. Yao, Y.M. Jiang, J. Shi, F.A. Tomas-Barberan, N. Datta, R. Singanusong, et al., Flavonoids in food and their health benefits, Plant Foods Hum. Nutr. 59 (2004) 113–122.

[26] A.P. Neilson, A.S. Hopf, B.R. Cooper, M.A. Pereira, J.A. Bomser, M.G. Ferruzzi, Catechin degradation with concurrent formation of homo- and heterocatechin dimers during *in vitro* digestion, J. Agric. Food Chem. 55 (2007) 8941–8949.

[27] A.P. Neilson, J.C. George, E.M. Janle, R.D. Mattes, R. Rudolph, N.V. Matusheski, et al., Influence of chocolate matrix composition on cocoa flavan-3-ol bioaccessibility *in vitro* and bioavailability in humans, J. Agric. Food Chem. 57 (2009) 9418–9426.

[28] A.P. Neilson, T.N. Sapper, E.M. Janle, R. Rudolph, N.V. Matusheski, M.G. Ferruzzi, Chocolate matrix factors modulate the pharmacokinetic behavior of cocoa flavan-3-ol phase II metabolites following oral consumption by Sprague–Dawley rats, J. Agric. Food Chem. 58 (2010) 6685–6691.

[29] V. Crespy, C. Morand, C. Besson, N. Cotelle, H. Vezin, C. Demigne, et al., The splanchnic metabolism of flavonoids highly differed according to the nature of the compound, Am. J. Physiol. Gastrointest. Liver Physiol. 284 (2003) G980–G988.

[30] J.D. Lambert, S.M. Sang, C.S. Yang, Biotransformation of green tea polyphenols and the biological activities of those metabolites, Mol. Pharm. 4 (2007) 819–825.

[31] J.B. Vaidyanathan, T. Walle, Cellular uptake and efflux of the tea flavonoid (−)-epicatechin-3-gallate in the human intestinal cell line Caco-2, J. Pharmacol. Exp. Therap 307 (2003) 745–752.

[32] M. Silberberg, C. Morand, C. Manach, A. Scalbert, C. Remesy, Co-administration of quercetin and catechin in rats alters their absorption but not their metabolism, Life Sci. 77 (2005) 3156–3167.

[33] W.Y. Feng, Metabolism of green tea catechins: an overview, Curr. Drug Metab. 7 (2006) 755–809.

[34] M. Takano, R. Yumoto, T. Murakami, Expression and function of efflux drug transporters in the intestine, Pharmacol. Ther. 109 (2006) 137–161.

[35] G. Williamson, A.J. Day, G.W. Plumb, D. Couteau, Human metabolic pathways of dietary flavonoids and cinnamates, Biochem. Soc. Trans. 28 (2000) 16–22.

[36] R. Hackman, J. Polagruto, Q. Zhu, B. Sun, H. Fujii, C. Keen, Flavanols: Digestion, absorption and bioactivity, Phytochem. Rev 7 (2008) 195–208.

[37] M.K. Piskula, J. Terao, Accumulation of (−)-epicatechin metabolites in rat plasma after oral administration and distribution of conjugation enzymes in rat tissues, J. Nutr 128 (1998) 1172–1178.

[38] L.M.S. Chan, S. Lowes, B.H. Hirst, The ABCs of drug transport in intestine and liver: efflux proteins limiting drug absorption and bioavailability, Eur. J. Pharm. Sci. 21 (2004) 25–51.

[39] C. Hu, D.D. Kitts, Evaluation of antioxidant activity of epigallocatechin gallate in biphasic model systems in vitro, Mol. Cell. Biochem. 218 (2001) 147–155.

[40] J.B. Vaidyanathan, T. Walle, Transport and metabolism of the tea flavonoid (−)-epicatechin by the human intestinal cell line Caco-2, Pharm. Res 18 (2001) 1420–1425.

[41] T. Kohri, N. Matsumoto, M. Yamakawa, M. Suzuki, F. Nanjo, Y. Hara, et al., Metabolic fate of (−)-[4-3H]epigallocatechin gallate in rats after oral administration, J. Agric. Food Chem. 49 (2001) 4102–4112.

[42] B.T. Zhu, U.K. Patel, M.X. Cai, A.J. Lee, A.H. Conney, Rapid conversion of tea catechins to monomethylated products by rat liver cytosolic catechol-O-methyltransferase, Xenobiotica 31 (2001) 879–890.

[43] S.L. Abrahamse, W.J. Kloots, J.M.M. van Amelsvoort, Absorption, distribution, and secretion of epicatechin and quercetin in the rat, Nutr. Res. 25 (2005) 305–317.

[44] J.D. Lambert, M.J. Lee, H. Lu, X.F. Meng, J. Ju, J. Hong, et al., Epigallocatechin-3-gallate is absorbed but extensively glucuronidated following oral administration to mice, J. Nutr. 133 (2003) 4172–4177.

[45] B. Yang, K. Arai, F. Kusu, Determination of catechins in human urine subsequent to tea ingestion by high-performance liquid chromatography with electrochemical detection, Anal. Biochem 283 (2000) 77–82.

[46] T. Kohri, M. Suzuki, F. Nanjo, Identification of metabolites of (−)-epicatechin gallate and their metabolic fate in the rat, J. Agric. Food Chem. 51 (2003) 5561–5566.

[47] C.S. Yang, L.S. Chen, M.J. Lee, D. Balentine, M.C. Kuo, S.P. Schantz, Blood and urine levels of tea catechins after ingestion of different amounts of green tea by human volunteers, Cancer Epidemiol. Biomarkers Prev 7 (1998) 351–354.

[48] M. Harada, Y. Kan, H. Naoki, Y. Fukui, N. Kageyama, M. Nakai, et al., Identification of the major antioxidative metabolites in biological fluids of the rat with ingested (+)-catechin and (−)-epicatechin, Biosci. Biotechnol. Biochem. 63 (1999) 973–977.

[49] C. Manach, G. Williamson, C. Morand, A. Scalbert, C. Remesy, Bioavailability and bioefficacy of polyphenols in humans: I. Review of 97 bioavailability studies, Am. J. Clin. Nutr. 81 (2005) 230S–242S.

[50] V. Mai, J.G. Morris, Colonic bacterial flora: changing understandings in the molecular age, J. Nutr. 134 (2004) 459–464.

[51] S.H. Duncan, P. Louis, H.J. Flint, Cultivable bacterial diversity from the human colon, Lett. Appl. Microbiol. 44 (2007) 343–350.

[52] A.M. O'Hara, F. Shanahan, The gut flora as a forgotten organ, EMBO Rep 7 (2006) 688–693.

[53] M.B. Roberfroid, F. Bornet, C. Bouley, J.H. Cummings, Colonic microflora: Nutrition and health. Summary and conclusions of an International Life Sciences Institute (ILSI) [Europe] workshop held in Barcelona, Spain, Nutr. Rev. 53 (1995) 127–130.

[54] F. Guarner, J.-R. Malagelada, Gut flora in health and disease, Lancet 361 (2003) 512–519.

[55] J.L. Donovan, C. Manach, L. Rios, C. Morand, A. Scalbert, C. Remesy, Procyanidins are not bioavailable in rats fed a single meal containing a grapeseed extract or the procyanidin dimer B-3, Br. J. Nutr. 87 (2002) 299–306.

[56] J.L. Donovan, S. Kasim-Karakas, J.B. German, A.L. Waterhouse, Urinary excretion of catechin metabolites by human subjects after red wine consumption, Br. J. Nutr. 87 (2002) 31–37.

[57] M.J. Lee, P. Maliakal, L.S. Chen, X.F. Meng, F.Y. Bondoc, S. Prabhu, et al., Pharmacokinetics of tea catechins after ingestion of green tea and (−)-epigallocatechin-3-gallate by humans: formation of different metabolites and individual variability, Cancer Epidemiol. Biomarkers Prev. 11 (2002) 1025–1032.

[58] S.M. Henning, Y.T. Niu, N.H. Lee, G.D. Thames, R.R. Minutti, H.J. Wang, et al., Bioavailability and antioxidant activity of tea flavanols after consumption of green tea, black tea, or a green tea extract supplement, Am. J. Clin. Nutr. 80 (2004) 1558–1564.

[59] C. Auger, W. Mullen, Y. Hara, A. Crozier, Bioavailability of poluphenon E flavan-3-ols in humans with an ileostomy, J. Nutr. 138 (2008) 1535–1542.

[60] S. Baba, N. Osakabe, M. Natsume, J. Terao, Absorption and urinary excretion of procyanidin B2 epicatechin-(4 beta-8)-epicatechin in rats, Free Radic. Biol. Med. 33 (2002) 142–148.

[61] C. Tsang, C. Auger, W. Mullen, A. Bornet, J.M. Rouanet, A. Crozier, et al., The absorption, metabolism and excretion of flavan-3-ols and procyanidins following the ingestion of a grape seed extract by rats, Br. J. Nutr. 94 (2005) 170–181.

[62] M.M. Appeldoorn, J.P. Vincken, H. Gruppen, P.C.H. Hollman, Procyanidin dimers A1, A2, and B2 are absorbed without conjugation or methylation from the small intestine of rats, J. Nutr. 139 (2009) 1469–1473.

[63] T. Shoji, S. Masumoto, N. Moriichi, H. Akiyama, T. Kanda, Y. Ohtake, et al., Apple procyanidin oligomers absorption in rats after oral administration: Analysis of procyanidins in plasma using the Porter method and high-performance liquid chromatography/tandem mass spectrometry, J. Agric. Food Chem 54 (2006) 884–892.

[64] R.R. Holt, S.A. Lazarus, M.C. Sullards, Q.Y. Zhu, D.D. Schramm, J.F. Hammerstone, et al., Procyanidin dimer B2 epicatechin-(4 beta-8)-epicatechin in human plasma after the consumption of a flavanol-rich cocoa, Am. J. Clin. Nutr. 76 (2002) 798–804.

[65] T. Kohri, M. Suzuki, F. Nanjo, Identification of metabolites of (−)-epicatechin gallate and their metabolic fate in the rat, J. Agric. Food Chem. 51 (2003) 5561–5566.

[66] T. Kohri, F. Nanjo, M. Suziki, R. Seto, N. Matsumoto, M. Yamakawa, et al., Synthesis of (−)-4-H-3 epigallocatechin gallate and its metabolic fate in rats after intravenous administration, J. Agric. Food Chem. 49 (2001) 1042–1048.

[67] U. Justesen, E. Arrigoni, B.R. Larsen, R. Amado, Degradation of flavonoid glycosides and aglycones during in vitro fermentation with human faecal flora, Lebensmittel-Wissenschaft Technol 33 (2000) 424–430.

[68] A.L. Simons, M. Renouf, S. Hendrich, P.A. Murphy, Human gut microbial degradation of flavonoids: Structure − function relationships, J. Agric. Food Chem. 53 (2005) 4258–4263.

[69] N.P. Das, L.A. Griffith, Studies on flavonoid metabolism: Metabolism of (+)-catechin in guinea pig, Biochem. J. 110 (1968) 449.

[70] N.P. Das, L.A. Griffith, Studies on flavonoid metabolism: Metabolism of (+)-14C catechin in rat and guinea pig, Biochem. J. 115 (1969) 831.

[71] J. Winter, L.H. Moore, V.R. Dowell, V.D. Bokkenheuser, C-ring cleavage of flavonoids by human intestinal bacteria, Appl. Environ. Microbiol. 55 (1989) 1203–1208.

[72] L. Bravo, R. Abia, M.A. Eastwood, F. Sauracalixto, Degradation of polyphenols (catechin and tannic-acid) in the rat intestinal tract: effect on colonic fermentation and fecal output, Br. J. Nutr. 71 (1994) 933–946.

[73] X. Tzounis, J. Vulevic, G.G.C. Kuhnle, T. George, J. Leonczak, G.R. Gibson, et al., Flavanol monomer-induced changes to the human faecal microflora, Br. J. Nutr. 99 (782–792) (2008).

[74] H.C. Lee, A.M. Jenner, C.S. Low, Y.K. Lee, Effect of tea phenolics and their aromatic fecal bacterial metabolites on intestinal microbiota, Res. Microbiol. 157 (2006) 876–884.

[75] M.P. Gonthier, V. Cheynier, J.L. Donovan, C. Manach, C. Morand, I. Mila, et al., Microbial aromatic acid metabolites formed in the gut account for a major fraction of the polyphenols excreted in urine of rats fed red wine polyphenols, J. Nutr. 133 (2003) 461–467.

[76] Y.-T. Lin, S.-L. Hsiu, Y.-C. Hou, H.-Y. Chen, P.-D.L. Chao, Degradation of flavonoid aglycones by rabbit, rat and human fecal flora, Biol. Pharm. Bull. 26 (2003) 747–751.

[77] L.Y. Rios, M.-P. Gonthier, C. Remesy, I. Mila, C. Lapierre, S.A. Lazarus, et al., Chocolate intake increases urinary excretion of polyphenol-derived phenolic acids in healthy human subjects, Am. J. Clin. Nutr. 77 (2003) 912–918.

[78] K. Gao, A. Xu, C. Krul, K. Venema, Y. Liu, Y. Niu, et al., Of the major phenolic acids formed during human microbial fermentation of tea, citrus, and soy flavonoid supplements, only 3,4-dihydroxyphenylacetic acid has antiproliferative activity, J. Nutr. 136 (2006) 52–57.

[79] R. Abia, S.C. Fry, Degradation and metabolism of C-14-labelled proanthocyanidins from carob (Ceratonia siliqua) pods in the gastrointestinal tract of the rat, J. Sci. Food Agric 81 (2001) 1156–1165.

[80] S. Veeriah, T. Hofmann, M. Glei, H. Dietrich, F. Will, P. Schreier, et al., Apple polyphenols and products formed in the gut differently inhibit survival of human cell lines derived from colon adenoma (LT97) and carcinoma (HT29), J. Agric. Food Chem. 55 (2007) 2892–2900.

[81] M. Urpi-Sarda, M. Monagas, N. Khan, R.M. Lamuela-Raventos, C. Santos-Buelga, E. Sacanella, et al., Epicatechin, procyanidins, and phenolic microbial metabolites after cocoa intake in humans and rats, Anal. Bioanal. Chem. 394 (2009) 1545–1556.

[82] M.P. Gonthier, J.L. Donovan, O. Texier, C. Felgines, C. Remesy, A. Scalbert, Metabolism of dietary procyanidins in rats, Free Radic. Biol. Med. 35 (2003) 837–844.

[83] A.M. Aura, I. Mattila, T. Seppanen-Laakso, J. Miettinen, K.M. Oksman-Caldentey, M. Oresic, Microbial metabolism of catechin stereoisomers by human faecal microbiota: comparison of targeted analysis and a non-targeted metabolomics method, Phytochem. Lett 1 (2008) 18–22.

[84] S. Deprez, C. Brezillon, S. Rabot, C. Philippe, I. Mila, C. Lapierre, et al., Polymeric proanthocyanidins are catabolized by human colonic microflora into low-molecular-weight phenolic acids, J. Nutr. 130 (2000) 2733–2738.

[85] K. Kahle, W. Huemmer, M. Kempf, W. Scheppach, T. Erk, E. Richling, Polyphenols are intensively metabolized in the human gastrointestinal tract after apple juice consumption, J. Agric. Food Chem. 55 (2007) 10605–10614.

[86] S. Stoupi, G. Williamson, J.W. Drynan, D. Barron, M.N. Clifford, Procyanidin B2 catabolism by human fecal microflora: partial characterization of "dimeric" intermediates, Arch. Biochem. Biophys. 501 (2010) 73–78.

[87] S. Stoupi, G. Williamson, J.W. Drynan, D. Barron, M.N. Clifford, A comparison of the in vitro biotransformation of (−)-epicatechin and procyanidin B2 by human faecal microbiota, Mol. Nutr. Food Res. 54 (2009) 747–759.

[88] G. van't Slot, H.-U. Humpf, Degradation and metabolism of catechin, epigallocatechin-3-gallate (EGCG), and related compounds by the intestinal microbiota in the pig cecum model, J. Agric. Food Chem 57 (2009) 8041–8048.

[89] M. Sharma, L. Li, J. Celver, C. Killian, A. Kovoor, N.P. Seeram, Effects of fruit ellagitannin extracts, ellagic acid, and their colonic metabolite, urolithin A, on Wnt signaling, J. Agric. Food Chem. 58 (2009) 3965–3969.

[90] S.G. Kasimsetty, D. Bialonska, M.K. Reddy, G. Ma, S.I. Khan, D. Ferreira, Colon cancer chemopreventive activities of pomegranate ellagitannins and urolithins, J. Agric. Food Chem. 58 (2010) 2180–2187.

[91] A. Gonzalez-Sarrias, M. Larrosa, F.A. Tomas-Barberan, P. Dolara, J.C. Espin, NF-kB-dependent anti-inflammatory activity of urolithins, gut microbiota ellagic acid-derived metabolites, in human colonic fibroblasts, Br. J. Nutr. 104 (2010) 503–512.

[92] D. Bialonska, S.G. Kasimsetty, S.I. Khan, D. Ferreira, Urolithins, intestinal microbial metabolites of pomegranate ellagitannins, exhibit potent antioxidant activity in a cell-based assay, J. Agric. Food Chem. 57 (2009) 10181–10186.

[93] M. Larrosa, A. González-Sarrías, M.J. Yáñez-Gascón, M.V. Selma, M. Azorín-Ortuño, S. Toti, et al., Anti-inflammatory properties of a pomegranate extract and its metabolite urolithin-A in a colitis rat model and the effect of colon inflammation on phenolic metabolism, J. Nutr. Biochem. 21 (2010) 717–725.

[94] S. Lu, L. Li, Carotenoid metabolism: Biosynthesis, regulation, and beyond, J. Integrative Plant Biol. 50 (2008) 778–785.

[95] J.J.M. Castenmiller, C.E. West, Bioavailability and bioconversion of carotenoids, Annu. Rev. Nutr. 18 (1998) 19–38.

[96] D. DellaPenna, B.J. Pogson, Vitamin synthesis in plants: Tocopherols and carotenoids, Annu. Rev. Plant Biol. 57 (2006) 711–738.

[97] C.K. Sen, S. Khanna, S. Roy, Tocotrienols: Vitamin E beyond tocopherols, Life Sci. 78 (2006) 2088–2098.

[98] M.L. Colombo, An update on vitamin E, tocopherol and tocotrienol: Perspectives, Molecules 15 (2010) 2103–2113.

[99] C. Schneider, Chemistry and biology of vitamin E, Mol. Nutr. Food Res. 49 (2005) 7–30.

[100] E. Fernandez-Garcia, I. Carvajal-Lerida, M. Jaren-Galan, J. Garrido-Fernandez, A. Perez-Galvez, D. Hornero-Mendez,

Carotenoids bioavailability from foods: from plant pigments to efficient biological activities, Food Res. Int. 46 (2012) 438−450.

[101] S. Goltz, M.G. Ferruzzi, Factors affecting carotenoid bioavailability: Dietary fat and fiber, in: S. Tanumihardjo (Ed.), Carotenoids and Human Health, Spinger, New York, 2012.

[102] E. Kotake-Nara, A. Nagao, Absorption and metabolism of xanthophylls, Marine Drugs 9 (2011) 1024−1037.

[103] E.H. Harrison, Mechanisms involved in the intestinal absorption of dietary vitamin A and provitamin A carotenoids, Biochim. Biophys. Acta 1821 (2012) 70−77.

[104] M.J. Brown, M.G. Ferruzzi, M.L. Nguyen, D.A. Cooper, A.L. Eldridge, S.J. Schwartz, et al., Carotenoid bioavailability is higher from salads ingested with full-fat than with fat-reduced salad dressings as measured with electrochemical detection, Am. J. Clin. Nutr. 80 (2004) 396−403.

[105] E. Reboul, M. Richelle, E.Ø. Perrot, C. Desmoulins-Malezet, V. Pirisi, P. Borel, Bioaccessibility of carotenoids and vitamin E from their main dietary sources, J. Agric. Food Chem. 54 (2006) 8749−8755.

[106] T. Huo, M.G. Ferruzzi, S.J. Schwartz, M.L. Failla, Impact of fatty acyl composition and quantity of triglycerides on bioaccessibility of dietary carotenoids, J. Agric. Food Chem. 55 (2007) 8950−8957.

[107] E.G. Kean, B.R. Hamaker, M.G. Ferruzzi, Carotenoid bioaccessibility from whole grain and degermed maize meal products, J. Agric. Food Chem. 56 (2008) 9918−9926.

[108] A.R. Kohut, M.L. Failla, B.A. Watkins, M.G. Ferruzzi, The impact of lipid quantity and type on carotenoid bioaccessibility from vegetables, FASEB J. 21 (2007) A350.

[109] M.G. Ferruzzi, J.L. Lumpkin, S.J. Schwartz, M. Failla, Digestive stability, micellarization, and uptake of beta-carotene isomers by Caco-2 human intestinal cells, J. Agric. Food Chem. 54 (2006) 2780−2785.

[110] T.Y. Huo, M.G. Ferruzzi, M.A. Belury, S.J. Schwartz, M.L. Failla, Impact of amount and triglyceride (TG) structure on micellarization of dietary carotenoids during simulated digestion, FASEB J. 21 (2007) A730−A731.

[111] K. Anwar, J. Iqbal, M.M. Hussain, Mechanisms involved in vitamin E transport by primary enterocytes and in vivo absorption, J. Lipid Res. 48 (2007) 2028−2038.

[112] J. Iqbal, M.M. Hussain, Intestinal lipid absorption, Am. J. Physiol. Endocrinol. Metab. 296 (2009) E1183−E1194.

[113] A. Rigotti, Absorption, transport, and tissue delivery of vitamin E, Mol. Aspects Med. 28 (2007) 423−436.

[114] L. Brisson, S. Castan, H. Fontbonne, C. Nicoletti, A. Puigserver, E.H. Ajandouz, Alpha-tocopheryl acetate is absorbed and hydrolyzed by Caco-2 cells: comparative studies with alpha-tocopherol, Chem. Phys. Lipids 154 (2008) 33−37.

[115] R. Wajda, J. Zirkel, T. Schaffer, Increase of bioavailability of coenzyme Q(10) and vitamin E, J. Medicinal Food 10 (2007) 731−734.

[116] Y. O'Callaghan, N. O'Brien, Bioaccessibility, cellular uptake and transepithelial transport of alpha-tocopherol and retinol from a range of supplemented foodstuffs assessed using the caco-2 cell model, Int. J. Food Sci. Technol. 45 (2010) 1436−1442.

[117] E. Reboul, P. Borel, Proteins involved in uptake, intracellular transport and basolateral secretion of fat-soluble vitamins and carotenoids by mammalian enterocytes, Prog. Lipid Res. 50 (2011) 388−402.

[118] P. Anand, A.B. Kunnumakkara, R.A. Newman, B.B. Aggarwal, Bioavailability of curcumin: problems and promises, Mol. Pharm. 4 (2007) 807−818.

[119] A. Shehzad, F. Wahid, Y.S. Lee, Curcumin in cancer chemoprevention: Molecular targets, pharmacokinetics, bioavailability, and clinical trials, Arch. Pharmazie 343 (2010) 489−499.

[120] T. Hamaguchi, K. Ono, M. Yamada, Review: Curcumin and Alzheimer's disease, CNS Neurosci. Ther. 16 (2010) 285−297.

[121] S. Bisht, A. Maitra, Systemic delivery of curcumin: 21st century solutions for an ancient conundrum, Curr. Drug Discov. Technol. 6 (2009) 192−199.

[122] C.R. Ireson, D.J.L. Jones, S. Orr, M.W.H. Coughtrie, D.J. Boocock, M.L. Williams, et al., Metabolism of the cancer chemopreventive agent curcumin in human and rat intestine, Cancer Epidemiol. Biomarkers Prev. 11 (2002) 105−111.

[123] R.A. Sharma, W.P. Steward, A.J. Gescher, Pharmacokinetics and pharmacodynamics of curcumin, Adv. Exp. Med. Biol. 595 (2007) 453−470.

[124] E. Burgos-Morón, J.M. Calderón-Montaño, J. Salvador, A. Robles, M. López-Lázaro, The dark side of curcumin, Int. J. Cancer 126 (2010) 1771−1775.

[125] B.T. Kurien, R.H. Scofield, Oral administration of heat-solubilized curcumin for potentially increasing curcumin bioavailability in experimental animals, Int. J. Cancer 125 (2009) 1992−1993.

[126] J. Shaikh, D.D. Ankola, V. Beniwal, D. Singh, M.N.V.R. Kumar, Nanoparticle encapsulation improves oral bioavailability of curcumin by at least 9-fold when compared to curcumin administered with piperine as absorption enhancer, Eur. J. Pharm. Sci. 37 (2009) 223−230.

[127] M.J. Kang, J.Y. Cho, B.H. Shim, D.K. Kim, J. Lee, Bioavailability enhancing activities of natural compounds from medicinal plants, J. Med. Plants Res. 3 (2009) 1204−1211.

[128] A. Khajuria, N. Thusu, U. Zutshi, Piperine modulates permeability characteristics of intestine by inducing alterations in membrane dynamics: influence on brush border membrane fluidity, ultrastructure and enzyme kinetics, Phytomedicine 9 (2002) 224−230.

PART C

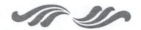

OVERWEIGHT AND OBESITY

CHAPTER

23

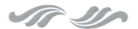

Genetics of Human Obesity

Janis S. Fisler, Craig H. Warden

University of California at Davis, Davis, California

I INTRODUCTION

Complex and incompletely defined interactions between the environment and genetics determine each individual's height and weight, as well as other human quantitative traits.[1] The result is a population in which individuals vary widely for height and weight, but no one factor can be identified as controlling either trait. In humans, long-term adult weight is relatively stable, as evidenced by the difficulty of sustaining intentional weight loss and the automatic return to previous weight following brief periods of overeating. This drive to constancy of body weight is due to both behavioral and physiological alterations that accompany weight change. Convincing evidence of the biological basis of the regulation of body fat stores comes from the identification of more than 50 single-gene mutations and Mendelian[2] syndromes that result in spontaneous massive obesity or in adipose tissue atrophy.

Most human obesity, however, is not due to mutations in single genes but is inherited as a complex, multigenic, quantitative trait influenced by many genetic and environmental variables. There are likely to be interactions among genes and between genes and environmental factors such that some alleles of one gene will not cause obesity unless specific alleles of another gene or environmental pressures are present. Genetic heterogeneity[3] and incomplete penetrance[4] of the trait also make dissection of complex phenotypes

difficult. Expression of an obesity gene may also be age or gender dependent. Thus, identification of all the genes promoting human obesity is not a trivial task.

Genetics is a rapidly progressing field, and knowledge of the genetic basis for obesity is expanding exponentially. Therefore, the reader should use this chapter only as the starting point for an understanding of this exciting body of knowledge.

II GENETIC EPIDEMIOLOGY OF HUMAN OBESITY

Genetic epidemiology of human obesity is the study of the relationships of the various factors determining the frequency and distribution of obesity in the population. Such studies of obesity are limited in that they do not examine DNA and rarely directly measure the amount or location of body fat. However, genetic epidemiology studies do provide information as to whether there is a genetic basis for the trait, whether a major gene is involved in the population, whether inheritance is maternal or paternal, and whether expression of the trait is gender or age dependent.

Genetic epidemiology studies of human obesity employ a variety of designs and statistical methods, each giving somewhat different heritability[5] estimates for obesity. For a discussion of genetic epidemiology

---

[1]A quantitative trait is one that varies over a continuous range, such as body weight and height, and is controlled by multiple genes.

[2]A Mendelian trait is one that is controlled by a single gene.

[3]Genetic heterogeneity refers to similar phenotypes caused by mutations in more than one gene.

[4]Incomplete penetrance means that not all individuals who have the gene mutation develop the phenotype.

[5]Genetic heritability is the percentage of interindividual variation in a trait that is explained by genetic factors.

Nutrition in the Prevention and Treatment of Disease, Third Edition.
DOI: http://dx.doi.org/10.1016/B978-0-12-391884-0.00023-8

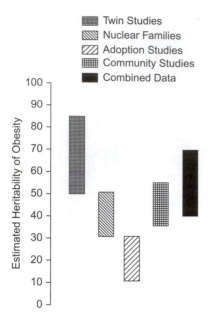

FIGURE 23.1 Heritability of obesity as determined by different study types. Data for studies of twins, nuclear families, and adoption studies are taken from Bouchard *et al.* [1]. Data for community-based studies are taken from Herbert *et al.* [143]. Range of heritability estimated from all study types is taken from Comuzzie and Allison [5].

methods employed in the study of obesity, see Bouchard *et al.* [1].

The heritability estimates for human obesity are derived from a large number of studies of adoptees, twins, families, or communities. Population or family studies tend to have lower, and twin studies to have higher, heritability for body mass index (BMI).[6] Heritability of BMI has been estimated from adoption studies to be as low as 10% and from twin studies to be as high as 85% [1,2] (Figure 23.1). In a pediatric twin study, genetic influences contributed 75–80% in the percentage of body fat [3]. The heritability estimate for BMI in a study of childhood obesity in an Hispanic population was 40% and, in that study, heritability of diet and physical activity phenotypes ranged from 32% to 69% [4]. By using data from all types of studies, it is estimated that 40–70% of the within-population variation in obesity is due to genetic variation [5] (Figure 23.1). Most studies indicate that familial environment has only a minor impact on obesity.

Genes implicated in obesity can have major, minor, or multigenic effects. A major gene is a single gene that has a large effect on the phenotype. Mode of transmission[7]

may be recessive, co-dominant, or dominant. Multigenic effects are due to many genes, each with a small effect on the phenotype.

III WHY DOES IT MATTER?

Not that long ago, it was possible to list all the genes causing Mendelian forms of obesity in a table of one to a few pages. Recent years have witnessed an explosion in the number of genes known to cause Mendelian forms of obesity and an even bigger explosion in the number of genes associated with obesity. To date, Mendelian obesity has been associated with missense mutations, copy number variants, deletions, and imprinted loci.

Two groups have attempted to estimate the total number of obesity genes. Reed *et al.* [6] used mouse models to estimate that approximately one-third of all knockouts have weight phenotypes suggesting that there are thousands of obesity genes. Speliotes *et al.* [7] used an association study with 249,796 people to determine that including the 270 genes with even slight but not genome-wide significant associations could account for only 4.5% of total heritability. Thus, two large-scale efforts, one in mice and the other in humans, estimate that the total number of obesity genes may be in the thousands. If this is the case, then why does finding obesity genes matter?

Data from other diseases are consistent with the hypothesis that the genetic causes of obesity will not be randomly distributed members of the entire collection of human alleles but are much more likely to be members of a much smaller number of networks or pathways [8–10]. It is likely that overall activity of these networks can be altered at one or a few control points and knowledge of network biology can be used to identify new targets for treatment. The nature of the mutation, whether deletion, missense, or copy number variant, will provide information on whether more or less of a gene or expressed sequence will promote weight loss.

IV THE SEARCH FOR OBESITY GENES

A Mapping of Loci in Animals

Animal models have been very important in the dissection of complex traits [11]. Quantitative trait locus

---

[6]Body mass index is calculated as body weight divided by height squared and is a commonly used surrogate for percentage body fat. A BMI of 25–30 is termed "overweight," BMI > 30 is termed "obese," and BMI > 40 is "morbidly obese."

[7]If a mutation has a recessive transmission, both copies of the gene must be defective to produce the phenotype. Codominant is inheritance in which two alleles of a pair of genes both have full phenotype expression causing individuals with two defective genes to be more obese than those with only one defective gene. With a dominant mode of transmission, only one defective gene need be present to express the phenotype.

(QTL)[8] mapping is a method for mapping Mendelian factors that underlie complex traits, in virtually any animal model, by using genetic linkage maps[9] (for discussion, see [11,12]). An advantage of linkage mapping is that no prior knowledge or assumptions are needed about the underlying genes. QTLs are regions of DNA containing one or more genes that affect the trait of interest. As of October 2005 (when the last Obesity Gene Map was compiled), 408 animal QTLs were linked variously to body weight, body fat, energy expenditure, food intake, leptin levels, or weight gain [13]. A number of these QTLs identified in separate crossbreeding experiments of different strains are overlapping, and it is likely that the same underlying gene is responsible for these overlapping QTLs. Many of these QTLs have pleiotropic effects.[10]

B From Mouse to Human

QTLs are valuable for identifying candidate genes to be further evaluated by gene targeting experiments in mice or by linkage studies or association studies of the candidate genes in humans. Because of the evolutionary relationship between mice and humans, many ancestral chromosomal segments have been retained where the same genes occur in the same order within discrete regions of chromosome. These regions of homology may include many hundreds to thousands of genes in the same orders, although some regions of homology are made more complex by chromosomal rearrangements within the region of homology. Because regions of homology between mouse and human chromosomes are well-defined, the identification of a gene in the mouse frequently gives the chromosomal location of the same gene in the human. For example, to test whether an obesity QTL on mouse chromosome 2 contributes to human obesity, linkage analysis between markers located within the homologous region on human chromosome 20 and measures of obesity was performed in more than 150 French Canadian families: A locus on 20q13 that contributes to body fat and fasting insulin was found [14]. This locus was later confirmed in a second population group [15].

C Linkage Studies in Humans

Linkage studies in humans are conducted with large extended families or with nuclear families. A conceptually simple and practical method is the nonparametric sib-pair linkage method that provides statistical evidence of linkage between a quantitative phenotype and a genetic marker [1,16,17]. The method is based on the concept that siblings who share a greater number of variants (alleles) (1 or 2) identical by descent[11] at a linked marker locus[12] should also share more alleles at the phenotypic locus of interest and should be phenotypically more similar than siblings who share fewer marker alleles (0 or 1). The method has been expanded to use data from multiple markers, allowing higher resolution mapping. Linkage studies do not identify any specific gene but are useful in identifying candidate genes for further study.

D The Candidate Gene Approach

Linkage studies in both rodents and humans have identified many chromosomal regions (QTLs) associated with obesity and related phenotypes. The candidate gene approach tests variants of a gene potentially contributing to the phenotype.

1 Association Studies of Candidate Genes in Humans

A positional candidate gene is identified both by its location in a chromosomal region that has significant linkage to obesity in family studies and because its biological functions are generally consistent with a role in body weight regulation. Association studies then examine the correlation of a genetic variant (allele) within that gene with the phenotype of interest. It is assumed that variants within a gene's coding region alter gene function, although proof of that requires gene-targeting experiments in cell or animal models. Although the candidate gene approach may allow identification of a gene with small effect, these studies have the disadvantage that an understanding of the biology of the gene is necessary.

---

[8]A QTL is a chromosomal region in which alleles are linked to variation of a quantitative trait.

[9]Genetic linkage is the tendency for regions of a chromosome to be inherited together. Linkage maps show the positions of known markers or genes relative to each other within a linkage group.

[10]Pleiotropy means that one gene has a primary effect on more than one phenotype.

[11]Identical by descent is in contrast to identical by state. Two siblings sharing the same allele are identical by descent if you know that it is the same allele inherited from the same parent. They are identical by state if they have the same allele but you do not know if they are derived from the same parental haplotype.

[12]A locus is any segment of DNA that is measurable in genetic analysis. A locus may be within a gene or may be a DNA sequence of no known function. A linkage map represents a set of loci on a single chromosome in which all members of the set are linked either directly or indirectly with all other members of the set. Linkage in humans refers to the cosegregation of a genetic marker and a trait together in families.

Association studies are generally carried out in unrelated individuals and are frequently designed as case—control studies. Although case—control studies remain a powerful tool in some areas, they are less powerful for genetic studies due to methodological issues that complicate analyses in complex populations such as those found in the United States. Therefore, many association studies are now conducted in isolated populations, such as occur in Finland and Quebec. For a discussion of difficulties with replication in association studies, see Herbert *et al.* [18].

2 Insertion/Deletion Studies in Rodents

Candidate genes are often tested in rodent studies. Expression of genes can be altered in the mouse by targeted insertion or deletion in the whole animal or by strategies that cause gene deficiencies in only those tissues of interest [19,20]. The development of obesity models with under- or overexpression of a gene not only confirms that the gene contributes to obesity but also provides a model to investigate the resulting phenotype, including energy balance, feeding and activity behaviors, and fat and carbohydrate metabolism.

A confounding factor in many gene deletion studies is the redundancy of gene function. For example, deletion of the β_1-adrenergic receptor only shows an obesity phenotype if there are also mutations in both β_2- and β_3-adrenergic receptors [21]. Other confounders are gene—gene interactions, requiring mutations in two or even three independent genes to have the phenotype expressed, and gene—environment interactions such as the necessity of a high-fat diet for obesity to develop.

E Genome-Wide Association Studies

In recent years, a new approach to associations studies, one in which whole genome SNP maps[13] are used to identify chromosomal regions influencing traits anywhere in the genome, has gained prominence due to technologies that allow genotyping hundreds of thousands of SNPs across the genome at reasonable cost. Genome-wide association studies (GWAS) examine markers throughout the genomes of individuals to identify associations between those markers and diseases or specific traits, often comparing genomes of cases (disease) with controls (no disease). This approach has the same advantage as linkage studies in that no prior assumptions about the identity of the underlying genes need to be made. Also, the overall data can be statistically evaluated to identify the most significant results, including gene—gene interactions. However, whole genome association studies also have several disadvantages. Whole genome studies necessarily restrict the number of markers to genotype per gene, whereas a more limited association study can investigate a greater number of markers within target genes. In addition, there are greater statistical problems with whole genome studies. GWAS have successfully identified common variants involved in many diseases, including obesity. It is important to remember that GWAS associate diseases or traits with regions of the genome but not with specific genes.

F The Problem of Missing Heritability

As indicated in Section II, as much as 70% of human obesity may be genetic. Yet, to date, less than 10% of that variability has been identified [22]. The gene most strongly associated with human obesity, the fat mass and obesity-associated gene (*FTO*), only contributes approximately 1% of the variance in BMI [23]. The problem of the missing heritability is true not only for obesity but also for most common genetically complex traits and diseases. For example, height is estimated to be 80—90% heritable, yet large-scale population studies have identified less than 10% of height's heritability [24].

A number of proposals regarding where this missing heritability is to be found have been debated [24—26]. These explanations involve complex genetic inheritance or structure, including the presence of rare variants, variants with low penetrance, copy number variants, parent-of-origin effects, epigenetic tags, and epistasis (gene $\times$ gene interaction), none of which are readily identified by GWAS.

1 Rare Variants

Rare variants are likely to be missed by the GWAS approach despite the fact that they may have larger effects than common variants [22,27,28]. Rare variants having a strong effect in severe obesity [29,30] and in cannabinoid metabolism [27] have been identified. Cohorts with extreme phenotypes of obesity [29,30] or thinness [31] may be enriched with highly penetrant but rare alleles. It is also possible that there are moderately penetrant but fairly rare variants or common very low penetrant variants that are also missed by GWAS [24].

2 Copy Number Variants

Variability in genome structure, specifically copy number variants (CNVs), might also be responsible for some missing heritability [24]. CNVs are stretches of DNA of variable numbers of base pairs that are duplicated or deleted, that differ between individuals, and that commonly arise in an individual with no family history of the mutation. Because of the repetitive nature

---

[13]SNP (single nucleotide polymorphism) maps are dense maps of the genome containing as many as 500,000 SNPs used in high-resolution genotyping.

of CNVs, they are not measured by most current genotyping methods. CNVs were shown to contribute to severe early onset obesity, frequently associated with developmental delay, in several studies [32,33].

3 Parent-of-Origin Effects

Imprinting occurs when there is differential expression of a gene depending on whether it was inherited from the mother or the father. The best known parent-of-origin effect in obesity is the Prader–Willi syndrome, a Mendelian disorder due to paternal imprinting (see Section IX). Using a large population of Icelanders, it was observed that an allele that confers risk of type 2 diabetes when paternally inherited is protective when maternally inherited [34].

Maternal genetic effects occur when maternal genotype influences phenotypes of progeny independent of progeny genotype [35]. Maternal effects have mostly been identified in rodents, in which nursing or grooming behavior, or food intake or obesity of the dam, influences the phenotype of the progeny.

4 Epigenetics

Epigenetic tags are alterations to DNA that change gene expression without changing the underlying DNA sequence. Common epigenetic tags are those resulting from DNA methylation[14] or histone deacetylation.[15] Epigenetic tags generally suppress gene expression and may be inherited. Rodent studies have shown paternal transgenerational effects of environment on food intake and body weight [36] or on diabetes [37,38] of progeny. In the study by Ng et al. [37], the fathers' chronic high-fat diet promoted adult onset of a diabetes syndrome in their daughters even though the fathers had no continuing contact with the dams or progeny.

Studies of historical famine events show that children conceived during famine were small and underweight with increased risk for obesity as adults [39,40]. In the Chinese famine (1958–1961), only females developed obesity in later life [41]. DNA isolated from individuals decades after the famine showed abnormal DNA methylation [42].

5 Epistasis

Epistasis (gene–gene interaction) is where a gene or genes mask or amplify the effects of another gene or genes. Gene–gene interactions are likely a universal phenomenon in common human diseases and may be more important in determining the phenotype than the independent main effects of any one susceptibility gene [43,44]. A classic example of the effect of gene–gene interactions on a complex trait comes from mouse studies. The severity of diabetes in both Lep^{ob} (leptin) and $Lepr^{db}$ (leptin receptor) mutant[16] mice is determined by the genetic background upon which the mutation is expressed. Both Lep^{ob} and $Lepr^{db}$ mutations in C57BL/6 mice result in hyperinsulinemia and obesity, whereas these mutations in C57BLKs mice result in severe diabetes and early death [45].

Because gene–gene interactions are difficult to identify using traditional genetic studies in humans, little is known of these significant contributions to phenotypic variation in obesity. However, gene–gene interaction effects have been shown on BMI and waist circumference [46], extreme obesity [47], and on immune dysfunction in obesity [48]. Gene–gene interactions among variants of the β-adrenergic receptor genes (ADRB1, ADRB2, and ADRB3) contribute to longitudinal weight changes in African and Caucasian American subjects [49]. Epistasis affecting obesity was also found in African-derived populations in Brazil, where interactions between LEPR and ADRB2 polymorphisms as well as a third-order effect between LEPR, ADRB2 and INSIG2 were found [50]. A three-way gene–gene interaction has been reported to affect abdominal fat [51]. In the study of Feitosa et al. [46], blood lipid profile and dietary habits were found to be confounding effects in the analysis. Thus, it is possible to have both gene–gene and gene–environment interactions affecting the same pathway.

V GENE–ENVIRONMENT INTERACTIONS

Why some people in modern societies become obese, despite considerable effort and expense to avoid this condition, whereas others stay lean without such effort, appears to have a genetic basis [31,52]. Chronic overfeeding studies by Sims and colleagues [53,54] beginning in the 1960s showed interindividual differences in weight gain. Bouchard and colleagues [55] determined the response to changes in energy balance by submitting pairs of monozygotic twins either to positive energy balance induced by overeating or to negative energy balance induced by exercise training. During

---

[14]DNA methylation involves the addition of a methyl group to cytosine or adenine bases. Methyl groups are typically, but not always, removed in the zygote and can be transmitted to progeny.

[15]Histone deacetylation results in more tightly packed chromatin resulting in reduced transcription.

[16]The designations Lep^{ob}, $Lepr^{db}$, etc., represent mutations of the genes coding for leptin and the leptin receptor that occur in the *obese* mouse and the *diabetes* mouse, etc., respectively. The homologous genes in humans are designated LEP and LEPR. Standard nomenclature dictates that gene symbols are in italics, whereas the protein encoded by the gene is written in plain text.

100 days of overfeeding by 1000 kcal/day, significant intra-pair resemblance was observed for changes in body composition and this was particularly striking for changes in regional fat distribution and amount of visceral fat, with six times as much variance among as within twin pairs. During long-term energy deficit induced by exercise training, intra-pair resemblance was observed for changes in body weight, fat mass, percentage fat, and abdominal visceral fat [56]. One explanation for these differences is that some twin pairs were found to be better oxidizers of lipid, as evidenced by reduced respiratory quotient, during submaximal work than were other twin pairs [56].

An important component of the interindividual difference in response to overeating may be individual differences in spontaneous physical activity or "fidgeting" [57,58]. A large portion of the variability in total daily energy expenditure, independent of lean body mass, is due to fidgeting, which varies by more the sevenfold among subjects [58], is a familial trait, and is a predictor of future weight gain [59]. In a very elegant study of the fate of excess energy during overfeeding, Levine *et al.* [57] again demonstrated the considerable interindividual variation in susceptibility to weight gain. Two-thirds of the increases in total daily energy expenditure in nonobese subjects overfed by 1000 kcal/day for 8 weeks were due to increased spontaneous physical activity associated with fidgeting, maintenance of posture, and other daily activities of life independent of volitional exercise [57].

The genetic contributions to physical performance and to voluntary food intake and eating behavior are less well-known than for obesity. Nevertheless, the genes contributing to these phenotypes are being increasingly identified [13,60−62].

Studies on the genetics of eating behavior have examined restraint,[17] disinhibition,[18] and hunger as phenotypes as well as the physical ability to taste bitter, sweet, or umami flavors (for review, see [60]). Restraint, disinhibition, and bitter or sweet taste ability are all related to BMI. Meal size and selection also have heritable components. The fat mass and obesity-associated gene (*FTO*) may contribute to a preference for more energy-dense, high-fat foods and large meal size.

Hormones involved in eating behavior include ghrelin, CCK, and leptin (for review, see [60]). Ghrelin is produced by the stomach, functions to increase appetite, and has been associated with binge eating and obesity. CCK and leptin both promote satiety: CCK is more associated with meal size, whereas leptin is more associated with snacking behavior.

VI SINGLE-GENE OBESITY IN HUMANS

Cloning of the mouse obesity genes *Lep^{ob}*, *Lepr^{db}*, *Cpe^{fat}*, *Tub*, and *A^{y}* from naturally occurring mutant models between 1992 and 1996 led to an explosion of knowledge of the genetic causes of obesity. Obesity in these rodent models exhibits Mendelian segregation, indicating that the obesity is inherited as a single-gene mutation. With one exception, these mutations result in the loss of gene or protein function and are expressed only when both copies of the gene in an individual are defective. Therefore, obesity due to these mutations in humans would not be common. Nevertheless, these genes are of great interest because subtle mutations may contribute to common forms of obesity. Study of these genes led to the identification of the leptin−melanocortin pathway, the central regulator of energy homeostasis.

Nine genes have been reliably shown to cause spontaneous Mendelian obesity in humans: brain-derived neurotrophic factor (gene abbreviation *BDNF*), leptin (*LEP*), leptin receptor (*LEPR*), melanocortin 3 receptor (*MC3R*), melanocortin 4 receptor (*MC4R*), neurotrophic tyrosine kinase receptor type 2 (*NTRK2*), proopiomelanocortin (*POMC*), proprotein convertase subtilisin/kexin type 1 (*PCSK1*), and single-minded homolog 1 (*SIM1*) (Table 23.1). Mutations in these genes in humans are associated with severe obesity, beginning in childhood, and may include developmental, endocrine, and behavioral disorders.

Most of the single-gene obesities reported in Table 23.1 are rare, with each reported in only a few cases or families. The exceptions are *MC4R* [63] and perhaps *NTRK2* [64], where for each gene more than 100 obese cases have been shown to harbor a mutation. These single-gene mutations result in severe obesity, and as more such individuals are studied, additional cases will surely be identified. For a description of the most common single-gene obesity disorders and syndromes, see [65].

VII THE LEPTIN−MELANOCORTIN PATHWAY

The genes listed in Table 23.1 are components of the leptin−melanocortin pathway that functions to control whole body energy balance. The mutations of this pathway that are known to cause obesity are highlighted in Figure 23.2. Leptin is secreted by adipocytes and its concentration in blood is therefore proportional to fat

---

[17]Restrained eaters chronically restrict food intake, but loss of control can result in binge eating.

[18]Disinhibition is a lack of restraint in eating behavior.

TABLE 23.1 Single-Gene Mutations, Causing Uncomplicated Obesity, in Components of the Hypothalamic Leptin–Melanocortin Pathway in Humans

Gene name	Chromosomal locus	Function of gene product relative to obesity
Brain-derived neurotrophic factor (*BDNF*)[a]	11p13	Necessary for survival of striated neurons in the brain. Regulates eating behavior including anorexia and bulimia. *BDNF* and its receptor *NTRK2* are downstream components of the *MC4R*-mediated control of energy balance.
Leptin (*LEP*)[b]		...n adipocytes that plays a critical role in regulation of body weight ...ke and stimulating energy expenditure. Causes autosomal ...ypogonadism.
		...toreceptor to suppress activity of POMC neurons. Inhibits feed
		...R mutations affect appetite, cause severe obesity, and increased ...th, and bone mass. Causes autosomal dominant obesity.
		...ved neurotrophic factor (BDNF). Decreased expression causes ...vere early onset obesity and developmental delay.
		...drenocorticotropin, MC, β-isotropin, and β-endorphin.
		...rtase that cleaves POMC (also cleaves proinsulin to insulin). ...sity and impaired prohormone processing.
		...t is essential for the development of the paraventricular nucleus ...lutation results in severe obesity.

...gov/omim).
...n.nih.gov/omim).

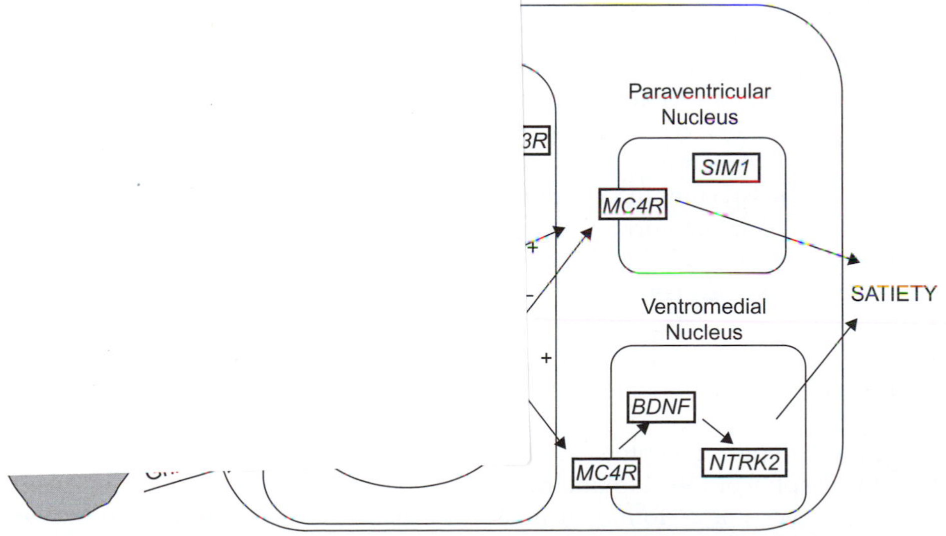

FIGURE 23.2 Simplified schematic, not showing transcription factors or enzymes, of the leptin–melanocortin pathway in the hypothalamus. Mutations of genes in bold are known to cause monogenic obesity in humans. This pathway is an essential component of the central control of energy homeostasis, propagating the signals that result in satiety. Leptin is secreted from adipocytes, crosses the blood–brain barrier, and activates leptin receptors. This activation stimulates POMC neurons producing melanocortins that activate melanocortin 4 receptors (MC4R) in the paraventricular and ventromedial nuclei, resulting in satiety. Melanocortin 3 receptor (MC3R) is an autoregulator of the POMC system. MC3R also affects obesity independently of its autoregulation of the POMC system, but whether it acts through the same pathway as MC4R is not known. SIM1 is essential for development of the paraventricular nucleus. Brain-derived neurotrophic factor and its receptor, neurotrophic tyrosine kinase receptor type 2, are part of the MC4R cascade leading to satiety. When stimulated by ghrelin receptors in the arcuate nucleus, agouti-related protein inhibits MC4R activity. AgRP, agouti-related protein; BDNF, brain-derived neurotrophic factor; CART, cocaine- and amphetamine-related transcript; GHR, ghrelin receptor; INSR, insulin receptor; LEP, leptin; LEPR, leptin receptor; α-MSH, α-melanocyte-stimulating hormone; β-MSH, β-melanocyte-stimulating hormone; NPY, neuropeptide Y; NTRK2, neurotrophic tyrosine kinase receptor type 2; PCSK1, proprotein convertase subtilisin/kexin type 1; POMC, proopiomelanocortin; SIM1, single-minded homolog 1 (*Drosophila*). Figure adapted from data from Mutch and Clement [69] and Xu *et al.* [144].

mass. Leptin crosses the blood−brain barrier and activates leptin receptors on the surface of neurons in the arcuate nucleus of the hypothalamus. This activation stimulates proprotein convertase (product of *PCSK1*) to cleave proopiomelanocortin (product of *POMC*) into the melanocortins including α-melanocyte-stimulating hormone (α-MSH), the primary ligand for melanocortin receptors and activation of downstream signaling to regulate energy balance. (For reviews of the leptin−melanocortin pathway and downstream signaling in obesity, see [2,66−70].)

A Leptin and Leptin Receptor Deficiencies

Cloning and characterization of the mouse *Lep^ob* gene identified its protein product, leptin, a hormone that is secreted from adipose tissue [71]. Leptin circulates in the blood [72], crosses the blood−brain barrier [73], and binds to its receptor in the hypothalamus to regulate food intake and energy expenditure [74]. Thus, leptin functions as an afferent signal in a negative feedback loop to maintain constancy of body fat stores.

Leptin clearly has a broader physiological role than just the regulation of body fat stores. Leptin deficiency results in many of the abnormalities seen in starvation, including reduced body temperature, reduced activity, decreased immune function, and infertility. (For reviews of the physiological role of leptin, see [74−76].)

Known mutations in leptin causing spontaneous massive obesity in humans are autosomal recessive and are rare. However, two highly consanguineous[19] families were identified that carry mutations in *LEP* [2,63]. Replacement with human recombinant leptin in children with severe leptin deficiency normalizes food intake and body composition [75]. Studies of long-term replacement therapy in patients with congenital leptin deficiency show that leptin regulates many body functions, including the endocrine system, energy balance, the adipoinsular axis, inflammation, and immunity [77].

Leptin acts through the leptin receptor, a single transmembrane domain receptor of the cytokine receptor family [78]. The leptin receptor is found in many tissues in several alternatively spliced forms, raising the possibility that leptin affects many tissues in addition to the hypothalamus. (For additional discussion of the leptin receptor, see [68,76].) As with the *LEP* gene, an autosomal recessive mutation in the human leptin receptor gene (*LEPR*) that results in a truncated leptin receptor was discovered in homozygosity[20] in a consanguineous family [63]. In a study of 300 subjects with severe early onset obesity (before age 10 years), eight families (two of which were nonconsanguineous) were identified in which severe obesity segregated with mutations in *LEPR* [79]. Individuals homozygous for these mutations were hyperphagic, had delayed or no pubertal development, had defects in immune function, and were hyperinsulinemic and hyperleptinemic consistent with the degree of obesity. This phenotype is similar to that seen in individuals with mutation of the leptin gene. Heterozygotes for *LEP* and *LEPR* mutations have increased fat mass but are not morbidly obese.

B Mutations in the Melanocortin System

Sequential cleavage of the precursor protein proopiomelanocortin (product of *POMC*) generates the melanocortin peptides adrenocorticotrophin (ACTH), the melanocyte-stimulating hormones (α-, β-, and δ-MSH), and the opioid receptor ligand β-endorphin (for review, see [68]). α-MSH plays a central role in the regulation of food intake by the activation of the brain melanocortin 4 receptor (product of *MC4R*). The dual role of α-MSH in regulating food intake and influencing hair pigmentation predicts that the phenotype associated with a defect in *POMC* function would include obesity, alteration in pigmentation (e.g., red hair and pale skin in Caucasians), and ACTH deficiency. The observations of these symptoms in two probands[21] led to the identification of three separate mutations within their *POMC* genes [80]. Another *POMC* variant in a region encoding β-MSH results in severe early onset obesity, hyperphagia, and increased linear growth—a phenotype much like that seen with mutations in *MC4R* [81]. Heterozygosity[22] for a *POMC* mutation having subtle effects on proopiomelanocortin expression and function was shown to influence susceptibility to obesity in a large family of Turkish origin [67].

A wide variety of hormones, enzymes, and receptors are initially synthesized as large inactive precursors. To release the active hormone, enzyme, or receptor, these precursors must undergo limited proteolysis by

---

[19]Consanguineous families result when individuals with common ancestry reproduce. If an allele is rare and if two copies (homozygocity) of a mutation are required for the phenotype to be expressed, then homozygotes are usually found only in highly consanguineous (inbred) families.

[20]Homozygosity refers to having the same alleles of a gene on the two chromosomes.

[21]A proband is the index case, the person through whom the pedigree (family) was ascertained.

[22]Heterozygosity refers to having different alleles of a gene on the two chromosomes.

TABLE 23.1 Single-Gene Mutations, Causing Uncomplicated Obesity, in Components of the Hypothalamic Leptin—Melanocortin Pathway in Humans

Gene name	Chromosomal locus	Function of gene product relative to obesity
Brain-derived neurotrophic factor (BDNF)[a]	11p13	Necessary for survival of striated neurons in the brain. Regulates eating behavior including anorexia and bulimia. BDNF and its receptor NTRK2 are downstream components of the MC4R-mediated control of energy balance.
Leptin (LEP)[b]	7q31.3	Hormone secreted from adipocytes that plays a critical role in regulation of body weight by inhibiting food intake and stimulating energy expenditure. Causes autosomal recessive obesity and hypogonadism.
Leptin receptor (LEPR)[b]	1p31	Receptor for leptin.
Melanocortin 3 receptor (MC3R)[b]	20q13.2	Receptor for MC[c] as autoreceptor to suppress activity of POMC neurons. Inhibits feed efficiency.
Melanocortin 4 receptor (MC4R)[b]	18q22	Receptor for MC. MC4R mutations affect appetite, cause severe obesity, and increased lean mass, linear growth, and bone mass. Causes autosomal dominant obesity.
Neurotrophic tyrosine kinase receptor type 2 (NTRK2)[b]	9q22.1	Receptor for brain-derived neurotrophic factor (BDNF). Decreased expression causes hyperphagia, causes severe early onset obesity and developmental delay.
Proopiomelanocortin (POMC)[b]	2p23.3	Precursor molecule of adrenocorticotropin, MC, β-isotropin, and β-endorphin.
Proprotein convertase subtilisin/ kexin type 1 (PCSK1)[b]	5q15—q21	Neuroendocrine convertase that cleaves POMC (also cleaves proinsulin to insulin). Mutation results in obesity and impaired prohormone processing.
Single-minded homolog 1 (SIM1)[b]	6q16.3—q21	Transcription factor that is essential for the development of the paraventricular nucleus of the hypothalamus. Mutation results in severe obesity.

[a]Data from Gray et al. [85] and Online Mendelian Inheritance in Man (http://www.ncbi.nlm.nih.gov/omim).
[b]Data from Rankinen et al. [61] and Online Mendelian Inheritance in Man (http://www.ncbi.nlm.nih.gov/omim).
[c]MC = α-MSH, β-MSH, and δ-MSH

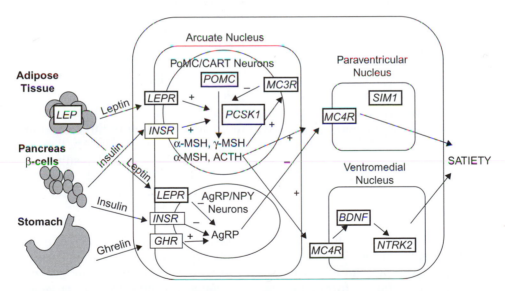

FIGURE 23.2 Simplified schematic, not showing transcription factors or enzymes, of the leptin—melanocortin pathway in the hypothalamus. Mutations of genes in bold are known to cause monogenic obesity in humans. This pathway is an essential component of the central control of energy homeostasis, propagating the signals that result in satiety. Leptin is secreted from adipocytes, crosses the blood—brain barrier, and activates leptin receptors. This activation stimulates POMC neurons producing melanocortins that activate melanocortin 4 receptors (MC4R) in the paraventricular and ventromedial nuclei, resulting in satiety. Melanocortin 3 receptor (MC3R) is an autoregulator of the POMC system. MC3R also affects obesity independently of its autoregulation of the POMC system, but whether it acts through the same pathway as MC4R is not known. SIM1 is essential for development of the paraventricular nucleus. Brain-derived neurotrophic factor and its receptor, neurotrophic tyrosine kinase receptor type 2, are part of the MC4R cascade leading to satiety. When stimulated by ghrelin receptors in the arcuate nucleus, agouti-related protein inhibits MC4R activity. AgRP, agouti-related protein; BDNF, brain-derived neurotrophic factor; CART, cocaine- and amphetamine-related transcript; GHR, ghrelin receptor; INSR, insulin receptor; LEP, leptin; LEPR, leptin receptor; α-MSH, α-melanocyte-stimulating hormone; β-MSH, β-melanocyte-stimulating hormone; NPY, neuropeptide Y; NTRK2, neurotrophic tyrosine kinase receptor type 2; PCSK1, proprotein convertase subtilisin/kexin type 1; POMC, proopiomelanocortin; SIM1, single-minded homolog 1 (Drosophila). Figure adapted from data from Mutch and Clement [69] and Xu et al. [144].

mass. Leptin crosses the blood—brain barrier and activates leptin receptors on the surface of neurons in the arcuate nucleus of the hypothalamus. This activation stimulates proprotein convertase (product of *PCSK1*) to cleave proopiomelanocortin (product of *POMC*) into the melanocortins including α-melanocyte-stimulating hormone (α-MSH), the primary ligand for melanocortin receptors and activation of downstream signaling to regulate energy balance. (For reviews of the leptin—melanocortin pathway and downstream signaling in obesity, see [2,66—70].)

A Leptin and Leptin Receptor Deficiencies

Cloning and characterization of the mouse *Lep^ob* gene identified its protein product, leptin, a hormone that is secreted from adipose tissue [71]. Leptin circulates in the blood [72], crosses the blood—brain barrier [73], and binds to its receptor in the hypothalamus to regulate food intake and energy expenditure [74]. Thus, leptin functions as an afferent signal in a negative feedback loop to maintain constancy of body fat stores.

Leptin clearly has a broader physiological role than just the regulation of body fat stores. Leptin deficiency results in many of the abnormalities seen in starvation, including reduced body temperature, reduced activity, decreased immune function, and infertility. (For reviews of the physiological role of leptin, see [74—76].)

Known mutations in leptin causing spontaneous massive obesity in humans are autosomal recessive and are rare. However, two highly consanguineous[19] families were identified that carry mutations in *LEP* [2,63]. Replacement with human recombinant leptin in children with severe leptin deficiency normalizes food intake and body composition [75]. Studies of long-term replacement therapy in patients with congenital leptin deficiency show that leptin regulates many body functions, including the endocrine system, energy balance, the adipoinsular axis, inflammation, and immunity [77].

Leptin acts through the leptin receptor, a single transmembrane domain receptor of the cytokine receptor family [78]. The leptin receptor is found in many tissues in several alternatively spliced forms, raising the possibility that leptin affects many tissues in addition to the hypothalamus. (For additional discussion of the leptin receptor, see [68,76].) As with the *LEP* gene, an autosomal recessive mutation in the human leptin receptor gene (*LEPR*) that results in a truncated leptin receptor was discovered in homozygosity[20] in a consanguineous family [63]. In a study of 300 subjects with severe early onset obesity (before age 10 years), eight families (two of which were nonconsanguineous) were identified in which severe obesity segregated with mutations in *LEPR* [79]. Individuals homozygous for these mutations were hyperphagic, had delayed or no pubertal development, had defects in immune function, and were hyperinsulinemic and hyperleptinemic consistent with the degree of obesity. This phenotype is similar to that seen in individuals with mutation of the leptin gene. Heterozygotes for *LEP* and *LEPR* mutations have increased fat mass but are not morbidly obese.

B Mutations in the Melanocortin System

Sequential cleavage of the precursor protein proopiomelanocortin (product of *POMC*) generates the melanocortin peptides adrenocorticotrophin (ACTH), the melanocyte-stimulating hormones (α-, β-, and δ-MSH), and the opioid receptor ligand β-endorphin (for review, see [68]). α-MSH plays a central role in the regulation of food intake by the activation of the brain melanocortin 4 receptor (product of *MC4R*). The dual role of α-MSH in regulating food intake and influencing hair pigmentation predicts that the phenotype associated with a defect in *POMC* function would include obesity, alteration in pigmentation (e.g., red hair and pale skin in Caucasians), and ACTH deficiency. The observations of these symptoms in two probands[21] led to the identification of three separate mutations within their *POMC* genes [80]. Another *POMC* variant in a region encoding β-MSH results in severe early onset obesity, hyperphagia, and increased linear growth—a phenotype much like that seen with mutations in *MC4R* [81]. Heterozygosity[22] for a *POMC* mutation having subtle effects on proopiomelanocortin expression and function was shown to influence susceptibility to obesity in a large family of Turkish origin [67].

A wide variety of hormones, enzymes, and receptors are initially synthesized as large inactive precursors. To release the active hormone, enzyme, or receptor, these precursors must undergo limited proteolysis by

---

[19]Consanguineous families result when individuals with common ancestry reproduce. If an allele is rare and if two copies (homozygocity) of a mutation are required for the phenotype to be expressed, then homozygotes are usually found only in highly consanguineous (inbred) families.

[20]Homozygosity refers to having the same alleles of a gene on the two chromosomes.

[21]A proband is the index case, the person through whom the pedigree (family) was ascertained.

[22]Heterozygosity refers to having different alleles of a gene on the two chromosomes.

specific convertases. An example is the clipping of proopiomelanocortin by proprotein convertase subtilisin/kexin type 1, also known as prohormone convertase-1 (product of *PCSK1*). A recessive mutation of the gene producing carboxypeptidase E, a homologous enzyme active in the processing and sorting of prohormones, causes obesity in the *Cpe^fat* mouse. Mutations in the human homolog *PCSK1* were found in individuals with extreme childhood obesity and elevated proinsulin and proopiomelanocortin concentrations but very low insulin levels (for review, see [63]). Because the human cases and the *Cpe^fat* mouse share similar phenotypes, it can be inferred that molecular defects in prohormone conversion represent a generic mechanism for obesity.

The agouti protein, identified in the yellow obese (*A^y*) mouse, inhibits binding of α-MSH to melanocortin receptors. Obesity and yellow coat color in the *A^y* mouse result from expressing agouti in all tissues, not just in skin, which is the normal condition. Two melanocortin receptors (*MC3R* and *MC4R*) are highly expressed in the hypothalamus, a region of the brain intimately involved in appetite regulation.

Mutations in *MC4R*, the gene encoding melanocortin receptor-4, are found in various ethnic groups and cause the most common form of monogenic obesity in humans. The global presence of obesity-specific *MC4R* mutations is estimated to vary from 2% to 6 % among population groups [68,82]. *MC4R*-linked obesity in humans is dominantly inherited with incomplete penetrance. Subjects with MC4R deficiency are obese from an early age. Adrenal function is not impaired, but severe hyperinsulinemia is present in the MC4R-deficient subjects. Sexual development and fertility are normal. Affected subjects are hyperphagic and have increased linear growth, similar to that which occurs in heterozygous MC4R-deficient mice. MC4R-deficient humans also have increased lean mass and bone mineral density and mild central hypothyroidism. Female haploinsufficiency[23] carriers are heavier than male carriers in their families, a pattern also seen in Mc4r-deficient mice. These data are strong evidence for dominantly inherited obesity, not associated with infertility, due to haploinsufficiency mutations in *MC4R*.

Mutation of a second melanocortin receptor, *MC3R*, is also shown to cause single-gene obesity [61]. MC3R acts as an autoreceptor indicating the tight regulation of the melanocortin system in energy balance. MC3R also modifies energy balance by decreasing feed

efficiency. Mutations in *MC3R* are not as common as in *MC4R* and do not result in an autosomal dominant form of obesity but may be important contributors to susceptibility to obesity. Two variants of the *MC3R* gene interacted with diet to affect weight loss success in an Italian clinic treating severe childhood obesity [83].

Three genes important in downstream signaling of the melanocortin system have also been shown to cause single-gene obesities. Single-minded homolog 1, product of *SIM1*, is a regulator of neurogenesis and is essential to the development of the paraventricular nucleus of the hypothalamus [61,84]. Brain-derived neurotrophic factor, product of *BDNF*, and its receptor, neurotrophic tyrosine kinase receptor type 2, product of *NTRK2*, are involved in signaling in the ventromedial nucleus of the hypothalamus and contribute to memory and learning [64]. Bdnf-deficient rodents are hyperphagic and obese. Case reports associate mutation in *BDNF* or *NTRK2* with massive obesity and impaired cognitive function [85].

VIII ASSOCIATION OF SUSCEPTIBILITY GENES WITH OBESITY PHENOTYPES

A number of genes, with variants that may alter gene product function, are believed to contribute to common obesity and its co-morbidities. Obesity frequently clusters with insulin resistance, hyperlipidemia, and hypertension [86]. This clustering might arise by any of several mechanisms: Obesity might promote co-morbidities, co-morbidities might promote obesity, or some genes might promote the development of both obesity and its co-morbidities. The more promising candidates are described in Table 23.2, and several are discussed here to emphasize the difficulty in interpreting such studies.

Two genes causing single-gene obesity in humans have been implicated in common obesity using association studies. The *LEPR* gene is associated with obesity in multiple studies, including one of severe obesity in children [87]. Populations from the Pacific Island of Nauru have some of the highest rates of obesity and non-insulin-dependent diabetes mellitus in the world. In Nauruan males, specific combinations of alleles in the *LEP* and *LEPR* genes are associated with increased risk for development of insulin resistance [88]. However, a meta-analysis[24] of 48 studies found that polymorphisms in *LEP* and *LEPR* were not associated with obesity susceptibility [89]. Some of the included

---

[23]Haploinsufficiency occurs when a gene, or a group of genes, is present in too few or too many copies. In autosomes (all but the X and Y chromosomes), one copy of each gene is inherited from each parent. The presence of extra chromosomal material or lack of chromosomal material alters gene dosage, causing abnormalities in gene function.

[24]Meta-analysis is a statistical tool for pooling data from many studies into a single analysis, thus greatly increasing the statistical power of the analysis.

studies examined BMI as a continuous variable, others as a cutoff variable for case—control studies, and still others examined specific populations. Differences in study design and sample size may contribute to the inconsistent results.

Three genes consistently and strongly associated with common obesity are *MC4R*, *FTO*, and *PPARγ* (for reviews, see [90,91]). *MC4R*, a component of the melanocortin pathway, plays a role in both monogenic and common multigenic obesity. Genetic variation near *MC4R* is associated with increased snacking behavior and hunger scores in several European populations [92].

The *FTO* gene was first identified through GWAS [93] and consistently shown to be associated with human obesity [90]. The function of FTO is unknown, although mouse studies suggest it is a 2-oxoglutarate-dependent oxygenase that catalyzes nucleic acid demethylation [94]. *FTO* is highly expressed in the hypothalamus, a primary site for the regulation of energy balance and satiety [93]. *FTO* variants interact with fat and carbohydrate intakes to affect BMI [95]. In a cohort of predominantly white female morbidly obese subjects (mean BMI = 51), mean BMI of subjects homozygous for the *FTO* obesity variant did not differ from that of nonhomozygotes [96]. However, subjects who had *FTO* obesity variants paired with certain variants of the insulin-induced gene 2 (*INSIG2*) had significantly higher BMIs than other genotype groups [96]. *FTO* variants have also been examined for interaction with physical activity, but studies to date are not consistent [91].

The combined effect of *MC4R* and *FTO* risk alleles was assessed in two European populations. Subjects with three or four risk alleles of these two genes, which occurred in 7—10% of the populations, had a threefold increased risk of developing childhood obesity, although the combined effect of these genes was more modest in adults [97].

Adiponectin, like leptin, is a hormone secreted by adipocytes. Adiponectin (product of *ADIPOQ*) regulates energy balance and glucose and lipid metabolism. *ADIPOQ* has been associated with obesity, BMI, abdominal fat, and metabolic rate in Hispanic, Japanese, and Caucasian populations [61,98]. The meta-analysis by Yu *et al*. [89], which found no association of *LEP* or *LEPR* with obesity susceptibility, did find that polymorphisms of *ADIPOQ* were significantly associated with increased risk of obesity.

The β_2-adrenergic receptor (product of *ADRB2*) is a major lipolytic receptor in human adipose tissue and, thus, plays a significant role in lipid mobilization. Several polymorphisms have been identified and their frequencies compared between lean and obese subjects. These variants were associated with BMI and blood triglycerides in both Swedish and Japanese populations [99—101]. Swedish women with two copies of a common

polymorphism, Glu27, were approximately 10 times more likely to be obese than those with the wild-type *ADRB2* gene, with approximately 20 kg excess body fat and a 50% increase in fat cell size. Another variant of the *ADRB2* gene, Gly16, was associated with improved adipocyte β_2-adrenergic receptor function. The frequency of the Glu27 allele carriers varies widely, being low in Asians, Pacific Islanders, and American Indians and high in European populations [102]. A meta-analysis found that the presence of the Glu27 allele of *ADRB2* was a risk factor for obesity only in the populations with low Glu27 allele frequency [102]. Thus, genetic variability in the human *ADRB2* gene may be a significant contributor to obesity in some populations.

The β_3-adrenergic receptor (product of *ADRB3*) is expressed in adipose tissue and is involved in the regulation of lipolysis and thermogenesis. Disruption of the *Adrb3* gene in mice results in moderate obesity [103]. This potential relevance to human obesity led to an initial positive report in 1995 of an association between *ADRB3* and obesity followed by numerous studies with conflicting results (for review, see [104]). A meta-analysis combining 23 studies and 7399 subjects concluded that the *ADRB3* gene variant is not significantly associated with BMI [104]. The possible association of the variant with diabetes phenotypes was not examined in the meta-analysis. Thus, whether the *ADRB3* gene contributes to obesity or diabetes phenotypes is still subject to debate.

Peroxisome proliferator-activated receptor (PPAR) γ (product of *PPARG*) is a member of the nuclear hormone receptor subfamily of transcription factors that includes T3 and vitamin D_3 receptors. PPARs regulate expression of genes involved in, among other things, adipocyte differentiation, lipid metabolism, and energy balance (for review, see [105]). Due to combined effects on both fat and muscle, activation of PPARγ improves insulin sensitivity and glucose metabolism, and it decreases blood triglyceride levels. Three association studies have implicated *PPARG* in obesity and insulin resistance phenotypes. Four of 121 obese German subjects had a missense mutation in *PPARG* compared to none in 237 normal-weight individuals [106]. All of the subjects with the mutant allele were severely obese. The mutant gene was then overexpressed in mouse fibroblasts, which led to the accelerated differentiation of the cells into adipocytes with greater accumulation of triglyceride than seen with wild-type *PPARG*. One gene variant interacts with fat intake to affect BMI and waist circumference [107,108], although a diet high in olive oil reversed the negative effect [109]. A different mutation of the *PPARG* gene was identified in Finnish populations and was found to be associated with lower BMI, lower fasting insulin levels, and greater insulin sensitivity [110].

TABLE 23.2 Association of Candidate Susceptibility Genes with Obesity Phenotypes

Gene name	Chromosomal locus[a]	Phenotypes associated with different gene variants
Adipocyte, C1Q (adiponectin) (ADIPOQ)[a,b,c]	3q27	Obesity, BMI, abdominal fat, type 2 diabetes
β$_2$-adrenergic receptor (ADRB2)[a,b,d]	5q31–q32	Mild obesity, severe obesity with high-fat diet, BMI, abdominal fat, lipolysis, leptin
β$_3$-adrenergic receptor (ADRB3)[a,b]	8p12	Mild obesity, severe obesity with high-fat diet, BMI, % body fat, abdominal fat, weight change, lipolysis
Fat mass and obesity-associated gene (FTO)[a,e]	16q12.2	BMI
Glucocorticoid receptor (GCCR or NR3C1)[a,b]	5q31	BMI, abdominal obesity, leptin
Glucosamine-6-phosphate deaminase 2 (GNPDA2)[a,b,e]	4p12	BMI
Guanine nucleotide-binding protein, β$_3$ (GNB3)[a,b]	12p13	Obesity, BMI, % body fat, lipolysis, weight gain
5-Hydroxytryptamine receptor 2C (HTR2C)[a,b]	Xq24	Maturity onset obesity, BMI, weight change
Interleukin-6 (IL-6)[a,b]	7p21	Early adulthood onset obesity, BMI, abdominal fat, weight change, energy expenditure, type 2 diabetes
Insulin (INS)[a,b]	11p15.5	Obesity, BMI, abdominal fat, type 2 diabetes
Insulin-induced gene 2 (INSIG2)[a,f,g]	2q14.2	Extreme BMI
Leptin receptor (LEPR)[a,b]	1p31	Obesity, BMI, % body fat, abdominal fat, weight change, energy expenditure, leptin, glucose and insulin metabolism
Lipase, hormone-sensitive (LIPE)[a,b]	19q13.2	Obesity, BMI, % body fat, abdominal fat, lipolysis
Melanocortin 4 receptor (MC4R)[a,b,e,g]	18q22	Obesity, BMI, % body fat, weight change, energy expenditure
Mitochondrial carrier homolog 2 (MTCH2)[a,b,e]	11p11.2	BMI
Neuronal growth regulator 1 (NEGR1)[a,b,e]	1p31.1	BMI
Peroxisome proliferator-activated receptor γ (PPARG)[a,b,h]	3p25	Severe obesity, BMI, % body fat, abdominal fat, weight change, leptin, lipid oxidation, insulin resistance
Transmembrane protein 18 (TMEM18)[a,e]	2p25.3	BMI
Tumor necrosis factor (TNF)[a,b,c]	6p21.3	Obesity, BMI, % body fat, abdominal fat, insulin resistance
Uncoupling protein 1 (UCP1)[a,b]	4q28–q31	Obesity, BMI, % body fat, abdominal fat, weight change, energy expenditure
Uncoupling protein 2 (UCP2)[a,b,i]	11q13	Obesity, BMI, % body fat, energy expenditure, glucose and lipid oxidation
Uncoupling protein 3 (UCP3)[a,b,i]	11q13	Severe obesity, BMI, % body fat, energy expenditure, lipid oxidation, leptin, type 2 diabetes

[a]From Online Mendelian Inheritance in Man (http://www.ncbi.nlm.nih.gov/omim).
[b]From Rankinen et al. [13].
[c]From Yu et al. [89].
[d]From Jalba et al. [102].
[e]From Willer et al. [145].
[f]From Chu et al. [96].
[g]From Still et al. [142].
[h]From Gouda et al. [146].
[i]From Xu et al. [119].

Uncoupling proteins 2 and 3 (products of *UCP2* and *UCP3*, respectively) are structurally related to uncoupling protein 1, a mitochondrial protein found in brown fat that plays an important role in generating heat and burning calories without the production of adenosine triphosphate. Uncoupling protein 1 is critical in the maintenance of body temperature of newborn humans, but it is unlikely to be significantly involved in weight regulation because brown fat is normally atrophied in adult humans. *UCP2* is widely expressed in human tissues, whereas *UCP3* is expressed only in skeletal muscle. In a large French Canadian study, *UCP2* and *UCP3* were linked with resting metabolic rate, BMI, percentage of body fat, and fat mass [111]. Several groups, therefore, examined polymorphisms within the coding regions of both *UCP2* and *UCP3* with mixed results.

Polymorphisms in *UCP2* were associated with metabolic rate [112] and BMI [113], but other studies failed to find a relationship between *UCP2* variants and energy expenditure, obesity, or insulin resistance [114,115]. A mutation and two missense polymorphisms in the *UCP3* gene were identified in two severely obese probands of African descent [116]. The gene variants were not found in the Caucasian population. The variants were transmitted in a Mendelian manner; however, they were not consistently associated with obesity in other family members. Individuals who carried one copy of the exon 6-splice polymorphism were found to have only 50% the capacity to oxidize fat and had elevated respiratory quotients (RQs), even though they were not obese. These data indicate that *UCP3* could alter the availability in the cell of fatty acids for oxidation, promoting fat storage. High RQ and low fat oxidation were previously identified risk factors for future weight gain in Pima Indians [117] and African Americans [118]. Thus, *UCP3* is a potentially important obesity gene in certain population groups.

A recent meta-analysis examined the association of *UCP2* and *UCP3* polymorphisms with the risks of type 2 diabetes [119]. No association was seen in Europeans. However, polymorphisms in both *UCP2* and *UCP3* may increase risk of type 2 diabetes in Asian populations [119].

IX RARE GENETIC SYNDROMES WITH OBESITY AS A PROMINENT FEATURE

More than 50 identified genes associated with rare Mendelian syndromes in which obesity is a prominent

clinical feature are described in the Online Mendelian Inheritance in Man (OMIM) database.[25] Among the better known of these syndromes are Prader–Willi syndrome, Bardet–Biedl syndromes, Cohen syndrome, and Alstrom syndrome. The pathophysiologic mechanisms leading to obesity in these syndromes are largely unknown. One gene, *SIM1*, causes single-gene obesity (see Table 23.1) and is also involved in a Prader–Willi-like syndrome associated with chromosome 6. The characteristic features of these syndromes were reviewed [65,120].

With an incidence of approximately 1 in 25,000 births, the most common of the Mendelian syndromes is the autosomal dominant Prader–Willi syndrome, which results from a microdeletion of paternal chromosome 15q11–q13 or, more rarely, as a result of maternal disomy[26] of chromosome 15. In addition to obesity, Prader–Willi syndrome is characterized by hypotonic musculature, mental retardation, hypogonadism, short stature, and small hands and feet (for review, see [121,122]). Aberrant behavior, including hyperphagia and aggressive food seeking, makes management of these patients difficult.

The better known of the autosomal recessive Mendelian obesity syndromes are Bardet–Biedl syndromes and Alstrom syndrome. Bardet–Biedl syndromes are associated with variants in genes at 17 separate loci but are all characterized by mental retardation, pigmentary retinopathy, polydactyly, obesity, and hypogonadism. It is therefore apparent that mutation in multiple genes can result in the same phenotype. The gene coding for BBS2 may predispose males carrying only one copy of the gene to obesity and may explain approximately 3% of severely overweight males [123]. Of interest, BBS2 parents of both sexes were significantly taller than U.S. individuals of comparable age [123].

In addition to obesity, Alstrom syndrome (causative gene *ALMS1*) is characterized by retinitis pigmentosa leading to blindness, insulin resistance, diabetes, and deafness, but it does not involve mental retardation or polydactyly (for review, see [124]). Onset of obesity is usually between 2 and 10 years of age and can range from mild to severe.

Cohen syndrome is a rare autosomal recessive disorder resulting from mutations of a gene (*COH1*) on 8q22.2. The syndrome expresses as truncal obesity, hypotonia, psychomotor deficiencies, ocular abnormalities, and characteristic facial features. Mutations in some patients with Cohen syndrome involve CNVs [125].

---

[25]The OMIM database is available at http://www.ncbi.nlm.nih.gov/omim. This database, a catalog of human genes and genetic disorders, is authored and edited by Dr. Victor A. McKusick and colleagues at Johns Hopkins University and elsewhere and developed for the World Wide Web by the National Center for Biotechnology Information.

[26]Maternal disomy is inheritance of an extra maternal chromosome or part thereof.

X CLINICAL IMPLICATIONS OF THE DISCOVERY OF OBESITY GENES

The discoveries of human obesity genes will ultimately have broad implications for clinical practice. The best known of the monogenic, nonsyndromic obesities are those involving *LEP* and *LEPR* mutations, both extremely rare, and *MC4R* mutations, the most common known cause of nonsyndromic, monogenic obesity. For the more infrequent obesity gene mutations, there is little information on the physiological impacts of these mutations except for obesity. Thus, methods for their diagnosis and the implications of their discovery for treatment have not been discussed in-depth.

A Diagnosis of Obesity Disorders

Until recently, only the rare Mendelian, syndromic mutations, such as Prader—Willi and Bardet—Biedl syndromes, were known to cause heritable obesity. These disorders are easily recognized, both by a wide spectrum of phenotypes [65,120] and by the use of cytogenetics assays that are widely available. However, the Mendelian, nonsyndromic obesity disorders are not so easily diagnosed because obesity is often the only apparent phenotype and clinical assays for known obesity gene mutations are currently not practical. It is estimated that 2—7% of morbidly obese patients have mutations in *MC4R* [126—129]; 3% have mutations in *PPARG* [106,130]; and an unknown, but smaller, percentage have mutations in other obesity genes, including *POMC* [131] and *NTRK2* [64]. Thus, only approximately 1 in 10 morbidly obese patients has a known mutation that explains the obesity, and molecular assays for the currently known Mendelian obesities would be negative in the majority of morbidly obese patients. Also, there are several known distinct mutations in each of these genes. Thus, no clinical laboratories yet provide diagnosis of these mutations; rather, they have only been diagnosed by research laboratories, which are not licensed to provide patient information. However, inability to make specific molecular diagnosis does not mean that one cannot identify people with increased risk for genetic obesity, and this may influence choices or approaches to treatment.

Several criteria can be used to estimate individual risks for genetic obesity (Table 23.3). Currently, due to lack of data, these estimates do not produce any quantitative values revealing individual risk that obesity is monogenic.

A strong family history of obesity is consistent with the presence of an obesity gene shared among family members.

TABLE 23.3 Evaluation of Suspected Monogenic Etiology for Severe Obesity[a]

Characteristic	Phenotype indicative of genetic etiology
Family history	Having first-degree relatives with severe obesity
Age of onset	Normal birth weight but age of onset of obesity before age 10 years
Hyperphagia	Hyperphagia developing within first year of life and aggressive food-seeking behavior
Low ACTH or high proinsulin levels	Mutation in *POMC* or *PCSK1*
Frequent infections	Mutation in *POMC* (ACTH), *LEP*, or *LEPR*
Very low leptin levels	Homozygous mutations in *LEP*
Delayed puberty, lack of growth spurt	Homozygous mutations in *LEP* or *LEPR*
Red hair segregating with obesity	Mutation in *POMC*
Severe hyperinsulinemia, acanthosis nigricans	Mutation in *MC4R*
Accelerated linear growth, increased bone mass	Mutation in *MC4R*
Delayed language skills, impaired short-term memory	Mutation in *NTRK2* or *BDNF*
Developmental delay, mental retardation	Prader—Willi, Bardet—Biedl, or other genetic syndrome
Visual and hearing impairments	Bardet—Biedl or other genetic syndrome
Polydactyly or small hands and feet	Bardet—Biedl or Prader—Willi syndromes, respectively

[a]*For a complete algorithm for the assessment of a severely obese individual, see Farooqi* [65].
BDNF, brain-derived neurotrophic factor; *LEP*, leptin; *LEPR*, leptin receptor; *MC4R*, melanocortin 4 receptor; *NTRK2*, neurotrophic tyrosine kinase receptor type 2; *PCSK1*, proprotein convertase subtilisin/kexin type 1; *POMC*, proopiomelanocortin.
Data adapted from [65,79,133,138].

The earlier the age of onset of obesity and the more extreme, the more likely that there is a genetic basis for the obesity. Extreme trait values are more likely to be genetic for many complex diseases simply because extremes tend to result from the actions of severe mutations or from mutations in genes that have larger effects [132]. Children with single-gene obesity are normal weight at birth, but severe early hyperphagia, often associated with aggressive food-seeking behavior, results in rapid weight gain, usually beginning in the first year of life. Severe obesity in children has been variously defined as a standard deviation score for BMI of more than 2.5 [133] or 3 [79] relative to the appropriate reference population.

Few diagnostic tools are available for the medical evaluation of patients suspected of having monogenic obesity. The only screening tests available are for endocrine abnormalities. Leptin should be measured. Very low or very high serum leptin levels will indicate mutation in *LEP* or *LEPR*, respectively. However, lack of very high leptin levels cannot rule out homozygous mutations in *LEPR* [79]. A subset of obese individuals have inappropriately low leptin levels for their fat mass, suggesting a less severe defect in leptin regulation [134]. ACTH and proinsulin should be measured to indicate defects in *POMC* or in prohormone processing. Insulin should be measured to evaluate the appropriateness of the degree of hyperinsulinemia because this may indicate an *MC4R* mutation.

Physical appearance provides evidence of *POMC* mutations or the syndromic obesities. *POMC* defects can cause red hair and obesity [80], although most red hair results from mutations in melanocortin 1 receptor (*MC1R*) [135], which does not influence obesity. Thus, red hair is only informative when red hair and obesity co-segregate within a family. Prader–Willi, Bardet–Biedl, and other syndromic obesities can be diagnosed by a variety of characteristic phenotypes, such as small hands and feet, polydactyly, and mental retardation, as well as by cytogenetic assays. Thus, one should rule out these diagnoses by phenotype determination and by absence of characteristic chromosomal abnormalities.

B Implications of Obesity Genes for Obesity Treatment

The implications of the discovery of obesity genes for diet, behavioral, and drug therapy of obese humans remains to be determined. Currently, there are no specific treatments available, with the exception of leptin, for monogenic obesities. Patients with monogenic obesity will probably be more difficult to treat than those with multigenic obesity because individuals with monogenic obesity will likely have strong food-seeking behavior and may have physiological resistance to fat loss. Also, unfortunately, the genetic markers associated with common obesity in candidate gene or genome-wide studies have poor predictive power.

The identification and characterization of gene products associated with obesity have, however, provided novel pathways that can be targeted for drug intervention. A potential drug target identified by the cloning of obesity genes is the melanocortin-4 receptor. Development of safe and effective drugs such as a small-molecule, α-MSH-like agonist for the melanocortin

receptor to increase satiety, or stimulators of the expression of *UCP2* or *UCP3* to enhance energy expenditure, is currently being done [136]. Unfortunately, centrally acting anti-obesity drugs may have significant adverse effects [137].

Currently, lifestyle changes that may promote weight loss and improve metabolic fitness and quality of life should be recommended [138]. Drugs should also be considered, but whether currently available drug therapies, such as the appetite suppressant phentermine or an inhibitor of fat absorption, orlistat, are more or less effective in individuals with single-gene obesity than those with multigenic obesity is unknown.

When lifestyle changes and pharmaceutical approaches are inadequate to ameliorate morbidity, surgical treatment of the obesity may be considered. There is concern that individuals with aggressive food-seeking behavior, as frequently seen in monogenic obesities, may be poor candidates for bariatric surgery. Heterozygous mutations in *MC4R* are the most common form of monogenic obesity. In a study of four such patients, maximal weight loss following Roux-en-Y gastric bypass did not differ from controls [139]. However, one subject with complete MC4R deficiency showed poor weight loss results to gastric banding [140].

In a study of 11 obesity candidate genes in 1443 Swedish obese subjects treated with either gastric banding or bypass, only *FTO* was strongly associated with maximal weight loss, and then only in patients who received a banding procedure: minor allele carriers lost 3 kg less than common allele homozygotes [141]. In subjects who received gastric bypass, minor and common alleles for *FTO* did not predict weight loss outcome. Also, none of the markers for obesity genes were associated with weight regain during a 6-year follow-up [141]. In a similar sized study of Caucasian patients from the northeastern United States, four candidate genes (*FTO*, *INSIG2*, *MC4R*, and *PCSK1*) were associated with BMI and weight loss outcome following Roux-en-Y gastric bypass [142]. There was a direct relationship between the number of obesity SNP alleles or number of homozygous alleles and initial BMI. Subjects with a higher burden of obesity SNP alleles or homozygous pairs had a reduced weight loss in the 30 months following gastric bypass [142].

The effect of obesity gene variants on treatment (diet, drug, or surgery) outcomes is certainly an important area for future research.

References

[1] C. Bouchard, L. Perusse, T. Rice, D.C. Rao, The genetics of human obesity, in: G.A. Bray, C. Bouchard, W.P.T. James (Eds), Handbook of Obesity, Dekker, New York, 1998, pp. 157–190.

[2] S. O'Rahilly, S. Farooqi, Genetics of obesity, Philos. Trans. R. Soc. London B 361 (2006) 1095–1105.

[3] M.S. Faith, A. Pietrobelli, C. Nunez, M. Heo, S.B. Heymsfield, D.B. Allison, Evidence for independent genetic influences on fat mass and body mass index in a pediatric twin sample, Pediatrics 104 (1999) 61–67.

[4] N.F. Butte, G. Cai, S.A. Cole, A.G. Comuzzie, Viva la familia study: genetic and environmental contributions to childhood obesity and its comorbidities in the Hispanic population, Am. J. Clin. Nutr. 84 (2006) 646–654.

[5] A.G. Comuzzie, D.B. Allison, The search for human obesity genes, Science 280 (1998) 1374–1377.

[6] D.R. Reed, M.P. Lawler, M.G. Tordoff, Reduced body weight is a common effect of gene knockout in mice, BMC Genetics 9 (2008) 4.

[7] E.K. Speliotes, C.J. Willer, S.I. Berndt, K.L. Monda, G. Thorleifsson, A.U. Jackson, et al., Association analyses of 249,796 individuals reveal 18 new loci associated with body mass index, Nat. Genet. 42 (2010) 937–948.

[8] X. Yang, J.L. Deignan, H. Qi, J. Zhu, S. Qian, J. Zhong, et al., Validation of candidate causal genes for obesity that affect shared metabolic pathways and networks, Nat. Genet. 41 (2009) 415–423.

[9] D.M. Greenawalt, R. Dobrin, E. Chudin, I.J. Hatoum, C. Suver, J. Beaulaurier, et al., A survey of the genetics of stomach, liver, and adipose gene expression from a morbidly obese cohort, Genome Res. 21 (2011) 1008–1016.

[10] H. Zhong, X. Yang, L.M. Kaplan, C. Molony, E.E. Schadt, Integrating pathway analysis and genetics of gene expression for genome-wide association studies, Am. J. Hum. Genet. 86 (2010) 581–591.

[11] C.H. Warden, J.S. Fisler, Molecular genetics of obesity, in: G.A. Bray, C. Bouchard, W.P.T. James (Eds), Handbook of Obesity, Dekker, New York, 1998, pp. 223–242.

[12] L.M. Silver, Mouse Genetics, Oxford University Press, New York, 1995.

[13] T. Rankinen, A. Zuberi, Y.C. Chagnon, S.J. Weisnagel, G. Argyropoulos, B. Walts, et al., The human obesity gene map: the 2005 update, Obesity (Silver Spring) 14 (2006) 529–644.

[14] A.V. Lembertas, L. Perusse, Y.C. Chagnon, J.S. Fisler, C.H. Warden, D.A. Purcell-Huynh, et al., Identification of an obesity quantitative trait locus on mouse chromosome 2 and evidence of linkage to body fat and insulin on the human homologous region 20q, J. Clin. Invest. 100 (1997) 1240–1247.

[15] J.H. Lee, D.R. Reed, W.D. Li, W. Xu, E.J. Joo, R.L. Kilker, et al., Genome scan for human obesity and linkage to markers in 20q13, Am. J. Hum. Genet. 64 (1999) 196–209.

[16] J.K. Haseman, R.C. Elston, The investigation of linkage between a quantitative trait and a marker locus, Behav. Genet. 2 (1972) 3–19.

[17] L. Kruglyak, E.S. Lander, High-resolution genetic mapping of complex traits, Am. J. Hum. Genet. 56 (1995) 1212–1223.

[18] A. Herbert, N.P. Gerry, M.B. McQueen, I.M. Heid, A. Pfeufer, T. Illig, et al., Response to comments on "A common genetic variant is associated with adult and childhood obesity," Science 315 (2007) 187e.

[19] S. Glaser, K. Anastassiadis, A.F. Stewart, Current issues in mouse genome engineering, Nat. Genet. 37 (2005) 1187–1193.

[20] J.E. McMinn, S.M. Liu, H. Liu, I. Dragatsis, P. Dietrich, T. Ludwig, et al., Neuronal deletion of Lepr elicits diabesity in mice without affecting cold tolerance or fertility, Am. J. Physiol. Endocrinol. Metab. 289 (2005) E403–E411.

[21] E.S. Bachman, H. Dhillon, C.Y. Zhang, S. Cinti, A.C. Bianco, B.K. Kobilka, et al., betaAR signaling required for diet-induced thermogenesis and obesity resistance, Science 297 (2002) 843–845.

[22] D.B. Goldstein, Common genetic variation and human traits, N. Engl. J. Med. 360 (2009) 1696–1698.

[23] T.M. Frayling, N.J. Timpson, M.N. Weedon, E. Zeggini, R.M. Freathy, C.M. Lindgren, et al., A common variant in the FTO gene is associated with body mass index and predisposes to childhood and adult obesity, Science 316 (2007) 889–894.

[24] B. Maher, Personal genomes: the case of the missing heritability, Nature 456 (2008) 18–21.

[25] E.E. Eichler, J. Flint, G. Gibson, A. Kong, S.M. Leal, J.H. Moore, et al., Missing heritability and strategies for finding the underlying causes of complex disease, Nat. Rev. Genet. 11 (2010) 446–450.

[26] H.H. Heng, Missing heritability and stochastic genome alterations, Nat. Rev. Genet. 11 (2010) 813.

[27] G. Bhatia, V. Bansal, O. Harismendy, N.J. Schork, E.J. Topol, K. Frazer, et al., A covering method for detecting genetic associations between rare variants and common phenotypes, PLoS Comput. Biol. 6 (2010) e1000954.

[28] T.A. Manolio, F.S. Collins, N.J. Cox, D.B. Goldstein, L.A. Hindorff, D.J. Hunter, et al., Finding the missing heritability of complex diseases, Nature 461 (2009) 747–753.

[29] A.I. Blakemore, D. Meyre, J. Delplanque, V. Vatin, C. Lecoeur, M. Marre, et al., A rare variant in the visfatin gene (NAMPT/PBEF1) is associated with protection from obesity, Obesity 17 (2009) 1549–1553.

[30] R.G. Walters, S. Jacquemont, A. Valsesia, A.J. de Smith, D. Martinet, J. Andersson, et al., A new highly penetrant form of obesity due to deletions on chromosome 16p11.2, Nature 463 (2010) 671–675.

[31] C.M. Bulik, D.B. Allison, The genetic epidemiology of thinness, Obes. Rev. 2 (2001) 107–115.

[32] E.G. Bochukova, N. Huang, J. Keogh, E. Henning, C. Purmann, K. Blaszczyk, et al., Large, rare chromosomal deletions associated with severe early-onset obesity, Nature 463 (2010) 666–670.

[33] J.T. Glessner, J.P. Bradfield, K. Wang, N. Takahashi, H. Zhang, P.M. Sleiman, et al., A genome-wide study reveals copy number variants exclusive to childhood obesity cases, Am. J. Hum. Genet. 87 (2010) 661–666.

[34] A. Kong, V. Steinthorsdottir, G. Masson, G. Thorleifsson, P. Sulem, S. Besenbacher, et al., Parental origin of sequence variants associated with complex diseases, Nature 462 (2009) 868–874.

[35] C.H. Warden, J.S. Fisler, Obesity: from animal models to human genetics to practical applications, Prog. Mol. Biol. Transl. Sci. 94 (2010) 373–389.

[36] S.N. Yazbek, S.H. Spiezio, J.H. Nadeau, D.A. Buchner, Ancestral paternal genotype controls body weight and food intake for multiple generations, Hum. Mol. Genet. 19 (2010) 4134–4144.

[37] S.F. Ng, R.C. Lin, D.R. Laybutt, R. Barres, J.A. Owens, M.J. Morris, Chronic high-fat diet in fathers programs beta-cell dysfunction in female rat offspring, Nature 467 (2010) 963–966.

[38] M.K. Skinner, Metabolic disorders: Fathers' nutritional legacy, Nature 467 (2010) 922–923.

[39] F. Ahmed, Epigenetics: tales of adversity, Nature 468 (2010) S20.

[40] L.C. Schulz, The Dutch Hunger Winter and the developmental origins of health and disease, Proc. Natl. Acad. Sci. USA 107 (2010) 16757–16758.

[41] Y. Wang, X. Wang, Y. Kong, J.H. Zhang, Q. Zeng, The Great Chinese Famine leads to shorter and overweight females in Chongqing Chinese population after 50 years, Obesity 18 (2010) 588–592.

[42] E.W. Tobi, L.H. Lumey, R.P. Talens, D. Kremer, H. Putter, A.D. Stein, et al., DNA methylation differences after exposure to prenatal famine are common and timing- and sex-specific, Hum. Mol. Genet. 18 (2009) 4046–4053.

[43] J.H. Moore, The ubiquitous nature of epistasis in determining susceptibility to common human diseases, Hum. Hered. 56 (2003) 73–82.

[44] C.H. Warden, N. Yi, J. Fisler, Epistasis among genes is a universal phenomenon in obesity: evidence from rodent models, Nutrition 20 (2004) 74—77.

[45] K.P. Hummel, D.L. Coleman, P.W. Lane, The influence of genetic background on expression of mutations at the diabetes locus in the mouse: I. C57BL-KsJ and C57BL-6J strains, Biochem. Genet. 7 (1972) 1—13.

[46] M.F. Feitosa, K.E. North, R.H. Myers, J.S. Pankow, I.B. Borecki, Evidence for three novel QTLs for adiposity on chromosome 2 with epistatic interactions: The NHLBI Family Heart Study, Obesity 17 (2009) 2190—2195.

[47] C. Dong, S. Wang, W.D. Li, D. Li, H. Zhao, R.A. Price, Interacting genetic loci on chromosomes 20 and 10 influence extreme human obesity, Am. J. Hum. Genet. 72 (2003) 115—124.

[48] C.F. Skibola, E.A. Holly, M.S. Forrest, A. Hubbard, P.M. Bracci, D.R. Skibola, et al., Body mass index, leptin and leptin receptor polymorphisms, and non-Hodgkin lymphoma, Cancer Epidemiol. Biomarkers Prev. 13 (2004) 779—786.

[49] D.L. Ellsworth, S.A. Coady, W. Chen, S.R. Srinivasan, E. Boerwinkle, G.S. Berenson, Interactive effects between polymorphisms in the beta-adrenergic receptors and longitudinal changes in obesity, Obes. Res. 13 (2005) 519—526.

[50] C.B. Angeli, L. Kimura, M.T. Auricchio, J.P. Vicente, V.S. Mattevi, V.M. Zembrzuski, et al., Multilocus analyses of seven candidate genes suggest interacting pathways for obesity-related traits in Brazilian populations, Obesity 19 (2011) 1244—1251.

[51] O. Ukkola, L. Perusse, Y.C. Chagnon, J.P. Despres, C. Bouchard, Interactions among the glucocorticoid receptor, lipoprotein lipase and adrenergic receptor genes and abdominal fat in the Quebec Family Study, Int. J. Obes. Relat. Metab. Disord. 25 (2001) 1332—1339.

[52] E. Ravussin, E. Danforth Jr., Beyond sloth—Physical activity and weight gain, Science 283 (1999) 184—185.

[53] E.A. Sims, E. Danforth Jr., E.S. Horton, G.A. Bray, J.A. Glennon, L.B. Salans, Endocrine and metabolic effects of experimental obesity in man, Recent Prog. Horm. Res. 29 (1973) 457—496.

[54] E.A. Sims, R.F. Goldman, C.M. Gluck, E.S. Horton, P.C. Kelleher, D.W. Rowe, Experimental obesity in man, Trans. Assoc. Am. Physicians 81 (1968) 153—170.

[55] C. Bouchard, A. Tremblay, J.P. Despres, A. Nadeau, P.J. Lupien, G. Theriault, et al., The response to long-term overfeeding in identical twins, N. Engl. J. Med. 322 (1990) 1477—1482.

[56] C. Bouchard, A. Tremblay, J.P. Despres, G. Theriault, A. Nadeau, P.J. Lupien, et al., The response to exercise with constant energy intake in identical twins, Obes. Res. 2 (1994) 400—410.

[57] J.A. Levine, N.L. Eberhardt, M.D. Jensen, Role of nonexercise activity thermogenesis in resistance to fat gain in humans, Science 283 (1999) 212—214.

[58] E. Ravussin, S. Lillioja, T.E. Anderson, L. Christin, C. Bogardus, Determinants of 24-hour energy expenditure in man: methods and results using a respiratory chamber, J. Clin. Invest. 78 (1986) 1568—1578.

[59] F. Zurlo, R.T. Ferraro, A.M. Fontvielle, R. Rising, C. Bogardus, E. Ravussin, Spontaneous physical activity and obesity: cross-sectional and longitudinal studies in Pima Indians, Am. J. Physiol. 263 (1992) E296—E300.

[60] E.R. Grimm, N.I. Steinle, Genetics of eating behavior: established and emerging concepts, Nutr. Rev. 69 (2011) 52—60.

[61] T. Rankinen, M.S. Bray, J.M. Hagberg, L. Perusse, S.M. Roth, B. Wolfarth, et al., The human gene map for performance and health-related fitness phenotypes: the 2005 update, Med. Sci. Sports Exerc. 38 (2006) 1863—1888.

[62] C.H. Warden, J.S. Fisler, Gene-nutrient and gene-physical activity summary—Genetics viewpoint, Obesity 16 (Suppl. 3) (2008) S55—S59.

[63] I. Farooki, S. O'Rahilly, Genetics of obesity in humans, Endocr. Rev. 27 (2006) 710—718.

[64] J. Gray, G. Yeo, C. Hung, J. Keogh, K. Banerjee, et al., Functional characterization of human NTRK2 mutations identified in patients with severe early-onset obesity, Int. J. Obes. (London) 31 (2007) 359—364.

[65] I.S. Farooqi, Genetic and hereditary aspects of childhood obesity, Best Pract. Res. Clin. Endocrinol. Metab. 19 (2005) 359—374.

[66] R.A. Adan, B. Tiesjema, J.J. Hillebrand, S.E. la Fleur, M.J. Kas, M. de Krom, The MC4 receptor and control of appetite, Br. J. Pharmacol. 149 (2006) 815—827.

[67] I.S. Farooqi, S. Drop, A. Clements, J.M. Keogh, J. Biernacka, S. Lowenbein, et al., Heterozygosity for a POMC-null mutation and increased obesity risk in humans, Diabetes 55 (2006) 2549—2553.

[68] Y.S. Lee, The role of leptin-melanocortin system and human weight regulation: lessons from experiments of nature, Ann. Acad. Med. Singapore 38 (2009) 34—44.

[69] D.M. Mutch, K. Clement, Unraveling the genetics of human obesity, PLoS Genet. 2 (2006) e188.

[70] J.M. Zigman, J.K. Elmquist, Minireview: from anorexia to obesity—The yin and yang of body weight control, Endocrinology 144 (2003) 3749—3756.

[71] Y. Zhang, R. Proenca, M. Maffei, M. Barone, L. Leopold, J.M. Friedman, Positional cloning of the mouse obese gene and its human homologue, Nature 372 (1994) 425—432.

[72] J.L. Halaas, K.S. Gajiwala, M. Maffei, S.L. Cohen, B.T. Chait, D. Rabinowitz, et al., Weight-reducing effects of the plasma protein encoded by the obese gene, Science 269 (1995) 543—546.

[73] P.L. Golden, T.J. Maccagnan, W.M. Pardridge, Human blood—brain barrier leptin receptor: binding and endocytosis in isolated human brain microvessels, J. Clin. Invest. 99 (1997) 14—18.

[74] M.M. Cohen Jr., Role of leptin in regulating appetite, neuroendocrine function, and bone remodeling, Am. J. Med. Genet. A 140 (2006) 515—524.

[75] I.S. Farooqi, S. O'Rahilly, Leptin: a pivotal regulator of human energy homeostasis, Am. J. Clin. Nutr. 89 (2009) 980S—984S.

[76] J.M. Friedman, J.L. Halaas, Leptin and the regulation of body weight in mammals, Nature 395 (1998) 763—770.

[77] G. Paz-Filho, M.L. Wong, J. Licinio, Ten years of leptin replacement therapy, Obes. Rev. 12 (2011) e315—e323.

[78] L.A. Tartaglia, M. Dembski, X. Weng, N. Deng, J. Culpepper, R. Devos, et al., Identification and expression cloning of a leptin receptor, OB-R, Cell 83 (1995) 1263—1271.

[79] I.S. Farooqi, T. Wangensteen, S. Collins, W. Kimber, G. Matarese, J.M. Keogh, et al., Clinical and molecular genetic spectrum of congenital deficiency of the leptin receptor, N. Engl. J. Med. 356 (2007) 237—247.

[80] H. Krude, H. Biebermann, W. Luck, R. Horn, G. Brabant, A. Gruters, Severe early-onset obesity, adrenal insufficiency and red hair pigmentation caused by POMC mutations in humans, Nat. Genet. 19 (1998) 155—157.

[81] Y.S. Lee, B.G. Challis, D.A. Thompson, G.S. Yeo, J.M. Keogh, M.E. Madonna, et al., A POMC variant implicates beta-melanocyte-stimulating hormone in the control of human energy balance, Cell Metab. 3 (2006) 135—140.

[82] C. Lubrano-Berthelier, B. Dubern, J.M. Lacorte, F. Picard, A. Shapiro, S. Zhang, et al., Melanocortin 4 receptor mutations in a large cohort of severely obese adults: prevalence, functional classification, genotype—phenotype relationship, and lack of association with binge eating, J. Clin. Endocrinol. Metab. 91 (2006) 1811—1818.

[83] N. Santoro, L. Perrone, G. Cirillo, P. Raimondo, A. Amato, C. Brienza, et al., Effect of the melanocortin-3 receptor C17A and G241A variants on weight loss in childhood obesity, Am. J. Clin. Nutr. 85 (2007) 950–953.

[84] C.C. Hung, J. Luan, M. Sims, J.M. Keogh, C. Hall, N.J. Wareham, et al., Studies of the SIM1 gene in relation to human obesity and obesity-related traits, Int. J. Obes. (London) 31 (2007) 429–434.

[85] J. Gray, G.S. Yeo, J.J. Cox, J. Morton, A.L. Adlam, J.M. Keogh, et al., Hyperphagia, severe obesity, impaired cognitive function, and hyperactivity associated with functional loss of one copy of the brain-derived neurotrophic factor (BDNF) gene, Diabetes 55 (2006) 3366–3371.

[86] A. Must, J. Spadano, E.H. Coakley, A.E. Field, G. Colditz, W.H. Dietz, The disease burden associated with overweight and obesity, JAMA 282 (1999) 1523–1529.

[87] H. Roth, T. Korn, K. Rosenkranz, A. Hinney, A. Ziegler, J. Kunz, et al., Transmission disequilibrium and sequence variants at the leptin receptor gene in extremely obese German children and adolescents, Hum. Genet. 103 (1998) 540–546.

[88] A.M. de Silva, K.R. Walder, T.J. Aitman, T. Gotoda, A.P. Goldstone, A.M. Hodge, et al., Combination of polymorphisms in OB-R and the OB gene associated with insulin resistance in Nauruan males, Int. J. Obes. Relat. Metab. Disord. 23 (1999) 816–822.

[89] Z. Yu, S. Han, X. Cao, C. Zhu, X. Wang, X. Guo, Genetic polymorphisms in adipokine genes and the risk of obesity: a systematic review and meta-analysis, Obesity 20 (2012) 396–406.

[90] K.A. Fawcett, I. Barroso, The genetics of obesity: FTO leads the way, Trends Genet. 26 (2010) 266–274.

[91] C. Razquin, A. Marti, J.A. Martinez, Evidences on three relevant obesogenes: MC4R, FTO and PPARgamma. Approaches for personalized nutrition, Mol. Nutr. Food Res. 55 (2011) 136–149.

[92] F. Stutzmann, S. Cauchi, E. Durand, C. Calvacanti-Proenca, M. Pigeyre, A.L. Hartikainen, et al., Common genetic variation near MC4R is associated with eating behaviour patterns in European populations, Int. J. Obes. 33 (2009) 373–378.

[93] T.M. Frayling, N.J. Timpson, M.N. Weedom, E. Zeggini, R.M. Freathy, C.M. Lindgren, et al., A common variant in the FTO gene is associated with body mass index and predisposes to childhood and adult obesity, Science 316 (2007) 889–894.

[94] T. Gerken, C.A. Girard, Y.C. Tung, C.J. Webby, V. Saudek, K.S. Hewitson, et al., The obesity-associated FTO gene encodes a 2-oxoglutarate-dependent nucleic acid demethylase, Science 318 (2007) 1469–1472.

[95] E. Sonestedt, C. Roos, B. Gullberg, U. Ericson, E. Wirfalt, M. Orho-Melander, Fat and carbohydrate intake modify the association between genetic variation in the FTO genotype and obesity, Am. J. Clin. Nutr. 90 (2009) 1418–1425.

[96] X. Chu, R. Erdman, M. Susek, H. Gerst, K. Derr, M. Al-Agha, et al., Association of morbid obesity with FTO and INSIG2 allelic variants, Arch. Surg. 143 (2008) 235–240.

[97] S. Cauchi, F. Stutzmann, C. Cavalcanti-Proenca, E. Durand, A. Pouta, A.L. Hartikainen, et al., Combined effects of MC4R and FTO common genetic variants on obesity in European general populations, J. Mol. Med. 87 (2009) 537–546.

[98] R.J. Loos, S. Ruchat, T. Rankinen, A. Tremblay, L. Perusse, C. Bouchard, Adiponectin and adiponectin receptor gene variants in relation to resting metabolic rate, respiratory quotient, and adiposity-related phenotypes in the Quebec Family Study, Am. J. Clin. Nutr. 85 (2007) 26–34.

[99] S. Ishiyama-Shigemoto, K. Yamada, X. Yuan, F. Ichikawa, K. Nonaka, Association of polymorphisms in the beta2-adrenergic receptor gene with obesity, hypertriglyceridaemia, and diabetes mellitus, Diabetologia 42 (1999) 98–101.

[100] V. Large, L. Hellstrom, S. Reynisdottir, F. Lonnqvist, P. Eriksson, L. Lannfelt, et al., Human beta-2 adrenoceptor gene polymorphisms are highly frequent in obesity and associate with altered adipocyte beta-2 adrenoceptor function, J. Clin. Invest. 100 (1997) 3005–3013.

[101] Y. Mori, H. Kim-Motoyama, Y. Ito, T. Katakura, K. Yasuda, S. Ishiyama-Shigemoto, et al., The Gln27Glu beta2-adrenergic receptor variant is associated with obesity due to subcutaneous fat accumulation in Japanese men, Biochem. Biophys. Res. Commun. 258 (1999) 138–140.

[102] M.S. Jalba, G.G. Rhoads, K. Demissie, Association of codon 16 and codon 27 beta 2-adrenergic receptor gene polymorphisms with obesity: a meta-analysis, Obesity 16 (2008) 2096–2106.

[103] V.S. Susulic, R.C. Frederich, J. Lawitts, E. Tozzo, B.B. Kahn, M.E. Harper, et al., Targeted disruption of the beta 3-adrenergic receptor gene, J. Biol. Chem. 270 (1995) 29483–29492.

[104] D.B. Allison, M. Heo, M.S. Faith, A. Pietrobelli, Meta-analysis of the association of the Trp64Arg polymorphism in the beta3 adrenergic receptor with body mass index, Int. J. Obes. Relat. Metab. Disord. 22 (1998) 559–566.

[105] S.D. Clarke, P. Thuillier, R.A. Baillie, X. Sha, Peroxisome proliferator-activated receptors: a family of lipid-activated transcription factors, Am. J. Clin. Nutr. 70 (1999) 566–571.

[106] M. Ristow, D. Muller-Wieland, A. Pfeiffer, W. Krone, C.R. Kahn, Obesity associated with a mutation in a genetic regulator of adipocyte differentiation, N. Engl. J. Med. 339 (1998) 953–959.

[107] A. Memisoglu, F.B. Hu, S.E. Hankinson, J.E. Manson, I. De Vivo, W.C. Willett, et al., Interaction between a peroxisome proliferator-activated receptor gamma gene polymorphism and dietary fat intake in relation to body mass, Hum. Mol. Genet. 12 (2003) 2923–2929.

[108] J. Robitaille, J.P. Despres, L. Perusse, M.C. Vohl, The PPAR-gamma P12A polymorphism modulates the relationship between dietary fat intake and components of the metabolic syndrome: results from the Quebec Family Study, Clin. Genet. 63 (2003) 109–116.

[109] C. Razquin, J. Alfredo Martinez, M.A. Martinez-Gonzalez, D. Corella, J.M. Santos, A. Marti, The Mediterranean diet protects against waist circumference enlargement in 12Ala carriers for the PPARgamma gene: 2 years' follow-up of 774 subjects at high cardiovascular risk, Br. J. Nutr. 102 (2009) 672–679.

[110] S.S. Deeb, L. Fajas, M. Nemoto, J. Pihlajamaki, L. Mykkanen, J. Kuusisto, et al., A Pro12Ala substitution in PPARgamma2 associated with decreased receptor activity, lower body mass index and improved insulin sensitivity, Nat. Genet. 20 (1998) 284–287.

[111] C. Bouchard, L. Perusse, Y.C. Chagnon, C. Warden, D. Ricquier, Linkage between markers in the vicinity of the uncoupling protein 2 gene and resting metabolic rate in humans, Hum. Mol. Genet. 6 (1997) 1887–1889.

[112] K. Walder, R.A. Norman, R.L. Hanson, P. Schrauwen, M. Neverova, C.P. Jenkinson, et al., Association between uncoupling protein polymorphisms (UCP2-UCP3) and energy metabolism/obesity in Pima Indians, Hum. Mol. Genet. 7 (1998) 1431–1435.

[113] P.G. Cassell, M. Neverova, S. Janmohamed, N. Uwakwe, A. Qureshi, M.I. McCarthy, et al., An uncoupling protein 2 gene variant is associated with a raised body mass index but not Type II diabetes, Diabetologia 42 (1999) 688–692.

[114] M. Klannemark, M. Orho, L. Groop, No relationship between identified variants in the uncoupling protein 2 gene and energy expenditure, Eur. J. Endocrinol. 139 (1998) 217–223.

[115] S.A. Urhammer, L.T. Dalgaard, T.I. Sorensen, A.M. Moller, T. Andersen, A. Tybjaerg-Hansen, et al., Mutational analysis of the coding region of the uncoupling protein 2 gene in obese NIDDM patients: impact of a common amino acid polymorphism on juvenile and maturity onset forms of obesity and insulin resistance, Diabetologia 40 (1997) 1227–1230.

[116] G. Argyropoulos, A.M. Brown, S.M. Willi, J. Zhu, Y. He, M. Reitman, et al., Effects of mutations in the human uncoupling protein 3 gene on the respiratory quotient and fat oxidation in severe obesity and type 2 diabetes, J. Clin. Invest. 102 (1998) 1345–1351.

[117] E. Ravussin, Metabolic differences and the development of obesity, Metabolism 44 (1995) 12–14.

[118] J.M. Jakicic, R.R. Wing, Differences in resting energy expenditure in African-American vs Caucasian overweight females, Int. J. Obes. Relat. Metab. Disord. 22 (1998) 236–242.

[119] K. Xu, M. Zhang, D. Cui, Y. Fu, L. Qian, R. Gu, et al., UCP2 -866G/A and Ala55Val, and UCP3 -55C/T polymorphisms in association with type 2 diabetes susceptibility: a meta-analysis study, Diabetologia 54 (2011) 2315–2324.

[120] G.A. Bray, Classification and evaluation of the overweight patient, in: G.A. Bray, C. Bouchard, W.P.T. James (Eds), Handbook of Obesity, Dekker, New York, 1989, pp. 831–854.

[121] R. Couper, Prader–Willi syndrome, J. Paediatr. Child Health 35 (1999) 331–334.

[122] N.L. Khan, N.W. Wood, Prader–Willi and Angelman syndromes: update on genetic mechanisms and diagnostic complexities, Curr. Opin. Neurol. 12 (1999) 149–154.

[123] J.B. Croft, D. Morrell, C.L. Chase, M. Swift, Obesity in heterozygous carriers of the gene for the Bardet–Biedl syndrome, Am. J. Med. Genet. 55 (1995) 12–15.

[124] J.D. Marshall, R.T. Bronson, G.B. Collin, A.D. Nordstrom, P. Maffei, R.B. Paisey, et al., New Alstrom syndrome phenotypes based on the evaluation of 182 cases, Arch. Intern. Med. 165 (2005) 675–683.

[125] N. Rivera-Brugues, B. Albrecht, D. Wieczorek, H. Schmidt, T. Keller, I. Gohring, et al., Cohen syndrome diagnosis using whole genome arrays, J. Med. Genet. 48 (2011) 136–140.

[126] A. Hinney, A. Schmidt, K. Nottebom, O. Heibult, I. Becker, A. Ziegler, et al., Several mutations in the melanocortin-4 receptor gene including a nonsense and a frameshift mutation associated with dominantly inherited obesity in humans, J. Clin. Endocrinol. Metab. 84 (1999) 1483–1486.

[127] M. Sina, A. Hinney, A. Ziegler, T. Neupert, H. Mayer, W. Siegfried, et al., Phenotypes in three pedigrees with autosomal dominant obesity caused by haploinsufficiency mutations in the melanocortin-4 receptor gene, Am. J. Hum. Genet. 65 (1999) 1501–1507.

[128] C. Vaisse, K. Clement, B. Guy-Grand, P. Froguel, A frameshift mutation in human MC4R is associated with a dominant form of obesity, Nat. Genet. 20 (1998) 113–114.

[129] G.S. Yeo, I.S. Farooqi, S. Aminian, D.J. Halsall, R.G. Stanhope, S. O'Rahilly, A frameshift mutation in MC4R associated with dominantly inherited human obesity, Nat. Genet. 20 (1998) 111–112.

[130] R. Valve, K. Sivenius, R. Miettinen, J. Pihlajamaki, A. Rissanen, S.S. Deeb, et al., Two polymorphisms in the peroxisome proliferator-activated receptor-gamma gene are associated with severe overweight among obese women, J. Clin. Endocrinol. Metab. 84 (1999) 3708–3712.

[131] J.E. Hixson, L. Almasy, S. Cole, S. Birnbaum, B.D. Mitchell, M.C. Mahaney, et al., Normal variation in leptin levels in associated with polymorphisms in the proopiomelanocortin gene, POMC, J. Clin. Endocrinol. Metab. 84 (1999) 3187–3191.

[132] E.S. Lander, N.J. Schork, Genetic dissection of complex traits, Science 265 (1994) 2037–2048.

[133] I.S. Farooqi, S. O'Rahilly, New advances in the genetics of early onset obesity, Int. J. Obes. (London) 29 (2005) 1149–1152.

[134] J. Hager, K. Clement, S. Francke, C. Dina, J. Raison, N. Lahlou, et al., A polymorphism in the 5′ untranslated region of the human ob gene is associated with low leptin levels, Int. J. Obes. Relat. Metab. Disord. 22 (1998) 200–205.

[135] J.S. Palmer, D.L. Duffy, N.F. Box, J.F. Aitken, L.E. O'Gorman, A.C. Green, et al., Melanocortin-1 receptor polymorphisms and risk of melanoma: Is the association explained solely by pigmentation phenotype? Am. J. Hum. Genet. 66 (2000) 176–186.

[136] Z. Xiang, B. Proneth, M.L. Dirain, S.A. Litherland, C. Haskell-Luevano, Pharmacological characterization of 30 human melanocortin-4 receptor polymorphisms with the endogenous proopiomelanocortin-derived agonists, synthetic agonists, and the endogenous agouti-related protein antagonist, Biochemistry 49 (2010) 4583–4600.

[137] P.J. Nathan, B.V. O'Neill, A. Napolitano, E.T. Bullmore, Neuropsychiatric adverse effects of centrally acting antiobesity drugs, CNS Neurosci. Ther. 17 (2010) 490–505.

[138] W.H. Dietz, T.N. Robinson, Clinical practice: overweight children and adolescents, N. Engl. J. Med. 352 (2005) 2100–2109.

[139] I.R. Aslan, G.M. Campos, M.A. Calton, D.S. Evans, R.B. Merriman, C. Vaisse, Weight loss after Roux-en-Y gastric bypass in obese patients heterozygous for MC4R mutations, Obes. Surg. 21 (2011) 930–934.

[140] I.R. Aslan, S.A. Ranadive, B.A. Ersoy, S.J. Rogers, R.H. Lustig, C. Vaisse, Bariatric surgery in a patient with complete MC4R deficiency, Int. J. Obes. 35 (2011) 457–461.

[141] M.A. Sarzynski, P. Jacobson, T. Rankinen, B. Carlsson, L. Sjostrom, C. Bouchard, et al., Associations of markers in 11 obesity candidate genes with maximal weight loss and weight regain in the SOS bariatric surgery cases, Int. J. Obes. 35 (2011) 676–683.

[142] C.D. Still, G.C. Wood, X. Chu, R. Erdman, C.H. Manney, P.N. Benotti, et al., High allelic burden of four obesity SNPs is associated with poorer weight loss outcomes following gastric bypass surgery, Obesity 19 (2011) 1676–1683.

[143] A. Herbert, N.P. Gerry, M.B. McQueen, I.M. Heid, A. Pfeufer, T. Illig, et al., A common genetic variant is associated with adult and childhood obesity, Science 312 (2006) 279–283.

[144] B. Xu, E.H. Goulding, K. Zang, D. Cepoi, R.D. Cone, K.R. Jones, et al., Brain-derived neurotrophic factor regulates energy balance downstream of melanocortin-4 receptor, Nat. Neurosci. 6 (2003) 736–742.

[145] C.J. Willer, et al., Six new loci associated with body mass index highlight a neuronal influence on body weight regulation, Nat. Genet. 41 (2009) 25–34.

[146] H.N. Gouda, et al., The association between peroxisome proliferator-activated receptor-gamma2 (PPARG2) Pro12Ala gene variant and type 2 diabetes mellitus: a HuGE review and meta-analysis, Am. J. Epidemiol. 171 (2010) 645–655.

Obesity: Overview of Treatments and Interventions

Helen M. Seagle*, Holly R. Wyatt†, James O. Hill†

*Children's Hospital of Colorado, Anschutz Medical Campus, Denver, Colorado †University of Colorado, Anschutz Medical Campus, Denver, Colorado

I INTRODUCTION

Obesity is a pervasive disease: In 2008, 1.5 billion adults worldwide were overweight and approximately 500 million adults were obese, and in 2010 nearly 43 million children younger than 5 years were overweight [1]. In the United States, 68% of the population is either overweight or obese, and this disease affects all age, sex, and race/ethnic groups [2]. The prevalence of overweight and obesity increased dramatically toward the end of the 20th century; in 1960, only one-third of the U.S. population was overweight [2]. Because excess weight is associated with a higher prevalence of diseases such as diabetes, cardiovascular diseases, and osteoarthritis [3], the burden of obesity is high. Policymakers as well as health care providers are faced with the dilemma of managing this obesity epidemic and preventing this situation from worsening [4].

This chapter provides a broad overview of weight-management interventions. We start with clinical assessment and the relevance of excess fat accumulation and then review specific interventions. These range from relatively low risk (e.g., lifestyle modifications) to higher risk but potentially a higher benefit for those individuals more compromised by their higher body weights. Ultimately, we encourage the reader to think about the treatment of obesity not just from an acute weight-loss perspective but also from the perspective of both prevention of weight gain and prevention of weight regain following the acute weight-loss phase.

II ASSESSMENT OF OVERWEIGHT AND OBESITY

The National Heart, Lung, and Blood Institute (NHLBI) outlined the identification and evaluation of overweight and obesity in its 1998 clinical guidelines (these are currently being revised) [5]. A careful assessment of weight status, the presence of co morbidities, as well as readiness for change is necessary to determine the appropriate treatment approach for an individual [5]. An obese person with two or three co-morbidities would receive greater benefit from a more aggressive approach than an overweight person suffering no medical impact from excess body fat. Obesity treatment is one arena in which a one-size-fits-all approach does not ensure success.

Obesity is characterized by the accumulation of excess body fat. Although accurate methods to measure body fat exist, they are expensive and impractical in most clinical settings. Body weight has traditionally been used as a surrogate measure of excess body fat. In the past, the classification of obese or overweight was based on ideal body weight tables established by the Metropolitan Life Insurance Company [6]. These insurance tables estimated an "ideal" weight for a given height, frame size, and gender based on collected mortality data. Overweight and obesity were then defined as some percentage above the estimated ideal body weight. Although widely used, these tables were criticized for being derived from populations with body fat contents that did not reflect those of the general public, for using frame size (an arbitrary assessment), and for

Nutrition in the Prevention and Treatment of Disease, Third Edition.
DOI: http://dx.doi.org/10.1016/B978-0-12-391884-0.00024-X

ft/in lbs.	4'10"	4'11"	5'0"	5'1"	5'2"	5'3"	5'4"	5'5"	5'6"	5'7"	5'8"	5'9"	5'10"	5'11"	6'0"	6'1"	6'2"	6'3"	6'4"
120	25	24	23	23	22	21	21	20	19	19	18	18	17	17	16	16	15	15	15
125	26	25	24	24	23	22	22	21	20	20	19	18	18	17	17	17	16	16	15
130	27	26	25	25	24	23	22	22	21	20	20	19	19	18	18	17	17	16	16
135	28	27	26	26	25	24	23	23	22	21	21	20	19	19	18	18	17	17	16
140	29	28	27	27	26	25	24	23	23	22	21	21	20	20	19	19	18	18	17
145	30	29	28	27	27	26	25	24	23	23	22	21	21	20	20	19	19	18	18
150	31	30	29	28	27	27	26	25	24	24	23	22	22	21	20	20	19	19	18
155	32	31	30	29	28	28	27	26	25	24	24	23	22	22	21	20	20	19	19
160	34	32	31	30	29	28	28	27	26	25	24	24	23	22	22	21	21	20	19
165	35	33	32	31·	30	29	28	28	27	26	25	24	24	23	22	22	21	21	20
170	36	34	33	32	31	30	29	28	27	27	26	25	24	24	23	22	22	21	21
175	37	35	34	33	32	31	30	29	28	27	27	26	25	24	24	23	23	22	21
180	38	36	35	34	33	32	31	30	29	28	27	27	26	25	24	24	23	22	22
185	39	37	36	35	34	33	32	31	30	29	28	27	27	26	25	24	24	23	22
190	40	38	37	36	35	34	33	32	31	30	29	28	27	27	26	25	24	24	23
195	41	39	38	37	36	35	34	33	32	31	30	29	28	27	27	26	25	24	24
200	42	40	39	38	37	36	34	33	32	31	30	30	29	28	27	26	26	25	24
205	43	41	40	39	38	36	35	34	33	32	31	30	29	29	28	27	26	26	25
210	44	43	41	40	38	37	36	35	34	33	32	31	30	29	29	28	27	26	26
215	45	44	42	41	39	38	37	36	35	34	33	32	31	30	29	28	28	27	26
220	46	45	43	42	40	39	38	37	36	35	34	33	32	31	30	29	28	27	27
225	47	46	44	43	41	40	39	38	36	35	34	33	32	31	31	30	29	28	27
230	48	47	45	44	42	41	40	38	37	36	35	34	33	32	31	30	30	29	28
235	49	48	46	44	43	42	40	39	38	37	36	35	34	33	32	31	30	29	29
240	50	49	47	45	44	43	41	40	39	38	37	36	35	34	33	32	31	30	29
245	51	50	48	46	45	43	42	41	40	38	37	36	35	34	33	32	32	31	30
250	52	51	49	47	46	44	43	42	40	39	38	37	36	35	34	33	32	31	30
255	53	52	50	48	47	45	44	43	41	40	39	38	37	36	35	34	33	32	31
260	54	53	51	49	48	46	45	43	42	41	40	38	37	36	35	34	33	33	32

FIGURE 24.1   Body mass index using height in feet and inches and weight in pounds.

being based on mortality outcomes alone without evaluating morbidity data [5].

A Clinical Assessment of Body Fat

1 Body Mass Index

The use of body mass index (BMI) has replaced the insurance tables and has become the recommended method to estimate body fat and to define both overweight and obesity in a clinical setting [1,5]. BMI is determined by weight in kilograms divided by height in meters squared ($BMI = kg/m^2$). The formula—weight (pounds)/height (inches)$^2 \times 704.5$—can be used to convert height in inches and weight in pounds directly into BMI units [7]. Figure 24.1 converts measures of height and weight into BMI units.

BMI is a better estimate of body fat than body weight [5,8] and has advantages over the ideal body weight estimation that preceded it. Unlike the ideal body weight tables that were based on mortality data alone, BMI correlates with morbidity. The relationship between a given BMI and the risk of both mortality and morbidity has been assessed in several large epidemiological studies [9–11]. BMI does not require a subjective assessment for frame size, and the same formula is used for both men and women (unlike the insurance tables, which were specific for gender). However, there are limitations to the usefulness of the BMI. It may overestimate total body fat in persons who are very muscular (e.g., elite athletes) and may underestimate body fat in persons who have lost muscle mass (e.g., the elderly). In addition, BMI inaccurately reflects body fat in edematous states or in individuals who are less than 5 feet tall. Therefore, clinical judgment is necessary for the interpretation of BMI on an individual client basis.

Despite these limitations, the correlation between BMI and excess body fat in the general population is good [12]. Both the National Institutes of Health and the World Health Organization have defined overweight as a BMI of 25.0–29.9 kg/m^2 and obesity as a BMI of 30 kg/m^2 or greater [1,5]. These BMI cutoffs were determined using studies evaluating the relationship between BMI and mortality and morbidity risk [9,10]. In general, morbidity and mortality risk increases as BMI rises, but this relationship is curvilinear. Increases in BMI between 20 and 25 kg/m^2 alter the morbidity and mortality risk less than increases in BMI greater than 25 kg/m^2. For example, in the Nurses' Health Study, relative to a woman with a BMI less than 21 kg/m^2, heart disease risk was 1.8 times greater for women with a BMI between 25 and 29 kg/m^2 but 3.3 times greater for women with a BMI greater than 29 kg/m^2 [9,13]. Gender does not alter this relationship; therefore, the same cutoff points are used to define obesity (BMI > 30 kg/m^2) and overweight (BMI = 25.0–29.9 kg/m^2) in both men and women [14].

2 Waist Circumference

The waist circumference as a measure of visceral adiposity can complement the BMI for assessing disease risk. Excess fat located in the intra-abdominal region (visceral fat) is associated with a greater disease risk than fat located in other areas [15]. Abdominal fatness is an independent risk factor (even when BMI is not increased) and is predictive of co-morbidities and mortality [15,16]. A high BMI alerts the provider that a client is carrying too much body fat, whereas a high waist circumference signals that a significant amount of the excess fat is visceral fat. High risk is defined by a waist circumference greater than 40 in. (102 cm) for men and greater than 35 in. (88 cm) for women [5]. The power of waist circumference to predict disease risk may vary by ethnicity and age [12] because waist circumference is a better disease risk indicator than BMI in Asian Americans and in older individuals. For this reason, waist circumference cutoffs may need to be adjusted in the future based on age and ethnicity. Sex-specific cutoffs for waist circumference can be used for adults with a BMI less than 35 kg/m^2. In individuals with a BMI greater than 35 kg/m^2, a waist circumference does not confer additional disease risk and therefore it is not necessary to measure waist circumference in clients with BMI greater than 35 kg/m^2. Figure 24.2 illustrates an appropriate technique to measure waist circumference.

3 Weight Gain

Several long-term cohort studies have shown that during the past few decades, the average U.S. adult gained approximately 1 pound each year or approximately 10 pounds each decade [17]. In addition to BMI and the waist circumference measurement, providers should assess increases in a client's weight over time.

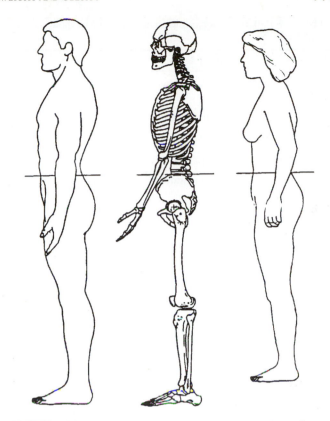

FIGURE 24.2 Measuring tape position for waist circumference. Source: *Adapted from North American Association for the Study of Obesity [22].*

Even at a healthy BMI, clients with a weight gain of more than 2.2 pounds (1 kg) per year or more than 22 pounds (10 kg) overall have an increased disease risk [9]. Providers should identify clients who are gaining weight from one year to the next and provide appropriate interventions to prevent further gain.

B Assessment of Co-morbidities and Risk Factors

Patients should be assessed for the presence of both weight-related co-morbidities and concomitant cardiovascular risk factors. Some obesity-associated diseases and cardiovascular risk factors will place the patient in a very high risk category, and the aggressiveness of the obesity treatment should be increased. Patients are considered to be at very high risk if they have existing co-morbidities such as coronary heart disease, atherosclerotic diseases, type 2 diabetes mellitus, or sleep apnea. This includes patients with a history of myocardial infarction, angina pectoris, heart surgery, or angioplasty. Many obese patients may have "silent" co-morbidities such as hyperlipidemia or hypertension. Obese patients should always have a blood

TABLE 24.1   Criteria for Clinical Diagnosis of Metabolic Syndrome by NCEP[a]

Risk factor	Defining level
Abdominal obesity	Waist circumference
Men	>102 cm (>40 in.)
Women	>88 cm (>35 in.)
Triglycerides	≥150 mg/dl or
	On drug treatment for ↑ triglycerides
HDL cholesterol	
Men	<40 mg/dl
Women	<50 mg/dl or
	On drug treatment for ↓ HDL
Blood pressure	≥130 mm Hg systolic or
	≥85 mm Hg diastolic or
	On drug treatment for history of high blood pressure
Fasting glucose	≥100 mg/dl or
	On drug treatment for ↑ glucose

[a]*Any three of the five risk factors constitute diagnosis of metabolic syndrome.*

pressure measurement with an appropriate-sized cuff and complete cardiovascular exam. Physical examination signs of high cholesterol, such as xanthomas, arcus cornelius, and xanthelasma, should be evaluated along with signs of retinopathy, neuropathy, and other signs of type 2 diabetes.

A key part of the health risk assessment during an office visit is determining the patient's risk of developing type 2 diabetes and cardiovascular disease. The National Cholesterol Education Program (NCEP) Adult Treatment Panel III encourages the identification of a constellation of risk factors (Table 24.1) that, when found in the same individual, can be diagnosed as the metabolic syndrome [18]. The purpose of identifying these risk factors is to prevent cardiovascular disease in a population group thought to be at high risk for developing the diseases in the future. Patients who have three or more of the listed cardiovascular risk factors can be classified as having the metabolic syndrome by NCEP guidelines. Weight reduction, healthy diet, and physical activity are critical components of a treatment plan for these individuals [18].

C   Assessment of Readiness

After assessing the patient's need for weight reduction, the health care provider must assess the patient's readiness to participate in treatment. Even when a patient is in the very high risk category, he or she may not be ready to make a commitment to weight reduction. Providers should assess if the patient recognizes the need for weight loss and is willing (and able) to sustain a weight-loss effort. Brownell developed a series of questions that can be used to help assess a patient's readiness to accept and participate in a long-term treatment plan [19,20]. Patients who are not ready and believe they are unable to make the commitment to treatment should not begin a weight-loss program. Goals for these patients may be simply encouraging them to think about what it would take in their lives to make a commitment. Preventing further weight gain rather than an immediate weight loss may be more appropriate for these patients.

D   Selecting Treatment Options

Although obesity is a complex disease of multifactorial origins, there is simplicity in the underlying model of body weight change. The energy balance equation dictates that in order for body weight to change, there must be an energy imbalance. Either a change in energy intake or a change in energy output must occur so that body stores of energy are altered, causing a change in total body weight [21]. Therefore, obesity treatments must focus on diminishing energy intake (e. g., diet, medications, and surgery), increasing energy output (e.g., physical activity), or a combination of both (e.g., behavior modification addressing changes in dietary intake and physical activity). In addition, both weight-gain prevention and weight maintenance must also be included in any intervention addressing overweight and obesity [5].

Many options are available for treating overweight and obese individuals. For each patient, the risks of each treatment option must be weighed against the benefit of the potential weight loss produced by that treatment. This risk:benefit assessment must take into account a patient's BMI, waist circumference, and the presence of co-morbidities and cardiovascular risk factors. Patients with a higher BMI or with existing obesity-related diseases are at more risk from their excess weight, and therefore more aggressive treatments such as pharmacotherapy and surgery become appropriate options. For each patient, there is a level of obesity at which the risk of the treatment is outweighed by the benefit the patient would receive from a long-term reduction in weight. Each treatment plan must be tailored to meet the BMI and risk:benefit assessment for each patient. Table 24.2 shows recommended treatment options based on BMI and the presence or absence of a serious health complication [22].

TABLE 24.2 Selecting Treatment Options Based on BMI and Co-morbidities

Body mass index	Co-morbidities present[a]	Diet	Exercise	Behavioral therapy	Pharmacotherapy	Surgery
25—26.9	No	−[b]	−[b]	−[b]	−	−
	Yes	+	+	+	−	−
27—29.9	No	−[b]	−[b]	−[b]	−	−
	Yes	+	+	+	+	−
30—34.9	No	+	+	+	+	−
	Yes	+	+	+	+	−
35—39.9	No	+	+	+	+	−
	Yes	+	+	+	+	+
>40	No	+	+	+	+	+
	Yes	+	+	+	+	+

[a]Co-morbidities include hypertension, sleep apnea, dyslipidemia, coronary heart disease, and type 2 diabetes.
[b]Prevention of weight gain with diet, exercise, and behavioral therapy is indicated.
+ indicates appropriate treatment option; − indicates inappropriate treatment option.
Source: Based on National Institutes of Health (1998). "NIH Clinical Guidelines on the Identification, Evaluation, and Treatment of Overweight and Obesity in Adults: The Evidence Report." National Institutes of Health, Bethesda, MD.

E Appropriate Goal Setting

The evidence-based NHLBI clinical guidelines for obesity treatment set the following general goals for weight loss and management: (1) to prevent further weight gain, (2) to reduce body weight, and (3) to maintain a lower body weight long term [5]. Traditionally, the goal of obesity treatment was to achieve an ideal body weight, and for many people this meant losing extremely large amounts of weight. However, a reduction to ideal body weight is not necessary for health improvement and risk reduction. Clinical studies indicate that moderate weight reduction (i.e., 5—10% of the initial body weight) can correct or ameliorate many of the metabolic abnormalities associated with obesity and that small weight losses are associated with improvements in hypertension, dyslipidemia, and type 2 diabetes mellitus [23—25]. Prescribing a weight-loss goal of 5—10% sets a reasonable and achievable goal that may be more easily maintained. Unfortunately, many patients are not satisfied with weight reduction in this range, and the provider must work closely with the patient to help set realistic expectations and provide guidance in this area [26].

III LIFESTYLE MODIFICATION

Lifestyle modification—that is, the modification of a person's daily diet and physical activity—is the cornerstone of obesity treatment programs. For most people, this treatment incurs no side effects, has minimal cost, and, if the lifestyle changes can be maintained, has great potential for long-term effectiveness [27]. In addition to creating changes in diet and physical activity patterns, the lifestyle modification component of obesity interventions also usually includes behavioral treatment to enhance the long-term effectiveness of the program.

A Dietary Modification

National surveys indicate that approximately 30% of U.S. adults are currently trying to lose weight [28] and approximately 50% report having tried to lose weight in the past year [29]. Most people report modifying their diet in some way to achieve their goals [28,29]. Because the prevalence of overweight and obesity is also at an all-time high, this interest in dieting and attempts to modify diet appear to be contradictory. This contradiction underscores the difficulty people face in making seemingly simple changes to their dietary intake in an environment that encourages easy overconsumption of energy.

1 Creating an Energy Deficit

The universal component of dietary interventions for weight loss is the creation of an energy deficit [1,5]. Most recommendations encourage a slow rate of weight loss through an energy deficit (energy output minus energy intake) of 500—1000 kcal/day [5]. This recommendation is aimed to produce an approximately 1-pound weight loss per week, although the rate of weight loss will slow due to compensatory declines in energy expenditure. Typically, the composition of the weight loss is approximately 25% fat-free mass and 75% fat mass. Metabolically, the more obese person can handle a greater energy deficit, as demonstrated by a lower protein oxidation rate during fasting, than can a lean person [30]. It is important to monitor the rate of weight loss during the active weight-loss phase. Initially, particularly at the greater energy deficits, diuresis may occur and weight will drop quickly. However, after this initial drop in weight, the rate of weight loss will slow and should not be greater than 1% body weight per week [31]. An energy deficit of 500−1000 kcal/day should produce an approximately 10% body weight reduction over 6 months [5].

Many health care providers prescribe a standard weight-loss diet of a preset calorie level (e.g., 1200 or 1500 kcal/day). This approach has the advantage of allowing the health care provider to give out preprinted diet plans already designed to achieve the calculated energy level. The disadvantages of this approach include inappropriately low energy intakes (i.e., >1000 kcal/day deficits) in very large individuals with high energy requirements, and diet plans that are not tailored to an individual's lifestyle. To avoid inappropriate energy deficits, it is useful to estimate a person's energy expenditure and subtract 500−1000 kcal/day (the greater energy deficit should be reserved for heavier individuals). Estimating a person's energy expenditure based on sex, body weight, and age [32] is preferable to using self-reported food intakes, which are notoriously unreliable, particularly among obese subjects [33,34]. Alternatively, as a general rule, an appropriate energy level can be determined by assigning 12 kcal per pound of current body weight and then subtracting 500−1000 calories to create an energy deficit. The NHLBI clinical guidelines recommend 1000−1200 kcal/day for women and 1200−1500 kcal/day for men [5]. Alternatively, calorie goals could be based on body weight as in the Look AHEAD trial [35], which used 114 kg (250 pounds) as a cut point for determining whether someone followed a 1200−1500 kcal/day diet plan (i.e., if less than 114 kg) or a 1500−1800 kcal/day diet plan (i.e., if 114 kg or greater).

Decreasing one's food consumption without ensuring an intake of a variety of foods may compromise a person's nutrient intake, particularly of calcium, iron, and vitamin E. At energy intakes below 1200 kcal/day, it is difficult to consume an adequate intake of essential vitamins and minerals. Multivitamin and mineral supplements are recommended for intakes below 1200 kcal/day and for individuals whose food choices limit their abilities to consume a satisfactory nutrient intake.

2 Very Low Calorie/Energy Diets

Some dietary regimens, such as very low-calorie diets (VLCDs), establish a greater than 1000 kcal/day energy deficit. A VLCD is typically a liquid formulation that contains up to 800 kcal/day (3350 kJ/day)

[36,37]. VLCDs are enriched in protein of high biological value (0.8−1.5 g/kg of ideal body weight per day) and are supplemented with essential vitamins, minerals, electrolytes, and fatty acids. A typical VLCD program lasts for 12−16 weeks, and the liquid formula completely replaces all usual foods. A structured period of refeeding usually occurs after a VLCD, with solid foods slowly being reintroduced into the patient's diet.

The purpose of VLCDs is to quickly achieve large weight loss while providing adequate nutrition and preserving lean body mass. The mean weight loss for a 12- to 16-week program (including the long-term weight loss of dropouts) is approximately 20 kg [38,39]. Weight losses on VLCDs are greater for men than for women [38], and heavier people lose more weight than do lighter people [40]. It has been hypothesized that beyond the greater than usual energy deficit, the form of these diets is an important factor in the effectiveness of a VLCD to produce a weight loss [38,40]. That is, the structured feeding regimen of a VLCD encourages excellent adherence to the low-calorie plan; a person does not have to make food choices and refrains from making impulsive high-calorie selections. Although effective at producing a quick weight loss, VLCDs have not proven to be effective for long-term weight-loss maintenance. A meta-analysis evaluating six randomized controlled trials of VLCD versus low-calorie diets showed similar long-term weight losses (6.3 ± 3.2% vs. 5.0 ± 4.0%, $p > 0.2$) despite significantly greater short-term weight loss with VLCD (16.1 ± 1.6% vs. 9.7 ± 2.4%, $p = 0.0001$) [41]. Other disadvantages of VLCDs include the expense of the programs and the side effects of the quick weight loss. The most serious side effects include hyperuricemia, gout, gallstones, and cardiac complications. These serious side effects underscore the need for: (1) Appropriate medical assessment for patients entering a program; (2) use of VLCDs in only obese patients (i.e., BMI > 30), especially those individuals with co-morbid conditions that would be responsive to weight loss (e.g., diabetes, sleep apnea, or presurgery); and (3) ongoing medical supervision during the course of the program [36]. The NIH clinical guidelines do not recommend VLCDs for use in obesity treatment [5].

3 Meal Replacements

Meal replacements differ from VLCDs in that they are designed to replace only one or two of the day's meals rather than the whole day's intake, and they are sold over-the-counter. The advantage of a meal replacement is that it can replace a person's most problematic meal of the day with a product (e.g., drink and bar) of a known energy and macronutrient content, thus helping to achieve a targeted energy intake goal. Few studies have specifically evaluated the efficacy of meal replacement for weight loss [42]. A 27-month study [43] showed a significantly greater weight loss in people following a low-calorie plan utilizing two meal replacement drinks per day versus people following a conventional low-calorie plan (11.3 ± 6.8 vs. 5.9 ± 5.0% of initial body weight, $p < 0.0001$). A meta-analysis of six randomized controlled trials indicated a significantly greater weight loss in subjects using meal replacements (7 or 8% body weight) versus a conventional reduced-calorie meal plan (3–7% body weight) at both 3-month and 12-month time points [44]. Meal replacements have been used effectively in large clinical trials such as Look AHEAD [35].

Meal replacement drinks may be useful for weight maintenance or weight-gain prevention. A study conducted in rural Wisconsin evaluated the efficacy of meal replacement drink treatment against the backdrop of weight gain experienced by matched controls over a 5-year period [45]. A total of 134 men and women participated in a self-management meal replacement drink program that included a 3-month active weight-loss phase (two meal replacement drinks per day with weekly weigh-ins) and a maintenance phase (self-monitoring of weight and use of a meal replacement drink if weight gain occurred). During the same 5-year period, 86% of the meal replacement drink participants were at least weight stable (<0.8 kg weight gain), whereas only 25% of the matched controls had prevented weight gain [45]. However, further research is required to verify the efficacy of this treatment for weight loss and weight-loss maintenance.

4 Macronutrient Composition

A negative energy balance is the most important factor affecting the amount, rate, and composition of weight loss. However, further dietary guidance beyond just eating fewer calories is necessary to address the dietary implications of obesity co-morbidities, such as diabetes and cardiovascular disease, as well as the long-term adherence to a new lower calorie regimen.

People typically eat a constant daily weight of food in feeding experiments regardless of the type of diet consumed [46]. Restricting or limiting this daily constant likely leads to hunger and dietary dissatisfaction; therefore, the manipulation of the energy density (energy/food weight) of foods and diets has been of interest as a mechanism to decrease energy intake without changing daily food weight [47]. Dietary energy density is typically manipulated by increasing water-rich foods such as fruits and vegetables (which increase the food volume without increasing dietary energy) and decreasing the frequency of high-fat foods (fat is the most energy-dense macronutrient). Laboratory studies have demonstrated that people consume fewer calories when presented with low-energy-dense foods versus higher energy-dense foods [47,48]. The DASH dietary pattern containing 9–12 daily servings of fruits and vegetables and total fat goals (total and saturated fat) of ≤25 and ≤7% of total caloric intake was associated with weight loss over a 6-month period as evaluated in the PREMIER trial [49]. Participants with the largest change in energy density lost more weight (5.9 kg) than did those in the middle (4.0 kg) or lowest (2.4 kg) energy density change tertile [49]. This weight-loss pattern was also demonstrated in obese women following a low-energy-dense diet plan for 1 year with larger weight losses (7.9 ± 0.9 vs. 6.4 ± 0.9 kg, $p = 0.002$), and less hunger ($p = 0.003$) was demonstrated in women assigned to a low-energy-dense diet incorporating fat reduction as well as fruit and vegetable increases versus fat reduction only [50].

A low-fat diet (<30% energy from fat) is currently the typical recommended macronutrient guideline for weight loss [5]. Because diabetes and cardiovascular disease are frequent co-morbidities of obesity, it is also recommended to modify the fat content of the diet to be low in saturated and trans fatty acids and higher in monounsaturated fats [51]. The effectiveness of low-fat, low-calorie diets in combination with lifestyle counseling and activity has been demonstrated in multicenter clinical trials in which, in addition to 5–10% weight loss, the reduction or prevention of co-morbidities such as diabetes or hypertension has also been documented [52–56]. Because of its greater energy density than either protein or carbohydrate (9 vs. 4 kcal/g) and its possible weak effect on both satiation (process controlling meal size) and satiety (process controlling subsequent hunger and eating) [57], for a long time fat was considered the most important macronutrient to control in weight-loss interventions. However, carefully controlled trials have evaluated the efficacy of weight-loss diets manipulated for protein content and/or carbohydrate content. Typically, more weight loss occurs with low-carbohydrate diets in the first 6 months compared to low-fat diets, although this weight-loss difference does not persist by 12 months [58–62] or at 2 years [63,64]. Concerns regarding an increase in cardiovascular risks with these low-carbohydrate diets do not appear to be as problematic as first thought [60,63,64]. These studies have underscored the need to better understand factors that impact study attrition rates as well as individual adherence to any type of weight-loss diet because these two parameters impacted the interpretation of these trial outcomes [60,61,65]. Regardless of macronutrient composition, translating dietary prescriptions to specific food group guidance, while acknowledging food preferences and barriers to compliance, will likely always be important for both client satisfaction and long-term success.

5 *The Nondiet Approach*

There has been a movement toward replacing restrictive diet approaches and unrealistic weight goals with promotion of healthful food choices and size acceptance. Proponents cite two rationales for adopting this approach: (1) There is no long-term effective strategy for treating obesity and (2) pressure to be thin impairs the psychological and social well-being of both people who are overweight and those who are not [66]. The focus of the nondiet approach is to encourage people to improve their self-acceptance (self-image) regardless of their current weight and to adopt healthy practices to promote physical well-being (e.g., promoting fitness and healthful food choices). Few studies have carefully evaluated the result of the nondiet approaches on weight loss or the reduction of comorbidities associated with obesity [67]. Repeated weight loss (also termed "weight cycling") does not appear to be associated with psychopathology or changes in weight- and eating-related constructs [68]. However, it is apparent that more research is needed to conclusively determine the psychological effect of repeated episodes of dieting and weight loss.

B Physical Activity Modification

Physical activity is important for improving health-related outcomes across many disease states, including heart disease, cancer, and diabetes (i.e., frequent comorbidities to obesity) [69]. In general, physical activity has been used as a key component of obesity treatment. However, studies examining physical activity per se for weight loss have found only modest reductions in body weight using this strategy [70]. Weight losses in the range of 0.09–0.10 kg/week have been reported when exercise is used alone compared to a no-treatment control group [70,71]. Exceptions to this trend have been reported with extreme levels of exercise as is seen in military-type training. Combining exercise with dietary restriction produces only a slight increase in weight loss over dietary restriction alone [70]. In general, groups using diet restriction plus exercise lost more weight than the diet-alone condition, but the magnitude of the difference was not significant in most studies.

A possible explanation for the relatively modest effect of physical activity on weight loss is that the energy cost of exercise is minimal compared to potential changes in energy intake. A person who exercises for 30 minutes 5 days a week may burn only 1000 kcal more per week depending on the individual's size, his or her fitness level, and the intensity of the exercise. In comparison, a person may consume an extra 1000 kcal in one or two unplanned snacks and easily negate the energy expended in exercise for the entire week.

Although its impact on weight loss may be minimal, physical activity appears to have a crucial role in the long-term maintenance of a weight loss (i.e., the prevention of weight regain). Many correlation studies show a strong association between self-reported exercise at follow-up and maintenance of a weight loss [70]. Studies using doubly labeled water suggest physical activity of 11 or 12 kcal/kg/day may be necessary to prevent weight regain following a weight loss [72].

Data from the National Weight Control Registry (NWCR) also support the concept that high levels of physical activity are crucial in preventing weight regain following a weight loss. The NWCR is a registry of individuals who have maintained a minimum of a 30-pound weight loss for at least 1 year. These individuals report using a variety of methods to lose weight initially, but more than 90% report exercise as a key element in maintaining the loss long term. They report expending, on average, 2682 kcal/week in physical activity [27]. This is approximately the equivalent of walking 4 miles 7 days a week, and many report much higher levels. This suggests that although physical activity may not have been essential for weight loss in these subjects, they believe it to be essential in prevention of weight regain.

Pedometers and step counters are small devices used to promote physical activity and are often included in weight-loss interventions. Pedometers promote awareness of a person's current level of activity and provide easy feedback on goals for increasing physical activity. Although 10,000 steps per day is frequently recommended to provide health benefits [73], when it comes to physical activity, more is better, and any increase in steps per day should be encouraged. In fact, increases of 2000 steps per day will help to prevent weight gain in most people [74].

C Behavior Modification

Behavior modification, a fundamental component of obesity interventions, helps patients develop a skill set to achieve a healthier weight. That skill set builds on the specific information about what to change and helps people on the "how" to change. Behavioral modification treatment is goal-directed (e.g., clear, measurable goals based on behaviors such as "walk for 20 minutes daily"), process-oriented (e.g., patients are encouraged to identify strategies to overcome anticipated barriers as well as learn from setbacks), and advocates small changes so a person can build on successive successful experiences with change [75]. The key behavioral modification components utilized in obesity treatment include self-monitoring, stimulus control, and relapse-prevention strategies.

Self-monitoring commonly includes the systematic recording of food intake and exercise activities. Consistent self-monitoring, particularly of food intake, is associated with improved obesity treatment outcome [76,77], even during high-risk periods such as holidays [78]. In addition to the self-monitoring of behaviors (e.g., minutes exercised and food choices), regular body weighing (i.e., self-monitoring of an outcome) is also associated with obesity treatment success. Findings from the NWCR reveal that 44% of these successful weight losers weigh themselves daily and an additional 31% weigh themselves at least weekly [27]. In a randomized clinical trial evaluating an intervention to prevent weight regain in successful weight losers, daily weighing was associated with an 82% reduction in risk of weight regain [79] and was not associated with adverse psychological effects [80]. Stimulus control involves the identification and modification of environmental cues associated with overeating and sedentary activity and is widely accepted as clinically effective [81]. Relapse-prevention strategies involve training patients to prepare for lapses in the weight-loss process and to utilize coping strategies to prevent complete relapse of behavior change efforts [82].

The behavior modification package includes many variations of diet, physical activity, behavior modification delivery, and treatment structure, making it difficult to evaluate the efficacy of behavior modification per se [83]. However, it is generally accepted that participants treated with a comprehensive behavior modification approach lose 8—10% of initial body weight over 16—26 weeks [4,81], as demonstrated in both the Diabetes Prevention Program and Look AHEAD multicenter randomized control trials [53,56]. The behavior modification interventions delivered in the Diabetes Prevention Program and Look AHEAD trials have been described as exemplars of behavioral treatment programs [81]: Intervention materials from both of these programs are in the public domain [84,85]. Behavior modification is typically delivered in the cost-efficient format of groups providing opportunities for social support, although there has been minimal systematic assessment of the group process specifically for obesity intervention [86,87]. A variety of important questions including optimal number of group participants, frequency and length of meetings, critical group leader skills, and strategies to identify the optimal candidates for group-based interventions have not been thoroughly investigated. Most behavioral techniques utilized in a group setting can be effectively incorporated into weight-loss counseling provided individually [4,88]. More information about specific behavior change and motivational interviewing techniques can be found in Chapters 9 and 10.

IV PHARMACEUTICAL INTERVENTION

A Background

Diet, physical activity, and behavior modification are key components of obesity management, but in the mid-1990s pharmaceutical intervention also became a valued therapeutic option (Table 24.3). Previously, there was a long history of pharmaceutical weight-loss intervention (both with and without medical supervision) including such drugs as laxatives, diuretics, thyroxin, and amphetamines with very little evidence of efficacy or safety. The U.S. Food and Drug Administration's (FDA) neuropharmacology division reviewed weight-loss medications (mainly appetite suppressants) up until the 1990s, and core safety concerns were the medications' abuse and addiction potential. In 1992, weight-loss medication oversight was moved to the FDA's metabolic and endocrine division, and the evaluation process began to change. In 1996, the FDA issued guidance on clinical trial treatment design and evidentiary standards that was more reflective of the chronic disease model that the medical community had started to embrace for obesity treatment. Clinical trials now focused on patients at high risk for metabolic sequelae—that is, patients with a BMI greater than 27 with co-morbidities or with a BMI less than 30 with or without co-morbidities. Duration of phase 3 trials was outlined: First-year placebo-controlled "proof of principle of efficacy" as well as second-year open-label durable efficacy and safety in long-term use were required. This guidance marked a perspective shift from medications being merely for short-term weight loss to being part of a long-term obesity treatment with outcomes focused on prevention or amelioration of co-morbidities as well as weight-regain prevention.

Since 1996, the FDA has approved dexfenfluramine, sibutramine, and orlistat but has subsequently withdrawn approval for dexfenfluramine (secondary to concerns for valvular heart disease) and sibutramine (secondary to increased cardiovascular risks). Rimonbant, a selective cannabinoid-1 receptor blocker that until recently was used widely in Europe but awaited FDA approval, has also been withdrawn due to concerns of increased risks for depression and suicidal ideation. In addition, since 2010 three promising obesity drugs (Contrave, Qnexa, and Locarserin) have been denied FDA approval without further extensive safety and effectiveness data. This has left a handful of short-term medications with insufficient data on long-term effectiveness and safety as well as only one medication approved for long-term weight loss. There is concern that pharmaceutical companies will

TABLE 24.3 Pharmaceutical Interventions Used in Obesity Treatment

Drug	Mechanism of action	Administration	Daily dose range (mg)	FDA approval for use
Benzphetamine	Stimulates NE release	Start with 25 mg qd; max dose 25–50 mg po tid	25–150	Short term
Phendimetrazine	Stimulates NE release	35 mg po tid before meals or 105 mg SR qd	35–105	Short term
Diethylpropion	Stimulates NE release	25 mg po tid or 75 mg SR qd	25–75	Short term
Mazindol	Blocks NE reuptake	Start with 1 mg po qd; max dose 1 mg po tid with meals	1–3	Short term
Phentermine	Stimulates NE release	15, 30, or 37.5 mg po qd in the AM	15–37.5	Short term
Orlistat	Lipase inhibitor	120 mg taken with each meal po tid	120–360	Long term
		60 mg taken with meal po tid	60–180	OTC

po, by mouth; qd, once a day; tid, three times a day; NE, norepinephrine; SR, slow-release capsule.

withdraw from investing in new obesity drug development due to perceived high regulatory hurdles and the obesity treatment field will be left with only surgical intervention for patients who have failed lifestyle interventions [89].

B Risk:Benefit Ratio

1 Selecting Patients for Pharmacotherapy

Weight-loss medications should be prescribed in combination with a diet, exercise, and behavioral modification program. Medications are not a substitute for but, rather, an adjunct to lifestyle intervention, providing additional benefit by helping patients adhere to the necessary diet and exercise changes. For some individuals, diet and exercise alone may be enough to produce a 10% weight loss and long-term maintenance. For others, medications may provide a necessary additional intervention to allow weight-loss success.

Evaluating pharmacotherapy as an option for a patient occurs after the clinical assessment and the evaluation of co-morbidities. The risk of the potential side effects of the medication must be carefully weighed against the benefits of the weight loss as a result of the treatment. The risk of not losing weight or even gaining weight must also be considered. In addition, many clinicians require that patients attempt weight loss in a structured program of diet, exercise, and behavioral modification before being considered for pharmacotherapy [4]. In addition to BMI, other factors such as a high waist circumference, recent weight gain, family history, and the presence of co-morbidities become important considerations in the decision to treat with weight-loss medications.

Use of medications for a cosmetic weight loss of just a few pounds in a lean person is not appropriate. The risk of the medication in this case is not outweighed by the benefit because a reduction in weight at a lean weight (BMI < 25 kg/m^2) is not associated with significant improvement in health risks. Currently, the evidence and the NHLBI guidelines justify the use of a weight-loss medication in patients with BMIs greater than 30 kg/m^2 or greater than 27 kg/m^2 if co-morbidities such as hypertension or diabetes are present [5].

2 Predictors of Efficacy

It is important that the weight loss expected from pharmaceutical intervention is neither under- nor overstated [90]. Most patients have an unrealistic view of how much weight they can lose, and a weight loss as low as 15% may be viewed as a failure [26]. Currently available medications seldom produce greater than 10% weight loss even in combination with a robust lifestyle intervention.

Not every patient responds to drug therapy. Therefore, it is important to monitor patients on weight-loss medications not only for potential side effects but also for the efficacy of the medication. Clinical trials have shown that initial responders tend to continue to lose weight, whereas initial nonresponders continue to be nonresponders. The initial rate of weight loss frequently predicts subsequent weight loss. If the patient does not lose weight or maintain a previous weight loss with the medication, the medication should be discontinued. In this case, the risk of the medication is not outweighed by the weight loss because there has not been a reduction in weight. As a general guideline, patients who do not lose 1% of body weight during their first month of treatment should discontinue treatment [91].

C Medications Approved for Short-Term Use in Weight Loss

There are several FDA-approved (pre-1996) medications for short-term use (<3 months), including phendimetrazine, phentermine, and diethylpropion. These are noradrenergic or sympathomimetic drugs that either stimulate release or block reuptake of norepinephrine. Sympthomimetic drugs are scheduled by the Drug Enforcement Agency indicating the potential for abuse. Side effects may include restlessness, dizziness, insomnia, euphoria, dysphoria, tremor, headache, dry mouth, asthenia, and constipation. In general, these medications produced more weight loss than placebo in most short-term clinical trials, but the magnitude of the weight loss was variable [92,93]. Large clinical trials evaluating these drugs for efficacy and safety in long-term obesity treatment are scarce, and the FDA has not approved their use for longer than 3 months. Despite the lack of long-term safety and efficacy data, these medications are frequently used by bariatric physicians [94] sometimes at higher doses and for longer treatment periods than those approved by the FDA. It is speculated that the cost of these older generic medications makes them a relatively cheap intervention in a health care environment in which obesity treatments are not always covered by third-party payers [94].

D Medications Approved for Long-Term Use

1 Orlistat

The FDA approved the use of orlistat for the long-term treatment of obesity in 1999. Orlistat is a minimally absorbable agent (<1%) that works in the gastrointestinal tract by blocking gastrointestinal lipases and reducing the subsequent absorption of ingested fat by approximately 30% [95]. Orlistat has been studied in 1- and 2-year clinical trials [96—98]. In general, the orlistat-treated groups lost more weight and had a higher percentage of subjects able to achieve a 10% weight loss than subjects in the placebo-treated group [99]. In a large study that evaluated more than 600 patients, 38.8% of the patients in the orlistat group achieved a 10% or greater weight loss compared to only 17.7% in the placebo group [100]. Orlistat has also been studied in a 4-year double-blind placebo-controlled study of more than 3000 patients undergoing intensive lifestyle intervention and randomized to receive either 120 mg Orlistat or placebo three times daily for 4 years [101]. After 4 years of treatment, 26% of the orlistat-treated patients lost at least 10% of baseline body weight versus only 16% of the placebo-treated group. Orlistat's use for weight-loss maintenance has been evaluated in 2-year studies. In these studies, a hypocaloric diet in combination with orlistat was used for weight loss in the first year, and then a eucaloric diet with orlistat or placebo was used in the second year to evaluate weight-loss maintenance. In a large study by Davidson and co-

workers [97], almost twice as many subjects (34.1%) in the orlistat group were able to maintain a greater than 10% weight loss for the 2-year period compared to the placebo group (17%) [97]. Similar results indicate that mean body weight regain is less with orlistat treatment than placebo (32.4 vs. 56.0% for orlistat and placebo, respectively) [96]. In these clinical trials, orlistat was used in combination with either a low-fat hypocaloric diet for weight loss or a eucaloric diet for weight maintenance, and a portion of the benefit seen in these trials must be attributable to that diet.

The optimal dosing of orlistat is 120-mg po tid with meals that contain fat. Higher doses do not have any additional efficacy in weight loss and may result in more adverse events [102]. Orlistat is minimally absorbed; therefore, any systemic adverse events would be expected to be negligible. Orlistat should be used with a diet that is less than 30% energy from fat to prevent adverse side effects that include oily stools, oily spotting, flatus with discharge, fecal urgency, and fecal incontinence [102]. These events are due to the drug inhibiting fat absorption rather than a direct effect of the drug. Patients should be advised to maintain a low-fat diet while using the medication because these side effects increase with diets that have more than 30% energy from fat. In general, these events tend to decrease over time.

Mean plasma levels of vitamins A, D, E, and β-carotene were monitored during the trials. In general, plasma levels of these vitamins decreased but remained in the reference ranges [100,102]. However, in the United States, a multivitamin supplement is recommended for patients prescribed orlistat and should be taken 2 hours before or after the dose of orlistat.

Over-the-counter (OTC) orlistat (sold as Alli in the United States) is the identical molecular compound of the prescription-strength orlistat; however, it is provided in a 60-mg capsule rather than the 120-mg capsule. Dosing is one 60-mg capsule three times a day with meals. OTC orlistat represents a change in the scheduling of orlistat from a 120-mg prescription compound requiring a medical physician to write a prescription to an OTC status that will allow patients to buy the medication without a medical consultation or oversight. Its OTC indication promotes weight loss in overweight adults when used along with a reduced-energy and low-fat diet. The OTC 60-mg dose of orlistat inhibits absorption of approximately 25% of ingested fats [103]. In contrast, the prescription dose of 120 mg blocks the absorption of approximately 30% of the fat consumed in a meal that contains approximately 30% fat. Similar to the 120-mg orlistat studies, significantly greater weight loss was observed with an orlistat dosage of 60 mg plus diet compared to placebo plus diet in overweight and obese patients [103–105]. Weight losses in the range of 4.8–9.7% were reported with the 60-mg OTC dose at 1 year.

E Medications Not Approved for Long-Term Weight Loss

Fluoxetine and bupropion (FDA-approved antidepressants) have been evaluated in several weight-loss trials [24,106,107]. Patients taking fluoxetine in doses greater than 60 mg/day have shown more weight loss than those using placebo in clinical trials. However, the long-term efficacy of fluoxetine is questionable because weight regain while continuing the medication was also demonstrated [24,106]. Bupropion is approved for the treatment of depression and for smoking cessation. Several clinical trials have evaluated its weight-loss potential. One study randomized 327 subjects to bupropion 300 mg/day, buproprion 400 mg/day, or placebo [107]. Weight loss at 6 months was 5 ± 1%, 7.2 ± 1%, and 10.1 ± 1% for the placebo, 300-mg, and 400-mg groups, respectively ($p < 0.0001$). Although bupropion is not approved for weight loss, if a person is clinically depressed, it may be an appropriate antidepressant (if medication is indicated), especially in the overweight person already trying to lose weight. Neither fluoxetine nor bupropion have FDA approval for weight loss.

Zonisamide and topiramate (FDA-approved antiepileptic drugs) have demonstrated weight loss in clinical trials designed for the treatment of epilepsy. The FDA has not approved either drug for weight loss. Zonisamide is an antiepileptic drug that has serotonergic and dopaminergic activity in addition to inhibiting sodium and calcium channels. Zonisamide has been studied in one 16-week trial in obese subjects for weight loss with favorable results [108]. Topiramate has been evaluated for weight loss, binge-eating treatment, and the Prader–Willi syndrome [109–114]. Initial studies reported weight loss in the range of 6–10%. Adverse events in these trials included paresthesias, somnolence, difficulty concentrating, and difficulty with memory. Several large studies were terminated early because a time-release formula was developed and it was hoped this new preparation would minimize the adverse event profile of the drug. There is no indication that the time-release preparation succeeded in alleviating the side effect profile, and the development of the program to pursue the indication from the FDA for obesity treatment was terminated by the sponsor in December of 2004. This decision was probably related to the associated adverse events. Topiramate, however, is still available as an antiepileptic drug.

F Medications Combined with Lifestyle Modification

It is important to emphasize that weight-loss medications should be prescribed in combination with diet, exercise, and a behavioral modification program. Medications are not a substitute for but, rather, an adjunct to lifestyle intervention providing additional benefit by helping patients adhere to the necessary diet and exercise changes. For some individuals, diet and exercise alone may be enough to produce a 10% weight loss and long-term maintenance. For others, medications may provide a necessary additional intervention to allow weight-loss success.

V SURGICAL TREATMENT

Although the prevalence of obesity (BMI > 30) increased 24% from 2000 to 2005, the prevalence of a BMI greater than 40 and of a BMI greater 50 increased two and three times faster, respectively, during the same period [115]. For people in these BMI categories, surgical intervention is considered the most effective treatment for weight loss and long-term weight maintenance. Increasingly, more people are considering surgery to reduce body weight: From 1998 to 2004, the total number of bariatric surgeries increased ninefold in the United States from 13,386 to 121,055 [116]. Surgery, with its inherent permanence, clearly has an advantage in long-term success [117]. Similar to pharmacotherapy, the use of a surgical intervention in obesity requires a case-by-case risk:benefit analysis. Patients with a low probability of success with nonsurgical interventions and who meet BMI criteria may be appropriate candidates for surgery. Patients who have been determined to have acceptable operative risks should be well informed about the procedure, the benefits and the risks, as well as the potential impact on their lifestyles. A commitment to long-term follow-up is also essential. It is recommended that surgeries be performed in high-volume clinics because the prevention of postoperative complications depends not only on the technical expertise of the surgeon but also on the careful preoperative assessment, screening, and minimization of preoperative risk [118]. See Chapter 25 for further discussion on surgical interventions for weight loss.

VI SPECIAL ISSUES IN THE TREATMENT OF PEDIATRIC OBESITY

Obesity is the most common pediatric nutrition-related problem, impacting one in six children in the

United States [119]. There are significant racial and ethnic disparities in obesity prevalence, with Hispanic boys and non-Hispanic black girls at much greater risk than their white counterparts [119]. Obese children tend to become obese adults and face an increased lifetime risk of diabetes and cardiovascular diseases [120,121]. In addition, even during childhood and adolescence, disorders such as hyperlipidemia, hypertension, and abnormal glucose tolerance occur with increased frequency in overweight and obese children [122]. In addition to the metabolic sequelae, significant negative psychosocial consequences of obesity are observed in this population, and obese children frequently face stigmatization in their daily school setting [122,123]. Strategies to address this staggering public health problem must be tailored to address the special needs of a pediatric population.

As in adults, obesity in children is characterized by the accumulation of excess body fat. However, the assessment for weight-related health risk is different for children than it is for adults. Because children's body fat levels change with age and are different between girls and boys, BMI requires age and sex adjustments in children (ages 2 years or older) and must be plotted on sex-specific BMI-for-age growth charts [124]. Obesity is defined as a BMI above the 95th percentile (reflecting a high health risk from excess body fat) and overweight as a BMI between the 85th and 95th percentiles (lower risk, although risk varies depending on BMI trajectory, family history, and other clinical factors). Severe obesity in childhood is defined by the 99th percentile and denotes those individuals with an extremely high risk of obesity-related co-morbidities. Instead of BMI, weight-for-recumbent length is used in infants and toddlers younger than 2 years because recumbent length is a more appropriate assessment of height in this age group. In 2007–2008, 9.5% of infants and toddlers were at or above the 95th percentile for weight-for-recumbent length [119]. Although the terms "obesity" and "overweight" are appropriate in the medical literature, they are not acceptable for discussions with families. Research shows that parents view terms such as "obese," "extremely obese," and "fat" as the most stigmatizing, blaming, and least motivating terms when used in the context of their children. Instead, "weight," "unhealthy weight," and "weight problem" are preferable terms for a health care provider to describe a child's excess weight and are more helpful in a conversation to engage a parent to consider behavioral changes [125].

Expert committee recommendations [126] encourage a universal assessment of obesity risk in children so that anticipatory guidance on healthy behaviors can be provided as part of a prevention strategy as well as early intervention initiated when necessary. BMI measurement and weight status categorization at annual well-child visits is the first step in obesity assessment. A review of BMI trajectory is informative because the child who crosses major percentile lines upward may be at risk of moving into the overweight or obese categories [127]. Identification of obesity in first-degree relatives (i.e., parents and siblings) is useful because parental obesity is a strong risk factor for a child's obesity persisting in adulthood, especially for young children [128]. Documentation of family history of cardiovascular disease and type 2 diabetes in first-degree or second-degree relatives (i.e., grandparents, uncles, aunts, and half-siblings) should also be integrated into the weight assessment. Depending on the presence of risk factors, children in the overweight and obese categories should be screened with a fasting lipid profile, fasting glucose, and liver enzyme levels (i.e., ALT and AST) starting at 10 years of age [126,127]. Obstructive sleep apnea, asthma, nonalcoholic fatty liver disease, type 2 diabetes, lipid level abnormalities, and orthopedic conditions such as Blount disease and slipped capital femoral epiphysis are medical conditions occurring more often in obese children, so an obesity-focused medical assessment is warranted to ensure that these related conditions are treated appropriately [126]. As part of the universal assessment for obesity risk, health care providers should also routinely assess dietary and physical activity patterns in all children regardless of weight (e.g., frequency of eating out, consumption of sweetened beverages, hours of screen time, and time spent in moderate physical activity [126]) to determine if there are any modifiable behaviors that promote energy imbalance. Specific dietary and physical activity behaviors to address are listed in Table 24.4.

Treatment recommendation goals for pediatric obesity are different than those for adult obesity. In general, because children are still growing linearly with increases in lean body mass, slowing weight gain (especially in younger children) or preventing further weight gain can improve weight status. For children in the severely obese category (i.e., BMI for age > 99th percentile), weight loss of 1 pound per month (ages 2–5 years) and up to 2 pounds per week (6 years or older) may be an appropriate weight goal to improve weight status [126]. In addition, any treatment aimed at regulating body weight and body fat must also provide adequate nutrition for the growth and development of the child.

Treatment programs of intensity greater than what can be achieved in a typical pediatric office are important for those children not responding to healthy eating and physical activity messages or those children whose health is most compromised by their weight. Such lifestyle interventions still address the dietary and

24 OBESITY OVERVIEW OF TREATMENTS AND INTERVENTIONS

physical activity behaviors as listed in Table 24.4 but provide increased frequency of contact, additional structure (e.g., planned diet, supervised activity, use of logs to monitor new behaviors, and planned reinforcement for achieving targeted behaviors) and support (e.g., assistance with parenting skills and referral for additional psychosocial therapy) [126]. A meta-analysis of randomized controlled trials found that lifestyle interventions for pediatric obesity produced significant treatment effects compared with no-treatment/waitlist control groups [129]. Analysis of change scores showed that treatment groups had a reduction of approximately 8% overweight, whereas no-treatment groups showed approximately 2% increases in overweight, highlighting the fact that an overweight or obese child receiving no treatment is most likely to continue to gain weight [129]. Further review indicates that lifestyle interventions can be effective under a variety of conditions and are not limited to controlled efficacy studies [130]. However, there are still many opportunities to understand and improve pediatric obesity programs, such as identifying specific factors that can improve program adherence and tailoring treatment approaches to best meet the needs of diverse populations [131,132]. An intensive, family-based lifestyle weight management program developed for the lifestyle arm of a multicenter clinical trial comparing treatments for 10- to 17-year-olds with type 2 diabetes (TODAY study) illustrates the behavior change strategies used in pediatric obesity interventions [133]. This intervention was designed to decrease the baseline weight of a youth by 7–10% (or the equivalent for children who are growing in height) through changes in eating and physical activity habits and also to sustain these changes through ongoing treatment contact. The TODAY study lifestyle intervention materials are available in the public domain [134].

TABLE 24.4 Strategies to Prevent or Control Overweight in Children and Adolescents

Increased physical activity

  Accumulate at least 60 minutes per day

Reduced television viewing

  Limit to screen time to <2 hours per day

No TV in child's bedroom

Reduced intake of sugar-sweetened beverages

Increased consumption of fruit and vegetables

  5 or more servings per day

Family meals eaten together where possible

Limit number of meals eaten outside the home

Parental involvement is essential for dietary changes to be effective because parental attitudes, purchase, and presentation of food as well as modeling of eating behavior can impact a child's intake [135]. Some child-feeding practices can have negative (and unintended) effects on a child's food preferences and ability to control food intake [136]. For example, stringent parental control can increase a child's preference for high-energy-dense foods and limit a child's acceptance of a wide variety of foods [136]. Parental support involves being a positive role model for healthful feeding behavior as well as providing a wide array of healthful food choices in a supportive eating context [137]. However, there are still many gaps in our understanding of how to effectively engage parents and assist them in making changes in the home food environment and adhere to behavior change strategies [132]. Finally, because the potential for the emergence of eating disorders is high in children and adolescents, dietary modifications must occur in the context of the promotion of realistic body weight goals, positive self-esteem, and body image satisfaction.

Increasing daily physical activity, regardless of weight status, is as important for children as it is for adults. Like adults, however, children live in an environment that appears to encourage underactivity [138], especially with sedentary activities such as television viewing, video game playing, or Internet surfing taking prominence in many children's lives. Physical activity interventions in the treatment of pediatric obesity in addition to promoting daily physical activity (at least 60 minutes per day) often include decreasing sedentary behaviors such as removing the TV from a child's bedroom and limiting screen time to no more than 1 or 2 hours per day [139,140]. Studies have shown this approach to be effective both in increasing physical activity and in producing relative changes in BMI [139,140]. In addition, because children are more likely to continue being active if they are able to choose their own activity, providing a choice of activities appears to be superior to providing a specific exercise prescription [139]. Exposing children to enjoyable physical activities can promote skill mastery and a lifelong love of being physically active. For overweight children, it is important that this exposure is appropriate: Activities that can be easily mastered with gradual increases in volume and intensity should be considered so that negative consequences of participation are avoided [131]. An obesity-focused medical assessment will identify factors such as joint pain or gait changes that may require exercise modification to ensure success in physical activity participation.

The school environment, with its continuous and intensive contact with children, presents a unique opportunity for obesity prevention through both education and environment changes. Schools have the necessary resources to promote physical activity (e.g., gym equipment and playing fields), they provide at least one meal a day where children can be exposed to healthful food choices, and many schools have access to school nurses or health clinics, which could potentially provide services to overweight children [141]. The effectiveness of school-based programs for the prevention of obesity has been modest, but the results are encouraging and are worthy of more research [142,143]. Program components such as ensuring that sufficient time and resources are devoted to a comprehensive intervention, a focus on policy changes (appropriate for the local school culture) rather than only on individual behavior changes, and that school stakeholders are engaged and committed are key to successful implementation [143]. These components were integral to an obesity prevention program delivered in an inner-city school district that resulted in a 50% reduction in the incidence of overweight: 7.5% of the children in the intervention schools versus 15% in the control schools became overweight after 2 years [144]. The Centers for Disease Control and Prevention's School Health Index is a tool to assist schools in assessing and planning for policies and practices to promote healthful eating, physical activity, and other health-related practices that can be used as part of an obesity prevention intervention [145]. Because weight-based stigmatization is prevalent within the school environment, it is essential that school-based policies prohibit weight-based victimization and that any initiative to address childhood obesity within the school does not impose further stigmatization on overweight and obese youth [123].

VII ACUTE WEIGHT LOSS VERSUS MAINTAINING LONG-TERM WEIGHT LOSS

Effective weight management comprises both a weight-loss phase and a weight-loss maintenance phase. Most people are relatively successful at achieving a short-term weight loss, but few people can sustain that weight loss over long periods of time. Although experts now acknowledge that obesity is not an acute disorder that is "cured" by a single short-term intervention, the public is still focused much more on achieving weight loss than on maintaining the weight loss. This is evidenced by the use of popular diets that advocate dietary changes that produce weight loss but that are difficult to maintain over time. Although a large number of resources are available to help people lose weight, there are few to help people keep the weight off. Considering weight loss as a different

process than weight-loss maintenance may help us develop different strategies and tools for each phase.

If weight loss and weight-loss maintenance are considered as separate processes, we can consider how strategies for each phase might vary. Many different dietary strategies (e.g., following low-fat, low-carbohydrate, or low-energy-dense diets) can produce weight loss [59]. Furthermore, physical activity added to food restriction does not add much to the amount of weight loss [70]. High levels of physical activity seem to be critical for most people to maintain a substantial weight loss [27,72]. The composition of the diet may be less important, although much data favor a low-fat diet for weight-loss maintenance [27]. It is not surprising that physical activity is important for weight-loss maintenance. Weight loss is accompanied by a decline in energy requirements so that the amount of energy needed to achieve energy balance is lower after weight loss than before. Keeping weight off by diet alone means continuous food restriction for most people, and this seems to be difficult. Increasing physical activity increases total energy requirements and can allow energy intake to be sufficiently high to avoid chronic hunger.

The real challenge in weight management lies in the prevention of weight gain after weight loss, not in the accomplishment of weight loss. Thus, a treatment plan for obesity cannot just involve a plan for producing negative energy balance but must also involve a plan for achieving and maintaining energy balance at a new, lower body weight. Treatments that produce the largest degree of negative energy balance will produce the most weight loss, but these treatments may not be easy to maintain chronically. Similarly, the treatments that most effectively maintain a weight loss may not be effective in producing weight loss. The best overall treatment for an obese individual may incorporate treatments for acute weight loss paired with a different treatment in the weight maintenance phase. Potentially, weight-loss medications may have their greatest role in helping obese individuals maintain a weight loss achieved by different interventions (e.g., diet and exercise) that may be difficult to maintain at the necessary level for long periods of time.

VIII THE FUTURE OF WEIGHT MANAGEMENT

The most efficient way to address obesity is in preventing excess weight gain from ever occurring; therefore, health care professionals should consider addressing prevention of weight gain in all patients. Because the entire U.S. population has been in a gradual weight-gain state, a first goal for all patients should be not to gain additional weight. This would apply to patients whether they are currently at a healthy weight, overweight, or obese. In children, this goal can be translated to preventing excessive weight gain. Hill *et al.* [74] suggested that modifying the energy balance by only 100 kcal/day could prevent weight gain in 90% of adults. Wang *et al.* [146] found that approximately 150 kcal/day could prevent excessive weight gain in most children.

Once individuals are obese, the real challenge is not in producing weight loss but in preventing weight gain after weight loss. It seems that larger lifestyle changes are required to prevent weight gain after weight loss than to prevent weight gain from occurring in the first place. There has been surprisingly little research on obesity prevention, and to date, prevention efforts have met with modest success at best. Although obesity prevention can be targeted as a high priority, there is much to learn about how to do it effectively.

It is becoming clear that preventing weight gain requires attention not only to individual behavior change but also to the larger environmental and societal factors that ultimately influence an individual's behavior. The current environment in the United States promotes weight gain and obesity by encouraging excessive food consumption and discouraging physical activity. We live in an environment that has an abundance of cheap, good-tasting, energy-dense foods but requires little physical exertion for day-to-day living. It is difficult for individuals in this environment to consistently maintain behaviors that would support a healthy body weight.

Making the permanent changes in diet and physical activity needed to achieve and sustain a healthy body weight requires a desire and commitment to change: How can we better instigate that desire in people? Similarly, how can we create the motivation to create the changes necessary in our physical and social environments? As we are learning more about "what to do," we cannot ignore the "why do people want to do it" question.

Reducing obesity levels will require concerted efforts to address behavior and the environment. At the same time, an appreciation of the biology of obesity is needed because the interventions that work with and not against human biology may be more successful. Despite the daunting nature of this task, the rapidity of the increase in obesity underscores the urgency to address the issue.

References

[1] World Health Organization (2011). "Obesity and Overweight Fact Sheet." Available at <http://www.who.int/mediacentre/factsheets/fs311/en/index.html>. Accessed September 2011.

[2] K.M. Flegal, M.D. Carroll, C.L. Ogden, L.R. Curtin, Prevalence and trends in obesity among U.S.: 1999–2008, JAMA 303 (2010) 235–241.

[3] A. Must, J. Spadano, E.H. Coakley, A.E. Field, G. Colditz, W.H. Dietz, The disease burden associated with overweight and obesity, JAMA 282 (1999) 1523–1529.

[4] J.L. Pomeranz, K.D. Brownell, Advancing public health obesity policy through state attorneys general, Am. J. Public Health 19 (2011) 74–82.

[5] National Heart, Lung, and Blood Institute, Obesity Education Initiative Expert Panel, Clinical guidelines on the identification, evaluation, and treatment of overweight and obesity in adults: the evidence report, Obes. Res. 6 (Suppl. 2) (1998) 51S–209S.

[6] Metropolitan Life Insurance Company, Metropolitan height and weight tables, Stat. Bull. Met. Life Ins. Co. 64 (1983) 2.

[7] S. Stensland, S. Margolis, Simplifying the calculation of body mass index for quick reference, J. Am. Diet. Assoc. 90 (1990) 1372.

[8] S.B. Heymsfield, D.B. Allison, S. Heshka, R.N. Pierson, Handbook of Assessment Methods for Eating Behavior and Weight Related Problems: Measures, Theory, and Research, Sage, Thousand Oaks, CA, 1995, pp. 515–560.

[9] J.E. Manson, W.C. Willett, M.J. Stampfer, G.A. Colditz, D.J. Hunter, S.E. Hankinson, et al., Body weight and mortality among women, N. Engl. J. Med. 333 (1995) 677–685.

[10] E.A. Lew, L. Garfinkel, Variations in mortality by weight among 750,000 men and women, J. Chronic Dis. 32 (1979) 563–576.

[11] T. Gordon, J.T. Doyle, Weight and mortality in men: The Albany Study, Int. J. Epidemiol. 17 (1988) 77–81.

[12] D. Gallagher, M. Visser, D. Sepulveda, R.N. Pierson, T. Harris, S.B. Heymsfield, How useful is body mass index for comparison of body fatness across age, sex, and ethnic groups? Am. J. Epidemiol. 143 (1996) 228–239.

[13] G.A. Bray, Health hazards of obesity, Endocrinol. Metab. Clin. North Am. 4 (1996) 907–919.

[14] J. Seidel, Epidemiology: Definition and classification of obesity, in: P.G. Kopleman, M.J. Stock (Eds), Clinical Obesity, Blackwell, Malden, MA, 1998, pp. 1–17.

[15] J.P. Despres, S. Moorjani, P.J. Lupien, A. Tremblay, A. Nadeau, C. Bouchard, Regional distribution of body fat, plasma lipoproteins, and cardiovascular disease, Arteriosclerosis 10 (1990) 497–511.

[16] S. Lemieux, D. Prud'homme, C. Bouchard, A. Tremblay, J.P. Despres, A single threshold value of waist girth identifies normal-weight and overweight subjects with excess visceral adipose tissue, Am. J. Clin. Nutr. 64 (1996) 685–693.

[17] C.E. Lewis, D.R. Jacobs, H. McCreath, C.I. Kiefe, P.J. Schreiner, D.E. Smith, et al., Weight gain continues in the 1990s: 10 year trends in weight and overweight from the CARDIA study, Am. J. Epidemiol. 151 (2000) 1172–1181.

[18] Expert Panel on Detection, Evaluation and Treatment of High Blood Cholesterol in Adults, Executive summary of the third report of the National Cholesterol Education Program (NCEP) Expert Panel on the Detection, Evaluation and Treatment of High Blood Cholesterol in Adults (Adult Treatment Panel III)., JAMA 285 (2001) 2486–2497.

[19] K.D. Brownell, Dieting readiness, Weight Control Digest 1 (1990) 1–9.

[20] G.A. Bray, The dieting readiness test, Contemporary Diagnosis and Management of Obesity, Handbooks in Health Care, Newtown, PA, 1998 (pp. A1–A7).

[21] J.O. Hill, Energy metabolism and obesity, in: B. Drazin, R. Rizza (Eds.), Clinical Research in Diabetes and Obesity, Vol. II: Diabetes and Obesity, Humana Press, Totowa, NJ, 1997, pp. 3–12.

[22] North American Association for the Study of Obesity, The Practical Guide to the Identification, Evaluation, and Treatment of Overweight and Obese Adults, National Institutes of Health, National Heart, Lung, and Blood Institute, Bethesda, MD, 1998.

[23] R. Wing, R. Koeske, Z.L. Epstein, M.P. Norwalk, W. Gooding, D. Becker, Long-term effects of modest weight loss in type II diabetic patients, Arch. Intern. Med. 147 (1987) 1749–1753.

[24] D.J. Goldstein, A.H. Rampey, P.J. Roback, M.G. Wilson, S.H. Hamilton, M.E. Sayler, et al., Efficacy and safety of long-term fluoxetine treatment of obesity: maximizing success, Obes. Res. 3 (Suppl. 4) (1995) 481S–490S.

[25] A.M. Dattilo, P.M. Kris-Etherton, Effects of weight reduction on blood lipids and lipoproteins: a meta-analysis, Am. J. Clin. Nutr. 56 (1992) 320–328.

[26] G.D. Foster, T.A. Wadden, R.A. Vogt, G. Brewer, What is a reasonable weight loss? Patients' expectations and evaluations of obesity treatment outcomes, J. Consult. Clin. Psychol. 65 (1997) 79–85.

[27] M.L. Klem, R.R. Wing, M.T. McGuire, H.M. Seagle, J.O. Hill, A descriptive study of individuals successful at long-term maintenance of substantial weight loss, Am. J. Clin. Nutr. 66 (1997) 239–246.

[28] J. Kruger, D.A. Galuska, M.K. Serdula, D.A. Jones, Attempting to lose weight: specific practices among U.S. adults, Am. J. Prev. Med. 26 (5) (2004) 402–406.

[29] A. Tatiana, M.W. Long, K.E. Henderson, G.M. Grode, Trying to lose weight: diet strategies among Americans with overweight or obesity in 1996 and 2003, J. Am. Diet. Assoc. 110 (2010) 535–542.

[30] M. Elia, R.J. Stubbs, C.J.K. Henry, Differences in fat, carbohydrate, and protein metabolism between lean and obese subjects undergoing total starvation, Obes. Res. 7 (1999) 597–604.

[31] T.B. VanItallie, Treatment of obesity: Can it become a science? Obes. Res. 7 (1999) 605–606.

[32] Food and Agricultural Organization/World Health Organization/United Nations University, Report of a Joint Expert Consultation: Energy and Protein Requirement of Adults, World Health Organization, Geneva, 1985 (Technical Report No. 724).

[33] D.A. Schoeller, L.G. Bandini, W.H. Dietz, Inaccuracies in self-reported intake identified by comparison with the doubly labeled water method, Can. J. Physiol. Pharmacol. 68 (1989) 941–949.

[34] S.W. Lichtman, K. Pisarska, E.R. Berman, M. Pestone, H. Dowling, E. Offenbacher, et al., Discrepancy between self-reported and actual caloric intake and exercise in obese subjects, N. Engl. J. Med. 327 (1992) 1893–1898.

[35] The Look AHEAD Research Group, The Look AHEAD study: A description of the lifestyle intervention and the evidence supporting it, Obesity 14 (2006) 737–752.

[36] National Task Force on the Prevention and Treatment of Obesity, Very low-calorie diets, JAMA 270 (1993) 967–974.

[37] W.H.M. Saris, Very-low-calorie diets and sustained weight loss, Obes. Res. 9 (2001) 295S–301S.

[38] T.A. Wadden, Treatment of obesity by moderate and severe caloric restriction: Results of clinical research trials, Ann. Intern. Med. 119 (1993) 688–693.

[39] J.W. Anderson, E.C. Konz, R.C. Frederich, C.L. Wood, Long-term weight-loss maintenance: a meta-analysis of U.S. studies, Am. J. Clin. Nutr. 74 (2001) 579–584.

[40] R.R. Wing, Don't throw out the baby with the bathwater: a commentary on very-low-calorie diets, Diabetes Care 15 (1992) 293–296.

[41] A.G. Tsai, T.A. Wadden, The evolution of very-low-calorie diets: an update and meta-analysis, Obes. Res. 14 (2006) 1283–1293.

[42] D. Heber, J.M. Ashley, H.J. Wang, R.M. Elashoff, Clinical evaluation of a minimal intervention meal replacement regimen for weight reduction, J. Am. Coll. Nutr. 13 (1994) 608–614.

[43] H.H. Ditschuneit, M. Flechtner-Mors, T.D. Johnson, G. Adler, Metabolic and weight-loss effects of a long-term dietary intervention in obese patients, Am. J. Clin. Nutr. 69 (1999) 198–204.

[44] S.B. Heymsfield, C.A. van Mierlo, H.C. van der Knaap, M. Heo, H.I. Frier, Weight management using a meal replacement strategy: meta and pooling analysis from six studies, Int. J. Obes. 27 (2003) 537–549.

[45] D. Quinn Rothacker, Five-year self-management of weight using meal replacements: comparison with matched controls in rural Wisconsin, Nutrition 16 (2000) 344–348.

[46] L. Lissner, D.A. Levitsky, B.J. Strupp, H.J. Kalkwarf, D.A. Roe, Dietary fat and the regulation of energy intake in human subjects, Am. J. Clin. Nutr. 46 (1987) 886–892.

[47] E.A. Bell, V.A. Castellanos, C.L. Pelkman, M.L. Thorwart, B.J. Rolls, Energy density of foods affects energy intake in normal-weight women, Am. J. Clin. Nutr. 67 (1998) 412–420.

[48] B.J. Rolls, L.S. Roe, J.S. Meengs, Reductions in portion size and energy density of foods are additive and lead to sustained decreases in energy intake, Am. J. Clin. Nutr. 83 (2006) 11–17.

[49] J.H. Ledikwe, B.J. Rolls, H. Smiciklas-Wright, D.C. Mitchell, J.D. Ard, C. Champagne, et al., Reductions in dietary energy density are associated with weight loss in overweight and obese participants in the PREMIER trial, Am. J. Clin. Nutr. 85 (2007) 1212–1221.

[50] J.A. Ello-Martin, L.S. Roe, J.H. Ledikwe, A.M. Beach, B.J. Rolls, Dietary energy density in the treatment of obesity: a year-long trial comparing 2 weight-loss diets, Am. J. Clin. Nutr. 85 (2007) 1465–1477.

[51] A.H. Lichtenstein, L.J. Appel, M. Brands, M. Carnetho, S. Daniels, H.A. Franch, et al., Diet and lifestyle recommendations revision 2006: a scientific statement from the American Heart Association Nutrition Committee, Circulation 114 (2006) 82–96.

[52] Finnish Diabetes Prevention Study Group, Sustained reduction in the incidence of type 2 diabetes by lifestyle intervention: follow-up of the Finnish Diabetes Prevention Study, Lancet 368 (2006) 1673–1679.

[53] Diabetes Prevention Program Research Group, Reduction in the incidence of type 2 diabetes with lifestyle intervention or metformin, N. Engl. J. Med. 346 (2002) 393–403.

[54] The Look AHEAD Research Group, Reduction in weight and cardiovascular disease risk factors in individuals with type 2 diabetes: one-year results of the Look AHEAD trial, Diabetes Care 30 (2007) 1374–1383.

[55] L.J. Appel, C.M. Champagne, D.W. Harsha, L.S. Cooper, E. Obarzanek, P.J. Elmer, , et al. Writing Group of the PREMIER Collaborative Research Group, Effects of the comprehensive lifestyle modification on blood pressure control: main results of the PREMIER clinical trial, JAMA 289 (2003) 2083–2093.

[56] The Look AHEAD Research Group, Long-term effects of a lifestyle intervention on weight and cardiovascular risk factors in individuals with type 2 diabetes mellitus, Arch. Intern. Med. 170 (2010) 1566–1575.

[57] J.E. Blundell, R.J. Stubbs, High and low carbohydrate and fat intakes: limits imposed by appetite and palatability and their implications for energy balance, Eur. J. Clin. Nutr. 53 (1999) S148–S165.

[58] B.J. Brehm, R.J. Seeley, S.R. Daniels, D.A. D'Alessio, A randomized trial comparing a very low carbohydrate diet and a calorie-restricted low fat diet on body weight and cardiovascular risk factors in healthy women, J. Clin. Endocrinol. Metab. 88 (2003) 1617–1623.

[59] G.D. Foster, H.R. Wyatt, J.O. Hill, B.G. McGuckin, C. Brill, S. Mohammed, et al., A multi-center, randomized, controlled clinical trial of the Atkins diet, N. Engl. J. Med. 348 (2003) 282–290.

[60] A.J. Nordmann, A. Nordmann, M. Briel, U. Keller, W.S. Yancy, B. J. Brehm, et al., Effects of low-carbohydrate vs. low-fat diets on weight loss and cardiovascular risk factors: a meta-analysis of randomized controlled trials, Arch. Intern. Med. 166 (2006) 285–293.

[61] M.L. Dansinger, J.A. Gleason, J.L. Griffith, H.P. Selker, E.J. Schaefer, Comparison of the Atkins, Ornish, Weight Watchers, and Zone diets for weight loss and heart disease risk reduction: a randomized trial, JAMA 293 (2005) 43–53.

[62] C.D. Gardner, A Kiazand, S. Alhassan, S. Kim, R.S. Stafford, R.R. Balise, et al., Comparison of the Atkins, Zone, Ornish and LEARN diet for change in weight and related risk factors among overweight premenopausal women, JAMA 297 (2007) 969–977.

[63] F.M. Sacks, G.A. Bray, V.J. Carey, S.R. Smith, D.H. Ryan, S.D. Amon, et al., Comparison of weight-loss diets with different compositions of fat, protein, and carbohydrates, N. Engl. J. Med. 260 (2009) 859–873.

[64] G.D. Foster, H.R. Wyatt, J.O. Hill, A.P. Makris, D.L. Rosenbaum, C. Brill, et al., Weight and metabolic outcomes after 2 years on a low-carbohydrate versus low-fat diet, Ann. Intern. Med. 153 (2010) 147–157.

[65] D. Arterburn, The BBC diet trials: reality television and academic researchers jointly tackle the weight loss industry, BMJ 332 (2006) 1284–1285.

[66] J.P. Ikeda, D. Hayes, E. Satter, E.S. Parham, K. Kratina, M. Woolsey, et al., A commentary on the new obesity guidelines from NIH, J. Am. Diet. Assoc. 99 (1999) 918–919.

[67] L. Higgins, W. Gray, What do anti-dieting programs achieve? A review of research, Aust. J. Nutr. Diet. 56 (1999) 128–136.

[68] G.D. Foster, D.B. Sarwer, T.A. Wadden, Psychological effects of weight cycling in obese persons: a review and research agenda, Obes. Res. 5 (1997) 474–488.

[69] U.S. Department of Health and Human Services (2008). "Physical Activity Guidelines for Americans." Available at <http://www.health.gov/paguidelines/guidelines/default.aspx>. Accessed 01.02.2012.

[70] J.E. Donnelly, S.N. Blair, J.M. Jakcic, M.M. Manore, J.W. Rankin, B. K. Smith, American College of Sports Medicine Position Stand: appropriate physical activity intervention strategies for weight loss and prevention of weight regain for adults, Med. Sci. Sports Exer. 41 (2009) 459–471.

[71] J.J. Zachwieja, Exercise as treatment for obesity, Endocrinol. Metab. Clin. North Am. 25 (4) (1996) 965–988.

[72] D.A. Schoeller, K. Shay, R.F. Kushner, How much physical activity is needed to minimize weight gain in previously obese women? Am. J. Clin. Nutr. 66 (1997) 551–556.

[73] J.M. Jakicic, A.D. Otto, Treatment and prevention of obesity: What is the role of exercise? Nutr. Rev. 64 (2006) S57–S61.

[74] J.O. Hill, H.R. Wyatt, G.W. Reed, J.C. Peters, Obesity and the environment: Where do we go from here? Science 299 (2003) 853–855.

[75] G.D. Foster, A.P. Makris, B.A. Bailer, Behavioral treatment of obesity, Am. J. Clin. Nutr. 82 (2005) 230s–235s.

[76] K.N. Boutelle, D.S. Kirshenbaum, Further support for consistent self-monitoring as a vital component of successful weight control, Obes. Res. 6 (1998) 219–224.

[77] K.J. Streit, N.H. Stevens, V.J. Stevens, J. Rossner, Food records: a predictor and modifier of weight change in a long-term weight loss program, J. Am. Diet. Assoc. 91 (1991) 213–216.

[78] K.N. Boutelle, D.S. Kirshenbaum, R.C. Baker, M.E. Mitchell, How can obese weight controllers minimize weight gain during high risk holiday season? By self-monitoring very consistently, Health Pyschol. 18 (1999) 364–368.

[79] R.R. Wing, D.F. Tate, A.A. Gorin, H.A. Raynor, J.L. Fava, Can we STOP weight regain? Results of a randomized trial, N. Engl. J. Med. 355 (2006) 1563–1571.

[80] R.R. Wing, D.F. Tate, A.A. Gorin, H.A. Raynor, J.L. Fava, "STOP Regain": Are there negative effects of daily weighing? J. Consult. Clin. Psychol. 75 (2007) 652–656.

[81] M.L. Butryn, V. Webb, T.A. Wadden, Behavioral treatment of obesity, Psychiatr. Clin. North Am. 34 (2011) 841–859.

[82] J.P. Foreyt, W.S. Poston II, The role of the behavioral counselor in obesity treatment, J. Am. Diet. Assoc. 98 (1998) S27–S30.

[83] B. Van Dorsten, E.M. Lindley, Cognitive and behavioral approaches in the treatment of obesity, Endocrinol. Metab. Clin. North Am. 37 (2008) 905–922.

[84] Look AHEAD (2012). "Lifestyle Intervention—Year 1." Available at <https://www.lookaheadtrial.org/public/dspMaterials.cfm>. Accessed January 2012.

[85] Diabetes Prevention Program (1996). "DPP Lifestyle Materials for Sessions 1–16: Standard Participant Handouts." Available at <http://www.bsc.gwu.edu/dpp/lifestyle/dpp_part.html>. Accessed January 2012.

[86] J. Hayaki, K.D. Brownell, Behaviour change in practice: group approaches, Int. J. Obes. 20 (1996) S27–S30.

[87] D.A. Renjilian, M.G. Perri, A.M. Nezu, W.F. McKelvey, R.L. Sherner, S.D. Anton, Individual versus group therapy for obesity: effects of matching participants to their treatment preferences, J. Consult. Clin. Psychol. 69 (2001) 717–721.

[88] A. Frank, A multidisciplinary approach to obesity management: the physician's role and team care alternatives, J. Am. Diet. Assoc. 98 (1998) S44–S48.

[89] J. Jordan, M. Schlaich, J. Redon, K. Narkiewicz, F.C. Luft, G. Grassi, et al. for the European Society of Hypertension Working Group on Obesity and the Australian and New Zealand Obesity Society, European Society of Hypertension Working Group on Obesity: obesity drugs and cardiovascular outcomes, J. Hypertens. 29 (2011) 189–193.

[90] G.A. Bray, D.H. Ryan, Drug treatment of the overweight patient, Gastroenterology 132 (2007) 2239–2252.

[91] A. Astrup, H.L. Hansen, C. Lundsgaard, S. Toubro, Sibutramine and energy balance, Int. J. Obes. 22 (Suppl. 1) (1998) S30–S35.

[92] D.H. Ryan, Medicating the obese patient, Endocrinol. Metab. Clin. North Am. 25 (1996) 989–1004.

[93] G.A. Bray, F.L. Greenway, Current and potential drugs for treatment of obesity, Endocrinol. Rev. 20 (6) (1999) 805–875.

[94] E.J. Hendricks, R.B. Rothman, F.L. Greenway, How physician obesity specialists use drugs to treat obesity, Obesity 17 (2009) 1730–1735.

[95] J. Zhi, A.T. Melia, R. Guerciolini, J. Chung, J. Kingberg, J.R. Hauptman, Retrospective population-based analysis of the dose–response (fecal fat excretion) relationship of orlistat in normal and obese volunteers, Clin. Pharmacol. Ther. 56 (1994) 82–85.

[96] J.O. Hill, J. Hauptman, J.W. Anderson, K. Fujioka, P.M. O'Neil, D.K. Smith, et al., Orlistat, a lipase inhibitor, for weight maintenance after conventional dieting: A 1-y study, Am. J. Clin. Nutr. 69 (1999) 1108–1116.

[97] M.H. Davidson, J. Hauptman, M. Di Girolamo, J.P. Foreyt, C. H. Halsted, D. Heber, et al., Weight control and risk factor reduction in obese subjects treated with orlistat: a randomized, controlled trial, JAMA 281 (1999) 235–242.

[98] W.P.T. James, A. Avenell, J. Broom, J. Whitehead, A one-year trial to assess the value of orlistat in the management of obesity, Int. J. Obes. Metab. Disord. 21 (Suppl) (1997) 24–30.

[99] J.O. Hill, H.R. Wyatt, The efficacy of orlistat (Xenical) in promoting weight loss and preventing weight regain, Curr. Prac. Med. 2 (11) (1999) 228–231.

[100] L.M. Sjostrom, A. Rissanen, T. Andersen, M. Boldrin, A. Golay, H.P. Koppeschaar, , et al.for the European Multi-Center Orlistat Study Group, Randomised placebo-controlled trial of orlistat for weight loss and prevention of weight regain in obese patients, Lancet 352 (1998) 167–172.

[101] J.S. Torgerson, M.N. Boldrin, J. Hauptman, L. Sjostrom, XENical in the prevention of Diabetes in Obese Subjects (XENDOS) study, Diabetes Care 27 (2004) 155–161.

[102] L.F. Van Gaal, J.I. Broom, G. Enzi, H. Toplak, for the Orlistat Dose-Ranging Group, Efficacy and tolerability of orlistat in the treatment of obesity: a 6-month dose ranging study, Eur. J. Clin. Pharmacol. 54 (1998) 125–132.

[103] J. Anderson, S. Schwartz, J. Hauptman, M. Boldrin, M. Rossi, V. Bansal, et al., Low-dose orlistat effects on body weight on mildly to moderately overweight individuals: a 16-week, double-blind, placebo-controlled trial, Ann. Pharmacol. 40 (2006) 1717–1723.

[104] S. Rossner, L. Sjostrom, R. Noack, E. Meinders, G. Noseda, Weight loss, weight maintenance, and improved cardiovascular risk factors after 2 years treatment with orlistat for obesity, Obes. Res. 8 (2000) 49–61.

[105] J. Hauptman, C. Lucas, M.N. Boldrin, H. Collins, K. Segal, for the Orlistat Primary Care Study, Orlistat in the long-term treatment of obesity in the primary care setting, Arch. Fam. Med. 9 (2000) 160–167.

[106] L.L. Darga, L. Carroll-Michals, S.J. Botsford, C.P. Lucas, Fluoxetine's effects on weight loss in obese subjects, Am. J. Clin. Nutr. 54 (1991) 321–325.

[107] J.W. Anderson, F.L. Greenway, K. Fujioka, K.M. Gadde, J. McKenney, P.M. O'Neil, Bupropion SR enhances weight loss: a 48-week double blinded, placebo controlled trial, Obes. Res. 10 (2002) 633–641.

[108] K.M. Gadde, D.M. Franciscy, H.R. Wagner II, K.R. Krishnan, Zonisamide for weight loss in obese adults: a randomized controlled trial, JAMA 289 (2003) 1820–1825.

[109] G.A. Bray, P. Hollander, S. Klein, R. Kushner, B. Levy, M. Fitchet, et al., A 6 month randomized placebo controlled dose ranging study of topiramate for weight loss in obesity, Obes. Res. 11 (2003) 722–733.

[110] J. Wilding, L.F. Van Gaal, A. Rissanen, F. Vercruysse, M. Fitchet, A randomized double-blinded placebo-controlled study of the long-term efficacy and safety of topiramate in the treatment of obese subjects, Int. J. Obes. Rel. Metab. Disord. 28 (2004) 1399–1410.

[111] A. Astrup, I. Caterson, P. Zelissen, B Guy-Grand, M. Carruba, B. Levy, et al., Topiramate: long-term maintenance of weight loss induced by a low calorie diet in obese subjects, Obes. Res. 12 (2004) 1658–1669.

[112] N.A. Shapira, T.D. Goldsmith, S.L. McElroy, Treatment of binge eating disorder with topiramate: a clinical case series, J. Clin. Psychiatry 61 (2000) 368–372.

[113] S.L. McElroy, L.M. Arnold, N.A. Shapira, P.E. Keck Jr., N.R. Rosenthal, M.R. Karim, et al., Topiramate in the treatment of binge eating disorder associated with obesity: a randomized placebo controlled trial, Am. J. Psychiatry 160 (2003) 255–261.

[114] S.A. Smathers, J.G. Wilson, M.A. Nigro, Topiramate effectiveness in Prader–Willi syndrome, Pediatr. Neurol. 28 (2003) 130–133.

[115] R. Sturm, Increases in morbid obesity in the USA: 2000–2005, Public Health 121 (2007) 492–496.

[116] Y. Zhao, W. Encinosa, Bariatric Surgery Utilizatation and Outcomes in 1998 and 2004, Agency for Healthcare Research and Quality, Rockville, MD, 2007 (Statistical Brief No. 23).

[117] J. Colquitt, A. Clegg, E. Lovemen, P. Royle, M.K. Sidhu, Surgery for morbid obesity, Cochrane Database Syst. Rev. 4 (2005) CD003641.

[118] R. Kuruba, L.S. Koche, M.M. Murr, Pre-operative assessment and perioperative care of patients undergoing bariatric surgery, Med. Clin. North Am. 91 (2007) 339–351.

[119] C.L. Ogden, K.M. Flegal, M.D. Carroll, C.L. Johnson, Prevalence and trends in overweight among U.S. children and adolescents, 1999–2000, JAMA 288 (2002) 1728–1732.

[120] Institute of Medicine, Progress in Preventing Childhood Obesity: How Do We Measure Up? Government Printing Office, Washington, DC, 2006 (Report brief).

[121] S.R. Daniels, D.K. Arnett, R.H. Eckel, S.S. Gidding, L.L. Hayman, S. Kumanyika, et al., Overweight in children and adolescents: pathophysiology, consequences, prevention, and treatment, Circulation 111 (2005) 1999–2012.

[122] N.F. Krebs, J.H. Himes, D. Jacobsen, T.A Nicklas, P. Guilday, D. Styne, Assessment of child and adolescent overweight and obesity, Pediatrics 120 (2007) S193–S228.

[123] R.M.. Puhl, J. Luedicke, C. Heuer, Weight-based victimization toward overweight adolescents: observations and reactions of peers, J. School Health 81 (2011) 696–703.

[124] Centers for Disease Control and Prevention (2010). "CDC Growth Charts." Available at <http://www.cdc.gov/growthcharts/cdc_charts.htm>. Accessed January 2012.

[125] R.M. Puhl, J.L. Peterson, J. Luedicke, Parental perceptions of weight terminology that providers use with youth, Pediatrics 120 (2011) 786–793.

[126] S.E. Barlow, the Expert Committee, Expert committee recommendations regarding the prevention, assessment, and treatment of child and adolescent overweight and obesity: summary report, Pediatrics 120 (2007) S164–S192.

[127] W.H. Dietz, T.N. Robinson, Overweight children and adolescents, N. Engl. J. Med. 352 (2005) 2100–2109.

[128] R.C. Whitaker, J.A. Wright, M.S. Pepe, K.D. Seidel, W.H. Dietz, Predicting obesity in young adulthood from childhood and parental obesity, N. Engl. J. Med. 337 (1997) 869–873.

[129] D.E. Wilfley, T.L. Tibbs, D.J. Van Buren, K.P. Reach, M.S. Walker, L.H. Epstein, Lifestyle interventions in the treatment of childhood overweight: a meta-analytic review of randomized controlled trials, Health Psychol. 26 (2007) 521–532.

[130] K.M. Kitzman, W.T. Dalton, C.M. Stanley, B.M. Beech, T.P. Reeves, J. Buscemi, et al., Lifestyle interventions for youth who are overweight: a meta-analytic review, Health Psychol. 29 (2010) 91–101.

[131] S.R. Daniels, M.S. Jacobsen, B.W. McCrindle, R.H. Eckel, B.M. Sanner, American Heart Association childhood obesity research summit: executive summary, Circulation 119 (2009) 2114–2123.

[132] M.S. Faith, L. Van Horn, L.J. Appel, L.E. Burke, J.S. Carson, H. A. Franch, et al., A scientific statement from the American Heart Association: evaluating parents and adult caregivers as "agents of change" for treating obese children: evidence for parent behavior change strategies and research gaps, Circulation 125 (2012) 1186–1207.

[133] TODAY Study Group, Design of a family-based lifestyle intervention for youth with type 2 diabetes: the TODAY study, Int. J. Obes. 34 (2010) 217–226.

[134] TODAY Study Group (2010). "Treatment Options for Type 2 Diabetes in Adolescents and Youth." Available at <https://today.bsc.gwu.edu/web/today/home>. Accessed January 2012.

[135] L.D. Ritchie, P.B. Crawford, D.M. Hoelscher, M.S. Sothern, Position of the American Dietetic Association: individual-, family-, school-, and community-based interventions for pediatric overweight, J. Am. Diet. Assoc. 106 (2006) 925–945.

[136] L.L. Birch, J.O. Fisher, Development of eating behaviors among children and adolescents, Pediatrics 101 (1998) 539–549.

[137] E.M. Satter, Internal regulation and the evolution of normal growth as the basis for prevention of obesity in children, J. Am. Diet. Assoc. 96 (1996) 860–864.

[138] J.O. Hill, J.C. Peters, Environmental contributions to the obesity epidemic, Science 280 (1998) 1371–1374.

[139] L.H. Epstein, R.A. Paluch, C.C. Gordy, J. Dorn, Decreasing sedentary behaviors in treating pediatric obesity, Arch. Pediatr. Adolesc. Med. 154 (2000) 220–226.

[140] T.N. Robinson, Reducing children's television viewing to prevent obesity, JAMA 282 (1999) 1561–1567.

[141] M. Story, School-based approaches for preventing and treating obesity, Int. J. Obes. 22 (1999) S43–S51.

[142] P.J. Veugelers, A.L. Fitzgerald, Effectiveness of school programs in preventing childhood obesity: a multilevel comparison, Am. J. Public Health 95 (2005) 432–435.

[143] G.D. Foster, E.G. Ford, L. Rosen, S. Solomon, A. Virus, School-based prevention of childhood overweight and obesity, in: C.A. Nonas, G.D. Foster (Eds), Managing Obesity: A Clinical Guide, second ed., American Dietetic Association, Chicago, 2009, pp. 241–259.

[144] G.D. Foster, S. Sherman, K.E. Borradaile, K.M. Grundy, S.S. Vander Veur, J. Nachmani, et al., A policy-based school intervention to prevent overweight and obesity, Pediatrics 121 (2008) 794–802.

[145] Centers for Disease Control and Prevention (2012). "Adolescent and School Health: School Health Index." Available at <http://www.cdc.gov/HealthyYouth/shi>. Accessed January 2012.

[146] Y.C. Wang, S.L. Gortmaker, A.M. Sobol, K.M. Kuntz, Estimating the energy gap among U.S. children: a counterfactual approach, Pediatrics 118 (2006) 1721–1733.

CHAPTER

25

Surgery for Severe Obesity

Robert F. Kushner, Holly Herrington

Northwestern University Feinberg School of Medicine, Chicago, Illinois

I INTRODUCTION

Various expert panels have endorsed bariatric surgery as an acceptable weight-loss option for patients with a body mass index (BMI) $\geq 40\,kg/m^2$ or those with a BMI $\geq 35\,kg/m^2$ who have co-morbid conditions [1–4]. An international survey of 36 nations or national groups estimated that more than 344,000 bariatric surgery operations were performed in 2008; 220,000 of these operations were performed in the United States or Canada [5]. The exponential growth in procedures is due to several factors, including: improved surgical techniques, reduction in the postoperative mortality rate, significant improvement in obesity-related co-morbid conditions [4], increased media attention, and increased profitability. The upsurge in surgical procedures also reflects the increasing prevalence of severe obesity in the United States. Between 1986 and 2000, the prevalence of severe obesity (BMI $\geq 40\,kg/m^2$) quadrupled from approximately 1 in 200 adult Americans to 1 in 50; the prevalence of a BMI ≥ 50 increased by a factor of 5, from approximately 1 in 2000 to 1 in 400 [6]. Nearly 6% of adult Americans are considered severely obese, with prevalence figures reaching 14% for African American women [7]. Many of the weight-loss surgeries, most notably the combined restrictive–malabsorptive surgical procedures, place patients at high risk for development of both macro- and micronutrient deficiencies unless they are properly counseled and supplemented. Because most of the deficiencies can be identified early at a preclinical stage, early treatment will prevent or reduce symptoms and deficiency syndromes. Although bariatric surgery does not cure obesity, it is considered a significant tool for weight loss and maintenance of weight loss. As such, patients are at risk to experience weight regain several years following surgery. This chapter reviews the most commonly performed weight-loss procedures, the importance of preoperative and postoperative management, the identification and management of nutritional deficiencies that may occur following bariatric surgery, and factors associated with weight regain.

II BARIATRIC SURGICAL PROCEDURES

A Mechanisms of Action

Bariatric surgery results in weight loss and improvement of multiple co-morbid conditions. Depending on the surgical procedure performed, weight loss primarily occurs by reducing caloric intake, altering gastrointestinal physiology, and/or reducing nutrient absorption. Weight stability is achieved when caloric intake matches caloric expenditure. In contrast, improvement in co-morbid conditions is due to multiple interacting factors that are incompletely understood and effect changes in metabolism, pressure dynamics, and mechanics. Whereas some of the changes are brought about by diet and weight loss alone, others are the result of anatomical and physiological changes of the gastrointestinal tract. The loss of fat mass, particularly visceral fat, is associated with multiple metabolic, adipokine, and inflammatory changes that include improved insulin sensitivity and glucose disposal, reduced free fatty acid flux, increased adiponectin levels, and decreased interleukin-6, tumor necrosis factor-α, and high-sensitivity C-reactive protein levels. Loss of visceral fat may also reduce intra-abdominal pressure that may be related to urinary incontinence, gastroesophageal reflux, and hypoventilation [8]. Metabolic effects resulting from bypassing the foregut include altered responses of ghrelin, glucagon-like peptide-1 (GLP-1), and peptide YY_{3-36} —gut hormones involved in glucose regulation and appetite control [9].

Nutrition in the Prevention and Treatment of Disease, Third Edition.
DOI: http://dx.doi.org/10.1016/B978-0-12-391884-0.00025-1

Fluid and hemodynamic changes related to hypertension include diuresis, naturesis, reduced total body water and blood volume, and decreased indices of sympathetic activity. Mechanical improvements include less weight bearing on joints, improved lung compliance, and reduced bulky fatty tissue around the neck to relieve obstruction to breathing. Depending on the co-morbid condition, some or all of these changes may be responsible for improvement or resolution of the co-morbidity.

B Weight-Loss Surgeries

Weight-loss surgeries are classified into three categories: restrictive, restrictive—malabsorptive, and malabsorptive (Figure 25.1).

1 Restrictive Surgeries

Restrictive procedures limit the amount of food the stomach can hold and slow the rate of gastric emptying. The vertical banded gastroplasty (VBG) is the prototype of this category but is no longer performed due to limited effectiveness in long-term trials. Laparoscopic adjustable gastric banding (LAGB) has replaced the VBG as the most commonly performed restrictive operation. The first banding device, the LAP-BAND, was approved for use in the United States in 2001. A second device, the REALIZE band, was approved in the United States in 2007. In contrast to previous devices, the diameter of these bands is adjustable by way of their connection to a reservoir that is implanted under the skin. Injection or removal of saline into the reservoir tightens or loosens the band's internal diameter, respectively, thus changing the size of the gastric opening. Because there is no rerouting of the intestine with LAGB, the risk for developing nutritional deficiencies is entirely dependent on the patient's diet and eating habits. The third and most recently described restrictive procedure is the laparoscopic sleeve gastrectomy (LSG). In this procedure, the stomach is restricted by stapling and dividing it vertically and removing approximately 80% of the greater curvature, leaving a slim "banana-shaped" remnant stomach along the lesser curvature.

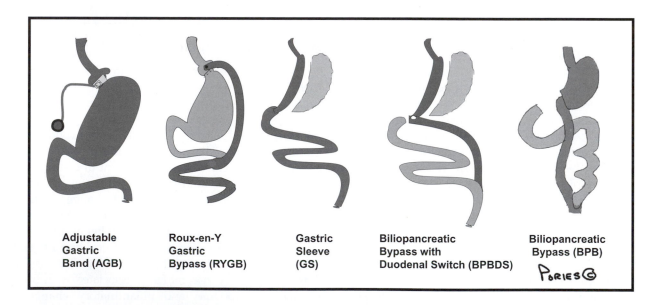

Adjustable Gastric Band (AGB) · Roux-en-Y Gastric Bypass (RYGB) · Gastric Sleeve (GS) · Biliopancreatic Bypass with Duodenal Switch (BPBDS) · Biliopancreatic Bypass (BPB)

PoriesⒼ

Doctor Robert Kushner has unlimited use of this drawing rendered by me and may publish it with his articles. I retain the copyright. October 11, 2011

Walter J. Pories

FIGURE 25.1   The five commonly accepted bariatric operations: laparoscopic adjustable gastric banding (AGB), Roux-en-Y gastric bypass (RYGB), laparoscopic gastric sleeve (GS), biliopancreatic bypass with duodenal switch (BPBDS), and biliopancreatic bypass (BPB). Source: *Reproduced with permission from Walter D. Pories. See color plate.*

2 Restrictive–Malabsorptive Surgeries

The restrictive–malabsorptive bypass procedure combines the elements of gastric restriction and selective malabsorption. The Roux-en-Y gastric bypass (RYGB) is the most commonly performed procedure. It involves formation of a 10- to 30-ml proximal gastric pouch by either surgically separating or stapling the stomach across the fundus. Outflow from the pouch is created by performing a narrow (10 mm) gastrojejunostomy. The distal end of jejunum is then anastomosed 50–150 cm below the gastrojejunostomy. "Roux-en-Y" refers to the Y-shaped section of small intestine created by the surgery; the Y is created at the point where the pancreobiliary conduit (afferent limb) and the Roux (efferent) limb are connected. "Bypass" refers to the exclusion or bypassing of the distal stomach, duodenum, and proximal jejunum. RYGB may be performed with an open incision or laparoscopically.

3 Malabsorptive Surgeries

There are two malabsorptive procedures. In the biliopancreatic diversion (BPD), a subtotal gastrectomy is performed, leaving a much larger gastric pouch compared with the RYGB. The small bowel is divided 250 cm proximal to the ileocecal valve and connected directly to the gastric pouch, producing a gastroileostomy. The remaining proximal limb (biliopancreatic conduit) is then anastomosed to the side of the distal ileum 50 cm proximal to the ileocecal valve. In this procedure, the distal stomach, duodenum, and entire jejunum are bypassed, leaving only a 50-cm distal ileum common channel for nutrients to mix with pancreatic and biliary secretions. The biliopancreatic diversion with duodenal switch (BPDDS) is a variation of the BPD that preserves the first portion of the duodenum. In this procedure, a vertical subtotal gastrectomy is performed and the duodenum is divided just beyond the pylorus. The distal small bowel is connected to the short stump of the duodenum, producing a 75- to 100-cm ileal–duodenal "common channel" for the absorption of nutrients. The other end of the duodenum is closed, and the remaining small bowel is connected onto the enteral limb approximately 75–100 cm from the ileocecal valve.

III CLINICAL ASPECTS

A Weight Loss

Several meta-analyses and systematic reviews of bariatric surgery outcomes have been conducted [10–12]. In general, weight loss is greatest with the malabsorptive procedures (BPD and BPDDS), followed by the restrictive–malabsorptive procedure (RYGB), and least with the restrictive procedures (LAGB and LSG). The percentage excess weight loss at 3–6 years is 62–81, 53–77, and 45–72% for each surgical type, respectively [13]. The trajectory of weight loss also differs between procedure types. Whereas the rate of weight loss is slower with LAGB, with maximal weight loss achieved after 2 or 3 years, maximal weight loss with RYGB is achieved at 12–18 months.

B Effects on Co-morbidities

A meta-analysis of controlled clinical trials comparing bariatric surgery versus no surgery showed that surgery was associated with a reduced odds ratio (OR) risk of global mortality (OR = 0.55), cardiovascular mortality (OR = 0.58), and all-cause mortality (OR = 0.70) [14]. Significant improvement in multiple obesity-related co-morbid conditions has been reported, including type 2 diabetes, hypertension, dyslipidemia, obstructive sleep apnea, and quality of life [15,16]. The beneficial effect of weight-loss surgery on type 2 diabetes is particularly striking. Observational studies have demonstrated a 60–80% rate of diabetes resolution with surgery [17,18]. Rates are greater following BPD or RYGB than following LAGB, and the extent of remission is influenced by the amount of weight loss, weight regain, duration of diabetes, and the presurgery hypoglycemic therapy requirements [19]. The mechanisms of the greater antidiabetic effect following RYGB are primarily thought to involve caloric restriction and enhanced release of the incretins GLP-1 and glucose insulinotropic polypeptide (GIP), affecting both insulin secretion and sensitivity [17].

IV PREOPERATIVE ASSESSMENT

A Overview

All patients who are considering weight-loss surgery should undergo a comprehensive assessment by a multidisciplinary team of health care providers that includes a physician, registered dietitian, and mental health care professional [13,20]. Preparation for surgery commonly spans 3–12 months depending on the patient's medical condition and criteria for insurance approval. During the preoperative process, patients are typically instructed on healthy eating and physical activity patterns, behavioral strategies to implement the lifestyle changes, and the importance of stress reduction and social support for long-term success. Specific dietary and nutritional recommendations pertinent to the surgical procedures include use of protein supplements, consumption of multiple meals and snacks, and slowing the rate of eating. Patients are seen either individually or in small groups. Many centers offer panel discussions between candidate patients and patients who have already undergone a procedure to provide a peer-to-peer discussion of risks, benefits, and challenges of life after bariatric surgery. Evidence-based recommendations for "best practice" patient care have been published [13,21].

B Indications for Bariatric Surgery

According to the 1991 National Institutes of Health Consensus Development Conference Panel on bariatric surgery [1], patients with a BMI $\geq 40 \, kg/m^2$ or those with a BMI $\geq 35 \, kg/m^2$ who have associated high-risk co-morbid conditions such as cardiopulmonary disease or type 2 diabetes could be considered surgical candidates. Consequently, Medicare and other third-party insurance payers have followed these criteria for reimbursement qualifications. The LAP-BAND system (Allergan, Irvine, CA), one of the LAGB products used in the United States, has been approved by the U.S. Food and Drug Administration for those with a BMI $\geq 30 \, kg/m^2$ with a related health condition. In addition to BMI and the presence of co-morbid conditions, other patient-related factors, such as psychosocial health, adherence, expectations, and past weight loss attempts, are taken into consideration. Contraindications include an extremely high operative risk, active substance abuse, or a major psychopathological condition such as major depressive disorder, schizophrenia, or bulimia.

C Medical Assessment

All patients need to undergo a comprehensive medical assessment prior to bariatric surgery. The purpose is to identify and optimally control medical problems prior to surgery. Patients with symptoms suggestive of obstructive sleep apnea (loud snoring, nighttime awakening, and morning and daytime sleepiness) should undergo a polysomnogram with initiation of continuous positive airway pressure (CPAP) if necessary. Patients with signs and symptoms of coronary artery disease or at high risk for cardiovascular disease should have a cardiac stress test performed. The two most common co-morbidities that require preoperative control are diabetes and hypertension. Many patients may require initiation of medications to control blood glucose and blood pressure levels, respectively. Patients should discontinue cigarette smoking at least 2 months prior to surgery to reduce respiratory complications. Due to the rapid change in patients' medical conditions after surgery, patients need to be closely managed postoperatively for medication dose adjustments.

D Dietary Assessment

Dietary management begins preoperatively through a series of assessments and screenings to determine the patient's current nutritional status, diet, education, existing medical conditions, and any potential psychological or physical behaviors that would impede the patient's weight-loss success postsurgery [13]. Nutrition management is closely related to the patient's weight-loss success; therefore, it is imperative to have a registered dietitian or other qualified nutrition expert as part of the comprehensive team. Nutrition assessment prior to bariatric surgery includes the current dietary intake, past weight-loss attempts, existing nutrient deficiencies, restaurant meal intake, and any disordered eating patterns. In addition to these basic questions, the comprehensive nutrition assessment also includes review of the patient's weight history, laboratory values and co-morbidities, general nutrition knowledge, motivation for behavior change, coping mechanisms, and social or economic concerns. The nutrition professional should develop dietary plans for both pre- and postsurgical success [22].

E Psychological Assessment

Psychological assessment should be performed by a licensed mental health professional prior to surgery. The evaluation serves two purposes: identification of potential contraindications to surgery, such as substance abuse or poorly treated depression or schizophrenia, and identification of potential postoperative problems, such as inability to adhere to behavioral changes needed for a successful outcome [13]. Patients presenting with depressive symptoms, anxiety, low self-esteem, or relationship issues often benefit from preoperative intervention and/or a delay in surgery.

V THE ROLE OF PREOPERATIVE WEIGHT LOSS

Although it is reasonable to encourage weight loss prior to surgery, the literature is conflicting regarding the benefit of mandating preoperative weight loss as a criterion to undergo surgery. The primary rationale for requiring routine preoperative weight loss is to decrease the short-term operative morbidity and mortality. Furthermore, the patient's motivation for and ability to adhere to the dietary restrictions considered essential for a successful surgical outcome could be assessed. Whereas 5–10% preoperative weight loss has been shown in some studies to reduce postoperative complications, hospital length of stay, and operating room time and improve 1-year weight loss, other studies have not shown a benefit in longer term weight-loss outcomes. An additional compelling reason to endorse preoperative weight loss is to optimize the operative field by reducing liver volume and visceral adipose tissue (VAT). Two prospective studies have confirmed the benefit of prescribing a very low-calorie liquid diet for 9–12 weeks on preoperative loss of body weight, VAT and subcutaneous adipose tissue, liver volume, and co-morbid risk factors [23,24]. Based on the existing literature, it is reasonable to include preoperative weight loss as an expectation during the preoperative period [25].

VI POSTOPERATIVE MANAGEMENT

A Medical and Surgical Considerations

Patients who have undergone weight-loss surgery require ongoing postoperative care. Medical monitoring includes frequent assessment of preexisting co-morbid conditions along with evaluation for postoperative complications. Patients with diabetes need to closely monitor their blood glucose levels because rapid resolution of diabetes frequently occurs following the RYGB and BPDDS procedures. Anti-diabetes medications are commonly reduced by half upon discharge from the hospital, and sulfonylurea agents—medications that may cause hypoglycemia—are discontinued entirely. Further reductions in anti-diabetes medications are made based on glucose control. Similarly, anti-hypertensive medications may need adjustment as blood pressure falls. Diuretic agents are discontinued upon discharge from the hospital because they may lead to dehydration and electrolyte abnormalities. Patients with obstructive sleep apnea will frequently experience an improvement in sleep quality and reduction in apneic–hypopneic episodes. A repeat sleep study and re-titration of CPAP is often performed 6 months postoperatively. Other preexisting medical problems, such as osteoarthritis, gastroesophageal reflux disease, urinary incontinence, asthma, heart disease, and hyperlipidemia, are managed according to symptoms or laboratory values [13,26].

Postoperative surgical care is necessary to ensure wound healing, surveillance for surgical complications, and, for patients who underwent LAGB, periodic tightening of the adjustable band. Food entrapment or vomiting suggests that the band is too tight and a need for loosening. Complications of the LAGB may include band slippage or erosion or fracture of the port and tubing. Complications from the RYGB procedure may include stenosis of the gastric outlet secondary to ulceration or scaring of the gastro-jejunal anastomosis. These complications are routinely treated by prescription of an acid blocker and endoscopic dilation under light sedation. Intestinal obstruction can occur after the RYGB or malabsorptive operations and requires urgent surgical intervention [13]. For these reasons, all patients should follow up with a physician who is knowledgeable about bariatric surgery.

B Diet Progression Post Bariatric Surgery

The primary focus of nutritional care after bariatric surgical procedures is to facilitate weight loss while reducing nutritional deficiencies, promote early satiety, and reduce occurrences of reflux and dumping syndrome (for patients who underwent RYGB). Patients receiving surgery require appropriate energy and nutritional needs to maintain a healthy body composition and avoid loss of muscle mass. A postsurgical diet is modified for food texture and consistency, volume; and frequency of meals and may be adjusted depending on food intolerances or nutrient deficiencies [15].

After bariatric surgery, food intake is suspended until gastrointestinal (GI) tract function returns. Once GI tract function is regained, liquids are initiated, followed by a slow progression to solid foods as tolerated for volume and consistency [16]. A multiphase diet progression can help the patient transition from liquid to solid diets while maximizing weight loss and nutrient intake. Because there are a wide variety of nutrition therapy protocols, there is no standardization of diet stages and diet progression. Each postdietary protocol will vary in terms of the length of time patients remain on each stage of the postsurgical diet and what types of fluids and foods are recommended at each diet stage. Diet progression is usually advised at the discretion of the dietitian [22].

1 Clear Liquid Diet

A clear liquid diet is the initial diet stage following the first 24-48 hours after bariatric surgery. It is during this phase that gastrointestinal motility is restored to the gut. Bariatric clear liquid diets should have no concentrated sweets and should provide electrolytes and energy. These clear liquids consist of any food that is liquid at room temperature and that leaves a minimal amount of residue in the GI tract. Examples of clear liquids that are acceptable are broth, coffee, tea, sugar-free gelatin, or any beverage with a sugar substitute. Patients should consume 48–64 ounces of total fluids per day [13].

2 Full Liquid Diet

After 24–48 hours on clear liquids, the patient is then progressed to a full liquid diet. All liquids should remain sugar-free or low sugar (<15 g sugar per serving). Full liquid diets are intended to increase texture and gastric residue to the GI tract and to provide the patient with more energy and nutrients [20]. The restrictive intake is similar to that of a very low-calorie diet. Patients should continue to consume 48–64 ounces of liquid per day: ≥24–32 ounces of clear liquids plus 24–32 ounces of any combination of full liquids. Examples of full liquids include milk or nonfat milk powder, soy milk mixed with a whey protein supplement, light yogurt blended, strained soups, and other beverages that contain solutes. Full liquid diets can last 10–14 days. At this stage, patients will also begin protein and vitamin supplementation [13].

3 Pureed Diet

The third diet stage post bariatric surgery is pureed consistency. The pureed diet is typically made up of foods that have been blended with water or other liquid to result in an applesauce or baby food-like consistency. The purpose of a pureed diet is to increase the gut tolerance of gastric residue from solute and fibers. This phase of the diet emphasizes protein intake as well, and protein supplements may be introduced to further increase the amounts of protein consumed. Patients should introduce proteins into the diet over four to six small meals per day. Tolerance for protein foods may be limited to only a few tablespoons at each meal or snack. Patients who have undergone the LAGB procedure will experience hunger at this stage, and this is common within 1 week postoperatively. Patients who have undergone the BPDDS procedure should aim to consume 60 g or more of protein per day at this stage. Patients are encouraged to increase protein intake as tolerated. Pureed diets generally last 10–14 days [13,22].

4 Mechanically Altered Soft Diet

The transition from pureed foods to a general diet is the fourth stage of a postsurgical diet. Mechanically altered soft diets include "soft" foods that are easy to chew and will easily pass through the modified gastric pouch to the jejunum (RYGB) or will easily pass through the gastric band (LAGB). Food should be chewed thoroughly, until it is in liquid form, because large food particles may become obstructed above the stoma of the band [13]. Soft foods can include any general food that has been chopped, mashed, or pureed or can include easily broken down foods such as eggs or canned fish. Patients will generally remain on this altered "soft" diet for 14 days [22].

After this dietary phase, the patient is transitioned to a general diet, with emphasis placed on portion sizes, protein intake, and restriction of dietary components such as sugar and fat. Throughout the diet phases, patients should refrain from eating and drinking at the same time and to wait at least 30 minutes

after meals to resume drinking fluids. A healthy diet consisting of adequate protein, fruits, vegetables, and whole grains should be consumed. Volume of food will increase as food is tolerated. Patients should avoid consumption of refined carbohydrates, concentrated sweets, rice, bread, and pasta. A patient's intake will generally range from 800 to 1200 kcal per day (depending on body weight and surgical procedure) in the first 6 months following bariatric surgery [13].

C Foods to Avoid or Delay Reintroduction

When patients progress to the soft and general diets, they are typically advised to avoid or delay introducing certain foods back into their diet. It is generally recommended to avoid certain foods and beverages that may cause gastric irritation, intolerances, obstruction, or alter the rate of weight loss. Nutritional impairment may occur in patients after bariatric surgery for two main reasons: (1) inadequate food intake related to anorexia or dumping syndrome and (2) malabsorption of ingested food and nutrients.

D Dumping Syndrome

Dumping syndrome is a complex physiologic response to the presence of certain liquids or solids, or larger amount of liquids or solids, in the proximal small intestine. Gastric dumping has been reported in approximately 70–76% of patients who have undergone a RYGB procedure [20]. Dumping syndrome occurs as a result of rapid gastric emptying and gastrointestinal and systemic responses to a meal. Symptoms of dumping include abdominal pain and cramping, nausea and vomiting, flushing, tachycardia, and syncope [27]. Symptoms may occur within 10 minutes and up to 3 hours after eating, when food is rapidly transported (or "dumped") into the small intestine. Symptoms can be present in stages. In the first stage of dumping, the patient may experience abdominal fullness or nausea within 10 minutes of eating. These symptoms may be a result of small bowel distention accompanied by a small fluid shift from systemic circulation into the small intestine resulting from ingesting hypertonic foods such as carbohydrates or concentrated sugars.

The second stage of dumping syndrome may be experienced between 20 minutes and 1 hour after eating. Bloating, flatulence, abdominal pain, and/or cramping or diarrhea may occur. These symptoms are related to the increased malabsorption or fermentation of carbohydrates in the colon.

The third stage of dumping syndrome may occur from 1 to 3 hours after eating. Symptoms include perspiration, feelings of anxiousness or weakness, shakiness or hunger, and difficulty concentrating. These symptoms are a result of reactive hypoglycemia from rapid delivery of carbohydrates in the small intestine. Carbohydrate hydrolysis and absorption results in a rise in insulin levels accompanied by a drop in blood glucose and secretion of peptides GIP and GLP-1 [16].

Dietary recommendations for patients experiencing dumping syndrome will vary depending on each patient's diet and severity of symptoms. Recommendations to relieve symptoms of dumping syndrome include eating small meals spread throughout the day to improve absorption and to decrease dramatic fluid shifts. Meals should be high in protein, contain moderate levels of fat, and should be devoid of refined or "simple" carbohydrates. Proteins and fats are hydrolyzed more slowly into osmotically active substances, whereas simple carbohydrates in the forms of lactose, sucrose, and dextrose are hydrolyzed rapidly. Complex carbohydrates and foods high in fiber content slow GI transit time and increase viscosity, but caution should be taken to avoid ingesting large amounts of high-fiber foods until tolerated. If fiber supplements are instituted, patients should be cautious with large supplements in the form of pills because gastric narrowing, especially following the LAGB procedure, may make it difficult for supplements to pass through narrowed gastric openings; patients should also be cautious if they are experiencing dysmotility [16].

VII NUTRIENTS

A Micronutrient and Macronutrient Deficiencies

Postoperative nutritional care is vital to the bariatric patient. Nutritional impairment following bariatric surgery can occur due to inadequate food intake, excessive vomiting, or malabsorption of nutrients. Malabsorptive and restrictive bariatric procedures result in a deficiency of vital macronutrients and micronutrients that are necessary to maintain body processes. Due to the altered anatomy resulting from RYGB, BPD, and BPDDS procedures, micronutrient and macronutrient deficiencies are to be expected. Micronutrients (vitamins and trace elements) are essential to the human body, in very small quantities, and are necessary for proper cell growth and metabolism. Macronutrients (protein, fat, and carbohydrate) are needed in much larger quantities. Nutrient deficiency will increase depending on the severity of malabsorption (Table 25.1).

1 Micronutrient Deficiencies

Malabsorption of crucial micronutrients may occur after bariatric surgery for many reasons. A patient may become deficient in micronutrients due to limited food intake or poor food choices, malabsorption from altered anatomy, or from persistent nausea and vomiting that are common after all bariatric procedures in the early postoperative period.

It is believed that malabsorptive procedures (BPDDS) cause weight loss due to malabsorption of macronutrients. As much as 25% of protein and 72% of fats are not absorbed. Fat-soluble vitamins such as A, D, E, K, and zinc rely on fat metabolism for absorption and may be affected after a malabsorptive procedure [28]. Nutrient deficiencies occurring after RYGB may result from either malabsorption or inadequate dietary intake. After bypassing the stomach, duodenum, and portions of the jejunum and ileum, malabsorption of key micronutrients such as thiamin, iron, folate, vitamin B_{12}, calcium, and vitamin D may occur.

A common misconception may be that nutrient deficiencies are not present in a restrictive procedure (LAGB) because no changes are made to the absorptive pathway. However, nutritional deficiencies may also occur in these patients due to low nutrient intake, poor food choices, food intolerances, and limited portion sizes. The following sections examine the specific micronutrients that a patient is likely to be deficient in following bariatric surgery.

a THIAMIN

Thiamin (vitamin B_1) is a water-soluble vitamin that is absorbed in the jejunum. Without regular and sufficient intake of thiamin, the brain, heart, muscle, liver, and kidneys can rapidly become depleted of thiamin stores. The half-life of thiamin in the body is only 9—18 days, meaning that a person can become deficient in thiamin stores over a very small period of time. Thiamin stores in the body are relatively small and replenishment must occur daily. A deficiency in thiamin levels for a week, accompanied by persistent vomiting, can rapidly deplete thiamin stores.

Excessive and/or persistent vomiting, combined with a restricted food intake, low nutrient intake, and malabsorption, can cause an acute deficiency of thiamin in patients undergoing bariatric surgery. Symptoms of thiamine deficiency usually present within 1—3 months but may present sooner if the patient had an underlying thiamine deficiency prior to surgery. Thiamin deficiency is characterized by anorexia and weight loss as well as cardiac and neurologic complications that will eventually manifest into one of two conditions: Wernicke—Korsakoff syndrome (WKS) and beriberi.

TABLE 25.1 Recommended Laboratory Tests and Frequency of Routine Biochemical Surveillance

Procedure	Recommended frequency of biochemical surveillance	Recommended laboratory tests
LAGB, RYGB, and SG	First year: every 3–6 months	CBC, electrolytes, glucose, iron studies, ferritin, vitamin B_{12}, liver function, lipids, 25-hydroxyvitamin D
	Thereafter: annually	As needed: intact PTH, thiamine, RBC folate, MMA, HCy
BPDDS	First year: every 3 months	Every 3–6 months: CBC, electrolytes, glucose, iron studies, ferritin, vitamin B_{12}, RBC folate, liver function, albumin, prealbumin, lipids
	Thereafter: every 3–6 months	Every 6–12 months: 25-hydroxyvitamin D, vitamin A, vitamin E, vitamin K, INR, intact PTH
		Every 12 months: urine N-telopeptide, metabolic stone evaluation (24-hour urine calcium, citrate, uric acid, and oxalate), zinc and selenium
		As needed: osteocalcin, carnitine, essential fatty acid chromatography

BPDDS, bilipancreatic diversion with duodenal switch; CBC, complete blood count; HCy, homocysteine; INR, international normalized ratio; LAGB, laparoscopic adjustable gastric banding; MMA, methylmalonic acid; PTH, parathyroid hormone; RBC, red blood cell; RYGB, Roux-en-Y gastric bypass; SG, sleeve gastrectomy.
Source: *Adapted from Mechanick* et al. [13].

WKS, or Wernicke's encephalopathy, is the most common condition that results from severe, acute thiamine deficiency, and it is characterized by ataxia, nystagmus and double vision, general disorientation, and confusion. Korsakoff syndrome is characterized by impaired memory, inability to form new memories, and even hallucinations. If left untreated, it may eventually lead to permanent alterations in the brain [29].

Beriberi, either "wet" or "dry," can also develop as a result of thiamin deficiency. Wet beriberi affects the cardiovascular system. Symptoms include tachycardia, shortness of breath, and swelling of the lower legs; it may progress to congestive heart failure with acidosis. Without thiamin, pyruvate cannot enter the tricarboxylic cycle, resulting in energy deprivation to the heart muscle, thus causing heart failure [16]. Dry beriberi affects the nervous system; symptoms include difficulty walking, loss of muscle function, paralysis, and mental confusion [29].

To prevent thiamin deficiencies from either low dietary intake or malabsorption, patients undergoing bariatric surgery should be supplemented with thiamin. A multivitamin containing 100% of the daily value should be adequate for most patients; patients who are experiencing extreme nausea and vomiting may require additional thiamine supplementation. If a patient is experiencing symptoms of thiamin deficiency, it is recommended to give oral doses of 20–30 mg/day until symptoms resolve. Patients with WKS are generally administered more than 100 mg/day intravenously for several days [22].

b IRON

Iron deficiency is more commonly found after RYGB and BPDDS procedures due to the altered anatomy of the intestinal tract, specifically diversion of the duodenum where iron is primarily absorbed. Deficiency can also result from decreased food intake and/or lack of gastric acid. A decrease in hydrochloric acid (HCl) in the stomach pouch after RYGB procedures can affect the reduction of ferric iron into the absorbable ferrous state. Malabsorption of iron coincides with a decreased intake of iron-containing foods such as meats, grains, and vegetables, which may be difficult for patients to tolerate. In addition, women may experience a depletion of iron stores more often than men due to menstrual blood losses.

Iron deficiency anemia occurs when iron stores are depleted. Symptoms may include fatigue and reduced capacity for exercise tolerance. To prevent iron deficiency, all patients should be evaluated prior to surgery to determine any preexisting diminished iron stores. Serum ferritin is the most sensitive indicator of iron status and is recommended for diagnosing early iron deficiency [30]. The concentration of serum ferritin reflects the size of the storage iron compartment, with each microgram/liter representing 8–10 mg of storage iron [31]. Postsurgical patients should supplement with daily multivitamin–mineral supplements. Orally administered ferrous sulfate, fumarate, or gluconate may be needed (320 mg twice a day) to prevent iron deficiency in patients who have undergone BPDDS [1]. Menstruating women and adolescents of both sexes may need additional supplementation [22]. Note that iron supplementation can be inhibited in the presence of calcium supplementation, especially calcium carbonate, calcium citrate, or calcium phosphate. Vitamin C may increase the absorption of iron; patients should be encouraged to increase their intake of citrus fruits or vitamin C supplements. The risk for iron deficiency decreases over time as the patient is able to increase his or her food intake and experiences less food intolerance [13].

c VITAMIN B$_{12}$ AND FOLATE

Malabsorptive and restrictive bariatric surgical procedures interfere with several key processes of vitamin B$_{12}$ absorption. Postsurgical RYGB patients have a decrease in the production of hydrochloric acid, which will increase the risk of becoming deficient in B$_{12}$ through a number of factors. Post RYGB patients no longer have the ability to release vitamin B$_{12}$ from protein foods because pepsinogen cannot be converted into pepsin due to the lack of HCl. Decreased production of intrinsic factor (IF) by the parietal cells in the stomach will also prevent vitamin B$_{12}$ from being absorbed. The parietal cells that excrete acid and IF, as well as the cells that excrete pepsinogen, are located primarily in the fundus and body of the stomach, which are bypassed after RYGB.

Deficiency of vitamin B$_{12}$ and folate is seen more commonly in patients who have undergone RYGB or BPDDS than in those who have had an LAGB procedure because LAGB does not alter gastric function (secretion of gastric acid and a subsequent increased availability of IF). However, patients having LAGB may still become deficient in B$_{12}$ stores as a result of low tolerances of animal protein foods. Symptoms of B$_{12}$ deficiency may not present initially, and it can take months or years for a patient to begin showing signs of deficiency. Symptoms may include numbness or tingling in the lower extremities, changes in gait or motor skills, loss of concentration, memory loss or disorientation, and symptoms associated with macrocytic anemia. Vitamin B$_{12}$ status is most commonly and easily assessed by serum or plasma vitamin levels. The concentration of B$_{12}$ in the serum or plasma reflects both the B$_{12}$ intake and stores. However, a more sensitive biochemical indicator of deficiency is elevation of serum homocysteine and methylmalonic acid levels, which rise when the supply of B$_{12}$ is low and virtually confirm the diagnosis.

Typically, only patients receiving RYGB and BPDDS are supplemented with vitamin B$_{12}$, although all patients undergoing bariatric surgery should be routinely screened. Providing 350—500 µg through high-dose supplements via oral, injectable (intramuscular), nasal, or sublingual routes is recommended [16].

Folate deficiency is not as commonly observed as B$_{12}$ or iron deficiency, but patients who become anemic should be screened for a folate deficiency. Folate deficiency may occur as a result of inadequate dietary intake, noncompliance with multivitamin supplementation, malabsorption, and medications. Folate is typically absorbed in the small intestine, which is bypassed following RYGB. Folate deficiencies can also be seen in patients with a LAGB due to low food volume intake of dietary folic acid. Folic acid stores can begin to diminish within a few months postoperatively and will present symptoms such as macrocytic anemia and mental confusion such as forgetfulness or paranoia.

Multivitamin and dietary sources such as dark green leafy vegetables, fruits, organ meats, and fortified grain products can replenish folic acid stores in the body. Daily multivitamin supplementation is imperative for all patients undergoing restrictive—malabsorptive bariatric surgery. Supplementations of folic acid between 800 and 1000 µg/day, which is commonly found in most multivitamins, can correct or prevent folate deficiency in most patients [32]. Supplementation exceeding 1000 µg per day is not recommended because this can potentially mask a B$_{12}$ deficiency. Folic acid deficiency in pregnant women is associated with an increased risk of neural tube defects in newborns. Women of childbearing age or who are seeking to become pregnant post bariatric surgery should carefully monitor their intake of folic acid [22].

d CALCIUM AND VITAMIN D

Calcium and vitamin D are typically grouped together because a deficiency in one or both of these may lead to metabolic bone disease, increased bone turnover, secondary hyperparathyroidism, undermineralized bone, and bone loss [15]. A reduction in bone mineral density and bone mineral content generally accompanies weight loss; it is crucial to differentiate between the effects of weight loss and the malabsorptive consequences of bariatric surgery [29,33]. A deficiency of calcium and vitamin D may result from a decrease in calcium- and vitamin D-rich dairy foods related to intolerance or from a reduction in intestinal absorption resulting from surgical bypass of the duodenum, proximal jejunum, and ileum. Calcium and vitamin D deficiencies are more prevalent in patients receiving malabsorptive procedures such as RYGB or BPDDS due to bypassing the stomach, absorption sites of the intestine, and poor mixing of bile salts [22]. Patients undergoing LAGB can still experience calcium and vitamin D deficiencies due to poor food intake, usually related to intolerances to dairy products.

Although low levels of calcium and vitamin D are associated with each other, decreased vitamin D is not necessarily indicative of low serum calcium levels. When serum calcium levels decrease, the parathyroid gland produces excessive parathyroid hormone (PTH), resulting in a condition known as secondary hyperparathyroidism. In this state, the kidneys convert 25-hydroxyvitamin D into the active form of vitamin D

TABLE 25.2 Recommended Micronutrient Supplementation after Bariatric Surgery[a]

Supplement	Dose and frequency
Multivitamin	Once or twice daily
Calcium citrate (after RYGB, SG, or BPD/DS)	1200–2000 mg/day in two or three divided doses
Calcium citrate or carbonate (after LAGB only)	1200 mg/day in two divided doses
Vitamin D (in calcium supplement or separate)	1000–2000 IU/day
Elemental iron (for menstruating women)	40–65 mg/day
Vitamin B$_{12}$ (after RYGB, SG, or BPDDS only)	≥350 μg/day oral
	Or 500 μg every week intranasally
	Or 1000 μg/month intramuscularly
	Or 3000 μg every 6 months intramuscularly

[a]*Patients with micronutrient deficiency states will require additional supplementation as indicated.*
BPDDS, bilipancreatic diversion with duodenal switch; LAGB, laparoscopic adjustable gastric banding; RYGB, Roux-en-Y gastric bypass; SG, sleeve gastrectomy.
Source: *Adapted from Mechanick et al. [13].*

(1,25-dihydroxycholecalciferol), stimulating the intestine to increase absorption of calcium. If dietary calcium is limited or intestinal absorption is impaired, calcium levels are maintained by increased bone resorption and in conservation of calcium by way of the kidneys. In the case of secondary hyperparathyroidism, calcium deficiency can remain hidden until the patient develops osteoporosis or osteomalcia [8].

Calcium and vitamin D deficiency following malabsorptive procedures is predictable, but a patient's levels should also be examined preoperatively. Patients with a high BMI may be subject to develop vitamin D deficiency due to increased uptake and storage of vitamin D in adipose tissue and less exposure to sunlight [22,34,35]. Severely obese patients should be screened for vitamin D deficiency and abnormalities in bone density prior to bariatric surgery. Serum 25(OH) vitamin D is the best indicator for determining adequacy of vitamin D intake because it represents the combination of cutaneous production of vitamin D and the oral ingestion of both vitamin D$_2$ (ergocalciferol or plant-based vitamin D) and vitamin D$_3$.

Patients who have undergone RYGB or BPDDS should take oral supplements of calcium, ergocalciferol (vitamin D$_2$), or cholecalciferol (vitamin D$_3$) to prevent or minimize decreased levels of calcium and vitamin

D. If a patient is experiencing severe vitamin D depletion or malabsorption, oral doses of vitamin D$_2$ or vitamin D$_3$ may be increased to 50,000–150,000 IU. In severe cases, calcitriol (1,25-dihydroxyvitamin D) may be administered orally [13].

To replenish or prevent deficiency in calcium stores, oral calcium citrate with vitamin D should be supplemented at dosage levels of 1200–2000 mg daily (+400–800 IU/day vitamin D) [13]. It is preferable to supplement with calcium citrate instead of calcium carbonate because calcium carbonate is poorly absorbed in a low-acid environment, such as occurs with the small stomach area that remains after RYGB. In addition, calcium citrate has been shown to decrease markers of bone resorption and does not increase PTH or calcium excretion [36]. Table 25.2 provides a listing of the recommended supplements and dosage following bariatric surgery.

e VITAMINS A, E, AND K

Patients who have undergone malabsorptive procedures are at increased risk of developing deficiencies of fat-soluble vitamins. After BPDDS, intestinal dietary fat absorption is decreased as a result of delays in the mixing of gastric and pancreatic enzymes with bile in the ileum [37]. BPDDS surgery decreases fat absorption up to 72% [28]. Fat-soluble vitamin deficiencies can also be present in RYGB and LAGB patients, typically resulting from poor nutritional intake.

Fat-soluble vitamins are passively absorbed in the upper small intestine. Dietary fat digestion and micellation of triglycerides are necessary for fat-soluble vitamin absorption. Transportation of fat-soluble vitamins to body tissues is dependent on chylomicrons and lipoproteins. Surgical procedures that alter the changes in fat digestion will result in the digestion, absorption, and transport of fat-soluble vitamins [22].

Vitamin A deficiencies after bariatric surgery, although not common following RYGB or LAGB, usually result from poor nutritional intake, incomplete digestion, malabsorption, and impaired hepatic release of vitamin A [27]. Clinical manifestations of vitamin A deficiencies include impaired vision, night blindness (nyctalopia), and xerophthalmia [16]. Supplementation of vitamin A is not usually required after RYG or LAGB, but routine screening 6 and 12 months postoperatively is recommended following BPDDS [13,15]. If deficiencies are discovered, supplementation may be provided with vitamin A alone or in combination with other fat-soluble vitamins [13].

Vitamin K and vitamin E deficiencies are rare following bariatric surgery procedures, especially among patients who are taking a daily supplement regimen of one or two multivitamins that contain vitamin K and E [15]. Deficiency of vitamin K is more prevalent following BPDDS, and levels should be assessed if the patient is experiencing hepatopathy, coagulopathy, or osteoporosis [13].

f ZINC, COPPER, AND TRACE ELEMENTS

Zinc is dependent on fat absorption for metabolism and may be compromised after RYGB or BPDDS. Clinical manifestations of zinc deficiency include alopecia, delayed wound healing, skin lesions, immune deficiencies, and hypogeusia. Impaired zinc absorption is also associated with intestinal diseases such as Crohn's disease or pancreatic insufficiency [16]. Inadequate zinc levels may also be related to poor dietary intake of zinc-containing foods, especially animal products including red meat and poultry as well as dairy products. A protein-rich diet promotes zinc absorption by forming zinc–amino acid chelates (the more absorbable form of zinc). There is insufficient research to support specific recommendations regarding zinc supplementation. A daily multivitamin supplement containing 8–11 mg of zinc is adequate in preventing zinc deficiencies [13].

Copper may inhibit zinc absorption because it competes for the same carrier protein as zinc [16]. Deficiencies in copper present similarly as deficiencies of B_{12} and can result in anemia and myelopathy. Copper is absorbed by the stomach and proximal gut but is not routinely measured in patients who have undergone RYGB or BPDDS. In patients who present with symptoms of neuropathy but have normal levels of B_{12}, copper levels should be examined. Daily multivitamin supplements containing 2 mg should be adequate to prevent copper depletion in postsurgical bariatric patients.

There are insufficient data supporting the need to monitor trace elements (selenium and magnesium) after bariatric surgery. However, selenium levels should be checked in patients who have undergone BPDDS who present with unexplained anemia, fatigue, persistent diarrhea, cardiomyopathy, or metabolic bone disease [13,15]. Daily supplementation with a multivitamin that contains these trace elements should be sufficient to prevent any deficiencies of trace elements [22].

2 Macronutrients

Unlike micronutrients that are needed in small quantities, macronutrients (protein, fat, and carbohydrates) are needed in larger amounts to maintain homeostasis in the body. Malabsorptive procedures such as BPDDS can result in as much as 25% of protein and 72% of fat being malabsorbed [22]. Nutritional deficiencies of macronutrients are mostly a result of poor dietary intake as opposed to malabsorption following RYBG and LAGB.

Protein malnutrition (PM) is the most severe macronutrient complication following malabsorptive procedures [20]. The small pouch capacity following RYGB and LAGB does not play a large role in protein digestion because protein is mostly digested in the small intestine [22]. All bariatric surgery patients are at increased risk of developing PM or protein-energy malnutrition (PEM) postsurgically as a consequence of decreased dietary intake or maladaptive eating behaviors [27]. PM is typically a result of decreased dietary intake, anorexia, vomiting, diarrhea, food intolerance, fear of weight gain, socioeconomic status, or other reasons that may cause a patient to avoid protein intake and limit intake of calories. However, patients who have the BPDDS procedure are at a greater risk of developing PM/PEM due to a greater degree of malabsorption [22].

Unlike vitamins and minerals, which can be stored in the body and supplemented once per day, the body does not have the ability to store a daily supply of protein [27]. After enduring a low-protein intake for a few days, the body will adjust to the negative nitrogen balance; fat and muscle breakdown from hypoinsulinemia supplies necessary amino acids, gluconeogenesis and fatty acid oxidation supply energy to vital organs, and protein is spared as the body enters ketosis. Weight loss occurs as a result of water losses from metabolism of liver and muscle glycogen stores and from breakdown of muscle mass and adipose tissue. Without adequate intake of protein, patients will experience decreased hepatic proteins, muscle wasting, weakness, and alopecia. PEM is also associated with anemia from lack of iron, B_{12}, folate, and copper [22].

If the patient is consuming a diet low in protein but high in carbohydrate and fat, muscle breakdown will be inhibited, resulting in decreased visceral protein synthesis. In severe cases, fat stores will be preserved, lean body mass will be decreased, and extracellular water will be accumulated (PM edema) [22].

PM is typically detected 3–6 months following surgery and is mostly related to poor nutritional intake and food intolerance to protein-rich foods. Weight loss following bariatric surgery or any very low-calorie diet will result in loss of muscle mass. It is necessary to regularly assess patients postoperatively regarding protein intake and to provide dietary counseling on consumption of protein-rich foods as well as protein supplements. All patients undergoing bariatric surgery should consume a diet high in protein-rich foods, especially those of high biologic value.

Protein requirements for adults correspond with body weight and are usually represented as a percentage of energy intakes [27]. The accepted protein intake should be 10–35% of total energy [20] or in a range of

80–120 g/day for patients with BPDDS and ≥60 g/day for patients with RYGB [13]. In proportion to body weight, dietary protein should be established first, and then carbohydrate and fat should be added as determined by energy needs [27].

In the initial months following bariatric surgery, patients will be limited in the amount of dietary protein consumed through solid foods due to decreased stomach pouch capacity and decreased meal sizes. Liquid protein supplementation can be used to compliment a patient's dietary consumption of proteins. Modular protein supplements vary in terms of convenience, texture, taste, price, and amino acid profile. Patients should consume protein supplements that provide the nine essential amino acids (histidine, isoleucine, leucine, lysine, methionine, phenylalanine, threonine, tryptophan, and valine). Modular protein supplements are protein concentrations derived from various sources: complete proteins (milk, soy, or eggs), collagen, combinations of nonessential amino acids, or hybrids of collagen and complete proteins and amino acids [22].

Generally, PM/PEM can be avoided or reduced by increasing protein-rich foods in the diet or with the addition of modular protein supplements. However, some patients may experience severe PM/PEM that is not responsive to supplementation. Parenteral nutrition should be considered for these patients [13].

VIII LONG-TERM CONCERNS

A Weight Regain

Although clinicians commonly see bariatric surgery patients regain some weight postoperatively, the prevalence and incidence of weight regain has not been well characterized. Using cross-sectional data, weight regain has been estimated to occur in 20–35% of patients, depending on the procedure performed and duration of time following surgery [12,27,38,39]. The causes of weight regain are likely to be multifactorial, similar to those for patients who regain weight after nonsurgical approaches. Table 25.3 provides a categorical list of potential etiologies that should be explored with all patients who present with weight regain. The physiological and behavioral (diet and physical activity) causes are common to surgical and nonsurgical patients. Depending on the patient's age and gender, a through history should be performed that reviews all of these reasons followed by appropriate counseling. In contrast, the anatomical factors for weight regain result directly from either malfunction or disruption of the surgical procedure. These causes

TABLE 25.3 Etiological Factors for Weight Regain Following Bariatric Surgery

Anatomical

  LAGB malfunction or mismanagement

    Band or port breakage, band too lose

  RYGB

    Pouch enlargement

    Gastrojejunal anastomosis dilation

    Gastrogastric fistula

Physiological

  Pregnancy

  Menopause

  Weight-gaining medications

  Smoking cessation

  Endocrine disorder: hypothyroidism, Cushing's disease

  Intestinal or hormonal adaptation

Behavioral

  Dietary

    Unhealthy eating patterns, grazing, nibbling, mindless eating

    Consumption of high-energy foods and beverages

    Loss of dumping syndrome symptoms

    Loss of control over urges, binges

    Reduced vigilance

  Physical activity

    Reduced leisure time activity

    Increased sedentary behaviors

    Insufficient moderate- and vigorous-intensity exercise

    Development of physical limitations to exercise

need to be evaluated by an imaging procedure or upper endoscopy. Additional studies are needed to better understand the frequency, etiology, and treatment for weight regain.

IX CONCLUSIONS

Bariatric surgery is an effective and acceptable treatment for individuals with severe obesity who are at risk for or have complications associated with obesity. Several surgical procedures are available with variable risk and weight-loss outcomes. However, regardless of the procedure performed, surgery is considered a tool that is adjunctive to choosing a healthy, calorie-controlled diet and engaging in daily physical activity. The goals of dietary treatment and nutrition education are to facilitate weight loss and reduce the risk of nutritional deficiencies. Bariatric surgery necessitates dietary modification of food texture, consistency, volume (of both solids and liquids), frequency and duration of meals, and adjustments for food intolerances and potential nutrient deficiencies. In order to maximize successful outcomes, all patients should be monitored and managed by a multidisciplinary team of health care providers knowledgeable in bariatric surgical care.

References

[1] Consensus Development Conference Panel, NIH conference: Gastrointestinal surgery for severe obesity, Ann. Intern. Med. 115 (12) (1991) 956–961.

[2] National Heart, Lung, and Blood Institute and National Institute for Diabetes and Digestive and Kidney Diseases, Clinical guidelines on the identification, evaluation, and treatment of overweight and obesity in adults: the evidence report, Obes. Res. 6 (Suppl. 2) (1998) 51S–210S.

[3] National Heart, Lung, and Blood Institute and North American Association for the Study of Obesity, Practical Guide on the Identification, Evaluation, and Treatment of Overweight and Obesity in Adults, National Institutes of Health, Bethesda, MD, 2000 (NIH Publicatio 00-4084).

[4] H. Buchwald, Bariatric surgery for morbid obesity: Health implications for patients, health professionals, and third-party payers, J. Am. Coll. Surg. 200 (2005) 593–604.

[5] H. Buchwald, D.M. Oien, Metabolic/bariatric surgery worldwide, Obes. Surg. 19 (12) (2008) 1605–1611.

[6] R. Sturm, Increase in clinically severe obesity in the United States, 1998–2000, JAMA 163 (2003) 2146–2148.

[7] K.M. Flegal, M.D. Carroll, C.L. Ogden, L.R. Curtin, Prevalence and trends in obesity among U.S. adults, 1999–2008, JAMA 303 (2010) 235–241.

[8] H. Sugerman, A. Windsor, M. Bessos, J. Kellum, H. Reines, E. DeMaria, Effects of surgically induced weight loss on urinary bladder pressure, sagittal abdominal diameter and obesity comorbidity, Int. J. Obes. 22 (1998) 230–235.

[9] D.E. Cummings, J. Overduin, K.E. Foster-Schubert, Gastric bypass for obesity: mechanisms of weight loss and diabetes resolution, J. Clin. Endocrinol. Metab. 89 (6) (2004) 2608–2615.

[10] H. Buchwald, Y. Avidor, E. Braunwald, M.D. Jenson, W. Pories, K. Fahrbach, et al., Bariatric surgery: a systematic review and meta-analysis, JAMA 292 (2004) 1724–1737.

[11] M.A. Maggard, L.R. Shugarman, M. Suttorp, M. Maglione, H.J. Sugerman, E.H. Livingston, et al., Meta-analysis: surgical treatment of obesity, Ann. Intern. Med. 142 (2005) 547–559.

[12] P.E. O'Brien, T. McPhail, T.B. Chaston, J.B. Dixon, Systematic review of medium-term weight loss after bariatric operations, Obes Surg. 16 (2006) 1032–1040.

[13] J.I. Mechanick, R.F. Kushner, J.M. Sugarman, M. Gonzalez-Campoy, M. Collazo-Clavell, S. Guven, et al., American Association of Clinical Endocrinologists, The Obesity Society, and American Society for Metabolic and Bariatric Surgery medical guidelines for clinical practice for the perioperative nutritional, metabolic and nonsurgical support of the bariatric patient, Obesity 17 (Suppl. 1) (2009) S1–S70.

[14] A.E. Pontiroli, A. Morabito, Long-term prevention of mortality in morbid obesity through bariatric surgery: a systematic review and meta-analysis of trials performed with gastric banding and gastric bypass, Ann. Surg. 253 (3) (2011) 484–487.

[15] M.M. McMahon, M.G. Sarr, M.M. Clark, M.M. Gall, J. Knoetgen, F.J. Service, et al., Clinical management after bariatric surgery: value of a multidisciplinary approach, Mayo Clin. Proc. 81 (2006) S34–S45.

[16] L.K. Mahan, S. Escott-Stump, Krause's Food, Nutrition and Diet Therapy, eleventh ed., Elsevier, New York, 2001.

[17] M.L. Vetter, S. Cardillo, M.R. Richels, N. Iqbal, Narrative review: effect of bariatric surgery on type 2 diabetes mellitus, Ann. Intern. Med. 150 (2009) 94–103.

[18] H. Buchwald, R. Estok, K. Fahrbach, D. Banel, M.D. Jensen, W.J. Pories, et al., Weight and type 2 diabetes after bariatric surgery: systematic review and meta-analysis, Am. J. Med. 122 (2009) 248–256.

[19] International Diabetes Federation (2011). "Bariatric Surgical and Procedural Interventions in the Treatment of Obese Patients with Type 2 Diabetes: A Position Statement from the International Diabetes Federation Taskforce on Epidemiology and Prevention." Available at <http://www.idf.org/webdata/docs/IDF-Position-Statement-Bariatric-Surgery.pdf>. Accessed September 2011.

[20] American Dietetic Association, Manuel of Clinical Dietetics, sixth ed., American Dietetic Association, Chicago, 2000.

[21] G.L. Blackburn, M.M. Hutter, A.M. Harvey, C.M. Apovian, H.R. Boulton, S. Cummings, et al., Expert Panel on Weight Loss Surgery: executive report update, Obesity 17 (5) (2009) 842–862.

[22] L. Aills, J. Blankenship, C. Buffington, M. Furtado, J. Parrott, ASMBS Allied Health nutritional guidelines for the surgical weight loss patient, Surg. Obes. Relat. Dis. 4 (2008) S73–S108.

[23] S.L. Colles, J.B. Dixon, P. Marks, B.J. Strauss, P.E. O'Brien, Preoperative weight loss with a very-low-energy diet: quantitation of changes in liver and abdominal fat by serial imaging, Am. J. Clin. Nutr. 84 (2006) 304–311.

[24] J. Collins, C. McCloskey, R. Tichner, B. Goodpaster, M. Hoffman, D. Hauser, et al., Preoperative weight loss in high-risk superobese bariatric patients: a computed tomography-based analysis, Surg. Obes. Relat. Dis. 7 (2011) 480–485.

[25] M. Livhits, C. Mercado, R. Yermilov, J.A. Parikh, E. Dutson, A. Mehran, et al., Does weight loss immediately before bariatric surgery improve outcomes: a systematic review, Surg. Obes. Relat. Dis. 5 (2009) 713–721.

[26] P. Frank, P.F. Crooks, Short- and long-term surgical follow-up of the postbariatric surgery patient, Gastroenterol. Clin. North Am. 39 (2010) 135–146.

[27] D. Heber, F.L. Greenway, L.M. Kaplan, E. Livingston, J. Salvador, C. Still, Endocrine and nutritional management of the post-bariatric surgery patient: An Endocrine Society clinical practice guideline, J. Clin. Endocrinol. Metab. 95 (11) (2010) 4823–4843.

[28] N. Scopinaro, G.F. Adami, G.M. Marinari, E. Gianetta, E. Traverso, D. Friedman, et al., Biliopancreatic diversion, World J. Surg. 22 (1998) 936–946.

[29] R.F. Kushner, D.H. Bessesen, Treatment of the Obese Patient, Humana Press, Totowa, NJ, 2007 (pp. 379–394).

[30] E.M. Ross, Evaluation and treatment of iron deficiency in adults, Nutr. Clin. Care 5 (2002) 220–224.

[31] J.L. Beard, H. Dawson, D.J. Pinero, Iron metabolism: a comprehensive review, Nutr. Rev. 54 (1996) 295–317.

[32] R.E. Brolin, R.C. Gorman, L.M. Milgrim, H.A. Kenler, Multivitamin prophylaxis in prevention of post-gastric bypass vitamin and mineral deficiencies, Int. J. Obes. 15 (10) (1991) 661–667.

[33] M.D. Van Loan, H.L. Johnson, T.F. Barberi, Effect of weight loss on bone mineral content and bone mineral density in obese women, Am. J. Clin. Nutr. 67 (1998) 734—738.

[34] C.K. Buffington, B. Walker, G.S. Cowan, Vitamin D deficiency in the morbidly obese, Obes. Surg. 3 (4) (1993) 421—424.

[35] J. Wortsman, L.Y. Matsuoka, T.C. Chen, Z. Lu, M.F. Holick, Decreased bioavailability of vitamin D in obesity, Am. J. Nutr. 72 (3) (2000) 690—693.

[36] A.M. Kenny, K.M. Prestwood, B. Biskup, Comparison of the effects of calcium loading with calcium citrate or calcium carbonate on bone turnover in postmenopausal women, Osteoporos Int. 4 (2004) 290—294.

[37] G.H. Slater, C.J. Ren, N. Seigel, Serum fat soluble vitamin deficiency and abnormal calcium metabolism after malabsorptive bariatric surgery, J. Gastrointest. Surg. 8 (2004) 48—55.

[38] M. Shah, V. Simha, A. Garg, Long-term impact of bariatric surgery on body weight, comorbidities, and nutritional status, J. Clin. Endocrinol. Metab. 91 (11) (2006) 4223—4231.

[39] L. Sjorstrom, K. Narbro, C.D. Sjorstrom, K. Karason, B. Larsson, H. Wedel, , et al.for the Swedish Obese Subjects Study, Effects of bariatric surgery on mortality in Swedish obese subjects, N. Engl. J. Med. 357 (2007) 741—752.

CHAPTER

26

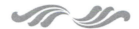

Behavioral Risk Factors for Overweight and Obesity
Diet and Physical Activity

Nancy E. Sherwood, Meghan M. Senso, Claire K. Fleming, Alison M. Roeder

HealthPartners Research Foundation, Minneapolis, Minnesota

I INTRODUCTION

Obesity is a significant problem that affects children, adolescents, and adults across gender, race, and socioeconomic strata [1−8]. Comprehensive data of trends since the 1960s in the prevalence of obesity provided by the National Health and Nutrition Examination Surveys (NHANES) show that the percentage of obese adults has increased over time during the past three decades, with the most recent data suggesting that the obesity rates may have stabilized. Results from NHANES 2007−2008 indicate that two-thirds of U.S. adults aged 20 years or older are either overweight or obese, with an estimated 34.2% classified as overweight ($25 \text{ kg/m}^2 \leq$ body mass index (BMI) $< 30 \text{ kg/m}^2$), 33.8% considered obese (BMI $\geq 30 \text{ kg/m}^2$), and 5.7% in the extremely obese (BMI $\geq 40 \text{ kg/m}^2$) category [9]. Although the prevalence of obesity among adults aged 20−74 years more than doubled between 1960−1962 and 2007−2008, from 13.4% to 34.3%, and the prevalence of severe obesity increased from 0.9% in 1960−1962 to 6% in 2007−2008, the prevalence of overweight remained stable during this same time period.

Prevalence rates of obesity and overweight among children and adolescents have also increased dramatically since the mid-1960s. Results from NHANES 2007−2008 indicated that 31.7% of U.S. children and adolescents aged 2−19 years are overweight ($\geq$85th percentile of BMI for age and gender), with 16.9% in the obese ($\geq$95th percentile of BMI for age and gender) category. The rates of obesity have approximately quadrupled for 6- to 19-year-olds from the mid-1960s through 2007−2008. NHANES data from the early

1970s suggest that the obesity rate among 2- to 5-year-old children has approximately doubled from 5 to 10%. The high prevalence of obesity among children is of particular concern given that childhood-onset overweight and obesity often tracks with adult obesity [10−12].

Concerning racial, ethnic, and socioeconomic disparities in the prevalence of overweight and obesity in children and adults have also been observed. Among both children and adults, Hispanic, non-Hispanic African American, and American Indian/Native Alaskan males and females are at particularly high risk for obesity [13−16]. From 2003 to 2007, obesity prevalence increased by 10% for all U.S. children but increased by 23−33% for children in low-education, low-income, and higher unemployment households. Moreover, children from low-income and low-education households had 3.4−4.3 times higher odds of obesity than did children from higher socioeconomic households. An inverse association between obesity and socioeconomic status has also been observed in adult populations [17].

The alarming increase in the prevalence of obesity during the past few decades has raised concerns about associated health risks for children, adolescents, and adults. Persistence of this trend could lead to substantial increases in the number of people affected by obesity-related health conditions and premature mortality. The health risks associated with obesity are numerous and include hypertension, type 2 diabetes mellitus, dyslipidemia, stroke, gallbladder disease, osteoarthritis, sleep apnea, respiratory problems, and certain cancers (e.g., endometrial, breast, prostate, and colon)

Nutrition in the Prevention and Treatment of Disease, Third Edition.
DOI: http://dx.doi.org/10.1016/B978-0-12-391884-0.00026-3

[18–26]. Obesity is also associated with psychosocial problems such as binge eating disorders and depression for some individuals [27,28]. Individuals who are obese are also adversely impacted by social bias and discrimination [29,30]. The economic burden of obesity is sizable because of its impact on individual health, costs to society due to lost productivity, premature mortality, treatment costs [31–36]. In 2008, the per-person direct medical cost of being overweight was $266 and of obesity was $1,723, with the aggregate national cost of overweight and obesity estimated to be $113.0 billion [31]. The adverse health consequences of obesity and associated health care costs are not limited to adults [37–40].

Obesity and being overweight are multidetermined chronic problems resulting from complex interactions between genes and an environment characterized by energy imbalance due to sedentary lifestyles and ready access to an abundance of food [41]. Research suggests that obesity runs in families and that some individuals are more vulnerable than others to weight gain and developing obesity [42–44]. Various mechanisms through which genetic susceptibility to weight gain has been proposed include low resting metabolic rate, low level of lipid oxidation rate, low fat-free mass, and poor appetite control [45–47]. Genetic research holds considerable promise for understanding the development of obesity and identifying those at risk of obesity. However, the rapid increase in rates of obesity has occurred over too brief a time period for there to have been significant genetic changes in the population. Although body weight is primarily regulated by a series of physiological processes, it is also influenced by behavioral and environmental factors. Recent epidemiological trends in obesity have been linked to behavioral and environmental changes that have occurred in recent years. The higher proportion of fat and the higher energy density of the diet in combination with reductions in physical activity levels and increases in sedentary behavior have been implicated as significant contributors to the obesity epidemic [41]. It is important to note that these dietary and activity behavioral risk factors are modifiable and can be targets for change in obesity prevention and treatment efforts.

Understanding the determinants of obesity and developing appropriate prevention and treatment strategies requires an in-depth examination of behavioral risk factors for obesity. This chapter reviews available data regarding behavioral and environmental determinants of dietary intake and physical activity and discusses implications for future public health research and intervention. The review focuses on behavioral risk factors for obesity in both children and adults.

II PHYSICAL ACTIVITY

This section examines the role of physical activity in the development of obesity. Multiple factors that influence physical activity levels are discussed, including sedentary behavior, psychological variables such as self-efficacy and social support, and environmental and societal influences. Prominent among the health benefits associated with a physically active lifestyle is the protective effect of physical activity on obesity. An abundance of cross-sectional research shows that lighter individuals are more active than heavier individuals, and prospective research indicates that changes in physical activity level are associated with changes in body weight in the direction predicted by the energy balance equation [48–51]. The majority of studies conducted in children also find that physical activity levels and body weight are negatively associated [52–54]. Exercise has also been shown to improve short- and long-term weight loss in experimental studies in both children and adults [55–57] and is a key factor in successful weight loss maintenance [58,59].

A Prevalence of Leisure-Time Physical Activity in Adults

The 2008 U.S. Department of Health and Human Services Physical Activity Guidelines recommend that adults engage in 150 min a week of moderate-intensity or 75 min a week of vigorous-intensity aerobic physical activity (or an equivalent combination of moderate- and vigorous-intensity aerobic physical activity) to obtain substantial health benefits. An approximate doubling of these amounts is recommended to obtain additional health benefits, and two or more weekly muscle-strengthening activities are recommended in addition to aerobic activity. Despite the benefits of physical activity for body weight regulation and health, we are in the midst of a sedentary behavior epidemic. Data from the 2008 National Health Interview Survey (NHIS) indicated that less than half of adults (47% of men and 40% of women) were active at recommended levels. Approximately one-third of men and one-fourth of women were considered "highly active," with approximately 14 and 16% of men and women, respectively, considered sufficiently active [60]. Of concern, 34% of men and 38% of women were considered inactive. Demographic differences in physical activity levels have been well documented. Across the three United States surveillance systems that monitor physical activity levels—the NHIS, NHANES, and the Behavioral Risk Factor Surveillance System—men tend to be more active than women; younger adults are more likely to be active than older adults, with the lowest levels of activity observed among those 65 years or older; and non-Hispanic whites are more likely to be active than other racial and/or ethnic groups [61]. Socioeconomic disparities in physical activity are also observed, with education and income positively associated with physical activity level [60,62].

B Prevalence of Leisure-Time Physical Activity in Youth

Although estimates of physical activity levels among younger people tend to be higher than self-reports by adults, the prevalence of regular physical activity is still surprisingly low. The availability of data on physical activity patterns and prevalence varies as a function of child age group. Representative survey data on the physical activity patterns of young children are not available, in part because of methodological difficulties in collecting such data from children. Young children are limited in their ability to accurately recall their activity patterns, and the unplanned, unstructured nature of children's physical activity patterns does not lend itself well to the self-report format employed in large-scale surveys. Increasingly, accelerometry is used to estimate children's physical activity levels, with Actigraphs used to measure physical activity in NHANES beginning in 2003.

The Centers for Disease Control and Prevention (CDC)'s Youth Media Campaign Longitudinal Survey (YMCLS), a nationally representative survey of children aged 9–13 years and their parents, was conducted between 2002 and 2006 [63,64]. Data from the 2002 survey found that 61.5% of children aged 9–13 years did not participate in any organized physical activity during their non-school hours and that 22.6% did not engage in any free-time physical activity. Between 2002 and 2006, physical activity levels reported on the YMCLS remained stable or slightly increased. Examination of 2003–2004 and 2005–2006 NHANES physical activity data measured by accelerometry among 6- to 19-year-olds showed that 6- to 11-year-olds spent more than twice as much time (88 min per day) engaged in moderate to vigorous physical activity compared to 12- to 15-year-olds and 16- to 19-year-olds, who engaged in 33 and 26 min/day, respectively [65]. Data from the Youth Risk Behavior Surveillance Surveys (YRBS) among U.S. high school students showed that in 2007, slightly more than one-third of young people reported any kind of physical activity that increased their heart rate and made them

breathe hard some of the time for a total of at least 60 min per day on 5 of the 7 days preceding the survey [66]. 2007 YRBS data also showed that slightly less than one-third of adolescents participated in insufficient amounts of physical activity. Similar to patterns observed among adults, across multiple national surveys, physical activity levels tend to be higher among boys compared to girls and higher among non-Hispanic white youth compared to black and Hispanic youths. Moreover, activity levels predictably decline as children transition into adolescence.

C Sedentary Behavior

Although low levels of leisure-time physical activity likely contribute to the epidemic of obesity, it is noteworthy that among adults, leisure-time activity has remained stable or increased since the mid-1980s, the period during which the prevalence of obesity increased [67]. The past century, however, has produced dramatic changes in physical activity patterns in the United States. Machines with motors have replaced human labor in virtually every aspect of life so that the energy expenditure now required for daily life is a fraction of what it was a generation or two ago. The consequences of this dramatic change are far reaching and only now are beginning to be carefully studied. It is likely that increases in sedentary activities such as television watching and computer use and decreases in lifestyle, household, and occupational activity that have been less carefully measured have contributed to reductions in overall energy expenditure at the population level. Examination of data from the U.S. Bureau of Labor Statistics and NHANES estimates that during the past 50 years, occupation-related energy expenditure has decreased by more than 100 calories per day [68]. Television viewing is a major source of inactivity and has received considerable attention as a risk factor for obesity. In addition to potentially contributing to lower energy expenditure by displacing time potentially spent in more active pursuits, television viewing has been hypothesized to contribute to excess energy intake [69]. Television watching can serve as a cue for eating given the numerous references to food and commercials for food—often high-fat, high-energy foods—on television [70]. According to data provided by A.C. Nielsen Company, the average household television set is turned on for more than 7 hr per day [71]. Survey data estimating the frequency of television watching are necessary, however, because television viewing is not necessarily the primary activity when the television set is turned on. Data from the Americans' Use of Time study show that free time spent watching television increased from approximately 10.4 hr per week in 1965 to approximately 18.9 hr in 2010 [72]. Nielsen data indicate that the amount of time per day adults spend watching television is closer to 5 hr per day. Increasingly, adults are watching "time-shifted" television and simultaneously watching television while using the Internet.

The high frequency of television viewing and other "screen time" amongst the young is disturbing. A review of the literature indicates that boys and girls are watching 1.5–3.7 and 1.4–3.0 hr of television per day, respectively [73]. The American Academy of Pediatrics (AAP) recommends that children older than the age of 2 years watch no more than 2 hr of "screen time" per day. Examination of NHANES data (2001–2006) indicated that nearly half (47%) of the children and adolescents spent ≥2 hr per day total screen time, largely driven by time spent viewing television [74]. Examination of media use data in younger children, including toddlers and infants, is also concerning. Despite the fact that the AAP discourages media use and screen time for children younger than the age of 2 years, a telephone survey conducted in Washington and Minnesota indicated that approximately 40% of children regularly watched television, DVDs, or videos by 3 months of age, with approximately 90% of children regularly experiencing screen time by 24 months of age [75]. Examination of data from the National Longitudinal Survey of Youth (1990–1998) indicated that almost one-fifth of 0- to 11-month-olds and almost half of 12- to 23-month-olds watched more television than the AAP recommends [76]. Demographic factors associated with higher screen time in younger children include lower levels of parent education [76] and race/ethnicity, with African American and Hispanic children tending to watch more television than non-Hispanic white children [76,77].

Cross-sectional research has shown that there is a consistently strong positive relationship between television watching and obesity in children [70,78–84] and adults [85–89]. Although it has been hypothesized that television watching influences obesity by replacing time that could otherwise be spent engaging in more active pursuits, data suggest that this relationship may not always be so simple (i.e., increases in sedentary behavior may result in decreases in physical activity, but physical activity does not necessarily increase in the context of reductions in sedentary activity) [90] and that physical activity and television viewing are often independent predictors of obesity [78]. Additional hypotheses regarding associations between television watching and obesity implicate increases in energy intake linked with television watching. The 2005 Institute of Medicine report focused on food marketing to children concluded that there is strong evidence that television advertising influences children's food preferences and requests, short-term food consumption patterns, and possibly usual dietary intake, and that exposure to advertising is associated with adiposity in children [91].

Despite the fact that relationships between sedentary behavior and obesity are somewhat unclear, intervention research with children and adolescents focused on reducing sedentary behavior shows promise as an obesity prevention and treatment strategy. The work of Epstein *et al.* [92–95] has figured prominently in the literature on decreasing sedentary activity as a strategy for promoting weight loss and higher levels of physical activity. According to Epstein, the principles of behavioral economics or behavioral choice theory can be applied to sedentary individuals who, given the opportunity to choose between sedentary and physically active alternatives, will consistently choose the sedentary alternative. Choice of a given alternative—in this case, sedentary behavior—depends on the behavioral "cost" of that choice. Epstein argues and has demonstrated empirically in the laboratory that reducing the accessibility of sedentary behaviors or increasing the cost of being sedentary are both methods for reducing sedentary behavior. Epstein and colleagues [93] have also demonstrated that obese children participating in family-based weight control programs show the best changes when they are reinforced for being less sedentary as opposed to being reinforced for being more active. Epstein and colleagues also demonstrated that an intervention designed to reduce television viewing and computer use was effective in reducing sedentary behavior, BMI z-score, and energy intake [92]. Of interest, reductions in television viewing were associated with reductions in dietary intake but not associated with change in physical activity.

Interventions focused on the reduction of sedentary behavior among youths have been conducted in multiple settings, including school [96–100], clinic [101,102], and community/home-based interventions [92,93,103–107]. However, a meta-analysis including 13 well-designed trials found that the interventions did not have strong significant effects on reductions in screen time or reductions in BMI [108]. The authors did indicate that screen time interventions focused on preschool-age children were more likely to have an effect. An innovative household-based obesity prevention intervention that targeted household-level weight gain and screen time reported promising findings [107]. The "Take Action" study randomized 99 households to either the intervention or the control group and followed them for 1 year. The intervention included six face-to-face group sessions, placement of a TV locking device on all home TVs, and home-based intervention activities. Although no significant intervention effects were observed for household BMI z-score, intervention households significantly reduced TV viewing.

D Self-Efficacy for Physical Activity

Self-efficacy is an individual's belief in his or her ability to successfully engage in a given behavior. It is theorized to influence the activities that individuals choose to approach, the effort expended on such activities, and the degree of persistence demonstrated in the face of failure or aversive stimuli [109]. Exercise self-efficacy is the degree of confidence an individual has in his or her ability to be physically active in a number of specific/different circumstances or, in other words, efficacy to overcome barriers to exercise [110]. Exercise self-efficacy is one of the strongest and most consistent predictors of exercise behavior in adults [111–116]. Among adults, self-efficacy is thought to be particularly important in the early stages of exercise [113]. In the early stage of an exercise program, exercise frequency is related to one's general beliefs regarding physical abilities and one's confidence that continuing to exercise in the face of barriers will pay off. Self-efficacy is also important among those who are already physically active and face the inevitable barriers to remaining active [116]. Self-efficacy has also been shown to be highly related to physical activity in youth [117–120]. In a systematic review examining determinants of change in physical activity in youth, self-efficacy was associated with smaller declines in physical activity among 10- to 18-year-olds [121]. Another study examining predictors of being persistently active during the transition from adolescence to adulthood found that perceived sports competency, specifically among females, was a strong predictor [122].

E Exercise History

Prior history of physical activity should positively influence future physical activity behavior by promoting and shaping self-efficacy for exercise and by developing physical activity skills. The observed relationship between exercise history and exercise behavior varies, however, depending on how exercise history is defined and the time period during which physical activity behavior is "tracked." Physical activity has been shown to track moderately well across childhood and adolescence [123] and in adulthood [124]. A systematic review of 27 papers from 16 different cohorts that included baseline age ranges from 8 to 10 years, with follow-up duration ranging from 5 to 55 years, suggested that physical activity tends to track more strongly in boys compared to girls, at older ages, and

tracks less strongly with increasing years of follow-up [125]. Youths who participate in sports tend to be more likely to be physically active as young adults [126,127]. Interestingly, there is an emerging literature suggesting that sedentary activities such as television viewing and video game use also track across childhood [128]. The perception of the exercise experience as a child may be as important as the amount of childhood exercise. One study found that recalling being forced to exercise as a child was associated with lower levels of physical activity in adulthood [129]. A child's enjoyment of physical activity [130,131] and enjoyment of physical education experiences [132] are significant predictors of physical activity levels. Creating positive environments for physical activity for youth is likely a key factor in promoting higher levels of physical activity as a lifestyle habit.

F Social Support

Social support is another strong correlate of physical activity for both youths [133–142] and adults [143–150]. Adults who engage in regular exercise report more support for activity from people in their home, work, and social environments. Instrumental support may be particularly important for initiation efforts among sedentary adults [151]. Carron et al. [152] examined six major sources of social influence on physical activity, including important others such as physicians or work colleagues, family member, exercise instructors or other in-class professionals, co-exercisers, and members of exercise groups, in a comprehensive review. The authors concluded that social influence generally has a small to moderate effect on exercise behavior. Moderate to large effect sizes were found for family support and attitudes about exercise, important others and attitudes about exercise, and family support and compliance behavior. More recently, there has been increased examination of how social support may interact with other factors to influence physical activity. For example, a study found that social support influenced self-regulation behaviors associated with higher levels of physical activity both directly and indirectly through self-efficacy [153]. Another study found that social encouragement influenced exercise behavior through motivational variables [154]. Further investigation of the pathways through which social support influences physical activity is important for developing effective interventions that capitalize on social influences.

Positive family environments and family support for physical activity is a robust correlate of physical activity for both boys and girls [134,136–139,141,142]. A comprehensive review of the literature examining the relationship between parental social support and youth physical activity identified two overarching categories of support, tangible and intangible [155]. Within these overarching categories, subcategories were identified. Tangible support included instrumental support, such as purchasing equipment, payment of fees, and transportation, and conditional support, which included either involvement of the parent in the activity or being physically present but not directly participating in the activity. Intangible support included motivational support, such as providing encouragement and praise, and informational support. Across the 80 reviewed studies, the majority demonstrated positive associations between the various types of parental support and physical activity. Peer support has also been shown to be a strong correlate of youth physical activity level, with the influence of peers increasing over time [134,135,140,156].

G Barriers to Physical Activity

1 Time

Among adults, time constraints are the most frequent barriers to exercise and are reported by both sedentary and active individuals across diverse populations with respect to age, race/ethnicity, and gender [157–163]. Even among regular exercisers, scheduling efficacy remains an important and significant predictor of adherence [110]. Therefore, to maintain exercise adherence, regular exercisers have to become adept at dealing with time as a barrier. The time barrier may be a particular problem for certain population subgroups. For example, time spent caring for children may make it difficult for parents to maintain a regular physical activity program [163].

Several physical activity intervention approaches geared toward addressing the time barrier have been developed in recent years. These include strategies to help people fit exercise and physical activity into their lives without necessarily having to engage in center- or gym-based activities, such as home-based programs, using phone- [164–166], mail- [167,168], or technology-based [167,169–171] delivery modalities (e.g., web-based options and smart phones). Another strategy to address the time barrier has been to focus on the potential health benefits of integrating multiple short bouts (<10 min) of physical activity throughout the day. A systematic review of the evidence for the effectiveness of short activity bouts that are incorporated into organizational routines in schools and work settings concluded that interventions that integrate physical activity into organizational routines have shown modest but consistent benefits [172].

2 Access and Environmental Factors and the "Built Environment"

Another barrier that has received increasing attention in recent years is access to exercise facilities, including parks and recreational facilities and safe and attractive places to walk and play outside. The burgeoning literature on the linkages between the built environment and physical inactivity and obesity has increasingly recognized the complexity in measuring the various aspects of the environment that are thought to be important. Brownson *et al.* [173] categorize measurement of the built environment in the following ways: (1) perceived measures obtained by telephone interview or self-administered questionnaires, (2) observational measures obtained using systematic observational methods (audits), and (3) archival data sets that are often layered and analyzed with geographic information systems. An extensive review of this literature is beyond the scope of this chapter; however, comprehensive reviews are available [174]. Distance between individuals' homes and recreational and exercise facilities and/or density of such facilities has been shown to be negatively correlated with exercise behavior in adults [175]. Depending on an individual's activity preference, access to exercise facilities may or may not be related to exercise levels. For individuals who prefer exercises such as walking or running, which can be done anywhere, access to facilities may be less relevant. In addition, for those who exercise with home equipment, which could include stationary bikes, treadmills, and even exercise videos, access to facilities may also not affect exercise adherence. Regardless, the extent to which environments are conducive to physical activity likely has a strong impact on population activity levels (e.g., walking/biking paths and safe streets). In addition to objective measures of availability, perceived availability and perceived safety are important [174].

Physical activity among youths appears to be particularly strongly influenced by environmental factors [174,176]. The amount of time children spend playing outside has been shown to be a strong correlate of physical activity levels in some [177,178] but not all [79]. Clearly, children who live in neighborhoods in which play spaces are not adequate are going to have more difficulty achieving recommended levels of physical activity. Inequality in availability of physical activity facilities and access to safe play spaces may contribute to ethnic and socioeconomic disparities in physical activity and overweight patterns among youth. Use of after-school time for sports and physical activity, access to community sports activities, and frequency of parents transporting children to activity locations have all been shown to be correlates of physical activity in boys and girls [179–183]. The extent to which families have time and resources to support their children in physical activity pursuits will also have a strong impact on children's activity levels. Anecdotal reports suggest that children spend less time in unstructured physical activities (e.g., neighborhood pick-up games, hide and seek, and tag) than in previous years. In contrast, there appears to have been an increase in community-organized sports (e.g., traveling soccer and basketball teams) that require increased parental time, involvement, and financial resources. These factors may potentially contribute to decreases in physical activity and increased socioeconomic differences in physical activity and obesity risk among youths and are an area worthy of further exploration.

3 Overweight and/or Discomfort with Physical Activity

Clearly, body weight and physical activity are inextricably linked. Although it is clear that increasing physical activity is an important factor in regulating body weight, weight status may serve as a barrier to physical activity. This is due in part to physical activity being less pleasurable (e.g., it is uncomfortable for people to exercise when they are heavier) and in part because of embarrassment (e.g., individuals report feeling embarrassed about being seen in public in exercise clothes, at gyms, due to weight status and societal reactions toward overweight individuals). However, weight status can also be a motivator for initiating exercise. One of the most common reasons adults give for exercising is weight control, and physical activity is one of the strongest correlates of successful weight loss and maintenance [184]. Physical activity promotion programs, however, need to be modified to address the needs of overweight youths and adults. Longitudinal data on adolescents indicate that body dissatisfaction predicts lower levels of physical activity, suggesting a need for physical activity interventions that help individuals feel more comfortable with their bodies, regardless of their weight status.

III DIETARY INTAKE FACTORS

This section examines the role of dietary factors in the development of overweight and obesity. Multiple factors that influence food intake are discussed, including total energy intake, specific eating patterns, and environmental and societal influences.

A Energy Intake

Laboratory experiments in animals and human clinical studies have repeatedly shown that the level of fat and energy intake in the diet is strongly and positively related to excess body weight. Examination of secular trends in self-reported overall eating frequency and energy density of diets suggests that increases in food consumption roughly parallel the pattern of obesity increase observed in the United States during the past 30 years [185]. Examination of trends in the frequency of eating episodes, meal and snack consumption, quantity of food consumed, and the energy density of foods reported by U.S. adults using data from four consecutive NHANES showed that the quantity of foods and their energy density increased beginning in NHANES III (1988–1994), although the increases were not large. Between 1971 and 2000, average energy intake increased from 2450 to 2618 kcal ($p < 0.01$) among men and from 1542 to 1877 kcal among women ($p < 0.01$). Cross-sectional nationally representative data from the Nationwide Food Consumption Survey (1977–1978), Continuing Survey of Food Intakes of Individuals (CSFII) (1989–1991), and NHANES (1994–1998 and 2003–2006) for adults (aged ≥ 19 years) suggest an increase in total energy intake of approximately 570 kcal/day between 2003 and 2006 [186].

Secular trends in energy intakes of youth aged 2–19 years have also been examined. Data from NHANES found that mean energy intake changed little from the 1970s to 1988–1994, except for an increase among adolescent girls. Between NHANES II and NHANES III, mean energy intake increased 1–4% among most age groups younger than age 20 years; mean intakes declined 3% for ages 6–11 years and increased 16% in females ages 16–19 years [187]. Among adolescent girls, energy intake increased by 225 calories. The increase between surveys for black females aged 12–19 years was slightly larger at 249 calories. Examination of dietary data from the NHANES 1988–1994, 1999–2002, and 2003–2008 showed no increase in total energy intake over time [188]. However, examination of data for children aged 2–18 years from the 1977–1978 Nationwide Food Consumption Survey, the 1989–1991 and 1994–1998 CSFII, and the 2003–2006 NHANES showed an increase in energy intake of approximately 179 kcal/day between 1977 and 2006 [189]. The inconsistencies in secular-trend surveys have been attributed to a number of factors, including weaknesses in the study design, methodological flaws, confounders, and random or systematic measurement error in the dietary data [36]. For example, the procedural changes between NHANES II and III in dietary survey methodologies, survey food coding, and nutrient composition databases make comparisons between the two surveys difficult.

B Underreporting of Food Intake

In contrast to measures of body weight, dietary intake is difficult to measure accurately.

Underreporting must be considered when interpreting dietary survey data. Studies have documented that food consumption is underreported by approximately 20–25% by people participating in dietary studies and occurs more often in women, overweight persons, and weight-conscious persons. Discrepancies between reported energy intakes and measured energy expenditures (with the doubly labeled water method) of 20–50% have been described in overweight individuals [190,191]. The systematic bias of underreporting in both overweight and non-overweight individuals may be due to socially desirable responses, poor memory for foods consumed, lack of awareness of food consumed, difficulty with portion size estimation, or undereating (consuming less food than usual because of the requirement to record food intake). A study of underreporting of habitual food intake in obese men found that approximately 70% of the total underreporting was due to a diminished intake of food during the reporting period; that is, subjects changed their food patterns during the recording period [191]. Selective underreporting of fat intake was also found. The magnitude of underestimations observed in various studies indicates the considerable error in dietary intake data and highlights the need for improved techniques of data collection [192].

C Sugar-Sweetened Beverages

Sugar-sweetened beverages (SSBs) include all sodas, fruit drinks, sport drinks, low-calorie drinks, and other beverages that contain added caloric sweeteners, such as sweetened tea. Consumption of SSBs has received increasing attention in recent years as playing a role in the obesity epidemic for several reasons. First, examination of national dietary intake data trends suggests that adults and children are consuming significantly greater amounts of SSBs than in previous years. Nielsen and Popkin [193] examined nationally representative data from the 1977–1978 Nationwide Food Consumption Survey, the 1989–1991 and 1994–1996 (also for children aged 2–9 years in 1998) CSFII, and the 1999–2001 NHANES and found that across all age groups, sweet consumption increased with energy intake from sweetened beverages by 135%. The majority of findings derived from large cross-sectional studies and prospective cohort studies with long periods of follow-up indicate that there is a positive association between SSB intake and unhealthy weight gain and obesity in both children and adults [194,195]. Moreover, there is emerging evidence that reducing consumption of SSBs may result in reductions in body mass index in youths and adults [196,197].

D Eating Away from Home and Fast Food

During the past 30 years, one of the most noticeable changes in eating patterns of Americans has been the increased popularity of eating out. The proportion of meals and snacks eaten away from home increased by more than two-thirds between 1977–1978 and 1995, rising from 16% of all meals and snacks in 1977–1978 to 27% in 1995 [198]. In 1999–2000, U.S. adults reported consuming an average of almost three commercially prepared meals each week, an 11% increase compared to the number of commercially prepared meals reported in 1987 and 1992 [199]. According to the U.S. Department of Agriculture (USDA), the percentage of daily caloric intake from food purchased and/or eaten away from home increased from 18 to 32% between the late 1970s and the mid-1990s; food away from home includes foods obtained at restaurants, fast-food places, school cafeterias, and vending machines. A number of factors account for the increasing trend in eating out, including a growing number of working women (75% of women 25–50 years old are in the workforce), more two-earner households, higher incomes, a desire for convenience foods because of busy lifestyles and little time for preparing meals, more fast-food outlets offering affordable food, smaller families, and increased advertising and promotion by large food-service chains and fast-food outlets [198]. The trend toward eating away from home more frequently has also been observed among adolescents and young adults [200]. Data from the 1977–1978 Nationwide Food Consumption Survey, 1989–1991 and 1994–1998 CSFII, and 2003–2006 NHANES for children aged 2–18 year indicate that the percentage of daily energy eaten away from home increased from 23.4 to 33.9% from 1977 to 2006 [189]. Of concern, the study authors also reported that the percentage of energy from fast food increased to surpass food intake in the school setting. Fast-food intake was also the largest contributor to food prepared away from home across all age groups.

The trend in eating out may be related to the observed increase in energy intake among Americans because food away from home is generally higher in energy and fat than food consumed at home. Many table-service restaurants provide 1000–2000 calories per meal, amounts equivalent to 35–100% of a full day's energy requirement for most adults [201]. Consumers may view food differently when eating out than when eating at home. Consumers may view eating away from home as an exception to their usual dietary patterns, regardless of how frequently it occurs, and an opportunity to "splurge." The most recent estimates from the USDA suggest that for the average consumer, eating one meal away from home each week translates to roughly 2 extra pounds each year; it is estimated that one meal eaten away from home increases daily energy intake by approximately 134 calories [202]. Eating out in fast-food restaurants, specifically, has been implicated as a risk factor for obesity. In both youth and adult populations, frequency of fast food consumption has been positively associated with BMI and obesity [186,203–205].

E Portion Size

It has been suggested that food portion sizes in food service establishments have become larger and thereby have increased energy intake, which may lead to obesity. However, empirical data to support this association have only just begun to emerge. It is noticeable that many restaurants, especially fast-food restaurants, in recent years have been offering large and extra-large portion sizes of products and meals at low cost. A comparison of food service portion sizes during the past 30 years is remarkable. Putnam [206] reports that the typical fast-food outlet's hamburger in 1957 contained slightly more than 1 ounce of cooked meat, compared with up to 6 ounces in 1997. Soda pop was 8 ounces in 1957, compared with 32–64 ounces in 1997. A theater serving of popcorn was 3 cups in 1957, compared with 16 cups (medium-size popcorn) in 1997. A muffin was less than 1.5 ounces in 1957, compared with 5–8 ounces in 1997.

Smiciklas-Wright *et al.* [207] examined data from the CSFII in 1989–1991 and 1994–1996 to compare quantities of a variety of foods consumed per eating occasion. In 1994–1996, all persons aged 2 years or older reported consuming larger amounts of soft drinks, tea, coffee, and ready-to-eat cereal and smaller amounts of margarine, mayonnaise, chicken, macaroni and cheese, and pizza. Nielsen and Popkin [208] used data from the Nationwide Food Consumption Survey (1977–1978) and the CSFII (1989–1991, 1994–1996, and 1998) to examine trends in average portion sizes consumed from specific food items (salty snacks, desserts, soft drinks, fruit drinks, French fries, hamburgers, cheeseburgers, pizza, and Mexican food) and whether portion sizes consumed varied by eating location (home, restaurant, or fast food). Food portion sizes increased both inside and outside the home for all categories except pizza between 1977 and 1996. The energy intake and portion size of salty snacks, soft drinks, hamburgers, French fries, and Mexican food increased by 93, 49, 97, 68, and 133 kcal, respectively, with portion sizes the largest at fast-food restaurants. In a more recent analysis of data from the Nationwide Food Consumption Survey (1977–1978), CSFII (1989–1991), and NHANES (1994–1998 and 2003–2006) for adults older than 19 years of age, Duffey and Popkin [186]

examined the role of portion size in relation to change in total energy intake over time and found that portion size and number of eating and/or drinking occasions were the strongest predictors of total energy intake.

F Food Marketing

Although multiple factors influence eating behaviors, one particularly powerful influence is food marketing. During the past few decades, U.S. children and adolescents have increasingly been targeted with intensive and aggressive forms of food marketing and advertising practice [209,210]. Multiple techniques and channels are used to reach youths, beginning when they are toddlers, to foster brand building and influence product purchase behavior. The Kaiser Family Foundation [211] released the largest study conducted on TV food advertising to children. The study found that children ages 8–12 years see the most food ads on TV, an average of 21 ads a day or more than 7600 per year. The majority of the ads were for candy, snacks, sugared cereals, and fast foods; none of the 8854 ads reviewed was for fruits and vegetables. Food marketing to children now extends beyond TV and is widely prevalent on the Internet [212,213]; it is expanding rapidly into an ever present digital media culture of new techniques including cell phones, instant messaging, video games, and three-dimensional virtual worlds [214].

The Institute of Medicine conducted a systematic review of the evidence and concluded that food and beverage marketing practices geared to children and youths are out of balance with recommended healthful diets and contribute to an environment that puts youths' health at risk [215]. The report set forth recommendations for different segments of society to guide the development of effective marketing strategies that promote healthier food, beverages, and meals for children and youths. Among the major recommendations for the food, beverage, and restaurant industries was that industry should shift its advertising and marketing emphasis to child- and youth-oriented foods and beverages that are healthier. If voluntary efforts related to children's television programming are unsuccessful in shifting the emphasis away from high-energy and low-nutrient foods and beverages to healthful foods and beverages, then Congress should enact legislation mandating the shift. Advocacy and public health groups are also calling on the Federal Trade Commission, the Federal Communications Commission, and Congress to work together with industry to develop a new set of rules governing the marketing of food and beverages to children—rules that take into account the full spectrum of advertising and marketing practices across all media and apply to all children, including adolescents. A synthesis of the evidence regarding progress the food industry has made in this regard concludes that to date, food and beverage companies have made moderate progress, whereas other industry stakeholders, such as restaurant companies, trade associations, entertainment companies, and the media, have not [216].

G Eating and Dietary Practices

The majority of research examining the potential role of diet in the etiology of obesity has focused on associations between obesity and dietary intake (e.g., intake of energy and portion size). As previously discussed, findings from this large body of research leave many questions unanswered. Fewer studies have examined associations between obesity and eating practices such as meal patterns, dieting, and binge eating. In this section, we highlight some of the research that examines associations between specific eating practices and obesity; identify questions that remain unanswered; and make some recommendations based on this body of research for future studies and for interventions aimed at obesity prevention/treatment.

1 Meal Patterns

Concerns about skipping meals exist in that meals are important for ensuring an adequate nutrient intake, for socializing (if eaten with family and/or friends), and for avoiding hunger, which may then lead to binge-eating episodes. Meal skipping has been found to be higher among overweight adolescents than among their normal-weight peers, with breakfast being the most common meal skipped. In a cross-sectional study of more than 8000 adolescents, usual breakfast consumption was reported by 53% of normal-weight youth, 48% of overweight youth (85th–95th percentile), and 43% of obese youth (BMI > 95th percentile) [217]. Because of the cross-sectional nature of these findings, it is not clear whether breakfast skipping leads to obesity (e.g., in that it may be associated with higher energy intake at later times in the day) or, rather, that breakfast skipping was a consequence of obesity (e.g., meals are being skipped for weight-control purposes). A review of the literature summarized the results of 47 studies examining the association of breakfast consumption with nutritional adequacy (9 studies), body weight (16 studies), and academic performance (22 studies) in children and adolescents and concluded that children who reported eating breakfast on a consistent basis tended to have nutritional profiles superior to those of their breakfast-skipping peers [218]. Breakfast eaters generally consumed more daily energy yet were less likely to be overweight. The quality of the

breakfast meal is a key consideration, with consumption of ready-to-eat or cooked cereal typically associated with better nutrition and weight outcomes [219,220].

Meal skipping is frequently used as a weight-control method. Among adolescents and adults trying to control their weight, Neumark-Sztainer et al. [221] found that skipping meals was commonly reported; 18.6% of adult males and females, 22.8% of adolescent females, and 14.1% of adolescent males trying to control their weight reported skipping meals. An important question relates to the impact of skipping meals on overall energy and nutrient intake. In a study of women participating in a weight-gain prevention study, skipping meals for weight-control purposes was not associated with overall energy intake [222]. However, meal skippers reported higher percentages of total energy intake from fat and from sweets, lower percentages of total energy intake from carbohydrates, and lower fiber intakes than women who did not report meal skipping [222].

In summary, existing research suggests that meal skipping is associated with a poorer nutrient intake and with obesity status [221,222]. However, it is not clear whether meal skipping plays an etiological role in the onset of obesity or, rather, is a consequence of obesity. Additional prospective studies and evaluations of interventions aimed at decreasing meal skipping are needed to assess causality. However, in light of the inverse associations between meal skipping and nutrient intake, and the potential for leading to uncontrolled eating due to hunger, meal skipping should not be recommended as a weight-control strategy. Rather, careful planning of meals with nutrient-dense foods that are low in fat and energy should be encouraged.

2 Dieting Behaviors and Dietary Restraint

Research findings clearly indicate that overweight individuals are more likely to report engaging in dieting and other weight-control behaviors than are normal individuals. For example, in a large cross-sectional study of adolescents, dieting behaviors were reported by 17.5% of underweight girls (BMI < 15th percentile), 37.9% of healthy weight girls (BMI 15th–85th percentile), 49.3% of overweight girls (BMI 85th–95th percentile), and 52.1% of obese girls (BMI > 95th percentile) [223]. In a 5-year follow-up study on the same population, dieters were found to be at increased risk for weight gain and for being overweight, even after adjusting for baseline weight status [224]. Adolescents using unhealthy weight-control behaviors were at approximately three times the risk for being overweight 5 years later, suggesting that behaviors such as skipping meals, taking diet pills, and imposing strict dietary restrictions may be counterproductive to long-term weight management. Similarly, in a prospective study on adolescent girls by Stice and colleagues [225], baseline dieting behaviors and dietary restraint were found to be associated with obesity onset 4 years later. After controlling for baseline BMI values, the hazard for obesity onset during the 4-year study period was 324% greater for baseline dieters than for baseline non-dieters. For each unit increase on the restraint scale, there was a corresponding 192% increase in the hazard for obesity onset [225].

These findings suggest that for some individuals, self-reported dieting may be associated with a higher energy intake and not a lower energy intake as intended. One explanation for this is that self-reported "dieting" may represent a temporary change in eating behaviors, which may be alternated with longer term eating behaviors that are not conducive to weight control. Another explanation is that self-reported dieting and dietary restraint may be associated with increased binge-eating episodes resulting from excessive restraint, control, and hunger. Indeed, Stice and colleagues did report positive, albeit modest, associations between binge eating and both dieting behaviors ($r = 0.20$) and dietary restraint ($r = 0.20$). In an analysis aimed at addressing the somewhat perplexing question as to why dieting leads to weight gain, Neumark-Sztainer and colleagues [224] found that binge eating was an important mediating variable between dieting and weight gain over time in adolescents. Other researchers have also suggested that dietary restraint may lead to binge-eating behaviors [226], thereby placing individuals at risk for weight gain rather than the intended weight loss or maintenance [227].

3 Binge Eating

Overweight individuals are more likely to engage in binge-eating behaviors than are their normal-weight counterparts among youths and adults [228−230]. In a nonclinical sample of adult women enrolled in a weight-gain prevention program, binge eating was reported by 9% of normal-weight women and 21% of overweight women [231]. Furthermore, binge eating tends to be more prevalent among overweight individuals seeking treatment for weight loss. It is estimated that approximately 30% of participants seeking weight loss counseling engage in binge eating [232], with approximately 3.5−5% of the population meeting clinical criteria for binge eating disorder, the majority of whom are overweight or obese [28,233]. Factors contributing to the higher rates of binge eating among overweight individuals, compared to normal individuals, may include the following: greater appetites brought on by higher physiological needs of a larger body size, greater emotional disturbances (e.g., depressive symptoms) or different responses to stressful situations, greater exposure to stressful situations (e.g., related to weight stigmatization), increased weight preoccupation and dieting behaviors, and stronger dietary restraint.

In working with overweight individuals within health care and other settings, it is essential to be sensitive to the daily struggles overweight clients may face within thin-oriented societies. Overweight clients may be reluctant to share their binge-eating experiences; therefore, a nonjudgmental attitude on the part of the health care provider is critical. For some individuals, hunger resulting from dieting or meal skipping may be a major cause of binge eating, whereas for others, binge eating may be a response to stress. Some individuals may be experiencing cyclical patterns; for example, emotional stress leads to binge eating, which leads to further emotional stress, which leads to further binge eating. Strategies for avoiding binge eating should be linked to factors that appear to be leading to binge eating for each individual.

4 Family Influences on Dietary Intake and Eating Practices

A considerable amount of research has been devoted to the role of the family in the etiology, prevention, and treatment of obesity [234−236]. Family based obesity treatments were founded on the premise that the home environment and parenting practices are critical to the eating and activity behavior changes needed to successfully promote and sustain healthy body weight for children [237−239]. Epstein's parent−family based obesity treatment produced impressive results. At the 10-year follow-up, 33% of all children decreased their BMI by 20% or more from baseline, and 30% were no longer obese. Other work supports the idea of parent-focused child-obesity treatment. After 7 years of follow-up, obese children whose parents initially were intervened on for the child's obesity were significantly less likely to be obese compared to children who were themselves the target of the initial intervention (e.g., 30 vs. 69%) [239]. These results clearly suggest that targeting parents is of critical importance and can be more effective than targeting the child.

With regard to dietary intake and eating practices, questions arise as to how the family environment influences individual family members' eating behaviors and what parents and the family can do to improve eating behaviors of its members. The aim is clearly to provide for an environment in which healthful food is available, eaten in an enjoyable manner, and consumed in appropriate amounts. Most of the research in this area has focused on the influence of parents on their children's eating behaviors. Parents/caretakers may influence their children's dietary intake and eating practices via numerous channels. Some of the key channels include food availability within the home setting (including food purchasing, food preparation, and food accessibility), family meal patterns, infant and child feeding practices, role modeling of eating behaviors and body image attitudes, and verbal encouragement of specific eating practices. Research in the arena of adolescent health indicates that general family context variables are strongly associated with the emotional well-being of adolescents and with eating and other health-related behaviors [240].

The role of parenting in the promotion of healthy eating behavior and activity patterns has received increased attention in recent years. Research has focused on the role of domain-specific parenting styles, such as parent feeding practices, as well as the role of more general parenting styles and practices, such as authoritative versus permissive parenting. Both food-specific parenting and family variables such as the frequency of family meals [241] and positive parenting styles [242] have been shown to be related to eating patterns. Although there is ongoing work in this area, research to date suggests that providing a healthy home food environment, including the provision of healthy routines such as frequent family meals, is important, allowing for children to make choices within that environment regarding exactly what and how much to eat and thus allowing for the development of internal regulation of food intake.

IV SUMMARY AND PUBLIC HEALTH RECOMMENDATIONS

We have reviewed the literature on key physical activity and diet-related risk factors for obesity in children and adults. Highlights of the review from the physical activity domain include (1) the importance of addressing the influence of both leisure-time physical activity and sedentary behavior to total energy expenditure, (2) the importance of fostering both self-efficacy and social support for physical activity to promote higher levels of physical activity, and (3) the influence of environmental factors on physical activity levels. Highlights related to dietary intake include (1) recognizing the contribution of total energy intake to energy regulation; (2) the importance of accurately assessing portion size; (3) the influence of eating practices such as eating out, breakfast skipping, restrained eating, and binge eating on obesity; and (4) social and environmental factors that promote excess energy intake.

To effectively combat the public health problem of obesity, interventions and policies that target change in dietary intake and physical activity are necessary. Intervention efforts must take into account that dietary intake and physical activity are complex, multidetermined behaviors influenced by individual, social, and environmental factors [243]. There has been tremendous effort in recent years to address the public health problem of obesity. Examples include Call to Action issued by the Surgeon General in 2001, large initiatives funded and led by the Robert Wood Johnson Foundation (RWJF) to change public policies and community environments in ways that promote improved nutrition and increased physical activity, the National Institutes of Health Obesity Task Force and research initiatives, and the Let's Move! campaign and associated efforts initiated by First Lady Michelle Obama.

A report issued by Trust for America's Health and the RWJF (http://healthyamericans.org/reports/obesity2011/Obesity2011Report.pdf) provides important guidance for the next steps in addressing the obesity epidemic among children and adults. Table 26.1 outlines the multiple opportunities to address physical activity, nutrition, and healthy weight through health reform, including initiatives involving the Prevention and Public Health Fund; Community Transformation Grants; the National Prevention Strategy; the National

TABLE 26.1 Opportunities to Reduce Obesity through Health Reform

Prevention and Public Health Fund	The fund provides more than $16 billion in mandatory appropriations for prevention programs, including obesity-prevention activities, over the next 10 years.
Community Transformation Grants (CTGs)	These grants were awarded for the first time by the CDC in fiscal year 2011. Communities throughout the country will have the opportunity to bid competitively for grants to prevent obesity, make affordable nutritious foods more widely available, and provide safe places to be physically active.
National Prevention Strategy (NPS)	The NPS, released in the spring of 2011, establishes priorities and approaches to preventing health problems, including obesity and obesity-related illnesses.
National Prevention, Health Promotion, and Public Health Council	The Council brings together a wide range of federal departments and agencies to consider how their own policies can impact health. The Council has the opportunity to take a "Health in All Policies" approach encouraging policies that help to improve health when possible and avoiding policies that might unintentionally have a negative impact. For instance, the U.S. Department of Health and Human Services

(Continued)

TABLE 26.1   (Continued)

	(HHS) and the U.S. Department of Transportation could work collaboratively to ensure that new road construction not only keeps traffic flowing but also includes pedestrian sidewalks and preserves open green spaces.
Essential benefits and coverage of preventive services	All new group benefit plans will be required to cover any preventive service that has received an "A" or "B" rating from the U.S. Preventive Services Task Force (U.S.PSTF), including intensive obesity counseling. U.S.PSTF has given "B" recommendations that clinicians screen all Americans ages 6 years or older for obesity and offer or refer them to comprehensive, intensive behavioral interventions. In addition, insurance plans sold in the new state health insurance exchanges will be required to offer essential health benefits that will be defined by HHS. These can and should include coverage of services—both in clinics and offered by community providers—that are shown to reduce obesity and associated conditions (e.g., the Diabetes Prevention Program). In addition, there are new requirements for coverage of preventive services in the Medicare program. In November 2010, the Centers for Medicare and Medicaid Services (CMS) released a final rule implementing coverage of an annual wellness visit and new covered preventive services for Medicare beneficiaries starting in 2011. The number of Medicaid beneficiaries is expected to expand dramatically in 2014, as everyone below 133% of the federal poverty level will be eligible for coverage. This is likely to increase the number of obese and overweight people served by Medicaid, given the close tie of obesity to poverty. Medicaid will need to ensure that all appropriate clinical and community-based services are offered to patients as a means of containing the costs associated with chronic disease. CMS is now accepting proposals from states for the Medicaid Incentives for Prevention of Chronic Disease Program (MIPCDP). MIPCPD will reward Medicaid recipients who make an effort to stay healthy. The program must focus on tobacco cessation, controlling or reducing weight, lowering cholesterol, lowering blood pressure, or either avoiding the onset of or improving the management of diabetes.
Nutritional labeling	Chain restaurants or food establishments with at least 20 locations will be required to disclose calorie counts and other nutritional information for standard menu items. Vending machine operators that own or operate at least 20 machines have similar requirements. In August 2010, the U.S. Food and Drug Administration (FDA) released draft compliance guidance. Although this requirement was effective upon enactment of the Affordable Care Act (ACA), the FDA has indicated that it will not enforce this provision until regulations are finalized. The FDA released a proposed rule to this effect in April 2011.
Healthy Aging, Living Well Pilot	This pilot authorizes HHS, acting through CDC, to award grants to states and local health departments to conduct disease prevention pilot programs for Americans ages 55–64 years to help people stay healthier before they are eligible for Medicare. To date, Congress has not appropriated funds for this program.
Center for Medicare and Medicaid Innovation	The Center for Medicare and Medicaid Innovation (the "Innovation Center") examines, evaluates, and expands new policies and programs to improve the quality of care and lower the costs for Medicare, Medicaid, and Children's Health Insurance Program beneficiaries. The Innovation Center affords a unique opportunity to test new population-based approaches to helping patients prevent obesity and/or achieve and sustain weight loss. The Innovation Center was formally established in November 2010 and has already announced demonstration projects aimed at promoting greater use of the medical home model. A dedicated funding stream has been appropriated to carry out these new grant programs as they are being tested and evaluated. One division of the Innovation Center, the Community Improvement Care Models Group, is obligated to help fight the epidemics of obesity, smoking, and heart disease.
National Diabetes Prevention Program	The ACA authorized CDC to manage National Diabetes Prevention Program grants and create community-based model sites to help adults at high risk prevent type 2 diabetes. Although the grants component of the program has not yet been funded, the CDC Division of Diabetes Translation has already begun implementation by partnering with the Y and United HealthGroup to recognize sites that offer qualifying interventions. CDC also established the Diabetes Training and Technical Assistance Center at Emory University to support related training to ensure that sites implement interventions efficiently and effectively.
Children's Health Insurance Program Childhood Obesity Demonstration Project	From 2010 to 2014, the ACA provides $25 million in funding for the Childhood Obesity Demonstration Project, which was established through the Children's Health Insurance Program Reauthorization Act of 2009 (CHIPRA). HHS grants are aimed at fostering the development of comprehensive approaches to reducing childhood obesity. CHIPRA requires that grantees carry out community-based activities that operate through schools, the health delivery system, and community health workers.

Source: *http://healthyamericans.org/reports/obesity2011/Obesity2011Report.pdf.*

A. RWJF POLICY PRIORITIES TO REVERSE THE CHILDHOOD OBESITY EPIDEMIC

As part of its efforts to reverse the childhood obesity epidemic by 2015, the Robert Wood Johnson Foundation has outlined six broad policy priorities that evidence suggests will have the greatest and longest-lasting impact on our nation's children. There are likely a variety of policy pathways to achieve each priority. Some of these approaches, as recommended by the Centers for Disease Control, Institute of Medicine and other key governmental and research organizations, are listed below.

1. Ensure that all foods and beverages served and sold in schools meet or exceed the most recent Dietary Guidelines for Americans.

- ■ Finalize and implement updated nutrition standards for all food and beverages served and sold in schools.
- ■ Increase federal reimbursement for the National School Lunch Program.
- ■ Expand access to the School Breakfast Program.
- ■ Ensure schools have the resources they need to train cafeteria employees and replace outdated and broken kitchen equipment.

2. Increase access to affordable foods through new or improved grocery stores and healthier corner stores and bodegas.

- ■ Create incentive programs to attract supermarkets and grocery stores to underserved neighborhoods. These may include tax credits, grant and loan programs, and small business/economic development programs.
- ■ Introduce or modify land use policies and zoning regulations to promote, expand and protect potential sites for community gardens, mobile markets and farmers' markets. Potential sites may include vacant city-owned land or unused parking lots.

3. Increase the time, intensity and duration of physical activity, in both schools and out-of-school programs.

- ■ Require physical education (PE) in schools.
- ■ Implement a minimum standard of 150 minutes per week of PE in elementary schools and 225 minutes per week in middle schools and high schools.
- ■ Increase opportunities for physical activity in schools outside of PE, such as classroom activity breaks, intramural and inter-scholastic sports.

4. Increase physical activity by improving the built environment in communities.

- ■ Establish joint use agreements that will allow community residents to use school playing fields, playgrounds and recreation centers when schools are closed. If necessary, adopt regulatory and legislative policies to address liability issues that might block implementation.

- ■ Build and maintain parks and playgrounds that are safe and attractive for playing, and located close to residential areas.
- ■ Adopt community policing strategies that improve safety and security for park use, especially in higher-crime neighborhoods.
- ■ Plan, build, and maintain a network of sidewalks and street crossings that creates a safe and comfortable walking environment that connects to schools, parks, and other destinations.

5. Use pricing strategies – both incentives and disincentives – to promote the purchase of healthier foods.

- ■ Implement fiscal policies and local ordinances (e.g., taxes, incentives, land use and zoning regulations) that discourage the consumption of foods and beverages that are high in calories but low in nutrients.
- ■ Provide incentives through federal food assistance programs to help families purchase healthier options. Examples may include "double bucks" programs that match Supplemental Nutrition Assistance Program dollars spent on healthy foods.

6. Reduce youths' exposure to the marketing of unhealthy foods through regulation, policy, and effective industry self-regulation.

- ■ Adopt voluntary, industry-wide nutrition standards developed by the federal Interagency Working Group on food marketing and ensure that the definition of "marketing" includes marketing via social media (e.g., text messaging, Facebook, Twitter, etc.).
- ■ Adopt a research-based, industry-wide, front-of-package labeling system.
- ■ Eliminate advertising and marketing of calorie-dense, nutrient-poor foods and beverages near school grounds and public places frequently visited by youths.
- ■ Use zoning policies to limit the number of fast-food outlets near schools and other settings frequented by youths.
- ■ Set nutritional standards for children's meals that include a toy or other incentive item.
- ■ Limit advertising that directly appeals to children (e.g., celebrities, cartoon characters, toys, gifts, games, food packaging).

FIGURE 26.1 RWJF Policy Policy Priorities to Reverse the Childhood Obesity Epidemic. Source: *http://healthyamericans.org/reports/obesity2011/Obesity2011Report.pdf*. See color plate.

Prevention, Health Promotion, and Public Health Council; Essential Benefits and Coverage of Preventive Services; nutritional labeling; the Center for Medicare and Medicaid Innovation; the National Diabetes Prevention Program; and the Children's Health Insurance Program Childhood Obesity Demonstration Project. Figure 26.1 outlines policy priorities identified by the RWJF to address childhood obesity specifically, including policies to increase the availability and affordability of healthy food and physical activity opportunities in schools and communities and to reduce exposure to the marketing of unhealthy foods. The depth and breadth of these policy recommendations is an important indicator of increased recognition that the obesity epidemic will not be adequately addressed with single-setting interventions, focused on individual behavior change alone.

V CONCLUSION

The etiology of obesity is complex and encompasses a wide variety of social, behavioral, cultural, environmental, physiological, and genetic factors. To achieve these ambitious goals, considerable effort must be focused on helping individuals at the population level modify their diets and increase their physical activity levels, key behaviors involved in the regulation of body weight. Educational and environmental interventions that support diet and exercise patterns associated with healthy body weight must be developed and evaluated. Prevention of obesity should begin early in life and involve the development and maintenance of healthy eating and physical activity patterns. These patterns need to be reinforced at home, in schools, and throughout the community. Public health agencies, communities, government, health organizations, the media, and the food and health industry must form alliances if we are to combat obesity.

References

[1] C.L. Ogden, R.P. Troiano, R.R. Briefel, R.J. Kuczmarski, K.M. Flegal, C.L. Johnson, Prevalence of overweight among preschool children in the United States, 1971 through 1994, Pediatrics 99 (4) (1997) E1.

[2] R.P. Troiano, K.M. Flegal, Overweight children and adolescents: description, epidemiology, and demographics, Pediatrics 101 (3 Pt 2) (1998) 497–504.

[3] K.M. Flegal, M.D. Carroll, R.J. Kuczmarski, C.L. Johnson, Overweight and obesity in the United States: prevalence and trends, 1960–1994, Int. J. Obes. Relat. Metab. Disord. 22 (1) (1998) 39–47.

[4] C.L. Ogden, M.M. Lamb, M.D. Carroll, K.M. Flegal, Obesity and socioeconomic status in children and adolescents: United States, 2005–2008, NCHS Data Brief 51 (2010) 1–8.

[5] C.L. Ogden, M.M. Lamb, M.D. Carroll, K.M. Flegal, Obesity and socioeconomic status in adults: United States, 2005–2008, NCHS Data Brief 50 (2010) 1–8.

[6] C.L. Ogden, M.D. Carroll, L.R. Curtin, M.A. McDowell, C.J. Tabak, K.M. Flegal, Prevalence of overweight and obesity in the United States, 1999–2004, JAMA 295 (13) (2006) 1549–1555.

[7] C.L. Ogden, K.M. Flegal, M.D. Carroll, C.L. Johnson, Prevalence and trends in overweight among U.S. children and adolescents, 1999–2000, JAMA 288 (14) (2002) 1728–1732.

[8] A.A. Hedley, C.L. Ogden, C.L. Johnson, M.D. Carroll, L.R. Curtin, K.M. Flegal, Prevalence of overweight and obesity among U.S. children, adolescents, and adults, 1999–2002, JAMA 291 (23) (2004) 2847–2850.

[9] C.L. Ogden, M.D. Carroll, Prevalence of overweight, obesity, and extreme obesity among adults: United States, trends 1960–1962 through 2007–2008. (2010). Available at <http://www.cdc.gov/NCHS/data/hestat/obesity_adult_07_08/obesity_adult_07_08.pdf>.

[10] R.C. Whitaker, J.A. Wright, M.S. Pepe, K.D. Seidel, W.H. Dietz, Predicting obesity in young adulthood from childhood and parental obesity, N. Engl. J. Med. 337 (13) (1997) 869–873.

[11] P.R. Nader, M. O'Brien, R. Houts, et al., Identifying risk for obesity in early childhood, Pediatrics 118 (3) (2006) E594–E601.

[12] M. Juonala, C.G. Magnussen, G.S. Berenson, et al., Childhood adiposity, adult adiposity, and cardiovascular risk factors, N. Engl. J. Med. 365 (20) (2011) 1876–1885.

[13] K.M. Flegal, M.D. Carroll, C.L. Ogden, L.R. Curtin, Prevalence and trends in obesity among U.S. adults, 1999–2008, JAMA 303 (3) (2010) 235–241.

[14] C.L. Ogden, M.D. Carroll, L.R. Curtin, M.M. Lamb, K.M. Flegal, Prevalence of high body mass index in U.S. children and adolescents, 2007–2008, JAMA 303 (3) (2010) 242–249.

[15] S.E. Anderson, R.C. Whitaker, Prevalence of obesity among U.S. preschool children in different racial and ethnic groups, Arch. Pediatr. Adolesc. Med. 163 (4) (2009) 344–348.

[16] S.N. Hinkle, A.J. Sharma, S.Y. Kim, et al., Prepregnancy obesity trends among low-income women, United States, 1999–2008, Matern. Child Health J. (2011) (Epub ahead of print).

[17] L. McLaren, Socioeconomic status and obesity, Epidemiol. Rev. 29 (2007) 29–48.

[18] L. Lu, H. Risch, M.L. Irwin, et al., Long-term overweight and weight gain in early adulthood in association with risk of endometrial cancer, Int. J. Cancer 129 (5) (2011) 1237–1243.

[19] A.J. Flint, K.M. Rexrode, F.B. Hu, et al., Body mass index, waist circumference, and risk of coronary heart disease: a prospective study among men and women, Obes. Res. Clin. Pract. 4 (3) (2010) E171–E181.

[20] A.J. Flint, F.B. Hu, R.J. Glynn, et al., Excess weight and the risk of incident coronary heart disease among men and women, Obesity (Silver Spring) 18 (2) (2010) 377–383.

[21] S.K. Das, N.K. Sharma, S.J. Hasstedt, et al., An integrative genomics approach identifies activation of thioredoxin/thioredoxin reductase-1-mediated oxidative stress defense pathway and inhibition of angiogenesis in obese nondiabetic human subjects, J. Clin. Endocrinol. Metab. 96 (8) (2011) E1308–E1313.

[22] A.E. Field, E.H. Coakley, A. Must, et al., Impact of overweight on the risk of developing common chronic diseases during a 10-year period, Arch. Intern. Med. 161 (13) (2001) 1581–1586.

[23] A.R. Weinstein, H.D. Sesso, I.M. Lee, et al., Relationship of physical activity vs body mass index with type 2 diabetes in women, JAMA 292 (10) (2004) 1188–1194.

[24] C. Chamberlain, P. Romundstad, L. Vatten, D. Gunnell, R.M. Martin, The association of weight gain during adulthood with prostate cancer incidence and survival: a population-based cohort, Int. J. Cancer 129 (5) (2011) 1199–1206.

[25] L.P. Wallner, H. Morgenstern, M.E. McGree, et al., The effects of metabolic conditions on prostate cancer incidence over 15 years of follow-up: results from the Olmsted County Study, BJU Int. 107 (6) (2011) 929–935.

[26] K.M. Narayan, J.P. Boyle, T.J. Thompson, E.W. Gregg, D.F. Williamson, Effect of BMI on lifetime risk for diabetes in the U.S, Diabetes Care 30 (6) (2007) 1562–1566.

[27] A. Pan, Q. Sun, S. Czernichow, et al., Bidirectional association between depression and obesity in middle-aged and older women, Int. J. Obes. (London) (2011) (Epub ahead of print).

[28] J.I. Hudson, E. Hiripi, H.G. Pope Jr., R.C. Kessler, The prevalence and correlates of eating disorders in the National Comorbidity Survey Replication, Biol. Psychiatry 61 (3) (2007) 348–358.

[29] R.M. Puhl, C.A. Heuer, The stigma of obesity: a review and update, Obesity (Silver Spring) 17 (5) (2009) 941–964.

[30] N.H. Falkner, S.A. French, R.W. Jeffery, D. Neumark-Sztainer, N.E. Sherwood, N. Morton, Mistreatment due to weight: prevalence and sources of perceived mistreatment in women and men, Obes. Res. 7 (6) (1999) 572–576.

[31] A.G. Tsai, D.F. Williamson, H.A. Glick, Direct medical cost of overweight and obesity in the U.S.A: a quantitative systematic review, Obes. Rev. 12 (1) (2011) 50–61.

[32] Y.C. Wang, K. McPherson, T. Marsh, S.L. Gortmaker, M. Brown, Health and economic burden of the projected obesity trends in the U.S.A and the UK, Lancet 378 (9793) (2011) 815–825.

[33] D. Withrow, D.A. Alter, The economic burden of obesity worldwide: a systematic review of the direct costs of obesity, Obes. Rev. 12 (2) (2011) 131–141.

[34] E.A. Finkelstein, M. DiBonaventura, S.M. Burgess, B.C. Hale, The costs of obesity in the workplace, J. Occup. Environ. Med. 52 (10) (2010) 971–976.

[35] E. Finkelstein, I.C. Fiebelkorn, G. Wang, National medical spending attributable to overweight and obesity: how much, and who's paying? Health Affairs W3 (2003) 219–226.

[36] E.A. Finkelstein, J.G. Trogdon, J.W. Cohen, W. Dietz, Annual medical spending attributable to obesity: payer-and service-specific estimates, Health Aff. (Millwood) 28 (5) (2009) w822–w831.

[37] P.A. Estabrooks, S. Shetterly, The prevalence and health care use of overweight children in an integrated health care system, Arch. Pediatr. Adolesc. Med. 161 (3) (2007) 222–227.

[38] S.E. Hampl, C.A. Carroll, S.D. Simon, V. Sharma, Resource utilization and expenditures for overweight and obese children, Arch. Pediatr. Adolesc. Med. 161 (1) (2007) 11–14.

[39] L. Trasande, S. Chatterjee, The impact of obesity on health service utilization and costs in childhood, Obesity (Silver Spring) 17 (9) (2009) 1749–1754.

[40] L. Trasande, Y. Liu, G. Fryer, M. Weitzman, Effects of childhood obesity on hospital care and costs, 1999–2005, Health Aff. (Millwood) 28 (4) (2009) w751–w760.

[41] Anonymous, Obesity: preventing and managing the global epidemic. Report of a WHO consultation, World Health Organ. Tech. Rep. Ser. 894 (2000) i–xii,1–253.

[42] C. Bouchard, Childhood obesity: are genetic differences involved? Am. J. Clin. Nutr. 89 (5) (2009) 1494S–1501S.

[43] H. Choquet, D. Meyre, Genetics of obesity: What have we learned? Curr. Genomics 12 (3) (2011) 169–179.

[44] H. Choquet, D. Meyre, Molecular basis of obesity: current status and future prospects, Curr. Genomics 12 (3) (2011) 154–168.

[45] J. Wardle, S. Carnell, Appetite is a heritable phenotype associated with adiposity, Ann. Behav. Med. (2009) (Epub ahead of print).

[46] S. Carnell, J. Wardle, Appetitive traits in children. New evidence for associations with weight and a common, obesity-associated genetic variant, Appetite 53 (2) (2009) 260–263.

[47] S. Carnell, C.M. Haworth, R. Plomin, J. Wardle, Genetic influence on appetite in children, Int. J. Obes. (London) 32 (10) (2008) 1468–1473.

[48] N.E. Sherwood, R.W. Jeffery, S.A. French, P.J. Hannan, D.M. Murray, Predictors of weight gain in the Pound of Prevention study, Int. J. Obes. Relat. Metab. Disord. 24 (4) (2000) 395–403.

[49] K.H. Schmitz, D.R. Jacobs Jr., A.S. Leon, P.J. Schreiner, B. Sternfeld, Physical activity and body weight: associations over ten years in the CARDIA study. Coronary artery risk development in young adults, Int. J. Obes. Relat. Metab. Disord. 24 (11) (2000) 1475–1487.

[50] A.L. Hankinson, M.L. Daviglus, C. Bouchard, et al., Maintaining a high physical activity level over 20 years and weight gain, JAMA 304 (23) (2010) 2603–2610.

[51] K. Waller, J. Kaprio, U.M. Kujala, Associations between long-term physical activity, waist circumference and weight gain: a 30-year longitudinal twin study, Int. J. Obes. (London) 32 (2) (2008) 353–361.

[52] A. Must, L.G. Bandini, D.J. Tybor, S.M. Phillips, E.N. Naumova, W.H. Dietz, Activity, inactivity, and screen time in relation to weight and fatness over adolescence in girls, Obesity (Silver Spring) 15 (7) (2007) 1774–1781.

[53] A. Must, D.J. Tybor, Physical activity and sedentary behavior: a review of longitudinal studies of weight and adiposity in youth, Int. J. Obes. (London) 29 (Suppl. 2) (2005) S84–S96.

[54] D. Menschik, S. Ahmed, M.H. Alexander, R.W. Blum, Adolescent physical activities as predictors of young adult weight, Arch. Pediatr. Adolesc. Med. 162 (1) (2008) 29–33.

[55] D.F. Tate Jr., N.E. Sherwood, R.R. Wing, Long-term weight losses associated with prescription of higher physical activity goals: Are higher levels of physical activity protective against weight regain? Am. J. Clin. Nutr. 85 (4) (2007) 954–959.

[56] E.P. Whitlock, E.A. O'Connor, S.B. Williams, T.L. Beil, K.W. Lutz, Effectiveness of weight management interventions in children: a targeted systematic review for the U.S.PSTF, Pediatrics 125 (2) (2010) E396–E418.

[57] L.H. Epstein, Exercise in the treatment of childhood obesity, Int. J. Obes. Relat. Metab. Disord. 19 (Suppl. 4) (1995) S117–S121.

[58] R.R. Wing, J.O. Hill, Successful weight loss maintenance, Annu. Rev. Nutr. 21 (2001) 323–341.

[59] J.M. Jakicic, K.K. Davis, Obesity and physical activity, Psychiatr. Clin. North Am. 34 (4) (2011) 829–840.

[60] S.A. Carlson, J.E. Fulton, C.A. Schoenborn, F. Loustalot, Trend and prevalence estimates based on the 2008 physical activity guidelines for americans, Am. J. Prev. Med. 39 (4) (2010) 305–313.

[61] S.A. Carlson, D. Densmore, J.E. Fulton, M.M. Yore, H.W. Kohl III, Differences in physical activity prevalence and trends from 3 U.S. surveillance systems: NHIS, NHANES, and BRFSS, J. Phys. Act. Health 6 (Suppl. 1) (2009) S18–S27.

[62] M.C. Whitt-Glover, W.C. Taylor, G.W. Heath, C.A. Macera, Self-reported physical activity among blacks: estimates from national surveys, Am. J. Prev. Med. 33 (5) (2007) 412–417.

[63] M. Huhman, R. Lowry, S. Lee, J. Fulton, S.A. Carlson, C.D. Patnode, Physical activity and screen time: trends in U.S. children aged 9–13 years, 2002–2006, J. Phys. Act. Health (2011) (Epub ahead of print).

[64] J. Duke, M. Huhman, C. Heitzler, Physical activity levels among children aged 9–13 years—United States, 2002, MMWR Morb. Mortal. Wkly. Rep. 52 (33) (2003) 785–788.

[65] B.R. Belcher, D. Berrigan, K.W. Dodd, B.A. Emken, C.P. Chou, D. Spruijt-Metz, Physical activity in U.S. youth: effect of race/ethnicity, age, gender, and weight status, Med. Sci. Sports Exerc. 42 (12) (2010) 2211–2221.

[66] T.J. Zywicki, Institutional review boards as academic bureau-cracies: an economic and experiential analysis, Northwestern Univ. Law Rev. 101 (2) (2007) 861–896.

[67] U.S. Department of Health and Human Services, Physical Activity and Health: A Report of the Surgeon General, U.S. Department of Health and Human Services, Centers for Disease Control and Prevention, National Center for Chronic Disease Prevention and Health Promotion, Atlanta, GA, 1996.

[68] T.S. Church, D.M. Thomas, C. Tudor-Locke, et al., Trends over 5 decades in U.S. occupation-related physical activity and their associations with obesity, PLoS One 6 (5) (2011) E19657.

[69] V.C. Strasburger, Children, adolescents, obesity, and the media, Pediatrics 128 (1) (2011) 201–208.

[70] F.J. Zimmerman, J.F. Bell, Associations of television content type and obesity in children, Am. J. Public Health 100 (2) (2010) 334–340.

[71] Blog. What Consumers Watch: Nielsen's Q1 2010 Three Screen Report. Available at <http://blog.nielsen.com/nielsenwire/online_mobile/what-consumers-watch-nielsens-q1-2010-three-screen-report/>.

[72] American Time Use Survey. Available at <http://www.bls.gov/tus/charts/LEISURE.HTM/>, 2012 (accessed 02.03.12).

[73] R.R. Pate, J.A. Mitchell, W. Byun, M. Dowda, Sedentary behaviour in youth, Br. J. Sports Med. 45 (11) (2011) 906–913.

[74] S.B. Sisson, T.S. Church, C.K. Martin, et al., Profiles of sedentary behavior in children and adolescents: the U.S. National Health and Nutrition Examination Survey, 2001–2006, Int. J. Pediatr. Obes. 4 (4) (2009) 353–359.

[75] F.J. Zimmerman, D.A. Christakis, A.N. Meltzoff, Television and DVD/video viewing in children younger than 2 years, Arch. Pediatr. Adolesc. Med. 161 (5) (2007) 473–479.

[76] L.K. Certain, R.S. Kahn, Prevalence, correlates, and trajectory of television viewing among infants and toddlers, Pediatrics 109 (4) (2002) 634–642.

[77] V. Rideout, E. Hamel, The media family: electronic media in the lives of infants, toddlers, preschoolers, and their parents. Available at <http://www.kff.org/entmedia/7500.cfm/>, 2012 (accessed 02.03.12).

[78] A. Perez, D.M. Hoelscher, A.E. Springer, et al., Physical activity, watching television, and the risk of obesity in students, Texas, 2004–2005, Prev. Chronic Dis. 8 (3) (2011) A61.

[79] R.T. Kimbro, J. Brooks-Gunn, S. McLanahan, Young children in urban areas: links among neighborhood characteristics, weight status, outdoor play, and television watching, Soc. Sci. Med. 72 (5) (2011) 668–676.

[80] S.C. Ullrich-French, T.G. Power, K.B. Daratha, R.C. Bindler, M. M. Steele, Examination of adolescents' screen time and physical fitness as independent correlates of weight status and blood pressure, J. Sports Sci. 28 (11) (2010) 1189–1196.

[81] J.E. Fulton, X. Wang, M.M. Yore, S.A. Carlson, D.A. Galuska, C. J. Caspersen, Television viewing, computer use, and BMI among U.S. children and adolescents, J. Phys. Act. Health 6 (Suppl. 1) (2009) S28–S35.

[82] K.R. Laurson, J.C. Eisenmann, G.J. Welk, E.E. Wickel, D.A. Gentile, D.A. Walsh, Combined influence of physical activity and screen time recommendations on childhood overweight, J. Pediatr. 153 (2) (2008) 209–214.

[83] S. Gable, Y. Chang, J.L. Krull, Television watching and frequency of family meals are predictive of overweight onset and persistence in a national sample of school-aged children, J. Am. Diet. Assoc. 107 (1) (2007) 53–61.

[84] K.K. Davison, S.J. Marshall, L.L. Birch, Cross-sectional and longitudinal associations between TV viewing and girls' body mass index, overweight status, and percentage of body fat, J. Pediatr. 149 (1) (2006) 32–37.

[85] M.L. Granner, A. Mburia-Mwalili, Correlates of television viewing among African American and Caucasian women, Women Health 50 (8) (2010) 783–794.

[86] M. Shields, M.S. Tremblay, Sedentary behaviour and obesity, Health Rep. 19 (2) (2008) 19–30.

[87] S.A. Bowman, Television-viewing characteristics of adults: correlations to eating practices and overweight and health status, Prev. Chronic Dis. 3 (2) (2006) A38.

[88] K.M. Johnson, K.M. Nelson, K.A. Bradley, Television viewing practices and obesity among women veterans, J. Gen. Intern. Med. 21 (Suppl. 3) (2006) S76–S81.

[89] F.B. Hu, T.Y. Li, G.A. Colditz, W.C. Willett, J.E. Manson, Television watching and other sedentary behaviors in relation to risk of obesity and type 2 diabetes mellitus in women, JAMA 289 (14) (2003) 1785–1791.

[90] L.H. Epstein, J.N. Roemmich, R.A. Paluch, H.A. Raynor, Physical activity as a substitute for sedentary behavior in youth, Ann. Behav. Med. 29 (3) (2005) 200–209.

[91] Institute of Medicine. Food marketing to children and youth: Threat or opportunity?. (2008). Available at <http://www.iom.edu/Reports/2005/Food-Marketing-to-Children-and-Youth-Threat-or-Opportunity.aspx/>.

[92] L.H. Epstein, J.N. Roemmich, J.L. Robinson, et al., A randomized trial of the effects of reducing television viewing and computer use on body mass index in young children, Arch. Pediatr. Adolesc. Med. 162 (3) (2008) 239–245.

[93] L.H. Epstein, A.M. Valoski, L.S. Vara, et al., Effects of decreasing sedentary behavior and increasing activity on weight change in obese children, Health Psychol. 14 (2) (1995) 109–115.

[94] L.H. Epstein, R.A. Paluch, C.K. Kilanowski, H.A. Raynor, The effect of reinforcement or stimulus control to reduce sedentary behavior in the treatment of pediatric obesity, Health Psychol. 23 (4) (2004) 371–380.

[95] L.H. Epstein, J.N. Roemmich, R.A. Paluch, H.A. Raynor, Influence of changes in sedentary behavior on energy and macronutrient intake in youth, Am. J. Clin. Nutr. 81 (2) (2005) 361–366.

[96] T.N. Robinson, Reducing children's television viewing to prevent obesity: a randomized controlled trial, JAMA 282 (16) (1999) 1561–1567.

[97] S.L. Gortmaker, K. Peterson, J. Wiecha, et al., Reducing obesity via a school-based interdisciplinary intervention among youth: planet health, Arch. Pediatr. Adolesc. Med. 153 (4) (1999) 409–418.

[98] B.A. Dennison, T.J. Russo, P.A. Burdick, P.L. Jenkins, An intervention to reduce television viewing by preschool children, Arch. Pediatr. Adolesc. Med. 158 (2) (2004) 170–176.

[99] J. Salmon, K. Ball, C. Hume, M. Booth, D. Crawford, Outcomes of a group-randomized trial to prevent excess weight gain, reduce screen behaviours and promote physical activity in 10-year-old children: switch-play, Int. J. Obes. (London) 32 (4) (2008) 601–612.

[100] R.R. Kipping, C. Payne, D.A. Lawlor, Randomised controlled trial adapting U.S. school obesity prevention to England, Arch. Dis. Child 93 (6) (2008) 469–473.

[101] B.S. Ford, T.E. McDonald, A.S. Owens, T.N. Robinson, Primary care interventions to reduce television viewing in African-American children, Am. J. Prev. Med. 22 (2) (2002) 106–109.

[102] S.L. Escobar-Chaves, C.M. Markham, R.C. Addy, A. Greisinger, N.G. Murray, B. Brehm, The fun families study: intervention to reduce children's TV viewing, Obesity (Silver Spring) 18 (Suppl. 1) (2010) S99–S101.

C. OVERWEIGHT AND OBESITY

[103] L.H. Epstein, R.A. Paluch, C.C. Gordy, J. Dorn, Decreasing sedentary behaviors in treating pediatric obesity, Arch. Pediatr. Adolesc. Med. 154 (3) (2000) 220–226.

[104] C. Ni Mhurchu, V. Roberts, R. Maddison, et al., Effect of electronic time monitors on children's television watching: pilot trial of a home-based intervention, Prev. Med 49 (5) (2009) 413–417.

[105] T.N. Robinson, D.M. Matheson, H.C. Kraemer, et al., A randomized controlled trial of culturally tailored dance and reducing screen time to prevent weight gain in low-income African American girls: stanford GEMS, Arch. Pediatr. Adolesc. Med. 164 (11) (2010) 995–1004.

[106] M.K. Todd, M.J. Reis-Bergan, C.L. Sidman, et al., Effect of a family-based intervention on electronic media use and body composition among boys aged 8–11 years: a pilot study, J. Child Health Care 12 (4) (2008) 344–358.

[107] S.A. French, A.F. Gerlach, N.R. Mitchell, P.J. Hannan, E.M. Welsh, Household obesity prevention: take action—a group-randomized trial, Obesity (Silver Spring) 19 (10) (2011) 2082–2088.

[108] G. Wahi, P.C. Parkin, J. Beyene, E.M. Uleryk, C.S. Birken, Effectiveness of interventions aimed at reducing screen time in children: a systematic review and meta-analysis of randomized controlled trials, Arch. Pediatr. Adolesc. Med. 165 (11) (2011) 979–986.

[109] A. Bandura, Social Foundations of Thought and Action: A Social Cognitive Theory, Prentice Hall, Englewood Cliffs, NJ, 1986.

[110] K.A. DuCharme, L.R. Brawley, Predicting the intentions and behavior of exercise initiates using two forms of self-efficacy, J. Behav. Med. 18 (5) (1995) 479–497.

[111] S.M. White, T.R. Wojcicki, E. McAuley, Social cognitive influences on physical activity behavior in middle-aged and older adults, J. Gerontol. B Psychol. Sci. Soc. Sci. 67 (1) (2012) 18–26.

[112] E. McAuley, G.J. Jerome, D.X. Marquez, S. Elavsky, B. Blissmer, Exercise self-efficacy in older adults: social, affective, and behavioral influences, Ann. Behav. Med. 25 (1) (2003) 1–7.

[113] E. McAuley, The role of efficacy cognitions in the prediction of exercise behavior in middle-aged adults, J. Behav. Med. 15 (1) (1992) 65–88.

[114] E. McAuley, Self-efficacy and the maintenance of exercise participation in older adults, J. Behav. Med. 16 (1993) 103–113.

[115] E. McAuley, J. Katula, S.L. Mihalko, et al., Mode of physical activity and self-efficacy in older adults: a latent growth curve analysis, J. Gerontol. B Psychol. Sci. Soc. Sci. 54 (5) (1999) P283–P292.

[116] A.L. Crain, B.C. Martinson, N.E. Sherwood, P.J. O'Connor, The long and winding road to physical activity maintenance, Am. J. Health Behav. 34 (6) (2010) 764–775.

[117] R.K. Dishman, R.P. Saunders, R.W. Motl, M. Dowda, R.R. Pate, Self-efficacy moderates the relation between declines in physical activity and perceived social support in high school girls, J. Pediatr. Psychol. 34 (4) (2009) 441–451.

[118] R.W. Motl, R.K. Dishman, R.P. Saunders, M. Dowda, R.R. Pate, Perceptions of physical and social environment variables and self-efficacy as correlates of self-reported physical activity among adolescent girls, J. Pediatr. Psychol. 32 (1) (2007) 6–12.

[119] D.J. Barr-Anderson, D.R. Young, J.F. Sallis, et al., Structured physical activity and psychosocial correlates in middle-school girls, Prev. Med. 44 (5) (2007) 404–409.

[120] A. Fisher, J. Saxton, C. Hill, L. Webber, L. Purslow, J. Wardle, Psychosocial correlates of objectively measured physical activity in children, Eur. J. Public Health 21 (2) (2011) 145–150.

[121] C. Craggs, K. Corder, E.M. van Sluijs, S.J. Griffin, Determinants of change in physical activity in children and adolescents: a systematic review, Am. J. Prev. Med. 40 (6) (2011) 645–658.

[122] K.A. Jose, L. Blizzard, T. Dwyer, C. McKercher, A.J. Venn, Childhood and adolescent predictors of leisure time physical activity during the transition from adolescence to adulthood: a population based cohort study, Int. J. Behav. Nutr. Phys. Act. 8 (2011) 54.

[123] K.F. Janz, J.D. Dawson, L.T. Mahoney, Tracking physical fitness and physical activity from childhood to adolescence: the muscatine study, Med. Sci. Sports Exerc. 32 (7) (2000) 1250–1257.

[124] I. De Bourdeaudhuij, J. Sallis, C. Vandelanotte, Tracking and explanation of physical activity in young adults over a 7-year period, Res. Q. Exerc. Sport 73 (4) (2002) 376–385.

[125] A.M. Craigie, A.A. Lake, S.A. Kelly, A.J. Adamson, J.C. Mathers, Tracking of obesity-related behaviours from childhood to adulthood: a systematic review, Maturitas 70 (3) (2011) 266–284.

[126] M.C. Nelson, P. Gordon-Larsen, L.S. Adair, B.M. Popkin, Adolescent physical activity and sedentary behavior: patterning and long-term maintenance, Am. J. Prev. Med. 28 (3) (2005) 259–266.

[127] T.E. Makinen, K. Borodulin, T.H. Tammelin, O. Rahkonen, T. Laatikainen, R. Prattala, The effects of adolescence sports and exercise on adulthood leisure-time physical activity in educational groups, Int. J. Behav. Nutr. Phys. Act. 7 (2010) 27.

[128] S.L. Francis, M.J. Stancel, F.D. Sernulka-George, B. Broffitt, S.M. Levy, K.F. Janz, Tracking of TV and video gaming during childhood: Iowa bone development study, Int. J. Behav. Nutr. Phys. Act. 8 (2011) 100.

[129] W.C. Taylor, S.N. Blair, S.S. Cummings, C.C. Wun, R.M. Malina, Childhood and adolescent physical activity patterns and adult physical activity, Med. Sci. Sports Exerc. 31 (1) (1999) 118–123.

[130] M. Dowda, K.A. Pfeiffer, W.H. Brown, J.A. Mitchell, W. Byun, R.R. Pate, Parental and environmental correlates of physical activity of children attending preschool, Arch. Pediatr. Adolesc. Med. 165 (10) (2011) 939–944.

[131] R.R. Rosenkranz, G.J. Welk, T.J. Hastmann, D.A. Dzewaltowski, Psychosocial and demographic correlates of objectively measured physical activity in structured and unstructured after-school recreation sessions, J. Sci. Med. Sport 14 (4) (2011) 306–311.

[132] E. Garcia Bengoechea, C.M. Sabiston, R. Ahmed, M. Farnoush, Exploring links to unorganized and organized physical activity during adolescence: the role of gender, socioeconomic status, weight status, and enjoyment of physical education, Res. Q. Exerc. Sport 81 (1) (2010) 7–16.

[133] S.B. Gesell, E.B. Reynolds, E.H. Ip, et al., Social influences on self-reported physical activity in overweight Latino children, Clin. Pediatr. (Philadelphia) 47 (8) (2008) 797–802.

[134] K.A. King, J.L. Tergerson, B.R. Wilson, Effect of social support on adolescents' perceptions of and engagement in physical activity, J. Phys. Act. Health 5 (3) (2008) 374–384.

[135] M.W. Beets, K.H. Pitetti, L. Forlaw, The role of self-efficacy and referent specific social support in promoting rural adolescent girls' physical activity, Am. J. Health Behav 31 (3) (2007) 227–237.

[136] M.W. Beets, R. Vogel, L. Forlaw, K.H. Pitetti, B.J. Cardinal, Social support and youth physical activity: the role of provider and type, Am. J. Health Behav. 30 (3) (2006) 278–289.

[137] M. Dowda, R.K. Dishman, K.A. Pfeiffer, R.R. Pate, Family support for physical activity in girls from 8th to 12th grade in South Carolina, Prev. Med. 44 (2) (2007) 153–159.

[138] J. Kuo, C.C. Voorhees, J.A. Haythornthwaite, D.R. Young, Associations between family support, family intimacy, and neighborhood violence and physical activity in urban adolescent girls, Am. J. Public Health 97 (1) (2007) 101–103.

[139] C.D. Heitzler, S.L. Martin, J. Duke, M. Huhman, Correlates of physical activity in a national sample of children aged 9–13 years, Prev. Med. 42 (4) (2006) 254–260.

[140] S.C. Duncan, T.E. Duncan, L.A. Strycker, Sources and types of social support in youth physical activity, Health Psychol. 24 (1) (2005) 3–10.

[141] R.P. Saunders, R.W. Motl, M. Dowda, R.K. Dishman, R.R. Pate, Comparison of social variables for understanding physical activity in adolescent girls, Am. J. Health Behav. 28 (5) (2004) 426–436.

[142] D. Neumark-Sztainer, M. Story, P.J. Hannan, T. Tharp, J. Rex, Factors associated with changes in physical activity: a cohort study of inactive adolescent girls, Arch. Pediatr. Adolesc. Med. 157 (8) (2003) 803–810.

[143] E.S. Anderson-Bill, R.A. Winett, J.R. Wojcik, Social cognitive determinants of nutrition and physical activity among web-health users enrolling in an online intervention: the influence of social support, self-efficacy, outcome expectations, and self-regulation, J. Med. Internet Res. 13 (1) (2011) e28.

[144] C. Kim, L.N. McEwen, E.C. Kieffer, W.H. Herman, J.D. Piette, Self-efficacy, social support, and associations with physical activity and body mass index among women with histories of gestational diabetes mellitus, Diabetes Educ. 34 (4) (2008) 719–728.

[145] B.A. Fischer Aggarwal, M. Liao, L. Mosca, Physical activity as a potential mechanism through which social support may reduce cardiovascular disease risk, J. Cardiovasc. Nurs. 23 (2) (2008) 90–96.

[146] M. Bopp, S. Wilcox, M. Laken, L. McClorin, Physical activity participation in African American churches, J. Cult. Divers. 16 (1) (2009) 26–31.

[147] B. Resnick, D. Orwig, J. Magaziner, C. Wynne, The effect of social support on exercise behavior in older adults, Clin. Nurs. Res. 11 (1) (2002) 52–70.

[148] P.A. Spanier, K.R. Allison, General social support and physical activity: an analysis of the Ontario Health Survey, Can. J. Public Health 92 (3) (2001) 210–213.

[149] A.A. Eyler, R.C. Brownson, R.J. Donatelle, A.C. King, D. Brown, J.F. Sallis, Physical activity social support and middle- and older-aged minority women: results from a U.S. survey, Soc. Sci. Med. 49 (6) (1999) 781–789.

[150] R.K. Oka, A.C. King, D.R. Young, Sources of social support as predictors of exercise adherence in women and men ages 50 to 65 years, Womens Health 1 (2) (1995) 161–175.

[151] M. Kanu, E. Baker, R.C. Brownson, Exploring associations between church-based social support and physical activity, J. Phys. Act. Health 5 (4) (2008) 504–515.

[152] A.V. Carron, H.A. Hausenblaus, D. Mack, Social influence and exercise: a meta-analysis, J. Sports Med. Phys. Fitness 18 (1996) 1–16.

[153] E.S. Anderson, J.R. Wojcik, R.A. Winett, D.M. Williams, Social–cognitive determinants of physical activity: the influence of social support, self-efficacy, outcome expectations, and self-regulation among participants in a church-based health promotion study, Health Psychol. 25 (4) (2006) 510–520.

[154] J.M. Gabriele, M.S. Walker, D.L. Gill, K.D. Harber, E.B. Fisher, Differentiated roles of social encouragement and social constraint on physical activity behavior, Ann. Behav. Med. 29 (3) (2005) 210–215.

[155] M.W. Beets, B.J. Cardinal, B.L. Alderman, Parental social support and the physical activity-related behaviors of youth: a review, Health Educ. Behav. 37 (5) (2010) 621–644.

[156] C.C. Voorhees, D.J. Catellier, J.S. Ashwood, et al., Neighborhood socioeconomic status and non school physical activity and body mass index in adolescent girls, J. Phys. Act. Health 6 (6) (2009) 731–740.

[157] B.R. Williams, J. Bezner, S.B. Chesbro, R. Leavitt, The effect of a walking program on perceived benefits and barriers to exercise in postmenopausal African American women, J. Geriatr. Phys. Ther. 29 (2) (2006) 43–49.

[158] T. Osuji, S.L. Lovegreen, M. Elliott, R.C. Brownson, Barriers to physical activity among women in the rural Midwest, Women Health 44 (1) (2006) 41–55.

[159] G.R. Dutton, J. Johnson, D. Whitehead, J.S. Bodenlos, P.J. Brantley, Barriers to physical activity among predominantly low-income African-American patients with type 2 diabetes, Diabetes Care 28 (5) (2005) 1209–1210.

[160] J. Kowal, M.S. Fortier, Physical activity behavior change in middle-aged and older women: the role of barriers and of environmental characteristics, J. Behav. Med 30 (3) (2007) 233–242.

[161] K.E. Donahue, T.J. Mielenz, P.D. Sloane, L.F. Callahan, R.F. Devellis, Identifying supports and barriers to physical activity in patients at risk for diabetes, Prev. Chronic Dis. 3 (4) (2006) A119.

[162] D.X. Marquez, E.E. Bustamante, B.C. Bock, G. Markenson, A. Tovar, L. Chasan-Taber, Perspectives of Latina and non-Latina white women on barriers and facilitators to exercise in pregnancy, Women Health 49 (6) (2009) 505–521.

[163] A.G. Cramp, S.R. Bray, Understanding exercise self-efficacy and barriers to leisure-time physical activity among postnatal women, Matern. Child Health J. 15 (5) (2011) 642–651.

[164] B.C. Martinson, N.E. Sherwood, A.L. Crain, et al., Maintaining physical activity among older adults: 24-month outcomes of the keep active Minnesota randomized controlled trial, Prev. Med. 51 (1) (2010) 37–44.

[165] A.C. King, R. Friedman, B. Marcus, et al., Ongoing physical activity advice by humans versus computers: the community health advice by telephone (CHAT) trial, Health Psychol. 26 (6) (2007) 718–727.

[166] B.H. Marcus, M.A. Napolitano, A.C. King, et al., Telephone versus print delivery of an individualized motivationally tailored physical activity intervention: project STRIDE, Health Psychol. 26 (4) (2007) 401–409.

[167] B.H. Marcus, B.A. Lewis, D.M. Williams, et al., A comparison of Internet and print-based physical activity interventions, Arch. Intern. Med. 167 (9) (2007) 944–949.

[168] C.E. Short, E.L. James, R.C. Plotnikoff, A. Girgis, Efficacy of tailored-print interventions to promote physical activity: a systematic review of randomised trials, Int. J. Behav. Nutr. Phys. Act. 8 (2011) 113.

[169] A.C. King, D.K. Ahn, B.M. Oliveira, A.A. Atienza, C.M. Castro, C.D. Gardner, Promoting physical activity through hand-held computer technology, Am. J. Prev. Med. 34 (2) (2008) 138–142.

[170] M.A. Napolitano, M. Fotheringham, D. Tate, et al., Evaluation of an Internet-based physical activity intervention: a preliminary investigation, Ann. Behav. Med. 25 (2) (2003) 92–99.

[171] M. Grim, B. Hortz, R. Petosa, Impact evaluation of a pilot web-based intervention to increase physical activity, Am. J. Health Promot. 25 (4) (2011) 227–230.

[172] D.J. Barr-Anderson, M. AuYoung, M.C. Whitt-Glover, B.A. Glenn, A.K. Yancey, Integration of short bouts of physical activity into organizational routine a systematic review of the literature, Am. J. Prev. Med. 40 (1) (2011) 76–93.

[173] R.C. Brownson, C.M. Hoehner, K. Day, A. Forsyth, J.F. Sallis, Measuring the built environment for physical activity: state of the science, Am. J. Prev. Med. 36 (4 Suppl.) (2009) S99—S123.

[174] J.F. Sallis, M.F. Floyd, D.A. Rodriguez, B.E. Saelens, Role of built environments in physical activity, obesity, and cardiovascular disease, Circulation 125 (5) (2012) 729—737.

[175] A.V. Diez Roux, K.R. Evenson, A.P. McGinn, et al., Availability of recreational resources and physical activity in adults, Am. J. Public Health 97 (3) (2007) 493—499.

[176] D. Ding, J.F. Sallis, J. Kerr, S. Lee, D.E. Rosenberg, Neighborhood environment and physical activity among youth a review, Am. J. Prev. Med. 41 (4) (2011) 442—455.

[177] R.C. Klesges, L.H. Eck, C.L. Hanson, C.K. Haddock, L.M. Klesges, Effects of obesity, social interactions, and physical environment on physical activity in preschoolers, Health Psychol. 9 (4) (1990) 435—449.

[178] V. Cleland, D. Crawford, L.A. Baur, C. Hume, A. Timperio, J. Salmon, A prospective examination of children's time spent outdoors, objectively measured physical activity and overweight, Int. J. Obes. (London) 32 (11) (2008) 1685—1693.

[179] D. Fuller, C. Sabiston, I. Karp, T. Barnett, J. O'Loughlin, School sports opportunities influence physical activity in secondary school and beyond, J. School Health 81 (8) (2011) 449—454.

[180] A.R. Kurc, S.T. Leatherdale, The effect of social support and school- and community-based sports on youth physical activity, Can. J. Public Health 100 (1) (2009) 60—64.

[181] J.F. Sallis, J.E. Alcaraz, T.L. McKenzie, M.F. Hovell, Predictors of change in children's physical activity over 20 months: variations by gender and level of adiposity, Am. J. Prev. Med. 16 (3) (1999) 222—229.

[182] J.F. Sallis, J.J. Prochaska, W.C. Taylor, J.O. Hill, J.C. Geraci, Correlates of physical activity in a national sample of girls and boys in grades 4 through 12, Health Psychol. 18 (4) (1999) 410—415.

[183] S. Adkins, N.E. Sherwood, M. Story, M. Davis, Physical activity among African-American girls: the role of parents and the home environment, Obes. Res. 12 (Suppl.) (2004) 38S—45S.

[184] R.R. Wing, S. Phelan, Long-term weight loss maintenance, Am. J. Clin. Nutr. 82 (Suppl. 1.) (2005) 222S—225S.

[185] A.K. Kant, B.I. Graubard, Secular trends in patterns of self-reported food consumption of adult Americans: NHANES 1971—1975 to NHANES 1999—2002, Am. J. Clin. Nutr. 84 (5) (2006) 1215—1223.

[186] K.J. Duffey, B.M. Popkin, Energy density, portion size, and eating occasions: contributions to increased energy intake in the United States, 1977—2006, PLoS Med. 8 (6) (2011) e1001050.

[187] R.R. Briefel, C.L. Johnson, Secular trends in dietary intake in the United States, Annu. Rev. Nutr. 24 (2004) 401—431.

[188] A.K. Kant, B.I. Graubard, 20-Year trends in dietary and meal behaviors were similar in U.S. children and adolescents of different race/ethnicity, J. Nutr. 141 (10) (2011) 1880—1888.

[189] J.M. Poti, B.M. Popkin, Trends in energy intake among U.S. children by eating location and food source, 1977—2006, J. Am. Diet. Assoc. 111 (8) (2011) 1156—1164.

[190] D.A. Schoeller, How accurate is self-reported dietary energy intake? Nutr. Rev. 48 (10) (1990) 373—379.

[191] A.H. Goris, M.S. Westerterp-Plantenga, K.R. Westerterp, Undereating and underrecording of habitual food intake in obese men: selective underreporting of fat intake, Am. J. Clin. Nutr. 71 (1) (2000) 130—134.

[192] S.S. Jonnalagadda, D.C. Mitchell, H. Smiciklas-Wright, et al., Accuracy of energy intake data estimated by a multiple-pass, 24-hour dietary recall technique, J. Am. Diet. Assoc. 100 (3) (2000) 303—311.

[193] S.J. Nielsen, B.M. Popkin, Changes in beverage intake between 1977 and 2001, Am. J. Prev. Med. 27 (3) (2004) 205—210.

[194] V.S. Malik, M.B. Schulze, F.B. Hu, Intake of sugar-sweetened beverages and weight gain: a systematic review, Am. J. Clin. Nutr. 84 (2) (2006) 274—288.

[195] N.J. Olsen, B.L. Heitmann, Intake of calorically sweetened beverages and obesity, Obes. Rev. 10 (1) (2009) 68—75.

[196] C.B. Ebbeling, H.A. Feldman, S.K. Osganian, V.R. Chomitz, S.J. Ellenbogen, D.S. Ludwig, Effects of decreasing sugar-sweetened beverage consumption on body weight in adolescents: a randomized, controlled pilot study, Pediatrics 117 (3) (2006) 673—680.

[197] D.F. Tate, G. Turner-McGrievy, E. Lyons, et al., Replacing caloric beverages with water or diet beverages for weight loss in adults: main results of the choose healthy options consciously everyday (CHOICE) randomized clinical trial, Am. J. Clin. Nutr. 95 (2012) 555—563.

[198] B.H. Lin, J. Guthrie, E. Frazao, Nutrient contribution of food eaten away from home, in: E. Frazao (Ed.), America's Eating Habits: Changes and Consequences, U.S.DA, Washington, DC, 1998.

[199] A.K. Kant, B.I. Graubard, Eating out in America, 1987—2000: trends and nutritional correlates, Prev. Med. 38 (2) (2004) 243—249.

[200] S.J. Nielsen, A.M. Siega-Riz, B.M. Popkin, Trends in food locations and sources among adolescents and young adults, Prev. Med. 35 (2) (2002) 107—113.

[201] M. Nestle, M.F. Jacobson, Halting the obesity epidemic: a public health policy approach, Public Health Rep. 115 (1) (2000) 12—24.

[202] J. Todd, L. Mancino, B.H. Lin, The impact of food away from home on adult diet quality, in:ERR-90, U.S. Department of Agriculture, Economic Research Service, Washington, DC, 2010.

[203] S.A. French, L. Harnack, R.W. Jeffery, Fast food restaurant use among women in the pound of prevention study: dietary, behavioral and demographic correlates, Int. J. Obes. Relat. Metab. Disord. 24 (10) (2000) 1353—1359.

[204] L. Frank, J. Kerr, B. Saelens, J. Sallis, K. Glanz, J. Chapman, Food outlet visits, physical activity and body weight: variations by gender and race-ethnicity, Br. J. Sports Med. 43 (2) (2009) 124—131.

[205] J. Boone-Heinonen, P. Gordon-Larsen, C.I. Kiefe, J.M. Shikany, C.E. Lewis, B.M. Popkin, Fast food restaurants and food stores: longitudinal associations with diet in young to middle-aged adults: The CARDIA study, Arch. Intern. Med. 171 (13) (2011) 1162—1170.

[206] J. Putnam, U.S. food supply providing more food and calories, Food Rev. 22 (1999) 2—12.

[207] H. Smiciklas-Wright, D.C. Mitchell, S.J. Mickle, J.D. Goldman, A. Cook, Foods commonly eaten in the United States, 1989—1991 and 1994—1996: Are portion sizes changing? J. Am. Diet. Assoc. 103 (1) (2003) 41—47.

[208] S. Nielsen, B. Popkin, Patterns and trends in food portion sizes, 1977—1998, JAMA 289 (4) (2003) 450—453.

[209] M. Story, S. French, Food advertising and marketing directed at children and adolescents in the U.S, Int. J. Behav. Nutr. Phys. Act. 1 (1) (2004) 3.

[210] J.L. Harris, M.B. Schwartz, K.D. Brownell, Marketing foods to children and adolescents: licensed characters and other promotions on packaged foods in the supermarket, Public Health Nutr 13 (3) (2010) 409—417.

[211] Kaiser Family Foundation. Food for thought: Television food advertising to children in the United States. (2007). Available

at <http://www.kff.org/entmedia/upload/7618.pdf/> (accessed 02.03.12).

[212] J. Brady, R. Mendelson, A. Farrell, S. Wong, Online marketing of food and beverages to children: a content analysis, Can. J. Diet. Pract. Res. 71 (4) (2010) 166−171.

[213] J. Culp, R.A. Bell, D. Cassady, Characteristics of food industry web sites and "advergames" targeting children, J. Nutr. Educ. Behav. 42 (3) (2010) 197−201.

[214] J. Chester, K. Montgomery, Interactive Food and Beverage Marketing: Targeting Children and Youth in the Digital Age, Berkeley Media Studies Group, Berkeley, CA, 2007.

[215] Institute of Medicine, Food Marketing to Children: Threat or Opportunity? National Academies Press, Washington, DC, 2006.

[216] V.I. Kraak, M. Story, E.A. Wartella, J. Ginter, Industry progress to market a healthful diet to American children and adolescents, Am. J. Prev. Med. 41 (3) (2011) 322−333.

[217] K. Boutelle, D. Neumark-Sztainer, M. Story, M. Resnick, Weight control behaviors among obese, overweight, and nonoverweight adolescents, J. Pediatr. Psychol. 27 (6) (2002) 531−540.

[218] G.C. Rampersaud, M.A. Pereira, B.L. Girard, J. Adams, J.D. Metzl, Breakfast habits, nutritional status, body weight, and academic performance in children and adolescents, J. Am. Diet. Assoc. 105 (5) (2005) 743−762.

[219] B.A. Barton, A.L. Eldridge, D. Thompson, et al., The relationship of breakfast and cereal consumption to nutrient intake and body mass index: the national heart, lung, and blood institute growth and health study, J. Am. Diet. Assoc. 105 (9) (2005) 1383−1389.

[220] S. Cho, M. Dietrich, C.J. Brown, C.A. Clark, G. Block, The effect of breakfast type on total daily energy intake and body mass index: results from the third national health and nutrition examination survey (NHANES III), J. Am. Coll. Nutr. 22 (4) (2003) 296−302.

[221] D. Neumark-Sztainer, C.L. Rock, M.D. Thornquist, L.J. Cheskin, M.L. Neuhouser, M.J. Barnett, Weight-control behaviors among adults and adolescents: associations with dietary intake, Prev. Med. 30 (5) (2000) 381−391.

[222] D. Neumark-Sztainer, S.A. French, R.W. Jeffery, Dieting for weight loss: associations with nutrient intake among women, J. Am. Diet. Assoc. 96 (11) (1996) 1172−1175.

[223] D. Neumark-Sztainer, M. Story, N.H. Falkner, T. Beuhring, M.D. Resnick, Sociodemographic and personal characteristics of adolescents engaged in weight loss and weight/muscle gain behaviors: Who is doing what? Prev. Med 28 (1) (1999) 40−50.

[224] D. Neumark-Sztainer, M. Wall, J. Guo, M. Story, J. Haines, M. Eisenberg, Obesity, disordered eating, and eating disorders in a longitudinal study of adolescents: How do dieters fare 5 years later? J. Am. Diet. Assoc. 106 (4) (2006) 559−568.

[225] E. Stice, R.P. Cameron, J.D. Killen, C. Hayward, C.B. Taylor, Naturalistic weight-reduction efforts prospectively predict growth in relative weight and onset of obesity among female adolescents, J. Consult Clin. Psychol. 67 (6) (1999) 967−974.

[226] C.P. Herman, J. Polivy, From dietary restraint to binge eating: attaching causes to effects, Appetite 14 (2) (1990) 123−125,142−143.

[227] D. Neumark-Sztainer, M. Wall, J. Haines, M. Story, M.E. Eisenberg, Why does dieting predict weight gain in adolescents? Findings from project EAT-II: A 5-year longitudinal study, J. Am. Diet. Assoc. 107 (3) (2007) 448−455.

[228] S.A. French, R.W. Jeffery, N.E. Sherwood, D. Neumark-Sztainer, Prevalence and correlates of binge eating in a nonclinical sample of women enrolled in a weight gain prevention program, Int. J. Obes. Relat. Metab. Disord. 23 (6) (1999) 576−585.

[229] A.E. Field, C.A. Camargo Jr., C.B. Taylor, et al., Overweight, weight concerns, and bulimic behaviors among girls and boys, J. Am. Acad. Child Adolesc. Psychiatry 38 (6) (1999) 754−760.

[230] M.A. Napolitano, S. Himes, Race, weight, and correlates of binge eating in female college students, Eat. Behav. 12 (1) (2011) 29−36.

[231] S.A. French, R.W. Jeffery, N.E. Sherwood, D. Neumark-Sztainer, Prevalence and correlates of binge eating in a nonclinical sample of women enrolled in a weight gain prevention program, Int. J. Obes. Relat. Metab. Disord. 23 (6) (1999) 576−585.

[232] M. de Zwaan, Binge eating disorder and obesity, Int. J. Obes. Relat. Metab. Disord. 25 (Suppl. 1) (2001) S51−S55.

[233] R.A. Grucza, T.R. Przybeck, C.R. Cloninger, Prevalence and correlates of binge eating disorder in a community sample, Compr. Psychiatry 48 (2) (2007) 124−131.

[234] L.L. Birch, K.K. Davison, Family environmental factors influencing the developing behavioral controls of food intake and childhood overweight, Pediatr. Clin. North Am. 48 (4) (2001) 893−907.

[235] L.L. Birch, A.K. Ventura, Preventing childhood obesity: What works? Int. J. Obes. (London) 33 (Suppl. 1) (2009) S74−S81.

[236] K.W. Bauer, D. Neumark-Sztainer, J.A. Fulkerson, P.J. Hannan, M. Story, Familial correlates of adolescent girls' physical activity, television use, dietary intake, weight, and body composition, Int. J. Behav. Nutr. Phys. Act. 8 (2011) 25.

[237] L.H. Epstein, A. Valoski, R.R. Wing, J. McCurley, Ten-year follow-up of behavioral, family-based treatment for obese children, JAMA 264 (19) (1990) 2519−2523.

[238] M. Golan, V. Kaufman, D.R. Shahar, Childhood obesity treatment: targeting parents exclusively v. parents and children, Br. J. Nutr. 95 (5) (2006) 1008−1015.

[239] M. Golan, S. Crow, Targeting parents exclusively in the treatment of childhood obesity: long-term results, Obes. Res. 12 (2) (2004) 357−361.

[240] J.M. Berge, M. Wall, K. Loth, D. Neumark-Sztainer, Parenting style as a predictor of adolescent weight and weight-related behaviors, J. Adolesc. Health 46 (4) (2010) 331−338.

[241] D. Neumark-Sztainer, N.I. Larson, J.A. Fulkerson, M.E. Eisenberg, M. Story, Family meals and adolescents: What have we learned from Project EAT (Eating Among Teens)? Public Health Nutr. (2010) 1−9.

[242] J.M. Berge, M. Wall, D. Neumark-Sztainer, N. Larson, M. Story, Parenting style and family meals: cross-sectional and 5-year longitudinal associations, J. Am. Diet. Assoc. 110 (7) (2010) 1036−1042.

[243] K.K. Davison, L.L. Birch, Childhood overweight: a contextual model and recommendations for future research, Obes. Rev. 2 (3) (2001) 159−171.

27

Snacking and Energy Balance in Humans

Richard Mattes, Sze-Yen Tan

Purdue University, West Lafayette, Indiana

I DEFINITIONS OF SNACKING

The health effects of snacking are controversial. It has been implicated in undesirable outcomes such as weight gain and obesity [1–7] but also recognized for healthful effects, including the contribution of nutrients to the diet [8]. One of the principal obstacles to determining the veracity of either view is the lack of a widely agreed upon definition of the term. Many have been proposed, including ones based on: (1) The time of day food is consumed, (2) portion size, (3) time and portion size, (4) the number of eating events per day, (5) consumer self-report, (6) type of food and its nutrient profile, and (7) where eating occurs. The first four criteria are favored by researchers engaged in clinical trials. They can be objectively defined and measured. The latter three are more subjective and frequently employed in survey research in which detailed quantization may not be feasible. Although often used interchangeably, these definitions actually address different dimensions of snacking with uncharacterized associations between them. No single definition adequately encompasses the different dimensions, and no effort has been made to derive a multivariate solution. Thus, at this time, it is critical that the strengths and weaknesses of different definitions be understood so that appropriate inferences can be drawn from the data collected from each. The most common definitions are elaborated here.

A Time of Day

One common approach defines snacking as the consumption of foods at certain times of day. Most commonly, in the United States, these are intervals during midmorning, midafternoon, and the evening [9]. This definition provides some consistency for data analysis by avoiding ambiguously or capriciously quantified food attributes such as form, nutrient profile, or portion size. However, this approach is subject to error for populations with different lifestyles and eating patterns. Cross-culturally, the main eating event in the United States tends to occur at approximately 6:00 pm, whereas it may occur at 10:00 pm in Spain. Thus, from a U.S. perspective, the eating event viewed as supper in Spain would be defined as a snack in the United States. This definition also has drawbacks for within-culture assessments. Eating events occurring at certain times of the day can be altered by various daily constraints (e.g., appointments) or their relaxation (e.g., sleeping later on weekends), leading to misclassification (eating early or late may shift meals to snacks and vice versa). Furthermore, individuals who choose to eat small and frequent-meals as well as shift workers, who may not consume meals at hours reflecting the customs of the larger population, will also add noise to measurements based on strict time-of-day criteria.

B Portion Size

Portion size is a common criterion for defining a snack. It is assumed that the portion size of a snack will be smaller than that of a meal. This metric is most straightforward when centered on a single food, but it can also be calculated by summing the energy of two or more foods that are consumed together. In either case, it is necessary to define the time intervals for clustering certain items and partitioning others to other eating events. This circumvents limitations attributable to defining what time of day a snack or meal occurs, but it still requires an arbitrary criterion for differentiating meals from snacks. It is not uncommon for people to engage in eating events that they consider a snack that contain more energy than eating events they term a meal. This is not an issue if there is no interest in melding the definition with cultural norms. However, if the goal is to objectify and measure a cultural practice, this is potentially problematic. Definitions based on portion size are also subject to time trends. Portion size of snacks may increase with rising daily energy intakes and portion sizes [10,11], complicating the interpretation of findings from the literature.

C Time and Portion Size

As already noted, definitions of snacks based only on time of day or portion size have limitations that require drawing on the other for better resolution. Consequently, many researchers use the two criteria in conjunction. That is, the definition of snacking should consider the intervals between two eating occasions and the energy content of the foods consumed within an eating event [12]. By this definition, a snack is defined as a food or a group of foods, not more or less than a predetermined portion size, consumed after a certain period of time following other eating events of defined portion size. Although this can create objectively measured data, it is based on arbitrary criteria that are defined by the researcher rather than an observed cultural pattern. To protect against false conclusions, researchers may use several sets of criteria to determine whether this changes their interpretation of the data [13]. This approach may not be feasible with survey data because the necessary level of time and portion size detail is often not available (e.g., with food frequency questionnaires).

D Eating Events

Characteristics of eating events can be another basis for defining snacks. Unlike regular meals (breakfast/brunch, lunch, and dinner/supper), snacking is assumed to be less structured and regular. Meal times are proposed to follow a relatively fixed routine, especially during the week, whereas snacks, if eaten, may occur at different times and places. In addition, snack consumption may range from regular to occasional, but meals are less commonly missed. Despite the popular view that breakfast is often skipped with adverse nutritional consequences [14], based on National Health and Nutrition Examination Survey (NHANES) data, it is still regularly consumed by approximately 83% of the population [15]. Nevertheless, based on these assumptions, foods eaten outside predefined meal times are viewed as snacks. It is worth noting that this approach is usually self-defined by the respondents [16]. Because more than one food may be consumed as a snack, all

foods consumed within a defined interval are combined as a single snacking occasion [17]. The "eating events" approach is very similar to the "time of day" definition, except that it provides more flexibility because meals do not have to be eaten within certain periods of time during a day. Thus, this definition can be used for individuals with different lifestyles and cultural backgrounds. However, this also results in different definitions applied across individuals or cultures, hampering comparative analyses. It also requires a researcher-imposed set of criteria, and no consensus on metrics exists.

E Self-Described by Consumers

Self-report is a commonly used approach in epidemiological studies. Study participants are asked to identify or report foods that are consumed as part of a meal or as a snack. Examples of studies that have used this approach are the Continuing Survey of Food Intake by Individuals (CSFII) and Nationwide Food Consumption Surveys [18,19]. This approach has strong cultural consonance but largely defies objective documentation. The basis of a decision by any respondent is not known; possibilities may include portion size, food type, time of day, consumption location, or some combination of these. Respondents may also be reporting based on perceived cultural norms rather than their own dietary practices. If their criterion was based, in whole or part, on food type, it is unclear how a respondent would report foods eaten once as a meal and a second time as a snack (e.g., eating "leftovers" from a meal at a non-meal time). If their criterion was based more on portion size, it is unclear how to average across individuals where one individual's meal could be another's snack and vice versa. Thus, the data generated from this approach, although potentially informative, should be interpreted as more qualitative than some of the other measures.

F Type of Food

The nutrient profile of foods has also been used to classify snacks, although there is no consensus on criteria. Often, there is an assumption that snacks are lower in nutrient density and higher in energy density. However, this view faces multiple challenges. Some foods have mixed profiles in which they provide important nutrients but also high energy density (e.g., ice cream). Others may have high energy density but because of other properties do not promote positive energy balance or weight gain (e.g., nuts [20]). Still others may be regarded as healthy but actually contain few nutrients (some fruit juices). Finally, it is not clear what distinguishes a snack item from a meal item by this definition alone because foods along the continuum of healthfulness may be consumed with meals or as snacks. Approximately half of the foods commonly regarded as snacks based on cultural norms (e.g., corn chips, potato chips, and confections) are consumed with meals [19]. Several systems have been proposed to identify high-quality snacks [21,22], but the criteria have varied, with none emerging as a common basis.

G Where Food is Consumed

Snacks may also be defined by where they are consumed. If a meal is assumed to be eaten at a fixed place such as a table in the home or restaurant, foods that are consumed elsewhere are, by default, considered snacks. This definition avoids issues related to food type, nutrient content, time of day, and portion size and is easily distinguished from a meal. However, with a premium on convenience (e.g., take-out meals from grocery stores and cup holders in cars), it is now common to eat a meal or snack in many venues. Indeed, the American Time Use Survey indicates that Americans spend approximately twice as much time engaged in secondary eating and drinking than in primary eating [23], the distinction being that secondary eating and drinking occurs when individuals indicate another activity is their primary focus (e.g., driving, reading, and watching television). Related to this definition is a potential influence of the social environment. The number and types of others present can influence ingestive behavior. For example, snacking frequency in children and adults may be increased when they socialize with their family or friends [24,25]. Given the high and increasing mobility of eating options, this definition would seem to have limited utility.

In summary, there is no single, widely accepted definition of snacking. Each approach holds advantages and disadvantages. The selection of a definition depends mainly on the study objectives and the feasibility of collecting different types of data. The critical point is that findings based on one definition cannot be readily extrapolated to those of another study using a different definition and that no single measure is broadly representative.

II PREVALENCE OF SNACKING

Trends in snacking behavior in the United States are available from several nationally representative samples of the population, such as CSFII [26] and "What We Eat in America," NHANES [15]. All are based on participant self-report using their own internal definition of snacking. These sources support a multifaceted increase in snacking. First, the percentage of the population that snacks has grown monotonically since the late 1970s in the adult population and in selected age-defined subgroups (19—39, 40—59, and >60 years old) [17]. However, this aspect of the trend will cease because virtually everyone in the population now reports snacking. Growth continues, however, as measured by the number of snacks consumed per day. In 2008, approximately 65% of U.S. adults consumed two or more snacks per day compared to 73% who reported snacking one or fewer times per day in 1977—1978 [15]. The mean number of snacks consumed per day increased from 1.0 to 2.2 during the past three decades. Almost 30% of the U.S. adult population derives 30% or more of their daily energy from snacks. The energy content of snacks has increased as well, from 144 to 219 kcal/snack, during the past three decades. Similar trends are reported in adolescents [15]. The proportion of snackers increased from 61 to 83% between the late 1970s and 2006, and the mean snacking frequency increased from 1.0 to 1.7 times per day. For both adolescents and adults, snacks now account for approximately one-fourth of daily energy intake, and daily snack frequency is positively associated with daily energy intake. Importantly, NHANES 2007—2008 data show that the proportions of adolescents and adults consuming snacks were the highest among those who ate three regular meals a day compared to those who consumed only one or two meals a day. The highest percentages fell in the groups consuming two or three snacks a day. This suggests that the higher prevalence and frequency of snacking may not be well explained by a change in the eating patterns that shifted from three main meals to more frequent meals per day. Results from a few studies indicate that secondary eating is becoming a major contributor of total daily energy intake, and high television viewership in children and young adults is linked to a higher possibility of snacking, especially on high-fat and high-energy foods [27,28]. Interestingly, one study that included 74 overweight women found that an increase in energy and fat consumption occurred only when foods were eaten as snacks but not as meals during television watching [29].

III TYPES OF SNACKS CONSUMED

Snacking encompasses a variety of food groups, including, in descending order, alcoholic beverages, sweetened beverages, savory snacks, candies, baked goods, fruit and fruit juice, dairy desserts, nuts and seeds, cookies, and milk and milk drinks in adults [15]. The portion size and energy density of energy-yielding beverages has increased in the past three decades [30], contributing to approximately 50% of snack energy in males and 40% in females. Moreover, the time spent engaged in secondary drinking exceeds the total time spent reported for primary eating and drinking combined on a daily basis [23]. These latter trends are of particular importance because of evidence that drinking energy elicits weak appetitive and compensatory dietary responses [31]. Consequently, drinking tends to add energy to the diet rather than displace other energy sources, resulting in greater energy intake [32,33].

IV SNACKING AND ENERGY BALANCE

Total energy intake is a function of eating frequency and the energy content of eating events. Stable energy intake can be achieved over wide ranges of variation in one component by precise offsetting adjustments in the other. That is, eating multiple meals daily may not promote weight gain if they are low in energy, nor will eating larger meals as long as they are not frequent. Similarly, purposefully increasing (perhaps to better control appetite or moderate swings in blood sugar) or decreasing (with the intent to lower intake) eating frequency will not necessarily result in lower energy consumption if portion size is not also controlled. Acute feeding trials and common experience reveal that energy intake is not stable within meals for most individuals. For example, there are multiple demonstrations that intake within a meal is influenced by the portion size in both children [34] and adults [35]. However, there are also data indicating that compensation occurs between eating events in both children [36] and adults [37,38] and occurs comparably in lean and obese individuals. Large eating events are generally followed by smaller eating events so that by the end of the day, intake is relatively precise. Precision, however, is a measure of reliability or constancy and does not speak to the issue of accuracy. Accuracy, in the current context, refers to energy balance. Consistent positive or negative energy balance results in weight gain or loss, respectively. As noted previously, in the current environment, both the number of eating occasions and their energy content have increased during the past 30+ years. This poses a particular challenge for maintenance of energy balance. In one study, it was demonstrated that a mandatory snack, consumed over a 2-week period, increased energy balance because energy from the snack was only partially compensated [39]. Although both eating frequency and portion size have changed, the larger shift appears to have occurred in eating frequency [1,40], particularly attributable to snacks [41].

V SNACKING AND OVERWEIGHT AND OBESITY

The evidence relating snacking with body weight or body mass index (BMI) is mixed in children (Table 27.1) and adults (Table 27.2). Some studies report that a higher BMI is associated with a lower eating frequency [42–45], whereas others have observed that increased snacking frequency is directly associated with energy intake and body weight [7]. These seemingly contradictory findings may stem from underreporting of snacks by study participants. However, some studies that specifically targeted high-energy snack items also arrived at the conclusion that snacking is inversely correlated with body weight in adolescents [46,47]. This section revisits the debate on the contribution of snacking to daily energy intake and how it relates to the weight status of adolescents and adults.

A Possible Explanations for the Inconsistent Findings between Snacking and BMI

A number of methodological and analytical issues may account for the inconsistent associations between snacking frequency and BMI. The first relates to variations in the study populations and in the definition of snacking used for data analysis. For example, a study in children that demonstrated a positive association between snacking and weight analyzed the data by adding a "sedentary lifestyle" dimension in addition to snacking [48], rendering it impossible to determine an independent effect of snacking. Among some trials with adults [6,7,49] and children [50], a positive association between snacking and body weight was found only in obese participants. A greater risk for weight gain among the obese has been reported under various conditions, including beverage consumption [51]. The basis for this differential risk is not known.

Second, snacking may only be associated with BMI as a marker for lifestyle factors that may variously influence energy balance. For example, it is possible that snacking is associated with increased physical activity, especially if foods such as protein bars and sport drinks are considered snacks [52]. Higher frequency of snacking on these foods therefore implies higher physical activity levels—hence the absence of a positive association between BMI and snacking. Without knowledge of what these contributors are and with a high likelihood that different studies will measure different population subgroups (e.g., lean vs. obese), associations will be variable. Snacking also directly determines the frequency of exposures to the sensory properties of foods and creates metabolic expectations that, in fact, alter digestive, absorptive, and metabolic

TABLE 27.1 Relationship between Snacking and Body Weight in Children

Study	Population	Study design	Results
Locard et al., 1992 [50]	327 obese and 704 non-obese	Case–control	Positive association in obese children
Lioret et al., 2008 [48]	748 (aged 3–11 years)	Cross-sectional	Positive association in younger overweight children
Tanasescu et al., 2000 [161]	29 obese and 24 non-obese (aged 7–10 years)	Case–control	No association
Crooks, 2003 [162]	54 elementary school children	Cross-sectional	No association
Kant, 2003 [3]	4,852 (aged 8–18 years)	Cross-sectional	No association
Nicklas et al., 2003 [163]	1,562 boys (aged 10 years)	Cross-sectional	No association
Field et al., 2004 [164]	8,203 girls and 6,774 boys (aged 9–14 years)	Prospective	No association
Huang et al., 2004 [165]	1,995 (aged 3–19 years)	Cross-sectional	No association
Nicklas et al., 2004 [166]	1,584 (aged 10 years)	Cross-sectional	No association
Phillips et al., 2004 [167]	196 girls (aged 8–12 years)	Prospective	No association
Colapinto et al., 2007 [168]	4,966 elementary school children	Cross-sectional	No association
Barker et al., 2000 [169]	328 schoolgirls (aged 14–16 years)	Cross-sectional	Inverse association
Snoek et al., 2007 [46]	10,087 (aged 11–16 years)	Cross-sectional	Inverse association
Li and Wang, 2008 [47]	181 (aged 10–14 years)	Prospective	Inverse association
Franko et al., 2008 [170]	2,375 girls (aged 9–10 years)	Prospective	Inverse association
Keast et al., 2010 [171]	5,811 adolescents (aged 12–18 years)	Cross-sectional	Inverse association

processes related to energy balance [31,53–55]. The types of food selected may also influence their impact on body weight. An estimated 5–20% of the energy from whole nuts is not bioaccessible, whereas the energy absorbed from nut butter is higher [56]. How foods are prepared is another factor, with cooked high-starch or high-protein items yielding more bio-available energy [57].

A third explanation stems from collecting only coarse data on snack energy intake. When snacking is measured with an unvalidated questionnaire (e.g., [58]), it is not known how well individual participant snacking habits are captured. Confronted with response options that do not permit accurate responses, participants may lose motivation, potentially resulting in biased outcomes. In one published study, only 22% of all participants reported on their snacking habits, although the basis for this poor yield is not known. Alternatively, some trials only obtain self-reported estimates of eating patterns without information on actual food choice (e.g., [59]), leading to a poorly defined predictor variable.

Fourth, the diversity of descriptors is large, and correlations between them are unknown. Examples of reported outcomes include the time of eating [60], percentage of energy consumed as snacks [61], nutrient composition of snacks [62], and the types of foods consumed as snacks [63].

Fifth, a critical issue in establishing a causal relationship between snacking and BMI is clearly characterizing the directionality of the relationship. It may be that increased eating frequency through snacking leads to positive energy balance and weight gain. Alternatively, individuals who are overweight or obese for some other reasons may choose to reduce the number of eating events in their diet as a means to curb energy intake. In correlation analyses, this would appear as a negative association. Reducing eating events is a common approach for weight management [64] and could lead to a misinterpretation of the relationship.

A sixth explanation for variable results relates to the low reliability of eating frequency reported by the participants [65]. A fluctuation in the snacking frequency may be due to the nature of snacking, which is often less structured than meals. The low reproducibility in the assessment of eating frequency is especially relevant to cross-sectional studies that examine intake patterns over only a day. This methodological limitation would tend to obscure true relationships (Type II errors) rather than generating false-positive or -negative observations [43].

TABLE 27.2 Relationship between Snacking and Body Weight in Adults

Study	Population	Study design	Results
Bertéus Forslund et al., 2002 [6]	83 obese and 94 lean women	Case—control	Positive association
Bertéus Forslund et al., 2005 [7]	4,429 obese and 1,092 lean adults	Case—control	Positive association
Scherwitz and Kesten, 2005 [58]	5,256 adults	Cross-sectional	Positive association
McCarthy et al., 2006 [49]	1,379 (aged 18—64 years)	Cross-sectional	Positive association
Howarth et al., 2007 [172]	2,685 (aged 20—90 years)	Cross-sectional	Positive association
Keski-Rahkonen et al., 2007 [59]	2,060 men and 233 women	Cross-sectional	Positive association
Bes-Rastrollo et al., 2010 [173]	10,162 university graduates	Prospective	Positive association
Edelstein et al., 1992 [174]	2,034 (aged 50—89 years)	Cross-sectional	No association
Basdevant et al., 1993 [61]	273 obese women	Cross-sectional	No association
Summerbell et al., 1996 [42]	187 adults	Cross-sectional	No association
Whybrow and Kirk, 1997 [60]	44 women (aged 17—26 years)	Cross-sectional	No association
Drummond et al., 1998 [175]	47 women (aged 20—55 years)	Cross-sectional	No association
Kant, 2000 [62]	15,611 (20 years or older)	Cross-sectional	No association
Neuhouser et al., 2000 [63]	982 adults	Cross-sectional	No association
Titan et al., 2001 [176]	7,776 women (aged 45—75 years)	Cross-sectional	No association
Hampl et al., 2003 [177]	1,756 men and 1,511 women	Cross-sectional	No association
Kant and Graubard, 2006 [178]	39,094 (aged 25—74 years)	Cross-sectional	No association
Fabry et al., 1964 [179]	379 adults	Cross-sectional	Inverse association
Metzner et al., 1977 [45]	1,000 men and 1,000 women (aged 35—69 years)	Cross-sectional	Inverse association
Charzewska et al., 1981 [180]	886 adults	Cross-sectional	Inverse association
Kant et al., 1995 [65]	7,147 adults	Cross-sectional	Inverse association
Drummond et al., 1998 [175]	48 men (aged 20—55 years)	Cross-sectional	Inverse association
Wahlqvist et al., 1999 [181]	145 men and 148 women (aged >70 years)	Cross-sectional	Inverse association
Titan et al., 2001 [176]	6,890 men (aged 45—75 years)	Cross-sectional	Inverse association
Ruidavets et al., 2002 [182]	300 men (aged 45—64 years)	Cross-sectional	Inverse association
Ma et al., 2003 [44]	499 (aged 20—70 years)	Cross-sectional	Inverse association

An additional explanation for inconsistent results stems from the well-documented problem of underreporting of dietary intake by study participants, especially among overweight and obese adults. There are also indications that underreporting of snacks is especially common [66]. The extent of underreporting is not routinely determined in studies that investigate the relationship between eating frequency and body weight status. This problem would tend to result in the absence of or an inverse relationship. In a critical review of an early, influential study reporting a positive association between eating frequency and BMI, underreporting was observed in stepwise proportion to eating frequency [43]. The problem of underreporting as it pertains to eating frequency has been critically assessed [67]. In a review of 20 studies, only 3 observed a positive association, whereas 10 reported a negative association. However, using cutoffs of estimated energy intakes required to maintain body weight, participants in some studies could be classified as plausible and implausible reporters [68]. In studies of adults and children that originally reported an inverse association between eating frequency and BMI, this relationship was diminished or reversed when underreporters were excluded [42,69,70]. In addition, reassessment of CSFII data on 6499 individuals from 1994 to 1996 revealed that the lack of association between eating frequency, energy intake, and BMI was likely attributable to underreporting. Positive associations were revealed when implausible reporters were excluded from the analyses [69]. Collectively, these findings lend more weight to the view that eating frequency is positively associated with BMI.

VI SNACKING AND WEIGHT LOSS OR MAINTENANCE

Given questions about eating frequency and the accuracy of the reciprocity with portion size, possible changes of the efficiency of energy use, appetite regulation, and energy expenditure, questions also remain about whether a reduction in eating events will aid weight management. Although there is one study that reported smaller weight loss percentage among mid-morning snackers [71], the literature is not highly supportive. Part of the evidence challenging a beneficial role stems from trials of purposeful addition or subtraction of eating events from an individual's diet. In one such study of weight-stable individuals [72], data from 3-day food records revealed total energy intake declined significantly initially after the omission of a snack from a traditional three-meal—one-gouter (similar to a snack) diet for 28 days. However, the reduction in energy intake failed to translate into a lower body weight, and fat mass percentage actually increased. Conversely, body weight and fat mass were unaffected by the addition of an eating event in traditional three-meal eaters.

Counterintuitive results have also been reported from a trial imposing a 12-week 750-kcal energy-restriction diet in adults. Breakfast eaters were asked to continue or to omit their regular breakfast, whereas breakfast skippers were asked to continue to omit breakfast or to add this eating event [73]. The exclusion of breakfast among regular breakfast eaters resulted in a weight loss that was approximately 2.7 kg greater than that of regular breakfast eaters who continued to eat this meal. This would suggest a primary role for reduced eating frequency except weight loss was also 1.7 kg greater in the group of breakfast skippers who added a breakfast meal compared to those who continued to skip that meal. Participants who included a breakfast, especially among the breakfast skippers, offset the energy consumed at breakfast in the subsequent meals. The researchers concluded that the participants who had to make the most substantial changes (from breakfast eaters to breakfast skippers or the reverse) in their diet patterns achieved better weight loss outcomes. Thus, the driving force for weight change was disruption of customary dietary patterns.

There is little controversy that under nonpathological conditions, energy restriction is the primary independent determinant of weight loss [74,75]. The importance of manipulating the number of eating occasions may be limited when a diet is planned and total

energy intake is fixed at a level lower than energy need. Under such conditions, there are many reports of weight loss independent of eating frequency [76—82]. However, where experimental controls are not strong and ingestive behavior is more variable, the data suggest that the relationship between eating frequency and BMI is influenced by whether all of the eating events are planned or customary compared to spontaneous. This idea was incorporated into a theoretical model, in which it was hypothesized that the inclusion of snacks may pose a moderate to high risk of overeating when a diet is not planned [41]. Within a planned-diet, the risk of overeating remains low even when the snacking frequency is higher. Given the strong literature related to beverage energy intake and its weak appetitive effects, we build on this model and suggest that the level of risk for positive energy balance and weight gain increases if eating events have higher proportional energy content from beverages (Figure 27.1).

In summary, the question of whether or not one should reduce eating events to help maintain or lose weight depends on how the diet is planned. Without proper planning, simply reducing the eating frequency may not provide additional benefits in reducing total energy intake and in assisting weight management.

VII THE ROLE OF SNACKS IN A HEALTHY DIET

Accepting that current trends in eating frequency [17] reflect consumer preferences, the question becomes how snacks can be incorporated into the diet while meeting weight management goals. A number of considerations are outlined here.

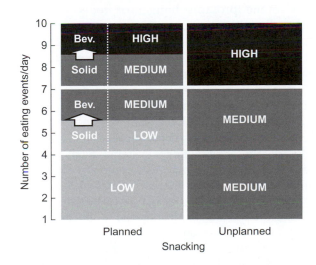

FIGURE 27.1 Risk of weight gain by planned or unplanned snacking, including beverages and solid foods.

A Timing of Snacking

Studies of the mechanisms responsible for snacking have been dominated by a biobehavioral approach that hypothesizes that food intake is driven by appetite, and appetite is regulated by biochemical parameters such as blood glucose, insulin, and leptin concentrations detected peripherally or centrally [83]. Thus, it has been proposed that providing snacks to offset swings in these bioactive compounds may prolong the intervals between eating events and reduce energy intake at eating events. Despite the theoretical appeal of the approach, it has not proven reliable for predicting human ingestive behavior [84]. There are multiple explanations. First, eating often occurs in the absence of hunger [85], it is not always feasible to eat when hungry, and often the sensation is purposefully overridden for reasons such as desired weight loss. Second, many trials use a preload testing paradigm in which individuals are administered some fixed load or intervention followed by assessments of appetitive sensations and intake at a subsequent eating event. The latter outcome is typically measured at a set time to standardize the procedure, but this does not reflect customary behavior and may result in misleading conclusions. Some food or meal constituent may appear to lead to reduced energy intake when study participants are required to eat when they would not have chosen to do so on their own, but the constituent may fail to reflect an effect when individuals are allowed to spontaneously request their next eating event [85,86], as is usually the case under more naturalistic eating conditions. Third, the relationship between putative appetite hormones and appetite sensations is variable. For example, several reports note that changes of hunger precede shifts of ghrelin [86,87], a reported orexigenic hormone, thus raising questions regarding whether the hormone prompts hunger or reflects it. Fourth, nearly all gut satiety peptides are associated with meal size rather than eating frequency, and given that the latter can compensate for changes of the former, this is an incomplete picture of the regulatory system. Similarly, dynamic changes in circulating hormones (e.g., insulin and bombesin) or metabolites (e.g., oleyethanolamide) act primarily to influence eating initiation, but less so on meal size. Thus, assessments of these regulatory systems also present an incomplete account of ingestive behavior. Studies combining the two complimentary systems are lacking. Given these constraints, it is not surprising that even well-executed trials exploring the importance of the timing of snacks on energy intake have yielded little support for an effect. This is exemplified by a crossover study of 11 young, lean men [88]. Following basal assessment of customary patterns of appetitive sensations, isoenergetic afternoon snacks were provided to participants at three time points (on three separate days) after ingestion of a standard lunch: (1) 5 minutes before blood glucose peaked, as observed in the basal session; (2) 40 minutes after blood glucose peaked; and (3) 2 hours before usual dinner time. The researchers found no effects of snacks given at any time point on the latency of dinner request compared to when no snack was provided. In addition, hunger ratings did not decrease, and the total energy intake was significantly higher when snacks were provided under these three conditions. Thus, snacking timed to match biochemical indices failed to delay subsequent meal, and dietary compensation for the snacks was not observed.

B Nutrient Composition of Snacks

The macronutrient composition of snacks not only determines their energy content but also reportedly impacts appetitive sensations. It is widely held that there is a hierarchical effect of different macronutrients on satiety, in the order of protein > carbohydrate > fat [89]. However, such effects are not robust. Many studies reporting strong satiating effects of high-protein meals provided the protein is in a solid food vehicle. (For a summary of these studies, see [90]), and this effect is similar for various proteins such as animal or plant sources [91−94, 183]. In contrast there is a loss of strong satiety effects from protein when protein is delivered in beverage form [95−100].

With carbohydrate, fructose, as a single nutrient, yields higher satiety than sucrose [101], but this effect diminishes when they are provided in a food matrix containing other types of starch [102,103]. Simple sugars are considerably more satiating than starch, which promotes satiety over a longer period of time [104]. This is consistent with the observation that low glycemic index foods prolong food latency [105], but even this effect may be due to other food properties. Finally, some studies report increased satiety following preloads of unsaturated fat [106], especially polyunsaturated fats [107], whereas others do not note such an effect [108−110]. Studies that compare the satiety effects of snacks of various macronutrient compositions are limited. Two studies that provided participants with isoenergetic high-protein, -carbohydrate, or -fat afternoon snacks demonstrated that high-protein snacks prolonged the interval between preload ingestion and the subsequent meal (dinner), but energy from all snacks was not compensated, resulting in higher total energy intake [111,112]. Macronutrient composition likely influences a snack's satiety properties, but additional study is required to determine how to optimize these effects.

C Fruits and Vegetables

Fruits and vegetables are one of the core food groups in the *Dietary Guidelines for Americans* [113]. They are generally considered healthy foods because of their higher nutrient and lower energy density properties. However, arguments have been made that such foods either promote [114,115] or fail to adequately sustain satiety [57], leaving open questions about their role as snacks. In the Prostate, Lung, Colorectal, and Ovarian Cancer (PLOC) screening trial, a lower BMI was observed with higher fruit and vegetable intake in more than 32,000 respondents [116]. However, this may be due to an overall healthier lifestyle led by the respondents. A greater proportion of those in the highest quintile of fruit and vegetable consumption were more physically active, defined as engaging in strenuous physical activity for more than 1 hour per week. This quintile also included fewer smokers and alcohol drinkers. Thus, the lower BMI may not necessarily be a result of higher fruit and vegetable intakes alone. The European Prospective Investigation into Cancer and Nutrition (EPIC) study revealed that BMI did not differ between the highest and the lowest quartiles of fruit and vegetable intake [117]. Observations that fruits and vegetables play minimal roles in regulating body weight are further supported by data from the Nurses Health Study, in which BMI was stable across the quintiles of fruit and vegetable consumption (analyzed separately or combined) [118]. Interestingly, in this study, energy consumption increased as fruit and vegetable consumption increased from the first to the fifth quintile, perhaps reflecting their weak effect on sustaining satiety. Administering generic advice to increase fruit and vegetable consumption to a population of more than 3000 women in the Women's Healthy Eating and Living (WHEL) trial led to substantive changes in their consumption. However, minimal effects were noted on body weight, and there was no difference in body weight between those receiving counseling and those in the control group throughout the 72-month observation period [119].

Other work indicates that advice to increase fruit and vegetable intake can exacerbate weight gain. In a study that manipulated fruit and vegetable intake, with or without reducing dietary fat intake, weight gain was reported in groups that were randomized into the high fruit and vegetable consumption group. Individuals in the low fruit and vegetable group lost weight [120]. In a study in which participants were followed up after a weight loss trial using low energy density strategies, weight regain was observed among individuals who consumed more fruits compared to those who successfully maintained their weight [121]. Overweight and obese individuals were especially vulnerable to weight gain following the addition of fruits and vegetables into the diet [122]. Taken together, this literature suggests that if fruits and vegetables are recommended as snacks, it will be important to include advice that this must be done in an energy-balanced or energy-reduced total diet plan. Spontaneous reductions of energy intake may not occur by simply recommending adding fruits and vegetables to a customary diet.

D Food Form

Hunger drives food-seeking behaviors to meet needs, whereas thirst initiates the ingestion of fluids to meet hydration needs [123,124]. Physiologically, drinking is more tightly regulated than eating because thirst is a more salient signal [125]. Daily hunger ratings generally exhibit a bimodal pattern, but thirst sensations are typically stronger and stable throughout the day [126]. Beverages are mostly ingested in conjunction with eating, and a majority of beverages contain energy [127]. Beverages contribute as much as 25% of total daily energy intake, and up to 50% of energy we consume from snacks comes in beverage form [15].

The positive relationship between energy-containing beverage consumption and body weight and BMI is observed in most epidemiological studies (for reviews, see [51] and [128]), although not in all studies [129–131]. Epidemiological studies usually measure exposure (beverage consumption) and health outcomes (weight status) at a given time point, but they cannot verify a causality relationship. Prospective and randomized studies provide more robust evidence in establishing a causal effect of beverage consumption on body weight. As found in a systematic review and meta-analysis of prospective studies, the inclusion of energy-yielding beverages increases body weight in a dose-dependent manner, whereas the exclusion of these beverages leads to weight reduction or stability in overweight individuals.

The obesogenic effects of energy-containing beverages can be due to differences in cognitive, oral, digestive, and absorptive processes for fluid and solid food forms. Appetitive responses to foods and beverages are influenced by the perception (expected energy content) of foods [132–134], consumption rates [135], oral exposure and mastication [136,137], and gastric distention and gastrointestinal tract transit [138,139]. As measured by these parameters, solid foods increase satiety more than their semisolid and liquid forms [140], leading to a lower subsequent intake [32,33]. On the other hand, beverages elicit weaker dietary compensation than solid foods, especially in overweight individuals [122].

The pursuit of mechanistic explanations to the differential satiety effects of solid and beverage food forms is ongoing, and biomarkers such as gut peptides (i.e., ghrelin, glucagon-like peptide 1, cholecystokinin, and peptide YY) are routinely used as part of a standard testing protocol to objectively measure appetite [141]. Our study observed that just the belief that test foods will be solid or liquid in people's stomachs altered endocrine responses in a manner consistent with lower satiety value for the fluid [31]. More mechanistic evidence will emerge in the near future, and it will help in the understanding of how food forms can affect body weight and other health outcomes. At this stage, evidence appears to favor solid foods as the preferred snack choice to manage energy intake due to their greater satiety effects.

E Portion Control and Energy Density

Larger portion size generally predicts higher energy intake [142], but when the portion size of foods is fixed, the energy density of food is positively related to energy intake [143,144] and lower food reinforcement in overweight adults [145,146]. In response to this evidence and consumers' desire to better manage their body weight, the food industry has made available portion-controlled snacks, particularly of high energy-dense items. Data on whether this approach has achieved its intended goal are limited. One trial observed that a reduction in portion size led to lower energy intake of unrestrained eaters [147]. Smaller portion sizes had no impact on the energy intake of people already attempting to moderate their energy consumption (i.e., restrained eaters) [148]. Another study observed the combined effects of energy density and portion size, in which significantly higher energy intake was observed when individuals were provided with a high energy density entrée and at a larger portion size [149].

One danger of formulating recommendations based on energy density is that there are many inconsistencies in responses based on the classification. For example, as noted previously, beverages may be especially problematic for promoting positive energy balance and weight gain, but they are among the lowest energy-dense products consumed (energy density scores typically of 0−0.6 kcal/g). In contrast, nuts are high-energy foods due to their high fat and low water content. However, epidemiological and prospective evidence does not support that they increase the risk of weight gain [150−153]. This may be due to their strong satiety properties and the fact that the energy from nuts is not efficiently absorbed [154]. The combined effects of compensatory reductions of energy intake and poor efficiency of energy absorption account for approximately 80% of the energy they contribute to the diet [155].

VIII CONCLUSIONS AND RECOMMENDATIONS

The evidence linking higher eating frequency to higher energy intake is strong but not uniform, and whether snacking contributes to weight gain requires consideration of the definition of snacking used, characteristics of the consumers and their customary dietary patterns, as well as properties of the snack foods and beverages ingested.

Although spontaneous snacking may pose a risk for weight gain, this is only one dimension of the health effects of snack foods. They also provide a substantial proportion of nutrients to the diets of both children and adults in the United States. They contribute to daily intake of vitamin E [156], dietary fiber, iron, folic acid, vitamin C [157], and monounsaturated fats [158]. In 2005 and 2006, snacks contributed 19% of grains, 12% of vegetables, 38% of fruits, 17% of dairy, 11% of meat and beans, and 32% of oil intake in adolescents based on the daily recommendations by MyPyramid [15]. They are also important sources of energy [16], vitamin A, vitamin C, vitamin E, copper, potassium, and selenium for older adults in the United States, a group at higher risk for malnutrition [159]. Furthermore, serum total cholesterol, low-density lipoprotein cholesterol, and insulin levels tended to be lower among people who were nibblers than those who ate three regular meals [160].

We propose that the risk of gaining weight by snacking is low when such eating events are part of an energy-balanced diet. During weight loss, energy restriction overrides the effects of eating frequency. The composition and timing of snacking appear to have minimal effect on energy balance, and fruits and vegetables are not necessarily superior to other snack foods. However, the physical form of snacks may be critical where solid foods are preferred when energy moderation is the goal.

References

[1] C. Zizza, A.M. Siega-Riz, B.M. Popkin, Significant increase in young adults' snacking between 1977−1978 and 1994−1996 represents a cause for concern!, Prev. Med. 32 (2001) 303−310.

[2] R. Sturm, Childhood obesity: what we can learn from existing data on society trends, Part 2, Prev. Chronic Dis. 2 (2005) A20.

[3] A.K. Kant, Reported consumption of low-nutrient-density foods by American children and adolescent: nutritional and health correlates, NHANES III, 1988 to 1994, Arch. Pediatr. Adolesc. Med. 157 (2003) 789−796.

[4] B.M. Nielsen, K.S. Bjornsbo, I. Tetens, B.L. Heitmann, Dietary glycaemic index and glycaemic load in Danish children in relation to body fatness, Br. J. Nutr. 94 (2005) 992−997.

[5] S.B. Templeton, M.A. Marlette, M. Panemangalore, Competitive foods increase the intake of energy and decrease the intake of

certain nutrients by adolescents consuming school lunch, J. Am. Diet. Assoc. 105 (2005) 215–220.

[6] H. Bertéus Forslund, A.K. Lindroos, L. Sjostrom, L. Lissner, Meal patterns and obesity in Swedish women: a simple instrument describing usual meal types, frequency and temporal distribution, Eur. J. Clin. Nutr. 56 (2002) 740–747.

[7] H. Bertéus Forslund, J.S. Torgerson, L. Sjostrom, A.K. Lindroos, Snacking frequency in relation to energy intake and food choices in obese men and women compared to a reference population, Int. J. Obes. 29 (2005) 711–719.

[8] R.S. Sebastian, L.E. Cleveland, J.D. Goldman, Effect of snacking frequency on adolescents' dietary intakes and meeting national recommendations, J. Adolesc. Health 42 (2008) 503–511.

[9] D. Gregori, C. Maffeis, Snacking and obesity: urgency of a definition to explore such a relationship, J. Am. Diet. Assoc. 107 (2007) 562.

[10] I.L. Berstein, J.C. Zimmerman, C.A. Czeisler, E.D. Weitzman, Meal patterns in "free-running" humans, Physiol. Behav. 27 (1981) 621–623.

[11] A. McBride, A. Wise, G. McNeill, W.P. James, The pattern of food consumption related to energy intake, J. Hum. Nutr. Diet. 3 (1990) 27–32.

[12] J.M. De Castro, The effects of the spontaneous ingestion of particular foods or beverages on the meal pattern and overall nutrient intake of humans, Physiol. Behav 53 (1993) 1133–1144.

[13] A. Rangan, D. Hector, D. Randall, T. Gill, K. Webb, Monitoring consumption of "extra" foods in the Australian diet: comparing two sets of criteria for classifying foods as "extras", Nutr. Diet. 64 (2007) 261–267.

[14] A. Keski-Rahkonen, J. Kaprio, A. Rissanen, M. Virkkunen, R.J. Rose, Breakfast skipping and health-compromising behaviors in adolescents and adults, Eur. J. Clin. Nutr. 57 (2003) 842–853.

[15] U.S. Department of Agriculture, Agricultural Research Service, What We Eat in America, U.S. Department of Agriculture, Washington, DC, 2011.

[16] C. Zizza, F.A. Tayie, M. Lino, Benefits of snacking in older Americans, J. Am. Diet. Assoc. 107 (2007) 800–806.

[17] C. Piernas, B.M. Popkin, Snacking increased among U.S. adults between 1977 and 2006, J. Nutr. 140 (2006) 325–332.

[18] L. Jahns, A.M. Siega-Riz, B.M. Popkin, The increasing prevalence of snacking among U.S. children from 1977 to 1996, J. Pediatr. 138 (2001) 493–498.

[19] S.J. Nielsen, A.M. Siega-Riz, B.M. Popkin, Trends in energy intake in U.S. between 1977 and 1996: similar shifts seen across age groups, Obes. Res. 10 (2002) 370–378.

[20] S. Rajaram, J. Sabate, Nuts, body weight and insulin resistance, Br. J. Nutr. 96 (2006) S79–S86.

[21] A.K. Kant, Indexes of overall diet quality: a review, J. Am. Diet. Assoc. 96 (1996) 785–791.

[22] C.J. Lackey, K.M. Kolasa, Healthy eating: Defining the nutrient quality of foods, Nutr. Today 39 (2004) 26–29.

[23] U.S. Department of Labor, American time use survey—2010 results, Bureau of Labor Statistics, U.S. Department of Labor, Washington, DC, 2011.

[24] N. Stroebele, J.M. De Castro, Effect of ambience on food intake and food choice, Nutrition 20 (2004) 821–838.

[25] G. Savige, A. MacFarlane, K. Ball, A. Worseley, D. Crawford, Snacking behaviours of adolescents and their association with skipping meals, Int. J. Behav. Nutr. Phys. Activity 4 (2007) 36.

[26] U.S. Environmental Protection Agency, Analysis of Total Food Intake and Composition of Individual's Diet Based on USDA's 1994–1996, 1998 Continuing Survey of Food Intakes by Individuals (CSFII), U.S. Environmental Protection Agency, National Center for Environmental Assessment, Washington, DC, 2007 (EPA/600/R-05/062F).

[27] L.A. Francis, Y. Lee, L.L. Birch, Parental weight status and girls' television viewing, snacking, and body mass indexes, Obes. Res. 11 (2003) 143–151.

[28] M. Thomson, J.C. Spence, K. Raine, L. Laing, The association of television viewing with snacking behavior and body weight of young adults, Am. J. Health Promot. 22 (2008) 329–335.

[29] S.A. Gore, J.A. Foster, V.G. DiLillo, K. Kirk, D.S. West, Television viewing and snacking, Eating Behav. 4 (2003) 399–405.

[30] K.J. Duffey, B.M. Popkin, Energy density, portion size, and eating occasions: contributions to increased energy intake in the United States, 1977–2006, PLos Med. 8 (2011) E1001050.

[31] B.A. Cassady, R.V. Considine, R.D. Mattes, Beverage consumption, appetite, and energy intake: what did you expect? Am. J. Clin. Nutr. 95 (2012) 587–593.

[32] D.M. Mourao, J. Bressan, W.W. Campbell, R.D. Mattes, Effects of food form on appetite and energy intake in lean and obese young adults, Int. J. Obes. 31 (2007) 1688–1695.

[33] D.P. DiMeglio, R.D. Mattes, Liquid versus solid carbohydrate: effects on food intake and body weight, Int. J. Obes. 24 (2000) 794–800.

[34] B.J. Rolls, D. Engell, L.L. Birch, Serving portion size influences 5-year-old but not 3-year-old children's food intakes, J. Am. Diet. Assoc. 100 (2000) 232–234.

[35] D.A. Levitsky, T. Youn, The more food young adults are served, the more they overeat, J. Nutr. 134 (2004) 2546–2549.

[36] L.L. Birch, S.L. Johnson, G. Andresen, J.C. Peters, M.C. Schulte, The variability of young children's energy intake, N. Engl. J. Med. 324 (1991) 232–235.

[37] F. McKiernan, J.H. Hollis, R.D. Mattes, Short-term dietary compensation in free-living adults, Physiol. Behav. 93 (2008) 975–983.

[38] M. Viskaal-van Dongen, F.J. Kok, C. De Graaf, Effects of snack consumption for 8 weeks on energy intake and body weight, Int. J. Obes. 34 (2010) 319–326.

[39] S. Whybrow, C. Mayer, T.R. Kirk, N. Mazlan, R.J. Stubbs, Effects of two week's mandatory snack consumption on energy intake and energy balance, Obesity 15 (2007) 673–685.

[40] D.M. Cutler, E.L. Glaeser, J.M. Shapiro, Why have Americans become more obese? J. Econ. Perspect. 17 (2003) 93–118.

[41] M.A. McCrory, W.W. Campbell, Effects of eating frequency, snacking, and breakfast skipping on energy regulation: symposium overview, J. Nutr. 141 (2011) 144–147.

[42] C.D. Summerbell, R.C. Moody, J. Shanks, M.J. Stock, C. Geissler, Relationship between feeding pattern and body mass index in 220 free-living people in four age groups, Eur. J. Clin. Nutr. 50 (1996) 513–519.

[43] F. Bellisle, R. McDevitt, A.M. Prentice, Meal frequency and energy balance, Br. J. Nutr. 77 (1997) S57–S70.

[44] Y. Ma, E.R. Bertone, E.J.I. Stanek, G.W. Reed, J.R. Hebert, N.L. Cohen, et al., Association between eating patterns and obesity in a free-living U.S. adult population, Am. J. Epidemiol. 158 (2003) 85–92.

[45] H.L. Metzner, D.E. Lamphiear, N.C. Wheeler, F.A. Larkin, The relationship between frequency of eating and adiposity in adult men and women in the Tecumseh Community Health Study, Am. J. Clin. Nutr. 30 (1977) 712–715.

[46] H.M. Snoek, T. Van Strien, J.M. Janssens, R.C. Engels, Emotional, external, restrained eating and overweight in Dutch adolescents, Scand. J. Psychol. 48 (2007) 23–32.

[47] J. Li, Y. Wang, Tracking of dietary intake patterns is associated with baseline characteristics of urban low-income African-American adolescents, J. Nutr. 138 (2008) 94–100.

[48] S. Lioret, M. Touvier, L. Lafay, J.L. Volatier, B. Maire, Dietary and physical activity patterns in French children are related to

overweight and socioeconomic status, J. Nutr. 138 (2008) 101–107.

[49] S.N. McCarthy, P.J. Robson, M.B. Livingstone, M. Kiely, A. Flynn, G.W. Cran, et al., Associations between daily food intake and excess adiposity in Irish adults: towards the development of food-based dietary guidelines for reducing the prevalence of overweight and obesity, Int. J. Obes. 30 (2006) 993–1002.

[50] E. Locard, N. Mamelle, A. Bilette, M. Miginiac, F. Munoz, S. Rey, Risk factors of obesity in a five year old population: parental versus environmental factors, Int. J. Obes. Relat. Metab. Disord. 16 (1992) 721–729.

[51] V.S. Malik, M.B. Schulze, F.B. Hu, Intake of sugar-sweetened beverages and weight gain: a systematic review, Am. J. Clin. Nutr. 84 (2006) 274–288.

[52] S. Drummond, N. Crombie, T. Kirk, A critique of the effects of snacking on body weight status, Eur. J. Clin. Nutr. 50 (1996) 779–783.

[53] M.A. Zafra, F. Molina, A. Puerto, The neural/cephalic phase reflexes in the physiology of nutrition, Neurosci. Biobehav. Rev. 30 (2006) 1032–1044.

[54] M.L. Power, J. Schulkin, Anticipatory physiological regulation in feeding biology: cephalic phase responses, Appetite 50 (2008) 194–206.

[55] R.D. Mattes, Orosensory considerations, Obesity (Silver Spring) 14 (Suppl. 4) (2006) 164S–167S.

[56] C.J. Traoret, P. Lokko, A.C. Cruz, C.G. Oliveira, N.M. Costa, J. Bressan, et al., Peanut digestion and energy balance, Int. J. Obes. (London) 32 (2008) 322–328.

[57] R.N. Carmody, G.S. Weintraub, R.W. Wrangham, Energetic consequences of thermal and nonthermal food processing, Proc. Natl. Acad. Sci. USA 108 (2011) 19199–19203.

[58] L. Scherwitz, D. Kesten, Seven eating styles linked to overeating, overweight, and obesity, Explore 1 (2005) 342–359.

[59] A. Keski-Rahkonen, C.M. Bulik, K.H. Pietilainen, R.J. Rose, J. Kaprio, A. Rissanen, Eating styles, overweight and obesity in young adult twins, Eur. J. Clin. Nutr. 61 (2007) 822–829.

[60] S. Whybrow, T.R. Kirk, Nutrient intakes and snacking frequency in female students, J. Hum. Nutr. Diet. 10 (1997) 237–244.

[61] A. Basdevant, C. Craplet, B. Guy-Grand, Snacking patterns in obese French women, Appetite 21 (1993) 17–23.

[62] A.K. Kant, Consumption of energy-dense, nutrient-poor foods by adult Americans: nutritional and health implications. The third National Health and Nutrition Examination Survey, 1988–1994, Am. J. Clin. Nutr. 72 (2000) 929–936.

[63] M.L. Neuhouser, R.E. Patterson, A.R. Kistal, C.L. Rock, D. Neumark-Sztainer, M.D. Thornquist, et al., Do consumers of savory snacks have poor-quality diets? J. Am. Diet. Assoc. 100 (2000) 576–579.

[64] R.R. Wing, J.O. Hill, Successful weight loss maintenance, Annu. Rev. Nutr. 21 (2001) 323–341.

[65] A.K. Kant, A. Schatzkin, B.I. Graubard, R. Ballard-Barbash, Frequency of eating occasions and weight change in the NHANES I Epidemiologic Follow-Up Study, Int. J. Obes. Relat. Metab. Disord. 19 (1995) 468–474.

[66] S.D. Poppitt, D. Swann, A.E. Black, A.M. Prentice, Assessment of selective under-reporting of food intake by both obese and non-obese women in a metabolic facility, Int. J. Obes. Relat. Metab. Disord. 22 (1998) 303–311.

[67] M.A. McCrory, N.C. Howarth, S.B. Roberts, T.T.-K. Huang, Eating frequency and energy regulation in free-living adults consuming self-selected diets, J. Nutr. 141 (2011) 148S–153S.

[68] M.A. McCrory, C.L. Hajduk, S.B. Roberts, Procedures for screening out inaccurate reports of dietary energy intake, Public Health Nutr. 5 (2002) 873–882.

[69] T.T.-K. Huang, S.B. Roberts, N.C. Howarth, M.A. McCrory, Effects of screening out implausible energy intake reports on relationships between diet and BMI, Obes. Res. 13 (2005) 1205–1217.

[70] T.T.-K. Huang, N.C. Howarth, B.-H. Lin, S.B. Roberts, M.A. McCrory, Energy intake and meal portions: Associations with BMI percentile in U.S. children, Obes. Res. 12 (2004) 1875–1885.

[71] A. Kong, S.A.A. Beresford, C.M. Alfano, K.E. Foster-Schubert, M.L. Neuhouser, D.B. Johnson, et al., Associations between snacking and weight loss and nutrient intake among postmenopausal overweight to obese women in a dietary weight-loss intervention, J. Am. Diet. Assoc. 111 (2011) 1898–1903.

[72] D. Chapelot, C. Marmonier, R. Aubert, C. Allegre, N. Gausseres, M. Fantino, et al., Consequences of omitting or adding a meal in man on body composition, food intake, and metabolism, Obesity 14 (2006) 215–227.

[73] D.G. Schlundt, J.O. Hill, T. Sbrocco, J. Pope-Cordle, T. Sharp, The role of breakfast in the treatment of obesity: a randomized clinical trial, Am. J. Clin. Nutr. 55 (1992) 645–651.

[74] F.M. Sacks, G.A. Bray, V.J. Carey, S.R. Smith, D.H. Ryan, S.D. Anton, et al., Comparison of weight-loss diets with different compositions of fat, protein, and carbohydrates, N. Engl. J. Med. 360 (2009) 859–873.

[75] K.E. Piehowski, A.G. Preston, D.L. Miller, S.M. Nickols-Richardson, A reduced-calorie dietary pattern including a daily sweet snack promotes body weight reduction and body composition improvements in premenopausal women who are overweight and obese: a pilot study, J. Am. Diet. Assoc. 111 (2011) 1198–1203.

[76] J.S. Garrow, M. Durrant, S. Blaza, D. Wilkins, O. Royston, S. Sunkin, The effect of meal frequency and protein concentration on the composition of the weight lost by obese subjects, Br. J. Nutr. 45 (1981) 5–15.

[77] C.M. Young, S.S. Scanlon, C.M. Topping, V. Simko, L. Lutwak, Frequency of feeding, weight reduction and body composition, J. Am. Diet. Assoc. 59 (1971) 466–472.

[78] W.M. Bortz, A. Wroldsen, B. Issekutz, K. Rodahl, Weight loss and frequency of feeding, N. Engl. J. Med. 274 (1966) 376–379.

[79] B. Finkelstein, B.A. Fryer, Meal frequency and weight reduction of young women, Am. J. Clin. Nutr. 24 (1971) 465–468.

[80] G. Debry, R. Azouaou, I. Vassilitch, G. Mottaz, Ponderal losses in obese subjects submitted to restricted diets differing by nibbling and by lipid and carbohydrate, in: M. Apfelbaum (Ed.), Energy Balance in Man, Masson, Paris, 1973, pp. 305–310.

[81] W.P.H.G. Verboeket-van de Venne, K.R. Westerterp, Frequency of feeding, weight reduction and energy metabolism, Int. J. Obes. 17 (31–36) (1993).

[82] J.D. Cameron, C. Marie-Josee, E. Doucet, Increased meal frequency does not promote greater weight loss in subjects who were prescribed an 8-week equi-energetic energy-restricted diet, Br. J. Nutr 103 (2010) 1098–1101.

[83] D. Chapelot, C. Marmonier, R. Aubert, N. Gausseres, J. Louis-Sylnestre, A role for glucose and insulin preprandial profiles to differentiate meals and snacks, Physiol. Behav. 80 (2004) 721–731.

[84] R.D. Mattes, J. Hollis, D. Hayes, A.J. Stunkard, Appetite: measurement and manipulation misgivings, J. Am. Diet. Assoc. 105 (2005) S87–S97.

[85] F. Rutters, A.G. Nieuwenhuizen, S.G.T. Lemmens, J.M. Born, M.S. Westerterp-Plantenga, Acute stress-related changes in eating in the absence of hunger, Obesity 17 (2008) 72–77.

[86] J.M. Frecka, R.D. Mattes, Possible entrainment of ghrelin to habitual meal patterns in humans, Am. J. Physiol. Gastrointest. Liver Physiol. 294 (2008) G699–G707.

[87] S.G.T. Lemmens, E.A. Martens, A.D. Kester, M.S. Westerterp-Plantenga, Changes in gut hormone and glucose concentrations

in relation to hunger and fullness, Am. J. Clin. Nutr. 94 (2011) 717–725.

[88] C. Marmonier, D. Chapelot, J. Louis-Sylnestre, Metabolic and behavioral consequences of a snack consumed in a satiety state, Am. J. Clin. Nutr. 70 (1999) 854–866.

[89] J. Stubbs, A. Raben, M.S. Westerterp-Plantenga, Macronutrient metabolism and appetite, in: M.S. Westerterp-Plantenga, A.B. Steffens, A. Tremblay (Eds), Regulation of Foods Intake and Energy Expenditure, Edra, Milan, 1999, pp. 59–84.

[90] T.L. Halton, F.B. Hu, The effects of high protein diets on thermogenesis, satiety and weight loss: a critical review, J. Am. Coll. Nutr. 23 (2004) 373–385.

[91] S. Borzoei, M. Neovius, B. Barkeling, A. Teixeira-Pinto, S. Rössner, A comparison of effects of fish and beef protein on satiety in normal weight men, Eur. J. Clin. Nutr. 60 (2006) 897–902.

[92] V. Lang, F. Bellisle, J.M. Oppert, C. Craplet, F.R. Bornet, G. Slama, et al., Satiating effect of proteins in healthy subjects: a comparison of egg, albumin, casein, gelatin, soy protein, pea protein, and wheat gluten, Am. J. Clin. Nutr. 67 (1998) 1197–1204.

[93] V. Lang, F. Bellisle, C. Alamowitch, C. Craplet, F.R. Bornet, G. Slama, et al., Varying the protein source in mixed meal modifies glucose, insulin and glucagon kinetics in healthy men, has weak effects on subjective satiety and fails to affect food intake, Eur. J. Clin. Nutr. 53 (1999) 959–965.

[94] J.A. Gilbert, N.T. Bendsen, A. Tremblay, A. Astrup, Effect of protein from different sources on body composition, Nutr. Metab. Cadiovasc. Dis 21 (2011) B16–B31.

[95] J.D. Latner, M. Schwartz, The effects of a high-carbohydrate, high-protein or balanced lunch upon later food intake and hunger ratings, Appetite 33 (1999) 119–128.

[96] A.A. Geliebter, Effects of equicaloric loads of protein, fat and carbohydrate on food intake in the rat and man, Physiol. Behav. 22 (1979) 267–273.

[97] M.J.I. Martens, S.G.T. Lemmens, J.M. Born, M.S. Westerterp-Plantenga, A solid high-protein meal evokes stronger hunger suppression than a liquefied high-protein meal, Obesity 19 (2011) 522–527.

[98] T.C. Lambert, A.J. Hill, J.E. Blundell, Investigating the satiating effect of protein with disguised liquid preloads, Appetite 12 (1989) 220.

[99] C. De Graaf, T. Hulshof, J.A. Westrate, P. Jas, Short-term effects of different amounts of protein, fats, and carbohydrate in a midday meal, Am. J. Clin. Nutr. 55 (1992) 33–38.

[100] R. Mattes, Beverages and positive energy balance: the menace is the medium, Int. J. Obes. 30 (2006) S60–S65.

[101] J. Rodin, Comparative effects of fructose, aspartame, glucose and water preloads on calorie and macronutrient intake, Am. J. Clin. Nutr. 51 (1990) 428–435.

[102] J. Rodin, Effects of pure sugar vs. mixed starch fructose loads on food intake, Appetite 17 (1991) 213–219.

[103] S.L. Stewart, R. Black, T.M.S. Wolever, G.H. Anderson, The relationship between the glycaemic response to breakfast cereals and subjective appetite and food intake, Nutr. Res. 17 (1997) 1249–1260.

[104] J.M.M. van Amelsvoort, J.A. Westrate, Amylose-amylopectin ratio in a meal affects post-prandial variables in male volunteers, Am. J. Clin. Nutr. 55 (1992) 712–718.

[105] S.D. Ball, K.R. Keller, L.J. Moyer-Mileur, Y.-W. Ding, D. Donaldson, W.D. Jackson, Prolongation of satiety after low versus moderately high glycemic index meals in obese adolescents, Pediatrics 111 (2003) 488–494.

[106] J. Maljaars, E.A. Romeyn, E. Haddeman, H.P.F. Peters, A.A.M. Masclee, Effect of fat saturation on satiety, hormone release, and food intake, Am. J. Clin. Nutr. 89 (1019–1024) (2009).

[107] C.L. Lawton, H.J. Delargy, J. Brockman, F.C. Smith, J.E. Blundell, The degree of saturation of fatty acids influences post-ingestive satiety, Br. J. Nutr. 83 (2000) 473–482.

[108] S.D. Poppitt, C.M. Strik, A.K. MacGibbon, B.H. McArdle, S.C. Budgett, A.T. McGill, Fatty acid chain length, postprandial satiety and food intake in lean men, Physiol. Behav. 101 (2010) 161–167.

[109] M.M.J.W. Kamphuis, M.S. Westerterp-Plantenga, W.H.M. Saris, Fat-specific satiety in humans for fat high in linoleic acid vs fat high in oleic acid, Eur. J. Clin. Nutr. 55 (2001) 499–508.

[110] C.G. MacIntosh, S.H.A. Holt, J.C. Brand-Miller, The degree of fat saturation does not alter glycemic, insulinemic or satiety responses to a starchy staple in healthy men, J. Nutr 133 (2003) 2577–2580.

[111] C. Marmonier, D. Chapelot, M. Fantino, J. Louise-Sylvestre, Snacks consumed in a nonhungry state have poor satiating efficiency: influence of snack composition on substrate utilization and hunger, Am. J. Clin. Nutr. 76 (2002) 518–528.

[112] C. Marmonier, D. Chapelot, J. Louis-Sylvestre, Effects of macronutrient content and energy density of snacks consumed in a satiety state on the onset of the next meal, Appetite 34 (2000) 161–168.

[113] U.S. Department of Agriculture and U.S. Department of Health and Human Services, Dietary Guidelines for Americans, seventh ed., U.S. Government Printing Office, Washington, DC, 2010.

[114] A. Drewnowski, Energy density, palatability, and satiety: implications for weight control, Nutr. Rev. 56 (1998) 347–353.

[115] S.D. Poppitt, D.N. McCormack, R. Buffenstein, Short-term effects of macronutrient preloads on appetite and energy intake in lean women, Physiol. Behav. 64 (1998) 279–285.

[116] A.E. Millen, A.F. Subar, B.I. Graubard, U. Peters, R.B. Hayes, J. L. Weissfeld, et al., Fruit and vegetable intake and prevalence of colorectal adenoma in a cancer screening trial, Am. J. Clin. Nutr. 86 (2007) 1754–1764.

[117] U. Nothlings, M.B. Schulze, C. Weikert, H. Boeing, Y.T. van der Schouw, C. Bamia, et al., Intake of vegetables, legumes, and fruit, and risk for all-cause, cardiovascular, and cancer mortality in a European diabetic population, J. Nutr. 138 (2008) 775–781.

[118] K. He, F.B. Hu, G.A. Colditz, J.E. Manson, W.C. Willett, S. Liu, Changes in intake of fruits and vegetables in relation to risk of obesity and weight gain among middle-aged women, Int. J. Obes. 28 (2004) 1569–1574.

[119] J.P. Pierce, L. Natarajan, B.J. Caan, B.A. Parker, E.R. Greenberg, S.W. Flatt, et al., Influence of a diet very high in vegetables, fruit, and fiber and low in fat on prognosis following treatment for breast cancer: the Women's Healthy Eating and Living (WHEL) randomized trial, J. Am. Med. Assoc. 298 (2007) 289–298.

[120] Z. Djuric, K.M. Poore, J.B. Depper, V.E. Uhley, S. Lababidi, C. Covington, et al., Methods to increase fruit and vegetable intake with and without a decrease in fat intake: compliance and effects on body weight in the nutrition and breast health study, Nutr. Cancer 43 (2002) 141–151.

[121] L.F. Greene, C.Z. Malpede, C.S. Henson, K.A. Hubbert, D.C. Heimburger, J.D. Ard, Weight maintenance 2 years after participation in a weight loss program promoting low-energy density foods, Obesity (Silver Spring) 14 (2006) 1795–1801.

[122] J.A. Houchins, J.R. Burgess, W.W. Campbell, J.R. Daniel, M.G. Ferruzzi, G.P. McCabe, et al., Beverages and solid fruits and vegetables: Effects on energy intake and body weight, Obesity (2011) (Epub ahead of print).

[123] J. LeMagnen, Hunger and food palatability in the control of feeding behavior, in: Y. Katsubi, M. Sato, S.F. Tobogi, Y. Oomura (Eds), Food Intake and Chemical Senses, University Park Press, Baltimore, 1977, pp. 263–280.

[124] M.R. Rosenzweig, The mechanisms of hunger and thirst, in: F. M. Toates (Ed.), Biological Foundations of Behaviour, Open University Press, Philadelphia, 1986, pp. 73–143.

[125] E.M. Stricker, Biological bases if hunger and satiety: Therapeutic implications, Nutr. Rev. 42 (1984) R333–R340.

[126] F. McKiernan, J.A. Houchins, R.D. Mattes, Relationships between human thirst, hunger, drinking, and feeding, Physiol. Behav. 94 (2008) 700–708.

[127] F. McKiernan, J.H. Hollis, G.P. McCabe, R.D. Mattes, Thirst-drinking, hunger-eating; Tight coupling? J. Am. Diet. Assoc. 109 (2009) 486–490.

[128] F.B. Hu, V.S. Malik, Sugar-sweetened beverages and risk of obesity and type 2 diabetes: Epidemiologic evidence, Physiol. Behav. 100 (2010) 47–54.

[129] R. Rajeshwari, S.-J. Yang, T.A. Nicklas, G.S. Berenson, Secular trends in children's sweetened-beverage consumption (1973–1994): the Bogalusa Heart Study, J. Am. Diet. Assoc. 105 (2005) 208–214.

[130] S.Z. Sun, M.W. Empie, Lack of findings for the association between obesity risk and usual sugar-sweetened beverage consumption in adults: a primary analysis of databases of CSFII-1989–1991, CSFII-1994–1998, NHANES III, and combined NHANES 1999–2002, Food Chem. Toxicol. 45 (2007) 1523–1536.

[131] L.G. Bandini, D. Vu, A. Must, H. Cyr, A. Goldberg, Comparison of high-calorie, low-nutrient dense food consumption among obese and non-obese adolescents, Obes. Res. 7 (1999) 438–443.

[132] R. Mattes, Soup and satiety, Physiol. Behav. 83 (2005) 739–747.

[133] M. Potier, G. Fromentin, A. Lesdema, R. Benamouzig, D. Tome, A. Marsset-Baglieri, The satiety effect of disguised liquid preloads administered acutely and differing in their nutrient content tended to be weaker for lipids but did not differ between proteins and carbohydrates in human subjects, Br. J. Nutr. 104 (2010) 1406–1414.

[134] O.W. Wooley, S.C. Wooley, R.B. Dunham, Can calories be perceived and do they affect hunger in obese and nonobese humans? J. Comp. Physiol. Psychol 80 (1872) 250–258.

[135] H.R. Kissileff, Effects of physical state (liquid–solid) of foods on food intake: procedural and substantive contributions, Am. J. Clin. Nutr. 42 (1985) 956–965.

[136] C. de Graaf, Why liquid energy results in overconsumption, Proc. Nutr. Soc. 70 (2011) 162–170.

[137] T. Fujise, H. Yoshimatsu, M. Kurokawa, A. Oohara, M. Kang, M. Nakata, et al., Satiation and masticatory function modulated by brain histamine in rats, Proc. Soc. Exp. Biol. Mol. 217 (1998) 228–234.

[138] H.P.F. Peters, D.J. Mela, The role of gastrointestinal tract in satiation, satiety, and food intake: evidence from research in humans, in: R.B.S. Harris, R.D. Mattes (Eds), Appetite and Food Intake, CRC Press, Boca Raton, FL, 2008, pp. 187–211.

[139] J.A. Siegel, J.-L. Urbain, L.P. Adler, N.D. Charkes, A.H. Maurer, B. Krevsky, et al., Biphasic nature of gastric emptying, Gut 29 (1988) 85–89.

[140] H.J. Leidy, J.W. Apolzan, R.D. Mattes, W.W. Campbell, Food form and portion size affect postprandial appetite sensations and hormonal responses in healthy, nonobese, older adults, Obesity 18 (2010) 293–299.

[141] T.H. Moran, Gut peptides in the control of food intake: 30 years of ideas, Physiol. Behav. 82 (2004) 175–180.

[142] M.T. Kelly, J.M.W. Wallace, P.J. Robson, K.L. Rennie, R.W. Welch, M.P. Hannon-Fletcher, et al., Increased portion size leads to a sustained increase in energy intake over 4d in normal-weight and overweight men and women, Br. J. Nutr. 102 (2009) 470–477.

[143] A.A. Devitt, R.D. Mattes, Effects of food unit size and energy density on intake in humans, Appetite 42 (2004) 213–220.

[144] B.J. Rolls, L.S. Roe, J.S. Meengs, Reductions in portion size and energy density of foods are additive and lead to sustained decreases in energy intake, Am. J. Clin. Nutr. 83 (2006) 11–17.

[145] J.L. Temple, A.M. Bulkley, R.L. Badawy, N. Krause, S. McCann, L.H. Epstein, Differential effects of daily snack food intake on the reinforcing value of food in obese and nonobese women, Am. J. Clin. Nutr. 90 (2009) 304–313.

[146] E.N. Clark, A.M. Dewey, J.L. Temple, Effects of daily snack food intake on food reinforcement depend on body mass index and energy density, Am. J. Clin. Nutr. 91 (2010) 300–308.

[147] H.A. Raynor, R.R. Wing, Package unit size and amount of food: Do both influence intake? Obesity 15 (2007) 2311–2319.

[148] M.L. Scott, S.M. Nowlis, N. Mandel, A.C. Morales, The effects of reduced food size and package size on the consumption behavior of restrained and unrestrained eaters, J. Consumer Res. 35 (2008) 391–405.

[149] J.O. Fisher, T.V.E. Kral, Super-size me: portion size effects on young children's eating, Physiol. Behav. 94 (2008) 39–47.

[150] M.A. Martinez-Gonzalez, M. Bes-Rastrollo, Nut consumption, weight gain and obesity: epidemiological evidence, Nutr. Metab. Cadiovasc. Dis. 21 (2011) S40–S45.

[151] M. Bes-Rastrollo, J. Sabate, E. Gomez-Gracia, A. Alonso, J.A. Martinez, M.A. Martinez-Gonzalez, Nut consumption and weight gain in a Mediterranean cohort: the SUN study, Obesity 15 (2007) 107–116.

[152] M. Bes-Rastrollo, N.M. Wedick, M.A. Martinez-Gonzalez, T.Y. Li, L. Sampson, F.B. Hu, Prospective study of nut consumption, long-term weight change, and obesity risk in women, Am. J. Clin. Nutr. 89 (2009) 1913–1919.

[153] J. Sabate, Nut consumption and body weight, Am. J. Clin. Nutr. 78 (2003) 647S–650S.

[154] B.A. Cassady, J.H. Hollis, A.D. Fulford, R.V. Considine, R.D. Mattes, Mastication of almonds: effects of lipid bioaccessibility, appetite, and hormone response, Am. J. Clin. Nutr. 89 (2009) 794–800.

[155] J.H. Hollis, R.D. Mattes, Effect of increased dairy consumption on appetitive ratings and food intake, Obesity (Silver Spring) 15 (2007) 1520–1526.

[156] S.A. Talegawkar, E.J. Johnson, T. Carithers, H.A. Taylor Jr., M. L. Bogle, K.L. Tucker, Total alpha-tocopherol intakes are associated with serum alpha-tocopherol concentrations in African American adults, J. Nutr. 137 (2007) 2297–2303.

[157] B.C. Stroehla, L.H. Malcoe, E.M. Velie, Dietary sources of nutrients among rural Native American and white children, J. Am. Diet. Assoc. 105 (2005) 1908–1916.

[158] T.A. Nicklas, J.S. Hampl, C.A. Taylor, V.J. Thompson, W.C. Heird, Monounsaturated fatty acid intake by children and adults: temporal trends and demographic differences, Nutr. Rev. 62 (2004) 132–141.

[159] C. Zizza, D.D. Arsiwalla, K.J. Ellison, Contribution of snacking to older adults' vitamin, carotenoid, and mineral intakes, J. Am. Diet. Assoc. 10 (2010) 768–772.

[160] D.A.J. Jenkins, A. Khan, A.L. Jenkins, R. Illingworth, A.S. Pappu, T.M.S. Wolever, et al., Effect of nibbling versus gorging on cardiovascular risk factors: Serum uric acid and blood lipids, Metabolism 44 (1995) 549–555.

[161] M. Tanasescu, A.M. Ferris, D.A. Himmelgreen, N. Rodriguez, R. Perez-Escamilla, Biobehavioral factors are associated with obesity in Puerto Rican children, J. Nutr. 130 (2000) 1734–1742.

[162] D.L. Crooks, Trading nutrition for education: nutritional status and the sale of snack foods in an eastern Kentucky school, Med. Anthropol. Q. 17 (2003) 182–199.

[163] T.A. Nicklas, S.J. Yang, T. Baranowski, I. Zakeri, G. Berenson, Eating patterns and obesity in children: the Bogalusa Heart Study, Am. J. Prev. Med. 25 (2003) 9–16.

[164] A.E. Field, S.B. Austin, M.W. Gillman, B. Rosner, H.R. Rockett, G.A. Colditz, Snack food intake does not predict weight change among children and adolescents, Int. J. Obes. Relat. Metab. Disord. 28 (2004) 1210–1216.

[165] T.T.-K. Huang, N.C. Howarth, B.H. Lin, S.B. Roberts, M.A. McCrory, Energy intake and meal portions: Associations with BMI percentile in U.S. children, Obes. Res. 12 (2004) 1875–1885.

[166] T.A. Nicklas, D. Demory-Luce, S.J. Yang, T. Baranowski, I. Zakeri, G. Berenson, Children's food consumption patterns have changed over two decades (1973–1994): the Bogalusa Heart Study, J. Am. Diet. Assoc. 104 (2004) 1127–1240.

[167] S.M. Phillips, L.G. Bandini, E.N. Naumova, H. Cyr, S. Colclough, W.H. Dietz, et al., Energy-dense snack food intake in adolescence: longitudinal relationship to weight and fatness, Obes. Res. 12 (2004) 461–472.

[168] C.K. Colapinto, A. Fitzgerald, L.J. Taper, P.J. Veugelers, Children's preference for large portions: prevalence, determinants, and consequences, J. Am. Diet. Assoc. 107 (2007) 1183–1190.

[169] M. Barker, S. Robinson, C. Wilman, D.J. Barker, Behaviour, body composition and diet in adolescent girls, Appetite 35 (2000) 161–170.

[170] D.L. Franko, R.H. Striegel-Moore, D. Thompson, S.G. Affenito, G.B. Schreiber, S.R. Daniels, et al., The relationship between meal frequency and body mass index in black and white adolescent girls: more is less, Int. J. Obes. 32 (2008) 23–29.

[171] D.R. Keast, T.A. Nicklas, C.E. O'Neil, Snacking is associated with reduced risk of overweight and reduced abdominal obesity in adolescents: National Health and Nutrition Examination Survey (NHANES) 1999–2004, Am. J. Clin. Nutr. 92 (2010) 428–435.

[172] N.C. Howarth, T.T.-K. Huang, S.B. Roberts, B.H. Lin, M.A. McCrory, Eating patterns and dietary composition in relation to BMI in younger and older adults, Int. J. Obes. 31 (2007) 675–684.

[173] M. Bes-Rastrollo, A. Sanchez-Villegas, F.J. Basterra-Gortari, J.M. Nunez-Cordoba, E. Toledo, M. Serrano-Martinez, Prospective study of self-reported usual snacking and weight gain in a Mediterranean cohort: The SUN project, Clin. Nutr. 29 (2010) 323–330.

[174] S.L. Edelstein, E.L. Barrett-Connor, D.L. Wingard, B.A. Cohn, Increased meal frequency associated with decreased cholesterol concentrations: Rancho Bernardo, CA 1984–1987, Am. J. Clin. Nutr. 55 (1992) 664–669.

[175] S.E. Drummond, N.E. Crombie, M.C. Cursiter, T.R. Kirk, Evidence that eating frequency is inversely related to body weight status in male, but not female, non-obese adults reporting valid dietary intakes, Int. J. Obes. Relat. Metab. Disord. 22 (1998) 105–112.

[176] S.M. Titan, S. Bingham, A. Welch, R. Luben, S. Oakes, N. Day, et al., Frequency of eating and concentrations of serum cholesterol in the Norfolk population of the European Prospective Investigation into Cancer (EPIC–Norfolk): Cross-sectional study, Br. Med. J. 323 (2001) 1286–1288.

[177] J.S. Hampl, C.L. Heaton, C.A. Taylor, Snacking patterns influence energy and nutrient intakes but not body mass index, J. Hum. Nutr. Diet. 16 (2003) 3–11.

[178] A.K. Kant, B.I. Graubard, Secular trends in patterns of self-reported food consumption of adult Americans: NHANES 1971–1975 to NHANES 1999–2002, Am. J. Clin. Nutr. 84 (2006) 1215–1223.

[179] P. Fabry, J. Fodor, Z. Hejl, T. Braun, K. Zvolankova, The frequency of meals: its relation to overweight, hypercholesterolaemia, and decreased glucose-tolerance, Lancet 2 (1964) 614–615.

[180] J. Charzewska, W.J.B. Kulesza, Z. Chwojnowska, Relationship between obesity or overweight development and the frequency of meals, their distribution during the day and consumption of atherogenic food products, Zywienie Czlowieka 8 (1981) 217–227.

[181] M.L. Wahlqvist, A. Kouris-Blazos, N. Wattanapenpaiboon, The significance of eating patterns: an elderly Greek case study, Appetite 32 (1999) 23–32.

[182] J.B. Ruidavets, V. Bongard, V. Bataille, P. Gourdy, J. Ferrieres, Eating frequency and body fatness in middle-aged men, Int. J. Obes. Relat. Metab. Disord. 26 (2002) 1476–1483.

[183] S.-Y. Tan, M.J. Batterham, L.C. Tapsell, Energy expenditure does not differ, but protein oxidation rates appear lower in meals containing predominantly meat versus soy sources of protein, Obesity Facts 3 (2010) 101–104.

PART D

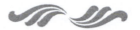

CARDIOVASCULAR DISEASE

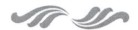

Genetic Influences on Blood Lipids and Cardiovascular Disease Risk

Jose M. Ordovas[*], *Martha Guevara-Cruz*[†]

[*]Jean Mayer U.S. Department of Agriculture Human Nutrition Research Center on Aging at Tufts University, Boston, Massachusetts; Centro Nacional Investigaciones Cardiovasculares (CNIC), Madrid, Spain; and Instituto Madrileno de Estudios Avanzados en Alimentación (IMDEA-FOOD), Madrid, Spain [†]Jean Mayer U.S. Department of Agriculture Human Nutrition Research Center on Aging at Tufts University, Boston, Massachusetts; and Department of Fisiologia de la Nutricion, Instituto Nacional de Ciencias Médicas y Nutrición Salvador Zubirán (INCMNSZ), Mexico City, Mexico

I INTRODUCTION

The major public health concerns in the developed world (i.e., cardiovascular disease, cancer, and diabetes) have both genetic and environmental causes. The interface between public health and genetics involves working toward an understanding of how genes and the environment act together to cause these diseases and how the environment (e.g., diet), rather than genes, might be manipulated to help prevent or delay the onset of disease.

Cardiovascular disease (CVD), the leading cause of mortality in most industrialized countries, is a multifactorial disease that is associated both with nonmodifiable risk factors, such as age, gender, and genetic background, and with modifiable risk factors, including elevated total and low-density lipoprotein cholesterol (LDL-C) levels, as well as reduced high-density lipoprotein cholesterol (HDL-C) level. Heritability estimates for blood lipids are high—approximately 40–60% for HDL-C, 40–50% for LDL-C, and 35–48% for triglycerides (TG) [1].

Traditionally, the major emphasis of public health measures has been on lowering serum cholesterol, which has long been recognized as an important risk factor for the development and progression of atherosclerotic vascular disease; multiple clinical studies for the past 30 years have demonstrated the benefits of this approach. In view of these findings, the National Heart, Lung, and Blood Institute convened the National Cholesterol Education Program Adult Treatment Panel I (NCEP ATP I) [2]. This panel and similar panels throughout the world have set the standards for lowering lipid profiles in clinical practice. Subsequent revisions of these standards (NCEP ATP II and III) [3,4] have placed a greater focus on LDL, and target LDL levels are based on patient risk of subsequent coronary disease events. Since the publication of the NCEP ATP III guidelines, several large-scale clinical trials of cholesterol-lowering treatments have been conducted, the findings of which may be used to further refine current clinical practice standards [5,6]. Although most of the evidence that lowering serum LDL-C can reduce CVD morbidity and mortality comes from pharmacological interventions, the NCEP has emphasized that therapeutic lifestyle change should be the primary treatment for lowering cholesterol, and drug therapies should be reserved for cases in which lifestyle modification is ineffective. The lifestyle modifications advocated include dietary changes, increased physical activity, and weight management. The recommended dietary changes to reduce LDL-C include restriction of saturated fat to less than 7% of total caloric intake, restriction of cholesterol to less than 200 mg/day, increased viscous fiber intake (10–24 g/day), and increased plant stanol/sterol intake (2 g/day) [4]. However, it is not known how many individuals can achieve the recommended levels of serum lipids using this approach, in large part because it is currently impossible to predict plasma lipid response to dietary changes in individual patients [7,8].

Nutrition in the Prevention and Treatment of Disease, Third Edition.
DOI: http://dx.doi.org/10.1016/B978-0-12-391884-0.00028-7

Other pharmacological approaches to CVD risk reduction have been investigated, including treatments to lower serum TG and raise HDL-C. Fibrate drugs are most commonly used to lower TG. Fenofibrate therapy has been associated with changes of −25 to −59% in TG, −33 to +1% in LDL-C, and +1 to +34% in HDL-C in CVD patients [9]. The largest reduction of CVD risk by fenofibrate has been detected in patients with marked dyslipidemia, a feature of metabolic syndrome (MetS), in whom a 27% relative risk reduction was found in the Fenofibrate Intervention and Event Lowering in Diabetes study [10,11]; therefore, fenofibrate would be expected to have large beneficial effects in MetS patients. The use of fenofibrate in the management of lipoprotein disorders dates back to the mid-1960s. However, their prominence has lessened throughout the years because of unimpressive results in major clinical trials, safety concerns, and the emergence of 3-hydroxy-3-methylglutaryl coenzyme A reductase inhibitors (statins). Moreover, the general trial results with these agents have been confusing, with varying cardiovascular benefits [12−14] depending on the dyslipidemia status [15].

The epidemiologic, experimental, and circumstantial evidence implicating low HDL-C as a major risk factor for CVD has driven considerable research on this lipoprotein fraction; it is hoped that raising HDL-C may further reduce CVD risk beyond what can be achieved with the use of statins. However, doubts about the clinical benefits of treatments to enhance plasma HDL-C levels have been raised by the premature termination of a large phase III trial with torcetrapib, the most potent and furthest-developed HDL-C-raising compound, which was discontinued because of excess mortality in patients receiving the drug [16]. The causes of torcetrapib failure are unknown and may be related to the drug's mode of action, to toxic off-target effects of the drug, or both. However, the failure of torcetrapib does not mean that targeting HDL in CVD prevention is no longer a research goal. Other HDL-C-raising therapies that act through similar or disparate molecular mechanisms are in various stages of preclinical and clinical development [17,18].

The considerable interindividual variation in lipid response, cardiovascular event response, and adverse events observed following these therapies has brought considerable attention to the concept of more targeted therapies based on genetic information. Pharmacogenomics (or pharmacogenetics) involves the search for and identification of genetic variants that influence patient response to drug therapy. During approximately the past decade, some progress has been made in our understanding of the variable efficacy of statin therapy [19]. Similarly, there is evidence that fenofibrate treatment improves the lipid profile, but there is significant interindividual variability in lipid response to fenofibrate, which may be mediated by specific genes [20,21]. Important limitations and issues in pharmacogenetics have been raised, however, which need to be resolved before its clinical application.

Regarding the connection between diet and plasma cholesterol concentration, several studies during the first half of the 20th century demonstrated that serum cholesterol could be modified by the composition of dietary fat [22,23]. Studies by Keys and colleagues [24] and Hegsted et al. [25] provided the first quantitative estimates of the relative effects of the various classes of dietary fatty acids and the amount of dietary cholesterol on serum cholesterol changes. Later, other predictive algorithms were developed, including predictions of LDL-C and HDL-C responses [26−28]. The relationships between dietary changes and serum lipid changes are well founded and predictable for groups. However, a striking variability in the response of serum cholesterol to diet between subjects was reported as early as 1933 [29], and this variability has been the subject of multiple reports. In some individuals, plasma total lipid and LDL-C levels dramatically decrease following the consumption of lipid-lowering diets, whereas they remain unchanged in others [27,30−34]. Multiple studies in animal models and in humans have shown that serum lipoprotein response to dietary manipulation has a significant genetic component [35−40]. Genetic variability could therefore have a significant impact on the success of public health policies and individual therapeutic interventions. Moreover, it could be partially responsible for the apparent lack of hard end point benefits shown by many dietary studies aimed at decreasing CVD [41−43].

As indicated previously, the success of CVD risk-reducing strategies has traditionally been measured based on their effects on plasma lipids and, specifically, lipoprotein levels. Lipoproteins are macromolecular complexes of lipids and proteins that originate mainly from the liver and intestine and are involved in the transport and redistribution of lipids in the body. Lipid and lipoprotein metabolism can be viewed as complex biological pathways containing multiple steps. Lipid homeostasis is achieved by the coordinated action of hundreds of gene products, including nuclear factors, binding proteins, apolipoproteins, enzymes, and receptors. Lipid metabolism is also closely linked to energy metabolism and is subject to many hormonal controls that are essential for adjustment to environmental and internal conditions. Genetic variability within candidate genes involved in lipoprotein metabolism has been associated with abnormal lipid metabolism and plasma lipoprotein profiles that may contribute to the pathogenesis of atherosclerosis. This complex regulatory network can be dissected into three major pathways (Figure 28.1). The exogenous lipoprotein pathway describes the metabolism of lipoproteins synthesized in the intestine following dietary fat intake, the endogenous pathway involves the metabolism of lipoproteins involved in the transport of liver lipids to peripheral tissues, and the reverse cholesterol transport pathway describes the process by which excess peripheral lipids (primarily cholesterol) are transported to the liver for catabolism. Our knowledge about how variants in candidate genes involved in each of these three interrelated processes affect dietary response and cardiovascular risk is discussed next.

A Exogenous Lipoprotein Pathway

The exogenous lipoprotein pathway begins in the enterocyte with the synthesis of chylomicron particles. Dietary fats absorbed in the intestine are packaged into large, triglyceride-rich chylomicrons for delivery to sites of lipid metabolism or storage. During their transit to the liver, these particles interact with lipoprotein lipase (LPL) and undergo partial lipolysis to form

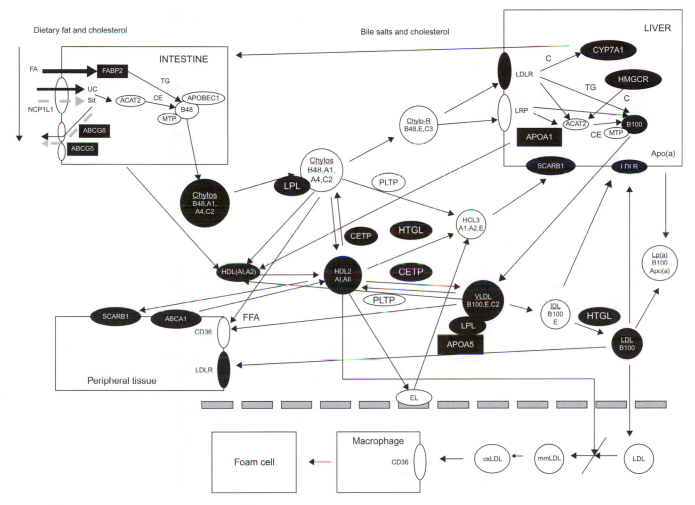

FIGURE 28.1 Human lipoprotein metabolism. A1, apolipoprotein A-I; A2, apolipoprotein A-II; A4, apolipoprotein A-IV; A5, apolipoprotein A-V; ABCA1, ATP binding cassette, subfamily A, member 1; ABCG5, ATP binding cassette, subfamily G, member 5; ABCG8, ATP binding cassette, subfamily G, member 8; ACAT2, cytosolic acetoacetyl-CoA thiolase; apo, apolipoprotein; APOBEC1, apolipoprotein B mRNA editing enzyme; B100, apolipoprotein B-100; B48, apolipoprotein B-48; C2, apolipoprotein C-II; C3, apolipoprotein C-III; CE, cholesteryl esters; CD36, CD36 antigen; CETP, cholesteryl ester transfer protein; Chylos, chylomicron; Chilo-R, chylomicron remnants; CYP7A1, cholesterol-7-alpha-hydroxylase; E, apolipoprotein E; FA, fatty acids; FABP2, intestinal fatty acid binding protein; FFA, free fatty acids; HDL, high-density lipoprotein; HMGCR, 3-hydroxy-3-methylglutaryl-CoA reductase; HTGL, hepatic triglyceride lipase; IDL, intermediate-density lipoproteins; LDL, low-density lipoprotein; LDLR, LDL receptor; Lp(a), lipoprotein (a); LPL, lipoprotein lipase; mmLDL, minimally modified LDL; MTP, microsomal triglyceride transfer protein; NPC1L1, Niemann–Pick C1-like 1; oxLDL, oxidized LDL; PLTP, phospholipid transfer protein; SCARB1, scavenger receptor type I B; Sit, sitosterol; TG, triglycerides; UC, unesterified cholesterol; VLDL, very low-density lipoprotein. Those components of the lipoprotein pathway highlighted in the chapter are indicated with white font over black background.

chylomicron remnants. These chylomicron remnants pick up apolipoprotein E (APOE) and a cholesteryl ester from HDL, after which they are taken up by the liver in a process that is mediated by the interaction of APOE with hepatic receptors. In most people, this occurs quickly, and chylomicrons are not usually present in the blood after prolonged fasting. However, there is dramatic variability in postprandial lipoprotein metabolism, which is determined in part by genetic factors, and this variability could be highly relevant to achieving a more precise definition of individualized CVD risk [44,45]. The most relevant candidate genes involved in this metabolic pathway and their known associations with plasma lipid levels and dietary response are described later.

B Endogenous Lipoprotein Metabolism

Hepatocytes synthesize and secrete triglyceride-rich very low-density lipoprotein (VLDL), which may be converted first to intermediate-density lipoproteins and then to LDL through lipolysis by a mechanism involving LPL, similar to that described for the exogenous lipoprotein pathway. The excess surface components are usually transferred to HDL. Some of these remnants may be taken up by the liver, whereas others are further lipolyzed to become LDL, which, in humans, contains APOB as its only apolipoprotein. This pathway uses many of the same genes as the exogenous pathway. The LDL receptor is primarily responsible for the catabolism of LDL particles in the liver and peripheral tissues. Another important factor in endogenous lipoprotein metabolism is the HMG-CoA reductase gene, which encodes a key enzyme in *de novo* cholesterol synthesis.

C Reverse Cholesterol Transport

Both the liver and the intestine synthesize HDL. In its precursor form, HDL is disc-shaped, and it matures in the circulation as it picks up unesterified cholesterol from cell membranes (see the later discussion of the ATP binding cassette-1), other lipids (phospholipids and TG), and proteins from TRL as these particles undergo lipolysis. The cholesterol is esterified by lecithin—cholesterol acyltransferase (LCAT), and the small HDL3 particle becomes a larger HDL2 particle. The esterified cholesterol is either delivered to the liver or transferred by the action of the cholesterol ester transfer protein (CETP) to TRL in exchange for TG. The liver may then take up cholesterol via receptors specific for these lipoproteins, or it can be delivered to the peripheral tissues. The TG received by HDL2 is hydrolyzed by hepatic lipase, and the particle is converted

back to HDL3, completing the HDL3 cycle in plasma. In the liver, cholesterol can be excreted directly into bile, converted to bile acids, or reused for lipoprotein production.

However, CVD has a multifactorial etiology in which a complex combination of environmental, genetic, and clinical risk factors seem to play determinant roles [46,47]. The complex architecture of this disease and its genetic basis [48] are still poorly understood, and some discrepancies remain in estimates of the heritability of numerous CVD-related quantitative traits (QTs) [49]. The identification and validation of genetic variants that promote CVDs and related QTs may lead to a better understanding of the pathogenesis of these diseases and to the identification of novel disease-associated biological pathways and risk factors.

During approximately the past two decades, the genetics of chronic diseases and related QTs have been assessed by candidate gene approaches [50]. Twin and family studies have been used to estimate heritability, whereas population-based studies are used to identify variants that are associated with specific phenotypes and to explore interactions between genetic and environmental factors. Candidate genes are those considered to influence complex phenotypes due to their participation in related biological pathways or due to their location near a region of interest [50]. This hypothesis-driven research has provided the foundation for the development of genetic CVD risk profiles [51]. However, since 2007, genome-wide association studies (GWAS) have revolutionized the research of chronic diseases such as CVDs and their associated QTs [52–54]. Recent technological advances have enabled the rapid and accurate assessment of millions of single-nucleotide polymorphisms (SNPs) in large populations, and many new GWAS have been conducted for different CVD phenotypes and related traits. These studies have identified hundreds of genetic factors, some of which have been frequently replicated, albeit with small individual effects. Moreover, GWAS have revealed previously unsuspected pathological pathways [55,56]. Nevertheless, the causal variants identified by GWAS are insufficient to explain the high heritability of different CVD phenotypes. Additional studies are required to further refine the prevention, diagnosis, treatment, and prognosis of CVD patients based on genetic factors [57].

II REPRESENTATIVE GENOME-WIDE ASSOCIATION STUDIES

Lipid measures represent excellent secondary phenotypes for the genetic investigation by many

GWAS of CVD, and relatively large sample sizes can be obtained to study these traits. Here, we discuss the main features of several GWAS using lipid measures.

Sabatti *et al.* [58] reported GWAS results for nine quantitative metabolic traits (HDL-C, LDL-C, TG, glucose, insulin, C-reactive protein, body mass index, and systolic and diastolic blood pressure) in the Northern Finland Birth Cohort of 1966 (NFBC1966), which was drawn from the most genetically isolated regions of Finland. This study replicated most previously reported gene associations and identified nine new associations, several of which highlighted genes with metabolic functions: HDL-C with *NR1H3* (LXRA), LDL-C with *AR* and *FADS1−FADS2*, glucose with *MTNR1B*, and insulin with *PANK1*. Two of these new associations emerged after adjusting results for body mass index. Gene−environment interaction analyses suggested additional associations that will require validation in larger samples. These loci, even when combined with quantified environmental exposures, explain little of the trait variation in NFBC1966. However, the association between LDL-C and an infrequent variant in *AR* suggests that cohort studies have the potential to identify associations with both common, low-impact and rare, high-impact quantitative trait loci.

In another study, Aulchenko *et al.* [59] reported the first GWA analysis of loci affecting total cholesterol (TC), LDL-C, HDL-C, and triglycerides sampled randomly from 16 population-based cohorts and genotyped using mainly the Illumina HumanHap300-Duo platform. Their study included a total of 17,797−22,562 persons aged 18−104 years and from geographic regions from the Nordic countries to southern Europe. They established 22 loci associated with serum lipid levels at a genome-wide significance level, including 16 loci that had been identified by previous GWAS. The 6 loci newly identified in this cohort were *ABCG5*, *TMEM57*, the *CTCF−PRMT8* region, *DNAH1*, *FADS3−FADS2*, and the *MADD−FOLH1* region. The effect sizes differed significantly by sex for 3 loci. Genetic risk scores based on lipid loci explained up to 4.8% of the variation in lipid profile and were associated with increased intima media thickness and coronary heart disease incidence.

To dissect the polygenic basis of these traits, Kathiresan *et al.* [60] conducted GWAS in 19,840 individuals and replicated it in up to 20,623 individuals. They identified 30 distinct loci associated with lipoprotein concentrations, including 11 loci that reached genome-wide significance. The 11 newly defined loci include common variants associated with LDL cholesterol near *ABCG8*, *MAFB*, *HNF1A*, and *TIMD4*; with HDL cholesterol near *ANGPTL4*,

FADS1−FADS2–FADS3, *HNF4A*, *LCAT*, *PLTP*, and *TTC39B*; and with triglycerides near *AMAC1L2*, *FADS1−FADS2−FADS3*, and *PLTP*. The proportion of individuals exceeding clinical cutoff points for high LDL cholesterol, low HDL cholesterol, and high TGs varied according to an allelic dosage score. These results suggest that the cumulative effect of multiple common variants contributes to polygenic dyslipidemia.

Ma *et al.* [61] reported single-locus and epistatic SNP effects on TC and HDL-C using Framingham Heart Study (FHS) data. Single-locus effects and pairwise epistasis effects of 432,096 SNP markers were tested for their significance on log-transformed TC and HDL-C levels. Twenty-nine additive SNP effects reached single-locus genome-wide significance ($p < 7.2 \times 10^{-8}$), and no dominant effect reached genome-wide significance. Two new gene regions were detected: The *RAB3GAP1−R3HDM1−LCT−MCM6* region of chr02 for TC was identified by 6 new SNPs, and the *OSBPL8−ZDHHC17* region (chr12) for HDL-C was identified by 1 new SNP. The remaining 22 single-locus SNPs identified confirmed previously reported genes or gene regions. For TC, 3 SNPs identified two gene regions that were tightly linked with previously reported TC-associated genes, including rs599839 10 bases downstream of *PSRC1* and 3.498 kb downstream of *CELSR2*, rs4970834 in *CELSR2*, and rs4245791 in *ABCG8*. The association of HDL-C with *LPL* was confirmed by 12 SNPs 8−45 kb downstream, with *CETP* by 2 SNPs 0.5−11 kb upstream, and with the *LIPG−ACAA2* region by 5 SNPs in this region. Two epistasis effects on TC and 13 epistasis effects on HDL-C reached the significance of "suggestive linkage." The most significant epistasis effect ($p = 5.72 \times 10^{-13}$) was a dominant × dominant effect of HDL-C between *LMBRD1* (chr06) and the *LRIG3* region (chr12) and was close to reaching "significant linkage"; this pair of gene regions had 6 other D × D effects with "suggestive linkage." Genome-wide association analysis of the FHS data detected two novel gene regions with genome-wide significance, detected epistatic SNP effects on TC and HDL-C with the significance of suggestive linkage in seven pairs of gene regions, and confirmed the association of some previously reported gene regions with TC and HDL-C.

Teslovich *et al.* [62] identified additional common variants associated with plasma TC, LDL-C, HDL-C, and TG concentrations. They performed a meta-analysis of 46 lipid GWAS. These studies together comprised more than 100,000 individuals of European descent from the United States, Europe, and Australia. They reported 95 significantly associated loci ($p < 5 \times 10^{-8}$), with 59 showing genome-wide significant association with lipid traits for the first time. The newly reported associations include SNPs near known lipid regulators (e.g., *CYP7A1*, *NPC1LA*, and *SCARB1*) and in many loci not previously implicated in lipoprotein metabolism. The 95 loci contribute not only to normal variation in lipid traits but also to extreme lipid phenotypes, and they affect lipid traits in three non-European populations (East Asians, South Asians, and African Americans). That study also identified several novel loci associated with plasma lipids that are also associated with CVD. Finally, it validated the functions of three novel genes—*GALNT2*, *PPP1R3B*, and *TTC39B*—with experiments in mouse models. Taken together, Teslovich *et al.*'s findings provide the foundation for a broader biological understanding of lipoprotein metabolism and identify new therapeutic opportunities for the prevention of coronary artery disease (CAD).

Waterworth *et al.* [63] conducted a meta-GWAS to identify novel genetic determinants of low LDL-C, HDL-C, and TGs. They combined GWAS data from eight studies, which included up to 17,723 participants and associated information on circulating lipid concentrations. They performed independent replication studies in up to 37,774 participants from eight populations and also in a population of Indian Asian descent. They also assessed the associations between SNPs at lipid loci and CVD risk in up to 9633 cases and 38,684 controls. They identified four novel genetic loci that showed reproducible associations with lipid levels, including a potential functional SNP in the *SLC39A8* gene for HDL-C, an SNP near the *MYLIP/GMPR* and *PPP1R3B* genes for LDL-C, and an SNP at the *AFF1* gene for triglycerides. SNPs at the *CELSR2–APOB–APOE–APOC1–APOC4–APOC2* cluster, *LPL–ZNF259–APOA5–APOA4–APOC3–APOA1* cluster, and *TRIB1* locus showed strong statistical association with one or more lipid traits and were also associated with CVD risk.

Lettre *et al.* [64] identified common genetic polymorphisms associated with CVD and its risk factors (LDC and HDL-C, hypertension, smoking, and type 2 diabetes) in individuals of African ancestry through a GWAS in 8090 African Americans from five population-based cohorts. They confirmed 17 loci that had previously been associated with CVD or its risk factors in Caucasians. For 5 of these regions (CHD: *CDKN2A/CDKN2B*; HDL-C: *FADS1–FADS3*, *PLTP*, *LPL*, and *ABCA1*), the authors were able to use the distinct linkage disequilibrium patterns in African Americans to identify DNA polymorphisms that were more strongly associated with the phenotypes than the previously reported index SNPs found in Caucasian populations. They also developed a new approach for association testing in admixed populations using allelic and local ancestry variation.

GWAS have identified a number of SNPs associated with serum lipid level in populations of European descent. The individual and the cumulative effects of these SNPs on blood lipids are largely unclear in the U.S. population. Chang *et al.* [65] used data from the second phase of the Third National Health and Nutrition Examination Survey (NHANES III), a nationally representative survey of the U.S. population, to examine associations of 57 GWAS-identified or well-established lipid-related genetic loci with plasma concentrations of HDL-C, LDL-C, TC, and TG. They used multivariable linear regression to examine single SNP associations and the cumulative effect of multiple SNPs on blood lipid levels. Analyses were conducted in adults for each of the three major racial/ethnic groups in the U.S.: non-Hispanic whites ($n = 2296$), non-Hispanic blacks ($n = 1699$), and Hispanics ($n = 1713$). The allele frequencies of all SNPs varied significantly by race/ethnicity, except rs3764261 in *CETP*. Individual SNPs had small effects on lipid levels, but the effects were consistent across racial/ethnic groups for most SNPs. More GWAS-validated SNPs were replicated in non-Hispanic whites (<67%) than in non-Hispanic blacks (<44%) or Hispanics (<44%). Genetic risk scores were strongly associated with increased lipid levels in each race/ethnic group. The combination of all SNPs into a weighted explained no more than 11% of the total variance in blood lipid levels. The authors concluded that the combined association of SNPs, used to generate a genetic risk score, was strongly correlated with blood lipid measures in all major race/ethnic groups in the United States and that this knowledge could help in identifying subgroups of patients at high risk for an unfavorable lipid profile.

GWAS were never designed to interrogate actual underlying causal variants; rather, they are used to "tag" the approximate locations of disease variants, typically down to a few hundred kilobases. The development of GWAS methodology may have transformed our ability to discover key genetic factors that are involved in the pathogenesis of cardiovascular disease, but this only represents the first step in a much longer process. The genes and pathways uncovered using the GWAS approach are likely to be fundamental to disease biology, so it will be crucial to determine how these variants affect the expression and function of the gene products through molecular biology approaches. Therefore, we compiled a list of genes identified by GWAS and additional evidence of their association with lipids. We found 118 loci potentially associated with serum lipid levels that were identified in different GWAS and were also implicated in previously known Mendelian forms of lipid disorders, previously published in candidate gene association studies, or identified through the examination of metabolic phenotypes of knockout mice maintained by the Jackson Laboratory. These genes are described in Table 28.1.

We identified 118 loci that showed genome-wide significant associations with at least one of the four traits tested (LDL-C, TG, HDLC, and TC). Among these loci, 53 demonstrated genome-wide association with LDL-C, 45 with TG, 56 with HDL-C, and 57 with TC. Only 2 genes in all GWAS had the same effects on HDL-C—the *LPL* and *CETP* genes. The genes most frequently identified in GWAS for LDL-C were *PCSK9*, *CELSR2*, *APOB*, *ABCG5/8*, *HMGCR*, *LDLR*, *APOE−APOC1−APOC4−APOC2*, and *NSRF*; *CILP2* and *NCAN* were also identified in multiple LDL association studies. The genes most frequently identified in GWAS for TG were *APOB*, *GCKR*, *ANGPTL3−DOCK7−ATG4C*, *MLXIPL*, *LPL*, *FADS1−FADS2−FADS3*, and *APOA−APOC3−APOA4*. The genes most frequently identified in GWAS for HDL-C was were *GALNT2*, *LPL*, *ABCA1*, *FADS1−FADS2−FADS3*, *MVK*, *LIPC*, *CETP*, *LCAT*, and *LIPG*. Finally, the genes most frequently identified in GWAS for TC were *CELS42*, *APOB*, *ABCA5G/8*, *LIPG*, and *LDLR* (Table 28.2).

It is now clear that many of these genes are novel and were not investigated by previous candidate gene studies. Larger sample sizes and additional meta-analyses of GWAS data sets will uncover further loci that make up the remaining genetic component of these diseases, albeit with increasingly smaller effect sizes. Indeed, investigators will need to work on large, high-throughput sequencing efforts involving thousands of DNA samples from affected subjects and a similar number of controls to identify new disease-associated loci.

Ultimately, one of the major challenges going forward will be to determine how these recently uncovered variants affect the expression and function of gene products using molecular biology approaches. Detailed genotype−phenotype studies will be required to determine the mechanisms involved and how these loci potentially interact with and are involved in other disorders. Only by uncovering the functional context of these genetic variants and understanding their interactions can these findings be truly translated in to meaningful benefits for patient care.

III DEVELOPMENT OF CARDIOVASCULAR SCORE

Measures of cardiovascular risk, such as the Framingham score, have long been used in public health research and practice [67−70]. These risk scores play an important role in screening programs to identify susceptible individuals before the onset of clinical symptoms and facilitate primary prevention [71].

Cardiovascular risk scores are also used in epidemiological research, namely as measures of exposure, as stratification variables, or as measures of potential confounders [72,73].

The predictive ability of existing cardiovascular risk scores varies greatly between populations and is particularly low for ethnic minorities [74]. This variability merits further investigation; most current cardiovascular risk measures are based on cohorts from high-income Western countries [75,76], and their generalizability to populations from low- or middle-income countries or ethnically and economically diverse communities in high-income countries is limited.

In addition, low LDL-C and high HDL-C, TG, and TC concentrations are important and heritable risk factors for cardiovascular disease. Although GWAS of circulating lipid levels have identified numerous disease-associated loci, a substantial portion of the heritability of these traits remains unexplained. Evidence of unexplained genetic variance can be detected by combining multiple independent markers into additive genetic risk scores. These polygenetic scores, which were constructed using results from the ENGAGE Consortium GWAS on serum lipids [59], were used to predict lipid levels in an independent population-based study, the Rotterdam Study II. This study also tested for evidence of a shared genetic basis for different lipid phenotypes. The polygenetic score approach was used to identify an alternative genome-wide significance threshold for subsequent pathway analysis, and the results of that analysis were compared with those based on the classical genome-wide significance threshold. Demirkan *et al.* [77] provide evidence suggesting that many loci that influence circulating lipid levels remain undiscovered. Cross-prediction models suggested a small overlap between the polygenic backgrounds involved in determining LDL-C, HDL-C, and TG levels. Pathway analysis utilizing the best polygenetic score for TC uncovered extra information compared with a model that used only genome-wide significant loci. These results suggest that the genetic architecture of circulating lipid involves many undiscovered variants with small effects. Thus, increasing GWAS sample sizes will enable the identification of novel variants that regulate lipid levels.

Using prediction modeling, Demirkan *et al.* [77] explain up to 4.8% of the variance in HDL-C, 2.6% in LDL-C, 3.8% in TG, and 2.7% in TC. However, these proportions are much lower than those identified by the Global Lipid Genetics Consortium, which were estimated to explain 12.4% (TC), 12.2% (LDL-C), 12.1% (HDL-C), and 9.6% (TG) of the variance in the FHS sample, as reported by Teslovich *et al.* [62]. This is expected because increases in sample size lead to better estimation of SNP effect sizes.

TABLE 28.1 List of Genes Identified in GWAS with Additional Evidence of Association with Lipid Traits

Locus[a]	Chr	Lead SNP	Lead trait[b]	Other traits[c]	Alleles/MAF[d]	Effect size[e]	p	eQTL[f]	CVD[g]	Ethnic[h]	Knockout mouse phenotype (pathway)[i]	Candidate gene association[j]	Mendelian lipid disorders[k]
LDLRAP1	1	rs12027135	TC	LDL	T/A/0.45	−1.22	4×0^{-11}	Y		+++?	Elevated LDL-C (CMP, SMP)		Familial hypercholest-erolemia
PABPC4	1	rs4460293	HDL		A/G/0.23	−0.48	4×10^{-10}	Y		++++			
PCSK9	1	rs2479409	LDL	TC	A/G/0.30	2.01	2×10^{-28}			++++	Decreased plasma cholesterol (CMP, SMP)	X	Autosomal-dominant hypercholest-erolemia
ANGPTL3	1	rs2131925	TG	TC, LDL	T/G/0.32	−4.94	9×10^{-43}	Y		++++	Decreased plasma lipids (CMP)		
EVI5	1	rs7515577	TC		A/C/0.21	−1.18	3×10^{-8}			+++?			
SORT1	1	rs629301	LDL	TC	T/C/0.22	−5.65	1×10^{-17}	Y	Y	++++			
ZNF648	1	rs1689800	HDL		A/G/0.35	−0.47	3×10^{-10}			+++-			
MOSC1	1	rs2242442	TC	LDL	T/C/0.32	−1.39	6×10^{-13}			+++?			
GALNT2	1	rs4846914	HDL	TG	A/G/0.40	−0.61	4×10^{-21}			++++			
IRF2BP2	1	rs514230	TC	LDL	T/A/0.48	−1.36	5×10^{-14}			+++?			
TMEM57	1	rs10903129	TC	HDL, LDL, TG	G/A/0.54	0.061	5×10^{-10}						
DOCK7	1	rs1167998	TC	TG	A/C/0.32	−0.073	6.4×10^{-10}						
ANGPTL3-DOCK7-ATG4C	1	rs1748195	TG	LDL	A/G/0.30	−0.08	1.60×10^{-4}						
CELSR2	1	rs646776	LDL	TC	G/T/0.21	−0.23	2×10^{-42}						
CR1L	1	rs4844614	LDL		G/A/0.32	−0.155	2.19×10^{-12}				Complete lethality during fetal growth and development		
PSRC1	1	rs599839	LDL		A/G/0.22	0.174	8.72×10^{-14}						

D. CARDIOVASCULAR DISEASE

Gene	Chr	SNP			Allele/Freq	Effect	P-value		+/−		Phenotype		Disease
APOB	2	rs1367117	LDL	TC	G/A/ 0.30	4.05	4×10^{-114}		++++		Embryonic lethal, heterozygotes have decreased plasma cholesterol, hypobetalipoproteinemia (CMP, LT, RN)	X	Hypobetalipo-proteinemia
		rs1042034	TG	HDL	T/C/ 0.22	−5.99	1×10^{-45}		+−++				
GCKR	2	rs1260326	TG	TC	C/T/ 0.41	8.76	6×10^{-133}	Y	++++		Insulin resistance (CHMP, RN)		
ABCG5/8	2	rs4299376	LDL	TC	T/G/ 0.30	2.75	2×10^{-47}		++++		Sitosterolemia (LT)	X	Sitosterolemia
RAB3GAP1	2	rs7570971	TC		C/A/ 0.34	1.25	2×10^{-8}		+−??		Abnormal excitatory postsynaptic currents		
											Abnormal neurotransmitter secretion		
											Enhanced paired pulse facilitation (BD)		
COBLL1	2	rs10195252	TG		T/C/ 0.40	−2.01	2×10^{-10}	Y	++++				
		rs12328675	HDL		T/C/ 0.13	0.68	3×10^{-10}		++?+				
IRS1	2	rs2972146	HDL	TG	T/G/ 0.37	0.46	3×10^{-9}	Y	++++	Y	Decreased circulating HDL cholesterol		
											Increased circulating free fatty acids		
											Increased circulating triglycerides		
											Insulin resistance (ISP)		
R3HDM1	2	rs12465802	LDLC		A/G/ 0.44	0.117	2.63×10^{-8}						
LCT	2	rs2322660	LDL		C/T/ 0.35	−0.12	2.42×10^{-8}						
MCM6	2	rs309180	LDL		G/A/ 0.36	−0.119	2.43×10^{-8}						
RAF1	3	rs2290159	TC		G/C/ 0.22	−1.42	4×10^{-9}		+++?		Abnormal liver sinusoid morphology (A)		
MSL2L1	3	rs645040	TG		T/G/ 0.22	−2.22	3×10^{-8}		++−+				
KLHL8	4	rs442177	TG		T/G/ 0.41	−2.25	9×10^{-12}		++++				

D. CARDIOVASCULAR DISEASE

(Continued)

TABLE 28.1 (Continued)

Locus[a]	Chr	Lead SNP	Lead trait[b]	Other traits[c]	Alleles/ MAF[d]	Effect size[e]	p	eQTL[f]	CVD[g]	Ethnic[h]	Knockout mouse phenotype (pathway)[i]	Candidate gene association[j]	Mendelian lipid disorders[k]
SLC39A8	4	rs13107325	HDL		C/T/ 0.07	−0.84	7×10^{-11}	Y		+ − ? −			
AFF1	4	rs442177	TG		A/C/ 0.60	0.014	1.5×10^{-7}				Partial postnatal lethality		
ARL15	5	rs6450176	HDL		G/A/ 0.26	−0.49	5×10^{-8}			− ?? +			
MAP3K1	5	rs9686661	TG		C/T/ 0.20	2.57	1×10^{-10}			+ + + +	Abnormal heart left ventricle morphology (A)		
HMGCR	5	rs12916	TC	LDL	T/C/ 0.39	2.84	9×10^{-47}			+ + + ?	Complete embryonic lethality before turning of embryo (A, CMP)	X	
TIMD4	5	rs6882076	TC	LDL, TG	C/T/ 0.35	−1.98	7×10^{-28}			+ + + ?			
C5ORF35	5	rs6867983	TG		C/T/ 0.14	0.014	6.1×10^{-6}						
RNF130	5	rs13161895	LDL		C/T/ 0.08	0.151	2.3×10^{-5}						
MYLIP	6	rs3757354	LDL	TC	C/T/ 0.22	−1.43	1×10^{-11}			+ − − +			
HFE	6	rs1800562	LDL	TC	G/A/ 0.06	−2.22	6×10^{-10}			+ + ? +			
HLA	6	rs3177928	TC	LDL	G/A/ 0.16	2.31	4×10^{-19}	Y		+ + + ?			
		rs2247056	TG		C/T/ 0.25	−2.99	2×10^{-15}			+ + + −			
C6orf106	6	rs2814944	HDL		G/A/ 0.16	−0.49	4×10^{-9}	Y		+ + + −			
		rs2814982	TC		C/T/ 0.11	−1.86	5×10^{-11}		Y	− − + ?			
FRK	6	rs9488822	TC	LDL	A/T/ 0.35	−1.18	2×10^{-10}	Y		+ + + ?	Decreased circulating triiodothyronine (RPT)		
CITED2	6	rs605066	HDL		T/C/ 0.42	−0.39	3×10^{-8}			+ + − +	Abnormal heart development (RES)		

Chr	Gene	rs ID	Trait 1	Trait 2	Allele/Freq	Beta	p-value		+/−	Phenotype	Disease	
6	LPA	rs1564348	LDL	TC	T/C/0.17	−0.56	2×10^{-17}	Y	++?+	Decreased total body fat, hemorrhage		
		rs1084651	HDL		G/A/0.16	1.95	3×10^{-8}		++?+			
6	IGF2R	rs456598	LDL		A/G/0.87	−0.015	8.4×10^{-7}			Complete prenatal lethality (A, RAMP)		
7	DNAH11	rs12670798	TC	LDL	T/C/0.23	1.43	9×10^{-10}		+++?	Abnormal heart morphology (AG)		
7	NPC1L1	rs2072183	TC	LDL	G/C/0.25	2.01	3×10^{-11}		+−+?	Increased cholesterol level (CMP, LT, STMP)		
7	TYW1B	rs13238203	TG		C/T/0.04	−7.91	1×10^{-9}		+???			
7	MLXIPL	rs17145738	TG	HDL	C//T/0.12	−9.32	6×10^{-58}	Y	++++	Decreased circulating cholesterol and free fatty acids (GL)		
7	KLF14	rs4731702	HDL		C/T/0.48	0.59	1×10^{-15}	Y	++++			
8	PPP1R3B	rs9987289	HDL	TC, LDL	G/A/0.09	−1.21	6×10^{-25}	Y	+++			
8	PINX1	rs11776767	TG		G/C/0.37	2.01	1×10^{-8}		−+++	Complete embryonic lethality during organogenesis (MMPC)		
8	NAT2	rs1495741	TG	TC	A/G/0.22	2.85	5×10^{-14}	Y	−+++	Abnormal xenobiotic pharmacokinetics		
8	LPL	rs12678919	TG	HDL	A/G/0.12	−13.64	2×10^{-115}	Y	++++	Decreased circulating HDL-C and LDL-C, increased circulating TG and VLDL (LMP)	LPL deficiency	X
8	CYP7A1	rs2081687	TC	LDL	C/T/0.35	1.23	2×10^{-12}		+++?	Nearly absent cholesterol absorption (CMP, STMP)	Hypercholesterolemia	X
8	TRPS1	rs2293889	HDL		G/T/0.41	−0.44	6×10^{-11}		++++	Complete neonatal lethality (RPT)	Trichorhinophalangeal syndrome, type 1	
		rs2737229	TC		A/C/0.30	−1.11	2×10^{-8}		++−?			
8	TRIB1	rs2954029	TG	TC, LDL, HDL	A/T/0.47	−5.64	3×10^{-55}	Y	++++			
8	PLEC1	rs11136341	LDL	TC	A/G/0.40	1.4	4×10^{-13}		++++	Abnormal heart morphology (RN)		

(Continued)

D. CARDIOVASCULAR DISEASE

TABLE 28.1 (Continued)

Locus[a]	Chr	Lead SNP	Lead trait[b]	Other traits[c]	Alleles/MAF[d]	Effect size[e]	p	eQTL[f]	CVD[g]	Ethnic[h]	Knockout mouse phenotype (pathway)[i]	Candidate gene association[j]	Mendelian lipid disorders[k]
XKR6-AMAC1L2	8	rs7819412	TG		A/G/0.48	−0.04	3×10^{-8}						
TTC39B	9	rs581080	HDL	TC	C/G/0.18	−0.65	3×10^{-12}			+ − + +			
ABCA1	9	rs1883025	HDL	TC	C/T/0.25	−0.94	2×10^{-33}			+ + + +	Nearly absent HDL-C (LT, CMP)	X	Tangier disease
AB0	9	rs9411489	LDL	TC	C/T/0.20	2.24	6×10^{-13}		Y	????			
JMJD1C	10	rs10761731	TG		A/T/0.43	−2.38	3×10^{-12}			+ + + +			
CYP26A1	10	rs2068888	TG		G/A/0.46	−2.28	2×10^{-8}			+ + + +	Abnormal heart morphology (RAMP)		
GPAM	10	rs2255141	TC	LDL	G/A/0.30	1.14	2×10^{-10}			+ + + ?	Decreased circulating insulin, cholesterol, and TG and decreased liver triglycerides (FAMP)		
AMPD3	11	rs2923084	HDL		A/G/0.17	−0.41	5×10^{-8}			+ + − +			
SPTY2D1	11	rs10128711	TC		C/T/0.28	−1.04	3×10^{-8}	Y		+ − + ?			
LRP4	11	rs3136441	HDL		T/C/0.15	0.78	3×10^{-18}	Y		+ + + ?	Abnormal postnatal growth (incisor and limbs) (RPT)		
FADS1-2-3	11	rs174546	TG	HDL, TC, LDL	C/T/0.34	3.82	5×10^{-24}	Y		+ + + +	Increased liver TG (FAMP, LT)		
APOA1	11	rs964184	TG	TC, HDL, LDL	C/G/0.13	16.95	7×10^{-240}		Y	+ + + +	Decreased cholesterol efflux and increased circulating TG (CMP, LT)	X	ApoA-1 deficiency
UBASH3B	11	rs7941030	TC	HDL	T/C/0.38	0.97	2×10^{-10}			+ + + ?			
ST3GAL4	11	rs11220462	LDL	TC	G/A/0.14	1.95	1×10^{-15}	Y		+ + + +	Abnormal platelet physiology		

Chr	Gene	rsID	Trait 1	Trait 2	Allele/Freq	Beta	P-value	Signs	Y	Phenotype	X
11	APOA1/APOC3/APOA4	rs12277004	TG	LDL, TC	C/C/0.93	−0.181	5.4×10^{-13}			Increased susceptibility to atherosclerosis	X
11	MADD-FOLDH	rs7395662	HDL	LDC, TC, TG	A/G/0.61	−0.073	6.0×10^{-11}	+++		Decreased circulating HDL and cholesterol	
11	NR1H3	rs2167079	HDL		G/A/0.41	0.04	5.13×10^{-8}				
12	PDE3A	rs7134375	HDL		C/A/0.42	0.4	4×10^{-8}	+++		Female infertility (RES)	
12	LRP1	rs11613352	TG	HDL	C/T/0.23	−2.7	4×10^{-10}	++?+		Complete embryonic lethality during organogenesis (A, LT)	
12	MVK	rs8134504	HDL		T/C/0.47	−0.44	7×10^{-15}	++?+	Y		
12	BRAP	rs11065987	TC	LDL	A/G/0.42	−0.96	7×10^{-12}	++??			
12	HNF1A	rs1169288	TC	LDL	A/C/0.33	1.42	1×10^{-14}	+++?	Y	Abnormal pancreatic islet morphology and increased cholesterol (CMP, FAMP, HIR)	
12	SBNO1	rs4759375	HDL		C/T/0.06	0.86	7×10^{-9}	+??+			
12	ZNF664	rs4765127	HDL	TG	G/T/0.34	0.44	3×10^{-10}	−+−+			
12	SCARB1	rs838880	HDL		T/C/0.31	0.61	3×10^{-14}	++−?		Increased susceptibility to atherosclerosis and increased circulating cholesterol (CMP, LT)	X
12	MMAB	rs2338104	HDL		G/C/0.45	−0.07	1×10^{-10}				
12	OSBPL8/ZDHHC17	rs17259942	HDL		A/G/0.12	0.168	8.61×10^{-8}				
14	NYNRIN	rs8017377	LDL		G/A/0.47	1.14	5×10^{-11}	+−++			
15	CAPN3	rs2412710	TG		G/A/0.02	7	2×10^{-8}	+??−		Dilated cardiomyopathy (RES); Muscular dystrophy, Limb−Girdle, type 2A:LGMD2A	

D. CARDIOVASCULAR DISEASE

(Continued)

TABLE 28.1 (Continued)

Locus[a]	Chr	Lead SNP	Lead trait[b]	Other traits[c]	Alleles/MAF[d]	Effect size[e]	p	eQTL[f]	CVD[g]	Ethnic[h]	Knockout mouse phenotype (pathway)[i]	Candidate gene association[j]	Mendelian lipid disorders[k]
FRMD5	15	rs2929282	TG		A/T/ 0.05	5.13	2×10^{-11}	Y		+ − − −			
LIPC	15	rs1532085	HDL	TC, TG	G/A/ 0.39	1.45	3×10^{-96}	Y		+ + + +	Increased circulating TG, HDL cholesterol and LDL cholesterol (CMP, FAMP, LMP)	X	Hepatic lipase deficiency
LACTB	15	rs2652834	HDL		G/A/ 0.20	−0.39	9×10^{-9}	Y		+ ???			
GCOM1	15	rs937254	HDL		G/A/ 0.57	0.077	5.4×10^{-6}						
CTF1	16	rs11649653	TG		C/G/ 0.40	−2.13	3×10^{-8}	Y		+ ?? −	Motor neuron degeneration (BD)		
CETP	16	rs3764261	HDL	TC, LDL, TG	C/A/ 0.32	3.39	7×10^{-380}			+ + + +	Decreased cholesterol and TG (involves transgenes)		CETP deficiency
LCAT	16	rs16942887	HDL		G/A/ 0.12	1.27	8×10^{-33}	Y		+ + + +	Decreased circulating HDL cholesterol (CMP, LMP, STMP)		LCAT deficiency (very low HDL)
HPR	16	rs2000999	TC	LDL	G/A/ 0.20	2.34	3×10^{-24}			+ + + ?			
CMIP	16	rs2925979	HDL		C/T/ 0.30	−0.45	2×10^{-11}			+ + + +			
CTCF-PRMTB	16	rs2271293	HDL		A/G/ 0.87	−0.129	8.3×10^{-16}						
STARD3	17	rs11869286	HDL		C/G/ 0.34	−0.48	1×10^{-13}	Y		+ + + +	Increased liver cholesterol (LT, STMP)		
OSBPL7	17	rs7206971	LDL	TC	G/A/ 0.49	0.78	2×10^{-8}	Y		+ + − +			
ABCA8	17	rs4148008	HDL		C/G/ 0.32	−0.42	2×10^{-10}			+ + + +			
PGS1	17	rs4129767	HDL		A/G/ 0.49	−0.39	8×10^{-9}			+ + + +			
LIPG	18	rs7241918	HDL	TC	T/G/ 0.17	−1.31	3×10^{-49}	Y		+ + + +	Abnormal vascular endothelial cell physiology and increased circulating HDL cholesterol (LMP)		
MC4R	18	rs12967135	HDL		G/A/ 0.23	−0.42	7×10^{-9}			+ + + +	Increased circulating leptin and hyperglycemia (HIR)		
ANGPTL4	19	rs7255436	HDL		A/C/ 0.47	−0.45	3×10^{-8}	Y		+ + + +	Decreased circulating cholesterol and TG (A)		

D. CARDIOVASCULAR DISEASE

Gene	Chr	SNP	Trait	Trait	Allele/Freq	β	P-value		Phenotype		Disease	Signs
LDLR	19	rs6511720	LDL	TC	G/T/0.11	−6.99	4×10^{-117}	Y	Elevated LDL-C (LT, CMP, LMP, STMP)	X	Homozygous familial hypercholesterolemia	++ ? +
LOC55908	19	rs737337	HDL		T/C/0.08	−0.64	3×10^{-9}					+ + + +
CILP2	19	rs10401969	TC	TG, LDL	T/C/0.07	−4.74	3×10^{-38}	Y				+ + + ?
APOE	19	rs4420638	LDL	TC, HDL	A/G/0.17	7.14	9×10^{-147}	Y	Hypercholesterolemia and atherosclerotic lesions (LT, CMP, LMP, RN)	X	Familial dysbetalipo-proteinemia (elevated chylomicrons and VLDL remnants)	+ + + +
		rs439401	TG		C/T/0.36	−5.5	1×10^{-30}	Y				+ + + ?
FLJ36070	19	rs492602	TC		A/G/0.49	1.27	2×10^{-10}					+ − + ?
LILRA3	19	rs386000	HDL		G/C/0.20	0.83	4×10^{-16}	Y				+ − + −
NCAN	19	rs2304130	TC	TG, LDL	A/G/0.07	−0.153	2.0×10^{-15}					
TOMM40-APOE	19	rs157580	TC	TG	A/G/0.33	−0.09	5.1×10^{-17}					
APOE-APOC1-APOC4-APOC2	19	rs4420638	LDL		A/G/0.16	0.29	4×10^{-27}					
ERGIC3	20	rs2277862	TC		C/T/0.15	−1.19	4×10^{-10}	Y				+ + + ?
MAFB	20	rs2902940	TC	LDL	A/G/0.29	−1.38	6×10^{-11}		Complete neonatal lethality (DNAD, BD)			− − + ?
TOP1	20	rs6029526	LDL	TC	T/A/0.47	1.39	4×10^{-19}	Y	Complete embryonic lethality before implantation (DNAI)			+ + + +
HNF4A	20	rs1800961	HDL	TC	C/T/0.03	−1.88	1×10^{-15}		Complete embryonic lethality (LMP, DNAD, RN, STMP)			+ + + −

D. CARDIOVASCULAR DISEASE

(Continued)

TABLE 28.1 (Continued)

Locus[a]	Chr	Lead SNP	Lead trait[b]	Other traits[c]	Alleles/MAF[d]	Effect size[e]	p	eQTL[f]	CVD[g]	Ethnic[h]	Knockout mouse phenotype (pathway)[i]	Candidate gene association[j]	Mendelian lipid disorders[k]
PLTP	20	rs6065906	HDL	TG	T/C/ 0.18	−0.93	2×10^{-22}			+ − + +	Decreased circulating HDL cholesterol and increased LDL and VLDL-C (LT)		
UBE2L3	22	rs181362	HDL		C/T/ 0.20	−0.46	1×10^{-8}	Y		+ + + +			
PLA2G6	22	rs5756931	TG		T/C/ 0.40	−1.54	4×10^{-8}			+ ?? +	Neurodegeneration with brain iron accumulation 2A: NIA2A (LMP)		

[a]Locus: either a plausible biological candidate gene at the identified locus or the annotated gene closest to the lead SNP.

[b]Lead trait: the lipid trait with best p value among all four traits.

[c]Other traits: additional lipid traits with $p < 5 \times 10^{-9}$.

[d]Alleles/MAF: the major allele, minor allele, and minor allele frequency (MAF) within the combined cohort.

[e]Effect size: mg/dl for the lead trait, modeled as an additive effect of the minor allele. p values are listed for the lead trait.

[f]In the eQTL column, "Y" indicates that the lead SNP has an eQTL with at least one gene within 500 kb, with $p < 5 \times 10^{-8}$ in at least one of the three tissues tested (liver, omental fat, and subcutaneous fat).

[g]In the CVD column, "Y" indicates that the lead SNP meets the prespecified statistical significance threshold of $p < 0.001$ for association with CVD and concordance between the direction of lipid effect and the change in CVD risk.

[h]In the "ethnic" column, "+" indicates a concordant effect of the variant between the primary meta-analysis cohort and the European or non-European group, "−" indicates a discordant effect on the lead trait, and "?" indicates data not available for the group. In order, the ethnic groups are European, East Asian, South Asian, and African American [62].

[i]Knockout mouse phenotype: gene examined in regard to metabolic phenotypes and pathways (xx) of knockout mice maintained by the Jackson laboratory. Pathways: A, apoptosis; AG, axon guidance; BD, brain development; CMP, cholesterol metabolic process; GL, glycolysis; HIR, humoral immune response; ISP, insulin signaling pathway; JNK, JNK cascade; LMP, lipid metabolic process; LT, lipid transport; MIT, metal ion transport; MMPC, mitotic metaphase plate congression; PPT, regulation of protein transport; RES, response to extracellular stimulus; RN, response to nutrient; RNL, response to nutrient levels; SMP, sterol metabolic process.

[j]Candidate gene association: gene examined in previously published candidate gene association studies.

[k]Mendelian lipid disorders: literature survey of previously known Mendelian form of lipid disorders [66].Chr, chromosome.

TABLE 28.2 Replication of Genetic Associations with Lipid Levels across Public GWASs

Locus[a]	Chr	LDL-C	TG	HDL-C	TC
LDLRAP1	1	1	1		
PABPC4	1			1	
PCSK9	1	1, 3, 4, 5, 6, 8			1
ANGPTL3	1	1	1, 3, 4		1
EVI5	1				1
SORT1	1	1, 4			1
ZNF648	1			1	
MOSC1	1	1			1
GALNT2	1		1, 4, 8	1, 3, 4, 5, 6, 8	
IRF2BP2	1	1			1
TM3M57	1	2	2	2	2
ANGPTL3-DOCK7-ATG4C	1	6, 8	2, 3, 4, 5, 8		8
CELSR2	1	2, 3, 4, 5, 6, 8			2, 7, 8
CR1L	1	4			
PSRC1	1	7, 8			
APOB	2	1, 3, 4, 5, 6, 8	1, 2, 3, 4, 5, 8	1, 2, 5	1, 2, 8
GCKR	2	8	1, 2, 3, 4, 5, 8		1
ABCG5/8	2	1, 2, 3, 7, 8	2	2	1, 2, 8
RAB3GAP1	2	7			1
COBLL1	2		1		
IRS1	2		1	1	
R3HDM1	2	7			
LCT	2	7			
MCM6	2	7			
RAF1	3				1
MSL2L1	3		1		
KLHL8	4		1		
SLC39A8	4			1, 5	
AFF1	4		5		
ARL15	5			1	
MAP3K1	5		1		
HMGCR	5	1, 2, 3, 4, 5, 8			1, 2
TIMD4	5	1, 3, 8	1		1
C5ORT35	5		5		
RNF130	5	6			
MYLIP	6	1, 5			1
HFE	6	1			1

(Continued)

TABLE 28.2 (Continued)

Locus[a]	Chr	LDL-C	TG	HDL-C	TC
HLA	6	1	1		1
C6orf106	6			1	1
FRK	6	1			1
CITED2	6			1	
LPA	6	1		1	1
IGF2R	6	5			
DNAH11	7	1, 2	2	2	1, 2
NPC1L1	7	1			1
TYW1B	7		1		
MLXIPL	7		1, 2, 3, 4, 5, 8	1	
KLF14	7			1	
PPP1R3B	8	1, 5		1, 6	1
PINX1	8		1		
NAT2	8		1		1
LPL	8		1, 2, 3, 4, 5, 7, 8	1, 2, 3, 4, 5, 6, 7, 8	
CYP7A1	8	1			1
TRPS1	8			1	
TRIB1	8	1, 5	1, 3, 4, 8	1	1, 2
PLEC1	8	1			1
XKR6-AMAC1L2	8		3		
TTC39B	9			1, 3, 5, 8	1
ABCA1	9			1, 2, 3, 4, 5, 6, 8	1, 2
AB0	9	1			1
JMJD1C	10		1		
CYP26A1	10		1		
GPAM	10	1			1
AMPD3	11			1	
SPTY2D1	11				1
LRP4	11			1	
FADS1-2-3	11	1, 2, 4	1, 2, 3, 5, 8	1, 2, 3, 5, 6, 8	1, 2
APOA1/APOC3/APOA4	11	5	2, 3, 4, 5, 8	3, 4, 5, 8	
APOA1	11	1	1	1	1
UBASH3B	11			1	1
ST3GAL4	11	1			1
MADD-FOLH1	11	2	2	2	2
NR1H3	11			4	
PDE3A	12			1	

(Continued)

TABLE 28.2   (*Continued*)

Locus[a]	Chr	LDL-C	TG	HDL-C	TC
LRP1	12		1	1	
MVK	12			1, 3, 4, 5, 8	
BRAP	12	1			1
HNF1A	12	1, 3, 8			1
SBNO1	12			1	
ZNF664	12		1	1	
SCARB1	12			1	
MMAB	12			3, 4, 5, 8	
OSBPL8-ZDHHC17	12			7	
NYNRIN	14	1			
CAPN3	15		1		
FRMD5	15		1		
LIPC	15		1	1, 2, 3, 4, 5, 6, 8	1, 2
LACTB	15			1	
GCOM1	15			6	
CTF1	16		1		
CETP	16	1, 2, 8	1, 2, 5	1, 2,3, 4, 5, 6, 7, 8	1
LCAT	16			1, 3, 4, 5, 6, 8	
HPR	16	1			1
CMIP	16			1	
CTCF-PRMT8	16			2	
STARD3	17			1	
OSBPL7	17	1			1
ABCA8	17			1	
PGS1	17			1	
LIPG	18			1, 2, 3, 4, 5, 7, 8	1, 2, 8
MC4R	18			1	
ANGPTL4	19			1, 3, 8	
LDLR	19	1, 2, 3, 4, 5, 6, 8			1, 2, 8
LOC55908	19			1	
CILP2	19	1, 3, 4, 5	1, 3, 5, 8		1
APOE	19	1,8	1	1	1,8
FLJ36070	19				1
LILRA3	19			1	
NCAN	19	2, 3, 4, 8	2, 3, 8		2
TOMM40-APOE	19	2	2, 8		2, 8
APOE-APOC1-APOC4-APOC2	19	3, 4, 5, 6, 8	8		8

(*Continued*)

TABLE 28.2 (*Continued*)

Locus[a]	Chr	LDL-C	TG	HDL-C	TC
ERGIC3	20				1
MAFB	20	1, 3, 8			1
TOP1	20	1			1
HNF4A	20			1, 3, 8	1
PLTP	20		1, 3, 8	1, 3, 6, 8	
UBE2L3	22			1	
PLA2G6	22		1		

[a]*Each genes listed in the "locus" column is either a plausible biological candidate gene in the locus or the nearest annotated gene to the lead SNP.*
Chr, chromosome; GWAS: 1, Teslovich *et al.* [62]; 2, Aulchenko *et al.* [59]; 3, Kathiresan *et al.* [60]; 4, Sabbatti *et al.* [58]; 5, Waterworth *et al.* [63]; 6, Lettre *et al.* [64]; 7, Ma *et al.* [61]; 8, Chang *et al.* [65].

GWAS have yielded a wealth of information about the pathogenesis of dyslipidemia. Even as we continue to use these studies to uncover novel protein and gene variants involved in lipoprotein metabolism, a significant investment of effort and resources needs to be made to fully exploit the findings of these important studies. Further research may include the identification of less frequent variants with large effects, which may help us narrow down the genetic loci of interest and provide proof-of-concept of the potential benefits of modulating the functions of these proteins.

The GWASs reviewed here represent the culmination of years of groundwork, but the studies and results reported in this chapter only scratch the surface of the true potential of this approach. In addition to the obvious next steps of replication, signal refinement, and identification of causative variants, the definition of the biological roles of GWAS-identified genes in metabolic pathways will require substantial further research, including studies of these genes in model systems.

Acknowledgments

This work was supported by National Heart, Lung, and Blood Institute grant HL-54776, National Institute of Diabetes and Digestive and Kidney Diseases grant DK075030, and by contracts 53-K06-5-10 and 58-1950-9-001 from the U.S. Department of Agriculture Research Service.

References

[1] L.A. Weiss, L. Pan, M. Abney, C. Ober, The sex-specific genetic architecture of quantitative traits in humans, Nat. Genet. 38 (2006) 218–222.

[2] J.I. Cleeman, C. Lenfant, New guidelines for the treatment of high blood cholesterol in adults from the National Cholesterol Education Program: From controversy to consensus, Circulation 76 (1987) 960–962.

[3] National Cholesterol Education Program Expert Panel on Detection, Evaluation, and Treatment of High Blood Cholesterol in Adults, National Cholesterol Education Program: Second report of the Expert Panel on Detection, Evaluation, and Treatment of High Blood Cholesterol in Adults (Adult Treatment Panel II), Circulation 89 (1994) 1333–1445.

[4] National Cholesterol Education Program Expert Panel on Detection, Evaluation, and Treatment of High Blood Cholesterol in Adults, Third report of the National Cholesterol Education Program (NCEP) Expert Panel on Detection, Evaluation, and Treatment of High Blood Cholesterol in Adults (Adult Treatment Panel III) final report, Circulation 106 (2002) 3143–3421.

[5] S.M. Grundy, J.I. Cleeman, C.N. Merz, H.B. Brewer Jr., L.T. Clark, D.B. Hunninghake, et al., A summary of implications of recent clinical trials for the National Cholesterol Education Program Adult Treatment Panel III guidelines, Arterioscler. Thromb. Vasc. Biol. 24 (2004) 1329–1330.

[6] N.J. Stone, S. Bilek, S. Rosenbaum, Recent National Cholesterol Education Program Adult Treatment Panel III update: adjustments and options, Am. J. Cardiol. 96 (2005) 53E–59E.

[7] D. Corella, J.M. Ordovas, Integration of environment and disease into "omics" analysis, Curr. Opin. Mol. Ther. 7 (2005) 569–576.

[8] D. Corella, J.M. Ordovas, Nutrigenomics in cardiovascular medicine, Circ. Cardiovasc. Genet. 2 (2009) 637–651.

[9] G.M. Keating, K.F. Croom, Fenofibrate: a review of its use in primary dyslipidaemia, the metabolic syndrome and type 2 diabetes mellitus, Drugs 67 (2007) 121–153.

[10] R. Scott, R. O'Brien, G. Fulcher, C. Pardy, M. D'Emden, D. Tse, et al., Effects of fenofibrate treatment on cardiovascular disease risk in 9795 individuals with type 2 diabetes and various components of the metabolic syndrome: The Fenofibrate Intervention and Event Lowering in Diabetes (FIELD) study, Diabetes Care 32 (2009) 493–498.

[11] A.T. Kraja, M.A. Province, R.J. Straka, J.M. Ordovas, I.B. Borecki, D.K. Arnett, Fenofibrate and metabolic syndrome, Endocr. Metab. Immune Disord. Drug Targets. 10 (2010) 138–148.

[12] J.M. Backes, C.A. Gibson, J.F. Ruisinger, P.M. Moriarty, Fibrates: what have we learned in the past 40 years? Pharmacotherapy 27 (2007) 412–424.

[13] W.V. Brown, Expert commentary: the safety of fibrates in lipid-lowering therapy, Am. J. Cardiol. 99 (2007) 19C–21C.

[14] A.S. Wierzbicki, Fibrates after the FIELD study: some answers, more questions, Diab. Vasc. Dis. Res. 3 (2006) 166–171.

[15] M. Lee, J.L. Saver, A. Towfighi, J. Chow, B. Ovbiagele, Efficacy of fibrates for cardiovascular risk reduction in persons with atherogenic dyslipidemia: a meta-analysis, Atherosclerosis 217 (2011) 492–498.

[16] M.L. Bots, F.L. Visseren, G.W. Evans, W.A. Riley, J.H. Revkin, C.H. Tegeler, et al., Torcetrapib and carotid intima-media thickness in mixed dyslipidaemia (RADIANCE 2 study): a randomised, double-blind trial, Lancet 370 (2007) 153–160.

[17] M.A. Miyares, Anacetrapib and dalcetrapib: two novel cholesteryl ester transfer protein inhibitors, Ann. Pharmacother. 45 (2011) 84–94.

[18] S. Fazio, M.F. Linton, High-density lipoprotein therapeutics and cardiovascular prevention, J. Clin. Lipidol. 4 (2011) 411–419.

[19] G. Schmitz, A. Schmitz-Madry, P. Ugocsai, Pharmacogenetics and pharmacogenomics of cholesterol-lowering therapy, Curr. Opin. Lipidol. 18 (2007) 164–173.

[20] M.F. Feitosa, P. An, J.M. Ordovas, S. Ketkar, P.N. Hopkins, R.J. Straka, et al., Association of gene variants with lipid levels in response to fenofibrate is influenced by metabolic syndrome status, Atherosclerosis 215 (2011) 435–439.

[21] Y. Liu, J.M. Ordovas, G. Gao, M. Province, R.J. Straka, M.Y. Tsai, et al., Pharmacogenetic association of the APOA1/C3/A4/A5 gene cluster and lipid responses to fenofibrate: the Genetics of Lipid-Lowering Drugs and Diet Network Study, Pharmacogenet. Genomics 19 (2009) 161–169.

[22] J.T. Anderson, F. Grande, A. Keys, Essential fatty acids, degree of unsaturation, and effect of corn (maize) oil on the serum-cholesterol level in man, Lancet 272 (1957) 66–68.

[23] E.H. Ahrens Jr., Seminar on atherosclerosis: nutritional factors and serum lipid levels, Am. J. Med. 23 (1957) 928–952.

[24] A. Keys, J.T. Anderson, F. Grande, Prediction of serum-cholesterol responses of man to changes in fats in the diet, Lancet 273 (1957) 959–966.

[25] D.M. Hegsted, R.B. McGandy, M.L. Myers, F.J. Stare, Quantitative effects of dietary fat on serum cholesterol in man, Am. J. Clin. Nutr. 17 (1965) 281–295.

[26] R.P. Mensink, M.B. Katan, Effect of dietary fatty acids on serum lipids and lipoproteins: a meta-analysis of 27 trials, Arterioscler. Thromb. 12 (1992) 911–919.

[27] M.M. Cobb, H. Teitlebaum, Determinants of plasma cholesterol responsiveness to diet, Br. J. Nutr. 71 (1994) 271–282.

[28] D.M. Hegsted, L.M. Ausman, J.A. Johnson, G.E. Dallal, Dietary fat and serum lipids: an evaluation of the experimental data, Am. J. Clin. Nutr. 57 (1993) 875–883.

[29] R. Okey, Dietary blood and cholesterol in normal women, J. Biol. Chem. 99 (1933) 717–727.

[30] M.B. Katan, A.C. Beynen, J.H. de Vries, A. Nobels, Existence of consistent hypo- and hyperresponders to dietary cholesterol in man, Am. J. Epidemiol. 123 (1986) 221–234.

[31] D.R. Jacobs Jr., J.T. Anderson, P. Hannan, A. Keys, H. Blackburn, Variability in individual serum cholesterol response to change in diet, Arteriosclerosis 3 (1983) 349–356.

[32] M.A. O'Hanesian, B. Rosner, L.M. Bishop, F.M. Sacks, Effects of inherent responsiveness to diet and day-to-day diet variation on plasma lipoprotein concentrations, Am. J. Clin. Nutr. 64 (1996) 53–59.

[33] M.M. Cobb, N. Risch, Low-density lipoprotein cholesterol responsiveness to diet in normolipidemic subjects, Metabolism 42 (1993) 7–13.

[34] M. Lefevre, C.M. Champagne, R.T. Tulley, J.C. Rood, M.M. Most, Individual variability in cardiovascular disease risk factor responses to low-fat and low-saturated-fat diets in men: body mass index, adiposity, and insulin resistance predict changes in LDL cholesterol, Am. J. Clin. Nutr. 82 (2005) 957–963quiz 1145–1146

[35] M.C. Mahaney, J. Blangero, D.L. Rainwater, G.E. Mott, A.G. Comuzzie, J.W. MacCluer, et al., Pleiotropy and genotype by diet interaction in a baboon model for atherosclerosis: a multivariate quantitative genetic analysis of HDL subfractions in two dietary environments, Arterioscler. Thromb. Vasc. Biol. 19 (1999) 1134–1141.

[36] D.L. Rainwater, C.M. Kammerer, L.A. Cox, J. Rogers, K.D. Carey, B. Dyke, et al., A major gene influences variation in large HDL particles and their response to diet in baboons, Atherosclerosis 163 (2002) 241–248.

[37] D.L. Rainwater, C.M. Kammerer, K.D. Carey, B. Dyke, J.F. VandeBerg, W.R. Shelledy, et al., Genetic determination of HDL variation and response to diet in baboons, Atherosclerosis 161 (2002) 335–343.

[38] D.L. Rainwater, C.M. Kammerer, J.L. VandeBerg, Evidence that multiple genes influence baseline concentrations and diet response of Lp(a) in baboons, Arterioscler. Thromb. Vasc. Biol. 19 (1999) 2696–2700.

[39] D. Corella, J.M. Ordovas, Single nucleotide polymorphisms that influence lipid metabolism: Interaction with dietary factors, Annu. Rev. Nutr. 25 (2005) 341–390.

[40] J.M. Ordovas, D. Corella, Genetic variation and lipid metabolism: Modulation by dietary factors, Curr. Cardiol. Rep. 7 (2005) 480–486.

[41] L. Hooper, C.D. Summerbell, J.P. Higgins, R.L. Thompson, G. Clements, N. Capps, et al., Reduced or modified dietary fat for preventing cardiovascular disease, Cochrane Database Syst. Rev. (2001).

[42] E.J. Brunner, M. Thorogood, K. Rees, G. Hewitt, Dietary advice for reducing cardiovascular risk, Cochrane Database Syst. Rev. (2005).

[43] A. Astrup, J. Dyerberg, P. Elwood, K. Hermansen, F.B. Hu, M.U. Jakobsen, et al., The role of reducing intakes of saturated fat in the prevention of cardiovascular disease: where does the evidence stand in 2010? Am. J. Clin. Nutr. 93 (2011) 684–688.

[44] P. Perez-Martinez, J. Delgado-Lista, F. Perez-Jimenez, J. Lopez-Miranda, Update on genetics of postprandial lipemia, Atheroscler. Suppl. 11 (2010) 39–43.

[45] J.M. Ordovas, Genetics, postprandial lipemia and obesity, Nutr. Metab. Cardiovasc. Dis. 11 (2001) 118–133.

[46] M.T. Cooney, A. Dudina, R. D'Agostino, I.M. Graham, Cardiovascular risk-estimation systems in primary prevention: Do they differ? Do they make a difference? Can we see the future? Circulation 122 (2010) 300–310.

[47] G.H. Gibbons, C.C. Liew, M.O. Goodarzi, J.I. Rotter, W.A. Hsueh, H.M. Siragy, et al., Genetic markers: progress and potential for cardiovascular disease, Circulation 109 (2004) IV47–IV58.

[48] E.E. Eichler, J. Flint, G. Gibson, A. Kong, S.M. Leal, J.H. Moore, et al., Missing heritability and strategies for finding the underlying causes of complex disease, Nat. Rev. Genet. 11 (2010) 446–450.

[49] D. Levy, A.L. DeStefano, M.G. Larson, C.J. O'Donnell, R.P. Lifton, H. Gavras, et al., Evidence for a gene influencing blood pressure on chromosome 17: genome scan linkage results for longitudinal blood pressure phenotypes in subjects from the framingham heart study, Hypertension 36 (2000) 477–483.

[50] T.A. Pearson, T.A. Manolio, How to interpret a genome-wide association study, JAMA 299 (2008) 1335–1344.

[51] J.P. Casas, J. Cooper, G.J. Miller, A.D. Hingorani, S.E. Humphries, Investigating the genetic determinants of cardiovascular disease using candidate genes and meta-analysis of association studies, Ann. Hum. Genet. 70 (2006) 145–169.

[52] J. Hardy, A. Singleton, Genomewide association studies and human disease, N. Engl. J. Med. 360 (2009) 1759–1768.

[53] T.A. Manolio, Genomewide association studies and assessment of the risk of disease, N. Engl. J. Med. 363 (2010) 166–176.

[54] T.A. Manolio, L.D. Brooks, F.S. Collins, A HapMap harvest of insights into the genetics of common disease, J. Clin. Invest. 118 (2008) 1590–1605.

D. CARDIOVASCULAR DISEASE

[55] D. Levy, G.B. Ehret, K. Rice, G.C. Verwoert, L.J. Launer, A. Dehghan, et al., Genome-wide association study of blood pressure and hypertension, Nat. Genet. 41 (2009) 677–687.

[56] C.J. Willer, E.K. Speliotes, R.J. Loos, S. Li, C.M. Lindgren, I.M. Heid, et al., Six new loci associated with body mass index highlight a neuronal influence on body weight regulation, Nat. Genet. 41 (2009) 25–34.

[57] T.A. Manolio, F.S. Collins, N.J. Cox, D.B. Goldstein, L.A. Hindorff, D.J. Hunter, et al., Finding the missing heritability of complex diseases, Nature 461 (2009) 747–753.

[58] C. Sabatti, S.K. Service, A.L. Hartikainen, A. Pouta, S. Ripatti, J. Brodsky, et al., Genome-wide association analysis of metabolic traits in a birth cohort from a founder population, Nat. Genet. 41 (2009) 35–46.

[59] Y.S. Aulchenko, S. Ripatti, I. Lindqvist, D. Boomsma, I.M. Heid, P.P. Pramstaller, et al., Loci influencing lipid levels and coronary heart disease risk in 16 European population cohorts, Nat. Genet. 41 (2009) 47–55.

[60] S. Kathiresan, C.J. Willer, G.M. Peloso, S. Demissie, K. Musunuru, E.E. Schadt, et al., Common variants at 30 loci contribute to polygenic dyslipidemia, Nat. Genet. 41 (2009) 56–65.

[61] L. Ma, J. Yang, H.B. Runesha, T. Tanaka, L. Ferrucci, S. Bandinelli, et al., Genome-wide association analysis of total cholesterol and high-density lipoprotein cholesterol levels using the Framingham Heart Study data, BMC Med. Genet. 11 (2010) 55.

[62] T.M. Teslovich, K. Musunuru, A.V. Smith, A.C. Edmondson, I.M. Stylianou, M. Koseki, et al., Biological, clinical and population relevance of 95 loci for blood lipids, Nature 466 (2010) 707–713.

[63] D.M. Waterworth, S.L. Ricketts, K. Song, L. Chen, J.H. Zhao, S. Ripatti, et al., Genetic variants influencing circulating lipid levels and risk of coronary artery disease, Arterioscler. Thromb. Vasc. Biol. 30 (2010) 2264–2276.

[64] G. Lettre, C.D. Palmer, T. Young, K.G. Ejebe, H. Allayee, E.J. Benjamin, et al., Genome-wide association study of coronary heart disease and its risk factors in 8090 African Americans: the NHLBI CARe Project, PLoS Genet. 7 (2011) e1001300.

[65] M.H. Chang, R.M. Ned, Y. Hong, A. Yesupriya, Q. Yang, T. Liu, et al., Race/ethnic variation in the association of lipid-related genetic variants with blood lipids in the U.S. adult population, Circ. Cardiovasc. Genet. 4 (2011) 523–533.

[66] A.C. Edmondson, D.J. Rader, Genome-wide approaches to finding novel genes for lipid traits: the start of a long road, Circ. Cardiovasc. Genet. 1 (2008) 3–6.

[67] P. Brindle, A. Beswick, T. Fahey, S. Ebrahim, Accuracy and impact of risk assessment in the primary prevention of cardiovascular disease: a systematic review, Heart 92 (2006) 1752–1759.

[68] K. Eichler, M.A. Puhan, J. Steurer, L.M. Bachmann, Prediction of first coronary events with the Framingham score: a systematic review, Am. Heart J. 153 (2007) 722–731731.e1–8

[69] I. Tzoulaki, G. Liberopoulos, J.P. Ioannidis, Assessment of claims of improved prediction beyond the Framingham risk score, JAMA 302 (2009) 2345–2352.

[70] P.W. Wilson, Challenges to improve coronary heart disease risk assessment, JAMA 302 (2009) 2369–2370.

[71] World Health Organization, Prevention of Cardiovascular Disease: Guidelines for Assessment and Management of Cardiovascular Risk., World Health Organization, Geneva, 2007.

[72] P.G. Arbogast, L. Kaltenbach, H. Ding, W.A. Ray, Adjustment for multiple cardiovascular risk factors using a summary risk score, Epidemiology 19 (2008) 30–37.

[73] J. Grewal, S. Chan, J. Frohlich, G.B. Mancini, Assessment of novel risk factors in patients at low risk for cardiovascular events based on Framingham risk stratification, Clin. Invest. Med. 26 (2003) 158–165.

[74] R.B. D'Agostino Sr., S. Grundy, L.M. Sullivan, P. Wilson, Validation of the Framingham coronary heart disease prediction scores: Results of a multiple ethnic groups investigation, JAMA 286 (2001) 180–187.

[75] P.W. Wilson, R.B. D'Agostino, D. Levy, A.M. Belanger, H. Silbershatz, W.B. Kannel, Prediction of coronary heart disease using risk factor categories, Circulation 97 (1998) 1837–1847.

[76] R.M. Conroy, K. Pyorala, A.P. Fitzgerald, S. Sans, A. Menotti, G. De Backer, et al., Estimation of ten-year risk of fatal cardiovascular disease in Europe: the SCORE project, Eur. Heart J. 24 (2003) 987–1003.

[77] A. Demirkan, N. Amin, A. Isaacs, M.R. Jarvelin, J.B. Whitfield, H.E. Wichmann, et al., Genetic architecture of circulating lipid levels, Eur. J. Hum. Genet. 19 (2011) 813–819.

The Role of Diet in the Prevention and Treatment of Cardiovascular Disease

Ann Skulas-Ray, Michael Flock, Penny Kris-Etherton

Pennsylvania State University, University Park, Pennsylvania

I INTRODUCTION

Cardiovascular disease (CVD) remains the leading cause of death in the United States despite decades of research and consequent evolution of prevention and treatment guidelines [1]. Health care costs (both direct and indirect, such as lost work days and productivity) are expected to exceed $1 trillion annually by 2030 [2]. The role of nutrition is of paramount importance to reducing the burden of CVD despite advances in pharmacological and surgical management. Thus, the identification and implementation of dietary strategies with the greatest potential for reducing CVD risk are of major scientific and public health importance. Nutrition plays a key role in preventing and treating CVD by modifying multiple risk factors. This chapter focuses on nutritional strategies for optimizing lipids and lipoproteins as a means of reducing CVD risk. The effects of diet on other established and emerging risk factors are also addressed briefly. When whole-food, evidence-based approaches are utilized, risk factor reduction includes both the well-characterized CVD risk factors and emerging and yet to be discovered risk pathways.

A Cardiovascular Risk Factors

Risk factors are classified as nonmodifiable or modifiable [3]. Nonmodifiable risk factors include age, gender, and family history. Major modifiable CVD risk factors include elevated total cholesterol (TC), low-density lipoprotein cholesterol (LDL-C), and triglyceride (TG) levels; reduced high-density lipoprotein cholesterol (HDL-C) levels; hypertension; diabetes mellitus; and overweight and obesity.

Other increasingly important emerging CVD risk factors that may be modified by diet include inflammation and oxidative stress, as well as derangements in metabolism exemplified by elevations in insulin and glucose or altered lipoprotein properties—such as particle size—not traditionally assessed in a standard lipid panel. There is increasing appreciation of the importance of nonfasting TGs and levels of chylomicron remnants [4–7]. There is also a greater appreciation that cardiac membrane fatty acid composition may play a role in arrhythmias and sudden cardiac arrest [8–11]. In addition, physiological testing, such as noninvasive endothelial function tests, has been added to the panel of risk assessments available to clinicians and researchers [12]. Thus, there is great potential for diet to alter multiple cardiovascular risk factors.

The importance of reducing major risk factors is illustrated by data obtained from three large prospective studies (Chicago Heart Association Detection Project in Industry, Multiple Risk Factor Intervention Trial, and Framingham Heart Study) that reported that 87–100% of men and women (ages 18–59 years) with one or more major risk factors died from coronary heart disease (CHD) [13]. In addition, an analysis of 112,458 patients with CHD found that 80–90% of the participants had major CVD factors [14]. It is important to note, however, that other risk factors also contribute to the development of CVD. This is best illustrated by the evidence that approximately 35% of CVD occurs in individuals with a TC < 200 mg/dl [15]. Thus, modifying as many CVD risk factors as possible will have the greatest impact on decreasing CVD risk.

Nutrition in the Prevention and Treatment of Disease, Third Edition.
DOI: http://dx.doi.org/10.1016/B978-0-12-391884-0.00029-9

Of particular relevance to nutritional therapies is the finding that selective, pharmacological targeting of some CVD risk factors fails to improve CVD outcomes. This has been exemplified by trials of HDL-raising pharmaceuticals, such as torcetrapib [16], and the failure of fibrate therapy [17], niacin [18], and antioxidant vitamin supplements [19] to reduce morbidity and mortality. In addition, attempts to reduce CVD risk by glucose-lowering drug therapy have not produced anticipated reductions in CVD events [20−22]. The associations between factors along biochemical pathways are complex, and evidence supports that in many cases reductions in risk factors achieved by diet and lifestyle modification are superior to reductions achieved by pharmacological therapy. This is because not all markers of increased CVD risk are causative factors and, thus, correctable by drug therapy.

B The Role of Nutrition in Cardiovascular Disease

Strong evidence from epidemiologic, mechanistic, and interventional studies supports the role of nutrition in preventing and treating heart disease by reducing modifiable risk factors. Supported by a large evidence base, therapeutic lifestyle changes (TLC) have been developed and applied in medical settings [23,24]. TLC recommendations focus on LDL-C and blood pressure (BP) reduction [23,25,26], two major CVD risk factors that are also the targets of most pharmacological therapies. Current TLC recommendations call for restricting saturated fat and cholesterol intake and increasing physical activity [24]. These evidence-based recommendations promote dietary patterns associated with reduced CVD risk. In practice, however, a major concern is that patients may focus on meeting macronutrient recommendations while consuming a diet that is low in the bioactive compounds that characterize a healthy diet pattern. Moreover, focusing on cholesterol and BP alone fails to identify approximately half of the 1.3 million individuals who develop myocardial infarction (MI) each year without being at significant risk from these factors alone [27]. It is clear that additional risk factors, such as chronic inflammation and oxidative stress, are also involved. Current recommendations focus on whole-food approaches and dietary patterns that target both LDL-C and BP reductions while also achieving effects on other CVD risk factors.

Diet has been a cornerstone in the management of heart disease risk factors for more than 50 years. The American Heart Association (AHA) published its first dietary recommendations for CVD risk reduction in 1957 [28]. The AHA updates dietary recommendations routinely as new science emerges. Other organizations, such as the U.S. Department of Agriculture (USDA), U.S. Department of Health and Human Services, National Cholesterol Education Program (NCEP), Academy of Nutrition and Dietetics (AND), and the American Diabetes Association, continually update and publish diet and lifestyle recommendations to reduce risk of chronic diseases, including (or specific to) CVD. Traditionally, these organizations have made dietary recommendations based on targeted nutrient levels (e.g., <7 to <10% of calories from saturated fat). Recently, more food-based dietary recommendations have been made, and this change is most notable in the development of the *Dietary Guidelines for Americans 2010 (DGA 2010)* [29,30]. These food-based recommendations are supported by the macronutrient and micronutrient recommendations made by the National Academies (Dietary Reference Intakes (DRI)), as well as other organizations (e.g., NCEP). AND's Evidence Analysis Library on Disorders of Lipid Metabolism is an excellent summary of the literature about the role of diet on lipid and lipoprotein risk factors, including dietary recommendations for the management of CVD risk factors [31]. A food-based approach that integrates all nutrient recommendations is encouraged because it targets multiple CVD risk factors as well as many chronic diseases. Food-based approaches that encompass all dietary recommendations translate to greater health benefits.

Modifying macronutrient type and amount is a major focus of the dietary recommendations. Historically, recommendations have centered on modifying the type and amount of fat. Recently, modifying the type and amount of carbohydrate and protein to lower CVD risk has received greater attention. The reduction and replacement of saturated fatty acids (SFAs) and *trans* fatty acids (TFAs) with unsaturated fat or unrefined carbohydrate (i.e., whole grain, vegetable, and fruit sources) is one of the most widely accepted approaches to decrease some major CVD risk factors. In addition, the evidence base for dietary protein as a substitute for SFAs and TFAs has grown. The effects of the type and amount of protein on CVD are being evaluated in ongoing research. With respect to dietary carbohydrates, studies have explored the impact of dietary fiber, the glycemic index of carbohydrate-rich foods, and the glycemic load of the diet on CVD risk factors.

Dietary recommendations have been made for other nutrients based on the emerging evidence. These new CVD dietary recommendations are notable in that they do not address an essential nutrient deficiency and do not always produce quantifiable effects on standard risk markers. For example, the cardioprotective benefits of a diet rich in omega-3 fatty acids, both marine and plant based, have been studied intensively, leading to specific dietary recommendations from multiple organizations. Recommendations to increase vegetable and fruit consumption relate, in part, to the understanding that plant phytochemicals, such as phenolic antioxidants, potentially ameliorate oxidative stress and inflammation. Dietary recommendations for CVD are now focusing on dietary patterns that have the potential to optimize multiple risk factors, including traditional targets.

We are transitioning through an exciting era of discovery in which we are gaining a better understanding of how macronutrients, micronutrients, and other dietary bioactives affect CVD risk; thus, it is not unreasonable to speculate that we will identify even more effective dietary approaches for reducing CVD risk. This chapter reviews current dietary guidelines for minimizing CVD risk and the research that informs our current understanding of how dietary components affect CVD risk status via changes in plasma lipid and lipoproteins, emerging physiological risk factors, and overall CVD-related morbidity and mortality.

II FOOD-BASED GUIDANCE

Food-based dietary recommendations include strategies that target lipid and lipoprotein risk factors, but they also include dietary patterns that address a wide array of nonlipid and lipoprotein CVD risk factors. Emphasizing nutrient-dense foods provides a strategy for building a healthy diet that has greater cardiovascular benefits than are attainable simply by targeting nutrients. Dietary patterns that emphasize nutrient-dense foods deliver multiple characterized and yet-to-be characterized nutrients for CVD risk reduction. Intervention studies have identified several healthy dietary patterns that include nutrient-dense foods high in fiber and low in solid fats, added sugars, sodium, and refined grains. These specific dietary patterns and food-based recommendations are presented next.

A Dietary Guidelines and Recommendations

Evidence-based dietary guidelines for reducing risk of CVD (and other chronic diseases) have been established by the *DGA 2010* [30] and AHA's diet and lifestyle recommendations for CVD risk reduction [32]. Nutrient-dense foods—particularly those high in dietary fiber, vitamin D, calcium, and potassium—are encouraged. Foods high in solid fats (SFAs and TFAs), sodium, dietary cholesterol, added sugars, and refined grains should be limited. Vegetables, fruits, whole grains high in fiber, seafood, eggs, low-fat dairy, nuts,

lean meat, and poultry all prepared without solid fats and added sugars are considered "nutrient-dense foods" [30]. Table 29.1 shows recommended intakes of nutrient-dense foods that can improve lipid levels and BP when not exceeding energy needs. *DGA 2010* recommends consuming <10% of calories from SFA and reduction to <7% of calories to further reduce CVD risk [30]. TFA consumption should be as low as possible [30]. The AHA recommends limiting SFA to <7% of calories and TFA to <1% of calories [33]. Both *DGA 2010* and AHA encourage adults who drink alcohol to limit their consumption to one drink per day for women and up to two drinks per day for men [30]. AHA recommends sodium intake to be <1500 mg/day for all adults, excluding individuals at risk for losing large amounts of sodium through sweat [32], whereas *DGA 2010* recommends the current sodium goal be <2300 mg/day or 1500 mg/day depending on individual characteristics that may affect sodium sensitivity, such as age, body weight, race/ethnicity, and genetics [30]. Sodium intake of <1500 mg/day is recommended for older adults (>51 years), younger children (<8 years), African Americans, and individuals with hypertension, diabetes, or chronic kidney disease [30]. These population groups represent approximately 50% of the population. Increasing consumption of fruits and vegetables, rich in potassium, may help reduce and/or prevent sodium-induced hypertension.

B Recommended Dietary Patterns

Dietary guidelines made by *DGA 2010*, AHA, and other expert organizations focus on dietary patterns designed to prevent CVD and other chronic diseases. Evidence-based research shows that the TLC diet, Dietary Approaches to Stop Hypertension (DASH) diet, certain vegetarian diets (e.g., Portfolio diet and Ornish diet), and Mediterranean-style diets all reduce risk factors associated with CVD [30]. All dietary patterns are low in SFA, TFA, and dietary cholesterol, and are high in dietary fiber. In addition, they all meet current recommendations for sodium (<2300 mg/day). The key characteristics of each dietary pattern are discussed next.

1 Therapeutic Lifestyle Changes Diet

The NCEP recommends the TLC diet for individuals with elevated LDL-C, lipid disorders, CVD, diabetes, insulin resistance, and/or metabolic syndrome [24]. The TLC diet focuses on reducing SFA (<7% of calories) and cholesterol intake (<200 mg/day) to lower LDL-C. Additional guidelines for LDL-C lowering include increased soluble fiber (10–25 g/day) and plant sterol/stanols intake (2 g/day). The TLC diet can

TABLE 29.1   USDA Recommended Intake Amounts from Each Food Group or Subgroup at Various Calorie Levels[a]

Energy level of pattern[b]	Calories				
	1600	2000	2400	2800	3200
Fruits	1½ c	2 c	2 c	2½ c	2½ c
Vegetables	2 c	2½ c	3 c	3½ c	4 c
Dark green vegetables	1½ c/week	1½ c/week	2 c/week	2½ c/week	2½ c/week
Red/orange vegetables	4 c/week	5½ c/week	6 c/week	7 c/week	7½ c/week
Cooked dry beans and peas	1 c/week	1½ c/week	2 c/week	2½ c/week	3 c/week
Starchy vegetables	4 c/week	5 c/week	6 c/week	7 c/week	8 c/week
Other vegetables	3½ c/week	4 c/week	5 c/week	5½ c/week	7 c/week
Grains	5 oz. eq.	6 oz. eq.	8 oz. eq.	10 oz. eq.	10 oz. eq.
Whole grains	3 oz. eq.	3 oz. eq.	4 oz. eq.	5 oz. eq.	5 oz. eq.
Other grains	2 oz. eq.	3 oz. eq.	4 oz. eq.	5 oz. eq.	5 oz. eq.
Meat and beans	5 oz. eq.	5½ oz. eq.	6½ oz. eq.	7 oz. eq.	7 oz. eq.
Milk (low fat/skim)	3 c	3 c	3 c	3 c	3 c
Oils	22 g	27 g	31 g	36 g	51 g
Maximum SoFAS limit (% total calories)	121 (8%)	258 (13%)	330 (14%)	395 (14%)	596 (19%)

[a]*Food group amounts are shown in cup (c) or ounce equivalents (oz. eq.). Oils are shown in grams. Quantity equivalents for each food group are as follows:*

Grains: 1 oz. equivalent is ½ cup cooked rice, pasta, or cooked cereal; 1 oz. dry pasta or rice; 1 slice of bread; 1 small muffin (1 oz.); or 1 oz. ready-to-eat cereal.

Fruits and vegetables: 1 cup equivalent is 1 cup raw or cooked fruit or vegetable, 1 cup fruit or vegetable juice, or 2 cups leafy salad greens.

Meat and beans: 1 oz. equivalent is 1 oz. lean meat, poultry, fish; 1 egg; ¼ cup cooked dry beans; 1 tbsp peanut butter; or ½ oz. nuts/seeds.

Milk: 1 cup equivalent is 1 cup milk or yogurt, 1½ oz. natural cheese such as cheddar cheese, or 2 oz. of processed cheese.

[b]*Food intake patterns at 1000, 1200, and 1400 calories meet the nutritional needs of children ages 2–8 years. Patterns from 1600 to 3200 calories meet the nutritional needs of children 9 years of age or older and adults. If a child age 2–8 years needs more calories and, therefore, is following a pattern at 1600 calories or more, the recommended amount from the milk group can be 2 cups per day. Children ages 9 years or older and adults should not use the 1000-, 1200-, or 1400-calorie patterns.*

SoFAS, calories from solid fats and added sugars.

Source: Adapted from U.S. Department of Agriculture and U.S. Department of Health and Human Services (2010). "Dietary Guidelines for Americans 2010," 7th ed. U.S. Government Printing Office, Washington, DC.

be implemented as part of a variety of dietary patterns that achieve the recommended nutrient composition described in Table 29.2. As demonstrated in Table 29.3, the TLC diet is expected to reduce LDL-C by 20–30% relative to the typical American diet: approximately 8–10% by the reduction in SFA to <7% of calories, 3–5% by the reduction in dietary cholesterol to <200 mg, up to 5% by the addition of 5–10 g/day of viscous fiber, and 6–15% by the inclusion of 2 g/day of plant stanol/sterol esters [34].

2 DASH Diet

The DASH diet emphasizes increased intake of fruits, vegetables, and low-fat dairy foods while limiting intake of red meat and added sugars [35]. Whole grains, poultry, fish, and nuts are also emphasized. Clinical evidence has consistently demonstrated that the DASH diet reduces BP, TC, and LDL-C but also reduces HDL-C. It does not affect TG. Compared to a

typical American diet, the DASH diet reduced BP by −5.5/−3.0 mm Hg [35,36]. In the DASH trial [36], subjects consuming a DASH diet high in fruits, vegetables, and low-fat dairy products for 8 weeks had significantly greater reductions in TC (−13.7 mg/dl), LDL-C (−10.7 mg/dl), and HDL-C (−3.7 mg/dl) levels compared to individuals consuming the typical American control diet that is relatively low in fiber and high in SFA. Men experienced a greater reduction in TC and LDL-C compared to women [36]. Calculations using the Framingham risk equations estimated a reduction in the 10-year CHD risk by 18% compared to the control diet [37].

Consistent with the original DASH trial, a prospective cohort study of 88,517 women reported an association between DASH-style dietary patterns and CHD risk in women [38]. Dietary intake data were obtained via food frequency questionnaires administered seven times during 24 years of follow-up. A DASH score was

TABLE 29.2 Therapeutic Lifestyle Changes Diet Recommendations

Nutrient	Recommended intake	For a 2000-calorie diet
Total fat	25—35% of total calories	55—78 g/day
SFA	<7% of total calories	≤16 g/day
MUFA	≤20% of total calories	≤44 g/day
PUFA	≤10% of total calories	≤22 g/day
Carbohydrate[a]	50—60% of total calories	250—300 g/day
Viscous fiber	10—25 g/day	10—25 g/day
Protein	~15% of total calories	~75 g/day
Cholesterol	<200 mg/day	<200 mg/day
Plant sterols	2 g/day	2 g/day

[a]Carbohydrate intake should be derived predominately from foods rich in complex carbohydrates, including grains (especially whole grains), fruits, and vegetables.
Source: Adapted from National Cholesterol Education Program (2002). Third report of the National Cholesterol Education Program (NCEP) Expert Panel on Detection, Evaluation, and Treatment of High Blood Cholesterol in Adults (Adult Treatment Panel III) final report. Circulation **106**, 3143—3421.

TABLE 29.3 Approximate and Cumulative Low-Density Lipoprotein Cholesterol (LDL-C) Reduction Achievable by Therapeutic Lifestyle Changes

Dietary component	Dietary change	Approximate LDL-C reduction (%)
Saturated fat	<7% of calories	8—10
Dietary cholesterol	<200 mg/day	3—5
Weight reduction	Lose 10 lbs	5—8
OTHER LDL-LOWERING OPTIONS		
Viscous fiber	5—10 g/day	3—5
Plant sterol/stanol esters	2 g/day	6—15
Cumulative estimate		20—30

Source: Data from National Cholesterol Education Program [24] and Jenkins et al. [228].

calculated based on eight food and nutrient components (fruits, vegetables, whole grains, nuts and legumes, low-fat dairy, red and processed meats, sweetened beverages, and sodium). Women in the highest quintile for DASH scores had 24% lower CHD risk than women in the bottom quintile. The risk reduction was significant for both fatal and nonfatal CHD. In an examination of 5532 hypertensive adults within the NHANES III sample, a DASH-like diet was associated with 31% lower all-cause mortality compared to a typical American diet, but there were no differences in mortality risk due to CVD [39]. In addition to the

smaller sample size, a potential limitation of this study is that dietary intakes were estimated from a single 24-hour dietary recall. More epidemiologic studies with rigorous dietary intake data are needed to examine the effectiveness of a DASH-like diet in reducing CVD risk among various populations. Modifications of the DASH diet that replace some carbohydrate (CHO) with protein or unsaturated fat have achieved improved lipids, BP, and 10-year coronary heart disease risk [26]. The unfavorable effects of the unmodified DASH diet on HDL-C suggest either substitution of CHO or other concurrent strategies, such as increased aerobic exercise and weight loss, may optimize the effectiveness of the DASH diet for reducing CVD risk.

The Prudent dietary pattern is very similar to the DASH dietary pattern without a specific recommendation for increased low-fat dairy consumption. *DGAC 2010* classified the Prudent diet as a "DASH derivative." A Prudent dietary pattern is characterized by higher intake of vegetables, fruits, legumes, whole grains, fish, and poultry with decreased intake of foods characterizing the Western dietary pattern: red meat, processed meat, refined grains, sweets and dessert, French fries, and high-fat dairy products [40]. In prospective cohort studies examining 5872 to 72,113 subjects, higher Prudent diet scores were associated with lower risk of CVD [40—43] and all-cause mortality [40,42,43]. People in the highest quintile for adherence to the Prudent pattern had up to 50% lower risk of CVD mortality compared to those consuming the most Western dietary pattern[40,43]. Thus, a large body of evidence supports implementation of DASH, Prudent, and other DASH derivative dietary patterns for the reduction of CVD and total mortality.

3 Vegetarian Diets

Vegetarian diets emphasize fruits, vegetables, whole grains, legumes, nuts, seeds, and soy foods and include little or no animal products. Compared to nonvegetarians, vegetarians typically consume fewer calories, SFA, cholesterol, and sodium but more fiber and carbohydrates [30,44,45]. Overall, these characteristics may impart favorable effects on CVD risk factors. However, individuals choosing to consume vegetarian dietary patterns must be well informed to ensure adequate nutrient intake. Poorly planned vegetarian diets increase the potential for nutrient deficiencies and do not decrease CVD risk.

The Portfolio diet is a vegetarian diet designed to achieve maximal LDL-C-lowering effects. The diet includes plant sterols; viscous fibers primarily from oat, barley, and psyllium; soy protein (21 g/1000 kcal); and almonds (14 g/1000 kcal) [46,47]. In a controlled feeding study, hyperlipidemic subjects following a Portfolio diet (22% of calories as vegetable protein,

50.6% CHO, 27.0% fat (4.3% SFA, 11.8% monounsaturated fatty acid [MUFA], and 9.9% polyunsaturated fatty acid [PUFA]), 10 mg cholesterol per 1000 kcal, and 30.7 g fiber per 1,000 kcal) for 4 weeks reduced TC and LDL-C (22.4 and 29.0%, respectively) with no significant effect on HDL-C or TG [46]. A follow-up study demonstrated a greater cholesterol-lowering effect of a Portfolio diet than a Step II diet [47]. TC and LDL-C decreased by 9.9 and 12.1% ,respectively, on the Step II diet (a diet containing <7% of calories as SFA), whereas on a Portfolio diet TC and LDL-C decreased by 26.6 and 35.0%, respectively.

In a 1-year, free-living study of people with hypercholesterolemia, the LDL-C lowering effects of the Portfolio diet were more modest [48]. A 14% reduction in LDL-C was achieved after 12 weeks and sustained after 1 year (12.8%). Self-reported dietary compliance over 1 year correlated with LDL-C reduction ($r = -0.42$), illustrating the importance of adherence to achieve maximal diet effectiveness.

It was demonstrated that use of counseling to follow the Portfolio diet reduced LDL-C concentrations >13% more than low-SFA dietary advice during 6 months of follow-up [49]. An important finding of this study is that the intervention was equally effective regardless of whether participants received seven instructional sessions or only two instructional sessions during the course of the 6-month intervention. In addition, the percentage reduction in LDL-C was associated with dietary adherence as assessed by intake of plant sterols, viscous fibers, soy protein, and nuts. Therefore, the Portfolio diet is an effective option for lowering blood lipids in motivated people even when only minimal instruction about the diet is provided.

Striking reductions in LDL-C, angina, and stenosis have been demonstrated with a very low-fat vegetarian diet combined with comprehensive lifestyle changes [50–53]. In the Lifestyle Heart Trial, 48 patients with moderate to severe CVD were randomized to an intensive lifestyle intervention, including a whole-foods vegetarian diet with only 10% fat, or a usual care control group. The foods emphasized in this diet include beans and legumes, fruits, grains, and vegetables; however, all sources of fat are restricted, including vegetarian sources such as avocados, seeds, and oils. The additional lifestyle interventions included aerobic exercise, stress management training, smoking cessation, and group psychological support. Thirty-five participants completed the 5-year evaluation with similar compliance between groups (71% of intervention patients and 75% of control patients). The intervention group experienced significant reductions in arterial stenosis, 91% reduction in angina, less than half the number of cardiac events, and a 40% reduction in LDL-C. Although the feasibility of such marked dietary changes has been

questioned, this trial has demonstrated the efficacy of this strategy in high-risk patients, and Medicare has begun covering the Ornish plan. Additional criticism has been raised about the lack of distinction between different types of fats. However, in a low-fat, whole-food vegetarian diet, an unfavorable fatty acid profile is unlikely, although omega-3 fatty acids could be low. This low-fat, whole-food vegetarian diet combined with lifestyle strategies was the first dietary pattern shown to reverse arterial stenosis.

4 Mediterranean Diet

The Mediterranean diet represents an eating pattern of the countries in the broad geographical area surrounding the Mediterranean Sea. The Mediterranean-style diet emphasizes fruits, root vegetables, grains (mostly whole), legumes, nuts, seeds, and olive oil. Dairy products, fish, and poultry are consumed in low to moderate amounts, whereas red meat and eggs are limited. Wine is also consumed in low to moderate amounts in non-Islamic countries. Overall, Mediterranean-style diets tend to be low in SFA and high in MUFA.

Clinical and epidemiologic studies have reported benefits of a Mediterranean diet on CVD risk factors. The Seven Countries Study stimulated interest in the Mediterranean diet when it reported in the 1980s that the 15-year mortality rate from CVD in southern Europe was two or three times lower than that in northern Europe or the United States [54]. Several years later, the Lyon Diet Heart Study [55] was designed to test the effects of a Mediterranean diet versus a Western diet on the secondary prevention of MI. Subjects were randomized to consume a control diet or a Mediterranean-style diet containing higher amounts of α-linolenic acid for 104 weeks. Despite no alterations in blood lipids and having similar body mass index and BP as the control group, subjects consuming the Mediterranean-style diet had lower prevalence of cardiac death, nonfatal MI, fewer major secondary events, and decreased hospitalizations. Overall, subjects consuming the Mediterranean-style diet had a 50–70% lower risk of recurrent heart based on these outcomes [55]. It is perhaps the abundance of bioactive compounds in the Mediterranean-style diet that accounts for these decreases in CVD outcomes, in part, by favorable effects on vascular function, arrhythmia, and oxidative stress.

Additional studies have validated the findings of the Lyon Diet Heart Study. A systematic review of 12 prospective cohort studies reported that greater adherence to a Mediterranean diet was associated with a significant reduction in mortality from CVD and total mortality [56]. In addition, a meta-analysis of cohort studies found that greater adherence to a Mediterranean dietary pattern was protective against

TABLE 29.4 Dietary Patterns Associated with Reducing Cardiovascular Disease Risk

	Dietary pattern			
	TLC	DASH (Prudent)	Vegetarian[a]	Mediterranean
Emphasizes	Vegetables, fruits, whole grains, legumes, low-fat milk products, plant stanols/sterols	Vegetables, fruits, whole grains, low-fat milk products[b]	Plant foods—vegetables, fruits, whole grains, legumes, nuts, seeds, soy foods	Grains, vegetables, fruits, nuts, legumes, seafood, oils
Limits	Solid fats, added sugars	Red meats, sweets, sugar-containing beverages	Meat, poultry, fish, dairy, eggs, added sugars	Meat, added sugars

[a]*Foods may vary depending on the strictness and type of vegetarian diet. The Ornish Plan excludes nuts, seeds, and oils.*
[b]*The Prudent diet does not emphasize low-fat dairy.*
DASH, Dietary Approaches to Stop Hypertension; TLC, Therapeutic Lifestyle Changes.

CVD [57]. An analysis of 81,722 women in the Nurses' Health Study found that women with a highest quintile for the Mediterranean diet score (high intake of vegetables, fruits, nuts, whole grains, legumes, and fish; high ratio of MUFAs to SFAs; moderate intake of alcohol; and low intake of red and processed meat) experienced a 40% reduction in sudden cardiac death relative to women who had the diets least reflective of this pattern [58].

The Prevención con Dieta Mediterránea (PREDIMED) study is an ongoing multicenter clinical trial evaluating the efficacy of a Mediterranean diet on the primary prevention of CVD [59]. In 2003, the PREDIMED trial began randomizing participants 55–80 years of age with diabetes or three or more major CVD risk factors (hypertension, hypercholesterolemia, family history of heart disease, tobacco use, or overweight/obesity) to consume a low-fat diet, a Mediterranean diet with virgin olive oil (1 l/week), or a Mediterranean diet with tree nuts (hazelnuts, almonds, and walnuts; 30 g/day). After 3 months, subjects in the Mediterranean diet groups containing olive oil or nuts both had lower TC/HDL-C ratios (−0.38 and −0.26, respectively) compared to that of the low-fat group. In addition, the Mediterranean diet with nuts reduced fasting glucose (−5.4 mg/dl), systolic BP (−7.1 mm Hg), diastolic BP (−2.6 mm Hg), and TG concentrations (−13 mg/dl) relative to the low-fat diet [59]. The Mediterranean diet with olive oil also reduced fasting glucose (−7.0 mg/dl) and systolic and diastolic BP (−5.9 and −1.6 mm Hg, respectively), but it did not reduce TG concentrations compared to the low-fat diet. After 4 years of follow-up, both Mediterranean diets reduced the incidence of diabetes by 52% compared to a low-fat diet in individuals with high CVD risk [60]. Thus, the PREDIMED study has provided evidence that the Mediterranean diet is effective for improving multiple CVD risk factors. AHA and *DGA 2010* continue to promote the consumption of Mediterranean-style diet to lower CVD risk.

In conclusion, several evidence-based dietary patterns can be implemented to reduce CVD risk in accordance with the guidelines set forth by AHA and *DGA 2010*. Table 29.4 summarizes the key recommendations of TLC, DASH, vegetarian, and Mediterranean dietary patterns. Increased consumption of vegetables and fruits with decreased consumption of solid fats and added sugars is common to all recommended dietary patterns. The evidence base informing for the specific macronutrient components within these dietary patterns is discussed in further detail in the following sections.

III DIETARY FAT

The role of dietary fat in the onset and progression of CVD has been studied extensively throughout the years, focusing largely on the effects of different types of fatty acids on blood lipids and lipoproteins. Determining the ideal quantity and quality of dietary fat is an important consideration for CVD prevention and treatment. Table 29.5 summarizes recommended fat intakes identified by several expert organizations, as well as estimated intakes in the U.S. population. The DRIs, *DGA 2010*, and AND recommend 20–35% of energy from fat for adults (>19 years old) [61], whereas NCEP, AHA, the Food and Agriculture Organization of the United Nations, and the World Health Organization recommend 25–35% of calories from fat, particularly for the management of dyslipidemia [24].

Recommendations to restrict dietary calories from total fat have been an area of controversy. In the Women's Health Initiative Dietary Modification Trial [62], 19,541 subjects in the intervention group were instructed to follow a diet that was lower in total fat. The women reduced their calories from fat from 39 to 30%, substituting vegetables, fruits, and grains for fat. During 8 years of follow-up, there was no reduction in

TABLE 29.5 Current Intakes in the United States Compared to Recommended Intakes

Type of fat	U.S. adult intakes (%)[a]	Recommended intake (%)[a]				
		DGA 2010	AND	AHA	NCEP ATP III	FAO/WHO
Total fat	33–34	20–35	20–35	25–35	25–35	25–35
SFA	11	<10	<10	<7	<7	<10
TFA	2–3	[b]	[b]	<1	[b]	<1
MUFA	12–13	[c]	≤25	[c]	≤20	15–20
PUFA	<7	[c]	≤10	[c]	≤10	6–11

[a]*Percentage of daily calories.*
[b]*No amount specified, although advises to keep intake as low as possible.*
[c]*No amount specified, although supports guidelines made by other organizations.*
AND, Academy of Nutrition and Dietetics; AHA, American Heart Association; DGA, *Dietary Guidelines for Americans*; FAO, Food and Agriculture Organization of the United Nations; NCEP ATP III, National Cholesterol Education Program Adult Treatment Panel III; WHO, World Health Organization.

CVD (including specifically CHD and stroke), despite a 4 mg/dl reduction in LDL-C.

It is important to recognize that the type of fatty acids consumed markedly affects CVD risk. Certain SFAs and TFAs adversely affect lipid and lipoprotein levels, whereas unsaturated fatty acids (MUFA and PUFA) improve levels. Dietary intake data demonstrate that many Americans are not consuming the optimal amounts of dietary fat (Table 29.5). Therefore, reducing solid fat consumption (SFAs and TFAs) and incorporating more foods containing unsaturated fats likely would be beneficial for the population.

A Saturated Fatty Acids

A large body of epidemiologic, clinical, and animal evidence demonstrates that SFAs (specifically certain types of SFAs) increase lipid and lipoprotein levels. Therefore, lowering SFA intake is a primary focus of dietary interventions to lower LDL-C and CVD risk. Early predictive equations developed by Keys *et al.* [63] and Hegsted *et al.* [64] demonstrated that SFA raised TC levels compared to CHO and MUFA (which both had neutral effects), whereas PUFA lowered TC levels. The effect of SFA was twice as potent in raising TC as PUFA was in lowering TC. Several predictive equations reported that every 1% increase in energy from SFA increases LDL-C levels by approximately 1.28–1.74 mg/dl and HDL-C levels by 0.43–0.50 mg/dl [65–67]. However, individual SFAs have different effects on lipids and lipoproteins [68]. Regression analyses have shown that stearic acid (18:0) has a neutral effect on TC, LDL-C, and HDL-C [69], whereas myristic acid (14:0) is more hypercholesterolemic than lauric acid (12:0) and palmitic acid (16:0) [70]. Because most people consume SFA as a blend within food sources, practical recommendations targeting individual fatty acids cannot be made.

Evidence has demonstrated adverse associations of SFA intake on CVD incidence and mortality. Epidemiological studies demonstrated that SFA intake was significantly associated with TC and CVD incidence among different populations [71–73]. There is evidence that reductions in SFA at a population level can reduce CVD mortality. Finnish men experienced an 80% reduction in CVD mortality from 1972 to 2007 when SFA intake decreased from 22 to 13% of calories [74]. The significant change in CVD mortality among the Finnish men provides population-level evidence that decreasing SFA intake may reduce CVD risk.

Decreasing dietary SFA intake is typically associated with an increase in some other macronutrient. Therefore, the nutrient(s) consumed in place of SFA will play an important role in the blood lipid and lipoprotein responses, thereby affecting overall CVD risk. Clinical evidence demonstrates that replacing SFA with unsaturated fat (MUFA or PUFA) improves the blood lipid profile, resulting in a significant decrease in CVD risk [30]. Substituting SFA with MUFA [75–77], PUFA [76,78,79], or CHO [75] consistently reduces LDL-C. However, when SFA is replaced with CHO, HDL-C decreases and TG increases compared to MUFA or PUFA [75]. It has been estimated that each 5% energy increase in PUFA as a replacement for SFA decreases CVD events by 10% [80]. Isocalorically replacing CHO with different types of fatty acids has varying effects on the TC/HDL-C ratio, as shown in Figure 29.1 [81,82]. Collectively, clinical evidence strongly supports that replacing SFA and TFA with unsaturated fat improves the blood lipid profile and reduces CVD risk.

SFA has also been shown to have adverse effects on emerging CVD risk factors such as flow mediated

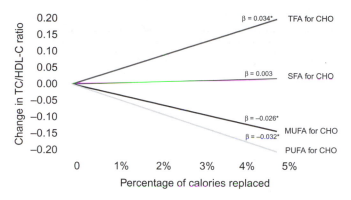

FIGURE 29.1 Changes in the TC/HDL-C ratio when carbohydrates are replaced isocalorically with SFA, MUFA, PUFA, and TFA. β reflects the change for each 1% energy replacement. *$p < 0.05$. Source: *Adapted from Micha and Mozaffarian [229]. See color plate.*

TABLE 29.6 Estimates of Relative Risk of Fatty Acids on Coronary Heart Disease Death and Events (Cohort Studies)

Type of fat	Relative risk (95% CI)			
	CHD death	p value	CHD events	p value
Total fat	0.94 (0.74–1.18)	0.583	0.93 (0.84–1.03)	0.177
TFA	1.32 (1.08–1.61)	0.006	1.25 (1.07–1.46)	0.007
SFA	1.14 (0.82–1.60)	0.431	0.93 (0.83–1.05)	0.269
MUFA	0.85 (0.60–1.20)	0.356	0.87 (0.74–1.03)	0.110
PUFA	1.25 (1.06–1.47)	0.009	0.97 (0.74–1.27)	0.825
n-3 LCPUFA	0.82 (0.71–0.94)	0.006	0.87 (0.71–1.10)	0.066

Source: *Adapted from Skeaff and Miller [92].*

dilation (FMD) of the brachial artery [18,83], cellular adhesion molecules [83,84], and hemostatic factors [85–87]. FMD is a measure of vascular reactivity commonly used to assess vascular endothelial function. Decreases in FMD are indicative of decreased vascular health, which increases risk for CVD. Both acute and chronic consumption of SFA have been shown to adversely affect FMD [18,83]. Cellular adhesion molecules (ICAM-1, sICAM-1, VCAM-1, P-selectin, and E-selectin) are compounds found on the blood vessel endothelium that bind leukocytes and initiate the leukocyte–endothelial cell adhesion cascade [88]. Increased levels of adhesion molecules increase risk of MI [89] and CVD [89,90]. The Atherosclerosis Risk in Communities (ARIC) [86] and the Dietary Effects on Lipoproteins and Thrombogenic Activity (DELTA) studies [87] both showed that a high SFA intake was associated with higher levels of factor VII coagulant activity, a key factor in blood clot formation. Collectively, these results indicate that SFA adversely affects emerging risk factors in addition to raising blood lipid levels.

Epidemiologic studies suggest that depending on the replacement nutrient, SFA may not be associated with CVD risk. A pooled analysis of 11 cohort studies from both the United States and Europe [91] reported that substitution of MUFA or CHO for SFA was associated with a greater risk of CVD events (hazard ratio (HR) 1.19 [95%confidence interval (CI): 1.00, 1.42] and HR 1.07 [95%CI: 1.01, 1.14], respectively), but not CVD death. In contrast, replacing SFA with PUFA reduced the risk of CHD death (HR 0.74 [95% CI: 0.61, 0.89]) and CHD events (HR 0.87 [95%CI: 0.77, 0.97]), suggesting that PUFA is the preferred SFA replacement. However, no discrimination was made between CHO sources and different glycemic indexes, which would be expected to significantly affect CHD risk [91]. The

authors also acknowledged that industrially modified TFA may not have been accurately accounted for in the analysis and thus included in MUFA estimates, which could explain the results reported for MUFA in this study [91]. Another systematic review of pooled prospective cohort studies also reported no significant relationship between SFA and CVD (relative risk (RR) 1.06 [95%CI: 0.96, 1.15]) but found strong evidence indicating an inverse association between MUFA and CHD risk (RR 0.80 [95%CI: 0.67, 0.93]) [57]. In contrast to the study by Jakobsen *et al.* [88] and other studies, PUFA was not related to CHD (RR 1.02 [95%CI: 0.81, 1.23]) in this analysis.

Skeaff and Miller [92] conducted a meta-analysis using results from prospective cohort and randomized controlled trials (RCTs) evaluating fatty acid associations with CHD risk. Table 29.6 shows the estimated relative risk of CVD associated with each fatty acid in the analysis. SFA intake was not significantly associated with CHD death (RR 1.14 [95% CI: 0.82–1.60]) or CHD events (RR 0.93 [95%CI: 0.83–1.05]). The authors concluded that the available evidence was unsatisfactory and unreliable due to inconsistent dietary assessment methods and the potential for regression dilution bias, the underestimation of an association due to variability, and/or measurement error. Moreover, several studies used a 24-hour recall to assess dietary intake, which is a relatively imprecise method to estimate long-term dietary habits. Another meta-analysis of prospective cohort studies conducted by Siri-Tarino *et al.* [93] also found no significant association between SFA and CHD (RR 1.07 [95% CI: 0.96, 1.19]). However, CHD was not defined nor separated into events versus deaths, in contrast to the report of Skeaff and Miller. Furthermore, a majority of the included studies used 24-hour recalls or similarly limited dietary assessment to determine SFA intake. The use of 24-hour recalls to assess long-term dietary habits by both Siri-Tarino *et al.*

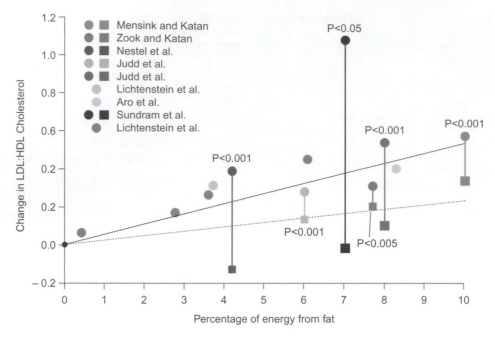

FIGURE 29.2 Results of randomized studies of the effects of a diet high in *trans* fatty acids (circles) or saturated fatty acids (squares) on the ratio of LDL cholesterol to HDL cholesterol. A diet with isocaloric amounts of *cis* fatty acids was used as the comparison group. The solid line indicates the best-fit regression for *trans* fatty acids. The dashed line indicates the best-fit regression for saturated fatty acids [100]. See color plate.

and Skeaff and Miller raises questions about the reliability of the results. In both analyses, SFA substitution was not evaluated. Therefore, identifying the specific nutrients (i.e., refined CHO or unsaturated fat) that would replace SFA is necessary to determine effects on CVD risk. More research is needed to clarify discrepancies about the association between SFA intake and CVD risk among recent epidemiologic studies.

B *Trans* Fatty Acids

1 *Industrial Trans Fatty Acids*

The adverse effects of TFAs on cardiovascular health have been demonstrated in clinical and epidemiologic trials. TFAs are classified as unsaturated fatty acids with at least one nonconjugated double bond having the *trans* stereochemistry. TFAs originate from industrial production or ruminant animals. Industrially synthesized TFAs increase TC and LDL-C similarly to SFAs and have additional negative effects on HDL-C levels, as shown in Figure 29.2 [94]. The effects of industrial TFAs on TC, LDL-C, HDL-C, and TG levels have been compared to those of other fatty acids using blood cholesterol-lowering predictive equations. A meta-analysis found that TFA intake consistently increases LDL-C and the TC/HDL-C ratio and consistently decreases HDL-C in both experimental and

observational studies [95]. These effects were most prominent when TFA intake was compared with intake of MUFA and PUFA. Collectively, evidence demonstrates that TFAs increase risk for CVD death and CVD events more than any other type of fatty acid [92]. Although naturally occurring ruminant TFA can also affect CVD risk, the amount consumed in the diet is minimal relative to industrial TFA. Therefore, *DGA 2010* recommends that total TFA consumption be as low as possible [30], whereas AHA recommends <1% of calories from TFAs to reduce CVD risk [96].

A controlled clinical trial conducted by Lichtenstein *et al.* [97] that evaluated the effects of different hydrogenated fats on lipids and lipoproteins found that diets highest in TFA content resulted in the least favorable blood lipid profile. The experimental diets provided 30% energy from total fat and differed only in the composition of this fat. Two-thirds of the fat was provided by soybean oil (<0.5 g TFA per 100 g fat), semiliquid margarine (<0.5 g), soft margarine (7.4 g), butter (1.25 g), shortening (9.9 g), or stick margarine (20.1 g). Although all vegetable fat diets resulted in lower TC, LDL-C, and HDL-C compared with the butter diet, stick margarine (containing the highest amount of TFA) decreased LDL-C the least and decreased HDL-C the most compared with the other vegetable fats. TFA also decreased LDL-C particle size in a dose-dependent manner ($p < 0.001$). The soybean oil diet (<0.5 g TFA)

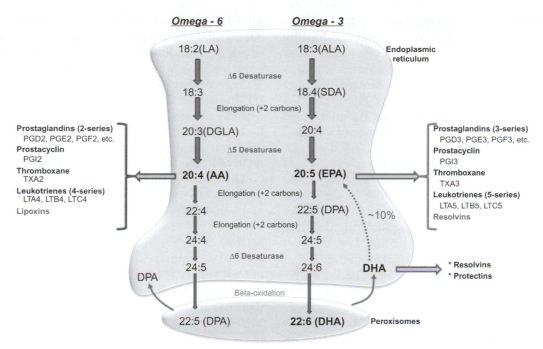

FIGURE 29.3 Biochemical pathway for the interconversion of n-6 and n-3 fatty acids. AA, arachidonic acid; ALA, α-linolenic acid; DGLA, dihomo-γ-linolenic acid; DHA, docosahexaenoic acid; DPA, docosapentaenoic acid; EPA, eicosapentaenoic acid; GLA, γ-linolenic acid; LA, linoleic acid; SDA, stearidonic acid [117]. Purple text = pro-resolution and maroon text = pro-inflammatory. See color plate.

elicited the greatest reduction in TC and LDL-C and the smallest reduction in HDL-C. A clinical trial by Judd *et al.* [98] found that replacing 8% of the calories from CHO with TFA increased TC and LDL-C by 5.8 and 10.1%, respectively. However, when 8% of the calories from CHO were replaced with a combination of TFA and stearic acid (1:1), TC and LDL-C increased by 5.6 and 8.7%, respectively. These studies demonstrate that increasing industrially synthesized TFA results in a dose-dependent increase in LDL-C and a decrease in HDL-C at high levels (higher than typical consumption, which is approximately 2.6% of calories), thereby increasing the TC/HDL-C ratio. Ascherio and Willett [99] demonstrated a linear dose-dependent relationship between TFA intake and the LDL-C/HDL-C ratio from intakes of 0.5–10% of total calories. The magnitude of this LDL-C/HDL-C ratio-raising effect was greater for TFA than it was for SFA (Figure 29.3). A 2% increase in TFA raised the LDL-C/HDL-C ratio by 0.1 unit, corresponding with a 53% increase in CHD risk [100].

2 Ruminant Trans Fatty Acids

Conjugated linoleic acid (CLA), an isomer of linoleic acid (n-6 FA), and vaccenic acid (C18:1 *trans*-11), a precursor to CLA, are present in ruminant fats in meat and dairy products. Vaccenic acid is metabolized to *cis*-9,*trans*-11 CLA in humans. The *cis*-9,*trans*-11 CLA isomer and vaccenic acid together form the majority of ruminant TFA in beef and dairy. The adjacent *cis* bond next to the *trans* bond may allow CLA to possess different characteristics relative to industrial TFA [101]. However, clinical studies on ruminant TFA have been limited compared to those on industrial TFA. In experimental animal studies, CLA isomers have been shown to decrease body fat, improve insulin sensitivity, and improve lipid profiles [102], whereas clinical evidence suggests that CLA may adversely affect the lipid profile. When healthy subjects are fed dairy products enriched with ruminant TFA, adverse effects on blood lipids and lipoproteins have been demonstrated [17,103]. Tricon *et al.* [103] evaluated the effects of dairy products enriched with *cis*-9,*trans*-11 CLA in healthy middle-aged men. Subjects consumed two diets containing milk, butter, and cheese for 6 weeks. The control diet provided 0.151 g/day of CLA, whereas the CLA-enriched diet provided 1.421 g/day. No significant effect on TC, LDL-C, or HDL-C was observed for either diet; however, the LDL-C/HDL-C ratio increased by 4% ($p = 0.023$) following the CLA-enriched diet relative to the control diet.

3 Ruminant versus Industrial Trans Fatty Acids

Several clinical studies have compared the effects of industrial TFA versus naturally occurring ruminant TFA on blood lipids and lipoproteins [104–106]. Wanders *et al.* [104] found that both industrial TFA and CLA consumption at approximately 7% of calories led to adverse lipid and lipoprotein effects in healthy adults. The TC/HDL-C ratio was 11.6% higher after the industrial TFA diet and 10.0% higher after the CLA diet compared to the oleic acid diet. Motard-Belanger et al. [106] compared high industrial and ruminant TFA diets (3.7% of calories) with a moderate ruminant TFA (1.5% of calories) and low total TFA (0.8% of calories) diet in healthy men. The high industrial TFA diets and the high ruminant TFA diets had similar adverse blood lipid effects, increasing LDL-C, decreasing HDL-C, and increasing the TC/HDL-C ratio relative to the lower TFA diets. However, the diet with only 1.5% of calories from ruminant TFA did not elicit significantly different blood lipids or lipoproteins than the low TFA (0.8% of calories) diet. Overall, this study demonstrated that high dietary intake of ruminant TFA had adverse effects on blood lipids, whereas moderate ruminant TFA intake (<1.5% of calories) had neutral effects.

Brouwer et al. [107] conducted a quantitative review of RCTs to determine the effects of both ruminant TFA and industrial TFA on HDL-C and LDL-C in humans. All classes of TFA (0.4–10.9% of energy) increased the LDL-C/HDL-C ratio when replacing cis MUFA. Most studies used supplements with an equal ratio of cis-9, trans-11 and trans-10,cis-12 CLAs (1.8 and 6.8 g/day). Although the difference was not significant, the effect of ruminant TFA was less than that of industrial TFA (0.038 vs. 0.055, $p = 0.37$). However, the amount of ruminant TFA provided in a majority of the studies greatly exceeded the intake typically consumed in usual diets (<2%) [30,108]. Maintaining a low SFA intake ensures low total consumption of ruminant TFA [108]. Industrially produced TFAs are consumed more commonly at amounts that may adversely affect CVD risk factors. Although it is possible that differences are present between metabolic effects of industrial and ruminant TFAs, at such small amounts consumed, there is currently no conclusive evidence to exclude ruminant TFA from total TFA reduction recommendations [108]. Therefore, total TFA intake should be the focus for dietary change rather than individual TFAs due to insufficient evidence suggesting differences among types of TFAs on the effect of CVD risk [30].

C Monounsaturated Fatty Acids

A strong body of evidence supports replacing SFA, TFA, or CHO with MUFA to improve blood lipids [30]. Both MUFAs and CHO significantly lower LDL-C levels when replacing SFA, but MUFAs also increase HDL-C, lower the TC/HDL-C ratio, and potentially decrease apolipoprotein B levels, the primary apolipoprotein in LDL-C [81,109]. Evidence also suggests that

MUFAs may lower susceptibility of spontaneous oxidation of LDL particles, protecting against oxidative stress and smooth muscle cell proliferation, thereby reducing their atherogenic potential [110–112].

A meta-analysis of 30 controlled trials by Cao et al. [113] reported that moderate-fat (~23.6% of calories as MUFA) and low-fat (~11.4% of calories as MUFA) diets had similar TC and LDL-C lowering effects, but the moderate-fat diet increased HDL-C and decreased TG relative to the low-fat diet [113]. A greater reduction in CVD risk was estimated after moderate-fat diets compared to low-fat diets for both men and women (−6.37 and −9.34%, respectively) [113].

DGA 2010 recommends that replacing SFA with MUFA or PUFA reduces CHD risk, whereas NCEP ATP III recommends that MUFA can make up to 20% of total energy [24,30]. The lower CVD prevalence associated with MUFA-rich diets (i.e., the Mediterranean diet) has been attributed typically to key foods high in MUFA, such as olive oil and nuts. Oleic acid (18:1), the main source of dietary MUFA, is a central component of vegetable oils and nuts, but the predominant sources of oleic acid in the typical American diet are grain-based desserts, meat, and poultry [30]. Therefore, the dietary source of MUFA may be important for its effects on CVD risk. Additional research is needed to evaluate different food sources of MUFA on CVD risk, as well as to compare MUFA and PUFA effects on the development of atherosclerosis.

Epidemiologic evidence for replacing SFA with MUFA is inconsistent with regard to CVD risk, as previously discussed. The pooled analysis of prospective cohort studies by Jakobsen et al. [91] reported a positive association between substituting MUFA in place of SFA and CHD events (HR 1.19 [95% CI: 1.00, 1.42]). In contrast, a similar analysis by Mente et al. [57] reported an inverse association between MUFA and CHD risk (RR 0.80 [CI: 0.67, 0.93]). Moreover, a prospective cohort study consisting of 5672 diabetic women reported that a 5% calorie replacement of MUFA for SFA was associated with a 37% lower CVD risk, larger than the 22% decrease associated with CHO replacement [114]. Although more studies are needed to clarify the importance of dietary MUFA source, current clinical evidence suggests that MUFA is a suitable substitution for SFA, TFA, and/or CHO to improve blood lipids and reduce CVD risk.

D Polyunsaturated Fatty Acids

PUFAs are long-chain fatty acids (18 carbons or more) that contain more than one double bond. There are two major classes of PUFAs that are defined by the position of the first double bond relative to the methyl terminus: omega-6 (n-6 FA) and omega-3 (n-3 FA) fatty acids. There is a large evidence base demonstrating benefits of dietary PUFA on CVD risk and multiple risk factors, but there is not yet consensus for optimal intakes of the individual fatty acids, especially linoleic acid.

Linoleic acid (LA; C18:2n-6) is the essential n-6 FA. The major source of LA in the diet is vegetable oil. Intakes of LA have increased from the 1930s (3% of calories) to the present (5 or 6% of calories) in the United States and Canada [115]. The adequate intake (AI) for LA is 17 and 12 g/day for men and women, respectively (19—50 years old) [29]. The acceptable macronutrient distribution range (AMDR) for n-6 FA (LA) is 5—10% of total calories. The lower range of the AMDR for LA is the AI. The upper range of PUFA intake has been set by both the DRI Committee and NCEP because it represents the upper range of PUFA consumption in the United States. The NCEP ATP III guidelines also recommend up to 10% of calories from PUFA [24]. Arachidonic acid (AA; C20:4n-6) is not essential, and it is found in animal products such as meat and egg yolks. Arachidonic acid is the precursor for bioactive compounds called eicosanoids (discussed later).

The two types of n-3 FAs, plant-derived and marine-derived, have unique benefits on CVD risk factors. α-Linolenic acid (ALA; C18:3n-3) is the major plant-derived n-3 FA and is an essential fatty acid. The two major marine-derived n-3 FAs are eicosapentaenoic acid (EPA; C20:5n-3) and docosahexaenoic acid (DHA; C22:6n-3). Fatty fish are the main source of EPA and DHA in the diet. These fatty acids are synthesized by cold-water organisms that are part of the food chain consumed by fish [116,117]. ALA, commonly found in flax/flaxseed oil, canola oil, walnuts/walnut oil, and soybean oil, can undergo a series of elongations and desaturations by the body to yield both EPA and DHA (Figure 29.3); however, these conversion rates are low, especially for the production of DHA [118—121]. The AI for ALA is 1.6 and 1.1 g/day, respectively, for men and women 19—50 years old. The AMDR for ALA is 0.6—1.2% of total energy. It is recommended that up to 10% of the AMDR for ALA can be consumed as EPA and/or DHA [29].

Dietary PUFAs have many physiological functions. EPA and AA serve as substrates for the production of lipid compounds called eicosanoids that have multiple effects on inflammatory and thrombotic pathways. For example, the balance of thromboxane and prostacyclin activity plays a key role in thrombosis and vascular function. There is also an established role of AA, EPA, and DHA as precursors for a variety of compounds that assist in the resolution of inflammatory processes termed lipoxins [122,123], resolvins, protectins, and maresins [124]. Thus, deficient intake of certain PUFAs, and consequently lower levels in the body, likely plays an important role in the development of chronic inflammation [125,126].

Increasing dietary PUFA improves blood lipid concentrations. Predictive equations developed by Keys [127] and Hegsted et al. [64] showed that a 1% increase in energy from PUFA resulted in a 0.9 mg/dl decrease in TC. Replacement of carbohydrate with PUFA increases HDL-C [81], but less than that observed for MUFA. PUFA also decreases the TC:HDL-C ratio (Figure 29.1). Three early controlled trials verified the cardioprotective effects of PUFA as observed by Keys and by Hegsted et al. [128]. The Oslo Heart Study [129], Finnish Mental Hospital Study [130], and Wadsworth Hospital and Veterans Administration Center in Los Angeles Study [131] all observed marked hypocholesterolemic effects of diets very high in PUFA from vegetable oils. Importantly, in three of these studies [129—131], the cholesterol-lowering response was associated with a reduction in the incidence of CVD (16—34%). The Nurses' Health Study also reported a dose—response relationship between PUFA intake and CVD risk, with the highest quintile of intake (6.4% of calories) conferring an approximately 30% reduction in risk [72].

Increased dietary ALA provides additional benefits beyond what has been demonstrated for total PUFA. Observational studies have shown cardioprotective effects of ALA on risk of coronary morbidity and mortality. The Nurses' Health Study reported a 30% reduction in relative risk of fatal CHD in individuals who consumed >1 g of ALA per day [132]. The Health Professionals Follow-Up Study, which included data from 45,722 U.S. health professionals (40—75 years old), reported that in men with low EPA and DHA intake (<100 mg/day), 1 g/day of ALA was associated with a 58% decrease in risk from nonfatal MI. However, no added benefit of ALA was observed when EPA and DHA intakes increased >100 mg/day [133]. In the Iowa Women's Health Study, the highest tertile of ALA intake was associated with a 15% reduction in total mortality [134]. Finally, in a secondary analysis of the 24-hour recall data from the Multiple Risk Factor Intervention Trial (MRFIT), a primary prevention study that examined the effects of reducing elevated serum cholesterol and diastolic BP along with smoking cessation on CHD mortality, it was observed that the highest quintile of ALA intake, 2.81 g/day, yielded a multivariate-adjusted relative risk for all-cause mortality of 0.67 [135].

The Lyon Diet Heart Study is the largest clinical trial to examine the effects of a diet high in ALA on CVD [136,137]. In this randomized secondary prevention trial, an AHA Step 1 Mediterranean dietary pattern (high in ALA) reduced cardiac death and nonfatal MI by approximately 70% and all coronary events by approximately 50%, despite no improvement in lipids and lipoproteins. The authors attributed the benefits to the 68% increase in ALA intake (~1.7 g/day; compared to the control group), whereas the AHA Science Advisory suggests that the other differences between the two diet groups may have played a role in the reduction in CVD risk observed in the Lyon Diet Heart Study [138]. For example, in the Lyon Diet Heart Study, subjects in the experimental group were instructed to adopt a Mediterranean-type diet that contained more bread, root vegetables and green vegetables, and fish; fruit at least once daily; less red meat (replaced with poultry); and margarine supplied by the study to replace butter and cream.

Despite the beneficial effects of ALA on coronary disease risk observed in observational studies and in the Lyon Diet Heart Study, some have questioned the cardiovascular benefits of plant-derived n-3 FAs, stating that there is "no high-quality evidence to support the beneficial effects of ALA" with respect to eliciting reductions in all-cause mortality, cardiac and sudden death, and stroke [139]. The majority of evidence comes from epidemiologic data and the one controlled clinical study conducted to date, which did not specifically evaluate ALA effects. More trials are needed to examine the unique effects of ALA on CVD outcomes to inform recommendations for optimal intake.

The 1970s marked the beginning of an extensive scientific evaluation of the role of marine n-3 FAs in the development of CVD. The seminal studies of Dyerberg *et al.* [140] noted that coronary atherosclerotic disease was rare in Greenland Eskimos and prevalent in a Danish population. These scientists attributed this difference in the incidence of CHD to the high intake of marine oils by the Eskimos and, in particular, EPA and DHA. During approximately the past 30 years, numerous studies have demonstrated that these fatty acids confer cardioprotective effects via multiple mechanisms of action. As shown in Figure 29.4, the effects of EPA and DHA on clinical outcomes (e.g., antiarrythmic, TG lowering, and BP lowering) occur in a time-dependent manner. Of importance is that the antiarrythmic effect occurs within months and is achieved at relatively low doses of EPA and DHA. This is important clinically because arrhythmias are the cause of sudden cardiac death, which is the leading cause of cardiac death in the United States [141]. The effects of EPA and DHA on lowering TG, heart rate, and blood pressure all occur within weeks to months at doses that are consistent with current dietary recommendations. Fish and/or fish oil consumption has been consistently shown to reduce CHD death (~35%), CHD sudden death (~50%), and ischemic stroke (~30%). Modest benefits

of fish and/or fish oil consumption have also been reported for nonfatal MI, delayed progression of atherosclerosis, recurrent ventricular tachyarrhythmias, and post-angioplasty restenosis [142].

Several large epidemiologic studies demonstrated that EPA and DHA intakes of 250–500 mg/day were associated with significant reductions in CHD mortality and sudden death [142]. Researchers have suggested that there is a threshold of effect because intakes more than 900 mg/day do not elicit a greater decrease in risk [133,142,143]. The beneficial effects of increased EPA and DHA intake in the prevention of CVD have been examined in both primary and secondary prevention studies.

In the MRFIT trial, individuals in the highest quintile of EPA and DHA had a 40% reduction in risk from cardiac death [144]. Data from the Nurses' Health Study showed that women in the highest quintile of EPA and DHA intake had a 31% lower risk of heart attack than those in the lowest quintile [145]. Participants in the Physicians Health Study who consumed fatty fish at least once a month had an approximately 50% reduction in risk of sudden death from MI; however, no associations between fish intake and reduction in incidence of MI were found [146]. Not all observational studies have demonstrated a benefit of an increased intake of EPA and DHA: A 6-year cohort study from Finland, which included 21,930 men, found no benefit of EPA and DHA or ALA in reducing cardiac death [147]. The researchers questioned the external validity of these findings because the subjects were mainly middle-aged, smoking men with high intakes of dietary fat. This study was also conducted in a population consuming fish high in mercury. Mercury levels can negatively impact CVD risk; mercury levels were not controlled for in the analysis.

Large RCTs have validated the use of marine n-3 in the secondary prevention of CVD. In these trials, patients with CHD were given dietary advice to consume at least two servings of fatty fish a week (200–400 g of fish) or given supplemental fish oil capsules (850 mg of EPA and DHA). These interventions resulted in a 21–29% reduction in all-cause mortality and 45% reduction in sudden death from MI [148–150]. This evidence is the basis for current recommendation for secondary prevention.

In addition, the first large-scale, prospective, randomized trial of combined treatment with a statin and EPA showed that the addition of EPA to statin therapy prevented major coronary events [151]. The Japan EPA Lipid Intervention Study (JELIS) tested the effects of long-term use of 1.8 g/day in addition to a statin in Japanese patients with hypercholesterolemia. Analysis of combined coronary event end points showed a significant 19% reduction with 1.8 g/day EPA. This study

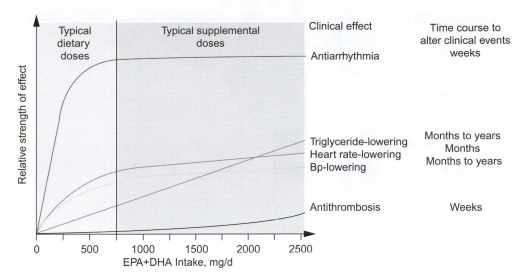

FIGURE 29.4 Schema of potential dose responses and time courses for altering clinical events of physiologic effects of fish or fish oil intake [142]. See color plate.

is also notable because the Japanese have much higher intakes of marine n-3 FAs relative to Americans. The results suggest that further risk reduction may occur at higher intakes of n-3 FA.

Clinical trials [152,153] have not replicated the earlier findings of Gruppo Italiano per lo Studio della Sopravvivenza nell'Infarto miocardico (GISSI) and JELIS. However, concerns have been expressed about several design aspects (e.g., lack of power and insufficient dosing) in these studies that have led to a lack of positive effects in the n-3 supplemented groups. Recommendations for n-3 intake (discussed further later) are unlikely to be affected by the results of these studies.

It is unlikely that there are benefits of fish oil supplementation in patients with implanted cardioverter/defibrillators (ICDs) and advanced congestive heart failure. Three fish oil supplementation trials have been conducted in people with ICDs with mixed results. One trial found a trend favoring the use of fish oil supplementation to prevent fatal ventricular arrhythmias; however, there was not enough statistical power to yield a significant result [154]. Another trial found that fish oil supplementation did not reduce the risk of ventricular fibrillation/ventricular tachycardia, and a potential adverse effect was seen in individuals with an ejection fraction less than 40% [155]. In the most recent trial, the Study on Omega-3 Fatty Acids and Ventricular Arrhythmia (SOFA), there was no protective effect attributed to fish oil supplementation in patients with ICDs [156]. Due to their effects of cardiac ion channels, n-3 FAs are not beneficial in the setting of pre-existing fibrotic damage despite their well-demonstrated anti-arrhythmic effects [157].

Fish oil also has a marked hypotriglyceridemic effect in individuals with normal or elevated TG levels ($\geq$2 mmol/l). In 21 studies that examined the effects of fish or fish oil on lipids and lipoproteins, EPA and DHA (0.1–5.4 g/day) reduced plasma TGs an average of 15% [158]. A dose–response relationship exists such that greater amounts of EPA and DHA result in greater reductions in TG values [158]. Individuals with elevated TG are more responsive to the TG-lowering effects of fish oil [159,160].

The effects of EPA and DHA consumption on LDL-C levels were evaluated by the Agency for Healthcare Research and Quality. Data from 15 randomized clinical trials showed that marine n-3 FA (ranging from 45 mg to 5.4 g of fish oil) consumption led to a net increase of 10 mg/dl in LDL-C [78]. The increase in LDL-C levels is thought to be due partly to an increase in LDL-C particle size. Research examining the effects on LDL-C particle size has shown both no change in size [161] and an increase in size [162,163]. It has been proposed that the change in LDL-C particle size relates to a patient's starting LDL-C particle size. Individuals with a pattern B phenotype, defined as having an increased amount of small dense LDL-C particles, respond to fish oil supplementation with an increase in LDL-C particle size, whereas individuals without this phenotype do not [161]. When a prescription level of EPA and DHA (3.4 g/day EPA + DHA) is added to statin therapy, the increase in LDL-C is attenuated [164]. Physical oversight is recommended for EPA and DHA doses exceeding 2 g/day for the reduction of TG concentrations [165].

One area of concern when recommending increased fish intake pertains to the issue of environmental

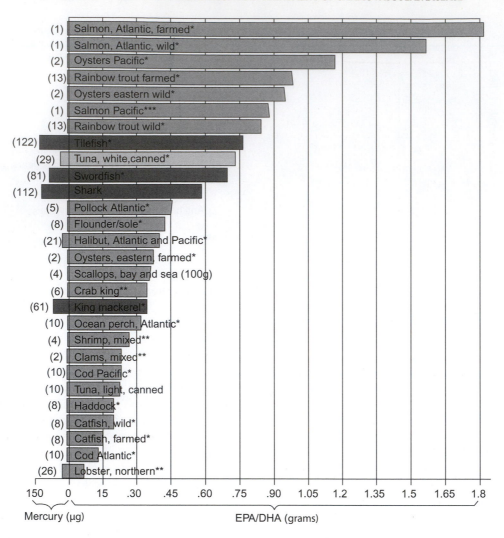

FIGURE 29.5   EPA/DHA intake and methylmercury intake exposure from one 3-ounce portion of seafood. *Cooked, dry heat; **cooked, moist heat; ***the EPA and DHA content in Pacific salmon is a composite from chum, Coho, and sockeye. Source: *Reprinted from Institute of Medicine [230] with permission by the National Academies of Sciences.* See color plate.

contaminants such as mercury. A majority of the fatty fish consumed are smaller with a shorter life span and thus have lower mercury concentrations than larger, longer lived fish such as shark and swordfish (Figure 29.5) [142]. Consumption of certain fish high in mercury, such as shark, tilefish, king mackerel, and swordfish, plays an important role in increased mercury accumulation in humans [166]. Therefore, emphasis on high n-3 FA fish (also low in mercury) is recommended.

The health benefits of oily fish consumption far outweigh the risks [142,167,168]. The best guidance is to follow U.S. Food and Drug Administration guidelines as well as state and local advisories for safe fish consumption because two studies observed higher risk for CVD with increased mercury intake [167,168]. Another strategy for increasing EPA and DHA

consumption is the use of fish oil supplements because they are cost-effective, convenient, and contain negligible quantities of environmental contaminants [169]. This is a strategy recommended for individuals who do not eat fish or those who need high doses of marine-derived n-3 FAs.

AHA has both food-based and nutrient-based recommendations (Table 29.7) [165] regarding n-3 FA, and specifically EPA and DHA. In a science advisory published in 2003, AHA made n-3 FA recommendations for individuals without heart disease, patients with documented CHD, and patients with hypertriglyceridemia. The AHA *Diet and Lifestyle Recommendations Revision 2006* recommends 500 mg/day of EPA and DHA for the primary prevention of CHD. This is equivalent to two servings (4 oz. each) of fatty fish weekly. The NCEP ATP III did not make specific n-3

TABLE 29.7 Summary of American Heart Association Recommendations for Omega-3 Fatty Acid Intake *Source*: Kris-Etherton *et al.* [165].

Population	Recommendation
Patients without documented coronary heart disease (CHD)	Eat a variety of (preferably fatty) fish at least twice a week. Include oils and foods rich in α-linolenic acid (flaxseed, canola, and soybean oils; flaxseed and walnuts).
Patients with documented CHD	Consume ~1 g of EPA + DHA per day, preferably from fatty fish. EPA + DHA in capsule form could be considered in consultation with the physician.
Patients who need to lower triglycerides	2−4 g of EPA + DHA per day provided as capsules under a physician's care.

FA recommendations but endorsed those made by the AHA in 2003 [24].

Several obstacles exist regarding recommended intakes of other PUFA, especially the n-6 FA LA. There is some concern that PUFAs may have adverse health effects due to their increased susceptibility for oxidation [170] and the potential impact that high intakes of LA may have on n-3 FA status and inflammation. However, many longer term clinical studies have shown that increased PUFA intakes lower CVD risk, and thus the impact of increased susceptibility to oxidation is unlikely in the context of a healthy dietary pattern [128,130,171].

Some have expressed concern that increased n-6 FA consumption will inhibit n-3 FA metabolism because n-3 and n-6 FAs share common enzymatic and metabolic pathways (Figure 29.4). The impact of increasing n-6 FA intake on n-3 FA metabolism is hypothesized to occur at two biological steps. First, an increase in LA levels can interfere with the formation of EPA from ALA because LA utilizes the same desaturase and elongase enzymes to form AA. The second is competition for the enzymes that produce eicosanoids and other oxygenated metabolites. AA, EPA, and DHA are all present in the lipid bilayers of cell membranes. It has been hypothesized that increased levels of dietary n-6 FAs lead to more n-6 FAs being used for eicosanoid synthesis, resulting in increased production of proinflammatory lipid mediators.

However, this evidence has been derived primarily from cell-based studies, and in humans, increased intakes of LA and AA have not been shown to increase inflammation [172]. This position also does not account for the finding that AA serves as the substrate for anti-inflammatory lipid mediators, including the pro-resolution products termed lipoxins [122,123]. The Health Professionals Follow-Up Study with 45,722 men reported that irrespective of background n-6 FA intake, increased consumption of n-3 FAs was associated with reduced CVD risk [173].

The importance of optimizing dietary n-3 FA intakes has been translated by some to an approach of targeting a lower dietary ratio of n-6 to n-3 FAs by reducing intake of LA [174−178]. Proponents call for a reduction in n-6 intake with substitution of dietary MUFA, specifically the substitution of olive and canola oils for cooking and dressings and avoidance of all high n-6 foods, such as vegetable oils, nuts, and seeds. There is a paucity of research examining dietary intake of n-6 FAs relative to diets higher in MUFA that has been able to account for the confounding associations of overall dietary patterns. In fact, much of the clinical evidence for the substitution of MUFA for LA has been derived from comparisons of the Mediterranean dietary pattern to a Western dietary pattern. In these comparisons, vegetable oils that are high in n-6 FAs are usually used in frying and preparation of foods that are relatively lower in fiber and plant antioxidants. In contrast, olive oil typically accompanies grains and vegetables in Mediterranean patterns. Olive oil contains additional antioxidants not present in refined vegetable oils, which contributes additional complexity to comparisons of dietary LA and oleic acid. Similarly, nuts that are high in LA are rich in many other bioactive compounds that have not been accounted for in these comparisons. It is likely that the ratio of n-6:n-3 FAs is not as important as the total amount of n-3 FAs [179]. Based on evidence to date, dietary advice should encourage increased consumption of ALA, EPA, and DHA, without instruction to limit intake of plant sources of omega-6 such as nuts and seeds.

Thus, advice to at-risk populations concerning fat intake should place emphasis on adopting evidenced-based dietary patterns, such as the Mediterranean diet, that are enriched with both plant and marine n-3 FAs rather than placing emphasis of restriction of LA because increased dietary PUFA significantly reduces CVD risk factors and CVD events. Because there are beneficial effects of PUFA intakes at 14−21% of calories, which is higher than the recommended intake range (5−10% of calories), more research is needed to determine the optimum level of PUFA in the diet [180].

In conclusion, intake of PUFA and long-chain n-3 FAs has been shown to have significant cardioprotective benefits in observational studies and clinical trials. This research supports current dietary recommendations for increased intake of oily fish as part of a diet that is also enriched with plant PUFA. The cardioprotective effects of ALA and LA, as well as optimal proportions of individual fatty acids, need to be clarified and explored further via randomized clinical trials.

IV DIETARY CARBOHYDRATE

DGA 2010 recommends limiting foods and beverages with added sugars and increasing consumption of unrefined sources of carbohydrate. AHA recommends that added sugar provide no more than 100 daily calories for women and 150 daily calories for men [181]. NCEP ATP III [24] recommends that 50–60% of energy be provided by carbohydrates. Many foods that are included in a high-carbohydrate diet, such as fruits and vegetables, whole grains, and legumes, contain bioactive compounds that favorably affect CVD risk. In this section, we discuss some areas of scientific investigation associated with carbohydrate and reduction of CVD risk: low carbohydrate diets, the role of glycemic index, dietary fiber, and soluble fiber.

A Glycemic Index and Glycemic Load

Carbohydrates are classified according to their blood glucose-raising effects, typically using the glycemic index. Low glycemic index foods, such as mature beans and green vegetables, elicit less of a glycemic response than high glycemic index foods, such as potatoes and ready-to-eat cereals. Glycemic load is defined as the mathematical product of the carbohydrate amount and glycemic index. The glycemic load is a measure of both type and amount of carbohydrates, whereas the glycemic index is a measure of only carbohydrate type. In general, foods high in soluble fiber have a low glycemic index. However, food preparation methods and consumption of other foods in the context of a mixed meal can alter the glycemic index.

Multiple studies of glycemic index and glycemic load illustrate the importance of considering not only the macronutrient composition of the diet but also the characteristics of carbohydrate consumed. Independent of weight loss, diets composed of low glycemic index foods increase insulin sensitivity [182,183] and decrease total serum cholesterol [183] and LDL-C [182] in individuals with type 2 diabetes. Furthermore, a review of 13 intervention studies that examined the effects of glycemic index on TGs, LDL-C, and TC:HDL-C ratio consistently showed the benefit of a lower glycemic diet [184]. In two analyses of data from the Nurses' Health Study, the glycemic load of the diet was strongly associated with CVD risk [185,186]. An additional analysis of healthy women demonstrated a strong correlation between high-sensitivity C-reactive protein and glycemic load [187]. This again suggests a relationship between the type and amount of carbohydrate consumed and cardiovascular disease, especially in adult women. In contrast, the Zutphen Elderly Study [188] found no relationship between a high glycemic index diet and CHD in elderly men. Thus, research suggests that reduction in glycemic load diet is efficacious for reducing CVD risk in women and individuals with insulin resistance.

B Dietary Fiber

An abundance of evidence demonstrates a beneficial association between dietary fiber intake and risk of CVD [189]. Dietary fiber is present in fruits, vegetables, whole-grains, and legumes. Fiber-fortified foods and supplements are also available that can be used to increase dietary fiber [190,191]. Soluble fiber, including oat bran, psyllium, guar gum, and pectin, has been shown to reduce CVD risk through its action on lipids and lipoproteins and glucose metabolism. Soluble fiber has numerous properties that mediate its cholesterol-lowering effects, such as binding bile acids and increasing gastrointestinal tract viscosity. In pooled data from 10 prospective cohort studies in the United States and Europe, each 10 g/day increment of dietary fiber yielded a 23% reduction in risk of coronary mortality and 14% reduction in all coronary events [192]. The association was strongest with cereal fiber compared to fruit/vegetable fiber. Increased fiber intake via whole grains has also been associated with improved insulin sensitivity [193].

The effects of different food sources of soluble fiber on lipids and lipoproteins have been studied. Incorporating 15–115 g of beans (navy or pinto) reduces both total and LDL-C by 15–23 and 13–24%, respectively [194]. Oats contain β-glucan, which has been shown to reduce total cholesterol along with fasting glucose and insulin [195]. Adding 3 g/day of oat β-glucan from oat cereal consumption to a weight-loss diet reduced LDL-C by 4.4% more than weight loss with consumption of low-fiber control foods [196]. A systematic review found a 5–10% reduction in LDL-C and total cholesterol from 3 g/day β-glucan [197]. In addition, soluble fiber has been shown to lower glucose and insulin levels in healthy individuals [198] and to favorably affect insulin sensitivity in individuals with diabetes [199] and moderate hypercholesterolemia [200].

C Dietary Carbohydrate and CVD Risk

Replacing calories from SFA with carbohydrates is one strategy for reducing SFA to decrease LDL-C. The resulting high-carbohydrate, low-fat diet, when not accompanied by weight loss, typically decreases HDL-C and increases TG, especially on low-fiber diets [201]. This is particularly problematic for people with insulin resistance and accompanying dyslipidemia characterized by low HDL-C and elevated TG [202]. A high-carbohydrate, low-fat diet has also been shown to increase plasma glucose and insulin in individuals with type 2 diabetes [203] and healthy women [204]. In the Women's Health Initiative Dietary Modification Trial [63], subjects in the intervention group who reduced their fat calories from 39 to 30% experienced no reduction in CVD risk.

Specific high-carbohydrate diets that emphasize high intake of vegetable, fruits, and whole grains, and thus have a high fiber content and low glycemic load, have been associated with improved CVD risk. As discussed previously, a vegetarian diet with an extreme reduction in fat (10% energy) and a high intake of minimally refined carbohydrate (70–80% energy) has been shown to be effective in achieving regression of plaque when combined with other intensive lifestyle changes (e.g., stress management and aerobic exercise) [51,205,206]. The OmniHeart Trial [26] and DASH Diet studies [36,207] both provided diets high in carbohydrate (58% of energy), and no significant increase in TG was observed. The effect of increasing carbohydrate intake on CVD risk is dependent on the source of dietary carbohydrate, and this is very important to consider when recommendations are made to replace fat intake with carbohydrate.

Carbohydrate restriction has become popular for weight loss and has also demonstrated success in reducing some CVD risk factors. Compared to a low-fat diet, a low-carbohydrate diet can elicit greater initial weight loss at 6 months (−7.3 vs. −3.1 lb); however, at 12 months, weight loss is the same for both diets [208,209]. Low-carbohydrate diets reduce TG levels and increase HDL-C [211]. In overweight or obese men, reductions in carbohydrate intake from 54 to 26% of total calories, in conjunction with controlled weight loss, reduced the proportion of small, dense LDL-C particles [210]. A low-carbohydrate diet can also improve clearance of TG-rich chylomicron remnants [211] that increase risk for coronary disease [212]. However, increased intake of SFA as part of a low-carbohydrate diet has detrimental effects on total cholesterol and LDL-C. In an examination of the Nurses' Health Study cohort, a low-carbohydrate diet was not associated with increased risk of CVD [186]. In fact, higher intake of vegetable fat and vegetable protein was associated with significantly reduced risk. These findings prompted a pooled re-examination of three studies in which 190 overweight women were provided advice about a Mediterranean diet and then followed for 2 years [213]. Women who had lower carbohydrate intake (45 vs. 58%) achieved greater reductions in body weight and TGs in addition to larger increases in adiponectin.

In conclusion, replacing high-glycemic carbohydrate sources with unrefined plant carbohydrate sources can be an effective strategy for reducing CVD risk. Thus, recommendations cannot be made for carbohydrate intake as a replacement for fat without considering the type of carbohydrate.

V DIETARY PROTEIN

Epidemiologic and controlled clinical studies have shown benefits of dietary protein on CVD risk, although some studies suggest an adverse relationship. Data from the Nurses' Health Study found that high protein intakes (up to 24% of total energy intake), which included animal and plant protein, were associated with a significantly reduced risk of CVD (RR = 0.75; 95% CI: 0.61, 0.92) [132]. Likewise, the OmniHeart Trial found that a high-protein diet (25% of energy intake) reduced the estimated 10-year risk (5.8% lower) for CHD compared with a high-CHO diet (58% of energy intake) [26]. However, in a 12-year follow-up study of middle-aged Swedish women participating in the Women's Lifestyle and Health Cohort, a diet low in carbohydrate and high in protein (assessed from protein and CHO intakes according to deciles of individual energy intake) was associated with higher total and CVD mortality [214]. In addition, in the Greek component of the European Prospective Investigation into Cancer and Nutrition, prolonged consumption of a low-carbohydrate, high-protein diet was associated with an increase in total mortality [215]. This study suggests that marked reductions in carbohydrate together with an increase in dietary protein are problematic.

There is uncertainty whether animal protein, particularly from red meat, affects CVD risk. In a prospective study that examined whether overall dietary patterns derived from a food frequency questionnaire (FFQ) predicted risk of CHD in men, a dietary pattern including red meat and processed meat was associated with a higher risk for CVD (RR adjusted for lifestyle variables and fat intake, 1.43; 95% CI: 1.01, 2.01) [216]. In contrast, the 2-year randomized Cholesterol Lowering Atherosclerosis Study found a reduction in new coronary artery lesions among those with increased dietary protein (lean meat and low-fat dairy) compared with subjects who decreased their protein intake [217]. The early work that reported associations between animal protein and CVD mortality [218] likely was confounded by correlations between protein intake and dietary SFA and cholesterol [219].

In an analysis of the Nurses' Health Study, intakes of both processed and unprocessed red meat—as well as high-fat dairy—were significantly associated with increased CHD risk [85]. Intake of poultry, fish, and nuts were associated with reduced risk. Each one serving per day of nuts reduced CHD risk by 22% in a multivariate model that adjusted for other potential risk factors. Each serving of red meat increased CHD risk by 16–19% in this adjusted model. Substituting one serving of red meat with nuts, low-fat dairy, poultry, or fish significantly reduced risk by 30, 13, 19, and 24%; respectively. In contrast, in an analysis that included 20 studies comprising more than 1 million people, consumption of processed meat, but not red (unprocessed) meat, was associated with a higher incidence of CHD [220]. This study finding suggests that the source of animal protein, leanness, and how it is processed prior to consumer consumption could impact its effect on CVD risk. More research is needed to establish whether consumption of unprocessed, and specifically lean, red meat is associated with CVD risk.

VI DIETARY CHOLESTEROL

Cholesterol plays an important role in steroid hormone and bile acid biosynthesis, and it serves as an integral component of cell membranes. There is no biological requirement for dietary cholesterol because all tissues synthesize sufficient amounts of cholesterol to meet metabolic and structural needs. The DRI report for macronutrients recommended that cholesterol intake be as low as possible because of the dose–response relationship between dietary cholesterol and total and LDL-C [65,221]. *DGA 2010* as well as AHA recommend <300 mg/day for normocholesterolemic individuals. *DGA 2010* and NCEP ATP III recommend <200 mg/day (less than one egg) for those at risk for CHD [29].

There is epidemiologic evidence demonstrating a relationship between dietary cholesterol and CVD risk [222]. Among Japanese women, one or two eggs per week was associated with a 12% lower all-cause death rate, with a trend toward a lower mortality due to stroke, ischemic heart disease, and cancer compared to women consuming one egg per day [222]. In contrast, in 117,933 subjects in the United States, no relationship was found between consumption of one egg or less per day and the risk of ischemic heart disease or stroke [223]. In the Framingham Heart Study, egg consumption was not associated with CHD [224] and was not related to serum cholesterol levels [225].

In a meta-analysis of 395 metabolic ward trials investigating the importance of dietary fatty acids and dietary cholesterol on serum TC, LDL-C, and HDL-C, it was found that isocaloric replacement of saturated fats (10% of dietary calories) by complex carbohydrates was associated with a decrease in TC by 20 mg/dl; and replacing carbohydrates by PUFA (5% calories) would further reduce TC by 5 mg/dl. A reduction of 200 mg/day in dietary cholesterol was associated with a further reduction in TC of 5 mg/dl. The sum of these isocaloric changes is a reduction in TC by 29 mg/dl (99% CI: 0.67, 0.85), a reduction in LDL-C by 24 mg/dl, and an increase in HDL-C by 4 mg/dl [65]. On the basis of this meta-analysis, dietary cholesterol elicits a small hypercholesterolemic effect that is less than that of saturated fat.

In a meta-analysis of 17 trials, consumption of dietary cholesterol increased the TC/HDL-C ratio by 0.02. Consuming approximately 200 mg/day of cholesterol (equivalent to one egg per day) increased the TC/HDL-C ratio by 0.04, TC by 4.3 mg/dl, LDL-C by 3.9 mg/dl, and HDL-C by 0.6 mg/dl [226]. This effect was independent of other dietary factors, such as the type and amount of fat.

Collectively, the evidence shows that dietary cholesterol does play a role in modifying CVD risk; however, the effects on total and LDL-C are modest. Nonetheless, decreasing dietary cholesterol would be expected to reduce the risk of CHD, especially in subgroups of individuals who are responsive to changes in cholesterol intake [227].

VII CONCLUSIONS

A food-based dietary pattern that meets current nutrient goals is recommended to reduce CVD risk by delivering the full complement of nutrients and dietary factors that target a broad array of health benefits, including beneficial effects on established CVD risk factors. This dietary pattern can be achieved in a variety of ways, but in general it promotes consumption of fruits, vegetables, whole grains, legumes (including soy products) or lean meat, low-fat/skim dairy products, oily fish, nuts and seeds, and liquid vegetable oils. Dietary sources of TFA, high-glycemic foods, and added sugars should be restricted. Implementation of this dietary pattern will impact multiple major CVD risk factors, including lipids and lipoproteins, blood pressure, and body weight, which can markedly decrease CVD risk. Thus, a healthful dietary pattern is important for the prevention and treatment of heart disease, and implementation of the food-based dietary recommendations that have been made by many organizations can have an important public health benefit.

References

[1] V.L. Roger, A.S. Go, D.M. Lloyd-Jones, R.J. Adams, J.D. Berry, T. M. Brown, et al., Heart disease and stroke statistics—2011 update: a report from the American Heart Association, Circulation 123 (2011) e18—e209.

[2] P.A. Heidenreich, J.G. Trogdon, O.A. Khavjou, J. Butler, K. Dracup, M.D. Ezekowitz, et al., Forecasting the future of cardiovascular disease in the United States: a policy statement from the American Heart Association, Circulation 123 (2011) 933—944.

[3] T.A. Pearson, The prevention of cardiovascular disease: have we really made progress? Health Aff. 26 (2007) 49—60.

[4] S. Bansal, J.E. Buring, N. Rifai, S. Mora, F.M. Sacks, P.M. Ridker, Fasting compared with nonfasting triglycerides and risk of cardiovascular events in women, JAMA 298 (2007) 309—316.

[5] J.J. Freiberg, A. Tybjaerg-Hansen, J.S. Jensen, B.G. Nordestgaard, Nonfasting triglycerides and risk of ischemic stroke in the general population, JAMA 300 (2008) 2142—2152.

[6] B.G. Nordestgaard, M. Benn, P. Schnohr, A. Tybjaerg-Hansen, Nonfasting triglycerides and risk of myocardial infarction, ischemic heart disease, and death in men and women, JAMA 298 (2007) 299—308.

[7] B.G. Nordestgaard, A. Langsted, J.J. Freiberg, Nonfasting hyperlipidemia and cardiovascular disease, Curr. Drug Targets 10 (2009) 328—335.

[8] W.S. Harris, The omega-3 index: from biomarker to risk marker to risk factor, Curr. Atheroscler. Rep. 11 (2009) 411—417.

[9] W.S. Harris, The omega-3 index: clinical utility for therapeutic intervention, Curr. Cardiol. Rep. 12 (2010) 503—508.

[10] W.S. Harris, The omega-3 index as a risk factor for coronary heart disease, Am. J. Clin. Nutr. 87 (2008) 1997S—2002S.

[11] W.S. Harris, Omega-3 fatty acids and cardiovascular disease: a case for omega-3 index as a new risk factor, Pharmacol. Res. 55 (2007) 217—223.

[12] A.A. Brown, F.B. Hu, Dietary modulation of endothelial function: implications for cardiovascular disease, Am. J. Clin. Nutr. 73 (2001) 673—686.

[13] P. Greenland, M.D. Knoll, J. Stamler, J.D. Neaton, A.R. Dyer, D. B. Garside, et al., Major risk factors as antecedents of fatal and nonfatal coronary heart disease events, JAMA 290 (2003) 891—897.

[14] U.N. Khot, M.B. Khot, C.T. Bajzer, S.K. Sapp, E.M. Ohman, S.J. Brener, et al., Prevalence of conventional risk factors in patients with coronary heart disease, JAMA 290 (2003) 898—904.

[15] W.P. Castelli, Lipids, risk factors and ischaemic heart disease, Atherosclerosis 124 (1996) S1—S9.

[16] M.H. Davidson, Update on CETP inhibition, J. Clin. Lipidol 4 (2010) 394—398.

[17] H.N. Ginsberg, M.B. Elam, L.C. Lovato, J.R. Crouse III, L.A. Leiter, P. Linz, et al., Effects of combination lipid therapy in type 2 diabetes mellitus, N. Engl. J. Med. 362 (2010) 1563—1574.

[18] AIM-HIGH investigators, The role of niacin in raising high-density lipoprotein cholesterol to reduce cardiovascular events in patients with atherosclerotic cardiovascular disease and optimally treated low-density lipoprotein cholesterol Rationale and study design. The Atherothrombosis Intervention in Metabolic Syndrome with Low HDL/High Triglycerides: impact on Global Health Outcomes (AIM-HIGH), Am. Heart J. 161 (2011) 471—477.

[19] G. Bjelakovic, D. Nikolova, L.L. Gluud, R.G. Simonetti, C. Gluud, Mortality in randomized trials of antioxidant supplements for primary and secondary prevention: systematic review and meta-analysis, JAMA 297 (2007) 842—857.

[20] H.C. Gerstein, M.E. Miller, S. Genuth, F. Ismail-Beigi, J.B. Buse, D.C. Goff Jr., et al., Long-term effects of intensive glucose lowering on cardiovascular outcomes, N. Engl. J. Med. 364 (2011) 818—828.

[21] H.C. Gerstein, M.E. Miller, R.P. Byington, D.C. Goff Jr., J.T. Bigger, J.B. Buse, et al., Effects of intensive glucose lowering in type 2 diabetes, N. Engl. J. Med. 358 (2008) 2545—2559.

[22] UK Prospective Diabetes Study Group, Intensive blood-glucose control with sulphonylureas or insulin compared with conventional treatment and risk of complications in patients with type 2 diabetes (UKPDS 33), Lancet 352 (1998) 837—853.

[23] R.M. Krauss, R.H. Eckel, B. Howard, L.J. Appel, S.R. Daniels, R.J. Deckelbaum, et al., AHA dietary guidelines: revision 2000: a statement for healthcare professionals from the Nutrition Committee of the American Heart Association, Circulation 102 (2000) 2284—2299.

[24] National Cholesterol Education Program, Third report of the National Cholesterol Education Program (NCEP) Expert Panel on Detection, Evaluation, and Treatment of High Blood Cholesterol in Adults (Adult Treatment Panel III) final report, Circulation 106 (2002) 3143—3421.

[25] L.J. Appel, T.J. Moore, E. Obarzanek, W.M. Vollmer, L.P. Svetkey, F.M. Sacks, et al., A clinical trial of the effects of dietary patterns on blood pressure: DASH Collaborative Research Group, N. Engl. J. Med. 336 (1997) 1117—1124.

[26] L.J. Appel, F.M. Sacks, V.J. Carey, E. Obarzanek, J.F. Swain, E.R. Miller III, et al., Effects of protein, monounsaturated fat, and carbohydrate intake on blood pressure and serum lipids: results of the OmniHeart randomized trial, JAMA 294 (2005) 2455—2464.

[27] N. Rifai, P.M. Ridker, High-sensitivity C-reactive protein: a novel and promising marker of coronary heart disease, Clin. Chem. 47 (2001) 403—411.

[28] I.H. Page, F.J. Stare, A.C. Corcoran, H. Pollack, C.F. Wilkinson Jr., Atherosclerosis and the fat content of the diet, J. Am. Med. Assoc. 164 (1957) 2048—2051.

[29] U.S. Department of Health and Human Services and U.S. Department of Agriculture, Dietary Guidelines for Americans., U.S. Government Printing Office, Washington, DC, 2005.

[30] U.S. Department of Agriculture and U.S. Department of Health and Human Services, Dietary Guidelines for Americans, 2010, seventh ed, U S Government Printing Office, Washington, DC, 2010.

[31] American Dietetic Association, Disorders of Lipid Metabolism: Evidence-Based Nutrition Practice Guideline, American Dietetic Association, Chicago, 2007.

[32] A.H. Lichtenstein, L.J. Appel, M. Brands, M. Carnethon, S. Daniels, H.A. Franch, et al., Diet and lifestyle recommendations revision 2006: a scientific statement from the American Heart Association Nutrition Committee, Circulation 114 (2006) 82—96.

[33] A.H. Lichtenstein, L.J. Appel, M. Brands, M. Carnethon, S. Daniels, H.A. Franch, et al., Summary of American Heart Association diet and lifestyle recommendations revision 2006, Arterioscler. Thromb. Vasc. Biol. 26 (2006) 2186—2191.

[34] Expert Panel on Detection, Evaluation, and Treatment of High Blood Cholesterol in Adults, Executive summary of the third report of the National Cholesterol Education Program (NCEP) Expert Panel on Detection, Evaluation, and Treatment of High Blood Cholesterol in Adults (Adult Treatment Panel III), JAMA 285 (2001) 2486—2497.

[35] L.J. Appel, T.J. Moore, E. Obarzanek, W.M. Vollmer, L.P. Svetkey, F.M. Sacks, et al., A clinical trial of the effects of dietary patterns on blood pressure, N. Engl. J. Med. 336 (1997) 1117—1124.

[36] E. Obarzanek, F.M. Sacks, W.M. Vollmer, G.A. Bray, E.R. Miller III, P.H. Lin, et al., Effects on blood lipids of a blood pressure-lowering diet: the Dietary Approaches to Stop Hypertension (DASH) trial, Am. J. Clin. Nutr. 74 (2001) 80−89.

[37] S.T. Chen, N.M. Maruthur, L.J. Appel, The effect of dietary patterns on estimated coronary heart disease risk, Circ. Cardiovasc. Qual. Outcomes 3 (2010) 484−489.

[38] T.T. Fung, S.E. Chiuve, M.L. McCullough, K.M. Rexrode, G. Logroscino, F.B. Hu, Adherence to a DASH-style diet and risk of coronary heart disease and stroke in women, Arch. Intern. Med. 168 (2008) 713−720.

[39] A. Parikh, S.R. Lipsitz, S. Natarajan, Association between a DASH-like diet and mortality in adults with hypertension: findings from a population-based follow-up study, Am. J. Hypertens. 22 (2009) 409−416.

[40] F.B. Hu, et al., Prospective study of major dietary patterns and risk of coronary heart disease in men, Am. J. Clin. Nutr. 72 (4) (2000) 912−921.

[41] T.T. Fung, E.B. Rimm, D. Spiegelman, N. Rifai, G.H. Tofler, W.C. Willett, et al., Association between dietary patterns and plasma biomarkers of obesity and cardiovascular disease risk, Am. J. Clin. Nutr. 73 (2001) 61−67.

[42] M. Osler, B.L. Heitmann, L.U. Gerdes, L.M. Jorgensen, M. Schroll, Dietary patterns and mortality in Danish men and women: a prospective observational study, Br. J. Nutr. 85 (2001) 219−225.

[43] C. Heidemann, M.B. Schulze, O.H. Franco, R.M. van Dam, C.S. Mantzoros, F.B. Hu, Dietary patterns and risk of mortality from cardiovascular disease, cancer, and all causes in a prospective cohort of women, Circulation 118 (2008) 230−237.

[44] D. Li, Chemistry behind vegetarianism, J. Agric. Food Chem. 59 (2011) 777−784.

[45] L. Duo, A.J. Sinclair, N.J. Mann, A. Turner, M.J. Ball, Selected micronutrient intake and status in men with differing meat intakes, vegetarians and vegans, Asia Pacific J. Clin. Nutr. 9 (2000) 18−23.

[46] D.J. Jenkins, C.W. Kendall, D. Faulkner, E. Vidgen, E.A. Trautwein, T.L. Parker, et al., A dietary portfolio approach to cholesterol reduction: combined effects of plant sterols, vegetable proteins, and viscous fibers in hypercholesterolemia, Metabolism 51 (2002) 1596−1604.

[47] D.J. Jenkins, C.W. Kendall, A. Marchie, D. Faulkner, E. Vidgen, K.G. Lapsley, et al., The effect of combining plant sterols, soy protein, viscous fibers, and almonds in treating hypercholesterolemia, Metabolism 52 (2003) 1478−1483.

[48] D.J. Jenkins, C.W. Kendall, D.A. Faulkner, T. Nguyen, T. Kemp, A. Marchie, et al., Assessment of the longer-term effects of a dietary portfolio of cholesterol-lowering foods in hypercholesterolemia, Am. J. Clin. Nutr. 83 (2006) 582−591.

[49] D.J. Jenkins, P.J. Jones, B. Lamarche, C.W. Kendall, D. Faulkner, L. Cermakova, et al., Effect of a dietary portfolio of cholesterol-lowering foods given at 2 levels of intensity of dietary advice on serum lipids in hyperlipidemia: a randomized controlled trial, JAMA 306 (2011) 831−839.

[50] N. Chainani-Wu, G. Weidner, D.M. Purnell, S. Frenda, T. Merritt-Worden, C. Pischke, et al., Changes in emerging cardiac biomarkers after an intensive lifestyle intervention, Am. J. Cardiol. 108 (2011) 498−507.

[51] C.R. Pischke, L. Scherwitz, G. Weidner, D. Ornish, Long-term effects of lifestyle changes on well-being and cardiac variables among coronary heart disease patients, Health Psychol. 27 (2008) 584−592.

[52] D. Ornish, L.W. Scherwitz, J.H. Billings, S.E. Brown, K.L. Gould, T.A. Merritt, et al., Intensive lifestyle changes for reversal of coronary heart disease, JAMA 280 (1998) 2001−2007.

[53] D. Ornish, S.E. Brown, L.W. Scherwitz, J.H. Billings, W.T. Armstrong, T.A. Ports, et al., Lifestyle changes and heart disease, Lancet 336 (1990) 741−742.

[54] A. Keys, A. Menotti, M.J. Karvonen, C. Aravanis, H. Blackburn, R. Buzina, et al., The diet and 15-year death rate in the seven countries study, Am. J. Epidemiol. 124 (1986) 903−915.

[55] M. de Lorgeril, S. Renaud, N. Mamelle, P. Salen, J.L. Martin, I. Monjaud, et al., Mediterranean alpha-linolenic acid-rich diet in secondary prevention of coronary heart disease, Lancet 343 (1994) 1454−1459.

[56] F. Sofi, F. Cesari, R. Abbate, G.F. Gensini, A. Casini, Adherence to Mediterranean diet and health status: Meta-analysis, BMJ 337 (2008) a1344.

[57] A. Mente, L. de Koning, H.S. Shannon, S.S. Anand, A systematic review of the evidence supporting a causal link between dietary factors and coronary heart disease, Arch. Intern. Med. 169 (2009) 659−669.

[58] S.E. Chiuve, T.T. Fung, K.M. Rexrode, D. Spiegelman, J.E. Manson, M.J. Stampfer, et al., Adherence to a low-risk, healthy lifestyle and risk of sudden cardiac death among women, JAMA 306 (2011) 62−69.

[59] R. Estruch, M.A. Martinez-Gonzalez, D. Corella, J. Salas-Salvado, V. Ruiz-Gutierrez, M.I. Covas, et al., Effects of a Mediterranean-style diet on cardiovascular risk factors: a randomized trial, Ann. Intern. Med. 145 (2006) 1−11.

[60] J. Salas-Salvadó, M. Bulló, N. Babio, M.A. Martínez-González, N. Ibarrola-Jurado, J. Basora, et al., Reduction in the incidence of type 2 diabetes with the Mediterranean diet: results of the PREDIMED-Reus nutrition intervention randomized trial, Diabetes Care 34 (2011) 14−19.

[61] Institute of Medicine, Dietary Reference Intakes for Energy, Carbohydrate, Fiber, Fat, Fatty Acids, Cholesterol, Protein, and Amino Acids (Macronutrients), The National Academies Press, Washington, DC, 2005.

[62] B.V. Howard, L. Van Horn, J. Hsia, J.E. Manson, M.L. Stefanick, S. Wassertheil-Smoller, et al., Low-fat dietary pattern and risk of cardiovascular disease: the Women's Health Initiative randomized controlled dietary modification trial, JAMA 295 (2006) 655−666.

[63] A. Keys, J.T. Anderson, F. Grande, Serum cholesterol response to changes in the diet: IV. Particular saturated fatty acids in the diet, Metabolism 14 (1965) 776−787.

[64] D.M. Hegsted, R.B. McGandy, M.L. Myers, F.J. Stare, Quantitative effects of dietary fat on serum cholesterol in man, Am. J. Clin. Nutr. 17 (1965) 281−295.

[65] R. Clarke, C. Frost, R. Collins, P. Appleby, R. Peto, Dietary lipids and blood cholesterol: quantitative meta-analysis of metabolic ward studies, BMJ 314 (1997) 112−117.

[66] D.M. Hegsted, L.M. Ausman, J.A. Johnson, G.E. Dallal, Dietary fat and serum lipids: an evaluation of the experimental data, Am. J. Clin. Nutr. 57 (1993) 875−883.

[67] R.P. Mensink, M.B. Katan, Effect of dietary fatty acids on serum lipids and lipoproteins: a meta-analysis of 27 trials, Arterioscler. Thromb. 12 (1992) 911−919.

[68] P.M. Kris-Etherton, S. Yu, Individual fatty acid effects on plasma lipids and lipoproteins: human studies, Am. J. Clin. Nutr. 65 (1997) 1628S−1644S.

[69] S. Yu, J. Derr, T.D. Etherton, P.M. Kris-Etherton, Plasma cholesterol-predictive equations demonstrate that stearic acid is neutral and monounsaturated fatty acids are hypocholesterolemic, Am. J. Clin. Nutr. 61 (1995) 1129−1139.

[70] H. Muller, B. Kirkhus, J.I. Pedersen, Serum cholesterol predictive equations with special emphasis on trans and saturated fatty acids: an analysis from designed controlled studies, Lipids 36 (2001) 783−791.

[71] A. Keys, Coronary heart disease in seven countries, Circulation 41 (1970) I1−I211.

[72] F.B. Hu, M.J. Stampfer, J.E. Manson, E. Rimm, G.A. Colditz, B. A. Rosner, et al., Dietary fat intake and the risk of coronary heart disease in women, N. Engl. J. Med. 337 (1997) 1491−1499.

[73] B.M. Posner, J.L. Cobb, A.J. Belanger, L.A. Cupples, R.B. D'Agostino, J. Stokes III, Dietary lipid predictors of coronary heart disease in men: the Framingham Study, Arch. Intern. Med. 151 (1991) 1181−1187.

[74] E. Vartiainen, T. Laatikainen, M. Peltonen, A. Juolevi, S. Männistö, J. Sundvall, et al., Thirty-five-year trends in cardio-vascular risk factors in Finland, Int. J. Epidemiol. 39 (2010) 504−518.

[75] L. Berglund, M. Lefevre, H.N. Ginsberg, P.M. Kris-Etherton, P. J. Elmer, P.W. Stewart, et al., Comparison of monounsaturated fat with carbohydrates as a replacement for saturated fat in subjects with a high metabolic risk profile: studies in the fasting and postprandial states, Am. J. Clin. Nutr. 86 (2007) 1611−1620.

[76] A.H. Lichtenstein, N.R. Matthan, S.M. Jalbert, N.A. Resteghini, E.J. Schaefer, L.M. Ausman, Novel soybean oils with different fatty acid profiles alter cardiovascular disease risk factors in moderately hyperlipidemic subjects, Am. J. Clin. Nutr. 84 (2006) 497−504.

[77] S. Yu-Poth, T.D. Etherton, C.C. Reddy, T.A. Pearson, R. Reed, G. Zhao, et al., Lowering dietary saturated fat and total fat reduces the oxidative susceptibility of LDL in healthy men and women, J. Nutr. 130 (2000) 2228−2237.

[78] E. Balk, M. Chung, A. Lichtenstein, P. Chew, B. Kupelnick, A. Lawrence, et al., Effects of omega-3 fatty acids on cardiovascu-lar risk factors and intermediate markers of cardiovascular dis-ease, Evidence Rep. Technol. Assess. 93 (2004) 1−6.

[79] I. Kralova Lesna, P. Suchanek, J. Kovar, P. Stavek, R. Poledne, Replacement of dietary saturated FAs by PUFAs in diet and reverse cholesterol transport, J. Lipid Res. 49 (2008) 2414−2418.

[80] D. Mozaffarian, R. Micha, S. Wallace, Effects on coronary heart disease of increasing polyunsaturated fat in place of saturated fat: a systematic review and meta-analysis of randomized con-trolled trials, PLoS Med. 7 (2010) e1000252.

[81] R.P. Mensink, P.L. Zock, A.D. Kester, M.B. Katan, Effects of die-tary fatty acids and carbohydrates on the ratio of serum total to HDL cholesterol and on serum lipids and apolipoproteins: a meta-analysis of 60 controlled trials, Am. J. Clin. Nutr. 77 (2003) 1146−1155.

[82] D. Mozaffarian, R. Clarke, Quantitative effects on cardiovascu-lar risk factors and coronary heart disease risk of replacing par-tially hydrogenated vegetable oils with other fats and oils, Eur. J. Clin. Nutr. 63 (Suppl. 2) (2009) S22−S33.

[83] J.B. Keogh, J.A. Grieger, M. Noakes, P.M. Clifton, Flow-medi-ated dilatation is impaired by a high-saturated fat diet but not by a high-carbohydrate diet, Arterioscler. Thromb. Vasc. Biol. 25 (2005) 1274−1279.

[84] AIM-HIGH investigators, The role of niacin in raising high-density lipoprotein cholesterol to reduce cardiovascular events in patients with atherosclerotic cardiovascular disease and opti-mally treated low-density lipoprotein cholesterol: baseline char-acteristics of study participants. The Atherothrombosis Intervention in Metabolic Syndrome with Low HDL/High Triglycerides: impact on Global Health Outcomes (AIM-HIGH) trial, Am. Heart J. 161 (2011) 538−543.

[85] A.M. Bernstein, Q. Sun, F.B. Hu, M.J. Stampfer, J.E. Manson, W. C. Willett, Major dietary protein sources and risk of coronary heart disease in women, Circulation 122 (2010) 876−883.

[86] E. Shahar, A.R. Folsom, K.K. Wu, B.H. Dennis, T. Shimakawa, M.G. Conlan, et al., Associations of fish intake and dietary n-3 polyunsaturated fatty acids with a hypocoagulable profile: the Atherosclerosis Risk in Communities (ARIC) study, Arterioscler. Thromb. 13 (1993) 1205−1212.

[87] H.N. Ginsberg, P. Kris-Etherton, B. Dennis, P.J. Elmer, A. Ershow, M. Lefevre, et al., Effects of reducing dietary saturated fatty acids on plasma lipids and lipoproteins in healthy subjects : the Delta Study, Protocol 1, Arterioscler. Thromb. Vasc. Biol. 18 (1998) 441−449.

[88] S.M. Albelda, C.W. Smith, P.A. Ward, Adhesion molecules and inflammatory injury, FASEB J. 8 (1994) 504−512.

[89] K.K. Ray, D.A. Morrow, A. Shui, N. Rifai, C.P. Cannon, Relation between soluble intercellular adhesion molecule-1, statin therapy, and long-term risk of clinical cardiovascular events in patients with previous acute coronary syndrome (from PROVE IT-TIMI 22), Am. J. Cardiol. 98 (2006) 861−865.

[90] I. Shai, T. Pischon, F.B. Hu, A. Ascherio, N. Rifai, E.B. Rimm, Soluble intercellular adhesion molecules, soluble vascular cell adhesion molecules, and risk of coronary heart disease, Obesity 14 (2006) 2099−2106.

[91] M.U. Jakobsen, E.J. O'Reilly, B.L. Heitmann, M.A. Pereira, K. Balter, G.E. Fraser, et al., Major types of dietary fat and risk of coronary heart disease: a pooled analysis of 11 cohort studies, Am. J. Clin. Nutr. 89 (2009) 1425−1432.

[92] C.M. Skeaff, J. Miller, Dietary fat and coronary heart disease: summary of evidence from prospective cohort and randomised controlled trials, Ann. Nutr. Metab. 55 (2009) 173−201.

[93] P.W. Siri-Tarino, Q. Sun, F.B. Hu, R.M. Krauss, Meta-analysis of prospective cohort studies evaluating the association of satu-rated fat with cardiovascular disease, Am. J. Clin. Nutr. 91 (2010) 535−546.

[94] R.P. Mensink, M.B. Katan, Effect of dietary trans fatty acids on high-density and low-density lipoprotein cholesterol levels in healthy subjects, N. Engl. J. Med. 323 (1990) 439−445.

[95] D. Mozaffarian, A. Aro, W.C. Willett, Health effects of trans-fatty acids: experimental and observational evidence, Eur. J. Clin. Nutr. 63 (Suppl. 2) (2009) S5−S21.

[96] D.M. Lloyd-Jones, Y. Hong, D. Labarthe, D. Mozaffarian, L.J. Appel, L. Van Horn, et al., Defining and setting national goals for cardiovascular health promotion and disease reduction: the American Heart Association's strategic impact goal through 2020 and beyond, Circulation 121 (2010) 586−613.

[97] A.H. Lichtenstein, L.M. Ausman, S.M. Jalbert, E.J. Schaefer, Effects of different forms of dietary hydrogenated fats on serum lipoprotein cholesterol levels, N. Engl. J. Med. 340 (1999) 1933−1940.

[98] J.T. Judd, D.J. Baer, B.A. Clevidence, P. Kris-Etherton, R.A. Muesing, M. Iwane, Dietary cis and trans monounsaturated and saturated FA and plasma lipids and lipoproteins in men, Lipids 37 (2002) 123−131.

[99] A. Ascherio, W.C. Willett, Health effects of trans fatty acids, Am. J. Clin. Nutr. 66 (1997) 1006S−1010S.

[100] A. Ascherio, M.B. Katan, P.L. Zock, M.J. Stampfer, W.C. Willett, Trans fatty acids and coronary heart disease, N. Engl. J. Med. 340 (1999) 1994−1998.

[101] G. Lawrence, The Fats of Life: Essential Fatty Acids in Health and Disease, Rutgers University Press, Piscataway, NJ, 2010.

[102] P.L. Mitchell, R.S. McLeod, Conjugated linoleic acid and ath-erosclerosis: studies in animal models, Biochem. Cell Biol. 86 (2008) 293−301.

[103] S. Tricon, G.C. Burdge, E.L. Jones, J.J. Russell, S. El-Khazen, E. Moretti, et al., Effects of dairy products naturally enriched with cis-9,trans-11 conjugated linoleic acid on the blood lipid profile in healthy middle-aged men, Am. J. Clin. Nutr. 83 (2006) 744−753.

[104] A.J. Wanders, I.A. Brouwer, E. Siebelink, M.B. Katan, Effect of a high intake of conjugated linoleic acid on lipoprotein levels in healthy human subjects, PLoS One 5 (2010) e9000.

[105] J.-M. Chardigny, F. Destaillats, C. Malpuech-Brugère, J. Moulin, D.E. Bauman, A.L. Lock, et al., Do trans fatty acids from industrially produced sources and from natural sources have the same effect on cardiovascular disease risk factors in healthy subjects? Results of the Trans Fatty Acids Collaboration (TRANSFACT) study, Am. J. Clin. Nutr. 87 (2008) 558–566.

[106] A. Motard-Bélanger, A. Charest, G. Grenier, P. Paquin, Y. Chouinard, S. Lemieux, et al., Study of the effect of trans fatty acids from ruminants on blood lipids and other risk factors for cardiovascular disease, Am. J. Clin. Nutr. 87 (2008) 593–599.

[107] I.A. Brouwer, A.J. Wanders, M.B. Katan, Effect of animal and industrial trans fatty acids on HDL and LDL cholesterol levels in humans: a quantitative review, PLoS One 5 (2010) e9434.

[108] W. Willett, D. Mozaffarian, Ruminant or industrial sources of trans fatty acids: Public health issue or food label skirmish? Am. J. Clin. Nutr. 87 (2008) 515–516.

[109] A. Garg, High-monounsaturated-fat diets for patients with diabetes mellitus: a meta-analysis, Am. J. Clin. Nutr. 67 (1998) 577S–582S.

[110] B. Gumbiner, C.C. Low, P.D. Reaven, Effects of a monounsaturated fatty acid-enriched hypocaloric diet on cardiovascular risk factors in obese patients with type 2 diabetes, Diabetes Care 21 (1998) 9–15.

[111] P. Reaven, S. Parthasarathy, B.J. Grasse, E. Miller, D. Steinberg, J.L. Witztum, Effects of oleate-rich and linoleate-rich diets on the susceptibility of low density lipoprotein to oxidative modification in mildly hypercholesterolemic subjects, J. Clin. Invest. 91 (1993) 668–676.

[112] C. Colette, C. Percheron, N. Pares-Herbute, F. Michel, T.C. Pham, L. Brillant, et al., Exchanging carbohydrates for monounsaturated fats in energy-restricted diets: effects on metabolic profile and other cardiovascular risk factors, Int. J. Obes. Relat. Metab. Disord. 27 (2003) 648–656.

[113] Y. Cao, D.T. Mauger, C.L. Pelkman, G. Zhao, S.M. Townsend, P.M. Kris-Etherton, Effects of moderate (MF) versus lower fat (LF) diets on lipids and lipoproteins: a meta-analysis of clinical trials in subjects with and without diabetes, J. Clin. Lipidol 3 (2009) 19–32.

[114] M. Tanasescu, E. Cho, J.E. Manson, F.B. Hu, Dietary fat and cholesterol and the risk of cardiovascular disease among women with type 2 diabetes, Am. J. Clin. Nutr. 79 (2004) 999–1005.

[115] K. Loss, C.K. Chow (Eds.), Fatty Acids in Foods and Their Health Implications, Dekker, New York, 2000.

[116] P.M. Kris-Etherton, D.S. Taylor, S. Yu-Poth, P. Huth, K. Moriarty, V. Fishell, et al., Polyunsaturated fatty acids in the food chain in the United States, Am. J. Clin. Nutr. 71 (2000) 179S–188S.

[117] A.P. Simopoulos, Omega-3 fatty acids in health and disease and in growth and development, Am. J. Clin. Nutr. 54 (1991) 438–463.

[118] L.M. Arterburn, E.B. Hall, H. Oken, Distribution, interconversion, and dose response of n-3 fatty acids in humans, Am. J. Clin. Nutr. 83 (2006) S1467–S1476.

[119] G.C. Burdge, Y.E. Finnegan, A.M. Minihane, C.M. Williams, S.A. Wootton, Effect of altered dietary n-3 fatty acid intake upon plasma lipid fatty acid composition, conversion of [13C]alpha-linolenic acid to longer-chain fatty acids and partitioning towards beta-oxidation in older men, Br. J. Nutr. 90 (2003) 311–321.

[120] G.C. Burdge, A.E. Jones, S.A. Wootton, Eicosapentaenoic and docosapentaenoic acids are the principal products of alpha-linolenic acid metabolism in young men, Br. J. Nutr. 88 (2002) 355–363.

[121] G.C. Burdge, S.A. Wootton, Conversion of alpha-linolenic acid to eicosapentaenoic, docosapentaenoic and docosahexaenoic acids in young women, Br. J. Nutr. 88 (2002) 411–420.

[122] C.N. Serhan, M. Hamberg, B. Samuelsson, Lipoxins: novel series of biologically active compounds formed from arachidonic acid in human leukocytes, Proc. Natl. Acad. Sci. USA 81 (1984) 5335–5339.

[123] N. Chiang, M. Arita, C.N. Serhan, Anti-inflammatory circuitry: lipoxin, aspirin-triggered lipoxins and their receptor ALX, Prostaglandins Leukot. Essent. Fatty Acids 73 (2005) 163–177.

[124] A. Ariel, C.N. Serhan, Resolvins and protectins in the termination program of acute inflammation, Trends Immunol. 28 (2007) 176–183.

[125] P.C. Calder, Polyunsaturated fatty acids, inflammatory processes and inflammatory bowel diseases, Mol. Nutr. Food Res. 52 (2008) 885–897.

[126] C.A. Hudert, K.H. Weylandt, Y. Lu, J. Wang, S. Hong, A. Dignass, et al., Transgenic mice rich in endogenous omega-3 fatty acids are protected from colitis, Proc. Natl. Acad. Sci. USA 103 (2006) 11276–11281.

[127] A. Keys, "Coronary Heart Disease in Seven Countries," Monograph No. 29., American Heart Association, New York, 1970.

[128] F.M. Sacks, M. Katan, Randomized clinical trials on the effects of dietary fat and carbohydrate on plasma lipoproteins and cardiovascular disease, Am. J. Med. 113 (Suppl. 9B) (2002) 13S–24S.

[129] P. Leren, The effect of plasma cholesterol lowering diet in male survivors of myocardial infarction: a controlled clinical trial, Acta Med. Scand. Suppl. 466 (1966) 1–92.

[130] O. Turpeinen, M.J. Karvonen, M. Pekkarinen, M. Miettinen, R. Elosuo, E. Paavilainen, Dietary prevention of coronary heart disease: the Finnish Mental Hospital Study, Int. J. Epidemiol. 8 (1979) 99–118.

[131] S. Dayton, M.L. Pearce, S. Hashimoto, L.J. Fakler, E. Hiscock, W.J. Dixon, A controlled clinical trial of a diet high in unsaturated fat: preliminary observations, N. Engl. J. Med. 266 (1962) 1017–1023.

[132] F.B. Hu, M.J. Stampfer, J.E. Manson, E. Rimm, G.A. Colditz, F.E. Speizer, et al., Dietary protein and risk of ischemic heart disease in women, Am. J. Clin. Nutr. 70 (1999) 221–227.

[133] D. Mozaffarian, W.T. Longstreth Jr., R.N. Lemaitre, T.A. Manolio, L.H. Kuller, G.L. Burke, et al., Fish consumption and stroke risk in elderly individuals: the Cardiovascular Health Study, Arch. Intern. Med. 165 (2005) 200–206.

[134] A.R. Folsom, Z. Demissie, Fish intake, marine omega-3 fatty acids, and mortality in a cohort of postmenopausal women, Am. J. Epidemiol. 160 (2004) 1005–1010.

[135] T. Dolecek, G. Granditis, Dietary polyunsaturated fatty acids and mortality in the Multiple Risk Factor Intervention Trial (MRFIT), World Rev. Nutr. Diet. 66 (1991) 205–216.

[136] M. de Lorgeril, S. Renaud, N. Mamelle, P. Salen, J. Martin, I. Monjaud, et al., Mediterranean alpha-linolenic acid-rich diet in secondary prevention of coronary heart disease, Lancet 343 (1994) 1454–1459.

[137] M. de Lorgeril, P. Salen, J.-L. Martin, I. Monjaud, J. Delaye, N. Mamelle, Mediterranean diet, traditional risk factors, and the rate of cardiovascular complications after myocardial infarction: final report of the Lyon Diet Heart Study, Circulation 99 (1999) 779–785.

[138] P. Kris-Etherton, R.H. Eckel, B.V. Howard, S. St. Jeor, T.L. Bazzarre, Lyon Diet Heart Study: benefits of a Mediterranean-Style, National Cholesterol Education Program/American

Heart Association Step I Dietary Pattern on Cardiovascular Disease, Circulation 103 (2001) 1823–1825.

[139] C. Wang, W.S. Harris, M. Chung, A.H. Lichtenstein, E.M. Balk, B. Kupelnick, et al., n-3 Fatty acids from fish or fish-oil supplements, but not α-linolenic acid, benefit cardiovascular disease outcomes in primary- and secondary-prevention studies: a systematic review, Am. J. Clin. Nutr. 84 (2006) 5–17.

[140] J. Dyerberg, H.O. Bang, N. Hjorne, Fatty acid composition of the plasma lipids in Greenland Eskimos, Am. J. Clin. Nutr. 28 (1975) 958–966.

[141] S. Richter, G. Duray, G. Gronefeld, C.W. Isreal, S.H. Hohnloser, Prevention of sudden cardiac death: lessons from recent controlled trials, Circ. J. 69 (2005) 625–629.

[142] D. Mozaffarian, E.B. Rimm, Fish intake, contaminants, and human health: evaluating the risks and the benefits, JAMA 296 (2006) 1885–1899.

[143] D.S. Siscovick, R.N. Lemaitre, D. Mozaffarian, The fish story: a diet-heart hypothesis with clinical implications: n-3 polyunsaturated fatty acids, myocardial vulnerability, and sudden death, Circulation 107 (2003) 2632–2634.

[144] Multiple Risk Factor Intervention Trial Research Group, Multiple risk factor intervention trial: risk factor changes and mortality results, JAMA 248 (1982) 1465–1477.

[145] F.B. Hu, L. Bronner, W.C. Willett, M.J. Stampfer, K.M. Rexrode, C.M. Albert, et al., Fish and omega-3 fatty acid intake and risk of coronary heart disease in women, JAMA 287 (2002) 1815–1821.

[146] M.C. Morris, J.E. Manson, B. Rosner, J.E. Buring, W.C. Willett, C.H. Hennekens, Fish consumption and cardiovascular disease in the Physicians' Health Study: a prospective study, Am. J. Epidemiol. 142 (1995) 166–175.

[147] P. Pietinen, A. Ascherio, P. Korhonen, A.M. Hartman, W.C. Willett, D. Albanes, et al., Intake of fatty acids and risk of coronary heart disease in a cohort of Finnish men: the alpha-tocopherol, beta-carotene cancer prevention study, Am. J. Epidemiol. 145 (1997) 876–887.

[148] Gruppo Italiano per lo Studio della Sopravvivenza nell'Infarto Miocardico, Dietary supplementation with n-3 polyunsaturated fatty acids and vitamin E after myocardial infarction: results of the GISSI-Prevenzione trial, Lancet 354 (1999) 447–455.

[149] L. Tavazzi, A.P. Maggioni, R. Marchioli, S. Barlera, M.G. Franzosi, R. Latini, et al., Effect of n-3 polyunsaturated fatty acids in patients with chronic heart failure (the GISSI-HF trial): a randomised, double-blind, placebo-controlled trial, Lancet 372 (2008) 1223–1230.

[150] M.L. Burr, A.M. Fehily, J.F. Gilbert, S. Rogers, R.M. Holliday, P.M. Sweetnam, et al., Effects of changes in fat, fish, and fibre intakes on death and myocardial reinfarction: diet and Reinfarction Trial (DART), Lancet 2 (1989) 757–761.

[151] M. Yokoyama, H. Origasa, M. Matsuzaki, Y. Matsuzawa, Y. Saito, Y. Ishikawa, et al., Effects of eicosapentaenoic acid on major coronary events in hypercholesterolaemic patients (JELIS): a randomised open-label, blinded endpoint analysis, Lancet 369 (2007) 1090–1098.

[152] B. Rauch, R. Schiele, S. Schneider, F. Diller, N. Victor, H. Gohlke, et al., OMEGA, a randomized, placebo-controlled trial to test the effect of highly purified omega-3 fatty acids on top of modern guideline-adjusted therapy after myocardial infarction, Circulation 122 (2010) 2152–2159.

[153] D. Kromhout, E.J. Giltay, J.M. Geleijnse, n-3 fatty acids and cardiovascular events after myocardial infarction, N. Engl. J. Med. 363 (2010) 2015–2026.

[154] A. Leaf, Y.F. Xiao, J.X. Kang, G.E. Billman, Membrane effects of the n-3 fish oil fatty acids, which prevent fatal ventricular arrhythmias, J. Membr. Biol. 206 (2005) 129–139.

[155] M.H. Raitt, W.E. Connor, C. Morris, J. Kron, B. Halperin, S.S. Chugh, et al., Fish oil supplementation and risk of ventricular tachycardia and ventricular fibrillation in patients with implantable defibrillators: a randomized controlled trial, JAMA 293 (2005) 2884–2891.

[156] I.A. Brouwer, P.L. Zock, A.J. Camm, D. Bocker, R.N. Hauer, E.F. Wever, et al., Effect of fish oil on ventricular tachyarrhythmia and death in patients with implantable cardioverter defibrillators: the Study on Omega-3 Fatty Acids and Ventricular Arrhythmia (SOFA) randomized trial, JAMA 295 (2006) 2613–2619.

[157] A. Leaf, J.X. Kang, Y.F. Xiao, Fish oil fatty acids as cardiovascular drugs, Curr. Vasc. Pharmacol. 6 (2008) 1–12.

[158] E.M. Balk, A.H. Lichtenstein, M. Chung, B. Kupelnick, P. Chew, J. Lau, Effects of omega-3 fatty acids on serum markers of cardiovascular disease risk: a systematic review, Atherosclerosis 189 (2006) 19–30.

[159] A.C. Skulas-Ray, P.M. Kris-Etherton, W.S. Harris, J.P. Vanden Heuvel, P.R. Wagner, S.G. West, Dose–response effects of omega-3 fatty acids on triglycerides, inflammation, and endothelial function in healthy persons with moderate hypertriglyceridemia, Am. J. Clin. Nutr. 93 (2011) 243–252.

[160] A.C. Skulas-Ray, S.G. West, M.H. Davidson, P.M. Kris-Etherton, Omega-3 fatty acid concentrates in the treatment of moderate hypertriglyceridemia, Expert Opin. Pharmacother. 9 (2008) 1237–1248.

[161] A.A. Rivellese, A. Maffettone, B. Vessby, M. Uusitupa, K. Hermansen, L. Berglund, et al., Effects of dietary saturated, monounsaturated and n-3 fatty acids on fasting lipoproteins, LDL size and post-prandial lipid metabolism in healthy subjects, Atherosclerosis 167 (2003) 149–158.

[162] A.M. Minihane, S. Khan, E.C. Leigh-Firbank, P. Talmud, J.W. Wright, M.C. Murphy, et al., ApoE polymorphism and fish oil supplementation in subjects with an atherogenic lipoprotein phenotype, Arterioscler. Thromb. 20 (2000) 1990–1997.

[163] T.A. Mori, V. Burke, I.B. Puddey, G.F. Watts, D.N. O'Neal, J.D. Best, et al., Purified eicosapentaenoic and docosahexaenoic acids have differential effects on serum lipids and lipoproteins, LDL particle size, glucose, and insulin in mildly hyperlipidemic men, Am. J. Clin. Nutr. 71 (2000) 1085–1094.

[164] M.H. Davidson, E.A. Stein, H.E. Bays, K.C. Maki, R.T. Doyle, R.A. Shalwitz, et al., Efficacy and tolerability of adding prescription omega-3 fatty acids 4 g/d to simvastatin 40 mg/d in hypertriglyceridemic patients: an 8-week, randomized, double-blind, placebo-controlled study, Clin. Ther. 29 (2007) 1354–1367.

[165] P.M. Kris-Etherton, W.S. Harris, L.J. Appel, Fish consumption, fish oil, omega-3 fatty acids, and cardiovascular disease, American Heart Association, Nutrition Committee, Circulation 106 (2002) 2747–2757.

[166] J.T. Salonen, K. Seppanen, K. Nyyssonen, H. Korpela, J. Kauhanen, M. Kantola, et al., Intake of mercury from fish, lipid peroxidation, and the risk of myocardial infarction and coronary, cardiovascular, and any death in eastern Finnish men, Circulation 91 (1995) 645–655.

[167] E. Guallar, M.I. Sanz-Gallardo, P. van't Veer, P. Bode, A. Aro, J. Gomez-Aracena, et al., Mercury, fish oils, and the risk of myocardial infarction, N. Engl. J. Med. 347 (2002) 1747–1754.

[168] J.K. Virtanen, S. Voutilainen, T.H. Rissanen, J. Mursu, T.-P. Tuomainen, M.J. Korhonen, et al., Mercury, fish oils, and risk of acute coronary events and cardiovascular disease, coronary heart disease, and all-cause mortality in men in eastern Finland, Arterioscler. Thromb. 25 (2005) 228–233.

[169] S.E. Foran, J.G. Flood, K.B. Lewandrowski, Measurement of mercury levels in concentrated over-the-counter fish oil

preparations: Is fish oil healthier than fish? Arch. Pathol. Lab. Med. 127 (2003) 1603−1605.

[170] Research Committee, Controlled trial of soya-bean oil in myocardial infarction, Lancet 2 (1968) 693−699.

[171] A. Kusumoto, Y. Ishikura, H. Kawashima, Y. Kiso, S. Takai, M. Miyazaki, Effects of arachidonate-enriched triacylglycerol supplementation on serum fatty acids and platelet aggregation in healthy male subjects with a fish diet, Br. J. Nutr. 98 (2007) 626−635.

[172] S.M. Grundy, What is the desirable ratio of saturated, polyunsaturated, and monounsaturated fatty acids in the diet? Am. J. Clin. Nutr. 66 (4) (1997) 988S−990S.

[173] D. Mozaffarian, Does alpha-linolenic acid intake reduce the risk of coronary heart disease? A review of the evidence, Alternative Therap. Health Med. 11 (2005) 24−30 quiz 31, 79

[174] P.C. Calder, The American Heart Association advisory on n-6 fatty acids: Evidence based or biased evidence? Br. J. Nutr. 104 (2010) 1575−1576.

[175] A.P. Simopoulos, The importance of the omega-6/omega-3 fatty acid ratio in cardiovascular disease and other chronic diseases, Exp. Biol. Med. 233 (2008) 674−688.

[176] C.E. Ramsden, J.R. Hibbeln, S.F. Majchrzak-Hong, All PUFAs are not created equal: absence of CHD benefit specific to linoleic acid in randomized controlled trials and prospective observational cohorts, World Rev. Nutr. Diet. 102 (2011) 30−43.

[177] C.E. Ramsden, J.R. Hibbeln, S.F. Majchrzak, J.M. Davis, n-6 fatty acid-specific and mixed polyunsaturate dietary interventions have different effects on CHD risk: a meta-analysis of randomised controlled trials, Br. J. Nutr. 104 (2010) 1586−1600.

[178] Ramsden, C. E., Hibbeln, J. R., and Lands, W. E. (2009). Letter to the Editor re: linoleic acid and coronary heart disease. Prostaglandins Leukot. Essent. Fatty Acids (2008), by W.S. Harris. Prostaglandins Leukot. Essent. Fatty Acids 80, 77; author reply 77−78.

[179] W.S. Harris, B. Assaad, W.C. Poston, Tissue omega-6/omega-3 fatty acid ratio and risk for coronary artery disease, Am. J. Cardiol. 98 (2006) 19i−26i.

[180] P.M. Kris-Etherton, W.S. Harris, Adverse effect of fish oils in patients with angina? Curr. Atheroscler. Rep. 6 (2004) 413−414.

[181] R.K. Johnson, L.J. Appel, M. Brands, B.V. Howard, M. Lefevre, R.H. Lustig, et al., Dietary sugars intake and cardiovascular health: a scientific statement from the American Heart Association, Circulation 120 (2009) 1011−1020.

[182] A.E. Jarvi, B.E. Karlstrom, Y.E. Granfeldt, I.E. Bjorck, N.G. Asp, B.O. Vessby, Improved glycemic control and lipid profile and normalized fibrinolytic activity on a low-glycemic index diet in type 2 diabetic patients, Diabetes Care 22 (1999) 10−18.

[183] T.M. Wolever, D.J. Jenkins, V. Vuksan, A.L. Jenkins, G.S. Wong, R.G. Josse, Beneficial effect of low-glycemic index diet in overweight NIDDM subjects, Diabetes Care 15 (1992) 562−564.

[184] D.S. Ludwig, The glycemic index: physiological mechanisms relating to obesity, diabetes, and cardiovascular disease, JAMA 287 (2002) 2414−2423.

[185] S. Liu, J.E. Manson, M.J. Stampfer, F.B. Hu, E. Giovannucci, G. A. Colditz, et al., A prospective study of whole-grain intake and risk of type 2 diabetes mellitus in U.S. women, Am. J. Public Health 90 (2000) 1409−1415.

[186] T.L. Halton, W.C. Willett, S. Liu, J.E. Manson, C.M. Albert, K. Rexrode, et al., Low-carbohydrate-diet score and the risk of coronary heart disease in women, N. Engl. J. Med. 355 (2006) 1991−2002.

[187] S. Liu, J.E. Manson, J.E. Buring, M.J. Stampfer, W.C. Willett, P. M. Ridker, Relation between a diet with a high glycemic load and plasma concentrations of high-sensitivity C-reactive protein in middle-aged women, Am. J. Clin. Nutr. 75 (2002) 492−498.

[188] R.M. van Dam, A.W. Visscher, E.J. Feskens, P. Verhoef, D. Kromhout, Dietary glycemic index in relation to metabolic risk factors and incidence of coronary heart disease: the Zutphen Elderly Study, Eur. J. Clin. Nutr. 54 (2000) 726−731.

[189] J.W. Anderson, T.J. Hanna, Impact of nondigestible carbohydrates on serum lipoproteins and risk for cardiovascular disease, J. Nutr. 129 (1999) 1457.

[190] J.W. Anderson, M.H. Davidson, L. Blonde, W.V. Brown, W.J. Howard, H. Ginsberg, et al., Long-term cholesterol-lowering effects of psyllium as an adjunct to diet therapy in the treatment of hypercholesterolemia, Am. J. Clin. Nutr. 71 (2000) 1433−1438.

[191] M.H. Davidson, K.C. Maki, J.C. Kong, L.D. Dugan, S.A. Torri, H.A. Hall, et al., Long-term effects of consuming foods containing psyllium seed husk on serum lipids in subjects with hypercholesterolemia [published erratum appears in Am. J. Clin. Nutr. 1998 Jun;67(6):1286] Am. J. Clin. Nutr. 67 (1998) 367−376.

[192] M.A. Pereira, E. O'Reilly, K. Augustsson, G.E. Fraser, U. Goldbourt, B.L. Heitmann, et al., Dietary fiber and risk of coronary heart disease: a pooled analysis of cohort studies, Arch. Intern. Med. 164 (2004) 370−376.

[193] A.D. Liese, A.K. Roach, K.C. Sparks, L. Marquart, R.B. D'Agostino Jr., E.J. Mayer-Davis, Whole-grain intake and insulin sensitivity: the Insulin Resistance Atherosclerosis Study, Am. J. Clin. Nutr. 78 (2003) 965−971.

[194] S.R. Glore, D. Van Treeck, A.W. Knehans, M. Guild, Soluble fiber and serum lipids: a literature review, J. Am. Diet. Assoc. 94 (1994) 425−436.

[195] M. Biorklund, A. van Rees, R.P. Mensink, G. Onning, Changes in serum lipids and postprandial glucose and insulin concentrations after consumption of beverages with beta-glucans from oats or barley: a randomised dose-controlled trial, Eur. J. Clin. Nutr. 59 (2005) 1272−1281.

[196] K.C. Maki, J.M. Beiseigel, S.S. Jonnalagadda, C.K. Gugger, M.S. Reeves, M.V. Farmer, et al., Whole-grain ready-to-eat oat cereal, as part of a dietary program for weight loss, reduces low-density lipoprotein cholesterol in adults with overweight and obesity more than a dietary program including low-fiber control foods, J. Am. Diet. Assoc. 110 (2010) 205−214.

[197] R.A. Othman, M.H. Moghadasian, P.J. Jones, Cholesterol-lowering effects of oat beta-glucan, Nutr. Rev. 69 (2011) 299−309.

[198] N.K. Fukagawa, J.W. Anderson, G. Hageman, V.R. Young, K.L. Minaker, High-carbohydrate, high-fiber diets increase peripheral insulin sensitivity in healthy young and old adults, Am. J. Clin. Nutr. 52 (1990) 524−528.

[199] J.W. Anderson, J.A. Zeigler, D.A. Deakins, T.L. Floore, D.W. Dillon, C.L. Wood, et al., Metabolic effects of high-carbohydrate, high-fiber diets for insulin-dependent diabetic individuals, Am. J. Clin. Nutr. 54 (1991) 936−943.

[200] J. Hallfrisch, D.J. Scholfield, K.M. Behall, Diets containing soluble oat extracts improve glucose and insulin responses of moderately hypercholesterolemic men and women, Am. J. Clin. Nutr. 61 (1995) 379−384.

[201] S. Yu-Poth, G. Zhao, T. Etherton, M. Naglak, S. Jonnalagadda, P.M. Kris-Etherton, Effects of the National Cholesterol Education Program's step I and step II dietary intervention programs on cardiovascular disease risk factors: a meta-analysis, Am. J. Clin. Nutr. 69 (1999) 632−646.

[202] R.A. DeFronzo, E. Ferrannini, Insulin resistance: a multifaceted syndrome responsible for NIDDM, obesity, hypertension, dyslipidemia, and atherosclerotic cardiovascular disease, Diabetes Care 14 (1991) 173−194.

[203] M. Parillo, A.A. Rivellese, A.V. Ciardullo, B. Capaldo, A. Giacco, S. Genovese, et al., A high-monounsaturated-fat/low-carbohydrate diet improves peripheral insulin sensitivity in non-insulin-dependent diabetic patients, Metabolism 41 (1992) 1373–1378.

[204] J. Jeppesen, P. Schaaf, C. Jones, M.Y. Zhou, Y.D. Chen, G.M. Reaven, Effects of low-fat, high-carbohydrate diets on risk factors for ischemic heart disease in postmenopausal women [published erratum appears in Am. J. Clin. Nutr. 1997 Aug;66 (2):437] Am. J. Clin. Nutr. 65 (1997) 1027–1033.

[205] D. Ornish, L.W. Scherwitz, J.H. Billings, K.L. Gould, T.A. Merritt, S. Sparler, et al., Intensive lifestyle changes for reversal of coronary heart disease, JAMA 280 (1998) 2001–2007.

[206] D. Ornish, S.E. Brown, L.W. Scherwitz, J.H. Billings, W.T. Armstrong, T.A. Ports, et al., Can lifestyle changes reverse coronary heart disease? The Lifestyle Heart Trial, Lancet 336 (1990) 129–133.

[207] D.W. Harsha, F.M. Sacks, E. Obarzanek, L.P. Svetkey, P.-H. Lin, G.A. Bray, et al., Effect of dietary sodium intake on blood lipids: results from the DASH-sodium trial, Hypertension 43 (2004) 393–398.

[208] M.L. Dansinger, J.A. Gleason, J.L. Griffith, H.P. Selker, E.J. Schaefer, Comparison of the Atkins, Ornish, Weight Watchers, and Zone diets for weight loss and heart disease risk reduction: a randomized trial, JAMA 293 (2005) 43–53.

[209] A.J. Nordmann, A. Nordmann, M. Briel, U. Keller, W.S. Yancy Jr., B.J. Brehm, et al., Effects of low-carbohydrate vs. low-fat diets on weight loss and cardiovascular risk factors: a meta-analysis of randomized controlled trials, Arch. Intern. Med. 166 (2006) 285–293.

[210] R.M. Krauss, P.J. Blanche, R.S. Rawlings, H.S. Fernstrom, P.T. Williams, Separate effects of reduced carbohydrate intake and weight loss on atherogenic dyslipidemia, Am. J. Clin. Nutr. 83 (2006) 1025–1031.

[211] J.S. Volek, M.J. Sharman, C.E. Forsythe, Modification of lipoproteins by very low-carbohydrate diets, J. Nutr. 135 (2005) 1339–1342.

[212] H.N. Ginsberg, New perspectives on atherogenesis: role of abnormal triglyceride-rich lipoprotein metabolism, Circulation 106 (2002) 2137–2142.

[213] K. Esposito, M. Ciotola, D. Giugliano, Low-carbohydrate diet and coronary heart disease in women, N. Engl. J. Med. 356 (2007) 750 author reply 750–752

[214] P. Lagiou, S. Sandin, E. Weiderpass, A. Lagiou, L. Mucci, D. Trichopoulos, et al., Low carbohydrate–high protein diet and mortality in a cohort of Swedish women, J. Intern. Med. 261 (2007) 366–374.

[215] A. Trichopoulou, T. Psaltopoulou, P. Orfanos, C.C. Hsieh, D. Trichopoulos, Low-carbohydrate–high-protein diet and long-term survival in a general population cohort, Eur. J. Clin. Nutr. 61 (2007) 575–581.

[216] F.B. Hu, E.B. Rimm, M.J. Stampfer, A. Ascherio, D. Spiegelman, W.C. Willett, Prospective study of major dietary patterns and risk of coronary heart disease in men, Am. J. Clin. Nutr. 72 (2000) 912–921.

[217] D.H. Blankenhorn, R.L. Johnson, W.J. Mack, H.A. el Zein, L.I. Vailas, The influence of diet on the appearance of new lesions in human coronary arteries, JAMA 263 (1990) 1646–1652.

[218] A.H. Terpstra, R.J. Hermus, C.E. West, The role of dietary protein in cholesterol metabolism, World Rev. Nutr. Diet. 42 (1983) 1–55.

[219] J. Stamler, Population studies. *In* "Nutrition, Lipids and Coronary Heart Disease", Raven Press, New York, 1979.

[220] R. Micha, S.K. Wallace, D. Mozaffarian, Red and processed meat consumption and risk of incident coronary heart disease, stroke, and diabetes mellitus: a systematic review and meta-analysis, Circulation 121 (2010) 2271–2283.

[221] Food and Nutrition Board, Institute of Medicine, Dietary Reference Intakes for Energy, Carbohydrate, Fiber, Fat, Fatty Acids, Cholesterol, Protein, and Amino Acids., National Academies Press, Washington, DC, 2002.

[222] Y. Nakamura, T. Okamura, S. Tamaki, T. Kadowaki, T. Hayakawa, Y. Kita, et al., Egg consumption, serum cholesterol, and cause-specific and all-cause mortality: The National Integrated Project for Prospective Observation of Non-communicable Disease and Its Trends in the Aged, 1980 (NIPPON DATA80), Am. J. Clin. Nutr. 80 (2004) 58–63.

[223] F.B. Hu, M.J. Stampfer, J.E. Manson, A. Ascherio, G.A. Colditz, F.E. Speizer, et al., Dietary saturated fats and their food sources in relation to the risk of coronary heart disease in women, Am. J. Clin. Nutr. 70 (1999) 1001–1008.

[224] T.R. Dawber, R.J. Nickerson, F.N. Brand, J. Pool, Eggs, serum cholesterol, and coronary heart disease, Am. J. Clin. Nutr. 36 (1982) 617–625.

[225] W.B. Kannel, T. Gordon, The Framingham Diet Study: Diet and the Regulations of Serum Cholesterol., U.S. Department of Health, Education, and Welfare, Washington, DC, 1970.

[226] R.M. Weggemans, P.L. Zock, M.B. Katan, Dietary cholesterol from eggs increases the ratio of total cholesterol to high-density lipoprotein cholesterol in humans: a meta-analysis, Am. J. Clin. Nutr. 73 (2001) 885–891.

[227] M. Kratz, Dietary cholesterol, atherosclerosis and coronary heart disease, Handb. Exp. Pharmacol. (2005) 195–213.

[228] D.J. Jenkins, C.W. Kendall, M. Axelsen, L.S. Augustin, V. Vuksan, Viscous and nonviscous fibres, nonabsorbable and low glycaemic index carbohydrates, blood lipids and coronary heart disease, Curr. Opin. Lipidol. 11 (2000) 49–56.

[229] R. Micha, D. Mozaffarian, Saturated fat and cardiometabolic risk factors, coronary heart disease, stroke, and diabetes: a fresh look at the evidence, Lipids 45 (2010) 893–905.

[230] Institute of Medicine, Seafood Choices: Balancing Benefits and Risks, National Academies Press, Washington, DC, 2006.

D. CARDIOVASCULAR DISEASE

Nutrition, Lifestyle, and Hypertension

Pao-Hwa Lin, Bryan C. Batch, Laura P. Svetkey

Duke University Medical Center, Durham, North Carolina

I INTRODUCTION

Approximately 30% of U.S. adults have hypertension,[1] a major risk factor for coronary heart disease, stroke, and premature death [1—3]. Furthermore, approximately 28% of U.S. adults have prehypertension,[2] which is also associated with a graded, increased risk of cardiovascular disease (CVD) and progression to hypertension [2—4]. Studies have shown that for every 20-mm Hg increase in systolic blood pressure (SBP) or 10-mm Hg increase in diastolic blood pressure (DBP), there is a doubling of mortality from ischemic heart disease (IHD) and stroke (Table 30.1) [2]. In industrialized societies, blood pressure (BP) increases with age: More than 50% of Americans ages 60—69 and more than three-fourths of those ages 70 or older are affected [5]. Hypertension is more common in African Americans [1]. Although the cause of hypertension is largely unknown, 1—5% of hypertension cases are due to a secondary underlying correctable condition.

In contrast to the prevalence in the United States, many non-Westernized, remote populations have a low prevalence of hypertension and do not experience an increase in BP with age [6,7]. Their protection from hypertension is often attributed to a very low salt intake [8—10], a rich potassium intake [9,11], being physically active [6], low alcohol consumption [9,12], and generally high plant food and fish consumption. Migration studies of indigenous populations also report increasing prevalence of hypertension with urbanization, providing additional evidence for a role

of environmental factors [13,14]. With urbanization, access to processed food increases, and fresh foods that were previously readily available become less affordable. In addition to other lifestyle changes, increases in body weight, sodium intake, dietary fat, and the ratio of urinary sodium to potassium have been observed during the process of acculturation [12—18]. Taken together, these observations support an important role of diet and lifestyle in BP and inspired much of the later research in this area.

In this chapter, we provide an overview of epidemiologic and clinical evidence for established and potential dietary factors for hypertension prevention and control. Because a comprehensive review of all individual trials in this area is beyond the scope of this chapter, when applicable, we review meta-analyses. Although meta-analyses are useful for evaluating consistency in the literature, they tend to weigh large studies more heavily [19,20], and it is rarely feasible to conduct subanalyses on potentially important modifying factors or to account for variable dietary adherence among studies.

The last two sections of this chapter are devoted to the review of several large-scale intervention trials. These trials include the whole diet-based controlled feeding trials such as the Dietary Approaches to Stop Hypertension (DASH) trial [21], DASH-Sodium [22], and OmniHeart [23] trials. In addition, large-scale multi-lifestyle intervention trials, including Trials of Hypertension Prevention (TOHP) I [24], TOHP II [25], and PREMIER [26], are also reviewed. Issues related to implementation of the current national guidelines are discussed. We

---

[1]The operational definition of hypertension is an SBP of 140 mm Hg or greater, a DBP of 90 mm Hg or greater, or current use of an antihypertensive medication. *Source: The Seventh Report of the Joint National Committee on Prevention, Detection, Evaluation, and Treatment of High Blood Pressure*[5]. A complete list of the classifications of high BP, used to guide treatment, is included in Appendix 1.

[2]Defined as an SBP of 120—139 mm Hg or a DBP of 80—89 mm Hg.

Nutrition in the Prevention and Treatment of Disease, Third Edition.
DOI: http://dx.doi.org/10.1016/B978-0-12-391884-0.00030-5

TABLE 30.1 Baseline Systolic BP and Age-Adjusted 10-Year Mortality from Cardiovascular Disease from the Multiple Risk Factor Intervention Trial[a]

Systolic BP (mm Hg)	n	Deaths	Rate per 1000	Relative risk	Excess deaths	% of all excess deaths
<110	21,379	202	10.5	1.0	0.0	0.0
110–119	66,080	658	11.0	1.0	33.0	1.0
120–129	98,834	1324	14.3	1.4	375.6	11.5
130–139	79,308	1576	19.8	1.9	737.6	22.6
140–149	44,388	1310	27.3	2.6	745.7	22.8
150–159	21,477	946	38.1	3.6	592.8	18.2
160–169	9,308	488	44.8	4.3	319.3	9.8
170–179	4,013	302	65.5	6.2	220.7	6.8
≥180	3,191	335	85.5	8.1	239.3	7.3

[a]Men free of history of myocardial infarction at baseline (N = 347,978); Multiple Risk Factor Intervention Trial primary screenees [4].
Source: Reprinted with permission from Stamler, J. (1991). BP and high BP: Aspects of risk. Hypertension 18(Suppl. 1), I95–I107.

conclude with a summary of qualitative and quantitative recommendations on dietary and lifestyle changes for the prevention and treatment of hypertension.

II INDIVIDUAL NUTRIENTS AND BLOOD PRESSURE

A Micronutrients

Micronutrients associated with BP tend to be highly correlated with each other because of similar food sources [27], thus limiting the interpretability of observational studies. For example, foods high in magnesium (e.g., nuts) are also high in fiber and potassium, making it virtually impossible to attribute associations with BP to the effects of a single nutrient. To isolate and test the effect of individual nutrients, intervention studies typically use dietary supplements. The use of supplements allows for any changes in BP seen as a result of the intervention to be attributed solely to the nutrient being examined. However, supplements may not be absorbed as well or have the same physiologic effects as when they are consumed in natural form. Varying levels of other dietary components may also modify the effectiveness of supplements.

1 Sodium

The mechanism by which a high sodium intake may affect BP is generally accepted to be related to sodium retention. Little research has been conducted on alternative mechanisms such as effects on vascular reactivity. It is clear that the association is influenced by genetics [28] and other dietary components [29,30]. A broad range of data supports the potential for sodium reduction to lower BP. Whether salt reduction should be broadly recommended to lower BP in individuals without hypertension has been the subject of much controversy [31,32]. Advocates propose that population-wide sodium reduction to 50–100 mmol/day (1150–2300 mg/day) would substantially lower the incidence of CVD in the general population [33,34]. Some express concern that sodium reduction may raise vasoconstrictive hormones and lipid levels [35] and increase BP in certain individuals [36,37]. However, the preponderance of evidence supports the safety and efficacy of moderate sodium reduction [38], which is part of the national recommendations for preventing and treating high BP.

Dietary sodium intake is not easily measured by standard dietary assessment methods because salt added at the table and during cooking is difficult to quantify and because processed foods vary widely in sodium content. Most often, 24-hour urine collections are used to assess daily sodium intake. Under stable conditions (e.g., adequate health, hydration, and no excessive sweating), 90–95% of dietary sodium is excreted in the urine [39]. Wide variations in day-to-day sodium excretion within individuals will weaken the correlation of single 24-hour urinary sodium levels with BP. This weakness may be minimized by collecting multiple samples in individuals or by increasing sample size in group analyses. Several investigators now employ statistical methods to correct for this source of error by using data from repeated collections in a subset of the study population [40,41]. Improperly collected urine samples and varying geographic conditions (e.g., climate) among populations [6] can introduce additional error. Despite these methodologic limitations, a relationship between dietary sodium intake and BP is well-established.

A OBSERVATIONAL STUDIES

Observations of a direct relationship between sodium intake and BP across populations support a causal role for sodium in hypertension [42,43]. The INTERSALT study measured the relationship between 24-hour urinary sodium excretion and BP in 10,079 men and women from 52 centers throughout the world [44]. Mean urinary sodium by center was positively associated with BP (Figure 30.1a, solid line). When excluding data from the four isolated, traditional populations in whom other unmeasured potentially relevant factors were of particular concern, the association disappeared (Figure 30.1A, dashed line). After adjusting for alcohol and body mass index (Figures 30.1B and C), a slightly positive relationship was again noted. The investigators also reported a strong positive relationship between sodium intake and

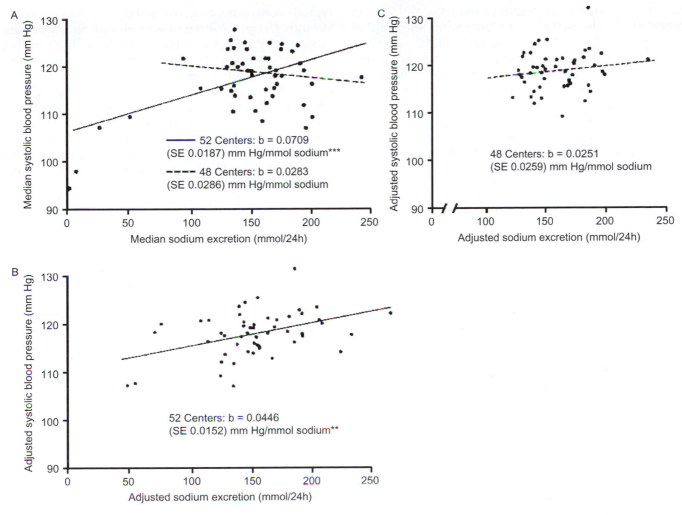

FIGURE 30.1 INTERSALT figure panel. Relationship between age and sex-standardized 24-hour urinary sodium excretion and systolic blood pressure from the INTERSALT study. (A) With and without including four remote populations, (B) also adjusted for alcohol intake and body mass index (52 centers), and (C) also adjusted for alcohol intake and body mass index (48 centers). *$p < 0.05$; **$p < 0.01$; ***$p < 0.001$ [44].

the slope of BP increase with age across populations [44], suggesting a role for sodium in age-related BP increase. In a re-analysis of the original INTERSALT data, corrected for measurement error due to use of single 24-hour urine collections, results were stronger: A 100-mmol/day (2300 mg sodium) increase in urinary sodium was associated with an increase in SBP of 3−6 mm Hg and DBP of 0−3 mm Hg [45]. In a meta-analysis of observational studies, Law *et al.* [46] reported somewhat stronger findings than INTERSALT, especially in the elderly and those with higher baseline BP, but diet and other confounders were not assessed in a standard manner across studies.

B INTERVENTIONAL STUDIES

The early observation of a large BP reduction in patients with severe hypertension consuming the Kempner rice diet [47] is often attributed to its low sodium content (7 mmol or 150 mg/day), although the diet was also rich in fruit, low in fat and protein, and supplemented with vitamins. The many trials of sodium reduction conducted since then have varied in design, population age, BP status, race and gender composition, amount and form of sodium provided, quantity and control of other nutrients in the diet, trial procedures (inpatient vs. outpatient), and degree of adherence to the diets. Several meta-analyses of clinical trials of sodium reduction have been published in the past two decades [33−35,48,49]. In a meta-analysis of 28 trials published by Midgley *et al.* [48], a reduction in urinary sodium by 100 mmol/day (2300 mg/day) was associated with a 3.7/0.9 mm Hg lower SBP/DBP in individuals with hypertension and 1.0/0.1 mm Hg BP reduction in nonhypertensives. A meta-analysis by Cutler and others [33] in 1997 of 78 published trials reported stronger results. In people with hypertension, a 100-mmol/day (2300 mg/day) reduction in sodium intake was associated with a reduction in SBP/DBP of 5.8/2.5 mm Hg; corresponding reductions were 2.3/1.4 mm Hg for nonhypertensives. Statistical approaches used to quantify the relationship between sodium and BP reduction may partly explain differing conclusions of these investigators.

The meta-analysis by Graudal and others [35] included 58 trials in individuals with hypertension and 56 trials in nonhypertensives. Despite greater mean reductions in sodium intake used to estimate the BP-lowering effect (a 118-mmol [2714−mg] sodium reduction in individuals with hypertension and a 160-mmol [3680−mg] reduction in nonhypertensives), their findings of a 3.9/1.9 mm Hg and 1.2/0.26 mm Hg BP reduction, respectively, were closer to those of Midgley *et al.* [48]. Graudal *et al.* and Midgley *et al.* included studies of short-term acute sodium reduction (which stimulates BP-regulating hormones), whereas Cutler *et al.* [33] excluded these studies. In two other meta-analyses, salt reduction was evaluated among trials of longer term [49,50]. Hooper *et al.* [50] reviewed only trials longer than 6 months, but the salt reduction achieved was smaller (on average by 87 mmol/day or 2000 mg/day). Thus, they found a smaller fall in BP and did not observe a dose−response to salt reduction. In one of the analyses [49], 20 salt reduction trials in hypertensives and 11 trials in nonhypertensives that were 4 weeks or longer were examined. The median reduction in urinary sodium was 78 mmol/day (1794 mg/day), and the mean reduction in SBP/DBP was 5.06/2.7 mm Hg among hypertensives. Corresponding findings among nonhypertensives were a reduction of urinary sodium of 74 mmol/day (1702 mg/day) and 2.03/0.99 mm Hg in SBP/DBP. There was a significant relationship between sodium reduction and BP. Despite variations in estimated effect size, all meta-analyses reported a direct relationship between sodium and BP, which was consistently significant in hypertensives. The estimate of the magnitude of the reduction varied at least partly because of statistical methods used and the choice of studies included in the meta-analyses.

The DASH-Sodium multicenter trial [22] provides more precise estimates of the magnitude of the effect of sodium reduction on BP. The study, funded by the National Heart, Lung, and Blood Institute, used a controlled feeding design to compare the effect of three sodium levels (resulting in urinary sodium excretion of 65, 107, and 142 mmol/day or 1495, 2461, and 3266 mg/day) on BP in adults with prehypertension or stage 1 hypertension. The sodium intervention was provided in conjunction with a typical U.S. (control) diet or the DASH dietary pattern (Appendix 2), and intake was precisely regulated—participants ate foods prepared in a metabolic kitchen. In the context of a typical American diet, reducing sodium intake to 107 mmol/day (2461 mg/day) reduced SBP/DBP significantly by 2.1/1.1 mm Hg. Reducing sodium further to 65 mmol/day (1495 mg/day) caused additional significant SBP/DBP reduction by 4.6/2.4 mm Hg. The effects of sodium were observed in participants with and in those without hypertension, African Americans and those of other races, and women and men. In addition, as noted later, the lowest sodium intake (65 mmol/day or 1495 mg/day) superimposed on the already effective DASH dietary pattern provided the most effective BP-lowering combination. Compared to the control diet with the highest sodium level, the DASH dietary pattern with the lowest sodium level reduced SBP significantly by 8.9 and 7.1 mm Hg, respectively, among participants with and without hypertension at baseline.

In addition to lowering BP, there is evidence that sodium reduction prevents hypertension incidence and cardiovascular events. Several long-term, randomized clinical trials have provided evidence that moderate sodium reduction with or without weight loss reduces the incidence of hypertension and cardiovascular events, especially in overweight participants [51]. In the Trial of Nonpharmacologic Interventions in the Elderly (TONE) [52], a 10-pound weight loss and dietary sodium reduction of 40 mmol/day (920 mg/day) were independently associated with approximately a 40% reduced risk of hypertension or cardiovascular event after medication withdrawal, compared with those receiving standard care. In the obese participants, the combined intervention was associated with a 53% reduced risk of hypertension or CVD event. In the TOHP II [53], overweight adults who were counseled to reduce sodium for 6 months achieved a 2.9/1.6 mm Hg BP reduction from sodium reduction alone and 4.0/2.8 mm Hg when coupled with weight loss. Although effects on average BP declined over time with recidivism, 20% reductions in hypertension incidence remained after 48 months of follow-up in each intervention group. Thus, combining sodium reduction with other lifestyle modifications such as weight loss is feasible and can increase effectiveness of BP control.

C SALT SENSITIVITY

Approximately 50% of individuals with hypertension and 25% of nonhypertensives are considered by some to be salt sensitive [54−56], defined arbitrarily as a mean arterial pressure reduction of at least 10 mm Hg or 10% with salt restriction. It is more common in the elderly and in African Americans [57]. Various protocols have been employed to diagnose salt sensitivity, including feeding low- and high-sodium diets and also a more rigorous protocol of saline infusion (to expand blood volume) followed by volume contraction with a low-sodium diet and administration of a diuretic [54]. The concept of salt sensitivity has been challenged [58]. Using the data collected in the DASH-Sodium trial, the variability and consistency of individual SBP responses to changes in sodium intake were examined. A total of 188 participants consumed a run-in (typical) diet at the higher sodium level and continued to eat the same diet at three sodium levels (higher, 142 mmol/day; intermediate, 107 mmol/day; and lower, 65 mmol/day) sequentially in random order for 30 days each. Changes in SBP from run-in to higher sodium (no sodium level change) ranged from −24 to +25 mm Hg and 8.0% of participants decreased 10 mm Hg or more. Comparing the higher versus lower sodium levels (78-mmol sodium difference), the range of SBP change was −32 to +17 mmHg, and 33.5% decreased 10 mm Hg or more. In addition, SBP change with run-in versus lower sodium was modestly correlated with SBP change with higher versus intermediate sodium; SBP change with higher versus lower sodium was similarly correlated with run-in versus intermediate sodium (combined Spearman $r = 0.27$, $p = 0.002$). These results show low-order consistency of response and confirm that identifying individuals as sodium responders or salt sensitive is difficult.

Even if the concept of a dichotomous trait in salt sensitivity is not useful, it is clear that there is a wide range of individual response to changes in sodium intake. The reasons why certain individuals respond differently to a sodium load are unclear but may be due to differences in the ability of the vascular system to adjust to a change in circulating blood volume and to blunted sodium excretion [59], abnormalities in kidney function, or the renin—angiotensin system. Physiologic abnormalities, such as low renin hypertension and abnormal modulation ("nonmodulation") of these hormones, predispose to salt sensitivity [60]. Sodium chloride-induced increases in BP may also be enhanced by a low calcium or potassium intake [30,61,62]. Genetic factors modulate the degree of salt sensitivity [63,64], but much work remains to explain the magnitude of heterogeneity observed. Ideally, future studies will identify markers of susceptibility to aid in targeting interventions.

Sodium is not the only factor that affects BP, as it appears to interact with body weight and levels of other nutrients in the diet. However, sodium reduction is likely to benefit most people. Because sodium is ubiquitous in the U.S. food supply, large reductions in intake are not easily attainable. For example, the TOHP I research group reported a mean decrease in sodium excretion of 44 mmol/day (1012 mg/day) after 18 months of intensive dietary counseling in a free-living population [65]. Only 20% of the population met the study goal of 60 mmol/day (1380 mg/day), but 56% were able to reduce sodium to less than 100 mmol/day (2300 mg/day). Counseling was least effective in men and in African Americans [65]. In the PREMIER clinical trial [26], a 6-month multi-lifestyle intensive intervention increased the proportion of participants who met the goal of less than 100 mmol/day in urinary sodium by approximately 18−28% compared to baseline. The control group, who received only a 30-minute advice session, also increased the corresponding figure by approximately 8%. All participants returned toward their baseline sodium intake levels at 18 months of follow-up. Thus, like all other lifestyle modifications, reducing sodium intake is no exception to the challenge of long-term maintenance. Seventy-five percent of sodium intake is derived from processed foods [66]; therefore, significant reductions in sodium intake will not be feasible on a population-wide basis unless sodium is reduced in processed and restaurant foods. Several countries, including the United Kingdom, Japan, and Finland, have successfully implemented population-wide sodium-reduction initiatives, and many other countries are in the process of implementing similar initiatives [67]. In 2009, the New York City Health Department began a national effort (National Salt Reduction Initiative) to reduce American's salt intake by 20% in 5 years [68]. The *Dietary Guidelines for Americans 2010* recommends that adults consume no more than 2300 mg sodium per day and those with a high risk for hypertension limit sodium to no more than 1500 mg per day [69]. Achieving such recommendations would certainly require the use of population-level strategies such as the initiatives mentioned previously and strategies at the individual level.

2 Potassium

The evidence for a role of potassium in lowering BP is relatively consistent across study types and is biologically plausible [70]. Potassium may lower BP through a direct vasodilatory role, alterations in the renin—angiotensin system [71], nitric oxide production [72], renal sodium handling, and/or natriuretic effects [73,74] (Figure 30.2).

A OBSERVATIONAL STUDIES

Epidemiologic observations support a role of dietary potassium in BP control [75]. Both potassium alone (inversely) and the sodium-to-potassium ratio (directly) have been associated with BP in cross-cultural studies [44]. Ophir *et al.* [75] noted that urinary potassium was the strongest discriminating feature related to low BP in vegetarian Seventh Day Adventists in Australia compared to nonvegetarians.

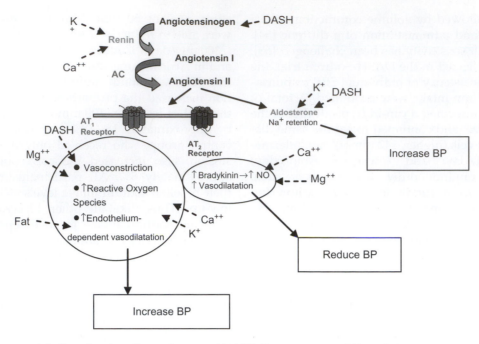

FIGURE 30.2 The potential effect of various dietary factors and DASH dietary pattern on BP regulation.

B INTERVENTIONAL STUDIES

Several meta-analyses have examined the effect of potassium supplementation on BP. In 1997, Whelton *et al.* [76] reviewed 33 randomized clinical trials of potassium and BP. These studies included mostly individuals with hypertension, some of whom were receiving antihypertensive medication. In all studies, potassium was provided as a supplement (median 75 mmol [2925 mg]), either superimposed on a controlled research diet or added to participants' usual diets. After excluding one outlier study, a high potassium intake was associated with 3.11/1.97 mm Hg reduction in SBP/DBP. Interestingly, greater BP reductions occurred in those with progressively higher urinary sodium excretion during follow-up (measured at the end of the study). This suggests that potassium is more effective at higher levels of sodium intake. Other research evidence also points to the interaction of potassium and sodium in BP [70]. In addition, results were significantly stronger in studies that included a high proportion of African Americans. This meta-analysis reached qualitatively similar conclusions to those of a 1991 analysis by Cappuccio *et al.*[77], with roughly a 50% overlap in studies included.

In a large intervention trial of U.S. female nurses (Nurses' Health Study II), Sacks and colleagues [78] administered supplemental potassium (40 mmol [1560 mg]), calcium (30 mmol [1200 mg]), magnesium (14 mmol [336 mg]), all three minerals, or placebo to women who reported habitually low intakes of these nutrients, for a 6-month period. Potassium,

administered alone, was the only intervention that reduced BP . The mild but significant reduction occurred even though the women were nonhypertensive (mean BP, 116/73 mm Hg).

Furthermore, two meta-analyses provide supporting evidence for an effect of potassium supplement on BP. Geleijnse *et al.* [79] examined 27 randomized trials with at least 2 weeks of follow-up among both hypertensives and nonhypertensives. They found that a median potassium supplementation of 44 mmol/day (1716 mg/day) was associated with a reduction of SBP/DBP by 2.42/1.57 mm Hg. This reduction was even greater among those who were hypertensive (3.51/2.51 mm Hg), but it was only borderline significant (~ 0.08). Dickinson *et al.* [80] reviewed 4 of the 27 trials in the Geleijnse study plus 2 other trials, all of which included at least 8 weeks of follow-up and only hypertensives. They found a large reduction in BP by potassium supplementation (11.2/5.0 mm Hg), but the reduction was not statistically significant, perhaps partially because of the heterogeneity of the trials. The authors stated that the heterogeneity of the trials was not explained by the varying dosage of potassium supplementation, study quality, or the baseline BP.

Strong support for the effect of dietary potassium on BP comes from the DASH trial as well. A fruit-and-vegetable diet, which contained increased amounts of potassium, magnesium, and fiber but was otherwise similar to the typical American control diet, significantly reduced SBP/DBP by 2.8/1.1 mm Hg [21]. Furthermore, the BP reduction was much greater among the African Americans (3.5/1.4 mm Hg) than among the non-African Americans (0.7/0.3 mm Hg), suggesting that African Americans may be more responsive to the BP effect of potassium.

Thus, research strongly supports the current Joint National Committee on Prevention, Detection, Evaluation, and Treatment of High Blood Pressure (JNC) recommendation of increasing potassium intake to 4700 mg/day for the prevention and control of high BP. Individuals should be encouraged to increase potassium intake by including more whole grains, fruits, vegetables, and low-fat dairy products.

3 Calcium

Although a modest BP-lowering effect of calcium is noted in some observational studies, results from intervention trials have been inconsistent. Studies showing the greatest effect have tended to use dietary sources of calcium (e.g., dairy products), in which several potentially confounding dietary factors also change [21]. In addition, the BP-lowering effect of calcium may be greater among those with a low habitual intake of calcium. Potential mechanisms by which calcium may affect BP include effects on plasma renin activity, endothelial function, or the production of nitric oxide (Figure 30.2).

A OBSERVATIONAL STUDIES

The higher calcium and magnesium content of "hard" water and its inverse relation to cardiovascular mortality [81] initially sparked epidemiologic investigation into the relation of both minerals to BP. Cutler and Brittain [82] reviewed 25 observational studies and showed only modest associations between calcium and BP. Because most studies used 24-hour recall methods to assess diet, random day-to-day variation may have obscured any relation with BP [82]. It is also worth noting that some low-BP populations have minimal calcium intakes [11]—more counterevidence to the link between calcium and BP. Cappuccio and others [83] later conducted a meta-analysis of 23 observational studies and found negligible associations for calcium with both SBP and DBP, although a re-analysis of the data resulted in a somewhat stronger inverse association [19]. A cross-sectional analysis of the NHANES III data showed that increasing calcium intake is significantly associated with a lower rate of age-related increase in SBP and pulse pressure [84]. Other cross-sectional studies have also shown a significant and inverse association between calcium intake [85,86] or dairy intake [87–89] and BP.

B INTERVENTIONAL STUDIES

In 1924, Addison and Clark [90] recorded the BP response to repeated administration and discontinuation of oral calcium supplements in a convenience sample of hospital outpatients and inpatients. They noted that BP decreased after 2 weeks of calcium supplementation and immediately rose with calcium discontinuation. It was not until much later in the century that the calcium hypothesis was tested in a more methodologically rigid manner in a number of intervention studies.

Several meta-analyses of calcium-intervention trials have been published since 1989 [91–96], all showing only a slight or negligible BP reduction, primarily of SBP, with calcium supplementation of approximately 1000 mg. Intervention studies using calcium from food sources have sometimes [96,97], but not always [97,98], been more effective, although these studies also involve changes in several other nutrients.

A randomized controlled trial of 732 postmenopausal women showed that calcium supplementation of 1 g per day significantly reduced SBP by 1 or 2 mm Hg at 6 months; however, this effect disappeared at 30 months despite continual calcium supplementation [99]. Two other small randomized trials did not find any significant effect of calcium supplementation on BP [100,101]. An interaction between calcium and other minerals in their effect on BP has been observed [102] such that calcium supplementation may prevent a salt-induced rise in BP in susceptible individuals. Inability to either control for sodium intake or stratify by level of sodium intake in most meta-analyses may obscure a relationship. Despite weak evidence for a role of calcium in BP, it is advisable for the public to consume adequate dietary calcium for the benefit of bone health. The Dietary Reference Intakes (DRIs) for calcium suggest an intake of 1000 mg/day for all adults and 1200 mg/day for women 51 years old or older and men 71 years old or older. This level of intake is similar to that tested in the DASH dietary pattern and may also promote BP health.

4 Magnesium

Adequate magnesium is required for the Na/K-ATPase pump, which regulates intracellular calcium—one of the critical determinants of vascular smooth muscle contraction [103] (Figure 30.2). In animal models, magnesium deficiency has been repeatedly shown to be associated with hypertension [104–106]. In humans, magnesium deficiency, although recognized rarely, is seen in severe malnutrition, in chronic alcoholism, and in association with malabsorption [103].

A OBSERVATIONAL STUDIES

As with calcium, one of the early suggestions for a role of magnesium in hypertension came from reports that water hardness (increased calcium and magnesium) was associated with lower cardiovascular mortality [81]. This finding was corroborated by Yang and

Chin [107]. Several cross-sectional [108] and prospective observational analyses [109,110] have found higher-magnesium diets to be associated with lower BP. However, interpretation of these results is limited by the fact that a high-magnesium diet tends to be high in other beneficial dietary factors as well. In a prospective study, magnesium intake was found to be inversely associated with risk for hypertension after adjustment for known risk factors among 28,349 participants of the Women's Health Study [111].

B INTERVENTIONAL STUDIES

Many intervention trials of magnesium supplementation have been conducted [24,78,112–122], and some have shown a beneficial effect on BP [112,113,118, 119,121]. Patients were magnesium depleted (due to diuretic treatment) in two of the studies [112,113], and in one study an effect was only seen in those with a low baseline intake of dietary magnesium [122]. Kawano et al. [120] found the greatest BP reduction with magnesium supplementation in older men on antihypertensive medications. More than half of these studies, however, found no BP-lowering effect with magnesium supplementation. In a meta-analysis of 12 randomized trials, magnesium supplement significantly reduced DBP only (by 2.2 mm Hg) but had no significant effect on SBP [122,123]. Overall, the quality of the included trials was poor, results varied, and thus the evidence was weak. In another meta-analysis of 9 randomized trials with diabetic participants, a median level of 360 mg/day magnesium supplementation did not have any significant effect on BP [123]. Thus, despite the potential role for magnesium in BP control, evidence from intervention trials has not been supportive. However, individuals are encouraged to consume adequate amount of magnesium from natural food sources as recommended by adopting the DASH eating pattern (see Section III.A.1).

B Macronutrients

Studies of macronutrients and BP are often subject to various design limitations. Thus, results can be difficult to interpret. For example, when a study is designed to examine the effect of the amount of fat intake on BP, alteration in fat intake under isocaloric conditions inevitably will change intake of protein and/or carbohydrate and may change the intake of other nutrients as well. As a result, it may be difficult to attribute the effect on BP to change in fat intake alone. In addition, the impact of macronutrients on BP potentially involves aspects of the absolute quantity and type of macronutrients consumed. Both aspects can affect BP independently, but they are not always distinguishable in research designs.

1 Protein

Despite evidence that high protein intake may promote renal injury, especially in those with existing kidney disease, the overall effect of protein on BP appears to be salutary. Although the exact mechanism(s) linking amount or type of protein to BP is unclear, possible explanations exist. First, an increase in protein intake may induce increases in renal plasma flow, renal size, glomerular filtration rate, and sodium excretion [124,125]. Second, the amino acid arginine may act as a vasodilator and contribute to BP lowering [126,127].

A OBSERVATIONAL STUDIES

Many observational studies have shown an inverse relationship between total dietary protein intake and BP [128]. Nevertheless, results have been mixed when studies examined animal and plant proteins separately. Cross-sectional studies conducted in rural Japanese and Chinese populations found only an inverse relationship between animal protein and BP [129,130]. In contrast, cohort studies conducted in the United States have shown an inverse association between the increase in SBP with aging and baseline intakes of plant protein but not animal protein [131,132]. Thus, there may be differential effects of animal and plant protein on BP, but the exact relationship is not clear.

B INTERVENTIONAL STUDIES

Evidence from randomized controlled trials suggests that an increased intake of protein, from both plant and animal sources, may lower BP. In a 6-week randomized three-period crossover trial in subjects with diagnosed hypertension, substitution of protein for carbohydrate led to a decrease in SBP of 3.5 mm Hg [23]. Hodgson et al. [133] demonstrated in a small trial that replacing carbohydrate with lean red meat while keeping total calorie and fat intake constant reduced SBP but not DBP. Although the reduction in SBP was statistically significant, the magnitude within the active intervention participants was quite small (−1.9 mm Hg using clinic BP and −0.6 mm Hg using ambulatory 24-hour BP). In contrast, using data collected from the PREMIER clinical trial, we found that dietary plant protein intake was inversely associated with both SBP and DBP in cross-sectional analyses at the 6-month follow-up ($p = 0.0009$ and $p = 0.0126$, respectively) [134]. An increase in plant protein intake from baseline to month 6 was marginally associated with a reduction of both SBP and DBP from baseline to month 6 ($p = 0.0516$ and $p = 0.082$, respectively), independent of change in body weight. Animal protein was not associated with BP or change in BP in PREMIER. Furthermore, among those with prehypertension, increased intake of plant protein was significantly associated with a lower risk of developing hypertension at 6 months. Note that many intervention trials employ different types or amounts of protein, and the delivery mechanism may differ as well, all of which contribute to variation in results. Most trials use protein supplements that include soy, vegetable, or animal protein and do not control for other nutrients.

Soy protein was hypothesized to reduce BP because it is rich in arginine, a potential vasodilator and a precursor for the vasodilator nitric oxide [126]. The results of numerous randomized controlled trials that supplemented soy protein have been mixed. In a 12-week randomized double-blind controlled trial, He *et al.* [135] demonstrated a decrease in SBP/DBP of 4.31/2.76 mm Hg soybean protein supplements compared to the placebo group. Furthermore, Rivas *et al.* [136] demonstrated that soy milk supplement significantly reduced SBP by 18.4 mm Hg in a 3-month randomized trial. In contrast, three randomized controlled trials [137−139] showed no difference in SBP or DBP between the soy protein-supplemented group and the placebo group. Note that some studies used milk supplements, which provide not only protein but also other nutrients that may affect BP. Thus, the BP responses cannot be attributed to protein alone.

Considering the available evidence, it is not advisable to use protein supplements as a dietary intervention to treat hypertension. Instead, ensuring an adequate protein intake on the basis of a healthy eating pattern may likely benefit BP. Furthermore, selecting protein from mainly plant sources may benefit overall cardiovascular health.

2 Dietary Fat

Numerous studies have investigated the relationship between dietary fat and BP. However, because of differences in study design, lack of adequate sample size, and other design limitations, the issue remains controversial. Both the absolute total intake of dietary fat and the relative fatty acid composition may independently relate to BP control. Research has suggested that increased intake of total fat and saturated fats may impair endothelial function, which may subsequently affect BP (Figure 30.2). Conversely, diets rich in omega-3 fatty acids may improve endothelial function and therefore may lower BP.

A OBSERVATIONAL STUDIES

Most observational studies have not found an association between total fat intake and BP [27,140−142]. However, two large studies [140−142] but not others [27,143] show a positive relationship between saturated fatty acids and BP. In addition, Hajjar and Kotchen [144] examined the NHANES III data and reported that the southern region of the United States, which consumed the highest amounts of monounsaturated and polyunsaturated fats, also had the highest SBP and DBP compared to other regions.

B INTERVENTIONAL STUDIES

Many studies have examined the impact of the amount or type of fat on BP. However, as discussed previously, any change in total fat intake often introduces changes in other dietary factors as well, leading to potential confounding. Thus, the BP responses may not be attributed solely to the change in fat intake. In a crossover randomized study, consumption of a single high-fat meal (42 g) was found to increase both SBP and DBP significantly more than did a low-fat meal (1 g) [145]. In 2000, Ferrara *et al.* [146] investigated the effect of monounsaturated versus polyunsaturated fat on BP in a 6-month double-blind randomized crossover study. The monounsaturated fat diet reduced SBP and DBP significantly more than did the polyunsaturated fat diet. Appel *et al.* [23] reported that substituting monounsaturated fats for saturated fats significantly reduced SBP by 2.9 mm Hg in a group of 191 subjects with prehypertension or stage 1 hypertension. This finding suggests that a high fat intake (37% energy) mainly provided as monounsaturated fat, in combination with other beneficial dietary factors, can lower BP effectively.

Many short-term intervention trials have been undertaken to determine whether supplementation of either fish or fish oil lowers BP. Because of variations in research design, participant criteria, dosage and type of supplements, and length of intervention, the results have been inconsistent. A meta-analysis of randomized controlled trials (36 of which included fish oil) explored the impact of fish oil intake on hypertension prevalence in five countries (Finland, Italy, The Netherlands, the United Kingdom, and the United States) [147]. Pooled meta-regression of data from these trials showed that a 4.1-g supplement of fish oil is associated with a 2.1/1.6 mm Hg decrease in SBP/DBP. Long-term studies are required to confirm the benefit of fish oil on BP lowering. Until such information is available, it is advisable to encourage greater fish consumption as part of a healthy diet rather than taking fish oil supplementation. Furthermore, it remains unclear how fat intake and various fatty acids affect BP and whether an interaction exists among these factors.

3 Carbohydrates

Although not well understood, carbohydrate may contribute to the development of essential hypertension through its glycemic effect. Kopp [148] suggests that consumption of a high glycemic index diet may create a chronic state of postprandial hyperinsulinemia, sympathetic nervous system overactivity, and vascular remodeling of renal vessels leading to chronic activation of the renin—angiotensin—aldosterone system and development of essential hypertension. Although logical, the relationship of a high-carbohydrate diet to high BP has not been consistent in all studies. Very few studies have been designed specifically to investigate the impact of the quantity or type of carbohydrate intake on BP. Nevertheless, studies of the relationship between fat intake and BP often alter intakes of both fat and carbohydrate while keeping protein intake constant. Thus, interpretation of the effect of fat intake on BP is potentially confounded by the effects of carbohydrate intake.

A OBSERVATIONAL STUDIES

Very few observational studies have specifically reported the relationship between carbohydrate intake and BP. Inevitably, examination of carbohydrate intake is often confounded by other nutrients or dietary factors. Using the NHANES III data, quintile of carbohydrate intake was not associated with the risk for increased SBP ($\geq$140 mm Hg) after adjustment for potential confounders and total sugar intake [149]. In fact, three cross-sectional studies, using NHANES 1999—2004 and 2003—2006 data, showed that sugary drinks or fructose consumption was positively associated with a higher BP [150—152]. In a secondary analysis of the PREMIER clinical trial data, reduction of sugary drink was also found to be associated with a decreased SBP/DBP. Together, these findings suggest a negative impact of simple carbohydrate intake on BP. Furthermore, a high intake of whole grain has been shown to be associated with a reduction of hypertension risk in the Women's Health Study [153] and the Health Professionals Follow-Up Study [154].

B INTERVENTIONAL STUDIES

No research study has been designed specifically to examine the impact of the amount of carbohydrate alone on BP. It is difficult to manipulate the amount of carbohydrate without changing intake of other nutrients if total energy is to be kept constant. However, in the context of whole dietary pattern change, both low- and high-carbohydrate intakes in combination with other dietary changes have been associated with BP lowering [21,23,149]. In a meta-analysis comparing high-carbohydrate to high-monounsaturated fat diets, the high-carbohydrate diet resulted in slightly higher SBP/DBP (2.6/1.8 mm Hg) while energy intake and weight were kept constant [155]. Thus, the impact of the amount of carbohydrate on BP is still inconclusive.

Some human studies have examined the impact of the type of carbohydrate on BP, but the research has been limited in number and yielded inconsistent results. In one study [156], SBP rose significantly 1

hour after ingestion of a sucrose or glucose solution but not after ingestion of fructose. On the contrary, a fructose drink, but not glucose, was found to significantly increase SBP/DBP within 2 hours in another study [157]. However, in an earlier study of patients with coronary artery disease, both SBP and DBP decreased after 4 days of a sucrose and fructose load at 4 g/kg/day but not glucose load [158]. In a study that was designed to examine the metabolic effect of sucrose in a group of overweight women, BP was not changed during the 6 weeks after consuming a hypocaloric diet with sucrose as the main source of carbohydrate [158,159].

Thus, it is unclear if the amount of carbohydrate alone or the type of carbohydrate affect BP. Future research designed specifically to examine these questions is needed to help clarify the roles of carbohydrate in BP control. Nevertheless, evidence is strong that consuming whole grains may benefit BP and overall cardiovascular health and should be encouraged as the main type of carbohydrate source.

4 Fiber

Fiber may indirectly lower BP through reduction of insulin levels [160]. Hyperinsulinemia is often associated with obesity, impaired glucose tolerance, and hypertension.

A OBSERVATIONAL STUDIES

Both cross-sectional [132,161] and prospective analyses [162] have demonstrated inverse associations between fiber and BP but have also noted a high correlation of fiber with other nutrients that can affect BP in a salutary manner. In a prospective 8-year study of 12,741 subjects, the highest quintile of total dietary fiber and nonsoluble dietary fiber intake was associated with an 11.6% lower risk of hypertension compared to that of the lowest quintile [161].

B INTERVENTIONAL STUDIES

Several interventional studies have examined the effect of fiber on BP, with most adding cereal fiber to the diet. These studies suggest that an average supplementation of 14 g fiber reduces SBP/DBP by approximately 1.6/2.0 mm Hg, respectively [160]. Similarly, a meta-analysis of 25 randomized controlled trials between 1966 and 2003 demonstrated that fiber supplementation (average 11.5 g/day) leads to a reduction in SBP/DBP of 1.13/1.26 mm Hg, respectively [163].

Thus, this evidence suggests a consistent small beneficial effect of fiber on BP. Individuals should be encouraged to increase fiber intake to the current recommended level not only for BP control but also possibly for other benefits to cardiovascular health. Such recommendation should be achieved by increasing fruits, vegetables, and whole grains based on the foundation of a healthy eating pattern rather than using a supplement.

5 Alcohol

The exact mechanism for an alcohol—BP association is not clear, but possibilities include stimulation of the sympathetic nervous system, inhibition of vascular relaxing substances, calcium or magnesium depletion, and increased intracellular calcium in vascular smooth muscle [164—166].

A OBSERVATIONAL STUDIES

Excessive alcohol consumption is associated with higher BP and higher prevalence of hypertension in observational studies [165]. Men who consume three or more drinks per day [167] and women who consume two or more drinks per day [168] may be at higher risk, but levels below this are not associated with increased risk. There is no consistent relationship between BP and type of alcohol consumed. Chronic, habitual intake may be more related to BP than recent intake . In one study, men who had quit drinking alcohol during an 18-year follow-up period experienced less age-related increase in BP than did those who did not quit drinking alcohol [169].

In a cohort study of 8334 participants from the Atherosclerosis Risk in Communities study [170], participants were free of hypertension at baseline and were followed for 6 years. Risk of incident hypertension was increased by 20% in those who consumed ≥210 g alcohol (78 oz. wine, 191 oz. beer, or 21 oz. liquor) per week compared to those who did not consume alcohol.

B INTERVENTIONAL STUDIES

The relatively few intervention studies of alcohol and BP have tended to be small and of short duration, and these are reviewed by Cushman *et al.* [164]. In 9 of 10 studies examined, SBP was significantly reduced after a reduction of one to six alcoholic beverages per day. The Prevention and Treatment of Hypertension Study (PATHS) [171] was designed to evaluate the long-term BP-lowering effect of reducing alcohol consumption in nondependent moderate drinkers (those who consumed more than three drinks per day). The goal of intervention was either two or fewer drinks daily or a 50% reduction in intake (whichever was less). After 6 months, the intervention group experienced a 1.2/0.7 mm Hg greater reduction in BP compared to the control group (not significant), and among hypertensives, this reduction was more modest. In this study, the intervention group reduced its intake by two alcoholic drinks per day, but the control group also lowered its alcohol intake during intervention so that the difference in intake between the groups was only 1.3 drinks/day. This small difference between the two groups may have limited the interpretation of the true BP effect of the intervention group. In addition, perhaps a greater reduction in alcohol consumption is necessary to identify a significant effect on BP. However, this level of reduction appears realistic in moderate alcohol drinkers and is similar to the absolute reduction achieved in a previous study [172].

In a study [173] of mainly heavier drinkers (more than 5 drinks/day), replacing alcohol with low-alcoholic substitutes resulted in a reduction of approximately five drinks per week and a greater reduction in BP (−4.8/3.3 mm Hg). Importantly, this intervention also reduced body weight of the participants by an average of 2.1 kg, which may explain the larger BP reduction than that observed in the PATHS trial. However, in a meta-analysis of 15 randomized controlled trials including a total of 2234 participants who drank an average of three to six drinks per day at baseline, the effect of alcohol reduction on BP was explored [174]. Reduced alcohol consumption, varying from 29 to 100% reduction from baseline, was associated with a significant reduction in mean SBP (3.31 mm Hg) and DBP (2.04 mm Hg), whereas the body weight was minimally changed (mean change, −0.56 kg). There was a dose—response relationship between the mean percentage of alcohol reduction and the mean percentage of BP reduction.

Thus, limiting alcohol consumption to the current recommendation of two or fewer drinks per day for men and one or fewer for women is supported by most research evidence and will likely improve BP. There is no need to recommend total abstinence; indeed, moderate alcohol consumption (compared to no alcohol intake) also has well-known benefits for overall CVD risk [175,176].

III OTHER DIETARY AND LIFESTYLE MODIFICATIONS

A Dietary Patterns

The previous sections on micro- and macronutrients highlight extensive confounding due to simultaneous changes in multiple nutrients. It is difficult to study (and change) one component of the diet without affecting others. Thus, it may be more appropriate to focus on dietary pattern rather than on individual micro- and macronutrients, and indeed there is extensive evidence that dietary pattern affects BP. For example, vegetarian groups in the United States and abroad have been observed to have lower BP than their nonvegetarian counterparts in many [177,178] but not all studies [179]. The term "vegetarian" comprises several heterogeneous groups [180], but in general, the diet tends to be high in whole grains, beans, vegetables, and sometimes fish, dairy products, eggs, and fruit [181]. Aspects of the vegetarian diet suggested to benefit BP include an ample amount of plant foods; a low intake of animal products [178] and a high intake of potassium, magnesium, fiber, and (sometimes) calcium [180,181]; a high ratio of polyunsaturated to saturated fat; and often a low sodium intake. However, as outlined previously, studies on individual nutrients have shown inconsistent results. Explanations for such inconsistencies may include the following: (1) The effect of individual nutrients may be too small to be detected, particularly when trials contain insufficient sample size and thus statistical power; (2) most intervention studies employed supplements of nutrients, which may function differently from nutrients in foods; (3) other dietary factors naturally occurring in foods that are not hypothesized to affect BP may also have an impact on BP; and (4) nutrients occurring in foods simultaneously may exert synergistic effects on BP. Clearly, differences in physical activity, stress, alcohol consumption, and other unmeasured factors may also contribute to a lower BP among vegetarians. However, when research participants were counseled to follow the vegetarian diet pattern in intervention studies, significant reductions in BP in both nonhypertensive [182] and mildly hypertensive [181] participants were reported.

Despite the clear BP effect of a vegetarian diet, it is not realistic to expect a wide-scale adoption of such dietary pattern. In addition, a vegetarian diet does not include all dietary factors associated with lower BP. Thus, the DASH multicenter trials were designed to test the impact of whole dietary patterns on BP simultaneously while controlling for multiple nutrients, weight, and dietary factors [21,22].

1 The DASH Dietary Pattern

The original DASH trial [21] was an 11-week randomized controlled feeding trial of 459 individuals with pre-hypertension or stage 1 hypertension. Three dietary patterns varying in amounts of fruits, vegetables, dairy products, meats, sweets, nuts and seeds and thus fats, cholesterol, fiber, calcium, potassium, and magnesium were tested (Table 30.2). In brief, the dietary patterns were (1) the control diet, which mimicked what most Americans were consuming at the time the trial was conducted; (2) a fruits and vegetables diet, which contained a macronutrient profile similar to that of the control diet except with a higher amount of fruits and vegetables; and (3) the DASH dietary pattern, which was higher in fruits, vegetables, and low-fat dairy products; lower in total and saturated fats and cholesterol; and rich in fiber, potassium, magnesium, and calcium. Sodium intake,

TABLE 30.2 Nutrient Target for the Three Dietary Patterns Tested in the DASH Trial

Item	Control diet nutrient target	Fruits-and-vegetables diet nutrient target	Combination diet nutrient target
Nutrients			
Fat (% kcal)	37	37	27
Saturated	16	16	6
Monounsaturated	13	13	13
Polyunsaturated	8	8	8
Carbohydrates (% kcal)	48	48	55
Protein (% kcal)	15	15	18
Cholesterol (mg/day)	300	300	150
Fiber (g/day)	9	31	31
Potassium (mg/day)	1700	4700	4700
Magnesium (mg/day)	165	500	500
Calcium (mg/day)	450	450	1240
Sodium (mg/day)	3000	3000	3000
Food groups (servings/day)			
Fruits and juices	1.6	5.2	5.2
Vegetables	2.0	3.3	4.4
Grains	8.2	6.9	7.5
Low-fat dairy	0.1	0.0	2.0
Regular-fat dairy	0.4	0.3	0.7
Nuts, seeds, and legumes	0.0	0.6	0.7
Beef, pork, and ham	1.5	1.8	0.5
Poultry	0.8	0.4	0.6
Fish	0.2	0.3	0.5
Fat, oils, and salad dressing	5.8	5.3	2.5
Snacks and sweets	4.1	1.4	0.7

body weight, and alcohol consumption were kept constant throughout the intervention.

The DASH dietary pattern reduced BP by 5.5/3.0 mm Hg more than the control group (both SBP and DBP, $p < 0.001$). The fruits and vegetables diet reduced BP by 2.8/1.1 mm Hg more than the control diet ($p < 0.001$ for SBP and $p = 0.07$ for DBP). The reductions in BP were significant after participants consumed the diets for 2 weeks and were sustained for the following

6 weeks (Figure 30.3). In addition, BP lowering was similarly effective in men and women and in younger and older persons, and it was particularly effective among African Americans and those who had high BP. These reductions occurred while body weight, sodium intake, alcohol consumption, and exercise patterns remained stable. Of note, sodium intake was not reduced and was identical in all treatment groups (3000 mg/day). Among the 133 participants with hypertension (SBP $\geq$ 140 mm Hg and/or DBP $\geq$ 90 mm Hg), the DASH dietary pattern lowered SBP and DBP by 11.4 and 5.5 mm Hg, respectively. These effects in hypertensives are similar to reductions seen with single drug therapy [183] and more effective than most of the other lifestyle modifications for BP reduction (Table 30.3).

Although the DASH trial was not designed to identify a specific nutrient(s) responsible for the BP-lowering effect, data from the fruits and vegetables group support the hypothesis that increasing potassium, magnesium, and dietary fiber intake reduces BP. In addition, by further lowering total and saturated fat and cholesterol, and increasing low-fat dairy products in the DASH dietary pattern, BP reduction was nearly doubled compared to that of the fruits and vegetables diet. Because whole food items rather than single nutrients were manipulated in this trial, other nutrients that were not controlled for in the study or other beneficial factors as yet unrecognized may also have contributed to the BP responses. Further research is needed to analyze the specific nutrients or factors responsible for the effect. Further details on DASH can be found in Appendix 2 and at the following website: <http://www.nhlbi.nih.gov/health/public/heart/hbp/dash/index.htm/>.

2 Variations of DASH Dietary Pattern

Although the DASH trial provided strong evidence of the efficacy of the DASH dietary pattern in reducing BP, this trial alone was not able to test all hypotheses related to dietary pattern and BP. As discussed previously,

research suggests that a high unsaturated fat intake and high protein intake may benefit BP. Thus, the OmniHeart study [23] was designed to further understand the impact on BP of macronutrient variations of the DASH dietary pattern. The dietary patterns tested were (1) the DASH dietary pattern with a slight reduction in total protein (called the carbohydrate diet, with 15% kcal protein instead of 18% tested in the original DASH trial), (2) the DASH dietary pattern with 10% of the carbohydrate energy replaced with unsaturated fats (called the unsaturated fat diet with mainly monounsaturated fats), and (3) the DASH dietary pattern with 10% of the carbohydrate energy replaced with protein (called the protein diet). A total of 164 adults with prehypertension or stage 1 hypertension were randomized into the three diets in a crossover manner for 6 weeks each. All three diets lowered BP significantly, but the protein and unsaturated fat diets significantly reduced SBP by 1.4 and 1.3 mm Hg more than the carbohydrate diet. The further reductions in BP were even greater among those who were hypertensive at baseline.

Thus, these studies have vigorously and consistently proven that whole dietary patterns such as the DASH dietary pattern or the two modified DASH patterns in the OmniHeart study are effective strategies for BP control. As noted previously, DASH in combination with reduced sodium intake lowers BP more than either intervention alone [22]. In addition, both DASH and OmniHeart studies demonstrate that benefits of adopting a whole dietary approach extend beyond BP to other health indicators such as lipids [23,184]. Thus, a nutritional approach to BP control that involves changes in overall dietary pattern appears to be superior to approaches that manipulate only a small number of nutritional factors.

B Weight Reduction and Multi-Lifestyle Modification

Weight loss alone is an effective strategy for BP reduction. Potential mechanisms for the effect of weight

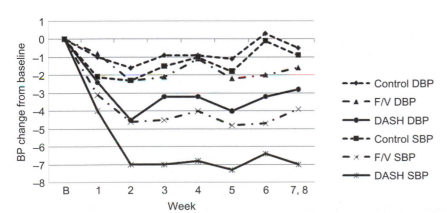

FIGURE 30.3 Mean changes in systolic and diastolic blood pressures from baseline during each intervention week, according to diet, for participants in the DASH study.

TABLE 30.3 Effect of Different Lifestyle Modification on Blood Pressure Reduction

Modification	Approximate SBP reduction (range)
Dietary sodium reduction	2–8 mm Hg
Moderation of alcohol consumption	2–4 mm Hg
Adopt DASH eating plan	8–14 mm Hg
Weight reduction	5–20 mm Hg/10-kg weight loss
Physical activity	4–9 mm Hg

Source: *Chobanian, A. V., Bakris, G. L., Black, H. R., et al. (2003). Seventh Report of the Joint National Committee on Prevention, Detection, Evaluation, and Treatment of High Blood Pressure. Hypertension 42(6), 1206–1252.*

loss on BP include suppression of sympathetic nervous system activity, lowered insulin resistance, normalization of BP regulating hormones [185], decreased body sodium stores, decreased blood volume and cardiac output, and reduction of salt sensitivity [186–188].

1 OBSERVATIONAL STUDIES

Several observational studies have reported a positive relationship between several indices of body weight or body fatness with BP [189–193].

2 INTERVENTIONAL STUDIES

Several large-scale clinical trials have been conducted to evaluate different lifestyle modification programs on BP, several of which provide evidence for a BP-lowering effect of weight loss. For example, in TOHP I [194], weight loss was found to be the most successful intervention in lowering BP compared to sodium reduction, stress management, or nutritional supplements (calcium, magnesium, or potassium). At the 6-month follow-up, men and women in the intervention group had lost 6.5 and 3.7 kg, respectively. This level of weight loss was achieved with a fairly rigorous counseling approach aimed at simultaneously reducing energy intake and increasing exercise [195]. At study termination, BP fell an average of 2.9/2.3 mm Hg overall (after subtracting the BP change in the control group). In this study, some recidivism occurred, and at 18 months, men had maintained a 4.7-kg reduction and women a 1.6-kg reduction. After 7 years of follow-up in a subset of study participants, the odds of developing hypertension were reduced by 77% in the weight-loss group [196], even though this group's long-term weight loss was nearly identical to that of the control group (4.9 and 4.5 kg, respectively).

As a follow-up to TOHP I, TOHP II [25] was conducted to examine the effects of weight loss and dietary sodium reduction alone and in combination on BP in overweight adults. The intervention lasted 3 years and included individual and group counseling meetings focusing on diet, exercise, and social support. The weight-loss intervention group ($n = 595$) achieved a mean reduction in weight from baseline to 6 months of 4.4 kg, 2.0 kg at 18 months, and 0.2 kg at 36 months. BP was significantly lower at all time points mentioned, and the greater the weight loss, the greater the BP reduction. At 36 months, every kilogram of weight loss was associated with a reduction of SBP/DBP of 0.35/0.45 mm Hg. Furthermore, this weight-loss intervention was associated with a 42% reduction in incident hypertension.

In a meta-analysis of 25 randomized controlled trials, weight loss of 1 kg was associated with approximately 1 mm Hg reduction in both SBP and DBP in individuals with prehypertension [197]. The largest of the trials included in this analysis, Trials of Hypertension Prevention [53], demonstrated a larger effect. In that trial, a behavioral weight-loss intervention in adults with prehypertension led to an average reduction in body weight of 4.4 pounds at 6 months, associated with an average reduction in BP of 3.7/2.7 mm Hg [195]. Thus, several studies demonstrate the BP-lowering effect of weight loss alone, and the evidence of an effect of weight loss on BP is strong and consistent. However, weight loss often involves change in dietary pattern, energy restriction, and increased physical activity. Implementing multiple simultaneous lifestyle changes may be an effective strategy for lowering BP.

In the PREMIER clinical trial [26], the effects on BP of two multicomponent lifestyle interventions compared to an advice-only control group were tested for 18 months. The two behavioral interventions were designed to stimulate adoption of what were at the time the well-established lifestyle guidelines for BP control (EST) or the well-established guidelines plus the DASH dietary pattern (EST + DASH). The well-established guidelines included weight loss if overweight (95% of participants), reducing sodium intake to less than 2300 mg/day, increasing physical activity to 180 minutes of moderate activity/week, and alcohol consumption not exceeding two drinks/day for men and one drink/day for women. A total of 810 individuals were randomized and completed the study. Participants in both intervention groups significantly reduced weight, improved fitness, and lowered sodium intake, and the EST + DASH group also increased fruit, vegetable, and dairy intake. Mean reduction in SBP, net of the control group, was 3.7 mm Hg ($p < 0.001$) in the EST group and 4.3 mm Hg ($p < 0.001$) in the EST + DASH group [26]. Each individual lifestyle modification was independently and significantly associated with SBP reduction at 6 and 18 months [198].

Overall, these studies demonstrate that individuals can make multiple dietary and lifestyle changes to reduce BP. Although the beneficial effect of lifestyle changes on BP may last beyond the intervention period, recidivism is often observed. Thus, it is important to develop and test strategies to help individuals maintain these changes long term.

IV CURRENT RECOMMENDATIONS AND IMPLEMENTATION

The JNC was appointed by the National Heart, Lung, and Blood Institute to provide evidenced-based clinical guidelines for the prevention and management of hypertension [5]. Current lifestyle guidelines include salt reduction, moderate alcohol consumption, weight loss if overweight, increased potassium intake, aerobic exercise, and following the DASH eating pattern. These lifestyle modifications are all recommended as part of the first-line therapy for low-risk individuals, defined as those without diabetes or CVD and with SBP less than 160 mm Hg and DBP less than 100 mm Hg. They are also recommended in combination with pharmacotherapy for high-risk individuals. These recommendations also apply to individuals with prehypertension in order to prevent the development of high BP.

Although much evidence indicates that diet and lifestyle modification can prevent and treat hypertension, reports suggest that approximately half of hypertensives are not well controlled (SBP/DBP < 140/90 mm Hg) [5,199]. The full potential of diet and lifestyle modification for treatment has likely not yet been realized both because dietary causes of hypertension have not been completely identified and because of poor adherence of both the clinicians and the public to the established medical and dietary guidelines. Despite data linking overweight and obesity to numerous adverse health outcomes including hypertension, clear guidelines for weight control, and a plethora of weight-loss programs, the obesity epidemic continues to grow. Similarly, despite clear and long-standing recommendations to reduce sodium intake to 2300 mg/day or less, the average intake remains above 3000 mg/day. Furthermore, according to the 1999—2000 NHANES survey [200,201], Americans are consuming far less than the nationally recommended amounts of fruit, vegetables, fiber, calcium, magnesium, and potassium—all of which are key components of the DASH dietary pattern [202].

Clearly, implementing dietary and lifestyle modifications is challenging. Lessons learned from past research indicate that behavioral intervention programs that result in successful behavior change are generally rooted in social cognitive theory [203] and techniques of behavioral self-management [204]. They are ideally constructed using the transtheoretical or stages-of-change model [205,206] and use motivational enhancement approaches [207,208]. These approaches emphasize the importance of the individual's ability to regulate behavior by setting goals, developing specific behavior change plans, monitoring progress toward the goals, and attaining skills necessary to reach the goals. Self-efficacy (one's confidence in performing a given behavior) and outcome expectancies (one's expectations concerning the outcome of that behavior) are critical mediators of behavior change [208,209]. The transtheoretical model recognizes that behavior change is a dynamic process of moving through different motivational stages of readiness for change. Different behavioral strategies may need to be emphasized at different times, depending on the individual's stage of change.

In addition, behavioral interventions conducted with small groups can take advantage of the economy of scale and the social support provided by a group of peers. In the PREMIER trial of lifestyle intervention for lowering BP, the behavioral strategies discussed previously were incorporated into an intervention consisting of frequent group sessions conducted by a trained interventionist. It is also important that any intervention program make efforts to create a culturally appropriate behavioral intervention. Such effort may include but is not limited to (1) having intervention encounters take place at a location in the community; (2) employing staff from the same cultural background as participants; (3) selecting foods, music, or examples from within the culture; and (4) involving staff of the same cultural background in program design and in consultation with the potential participants. Despite considerable understanding of the theory and practice of behavior change, additional research is needed to develop effective strategies for sustaining dietary and lifestyle change long term.

V SUMMARY

The evidence that diet modification can prevent and treat hypertension is strong, and recommendations are summarized in Table 30.4. In some cases, the effective intervention strategy and mechanisms involved are still being clarified. Because of various design limitations, inadequate statistical power, and measurement issues, studies of single nutrients, with the exception of sodium and potassium, have generally provided inconsistent results. However, when multiple nutrients or dietary factors are combined in a whole dietary strategy, as seen in the DASH and OmniHeart studies, BP is significantly and effectively reduced. Nutrients may have additive or interactive effects when provided together in whole foods. Thus, the current national

TABLE 30.4 Summary of Evidence Relating Dietary Factors with BP

Dietary factor	Strength of relationship with BP"	Direction of association	Potential mechanisms	Recommendations	Those most likely to benefit
Sodium	1A	Direct	Changes in blood volume and BP regulating hormones	< 65–100 mmol/day	Hypertensives, salt-sensitive individuals, African Americans, elderly, and those consuming typical American diet
Potassium	1A	Inverse	Vasodilatory; natriuretic	Increase potassium-rich foods	Those on high-salt diet
Calcium	2A	Inverse	Regulation of parathyroid hormone and intracellular calcium; natriuretic	2–3 reduced-fat dairy products/day	Possibly salt-sensitive individuals
Magnesium	2B	—	Modification of Na-K/ATPase activity	Maintain adequate magnesium intake	Those depleted in magnesium, for example, from diuretics
Protein	2A	Inverse	BP-related amino acid may act as vasodilator	Consume adequate protein (particularly plant sources); limit intake of high-fat animal protein	
Fat	1C	Direct for saturated fat, inverse for monounsaturated fats	Vasodilatory action of prostaglandins	Moderate total fat (include more monounsaturated fat sources); reduce saturated fat	
Carbohydrates	2B	—	Unclear	Consume more whole grains and less sugar	
Fiber	2B	—	Unclear, possible reduction of insulin levels	Increase fiber-rich foods for overall health benefits	Those who have insulin resistance or impaired glucose tolerance
Alcohol	IB	Direct	Unclear, possible role of sympathetic nervous system, inhibition of vascular relaxing substances, calcium and magnesium depletion	Moderate consumption: <2 drinks/day for men, <1 drink/day for women	Those consuming > 2–3 drinks/day
Body weight	1A	Direct	Lowering of blood volume, cardiac output, and insulin resistance; raising salt sensitivity	Maintain healthy weight; lose weight if overweight	Overweight individuals
Dietary patterns	1A	Depends on factor	Multiple mechanisms, as previous	DASH dietary pattern (see Appendix 2)	Those at risk for, or with, hypertension

1A, clear, consistent, and strong randomized controlled trial (RCT); IB, clear RCT but inconsistent results; 1C, clear, observational studies; 2A, unclear, consistent RCT—intermediate strength; 2B, unclear, RCT with inconsistent results; 2C, unclear, observational studies.

guideline of lifestyle modification for BP control includes the DASH pattern, sodium reduction, weight loss, increased physical activity, and consumption of alcohol in moderation. Concurrent adherence to several recommendations is likely to hold the greatest promise for preventing and treating hypertension and has been shown to be feasible. In addition to addressing unresolved nutritional hypotheses, future research should focus on strategies to motivate and maintain lifestyle changes for BP control. At both the population level and the individual level, success in dietary and lifestyle intervention relies on multiple levels of support ranging from clinicians to government agencies to private institutes and industries. In particular, partnering with industry to improve the nutritional quality of the food supply, such as reducing sodium and fat content of processed foods, and promoting foods and nutrients consistent with the DASH dietary pattern will play a critical role in implementing dietary and lifestyle modifications. Consistent efforts to educate and promote adherence to dietary and lifestyle guidelines by dietetic and other health care professionals are also instrumental to the prevention and management of hypertension.

APPENDIX 1

Classification of BP and Lifestyle Modification for Adults Ages 18 and Older[a]

Category	Systolic (mm Hg)	Diastolic (mm Hg)	Lifestyle/nutrition modification
Normal	<120	And <80	Encourage
Prehypertension	120–139	Or 80–89	Yes
Stage 1 hypertension	140–159	Or 90–99	Yes
Stage 2 hypertension	≥160	Or ≥100	Yes

[a]Based on the average of two or more properly measured, seated BP readings on each of two or more office visits.
Source: Chobanian, A. V., Bakris, G. L., Black, H. R., et al. (2003). Seventh Report of the Joint National Committee on Prevention, Detection, Evaluation, and Treatment of High Blood Pressure. Hypertension 42(6), 1206–1252.

APPENDIX 2. NATIONAL INSTITUTES OF HEALTH

The DASH Dietary Pattern

This eating plan is from the DASH clinical study. The research was funded by the National Heart, Lung, and Blood Institute (NHLBI), with additional support by the National Center for Research Resources and the Office of Research on Minority Health, all units of the National Institutes of Health. The final results of the DASH study appear in the April 17, 1997, issue of the *New England Journal of Medicine*. The results show that the DASH "combination diet" lowered BP and so may help prevent and control high BP. The DASH dietary pattern is rich in fruits, vegetables, and low-fat dairy foods and low in saturated and total fat. It is also low in cholesterol; high in dietary fiber, potassium, calcium, and magnesium; and moderately high in protein.

The DASH eating plan shown here is based on 2000 calories a day. Depending on your caloric needs, your number of daily servings in a food group may vary from those listed. Note that the servings listed here may be slightly different from those published previously due to the changes in serving sizes. For example, one serving of meat was defined previously as 3 oz., and the new definition is 1 oz.

Following the DASH Eating Plan

The DASH eating plan shown in Table 30.5 is based on 2000 calories a day. The number of daily servings in a food group may vary from those listed depending on your caloric needs. Use Tables 30.6 and 30.7 to help plan your menus, or take them with you when you go to the store.

DASH Dietary Pattern at Other Calorie Levels

The DASH eating plan used in the studies calls for a certain number of daily servings from various food groups. The number of servings you require may vary, depending on your caloric need; Table 30.8 gives the servings for 1600, 2600, and 3100 calories.

Getting Started with DASH

It is easy to adopt the DASH eating plan. Here are some ways to get started:

Change gradually.

- If you now eat one or two vegetables a day, add a serving at lunch and another at dinner.
- If you do not eat fruit now or have only juice at breakfast, add a serving to your meals or have it as a snack.
- Gradually increase your use of fat-free and low-fat milk and milk products to three servings a day. For example, drink milk with lunch or dinner instead of soda, sugar-sweetened tea, or alcohol. Choose fat-free (skim) or low-fat (1%) milk and milk products to reduce your intake of saturated fat, total fat, cholesterol, and calories and increase your calcium.
- Read Nutrition Facts label on margarines and salad dressings to choose those lowest in saturated fat. Some margarines are now *trans* fat free.

Treat meats as one part of the whole meal, instead of the focus.

- Limit lean meats to 6 ounces a day—all that's needed. Have only 3 oz. at a meal, which is approximately the size of a deck of cards.
- If you now eat large portions of meats, cut them back gradually—by a half or a third at each meal.
- Include two or more vegetarian-style (meatless) meals each week.
- Increase servings of vegetables, brown rice, whole wheat pasta, and cooked dry beans in meals. Try casseroles, whole wheat pasta, and stir-fry dishes, which have less meat and more vegetables, grains, and dry beans.

TABLE 30.5 The DASH Eating Plan

Food group	Daily servings	Serving sizes	Examples and notes	Significance of each food group to the DASH eating plan
Grains[a]	6–8	1 slice bread 1 oz. dry cereal ½ cup cooked rice, pasta, or cereal[b]	Whole wheat bread and rolls, whole wheat pasta, English muffin, pita bread, bagel, cereals, grits, oatmeal, brown rice, unsalted pretzels and popcorn	Major sources of energy and fiber
Vegetables	4–5	1 cup raw leafy vegetable ½ cup cut-up raw or cooked vegetable ½ cup vegetable juice	Broccoli, carrots, collards, green beans, green peas, kale, lima beans, potatoes, spinach, squash, sweet potatoes, tomatoes	Rich source of potassium, magnesium, and fiber
Fruits	4–5	1 medium fruit ¼ cup dried fruit ½ cup fresh, frozen, or canned fruit ½ cup fruit juice	Apples, apricots, bananas, dates, grapes, oranges, grapefruit, grapefruit juice, mangoes, melons, peaches, pineapples, raisins, strawberries, tangerines	Important sources of potassium, magnesium, and fiber
Fat-free or low-fat milk and milk products	2–3	1 cup fat-free milk or yogurt 1½ oz. cheese	Fat-free (skim) or low-fat (1%) milk, fat-free, low-fat, or reduced-fat cheese, fat-free or low-fat regular or frozen yogurt	Major sources of calcium and protein
Lean meats, poultry, fish	<6	1 oz. cooked meats, poultry, or fish 1 egg[c]	Select only lean; trim away visible fats; broil, roast, or poach; remove skin from poultry	Rich sources of protein and magnesium
Nuts, seeds, and legumes	4–5 per week	1/3 cup or 1½ oz. nuts 2 tbsp peanut butter 2 tbsp or ½ oz. seeds ½ cup cooked dry beans or peas	Almonds, filberts, mixed nuts, peanuts, walnuts, sunflower seeds, kidney beans, lentils, split peas	Rich sources of energy, fiber, magnesium, potassium, and protein

Food group	Servings	Serving sizes	Examples	Significance
Fats and oils[d]	2–3	1 tsp soft margarine; 1 tsp vegetable oil; 1 tbsp mayonnaise; 2 tbsp salad dressing	Soft margarine, vegetable oil (e.g., olive, corn, canola, or safflower), low-fat mayonnaise, light salad dressing	The DASH study had 27% of calories as fat, including fat in or added to foods
Sweets and added sugars	<5 per week	1 tbsp sugar; 1 tbsp jelly or jam; ½ cup sorbet, gelatin; 1 cup lemonade	Fruit-flavored gelatin, fruit punch, hard candy, jelly, maple syrup, sorbet and ices, sugar	Sweets should be low in fat

[a] Whole grains are recommended for most grain servings.
[b] Serving sizes vary from ½ to 1¼ cups, depending on cereal type. Check the product's Nutrition Facts label.
[c] Because eggs are high in cholesterol, limit egg yolk intake to no more than 4 per week; 1 egg white has the same protein content as 1 oz. of meat.
[d] Fat content changes serving counts for fats and oils. For example, 1 tbsp of regular salad dressing equals 1 serving; 1 tbsp of a low-fat dressing equals ½ serving; 1 tbsp of a fat-free dressing equals 0 servings.

TABLE 30.6 The DASH Dietary Pattern: Sample Menu (Based on 2000 Calories and 2300 mg Sodium per Day)

Food	Amount	Servings provided	Substitution to reduce sodium to 1500 mg
Breakfast			
Orange juice	1 C	2 fruits	
Low-fat milk	1 C	1 dairy	
Bran flake cereal	¾ C	1 grain	2 cups puffed wheat cereal
Banana	1 medium	1 fruit	
Whole wheat bread	1 slice	1 grain	
Soft margarine	1 tsp	1 fats and oils	1 tsp unsalted soft (tub) margarine
Beef barbeque sandwich			
Beef, eye of round, cooked	2 oz.	2 meats	
Barbeque sauce	1 tbsp		
Natural cheddar cheese, reduced fat	2 slices (1½ oz.)	1 dairy	1½ oz. natural cheddar cheese, reduced fat, low sodium
Hamburger bun	1 each	2 grains	
Romaine lettuce	1 large leaf	¼ vegetable	
Tomato	2 slices	½ vegetable	
New potato salad	1 C	2 vegetables	
Orange	1 medium	1 fruit	
Dinner			
Herbed baked cod	3 oz.	3 meats	
Brown rice	½ C	1 grain	
Spinach, sautéed from frozen with	1 C	2 vegetables	
Canola oil	1 tsp	1 fats and oils	
Almonds, slivered	1 tbsp	¼ nuts and seeds	
Cornbread muffin, made with oil	1 small	1 grain	
Soft margarine (tub)	1 tsp	1 fats and oils	1 tsp unsalted soft margarine
Snacks			
Fruit yogurt, fat-free, no added sugar	1 C	1 dairy	
Sunflower seeds, unsalted	1 Tbsp	½ nuts and seeds	
Graham cracker rectangles	2 large	1 grain	
Peanut butter	1 tbsp	½ nuts and seeds	

TABLE 30.7 Total Number of Servings in 2000 Calories/Day Menu

Food group	Servings
Grains	= 7
Vegetables	= 4
Fruits	= 4
Dairy foods	= 3
Meats, poultry, and fish	= 5
Nuts, seeds, and legumes	= 1¼
Fats and oils	= 3

Use fruits or other foods low in saturated fat, *trans* fat, cholesterol, sodium, sugar, and calories as desserts and snacks.

- Fruits and other lower fat foods offer great taste and variety. Use fruits canned in their own juice or packed in water. Fresh fruits require little or no preparation. Dried fruits are a good choice to carry with you or to have ready in the car.
- Try these snack ideas: unsalted rice cakes or nuts mixed with raisins, graham crackers, fat-free and low-fat yogurt and frozen yogurt, popcorn with no salt or butter added, and raw vegetables.

TABLE 30.8 DASH Eating Plan: Number of Daily Servings for Other Calorie Levels

Food group	Servings/day		
	1600 Calories/day	2600 Calories/day	3100 Calories/day
Grains[a]	6	10–11	12–13
Vegetables	3–4	5–6	6
Fruits	4	5–6	6
Fat-free or low-fat milk and milk products	2–3	3	3–4
Lean meats, poultry, and fish	3–4	6	6–7
Nuts, seeds, and legumes	0.5	1	1
Fats and oils	2	3	4
Sweets and added sugars	0	≤2	≤2

[a]Whole grains are recommended for most grain servings as a good source of fiber and other nutrients.

TABLE 30.9 DASH Dietary Pattern Assessment

Food group	DASH recommendation	What is a serving?	Your usual intake	Goal
Fruits	4–5 servings/day	1 medium fruit, ½ cup canned fruit, ¼ cup dried fruit, 6 oz. fruit juice		
Vegetables	4–5 servings/day	1 cup raw leafy vegetable, ½ cup cooked vegetable, 6 oz. vegetable juice		
Low-fat or fat-free dairy	2–3 servings/day	8 oz. milk, 1 cup yogurt or 1.5 oz. cheese		
Grains	6–8 servings/day	1 slice bread, ½ cup cooked rice, pasta, or cereal, preferably whole grain		
Meats, poultry, and fish	Less than 6 servings/day	1 oz. cooked meats, poultry, or fish		
Nuts, seeds, and legumes	4–5 servings/week or 0.5 serving/day	¼ cup nuts or seeds, ½ cup cooked legumes		
Sweets, sugared drinks	Less than ½ serving/day	12 oz. sugared drink, 1 tbsp sugar or syrup, 1 slice of cake/brownie/pie		

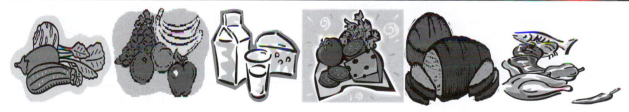

1. Write down your usual intakes of the following food groups using serving sizes defined below.
2. Compare your usual intakes to DASH recommendations and make goal/plans to move closer to DASH.

Other tips
- Choose whole grain foods for most grain servings to get added nutrients, such as minerals and fiber. For example, choose whole wheat bread or whole grain cereals.
- If you have trouble digesting milk and milk products, try taking lactase enzyme pills (available at drugstores and groceries) with the milk products, or buy lactose-free milk, which has the lactase enzyme already added to it.
- If you are allergic to nuts, use seeds or legumes (cooked dried beans or peas).
- Use fresh, frozen, or no-salt-added canned vegetables and fruits.

Source: National Heart, Lung, and Blood Institute (2006). *Your Guide to Lowering Your Blood Pressure with DASH*, NIH Publication No. 06–4082. U.S. Department of Health and Human Services, National Institutes of Health, Bethesda, MD..

For health care providers, Table 30.9 presents a tool for assessing how one's intake compares to the DASH dietary pattern and to make goals and plans in moving toward DASH.

To learn more about high BP, call 1-800-575-WELL or visit the NHLBI website at <http://www.nhlbi.nih.gov/hbp/bp/bp.htm/>. DASH is also online at <http://www.nhlbi.nih.gov/health/public/heart/hbp/dash/new_dash.pdf/> and <http://www.nih.gov/news/pr/apr97/Dash.htm/>.

References

[1] V.L. Burt, P. Whelton, E.J. Roccella, et al., Prevalence of hypertension in the U.S. adult population: results from the Third National Health and Nutrition Examination Survey, 1988–1991, Hypertens. 25 (1995) 305–313.

[2] J. Stamler, Blood pressure and high blood pressure: aspects of risk, Hypertens. 18 (Suppl. I) (1991) I95–I107.

[3] U.S. Department of Health and Human Services, Health, United States, 2006, with Chartbook on Trends in the Health of Americans, U.S. Government Printing Office, Washington, DC, 2006.

[4] J. Stamler, J.D. Neaton, D.N. Wentworth, Blood pressure (systolic and diastolic) and risk of fatal coronary heart disease, Hypertens. 13 (Suppl. I) (1989) I-2.

[5] A.V. Chobanian, G.L. Bakris, H.R. Black, et al., Seventh report of the joint national committee on prevention, detection, evaluation, and treatment of high blood pressure, Hypertens. 42 (6) (2003) 1206–1252.

[6] G.D. James, P.T. Baker, Human population biology and hypertension: evolutionary and ecological aspects of blood pressure, in: J.H. Laragh, B.M. Brenner (Eds.), Hypertension: Pathophysiology, Diagnosis and Management, Raven Press, New York, 1990, pp. 137–145.

[7] F.W. Lowenstein, Blood-pressure in relation to age and sex in the tropics and subtropics, Lancet 1 (1961) 389–392.

[8] L.B. Page, A. Damon, R.C. Moellering, Antecedents of cardiovascular disease in six Solomon Islands societies, Circ 49 (1974) 1132–1146.

[9] J.J.M. Carvalho, R.G. Baruzzi, P.F. Howard, et al., Blood pressure in four remote populations in the INTERSALT study, Hypertens. 14 (1989) 238–246.

[10] W.J. Oliver, E.L. Cohen, J.V. Neel, Blood pressure, sodium intake, and sodium related hormones in the Yanomamo Indians, a "no-salt" culture, Circ 52 (1975) 146–151.

[11] N.K. Hollenberg, G. Martinez, M. McCullough, et al., Aging, acculturation, salt intake, and hypertension in the Kuna of Panama, Hypertens. 29 (2) (1997) 171–176.

[12] N.R. Poulter, K.T. Khaw, B.E.C. Hopwood, et al., The Kenyan Luo migration study: observations on the initiation of a rise in blood pressure, BMJ 300 (1990) 967–972.

[13] J. He, G.S. Tell, Y.C. Tang, P.S. Mo, G.Q. He, Effect of migration on blood pressure: the Yi people study, Epidemiology 2 (1991) 88–97.

[14] I.A.M. Prior, Cardiovascular epidemiology in New Zealand and the Pacific, N. Z. Med. J. 80 (1974) 245–252.

[15] R.J. Eason, J. Pada, R. Wallace, A. Henry, R. Thornton, Changing patterns of hypertension, diabetes, obesity and diet among Melanesians and Micronesians in the Solomon Islands, Med. J. Aust. 146 (1987) 465–473.

[16] J.M. Hanna, D.L. Pelletier, V.J. Brown, The diet and nutrition of contemporary Samoans, in: P.T. Baker, J.M. Hanna, T.S. Baker (Eds.), The Changing Samoans: Behavior and Health in Transition, Oxford University Press, Oxford, 1986, pp. 275–296.

[17] P. Zimmet, L. Jackson, S. Whitehouse, Blood pressure studies in two Pacific populations with varying degrees of modernisation, N. Z. Med. J. 91 (1980) 249–252.

[18] J.S. Kaufman, E.E. Owoaje, S.A. James, C.N. Rotimi, R.S. Cooper, Determinants of hypertension in West Africa: contribution of anthropometric and dietary factors to urban–rural and socioeconomic gradients, Am. J. Epidemiol. 143 (12) (1996) 1203–1218.

[19] N.J. Birkett, Comments on a meta-analysis of the relation between dietary calcium intake and blood pressure, Am. J. Epidemiol 148 (3) (1998) 223–228.

[20] M.A. Stoto, Invited commentary on meta-analysis of epidemiologic data: the case of calcium intake and blood pressure, Am. J. Epidemiol 148 (3) (1998) 229–230.

[21] L.J. Appel, T.J. Moore, E. Obarzanek, et al., A clinical trial of the effects of dietary patterns on blood pressure, N. Engl. J. Med. 336 (1997) 1117–1124.

[22] F.M. Sacks, L.P. Svetkey, W.M. Vollmer, et al., Effects on blood pressure of reduced dietary sodium and the dietary approaches to stop hypertension (DASH) diet: DASH-Sodium Collaborative Research Group, N. Engl. J. Med. 344 (1) (2001) 3–10.

[23] L.J. Appel, F.M. Sacks, V.J. Carey, et al., Effects of protein, monounsaturated fat, and carbohydrate intake on blood pressure and serum lipids: Results of the OmniHeart randomized trial, J. Am. Med. Assoc. 294 (19) (2005) 2455–2464.

[24] M.E. Yamamato, W.B. Applegate, M.J. Klag, et al., Lack of blood pressure effect with calcium and magnesium supplementation in adults with high-normal blood pressure: results from phase I of the Trials of Hypertension Prevention (TOHP), Ann. Epidemiol. 5 (1995) 96–107.

[25] V.J. Stevens, E. Obarzanek, N.R. Cook, et al., Long-term weight loss and changes in blood pressure: results of the trials of hypertension prevention, phase II, Ann. Intern. Med. 134 (1) (2001) 1–11.

[26] L.J. Appel, C.M. Champagne, D.W. Harsha, et al., Effects of comprehensive lifestyle modification on blood pressure control: main results of the PREMIER clinical trial, JAMA 289 (16) (2003) 2083–2093.

[27] D. Reed, D. McGee, K. Yano, J. Hankin, Diet, blood pressure, and multicollinearity, Hypertens. 7 (1985) 405–410.

[28] F.C. Luft, J.Z. Miller, M.H. Weinberger, J.C. Christian, F. Skrabal, Genetic influences on the response to dietary salt reduction, acute salt loading, or salt depletion in humans, J. Cardiovasc. Pharmacol. 12 (Suppl. 3) (1988) S49–S55.

[29] J.R. Sowers, M.B. Zemel, P.C. Zemel, P.R. Standley, Calcium metabolism and dietary calcium in salt sensitive hypertension, Am. J. Hypertens. 4 (1991) 557–563.

[30] J.A. Cutler, The effects of reducing sodium and increasing potassium intake for control of hypertension and improving health, Clin. Exp. Hypertens. 21 (5–6) (1999) 769–783.

[31] D.A. McCarron, The dietary guideline for sodium: should we shake it up? yes!, Am. J. Clin. Nutr. 71 (2000) 1013–1019.

[32] N.M. Kaplan, The dietary guideline for sodium: should we shake it up? no, Am. J. Clin. Nutr. 71 (2000) 1020–1026.

[33] J.A. Cutler, D. Follmann, P.S. Allender, Randomized trials of sodium reduction: an overview, Am. J. Clin. Nutr. 65 (1997) 643S–651S.

[34] M.R. Law, C.D. Frost, N.J. Wald III, Analysis of data from trials of salt reduction, BMJ 302 (1991) 819–824.

[35] N.A. Graudal, A.M. Galloe, P. Garred, Effects of sodium restriction on blood pressure, renin, aldosterone, catecholamines, cholesterols, and triglyceride: a meta-analysis, JAMA 279 (17) (1998) 1383−1391.

[36] M.H. Alderman, B. Lamport, Moderate sodium restriction: do the benefits justify the hazards? Am. J. Hypertens. 3 (1990) 499−504.

[37] F.C. Luft, Sodium: complexities in a simple relationship, Hosp. Pract. (1988) 73−80.

[38] S.K. Kumanyika, J.A. Cutler, Dietary sodium reduction: is there cause for concern? J. Am. Coll. Nutr. 16 (3) (1997) 192−203.

[39] P. Pietinen, J. Tuomilehto, Estimating sodium intake in epidemiological studies, in: H. Kestleloot (Ed.), Epidemiology of Arterial Blood Pressure, Martinus Nijhoff, The Hague, The Netherlands, 1980, pp. 29−44.

[40] A.R. Dyer, P. Elliott, M. Shipley, Urinary electrolyte excretion in 24-hours and blood pressure in the INTERSALT study: II. Estimates of electrolyte−blood pressure associations corrected for regression dilution bias, Am. J. Epidemiol. 139 (1994) 940−951.

[41] C.D. Frost, M.R. Law, N.J. Wald, Analysis of observational data within populations, BMJ 302 (1991) 815−818.

[42] L. Dahl, Possible Role of Salt Intake in the Development of Hypertension, Springer-Verlag, Berlin, 1960.

[43] P. Elliott, Observational studies of salt and blood pressure, Hypertens. 17 (Suppl.) (1991) I-3.

[44] INTERSALT Cooperative Research Group, INTERSALT: an international study of electrolyte excretion and blood pressure: results for 24-hour urinary sodium and potassium excretion, BMJ 297 (1988) 319−328.

[45] J. Stamler, The INTERSALT study: background, methods, findings and implications, Am. J. Clin. Nutr. 65 (Suppl.) (1997) 626S−642S.

[46] M.R. Law, C.D. Frost, N.J. Wald, By how much does dietary salt reduction lower blood pressure? I. Analysis of observational data among populations, BMJ 302 (1991) 811−814.

[47] W. Kempner, Treatment of hypertensive vascular disease with rice diet, Am. J. Med. 4 (1948) 545−577.

[48] J.P. Midgley, A.G. Matthew, C.M.T. Greenwood, A.G. Logan, Effect of reduced dietary sodium on blood pressure, JAMA 275 (20) (1996) 1590−1597.

[49] F.J. He, G.A. MacGregor, Effect of longer-term modest salt reduction on blood pressure, Cochrane Database Syst. Rev. (3) (2004) CD004937.

[50] L. Hooper, C. Bartlett, G. Davey Smith, S. Ebrahim, Systematic review of long term effects of advice to reduce dietary salt in adults, BMJ 325 (7365) (2002) 628.

[51] A.V. Chobanian, M. Hill, National heart, lung, and blood institute workshop on sodium and blood pressure. A critical review of current scientific evidence, Hypertens. 35 (2000) 858−863.

[52] P.K. Whelton, L.J. Appel, M.A. Espeland, et al., Sodium reduction and weight loss in the treatment of hypertension in older persons: a randomized controlled trial of nonpharmacologic interventions in the elderly (TONE): TONE collaborative research group, JAMA 279 (11) (1998) 839−846.

[53] The Trials of Hypertension Prevention Collaborative Research Group, Effects of weight loss and sodium reduction intervention on BP and hypertension incidence in overweight people with high-normal blood pressure: the trials of hypertension prevention, phase II, Arch. Intern. Med. 157 (6) (1997) 657−667.

[54] M.H. Weinberger, J.Z. Miller, F.C. Luft, C.E. Grim, N.S. Fineberg, Definitions and characteristics of sodium sensitivity and blood pressure resistance, Hypertens. 8 (Suppl. II) (1986) II-127.

[55] T. Kawasaki, C.S. Delea, F.C. Bartter, H. Smith, The effect of high-sodium and low-sodium intakes on blood pressure and other related variables in human subjects with idiopathic hypertension, Am. J. Med. 64 (1978) 193−198.

[56] T. Fujita, W.L. Henry, F.C. Bartter, C.R. Lake, C.S. Delea, Factors influencing blood pressure in salt-sensitive patients with hypertension, Am. J. Med. 69 (1980) 334−344.

[57] F.C. Luft, M.H. Weinberger, Heterogeneous responses to changes in dietary salt intake: the salt-sensitivity paradigm, Am. J. Clin. Nutr. 65 (Suppl.) (1997) 612S−617S.

[58] E. Obarzanek, M.A. Proschan, W.M. Vollmer, et al., Individual blood pressure responses to changes in salt intake: Results from the DASH-Sodium trial, Hypertens. 42 (4) (2003) 459−467.

[59] B. Falkner, Sodium sensitivity: a determinant of essential hypertension, J. Am. Coll. Nutr. 7 (1) (1988) 35−41.

[60] G.H. Williams, N.K. Hollenberg, "Sodium-sensitive" essential hypertension: emerging insights into pathogenesis and therapeutic implications, in: S. Klahr, S.G. Massry (Eds.), Contemporary Nephrology, Plenum, New York, 1985 vol. 3, pp. 303−331.

[61] M.B. Zemel, J. Kraniak, P.R. Standley, J.R. Sowers, Erythrocyte cation metabolism in salt-sensitive hypertensive blacks as affected by dietary sodium and calcium, Am. J. Hypertens. 1 (1988) 386−392.

[62] T.A. Kotchen, J.M. Kotchen, Dietary sodium and blood pressure: interactions with other nutrients, Am. J. Clin. Nutr. 65 (1997) 708S−711S.

[63] L.P. Svetkey, T.J. Moore, D.G. Simons-Morton, et al., Angiotensinogen genotype and blood pressure response in the Dietary Approaches to Stop Hypertension (DASH) study, J. Hypertens. 19 (11) (2001) 1949−1956.

[64] S.C. Hunt, N.R. Cook, A. Oberman, et al., Angiotensinogen genotype, sodium reduction, weight loss, and prevention of hypertension: trials of hypertension prevention, phase II, Hypertens. 32 (1998) 393−401.

[65] S.K. Kumanyika, P.R. Hebert, J.A. Cutler, et al., Feasibility and efficacy of sodium reduction in the trials of hypertension prevention, phase I, Hypertens. 22 (1993) 502−512.

[66] National Heart, Lung, and Blood Institute, Implementing Recommendations for Dietary Salt Reduction, National Institutes of Health, Bethesda, MD, 1996 Publication No. 55−728N

[67] F.J. He, G.A. MacGregor, A comprehensive review on salt and health and current experience of worldwide salt reduction programmes, J. Hum. Hypertens. 23 (6) (2009) 363−384.

[68] New York City Department of Health and Mental Hygiene. Cutting Salt, Improving Health. Available at <http://home2.nyc.gov/html/doh/html/cardio/cardio-salt-initiative.shtml/>. Accessed October 2011.

[69] U.S. Department of Agriculture. Dietary Guidelines for Americans, 2010. <http://www.cnpp.usda.gov/dietaryguidelines.htm/>. Accessed October 2011.

[70] P.E. Ray, S. Suga, X.H. Liu, X. Huang, R.J. Johnson, Chronic potassium depletion induces renal injury, salt sensitivity, and hypertension in young rats, Kidney Int. 59 (5) (2001) 1850−1858.

[71] M.S. Zhou, H. Kosaka, H. Yoneyama, Potassium augments vascular relaxation mediated by nitric oxide in the carotid arteries of hypertensive Dahl rats, Am. J. Hypertens. 13 (6 Pt. 1) (2000) 666−672.

[72] F.C. Luft, M.H. Weinberger, C.E. Grim, N.S. Fineberg, Effects of volume expansion and contraction on potassium homeostasis in normal and hypertensive humans, J. Am. Coll. Nutr. 5 (1986) 357−369.

[73] M.B. Pamnani, X. Chen, F.J. Haddy, J.F. Schooley, Z. Mo, Mechanism of antihypertensive effect of dietary potassium in experimental volume expanded hypertension in rats, Clin. Exp. Hypertens. 22 (6) (2000) 555−569.

[74] I.M. Hajjar, C.E. Grim, V. George, T.A. Kotchen, Impact of diet on blood pressure and age-related changes in blood pressure in

the U.S. population: analysis of NHANES III, Arch. Intern. Med. 161 (4) (2001) 589–593.

[75] O. Ophir, G. Peer, J. Gilad, M. Blum, A. Aviram, Low blood pressure in vegetarians: the possible role of potassium, Am. J. Clin. Nutr. 37 (1983) 755–762.

[76] P.K. Whelton, J. He, J.A. Cutler, et al., Effects of oral potassium on blood pressure: meta-analysis of randomized controlled clinical trials, JAMA 277 (20) (1997) 1624–1632.

[77] F.P. Cappuccio, G.A. MacGregor, Does potassium supplementation lower blood pressure? a meta-analysis of published trials, J. Hypertens. 9 (1991) 465–473.

[78] F.M. Sacks, W.C. Willett, A. Smith, L.E. Brown, B. Rosner, T.J. Moore, Effect on blood pressure of potassium, calcium, and magnesium in women with low habitual intake, Hypertens. 31 (1) (1998) 131–138.

[79] J.M. Geleijnse, F.J. Kok, D.E. Grobbee, Blood pressure response to changes in sodium and potassium intake: a metaregression analysis of randomised trials, J. Hum. Hypertens. 17 (7) (2003) 471–480.

[80] H.O. Dickinson, D.J. Nicolson, F. Campbell, F.R. Beyer, J. Mason, Potassium supplementation for the management of primary hypertension in adults, Cochrane Database Syst. Rev. (3)) (2006) CD004641.

[81] M.D. Crawford, M.J. Gardner, J.N. Morris, Mortality and hardness of local water supplies, Lancet 1 (1968) 827–831.

[82] J.A. Cutler, E. Brittain, Calcium and blood pressure: an epidemiologic perspective, Am. J. Hypertens. 3 (1990) 137S–146S.

[83] F.P. Cappuccio, P. Elliott, P.S. Allender, J. Pryer, D.A. Follman, J.A. Cutler, Epidemiologic association between dietary calcium intake and blood pressure: a meta-analysis of published data, Am. J. Epidemiol. 142 (9) (1995) 935–945.

[84] I.M. Hajjar, C.E. Grim, T.A. Kotchen, Dietary calcium lowers the age-related rise in blood pressure in the United States: the NHANES III survey, J. Clin. Hypertens. 5 (2) (2003) 122–126.

[85] H. Schroder, E. Schmelz, J. Marrugat, Relationship between diet and blood pressure in a representative Mediterranean population, Eur. J. Nutr. 41 (4) (2002) 161–167.

[86] Y. Morikawa, H. Nakagawa, A. Okayama, et al., A cross-sectional study on association of calcium intake with blood pressure in Japanese population, J. Hum. Hypertens. 16 (2) (2002) 105–110.

[87] L. Djousse, J.S. Pankow, S.C. Hunt, et al., Influence of saturated fat and linolenic acid on the association between intake of dairy products and blood pressure, Hypertens. 48 (2) (2006) 335–341.

[88] R. Jorde, K.H. Bonaa, Calcium from dairy products, vitamin D intake, and blood pressure: the tromso study, Am. J. Clin. Nutr. 71 (6) (2000) 1530–1535.

[89] A. Alonso, V. Ruiz-Gutierrez, M.A. Martinez-Gonzalez, Monounsaturated fatty acids, olive oil and blood pressure: epidemiological, clinical and experimental evidence, Public Health Nutr. 9 (2) (2006) 251–257.

[90] W.L.T. Addison, H.G. Clark, Calcium and potassium chlorides in the treatment of arterial hypertension, Can. Med. Assoc. J. 15 (1924) 913–915.

[91] F.P. Cappuccio, A. Siani, P. Strazzullo, Oral calcium supplementation and blood pressure: an overview of randomized controlled trials, J. Hypertens. 7 (1989) 941–946.

[92] H.C. Bucher, R.J. Cook, G.H. Guyatt, et al., Effects of dietary calcium supplementation on blood pressure, JAMA 275 (13) (1986) 1016–1022.

[93] P.S. Allender, J.A. Cutler, D. Follmann, F.P. Cappuccio, J. Pryer, P. Elliott, Dietary calcium and blood pressure: a meta-analysis of randomized clinical trials, Ann. Intern. Med. 124 (1996) 825–831.

[94] L.E. Griffith, G.H. Guyatt, R.J. Cook, H.C. Bucher, D.J. Cook, The influence of dietary and nondietary calcium supplementation on blood pressure: an updated meta-analysis of randomized controlled trials, Am. J. Hypertens. 12 (1999) 84–92.

[95] L.A. van Mierlo, L.R. Arends, M.T. Streppel, et al., Blood pressure response to calcium supplementation: a meta-analysis of randomized controlled trials, J. Hum. Hypertens. 20 (8) (2006) 571–580.

[96] H.O. Dickinson, D.J. Nicolson, J.V. Cook, et al., Calcium supplementation for the management of primary hypertension in adults, Cochrane Database Syst. Rev. (2) (2006) CD004639.

[97] F.P. Cappuccio, The calcium antihypertension theory, Am. J. Hypertens. 12 (1999) 93–95.

[98] S.A. Kynast-Gales, L.K. Massey, Effects of dietary calcium from dairy products on ambulatory blood pressure in hypertensive men, J. Am. Diet. Assoc. 92 (1992) 1497–1501.

[99] I.R. Reid, A. Horne, B. Mason, R. Ames, U. Bava, G.D. Gamble, Effects of calcium supplementation on body weight and blood pressure in normal older women: a randomized controlled trial, J. Clin. Endocrinol. Metab. 90 (7) (2005) 3824–3829.

[100] C.A. Nowson, A. Worsley, C. Margerison, et al., Blood pressure response to dietary modifications in free-living individuals, J. Nutr. 134 (9) (2004) 2322–2329.

[101] R. Jorde, K. Szumlas, E. Haug, J. Sundsfjord, The effects of calcium supplementation to patients with primary hyperparathyroidism and a low calcium intake, Eur. J. Nutr. 41 (6) (2002) 258–263.

[102] S.F. Elmarsafawy, N.B. Jain, J. Schwartz, D. Sparrow, H. Nie, H. Hu, Dietary calcium as a potential modifier of the relationship of lead burden to blood pressure, Epidemiol. 17 (5) (2006) 531–537.

[103] T.J. Moore, The role of dietary electrolytes in hypertension, J. Am. Coll. Nutr. 8 (Suppl.) (1989) 1–12.

[104] R.M. Touyz, Q. Pu, G. He, et al., Effects of low dietary magnesium intake on development of hypertension in stroke-prone spontaneously hypertensive rats: role of reactive oxygen species, J. Hypertens. 20 (11) (2002) 2221–2232.

[105] D. Blache, S. Devaux, O. Joubert, et al., Long-term moderate magnesium-deficient diet shows relationships between blood pressure, inflammation and oxidant stress defense in aging rats, Free Radic. Biol. Med. 41 (2) (2006) 277–284.

[106] K. Kisters, F. Wessels, F. Tokmak, et al., Early-onset increased calcium and decreased magnesium concentrations and an increased calcium/magnesium ratio in SHR versus WKY, Magnes. Res. 17 (4) (2004) 264–269.

[107] C.Y. Yang, H.F. Chin, Calcium and magnesium in drinking water and risk of death from hypertension, Am. J. Hypertens. 12 (9) (1999) 894–899.

[108] M.R. Joffres, D.M. Reed, K. Yano, Relationship of magnesium intake and other dietary factors to blood pressure: the Honolulu heart study, Am. J. Clin. Nutr. 45 (1987) 469–475.

[109] A. Ascherio, E. Rimm, E.L. Giovannucci, et al., A prospective study of nutritional factors and hypertension among U.S. men, Circ. 86 (1992) 1475–1484.

[110] J.C.M. Witteman, W.C. Willett, M.J. Stampfer, et al., A prospective study of nutritional factors and hypertension among U.S. women, Circ. 80 (1989) 1320–1327.

[111] Y. Song, H.D. Sesso, J.E. Manson, N.R. Cook, J.E. Buring, S. Liu, Dietary magnesium intake and risk of incident hypertension among middle-aged and older U.S. women in a 10-year follow-up study, Am. J. Cardiol. 98 (12) (2006) 1616–1621.

[112] A.J. Reyes, W.P. Leary, T.N. Acosta-Barrios, W.H. Davis, Magnesium supplementation in hypertension treated with hydrochlorothiazide, Curr. Ther. Res. 36 (2) (1984) 332–340.

[113] F.P. Cappuccio, N.D. Markandu, G.W. Beynon, A.C. Shore, B. Sampson, G.A. MacGregor, Lack of effect of oral magnesium on high blood pressure: a double blind study, BMJ 291 (1985) 235–238.

[114] D.G. Henderson, J. Schierup, T. Schodt, Effect of magnesium supplementation on blood pressure and electrolyte concentrations in hypertensive patients receiving long term diuretic treatment, BMJ 293 (1986) 664–665.

[115] C.A. Nowson, T.O. Morgan, Magnesium supplementation in mild hypertensive patients on a moderately low sodium diet, Clin. Exp. Pharm. Physiol. 16 (1989) 299–302.

[116] P.C. Zemel, M.B. Zemel, M. Urberg, F.L. Douglas, R. Geiser, J.R. Sowers, Metabolic and hemodynamic effects of magnesium supplementation in patients with essential hypertension, Am. J. Clin. Nutr. 51 (1990) 665–669.

[117] M.P. Wirell, P.O. Wester, B.G. Stegmayr, Nutritional dose of magnesium in hypertensive patients on beta blockers lowers systolic blood pressure: a double-blind, cross-over study, J. Int. Med. 236 (1994) 189–195.

[118] J.C.M. Witteman, D.E. Grobbee, F.H.M. Derkx, R. Bouillon, A.M. de Bruijn, A. Hofman, Reduction of blood pressure with oral magnesium supplementation in women with mild to moderate hypertension, Am. J. Clin. Nutr. 60 (1994) 129–135.

[119] F.M. Sacks, L.E. Brown, L. Appel, N.O. Borhani, D. Evans, P. Whelton, Combinations of potassium, calcium, and magnesium supplements in hypertension, Hypertens. 26 (1) (1995) 950–956.

[120] Y. Kawano, H. Matsuoka, S. Takishita, T. Omae, Effects of magnesium supplementation in hypertensive patients: assessment by office, home, and ambulatory blood pressures, Hypertens. 32 (1998) 260–265.

[121] L. Lind, H. Lithell, T. Pollare, S. Ljunghall, Blood pressure response during long-term treatment with magnesium is dependent on magnesium status: a double-blind, placebo-controlled study in essential hypertension and in subjects with high-normal blood pressure, Am. J. Hypertens. 4 (1991) 674–679.

[122] H.O. Dickinson, D.J. Nicolson, F. Campbell, et al., Magnesium supplementation for the management of essential hypertension in adults, Cochrane Database Syst. Rev. (3) (2006) CD004640.

[123] Y. Song, K. He, E.B. Levitan, J.E. Manson, S. Liu, Effects of oral magnesium supplementation on glycaemic control in type 2 diabetes: a meta-analysis of randomized double-blind controlled trials, Diabet. Med. 23 (10) (2006) 1050–1056.

[124] M.E. Rosenberg, J.E. Swanson, B.L. Thomas, T.H. Hostetter, Glomerular and hormonal responses to dietary protein intake in human renal disease, Am. J. Physiol. 253 (2) (1987) F1083–F1090.

[125] J. Bergstrom, M. Ahlberg, A. Alvestrand, Influence of protein intake on renal hemodynamics and plasma hormone concentrations in normal subjects, Acta Med. Scand 217 (2) (1985) 189–196.

[126] S. Moncada, A. Higgs, The L-arginine–nitric oxide pathway, N. Engl. J. Med. 329 (27) (1993) 2002–2012.

[127] A. Palloshi, G. Fragasso, P. Piatti, et al., Effect of oral L-arginine on blood pressure and symptoms and endothelial function in patients with systemic hypertension, positive exercise tests, and normal coronary arteries, Am. J. Cardiol. 93 (7) (2004) 933–935.

[128] E. Obarzanek, P.A. Velletri, J.A. Cutler, Dietary protein and blood pressure, JAMA 275 (20) (1996) 1598–1603.

[129] Y. Yamori, M. Kihara, Y. Nara, et al., Hypertension and diet: multiple regression analysis in a Japanese farming community, Lancet 1 (8231) (1981) 1204–1205.

[130] B.F. Zhou, X.G. Wu, S.Q. Tao, et al., Dietary patterns in 10 groups and the relationship with blood pressure: collaborative study group for cardiovascular diseases and their risk factors, Chin. Med. J. (Engl.) 102 (4) (1989) 257–261.

[131] J. Stamler, K. Liu, K.J. Ruth, J. Pryer, P. Greenland, Eight-year blood pressure change in middle-aged men: relationship to multiple nutrients, Hypertens. 39 (5) (2002) 1000–1006.

[132] J. Stamler, A.W. Caggiula, G.A. Grandits, Relation of body mass and alcohol, nutrient, fiber, and caffeine intakes to blood pressure in the special intervention and usual care groups in the multiple risk factor intervention trial, Am. J. Clin. Nutr. 65 (1 Suppl.) (1997) 338S–365S.

[133] J.M. Hodgson, V. Burke, L.J. Beilin, I.B. Puddey, Partial substitution of carbohydrate intake with protein intake from lean red meat lowers blood pressure in hypertensive persons, Am. J. Clin. Nutr. 83 (4) (2006) 780–787.

[134] Y.F. Wang, W.S. Yancy Jr., D. Yu, C. Champagne, L.J. Appel, P.H. Lin, The relationship between dietary protein intake and blood pressure: results from the PREMIER study, J. Hum. Hypertens. 22 (11) (2008) 745–754.

[135] J. He, D. Gu, X. Wu, J. Chen, X. Duan, P.K. Whelton, Effect of soybean protein on blood pressure: a randomized, controlled trial, Ann. Intern. Med. 143 (1) (2005) 1–9.

[136] M. Rivas, R.P. Garay, J.F. Escanero, P. Cia Jr., P. Cia, J.O. Alda, Soy milk lowers blood pressure in men and women with mild to moderate essential hypertension, J. Nutr. 132 (7) (2002) 1900–1902.

[137] S. Kreijkamp-Kaspers, L. Kok, M.L. Bots, D.E. Grobbee, J.W. Lampe, Y.T. van der Schouw, Randomized controlled trial of the effects of soy protein containing isoflavones on vascular function in postmenopausal women, Am. J. Clin. Nutr. 81 (1) (2005) 189–195.

[138] M. Sagara, T. Kanda, M. Njelekera, et al., Effects of dietary intake of soy protein and isoflavones on cardiovascular disease risk factors in high risk, middle-aged men in Scotland, J. Am. Coll. Nutr. 23 (1) (2004) 85–91.

[139] H.J. Teede, D. Giannopoulos, F.S. Dalais, J. Hodgson, B.P. McGrath, Randomised, controlled, cross-over trial of soy protein with isoflavones on blood pressure and arterial function in hypertensive subjects, J. Am. Coll. Nutr. 25 (6) (2006) 533–540.

[140] J.T. Salonen, R. Salonen, M. Ihanainen, et al., Blood pressure, dietary fats, and antioxidants, Am. J. Clin. Nutr. 48 (5) (1988) 1226–1232.

[141] J.T. Salonen, J. Tuomilehto, A. Tanskanen, Relation of blood pressure to reported intake of salt, saturated fats, and alcohol in healthy middle-aged population, J. Epidemiol. Community Health 37 (1) (1983) 32–37.

[142] J. Stamler, P. Elliott, H. Kesteloot, et al., Inverse relation of dietary protein markers with blood pressure: findings for 10,020 men and women in the INTERSALT Study. INTERSALT cooperative research group. INTERnational study of SALT and blood pressure, Circ. 94 (7) (1996) 1629–1634.

[143] H.W. Gruchow, K.A. Sobocinski, J.J. Barboriak, Alcohol, nutrient intake, and hypertension in U.S. adults, JAMA 253 (11) (1985) 1567–1570.

[144] I. Hajjar, T. Kotchen, Regional variations of blood pressure in the United States are associated with regional variations in dietary intakes: the NHANES-III data, J. Nutr. 133 (1) (2003) 211–214.

[145] F. Jakulj, K. Zernicke, S.L. Bacon, et al., A high-fat meal increases cardiovascular reactivity to psychological stress in healthy young adults, J. Nutr. 137 (4) (2007) 935–939.

[146] L.A. Ferrara, A.S. Raimondi, L. d'Episcopo, L. Guida, A. Dello Russo, T. Marotta, Olive oil and reduced need for antihypertensive medications, Arch. Intern. Med. 160 (6) (2000) 837–842.

[147] J.M. Geleijnse, F.J. Kok, D.E. Grobbee, Impact of dietary and lifestyle factors on the prevalence of hypertension in western populations, Eur. J. Public Health 14 (3) (2004) 235–239.

D. CARDIOVASCULAR DISEASE

[148] W. Kopp, Pathogenesis and etiology of essential hypertension: role of dietary carbohydrate, Med. Hypotheses 64 (4) (2005) 782–787.

[149] E.J. Yang, H.K. Chung, W.Y. Kim, J.M. Kerver, W.O. Song, Carbohydrate intake is associated with diet quality and risk factors for cardiovascular disease in U.S. adults: NHANES III, J. Am. Coll. Nutr. 22 (1) (2003) 71–79.

[150] A.A. Bremer, P. Auinger, R.S. Byrd, Relationship between insulin resistance-associated metabolic parameters and anthropometric measurements with sugar-sweetened beverage intake and physical activity levels in U.S. adolescents: findings from the 1999–2004 national health and nutrition examination survey, Arch. Pediatr. Adolesc. Med. 163 (4) (2009) 328–335.

[151] S. Nguyen, H.K. Choi, R.H. Lustig, C.Y. Hsu, Sugar-sweetened beverages, serum uric acid, and blood pressure in adolescents, J. Pediatr. 154 (6) (2009) 807–813.

[152] D.I. Jalal, G. Smits, R.J. Johnson, M. Chonchol, Increased fructose associates with elevated blood pressure, J. Am. Soc. Nephrol. 21 (2010) 1543–1549.

[153] L. Wang, J.M. Gaziano, S. Liu, J.E. Manson, J.E. Buring, H.D. Sesso, Whole- and refined-grain intakes and the risk of hypertension in women, Am. J. Clin. Nutr. 86 (2) (2007) 472–479.

[154] A.J. Flint, F.B. Hu, R.J. Glynn, et al., Whole grains and incident hypertension in men, Am. J. Clin. Nutr. 90 (3) (2009) 493–498.

[155] M. Shah, B. Adams-Huet, A. Garg, Effect of high-carbohydrate or high-cis-monounsaturated fat diets on blood pressure: a meta-analysis of intervention trials, Am. J. Clin. Nutr. 85 (5) (2007) 1251–1256.

[156] R.E. Hodges, T. Rebello, Carbohydrates and blood pressure, Ann. Intern. Med. 98 (Part 2) (1983) 838–841.

[157] C.M. Brown, A.G. Dulloo, G. Yepuri, J.P. Montani, Fructose ingestion acutely elevates blood pressure in healthy young humans, Am. J. Physiol. Regul. Integr. Comp. Physiol. 294 (3) (2008) R730–R737.

[158] P.J. Palumbo, E.R. Briones, R.A. Nelson, B.A. Kottke, Sucrose sensitivity of patients with coronary-artery disease, Am. J. Clin. Nutr. 30 (1977) 394–401.

[159] R.S. Surwit, M.N. Feinglos, C.C. McCaskill, et al., Metabolic and behavioral effects of a high-sucrose diet during weight loss, Am. J. Clin. Nutr. 65 (1997) 908–915.

[160] J. He, P.K. Whelton, Effect of dietary fiber and protein intake on blood pressure: a review of epidemiologic evidence, Clin. Exp. Hypertens. 21 (5–6) (1999) 785–796.

[161] D. Lairon, N. Arnault, S. Bertrais, et al., Dietary fiber intake and risk factors for cardiovascular disease in French adults, Am. J. Clin. Nutr. 82 (6) (2005) 1185–1194.

[162] A. Ascherio, E.B. Rimm, E.L. Giovannucci, et al., A prospective study of nutritional factors and hypertension among U.S. men, Circ. 86 (5) (1992) 1475–1484.

[163] M.T. Streppel, L.R. Arends, P. van 't Veer, D.E. Grobbee, J.M. Geleijnse, Dietary fiber and blood pressure: a meta-analysis of randomized placebo-controlled trials, Arch. Intern. Med. 165 (2) (2005) 150–156.

[164] W.C. Cushman, J.A. Cutler, S.F. Bingham, et al., Prevention and treatment of hypertension study (PATHS): rationale and design, Am. J. Hypertens. 7 (1994) 814–823.

[165] S. MacMahon, Alcohol consumption and hypertension, Hypertens. 9 (1987) 111–121.

[166] M.R. Piano, The cardiovascular effects of alcohol: the good and the bad: how low-risk drinking differs from high-risk drinking, Am. J. Nurs. 105 (7) (2005) 89–9187

[167] A.L. Klatsky, G.D. Friedman, M.A. Armstrong, The relationships between alcoholic beverage use and other traits to blood pressure: a new Kaiser-Permanente study, Circ. 73 (1986) 628–636.

[168] J.C. Witteman, W.C. Willett, M.J. Stampfer, et al., Relation of moderate alcohol consumption and risk of systemic hypertension in women, Am. J. Cardiol. 65 (9) (1990) 633–637.

[169] T. Gordon, J.T. Doyle, Alcohol consumption and its relationship to smoking, weight, blood pressure, and blood lipids, Arch. Int. Med. 146 (1986) 262–265.

[170] F.D. Fuchs, L.E. Chambless, P.K. Whelton, F.J. Nieto, G. Heiss, Alcohol consumption and the incidence of hypertension: the atherosclerosis risk in communities study, Hypertens. 37 (5) (2001) 1242–1250.

[171] W.C. Cushman, J.A. Cutler, E. Hanna, et al., Prevention and Treatment of Hypertension Study (PATHS): effects of an alcohol treatment program on blood pressure, Arch. Intern. Med. 158 (1998) 1197–1207.

[172] P. Wallace, S. Cutler, A. Haines, Randomised controlled trial of general practitioner intervention in patients with excessive alcohol consumption, BMJ 297 (1988) 663–668.

[173] I.B. Puddey, M. Parker, L.J. Beilin, R. Vandongen, J.R.L. Masarei, Effects of alcohol and caloric restrictions on blood pressure and serum lipids in overweight men, Hypertens. 20 (1992) 533–541.

[174] X. Xin, J. He, M.G. Frontini, L.G. Ogden, O.I. Motsamai, P.K. Whelton, Effects of alcohol reduction on blood pressure: a meta-analysis of randomized controlled trials, Hypertens. 38 (5) (2001) 1112–1117.

[175] L.J. Beilin, Alcohol, hypertension and cardiovascular disease, J. Hypertens. 13 (1995) 939–942.

[176] E.B. Rimm, E.L. Giovannucci, W.C. Willett, et al., A prospective study of alcohol consumption and the risk of coronary disease in men, Lancet 338 (1991) 464–468.

[177] B. Armstrong, A.J. van Merwyk, H. Coates, Blood pressure in seventh-day adventist vegetarians, Am. J. Epidemiol. 105 (5) (1977) 444–449.

[178] F.M. Sacks, B. Rosner, E.H. Kass, Blood pressure in vegetarians, Am. J. Epidemiol. 100 (5) (1974) 390–398.

[179] M.L. Burr, C.J. Bates, A.M. Fehily, A.S. St. Leger, Plasma cholesterol and blood pressure in vegetarians, J. Hum. Nutr. 35 (6) (1981) 437–441.

[180] L.J. Beilin, I.L. Rouse, B.K. Armstrong, B.M. Margetts, R. Vandongen, Vegetarian diet and blood pressure levels: incidental or causal association? Am. J. Clin. Nutr. 48 (3 Suppl.) (1988) 806–810.

[181] B.M. Margetts, L.J. Beilin, R. Vandongen, B.K. Armstrong, Vegetarian diet in mild hypertension: a randomised controlled trial, Br. Med. J. (Clin. Res. Ed.) 293 (6560) (1986) 1468–1471.

[182] I.L. Rouse, L.J. Beilin, B.K. Armstrong, R. Vandongen, Blood-pressure-lowering effect of a vegetarian diet: controlled trial in normotensive subjects, Lancet 1 (8314–8315) (1983) 5–10.

[183] B.J. Materson, D.J. Reda, W.C. Cushman, et al., Single-drug therapy for hypertension in men: a comparison of six antihypertensive agents with placebo. The department of veterans affairs cooperative study group on antihypertensive agents, N. Engl. J. Med. 328 (13) (1993) 914–921.

[184] E. Obarzanek, F.M. Sacks, W.M. Vollmer, et al., Effects on blood lipids of a blood pressure-lowering diet: The Dietary Approaches to Stop Hypertension (DASH) trial, Am. J. Clin. Nutr. 74 (1) (2001) 80–89.

[185] H.P. Dustan, R.L. Weinsier, Treatment of obesity-associated hypertension, Ann. Epidemiol. 1 (4) (1991) 371–379.

[186] J. He, L.G. Ogden, S. Vupputuri, L.A. Bazzano, C. Loria, P.K. Whelton, Dietary sodium intake and subsequent risk of cardiovascular disease in overweight adults, JAMA 282 (21) (1999) 2027–2034.

[187] A.P. Rocchini, J. Key, D. Bondie, et al., The effect of weight loss on the sensitivity of blood pressure to sodium in obese adolescents, N. Engl. J. Med. 321 (9) (1989) 580–585.

[188] J.A. McKnight, T.J. Moore, The effects of dietary factors on blood pressure, Compr. Ther. 20 (9) (1994) 511–517.

[189] D. Spiegelman, R.G. Israel, C. Bouchard, W.C. Willett, Absolute fat mass, percent body fat, and body-fat distribution: which is the real determinant of blood pressure and serum glucose? Am. J. Clin. Nutr. 55 (6) (1992) 1033–1044.

[190] J. Stamler, Epidemiologic findings on body mass and blood pressure in adults, Ann. Epidemiol. 1 (4) (1991) 347–362.

[191] W.R. Harlan, A.L. Hull, R.L. Schmouder, J.R. Landis, F.E. Thompson, F.A. Larkin, Blood pressure and nutrition in adults: the national health and nutrition examination survey, Am. J. Epidemiol. 120 (1) (1984) 17–28.

[192] E.S. Ford, R.S. Cooper, Risk factors for hypertension in a national cohort study, Hypertens. 18 (5) (1991) 598–606.

[193] I.S. Okosun, T.E. Prewitt, R.S. Cooper, Abdominal obesity in the United States: prevalence and attributable risk of hypertension, J. Hum. Hypertens. 13 (7) (1999) 425–430.

[194] Anonymous, The effects of nonpharmacologic interventions on blood pressure of persons with high normal levels: results of the trials of hypertension prevention, phase I, JAMA 267 (9) (1992) 1213–1220.

[195] V.J. Stevens, S.A. Corrigan, E. Obarzanek, et al., Weight loss intervention in phase 1 of the trials of hypertension prevention: the TOHP collaborative research group, Arch. Intern. Med. 153 (7) (1993) 849–858.

[196] J. He, P.K. Whelton, L.J. Appel, J. Charleston, M.J. Klag, Long-term effects of weight loss and dietary sodium reduction on incidence of hypertension, Hypertens. 35 (2) (2000) 544–549.

[197] J.E. Neter, B.E. Stam, F.J. Kok, D.E. Grobbee, J.M. Geleijnse, Influence of weight reduction on blood pressure: a meta-analysis of randomized controlled trials, Hypertens. 42 (5) (2003) 878–884.

[198] P.J. Elmer, E. Obarzanek, W.M. Vollmer, et al., Effects of comprehensive lifestyle modification on diet, weight, physical fitness, and blood pressure control: 18-month results of a randomized trial, Ann. Intern. Med. 144 (7) (2006) 485–495.

[199] B.M. Egan, Y. Zhao, R.N. Axon, U.S. trends in prevalence, awareness, treatment, and control of hypertension, 1988–2008, JAMA 303 (20) (2010) 2043–2050.

[200] S.S. Casagrande, Y. Wang, C. Anderson, T.L. Gary, Have Americans increased their fruit and vegetable intake? the trends between 1988 and 2002, Am. J. Prev. Med. 32 (4) (2007) 257–263.

[201] Centers for Disease Control and Prevention, QuickStats: Age-Adjusted Kilocalorie and Macronutrient Intake among Adults Aged ≥20 Years, by Sex: National Health and Nutrition Examination Survey, United States, 2007–2008, Centers for Disease Control and Prevention, Bethesda, MD, 2011.

[202] P.B. Mellen, S.K. Gao, M.Z. Vitolins, D.C. Goff Jr., Deteriorating dietary habits among adults with hypertension: DASH dietary accordance, NHANES 1988–1994 and 1999–2004, Arch. Intern. Med. 168 (3) (2008) 308–314.

[203] A. Bandura, Social Foundations of Thought and Action: A Social Cognitive Theory, Prentice-Hall, Upper Saddle River, NJ, 1986.

[204] D.L. Watson, R.G. Tharp, Self-Directed Behavior: Self-Modification for Personal Adjustment, Wadsworth, Belmont, CA, 2002.

[205] J.O. Prochaska, C.C. DiClemente, Stages and processes of self-change of smoking: toward an integrative model of change, J. Consult. Clin. Psychol. 51 (3) (1983) 390–395.

[206] J.O. Prochaska, W.F. Velicer, J.S. Rossi, et al., Stages of change and decisional balance for 12 problem behaviors, Health Psychol. 13 (1) (1994) 39–46.

[207] W.R. Miller, S. Rollnick, Motivational Interviewing: Preparing People to Change Addictive Behavior, Guilford, New York, 1991.

[208] S. Rollnick, P. Mason, C. Butler, Health Behavior Change: A Guide for Practitioners, Churchill Livingstone, London, 1999.

[209] A. Bandura, The anatomy of stages of change, Am. J. Health Promot. 12 (1) (1997) 8–10.

PARTE

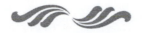

DIABETES MELLITUS

Obesity and the Risk for Type 2 Diabetes

Réjeanne Gougeon

McGill University, Crabtree Laboratory, Montreal, Canada

I INTRODUCTION

One of the medical consequences of obesity is development of type 2 diabetes mellitus. Epidemiological studies, both cross-sectional [1−12] and prospective [8,13−25], show a positive relationship between degree of obesity, notably of central adiposity [7,11,15,16,23,24,26], and the risk for diabetes. Two large prospective studies have examined the impact of obesity on the incidence of diabetes in women [27] and in men [22] and calculated that 77% of new cases in women and 64% in men could be prevented if body mass index (BMI; weight (kg)/height (m²)) were maintained below 25 kg/m². A follow-up study of a middle-aged Japanese population found that increases in BMI of 1, even within non-obese levels, increased the risk for diabetes by approximately 25% [28]. In the EPIC-Potsdam study, weight gain between ages 25 and 40 years was associated with higher risk of diabetes than weight gain in later life [29]. The magnitude of risk associated with adiposity was much greater than with lack of physical activity [24] or other risk factors such as smoking and poor dietary habits [25]. An increase in the prevalence of obesity in certain countries may explain the concurrent and projected increase in diabetes prevalence [30−32] termed "diabesity pandemic" [33]. Body fat mass also increases the risk of developing prediabetic conditions such as glucose intolerance and insulin resistance [6].

Despite these strong associations with diabetes, obesity does not appear to be an essential condition for type 2 diabetes to express itself in a genetically predisposed person. Indeed, 20−25% of type 2 diabetic persons are not obese [27,34,35], and 80% of individuals with elevated BMI and indicators of high intra-abdominal adiposity do not develop diabetes [27]. Low-risk lifestyle patterns that combined not smoking, regular physical activity, a healthful diet, and moderate alcohol consumption reduced risk for new-onset diabetes even among the obese and those with a family history of diabetes [25]. Dietary interventions such as adherence to the Mediterranean food pattern were shown to reduce risk for diabetes without changes in body weight [36]. However, the delaying of diabetes or improvement of its control with weight loss [25,33−44] indicates that obesity affects diabetes and its prevention and management. In a 30-year follow-up subanalysis of the Framingham Heart Study, the risk for cardiovascular disease was lower in normal-weight compared to obese women and men with type 2 diabetes [45].

This chapter (1) provides the current definitions and diagnostic criteria of obesity and diabetes; (2) examines some of the evidence that suggests a major role for excess adiposity in the etiology of diabetes and its complications; (3) examines some of the mechanisms that relate increased adiposity to diabetes; and (4) describes the contributions of weight loss and energy restriction in the treatment of the obese person at risk for diabetes, particularly through lifestyle interventions [46].

II DEFINITIONS AND CLASSIFICATIONS OF OBESITY AND DIABETES

A Obesity

Obesity, which affects one-third of the adult U.S. population [47], has been explained as the result of an imbalance between the intake of energy substrates and energy utilization [48]. This imbalance promotes the shunting of substrates into anabolic pathways for synthesis and storage of fat [48]. Obesity is a medical a condition when fat accumulation is excessive to an extent that it increases risk of ill health [49], especially if it is stored in the abdominal region [50]. The relationship between BMI and adverse health outcomes exists in all age groups, including those older than 75 years [51]. A World Health Organization (WHO) expert committee has proposed cutoff points (Table 31.1) for the classification of overweight and obesity [52] such that it would be possible to identify individuals or groups at risk and to compare weight status among populations. A classification can also provide a basis for the evaluation of interventions. BMI has been used to classify obesity in populations because it correlates with percentage of body fat and with mortality and morbidity. Furthermore, the values are the same for both sexes because the relationship between BMI and mortality is similar in men and women. Because women have a higher percentage of body fat for a comparable weight than men, this indicates that at least premenopausal women can carry fat better than can men. It has been suggested that they do so because their excess fat is mainly subcutaneous and peripherally distributed (thighs, buttocks, and breasts) compared with men, who store fat in the abdominal region [53].

A BMI of $30 \, kg/m^2$ does not always correspond to excess adiposity. A muscle builder may have a BMI of $30 \, kg/m^2$ that is associated with a large muscle mass. Ethnic groups with deviating body proportions, such as being very tall and thin, have healthy BMIs ranging from 17 to 22 and have excessive fat mass at a BMI of $25 \, kg/m^2$ [54].

Cutoff points have also been defined for waist circumference as a surrogate marker of abdominal fat mass [55] and as a strong predictor of metabolic co-morbidities [56]. A waist circumference of 94 cm (37 in.) or more in men and 80 cm (32 in.) or more in women indicates a need for concern [57], even in persons with a normal BMI, and that of 102 cm (40 in.) or more in men and 88 cm (35 in.) or more in women indicates a need for action and intervention [55]. The waist circumference is measured at the narrowest part of the torso, at midpoint between the lower border of the rib cage and the iliac crest, with a nonstretchable tape measure placed horizontal to the floor. It is considered a useful tool for initial screening and follow-up assessment of change. However, increased waist girths have been seen to relate to excess abdominal subcutaneous fat rather than intra-abdominal fat in very obese persons with a normal risk factor profile [58]. It has been suggested that accumulation of intra-abdominal fat may be a marker for a relative inability of subcutaneous fat to store excess energy intake; the overflow would also find its way into ectopic sites such as the liver and skeletal muscles [59]. Studies have shown an inverse association between hip circumference, a marker for subcutaneous fat, and the prevalence of undiagnosed diabetes in a large population-based survey [60]. These findings suggest that larger hips may have a protective effect possibly linked to greater muscle mass or femoral fat mass. Femoral fat has greater lipoprotein lipase activity and lower rates of lipolysis than does intra-abdominal fat, favoring fat uptake and storage, particularly in women [61]. In 2484 men and women, hip circumference was negatively associated with markers of glucose intolerance, independently of the waist circumference, which was positively associated with glucose intolerance [62].

B Diabetes Mellitus

In 2011, the International Diabetes Federation declared that 366 million people worldwide had diabetes mellitus, a prevalence posing a massive challenge to health care systems. Diabetes mellitus is a metabolic disorder characterized by elevated blood glucose concentrations and disturbances of carbohydrate, fat, and protein metabolism secondary to defective insulin secretion and/or action [63,64]. Asymptomatic diabetes, particularly type 2 diabetes mellitus, may be diagnosed when abnormal blood or urine glucose levels are found during routine testing. Exposure to chronic hyperglycemia is associated with pathologic and functional changes in organs such as the eyes, blood vessels, heart, kidneys, and nerves [64].

The classification of diabetes mellitus is based primarily on its clinical description and comprises four major types: type 1, type 2, other specific types, and gestational diabetes mellitus. All differ in their etiology. For example, type 1 diabetes, which is prone to ketoacidosis, is due to autoimmune or idiopathic destruction of the β cells of the pancreas—destruction that results in a deficiency in insulin secretion. Type 2 diabetes is due to metabolic abnormalities leading to a diminished response to the action of insulin, along with a defect in insulin secretion. Other types relate to genetic defects, pancreatopathy, or are first diagnosed during pregnancy (e.g., gestational diabetes) and may or may not subsequently develop into diabetes after parturition [65].

TABLE 31.1 Cutoff Points for Body Mass Index

BMI (kg/m²)	WHO classification of overweight in adults according to BMI
<18.5	Underweight
18.5–24.9	Normal range
25.0–29.9	Overweight, pre-obese at increased risk
30.0–34.9	Obese class I at high risk
35.0–39.9	Obese class II at very high risk
≥40.0	Obese class III at extremely high risk

The classification also includes prediabetes, a term used for impaired glucose tolerance and impaired fasting glucose, which place people at risk of developing diabetes and its complications [66]. Although diabetes is characterized by alterations of fat [67] and of protein metabolism [68,69], glucose impairment remains the hallmark of diabetes diagnosis and control.

Diagnostic criteria for diabetes mellitus [70] are summarized in Table 31.2 and those for prediabetes in Table 31.3. Criteria for the metabolic syndrome are given in Table 31.4.

The diagnosis of diabetes is made in (1) a person who shows symptoms of diabetes (polyuria, polydipsia, and unexplained weight loss) and has a plasma glucose concentration, taken at any time of day, ≥ 200 mg/dl (11.1 mmol/l); (2) a person who has a fasting plasma glucose concentration (FPG) ≥ 126 mg/dl (7.0 mmol/l), fasting meaning at least 8 hours after food consumption; (3) a person with a plasma glucose concentration ≥ 200 mg/dl (11.1 mmol/l) 2-hour post oral challenge of 75 g glucose, called an oral glucose tolerance test (OGTT); and (4) a person with an A1C $\geq 6.5\%$. These values are chosen because they best predict the development of microvascular diseases, such as retinopathy and nephropathy [64], although the thresholds for increased risk of macrovascular diseases also correspond with these values.

Categories of increased risk for diabetes or prediabetes have also been defined for individuals with (1) A1C results between 5.7 and 6.4%;(2) FPG between 100 and 125 mg/dl (5.6 and 6.9 mmol/l), which is referred to as impaired fasting glucose (IFG); or (3) 2-hour plasma glucose of an OGTT at or above 140 mg/dl (7.8 mmol/l) but below 200 mg/dl (11.1 mmol/l), which is referred to as impaired glucose tolerance.

The American Diabetes Association criteria recommend that testing should be done in individuals 45 years of age or older and, when results are normal, be repeated every 3 years thereafter. However, testing should be done at a younger age and more frequently in individuals with a BMI above 25 kg/m^2 because obese individuals are considered to be more at risk of having undiagnosed diabetes. The early detection and treatment of this disease could decrease mortality and minimize complications, especially those related to renal disease, peripheral vascular disease, and cardiovascular disease [63]. Thus, testing individuals at high risk becomes highly cost-effective and has implications in the prevention of diabetes [63]. Obese individuals— particularly those with IFG, IGT, and the metabolic

TABLE 31.2 Criteria for the Diagnosis of Diabetes

1. Symptoms of diabetes and a casual plasma glucose ≥ 200 mg/dl (11.1 mmol/l). Casual is defined as any time of day without regard to time since last meal. The classic symptoms of diabetes include polyuria, polydipsia, and unexplained weight loss.

or

2. FPG ≥ 126 mg/dl (7.0 mmol/l). Fasting is defined as no caloric intake for at least 8 hours.

or

3. 2-Hour plasma glucose ≥ 200 mg/dl (11.1 mmol/l) during an OGTT. The test should be performed as described by WHO using a glucose load containing the equivalent of 75 g anhydrous glucose dissolved in water.

or

4. A1C > 6.5%.

FPG, fasting plasma glucose; OGTT, oral glucose tolerance test.

TABLE 31.3 Plasma Glucose Levels for Diagnosis of IFG, IGT, and Diabetes

	FPG			2hPG in the 75-g OGTT		
	mmol/l	mg/dl		mmol/l	mg/dl	
IFG	5.6–6.9	100–125		NA		
IFG (isolated)	5.6–6.9	100–125	and	<7.8	<140	
IGT (isolated)	<5.6	<100	and	7.8–11.0	140–200	
IFG and IGT	5.6–6.9	100–125	and	7.8–11.0	140–200	
Diabetes	≥7.0	≥126	or	≥11.1	≥200	

2hPG, 2-hour plasma glucose; FPG, fasting plasma glucose; IFG, impaired fasting glucose; IGT, impaired glucose tolerance; NA, not applicable; OGTT, oral glucose tolerance test.

TABLE 31.4 Clinical Identification of the Metabolic Syndrome Using NCEP-ATP III Criteria [72]

Risk factor	Defining level[a]	
FPG	≥ 5.6 mmol/l	100 mg/dl
BP	$\geq 130/85$ mm Hg	
TG	≥ 1.7 mmol/l	>150 mg/dl
HDL-C		
Men	<1.04 mmol/l	<40 mg/dl
Women	<1.29 mmol/l	<50 mg/dl
Abdominal obesity	Waist circumference	
Men	>102 cm	
Women	>88 cm	

[a]*A diagnosis of metabolic syndrome is made when three or more of the five abnormalities are present.*

BP, blood pressure; FPG, fasting plasma glucose; HDL-C, high-density lipoprotein cholesterol; NCEP-ATP III, National Cholesterol Education Program Adult Treatment Panel III; TG, triglyceride.

syndrome, a condition characterized by a constellation of abnormalities that predicts diabetes beyond IGT alone [71] (see Table 31.4 for criteria)—are such individuals at high risk for diabetes and cardiovascular disease [64].

III WHY ARE THE OBESE AT RISK?

A Epidemiological Evidence

Obesity has been implicated as a risk factor for diabetes in cross-sectional [73–75] and longitudinal studies [76–84]. Population-based studies have shown strong associations between central adiposity, assessed by measurements of skinfolds on the trunk, and type 2 diabetes [82,85,86]. Ratios of waist-to-hip circumferences have been reported to be highly predictive of not only abnormal blood lipids and lipoproteins but also glucose intolerance [1–21,87–91]. A meta-analysis of prospective studies provided evidence that as upper body adiposity increased, in the presence of criteria of the metabolic syndrome, the risk of developing diabetes increased [92]. Elevated glucose [17,79,93] and insulin [17] concentrations were likewise associated with a greater risk for diabetes.

Hyperinsulinemia, an indirect indicator of insulin resistance, mediated the development of diabetes in subjects characterized by an unfavorable body fat distribution [94]. However, in other population studies carried out in whites [79], Nauruans [95], and Japanese [96], obesity remained an independent predictive factor after adjusting for glucose and insulin, indicating that it may act through other pathways than insulin action and secretion. Insulin and glucose concentrations may be better predictors of prediabetes, and their screening identifies persons who could benefit from intervention; more obese than lean persons show resistance to insulin action that can improve with weight loss and physical fitness, particularly if they are middle-aged. In a large cohort of Japanese adults, the effect of obesity on incident type 2 diabetes was greater among middle-aged than older adults [97], partly because the risk for diabetes was elevated in non-obese elderly, who show aging-associated increased visceral fat and physical inactivity. There is also evidence that duration of obesity in younger compared with older individuals is associated with a greater risk for diabetes [98].

Data from a cohort of 51,529 U.S. male health professionals, 40–75 years of age, followed during 5 years provided evidence that weight gain during adult life increases the risk of developing diabetes [22]. The risk was 77 times greater in men whose BMI was above 35 kg/m^2 than in lean men. In men who had gained more than 11 kg, the relative risk was amplified

according to their BMI at age 21 years by 6.3 with a BMI below 22, by 9.1 with a BMI of 22 or 23, and by 21.1 with a BMI above 24 kg/m^2. The data also suggested that waist circumference was a better predictor of diabetes than waist-to-hip ratio [22]. A high prevalence of diabetes has been found in populations that have a tendency for central adiposity and have been exposed to the Westernization of their lifestyle and its consequence—weight gain [99].

B Fetal Origins of Type 2 Diabetes and Obesity

Some individuals may be more prone to insulin resistance and diabetes with weight gain if they have been malnourished *in utero*. Maternal undernutrition forces the fetus to adapt during its development and drives a reprogramming of its endocrine—metabolic status to an extent that permanent changes occur in the structure and the physiology of its body [100]. These changes seen in low-birth-weight infants (normal range, 3000–4000 g) have been identified as contributing factors in adult life to chronic diseases such as type 2 diabetes, coronary heart disease, stroke, and hypertension [101–103]. It was first reported in England at the beginning of the 1990s that middle-aged adults who had low weights at birth and during infancy were at greater risk of type 2 diabetes and insulin resistance [103]. This association was confirmed in later studies in Europe and the United States [104–106] suggesting that fetal adaptations or developmental plasticity induced by malnutrition could explain insulin resistance in skeletal muscle [107]. In addition, prenatal exposure to the Dutch famine in 1944 was associated with glucose intolerance and insulin resistance in the offspring once adults, even if the famine had little effect on their birth weights [108].

These associations only applied to infants born of mothers without gestational diabetes. The infants of the latter, by contrast, tend to be of high birth weight (macrosomia) but also at higher risk for developing the metabolic syndrome and type 2 diabetes as adults [106].

In the Nurses' Health Study [106], the inverse association between birth weights and diabetes remained significant even after adjustment for adult adiposity. The increased relative risk was seen among lean, overweight, and obese women, indicating that *in utero* growth had independent effects from adult body weight on the risk for developing type 2 diabetes. However, the greatest risk remained in women of low birth weight who developed obesity as adults [106].

Data obtained from rat studies confirm human observations. Pregnant rats fed isoenergetic protein-restricted diets gave birth to offspring with low birth weights, reduced pancreatic β cell mass and islet vascularization, and an impaired insulin response [109,110]—conditions that were not restored by normal nutrition after birth [110]. These offspring experienced diabetic pregnancies, exposing their fetus to hyperglycemia and increasing their risk of becoming diabetic adults. These observations indicated that *in utero* environment affects endocrine function and, when deficient, contributes to insulin resistance and β cell dysfunction—factors that may lead to type 2 diabetes, especially in the presence of obesity [99].

C Maternal Obesity and Gestational Weight Gain

Maternal obesity has been shown to alter gestational metabolic adjustments and fetal growth and development [111,112]. It is associated with greater incidence of larger placentas and bigger babies [113], which are significant predictors of type 2 diabetes in the offspring [106,114]. Considering that one-third of pregnant women in the United States are obese [115], metabolic complications, preeclampsia, fetal anomalies, and poor pregnancy outcomes have become more prevalent [116]. Risk of gestational diabetes was reported to be up to eightfold in severe obesity [117] and to increase in women who had gained weight within 5 years prior to pregnancy [118]. Infants large or small for gestational age are more often seen in obese compared with normal-weight mothers and are at increased risk for diabetes and hypertension later in life [119]. Some of the factors implicated in maternal obesity, in addition to maternal overnutrition, are (1) maternal hypertension and its influence on placental size [119]; (2) a subclinical inflammatory state and elevated cytokine [120] and leptin levels [112]; and (3) an enhanced insulin resistance that exaggerates the pregnancy-associated increase in circulating plasma glucose, lipids, and amino acids, exposing the fetus to an excess of all fuel sources [121].

The evidence for poor long-term maternal and child outcomes of extremes of weight gains with pregnancy justified that the 1990 Institute of Medicine's (IOM) gestational weight gain guidelines be revised in 2009. Reduced gains of 5−9 kg were recommended in obese mothers [122]. However, less than one-third of pregnant women meet those recommendations [123]. Rather excessive gains (>19 kg) have become the common trend and account for a growing proportion of cesarean deliveries [124] and postpartum weight retention and obesity in mothers [125]. Oken *et al.* [115] reported, in a sample of 1044 mother−child pairs, a fourfold increased risk of having an overweight child at age 3 years in mothers whose gestational weight gain was adequate or excessive compared with mothers whose weight gain was inadequate based on the 1990 IOM guidelines. The increased risk was independent of parental BMI, maternal glucose tolerance, breast-feeding duration, fetal and infant growth, and child behaviors such as frequency of TV watching or fast-food consumption. Strategies for weight control should avoid strict energy and carbohydrate restrictions to prevent ketosis and associated metabolic complications and their negative effects on fetal cognitive development [111]. The dietary approach to treating maternal obesity must attempt to improve insulin sensitivity in the mother without reducing fetal glucose levels and compromising fetal growth. This is achieved by the consumption of dark green and orange vegetables, fruits, legumes, whole grain breads and cereals, carbohydrates with a low glycemic index [126], nuts, fish, low-fat meat and dairy products, and the use of oils such as canola oil for cooking and/or olive oil for salad dressing, while limiting added fat, sugar, and salt. Because motivation for dietary changes may be high during pregnancy, it is an opportune time to establish healthier eating habits and influence those of other family members, father included.

D Visceral Obesity, Inflammation, and Insulin Resistance: Major Predictors of Diabetes

Type 2 diabetes is a syndrome of diseases with different causes. For a minority of patients, they include mutations in some genes, such as the insulin receptor gene, that are associated with insulin resistance or in other genes that impair β cell functions, compromise the glucose-sensing mechanism in the β cell, and present as a mild form of the autoimmune disease [127,128]. However, not all individuals with identified mutations express the diabetic phenotype [129]. Four genes that predispose individuals to developing type 2 diabetes have been identified; two are involved in the development or function of insulin-secreting cells, and one is involved in the transport of zinc, a mineral required for regulation of insulin secretion [130]. The knowledge of specific genetic mutations associated with type 2 diabetes could help in the early identification of people with a genetic risk and in the development of better treatments. It has long been recognized that family history plays an important role in determining if one will develop diabetes. Most prospective studies of prediabetic individuals demonstrate that they are hyperinsulinemic [131] or have impaired insulin secretion—subtle abnormalities of β cell function that may be present before overt diabetes develops. The absence of rapid oscillations of insulin has been reported in first-degree relatives of patients with type 2 diabetes [132]. Other abnormalities include a greater proportion of proinsulin in plasma of patients with type 2 diabetes [133]. Impaired insulin secretion may reflect a genetic susceptibility to impaired glucose tolerance and type 2 diabetes [134,135], but for the majority of patients, the best predictor is insulin resistance.

Insulin resistance, which is characterized by hyperinsulinemia, is closely related to abdominal adiposity, and the inflammatory process is most marked in the visceral fat depot (Figure 31.1) [136–140]. A prospective study that followed second- and third-generation Japanese Americans for up to 10 years confirmed that the amount of intra-abdominal fat plays an important role in the development of diabetes [141]. In this study, visceral adiposity, measured by computed tomography, was predictive of diabetes incidence, regardless of age, sex, family history of diabetes, fasting insulin, insulin secretion, glycemia, and total and regional adiposity. By increasing the demand for insulin, insulin resistance becomes a risk factor for diabetes, causing glucose intolerance in subjects who have impaired insulin secretory capacity and a reduction in the glucose potentiation of insulin secretion [142]. Incremental insulin response to an oral glucose challenge, an assessment of insulin secretion, was depressed in an older generation, suggesting that a failure in β cell function preceded the onset of diabetes [143]. Insulin resistance was also associated with a blunted suppression of glucagon secretion by glucose in impaired glucose tolerance, suggesting that β cell dysfunction and local insulinopenia may exaggerate glucagon secretion because the α cell becomes less sensitive to glucose [142].

E Insulin Resistance in Non-Obese with Visceral Adiposity

The effects of nutrition and sedentary lifestyles on body composition and metabolic fitness are becoming the burden of non-obese as well. Normal-weight individuals are displaying a cluster of characteristics that predispose them to type 2 diabetes. Thirteen young women were identified in a cohort of 71 healthy non-obese women as being insulin insensitive to glucose [144]. The same women had a higher body fat percentage and visceral adiposity compared to the insulin-sensitive group. The energy expended in physical activity, measured by doubly labeled water methodology and indirect calorimetry, was less (2.7 ± 0.9 vs. 4.4 ± 1.5 MJ/day, $p = 0.01$) than that by the insulin-sensitive group. This study indicates that body fat and inactivity override body weight in determining glucose metabolism. Furthermore, there is evidence that there is a high prevalence of these individuals in the general population [145]. Although assessed from self-reported questionnaires, physical activity has been shown to relate negatively with the incidence of type 2 diabetes [146].

F Metabolic Alterations in Obesity that Predispose to Type 2 Diabetes Mellitus

Total fatness and a body fat distribution that reflects visceral fat cell hypertrophy [88,89] alter the metabolism of glucose. Both are associated with more insulin resistance than observed in obese individuals with lower body adiposity [147,148], greater breakdown of the stored fat in adipose cells [149], and elevated plasma nonesterified free fatty acid concentrations that can lead to impaired glucose tolerance [150–153] (Table 31.5).

TABLE 31.5 Metabolic Alterations in Obesity Related to Diabetes

1. α_2-Adrenoceptor activity in abdominal tissue of men that favors greater visceral adiposity
2. β_3-Adrenoceptor sensitivity in visceral fat that increases the lipolytic response to catecholamine
3. Strong relationship between insulin resistance and visceral adiposity
4. Inflammatory cytokines by enlarged adipocytes, altering insulin action
5. Reduction of hepatic insulin clearance in upper body obesity leading to hyperinsulinemia
6. Defects in intracellular glucose transporters
7. Less suppression of fat mobilization by insulin in visceral fat
8. Hypercortisolism in upper body obesity that favors lipolysis
9. Metabolic inflexibility of oxidation fuel selection in skeletal muscle
10. Endothelial dysfunction

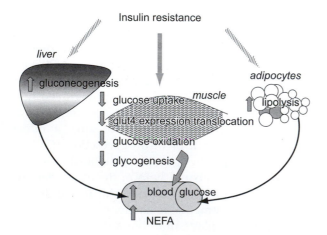

FIGURE 31.1 As fat mass and abdominal obesity increase, insulin sensitivity falls in skeletal muscle, leading to a decrease in glucose uptake, glucose oxidation, especially postprandially, and glycogen stores. In liver, less insulin clearance is contributing to hyperinsulinemia, and gluconeogenesis increases, as does glucose output. Enlarged visceral adipose tissue is associated with less response to the antilipolytic action of insulin and more response to the lipolytic action of catecholamines associated with increased nonesterified fatty acids (NEFA) in circulation.

1 Visceral Fat Alterations in Obesity

The extent of fat storage as triacylglycerol in adipocytes will depend on the balance between its formation and its mobilization. Both processes are under hormonal and nervous system regulation. Insulin plays a major role in suppressing the breakdown of triglycerides or lipolysis by lowering cyclic AMP concentrations [154], which causes a disphosphorylation of hormone-sensitive lipase, and—especially after food intake—by activating the enzyme lipoprotein lipase. Lipoprotein lipase releases fatty acids from chylomicrons and very low-density lipoproteins in the circulation. Half of these are taken up for storage [150]. Catecholamines can suppress lipolysis [155] via their action on α_2-adrenoceptors, but they mostly have the opposite effect of insulin and, by acting on β-adrenoreceptors, increase cyclic AMP and the phosphorylation of hormone-sensitive lipase, stimulating lipolysis and the release of fatty acids in the circulation [155].

Body fat distribution may be influenced by differences in lipoprotein lipase activity. In premenopausal women, lipoprotein lipase activity is higher in femoral and gluteal regions, in which fat cells are larger, compared with abdominal regions. These differences are not seen in men or in postmenopausal women [156]. A greater α_2 activity in the abdominal tissue of men may explain greater adiposity in that location [157].

Body fat distribution also affects the lipolytic response to the catecholamine norepinephrine, being greater in abdominal compared to gluteal and femoral adipose tissues, with abdominal adipocytes having greater β_3-adrenoceptor sensitivity. Receptor numbers are reported to be increased in obese subjects [158]. Because lipolysis is relatively more elevated in visceral fat cells, subjects with upper body obesity would be exposed to a greater release of free fatty acids into the portal system.

2 Insulin Sensitivity in Obesity

Insulin resistance is a major determinant of increased risk for impaired glucose tolerance, type 2 diabetes, and cardiovascular disease in obesity [159]. Studies measuring insulin sensitivity showed similar positive correlations between adiposity, whether measured as BMI or waist circumference, and the steady-state plasma glucose, an index of the capacity of a subject to dispose of a glucose challenge under insulin stimulus [88,160]. The correlation between insulin resistance and abdominal fat has been shown to be independent of total body fatness by some researchers [88,161,162], but others found that its relationship with visceral fat measured by imaging techniques did not explain it to a greater extent than did BMI [159]. Lower insulin-mediated glucose disposal by skeletal muscle

in premenopausal women was also shown with greater upper body fatness and related to the reduction in insulin-stimulated activity of glucose-6-phosphate independent form of glycogen synthase [163].

3 Inflammation and Insulin Resistance

Another factor that may explain why insulin resistance worsens in some obese individuals and not in others as their fat mass increases is the overproduction by specific adipocytes of proinflammatory cytokines such as tumor necrosis factor-α (TNF-α) and interleukin-6 (IL-6). These cytokines block the effect of insulin on glucose transport in skeletal muscle by producing nitric oxide in excess via the induction of the expression of inducible nitric oxide synthase [164,165]. TNF-α mRNA expression in adipose tissue and skeletal muscle correlates with BMI and plasma insulin levels. It inhibits the tyrosine kinase activity of the insulin receptor, altering its action and possibly leading to insulin resistance [166]. In visceral obesity, plasma levels of C-reactive protein, a marker of inflammation produced in the adipocyte, are elevated [167], whereas adiponectin concentrations are reduced [168]. Adiponectin improves insulin sensitivity by inhibiting the action of TNF-α on nuclear factor-κB [169]. Visceral fat cells appear more pathogenic. In fat tissue and liver, lipid accumulation activates inflammatory signaling pathways such that proinflammatory cytokines (TNF-α, IL-6, leptin, resistin, and chemokines) are produced and induce local insulin resistance. Systemic proinflammatory mediators cause insulin resistance in skeletal muscle and other tissues, such as the kidney. Thus, chronic subacute inflammation modulates metabolism in obesity, increasing the risk for insulin resistance and eventually type 2 diabetes (Figure 31.2).

Fractional hepatic clearance of insulin, postabsorptive and during stimulation by intravenous glucose or

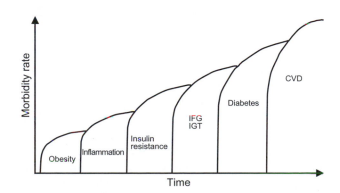

FIGURE 31.2 Probable progression from obesity, particularly visceral obesity, to cardiovascular disease via the inflammatory process, insulin resistance, impaired fasting glucose (IFG), impaired glucose tolerance (IGT), and type 2 diabetes mellitus. CVD, cardiovascular disease.

an oral glucose load, is reduced in upper body obesity compared with lower body obesity, despite indications that the portal plasma insulin levels do not differ [170].

Forty percent of the insulin secreted by the pancreas is removed by the liver. Less hepatic insulin extraction leads to greater peripheral insulin concentrations, a downregulation of insulin receptors, and insulin resistance [171]. This effect may be a consequence of elevated levels of free testosterone and decreased sex hormone-binding globulin [172] that characterize upper body obesity [90].

The transport of glucose into the adipose cell was reduced in obesity and more so in type 2 diabetes because of the depletion of intracellular glucose transporters and carriers for their recruitment to the plasma membrane of the cell [173]. Although the content in intracellular glucose transporters did not differ in the skeletal muscle of subjects who were obese compared with controls, the defect associated with impaired responsiveness to insulin was a loss in the functional activity of the transporters or a decrease in their translocation to the cell surface. The latter may be a consequence of long-term exposure to hyperglycemia in type 2 diabetes [174].

Visceral adipose tissue shows a greater response to lipolytic stimuli but is less sensitive to suppression of fat mobilization by insulin than subcutaneous adipose tissue. The elevated concentrations in insulin in upper body obesity will have a greater inhibitory effect on lipolysis in subcutaneous adipose tissue, and a proportionally greater amount of nonesterified fatty acids will be mobilized from visceral fat [175]. It is conceivable that more portal nonesterified fatty acids will be conducive to greater hepatic and skeletal muscle insulin resistance [176].

Upper body obesity is associated with hypercortisolism, characterized by increased degradation and clearance rates of cortisol that are compensated by increased production rates. Cortisol favors lipolysis by inhibiting the action of insulin and permitting that of catecholamines [177]. Because visceral fat shows a higher density of glucocorticoid receptors compared with subcutaneous fat, hypercortisolism in obesity may contribute to more portal nonesterified fatty acids and hepatic and skeletal muscle insulin resistance.

Plasma nonesterified fatty acid concentrations increase as fat mass increases [176]. Furthermore, as insulin action diminishes with obesity, suppression of nonesterified acids is decreased and their concentration in plasma is increased [171]. The larger supply of fatty acids to the liver, particularly if they are not totally suppressed after meals, is associated with accumulation of acetyl-CoA and inhibition of pyruvate carboxylase altering glucose utilization and stimulating gluconeogenesis and inappropriate hepatic glucose production. In muscle, maintaining or increasing plasma nonesterified fatty acid concentrations decreased insulin-stimulated glucose uptake. Using the euglycemic—hyperinsulinemic clamp and indirect calorimetry, lipid infusions produced a decrease in glucose oxidation and a greater decrease in glycogen synthesis [178]. These results indicated that in insulin-resistant states with increased lipid availability and oxidation, glucose oxidation was reduced. However, in fasting conditions, hyperglycemia in type 2 diabetes was shown to override the effect of increased lipid availability and to be associated with increased glucose oxidation in leg muscle. Normalization of the leg muscle hyperglycemia with a low dose of insulin increased fat oxidation [179]. There is evidence (reviewed in [180]) that postabsorptive skeletal muscle fat oxidation in insulin-resistant states is decreased. This decrease is explained by the presence in muscle of carbohydrate-derived malonyl-CoA, which inhibits carnitine palmitoyl transferase, blocking the entry of free fatty acids into the mitochondria [181]. Carnitine palmitoyl transferase activity has been shown to be reduced in the vastus lateralis muscle of insulin-resistant obese individuals [182]. The excess free fatty acids may increase long-chain acyl-CoA concentrations and diacylglycerol, leading to the accumulation of lipids in muscle—an effect conducive to alterations of insulin signaling and insulin action.

Human studies suggest that muscle lipid content in obesity could be a determinant of insulin insensitivity [183,184], independent of visceral fat [183]. Lipid accumulation in muscle is observed in trained athletes who are insulin sensitive but who have a great metabolic capacity for lipid utilization, which is not the case in muscles of sedentary individuals who are obese. Obese subjects appear to display what has been called metabolic inflexibility of oxidative fuel selection [180]. Compared with insulin-sensitive lean individuals, obese subjects have shown lower fat oxidation after an overnight fast, as indicated by higher leg respiratory quotient (RQ), and less capacity to switch to glucose in insulin-stimulated conditions, as indicated by an absence of increased leg RQ. Furthermore, high levels of free fatty acids may suppress insulin secretion, and their effect may be toxic to the β cells of the pancreas, becoming an important contributor to the pathogenesis of obesity-dependent type 2 diabetes [176]. Elevated nonesterified fatty acid concentration reduces hepatic insulin extraction, further increasing its serum concentration [176].

The prevalence of visceral fat measured by computed tomography correlated with endothelial dysfunction, independent of BMI, in otherwise healthy women who were obese [185]. Endothelial dysfunction was also closely associated with insulin insensitivity. The authors attributed these early alterations involved in the atherosclerotic process to elevated nonesterified fatty acid levels.

As long as the pancreas maintains sufficient insulin secretion to compensate for insulin resistance, glycemia remains within the normal range. Once the β cells fail to compensate, insulin response is decreased and glucose uptake by muscle diminished. Then, the liver oxidizes preferentially fatty acids, and gluconeogenesis is stimulated. The consequences are a conversion from normal to impaired glucose tolerance and, in genetically susceptible individuals, to diabetes [186].

G Associations among Psychological Stress, Diabetes, and Visceral Adiposity

Psychological stress can be associated with high cortisol and low sex steroid concentrations. These antagonize insulin action and cause visceral adiposity, factors that contribute to insulin resistance and the onset of type 2 diabetes mellitus. Psychological stress is known to aggravate glycemia in diabetes [187]. A greater prevalence of previously undetected diabetes was reported with more stressful events; the age- and sex-adjusted association between major life changes and diabetes was independent of family history of diabetes, physical activity, heavy alcohol use, or low level of education. There was no association between work-related stressful events and type 2 diabetes in this cross-sectional study. A weak positive association was found with waist-to-hip ratio, but visceral fat was not the main mediating factor between stress and diabetes [188]. It has been suggested that the link between stress and diabetes may be through other factors, such as the chronic stimulation of the autonomic nervous system and its resulting hyperglycemia [188,189]. The inflammatory consequences of psychological stress have been proposed as the link to insulin resistance and diabetes [190]. Psychological stress via stimulation of the major stress hormones norepinephrine and cortisol, the renin—angiotensin system, the proinflammatory cytokines, and free fatty acid fluxes produces an inflammatory response by activation of nuclear factor-κB in macrophages, visceral fat, and endothelial cells. This process leads to insulin resistance and, if maintained, to increased risk for diabetes.

H Improvement in Insulin Sensitivity with Weight Loss and Energy Intake Restriction

In obesity with diminished insulin action, any weight-loss treatment improves insulin sensitivity and fasting plasma glucose; these improvements are related to losses of abdominal fat [191,192]. Fujioka et al. [191] measured the changes in body fat distribution and those in metabolic disorders after an 8-week energy-restricted diet (800 kcal/day) in 40 women aged 38±9 (mean±SD)

years with uncomplicated obesity. Fourteen women were characterized, by computed tomography, as having visceral fat obesity rather than subcutaneous fat obesity. At week 8 of diet, the decrease in visceral fat volume correlated more with the changes in plasma glucose and in lipid profile than with the decreases in body weight, total fat, or subcutaneous fat volume, and these correlations were independent of total fat loss. The reduction in visceral fat was more pronounced than that in subcutaneous fat.

Another study [192] reported that the improvements in fasting plasma glucose and insulin sensitivity with weight loss related to losses of abdominal fat. This study was designed to distinguish, in 20 overweight subjects with or without type 2 diabetes, the effects of restricting energy intake by 50% before any substantial weight loss took place from those of a weight loss of 6.3±0.4 kg on glycemia, hepatic glucose production, and insulin action and secretion. On day 4 of energy restriction, a significant decrease in fasting hepatic glucose output and a greater insulin suppression of endogenous glucose production, measured during a hyperinsulinemic—euglycemic clamp, were observed in all subjects. Although the decrease in fasting glucose output was counteracted by a decrease in metabolic clearance rate of glucose, it resulted in a decrease in fasting plasma glucose. This decrease related to the decrease in carbohydrate intake. On day 4 of energy restriction, fat oxidation and the nonesterified fatty acid levels were increased. With substantial weight loss, at day 28 of energy restriction, plasma glucose was further decreased in the diabetic subjects only—a decrease associated with increased metabolic clearance rates. Fasting insulin concentrations were reduced compared with the values preceding weight loss, and insulin sensitivity was improved in both groups. These improvements were associated with a reduction in the abdominal fat depot. These data support a role for central adiposity in the alterations of glucose metabolism observed in obesity.

Loss of weight and visceral fat also improved endothelial dysfunction and vascular inflammatory markers when combined with exercise or secondary to gastric bypass surgery [193,194]. Dietary factors modulate endothelial function; not only have postprandial hyperglycemia and hypertriglyceridemia been shown to generate oxidative stress and endothelial dysfunction [195] but also meals high in dietary advanced glycation end products, formed from exposing foods, particularly meats, to high and dry heat (with frying, grilling, barbequing, or broiling for long durations), have been reported to induce acute impairment of vascular function [196]. These results provide evidence for the wisdom of using cooking techniques such as steaming, boiling, poaching, or stewing to minimize dietary sources of advanced glycation end products.

I Obesity and Treatment of Diabetes

The conclusions of the U.K. Prospective Diabetes Study [197] are that optimal diabetes control aiming at an A1C below 7.0% must be achieved if morbidity is to be significantly prevented. To do so, intensive therapy using insulin alone or combined with oral antihyperglycemic agents may be required. Results from the Finnish Multicenter Insulin Therapy Study, in which 100 insulin-treated type 2 diabetic individuals were followed for 12 months, showed that good glycemic control started to deteriorate after 3 months and more so in the obese subjects, the latter being attributed to their greater insulin resistance. Glycemic control was best achieved in the non-obese subjects whether with insulin alone or in combination with other therapeutic agents. However, the combination therapy was associated with less weight gain [198].

Obesity in persons with type 1 diabetes can affect their insulin requirements by reducing their insulin sensitivity. The consequences of increasing the insulin dosages can be further weight gain associated with the lipogenic effects of insulin and the additional eating in reaction to the hypoglycemic events often seen with intensive therapy [199]. Weight gain with insulin therapy is often associated with higher waist-to-hip ratios [197]. Given the associations between obesity and dyslipidemia, atherosclerosis and hypertension, intensive therapy of diabetes should aim at not producing weight gain [197].

IV CONCLUSION

Family history of diabetes and age are recognized risk factors for diabetes [18], but they cannot be controlled. Recommendations for prevention of diabetes address factors that can be controlled. Thus, it is crucial to screen early for persons at risk of developing diabetes using the recommended criteria for BMI, waist circumference, metabolic syndrome, and inflammatory markers. Tight control of glycemia in the person with diabetes is necessary to prevent microvascular complications [197], but fewer than half achieve such control [200]. Furthermore, the increased cardiovascular risk associated with the disease requires that therapeutic strategies be devised to correct the factors related to that risk, including elevated blood pressure, smoking, abnormal lipid profile, low physical activity, and obesity. Current data support that to reduce the incidence of diabetes, it is advisable to achieve a healthy weight when young and maintain it throughout life [22]. Prevention of overall obesity should be the result of a lifestyle that includes healthy eating habits favoring foods with a low energy density [201] and levels of physical activity associated with the maintenance of optimal fitness for age [202]. Innovative ways are especially needed to promote and achieve proficient physical activity and exercise habits in those who are obese and have diabetes [202].

References

[1] S.M. Haffner, M.P. Stern, H.P. Hazuda, J. Pugh, J.K. Patterson, Do upper-body and centralized adiposity measure different aspects of regional body-fat distribution? Relationship to non-insulin-dependent diabetes mellitus, lipids, and lipoproteins, Diabetes 36 (1987) 43—51.

[2] P.A. van Noord, J.C. Seidell, I. den Tonkelaar, E.A. Baanders-van Halewijn, I.J. Ouwehand, The relationship between fat distribution and some chronic diseases in 11,825 women participating in the DOM-project, Int. J. Epidemiol. 19 (1990) 564—570.

[3] E.T. Skarfors, K.I. Selinus, H.O. Lithell, Risk factors for developing non-insulin dependent diabetes: a 10 year follow up of men in Uppsala, BMJ 303 (1991) 755—760.

[4] K.M. Shelgikar, T.D. Hockaday, C.S. Yajnik, Central rather than generalized obesity is related to hyperglycaemia in Asian Indian subjects, Diabet. Med. 8 (1991) 712—717.

[5] G.K. Dowse, P.Z. Zimmet, H. Gareeboo, K. George, M.M. Alberti, J. Tuomilehto, et al., Abdominal obesity and physical inactivity as risk factors for NIDDM and impaired glucose tolerance in Indian, Creole, and Chinese Mauritians, Diabetes Care 14 (1991) 271—282.

[6] T.Y. Tai, L.M. Chuang, H.P. Wu, C.J. Chen, Association of body build with non-insulin-dependent diabetes mellitus and hypertension among Chinese adults: a 4-year follow-up study, Int. J. Epidemiol. 21 (1992) 511—517.

[7] M.I. Schmidt, B.B. Duncan, L.H. Canani, C. Karohl, L. Chambless, Association of waist—hip ratio with diabetes mellitus: strength and possible modifiers, Diabetes Care 15 (1992) 912—914.

[8] P.M. McKeigue, T. Pierpoint, J.E. Ferrie, M.G. Marmot, Relationship of glucose intolerance and hyperinsulinaemia to body fat pattern in south Asians and Europeans, Diabetologia 35 (1992) 785—791.

[9] B.J. Shaten, G.D. Smith, L.H. Kuller, J.D. Neaton, Risk factors for the development of type II diabetes among men enrolled in the usual care group of the Multiple Risk Factor Intervention Trial, Diabetes Care 16 (1993) 1331—1339.

[10] J.A. Marshall, R.F. Hamman, J. Baxter, E.J. Mayer, D.L. Fulton, M. Orleans, et al., Ethnic differences in risk factors associated with the prevalence of non-insulin-dependent diabetes mellitus: the San Luis Valley Diabetes Study, Am. J. Epidemiol. 137 (1993) 706—718.

[11] V.R. Collins, G.K. Dowse, P.M. Toelupe, T.T. Imo, F.L. Aloaina, R.A. Spark, et al., Increasing prevalence of NIDDM in the Pacific island population of Western Samoa over a 13-year period, Diabetes Care 17 (1994) 288—296.

[12] P. Chou, M.J. Liao, S.T. Tsai, Associated risk factors of diabetes in Kin-Hu, Kinmen, Diabetes Res. Clin. Pract. 26 (1994) 229—235.

[13] L.O. Ohlson, B. Larsson, K. Svardsudd, L. Welin, H. Eriksson, L. Wilhelmsen, et al., The influence of body fat distribution on the incidence of diabetes mellitus: 13.5 years of follow-up of the participants in the study of men born in 1913, Diabetes 34 (1985) 1055—1058.

[14] M. Modan, A. Karasik, H. Halkin, Z. Fuchs, A. Lusky, A. Shitrit, et al., Effect of past and concurrent body mass index on prevalence of glucose intolerance and type 2 (non-insulin-dependent) diabetes and on insulin response: the Israel Study of Glucose

Intolerance, Obesity and Hypertension, Diabetologia 29 (1986) 82−89.

[15] H. Lundgren, C. Bengtsson, G. Blohme, L. Lapidus, L. Sjostrom, Adiposity and adipose tissue distribution in relation to incidence of diabetes in women: results from a prospective population study in Gothenburg, Sweden, Int. J. Obes. 13 (1989) 413−423.

[16] S. Lemieux, D. Prud'homme, A. Nadeau, A. Tremblay, C. Bouchard, J.P. Despres, Seven-year changes in body fat and visceral adipose tissue in women: association with indexes of plasma glucose-insulin homeostasis, Diabetes Care 19 (1996) 983−991.

[17] S.M. Haffner, M.P. Stern, B.D. Mitchell, H.P. Hazuda, J.K. Patterson, Incidence of type II diabetes in Mexican Americans predicted by fasting insulin and glucose levels, obesity, and body-fat distribution, Diabetes 39 (1990) 283−288.

[18] G.A. Colditz, W.C. Willett, M.J. Stampfer, J.E. Manson, C.H. Hennekens, R.A. Arky, et al., Weight as a risk factor for clinical diabetes in women, Am. J. Epidemiol. 132 (1990) 501−513.

[19] W.C. Knowler, D.J. Pettitt, M.F. Saad, M.A. Charles, R.G. Nelson, B.V. Howard, et al., Obesity in the Pima Indians: its magnitude and relationship with diabetes, Am. J. Clin. Nutr. 53 (1991) 1543S−1551S.

[20] M.A. Charles, A. Fontbonne, N. Thibult, J.M. Warnet, G.E. Rosselin, E. Eschwege, Risk factors for NIDDM in white population: Paris prospective study, Diabetes 40 (1991) 796−799.

[21] P.A. Cassano, B. Rosner, P.S. Vokonas, S.T. Weiss, Obesity and body fat distribution in relation to the incidence of non-insulin-dependent diabetes mellitus: a prospective cohort study of men in the normative aging study, Am. J. Epidemiol. 136 (1992) 1474−1486.

[22] J.M. Chan, E.B. Rimm, G.A. Colditz, M.J. Stampfer, W.C. Willett, Obesity, fat distribution, and weight gain as risk factors for clinical diabetes in men, Diabetes Care 17 (1994) 961−969.

[23] Y. Wang, E.B. Rimm, M.J. Stampfer, W.C. Willett, F.B. Hu, Comparison of abdominal adiposity and overall obesity in predicting risk of type 2 diabetes among men, Am. J. Clin. Nutr. 81 (2005) 555−563.

[24] J.S. Rana, T.Y. Li, J.E. Manson, F.B. Hu, Adiposity compared with physical inactivity and risk of type 2 diabetes in women, Diabetes Care 30 (2007) 53−58.

[25] J.P. Reis, C.M. Loria, P.D. Sorlie, Y. Park, A. Hollenbeck, A. Schatzkin, Lifestyle factors and risk of new-onset diabetes: a population-based cohort study, Ann. Intern. Med. 6 (2011) 292−299.

[26] A.M. Wassink, Y. Van Der Graaf, S.S. Soedamah-Muthu, W. Spiering, F.L. Visseren, the Smart Study Group, Metabolic syndrome and incidence of type 2 diabetes in patients with manifest vascular disease, Diab. Vasc. Dis. Res. 5 (2008) 114−122.

[27] G.A. Colditz, W.C. Willett, A. Rotnitzky, J.E. Manson, Weight gain as a risk factor for clinical diabetes mellitus in women, Ann. Intern. Med. 122 (1995) 481−486.

[28] T. Nagaya, H. Yoshida, H. Takahashi, M. Kawai, Increases in body mass index, even within non-obese levels, raise the risk for type 2 diabetes mellitus: a follow-up study in a Japanese population, Diabet. Med. 22 (2005) 1107−1111.

[29] A. Schienkiewitz, M.B. Schulze, K. Hoffmann, A. Kroke, H. Boeing, Body mass index history and risk of type 2 diabetes: results from the European Prospective Investigation into Cancer and Nutrition (EPIC)−Potsdam Study, Am. J. Clin. Nutr. 84 (2006) 427−433.

[30] D. Ruwaard, R. Gijsen, A.I. Bartelds, R.A. Hirasing, H. Verkleij, D. Kromhout, Is the incidence of diabetes increasing in all age-groups in The Netherlands? Results of the second study in the Dutch Sentinel Practice Network, Diabetes Care 19 (1996) 214−218.

[31] K. Midthjell, O. Kruger, J. Holmen, A. Tverdal, T. Claudi, A. Bjorndal, et al., Rapid changes in the prevalence of obesity and known diabetes in an adult Norwegian population: the Nord-Trondelag Health Surveys: 1984−1986 and 1995−1997, Diabetes Care 22 (1999) 1813−1820.

[32] A.G. Mainous III, R. Baker, R.J. Koopman, S. Saxena, V.A. Diaz, C.J. Everett, et al., Impact of the population at risk of diabetes on projections of diabetes burden in the United States: an epidemic on the way, Diabetologia 50 (2007) 934−940.

[33] A. Astrup, N. Finer, Redefining type 2 diabetes: "Diabesity" or "obesity dependent diabetes mellitus"? Obes. Rev. 1 (2000) 57−59.

[34] D.R. Hadden, D.A. Montgomery, R.J. Skelly, E.R. Trimble, J.A. Weaver, E.A. Wilson, et al., Maturity onset diabetes mellitus: response to intensive dietary management, Br. Med. J. 3 (1975) 276−278.

[35] M.E. Lean, J.K. Powrie, A.S. Anderson, P.H. Garthwaite, Obesity, weight loss and prognosis in type 2 diabetes, Diabet. Med. 7 (1990) 228−233.

[36] J. Salas-Salvado, M. Bullo, M.A. Martinez-Gonzalez, N. Ibarrola-Jurado, J. Basora, R. Estruch, PREDIMED study investigators, et al., Reduction in the incidence of type 2 diabetes with the Mediterranean diet: results of the PREDIMED-Reus nutrition intervention randomized trial, Diabetes Care 34 (2011) 14−19.

[37] UK Prospective Diabetes Study, UK Prospective Diabetes Study 7: response of fasting plasma glucose to diet therapy in newly presenting type II diabetic patients, Metabolism 39 (1990) 909−912.

[38] B. Vessby, M. Boberg, B. Karlstrom, H. Lithell, I. Werner, Improved metabolic control after supplemented fasting in overweight type II diabetic patients, Acta Med. Scand. 216 (1984) 67−74.

[39] D.F. Williamson, E. Pamuk, M. Thun, D. Flanders, T. Byers, C. Heath, Prospective study of intentional weight loss and mortality in never-smoking overweight U.S. white women aged 40−64 years, Am. J. Epidemiol. 141 (1995) 1128−1141.

[40] J. Tuomilehto, J. Lindstrom, J.G. Eriksson, T.T. Valle, H. Hamalainen, P. Ilanne-Parikka, et al., Prevention of type 2 diabetes mellitus by changes in lifestyle among subjects with impaired glucose tolerance, N. Engl. J. Med. 344 (2001) 1343−1350.

[41] W.C. Knowler, E. Barrett-Connor, S.E. Fowler, R.F. Hamman, J.M. Lachin, E.A. Walker, et al., Reduction in the incidence of type 2 diabetes with lifestyle intervention or metformin, N. Engl. J. Med. 346 (2002) 393−403.

[42] C.L. Gillies, K.R. Abrams, P.C. Lambert, N.J. Cooper, A.J. Sutton, R.T. Hsu, et al., Pharmacological and lifestyle interventions to prevent or delay type 2 diabetes in people with impaired glucose tolerance: systematic review and meta-analysis, BMJ 334 (2007) 299.

[43] T. Saaristo, L. Moilanen, E. Korpi-Hyövältj, J. Saltevo, L. Niskanen, J. Jokelainen, et al., Lifestyle intervention for prevention of type 2 diabetes in primary health care: one-year follow-up of the Finnish National Diabetes Prevention Program (FIN-D2D), Diabetes Care 33 (2010) 46−51.

[44] R.R. Wing, the Look AHEAD Research Group, Benefits of modest weight loss in improving cardiovascular risk factors in overweight and obese individuals with type 2 diabetes, Diabetes Care 34 (2011) 1481−1486.

[45] C.S. Fox, M.J. Pencina, P.W. Wilson, N.P. Paynter, R.S. Vasan, R.B. D'Agostino Sr., Lifetime risk of cardiovascular disease among individuals with and without diabetes stratified by obesity status in the Framingham Heart Study, Diabetes Care 31 (2008) 1582−1584.

[46] M. Laakso, Prevention of type 2 diabetes, Curr. Mol. Med. 5 (2005) 365−374.

[47] C.L. Ogden, M.D. Carroll, K.M. Flegal, High body mass index for age among children and adolescents, JAMA 20 (2008) 2401−2405.

E. DIABETES MELLITUS

[48] M. Rosenbaum, R.L. Leibel, J. Hirsch, Obesity, N. Engl. J. Med. 337 (1997) 396–407.

[49] J.S. Garrow, Health implications of obesity, Obesity Related Diseases, Churchill Livingstone, London, 1988, pp. 1–16

[50] J. Vague, The degree of masculine differentiation of obesities: a factor determining predisposition to diabetes, atherosclerosis, gout, and uric calculous disease, Am. J. Clin. Nutr. 4 (1956) 20–34.

[51] J. Stevens, J. Cai, E.R. Pamuk, D.F. Williamson, M.J. Thun, J.L. Wood, The effect of age on the association between body-mass index and mortality, N. Engl. J. Med. 338 (1998) 1–7.

[52] World Health Organization, Physical Status: The Use and Interpretation of Anthropometry: Report of a WHO Expert Committee, World Health Organization, Geneva, 1995Technical Report Series No. 854

[53] J.C. Seidell, K.M. Flegal, Assessing obesity: classification and epidemiology, Br. Med. Bull. 53 (1997) 238–252.

[54] N.G. Norgan, P.R. Jones, The effect of standardising the body mass index for relative sitting height, Int. J. Obes. Relat. Metab. Disord. 19 (1995) 206–208.

[55] S. Lemieux, D. Prud'homme, C. Bouchard, A. Tremblay, J.P. Despres, A single threshold value of waist girth identifies normal-weight and overweight subjects with excess visceral adipose tissue, Am. J. Clin. Nutr. 64 (1996) 685–693.

[56] S. Klein, D.B. Allison, S.B. Heymsfield, D.E. Kelley, R.L. Leibel, C. Nonas, et al., Waist circumference and cardiometabolic risk: a consensus statement from Shaping America's Health: Association for Weight Management and Obesity Prevention; NAASO, The Obesity Society; the American Society for Nutrition; and the American Diabetes Association, Am. J. Clin. Nutr. 85 (2007) 1197–1202.

[57] M.E. Lean, T.S. Han, C.E. Morrison, Waist circumference as a measure for indicating need for weight management, BMJ 311 (1995) 158–161.

[58] I. Lemieux, V. Drapeau, D. Richard, J. Bergeron, P. Marceau, S. Biron, et al., Waist girth does not predict metabolic complications in severely obese men, Diabetes Care 29 (2006) 1417–1419.

[59] P.J. Miranda, R.A. DeFronzo, R.M. Califf, J.R. Guyton, Metabolic syndrome: definition, pathophysiology, and mechanisms, Am. Heart J. 149 (2005) 33–45.

[60] M.B. Snijder, P.Z. Zimmet, M. Visser, J.M. Dekker, J.C. Seidell, J. E. Shaw, Independent and opposite associations of waist and hip circumferences with diabetes, hypertension and dyslipidemia: the AusDiab Study, Int. J. Obes. Relat. Metab. Disord. 28 (2004) 402–409.

[61] M. Rebuffe-Scrive, L. Enk, N. Crona, P. Lonnroth, L. Abrahamsson, U. Smith, et al., Fat cell metabolism in different regions in women: effect of menstrual cycle, pregnancy, and lactation, J. Clin. Invest. 75 (1985) 1973–1976.

[62] M.B. Snijder, J.M. Dekker, M. Visser, J.S. Yudkin, C.D. Stehouwer, L.M. Bouter, et al., Larger thigh and hip circumferences are associated with better glucose tolerance: the Hoorn study, Obes. Res. 11 (2003) 104–111.

[63] World Health Organization, Prevention of Diabetes Mellitus: Report of a WHO Study Group, World Health Organization, Geneva, 1994Technical Report Series No. 844

[64] Expert Committee on the Diagnosis and Classification of Diabetes Mellitus, Report of the Expert Committee on the Diagnosis and Classification of Diabetes Mellitus, Diabetes Care 23 (Suppl. 1) (2000) S4–S19.

[65] M.P. Stern, Type II diabetes mellitus: interface between clinical and epidemiological investigation, Diabetes Care 11 (1988) 119–126.

[66] J.H. Fuller, M.J. Shipley, G. Rose, R.J. Jarrett, H. Keen, Coronary-heart-disease risk and impaired glucose tolerance: the Whitehall study, Lancet 1 (1980) 1373–1376.

[67] R.H. Unger, Lipotoxicity in the pathogenesis of obesity-dependent NIDDM: genetic and clinical implications, Diabetes 44 (1995) 863–870.

[68] K.S. Nair, J.S. Garrow, C. Ford, R.F. Mahler, D. Halliday, Effect of poor diabetic control and obesity on whole body protein metabolism in man, Diabetologia 25 (1983) 400–403.

[69] R. Gougeon, K. Styhler, J.A. Morais, P.J. Jones, E.B. Marliss, Effects of oral hypoglycemic agents and diet on protein metabolism in type 2 diabetes, Diabetes Care 23 (2000) 1–8.

[70] American Diabetes Association, Diagnosis and classification of diabetes mellitus, Diabetes Care 34 (Suppl. 1) (2011) S62–S69.

[71] C. Lorenzo, K. Williams, K.J. Hunt, S.M. Haffner, The National Cholesterol Education Program—Adult Treatment Panel III, International Diabetes Federation, and World Health Organization definitions of the metabolic syndrome as predictors of incident cardiovascular disease and diabetes, Diabetes Care 30 (2007) 8–13.

[72] S.M. Grundy, J.I. Cleeman, S.R. Daniels, K.A. Donato, R.H. Eckel, B.A. Franklin, et al., Diagnosis and management of the metabolic syndrome: an American Heart Association/National Heart, Lung, and Blood Institute scientific statement, Circulation 112 (2005) 2735–2752.

[73] H. King, P. Zimmet, L.R. Raper, B. Balkau, Risk factors for diabetes in three Pacific populations, Am. J. Epidemiol. 119 (1984) 396–409.

[74] H. King, R. Taylor, G. Koteka, H. Nemaia, P. Zimmet, P.H. Bennett, et al., Glucose tolerance in Polynesia: population-based surveys in Rarotonga and Niue, Med. J. Aust. 145 (1986) 505–510.

[75] D.G. McLarty, A.B. Swai, H.M. Kitange, G. Masuki, B.L. Mtinangi, P.M. Kilima, et al., Prevalence of diabetes and impaired glucose tolerance in rural Tanzania, Lancet 1 (1989) 871–875.

[76] J.H. Medalie, C.M. Papier, U. Goldbourt, J.B. Herman, Major factors in the development of diabetes mellitus in 10,000 men, Arch. Intern. Med. 135 (1975) 811–817.

[77] J.M. Stanhope, I.A. Prior, The Tokelau Island Migrant Study: prevalence and incidence of diabetes mellitus, N. Z. Med. J. 92 (1980) 417–421.

[78] W.C. Knowler, D.J. Pettitt, P.J. Savage, P.H. Bennett, Diabetes incidence in Pima Indians: contributions of obesity and parental diabetes, Am. J. Epidemiol. 113 (1981) 144–156.

[79] H. Keen, R.J. Jarrett, P. McCartney, The ten-year follow-up of the Bedford Survey (1962–1972): glucose tolerance and diabetes, Diabetologia 22 (1982) 73–78.

[80] W.J. Butler, L.D. Ostrander Jr., W.J. Carman, D.E. Lamphiear, Diabetes mellitus in Tecumseh, Michigan: prevalence, incidence, and associated conditions, Am. J. Epidemiol. 116 (1982) 971–980.

[81] B. Balkau, H. King, P. Zimmet, L.R. Raper, Factors associated with the development of diabetes in the Micronesian population of Nauru, Am. J. Epidemiol. 122 (1985) 594–605.

[82] S.M. Haffner, M.P. Stern, H.P. Hazuda, M. Rosenthal, J.A. Knapp, R.M. Malina, Role of obesity and fat distribution in non-insulin-dependent diabetes mellitus in Mexican Americans and non-Hispanic whites, Diabetes Care 9 (1986) 153–161.

[83] L.O. Ohlson, B. Larsson, P. Bjorntorp, H. Eriksson, K. Svardsudd, L. Welin, et al., Risk factors for type 2 (non-insulin-dependent) diabetes mellitus: thirteen and one-half years of follow-up of the participants in a study of Swedish men born in 1913, Diabetologia 31 (1988) 798–805.

[84] A.G. Schranz, Abnormal glucose tolerance in the Maltese: a population-based longitudinal study of the natural history of NIDDM and IGT in Malta, Diabetes Res. Clin. Pract. 7 (1989) 7–16.

[85] R. Feldman, A.J. Sender, A.B. Siegelaub, Difference in diabetic and nondiabetic fat distribution patterns by skinfold measurements, Diabetes 18 (1969) 478–486.

[86] S.K. Joos, W.H. Mueller, C.L. Hanis, W.J. Schull, Diabetes Alert Study: weight history and upper body obesity in diabetic and non-diabetic Mexican American adults, Ann. Hum. Biol. 11 (1984) 167–171.

[87] A.H. Kissebah, N. Vydelingum, R. Murray, D.J. Evans, A.J. Hartz, R.K. Kalkhoff, et al., Relation of body fat distribution to metabolic complications of obesity, J. Clin. Endocrinol. Metab. 54 (1982) 254–260.

[88] M. Krotkiewski, P. Bjorntorp, L. Sjostrom, U. Smith, Impact of obesity on metabolism in men and women: importance of regional adipose tissue distribution, J. Clin. Invest. 72 (1983) 1150–1162.

[89] D.J. Evans, R.G. Hoffmann, R.K. Kalkhoff, A.H. Kissebah, Relationship of androgenic activity to body fat topography, fat cell morphology, and metabolic aberrations in premenopausal women, J. Clin. Endocrinol. Metab. 57 (1983) 304–310.

[90] A.J. Hartz, D.C. Rupley, A.A. Rimm, The association of girth measurements with disease in 32,856 women, Am. J. Epidemiol. 119 (1984) 71–80.

[91] D.J. Evans, R.G. Hoffmann, R.K. Kalkhoff, A.H. Kissebah, Relationship of body fat topography to insulin sensitivity and metabolic profiles in premenopausal women, Metabolism 33 (1984) 68–75.

[92] A. Galassi, K. Reynolds, J. He, Metabolic syndrome and risk of cardiovascular disease: a meta-analysis, Am. J. Med. 119 (2006) 812–819.

[93] M.F. Saad, W.C. Knowler, D.J. Pettitt, R.G. Nelson, D.M. Mott, P.H. Bennett, The natural history of impaired glucose tolerance in the Pima Indians, N. Engl. J. Med. 319 (1988) 1500–1506.

[94] A.K. Diehl, M.P. Stern, Special health problems of Mexican-Americans: obesity, gallbladder disease, diabetes mellitus, and cardiovascular disease, Adv. Intern. Med. 34 (1989) 73–96.

[95] R.A. Sicree, P.Z. Zimmet, H.O. King, J.S. Coventry, Plasma insulin response among Nauruans: prediction of deterioration in glucose tolerance over 6 years, Diabetes 36 (1987) 179–186.

[96] T. Kadowaki, Y. Miyake, R. Hagura, Y. Akanuma, H. Kajinuma, N. Kuzuya, et al., Risk factors for worsening to diabetes in subjects with impaired glucose tolerance, Diabetologia 26 (1984) 44–49.

[97] H. Sasai, T. Sairenchi, H. Iso, F. Irie, E. Otaka, K. Tanaka, et al., Relationship between obesity and incident diabetes in middle-aged and older Japanese adults: the Ibaraki Prefectural Health Study, Mayo Clin. Proc. 85 (2010) 36–40.

[98] J.M. Lee, A. Gebremariam, S. Vijan, J.G. Gurney, Excess body mass index-years, a measure of degree and duration of excess weight, and risk for incident diabetes, Arch. Pediatr. Adolesc. Med. 166 (2012) 42–48.

[99] J. Wilding, G. WIlliams, Diabetes and obesity, in: P.G. Kopelman, M.J. Stock (Eds.), Clinical Obesity, Blackwell, Cambridge, UK, 1998, pp. 309–349.

[100] C. Kanaka-Gantenbein, Fetal origins of adult diabetes, Ann. N. Y. Acad. Sci. 205 (2010) 99–105.

[101] D.J.P. Barker, Mothers, Babies and Health in Later Life, second ed., Churchill Livingstone, Edinburgh, UK, 1998.

[102] D.J. Barker, Fetal origins of coronary heart disease, BMJ 311 (1995) 171–174.

[103] C.N. Hales, D.J. Barker, P.M. Clark, L.J. Cox, C. Fall, C. Osmond, et al., Fetal and infant growth and impaired glucose tolerance at age 64, BMJ 303 (1991) 1019–1022.

[104] H.O. Lithell, P.M. McKeigue, L. Berglund, R. Mohsen, U.B. Lithell, D.A. Leon, Relation of size at birth to non-insulin dependent diabetes and insulin concentrations in men aged 50–60 years, BMJ 312 (1996) 406–410.

[105] D.R. McCance, D.J. Pettitt, R.L. Hanson, L.T. Jacobsson, W.C. Knowler, P.H. Bennett, Birth weight and non-insulin dependent diabetes: thrifty genotype, thrifty phenotype, or surviving small baby genotype? BMJ 308 (1994) 942–945.

[106] J.W. Rich-Edwards, G.A. Colditz, M.J. Stampfer, W.C. Willett, M.W. Gillman, C.H. Hennekens, et al., Birthweight and the risk for type 2 diabetes mellitus in adult women, Ann. Intern. Med. 130 (1999) 278–284.

[107] K.M. Godfrey, P.D. Gluckman, M.A. Hanson, Developmental origins of metabolic disease: life course and intergenerational perspectives, Trends Endocrinol. Metab. 21 (2010) 199–205.

[108] A.C. Ravelli, J.H. van der Meulen, R.P. Michels, C. Osmond, D. J. Barker, C.N. Hales, et al., Glucose tolerance in adults after prenatal exposure to famine, Lancet 351 (1998) 173–177.

[109] A. Snoeck, C. Remacle, B. Reusens, J.J. Hoet, Effect of a low protein diet during pregnancy on the fetal rat endocrine pancreas, Biol. Neonate. 57 (1990) 107–118.

[110] S. Dahri, A. Snoeck, B. Reusens-Billen, C. Remacle, J.J. Hoet, Islet function in offspring of mothers on low-protein diet during gestation, Diabetes 40 (Suppl. 2) (1991) 115–120.

[111] J.C. King, Maternal obesity, metabolism, and pregnancy outcomes, Annu. Rev. Nutr. 26 (2006) 271–291.

[112] M.L. Power, J. Schulkin, Maternal obesity, metabolic disease, and allostatic load, Physiol. Behav. 106 (2012) 22–28.

[113] L.A. Williams, S.F. Evans, J.P. Newnham, Prospective cohort study of factors influencing the relative weights of the placenta and the newborn infant, BMJ 314 (1997) 1864–1868.

[114] D.J. Barker, The fetal origins of type 2 diabetes mellitus, Ann. Intern. Med. 130 (1999) 322–324.

[115] E. Oken, E.M. Taveras, K.P. Kleinman, J.W. Rich-Edwards, M. W. Gillman, Gestational weight gain and child adiposity at age 3 years, Am. J. Obstet. Gynecol. 196 (2007) 322.e1–322.e8.

[116] F. Galtier-Dereure, C. Boegner, J. Bringer, Obesity and pregnancy: complications and cost, Am. J. Clin. Nutr. 71 (2000) 1242S–1248S.

[117] S.Y. Chu, W.M. Callaghan, S.Y. Kim, C.H. Schmid, J. Lau, L.J. England, et al., Maternal obesity and risk of gestational diabetes mellitus, Diabetes Care 30 (2007) 2070–2076.

[118] M.M. Hedderson, M.A. Williams, V.L. Holt, N.S. Weiss, A. Ferrara, Body mass index and weight gain prior to pregnancy and risk of gestational diabetes mellitus, Am. J. Obstet. Gynecol. 198 (2008) 409.e1–409.e7.

[119] R.C. Whitaker, W.H. Dietz, Role of the prenatal environment in the development of obesity, J. Pediatr. 132 (1998) 768–776.

[120] A.S. Greenberg, M.S. Obin, Obesity and the role of adipose tissue in inflammation and metabolism, Am. J. Clin. Nutr. 83 (2006) 461S–465S.

[121] N.F. Butte, Carbohydrate and lipid metabolism in pregnancy: normal compared with gestational diabetes mellitus, Am. J. Clin. Nutr. 71 (2000) 1256S–1261S.

[122] Institute of Medicine, Weight Gain During Pregnancy: Reexamining the Guidelines, National Academies Press, Washington, DC, 2009.

[123] S.J. Herring, M.Z. Rose, H. Skouteris, E. Oken, Optimizing weight gain in pregnancy to prevent obesity in women and children, Diabetes Obes. Metab. 10 (2011) 1463.

[124] J.C. Rhodes, K.C. Schoendorf, J.D. Parker, Contribution of excess weight gain during pregnancy and macrosomia to the cesarean delivery rate, 1990–2000, Pediatrics 111 (2003) 1181–1185.

[125] A.M. Siega-Riz, K.R. Evenson, N. Dole, Pregnancy-related weight gain: a link to obesity? Nutr. Rev. 62 (2004) S105–S111.

[126] T.M. Wolever, C. Mehling, Long-term effect of varying the source or amount of dietary carbohydrate on postprandial plasma glucose, insulin, triacylglycerol, and free fatty acid concentrations in subjects with impaired glucose tolerance, Am. J. Clin. Nutr. 77 (2003) 612–621.

[127] D.F. Steiner, H.S. Tager, S.J. Chan, K. Nanjo, T. Sanke, A.H. Rubenstein, Lessons learned from molecular biology of insulin-gene mutations, Diabetes Care 13 (1990) 600–609.

[128] P. Froguel, H. Zouali, N. Vionnet, G. Velho, M. Vaxillaire, F. Sun, et al., Familial hyperglycemia due to mutations in glucokinase: definition of a subtype of diabetes mellitus, N. Engl. J. Med. 328 (1993) 697–702.

[129] S.I. Taylor, D. Accili, Y. Imai, Insulin resistance or insulin deficiency: which is the primary cause of NIDDM? Diabetes 43 (1994) 735–740.

[130] R. Sladek, G. Rocheleau, J. Rung, C. Dina, L. Shen, D. Serre, et al., A genome-wide association study identifies novel risk loci for type 2 diabetes, Nature 445 (2007) 881–885.

[131] B.C. Martin, J.H. Warram, A.S. Krolewski, R.N. Bergman, J.S. Soeldner, C.R. Kahn, Role of glucose and insulin resistance in development of type 2 diabetes mellitus: results of a 25-year follow-up study, Lancet 340 (1992) 925–929.

[132] S. O'Rahilly, R.C. Turner, D.R. Matthews, Impaired pulsatile secretion of insulin in relatives of patients with non-insulin-dependent diabetes, N. Engl. J. Med. 318 (1988) 1225–1230.

[133] D. Porte Jr., S.E. Kahn, Hyperproinsulinemia and amyloid in NIDDM: clues to etiology of islet beta-cell dysfunction? Diabetes 38 (1989) 1333–1336.

[134] J.E. Gerich, The genetic basis of type 2 diabetes mellitus: impaired insulin secretion versus impaired insulin sensitivity, Endocr. Rev. 19 (1998) 491–503.

[135] I. Vauhkonen, L. Niskanen, E. Vanninen, S. Kainulainen, M. Uusitupa, M. Laakso, Defects in insulin secretion and insulin action in non-insulin-dependent diabetes mellitus are inherited: metabolic studies on offspring of diabetic probands, J. Clin. Invest. 101 (1998) 86–96.

[136] W.M. Kohrt, J.P. Kirwan, M.A. Staten, R.E. Bourey, D.S. King, J.O. Holloszy, Insulin resistance in aging is related to abdominal obesity, Diabetes 42 (1993) 273–281.

[137] R.A. DeFronzo, E. Ferrannini, Insulin resistance: a multifaceted syndrome responsible for NIDDM, obesity, hypertension, dyslipidemia, and atherosclerotic cardiovascular disease, Diabetes Care 14 (1991) 173–194.

[138] J.C. Beard, W.K. Ward, J.B. Halter, B.J. Wallum, D. Porte Jr., Relationship of islet function to insulin action in human obesity, J. Clin. Endocrinol. Metab. 65 (1987) 59–64.

[139] R. Prager, P. Wallace, J.M. Olefsky, In vivo kinetics of insulin action on peripheral glucose disposal and hepatic glucose output in normal and obese subjects, J. Clin. Invest. 78 (1986) 472–481.

[140] B.E. Wisse, The inflammatory syndrome: the role of adipose tissue cytokines in metabolic disorders linked to obesity, J. Am. Soc. Nephrol. 15 (2004) 2792–2800.

[141] E.J. Boyko, W.Y. Fujimoto, D.L. Leonetti, L. Newell-Morris, Visceral adiposity and risk of type 2 diabetes: a prospective study among Japanese Americans, Diabetes Care 23 (2000) 465–471.

[142] H. Larsson, B. Ahren, Islet dysfunction in insulin resistance involves impaired insulin secretion and increased glucagon secretion in postmenopausal women with impaired glucose tolerance, Diabetes Care 23 (2000) 650–657.

[143] K. Samaras, L.V. Campbell, Increasing incidence of type 2 diabetes in the third millennium: is abdominal fat the central issue? Diabetes Care 23 (2000) 441–442.

[144] R.V. Dvorak, W.F. DeNino, P.A. Ades, E.T. Poehlman, Phenotypic characteristics associated with insulin resistance in metabolically obese but normal-weight young women, Diabetes 48 (1999) 2210–2214.

[145] N. Ruderman, D. Chisholm, X. Pi-Sunyer, S. Schneider, The metabolically obese, normal-weight individual revisited, Diabetes 47 (1998) 699–713.

[146] S.P. Helmrich, D.R. Ragland, R.W. Leung, R.S. Paffenbarger Jr., Physical activity and reduced occurrence of non-insulin-dependent diabetes mellitus, N. Engl. J. Med. 325 (1991) 147–152.

[147] L.B. Salans, J.L. Knittle, J. Hirsch, The role of adipose cell size and adipose tissue insulin sensitivity in the carbohydrate intolerance of human obesity, J. Clin. Invest. 47 (1968) 153–165.

[148] J.M. Olefsky, The insulin receptor: its role in insulin resistance of obesity and diabetes, Diabetes 25 (1976) 1154–1162.

[149] R.B. Goldrick, G.M. McLoughlin, Lipolysis and lipogenesis from glucose in human fat cells of different sizes: effects of insulin, epinephrine, and theophylline, J. Clin. Invest. 49 (1970) 1213–1223.

[150] P. Bjorntorp, C. Bengtsson, G. Blohme, A. Jonsson, L. Sjostrom, E. Tibblin, et al., Adipose tissue fat cell size and number in relation to metabolism in randomly selected middle-aged men and women, Metabolism 20 (1971) 927–935.

[151] P. Bjorntorp, Hazards in subgroups of human obesity, Eur. J. Clin. Invest. 14 (1984) 239–241.

[152] P.J. Randle, P.B. Garland, C.N. Hales, E.A. Newsholme, The glucose fatty-acid cycle: its role in insulin sensitivity and the metabolic disturbances of diabetes mellitus, Lancet 1 (1963) 785–789.

[153] M.P. Stern, J. Olefsky, J.W. Farquhar, G.M. Reaven, Relationship between fasting plasma lipid levels and adipose tissue morphology, Metabolism 22 (1973) 1311–1317.

[154] C.J. Smith, V. Vasta, E. Degerman, P. Belfrage, V.C. Manganiello, Hormone-sensitive cyclic GMP-inhibited cyclic AMP phosphodiesterase in rat adipocytes: regulation of insulin- and cAMP-dependent activation by phosphorylation, J. Biol. Chem. 266 (1991) 13385–13390.

[155] M. Lafontan, M. Berlan, Fat cell adrenergic receptors and the control of white and brown fat cell function, J. Lipid Res. 34 (1993) 1057–1091.

[156] M. Rebuffe-Scrive, P. Bjorntorp, Regional adipose tissue metabolism in man, Metabolic Complications of Human Obesity, Excerpta Medicine, Amsterdam, 1985, pp. 149–159

[157] M. Lafontan, L. Dang-Tran, M. Berlan, Alpha-adrenergic antilipolytic effect of adrenaline in human fat cells of the thigh: comparison with adrenaline responsiveness of different fat deposits, Eur. J. Clin. Invest. 9 (1979) 261–266.

[158] F. Lonnqvist, A. Thome, K. Nilsell, J. Hoffstedt, P. Arner, A pathogenic role of visceral fat beta 3-adrenoceptors in obesity, J. Clin. Invest. 95 (1995) 1109–1116.

[159] G.M. Reaven, Insulin resistance: the link between obesity and cardiovascular disease, Med. Clin. North Am. 95 (2011) 875–892.

[160] H.M. Farin, F. Abbasi, G.M. Reaven, Body mass index and waist circumference both contribute to differences in insulin-mediated glucose disposal in nondiabetic adults, Am. J. Clin. Nutr. 83 (2006) 47–51.

[161] D.G. Carey, A.B. Jenkins, L.V. Campbell, J. Freund, D.J. Chisholm, Abdominal fat and insulin resistance in normal and overweight women: direct measurements reveal a strong relationship in subjects at both low and high risk of NIDDM, Diabetes 45 (1996) 633–638.

[162] J.P. Despres, Abdominal obesity as important component of insulin-resistance syndrome, Nutrition 9 (1993) 452–459.

[163] D.J. Evans, R. Murray, A.H. Kissebah, Relationship between skeletal muscle insulin resistance, insulin-mediated glucose disposal, and insulin binding: effects of obesity and body fat topography, J. Clin. Invest. 74 (1984) 1515–1525.

[164] S. Bedard, B. Marcotte, A. Marette, Cytokines modulate glucose transport in skeletal muscle by inducing the expression of inducible nitric oxide synthase, Biochem. J. 325 (Pt. 2) (1997) 487–493.

[165] S. Kapur, S. Bedard, B. Marcotte, C.H. Cote, A. Marette, Expression of nitric oxide synthase in skeletal muscle: a novel role for nitric oxide as a modulator of insulin action, Diabetes 46 (1997) 1691–1700.

[166] G.S. Hotamisligil, B.M. Spiegelman, Tumor necrosis factor alpha: a key component of the obesity–diabetes link, Diabetes 43 (1994) 1271–1278.

[167] I. Lemieux, A. Pascot, D. Prud'homme, N. Almeras, P. Bogaty, A. Nadeau, et al., Elevated C-reactive protein: another component of the atherothrombotic profile of abdominal obesity, Arterioscler. Thromb. Vasc. Biol. 21 (2001) 961–967.

[168] M. Cote, P. Mauriege, J. Bergeron, N. Almeras, A. Tremblay, I. Lemieux, et al., Adiponectinemia in visceral obesity: impact on glucose tolerance and plasma lipoprotein and lipid levels in men, J. Clin. Endocrinol. Metab. 90 (2005) 1434–1439.

[169] S.E. Shoelson, J. Lee, A.B. Goldfine, Inflammation and insulin resistance, J. Clin. Invest. 116 (2006) 1793–1801.

[170] A.N. Peiris, R.A. Mueller, G.A. Smith, M.F. Struve, A.H. Kissebah, Splanchnic insulin metabolism in obesity: influence of body fat distribution, J. Clin. Invest. 78 (1986) 1648–1657.

[171] P.J. Campbell, M.G. Carlson, N. Nurjhan, Fat metabolism in human obesity, Am. J. Physiol. 266 (1994) E600–E605.

[172] A.H. Kissebah, D.J. Evans, A.N. Peiris, C.R. Wilson, Endocrine characteristics in regional obesities: Role of sex steroids, in: J. Vague, P. Bjorntorp, B. Guy-Grand, M. Rebuffe-Scrive, P. Vague (Eds.), Metabolic Complications for Human Obesities, Elsevier, Amsterdam, 1985, pp. 115–130.

[173] W.T. Garvey, L. Maianu, T.P. Huecksteadt, M.J. Birnbaum, J.M. Molina, T.P. Ciaraldi, Pretranslational suppression of a glucose transporter protein causes insulin resistance in adipocytes from patients with non-insulin-dependent diabetes mellitus and obesity, J. Clin. Invest. 87 (1991) 1072–1081.

[174] W.T. Garvey, J.M. Olefsky, S. Matthaei, S. Marshall, Glucose and insulin co-regulate the glucose transport system in primary cultured adipocytes: a new mechanism of insulin resistance, J. Biol. Chem. 262 (1987) 189–197.

[175] M. Rebuffe-Scrive, B. Andersson, L. Olbe, P. Bjorntorp, Metabolism of adipose tissue in intraabdominal depots of non-obese men and women, Metabolism 38 (1989) 453–458.

[176] G. Boden, Role of fatty acids in the pathogenesis of insulin resistance and NIDDM, Diabetes 46 (1997) 3–10.

[177] M. Cigolini, U. Smith, Human adipose tissue in culture: VIII. Studies on the insulin-antagonistic effect of glucocorticoids, Metabolism 28 (1979) 502–510.

[178] D.E. Kelley, M. Mokan, J.A. Simoneau, L.J. Mandarino, Interaction between glucose and free fatty acid metabolism in human skeletal muscle, J. Clin. Invest. 92 (1993) 91–98.

[179] D.E. Kelley, L.J. Mandarino, Hyperglycemia normalizes insulin-stimulated skeletal muscle glucose oxidation and storage in noninsulin-dependent diabetes mellitus, J. Clin. Invest. 86 (1990) 1999–2007.

[180] D.E. Kelley, L.J. Mandarino, Fuel selection in human skeletal muscle in insulin resistance: a reexamination, Diabetes 49 (2000) 677–683.

[181] W.W. Winder, J. Arogyasami, I.M. Elayan, D. Cartmill, Time course of exercise-induced decline in malonyl-CoA in different muscle types, Am. J. Physiol. 259 (1990) E266–E271.

[182] J.A. Simoneau, J.H. Veerkamp, L.P. Turcotte, D.E. Kelley, Markers of capacity to utilize fatty acids in human skeletal muscle: relation to insulin resistance and obesity and effects of weight loss, FASEB J. 13 (1999) 2051–2060.

[183] D.A. Pan, S. Lillioja, A.D. Kriketos, M.R. Milner, L.A. Baur, C. Bogardus, et al., Skeletal muscle triglyceride levels are inversely related to insulin action, Diabetes 46 (1997) 983–988.

[184] B.H. Goodpaster, F.L. Thaete, J.A. Simoneau, D.E. Kelley, Subcutaneous abdominal fat and thigh muscle composition predict insulin sensitivity independently of visceral fat, Diabetes 46 (1997) 1579–1585.

[185] G. Arcaro, M. Zamboni, L. Rossi, E. Turcato, G. Covi, F. Armellini, et al., Body fat distribution predicts the degree of endothelial dysfunction in uncomplicated obesity, Int. J. Obes. Relat. Metab. Disord. 23 (1999) 936–942.

[186] G.M. Reaven, The fourth musketeer—From Alexandre Dumas to Claude Bernard, Diabetologia 38 (1995) 3–13.

[187] R.S. Surwit, M.S. Schneider, M.N. Feinglos, Stress and diabetes mellitus, Diabetes Care 15 (1992) 1413–1422.

[188] J.M. Mooy, H. de Vries, P.A. Grootenhuis, L.M. Bouter, R.J. Heine, Major stressful life events in relation to prevalence of undetected type 2 diabetes: the Hoorn Study, Diabetes Care 23 (2000) 197–201.

[189] R.S. Surwit, M.N. Feinglos, Stress and autonomic nervous system in type II diabetes: a hypothesis, Diabetes Care 11 (1988) 83–85.

[190] P.H. Black, The inflammatory consequences of psychologic stress: relationship to insulin resistance, obesity, atherosclerosis and diabetes mellitus, type II, Med. Hypotheses 67 (2006) 879–891.

[191] S. Fujioka, Y. Matsuzawa, K. Tokunaga, T. Kawamoto, T. Kobatake, Y. Keno, et al., Improvement of glucose and lipid metabolism associated with selective reduction of intra-abdominal visceral fat in premenopausal women with visceral fat obesity, Int. J. Obes. 15 (1991) 853–859.

[192] T.P. Markovic, A.B. Jenkins, L.V. Campbell, S.M. Furler, E.W. Kraegen, D.J. Chisholm, The determinants of glycemic responses to diet restriction and weight loss in obesity and NIDDM, Diabetes Care 21 (1998) 687–694.

[193] K. Esposito, A. Pontillo, C. Di Palo, G. Giugliano, M. Masella, R. Marfella, et al., Effect of weight loss and lifestyle changes on vascular inflammatory markers in obese women: a randomized trial, JAMA 289 (2003) 1799–1804.

[194] E.J. Ramos, Y. Xu, I. Romanova, F. Middleton, C. Chen, R. Quinn, et al., Is obesity an inflammatory disease? Surgery 134 (2003) 329–335.

[195] A. Ceriello, C. Taboga, L. Tonutti, L. Quagliaro, L. Piconi, B. Bais, et al., Evidence for an independent and cumulative effect of postprandial hypertriglyceridemia and hyperglycemia on endothelial dysfunction and oxidative stress generation: effects of short- and long-term simvastatin treatment, Circulation 106 (2002) 1211–1218.

[196] M. Negrean, A. Stirban, B. Stratmann, T. Gawlowski, T. Horstmann, C. Gotting, et al., Effects of low- and high-advanced glycation endproduct meals on macro- and microvascular endothelial function and oxidative stress in patients with type 2 diabetes mellitus, Am. J. Clin. Nutr. 85 (2007) 1236–1243.

[197] UK Prospective Diabetes Study Group, Intensive blood-glucose control with sulphonylureas or insulin compared with conventional treatment and risk of complications in patients with type 2 diabetes (UKPDS 33): UK Prospective Diabetes Study (UKPDS) Group, Lancet 352 (1998) 837–853.

[198] H. Yki-Jarvinen, L. Ryysy, M. Kauppila, E. Kujansuu, J. Lahti, T. Marjanen, et al., Effect of obesity on the response to insulin therapy in noninsulin-dependent diabetes mellitus, J. Clin. Endocrinol. Metab. 82 (1997) 4037–4043.

E. DIABETES MELLITUS

[199] The Diabetes Control and Complications Trial Research Group, The effect of intensive treatment of diabetes on the development and progression of long-term complications in insulin-dependent diabetes mellitus: the Diabetes Control and Complications Trial Research Group, N. Engl. J. Med. 329 (1993) 977—986.

[200] M.I. Harris, R.C. Eastman, C.C. Cowie, K.M. Flegal, M.S. Eberhardt, Racial and ethnic differences in glycemic control of adults with type 2 diabetes, Diabetes Care 22 (1999) 403—408.

[201] J.H. Ledikwe, B.J. Rolls, H. Smiciklas-Wright, D.C. Mitchell, J.D. Ard, C. Champagne, et al., Reductions in dietary energy density are associated with weight loss in overweight and obese participants in the PREMIER trial, Am. J. Clin. Nutr. 85 (2007) 1212—1221.

[202] N.P. Pronk, R.R. Wing, Physical activity and long-term maintenance of weight loss, Obes. Res. 2 (1994) 587—599.

CHAPTER

32

The Role of Diet in the Prevention and Treatment of Diabetes

Judith Wylie-Rosett[*], *Linda M. Delahanty*[†]

[*]Albert Einstein College of Medicine, Bronx, New York [†]Massachusetts General Hospital Diabetes Center,
Boston, Massachusetts

I INTRODUCTION

The number of people in the United States with diabetes is estimated to be 25.8 million or 8.3% of the population based on the 2010 U.S. Census population estimates and diabetes prevalence data from the 2005−2008 National Health and Nutrition Examination Survey and the 2007−2009 National Health Interview Survey [1]. However, only 18.8 million of those with diabetes have diagnosed diabetes, and the other 7.0 million are unaware they have diabetes. The risk of having diabetes increases with age, and 26.9% of the U.S. population age 65 years or older has diabetes. In addition, 35% (79 million) of U.S. adults (≥20 years of age) are at high risk for developing diabetes and can be classified as having prediabetes [2]. If current trends continue, the Centers for Disease Control and Prevention (CDC) estimates that one-third of the U.S. adult population will have diabetes by 2050 [1,2].

Data from 216 countries were used to estimate the global prevalence of diabetes for 2010 and projections for 2030 [3]. The number of adults (age 20−79 years) with diabetes was estimated to be 285 million (6.4% of the world population) in 2010, with an increase to 439 million (7.7% of the world population) by 2030. The increase between 2010 and 2030 is expected to be 20% in developed economies and 69% in developing economies. Currently, approximately 70% of the world's population lives in low- and middle-income countries, where most of the increase in diabetes is expected to occur. Countries with a large population and rapid economic development are likely to carry the greatest diabetes burden. For example, China and India rank first

and second, respectively, for number of diabetes cases, with the U.S. ranking third. The projected number of adults with diabetes in 2030 is 87 million in India, 62 million in China, and 36 million in the United States [3].

The increased global diabetes burden appears to be the result of population aging and urbanization, with the associated changes in diet and physical activity. However, there is growing evidence that in some middle-income countries, especially India and China, the prevalence in rural areas is approaching that in urban areas, perhaps related to mechanization [4]. The estimated direct medical cost for prevention and treatment of diabetes worldwide was approximately $376 billion in 2010 and will exceed $490 billion by 2030 [5]. Total costs are substantially higher due to loss of productive years of life, particularly in developing countries. The effort to reduce the growing public health burden of diabetes in the United States and throughout the world includes goals for prevention as well as treatment.

This chapter provides an overview of criteria for diagnosing and classifying diabetes. Prevention of diabetes is addressed focusing on weight management and increased physical activity. The review of treatment focuses on medical nutrition therapy (MNT). Diabetes MNT for preventing complications focuses on the goal of achieving as close to normal metabolism as possible. Metabolic goals target controlling blood pressure and lipid levels as well as glycemic control. The role of MNT in treating diabetes complications is also addressed. The chapter concludes with an overview of programs and resources for preventing and treating diabetes.

Nutrition in the Prevention and Treatment of Disease, Third Edition.
DOI: http://dx.doi.org/10.1016/B978-0-12-391884-0.00032-9

II DIAGNOSTIC CRITERIA AND DIABETES CATEGORIES

Diagnostic tests and criteria used to identify individuals who are at risk for developing diabetes (prediabetes) or who have diabetes [6] are listed in Table 32.1. The classifications of diabetes include type 1, type 2, gestational, and secondary diabetes [6].

Type 1 diabetes, formerly known as insulin-dependent or juvenile diabetes, represents approximately 5–10% of known cases of diabetes [6]. Type 1 diabetes is characterized by severe insulin deficiency requiring exogenous insulin to prevent ketoacidosis, coma, and death. Population-based research in the United States from the SEARCH for Diabetes in Youth Study multicenter observational study of youth has assessed the incidence of clinically diagnosed diabetes [7]. Data from 2002 and 2003 suggest that approximately 15,000 youth are newly diagnosed with type 1 diabetes annually in the United States [7]. The incidence of type 1 diabetes is higher in whites than in other ethnic/racial groups, with the greatest discrepancy at younger ages [7].

Type 2 diabetes, formerly known as non-insulin-dependent or adult-onset diabetes, accounts the vast majority (90–95%) of diabetes cases [8]. Development of type 2 diabetes is associated with insulin resistance and inadequate pancreatic β cell compensatory insulin production [6]. Symptoms and signs associated with developing type 2 diabetes, which are usually more subtle than for type 1 diabetes, may be related to the presence of complications and include poor wound healing, blurred vision, recurrent gum or bladder infections, and changes in hand or foot sensation. Type 2 diabetes may remain undiagnosed for several years before a clinical diagnosis is made. Many individuals are asymptomatic, and their glucose elevation may be detected as the result of a routine blood test. Type 2 diabetes is rare in children younger than the age of 10 years, but it accounts for an increasing proportion of cases as age increases [7].

Gestational diabetes (GDM) is defined as hyperglycemia identified during pregnancy [8], but for many women undiagnosed type 2 diabetes may be identified during pregnancy. Therefore, the American Diabetes Association, in conjunction with the International Association of Diabetes and Pregnancy Study Groups (IADPSG), recommends that women diagnosed with diabetes at their first prenatal visit receive a diagnosis of overt diabetes (not GDM) and then only when the diabetes is resolved upon delivery should the diabetes be classified as gestational [9].

Approximately 7% of pregnancies are complicated by GDM. The American Diabetes Association recommends a risk assessment during the first prenatal visit for all women and that women deemed "very high risk" should be screened as soon as possible thereafter. Criteria for very high risk include severe obesity, history of GDM or large-for-gestational-age neonate, the presence of glycosuria, diagnosis of polycystic ovarian syndrome, and strong family history of type 2 diabetes. For other pregnant women, testing at 24–28 weeks of gestation is recommended. Diagnostic cut points for the fasting, 1-hour, and 2-hour post-glucose load tests were developed using data from the Hyperglycemia and Adverse Pregnancy Outcomes study [10].

TABLE 32.1   Assessment Methods and Criteria for Diabetes Diagnoses

Assessment method	At increased risk for diabetes (prediabetes)	Diagnostic for diabetes	Gestational diabetes (at least two of the following)
Hemoglobin A1c[a]	A1c 5.7–6.4%	≥ 6.5%	Not applicable
Fasting plasma glucose (FPG)	Impaired fasting glucose of 100–125 mg/dl (5.6–6.9 mmol/l)	FPG ≥ 126 mg/dl (7.0 mmol/l) (on two occasions)	FPG ≥ 95 mg/dl (5.3 mmol/l)
Oral glucose tolerance test, 75-g glucose load	Impaired glucose tolerance 2-hour glucose of 140–199 mg/dl (7.8–11.0 mmol/l)	2-Hour plasma glucose ≥ 200 mg/dl (11.1 mmol/l)	1-Hour plasma glucose ≥ 180 mg/dl (10.0 mmol/l)
			2-Hour plasma glucose ≥ 155 mg/dl (8.6 mmol/l)
			3-Hour plasma glucose ≥ 140 mg/dl (7.8 mmol/l)
Symptomatic	Not applicable	Symptoms of hyperglycemia or hyperglycemic crisis with random plasma glucose ≥ 200 mg/dl (11.1 mmol/l)	Not applicable

[a]National Glycohemoglobin Standardization Program certified and standardized to the Diabetes Control and Complications Trial assay.

The etiologies of secondary diabetes vary considerably [6]. Any disorder or compound that affects the function of the β cell in the pancreas can secondarily cause diabetes. Diabetes can also be secondary to endocrinopathies, leading to increased counterregulatory hormone production (e.g., acromegaly (excess growth hormone) and Cushing's syndrome (excess cortisol)). Pharmacological agents can also create insulin resistance or damage to the pancreatic β cells. Steroids and second-generation antipsychotic medications that increase insulin resistance and visceral fat may increase insulin requirements beyond endogenous capacity. Cystic fibrosis-related diabetes is the most common co-morbidity in people with cystic fibrosis. The addition of diabetes to cystic fibrosis is associated with poorer nutrition outcomes in addition to more severe inflammatory lung disease and greater mortality from respiratory failure, especially in women [6].

III MEDICAL NUTRITION THERAPY FOR DIABETES PREVENTION AND TREATMENT

The American Diabetes Association *2012 Standards of Medical Care* [8] state that "individuals who have prediabetes or diabetes should receive individualized medical nutrition therapy (MNT) as needed to achieve treatment goals, preferably provided by a registered dietitian (RD) familiar with the components of diabetes MNT." Medicare and other third-party payers require that MNT be administered by a licensed/certified RD or nutrition professional. The steps and strategies for MNT in the prevention and treatment of diabetes are listed in Table 32.2. The American Diabetes Association endorses eating a healthful dietary pattern high in fruits, vegetables, whole grains, and nuts; low sodium intake (for patients with diabetes and symptomatic heart failure, <2000 mg/day; in normotensive and hypertensive patients, <2300 mg/day); and, for most individuals, a modest amount of weight loss [8]. To date, there are no large-scale randomized, controlled trials of overall MNT recommendations and cardiovascular disease risk reduction in individuals with prediabetes or diabetes.

A Prevention of Diabetes

Prevention is an important strategy for reducing health care costs as well as the morbidity and mortality resulting from diabetes. Although there are no established approaches for prevention of type 1 diabetes, research is needed to provide a better understanding of environmental triggers as well as the potential role of immunosuppressive therapy and other possible approaches.

Strategies for the prevention of type 2 diabetes target intervention goals of weight loss and increased physical activity to reduce insulin resistance [11,12]. The evidence that a lifestyle intervention can prevent or delay type 2 diabetes is from randomized clinical trials conducted in people at high risk of developing the disease. The trials demonstrate the critical role of addressing excess body weight and physical inactivity [12−16].

The Da Qing Diabetes Prevention Study was a 6-year lifestyle intervention (diet, exercise, or diet plus exercise) in 577 adults with impaired glucose tolerance in China. The results of this study provided preliminary evidence that diet and exercise interventions can lower the conversion to overt diabetes [13]. The 20-year follow-up results showed that individuals in the combined intervention group had a 43% lower incidence of diabetes during the 20-year period and spent an average of 3.6 fewer years with diabetes compared to control group participants [17].

The Finnish Diabetes Prevention Study (FDPS) was a randomized, controlled, clinical trial in 522 individuals with impaired glucose tolerance randomized to either a control or an intervention group [11]. The lifestyle intervention involved a low-fat (<30% of calories from fat and <10% of calories from saturated fat), high-fiber (at least 15 g/1000 kcal) diet in conjunction with moderate-intensity exercise for at least 30 minutes/day [11]. After an average follow-up of 3.2 years, results of the FDPS showed a 58% reduction in the incidence of type 2 diabetes with lifestyle intervention [18]. There were small but significant reductions in total cholesterol, triglyceride, systolic blood pressure, and measurements of inflammation as well an an increase in high-density lipoprotein (HDL) cholesterol in the lifestyle intervention group but not in the control group [18]. Studies from the FDPS of candidate genes affecting energy metabolism showed the importance of genetic polymorphisms in defining responses to lifestyle interventions [19].

The Diabetes Prevention Program (DPP), which was a randomized, controlled, clinical trial conducted in 3234 ethnically diverse individuals with impaired glucose tolerance, randomized participants to one of three treatments: (1) standard lifestyle recommendations plus metformin, (2) standard lifestyle recommendations plus placebo, or (3) intensive lifestyle intervention [12]. The intensive lifestyle intervention was designed to achieve a 7% weight loss (based on initial body weight) and at least 150 minutes of moderate-intensity physical activity per week. The intervention goals included reducing energy intake (500−1000 fewer calories than the amount needed to maintain baseline weight) with a low-fat (25% of calories from fat) diet. The intensive lifestyle intervention program consisted of a 16-session core curriculum in which participants received individualized advice on how to reach their

TABLE 32.2 Medical Nutrition Therapy (MNT) Steps and Strategies by Class of Diabetes

---

MNT STEPS

---

1. Nutrition referral (physician): Include medical diagnoses and history, laboratory tests, medications, relative body weight, and other pertinent information.
2. Nutrition assessment (RD): Evaluate referring information, the patient's concerns/questions, and review patient's relevant knowledge, skills, and behavior.
3. Nutrition diagnosis (RD): Develop coded problem list for MNT intervention; for example, "Inconsistent carbohydrate intake and inadequate meal planning with meals and snacks varying from 0 to 150 g of carbohydrates on a regular basis."
4. Nutrition intervention (RD): Teach skills for planning meals and carbohydrate intake, develop goals collaboratively with patient related to inconsistent intake, ask patient about barriers to achieving goals, and develop problem-solving strategies with patient to address barriers.
5. Nutrition monitoring and evaluation (RD): Conduct ongoing review of biochemical factors such as A1c and serum lipid levels, as well as lifestyle factors such as dietary intake.

MNT STRATEGIES

Prediabetes

- If overweight, reduce calorie intake to achieve 5–10% weight loss.
- Increase moderate intensity physical activity to at least 150 minutes per week.
- Reduce and/or modify type of fat to achieve weight and lipid goals.

Type 1 diabetes

- Assess usual lifestyle, focusing on eating and physical activity habits, noting time schedule.
- Plan insulin therapy to match insulin action to lifestyle schedule—for example, starting with one unit of insulin for 15 g of carbohydrate.
- Monitor blood glucose levels while keeping lifestyle consistent to better assess how to match insulin to carbohydrate intake and physical activity.
- Adjust insulin and lifestyle to achieve blood glucose levels in the target range.
- Create algorithms for adjusting insulin for lifestyle flexibility (e.g., insulin to carbohydrate ratios) and to correct blood glucose levels that are not in the target range.

Type 2 diabetes

- If overweight, reduce calorie intake to achieve 5–10% weight loss.
- Increase physical activity.
- Monitor blood glucose to assess pattern of glycemic control.
- If postprandial glucose level is high, spread food intake throughout the day (using five or six small meals/snacks rather than having fewer larger ones).
- Reduce and/or modify type of fat to achieve weight and lipid goals.

Gestational diabetes

- Plan calorie intake to achieve desired weight gain based on desirable body weight.
- Balance carbohydrate intake throughout the day (usually 40–50% of calories).
- Monitor glucose approximately seven times per day; adjust intake to achieve glucose levels in target range.
- Add exogenous insulin if target glucose levels are not achieved by diet alone.

Secondary diabetes

- Assess interrelationship between primary disease(s) and its treatment in relation to the secondary diabetes to establish treatment priorities.
- Institute diabetes treatment as needed to avoid short- and long-term complications.

---

goals [20], with follow-up booster sessions to support maintenance of lifestyle changes.

After an average follow-up period of 2.8 years, the DPP results showed that the incidence of diabetes was reduced by 58% in the intensive lifestyle intervention group compared to 31% in the metformin group [12]. Further analysis revealed that weight loss was the dominant predictor of the observed reduced diabetes incidence: When adjusted for changes in diet and physical activity, each kilogram of weight loss resulted in a 16% reduction in diabetes risk [21]. Furthermore, lower percentage of calories from fat and increased physical activity accounted for the weight loss, indicating that it was through these intermediates that the diabetes risk reduction was accomplished [21]. However, participants in the intensive lifestyle intervention who did not achieve the 7% weight loss goal but did achieve the goal of 150 minutes of physical activity per week had a 44% reduction in the incidence of diabetes [21]. The intensive lifestyle treatment effects did not differ by sex, race, or ethnic group. Ten-year follow-up of the DPP found that the cumulative incidence of diabetes two Mediterranean diet groups compared to the low-fat group in the absence of significant changes in weight [25].

The HEALTHY study was a randomized, controlled, multicenter study of middle-school-aged children in the United States designed to reduce risk factors associated with developing type 2 diabetes [26]. The combined prevalence (intervention and control schools) of overweight and obesity in schools was decreased (primary outcome), but there were no differences in prevalence of overweight and obesity between intervention and control schools. However, the intervention schools had significantly greater decreases in BMI z-scores, percentage of students with a waist circumference at or above the 90th percentile, fasting insulin levels, and obesity prevalence [27]. The efficacy of the intervention in prevention of type 2 diabetes in youth will require additional participant follow-up and further testing.

B Diabetes Treatment

The overall goal of therapy for diabetes is to normalize metabolism (with emphasis on blood glucose and lipids, particularly low-density lipoprotein (LDL) cholesterol and blood pressure) in order to prevent diabetes-related complications [8]. Acute complications include hyperglycemia resulting in ketoacidosis in type 1 and hyperglycemic coma in type 2 diabetes and hypoglycemia in patients treated with insulin or medications that raise blood insulin levels [8]. Longer term complications include microvascular, macrovascular, and neuropathic complications [8]. Results from clinical trials in individuals with both type 1 and type 2 diabetes provide evidence that improving metabolic control (glycemia, blood pressure, and lipids) greatly reduces the development and progression rates for microvascular, macrovascular, and neuropathic complications [20,22,28–31]. The goals are sometimes referred to as the ABCs, with targets of A1c≤7%, blood pressure (systolic <130 mm Hg and diastolic <80 mm Hg), and LDL cholesterol <100 mg/dl (2.59 mmol/l) [8]. These clinical goals are typically achieved with a combination of nutrition and lifestyle interventions and medications. A range of oral medications, injectables, and insulins are available to manage glycemia in addition to nutrition and lifestyle recommendations (Tables 32.3 and 32.4). Type 1 diabetes is primarily managed with intensive insulin therapy. Due to the large number of treatment options for type 2 diabetes, evidence-based consensus algorithms are available to guide the initiation and adjustment of therapies for management of hyperglycemia in type 2 diabetes, particularly if life-style interventions fail to achieve or maintain metabolic goals because of failure to lose weight, weight regain,

remained the lowest in the intensive lifestyle intervention group [16].

Unlike the intensive lifestyle intervention, which was effective across the entire baseline body weight and fasting glucose ranges, metformin was ineffective in those with a body mass index (BMI) less than 30 kg/m² and minimally effective in those with a BMI less than 35 kg/m² or with a fasting glucose level less than 110 mg/dl (6.1 mmol/l). As in the FDPS, insulin sensitivity improved in the intensive lifestyle intervention group, with a smaller increase in the metformin group and no change in the placebo group. Insulin secretion decreased in all groups, but it was associated with improved β cell function only in the intensive lifestyle intervention group. The lifestyle intervention resulted in a lower prevalence and need for medical treatment of hypertension and dyslipidemia. The lifestyle intervention also lowered inflammatory biomarkers associated with increased cardiovascular risk.

Both the DPP and the FDPS asked participants to self-monitor their food intake [18,20,22]. In the FDPS, participants were asked to complete 3-day food records four times per year [18,22]; in the DPP, participants were asked to self-monitor their activity, food intake, calories, and fat grams daily during the first 24 weeks and then at least 1 week per month thereafter. In the DPP, the frequency of dietary self-monitoring was related to success at achieving both the physical activity goal and the weight loss goal. Moreover, participants who were 65 years old or older were more likely to complete self-monitoring records, report a lower percentage of calories from fat, and meet the activity and weight loss goals than were those who were younger than 45 years [23]. Thus, it is not surprising that older participants had a greater (71%) risk reduction in the development of diabetes with lifestyle intervention [12]. Lifestyle coaches in the DPP taught the participants to use a problem-solving approach to manage high-risk situations (stress, vacations, and eating out) and used a toolbox approach to deal with barriers to lifestyle change [20]. The DPP lifestyle intervention materials have been made available to all health care practitioners at http://www.bsc.gwu.edu/dpp/lifestyle/dpp_part.html. Diabetes prevention intervention materials for community programs are available at http://www.cdc.gov/diabetes/projects/prevention_program.htm. When translating the DPP lifestyle intervention into practice, it is important to provide clients with both the knowledge and the skills needed to make lifestyle changes. The skills of goal setting, self-monitoring, problem solving, relapse prevention, and managing high-risk situations were critical in facilitating the life-style change process [24].

A randomized trial (the PREDIMED study) observed a lower 4-year incidence of diabetes in the progressive disease, or a combination of other factors. The guidelines in consensus algorithm are based on clinical trials demonstrating the effectiveness and safety of the various treatment modalites and on clinical experience taking into account benefits, risks, and costs of treatment. Initial therapy with lifestyle intervention and metformin is recommended for patients with type 2 diabetes. Assessment of motivation to focus on weight loss and increased activity along with results of self-monitoring of blood glucose (SMBG) monitoring of blood glucose is important in determining the need for adjustment or advancement of the medication regimen. If glycemic targets are not achieved within 2 or 3 months or are not sustained, then rapid addition of medications and transition to new regimens including insulin is recommended [32].

1 Type 1 Diabetes

The Diabetes Control and Complications Trial (DCCT) was conducted in individuals with type 1 diabetes to compare the effects of intensive versus standard glycemic control. Intensive treatment reduced the mean A1c from 9 to 7.2%, and greater attention to dietary strategies accounted for almost one-fourth of the glycemic improvement [33,34]. The risk of development and progression of retinopathy, albuminuria, and neuropathy was reduced by between 50 and 75% over 8 years [33]. Reduction in the risk of complications was linearly related to the reduction in A1c, indicating that risk reduction can be achieved by improving glycemic control, even if a perfect or normal metabolic state is not achieved [35–37]. These accomplishments, as well as efforts to attenuate the two- or threefold increase in severe hypoglycemia and weight gain, were largely due to educational and nutritional strategies [34,38].

Longer term follow-up of the DCCT cohort in the Epidemiology of Diabetes Interventions and Complications study has documented a continued differential in the risk of microvascular (nephropathy and retinopathy) and macrovascular (cardiovascular disease) complications, even though A1c levels in the two groups were similar for the preceding 8 years [39,40].

Several types of insulin are available (Table 32.3), and they are often used in various combinations in order to match insulin action to the patient's lifestyle—for example, time and type and amount of food eaten. A typical approach in terms of insulin use is a "basal-bolus" regimen, either via subcutaneous insulin infusion (or pump therapy) or via multiple daily injections (MDIs) in which insulin is delivered as a bolus before meals in amounts matched to total carbohydrate intake, with basal insulin on board consistently over time. There are other approaches to MDI that utilize different types of insulin. Patients can either vary their insulin dose to match the amount of food consumed, with additional considerations for physical activity, or meals and physical activity can be held constant in order to match a constant dosing of insulin from day to day. Reduction of insulin dosage is the preferred method of preventing hypoglycemia during and/or after exercise, but this requires planning physical activity ahead of time. For unplanned exercise, increased carbohydrate intake may be needed.

In the DCCT, dietary behaviors associated with better glycemic control in the intensively treated group included adherence to an overall meal plan (timing

TABLE 32.3 Insulin Preparations: Onset, Peak, and Duration of Action

Insulin type	Brand name	Onset of action	Peak action	Duration of action
Very rapid acting				
Insulin aspart analog Insulin lispro analog	NovoLog Humalog	10–20 minutes	0.5–2.5 hours	3–5 hours
Regular insulin	Humulin R Novolin R	30–40 minutes	2–4 hours	5–7 hours
Intermediate acting				
NPH insulin	Humulin N Novolin N	1–3 hours	4–10 hours	14–24 hours
Lente insulin	Humulin L	2–4 hours	4–15 hours	16–24 hours
Long acting				
Ultralente insulin	Humulin U	3–4 hours	8–14 hours	18–24 hours
Insulin glargine	Lantus	1–2 hours	No peak	~24 hours

TABLE 32.4 Oral Antidiabetic Medication Categories: Mechanism of Action and Side Effects

Generic name	Brand name	Mechanism of action and side effects
Sulfonylureas		
Chlorpropamide (first generation)	Diabinese	**Stimulate the pancreatic β cells to secrete more insulin.**
		Hypoglycemia risk, especially when using chlorpropamide and glyburide compared to other sulfonylureas or in the elderly.
Glyburide (second generation)	Micronase, Diabeta, Glynase Pres Tab	Weight gain (approximately 2 kg) upon treatment initiation common.
		Higher doses should be avoided.
Glipizide (second generation)	Glucotrol, Glucotrol XL	
Glimepiride (third generation)	Amaryl	
Meglitinides (glinides)		
Repaglixnide	Prandin	**Stimulate β cell insulin secretion.**
Nateglinide	Starlix	Must be administered more frequently than sulfonylureas.
		Hypoglycemia risk, less than with sulfonylureas for nateglinide.
		Weight gain similar to sulfonylureas.
Biguanides[a]		
Metformin	Glucophage	**Reduce hepatic glucose output.**
		May have gastrointestinal side effects.
		May interfere with B_{12} absorption rarely resulting in anemia.
		Contraindicated in patients with renal dysfunction.
		Check creatinine clearance if older than 65 years of age.
α-Glucosidase inhibitors[a]		
Acarbose	Precose	**Decrease rate of digestion of carbohydrate-containing foods.**
Miglitol	Glyset	Gastrointestinal side effects, including gas and diarrhea.
Thiazolidinediones[a]		
Pioglitazone	Actos	**Enhance insulin sensitivity.**
		Fluid retention, with potential congestive heart failure in the elderly or other high-risk patients.
		Contraindicated in liver disease; check liver enzymes on an ongoing basis.
		May be associated with bladder cancer.
		Weight gain.
Dipeptidyl peptidase-4 inhibitors[a]		
Sitagliptin	Januvia	**Prevent breakdown of GLP-1.**
		Upper respiratory tract infection risk.

[a]Do not increase blood insulin levels and risk of hypoglycemia.

and amount of carbohydrate), appropriate treatment of hypoglycemia (avoiding excess consumption of carbohydrate to treat symptoms), prompt intervention for hyperglycemia (more insulin and/or less food), and consistent consumption of planned evening snacks [34]. The mean level of weight gain in the intensively treated group was reduced by 50% after the intervention staff focused on strategies to control weight gain.

Strategies to minimize potential for weight gain included discussing risk for weight gain prior to initiation of intensive therapy, proactively reducing calorie intake goals by 250–300 calories, adjusting insulin doses preferentially for anticipated increases in activity (rather than adding extra snacks), and avoiding excessive food consumption to prevent and treat hypoglycemia [38].

A strategy to avoid overtreating hypoglycemic symptoms involves (1) documenting that the symptoms are truly indicative of hypoglycemia (blood glucose below the normal fasting range of 70–120 mg/dl (3.89–6.67 mmol/l)), (2) treating the hypoglycemia with 15 g of carbohydrate, and (3) waiting for 15 minutes before eating more. This strategy is sometimes referred to as the 15/15 rule for hypoglycemia. Strategies to minimize the frequency of hypoglycemia focused on the importance of carbohydrate consistency and prioritizing reduction of fat intake when reducing calories to prevent weight gain and teaching tailored adjustment of insulin dose for activities of various intensities and durations based on blood glucose monitoring results [34].

The American Dietetic Association has established evidenced-based diabetes MNT for patients with type 1 diabetes [41]. In the randomized field test, specific guidelines for nutrition counseling were used by dietitians with 24 patients, and results were compared with those of 30 patients receiving "usual counseling" as the control treatment condition. The mean A1c in the guidelines-treated patient group was significantly reduced compared with the control group (1.0 vs. 0.3%) [42].

The Dose Adjustment for Normal Eating study demonstrated improvements in A1c, quality of life, psychological well-being, and satisfaction with treatment in individuals with type 1 diabetes, who learned to use glucose testing to better match insulin to carbohydrate intake despite an increase in the number of daily glucose tests and insulin injections [43]. The quality-of-life improvements were maintained at the 4 year follow-up, although the glycemic control improvements were maintained to a lesser extent [44].

2 Type 2 Diabetes

The United Kingdom Prospective Diabetes Study (UKPDS) examined the benefit of metabolic control (glucose and blood pressure) in patients newly diagnosed with type 2 diabetes [31,45–49]. Fundamentally, the UKPDS confirmed that the findings of the DCCT also apply to type 2 diabetes. There was a reduction in macrovascular and microvascular complications, and the best results were obtained in those individuals who achieved both glucose and blood pressure control. Similarly, there was a clear dose–response relationship between metabolic and blood pressure control and the risk of diabetes complications.

The Lifestyle Over and Above Drugs in Diabetes randomized, controlled trial in New Zealand examined the impact of intensive nutritional counseling over a period of 6 months in patients with type 2 diabetes ($n = 93$). Significant reductions in the intervention group were observed in A1c, weight, BMI, and waist circumference compared to the control group [50].

MNT for treatment of type 2 diabetes focuses on weight loss and physical activity to improve insulin sensitivity and metabolic control of glucose, lipids, and blood pressure. The American Diabetes Association algorithm for the management of type 2 diabetes indicates that medication—metformin unless contraindicated—be initiated at the time of diagnosis [51]. Many patients with type 2 diabetes take five or more medications to achieve blood glucose, blood pressure, and cholesterol goals, as well as low-dose aspirin. The impact of weight loss is most dramatically demonstrated by bariatric surgery, although the effects of bariatric surgery on diabetes appear to be largely independent of weight loss and may be due to changes in hormonal metabolism [52].

The Look-AHEAD (Action for Health in Diabetes) study, an ongoing multicenter, randomized, control trial of an intensive lifestyle intervention in 5145 patients with type 2 diabetes, found that a weight loss of 8.6% was associated with improved diabetes control, as indicated by reductions in diabetes medication use and A1c levels [53]. Four-year results of the Look-AHEAD study indicate that the improvements in weight (loss of 6.15%), fitness, and A1c observed in the intensive lifestyle intervention group compared to the control group were sustained [54]. The Look-AHEAD lifestyle intervention was adapted from the DPP intervention to meet the needs of people with diabetes and incorporated the use of meal replacements to provide structure and enhance weight loss results [55].

IV APPROACHES TO REDUCE COMPLICATIONS

The rates of cardiovascular disease and related complications such as heart attack and stroke are two to four times higher in adults with diabetes than in the general population [8]. Diabetes is also the leading cause of kidney failure, nontraumatic amputations, and new cases of blindness for U.S. adults. The ACCORD (Action to Control Cardiovascular Risk in Diabetes) study was a randomized, controlled trial that examined the effects of intensive glycemic control (target A1c $< 6\%$) versus standard glycemic control (target A1C between 7 and 7.9%) in 10,251 patients with extant diabetes on cardiovascular disease outcomes. The treatment arm receiving intensive control of blood pressure and lipids did not have a significant improvement over controls [56]. Results from two other large, randomized, controlled trials—the ADVANCE study and the Veterans Affairs Diabetes Trial—also found no significant reduction in cardiovascular disease risk with intensive glycemic control [28,57]. The results of these three trials indicate that intensive treatment may not provide any additional benefit, at least in the time period of treatment and populations observed in these studies [58].

The Look-AHEAD study also examined the effect of achieving and maintaining weight loss on cardiovascular risk reduction. One-year results of the intervention indicated that the clinically significant weight loss (8.6%) was associated with reductions in cardiovascular disease risk factors as indicated by blood pressure, triglycerides, HDL cholesterol, and urine albumin-to-creatinine ratio [53]. Reductions in C-reactive protein have also been observed [59]. Four-year results of the study indicate that the improvements in systolic blood pressure and HDL cholesterol levels observed in the intensive lifestyle intervention group compared to the control group were sustained [54].

V GESTATIONAL DIABETES

The nutrition treatment goal in GDM is to achieve and maintain euglycemia in order to improve pregnancy outcomes; reduce risks to the fetus/baby, such as macrosomia and perinatal complications; and perhaps reduce chances of fetal malnutrition, with subsequent increased risk for adult chronic diseases. Women with GDM actually have similar nutrition requirements as other pregnant women but are much more likely to also be overweight. Strategies to minimize the effects of carbohydrate on the 1-hour postprandial glucose level have included limiting carbohydrate to approximately 40% of energy intake and distributing intake across six feedings, with 10−15% for breakfast, 20−30% for lunch, 30−40% for dinner, and 10% for each of three between-meal snacks [60]. Research studies need to address dietary composition (amounts and types of carbohydrates and fats), weight gain, and energy and carbohydrate restriction.

VI NUTRIENT INTAKE CONSIDERATIONS

The American Diabetes Association and other diabetes organizations address nutrient intake in their nutritional recommendations [61−63]. The guidelines are similar; therefore, this section focuses on American Diabetes Association statements [61] and highlights a few additional recommendations developed by the European Association for the Study of Diabetes [62,63].

A Protein

The American Diabetes Association recommends basing protein intake for individuals with all classes of diabetes and normal renal function largely on the review by the Institute of Medicine to establish recommendations for the general public with 15−20% of energy intake from protein [54,64]. The European Association for the Study of Diabetes recommends 10−20% of energy intake from protein without established nephropathy [62]. Individuals who may need more than 20% of energy intake from protein include those in a catabolic state, those with growth needs (children, adolescents, and pregnant women), and individuals on very low-energy diets to achieve weight loss. Treatment recommendations for micro- or macroalbuminuria (chronic kidney disease) include reducing protein intake to 0.8−1.0 g/kg body weight/day [41,65] based on evidence that lowering protein intake is associated with improved renal function (urine albumin excretion rate and glomerular filtration rate) in select patients. The European Association for the Study of Diabetes recommends a reduction of protein intake to the lower end of this range (0.8 g/kg body weight/day) for individuals with type 1 diabetes and established nephropathy. Neither the American Diabetes Association nor the European Association for the Study of Diabetes make specific recommendations regarding the type of protein.

B Fat

Intake of fat can blunt and extend postprandial glycemic excursions. An evaluation of the intensively treated DCCT patients revealed that a higher intake of fat and saturated fat and lower intake of carbohydrate were associated with worse glycemic control, independent of exercise and BMI [66]. The American Diabetes Association recommends that all individuals with diabetes limit their saturated fat to less than 7% of total energy, minimize *trans* fat intake, and limit dietary cholesterol intake to less than 200 mg/day. In addition to these recommendations, the American Diabetes Association also recommends consumption of two or more servings of fish per week in order to increase intake of n-3 fatty acids, which may contribute to improved cardiometabolic risk factor outcomes [61]. Similar to the American Diabetes Association, the European Association for the Study of Diabetes recommends limiting saturated and *trans* fat intakes (<10% of total energy intake; <8% if LDL cholesterol is elevated), limiting total fat intake to less than 35% of total energy intake (<30% if overweight or obese), limiting cholesterol intake (<300 mg/day), and consuming two or three servings of fish per week [62].

C Carbohydrates

Dietary carbohydrate is the major determinant of postprandial glucose concentration and is therefore integral to glycemic control. The American Diabetes Association recognizes total carbohydrate as the major determinant of postprandial glucose concentration, with the type of carbohydrate as an additional determinant [61]. Although fructose has been shown to reduce postprandial hyperglycemia when it is substituted for sucrose or starch, the long-term consequences of high fructose intake on plasma lipids and other diabetic complications is unknown. A 2009 meta-analysis of 16 trials found that the effects of fructose intake on blood lipids in individuals with type 2 diabetes were mixed [67], and there is no recommendation to encourage use of fructose by the American Diabetes Association or the European Association for the Study of Diabetes [62,63]. The American Diabetes Association's nutrition recommendations indicate that glycemic control is not contingent on restricting sucrose and suggest that the decision about sugar consumption should be based on overall nutrition considerations [61]. Nonetheless, consumption of large quantities of sugars (e.g., high-fructose corn syrup in soft drinks and other beverages) is a major source of excess calories [68].

The concept of glycemic indexing of food was developed to compare the effects of the quality of carbohydrate while keeping the amount of carbohydrate standardized. The estimated glycemic load of foods, meals, and dietary patterns is calculated by multiplying the glycemic index by the amount of carbohydrate in each food and then totaling for all of the foods in a meal or dietary pattern. The role of the glycemic index and/or glycemic load lacks consensus recommendations, although modifying the type as well as the amount of carbohydrate can improve glycemic control [61]. A randomized trial conducted in children with type 1 diabetes achieved better A1c and quality-of-life outcomes with a flexible low-glycemic index diet than with a measured carbohydrate exchange diet [69]. Randomized controlled trials in individuals with type 2 diabetes have achieved mixed results: A 6-month trial found a moderate decrease in A1c [70], whereas a 1-year trial found no improvement in A1c [71]. A third trial found a decrease in A1c in both the low-glycemic diet group and the American Diabetes Association diet education group at 1 year [72]. Meta-analysis results have also been mixed; a review by Brand-Miller *et al.* [73] found significant decreases in A1c levels while on low-glycemic diets, whereas Anderson *et al.* [74] found no significant difference in A1c levels between a low- and high-glycemic diet. Taking this evidence into account, the American Diabetes Association and the European Association for the Study of Diabetes recognize that considering the glycemic index of carbohydrates may provide additional benefit over considering total carbohydrate alone, provided that the overall attributes of the carbohydrate are taken into account [61–63]. Both organizations

recommend dietary patterns that include carbohydrates from whole grain cereals, fruits, vegetables, legumes, and low-fat milk [61,62].

Findings from several randomized, controlled trials [75–77] indicate that fiber supplements (additional 4–19 g/day) do not improve glycemia or cardiovascular disease risk factors, and therefore the recommended dietary intake for the general public is also recommended for people with diabetes: 14 g per 1000 kcal by the American Diabetes Association and 20 g per 1000 kcal by the European Association for the Study of Diabetes [61,62]. In essence, given the many factors that can affect glucose metabolism, including those beyond nutrition per se (e.g., medicines and activity), it is often problematic to predict the exact plasma glucose response to specific carbohydrate-containing foods. Certainly, blood glucose self-monitoring and experience can help predict the glycemic effects of food products. Furthermore, a variety of methods can be used to estimate the nutrient content of meals, including carbohydrate counting, the exchange system, and experience. With emerging evidence of the relations between postprandial glycemia and cardiovascular disease [78], postprandial glucose levels are of increasing importance.

Fructose, mannitol, and sorbitol are often substituted for sucrose in "sugar-free" products. In experimental studies, these products can shift the balance from oxidation of fatty acids to esterification of fatty acids in the liver, which can in turn increase very low-density lipoprotein synthesis [41]. Although the effects on serum lipids are inconsistent, susceptible individuals may have a worsening of dyslipidemia. These sweeteners appear to offer no documented advantage in the management of diabetes over other carbohydrate sources.

Labeling of food products with regard to carbohydrate composition can be confusing. Food products may list the "net" or "impact" carbohydrate on the front of the label, a value considerably lower than the "total" carbohydrate listed on the nutrient facts panel. Fiber or fiber plus the sugar alcohols are usually subtracted to obtain the net or impact carbohydrate value, but there is no standardization. If patients with diabetes use these products, monitoring is needed to determine the effects on blood glucose [65].

Non-nutritive sweeteners, which are considered high-intensity sweeteners, are widely used as a replacement of various types of sugar in food and beverage products. An evidence-based review by the American Dietetic Association suggests that all approved intense sweeteners, also known as noncaloric and non-nutritive sweeteners (aspartame, saccharin, acesulfame K, sucralose, and stevia), have no adverse effects on diabetes management [41].

Alcohol can inhibit hepatic glucose production resulting in hypoglycemia if consumed without food when the diabetes treatment regimen includes insulin or sulfonylureas [41]. Conversely, consuming large amounts of alcohol can increase blood glucose levels during severe insulin deficiency. A systemic review found that alcohol intake, diabetes, hypertension, and hypertriglyceridemia are associated with increased risk of developing gout [64]. Alcohol intake can exacerbate pancreatitis, severe hypertriglyceridemia, severe neuropathy, myocardiopathy, or renal failure, which are co-morbidities associated with diabetes.

The Study to Help Improve Early Evaluation and Management of Risk Factors Leading to Diabetes findings [79] have demonstrated that for people with diabetes there is a significant gap between knowledge of nutrition and lifestyle recommendations (what to do) and how to incorporate these recommendations into lifestyle routines [80]. MNT is the process by which these evidence-based nutrition recommendations are translated into a plan that individuals can follow based on a thorough assessment of each person's lifestyle, capabilities, and motivation to change. The tools and techniques to facilitate behavior change are discussed in Chapter 10.

TABLE 32.5 Information Sources for Diabetes

Agency for Healthcare Research and Quality: http://www.ahrq.gov/browse/diabetes.htm

American Association of Diabetes Educators: http://www.diabeteseducator.org

American Diabetes Association: http://www.diabetes.org

Centers for Disease Control and Prevention: http://www.cdc.gov/diabetes, http://www.cdc.gov/nchs

Centers for Medicare & Medicaid Services: http://www.cms.hhs.gov

Health Resources and Services Administration: http://www.hrsa.gov

Indian Health Service: http://www.ihs.gov/PublicAffairs/IHSBrochure/diabetes.asp

International Diabetes Federation: http://www.idf.org/

Juvenile Diabetes Research Foundation International: http://www.jdrf.org

National Diabetes Education Program, a joint program of the National Institutes of Health and the Centers for Disease Control and Prevention: http://www.yourdiabetesinfo.org

National Diabetes Information Clearinghouse: http://www.diabetes.niddk.nih.gov

National Institute of Diabetes and Digestive and Kidney Diseases of the National Institutes of Health: http://www.niddk.nih.gov

U.S. Department of Health and Human Services, Office of Minority Health: http://minorityhealth.hhs.gov

U.S. Department of Veterans Affairs: http://www.healthquality.va.gov

U.S. Food and Drug Administration: http://www.fda.gov

VII COLLABORATIVE EFFORTS FOR DIABETES PREVENTION AND TREATMENT

In the United States, much effort within the voluntary, professional, academic, and private sectors is directed at addressing the challenges of diabetes. The National Diabetes Education Program (NDEP), a partnership of the National Institutes of Health and the CDC, tries to serve as a "coordinating entity" among more than 200 public and private organizations [81]. In addition, the CDCP's Division of Diabetes Translation is addressing community infrastructure and environmental issues to reduce the burden of diabetes, including public health surveillance systems for diabetes, applied translational research, state-based diabetes control programs, and public information [82]. The National Institutes of Health has also expanded the focus of research to address how environmental factors and community infrastructure are related to obesity and the risk of diabetes and other chronic diseases. Resources to address diabetes prevention and control are available from the website links listed in Table 32.5.

VIII CONCLUSION

The long-term goal of diabetes prevention and treatment is restoring metabolism as close to normal as possible in order to reduce the morbidity and mortality associated with diabetes. The focus for all classes of diabetes is on reducing cardiovascular risk factors such as hypertension and dyslipidemia. The distribution of macronutrient intake may vary based on a number of factors, including matching insulin to lifestyle in type 1 diabetes and weight loss in type 2 diabetes.

MNT is based on individual assessment and development of a personalized tailored evidence-based treatment plan. A registered dietitian who consults with the health care team and assesses the patient's needs is well positioned to develop a tailored treatment plan that considers overall health needs and individual capabilities with the goal of ameliorating the metabolic effects of diabetes and its complications.

References

[1] American Diabetes Association. "Diabetes Statistics." Available at <http://www.diabetes.org/diabetes-basics/diabetes-statistics>, (2011) (accessed September 2011).

[2] Centers for Disease Control and Prevention (2011). "Diabetes at a Glance—2011." Available at <http://www.cdc.gov/chronicdisease/resources/publications/aag/pdf/2011/Diabetes-AAG-2011-508.pdf>, (ccessed September 2011).

[3] J.E. Shaw, R.A. Sicree, P.Z. Zimmet, Global estimates of the prevalence of diabetes for 2010 and 2030, Diabetes Res. Clin. Pract. 87 (2010) 4–14.

[4] W. Yang, J. Lu, J. Weng, W. Jia, L. Ji, J. Xiao, et al., Prevalence of diabetes among men and women in China, N. Engl. J. Med. 362 (2010) 1090–1101.

[5] P. Zhang, X. Zhang, J. Brown, D. Vistisen, R. Sicree, J. Shaw, et al., Global healthcare expenditure on diabetes for 2010 and 2030, Diabetes Res. Clin. Pract. 87 (2010) 293–301.

[6] American Diabetes Association, Diagnosis and classifications of diabetes mellitus, Diabetes Care 35 (2012) S64–S71.

[7] A.D. Liese, R.B. D'Agostino Jr., R.F. Hamman, P.D. Kilgo, J.M. Lawrence, L.L. Liu, et al., The burden of diabetes mellitus among U.S. youth: prevalence estimates from the search for diabetes in youth study, Pediatr 118 (2006) 1510–1518.

[8] American Diabetes Association, Standards of medical care in diabetes—2012, Diabetes Care 35 (2012) S11–S63.

[9] A. Lapolla, M.G. Dalfra, E. Ragazzi, A.P. De Cata, D. Fedele, New International Association of the Diabetes and Pregnancy Study Groups (IADPSG) recommendations for diagnosing gestational diabetes compared with former criteria: a retrospective study on pregnancy outcome, Diabet. Med 28 (2011) 1074–1077.

[10] J. Leary, D.J. Pettitt, L. Jovanovic, Gestational diabetes guidelines in a HAPO world, Best Pract. Res. Clin. Endocrinol. Metab 24 (2010) 673–685.

[11] J. Tuomilehto, J. Lindstrom, J.G. Eriksson, T.T. Valle, H. Hamalainen, P. Ilanne-Parikka, et al., Prevention of type 2 diabetes mellitus by changes in lifestyle among subjects with impaired glucose tolerance, N. Engl. J. Med. 344 (2001) 1343–1350.

[12] W.C. Knowler, E. Barrett-Connor, S.E. Fowler, R.F. Hamman, J.M. Lachin, E.A. Walker, et al., Reduction in the incidence of type 2 diabetes with lifestyle intervention or metformin, N. Engl. J. Med. 346 (2002) 393–403.

[13] X.R. Pan, G.W. Li, Y.H. Hu, J.X. Wang, W.Y. Yang, Z.X. An, et al., Effects of diet and exercise in preventing NIDDM in people with impaired glucose tolerance: the Da Qing IGT and diabetes study, Diabetes Care 20 (1997) 537–544.

[14] J. Wylie-Rosett, W.H. Herman, R.B. Goldberg, Lifestyle intervention to prevent diabetes: intensive and cost effective, Curr. Opin. Lipidol. 17 (2006) 37–44.

[15] J. Lindstrom, P. Ilanne-Parikka, M. Peltonen, S. Aunola, J.G. Eriksson, K. Hemio, et al., Sustained reduction in the incidence of type 2 diabetes by lifestyle intervention: follow-up of the Finnish Diabetes Prevention Study, Lancet 368 (2006) 1673–1679.

[16] W.C. Knowler, S.E. Fowler, R.F. Hamman, C.A. Christophi, H.J. Hoffman, A.T. Brenneman, et al., 10-Year follow-up of diabetes incidence and weight loss in the diabetes prevention program—outcomes study, Lancet 374 (2009) 1677–1686.

[17] G. Li, P. Zhang, J. Wang, E.W. Gregg, W. Yang, Q. Gong, et al., The long-term effect of lifestyle interventions to prevent diabetes in the China Da Qing Diabetes prevention study: a 20-year follow-up study, Lancet 371 (2008) 1783–1789.

[18] M. Uusitupa, V. Lindi, A. Louheranta, T. Salopuro, J. Lindstrom, J. Tuomilehto, Long-term improvement in insulin sensitivity by changing lifestyles of people with impaired glucose tolerance: 4-year results from the Finnish Diabetes Prevention Study, Diabetes 52 (2003) 2532–2538.

[19] M. Uusitupa, Gene–diet interaction in relation to the prevention of obesity and type 2 diabetes: evidence from the Finnish Diabetes Prevention Study, Nutr. Metab. Cardiovasc. Dis 15 (2005) 225–233.

[20] Diabetes Prevention Program, Description of lifestyle intervention, Diabetes Care 25 (2002) 2165–2171.

[21] R.F. Hamman, R.R. Wing, S.L. Edelstein, J.M. Lachin, G.A. Bray, L. Delahanty, et al., Effect of weight loss with lifestyle intervention on risk of diabetes, Diabetes Care 29 (2006) 2102–2107.

[22] J. Lindstrom, A. Louheranta, M. Mannelin, M. Rastas, V. Salminen, J. Eriksson, et al., The Finnish Diabetes Prevention Study (DPS): lifestyle intervention and 3-year results on diet and physical activity, Diabetes Care 26 (2003) 3230–3236.

[23] R.R. Wing, R.F. Hamman, G.A. Bray, L. Delahanty, S.L. Edelstein, J.O. Hill, et al., Achieving weight and activity goals among Diabetes Prevention Program lifestyle participants, Obes. Res. 12 (2004) 1426–1434.

[24] L.M. Delahanty, D.M. Nathan, Implications of the Diabetes Prevention Program and look-AHEAD clinical trials for lifestyle interventions, J. Am. Diet Assoc. 108 (2008) S66–S72.

[25] J. Salas-Salvado, M. Bullo, N. Babio, M.A. Martinez-Gonzalez, N. Ibarrola-Jurado, J. Basora, et al., Reduction in the incidence of type 2 diabetes with the Mediterranean diet: results of the PREDIMED-REUS nutrition intervention randomized trial, Diabetes Care 34 (2011) 14–19.

[26] B. Gillis, C. Mobley, D.D. Stadler, J. Hartstein, A. Virus, S.L. Volpe, et al., Rationale, design and methods of the HEALTHY study nutrition intervention component, Int. J. Obes. 33 (Suppl. 4) (2009) S29–S36.

[27] G.D. Foster, B. Linder, T. Baranowski, D.M. Cooper, L. Goldberg, J.S. Harrell, et al., A school-based intervention for diabetes risk reduction, N. Engl. J. Med. 363 (2010) 443–453.

[28] A. Patel, S. MacMahon, J. Chalmers, B. Neal, L. Billot, M. Woodward, et al., Intensive blood glucose control and vascular outcomes in patients with type 2 diabetes, N. Engl. J. Med. 358 (2008) 2560–2572.

[29] D.R. Matthews, C.A. Cull, I.M. Stratton, R.R. Holman, R.C. Turner, UKPDS 26: sulphonylurea failure in non-insulin-dependent diabetic patients over six years: UK Prospective Diabetes Study (UKPDS) group, Diabet. Med 15 (1998) 297–303.

[30] R.C. Turner, H. Millns, H.A. Neil, I.M. Stratton, S.E. Manley, D.R. Matthews, et al., Risk factors for coronary artery disease in non-insulin dependent diabetes mellitus: United Kingdom Prospective Diabetes Study (UKPDS: 23), BMJ 316 (1998) 823–828.

[31] U.K. Prospective Diabetes Study Group, UKPDS 28: a randomized trial of efficacy of early addition of metformin in sulfonyl-urea-treated type 2 diabetes, Diabetes Care 21 (1998) 87–92.

[32] D.M. Nathan, J.B. Buse, M.B. Davidson, E. Ferrannini, R.R. Holman, R. Sherwin, et al., Medical management of hyperglycemia in type 2 diabetes: a consensus algorithm for the initiation and adjustment of therapy: a consensus statement of the American Diabetes Association and the European Association for the Study of Diabetes, Diabetes Care 32 (2009) 193–203.

[33] D.M. Nathan, Long-term complications of diabetes mellitus, N. Engl. J. Med. 328 (1993) 1676–1685.

[34] L.M. Delahanty, B.N. Halford, The role of diet behaviors in achieving improved glycemic control in intensively treated patients in the Diabetes Control and Complications Trial, Diabetes Care 16 (1993) 1453–1458.

[35] W.H. Herman, R.C. Eastman, The effects of treatment on the direct costs of diabetes, Diabetes Care 21 (Suppl. 3) (1998) C19–C24.

[36] R.C. Eastman, Cost-effectiveness of treatment of type 2 diabetes, Diabetes Care 21 (1998) 464–465.

[37] M.I. Harris, R.C. Eastman, Is there a glycemic threshold for mortality risk? Diabetes Care 21 (1998) 331–333.

[38] The Diabetes Control and Complications Trial research group, Weight gain associated with intensive therapy in the Diabetes Control and Complications Trial, Diabetes Care 11 (1988) 567–573.

[39] D.M. Nathan, P.A. Cleary, J.Y. Backlund, S.M. Genuth, J.M. Lachin, T.J. Orchard, et al., Intensive diabetes treatment and cardiovascular disease in patients with type 1 diabetes, N. Engl. J. Med. 353 (2005) 2643–2653.

[40] S. Genuth, W. Sun, P. Cleary, D.R. Sell, W. Dahms, J. Malone, et al., Glycation and carboxymethyllysine levels in skin collagen predict the risk of future 10-year progression of diabetic retinopathy and nephropathy in the Diabetes Control and Complications Trial and Epidemiology of Diabetes Interventions and Complications participants with type 1 diabetes, Diabetes 54 (2005) 3103–3111.

[41] M.J. Franz, M.A. Powers, C. Leontos, L.A. Holzmeister, K. Kulkarni, A. Monk, et al., The evidence for medical nutrition therapy for type 1 and type 2 diabetes in adults, J. Am. Diet. Assoc. 110 (2010) 1852–1889.

[42] K. Kulkarni, G. Castle, R. Gregory, A. Holmes, C. Leontos, M. Powers, et al., Nutrition practice guidelines for type 1 diabetes mellitus positively affect dietitian practices and patient outcomes: The Diabetes Care and Education Dietetic Practice Group, J. Am. Diet. Assoc. 98 (1998) 62–70.

[43] Dose Adjustment For Normal Eating (DAFNE) study group, Training in flexible, intensive insulin management to enable dietary freedom in people with type 1 diabetes: Dose Adjustment For Normal Eating (DAFNE) randomised controlled trial, BMJ 325 (2002) 746.

[44] J. Speight, S.A. Amiel, C. Bradley, S. Heller, L. Oliver, S. Roberts, et al., Long-term biomedical and psychosocial outcomes following DAFNE (Dose Adjustment for Normal Eating) structured education to promote intensive insulin therapy in adults with sub-optimally controlled type 1 diabetes, Diabetes Res. Clin. Pract. 89 (2010) 22–29.

[45] UK Prospective Diabetes Study (UKPDS) Group, Effect of intensive blood-glucose control with metformin on complications in overweight patients with type 2 diabetes (UKPDS 34): UK Prospective Diabetes Study (UKPDS) group, Lancet 352 (1998) 854–865.

[46] UK Prospective Diabetes Study (UKPDS) group, Intensive blood-glucose control with sulphonylureas or insulin compared with conventional treatment and risk of complications in patients with type 2 diabetes (UKPDS 33): UK Prospective Diabetes Study (UKPDS) group, Lancet 352 (1998) 837–853.

[47] UK Prospective Diabetes Study (UKPDS) group, Cost-effectiveness analysis of improved blood pressure control in hypertensive patients with type 2 diabetes (UKPDS 40): UK Prospective Diabetes Study group, BMJ 317 (1998) 720–726.

[48] UK Prospective Diabetes Study (UKPDS) group, Efficacy of atenolol and captopril in reducing risk of macrovascular and microvascular complications in type 2 diabetes (UKPDS 39): UK Prospective Diabetes Study group, BMJ 317 (1998) 713–720.

[49] UK Prospective Diabetes Study (UKPDS) group, Tight blood pressure control and risk of macrovascular and microvascular complications in type 2 diabetes (UKPDS 38): UK Prospective Diabetes Study group, BMJ 317 (1998) 703–713.

[50] K.J. Coppell, M. Kataoka, S.M. Williams, A.W. Chisholm, S.M. Vorgers, J.I. Mann, Nutritional intervention in patients with type 2 diabetes who are hyperglycaemic despite optimised drug treatment—Lifestyle Over and Above Drugs in Diabetes (LOADD) study: randomised controlled trial, BMJ 341 (2010) c3337.

[51] D.M. Nathan, J.B. Buse, M.B. Davidson, E. Ferrannini, R.R. Holman, R. Sherwin, et al., Management of hyperglycemia in type 2 diabetes: a consensus algorithm for the initiation and adjustment of therapy: update regarding thiazolidinediones: a consensus statement from the American Diabetes Association and the European Association for the Study of Diabetes, Diabetes Care 31 (2008) 173–175.

[52] H. Buchwald, Y. Avidor, E. Braunwald, M.D. Jensen, W. Pories, K. Fahrbach, et al., Bariatric surgery: a systematic review and meta-analysis, JAMA 292 (2004) 1724–1737.

[53] X. Pi-Sunyer, G. Blackburn, F.L. Brancati, G.A. Bray, R. Bright, J.M. Clark, et al., Reduction in weight and cardiovascular disease risk factors in individuals with type 2 diabetes: one-year results of the look AHEAD trial, Diabetes Care 30 (2007) 1374–1383.

[54] R.R. Wing, Long-term effects of a lifestyle intervention on weight and cardiovascular risk factors in individuals with type 2 diabetes mellitus: four-year results of the look AHEAD trial, Arch. Intern. Med 170 (2010) 1566–1575.

[55] L.M. Delahanty, Research charting a course for evidence-based clinical dietetic practice in diabetes, J. Hum. Nutr. Diet. 23 (2010) 360–370.

[56] F. Ismail-Beigi, T. Craven, M.A. Banerji, J. Basile, J. Calles, R.M. Cohen, et al., Effect of intensive treatment of hyperglycaemia on microvascular outcomes in type 2 diabetes: an analysis of the ACCORD randomised trial, Lancet 376 (2010) 419–430.

[57] W. Duckworth, C. Abraira, T. Moritz, D. Reda, N. Emanuele, P.D. Reaven, et al., Glucose control and vascular complications in veterans with type 2 diabetes, N. Engl. J. Med. 360 (2009) 129–139.

[58] J.S. Skyler, R. Bergenstal, R.O. Bonow, J. Buse, P. Deedwania, E.A. Gale, et al., Intensive glycemic control and the prevention of cardiovascular events: implications of the ACCORD, ADVANCE, and VA diabetes trials: a position statement of the American Diabetes Association and a scientific statement of the American College of Cardiology Foundation and the American Heart Association, Diabetes Care 32 (2009) 187–192.

[59] L.M. Belalcazar, D.M. Reboussin, S.M. Haffner, R.C. Hoogeveen, A.M. Kriska, D.C. Schwenke, et al., A 1-year lifestyle intervention for weight loss in individuals with type 2 diabetes reduces high c-reactive protein levels and identifies metabolic predictors of change: from the look AHEAD (Action for Health in Diabetes) study, Diabetes Care 33 (2010) 2297–2303.

[60] L. Jovanovic, Role of diet and insulin treatment of diabetes in pregnancy, Clin. Obstet. Gynecol. 43 (2000) 46–55.

[61] J.P. Bantle, J. Wylie-Rosett, A.L. Albright, C.M. Apovian, N.G. Clark, M.J. Franz, et al., Nutrition recommendations and interventions for diabetes: a position statement of the American Diabetes Association, Diabetes Care 31 (Suppl. 1) (2008) S61–S78.

[62] J.I. Mann, G. Riccardi, Evidence-based European guidelines on diet and diabetes, Nutr. Metab. Cardiovasc. Dis. 14 (2004) 332–333.

[63] J.I. Mann, I. De Leeuw, K. Hermansen, B. Karamanos, B. Karlstrom, N. Katsilambros, et al., Evidence-based nutritional approaches to the treatment and prevention of diabetes mellitus, Nutr. Metab. Cardiovasc. Dis. 14 (2004) 373–394.

[64] J.A. Singh, S.G. Reddy, J. Kundukulam, Risk factors for gout and prevention: a systematic review of the literature, Curr. Opin. Rheumatol. 23 (2011) 192–202.

[65] J. Wylie-Rosett, Paradigm shifts in obesity research and treatment: introduction, Obes. Res. 12 (Suppl. 2) (2004) 85S–87S.

[66] L.M. Delahanty, D.M. Nathan, J.M. Lachin, F.B. Hu, P.A. Cleary, G.K. Ziegler, et al., Association of diet with glycated hemoglobin during intensive treatment of type 1 diabetes in the Diabetes Control and Complications Trial, Am. J. Clin. Nutr. 89 (2009) 518–524.

[67] J.L. Sievenpiper, A.J. Carleton, S. Chatha, H.Y. Jiang, R.J. de Souza, J. Beyene, et al., Heterogeneous effects of fructose on blood lipids in individuals with type 2 diabetes: Systematic

review and meta-analysis of experimental trials in humans, Diabetes Care 32 (2009) 1930—1937.

[68] R.K. Johnson, L.J. Appel, M. Brands, B.V. Howard, M. Lefevre, R.H. Lustig, et al., Dietary sugars intake and cardiovascular health: a scientific statement from the American Heart Association, Circulation 120 (2009) 1011—1020.

[69] H.R. Gilbertson, J.C. Brand-Miller, A.W. Thorburn, S. Evans, P. Chondros, G.A. Werther, The effect of flexible low glycemic index dietary advice versus measured carbohydrate exchange diets on glycemic control in children with type 1 diabetes, Diabetes Care 24 (2001) 1137—1143.

[70] D.J. Jenkins, C.W. Kendall, G. McKeown-Eyssen, R.G. Josse, J. Silverberg, G.L. Booth, et al., Effect of a low-glycemic index or a high-cereal fiber diet on type 2 diabetes: a randomized trial, JAMA 300 (2008) 2742—2753.

[71] T.M. Wolever, A.L. Gibbs, C. Mehling, J.L. Chiasson, P.W. Connelly, R.G. Josse, et al., The Canadian Trial of Carbohydrates in Diabetes (CCD), a 1-y controlled trial of low-glycemic-index dietary carbohydrate in type 2 diabetes: no effect on glycated hemoglobin but reduction in C-reactive protein, Am. J. Clin. Nutr. 87 (2008) 114—125.

[72] Y. Ma, B.C. Olendzki, P.A. Merriam, D.E. Chiriboga, A.L. Culver, W. Li, et al., A randomized clinical trial comparing low-glycemic index versus ADA dietary education among individuals with type 2 diabetes, Nutrition 24 (2008) 45—56.

[73] J. Brand-Miller, S. Hayne, P. Petocz, S. Colagiuri, Low-glycemic index diets in the management of diabetes: a meta-analysis of randomized controlled trials, Diabetes Care 26 (2003) 2261—2267.

[74] J.W. Anderson, K.M. Randles, C.W. Kendall, D.J. Jenkins, Carbohydrate and fiber recommendations for individuals with diabetes: a quantitative assessment and meta-analysis of the evidence, J. Am. Coll. Nutr. 23 (2004) 5—17.

[75] D.J. Jenkins, C.W. Kendall, V. Vuksan, E. Vidgen, T. Parker, D. Faulkner, et al., Soluble fiber intake at a dose approved by the U.S. Food and Drug Administration for a claim of health benefits: serum lipid risk factors for cardiovascular disease assessed in a randomized controlled crossover trial, Am. J. Clin. Nutr. 75 (2002) 834—839.

[76] A.M. Flammang, D.M. Kendall, C.J. Baumgartner, T.D. Slagle, Y.S. Choe, Effect of a viscous fiber bar on postprandial glycemia in subjects with type 2 diabetes, J. Am. Coll. Nutr. 25 (2006) 409—414.

[77] D. Magnoni, C.H. Rouws, M. Lansink, K.M. van Laere, A.C. Campos, Long-term use of a diabetes-specific oral nutritional supplement results in a low-postprandial glucose response in diabetes patients, Diabetes Res. Clin. Pract. 80 (2008) 75—82.

[78] M.E. Tushuizen, M. Diamant, R.J. Heine, Postprandial dysmetabolism and cardiovascular disease in type 2 diabetes, Postgrad. Med. J. 81 (2005) 1—6.

[79] N.G. Clark, K.M. Fox, S. Grandy, Symptoms of diabetes and their association with the risk and presence of diabetes: findings from the Study to Help Improve Early Evaluation and Management of Risk Factors Leading to Diabetes (SHIELD), Diabetes Care 30 (2007) 2868—2873.

[80] J.R. Gavin, 3rd. Implications of SHIELD Study for Management of Diabetes and Individuals at Risk. Paper presented at the 71st Scientific Sessions of the American Diabetes Association, 24.06.2011

[81] C.M. Clark Jr., Reducing the burden of diabetes: The National Diabetes Education Program, Diabetes Care 21 (Suppl. 3) (1998) C30—C31.

[82] D. Murphy, T. Chapel, C. Clark, Moving diabetes care from science to practice: the evolution of the National Diabetes Prevention and Control Program, Ann. Intern. Med 140 (2004) 978—984.

C H A P T E R

33

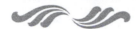

Nutritional Management for Gestational Diabetes

Maria Duarte-Gardea

The University of Texas at El Paso, El Paso, Texas

I INTRODUCTION

Gestational diabetes mellitus (GDM) is defined as carbohydrate intolerance of variable degree with onset or first recognition during pregnancy [1,2]. Exposure to maternal hyperglycemia conveys a risk for obesity and type 2 diabetes in the offspring, in addition to genetic predisposition, regardless of the type of maternal diabetes [3−6].

Nutrition management is an essential component in the overall medical care of the patient diagnosed with GDM, and it plays an important role in controlling blood glucose levels throughout pregnancy. Ideally, an interdisciplinary health care team that includes endocrinologists, obstetricians, diabetes educators, nurses, social workers, nutritionists, and other professionals works in collaboration with the common goal of assisting the pregnant woman to achieve normoglycemia beyond diagnosis and throughout delivery. Nutrition management consists of the implementation of a meal plan that provides adequate nutrition that promotes appropriate weight gain, normoglycemia, and the absence of kentonuria [7]. The meal plan provides additional calories to sustain weight gain and specific amounts and types of carbohydrates distributed throughout the day to achieve desirable blood glucose levels [8].

A nutrition assessment is initially obtained through medical and obstetrical history, anthropometric and laboratory data, and documentation of lifestyle and food preferences. This information is useful in the design of an individualized and culturally appropriate meal plan that contributes to achieving an ultimate goal of delivering a healthy infant. Due to the lack of consensus by different research groups on the

additional recommended caloric levels needed to sustain weight after diagnosis, an individualized meal plan should be prepared by the nutritionist.

The nutrition educational materials delivered and explained to the patient with GDM should be appropriate for the patient's educational level. During intervention, the nutritionist emphasizes lifestyle modifications aimed at reducing the possibility of developing diabetes later in life. In order to evaluate the patient's outcomes, frequent follow-up visits are required to monitor nutrient intake and parameters such as weight gain, blood glucose control, prevention of ketosis, compliance, and patient concerns and satiety.

Pregnancy complicated with diabetes represents an opportunity for the nutritionist and other health care providers to impact lifestyle patterns aimed toward habits that will be beneficial for the woman and her family.

A Prevalence

The prevalence of GDM varies worldwide and among different racial and ethnic groups within a country. Approximately 135,000 cases of GDM, representing on average 3−8% of all pregnancies, are diagnosed annually in the United States [1,9]. There is variability of GDM among members of certain ethnic groups (African American, Native American, Hispanic, South or East Asian, Pacific Islander, and Indigenous Australian) [10]. For example, the prevalence among Zuni Indians is 14.3% [11]. The prevalence of GDM among women with diverse ethnic backgrounds was examined between 1994 and 2002. It was reported that the prevalence of GDM among different ethnic groups

Nutrition in the Prevention and Treatment of Disease, Third Edition.
DOI: http://dx.doi.org/10.1016/B978-0-12-391884-0.00033-0

in the United States increased from 1.7 to 3.1% among non-Hispanic whites; from 2.8 to 5.4% in Hispanics, and from 2.9 to 5.4% in African Americans [12]. The prevalence of GDM among the Hispanic population in the United States ranges between 5 and 15% depending on the geographical location. The prevalence of GDM in Hispanic women of Mexican origin living in border communities ranges from 10 to 15% [13–15]. A similar trend has been reported for Canadian aboriginal populations. The prevalence in the inland communities was twice as high as that in the coastal communities (18.0 vs. 9.3%, $p = 0.002$) [16]. The increase in GDM prevalence may represent a major determinant of the recent increase in obesity among women of childbearing age, which may lead to further increases in GDM [12].

B Risk Factors

Risk factors associated with the development of GDM include age, obesity, family history of diabetes, and being member of a high-prevalence ethnic group. Risk can be classified as low, average, or high according to the criteria described later and should be determined during the first prenatal visit. Table 33.1 describes characteristics associated with low, average, and high risk for developing GDM. A patient identified as low risk for developing GDM does not require a routine screening. Patients with one or more characteristics in the average risk category should be screened for GDM between week 24 and week 28 of gestation. If any characteristic is present in the high-risk category, screening is performed as soon as possible. If GDM is not diagnosed, blood glucose testing should be repeated at 24–28 weeks or at any time the patient has symptoms or signs that are suggestive of hyperglycemia [10].

C Dietary Risk Factors

Several dietary factors have been found to be predisposing factors to develop GDM. One study examined the effects of dietary fat on GDM in nulliparous pregnant (NP) women with GDM ($n = 85$) compared with normal pregnant women ($n = 159$). Dietary assessments were conducted and evaluated in both groups. The analysis focused on carbohydrate, protein, and fat, especially on dietary fat subtypes. Fat intake in the GDM group was significantly higher than that in the NP group ($p < 0.05$), whereas carbohydrate and protein intakes in the GDM group were not significantly different compared with those of the NP group. Intake of polyunsaturated fatty acids in the GDM group was lower than that in the NP group, but intake of

TABLE 33.1   Risk Categories for Screening for Gestational Diabetes Mellitus (GDM)

Risk category	Characteristics
Low	• Not a member of an ethnic group with a higher prevalence of GDM • No known diabetes in first-degree relatives (parents, siblings) • Normal pre-pregnant body mass index • No previous history of abnormal glucose tolerance • No history of adverse pregnancy outcome associated with GDM (e.g., unexplained loss, macrosomia, or excessive sized infant)
Average	• 25 years of age • < 25 years of age and obese (i.e., 20% over desired body weight or body mass index >27 kg/m^2) • Family history of diabetes in first-degree relatives • Member of an ethnic/racial group of high prevalence (e.g., Hispanic-American, Native American, Asian-American, African-American, or Pacific Islander)
High	• Significant obesity • Family history of diabetes • GDM in previous pregnancy • History of glucose intolerance • Glucosuria • History of adverse pregnancy outcome associated with GDM

saturated fatty acids was higher in the GDM group. Although intake of monounsaturated fatty acids in the GDM group was higher than that in the NP group, there was no significant difference between the two groups. It was concluded that intake of high dietary fat, high saturated fatty acids, and low polyunsaturated fatty acids may be one of the high-risk factors for GDM [17].

In a large cohort prospective study of 13,110 U.S. women of reproductive age (The Nurses' Health Study II), the authors examined whether pregravid dietary fiber consumption from cereal, fruit, and vegetable sources and dietary glycemic load were related to GDM risk. Dietary fiber (source and amount), average glycemic index, and glycemic load were evaluated in accordance with the risk of developing GDM. It was concluded that dietary total fiber, particularly cereal and fruit fiber, was strongly and inversely associated with GDM risk. A multivariate analysis indicated that for each 10 g/day increment in total fiber, the risk of GDM was reduced by 26%. No significant associations were observed between vegetable fiber and GDM risk. Dietary glycemic load was significantly and positively associated with GDM risk after adjustment for nondietary and dietary covariates. The association between dietary glycemic index alone and GDM risk was not statistically significant.

Women with low cereal fiber intake and high glycemic load had a 2.15-fold (95% confidence interval,1.04−4.29) higher risk for GDM [18].

In summary, a diet high in total fat containing high saturated and low polyunsaturated fatty acids as well as low cereal fiber and high glycemic load has been associated with the risk of developing GDM [17,18].

II SCREENING AND DIAGNOSIS

According to the World Health Organization (WHO), women with a high risk for GDM (older women, those from high-risk ethnic groups, those with a personal history of glucose intolerance, those with a personal history of large for gestational age offspring, and those presenting elevated fasting or casual blood glucose levels) should be screened during the first trimester of pregnancy. Systematic testing should be performed between 24 and 28 weeks of pregnancy after an overnight fast with a 75-g oral glucose tolerance test (OGTT). Pregnant women who meet the WHO criteria for diabetes mellitus (fasting glucose ≥ 7.0 mmol/l (≥ 126 mg/dl) or 2-hour glucose ≥ 11.1 mmol/l (≥ 200 mg/dl)) or impaired glucose tolerance (IGT) (fasting glucose ≥ 7.0 mmol/l (≥ 126 mg/dl) or 2-hour post-glucose load ≥ 7.8 mmol/l (≥ 140 mg/dl) and <11.1 mmol/l (<200 mg/dl)) are classified as having GDM [19].

As the ongoing epidemic of obesity and diabetes has led to increased cases of type 2 diabetes in women of childbearing age, the number of pregnant women with undiagnosed type 2 diabetes has also increased. The American Diabetes Association recommends that women with risk factors for type 2 diabetes be screened at their initial prenatal visit using standard diagnostic criteria. Women who meet any of the following criteria should receive a diagnosis of overt, not gestational, diabetes: fasting plasma glucose level ≥ 126 mg/dl (7.0 mmol/l), 2-hour plasma glucose ≥ 200 mg/dl (11.1 mmol/l) during an OGTT, a random plasma glucose >200 mg/dl (11.1 mmol/l), or hemoglobin A1c$>6.5\%$. In 2009, an international expert committee that included representatives of the American Diabetes Association, the International Diabetes Federation, and the European Association for the Study of Diabetes recommended use of the hemoglobin A1c test to diagnose diabetes with a threshold of $>6.5\%$.

A new diagnosis criteria resulted from a consensus based on the Hyperglycemia and Adverse Pregnancy Outcomes study, a large-scale epidemiological study of approximately 25,000 pregnant women. The number of women who demonstrated risk of adverse maternal and neonatal outcomes continuously increased as a function of maternal glycemia at 24−28 weeks. In 2008

and 2009, the International Association of Diabetes and Pregnancy Study Groups, an international consensus group with representatives from multiple obstetrical and diabetes organizations including the American Diabetes Association, developed revised recommendations for diagnosing GDM. The group recommended screening for GDM at 24−28 weeks of gestation using a 75-g OGTT (as described by WHO using a glucose load containing 75 g anhydrous glucose dissolved in water), with plasma glucose measurement after fasting and at 1 and 2 hours. The result should be confirmed by repeat testing in the absence of unequivocal hyperglycemia. The test should be performed in the morning after an overnight fast of at least 8 hours. The diagnosis of GDM is made when any of the following plasma glucose values are exceeded [20]:

Fasting: >92 mg/dl (5.1 mmol/l)
1 hour: >180 mg/dl (10.0 mmol/l)
2 hours: >153 mg/dl (8.5 mmol/l)

In opposition to the new diagnosis criteria, other groups endorse the 50-g glucose challenge test followed by the 100-g glucose tolerance test as a more cost-effective, familiar, and possibly well-validated screening tool [21]. A 50-g oral glucose load is administered between weeks 24 and 28, without regard to time of day or time of last meal, to all pregnant women who have not been identified as having glucose intolerance, and venous plasma glucose is measured 1 hour later. A value of >130 mg/dl in venous plasma indicates a full diagnostic OGTT.

A Oral Glucose Tolerance Test

1. A 100-g glucose load is administered in the morning after overnight fast of at least 8 hours but not more than 14 hours and after at least 3 days of unrestricted diet (≥ 150 g carbohydrate) and physical activity.
2. Venous plasma glucose is measured after fasting and at 1, 2, and 3 hours. The subject should remain seated and not smoke during the test. Two or more of the following venous plasma concentrations must be met or exceeded for a positive diagnosis of GDM:
Fasting: ≥ 95 mg/dl or 5.3 mmol/l
1.hour: ≥ 180 mg/dl or 10.0 mmol/l
2.hours: ≥ 155 mg/dl or 8.6 mmol/l
3.hours: ≥ 140 mg/dl or 7.8 mmol/l

One abnormal value on the 100-g glucose load as well as significantly elevated (>185 mg/dl) glucose screens despite normal results have been associated with fetal macrosomia and may warrant management. If one abnormal value is seen during the 100-g 3-hour OGTT, it is recommended that the test be repeated approximately 1 month later. There is growing evidence that one abnormal value is sufficient to impact the health of the fetus. Hence, this is now the criterion used by most clinicians to initiate treatment. When the two-step approach is employed, a glucose threshold value >140 mg/dl (7.8 mmol/l) identifies approximately 80% of women with GDM, and the yield is further increased to 90% by using a cutoff of >130 mg/dl (7.2 mmol/l) [22,23]. A fasting glucose level >126 mg/dl or a causal plasma glucose >200 mg/dl that is confirmed on a subsequent day precludes the need for any glucose challenge.

III COMPLICATIONS

Perinatal morbidity and mortality in GDM are associated with uncontrolled blood glucose. When managed intensively, the risk of intrauterine fetal death is similar to that in normal pregnancies [24]. The severity of risk is associated with the degree of maternal hyperglycemia. Even mild blood glucose elevations, however, may cause fetal macrosomia. Whereas maternal glucose readily crosses the placenta, insulin does not. Elevated maternal blood glucose levels produce fetal hyperglycemia, which results in fetal hyperinsulinemia, lipogenesis, glycogen and protein synthesis, and subsequent macrosomia. In a prospective study that included 115 untreated women with borderline GDM by the broader criteria of Carpenter and Coustan, it was found that compared with normoglycemic controls, the untreated borderline GDM group had increased rates of macrosomia (28.7 vs. 13.7%, $p<0.001$) and cesarean delivery (29.6 vs. 20.2%, $p = 0.02$) [25]. In a retrospective case–control study of 970 women, infant and maternal morbidity was assessed in 114 mother–children pairs with an infant birth weight higher than the 90th percentile. The incidence of preeclampsia was 8.8 versus 2.7% in the peer group ($p = 0.002$), and neonatal jaundice was 16.7% in the undiagnosed GDM group versus 4.5% in the peer group ($p<0.0001$). Cord blood insulin levels were significantly elevated in comparison to those of the peer group of mothers without metabolic disorders and those who had eutrophic infants (8.4 mU/l (range, 3.0–100.0 mU/l) vs. 5.3 mU/l (range, 3.0–30.7 mU/l); $p = 0.01$). Cord blood insulin levels were above the normal range in 11.4% of all macrosomic infants [26].

Major complications of uncontrolled GDM have been associated with traumatic birth, shoulder dystocia, clavicular fracture, brachial palsy or other trauma injury, congenital anomalies, neonatal metabolic disorders, cardiomyopathy, neurological symptoms, renal vein thrombosis, hyaline membrane disease, neonatal respiratory distress syndrome, asphyxia, resuscitation

at delivery, and transient tachypnea [27]. In a retrospective case–control study of pregnant women with GDM, the relationship among unrecognized gestational diabetes and infant birth weight, delivery mode, and perinatal complications was evaluated in 297 women treated with diet, 76 treated with diet and insulin, and 16 with unrecognized GDM. Controlled confounding variables were maternal body mass index (BMI), weight gain, age, parity, and gestational age. It was found that shoulder dystocia occurred in 19% of the unrecognized group compared with 3% in the control group ($p<0.05$) and 3% in the diet group ($p<0.02$). The incidence of birth trauma in the unrecognized group (25%) was significantly greater than that in the control group (0%), diet group (0.3%), and insulin group (1%) ($p<0.001$). There were significantly higher rates of hyperbilirubinemia, hypocalcemia, polycythemia, and neonatal intensive care unit admission in the unrecognized compared to the control group (13 vs. 0%, $p<0.05$) [28].

In a case–control study of 555 women with untreated GDM, one or more of five indicators were measured (stillbirth, neonatal macrosomia/large for gestational age, neonatal hypoglycemia, erythrocytosis, and hyperbilirubinemia). It was reported that for every 10 mg/dl increment in fasting plasma glucose, there was an increased adverse outcome by 15% [29]. In addition to the clinical implications for the woman and her infant, GDM is an expensive health problem.

IV NUTRITION MANAGEMENT

Nutrition management represents the cornerstone of treatment during GDM for blood glucose control. The importance of nutrition management in GDM was documented when a randomized clinical trial reported a reduced risk of serious perinatal outcomes in a group of women who received individualized dietary advice by a qualified nutritionist, blood glucose monitoring, and insulin therapy as needed. Women in the intervention group had infants whose weight was significantly lower than that of infants of their counterparts [30]. Another study examining the impact of nutrition practice guidelines implemented by registered dietitians on pregnancy outcomes showed lower insulin use, reduced glycated hemoglobin, and lower birth weight [31].

According to the American Diabetes Association, all women with GDM should receive nutritional counseling by a registered dietitian, when possible. Individualization of medical nutrition therapy (MNT) depending on maternal weight and height is recommended. Macronutrient management should include the best mix of carbohydrate, protein, and fat adjusted

TABLE 33.2 Total Weight Gain and Mean Rate of Weight Gain for Each Body Mass Index Category

Pre-pregnancy BMI category	Total weight gain (kg)	First trimester (total kg)	Second trimester (kg/week)	Third trimester (kg/week)
Low (BMI < 18.5)	12.5−18	2.3	0.49	0.49
Normal (BMI 18.5−24.9)	11.5−16	1.6	0.44	0.44
High (BMI 25s29.9)	7−11.5	0.9	0.30	0.30
Obese (BMI > 29)	>7			

to meet metabolic goals and individual patient preferences. An individualized meal plan should include optimization of food choices to meet Recommended Dietary Allowances/dietary reference intake (DRI) for all micronutrients for pregnant women [20]. During nutrition management of GDM, specific caloric and nutrient recommendations are determined and subsequently modified as needed based on individual assessment and self-monitoring of blood glucose. Due to the continuous fetal draw of glucose from the mother, maintaining consistency of times and amounts of food eaten is important to avoid hypoglycemia. Plasma glucose monitoring and daily food records provide valuable information for insulin and meal plan adjustments [8].

A Weight Gain Recommendations

Total weight gain during pregnancy varies widely among women. The current weight gain recommendations from the Institute of Medicine are based on women's pre-pregnancy BMI. Table 33.2 displays recommendations for total weight gain for each BMI category and the recommended total weight for the first trimester and weekly weight gain for the second and third trimesters [32].

B Caloric Requirements

The energy allowance for pregnancy may be estimated by dividing the gross energy cost (80,000 kcal) by the approximate duration (250 days following the first month), yielding an average value of 300 kcal per day in addition to the allowance of nonpregnant females [33,34].

The caloric requirements are different for each trimester. During the first trimester, the energy needs are the same as those for a nonpregnant woman. An initial guideline for the first trimester is to use 30 kcal/kg of ideal pre-pregnant body weight. Energy requirements for the second and third trimesters are roughly assessed by multiplying actual maternal weight in kilograms by the recommended kilocalories per kilogram correspondent to each pre-pregnant (BMI) category. It is recommended to use 36 kcal/kg ideal body weight for the second trimester and 38 kcal/kg ideal body weight for the third trimester [35]. A number of studies have reported using different caloric recommendations either per actual body weight or pre-pregnant body weight. For example, Jovanic-Peterson's team reported that the euglycemic diet, in which 30 kcal/kg of current weight is recommended for normal pre-pregnant weight, 24 kcal/kg of current weight for overweight, and 12−15 kcal/kg for obese pregnant women during their second and third trimesters, provides sufficient energy needs without causing excessive weight gain or hyperglycemia [36]. It has been documented that when women with GDM follow the euglycemic diet, normal glycemia is achieved in 75−80% of cases. The diet reduces caloric intake to just above the ketonuric threshold [37]. Langer et al. [38] studied the relationship between pre-pregnant weight, treatment modality (diet and insulin), levels of glycemic control, and pregnancy outcome. Normal-weight women were prescribed 35 kcal/kg for actual maternal weight and obese women 25 kcal/kg. It was concluded that well-controlled gestational diabetes was associated with good outcomes in all maternal weight groups [38]. In that study, it was not clear whether overweight women were prescribed the same caloric level as obese women. In another study, Mexican American women with GDM who received culturally appropriate nutrition therapy were prescribed 37±3 kcal/kg for normal pre-pregnant weight (n = 42). Overweight (n = 46) and obese (n = 47) pregnant women were prescribed an average of 23±3 kcal/kg. At delivery, neonatal weights of normal-weight, overweight, and obese women were 3313±671, 3413±727, and 3448 ± 654 g, respectively. In that study and in contrast with other studies, the caloric prescription was based on pre-pregnant body weight for all BMI categories, whereas the majority of studies have based their requirements on current weight [39].

The energy requirements for pregnant adolescents (14−18 years) and adult women (19−50 years) are determined by using the estimated energy requirements (EER) formula [34]. This method is not applicable to overweight and obese women. Caloric requirement for overweight and obese women can be obtained using adjusted body weight in the Harris−Benedict formula and adding 150−300 kcal for the second and third trimesters [8]. Table 33.3 displays the EER formulas to determine energy requirements

TABLE 33.3 Energy Requirements for Pregnancy

Name _____   *Age* (**A**) _____

Gestational age _____ **weeks**

Pre-pregnancy Wt _____ kg

Pre-pregnancy BMI Category
Low (BMI < 18.5)
Normal (BMI 18.5–24.9)
High (BMI 25–29.9)
Obese (BMI > 29)

Height _____ m * 100 <u>cm</u> = _____ cm

                                         m

BMI _____ kg/m^2

Estimated Energy Requirements for Normal Pre-pregnant BMI

Energy$_{First\ Trimester}$ = EER + 0	EER = 354 − (6.91 * A) + PA * (9.36 * Wt kg + 726 * Ht m)
Energy$_{Second\ Trimester}$ = EER + 340	EER = 354 − (6.91 * A) + PA * (9.36 * Wt kg + 726 * Ht m) + 340
Energy$_{Third\ Trimester}$ = EER + 452	354 − (6.91 * A) + PA * (9.36 * Wt kg + 726 * Ht m) + 452

Source: Data from Reference 31.

Physical Activity Coefficient (PA)

Sedentary	Low Activity	Active	Very Active
1.0	1.12	1.27	1.45

Energy Requirements for High and Obese Pre-pregnant BMI for Second and Third Trimesters

Energy = [655 + (9.6 * AdBWt kg) + (1.8 * Ht cm) − (4.7 * A)] * PA + *X*

X = 150–300 kcal

Adjusted Body Weight (AdBWt)

AdBWt = [(actual body Wt − desirable body Wt) × 0.25] + desirable body Wt

for normal pre-pregnant BMI category for the second and third trimesters. It also displays formulas to determine energy requirements for the high pre-pregnant BMI category [8,34].

Independently of the method used to estimate caloric level, appetite, weight gain pattern, and ketone testing will indicate if adjustments of caloric recommendations are necessary.

C Carbohydrates

Carbohydrate is the primary nutrient affecting postprandial glucose levels, and it is the postprandial blood glucose concentration that has the most important role in macrosomia [40]. The amount and kind of carbohydrates eaten at meals and snacks are essential to maintaining optimal blood glucose and reducing the need for insulin while controlling maternal weight gain and infant birth weight [8]. In summary, it is recommended that carbohydrates be provided from a variety of food sources, such as fruits, vegetables, low-fat milk, and whole grains [7].

1 Total Carbohydrate Intake

In order to ensure provision of glucose to the fetal brain (approximately 33 g/day) and supply the glucose fuel requirement for the mother's brain independent of utilization of ketoacids (or other substrates), a minimum amount of 175 g/day of carbohydrates is necessary to prevent ketosis [34]. Carbohydrate recommendations vary from 40 to 45% of total daily calories [8,38,41,42]. An estimated amount of carbohydrates generally comprises approximately 40−45% of total daily calories or between 200 and 225 g of carbohydrates for a 2000-calorie meal plan. On the euglycemic diet, the amount of carbohydrate consumption is restricted to less than 40% of total calories, allowing 40% or more of calories to be fat and the remaining 20% to be protein [37]. Low-carbohydrate diets (<130 g/day) are not recommended [7].

2 Carbohydrate Distribution

The distribution of energy and carbohydrate in the meal plan should be based on a woman's eating habits and plasma glucose responses. A better glucose response is achieved when the total amount of carbohydrates is distributed throughout the day and limited at breakfast [7]. Peterson et al. [43] demonstrated this in a study in which the effect of the percentage of carbohydrate on glucose response to breakfast, lunch, and dinner was evaluated in subjects with GDM. Fourteen women were prescribed a diet with 24 kcal/kg of current pregnant weight/day (12.5% of calories at breakfast and 28% of calories at lunch and dinner, with the remaining calories divided among three snacks). Blood glucose response was measured four times a day. The glycemic response to a meal was highly correlated with the carbohydrate content of the meal. The glycemic response to carbohydrate content of a meal was more consistent for dinner ($r = 0.95$, $p < 0.001$), with greater variability at breakfast ($r = 0.75$, $p = 0.002$) and lunch ($r = 0.86$, $p = 0.001$). If the postprandial blood glucose were to remain <6.7 mmol/l (120 mg/dl), the following percentage of carbohydrate should be used at each meal: 33% at breakfast, 45% at lunch, and 40% at dinner [43].

Carbohydrate tolerance is often lower in the morning because high cortisol levels interfere with glucose clearance in the morning and are particularly high during pregnancy [37]. Post-breakfast hyperglycemia is prevented by limiting the total carbohydrate to less than 30 g and minimizing or avoiding fruit, fruit juice, and refined grain products [44]. The total amount of carbohydrate is generally distributed into three meals and two to four snacks. The amount of carbohydrates recommended for snacks is smaller than the amount recommended for meals [8,35,43,44]. An intake of 15–30 g of carbohydrates during breakfast is recommended based on higher levels of plasma cortisol and growth hormone in the morning affecting glucose levels [43]. This carbohydrate distribution throughout the day helps in the prevention of hunger, ketonuria, heartburn, and nausea [8]. A consistent amount of carbohydrates at meals and snacks will result in better glucose control and will facilitate insulin adjustments, if necessary [45]. An acceptable caloric distribution would be 10% of calories at breakfast, 30% at both lunch and dinner, and 30% distributed in between meals as snacks [43].

3 Type of Carbohydrate

Gestational diabetes is associated with increased carbohydrate sensitivity. To address this sensitivity, it is advised to use the glycemic index to customize the food plan.

Lock et al. [46] studied the applicability of the glycemic index concept in pregnancy. The study aimed to evaluate whether typical and uniform glycemic responses follow by the ingestion of foods in GDM. The postprandial curves of eight foods, such as raisins, dates, sweet corn, bananas, oranges, spaghetti, and green peas, were measured in 28 gestational diabetic subjects and compared to glycemic indices reported by other nonpregnant women. Each food contained 50 g of carbohydrate, with the exception of peas, which contained 25 g. Glucose (50 and 25 g) was the reference food. After bread ingestion, the glycemic excursion was similar in form but slightly blunted compared with glucose. The other test foods had earlier peaking and more blunted postprandial glucose curves. The glycemic index of bread (77.7 ± 5.0) was significantly higher than those of corn (51.8 ± 6.8), bananas (49.0 ± 5.5), oranges (46.6 ± 4.7), spaghetti (42.2 ± 7.3), and peas (35.1 ± 4.2). The glycemic indices of dates (61.6 ± 3.5) and raisins (65.7 ± 5.8) were also significantly higher than that of peas. There was a weak positive correlation between individual glycemic indices and the mean fasting glucose levels used in their calculation. In was concluded that during GDM, the glycemic indices were uniform after the ingestion of the foods and therefore pregnancy does not appear to alter the glycemic indices of the foods tested. In addition, there is a good correlation between glycemic indices reported in the literature for nonpregnant subjects.

In a study of pregnant (nondiabetic) women, the glycemic index was examined in relation to pregnancy outcome. It was found that glycemic index was positively and significantly related to maternal glycosylated hemoglobin and plasma glucose. It was also reported that pregnant women with low dietary glycemic index had reduced infant birth weight and approximately twofold increased risk of a small-for-gestational-age infant [47].

The glycemic response not only depends on dietary carbohydrates but also is influenced by other meal components. The glycemic index can be used as an adjunct for the fine-tuning of postprandial blood glucose responses [48]. Because many clinicians find that certain foods lead to a higher glycemic response causing a higher elevation in postprandial blood glucose [8], it is the general recommendation to restrict high glycemic index foods (e.g., highly processed breakfast cereals, instant potatoes, instant noodles, sugar, honey, molasses, corn syrup, candy, and sweetened beverages) and limit intake of fruit, fruit juice, and milk. Low glycemic index foods (e.g., whole wheat bread, old-fashioned oatmeal, bran cereal, nuts, legumes, and lentils) and protein foods are emphasized [46].

A randomized controlled trial investigating the effects of low glycemic index diet on pregnancy outcomes in gestational diabetes concluded that in intensively monitored women with GDM, a low glycemic index diet and a conventional high-fiber diet produce similar pregnancy outcomes [49].

4 Consistency of Carbohydrates

Consistency of carbohydrate intake is encouraged, specifically to prevent undereating and to assist with postprandial blood glucose evaluation. A consistent amount and type of carbohydrates at meals and snacks is recommended for better glucose control. Consistency of carbohydrates will facilitate insulin adjustments if necessary [8,44].

5 Dietary Fiber

Dietary fiber such as pectin and guar gum and that present in oatmeal products and beans has been found to produce a reduction in glycemic response and high insulin sensitivity. Specifically, it has been reported that vegetable fibers with a high viscosity reduce the levels of basal and postprandial glycemia in both normal and diabetic subjects. The value of glucomannan and guar in the treatment of excessive weight gain in pregnancy and GDM was studied [50]. Thirty-four patients were included in the study, of which 13 received glucomannan (3 g/day) and 21 guar (10 g/day). An OGTT was performed in all patients before and after therapy. A reduction of basal and post-OGTT glycemia values was observed in all subjects.

In the study by Reece et al. [51], non-insulin-requiring GDM patients were placed in three different fiber dose groups (moderate-fiber dose, 40–60 g; high-fiber dose, 70–80 g; and a normal fiber dose, ≤20 g). No significant difference was observed in the mean blood glucose and postprandial glucose levels among the three groups. It was concluded that a high intake of fiber (40–80 g/day) in GDM is not associated with an improved glucose response.

People with diabetes are advised to ingest a variety of fiber-containing foods. Higher fiber intake (<50 g) does not provide additional benefits [7]. An adequate intake of dietary fiber for pregnant women is 28 g/day. This amount of fiber should be enough to slow gastric emptying and result in a significant reduction in postprandial glucose [34].

6 Simple Carbohydrates and Nutritive Sweeteners

Limiting foods high in total carbohydrates, such as regular sodas, other sweetened beverages, candies, and desserts, may help in attaining glucose levels [8], although it has been demonstrated that the consumption of sucrose, the sweetener added to soft drinks and candies, does not compromise blood glucose when total carbohydrate content remains the same [52]. However, because of its low nutrient density, the consumption of foods containing high amounts of sucrose is not recommended. Other carbohydrate-containing foods such as whole grains are more nutrient dense. Foods that contain large amounts of sucrose, such as sweet rolls and cookies, often contain large amounts of fat [8]. Sugar alcohols and non-nutritive sweeteners should be consumed in accordance to the parameters established by the U.S. Food and Drug Administration (FDA). Fructose intake is not advised unless it is as a food constituent [7].

Sorbitol, Mannitol, and Xylitol are sugar alcohols supplying 4 kcal/g. They have less influence on blood glucose or insulin levels than does sugar because they are absorbed more slowly from the gastrointestinal tract. Because the slow, passive absorption of sugar alcohols can produce osmotic diarrhea, malabsorption, and abdominal discomfort, they should be avoided or used in limited amounts [52].

D Fat

Fat content in the diet of a pregnant woman usually ranges from 30 to 40% of total calories; however, large amounts of fat beyond total caloric needs should be avoided to prevent excessive weight gain, which in turn can result in further insulin resistance [53,54]. The acceptable macronutrient distribution range of fat is 20–35% of total energy, the same as for nonpregnant women [34].

The type of fat in the diet may play an important role in the glucose response to a meal, independent of the carbohydrate content. In the study by Ilic et al. [55], 10 GDM women well controlled on diet alone were randomized to receive a meal after overnight fast containing saturated fat (SF) or monounsaturated fat (MUFA). Blood was drawn at 0, 60, 120, and 180 minutes for plasma glucose, insulin, lipid profile, and free fatty acids. After 2 weeks, each patient received the other type of meal. The test meal was composed of 20% of the total daily caloric needs based on ideal body weight. The area under the curve showed a significantly lower glucose concentration for SF meal ($p = 0.001$). Serum insulin concentrations followed the glucose response, with the peak at the 60-minute time point and a significantly lower concentration at the 180-minute time point in the SF compared to the MUFA group. The study demonstrated that the addition of SF to the meal resulted in lower postprandial glucose and insulin than when the meal contained MUFA. Therefore, SF may be useful in controlling postprandial glucose [55].

In addition to total fat recommendations, DRIs have been formulated for essential polyunsaturated fatty acids (PUFAs). There is evidence that docosahexaenoic acid modulates insulin resistance and that it is vital for neurovisual development [56]. Consumption of omega-3 fatty acids in pregnant women continues to be below recommendations. In the study by Thomas *et al.* [57], the consumption of omega-3 fatty acids and fiber was increased in women with GDM after nutrition intervention. Adequate intake for omega-6 (PUFA) linoleic acid is 13 g/day, and that for omega-3 (PUFA) α-linolenic acid is 1.4 g/day [34].

Within the fat allowance, no more than 7—10% of total energy intake should come from saturated fat, *trans* fat should be reduced, and cholesterol intake should be less than 200 mg/day [7].

E Protein

The diet of well-nourished women in the preconception period and throughout most of pregnancy has a significant effect on birth weight, and proteins are the macronutrient that has the greatest influence. Cuco *et al.* [58] demonstrated that in a protein and fat model, a 1-g increase in maternal protein intake during preconception and in the 10th, 26th, and 38th weeks of pregnancy led to a significant increase in birth weight of 7.8—11.4 g. On the other hand, high intakes of protein and fat during pregnancy may impair development of the fetal pancreatic β cells and lead to insulin deficiency in the offspring [54]. In a case—control study of 2341 women with singleton pregnancy, three different levels of protein in the diet were associated with birth weight. Birth weight was 77 g lower ($p = -0.021$) in the low-protein group and 71 g lower ($p = 0.009$) in the high-protein group compared with the intermediate-protein group. Birth weight increased with protein levels up to 69.5 g/day and declined with higher protein intake. A high average prenatal protein consumption results in a significant depression of birth weight; in fact, a protein intake of more than 84 g/day on average is more detrimental than low protein intake. It appears that moderate protein intake is optimal during pregnancy [59].

The inclusion of protein in meals and snacks does not significantly affect blood glucose excursions; thus, it can be added for additional calories in place of carbohydrate foods [8]. The DRI for pregnancy for all age groups is 1.1 g/kg/day or 25 g additional protein [34]. This recommendation is easily met in meal plans for GDM when the carbohydrate is controlled to 40—45%. Protein generally comprises 20—25% of calories [8].

F Non-Nutritive Sweeteners

According to the American Dietetic Association position statement, the use of non-nutritive sweeteners in pregnancy must be based on well-designed and approved clinical investigation to ensure healthy pregnancy outcomes. Although no specific recommendations have been made regarding their use during pregnancy, moderation may be appropriate [52].

Aspartame (Equal or Nutrasweet) does not cross the placenta when consumed in usual amounts. It is useful in uncooked foods but unstable when heated. Women who have phenylketonuria (PKU) must restrict their phenylalanine intake. Because the amino acid phenylalanine is one of the metabolites of aspartame, women with PKU should avoid it. Maternal plasma levels of phenylalanine after ingestion of aspartame-containing foods, in normal amounts, are no higher than those after the ingestion of protein-containing meals [60]. Use of aspartame within FDA guidelines appears to be safe during pregnancy [52]. Acesulfame potassium (acesulfame-K; Sweet One and Sunette) is considered to be safe during pregnancy. Sucrolose (Splenda), which is derived from sucrose, is a high-intensity sweetener FDA approved as safe for human consumption. The FDA concluded that this sweetener does not pose carcinogenic, reproductive, or neurologic risk to human beings. Saccharin (Sweet'n Low) crosses the placenta and may remain in fetal tissue due to slow fetal clearance. The American Medical Association and the American Dietetic Association suggest careful use of saccharin in pregnancy. Many practitioners suggest avoidance of saccharin in pregnancy [52].

G Nutrient Intake Summary

Medical nutrition therapy remains the cornerstone of treatment for GDM and is best prescribed by a registered dietitian or a qualified individual with experience in the management of GDM. Nutrition recommendations for GDM, including gestational weight gain, calorie intake, and macronutrient composition and distribution, are based on limited scientific evidence [61]. Currently, nutrition practice guidelines for GDM recommend a carbohydrate-controlled meal plan with adequate nutrient content aimed to sustain maternal needs and fetal growth. In addition to practice guidelines, research findings associating macronutrients and caloric prescriptions to birth outcomes are also available. Using the current nutrition practice guidelines in combination with research findings can help the nutritionist to individualize a meal plan that will contribute to the delivery of a healthy infant. Table 33.3 displays formulas to calculate energy requirements for normal, high, and obese pre-pregnant BMI. These calculations may be used as initial baseline information. Table 33.4 summarizes the Institute of Medicine's micronutrient recommendations for pregnant women [34].

TABLE 33.4 Recommended Dietary Allowances and Adequate Intakes for Micronutrients

Micronutrient	≤ 18 years	Age 19–30 years	31–50 years
Thiamin (mg/day)[a]	1.4	1.4	1.4
Riboflavin (mg/day)[a,c]	1.4	1.4	1.4
Niacin (mg/day)[a]	18	18	18
Biotin (µg/day)[b]	30	30	30
Pantothenic acid (mg/day)[b]	6	6	6
Vitamin B$_6$ (mg/day)[a]	1.9	1.9	1.9
Folate (µg/day)[a,d]	600	600	600
Vitamin B$_{12}$ (µg/day)[a]	2.6	2.6	2.6
Choline (mg/day)[b]	450	450	450
Vitamin C (mg/day)[a]	80	85	85
Vitamin A (µg/day)[a,e]	750	770	770
Vitamin D (µg/day)[b,f]	5	5	5
Vitamin E (mg/day)[a,g]	15	15	15
Vitamin K (µg/day)[b]	75	90	90
Sodium (mg/day)[b]	1500	1500	1500
Chloride (mg/day)[b]	2300	2300	2300
Potassium (mg/day)[b]	4700	4700	4700
Calcium (mg/day)[b]	1300	1000	1000
Phosphorus (mg/day)[a]	1250	700	700
Magnesium (mg/day)[a]	400	350	360
Iron (mg/day)[a]	27	27	27
Zinc (mg/day)[a]	12	11	11
Iodine (µg/day)[a]	220	220	220
Selenium (µg/day)[a]	60	60	60
Copper (µg/day)[a]	1000	1000	1000
Manganese (mg/day)[b]	2.0	2.0	2.0
Fluoride (mg/day)[b]	3	3	3
Chromium (µg/day)[b]	29	30	30
Molybdenum (µg/day)[a]	50	50	50

[a]*Recommended Dietary Allowance (RDA).*
[b]*Adequate intake (AI).*
[c]*Niacin recommendations are expressed as niacin equivalents (NEs).*
[d]*Folate recommendations are expressed as dietary folate equivalents (DFEs).*
[e]*Vitamin A recommendations are expressed as retinol activity equivalents (RAE).*
[f]*Vitamin D recommendations are expressed as cholecalciferol and assume the absence of adequate exposure to sunlight.*
[g]*Vitamin E recommendations are expressed as α-tocoferol.*

V CLINICAL OUTCOMES

Nutrition management in combination with intensive monitoring can contribute to the delivery of a healthy infant. Frequent follow-up visits are needed in order to determine if the patient is achieving the clinical outcomes originally established by the medical team. The information obtained from blood glucose monitoring, food and physical activity records, ketone testing, hemoglobin A1c when available, weight gain patterns, as well as the patient's ability to understand and follow a meal plan will allow the practitioner to evaluate the level of glycemic control. That information may be necessary for meal plan adjustments and can be useful in identifying the need for and adjustments in insulin therapy.

A Blood Glucose Monitoring

The use of self-monitoring blood glucose (SMBG) allows the medical team to objectively evaluate the nutrition management recommended and reinforces selection of appropriate amounts and types of foods that are likely to produce normogylcemia. Blood glucose data allow evaluation of the glycemic response to meals and snacks and the determination of whether changes in macronutrient amount or distribution are needed [62].

Maternal metabolic surveillance should be directed at detecting hyperglycemia severe enough to increase risks to the fetus. Daily SMBG appears to be superior to intermittent office monitoring of plasma glucose. For women treated with insulin, limited evidence indicates that postprandial monitoring is superior to preprandial monitoring. However, the success of either approach depends on the glycemic targets that are set and achieved [10].

The initial daily testing schedule is five times per day: fasting and 1 hour after breakfast, lunch, and supper, and at bedtime. The frequency from daily to every third or fourth day may be used once control of blood glucose is established. Increased surveillance for pregnancies at risk for fetal demise is appropriate, particularly when fasting glucose levels exceed 105 mg/dl (5.8 mmol/l) or pregnancy progresses past term [10]. The self-monitored plasma glucose level recommendations from the Fifth International Workshop on Gestational Diabetes targeted maternal capillary glucose concentrations as follows: preprandial ≤ 95 mg/dl (5.3 mmol/l) and either 1-hour postmeal ≤ 140 mg/dl (8.8 mmol/l) or 2-hour postmeal ≤ 120 mg/dl (6.7 mmol/l) [10]. Many obstetricians use lower target glucose levels: fasting <95 mg/dl; 1-hour postprandial, 120 mg/dl; and 2-hour postprandial <120 mg/dl.

B Food Records

Detailed information recorded in food records is useful to make adjustments to the meal plan or to the insulin regimen. By keeping food records, the patient becomes aware of individual blood glucose response to particular types and amounts of foods. Food intake records also indicate the patient's level of understanding and compliance with the recommended meal plan.

C Urinary Ketone Testing

Urinary ketone tested on the first morning voided specimen may be useful in detecting insufficient caloric or carbohydrate intake in women treated with calorie restriction [10].

D Hemoglobin A1c

Periodic glycosylated hemoglobin determinations evaluate glycemic control over the previous 4–6 weeks because the attachment of glucose to hemoglobin occurs over the life span of the red blood cells. Levels greater than 7% (varies with individual laboratory) indicate suboptimal blood glucose control [63].

E Weight Gain Patterns

A weight gain grid in the medical records is useful and helps to evaluate weight gain progress. Weight gain monitoring is helpful to identify inadequate weight gain, which may be related to restriction of food intake. A guideline for weight gain recommendations is displayed in Table 33.2 [32].

VI PHARMACOLOGICAL AGENTS

Pharmacological therapy is prescribed by the physician and added to nutrition therapy when women with GDM do not achieve or maintain target blood glucose levels and/or when the rate of fetal growth is higher than normal [8,64].

A Insulin Therapy

Insulin therapy is recommended when nutrition therapy fails to maintain target glucose levels. The American Diabetes Association recommends the initiation of insulin therapy when unable to maintain a fasting blood glucose level of 105 mg/dl (5.8 mmol/l), a 1-hour postprandial glucose level ≤ 155 mg/dl (8.6 mmol/l), or a 2-hour postprandial glucose level ≤ 130 mg/dl (7.2 mmol/l) [10]. The amount of insulin to be administered for GDM in the first trimester is 0.6–0.8 U/kg body weight; in the second trimester, the insulin requirement is 1.0 U/kg body weight; and in the third trimester, the requirement is 1.2 U/kg body weight [65]. The total amount of insulin is distributed as follows: two-thirds in the morning and one-third in the evening. The morning dose is administered in two-thirds of intermediate-acting or neutral protamin Hagedorn (NPH) insulin and one-third of short-acting or regular insulin. The evening dose is divided in one-half of short-acting or regular insulin and one-half of intermediate-acting or NPH insulin [66].

If the postprandial glucose level is elevated, pre-meal rapid-acting insulin should be prescribed, beginning with a dose of 1 U per 10 g carbohydrate in the meal. If both fasting and postprandial glucose levels are elevated, or if a women's postprandial glucose levels can only be blunted when starvation ketosis occurs, a four-injections-per-day regimen should be prescribed. The latter can be based on combinations of NPH insulin and regular human insulin, timed to provide basal and meal-related insulin boluses. The total daily insulin dose for the four-injections regimen should be adjusted according to pregnant body weight and gestational week (0.7–1 U/kg/day); doses may need to be increased for the morbidity obese or when there is twin gestation [67].

B Oral Hypoglycemic Agents

There is evidence that oral hypoglycemic agents may be beneficial in GDM and that they can be used as alternatives for insulin. It has been demonstrated that the use of glyburide in GDM is effective in lowering fasting glucose [68–70]. Langer et al. [71] reported no significant differences between the use of glyburide and insulin in two groups of GDM with regard to maternal outcomes such as glycosylated hemoglobin, rate of preeclampsia, or cesarean section or neonatal complications, including neonatal intensive care unit admissions and risk of neonatal hypoglycemia. In addition, another study reported that women with GDM using glyburide had a higher risk of preeclampsia and their infants had an increased risk of phototherapy [72]. Although the use of glyburide has been suggested as a cost-effective, patient-friendly alternative modality to insulin therapy, more studies supporting maternal and neonatal safety are needed.

VII PHYSICAL ACTIVITY

Moderate exercise can be an important adjunctive therapy in the management of diabetes in pregnancy, particularly in GDM. Regular physical activity decreases the common discomforts associated with pregnancy without a negative effect on maternal or neonatal outcomes. Regular physical activity is also beneficial for reducing insulin resistance, postprandial hyperglycemia, and excessive weight gain. In combination with dietary management, planned physical activity of 30 minutes/day is recommended for all individuals capable of participating and after approval by health care provider [10]. The proper amount of physical activity for women with GDM should be individualized by the health care provider. [73]. To prevent hypoglycemia, exercise should be avoided in the fasting state and during periods of peak insulin activity. Energy and carbohydrate intake in a rapidly absorbed form should be adequate prior to exercise and be readily available during exercise. Blood glucose should be monitored before and after exercise.

VIII POSTPARTUM FOLLOW-UP

Glucose tolerance testing should be delayed until 6–12 weeks after delivery in GDM women who do not have diabetes immediately postpartum. A 2-hour, 75-g glucose tolerance test can be coordinated with the postpartum visit. If glucose levels are normal postpartum, reassessment of glycemia should be undertaken at a minimum of 3-year intervals. Women with impaired fasting glucose (<140 mg/dl) or IGT (≥140 to <200 mg/dl) in the postpartum period should be tested for diabetes annually. Due to the high risk for diabetes, these patients should receive MNT and be placed on an individualized exercise program [10].

IX PREVENTION

The risk for developing diabetes after GDM has been reported to be higher than 70%. Current recommendations for women with GDM aimed to prevent type 2 diabetes include receiving diet counseling, awareness of the benefits of weight reduction or weight maintenance, and participating in regular physical activity. In addition, lifestyle modification and pharmacological therapies (metformin, troglitazone, and pioglitazone) have been shown to reduce diabetes development by 50% or more [74].

It has been reported that dietary modifications including lowering fat and carbohydrate intake in combination with physical activity can reduce the risk of developing GDM in subsequent pregnancies [75,76]. An intervention study aimed at increasing physical activity and healthy behaviors through dietary changes improved body weight and glucose tolerance during a period of 2 or 3 years [77]. Another study documented that a diagnosis of diabetes could be prevented when diet and intense exercise reduced fasting glucose and body weight in a 2-month period [78]. In addition to the implementation of dietary modifications and increased physical activity, other studies have demonstrated that oral hypoglycemic agents can be used to prevent or delay a positive diagnosis of type 2 diabetes [79]. On the other hand, evidence indicates that a prepregnancy diet, particularly a diet with low fiber and high glycemic load, is associated with an increased risk of gestational diabetes [80].

Nutrition practice guidelines for GDM recommend a carbohydrate-controlled food plan aimed at promoting adequate nutrition, appropriate weight gain, normoglycemia, and the absence of ketonuria. The food plan should be individualized, culturally appropriate, and according to the patient's food preferences and lifestyle. Monitoring of blood glucose levels, ketones, food intake, and prescribed physical activity are crucial in evaluating the nutrition intervention. The proper nutrition management in combination with intensive monitoring can contribute to the delivery of a healthy infant.

X CONCLUSION

The diagnosis of GDM should initiate a long-term intervention and diagnostic process to minimize the risk of developing diabetes or to diagnose it early in the course of the disease [74]. Pregnancy complicated by diabetes represents a window of opportunity for the implementation of nutrition education and a physical activity program to modify lifestyle patterns toward healthier habits for the woman and her family. Furthermore, the prevention of diabetes and specifically of gestational diabetes could begin with a healthy lifestyle in the preconception stage.

References

[1] B.E. Metzger, D.R. Constan, Summary and recommendations of the Fourth International Workshop-Conference on Gestational Diabetes Mellitus: The Organizing Committee, Diabetes Care 21 (1998) B161–B167.

[2] T.A. Buchanan, A. Xiang, S.L. Kjos, R. Watanabe, What is gestational diabetes? Diabetes Care 30 (2007) S105–S111.

[3] D. Dabelea, The predisposition to obesity and diabetes in offspring of diabetic mothers, Diabetes Care 30 (2007) S169–S174.

[4] D. Dabelea, W.C. Knowler, D.J. Pettitt, Effect of diabetes in pregnancy on offspring: follow-up research in the Pima Indians, J. Matern. Fetal Med. 9 (2000) 83–88.

[5] D.J. Pettitt, W.C. Knowler, Diabetes and obesity in the Pima Indians: a crossgenerational vicious cycle, J. Obesity Weight Regul. 7 (1988) 61–65.

[6] B.L. Silverman, T. Rizzo, O.C. Green, N.H. Cho, R.J. Winter, E.S. Ogata, et al., Long-term prospective evaluation of offspring of diabetic mothers, Diabetes 40 (1991) S121–S125.

[7] American Diabetes Association, Nutrition recommendations and interventions for diabetes: a position statement of the American Diabetes Association, Diabetes Care 30 (2007) S48–S65.

[8] American Dietetic Association, "Medical Nutrition Therapy Evidence-Based Guide for Practice: Nutrition Practice Guidelines for Gestational Diabetes Mellitus" (CD-ROM), American Dietetic Association, Chicago, 2001.

[9] N.A. Beischer, J.N. Oats, O.A. Henry, M.T. Cedí, J.E. Walstab, Incidence and severity of gestational diabetes mellitus according to country of birth in women living in Australia, Diabetes 40 (1991) S35–S38.

[10] B.E. Metzger, T.A. Buchanan, D.R. Coustan, et al., Summary and recommendations of the Fifth International Workshop–Conference on Gestational Diabetes, Diabetes Care 30 (2007) S251–S260.

[11] H. King, Epidemiology of glucose intolerance and gestational diabetes in women of childbearing age, Diabetes Care 21 (1998) B9–B13.

[12] D. Dabelea, J.K. Snell-Bergeon, C.L. Hartsfield, K.J. Bischoff, R.F. Hamman, R.S. McDuffie, Increasing prevalence of gestational diabetes mellitus (GDM) over time and by birth cohort, Diabetes Care 28 (2005) 579–584.

[13] M.E. O'Brian, G. Gilson, Detection and management of gestational diabetes in an out-of-hospital birth center, J. Nurse Midwifery 32 (1987) 79–84.

[14] J. Mestman, Outcome of diabetes screening in pregnancy and perinatal morbidity in infants of mothers with mild impairment in glucose intolerance, Diabetes Care 3 (1980) 447–452.

[15] M. Duarte-Gardea, J.L. Gonzalez, Screening and diagnosis scheme for glucose intolerance and gestational diabetes in Hispanic women, American Diabetes Association 59th Scientific Sessions, 1999, Abstract 2071.

[16] S. Rodríguez, E. Robinson, K. Gary-Donald, Prevalence of gestational diabetes mellitus among James Bay Cree women in northern Quebec, Can. Med. Assoc. J. 160 (1999) 1293–1297.

[17] H. Ying, D.F. Wang, Effects of dietary fat on onset of gestational diabetes mellitus [in Chinese], Zhonghua Fu Chan Ke Za Zhi 41 (2006) 729–731.

[18] C. Zhang, S. Liu, C.G. Solomon, F.B. Hu, Dietary fiber intake, dietary glycemic load, and the risk for gestational diabetes mellitus, Diabetes Care 29 (2006) 2223–2230.

[19] World Health Organization, Definition, Diagnosis and Classification of Diabetes Mellitus and Its Complications: report of a WHO Consultation: Part 1, Diagnosis and Classification of Diabetes Mellitas. Available at <http://www.staff.ncl.ac.uk/philip.home/who_dmc.htm#DiagGDM>, 1999 (accessed 06.11).

[20] American Diabetes Association, Standards of medical care in diabetes—2011, Diabetes Care 34 (2011) S11–S61.

[21] J. Leary, D.J. Pettitt, L. Jovanovic, Gestational diabetes guidelines in HAPO world, Best Pract. Res. Clin. Endocrinol. Metab. 24 (2010) 673–685.

[22] American Diabetes Association, Gestational diabetes, Diabetes Care 27 (2004) S88–S90.

[23] B.E. Metzger, D.R. Coustan, et al., Summary and recommendations of the Fourth International Workshop Conference in Gestational Diabetes, Diabetes Care 21 (1988) B161–B167.

[24] American Diabetes Association, Position statement: Gestational diabetes mellitus, Diabetes Care 22 (1999) S74–S76.

[25] C.H. Naylor, M. Sermer, E. Chen, K. Sykora, Cesarean delivery in relation to birth weight and gestational glucose tolerance: pathophysiology or practice style? Toronto Trihospital Gestational Diabetes Investigators, JAMA 275 (1996) 1165–1179.

[26] W. Hunger-Dathe, K. Volk, A. Braun, A. Sammann, U.A. Muller, G. Peiker, et al., Perinatal morbidity in women with undiagnosed gestational diabetes in northern Thuringia in Germany, Exp. Clin. Endocrinol. Diabetes 113 (2005) 160–166.

[27] American Diabetes Association, Proceedings of the Fourth International Workshop-Conference on Gestational Diabetes Mellitus, Diabetes Care 21 (1998) B79.

[28] K.M. Adams, H. Li, R.L. Nelson, P.L. Ogburn Jr., D.R. Danilenko-Dixon, Sequelae of unrecognized gestational diabetes, Am. J. Obstet. Gynecol. 178 (1998) 1321–1332.

[29] O. Langer, Y. Yogev, O. Most, E.M.J. Xenakis, Gestational diabetes: the consequences of not treating, Am. J. Obstet. Gynecol. 192 (2005) 989–997.

[30] C.A. Crowther, J.E. Hiller, J.R. Moss, W.S. Jeffries, J.S. Robinson, Australian Carbohydrate Intolerance Study in Pregnant Women (ACHOIS): effect of treatment of gestational diabetes mellitus on pregnancy outcomes, N. Engl. J. Med. 16 (2005) 2477–2486.

[31] D. Reader, P. Splett, E.P. Gunderson, Diabetes care and education practice group: impact of gestational diabetes mellitus nutrition practice guidelines implemented by registered dietitians on pregnancy outcome, J. Am. Diet. Assoc. 106 (2006) 1426–1433.

[32] Institute of Medicine, "Nutrition during Pregnancy: Part 1. Weight Gain"; "Part 2. Nutrient Supplements.", National Academy of Sciences, Washington, DC, 1990.

[33] Institute of Medicine, Recommended Dietary Allowances, tenth ed., National Academy Press, Washington, DC, 1989.

[34] Institute of Medicine, Dietary Reference Intakes for Energy, Carbohydrates, Fiber, Fat, Fatty Acids, Cholesterol, Protein and Amino Acids (Macronutrients), National Academy Press, Washington, DC, 2002. Available at <http://www.iom.edu> Accessed March 2007.

[35] D. Thomas-Dobersen, Nutritional management of gestational diabetes and nutritional management of women with a history of gestational diabetes: two different therapies or the same? Clin. Diabetes 17 (1999). Available at<http://journal.diabetes.org/clinicaldiabetes/V17N41999/pg1%5b70%5dhtm>. Accessed October 2011

[36] L. Jovanic, American Diabetes Association's Fourth International Workshop–Conference on Gestational Diabetes Mellitus: Summary and Discussion—Therapeutic Interventions, Diabetes Care 21 (1998) B131–B137.

[37] L. Jovanovic, Controversies in the diagnosis and treatment of gestational diabetes, Cleve. Clin. J. Med. 67 (2000) 481–488.

[38] O. Langer, Y. Yogev, E. Xenakis, L. Brustman, Overweight and obese in gestational diabetes: the impact of pregnancy outcome, Am. J. Obst. Gynecol. 192 (2005) 1768–1776.

[39] M. Duarte-Gardea, J. Gonzalez, Outcomes of Nutrition Therapy in Mexican-American Women with Gestational Diabetes, Paper presented at the Overcoming Diabetes Health Disparities Conference, Nashville, TN, 2003November 2003

[40] L. Jovanovic, Y. Nakai, Successful pregnancy in women with type 1 diabetes: from preconception through postpartum care, Endocrinol. Metab. Clin. North Am. 35 (2006) 79–97.

[41] M. Romon, M.C. Nuttens, A. Vambergue, O. Verier-Mine, S. Biausque, C. Lemaire, et al., Higher carbohydrate intake is associated with decreased incidence of newborn macrosomia in women with gestational diabetes, J. Am. Diet. Assoc. 101 (2001) 897–902.

[42] A.M. Thomas, Y.M. Gutierrez, American Dietetic Association Guide to Gestational Diabetes Mellitus, American Dietetic Association, Chicago, 2005.

[43] C.M. Peterson, L. Jovanovic-Peterson, Y. Nakai, Percentage of carbohydrate and glycemic response to breakfast, lunch, and dinner in women with gestational diabetes, Diabetes 40 (1991) 172–174.

[44] E. Gunderson, Intensive nutrition therapy for gestational diabetes, Diabetes Care 20 (1997) 221–226.

[45] E.P. Gunderson, Gestational diabetes and nutritional recommendations, Curr. Diab. Rep. 4 (2004) 377–386.

[46] D.R. Lock, A. Bar-Eyal, H. Voet, Z. Madar, Glycemic indices of various foods given to pregnant diabetic subjects, Obstet. Gynecol. 71 (2000) 180−183.

[47] T.O. Scholl, X. Chen, C.S. Khoo, C. Lenders, The dietary glycemic index during pregnancy: Influence on infant birth weight, fetal growth, and biomarkers of carbohydrate metabolism., Am. J. Epidemiol. 159 (2004) 467−474.

[48] M.J. Franz, The argument against glycemic index: what are the other options? Nestle Nutr Workshop Ser. Clin. Perform Programme 11 (2006) 57−68.

[49] J.C. Louie, T.P. Markovic, N. Perera, D. Foote, P. Petocz, G.P. Ross, et al., A randomized controlled trial investigating the effect of low-glycemic diet on pregnancy outcomes in gestational diabetes, Diabetes Care 34 (2011) 2341−2346.

[50] F. Cesa, S. Mariani, A. Fava, R. Rauseo, H. Zanetti, The use of vegetable fiber in the treatment of pregnancy diabetes and/or excessive weight gain during pregnancy, Minerva Ginecol. 42 (1990) 271−274.

[51] E.A. Reece, Z. Hagay, D. Caseria, L.J. Gay, N. DeGennaro, Do fiber-enriched diabetic diets have glucose-lowering effects in pregnancy? Am. J. Perinatol. 10 (1993) 272−274.

[52] American Dietetic Association, Position of the American Dietetic Association: use of nutritive and nonnutritive sweeteners, J. Am. Diet. Assoc. 104 (1998) 255−275.

[53] American Diabetes Association, Nutrition recommendations and interventions for diabetes—2006: A position statement of the American Diabetes Association, Diabetes Care 29 (2006) 2140−2157.

[54] A.W. Shiell, D.M.. Campbell, M.H. Hall, D.J. Barker, Diet in late pregnancy and glucose-insulin metabolism of the offspring 40 years later, Br. J. Obstet. Gynecol. 107 (2000) 890−895.

[55] S. Ilic, L. Jovanovic, D.J. Pettitt, Comparison of the effect of saturated and monounsaturated fat on postprandial plasma glucose and insulin concentration in women with gestational diabetes mellitus, Am. J. Perinatal. 16 (1999) 489−495.

[56] R Uauy, A.R. Dangour, Nutrition in brain development and aging: role of essential fatty acids, Nutr. Rev. 64 (2006) S24−S33.

[57] B. Thomas, K. Ghebremeskel, C. Lowy, M. Crawford, B. Offley-Shore, Nutrient intake of women with and without gestational diabetes with a specific focus on fatty acids, Nutrition 22 (2006) 230−236.

[58] G. Cuco, V. Arija, R. Iranzo, J. Vila, M.T. Prieto, J. Fernandez-Ballart, Association of maternal protein intake before conception and throughout pregnancy with birth weight, Acta Obstet. Gynecol. Scand. 85 (2006) 413−421.

[59] N.L. Sloan, S.A. Lederman, J. Leighton, J.H. Himes, D. Rush, The effect of prenatal dietary protein intake on birth weight, Nutr. Res. 21 (2001) 129−139.

[60] R.M. Pitkin, Aspartame ingestion during pregnancy, in: L.D. Stegink, J.F. Filer (Eds.), Aspartame, Dekker, New York, 1984.

[61] D.M. Reader, Medical nutrition therapy and lifestyle interventions, Diabetes Care 30 (2007) S188−S193.

[62] American Diabetes Association, Position statement: Gestational diabetes, Diabetes Care 24 (2001) S77.

[63] M. Powers, Handbook of Diabetes Medical Nutrition Therapy, Aspen, Gaithersburg, MD, 1996.

[64] O. Langer, Maternal glycemic criteria for insulin therapy in gestational diabetes, Diabetes Care 21 (1998) S91−S98.

[65] S.G. Gabbe, C.R. Graves, Management of diabetes mellitus complicating pregnancy, Obstet. Gynecol. 102 (2003) 857−868.

[66] M.W. Jones, L.C. Stone, Management of women with gestational diabetes mellitus, J. Perinat. Neonat. Nurs. 11 (1998) 13−24.

[67] L. Jovanic, Achieving euglycaemia in women with gestational diabetes mellitus: current options for screening, diagnosis and treatment, Drugs 64 (2004) 1401−1417.

[68] S. Chamit, T. Denise, T. Moore, Prospective observational study to establish predictors of glyburide success in women with gestational diabetes mellitus, J. Perinatol. 24 (2004) 617−622.

[69] D.L. Conway, O. Gonzalez, D. Skiver, Use of glyburide for the treatment of gestational diabetes: the San Antonio experience, J. Matern. Fetal Neonatal Med. 15 (2004) 51−55.

[70] G.A. Ramos, G.F. Jabckoson, R.S. Kirby, J.Y. Ching, D.R. Field, Comparison of glyburide and insulin for the management of gestational diabetics with markedly elevated oral glucose challenge test and fasting hyperglycemia, J. Perinatol. 27 (2007) 262−267.

[71] O. Langer, D.L. Conway, M.D. Berkus, E.M. Xenakis, O. Gonzalez, A comparison of glyburide and insulin in women with gestational diabetes mellitus, N. Engl. J. Med. 343 (2003) 1134−1138.

[72] G.F. Jabckoson, G.A. Ramos, J.Y. Ching, R.S. Kirby, A. Ferrara, D.R. Field, Comparison of of glyburide and insulin for the management of gestational diabetes in a large managed care organization, Am. J. Obstet. Gynecol. 193 (2005) 118−124.

[73] National Institutes of Health, Eunice Kennedy Shriver National Institute of Child Health and Human Development, What Should I Do If I Have Gestational Diabetes. Available at: <http://www.nichd.nih.gov/publications/pubs/gest_diabetes/sub6.cfm>, 2006 (accessed 06.12).

[74] R.E. Ratner, Prevention of type 2 diabetes in women with previous gestational diabetes, Diabetes Care 30 (2007) S242−S245.

[75] R.G. Moses, J.L. Shand, L.C. Tapsell, The recurrence of gestational diabetes: Could dietary differences in fat intake be an explanation? Diabetes Care 20 (1997) 1647−1650.

[76] D.K. Tobias, C. Ahang, R.M. van Dam, K. Bowers, F.B. Hu, Physical activity before and during pregnancy and risk of gestational diabetes mellitus: A meta-analysis, Diabetes Care 34 (2011) 223−229.

[77] B.A. Swinburn, P.A. Metcalf, S.J. Lay, Long-term (5-year) effects of a reduced-fat diet intervention in individuals with glucose intolerance, Diabetes Care 24 (2001) 619−624.

[78] M. Duarte-Gardea, Case study: the prevention of diabetes through diet and intense exercise, Clin. Diabetes 22 (2004) 45−46.

[79] W.C. Knowler, E. Barret-Connor, S.E. Fowler, R.F. Hamman, J.M. Lachin, E.A. Walter, et al., Reduction in the incidence of type 2 diabetes with lifestyle intervention or metformin, N. Engl. J. Med. 346 (2002) 393−403the Diabetes Prevention Program Research Group

[80] C. Zhang, S. Liu, C.G. Solomon, F.B. Hu, Dietary fiber intake, dietary glycemic load, and the risk of gestational diabetes mellitus, Diabetes Care 29 (2006) 2223−2230.

PART F

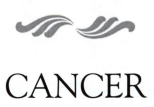

CANCER

Nutrition and Genetic Factors in Carcinogenesis

Jo L. Freudenheim

University at Buffalo, The State University of New York, Buffalo, New York

I INTRODUCTION

Cancer leads to the death of approximately 7.6 million people throughout the world each year, with more than 12.7 million new cases of cancer each year. In the United States alone, there are approximately 1.4 million new cases annually [1]; approximately 68% of those cancer patients survive for 5 years after diagnosis [2]. Therapies to cure cancer continue to improve, but prevention is clearly an essential strategy in ameliorating cancer-related morbidity and mortality.

Given differences in rates of cancer worldwide and given changes in rates of cancer among populations that migrate from one environment to another, it is generally agreed that the cause of most common cancers is, in large part, environmental factors with the potential to be controlled [3,4]. One likely component of the relevant environmental change is in diet alterations. An understanding of how dietary factors contribute to cancer etiology is an important part of understanding cancer prevention. There is accumulating evidence that this is a complicated process involving interactions of an individual's endogenous milieu, including his or her genetic makeup, with diet and other exogenous exposures.

In conceptualizing what causes cancer, it is crucial to understand that a cancer may have more than one cause. For example, both occupational exposures and diet could contribute to the etiology of one kind of cancer and even to the cancer of one individual, and either a change in the occupational exposure or a change in diet might prevent that cancer or reduce the risk. It is estimated that nutritional factors contribute to between 30 and 40% of tumors [3]. Genetic inheritance likely plays a role in many, if not all, cancers. Even when an exposure is clearly required for a particular kind of cancer, genetic factors often play a role in determining who, among exposed individuals, develops that cancer.

II BACKGROUND AND DEFINITIONS

Cancer is characterized by a number of changes in cells. Tumor cells have their own growth signals, do not respond to signals inhibiting growth, can replicate indefinitely (replicative immortality), can avoid programmed cell death (apoptosis), can alter energy metabolism, can avoid immune surveillance, can invade other tissues (metastasis), and can develop a blood supply for those metastases (angiogenesis). Inflammation and instability in the genome leading to mutations and other alterations are both key to the observed changes [5]. Cancer is characterized by the accumulation of genetic alterations such that there are these significant changes in the functioning of the cell.

Genes are the basic unit of heredity, with each gene having its own location in the DNA on a particular chromosome [6]. A *mutation* is a structural change in the base pair sequence of DNA, the chromosomal material that provides the code for gene expression [6]. In tumor cells, there are generally a number of mutations to the DNA. In addition, there may also be *epigenetic* changes. These are changes other than changes to the DNA base pair sequences. Like mutations, epigenetic changes can also affect gene structure, function, and expression. One such change is *altered DNA methylation*, the addition or loss of methyl groups on the DNA, which can affect gene expression. *Hypermethylation* to the promoter region of tumor suppressor genes leads to silencing of these genes. This change is common in tumors and may be as important a mechanism as mutation in carcinogenesis.

Nutrition in the Prevention and Treatment of Disease, Third Edition.
DOI: http://dx.doi.org/10.1016/B978-0-12-391884-0.00034-2

Other epigenetic changes include those such as methylation or acetylation of the *histones*, which are proteins associated with the DNA that affect folding [6]. There may also be alterations in copy number—that is, the number of copies of the same gene—altering the overall expression. In cancer cells, there may also be losses of sections of the genome or translocation of sections from one chromosome to another.

Genotype refers to an individual's genetic structure for a gene, based on his or her DNA [6]; it is the nucleic acid sequence of the DNA. Each individual has two copies of each gene, one inherited from each parent. From knowledge of genotype, it is possible to infer the amino acid sequence of the protein encoded by a gene. In some but not all cases, differences in genotype can provide information regarding protein activity. For example, genotype for the faster or slower version of a particular enzyme would influence the rate of the reaction catalyzed by that enzyme. Other factors besides genotype also influence actual enzyme activity, including the rate of transcription of the gene, available concentration of substrate, and the rates of synthesis and degradation of the enzyme. *Phenotype* refers to observable characteristics; it represents the expression of the genotype, with interactions with other genes and with the environment [6]. Examples of phenotype are height, body weight, and blood vitamin concentration.

Agreement between genotype and phenotype often is not exact, as described in more detail later. Phenotype may not be dependent on a single gene but, rather, the result of genotype of a number of different genes in a pathway, combined with the impact of external exposures. For example, height is influenced by several genes and by external factors including nutrition. In many instances, there are gene—gene interactions as well as gene—environment interactions. For example, a person may have the genotype for lower activity for a particular enzyme. However, there can be other exposures including dietary factors that induce a high level of expression of that enzyme. Phenotype would be the combination of the genotype and the other interactions. The measurement of phenotype is of interest because it gives an indication of the true level of exposure. Thus, for example, measurement of serum vitamin D might be more informative than measurement of genotype for several genes related to vitamin D status. In some cases, genotype is the preferable measurement. In particular, when study participants have a disease, genotype may give a better indication of lifetime exposure, whereas phenotype (gene expression) may be influenced by the disease process.

Penetrance of a genetic factor refers to the likelihood that those with a specific gene will exhibit a particular phenotype in given environmental circumstances [6]. A gene with very high penetrance is one for which virtually everybody with the gene has the expressed trait, whereas a gene with low penetrance is one for which there is a lower likelihood of the trait being expressed.

Some individuals are at greater risk for certain types of cancers. This increased risk can be related to differences in exposure to cancer-inducing or -protecting agents, to the individual's genetic makeup, or to a combination of these factors. Genetic factors vary widely with regard to the magnitude of their impact. Some inherited mutations greatly increase the risk of cancer; others cause smaller increases in risk. Some mutations may only increase risk in the presence of a particular exposure. Examples of inherited mutations with high penetrance are mutations identified in the *BRCA1* gene. Particular mutations in this gene have been shown to be strongly related to risk of breast and ovarian cancer. It is estimated that carriers of this genetic mutation have a 65% risk of breast cancer by age 70 years; that is, many, but not all, women with this mutation will develop breast cancer [7]. Relatively few individuals in the population carry this factor (estimates range between 1 in 2000 and 1 in 500). Therefore, although those with the gene are at high risk, only approximately 1—5% of women with breast cancer have this mutation [8—10].

There is a considerable range in the impact of genetic differences on phenotype. Other genetic variants that are more common and that have weaker effects on risk are referred to as *genetic polymorphisms*. A gene that is polymorphic has more than one form; its structure varies among individuals in a population. Many polymorphisms are silent, not affecting phenotype. Other polymorphisms can alter the effectiveness of a protein and/or may affect its interaction with other compounds including nutrients. The change in one nucleotide is referred to as a *single nucleotide polymorphism* (SNP). One or more polymorphisms are frequently found in genes. The frequency of the occurrence of a genetic polymorphism among individuals within a population can vary greatly depending on the origin of the population. Generally, polymorphisms have less impact on cancer risk than do highly penetrant mutations such as *BRCA1*. However, when they are common, they may still have a significant effect on the rate of disease in a population. Common polymorphisms may affect the response to an exposure so that their effect on risk is evident only when that exposure or exposures are present, referred to as a gene—environment interaction. For these types of gene—environment interactions, an understanding of both the genetic factor and the environmental exposure is important in order to understand disease etiology and prevention.

Several terms have been developed to describe the interaction of food components with genes. *Nutrigenomics* is the broadest term, describing the interaction of dietary components with genes. Included in this term is *nutrigenetics*, the study of the impact of genetic variation on the response to dietary components; *nutritional epigenetics*, the study of the effect of food-derived compounds on DNA structure other than base pairs—that is, on methylation and on chromatin structure; and *nutritional transcriptomics*, the study of the impact of dietary components on gene transcription. In addition, dietary components may affect protein structure post-translation; the study of these interactions is *nutritional proteomics* (Figure 34.1)[11,12].

III MECHANISMS OF DIET—GENE INTERACTIONS

A Overview of Interactions

In the exploration of the role of dietary factors in carcinogenesis, both essential nutrients and other compounds in foods with biological activity may be important. These interactions may operate in two directions. Genes can affect the action of these compounds of dietary origin (e.g., increasing or decreasing the amount needed for good nutritional status), and these compounds can affect the action of genes. To clearly understand these processes, several layers of complexity need to be taken into account. Individual bioactive food components may have more than one action, in some cases interacting with other food components and with more than one gene. Food composition can differ significantly, depending on growing conditions, genetic differences in the foodstuff, storage and cooking, and other food processing [13]. After consumption,

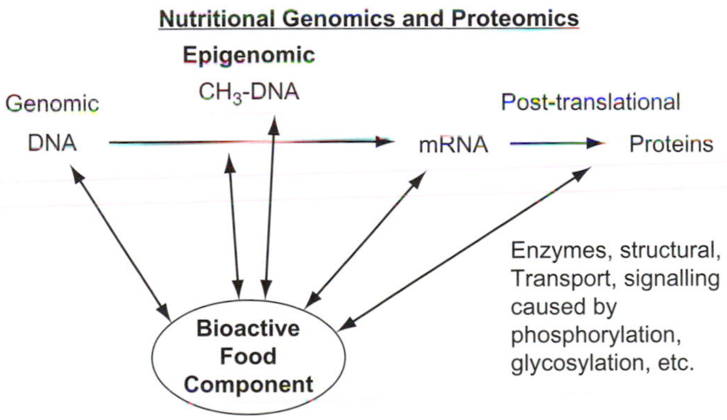

Nutritional Genomics and Proteomics

FIGURE 34.1 Bioactive food components may interact with genes and their products in a number of different ways, including interactions with the coding DNA, with other parts of the chromosome structure, with the messenger RNA, and with the protein product after translation. Source: *From Milner, J. A. "Molecular Targets for Bioactive Food Components." Copyright The American Society of Nutrition, Reprinted by permission from* The Journal of Nutrition, *volume 134, pp. 2492S—2498S, 2004.*

there can be interactions of a particular bioactive compound with other food constituents, with other environmental exposures (e.g., from air and water), and with genes. Furthermore, genes interact with each other. The resulting metabolic environment derives from these numerous interactions of factors of both endogenous and exogenous origin. In understanding the role of a particular food component, examination of its interactions with other food components and with one or more metabolic pathways may be necessary, as well as possible consideration of differing actions depending on dose or on tissue site.

Most of this complexity is only partially understood for most of the bioactive compounds that have been studied. Single food components and single foods have been studied in relation to single genes for cancer. A limited number of studies have examined the impact of a group of foods or of dietary patterns on risk or prognosis. There have been some studies of the association of multiple genes with blood levels of particular nutrients. These studies are essential first steps; there is much to be learned as the more complex systems of interactions are examined. Presented here is information about the impact of genetic variation on the availability and utilization of dietary compounds in relation to carcinogenesis and about the impact of diet on genetic factors in relation to carcinogenesis.

B Genetic Variation in Relation to Metabolism of Food Components

1 Carcinogen Metabolism

Regarding the impact of genetic variation on metabolism, one focus has been on genes that modulate the metabolism of carcinogens. These carcinogens include both compounds occurring naturally in foods and others that contaminate foods. If an individual has genetic variants that result in slower metabolism of a carcinogen, that individual will be more affected by a given dose of that carcinogen than would someone who can metabolize and excrete the carcinogen more rapidly. Conversely, if an individual has genetic variants that result in more rapid metabolism of a carcinogen, then he or she may be less affected by the same dose than someone who does not have that variant.

The enzymes related to carcinogen metabolism and excretion are divided into two groups: phase I and phase II. Phase I enzymes activate the compound, and phase II enzymes attach polar groups to the activated compound so that it will be more water soluble and can be excreted in the urine. Many of the phase I enzymes are in the cytochrome P-450 (CYP) family. Phase II enzymes include glutathione-*S*-transferases (GSTs) and *N*-acetyltransferase (NAT). In some cases, phase I activation leads to the production of compounds with greater carcinogenic potential. Often, foods contain procarcinogens, compounds that are carcinogenic after metabolic activation. The process of metabolic activation may vary depending on genetic factors. For example, heterocyclic amines are a group of compounds found in meat cooked at high temperatures, primarily "well-done" meat and fish. There is some, although inconsistent, evidence that the heterocyclic amines are associated with cancer. For example, there is evidence of an association between intake of these compounds from meat with risk of breast cancer [14] and with increased risk of advanced prostate cancer [15]. This association may depend on genetic factors. Metabolism and excretion of heterocyclic amines involve CYP1A2, N-acetyltransferases 1 and 2 (NAT1 and -2), and UDP-glucuronosyltransferases [16]. With regard to colorectal cancer, there is some, although inconsistent, evidence that individuals who eat well-cooked meat and who have the rapid version of the enzymes for both *CYP1A2* and *NAT2* are at increased risk [16]. Figure 34.2 illustrates the relationships between these phase I and phase II enzyme systems [17,18].

Other kinds of genetic variation may also affect association of nutrition and diet with cancer outcomes. Copy number variation—the number of copies an individual has of a particular gene—may also affect metabolism. For example, there is evidence that the number of copies of the amylase gene is correlated with the levels of the amylase protein in saliva [19]. Dietary intake of nutrients important in one-carbon metabolism may also impact DNA methylation. One study showed an association of folate and green vegetable intake with promoter methylation in sputum from apparently healthy smokers [20]. However, in another, there was no association of folate intake with DNA methylation of three particular genes in breast tumors [21]. Examination of methylation of all genes will be important in understanding the relationships, if any, between diet and altered DNA methylation.

2 Metabolism of Nutrients and Other Food Components

There can be significant genetic variation among individuals in the absorption, tolerance, transport, and excretion of nutrients and other bioactive food components as well as their metabolism [13,22]. All of these can alter effects of intake of the same amount of a food component by individuals with different genes. Furthermore, genetic factors may alter food preferences and therefore food consumption [23].

The impact of a particular genetic polymorphism may differ for different compounds and may even protect against cancer for one compound and increase risk for another. For example, the GSTs are phase II enzymes that catalyze transformation of carcinogens

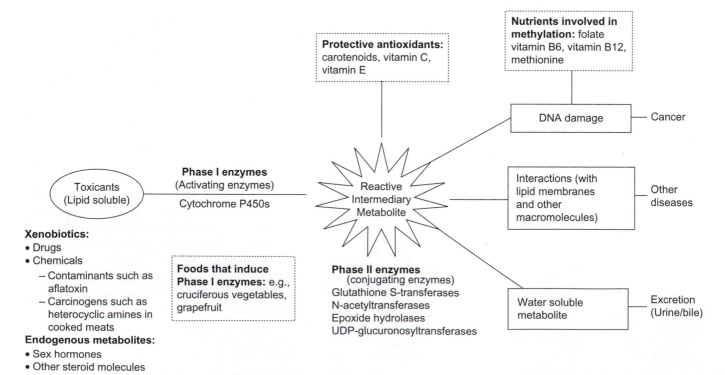

FIGURE 34.2 Interrelationship between the biotransformation enzyme systems. Source: *From Patterson, R. E., Eaton, D. L., and Potter, J. D. The genetic revolution: Change and challenge for the dietetics profession. Copyright The American Dietetic Association. Reprinted by permission from Journal of the American Dietetic Association, vol. 99, pp. 1412–1420, 1999.*

such as polycyclic aromatic hydrocarbons (PAHs) for excretion. For those with higher exposure to PAHs, including PAHs of dietary origin produced in the cooking of foods, the more rapid metabolism would be advantageous. Some of the GSTs also deactivate other phytochemicals that are thought to exert protective effects. Included in the latter group are the isothiocyanates from cruciferous vegetables, which are metabolized by GST, also resulting in their excretion [23].

Genetic variation in the pathway for a vitamin can affect the physiologic impact of intake of that vitamin. If a vitamin plays a role in cancer prevention, differences in the receptor for the vitamin could also affect the susceptibility of an individual to cancer. For example, there are commonly occurring genetic differences in the vitamin D receptor that may have functional significance. A number of studies have examined the association of those variants with risk of several cancers. In a meta-analysis, genetic variation in the receptor was associated with cancer risk [24]. In a genome-wide association study (GWAS) examining a large number of SNPs in association with vitamin D in blood, several genetic variants were found to be associated with circulating 25-hydroxyvitamin D [25].

There has been considerable exploration of genetic variants in the one-carbon metabolism pathway. Genetic variation in this pathway affects blood folate concentrations and folate transport and utilization. This genetic variation may also affect the synthesis of purines and pyrimidines for DNA synthesis and may affect gene methylation and thus the expression of genes. There is some, although not consistent, evidence of an association of variants in genes in this pathway and risk of several cancers [11]. However, in one study examining genetic variation of genes involved in one-carbon metabolism, there was no association with the prevalence of DNA methylation in breast tumors [26].

Another example of a gene that affects nutrient utilization is the *HFE* gene. This gene contains a variant, common among Europeans, that affects iron storage and is part of the etiology of hemochromatosis [27].

There is genetic variation in several of the enzymes involved in alcohol metabolism. For example, one variant in the gene for aldehyde dehydrogenase (ALDH2), which is carried by approximately 50% of Asians, results in greatly reduced clearance of acetaldehyde, a likely carcinogen. Those who are either heterozygous or homozygous for the variant experience an adverse reaction, an intense flushing, when they consume alcohol. This variant has been shown to be associated with both lower alcohol consumption and alcoholism [28]. In one study, there appeared to be an interaction between *ALDH* genotype, folate intake, and risk of oral and pharyngeal cancer [29].

C Interactions of Bioactive Food Components with Gene Functions in Relation to Carcinogenesis

1 Mutations and Metastasis

Nutrients and other bioactive food components appear to contribute both in positive and negative ways at every stage of the carcinogenic process, including DNA mutations and tumor metastasis. One mechanism for the occurrence of DNA mutations is the formation of DNA adducts with carcinogens. Carcinogens in foods, such as the PAHs described previously, are one potential source of these carcinogen adducts with DNA, binding to the DNA. Such adducts may interfere with DNA replication and result in mutations or deletions in DNA structure. Dietary factors may also affect the formation of adducts, such as those from smoking. For example, there is evidence that among smokers, adduct formation is inversely associated with β-carotene intake. Furthermore, genetic variation may also affect this association. The association between adduct formation and β-carotene intake appears to be limited to individuals who carry homozygous deletions for the gene for glutathione *S*-transferase (*GSTM1null*) [30].

There is evidence that reactive oxygen species from both exogenous and endogenous sources affect the rate of DNA mutations. Diet can affect exposure to reactive oxygen species both positively and negatively. Energy consumption is positively correlated with the number of oxidized DNA bases [3]. Antioxidant vitamins and other enzymes affected by genetic variation are part of the body's defense against these oxidative processes. Those who have genetically weaker defense systems against oxidation may benefit more from increased intake of antioxidant vitamins, such as vitamin C and vitamin E. For example, superoxide dismutase is important in the control of endogenously produced reactive oxygen species; manganese superoxide dismutase (MnSOD) is found in the mitochondria, an important location for production of oxidative species. The gene coding for MnSOD is polymorphic, and a study suggests that one variant of this gene may be associated with increased risk of premenopausal breast cancer but primarily among women with a low intake of antioxidant vitamins from fruits and vegetables [31].

Dietary factors may also influence genes that are related to metastasis. Catechins—found particularly in green tea but also in black tea, apples, and chocolate—can downregulate enzymes important in the development of metastases [32].

Genetic variation may also affect DNA repair. Although the data regarding this potential mechanism are rather limited, there is evidence of an effect of diet on these functions essential to the maintenance of DNA integrity [33].

2 Gene Induction

There are several ways in which bioactive food components may interact with genes. As noted previously, dietary factors may influence genetic functioning by causing mutations. They may also affect gene expression. For example, the *CYP1A2* gene can be induced by indole-3-carbinol found in cruciferous vegetables, by heterocyclic amines in cooked meats, and by PAHs found in grilled meat. *CYP1A2* is also inhibited by the compound naringenin, which is found in grapefruit [34]. Therefore, metabolism of heterocyclic amines by the enzyme encoded by this gene may depend not only on the genetic variant of *CYP1A2* that is carried by an individual but also on the individual's intake of these other food components that affect *CYP1A2* expression. Similarly, consumption of a diet that is low in fat and low in glycemic load was shown to be associated with alterations in gene expression in the prostate epithelium in humans [35].

Interactions with gene expression may be part of the normal functioning of the food component and of the gene, leading to either upregulation or downregulation of the gene expression. Vitamins A and D interact with the promoter regions of a number of genes, influencing their expression and thereby affecting a host of cellular functions, including cell proliferation and differentiation and DNA replication and repair [36]. A group of receptors called peroxisome proliferation-activated receptors (PPARs) affect the expression of genes important in fatty acid metabolism and tumorigenesis. One of these, PPARα, is activated by oxidized fats, affecting expression of genes important in fatty acid synthesis [37]. The intracellular energy balance can also affect gene expression [33]. A number of other nutrients and other food components have been shown to affect gene expression in cell culture, including vitamin E, biotin, zinc, flavones, and catechins [33].

3 Epigenetic Alterations

Alterations of DNA structure other than base pair changes can also affect gene expression. Important among these are DNA methylation and alterations in histones. There is evidence of possible contributions to carcinogenesis by both an overall decrease in DNA methylation (global hypomethylation) and an increase in the methylation (hypermethylation) of the promoters of certain genes, particularly tumor suppressor genes, thus silencing them. Dietary factors involved in one-carbon metabolism may affect this methylation. These factors include folate, vitamins B_6 and B_{12}, biotin, choline, and methionine. For example, alcohol can adversely affect folate status and therefore indirectly affect methyl availability. In addition to nutrients related to methyl availability, there is also evidence that genistein, coumestrol, and a high-fiber diet may all affect methylation patterns [38]. The mechanisms for both hypo- and hypermethylation are not well understood and may involve other factors of both exogenous and endogenous origin.

In addition to methylation changes, dietary factors may affect the histones. Inhibitors of histone deacetylators include butyrate (formed by the bacterial fermentation of fiber in the colon), diallyl disulfide (from plants in the allium family, including garlic), and sulforaphane from cruciferous vegetables [11]. Reservatrol, found in grapes and grape products, may affect carbonylation of histones.

Diet may also affect other epigenetic processes, impacting gene expression. In animal models, there is evidence of alterations in microRNA expression profiles of hepatocellular carcinomas for diets low in nutrients important in one-carbon metabolism—folic acid, methionine, and choline [39]. In lymphoblastoid cell lines, folate has been shown to affect global microRNA expression [40].

The fields of genetics in general and nutrigenetics in particular are changing rapidly; numerous discoveries are leading to major shifts in our understanding of the role of genetic factors in cancer risk and of the interaction of dietary and other exposures with those genetic factors. There is evidence that several pathways can affect diet and gene interactions and ultimately disease. However, in the next several years, other pathways of interaction will likely be identified, and some of the ones detailed here may be determined to be of lesser importance to humans. Because much of our understanding of gene–environment interactions in relation to cancer is based on relatively new information, it is important to recognize that much of the data are subject to reinterpretation and that an understanding of the methodological issues involved is key.

IV METHODOLOGICAL ISSUES

Data regarding interactions of diet and genes and cancer come from a number of sources, including studies of normal and tumor cells in culture, animal models, and human epidemiologic studies. Each of these study modalities has advantages and disadvantages. For cell culture studies, the concentration of an agent may be very important, and the studied concentration may or may not relate to physiological conditions in the tissue of interest. Also important to consider are the duration of the dosage and the type of cells used. Some cultured cells may also have characteristics different from what occurs *in vivo*.

Animal models are an important source of understanding of the underlying mechanisms of carcinogenesis. Again, however, in interpretation of findings, considerations of the dose and duration of administration of an agent are important, as is an understanding of differences between the physiology of a particular animal model and humans. In addition, the complex mix of exposures humans experience may be of importance and may not be replicated in laboratory animal or cell culture studies. Even when the animal model can provide very good information, there may be important caveats that inform the conclusions that can be made from the experiments. For example, there are numerous studies of the administration of high-fat diets to animals with increasing mammary tumor development. One limitation of such studies that is often not noted is that the observed increases in mammary tumors are found only when the high-fat diets are administered to virgin animals. In parous animals, the high-fat diets do not increase mammary tumors [41]. Such caveats are important in understanding the results from animal studies and may also, although not necessarily, inform our understanding of human disease processes. Epidemiologic studies have the advantage of being a study of human populations with gene frequencies and exogenous exposure levels at the pertinent levels. However, there are other concerns with studies of this kind.

In epidemiologic studies, an individual's genotype can be determined from DNA extracted from cells. The DNA is typically obtained from blood cells, from sloughed cells in saliva, or from sloughed cells from the inside of the mouth. For polymorphic genes, laboratory methods are used to identify which of the variants for a particular gene are carried by an individual based on the sequence of the DNA. Because the many mutations are correlated with each other, it may not be necessary to measure every variant in a particular gene. Rather, markers or tag SNPs can be measured that identify the group of variants in a gene. These variant groups that tend to travel together are referred to as haplotypes.

An individual's phenotype may also be measured. Phenotype may be the measure of some physical characteristic such as body weight, eye color, or blood concentration of a vitamin. Alternatively, phenotype may be measured as the response to an exposure. An individual ingests a measured amount of a substance (e.g., caffeine), and then blood or urine samples are collected for several hours or days to determine the rate of metabolism of that substance. Measurement of phenotype is advantageous in that it provides an indication of the sum of the processes involved and therefore an indication of the true exposure. As noted previously, phenotype may depend on more than one gene; it may reflect processes involved in absorption and excretion as well as metabolism. However, when comparisons are being made of individuals with and without a disease, the phenotype may be affected by the disease state and might not be reflective of the diseased individual's lifetime exposure. In studies that include people with disease, a determination of phenotype may be less useful than determination of a genotype, unless it can be shown that the phenotype does not change for those with the disease.

In epidemiology, the interaction of genes and diet may be assessed in case—control studies, in cohort and nested case—control studies, or in clinical trials. In case—control studies, cases, people with recently diagnosed disease, are compared to healthy controls from the same population. Statistical methods are used to determine whether there are systematic differences between those people who get the disease and those who do not. In a prospective cohort study, a population of exposed and unexposed individuals is identified and their exposure status measured. Those individuals are then followed to compare the rate of disease in the exposed and unexposed groups. Because cancer is relatively rare, these studies need to include thousands or even hundreds of thousands of individuals in order to examine diet in relation to cancer.

When blood has been collected from study participants, it is possible to determine genotype for the participants. In a cohort study, generally, a nested case—control study is conducted for analysis of gene—environment interactions. Individuals in the cohort with incident cancer (cases) are compared to a group of controls selected from the cohort. The controls are chosen to be similar to the cases for relevant characteristics such as age, race, and gender. Genotypes are then determined and the gene—environment interactions analyzed for this subset of the whole cohort. Environmental exposures are estimated from interview data or from other, more direct measures of exposure. In a clinical trial, study participants are randomly allocated to exposure category; in this case, a dietary intervention would be compared to the lack of that intervention. To examine diet—gene interactions, the effect of the intervention would be compared by genotype. It is possible to determine genotype in advance of randomization in order to group participants based on their genotype, to ensure that the number of participants with a particular genotype is the same in the intervention and control groups.

For both case—control and nested case—control studies, the examination of gene—diet interactions generally involves a few steps: (1) the examination of the association between risk of a particular cancer and the genetic factor(s) alone—genetic factors can be a single polymorphism with known functional significance, haplotypes within a gene, a group of genes in one or more pathways, or thousands of variants across the entire genome; (2) the examination of the association between risk of that cancer and the dietary factor(s) alone—dietary factors can be nutrients, single food components, foods, groups of bioactive agents, or dietary patterns; and (3) the examination of the gene—diet interactions. In some cases, there will be further examination of interaction with other exposures (e.g., exposure to hormone replacement therapy or body weight).

Although this is a relatively new area of research, in some clinical trials, the interaction of genes and environment is studied. The effect of a dietary intervention might be examined within and across groups to determine if one group is more susceptible to the intervention.

For all these study designs, there are some important methodological considerations. Many of these are the same considerations as for any epidemiologic study of diet and cancer [42]. A significant one is that, as in all epidemiology, conclusions about causality need to be derived from a synthesis of epidemiologic findings in a number of populations, animal research, and metabolic studies. No single epidemiologic study can be considered definitive and used to establish causality. In case—control and cohort studies, there is concern that the findings may not be causal but rather the result of confounding. That is, another factor may be correlated both with the exposure under study and with the disease and may be the causative agent. If the investigators are unaware of this confounding factor or they are unable to control for it sufficiently well, it might appear that the exposure under study is associated with disease simply because it is correlated with the second factor. The confounding factor can be an exogenous exposure or another genetic factor. When genes tend to be inherited together and therefore can confound an investigation of each of the genes, it is called linkage disequilibrium.

Confounding may occur, for example, in a study of diet and lung cancer. In many populations, individuals who smoke are also more likely to drink alcohol. Unless smoking is measured well and controlled for in an analysis, one might incorrectly assess the relation of alcohol to lung cancer because of the correlation between these two behaviors. That is, it might be difficult to determine if alcohol is associated with lung cancer because of the confounding by smoking. When studies are done in different populations in different cultures, the likelihood of confounding is diminished; it is less likely that the same correlations exist between behaviors. In addition, other sources of error may differ among studies, making a consistent finding more believable. Only with a randomized trial can a causal link be identified with certainty because of the randomization to intervention or control group.

However, even among clinical trials, differences in study results can occur because of differences in participant populations, so results need to be carefully interpreted. Clearly, it is only possible to randomize participants on some genotypes, and linkage disequilibrium can make determination difficult as to which gene or genes are important in the process being studied.

Because the technology to measure genotypes in large studies is relatively new, there are few hypotheses related to the interaction of diet and genetics in cancer etiology that have been examined in numerous studies. Many questions have been examined in only a single study. This is a rapidly expanding field. With further development of the field, it will be possible to begin to identify the most consistent and important associations. At all times, it is important to examine findings critically and to search for consistent findings from well-conducted studies.

A major concern in evaluating diet and genetic interactions in relation to risk of cancer is that studies need to have large numbers of participants in order to have sufficient power to examine risk within strata defined by genotype or by diet. Because of the need to examine interactions, large studies are required to provide a sufficient number of individuals within the group of interest. Even if the results are statistically significant, such findings can be unstable. That is, if the study were redone, findings may not be consistent. In particular, for genes with low frequencies, the number of participants required can be very large. Furthermore, to examine the interactions of more than one gene and more than one dietary or other exposure, the number of participants required may be exceedingly large. In evaluation of any study, it is important to consider the number of participants in each cell to make a determination of the likely stability of the findings.

Cancer is a multifactorial disease, and it is likely that several genetic factors are of importance even within a single causative pathway. Analysis of a single polymorphism or even of several genes in a pathway might not capture the total picture of variation in risk. Similarly, several nutrients are likely to be important even within a single causal pathway. As noted previously, the examination of gene—gene and gene—environment interactions can be seriously hampered by the required sample size.

Diet is also a complex set of exposures. A single food may include different factors with both carcinogenic and anticarcinogenic properties. Intakes of different nutrients are often highly correlated so that an association attributed to intake of one nutrient may in fact be the result of a causal relationship with a different nutrient. Finally, when there is evidence that a particular nutrient is related to a decrease in risk, it cannot be assumed that larger quantities of that nutrient would be even more protective. For example, whereas vitamin C has antioxidant properties at the level found in most foods, at higher intake levels, it may have pro-oxidant properties [43].

A final challenge in this field is in the measurement of dietary exposure. Much literature is available on the problems of measurement of diet for epidemiologic purposes [44]. Beyond those concerns, the study of gene—diet interactions in relation to cancer risk has led to an interest in a number of new bioactive compounds found in foods. For many of these compounds, the dietary instruments used in the past may not provide sufficient detail for assessment of intake of that compound. For example, the study of heterocyclic amines has led to the development of a questionnaire that specifically addresses the sources of these compounds because the information regarding intake on the existing questionnaires did not include the necessary detail to assess intake of heterocyclic amines [45]. Furthermore, nutrient composition databases may be limited and may need work in order to determine the composition for compounds that may relate to disease risk but that have not been previously analyzed.

V DIET—GENE INTERACTIONS AND CANCER

As described previously, there are a number of properties that distinguish a tumor. These properties contribute to the ability of a tumor to break loose from normal controls on growth and to invade tissues. Tumor cells have their own growth signals, they do not respond to signals inhibiting growth, they can replicate indefinitely and do not go into programmed cell death (apoptosis), they can invade other tissues (metastasis), and they can develop a blood supply for those metastases (angiogenesis) [5]. All of these pathways may be appropriate targets for cancer prevention. Given the nature of tumor biology, it is unlikely that there will be one food or compound that will prevent all cancers or even all of one kind of tumor; rather, the cumulative effect of a number of compounds may be important in prevention [46]. Many processes are important in carcinogenesis, including carcinogen metabolism, hormone regulation, cell differentiation, DNA repair, apoptosis, cell growth cycle, and inflammatory response. Nutrients and other bioactive food components may play a role in each of these processes (Figure 34.3) [47]. In this section, breast cancer is used as an example and data regarding diet and gene interactions for some of these processes for breast cancer are described. This area of research is rapidly changing, and our understanding of these relationships is likely to shift with further investigation. This overview is provided to give examples of the developing understanding.

A Carcinogen Metabolism

One example is metabolism of alcohol. There is consistent epidemiologic evidence that alcohol consumption is associated with a moderate increase in breast cancer risk [48]. Although there are several possible mechanisms to explain these observations, there is also evidence that the mechanism of this association involves gene—environment interactions in carcinogen metabolism. Alcohol is metabolized to acetaldehyde in the liver and in other tissues including breast tissue by a group of enzymes called alcohol dehydrogenases. Acetaldehyde has been identified as a likely carcinogen [49]. It may be that the exposure of breast tissue to acetaldehyde accounts for the increased risk associated with alcohol consumption. Several studies have examined the interaction of alcohol consumption and a common genetic variant in one isozyme of alcohol dehydrogenase in relation to risk of breast cancer. This variant affects how quickly acetaldehyde is formed from ingested ethanol. Some [50—52], but not all [53,54], studies found that there was more risk associated with alcohol consumption among women who also had the variant resulting in more rapid metabolism to acetaldehyde.

B Regulation of Hormones

There is considerable evidence that estrogen exposure is a strong risk factor for breast cancer [55]. Of interest is whether compounds of plant origins with estrogenic properties, called phytoestrogens, affect breast cancer risk. Among these is indole 3-carbinol, which is found in cruciferous vegetables after they are cooked or crushed. There is evidence from studies of breast cells in culture that this compound can affect the estrogen receptor, ER-α. It can alter the estrogen and the DNA binding regions of the ER, leading to decreased response to estrogen in estrogen-responsive cells [56]. Thus, the interaction of this dietary compound with DNA may affect breast cancer risk because of the dampening of response to estrogen.

C Cellular Differentiation

Genistein, a polyphenol found in soy, has been found to decrease mammary tumors in animal models. There is evidence that when genistein is ingested in the prepubertal rat, it can help to regulate mammary development and differentiation. An increase in differentiation of mammary tissue is observed, as are differences in cellular proliferation, apoptosis, and tumor suppressor expression. The effects of genistein on mammary development appear to be different and most beneficial with administration of this bioactive compound in young animals and may not have the same impact in older ones [57].

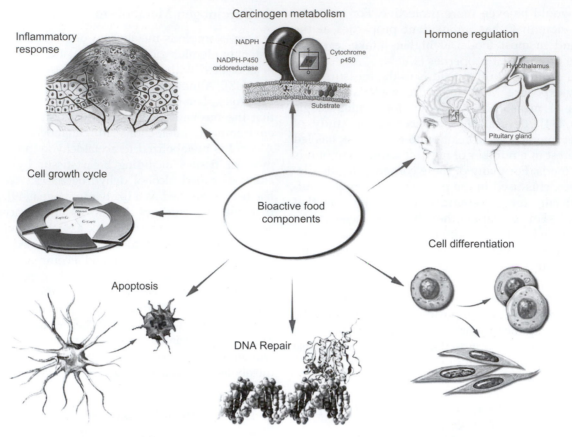

FIGURE 34.3 Interactions of bioactive food components with genes appear to be important mechanisms for carcinogenesis. Source: *From Trujillo, E., Davis, C., and Milner, J. "Nutrigenomics, Proteomics, Metabalomics and the Practice of Dietetics." Copyright The American Dietetic Association. Reprinted by permission from* Journal of the American Dietetic Association, *vol. 106, pp. 403–413, 2006.*

D DNA Repair

Repair of DNA errors resulting from exogenous exposures or from errors in replication is an important function of the cell. Errors in DNA repair may be important in the carcinogenic process. There are several different processes to maintain the integrity of the DNA. In one epidemiologic study, there was evidence of interaction of a variant in a gene in the excision repair pathway with intake of fruits and vegetables and risk of breast cancer. Among women with at least one copy of the apparently protective variant and who reported higher intake of fruits and vegetables, risk of breast cancer was lower than for women with lower intake or without the variant [58]. Another food compound that may also affect DNA repair is indole 3-carbinol. There is evidence that it may block DNA strand breaks. It can upregulate the *BRCA1* gene, which plays a role in DNA repair [56].

E Apoptosis

Programmed cell death or apoptosis is an important function in the maintenance of the integrity of tissues. Dietary factors may also affect apoptosis and may interact with genes that control it. For example, there is evidence that vitamin D can influence genes controlling apoptosis [59]. Other dietary factors may also play a role. In one study, overweight or obese postmenopausal women were placed on a low-fat, high-fiber diet and an exercise program. A comparison was made of the growth-promoting properties of serum from the women taken before and after the intervention evaluated in three different estrogen receptor-positive breast cancer cell lines. Among other changes, there was an increase in apoptosis for several different cell lines when the post-intervention serum was used as the growth medium [60]. Other dietary factors that may also affect the expression of genes important in apoptosis include organosulfur compounds from foods from the allium family, including garlic; polyphenols from green tea, chocolate, and chili peppers; and isothiocyanates from cruciferous vegetables [61].

VI FUTURE DIRECTIONS

Understanding of the role of genes in cancer and particularly the role of the interactions of diet with genes in this disease process is a rapidly expanding field of inquiry. Most of the available evidence remains somewhat preliminary, based on cell culture and animal studies or on a small number of epidemiologic studies. Our understanding of gene–diet interactions and how to study them is advancing rapidly, with tremendous potential implications for our understanding of the role of dietary factors in cancer etiology. Clearly, as the field progresses, extremely large studies will be needed to allow for the examination of multiple levels of interaction to fully understand the relevant etiological pathways.

In the future, genotype needs to be examined in metabolic studies to determine the short-term effects on intermediate outcome measures in healthy individuals. A great deal remains to be understood about the relation between genotype and phenotype for the genes that appear to be important in cancer risk. Furthermore, we need to understand the factors—both dietary and from other sources—that affect gene induction and the etiological pathways. More work must be performed to identify the relevant genes that make the most difference, likely those that are control points for metabolic pathways and that are also found sufficiently often in the population to have an impact. We are moving toward the examination of the role of diet in cancer etiology, examining effects within groups defined by genotype. Such studies may allow us to identify relationships that are important among particular groups of the population but that are not evident when the whole population is studied together.

There is little doubt that environmental factors are very important in causing cancer. It is not likely that genetic factors alone are sufficient to explain who will get the disease and who will not for most cancers. Important among the likely environmental factors are dietary factors. With increased understanding of the interactions of genetic and nutritional factors, it may eventually become possible to identify individuals with higher or lower requirements for particular nutrients or to identify individuals with greater sensitivity to agents such as alcohol. Furthermore, the elucidation of genetic factors in relation to diet will help us to truly understand the natural history of cancer and how best to prevent it.

References

[1] Ferlay, J., Shin, H. R., Bray, F., Forman, D., Mathers, C., and Parkin, D. M. (2008). Globocan 2008: Cancer Incidence and Mortality Worldwide, IARC CancerBase No. 10, version 1.2 [Internet]. International Agency for Research on Cancer, Lyon, France. Available at <http://globocan.iarc.fr/>. Accessed August 2011.

[2] American Cancer Society, Cancer Facts and Figures 2011, American Cancer Society, Atlanta, GA, 2011.

[3] World Cancer Research Fund/American Institute for Cancer Research, Food, Nutrition, Physical Activity and the Prevention of Cancer: A Global Perspective, American Institute for Cancer Research, Washington, DC, 2007.

[4] R.A. Weinberg, The Biology of Cancer., Garland, New York, 2007.

[5] D. Hanahan, R.A. Weinberg, Hallmarks of cancer: the next generation, Cell 144 (2011) 646–674.

[6] R.C. King, W.D. Stansfield, A Dictionary of Genetics., Oxford University Press, New York, 1997.

[7] A. Antoniou, P.D.P. Pharoah, S. Narod, et al., Average risks of breast and ovarian cancer associated with BRCA1 and BRCA2 mutations detected in case series unselected for family history: A combined analysis of 22 studies, Am. J. Hum. Genet. 72 (2003) 1117–1130.

[8] D.F. Easton, D. Ford, D.T. Bishop, Breast and ovarian cancer incidence in BRCA1-mutation carriers: Breast Cancer Linkage Consortium, Am. J. Hum. Genet. 56 (1995) 265–271.

[9] D.F. Easton, S.A. Narod, D. Ford, M. Steel, The genetic epidemiology of BRCA1: Breast Cancer Linkage Consortium [letter], Lancet 344 (1994) 761.

[10] B. Newman, H. Mu, L. Butler, R.C. Milliken, P.G. Moorman, M.-C. King, Frequency of breast cancer attributable to BRCA1 in a population based series of American women, JAMA 279 (1998) 915–921.

[11] C.D. Davis, N.G. Hord, Nutritional "omics" technologies for elucidating the role(s) of bioactive food components in colon cancer prevention, J. Nutr. 135 (2005) 2694–2697.

[12] J.A. Milner, Molecular targets for bioactive food components, J. Nutr. 134 (2004) 2492S–2498S.

[13] J. Kaput, Nutrigenomics: 2006 update, Clin. Chem. Lab. Med. 45 (2007) 279–287.

[14] H.M. Ochs-Balcom, G. Wiesner, R.C. Elston, A meta-analysis of the association of N-acetyltransferase gene (NAT2) variants with breast cancer, Am. J. Epidemiol. 166 (2007) 246–254.

[15] E.M. John, M.C. Stern, R. Sinha, J. Koo, Meat consumption, cooking practices, meat mutagens, and risk of prostate cancer, Nutr. Cancer 63 (2011) 525–537.

[16] A.J. Cross, R. Sinha, Meat related mutagens/carcinogens in the etiology of colorectal cancer, Environ. Mol. Mutagen. 44 (2004) 44–55.

[17] R.E. Patterson, D.L. Eaton, J.D. Potter, The genetic revolution: Change and challenge for the dietetics profession, J. Am. Diet. Assoc. 99 (1999) 1412–1420.

[18] C.L. Rock, J.W. Lampe, R.E. Patterson, Nutrition, genetics, and risks and cancer, Annu. Rev. Public Health 21 (2000) 47–64.

[19] G.H. Perry, N.J. Dominy, K.G. Claw, A.S. Lee, H. Fiegler, R. Redon, et al., Diet and the evolution of human amylase gene copy number variation, Nat. Genet. 39 (2007) 1256–1260.

[20] C.A. Stidley, M.A. Picchi, S. Leng, R. Willink, R.E. Crowell, K.G. Flores, et al., Multivitamins, folate, and green vegetables protect against gene promoter methylation in the aerodigestive tract of smokers, Cancer Res. 70 (2010) 568–574.

[21] M.H. Tao, J.B. Mason, C. Marian, S.E. McCann, M.E. Platek, A. Millen, et al., Promoter methylation of E-cadherin, p16, and RAR-β2 genes in breast tumors and dietary intake of nutrients important in one-carbon metabolism, Nutr. Caner. 63 (2011) 1143–1150.

[22] S.A. Ross, Evidence for the relationship between diet and cancer, Exp. Oncol. 32 (2010) 137–142.

[23] J.W. Lampe, Diet, genetic polymorphisms, detoxification and health risks, Altern. Ther. Health Med. 13 (2007) S108–S111.

[24] S. Raimondi, H. Johansson, P. Masonneruve, S. Gandini, Review and meta-analysis on vitamin D receptor polymorphisms and cancer risk, Carcinogenesis 30 (2009) 1170–1180.

[25] J. Ahn, K. Yu, R. Stolzenberg-Solomon, K.C. Simon, M.L. McCullough, L. Gallicchio, et al., Genome wide association

study of circulating vitamin D levels, Hum. Mol. Genet. 19 (2010) 1745–2739.

[26] M.H. Tao, P.G. Shields, J. Nie, C. Marian, C.B. Ambrosone, S.E. McCann, et al., DNA promoter methylation in breast tumors: No association with genetic polymorphisms in MTHFR and MTR, Cancer Epidemiol. Biomarkers Prev. 18 (2009) 998–1002.

[27] P.J. Stover, Influence of human genetic variation on nutritional requirements, Am. J. Clin. Nutr. 83 (Suppl) (2006) 436S–442S.

[28] D.P. Agarwal, Genetic polymorphisms of alcohol metabolizing enzymes, Pathol. Biol. 49 (2001) 703–709.

[29] K. Matsuo, M. Rossi, E. Negri, I. Oze, S. Hosono, H. Ito, et al., Folate, alcohol and aldehyde dehydrogenase 2 polymorphism and the risk of oral and pharyngeal cancer in Japanese, Eur. J. Cancer Prev. 21 (2012) 193–198.

[30] L.A. Mooney, D.A. Bell, R.M. Santella, A.M. Van Bennekum, R. Ottman, M. Paik, et al., Contribution of genetic and nutritional factors to DNA damage in heavy smokers, Carcinogenesis 18 (1997) 503–509.

[31] C.B. Ambrosone, J.L. Freudenheim, P.A. Thompson, E. Bowman, J.E. Vena, J.R. Marshall, et al., Manganese superoxide dismutase (MnSOD) genetic polymorphisms, dietary antioxidants and risk of breast cancer, Cancer Res. 59 (1999) 602–606.

[32] D. Mariappen, J. Winkler, V. Parthiban, M.X. Doss, J. Hescheler, A. Sachinidis, Dietary small molecules and large-scale gene expression studies: An experimental approach for understanding their beneficial effects on the development of malignant and non-malignant proliferative diseases, Curr. Med. Chem. 13 (2006) 1481–1489.

[33] J.C. Mathers, J.M. Coxhead, J. Tyson, Nutrition and DNA repair: Potential molecular mechanisms of action, Curr. Cancer Drug Targets 7 (2007) 425–431.

[34] R. Sinha, N. Caporaso, Diet, genetic susceptibility and human cancer etiology, J. Nutr. 129 (1999) 556S–559S.

[35] D.W. Lin, M.L. Neuhouser, J.M. Schenk, I.M. Coleman, S. Hawley, D. Gifford, et al., Low-fat, low glycemic load diet and gene expression in human prostate epithelium: A feasibility study using cDNA microarrays to assess the response to dietary intervention in target tissues, Cancer Epidemiol. Biomarkers Prev. 16 (2007) 2130–2154.

[36] R. Bouillon, G. Eelen, L. Verlinden, C. Mathieu, G. Carmeliet, A. Vestuyf, Vitamin D and cancer, J. Steroid Biochem. Mol. Biol. 102 (2006) 156–162.

[37] R. Ringsieis, K. Eder, Regulation of genes involved in lipid metabolism by dietary oxidized fat, Mol. Nutr. Food Res. 55 (2011) 109–121.

[38] S.A. Ross, Diet and DNA methylation interactions in cancer prevention, Ann. N. Y. Acad. Sci. 983 (2003) 197–207.

[39] H. Kutay, B. Shoumei, J. Datta, T. Motiwala, I. Pogribny, W. Frankel, et al., Downregulation of miR-122 in the rodent and human hepatocarcinomas, J. Cell. Biochem. 99 (2006) 671–678.

[40] C.J. Marsit, K. Eddy, K.T. Kelsey, MicroRNA responses to cellular stress, Cancer Res. 66 (2006) 10843–10848.

[41] C. Ip, Controversial issues of dietary fat and experimental mammary carcinogenesis, Prev. Med. 22 (1993) 728–737.

[42] J.L. Freudenheim, Study design and hypothesis testing: issues in the evaluation of evidence from nutritional epidemiology, Am. J. Clin. Nutr. 69 (1999) 1315S–1321S.

[43] Panel on Dietary Antioxidants and Related Compounds, Food and Nutrition Board, Institute of Medicine, Dietary Reference Intakes for Vitamin C, Vitamin E, Selenium and Carotenoids, National Academy Press, Washington, DC, 2000.

[44] W.C. Willett, Nutritional Epidemiology, second ed., Oxford University Press, New York, 1998.

[45] R. Sinha, N. Rothman, Exposure assessment of heterocyclic amines (HCAs) in epidemiologic studies, Mutat. Res. 376 (1997) 195–202.

[46] C.D. Davis, Nutritional interactions: credentialing of molecular targets for cancer prevention, Exp. Biol. Med. 232 (2007) 176–183.

[47] E. Trujillo, C. Davis, J. Milner, Nutrigenomics, proteomics, metabolomics and the practice of dietetics, J. Am. Diet. Assoc. 106 (2006) 403–413.

[48] S.A. Smith-Warner, D. Spiegelman, S.S. Yaun, P.A. van den Brandt, A.R. Folsom, R.A. Goldbohm, et al., Alcohol and breast cancer in women: a pooled analysis of cohort studies, JAMA 279 (1998) 535–540.

[49] International Agency for Research on Cancer, World Health Organization. IARC Monographs on the Evaluation of Carcinogenic Risks to Humans, International Agency for Research on Cancer Monographs, volumes 1–102, Lyon, France (2012). Available at <http://monographs.iarc.fr/>.

[50] J.L. Freudenheim, C.B. Ambrosone, K.B. Moysich, J.E. Vena, S. Graham, J.R. Marshall, et al., Alcohol dehydrogenase 3 genotype modification of the association of alcohol consumption with breast cancer, Cancer Causes Control 10 (1999) 369–377.

[51] M.B. Terry, M.D. Gammon, F.F. Zang, J.A. Knight, Q. Wang, J.A. Britton, et al., ADH3 genotype, alcohol intake and breast cancer risk, Carcinogenesis 27 (2006) 840–847.

[52] L.S. Benzon, U. Vogel, J. Christensen, R.D. Hansen, H. Wallin, K. Overvad, et al., Interaction between ADH1C Arg(272)Gln and alcohol intake in relation to breast cancer risk suggests that ethanol is the causal factor in alcohol related breast cancer, Cancer Lett. 295 (2010) 191–197.

[53] L.M. Hines, S.E. Hankinson, S.A. Smith-Warner, D. Spiegelman, K.T. Kelsey, G.A. Colditz, et al., A prospective study of the effect of alcohol consumption and ADH3 genotype on plasma steroid hormone levels and breast cancer risk, Cancer Epidemiol. Biomarkers Prev. 9 (2000) 1099–1105.

[54] K. Vishvanathan, R.M. Crum, P.T. Strickland, X. You, I. Ruscinski, S.I. Berndt, et al., Alcohol dehydrogenase polymorphisms, low-to-moderate alcohol consumption and risk of breast cancer, Alcohol Clin. Exp. Res. 31 (2007) 46–76.

[55] T.J. Key, P.N. Appleby, G.K. Reeves, et al., Body mass index, serum sex hormones, and breast cancer risk in postmenopausal women, J. Natl. Cancer Inst. 95 (2003) 1218–1226.

[56] Y.S. Kim, J.A. Milner, Targets for indole-3-carbinol in cancer prevention, J. Nutr. Biochem. 16 (2005) 65–73.

[57] T.G. Witsett, L.A. Lamartiniere, Genistein and reservatrol: Mammary cancer chemoprevention and mechanisms of action in the rat, Expert Rev. Anticancer Ther. 6 (2006) 1699–1706.

[58] J. Shen, M.D. Gammon, M.B. Terry, L. Wang, Q. Wang, F. Zhang, et al., Polymorphisms in XRCC1 modify the association between aromatic hydrocarbon-DNA adducts, cigarette smoking, dietary antioxidants and breast cancer, Cancer Epidemiol. Biomarkers Prev. 14 (2005) 336–342.

[59] M.F. Holick, Vitamin D deficiency, N. Engl. J. Med. 357 (2007) 266–281.

[60] R.J. Barnard, J.H. Gonzalez, M.E. Liva, T.H. Ngo, Effects of a low-fat, high-fiber diet and exercise on breast cancer risk factors in vivo and tumor cell growth and apoptosis, in vitro. Nutr. Cancer. 55 (2006) 28–34.

[61] K.R. Martin, Targeting apoptosis with dietary bio-active agents, Exp. Biol. Med. 231 (2006) 117–129.

Nutrition and Cancers of the Breast, Endometrium, and Ovary

Kim Robien[*], *Cheryl L. Rock*[†], *Wendy Demark-Wahnefried*[‡]

[*]University of Minnesota, Minneapolis, Minnesota, [†]University of California at San Diego, San Diego, California,
[‡]University of Alabama at Birmingham, Birmingham, Alabama

I INTRODUCTION

Carcinomas of the breast, endometrium, and ovary are hormone-related cancers that have biologic similarities. Among U.S. women, breast cancer is far more common than endometrial or ovarian cancers. In 2011, roughly 230,480 women were diagnosed with breast cancer, thus comprising approximately 30% of the incident cancers among females [1]. In contrast, cancers of the endometrium (uterine corpus) and ovary comprised approximately 6 and 3% of female cancers, respectively. Because of differences in treatment efficacy and usual stage at diagnosis, the mortality estimates for these cancers vary considerably. Breast cancer will be the cause of death for approximately 39,520 women during 2011 (approximately 15% of cancer-related deaths among U.S. females), whereas endometrial and ovarian cancers account for approximately 3 and 6% of cancer-related mortality among women, respectively [1].

Breast cancer occurs infrequently in men, although the incidence is rising. In 2011, an estimated 2140 men were diagnosed with breast cancer, and 450 men will die of this disease [1], accounting for more than 1% of all malignancies and cancer deaths in men. Men tend to have a less favorable breast cancer outcome compared to women, largely due to advanced stage at diagnosis. More than 40% of male breast cancer patients present with stage III or IV disease [2].

Estrogens likely play an important role in breast, endometrial, and ovarian cancers [3]. Normal cell proliferation and differentiation in these tissues is highly responsive to estrogens and the other gonadal hormones. In addition to the ovarian steroids, other growth factors and mitogens influenced by nutritional factors and dietary patterns also appear to play an important role in the initiation and promotion of breast cancer. Insulin and insulin-like growth factor 1 (IGF-1) are currently under active investigation, as well as the interactions of these factors with adiposity and weight gain [4].

Diet and/or nutritional status is presumed to play a major role in the risk and progression of these hormone-related cancers, either through influence on the hormonal milieu or gene expression or via direct effects. Compared to the amount of research on breast cancer, far fewer studies have examined the relationship between nutritional factors and risk and/or progression of endometrial and ovarian cancers. This chapter reviews and summarizes evidence on the relationships between nutritional factors and breast, endometrial, and ovarian cancers. Recent clinical and epidemiological studies are emphasized, with the goal of identifying clinically useful strategies for prevention and patient management.

II BREAST CANCER

A Nutritional Factors and Primary Breast Cancer Risk

1 Height, Weight, and Body Fat Distribution

During the past four decades, numerous studies have evaluated the association between height and breast cancer risk, including a meta-analysis by the

Nutrition in the Prevention and Treatment of Disease, Third Edition.
DOI: http://dx.doi.org/10.1016/B978-0-12-391884-0.00035-4

World Cancer Research Fund (WCRF)/American Institute for Cancer Research (AICR) confirming a strong association for both pre- and postmenopausal disease [5]. Furthermore, height has also been associated with increased mammographic density, which is considered a strong risk factor for breast cancer [6]. It is hypothesized that the observed associations between height and breast cancer are due to factors that promote growth rather than height. Height attainment during puberty and selected periods during childhood has also been investigated in relation to breast cancer risk [7,8]. Other studies have concentrated on birth size as a proxy for *in utero* exposure. A meta-analysis (17 cohort and 15 case−control) found a statistically significant increased risk of breast cancer among women who weighed 4.0 kg or more at birth (relative risk (RR) = 1.12; 95% confidence interval (CI), 1.00−1.25) compared to women with birth weights between 3.0 and 3.5 kg [9]. Birth length and head circumference obtained from birth record data were also found to be positively associated with breast cancer risk [9]. Other skeletal indices, such as increased elbow breadth (a frame size marker), femur and trunk length, and bone density, have also been associated with increased risk [10−12].

A clear discrepancy exists between adiposity and its apparent effect on risk for pre- versus postmenopausal disease. Leanness is an acknowledged risk factor for premenopausal breast cancer, whereas obesity serves as a strong risk factor for postmenopausal disease [5]. A meta-analysis of cohort studies reported a 15% decreased risk of premenopausal breast cancer and a 8% increased risk of postmenopausal breast cancer per 5 kg/m^2 difference in body mass index (BMI) [13]. These risks are modified by (1) relative chronicity within the broad categories of pre- versus postmenopause (i.e., younger obese postmenopausal women may be at greatest risk [14]), (2) hormone-replacement therapy use (which may mask associations between obesity and postmenopausal disease) [14,15], and (3) genetic variation [16,17]. Studies also indicate that obesity is a strong risk factor only for estrogen receptor (ER) and progesterone receptor (PR) positive breast cancer [18,19]. The relationship between obesity and breast cancer risk in men is similar to the relationship observed in postmenopausal breast cancer in women [20,21].

There are several hypothesized mechanisms by which overweight and obesity confer risk for male and postmenopausal female breast cancer [22]. A classic hypothesis involves the increased peripheral aromatization of androgens within the adipose tissue, thus yielding increased levels of circulating estrogens. Studies show that obese women have significantly higher circulating levels of total testosterone, estrone, and estradiol, as well as higher free levels of these hormones [23,24], thus providing support for this premise.

Obesity also results in increased circulating levels of insulin and insulin-like growth factors, which stimulate intracellular signaling pathways and enhance proliferation of cancer cells [25]. For premenopausal breast cancer, in which increased skeletal structure is associated with risk, the IGF-1 pathway has also been implicated as a potentially viable mechanism [26]. Studies are ongoing to determine the role of leptin, adiponectin, interleukin-6, tumor necrosis factor, and other potential mediating factors that may have an impact on carcinogenesis via inflammation [27].

Diabetes has been associated with risk of many cancers, including postmenopausal breast cancer, although the exact mechanisms are unclear [28]. In a prospective analysis of 12,792 cancer-free participants in the Atherosclerosis Risk in Communities study, nondiabetic women with elevated glycated hemoglobin levels (hazard ratio (HR) = 1.24; 95% CI, 1.07−1.44) and diabetic women (HR = 1.30; 95% CI, 1.06−1.60) were at increased risk of breast cancer compared to nondiabetic women with normal glycated hemoglobin levels [29]. Similarly, in the Women's Health Initiative (WHI) Observational Study, fasting insulin levels were found to be positively associated with breast cancer risk (HR = 1.46; 95% CI, 1.00−2.13 for highest vs. lowest quartile of insulin level; p-trend = 0.02) [30]. The observation that cancer incidence is lower among individuals with diabetes taking metformin [31], which suppresses hepatic gluconeogenesis and increases insulin sensitivity in peripheral tissues, has led to a number of clinical trials of metformin as a breast cancer chemopreventive agent that are currently underway [25].

Because body weight fluctuates throughout life, it is conceivable that risk may be modified by body weight status at differing ages. Birth weight greater than 4000 g was associated with a small but statistically significant increased risk of breast cancer compared to birth weights between 2500 and 2599 g (odds ratio (OR) = 1.24; 95% CI, 1.04−1.48) [32]. Other studies that have explored obesity during childhood suggest that it may be protective [33,34], with one study suggesting that this relationship is particularly significant among females with a positive family history of breast cancer [35]. An analysis from the Nurses' Health Study (NHS) II [36] suggests that an increased BMI at age 18 years may be the strongest protective factor for premenopausal disease. A possible explanation for this unanticipated finding is that obese teenage girls have significantly fewer ovulatory cycles and therefore lower circulating levels of both estrogen and progesterone [37]. Weight gain and increased body weight in adulthood have consistently been found to be associated with increased risk for postmenopausal cancer

[38–40], although risk may be altered by use of hormone therapy and ethnicity [41,42]. Data from the European Prospective Investigation into Cancer (EPIC) study indicate an 8% increase in risk for each 5-kg gain among non-hormone therapy users [41], which may be largely explained by the fact that as women age, their circulating levels of estrogen become more influenced by estrogens produced by adipose tissue than those produced by the ovary [22]. Weight gain during adulthood is also more likely to be deposited in an android versus gynoid pattern and hence may promote insulin resistance and the increased production of insulin and insulin-like growth factors [43]. A meta-analysis (three cohort and eight case–control studies) found that adult weight gain was associated with statistically significant increased risk of both ER^+/PR^+ and ER^-/PR^- breast cancers, although the risk was higher for ER^+/PR^+ breast cancers (summarized risk estimate (RE) = 2.03; 95% CI, 1.62–2.45) than ER^-/PR^- tumors (RE = 1.34; 95% CI, 1.06–1.63) [44].

In contrast, studies that have investigated weight loss have found a protective effect [45]. Parker and Folsom [46] found a risk reduction for postmenopausal breast cancer of approximately 19% among women who intentionally lost 20 pounds or more during adulthood. Among women carrying the BRCA1 mutation, weight loss of 10 pounds or more between the ages of 18 and 30 years was associated with a risk reduction of approximately 50% [47].

Studies consistently show that abdominal obesity (primarily assessed via waist:hip ratio) is associated with increased risk of postmenopausal breast cancer; however, a 2007 meta-analysis by the WCRF/AICR found that these associations disappear when analyses are controlled for BMI [13]. Associations between central obesity and increased risk may still exist for select populations, such as Asians [48].

2 Dietary Composition

In ecologic studies, a fivefold difference in breast cancer mortality rates has been observed across countries, and dietary patterns may be one of the environmental exposures that differ across these countries [49]. Also, risk for breast cancer increases on relocation from low-risk countries to high-risk countries, concurrent with the adoption of the dietary and lifestyle patterns of the new locale [50].

The possible link between dietary fat intake and breast cancer risk has received the most attention. However, fat intake, total energy consumption, and adiposity are inextricably linked; therefore, demonstrating an independent effect of total dietary fat per se is a challenge [51]. A meta-analysis of data from five cohort studies showed no statistically significant association between dietary fat and breast cancer risk (RR = 1.06; 95% CI, 0.99–1.14) [13].

Various feeding studies and small diet intervention trials have examined the effect of dietary fat reduction on serum estrogen levels. Low-fat diets were associated with an average 13% reduction in serum estradiol concentrations in a meta-analysis of several small feeding studies [52]. However, significant weight loss occurred in most studies in which serum estradiol was significantly reduced, and dietary fiber was also concurrently increased in 8 of the 13 studies included in the analysis. Thus, an energy deficit, weight loss, or increased fiber intake are just as likely as fat to promote a reduction in hormone levels.

In the WHI randomized controlled dietary modification trial, the impact of a low-fat diet (< 20% of energy intake) was tested in comparison to a usual care control group as a potential means of reducing risk of breast cancer in 48,835 postmenopausal women during an 8-year follow-up period [53]. Adherence was an issue in both study arms, with those in the intervention arm having higher fat intakes than planned, and those in the control arm reporting reductions in intake such that the difference in fat intake between the two study arms was not as great as anticipated (i.e., a difference of only 10.7% in year 1 and 8.1% in year 2). Results indicate a nonsignificant impact on risk (HR = 0.91; 95% CI, 0.83–1.01). Similarly, the Canadian Diet and Breast Cancer Prevention Trial, a multicenter randomized controlled study that tested whether a low-fat (15% of energy), high-carbohydrate diet intervention could reduce the incidence of breast cancer among women with extensive mammographic density, found that a sustained reduction in dietary fat intake did not reduce breast cancer risk, even though the intervention group was able to decrease dietary fat intake from 30 to 20% of total energy intake and maintained a dietary fat intake that was 9 or 10% lower than that of the comparison group throughout the study [54].

The effect of dietary carbohydrates on breast cancer risk has also been evaluated. A meta-analysis of eight cohort studies found no association between glycemic index (GI) (RR = 1.06; 95% CI, 0.98–1.15 for highest vs. lowest subgroup) or glycemic load (GL) (RR = 0.99; 95% CI, 0.94–1.06 for highest vs. lowest subgroup) and breast cancer risk [55]. A second systematic review and meta-analysis published the same year also found no statistically significant associations between GI or GL and breast cancer risk among pre- or postmenopausal women [56]. Despite the significant limitations of GI and GL determinations in general [57], these findings suggest that weight management may be more effective in decreasing breast cancer risk than modifying dietary carbohydrate intake.

Dietary fiber has been hypothesized to exert a protective effect against breast cancer by binding estrogen in the enterohepatic circulation and hindering reabsorption [58]. However, studies that have examined the relationship between fiber intake and risk for breast cancer have generally not found a significant protective effect [13].

Several studies have examined the association between vegetable and fruit intake and breast cancer risk. A meta-analysis (21 case–control and 5 cohort studies) found that high (vs. low) consumption of vegetables exhibited a significant protective effect (RR = 0.75; 95% CI, 0.66–0.85), whereas fruit consumption was not associated with breast cancer risk [59]. A subsequent pooled analysis including 7377 incident breast cancer cases from 8 prospective cohort studies found a small and only marginally significant protective effect of total fruit and vegetable intake (RR = 0.93; 95% CI, 0.86–1.00 for highest vs. lowest quintiles) [60]. Although the median period of follow-up was only 5.3 years, the relationship between vegetable and fruit intake and breast cancer risk also was not significant in the EPIC study [61].

Studies in which tissue concentrations of carotenoids (a marker of vegetable and fruit intake) have been quantified and analyzed suggest a protective effect of higher concentrations of these compounds. In a report from the New York University Women's Health Study [62], α- and β-carotene, lutein, and β-cryptoxanthin levels were inversely associated with breast cancer risk. Similarly, an analysis from the WHI using repeated measures of serum carotenoids, retinol, and tocopherols at years 1, 3, and 6 of the study also found that breast cancer risk was inversely associated with serum α- and β-carotene levels but positively associated with γ-tocopherol levels [63]. In a pooled analysis of 18 prospective cohort studies, α- and β-carotene and lutein/zeaxanthin intakes were inversely associated with risk of ER$^-$ breast cancers but not ER$^+$ breast cancers [64].

Cell culture studies indicate that retinoids and carotenoids affect cellular differentiation and also inhibit mammary cell growth [65]. Antioxidants, such as vitamin C, may reduce the risk for breast cancer by protecting against DNA damage and other free radical-induced cellular changes associated with neoplasia. Vegetables of the *Brassica* genus, such as broccoli, may favorably alter estrogen metabolism via the induction of cytochrome P450 enzymes [66].

Countries that consume greater amounts of soy and soy products, mainly Asian countries, have historically exhibited the lowest breast cancer mortality rates, compared with the United States and most European countries [67]. Thus, the role of soy and soy isoflavones in breast cancer prevention has been investigated in numerous laboratory and epidemiological studies, but the findings remain inconclusive [13]. Soy is a rich source of phytoestrogens; however, they can act as both estrogen agonists and antagonists [68]. The inconsistent findings between Asian and non-Hispanic white study populations suggest that lifelong or early life soy intake may be necessary in order to observe the breast cancer protective effects [69].

Alcohol intake has been consistently and positively associated with breast cancer risk in epidemiological studies. Pooled analysis of data from six cohort studies indicates that alcohol exhibits a dose–response relationship with risk for breast cancer, at least up to 60 g/day (RR = 1.41; 95% CI, 1.18–1.69, for 30–60 g/day vs. no alcohol) [70]. Another meta-analysis confirmed these findings of an increased risk for breast cancer overall (RR = 1.10; 95% CI, 1.06–1.14, per 10 g alcohol/day), and when stratified by premenopausal (RR = 1.09; 95% CI, 1.01–1.17) and postmenopausal (RR = 1.08; 95% CI, 1.05–1.11) breast cancer [13]. The proposed biologic mechanism is that alcohol intake promotes increased serum estrogen levels, which then increase breast cancer risk. Studies of other beverages, such as coffee and tea, have found no association with breast cancer risk [13,71,72].

Although an association between folate intake per se and breast cancer risk has not been observed consistently in epidemiological studies, results from several cohort studies suggest that dietary folate intake may influence breast cancer risk through an interaction with alcohol [73–75]. Alcohol is known to interfere with folate metabolism [76]. A meta-analysis of two prospective cohort studies and two case–control studies found that high dietary folate intake (compared to low folate intake) was protective against breast cancer among women who had moderate to high alcohol intake (summary estimate = 0.51; 95% CI, 0.41–0.63) but not among women who reported low or no alcohol intake [75].

Vitamin D is known to have antiproliferative activity in a variety of cell types [77] and thus may decrease cancer risk. Prospective cohort studies consistently report decreased risks of breast cancer with increased vitamin D intake despite the relatively low intake of dietary vitamin D of the populations studied [78]. However, results vary across studies depending on the menopausal status of the participants and tumor characteristics. The NHS [79] observed decreasing incidence of breast cancer with increased intake of dietary or supplemental vitamin D, but only among premenopausal women (RR = 0.72; 95% CI, 0.55–0.94). A report based on the Women's Health Study also found reduced risk of breast cancer with total vitamin D at levels beginning above 230 IU among pre- but not postmenopausal women [80]. Results were stronger for premenopausal women with ER^+/PR^+ or more advanced stage tumors. In the Cancer Prevention Study (CPS) II Nutrition Cohort of postmenopausal women [81], a weak inverse association was observed between dietary vitamin D and breast cancer (RR = 0.87; 95% CI, 0.75–1.00, comparing >300 IU to ≤100 IU/day). However, the vitamin D associations were somewhat stronger for women diagnosed with ER^+ tumors. Among postmenopausal women participating in the Iowa Women's Health Study (IWHS) [82], those consuming ≥ 800 IU of vitamin D from diet and supplements had an 11% reduced risk of breast cancer. Findings were stronger for women with ER^- or *in situ* tumors.

Because diet is a complex, multidimensional, chronic exposure [83], there has been interest in evaluating dietary patterns and adherence scores for dietary recommendations as measures of overall diet quality. In an analysis of the NHS data, compliance with the Dietary Approaches to Stop Hypertension (DASH) diet was inversely related to risk of ER^- breast cancers, but no association was observed for risk of ER^+ tumors [84]. Similarly, a dietary pattern high in fruits and salads was associated with a reduced risk of breast cancer, especially ER^- and PR^- breast cancers, among participants in the Melbourne Collaborative Cohort Study [85]. Among Chinese women participating in the Shanghai Breast Cancer Study, a Western diet pattern ("meat–sweet" pattern: shrimp, chicken, beef, pork, candy, and desserts) was associated with an increased risk of breast cancer in postmenopausal women, especially with ER^+ tumors [86].

To date, only one small case–control study has explored the association between intake of selected foods and male breast cancer [87]. No statistically significant associations were reported; however, study design issues (e.g., small sample size, use of death index to identify cases, and use of next-of-kin interviews to assess dietary intake among cases) limit the ability to draw conclusions from this study, and further research is needed.

B Nutritional Factors and Breast Cancer Recurrence, Progression, and Survival

Breast cancer mortality has been declining in recent years—a trend that has been attributed to earlier diagnosis and improvements in treatment [1]. A majority of all breast cancers are now diagnosed at a localized stage, with 98% 5-year relative survival rates [1]. As a result, there are increasing numbers of women in the population who are breast cancer survivors and at risk for breast cancer recurrence. Women who have been diagnosed with breast cancer have higher rates of mortality from other causes, such as cardiovascular disease and diabetes—co-morbid factors in which diet and nutritional status play an important role [88].

1 Obesity and Overweight

Weight is the nutritional factor associated most consistently with mortality. Although several studies suggest that overweight and obesity may be linked to increased recurrence or to progressive disease [89–92], findings are somewhat mixed with regard to these outcomes [93–95]. However, because overweight is associated with several other chronic diseases, data are fairly consistent regarding overall survival, for which normal-weight women demonstrate a significant advantage [96]. Findings by Pierce and colleagues [97] suggest that physical activity may be more important than weight in conferring a survival advantage; however, further study is needed. Compared to those who are overweight, normal-weight women experience significantly fewer surgical complications [98,99], less lymphedema [100,101], and fewer thromboembolic events while on hormonal therapy [102]. Studies exploring body fat distribution in relation to survival or co-morbid conditions have yielded mixed findings [96,103–105].

Weight gain after the diagnosis of breast cancer is a common occurrence and may be undesirable for several reasons. First, weight gain may negatively affect quality of life [106]. Second, weight gain may predispose women to other chronic conditions, such as hypertension, cardiovascular disease, diabetes, and impaired mobility [107]. Finally, weight gain may adversely affect disease-free survival. Kroenke and colleagues [108] found that breast cancer survivors who increased their BMI by 0.5–2 units had an RR of recurrence of 1.40 (95% CI, 1.02–1.92), and those who gained more than 2.0 BMI units had an RR of 1.53 (95% CI, 1.54–2.34); both groups also experienced significantly higher all-cause mortality. In contrast, Caan and colleagues [93] found no evidence of increased mortality with weight gain in a cohort of 3215 early stage breast cancer patients. More study is needed in this area, especially to determine the impact of weight-loss interventions on survival and other short- and long-term outcomes.

Reports of mean weight gain during chemotherapy vary considerably but typically range from 1 to 5 kg [109]. Some have reported that as many as 20% of women gain 5 kg or more [110]. Weight gain is most prevalent among premenopausal patients receiving adjuvant chemotherapy and may vary by treatment regimen, with anthracycline agents associated with greater gains [109,111,112]. Several groups have conducted weight-loss interventions among women with breast cancer, with success rates differing by type and duration of intervention. Differential effects were found for individual diet counseling by a dietitian, with one study showing significantly favorable effects on body weight status [113] and the other showing no effect [114]. Djuric and colleagues [115] found that counseling by a dietitian was most effective if combined with a structured group weight-loss program that included exercise. Behavioral interventions that utilize a comprehensive approach to energy balance by including both diet and exercise components may be more effective than interventions relying on either component alone. Goodwin *et al.* [116] found that exercise was the strongest predictor of weight loss among early stage breast cancer patients receiving a diet and exercise intervention during the time of treatment and extended throughout the year following diagnosis. Exercise (especially strength training exercise) may be of particular importance for cancer survivors because it is considered the cornerstone of treatment for sarcopenic obesity (gain of adipose tissue at the expense of lean body mass), a documented side effect of both chemotherapy and hormonal therapy [111].

2 Dietary Composition

Observational studies of the relationship between fat intake and survival after a breast cancer diagnosis have reported inconsistent findings, with some studies reporting inverse associations between survival and dietary fat intake at diagnosis [117−119], whereas others [120−122] have found no association.

Protective effects of vegetables and fruits and the micronutrients provided by these foods (e.g., vitamin C and carotenoids) have been observed in several of these cohort studies, with findings somewhat more consistent than those for dietary fat, although the strength of the association is modest. Several studies reported significant inverse associations between fruit and vegetable intake and risk of death [117,118], two found that risk of dying was nonsignificantly decreased in association with frequent vegetable consumption [123,124], and one found a significant inverse association in women with node-negative disease, who comprised 62% of that cohort (but not in the total group, which included women at all stages of invasive breast cancer) [121]. In the studies that found an inverse relationship with survival and intakes of vegetables, fruit, and related nutrients (β-carotene and vitamin C), the magnitude of the protective effect was a 20−90% reduction in risk for death. In a cohort study involving 1511 women previously diagnosed and treated for breast cancer, women in the highest quartile of plasma total carotenoid concentration had an estimated 43% reduction in risk for a new breast cancer event (recurrence or new primary) compared to women in the lowest quintile [125]. In the same cohort, breast cancer survivors who reported consuming five or more daily servings of vegetables and fruit and exercised at least at a moderate level 30 minutes nearly every day had a 50% reduction in risk associated with these healthy lifestyles [97]. An overall dietary pattern characterized by higher intakes of vegetables, fruit, whole grains, and low-fat dairy products was not related to all-cause or breast cancer mortality but was related to a significantly lower risk of mortality from other causes during a 20-year follow-up period in another cohort of 2619 women [126].

Although alcohol intake has been identified as a risk factor for primary breast cancer, the effect on breast cancer recurrence or survival is unclear, with studies reporting increased [127−130] or decreased [97,119,131,132] risk of death, as well as no association [121,133,134]. The Collaborative Women's Longevity Study ($N = 4441$) found a statistically significant trend toward lower risk of death with higher alcohol consumption (p-trend $= 0.01$) but no association with breast cancer-specific survival [119]. In contrast, the Life after Cancer Epidemiology (LACE) study ($N = 1897$) found that consuming three or more alcoholic drinks per week was associated with increased risk of breast cancer recurrence, especially among postmenopausal and overweight/obese women [130]. One study ($N = 472$ with a history of early stage breast cancer) found that beer intake was directly related to risk for recurrence (but not survival), and wine and hard liquor intake were unrelated to risk for either outcome [127].

Two multicenter randomized controlled intervention trials have tested whether diet modification can influence the risk for recurrence and overall survival following the diagnosis of early stage breast cancer. In the Women's Intervention Nutrition Study (WINS), which involved 2437 postmenopausal women randomized within 12 months of primary surgery, the primary dietary goal was a reduction in dietary fat intake (<15% energy from fat) [135]. Women in the intervention arm in WINS reported a reduction in fat intake (33.3 g/day vs. 51.3 g/day in the control group), which was associated with an average 6-pound weight loss. The HR of relapse events in the intervention group compared with the control group was 0.76 (95% CI, 0.60−0.98) after approximately 5 years of follow-up [136]. Results of secondary analysis suggest a greater protective effect among women with hormone receptor-negative breast cancers compared with women whose cancers were hormone receptor-positive. In the Women's Healthy Eating and Living (WHEL) study, the target population consisted of 3088 pre- and postmenopausal women who had been diagnosed with breast cancer within the preceding 4 years and who had completed initial therapies. The primary emphasis of the WHEL study diet intervention was on increased vegetable and fruit intake, with daily dietary goals of five vegetable servings, 16 ounces of vegetable juice or equivalent, three fruit servings, 15–20% energy intake from fat, and 30 g dietary fiber. Feasibility study reports and trial data from this study indicated excellent adherence [137,138], and increased intake of vegetables and fruit in the intensive intervention group was validated by plasma carotenoid concentrations [139]. Overall findings indicated no significant differences in risks for recurrence or survival in the intensive intervention versus the control group during a mean 7.3-year follow-up [140]. Notably, the study participants reported at baseline an average daily consumption of 7.3 servings of vegetables and fruit, which actually meets or exceeds current recommendations, so the WHEL study results mainly indicate that an extraordinarily high intake of vegetables and fruit does not appear to further reduce risk for recurrence.

The effect of dietary patterns on breast cancer recurrence and survival has been evaluated in several large cancer survivor cohorts. Higher adherence to a prudent diet pattern (high intakes of fruits, vegetables, whole grains, and poultry) was not associated with recurrence but was associated with significantly improved survival among participants in the LACE study [141]. In the NHS, higher intake of a prudent dietary pattern and lower intake of a Western dietary pattern was associated with lower risk of death unrelated to breast cancer [126]. These findings are not surprising given the known beneficial effects of the prudent diet pattern in the prevention of chronic disease, especially cardiovascular disease, for which breast cancer survivors are at increased risk [88].

III ENDOMETRIAL CANCER

Cancer of the endometrium (uterine corpus) is the most common invasive gynecologic cancer [142]. Similar to breast and ovarian cancers, endometrial cancer is most common after menopause and is more prevalent among non-Hispanic whites, although blacks have higher rates of mortality. Relative 5-year survival rates are 96, 68, and 17% for cancers diagnosed at local, regional, and distant stages, respectively [1].

Endometrial cancers are stratified histologically by responsiveness to estrogen, with the estrogen-dependent type I being most common (90% of cases) and the non-estrogen-dependent type II being less common (10% of cases) [143,144]. Type I tumors are typically low grade and have a good prognosis, whereas type II tumors are more aggressive, tend to be diagnosed in later stages, and are associated with poor prognosis [145]. High cumulative exposure to estrogen is the major risk factor for type I endometrial cancer, whereas exposure to progesterone is protective [1]. Hence, early menarche, late menopause, and nulliparity are risk factors for type I endometrial cancer, just as they are for breast and ovarian cancers [1]. However, unlike these cancers, risk factors for type I endometrial cancer also include tamoxifen use and factors associated with unopposed estrogens [146]. Risk factors for type II endometrial cancer are less well understood because most of the epidemiology study cohorts currently have too few cases to evaluate these tumors separately.

A Nutritional Factors and Endometrial Cancer Risk

1 Height, Weight, and Body Fat Distribution

The link between obesity and endometrial cancer risk is well-established. A 2007 meta-analysis of 23 cohort studies conducted by the WCRF/AICR found that endometrial cancer risk increased by 52% per 5 kg/m^2 increase in BMI [13]. Research suggests that biomarkers associated with adiposity, such as higher circulating levels of leptin and insulin-like growth factors and lower levels of adiponectin, may also be independently linked with increased endometrial cancer risk [142]. Data from two large cohort studies (EPIC and the AARP Diet and Health Study) suggest that waist circumferences greater than 88 cm and increased waist-to-hip ratio are associated with increased endometrial cancer risk, independent of body weight status [147,148]. Both studies also found that compared to women who are weight stable, those who gain at least 20 kg during adulthood have an increased risk that is roughly two or three times higher [147,148]. Given the strong associations between endometrial cancer and obesity and other markers of adiposity, it is somewhat surprising that intentional weight loss of ≥ 20 kg was found to be associated with a nonsignificant risk reduction of only 4% among women participating in the IWHS [46]. Although a BMI ≥ 30 was associated with increased risk of type II endometrial cancer (RR = 2.87; 95% CI, 1.59–5.16) in the CPS-II Nutrition Cohort [149], women with the non-estrogen-dependent type II endometrial cancer are less likely to be obese (OR = 0.45; 95% CI, 0.29–0.70) compared to women with type I endometrial cancer [150].

In the Netherlands Cohort Study (NCS; 226 cases within a cohort of 62,573), an increased risk of endometrial cancer (RR = 2.57; 95% CI, 1.32–4.99) was found for women who were at least 175 cm in height compared to those measuring 160 cm or less [151]. This association is similar and of the same magnitude as found between height and breast cancer, and it points to the potential role of growth factors and early nutritional status in the etiology of this disease.

2 Dietary Composition

Although obesity is clearly a strong risk factor for endometrial cancer, there is significantly less research available related to specific dietary components and risk of endometrial cancer. Several large cohort studies [152–154] found no associations with carbohydrate intake and either an absence or very weak association between GI or GL and endometrial cancer risk. However, these factors may increase risk for obese versus normal-weight women [152,153] or for nondiabetic women versus women with diabetes [154]. Similarly, two cohort studies found no association between dietary fat intake and endometrial cancer risk [155,156]. A meta-analysis conducted by a workgroup of the International Agency for Research on Cancer (World Health Organization) found no association between fruit and vegetable consumption and endometrial cancer risk (OR = 1.03; 95% CI, 0.9–1.17) [157]. Similarly, few associations for individual plant food constituents, such as lycopene or fiber, have been reported; however, a study by Horn-Ross and colleagues [158] suggests that isoflavones may be protective (RR = 0.59; 95% CI, 0.37–0.93 for highest vs. lowest quartiles). In this study, obesity was found to interact with phytoestrogen intake, suggesting a sevenfold increase in risk among obese women with the lowest intakes of phytoestrogens.

Whereas Jain *et al.* [155] found no association between folic acid intake and endometrial cancer risk in general among the Canadian National Breast Screening Study cohort, a report from the IWHS cohort [159] stratified endometrial cancer cases by histologic stage. No associations were observed for type I endometrial cancer; however, for type II endometrial cancer, dietary or supplemental folate, methionine, and vitamins B_2, B_6, and B_{12} were associated with increased risk [159].

Finally, although reports from case–control studies suggest a protective benefit of various foods, such as coffee [160] and fatty fish [161], or nutrients, such as vitamin C [162], calcium [160,163], and vitamin D [163], further research is necessary to corroborate these findings. Cohort studies have reported no association with endometrial cancer risk for vitamin A [155], serum retinol [164], vitamin C [155], or vitamin E [155].

Alcohol use has been shown to be associated with elevated circulating estrogen levels and reduced progesterone; however, a meta-analysis found no association between alcohol intake and endometrial cancer risk among cohort or case–control studies [13]. Small sample sizes, limited range of alcohol intake, and confounding factors (e.g., possible interaction with exogenous estrogens or factors such as age) may have limited the ability to detect associations [165,166]. In addition, no study to date has evaluated potential differences in risk by the two histologic subtypes. Thus, more research is needed to clarify the role of alcohol in the etiology of this cancer.

B Nutritional Factors and Endometrial Cancer Recurrence, Progression, and Survival

Comparatively little is known regarding nutritional issues after the diagnosis of endometrial cancer, although research on this topic is increasing. Data regarding the effect of obesity on recurrence, disease-free survival, and overall survival are conflicting. For example, obesity was found to be unassociated with recurrence in one study [167] but inversely associated with recurrence in two others [168,169]. Furthermore, in two studies conducted in the United States, obesity was associated with increased overall mortality [167,170], whereas in a smaller study conducted in Poland, it was found to be protective [171]. Thus, the only consensus regarding obesity and survivorship of endometrial cancer relates to co-morbid conditions, in which obesity was found to be associated with the increased prevalence of diabetes, hypertension, and pulmonary disease [168,170] and was also found to be consistently associated with poorer quality of life [172–174].

To date, no studies have investigated other nutritional issues beyond weight status in endometrial cancer survivors. However, the Survivors of Uterine Cancer Empowered by Exercise and Health Diet (SUCCEED) intervention study is currently underway and will evaluate the effect of a dietary intervention (2 cups fruit, 2.5 cups vegetables, three servings of low-fat dairy foods, and three servings whole grain foods per day) on quality of life and treatment outcomes [175].

IV OVARIAN CANCER

Ovarian cancer is the most lethal of the gynecologic cancers, being the fifth most common cause of cancer death among U.S. women despite having a relatively low incidence rate [1]. Women diagnosed with ovarian cancer typically present at an advanced stage of the disease because the early stages are asymptomatic. The established risk factors for ovarian cancer are older age (>50 years), low parity, never having used oral contraceptives, and having a family history of breast or ovarian cancer [176,177]. Although the etiology is still a focus of intense investigation, one theory is that increased ovulation or hormonal stimulation of ovarian epithelial cells plays a role in the development of ovarian cancer [178,179]. Prevention strategies for women at high risk include oral contraceptive use, tubal ligation, and prophylactic oophorectomy [180]. Relatively few studies on the relationship between nutritional factors and risk for ovarian cancer have been reported, and there is a dearth of research that examines how these factors may influence progression or survival after the diagnosis of ovarian cancer.

A Nutritional Factors and Ovarian Cancer Risk

1 Height, Weight, and Body Fat Distribution

Anthropometric factors have been studied extensively with regard to ovarian cancer risk but remain inconclusive. A pooled analysis of 12 prospective cohort studies (2036 ovarian cancer cases among 531,583 women) found that adult attained height of ≥ 170 cm (67 in.) was associated with an increased risk of ovarian cancer (RR = 1.38; 95% CI, 1.16−1.65) [181]. BMI was not associated with ovarian cancer risk in postmenopausal women, but premenopausal women with a BMI ≥ 30 kg/m^2 were at increased risk of ovarian cancer (RR = 1.72; 95% CI, 1.02−2.89) compared to women with a BMI between 18.5 and 23 kg/m^2 [181]. In contrast, the EPIC study (611 ovarian cancer cases among 226,798 women) found that BMI ≥ 30 kg/m^2 was associated with increased risk for all women combined (HR = 1.3; 95% CI, 1.05−1.68); however, when stratified by menopausal status, the observed increase in risk was only statistically significant among postmenopausal women [182]. Attained adult height, weight change during adulthood, and measures of body fat distribution (waist circumference, waist:hip ratio, or hip circumference) were not found to be associated with risk of ovarian cancer [182]. The findings suggest that the relationship between obesity and ovarian cancer risk may differ from the relationships observed between obesity and risk for either postmenopausal breast cancer or endometrial cancer.

2 Dietary Composition

Similar to the evidence for breast cancer, international comparisons of the incidence of ovarian cancer indicate a strong inverse relationship with per capita dietary fat consumption [183], and the hypothesis that dietary fat intake is associated with increased circulating estrogen concentrations (discussed previously) has stimulated several observational studies of the relationship between dietary fat intake and risk for ovarian cancer. However, a pooled analysis of 12 prospective cohort studies (2132 cases of epithelial ovarian cancer among 523,217 women) found no association between total fat, mono- or polyunsaturated fats, trans unsaturated fat, cholesterol, animal or vegetable fat, or egg

intake and ovarian cancer risk [184]. Similarly, data from the NCS (340 ovarian cancer cases among 62,573 postmenopausal women) found no association between total fat, saturated fat, mono- or polyunsaturated fat, or fat source (animal, plant, dairy, meat, or fish) and ovarian cancer risk; however, trans unsaturated fatty acid intake was found to be associated with increased risk of ovarian cancer (RR = 1.51; 95% CI, 1.04−2.20 for highest vs. lowest quintile) [185].

Dietary carbohydrate has been less well studied with respect to ovarian cancer risk. A report from the Canadian National Breast Screening Study (264 ovarian cancer cases among 49,613 women) found that GL was positively associated with ovarian cancer risk (HR = 1.72; 95% CI, 1.13−2.62); however, dietary carbohydrate, sugar intake, and GI were not associated with ovarian cancer risk [186]. A study from the Swedish Women's Lifestyle and Health Cohort (163 ovarian cancer cases among 47,140 women) found no association between dietary fiber and ovarian cancer risk [187].

A report from the NHS found that women who consumed at least 2.5 servings of vegetables and fruit as adolescents had a 46% reduction in risk for ovarian cancer [188], although adult vegetable and fruit intake was unrelated to ovarian cancer risk. A subsequent evaluation of specific dietary flavonoids in this same cohort found no association for total flavonoid intake; however, a statistically significant decrease in ovarian cancer risk was observed for the highest versus lowest quintile of kaempferol intake (RR = 0.75; 95% CI, 0.49−0.91) [189]. These findings were consistent with inverse associations with ovarian cancer observed for nonherbal tea and broccoli (the primary contributors of kaempferol intake in the cohort). Among participants in the California Teachers Study (280 ovarian cancer cases among 97,275 women), women consuming >3 mg/day of soy isoflavones had a significantly decreased risk of ovarian cancer (RR = 0.56; 95% CI, 0.33−0.96) compared to those consuming <1 mg total isoflavones/day [190]. Dietary carotenoids were not associated with ovarian cancer risk in two large prospective cohort studies [188,191].

One small prospective cohort study (35 cases and 67 controls) examined associations between serum concentrations of micronutrients and risk for ovarian cancer [192] using sera collected prior to diagnosis. It found no relationship between risk and serum retinol, β-carotene, lycopene, and lipid-adjusted α-tocopherol and γ-tocopherol concentrations, but serum selenium concentration was inversely associated with risk of ovarian cancer among cases diagnosed 4 or more years after blood collections (p-trend = 0.02) [192]. In contrast to these findings linking serum selenium to risk, another prospective study did not find an association between toenail selenium level and ovarian cancer risk

[193]. A large pooled analysis of data from seven prospective cohort studies found no association between serum 25-hydroxyvitamin D levels and ovarian cancer risk [194].

A meta-analysis of two cohort and seven case—control studies found no association between tea intake and ovarian cancer risk (RR = 0.84; 95% CI, 0.66—1.07) [195]; however, important limitations, such as lack of detailed assessment of type of tea consumed, frequency of tea consumption, and duration of tea intake, limit the ability to make a firm conclusion [196]. A meta-analysis of five cohort studies found a statistically significant decrease in risk of ovarian cancer with higher versus lower tea consumption (RR = 0.71; 95% CI, 0.55—0.93), and it also found a marginally increased risk for higher versus lower coffee consumption (RR = 1.32; 95% CI, 0.99—1.77) among four cohort studies [197]. A subsequent report from the IWHS (266 ovarian cancer cases among 29,060 postmenopausal women) supported those findings by observing that women who consumed five or more cups per day of caffeinated coffee were at increased risk of ovarian cancer compared to non-users (HR = 1.81; 95% CI, 1.10—2.95) [198].

B Nutritional Factors and Ovarian Cancer Recurrence, Progression, and Survival

Only a small number of studies have examined nutritional factors related to survival after an ovarian cancer diagnosis. A meta-analysis found no association between obesity at the time of diagnosis and subsequent prognosis [199]. Similarly, a retrospective review of 792 advanced ovarian cancer patients participating in a randomized clinical trial of cisplatin/paclitaxel versus carboplatin/paclitaxel found no association between pre-chemotherapy BMI and survival; however, weight gain during treatment was associated with a statistically significant improvement in overall survival (68.2 vs. 48.0 months for >5% increase vs. >5% decrease, $p = 0.01$) [200]. A study of 198 advanced ovarian cancer patients undergoing primary surgery and adjuvant chemotherapy found that weight change in the 6 months after completion of treatment had no effect on progression-free or overall survival [201].

In a prospective cohort study of 609 women with invasive epithelial ovarian cancer, a statistically significant survival advantage was observed for women who reported higher vegetable intake in general (HR = 0.75; 95% CI, 0.57—0.99) and cruciferous vegetables in particular (HR = 0.75; 95% CI, 0.57—0.98) [202]. A longitudinal study of 341 women with ovarian cancer found that women who consumed diets higher in total fruits at baseline had a significantly decreased likelihood of

death during the follow-up period (HR = 0.61; 95% CI, 0.38—0.98), whereas women who consumed diets high in meats (HR = 2.28; 95% CI, 1.34—3.89) or milk (HR = 2.15; 95% CI, 1.2—3.84) were at increased likelihood of death [203].

V SUMMARY AND CONCLUSION

Although a considerable amount of research has been devoted to understanding the effects of nutritional factors on the risk for breast cancer, much remains to be learned. More research on the relationships between these factors and risk for endometrial and ovarian cancers is sorely needed, and to date, few studies have examined how these factors may influence overall survival in women who have been diagnosed with hormone-related cancers. At this time, guidelines from the American Cancer Society [204,205] and the WCRF/AICR [13] form the basis of current dietary recommendations, with both groups emphasizing the importance of achieving and maintaining a healthy weight; eating a diet rich in vegetables, fruits, and whole grains; and limiting meat and alcohol consumption.

The risk for morbidity and mortality from causes other than breast, endometrial, and ovarian cancer should also be considered in dietary recommendations for women and men at risk for cancer and for cancer survivors, especially those diagnosed with early stage cancers [107]. For example, although evidence to support a link between fat intake and breast cancer risk and prognosis is inconsistent, limiting saturated fat intake is an established strategy to reduce risk for cardiovascular disease. Similarly, eating a diet with adequate dietary fiber has been associated with decreased risk of coronary heart disease and may contribute to overall health [206], irrespective of a specific link between fiber and hormone-related cancers. Diets that emphasize vegetables, fruit, whole grains, low-fat dairy foods, and lean meats and poultry have been associated with decreased risk of all-cause mortality [207].

References

[1] American Cancer Society, Cancer Facts & Figures 2011, American Cancer Society, Atlanta, 2011.

[2] I.S. Fentiman, A. Fourquet, G.N. Hortobagyi, Male breast cancer, Lancet 367 (2006) 595—604.

[3] A.H. Eliassen, S.E. Hankinson, Endogenous hormone levels and risk of breast, endometrial and ovarian cancers: prospective studies, Adv. Exp. Med. Biol. 630 (2008) 148—165.

[4] E.J. Gallagher, D. LeRoith, Minireview: IGF, insulin, and cancer, Endocrinology 152 (2011) 2546—2551.

[5] World Cancer Research Fund/American Institute for Cancer Research, Continuous Update Report Summary: Food, Nutrition and Physical Activity and the Prevention of Breast Cancer, World Cancer Research Fund/American Institute for Cancer Research, Washington, DC, 2010.

[6] D. Heng, F. Gao, R. Jong, E. Fishell, M. Yaffe, L. Martin, et al., Risk factors for breast cancer associated with mammographic features in Singaporean Chinese women, Cancer Epidemiol. Biomarkers Prev. 13 (2004) 1751–1758.

[7] M. Ahlgren, M. Melbye, J. Wohlfahrt, T.I. Sorensen, Growth patterns and the risk of breast cancer in women, Int. J. Gynecol. Cancer 16 (Suppl. 2) (2006) 569–575.

[8] B.L. De Stavola, I. dos Santos Silva, V. McCormack, R.J. Hardy, D.J. Kuh, M.E. Wadsworth, Childhood growth and breast cancer, Am. J. Epidemiol. 159 (2004) 671–682.

[9] S. Silva Idos, B. De Stavola, V. McCormack, Birth size and breast cancer risk: re-analysis of individual participant data from 32 studies, PLoS Med. 5 (2008) e193.

[10] L.A. Brinton, C.A. Swanson, Height and weight at various ages and risk of breast cancer, Ann. Epidemiol. 2 (1992) 597–609.

[11] D.A. Lawlor, M. Okasha, D. Gunnell, G.D. Smith, S. Ebrahim, Associations of adult measures of childhood growth with breast cancer: findings from the British Women's Heart and Health Study, Br. J. Cancer 89 (2003) 81–87.

[12] R. Mondina, G. Borsellino, S. Poma, M. Baroni, B. Di Nubila, P. Sacchi, Breast carcinoma and skeletal formation, Eur. J. Cancer 28A (1992) 1068–1070.

[13] World Cancer Research Fund/American Institute for Cancer Research, Food, Nutrition, Physical Activity, and the Prevention of Cancer: A Global Perspective, American Institute for Cancer Research, Washington, DC, 2007.

[14] L.M. Morimoto, E. White, Z. Chen, R.T. Chlebowski, J. Hays, L. Kuller, et al., Obesity, body size, and risk of postmenopausal breast cancer: the Women's Health Initiative (United States), Cancer Causes Control 13 (2002) 741–751.

[15] F. Modugno, K.E. Kip, B. Cochrane, L. Kuller, T.L. Klug, T.E. Rohan, et al., Obesity, hormone therapy, estrogen metabolism and risk of postmenopausal breast cancer, Int. J. Cancer 118 (2006) 1292–1301.

[16] L. Wasserman, S.W. Flatt, L. Natarajan, G. Laughlin, M. Matusalem, S. Faerber, et al., Correlates of obesity in postmenopausal women with breast cancer: comparison of genetic, demographic, disease-related, life history and dietary factors, Int. J. Obes. Relat. Metab. Disord. 28 (2004) 49–56.

[17] C. Liu, L. Liu, Polymorphisms in three obesity-related genes (LEP, LEPR, and PON1) and breast cancer risk: a meta-analysis, Tumour Biol. 32 (2011) 1233–1240.

[18] G.A. Colditz, B.A. Rosner, W.Y. Chen, M.D. Holmes, S.E. Hankinson, Risk factors for breast cancer according to estrogen and progesterone receptor status, J. Natl. Cancer Inst. 96 (2004) 218–228.

[19] R. Suzuki, T. Rylander-Rudqvist, W. Ye, S. Saji, A. Wolk, Body weight and postmenopausal breast cancer risk defined by estrogen and progesterone receptor status among Swedish women: a prospective cohort study, Int. J. Cancer 119 (2006) 1683–1689.

[20] L.A. Brinton, J.D. Carreon, G.L. Gierach, K.A. McGlynn, G. Gridley, Etiologic factors for male breast cancer in the U.S. Veterans Affairs medical care system database, Breast Cancer Res. Treat. 119 (2010) 185–192.

[21] J.R. Weiss, K.B. Moysich, H. Swede, Epidemiology of male breast cancer, Cancer Epidemiol. Biomarkers Prev. 14 (2005) 20–26.

[22] A.M. Lorincz, S. Sukumar, Molecular links between obesity and breast cancer, Endocr. Relat. Cancer 13 (2006) 279–292.

[23] A. McTiernan, K.B. Rajan, S.S. Tworoger, M. Irwin, L. Bernstein, R. Baumgartner, et al., Adiposity and sex hormones in postmenopausal breast cancer survivors, J. Clin. Oncol. 21 (2003) 1961–1966.

[24] S. Rinaldi, T.J. Key, P.H. Peeters, P.H. Lahmann, A. Lukanova, L. Dossus, et al., Anthropometric measures, endogenous sex steroids and breast cancer risk in postmenopausal women: a study within the EPIC cohort, Int. J. Cancer 118 (2006) 2832–2839.

[25] P.J. Goodwin, V. Stambolic, Obesity and insulin resistance in breast cancer: chemoprevention strategies with a focus on metformin, Breast 20 (Suppl. 3) (2011) S31–S35.

[26] E.S. Schernhammer, J.M. Holly, M.N. Pollak, S.E. Hankinson, Circulating levels of insulin-like growth factors, their binding proteins, and breast cancer risk, Cancer Epidemiol. Biomarkers Prev. 14 (2005) 699–704.

[27] C.M. Perks, J.M. Holly, Hormonal mechanisms underlying the relationship between obesity and breast cancer, Endocrinol. Metab. Clin. North Am. 40 (2011) 485–507, vii.

[28] C. La Vecchia, S.H. Giordano, G.N. Hortobagyi, B. Chabner, Overweight, obesity, diabetes, and risk of breast cancer: interlocking pieces of the puzzle, Oncologist 16 (2011) 726–729.

[29] C.E. Joshu, A.E. Prizment, P.J. Dluzniewski, A. Menke, A.R. Folsom, J. Coresh, et al., Glycated hemoglobin and cancer incidence and mortality in the Atherosclerosis in Communities (ARIC) study, 1990–2006, Int. J. Cancer (2011) [Epub ahead of print].

[30] M.J. Gunter, D.R. Hoover, H. Yu, S. Wassertheil-Smoller, T.E. Rohan, J.E. Manson, et al., Insulin, insulin-like growth factor-I, and risk of breast cancer in postmenopausal women, J. Natl. Cancer Inst. 101 (2009) 48–60.

[31] A. Decensi, M. Puntoni, P. Goodwin, M. Cazzaniga, A. Gennari, B. Bonanni, et al., Metformin and cancer risk in diabetic patients: a systematic review and meta-analysis, Cancer Prev. Res. (Philadelphia) 3 (2010) 1451–1461.

[32] S.K. Park, D. Kang, K.A. McGlynn, M. Garcia-Closas, Y. Kim, K.Y. Yoo, et al., Intrauterine environments and breast cancer risk: meta-analysis and systematic review, Breast Cancer Res. 10 (2008) R8.

[33] K.B. Michels, F. Xue, K.L. Terry, W.C. Willett, Longitudinal study of birthweight and the incidence of breast cancer in adulthood, Carcinogenesis 27 (2006) 2464–2468.

[34] H.J. Baer, G.A. Colditz, B. Rosner, K.B. Michels, J.W. Rich-Edwards, D.J. Hunter, et al., Body fatness during childhood and adolescence and incidence of breast cancer in premenopausal women: a prospective cohort study, Breast Cancer Res. 7 (2005) R314–R325.

[35] E. Weiderpass, T. Braaten, C. Magnusson, M. Kumle, H. Vainio, E. Lund, et al., A prospective study of body size in different periods of life and risk of premenopausal breast cancer, Cancer Epidemiol. Biomarkers Prev. 13 (2004) 1121–1127.

[36] K.B. Michels, K.L. Terry, W.C. Willett, Longitudinal study on the role of body size in premenopausal breast cancer, Arch. Intern. Med. 166 (2006) 2395–2402.

[37] B.A. Stoll, Impaired ovulation and breast cancer risk, Eur. J. Cancer 33 (1997) 1532–1535.

[38] K.L. Radimer, R. Ballard-Barbash, J.S. Miller, M.P. Fay, A. Schatzkin, R. Troiano, et al., Weight change and the risk of late-onset breast cancer in the original Framingham cohort, Nutr. Cancer 49 (2004) 7–13.

[39] A.H. Eliassen, G.A. Colditz, B. Rosner, W.C. Willett, S.E. Hankinson, Adult weight change and risk of postmenopausal breast cancer, JAMA 296 (2006) 193–201.

[40] J. Ahn, A. Schatzkin, J.V. Lacey Jr., D. Albanes, R. Ballard-Barbash, K.F. Adams, et al., Adiposity, adult weight change, and postmenopausal breast cancer risk, Arch. Intern. Med. 167 (2007) 2091–2102.

[41] P.H. Lahmann, M. Schulz, K. Hoffmann, H. Boeing, A. Tjonneland, A. Olsen, et al., Long-term weight change and breast cancer risk: the European Prospective Investigation into Cancer and Nutrition (EPIC), Br. J. Cancer 93 (2005) 582–589.

[42] M.L. Slattery, C. Sweeney, S. Edwards, J. Herrick, K. Baumgartner, R. Wolff, et al., Body size, weight change, fat distribution and breast cancer risk in Hispanic and non-Hispanic white women, Breast Cancer Res. Treat. 102 (2007) 85–101.

[43] B.A. Stoll, Upper abdominal obesity, insulin resistance and breast cancer risk, Int. J. Obes. Relat. Metab. Disord. 26 (2002) 747–753.

[44] A. Vrieling, K. Buck, R. Kaaks, J. Chang-Claude, Adult weight gain in relation to breast cancer risk by estrogen and progesterone receptor status: a meta-analysis, Breast Cancer Res. Treat. 123 (2010) 641–649.

[45] A. Howell, M. Chapman, M. Harvie, Energy restriction for breast cancer prevention, Recent Results Cancer Res. 181 (2009) 97–111.

[46] E.D. Parker, A.R. Folsom, Intentional weight loss and incidence of obesity-related cancers: the Iowa Women's Health Study, Int. J. Obes. Relat. Metab. Disord. 27 (2003) 1447–1452.

[47] J. Kotsopoulos, O.I. Olopado, P. Ghadirian, J. Lubinski, H.T. Lynch, C. Isaacs, et al., Changes in body weight and the risk of breast cancer in BRCA1 and BRCA2 mutation carriers, Breast Cancer Res. 7 (2005) R833–R843.

[48] A.H. Wu, M.C. Yu, C.C. Tseng, M.C. Pike, Body size, hormone therapy and risk of breast cancer in Asian-American women, Int. J. Cancer 120 (2007) 844–852.

[49] H.E. Kesteloot, J. Zhang, Differences in breast cancer mortality worldwide: unsolved problems, Eur. J. Cancer Prev. 15 (2006) 416–423.

[50] L.N. Kolonel, D. Altshuler, B.E. Henderson, The multiethnic cohort study: exploring genes, lifestyle and cancer risk, Nat. Rev. Cancer 4 (2004) 519–527.

[51] D.J. Hunter, Role of dietary fat in the causation of breast cancer: counterpoint, Cancer Epidemiol. Biomarkers Prev. 8 (1999) 9–13.

[52] A.H. Wu, M.C. Pike, D.O. Stram, Meta-analysis: dietary fat intake, serum estrogen levels, and the risk of breast cancer, J. Natl. Cancer Inst. 91 (1999) 529–534.

[53] R.L. Prentice, B. Caan, R.T. Chlebowski, R. Patterson, L.H. Kuller, J.K. Ockene, et al., Low-fat dietary pattern and risk of invasive breast cancer: the Women's Health Initiative Randomized Controlled Dietary Modification Trial, JAMA 295 (2006) 629–642.

[54] L.J. Martin, Q. Li, O. Melnichouk, C. Greenberg, S. Minkin, G. Hislop, et al., A randomized trial of dietary intervention for breast cancer prevention, Cancer Res. 71 (2011) 123–133.

[55] A.W. Barclay, P. Petocz, J. McMillan-Price, V.M. Flood, T. Prvan, P. Mitchell, et al., Glycemic index, glycemic load, and chronic disease risk: a meta-analysis of observational studies, Am. J. Clin. Nutr. 87 (2008) 627–637.

[56] H.G. Mulholland, L.J. Murray, C.R. Cardwell, M.M. Cantwell, Dietary glycaemic index, glycaemic load and breast cancer risk: a systematic review and meta-analysis, Br. J. Cancer 99 (2008) 1170–1175.

[57] F.X. Pi-Sunyer, Glycemic index and disease, Am. J. Clin. Nutr. 76 (2002) 290S–298S.

[58] C.J. Arts, C.A. Govers, H. van den Berg, M.G. Wolters, P. van Leeuwen, J.H. Thijssen, In vitro binding of estrogens by dietary fiber and the in vivo apparent digestibility tested in pigs, J. Steroid Biochem. Mol. Biol. 38 (1991) 621–628.

[59] S. Gandini, H. Merzenich, C. Robertson, P. Boyle, Meta-analysis of studies on breast cancer risk and diet: the role of fruit and vegetable consumption and the intake of associated micronutrients, Eur. J. Cancer 36 (2000) 636–646.

[60] S.A. Smith-Warner, D. Spiegelman, S.S. Yaun, H.O. Adami, W.L. Beeson, P.A. van den Brandt, et al., Intake of fruits and vegetables and risk of breast cancer: a pooled analysis of cohort studies, JAMA 285 (2001) 769–776.

[61] C.H. van Gils, P.H. Peeters, H.B. Bueno-de-Mesquita, H.C. Boshuizen, P.H. Lahmann, F. Clavel-Chapelon, et al., Consumption of vegetables and fruits and risk of breast cancer, JAMA 293 (2005) 183–193.

[62] P. Toniolo, A.L. Van Kappel, A. Akhmedkhanov, P. Ferrari, I. Kato, R.E. Shore, et al., Serum carotenoids and breast cancer, Am. J. Epidemiol. 153 (2001) 1142–1147.

[63] G.C. Kabat, M. Kim, L.L. Adams-Campbell, B.J. Caan, R.T. Chlebowski, M.L. Neuhouser, et al., Longitudinal study of serum carotenoid, retinol, and tocopherol concentrations in relation to breast cancer risk among postmenopausal women, Am. J. Clin. Nutr. 90 (2009) 162–169.

[64] X. Zhang, D. Spiegelman, L. Baglietto, W.L. Beeson, L. Bernstein, P.A. van den Brandt, et al., Carotenoid intakes and risk of breast cancer defined by estrogen receptor and progesterone receptor status: a pooled analysis of 18 prospective cohort studies, Am. J. Clin. Nutr. 95 (2012) 713–725.

[65] P. Prakash, N.I. Krinsky, R.M. Russell, Retinoids, carotenoids, and human breast cancer cell cultures: a review of differential effects, Nutr. Rev. 58 (2000) 170–176.

[66] J.H. Fowke, C. Longcope, J.R. Hebert, Brassica vegetable consumption shifts estrogen metabolism in healthy postmenopausal women, Cancer Epidemiol. Biomarkers Prev. 9 (2000) 773–779.

[67] B.E. Henderson, L. Bernstein, The international variation in breast cancer rates: an epidemiological assessment, Breast Cancer Res. Treat. 18 (Suppl. 1) (1991) S11–S17.

[68] H.B. Patisaul, W. Jefferson, The pros and cons of phytoestrogens, Front. Neuroendocrinol. 31 (2010) 400–419.

[69] M. Messina, A.H. Wu, Perspectives on the soy-breast cancer relation, Am. J. Clin. Nutr. 89 (2009) 1673S–1679S.

[70] S.A. Smith-Warner, D. Spiegelman, S.S. Yaun, P.A. van den Brandt, A.R. Folsom, R.A. Goldbohm, et al., Alcohol and breast cancer in women: a pooled analysis of cohort studies, JAMA 279 (1998) 535–540.

[71] G.L. Gierach, N.D. Freedman, A. Andaya, A.R. Hollenbeck, Y. Park, A. Schatzkin, et al., Coffee intake and breast cancer risk in the NIH-AARP diet and health study cohort, Int. J. Cancer 131 (2012) 452–460.

[72] D.A. Boggs, J.R. Palmer, M.J. Stampfer, D. Spiegelman, L.L. Adams-Campbell, L. Rosenberg, Tea and coffee intake in relation to risk of breast cancer in the Black Women's Health Study, Cancer Causes Control 21 (2010) 1941–1948.

[73] T.E. Rohan, M.G. Jain, G.R. Howe, A.B. Miller, Dietary folate consumption and breast cancer risk, J. Natl. Cancer Inst. 92 (2000) 266–269.

[74] T.A. Sellers, L.H. Kushi, J.R. Cerhan, R.A. Vierkant, S.M. Gapstur, C.M. Vachon, et al., Dietary folate intake, alcohol, and risk of breast cancer in a prospective study of postmenopausal women, Epidemiology 12 (2001) 420–428.

[75] S.C. Larsson, E. Giovannucci, A. Wolk, Folate and risk of breast cancer: a meta-analysis, J. Natl. Cancer Inst. 99 (2007) 64–76.

[76] C.H. Halsted, V. Medici, F. Esfandiari, Influence of alcohol on folate status and methionine, in: L.B. Bailey (Ed.), Folate in Health and Disease, CRC Press, Boca Raton, FL, 2010, pp. 429–448.

[77] A.V. Krishnan, D.L. Trump, C.S. Johnson, D. Feldman, The role of vitamin D in cancer prevention and treatment, Endocrinol. Metab. Clin. North Am. 39 (2010) 401–418.

[78] E.R. Bertone-Johnson, Prospective studies of dietary vitamin D and breast cancer: more questions raised than answered, Nutr. Rev. 65 (2007) 459–466.

[79] M.H. Shin, M.D. Holmes, S.E. Hankinson, K. Wu, G.A. Colditz, W.C. Willett, Intake of dairy products, calcium, and vitamin D and risk of breast cancer, J. Natl. Cancer Inst. 94 (2002) 1301–1311.

[80] J. Lin, J.E. Manson, I.M. Lee, N.R. Cook, J.E. Buring, S.M. Zhang, Intakes of calcium and vitamin D and breast cancer risk in women, Arch. Intern. Med. 167 (2007) 1050–1059.

[81] M.L. McCullough, C. Rodriguez, W.R. Diver, H.S. Feigelson, V. L. Stevens, M.J. Thun, et al., Dairy, calcium, and vitamin D intake and postmenopausal breast cancer risk in the Cancer Prevention Study II Nutrition Cohort, Cancer Epidemiol. Biomarkers Prev. 14 (2005) 2898–2904.

[82] K. Robien, G.J. Cutler, D. Lazovich, Vitamin D intake and breast cancer risk in postmenopausal women: the Iowa Women's Health Study, Cancer Causes Control 18 (2007) 775–782.

[83] A.K. Kant, Dietary patterns and health outcomes, J. Am. Diet. Assoc. 104 (2004) 615–635.

[84] T.T. Fung, F.B. Hu, S.E. Hankinson, W.C. Willett, M.D. Holmes, Low-carbohydrate diets, dietary approaches to stop hypertension-style diets, and the risk of postmenopausal breast cancer, Am. J. Epidemiol. 174 (2011) 652–660.

[85] L. Baglietto, K. Krishnan, G. Severi, A. Hodge, M. Brinkman, D. R. English, et al., Dietary patterns and risk of breast cancer, Br. J. Cancer 104 (2011) 524–531.

[86] X. Cui, Q. Dai, M. Tseng, X.O. Shu, Y.T. Gao, W. Zheng, Dietary patterns and breast cancer risk in the shanghai breast cancer study, Cancer Epidemiol. Biomarkers Prev. 16 (2007) 1443–1448.

[87] A.W. Hsing, J.K. McLaughlin, P. Cocco, H.T. Co Chien, J.F. Fraumeni Jr., Risk factors for male breast cancer (United States), Cancer Causes Control 9 (1998) 269–275.

[88] J.L. Patnaik, T. Byers, C. Diguiseppi, D. Dabelea, T.D. Denberg, Cardiovascular disease competes with breast cancer as the leading cause of death for older females diagnosed with breast cancer: a retrospective cohort study, Breast Cancer Res. 13 (2011) R64.

[89] S. Loi, R.L. Milne, M.L. Friedlander, M.R. McCredie, G.G. Giles, J.L. Hopper, et al., Obesity and outcomes in premenopausal and postmenopausal breast cancer, Cancer Epidemiol. Biomarkers Prev. 14 (2005) 1686–1691.

[90] M.K. Whiteman, S.D. Hillis, K.M. Curtis, J.A. McDonald, P.A. Wingo, P.A. Marchbanks, Body mass and mortality after breast cancer diagnosis, Cancer Epidemiol. Biomarkers Prev. 14 (2005) 2009–2014.

[91] A.R. Carmichael, Obesity and prognosis of breast cancer, Obes. Rev. 7 (2006) 333–340.

[92] M. Ewertz, M.B. Jensen, K.A. Gunnarsdottir, I. Hojris, E.H. Jakobsen, D. Nielsen, et al., Effect of obesity on prognosis after early-stage breast cancer, J. Clin. Oncol. 29 (2011) 25–31.

[93] B.J. Caan, J.A. Emond, L. Natarajan, A. Castillo, E.P. Gunderson, L. Habel, et al., Post-diagnosis weight gain and breast cancer recurrence in women with early stage breast cancer, Breast Cancer Res. Treat. 99 (2006) 47–57.

[94] S.M. Enger, L. Bernstein, Exercise activity, body size and premenopausal breast cancer survival, Br. J. Cancer 90 (2004) 2138–2141.

[95] B.J. Caan, M.L. Kwan, G. Hartzell, A. Castillo, M.L. Slattery, B. Sternfeld, et al., Pre-diagnosis body mass index, post-diagnosis weight change, and prognosis among women with early stage breast cancer, Cancer Causes Control 19 (2008) 1319–1328.

[96] M. Protani, M. Coory, J.H. Martin, Effect of obesity on survival of women with breast cancer: systematic review and meta-analysis, Breast Cancer Res. Treat. 123 (2010) 627–635.

[97] J.P. Pierce, M.L. Stefanick, S.W. Flatt, L. Natarajan, B. Sternfeld, L. Madlensky, et al., Greater survival after breast cancer in physically active women with high vegetable-fruit intake regardless of obesity, J. Clin. Oncol. 25 (2007) 2345–2351.

[98] V. Pinsolle, C. Grinfeder, S. Mathoulin-Pelissier, A. Faucher, Complications analysis of 266 immediate breast reconstructions, J. Plast. Reconstr. Aesthet. Surg. 59 (2006) 1017–1024.

[99] S.L. Spear, I. Ducic, F. Cuoco, N. Taylor, Effect of obesity on flap and donor-site complications in pedicled TRAM flap breast reconstruction, Plast. Reconstr. Surg. 119 (2007) 788–795.

[100] E.D. Paskett, M.J. Naughton, T.P. McCoy, L.D. Case, J.M. Abbott, The epidemiology of arm and hand swelling in premenopausal breast cancer survivors, Cancer Epidemiol. Biomarkers Prev. 16 (2007) 775–782.

[101] C. Shaw, P. Mortimer, P.A. Judd, A randomized controlled trial of weight reduction as a treatment for breast cancer-related lymphedema, Cancer 110 (2007) 1868–1874.

[102] A. Decensi, P. Maisonneuve, N. Rotmensz, D. Bettega, A. Costa, V. Sacchini, et al., Effect of tamoxifen on venous thromboembolic events in a breast cancer prevention trial, Circulation 111 (2005) 650–656.

[103] P.E. Abrahamson, M.D. Gammon, M.J. Lund, E.W. Flagg, P.L. Porter, J. Stevens, et al., General and abdominal obesity and survival among young women with breast cancer, Cancer Epidemiol. Biomarkers Prev. 15 (2006) 1871–1877.

[104] N.B. Kumar, A. Cantor, K. Allen, C.E. Cox, Android obesity at diagnosis and breast carcinoma survival: evaluation of the effects of anthropometric variables at diagnosis, including body composition and body fat distribution and weight gain during life span, and survival from breast carcinoma, Cancer 88 (2000) 2751–2757.

[105] M.J. Borugian, S.B. Sheps, C. Kim-Sing, I.A. Olivotto, C. Van Patten, B.P. Dunn, et al., Waist-to-hip ratio and breast cancer mortality, Am. J. Epidemiol. 158 (2003) 963–968.

[106] R.L. Helms, E.L. O'Hea, M. Corso, Body image issues in women with breast cancer, Psychol. Health Med. 13 (2008) 313–325.

[107] K. Robien, W. Demark-Wahnefried, C.L. Rock, Evidence-based nutrition guidelines for cancer survivors: current guidelines, knowledge gaps, and future research directions, J. Am. Diet. Assoc. 111 (2011) 368–375.

[108] C.H. Kroenke, W.Y. Chen, B. Rosner, M.D. Holmes, Weight, weight gain, and survival after breast cancer diagnosis, J. Clin. Oncol. 23 (2005) 1370–1378.

[109] C. Ingram, J.K. Brown, Patterns of weight and body composition change in premenopausal women with early stage breast cancer: has weight gain been overestimated? Cancer Nurs. 27 (2004) 483–490.

[110] M.L. Irwin, A. McTiernan, R.N. Baumgartner, K.B. Baumgartner, L. Bernstein, F.D. Gilliland, et al., Changes in body fat and weight after a breast cancer diagnosis: influence of demographic, prognostic, and lifestyle factors, J. Clin. Oncol. 23 (2005) 774–782.

[111] W. Demark-Wahnefried, B.L. Peterson, E.P. Winer, L. Marks, N. Aziz, P.K. Marcom, et al., Changes in weight, body composition, and factors influencing energy balance among premenopausal breast cancer patients receiving adjuvant chemotherapy, J. Clin. Oncol. 19 (2001) 2381–2389.

[112] G. Makari-Judson, C.H. Judson, W.C. Mertens, Longitudinal patterns of weight gain after breast cancer diagnosis: observations beyond the first year, Breast J. 13 (2007) 258–265.

[113] F. de Waard, R. Ramlau, Y. Mulders, T. de Vries, S. van Waveren, A feasibility study on weight reduction in obese post-menopausal breast cancer patients, Eur. J. Cancer Prev. 2 (1993) 233–238.

[114] C.L. Loprinzi, L.M. Athmann, C.G. Kardinal, J.R. O'Fallon, J.A. See, B.K. Bruce, et al., Randomized trial of dietician counseling to try to prevent weight gain associated with breast cancer adjuvant chemotherapy, Oncology 53 (1996) 228–232.

[115] Z. Djuric, N.M. DiLaura, I. Jenkins, L. Darga, C.K. Jen, D. Mood, et al., Combining weight-loss counseling with the Weight Watchers plan for obese breast cancer survivors, Obes. Res. 10 (2002) 657–665.

[116] P. Goodwin, M.J. Esplen, K. Butler, J. Winocur, K. Pritchard, S. Brazel, et al., Multidisciplinary weight management in locoregional breast cancer: results of a phase II study, Breast Cancer Res. Treat. 48 (1998) 53–64.

[117] A.J. McEligot, J. Largent, A. Ziogas, D. Peel, H. Anton-Culver, Dietary fat, fiber, vegetable, and micronutrients are associated with overall survival in postmenopausal women diagnosed with breast cancer, Nutr. Cancer 55 (2006) 132–140.

[118] T.E. Rohan, J.E. Hiller, A.J. McMichael, Dietary factors and survival from breast cancer, Nutr. Cancer 20 (1993) 167–177.

[119] J.M. Beasley, P.A. Newcomb, A. Trentham-Dietz, J.M. Hampton, A.J. Bersch, M.N. Passarelli, et al., Post-diagnosis dietary factors and survival after invasive breast cancer, Breast Cancer Res. Treat. 128 (2011) 229–236.

[120] G.A. Saxe, C.L. Rock, M.S. Wicha, D. Schottenfeld, Diet and risk for breast cancer recurrence and survival, Breast Cancer Res. Treat. 53 (1999) 241–253.

[121] M.D. Holmes, M.J. Stampfer, G.A. Colditz, B. Rosner, D.J. Hunter, W.C. Willett, Dietary factors and the survival of women with breast carcinoma, Cancer 86 (1999) 826–835.

[122] P.J. Goodwin, M. Ennis, K.I. Pritchard, J. Koo, M.E. Trudeau, N. Hood, Diet and breast cancer: evidence that extremes in diet are associated with poor survival, J. Clin. Oncol. 21 (2003) 2500–2507.

[123] M. Ewertz, S. Gillanders, L. Meyer, K. Zedeler, Survival of breast cancer patients in relation to factors which affect the risk of developing breast cancer, Int. J. Cancer 49 (1991) 526–530.

[124] B.N. Fink, M.M. Gaudet, J.A. Britton, P.E. Abrahamson, S.L. Teitelbaum, J. Jacobson, et al., Fruits, vegetables, and micronutrient intake in relation to breast cancer survival, Breast Cancer Res. Treat. 98 (2006) 199–208.

[125] C.L. Rock, S.W. Flatt, L. Natarajan, C.A. Thomson, W.A. Bardwell, V.A. Newman, et al., Plasma carotenoids and recurrence-free survival in women with a history of breast cancer, J. Clin. Oncol. 23 (2005) 6631–6638.

[126] C.H. Kroenke, T.T. Fung, F.B. Hu, M.D. Holmes, Dietary patterns and survival after breast cancer diagnosis, J. Clin. Oncol. 23 (2005) 9295–9303.

[127] J.R. Hebert, T.G. Hurley, Y. Ma, The effect of dietary exposures on recurrence and mortality in early stage breast cancer, Breast Cancer Res. Treat. 51 (1998) 17–28.

[128] M.G. Jain, R.G. Ferrenc, J.T. Rehm, S.J. Bondy, T.E. Rohan, M.J. Ashley, et al., Alcohol and breast cancer mortality in a cohort study, Breast Cancer Res. Treat. 64 (2000) 201–209.

[129] P.A. McDonald, R. Williams, F. Dawkins, L.L. Adams-Campbell, Breast cancer survival in African American women: is alcohol consumption a prognostic indicator? Cancer Causes Control 13 (2002) 543–549.

[130] M.L. Kwan, L.H. Kushi, E. Weltzien, E.K. Tam, A. Castillo, C. Sweeney, et al., Alcohol consumption and breast cancer recurrence and survival among women with early-stage breast cancer: the Life after Cancer Epidemiology study, J. Clin. Oncol. 28 (2010) 4410–4416.

[131] G.C. Barnett, M. Shah, K. Redman, D.F. Easton, B.A. Ponder, P. D. Pharoah, Risk factors for the incidence of breast cancer: do they affect survival from the disease? J. Clin. Oncol. 26 (2008) 3310–3316.

[132] K.W. Reding, J.R. Daling, D.R. Doody, C.A. O'Brien, P.L. Porter, K.E. Malone, Effect of prediagnostic alcohol consumption on survival after breast cancer in young women, Cancer Epidemiol. Biomarkers Prev. 17 (2008) 1988–1996.

[133] L.E. Holm, E. Nordevang, M.L. Hjalmar, E. Lidbrink, E. Callmer, B. Nilsson, Treatment failure and dietary habits in women with breast cancer, J. Natl. Cancer Inst. 85 (1993) 32–36.

[134] L. Dal Maso, A. Zucchetto, R. Talamini, D. Serraino, C.F. Stocco, M. Vercelli, et al., Effect of obesity and other lifestyle factors on mortality in women with breast cancer, Int. J. Cancer 123 (2008) 2188–2194.

[135] R.T. Chlebowski, G.L. Blackburn, I.M. Buzzard, D.P. Rose, S. Martino, J.D. Khandekar, et al., Adherence to a dietary fat intake reduction program in postmenopausal women receiving therapy for early breast cancer: the Women's Intervention Nutrition Study, J. Clin. Oncol. 11 (1993) 2072–2080.

[136] R.T. Chlebowski, G.L. Blackburn, C.A. Thomson, D.W. Nixon, A. Shapiro, M.K. Hoy, et al., Dietary fat reduction and breast cancer outcome: interim efficacy results from the Women's Intervention Nutrition Study, J. Natl. Cancer Inst. 98 (2006) 1767–1776.

[137] J.P. Pierce, S. Faerber, F.A. Wright, V. Newman, S.W. Flatt, S. Kealey, et al., Feasibility of a randomized trial of a high-vegetable diet to prevent breast cancer recurrence, Nutr. Cancer 28 (1997) 282–288.

[138] C.L. Rock, C. Thomson, B.J. Caan, S.W. Flatt, V. Newman, C. Ritenbaugh, et al., Reduction in fat intake is not associated with weight loss in most women after breast cancer diagnosis: evidence from a randomized controlled trial, Cancer 91 (2001) 25–34.

[139] C.L. Rock, S.W. Flatt, F.A. Wright, S. Faerber, V. Newman, S. Kealey, et al., Responsiveness of carotenoids to a high vegetable diet intervention designed to prevent breast cancer recurrence, Cancer Epidemiol. Biomarkers Prev. 6 (1997) 617–623.

[140] J.P. Pierce, L. Natarajan, B.J. Caan, B.A. Parker, E.R. Greenberg, S.W. Flatt, et al., Influence of a diet very high in vegetables, fruit, and fiber and low in fat on prognosis following treatment for breast cancer: the Women's Healthy Eating and Living (WHEL) randomized trial, JAMA 298 (2007) 289–298.

[141] M.L. Kwan, E. Weltzien, L.H. Kushi, A. Castillo, M.L. Slattery, B.J. Caan, Dietary patterns and breast cancer recurrence and survival among women with early-stage breast cancer, J. Clin. Oncol. 27 (2009) 919–926.

[142] A.N. Fader, L.N. Arriba, H.E. Frasure, V.E. von Gruenigen, Endometrial cancer and obesity: epidemiology, biomarkers, prevention and survivorship, Gynecol. Oncol. 114 (2009) 121–127.

[143] F.A. Tabassoli, P. Devilee (Eds.), Pathology and Genetics of Tumours of the Breast and Female Genital Organs, International Agency for Research on Cancer, Lyon, France, 2003.

[144] L.M. Duong, R.J. Wilson, U.A. Ajani, S.D. Singh, C.R. Eheman, Trends in endometrial cancer incidence rates in the United States, 1999–2006, J. Womens Health (Larchmt.) 20 (2011) 1157–1163.

[145] M. Llaurado, A. Ruiz, B. Majem, T. Ertekin, E. Colas, N. Pedrola, et al., Molecular bases of endometrial cancer: new roles for new actors in the diagnosis and the therapy of the disease, Mol. Cell. Endocrinol. 358 (2012) 244–255.

[146] G.E. Hale, C.L. Hughes, J.M. Cline, Endometrial cancer: hormonal factors, the perimenopausal "window of risk," and isoflavones, J. Clin. Endocrinol. Metab. 87 (2002) 3—15.

[147] S.C. Chang, J.V. Lacey Jr., L.A. Brinton, P. Hartge, K. Adams, T. Mouw, et al., Lifetime weight history and endometrial cancer risk by type of menopausal hormone use in the NIH-AARP diet and health study, Cancer Epidemiol. Biomarkers Prev. 16 (2007) 723—730.

[148] C. Friedenreich, A. Cust, P.H. Lahmann, K. Steindorf, M.C. Boutron-Ruault, F. Clavel-Chapelon, et al., Anthropometric factors and risk of endometrial cancer: the European Prospective Investigation into Cancer and Nutrition, Cancer Causes Control 18 (2007) 399—413.

[149] M.L. McCullough, A.V. Patel, R. Patel, C. Rodriguez, H.S. Feigelson, E.V. Bandera, et al., Body mass and endometrial cancer risk by hormone replacement therapy and cancer subtype, Cancer Epidemiol. Biomarkers Prev. 17 (2008) 73—79.

[150] A.S. Felix, J.L. Weissfeld, R.A. Stone, R. Bowser, M. Chivukula, R.P. Edwards, et al., Factors associated with Type I and Type II endometrial cancer, Cancer Causes Control 21 (2010) 1851—1856.

[151] L.J. Schouten, R.A. Goldbohm, P.A. van den Brandt, Anthropometry, physical activity, and endometrial cancer risk: results from the Netherlands Cohort Study, J. Natl. Cancer Inst. 96 (2004) 1635—1638.

[152] S.C. Larsson, E. Friberg, A. Wolk, Carbohydrate intake, glycemic index and glycemic load in relation to risk of endometrial cancer: a prospective study of Swedish women, Int. J. Cancer 120 (2007) 1103—1107.

[153] S.A. Silvera, T.E. Rohan, M. Jain, P.D. Terry, G.R. Howe, A.B. Miller, Glycaemic index, glycaemic load and risk of endometrial cancer: a prospective cohort study, Public Health Nutr. 8 (2005) 912—919.

[154] A.R. Folsom, Z. Demissie, L. Harnack, Glycemic index, glycemic load, and incidence of endometrial cancer: the Iowa Women's Health Study, Nutr. Cancer 46 (2003) 119—124.

[155] M.G. Jain, T.E. Rohan, G.R. Howe, A.B. Miller, A cohort study of nutritional factors and endometrial cancer, Eur. J. Epidemiol. 16 (2000) 899—905.

[156] A.S. Furberg, I. Thune, Metabolic abnormalities (hypertension, hyperglycemia and overweight), lifestyle (high energy intake and physical inactivity) and endometrial cancer risk in a Norwegian cohort, Int. J. Cancer 104 (2003) 669—676.

[157] (2003). "IARC Handbooks of Cancer Prevention: vol. 8. Fruits and Vegetables." International Agency for Research on Cancer, Lyon, France.

[158] P.L. Horn-Ross, E.M. John, A.J. Canchola, S.L. Stewart, M.M. Lee, Phytoestrogen intake and endometrial cancer risk, J. Natl. Cancer Inst. 95 (2003) 1158—1164.

[159] S. Uccella, A. Mariani, A.H. Wang, R.A. Vierkant, K. Robien, K. E. Anderson, et al., Dietary and supplemental intake of one-carbon nutrients and the risk of type I and type II endometrial cancer: a prospective cohort study, Ann. Oncol. 22 (2011) 2129—2136.

[160] P. Terry, H. Vainio, A. Wolk, E. Weiderpass, Dietary factors in relation to endometrial cancer: a nationwide case—control study in Sweden, Nutr. Cancer 42 (2002) 25—32.

[161] P. Terry, A. Wolk, H. Vainio, E. Weiderpass, Fatty fish consumption lowers the risk of endometrial cancer: a nationwide case—control study in Sweden, Cancer Epidemiol. Biomarkers Prev. 11 (2002) 143—145.

[162] W.H. Xu, Q. Dai, Y.B. Xiang, G.M. Zhao, Z.X. Ruan, J.R. Cheng, et al., Nutritional factors in relation to endometrial cancer: a report from a population-based case—control study in Shanghai, China, Int. J. Cancer 120 (2007) 1776—1781.

[163] E. Salazar-Martinez, E. Lazcano-Ponce, L.M. Sanchez-Zamorano, G. Gonzalez-Lira, D.E.L.R.P. Escudero, M. Hernandez-Avila, Dietary factors and endometrial cancer risk: results of a case—control study in Mexico, Int. J. Gynecol. Cancer 15 (2005) 938—945.

[164] P. Knekt, A. Aromaa, J. Maatela, R.K. Aaran, T. Nikkari, M. Hakama, et al., Serum vitamin A and subsequent risk of cancer: cancer incidence follow-up of the Finnish Mobile Clinic Health Examination Survey, Am. J. Epidemiol. 132 (1990) 857—870.

[165] E.V. Bandera, L.H. Kushi, S.H. Olson, W.Y. Chen, P. Muti, Alcohol consumption and endometrial cancer: some unresolved issues, Nutr. Cancer 45 (2003) 24—29.

[166] E. Weiderpass, J.A. Baron, Cigarette smoking, alcohol consumption, and endometrial cancer risk: a population-based study in Sweden, Cancer Causes Control 12 (2001) 239—247.

[167] V.E. von Gruenigen, C. Tian, H. Frasure, S. Waggoner, H. Keys, R.R. Barakat, Treatment effects, disease recurrence, and survival in obese women with early endometrial carcinoma: a Gynecologic Oncology Group study, Cancer 107 (2006) 2786—2791.

[168] E. Everett, H. Tamimi, B. Greer, E. Swisher, P. Paley, L. Mandel, et al., The effect of body mass index on clinical/pathologic features, surgical morbidity, and outcome in patients with endometrial cancer, Gynecol. Oncol. 90 (2003) 150—157.

[169] B. Anderson, J.P. Connor, J.I. Andrews, C.S. Davis, R.E. Buller, J.I. Sorosky, et al., Obesity and prognosis in endometrial cancer, Am. J. Obstet. Gynecol. 174 (1996) 1171—1179.

[170] V.M. Chia, P.A. Newcomb, A. Trentham-Dietz, J.M. Hampton, Obesity, diabetes, and other factors in relation to survival after endometrial cancer diagnosis, Int. J. Gynecol. Cancer 17 (2007) 441—446.

[171] Z. Studzijnski, W. Zajewski, Factors affecting the survival of 121 patients treated for endometrial carcinoma at a Polish hospital, Arch. Gynecol. Obstet. 267 (2003) 145—147.

[172] K.S. Courneya, K.H. Karvinen, K.L. Campbell, R.G. Pearcey, G. Dundas, V. Capstick, et al., Associations among exercise, body weight, and quality of life in a population-based sample of endometrial cancer survivors, Gynecol. Oncol. 97 (2005) 422—430.

[173] V.E. von Gruenigen, K.M. Gil, H.E. Frasure, E.L. Jenison, M.P. Hopkins, The impact of obesity and age on quality of life in gynecologic surgery, Am. J. Obstet. Gynecol. 193 (2005) 1369—1375.

[174] A.N. Fader, H.E. Frasure, K.M. Gil, N.A. Berger, V.E. von Gruenigen, Quality of life in endometrial cancer survivors: what does obesity have to do with it? Obstet. Gynecol. Int. 2011 (2011) 308609.

[175] V.E. von Gruenigen, H.E. Frasure, M.B. Kavanagh, E. Lerner, S. E. Waggoner, K.S. Courneya, Feasibility of a lifestyle intervention for ovarian cancer patients receiving adjuvant chemotherapy, Gynecol. Oncol. 122 (2011) 328—333.

[176] R.J. Edmondson, J.M. Monaghan, The epidemiology of ovarian cancer, Int. J. Gynecol. Cancer 11 (2001) 423—429.

[177] I.B. Runnebaum, E. Stickeler, Epidemiological and molecular aspects of ovarian cancer risk, J. Cancer Res. Clin. Oncol. 127 (2001) 73—79.

[178] H.A. Risch, Hormonal etiology of epithelial ovarian cancer, with a hypothesis concerning the role of androgens and progesterone, J. Natl. Cancer Inst. 90 (1998) 1774—1786.

[179] T. Riman, S. Nilsson, I.R. Persson, Review of epidemiological evidence for reproductive and hormonal factors in relation to the risk of epithelial ovarian malignancies, Acta Obstet. Gynecol. Scand. 83 (2004) 783—795.

[180] S.A. Narod, J. Boyd, Current understanding of the epidemiology and clinical implications of BRCA1 and BRCA2 mutations

for ovarian cancer, Curr. Opin. Obstet. Gynecol. 14 (2002) 19–26.

[181] L.J. Schouten, C. Rivera, D.J. Hunter, D. Spiegelman, H.O. Adami, A. Arslan, et al., Height, body mass index, and ovarian cancer: a pooled analysis of 12 cohort studies, Cancer Epidemiol. Biomarkers Prev. 17 (2008) 902–912.

[182] P.H. Lahmann, A.E. Cust, C.M. Friedenreich, M. Schulz, A. Lukanova, R. Kaaks, et al., Anthropometric measures and epithelial ovarian cancer risk in the European Prospective Investigation into Cancer and Nutrition, Int. J. Cancer 126 (2010) 2404–2415.

[183] B. Armstrong, R. Doll, Environmental factors and cancer incidence and mortality in different countries, with special reference to dietary practices, Int. J. Cancer 15 (1975) 617–631.

[184] J.M. Genkinger, D.J. Hunter, D. Spiegelman, K.E. Anderson, W. L. Beeson, J.E. Buring, et al., A pooled analysis of 12 cohort studies of dietary fat, cholesterol and egg intake and ovarian cancer, Cancer Causes Control 17 (2006) 273–285.

[185] A.M. Gilsing, M.P. Weijenberg, R.A. Goldbohm, P.A. van den Brandt, L.J. Schouten, Consumption of dietary fat and meat and risk of ovarian cancer in the Netherlands Cohort Study, Am. J. Clin. Nutr. 93 (2011) 118–126.

[186] S.A. Silvera, M. Jain, G.R. Howe, A.B. Miller, T.E. Rohan, Glycaemic index, glycaemic load and ovarian cancer risk: a prospective cohort study, Public Health Nutr. 10 (2007) 1076–1081.

[187] M. Hedelin, M. Lof, T.M. Andersson, H. Adlercreutz, E. Weiderpass, Dietary phytoestrogens and the risk of ovarian cancer in the Women's Lifestyle and Health Cohort study, Cancer Epidemiol. Biomarkers Prev. 20 (2011) 308–317.

[188] K.M. Fairfield, S.E. Hankinson, B.A. Rosner, D.J. Hunter, G.A. Colditz, W.C. Willett, Risk of ovarian carcinoma and consumption of vitamins A, C, and E and specific carotenoids: a prospective analysis, Cancer 92 (2001) 2318–2326.

[189] M.A. Gates, S.S. Tworoger, J.L. Hecht, I. De Vivo, B. Rosner, S. E. Hankinson, A prospective study of dietary flavonoid intake and incidence of epithelial ovarian cancer, Int. J. Cancer 121 (2007) 2225–2232.

[190] E.T. Chang, V.S. Lee, A.J. Canchola, C.A. Clarke, D.M. Purdie, P. Reynolds, et al., Diet and risk of ovarian cancer in the California Teachers Study cohort, Am. J. Epidemiol. 165 (2007) 802–813.

[191] L.H. Kushi, P.J. Mink, A.R. Folsom, K.E. Anderson, W. Zheng, D. Lazovich, et al., Prospective study of diet and ovarian cancer, Am. J. Epidemiol. 149 (1999) 21–31.

[192] K.J. Helzlsouer, A.J. Alberg, E.P. Norkus, J.S. Morris, S.C. Hoffman, G.W. Comstock, Prospective study of serum micronutrients and ovarian cancer, J. Natl. Cancer Inst. 88 (1996) 32–37.

[193] M. Garland, J.S. Morris, M.J. Stampfer, G.A. Colditz, V.L. Spate, C.K. Baskett, et al., Prospective study of toenail selenium levels and cancer among women, J. Natl. Cancer Inst. 87 (1995) 497–505.

[194] W. Zheng, K.N. Danforth, S.S. Tworoger, M.T. Goodman, A.A. Arslan, A.V. Patel, et al., Circulating 25-hydroxyvitamin D and risk of epithelial ovarian cancer: Cohort Consortium Vitamin D Pooling Project of Rarer Cancers, Am. J. Epidemiol. 172 (2010) 70–80.

[195] B. Zhou, L. Yang, L. Wang, Y. Shi, H. Zhu, N. Tang, et al., The association of tea consumption with ovarian cancer risk: a metaanalysis, Am. J. Obstet. Gynecol. 197 (2007) e1–e6594

[196] S.J. Oppeneer, K. Robien, Tea consumption and epithelial ovarian cancer risk: a systematic review of observational studies, Nutr. Cancer 63 (2011) 817–826.

[197] J. Steevens, L.J. Schouten, B.A. Verhage, R.A. Goldbohm, P.A. van den Brandt, Tea and coffee drinking and ovarian cancer risk: results from the Netherlands Cohort Study and a meta-analysis, Br. J. Cancer 97 (2007) 1291–1294.

[198] N.A. Lueth, K.E. Anderson, L.J. Harnack, J.A. Fulkerson, K. Robien, Coffee and caffeine intake and the risk of ovarian cancer: the Iowa Women's Health Study, Cancer Causes Control 19 (2008) 1365–1372.

[199] H.S. Yang, C. Yoon, S.K. Myung, S.M. Park, Effect of obesity on survival of women with epithelial ovarian cancer: a systematic review and meta-analysis of observational studies, Int. J. Gynecol. Cancer 21 (2011) 1525–1532.

[200] L.M. Hess, R. Barakat, C. Tian, R.F. Ozols, D.S. Alberts, Weight change during chemotherapy as a potential prognostic factor for stage III epithelial ovarian carcinoma: a Gynecologic Oncology Group study, Gynecol. Oncol. 107 (2007) 260–265.

[201] F.J. Backes, C.I. Nagel, E. Bussewitz, J. Donner, E. Hade, R. Salani, The impact of body weight on ovarian cancer outcomes, Int. J. Gynecol. Cancer 21 (2011) 1601–1605.

[202] C.M. Nagle, D.M. Purdie, P.M. Webb, A. Green, P.W. Harvey, C.J. Bain, Dietary influences on survival after ovarian cancer, Int. J. Cancer 106 (2003) 264–269.

[203] T.A. Dolecek, B.J. McCarthy, C.E. Joslin, C.E. Peterson, S. Kim, S.A. Freels, et al., Prediagnosis food patterns are associated with length of survival from epithelial ovarian cancer, J. Am. Diet. Assoc. 110 (2010) 369–382.

[204] L.H. Kushi, T. Byers, C. Doyle, E.V. Bandera, M. McCullough, A. McTiernan, et al., American Cancer Society Guidelines on Nutrition and Physical Activity for cancer prevention: reducing the risk of cancer with healthy food choices and physical activity, CA Cancer J. Clin. 56 (2006) 254–281, quiz 313–254

[205] C. Doyle, L.H. Kushi, T. Byers, K.S. Courneya, W. Demark-Wahnefried, B. Grant, et al., Nutrition and physical activity during and after cancer treatment: an American Cancer Society guide for informed choices, CA Cancer J. Clin. 56 (2006) 323–353.

[206] A. Wolk, J.E. Manson, M.J. Stampfer, G.A. Colditz, F.B. Hu, F.E. Speizer, et al., Long-term intake of dietary fiber and decreased risk of coronary heart disease among women, JAMA 281 (1999) 1998–2004.

[207] A.K. Kant, A. Schatzkin, B.I. Graubard, C. Schairer, A prospective study of diet quality and mortality in women, JAMA 283 (2000) 2109–2115.

36

Nutrition and Prostate Cancer

Song-Yi Park, Laurence N. Kolonel

University of Hawaii Cancer Center, Honolulu, Hawaii

I INTRODUCTION

In this chapter, we discuss the epidemiologic evidence for associations of dietary factors with prostate cancer risk and the potential for diet to play a role in prostate cancer prevention. We begin with some general background on the disease and its diagnosis, followed by a description of incidence patterns and risk factors for prostate cancer other than diet. The relationship of nutrition to prostate cancer includes foods and dietary constituents that have been associated with increased risk of the disease, as well as those that have been associated with decreased risk. Some findings from animal and *in vitro* studies, as well as possible mechanisms for the carcinogenic effects, are presented in support of the epidemiologic findings. We conclude with a few comments on genetic studies of prostate cancer.

A Normal Prostate Anatomy and Function

The normal adult prostate gland is a walnut-sized organ that surrounds the urethra and the neck of the bladder. The gland is composed of three distinct zones: peripheral, central, and transition. The peripheral zone is composed of left and right lobes that can be palpated during digital rectal examination. The transition zone is the region that enlarges in benign prostatic hyperplasia, which is common in older men [1]. The prostate gland is a male secondary sex organ that secretes one fluid component of semen. Prostatic fluid is essential for male fertility.

Normal growth and activity of the prostate gland is under the control of androgenic hormones. Circulating testosterone, primarily produced in the testes, diffuses into the prostate, where it is irreversibly converted by the enzyme steroid 5α-reductase type II to dihydrotestosterone (DHT), a metabolically more active form of the hormone. DHT binds to the androgen receptor, and this complex then translocates to the cell nucleus, where it activates selected genes [2].

B Pathology and Diagnosis of Prostate Cancer

Almost all prostate tumors are classified as adenocarcinomas (i.e., they arise from the glandular epithelial cells) and occur most commonly in the peripheral zone of the gland. Accordingly, they can often be felt by the physician during digital rectal examination. A unique feature of human prostate cancer is the high frequency of small, latent tumors in older men. A clear relationship between these occult tumors and those that become clinically apparent has not been established, although it is commonly assumed that the latter evolve from the former as a consequence of additional genetic mutations.

Generally, prostate cancer in its early stages is asymptomatic. Enlargement of the prostate gland (benign prostatic hyperplasia (BPH)) commonly begins after the age of 45 years, ultimately leading to urinary tract symptoms (difficult and frequent urination). Many cases of prostate cancer are diagnosed as a result of digital rectal examination performed when a man visits his physician for relief of these symptoms. (Suspicious lesions on examination may be confirmed by transrectal ultrasound, followed by a biopsy of the gland.) Since its approval by the U.S. Food and Drug Administration in 1986, the prostate-specific antigen (PSA) test has come into widespread use. This test is not specific for prostate cancer, however, and gives an abnormal result if there is any increased tissue growth in the gland, such as occurs in BPH. Because of its

Nutrition in the Prevention and Treatment of Disease, Third Edition.
DOI: http://dx.doi.org/10.1016/B978-0-12-391884-0.00036-6

sensitivity, the PSA test can lead to the diagnosis of very early, microscopic tumors. Although such lesions might never progress to clinical disease, surgical removal carries a risk of major complications (notably incontinence and/or impotence), leading to controversy regarding the proper use of PSA as a screening test for early prostate cancer [3,4]. Indeed, in its most recent review, the U.S. Preventive Services Task Force concluded that use of PSA as a screening modality has not resulted in any decrease in prostate cancer mortality and that, to the contrary, its use has led to more harm than good [5].

II DESCRIPTIVE EPIDEMIOLOGY OF PROSTATE CANCER

A Incidence and Mortality Trends

Prostate cancer is a common cancer among men in many Western countries, and it is the leading male incident cancer in the United States, where 240,890 new cases are projected for the year 2011 [6,7]. Incidence trends in the United States show a rather slow increase over most of the past 50 years, with a striking increase between 1989 and 1992, attributable in large measure to the widespread adoption of the PSA screening test, which first became available in the early 1980s [8,9]. After 1992, the incidence declined until approximately 1995, remained stable until 2000, and then declined again from 2000 to 2007 [10]. Moreover, mortality from prostate cancer is low relative to its incidence. This is because prostate cancer is generally well controlled by treatment (surgery, radiation, and androgen ablation) and occurs at relatively late ages so that even men who are not cured of the disease often die from other causes. Interestingly, a parallel increase in prostate cancer mortality did not occur during the period 1989–1992, presumably because most of the additional cases diagnosed would not otherwise have led to fatal outcomes.

B Risk Factors for Prostate Cancer

Few risk factors for prostate cancer have been established. Proposed factors are listed in Table 36.1. Age is the strongest risk factor. Prostate cancer incidence increases more sharply with age than does any other cancer; approximately 62% of cases in the United States are diagnosed in men 65 years of age or older [6,7].

Race/ethnicity is a second risk factor for prostate cancer. In the United States, the lowest incidence rates are seen among Korean and Vietnamese men, both relatively recent immigrant groups from Asia; the rates

TABLE 36.1 Proposed Risk Factors for Prostate Cancer

Category	Characteristic or exposure
Demographic	Age, ethnicity, geography
Genetic	Family history (father, brothers); rare high-penetrance genes; more common susceptibility genes
Occupational	Cadmium products, rubber industry, agricultural chemicals
Hormonal	Androgens (testosterone, dihydrotestosterone)
Lifestyle	Sexually transmitted agents, smoking, alcohol, vasectomy, physical activity, diet

are somewhat higher among Chinese, American Indian, Alaska Native, and Native Hawaiian men. Caucasian men have very high rates, but by far the highest incidence of this cancer is among African American men [11,12].

The incidence of prostate cancer varies widely in populations throughout the world (Figure 36.1). Indeed, of all common malignancies, this cancer shows the widest variation between low- and high-risk countries or populations. High rates are seen in developed, especially Western, countries, including the United States, Canada, areas of Europe, and Australasia. Low rates tend to occur in Asia, particularly China [6]. The highest reported rates in the world are among African Americans, whereas the lowest reported rates are among men in China. Interestingly, Chinese men in more developed areas of Asia (Singapore and Hong Kong) and Chinese men in the United States have much higher incidence rates than men in mainland China (see cross-hatched populations in Figure 36.1). Furthermore, immigrants from Japan to Brazil and the United States have higher rates than do men in Japan [13]. The incidence of prostate cancer in Japan increased approximately sixfold between 1975 and 2006 [14], although the actual incidence in Japan is still low compared with that of Japanese men in the United States.

Men with a first-degree male relative who has had prostate cancer are at a two- or threefold increased risk; whether this reflects an inherited predisposition for the disease or a shared environmental exposure has not been confirmed [15–17]. The search for high-penetrance, rare genes for prostate cancer has identified some candidates, although none has yet been confirmed; of even greater interest is the potential role in this disease of low-penetrance, highly prevalent susceptibility genes (discussed later).

Apart from these few established risk factors, the etiology of prostate cancer is unknown. Among the

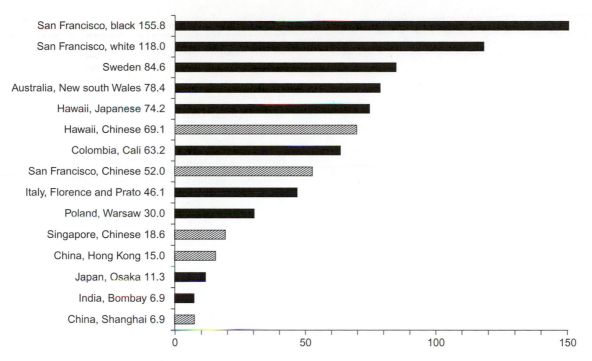

FIGURE 36.1   Prostate cancer incidence in selected populations, 1998–2002 (rates age-adjusted to the World Standard Population).

several potential causal agents, apart from diet, that have been proposed are (1) occupational exposures (rubber industry; manufacture of products containing cadmium, such as paints and batteries; and use of agriculture chemicals), (2) sexually transmitted agents (e.g., gonorrhea, syphilis, and human papillomavirus), (3) smoking, (4) alcohol use, (5) vasectomy, and (6) physical activity [18–24]. However, the evidence is not convincing for any of these exposures.

Although it is suspected that most exogenous factors affecting prostate cancer risk exert their influence by altering endogenous androgen levels [25,26], epidemiologic studies have not clearly established the role of androgens in prostate cancer. Some studies have supported a positive relationship of circulating androgen levels to prostate cancer risk [27–30], but others have not [31–36]. In a pooled analysis of 18 prospective studies, prediagnostic circulating levels of individual androgens were not associated with prostate cancer, whereas the sex hormone-binding globulin level was modestly inversely associated with prostate cancer [37]. Further studies are warranted to understand the role of androgens in tissue, androgen action in the prostate, and the relationship between tissue and blood levels of androgen in the causation of prostate cancer [38].

The most promising area of research, apart from genetics, on the etiology of prostate cancer pertains to diet.

III STUDIES OF DIET IN RELATION TO PROSTATE CANCER

A Origin of the Diet–Prostate Cancer Hypothesis

The descriptive patterns of prostate cancer, especially data showing very different rates of the disease in the same ethnic/racial group living in different geographic settings, as well as changing rates in migrants and their offspring [13], prompted investigators to seek environmental risk factors for this cancer. Diet became an important focus of this research because (1) geographic variations in food and nutrient intakes are known to be large [39] and (2) components of the diet can influence the levels of circulating androgens [40], which, as noted previously, are thought to play a role in prostate cancer risk. Many different dietary factors, including both foods and particular constituents of foods, have been proposed and studied. Some of these appear to increase risk, whereas others are possibly protective. These factors are listed in Table 36.2, and the supporting evidence is discussed in the following sections.

B Dietary Factors that Increase Risk

In 2007, the World Cancer Research Fund (WCRF) and the American Institute for Cancer Research (AICR)

TABLE 36.2 Proposed Dietary Risk Factors for Prostate Cancer

Increasing risk	Decreasing risk
Foods and Beverages	
Processed and red meat	Vegetables
Milk and dairy products	Fruits
Alcohol	Legumes
	Tea
Food Components	
Total energy	Vitamin D
Fat	Vitamin E
Calcium	Carotenoids
Zinc	Fructose
Cadmium	Selenium
	Isoflavonoids
Diet-Associated Factors	
Obesity, weight and height	Physical activity

produced an authoritative report, titled *Food, Nutrition, Physical Activity, and the Prevention of Cancer: A Global Perspective*, containing recommendations to reduce the risk of cancer [39]. These recommendations were based on comprehensive systematic literature reviews (SLRs) that were evaluated by an international panel of experts, including one of the present authors (LNK). The SLR for prostate cancer covered all major databases up to 2005, and it is available online at http://www.dietandcancerreport.org/expert_report/view_slrs.php [41]. Thus, in the following sections, we use the conclusions of the WCRF/AICR report as a starting point and then review the findings from recent studies to make an overall assessment of the literature. In its judgments, the WCRF/AICR expert panel graded the evidence in five categories: convincing, probable, limited—suggestive, limited—no conclusion, and substantial effect on risk unlikely. Recommendations were based only on the highest two categories.

1 Dietary Patterns

Foods are generally consumed in many combinations, and together they may have a greater impact on cancer risk than as individual components [42]. Thus, a dietary pattern approach that reflects the complexity of dietary intake may provide a more comprehensive assessment of the role of diet in cancer causation. Although many health outcomes have been associated with dietary patterns [43,44], only a few such studies have examined prostate cancer. Three case—control studies in Western countries found that dietary

patterns reflecting high consumption of meat and/or processed foods (referred to as a Western, processed, or traditional diet) were associated with an increased risk of total [45,46] or advanced prostate cancer [47]. One cohort study of U.S. health professionals reported that a Western pattern (including meat, refined grains, and high-fat dairy products) was suggestively associated with a greater risk of advanced prostate cancer among older men [48]. Another U.S. cohort study, based on a national population sample, found that a Southern dietary pattern (characterized by cornbread, grits, sweet potatoes, okra, beans, and rice) was related to a reduction in risk [49], whereas an Australian cohort reported no association between any dietary pattern and prostate cancer risk [50]. Thus, the evidence on dietary patterns and prostate cancer risk is too limited to draw any firm conclusion.

2 Foods and Beverages

A PROCESSED AND RED MEAT

The WCRF/AICR report concluded that there was only limited evidence from sparse and inconsistent studies suggesting that processed meat is a cause of prostate cancer [39]. The SLR found four cohort and six case—control studies that met the criteria for a meta-analysis as described in the SLR. All cohort studies reported increased risks with higher intake; the summary relative risk estimate was 1.11 (95% confidence interval (CI): 0.995, 1.25). However, the meta-analysis of case—control studies did not yield a positive summary risk. Since that SLR, two of five cohort studies found a positive association between processed meat and prostate cancer risk [51,52], whereas the remaining three studies did not [53—55]. Two population-based case—control studies [56,57] reported an increase in risk associated with processed meat, but one hospital-based study did not [58]. Thus, these findings continue to show inconsistencies and would be unlikely to change the conclusion of the WCRF/AICR report.

A great many epidemiologic studies have investigated associations between red meat consumption and prostate cancer risk. However, the findings are not consistent. The WCRF/AICR meta-analysis of seven cohort and five case—control studies produced nonsignificant summary risk estimates and led to no conclusion by the expert panel. Since that SLR, three case—control [57—59] and two cohort [51,52] studies have reported a positive association. However, several other studies, including five cohort studies [53—55,60,61] and one case—control study [56], did not reproduce this finding. Furthermore, a meta-analysis of 15 prospective studies did not support the association [62]. Thus, these newer data do not seem to alter the conclusion of the WCRF/AICR report on red meat.

Explaining a possible association with meat intake is not straightforward. Initially, positive findings were thought to reflect a high exposure to dietary fat, especially saturated fat, because meat and dairy products are the major contributors to fat intake in the Western diet. However, because the findings on dietary fat per se and prostate cancer are equivocal (discussed later), other explanations for an association with meat need to be considered. There are several possibilities. First, in the American diet, meat is a major source of zinc, which is essential for testosterone synthesis and may have other effects in the prostate (discussed later). Second, diets high in meat and other animal products may be relatively deficient in certain anticarcinogenic constituents found primarily in plant foods. Third, red meat contains high levels of heme iron, which is a source for free radical formation and oxidative damage to tissues [63]. Fourth, nitrates added as preservatives to processed meat may contribute to N-nitroso compound production and exposures. These compounds are suspected mutagens and carcinogens [64]. Heme also promotes the formation of N-nitroso compounds. Finally, and most intriguing, many meats are cooked at high temperatures, such as by pan frying, grilling, or barbecuing. Cooking meats at high temperatures can result in the formation of heterocyclic amines (HAs), which are potent carcinogens in animals, including the rat prostate [65,66]. Furthermore, when meats are cooked on charcoal grills, rendered fat is pyrolized by the coals, leading to the deposition of polycyclic aromatic hydrocarbons (PAHs), which are also carcinogenic in animals, on the outer surface of the meat [67]. Although an accurate assessment of dietary intake of HAs and PAHs is difficult, one study reported a positive association of prostate cancer with estimated intakes of very well-done meat and of a particular HA (PhIP) [68]. However, other studies that examined intake of well-done meat [69] or estimated HA and PAH intakes from cooked meat [52,54,57,70,71] in relation to risk of prostate cancer did not provide clear support for the hypothesis.

B MILK AND DAIRY PRODUCTS

The WCRF/AICR report concluded that there was limited evidence suggesting that milk and dairy products are a cause of prostate cancer. In the SLR, the summary relative risk estimate from a meta-analysis of 8 cohort studies was 1.06 (95% CI: 1.01, 1.11), whereas that from 8 case–control studies was not statistically significant. One cohort study produced a clear dose–response relationship between advanced/aggressive cancer risk and milk intake (relative risk = 1.30; 95% CI: 1.04, 1.61) [72]. Since the WCRF/AICR review, several case–control [73,74] and cohort [60,75–79] studies have found positive associations between the consumption of milk and other dairy products and the risk of prostate cancer. Nevertheless, other studies did not find this association [55,61,80–82]. A comprehensive overview of 21 cohort and 24 case–control studies provided no support for a causal role of dairy products in prostate cancer risk [83]. Thus, although several reports have appeared since the WCRF/AICR report, the evidence remains weak and inconclusive for a detrimental effect of milk and dairy products on prostate cancer risk.

A possible explanation for the positive association is an adverse effect on the prostate of the high fat, especially saturated fat, content of dairy products. Another prominent constituent of these foods is calcium, which has also been proposed as a risk factor for prostate cancer (discussed later). Finally, milk consumption may increase blood levels of insulin-like growth factor-I (IGF-I), which has been associated with increased prostate cancer risk in some studies [84].

C ALCOHOLIC BEVERAGES

The WCRF/AICR SLR was able to meta-analyze 8 cohort and 14 case–control studies from the 35 prospective and 64 case–control studies found, which yielded nonstatistically significant summary risk estimates. The expert panel determined, however, that the evidence was too limited for a firm conclusion as to whether alcohol consumption was associated with prostate cancer risk. Since the SLR, 2 case–control studies in Canada found a positive association for total alcohol intake [85,86], but one study in Italy did not [87]. Whereas a cohort study [88] observed a positive association, most cohort studies reported null results for alcohol and prostate cancer risk [89–93]. A meta-analysis showed a direct association from 14 population case–control studies but not from 14 cohort and 7 hospital case–control studies [94]. Thus, the new studies have added to the inconsistent findings, with most of the cohort studies null, and do not strengthen the evidence for an effect of alcohol on prostate cancer risk.

Some general mechanisms by which alcohol might enhance carcinogenesis have been proposed, including the activation of environmental nitrosamines, production of carcinogenic metabolites (acetaldehyde), immune suppression, and secondary nutritional deficiencies [95–97].

3 Nutrients and Other Food Constituents

A ENERGY

The findings from studies that have examined total energy intake in relation to prostate cancer are very inconsistent. No conclusion was made about energy intake in the WCRF/AICR report. The meta-analysis in the SLR of 10 cohort and 29 case—control studies showed no significant association. No study has reported the relationship between energy intake and prostate cancer since the SLR.

An experimental study in rodents (rats and mice) found that energy restriction reduced prostate tumor growth, possibly by inhibiting tumor angiogenesis [98].

B FAT

Dietary fat has been the most studied nutrient with regard to effects on prostate cancer risk. Detailed reviews on this topic have been published [99—101]. The SLR in the WCRF/AICR report yielded no significant association for total or saturated fat consumption, either as grams or as percentage energy, in a meta-analysis of seven cohort and 25 case—control studies. However, because the evidence was limited, the expert panel reached no conclusion about total and subtypes of dietary fat in relation to prostate cancer. Since that SLR, 2 case—control studies have reported that total fat intake was positively associated with the risk of prostate cancer [57,102], and one of them observed a stronger association for the advanced cases [57]. However, four cohort studies [53,61,103,104] and another case-control study [86] did not support the association. These findings are inconsistent, and those from the cohort studies are mostly null; thus, they do not provide additional support for an association between total or saturated fat consumption and prostate cancer risk.

Some epidemiologic studies examined dietary intakes of monounsaturated and polyunsaturated fat as well. The WCRF/AICR SLR included three cohort studies in the meta-analysis for monounsaturated fatty acids, with a summary relative risk estimate of 1.37 (95% CI: 1.10, 1.70), whereas the summary estimate from 13 case—control studies was not significant. The meta-analyses for dietary polyunsaturated fatty acids were based on two cohort and 13 case—control studies and did not show any association. Since the WCRF/AICR review, 1 case—control study has reported positive associations of monounsaturated and polyunsaturated fat with prostate cancer risk [102]. However, the majority of the recent studies found no association of either of these classes of fat with prostate cancer, including four cohort [53,61,103,104] and 2 case—control [86,105] studies. Thus, these recent studies do not provide support for an effect of total or subtypes of dietary fat on prostate cancer risk.

Several studies have also examined specific fatty acids (including several omega-3 and omega-6 polyunsaturated fatty acids), based either on dietary intake data or on biochemical measurements in blood or adipose tissue [99,106]. A few studies suggested that long-chain omega-3 fatty acids, such as eicosapentaenoic acid (EPA) and docosahexaenoic acid (DHA), were inversely associated with prostate cancer [107—110], although other studies did not reproduce this finding [53,103,111—113]. Additional support for these inverse findings was provided by studies of fatty fish intake (a good source of long-chain polyunsaturated fatty acids) that also showed inverse associations with prostate cancer risk [114—117]. The effect of α-linolenic acid (ALA) intake was examined in several studies, with some showing a positive association [108,111,118] and some no association [53,103,112,119]. A meta-analysis involving eight cohort and eight case—control studies that measured either ALA intake or blood/tissue concentrations supported the positive association with prostate cancer [120]. Finally, two studies reported that prediagnostic blood concentrations of *trans* fatty acids were associated with increased risk of prostate cancer [121,122]. Overall, these reports are not very consistent, and no firm conclusion regarding the role of specific fatty acids on the risk of prostate cancer can be reached on the basis of current data.

Some animal experiments have tested the fat—prostate cancer hypothesis. For example, a high-fat diet increased prostate cancer incidence and shortened the latency period in Lobund—Wistar rats treated with exogenous testosterone to induce the tumors [123]. Conversely, prostate tumor growth rate was reduced by a fat-free diet in Dunning rats [124] or by lowering dietary fat intake in athymic nude mice injected with LNCaP cells (a human prostate cancer cell line) [125,126]. With regard to specific types of fat, fish oils containing high levels of long-chain omega-3 fatty acids, such as EPA and DHA, generally suppressed prostate tumor growth in rodents, whereas omega-6 polyunsaturated fatty acids, such as linoleic and linolenic acids, promoted tumor growth [117,127,128]. However, because most animal studies have been conducted in rodents, whose prostate glands differ anatomically from that of the human, extrapolation of these findings to humans is particularly tenuous.

A number of plausible mechanisms by which dietary fat could increase cancer risk have been proposed. These include the formation of lipid radicals and hydroperoxides that can produce DNA damage, increased circulating androgen levels, decreased gap-junctional communication between cells, altered activity of signal transduction molecules, effects on eicosanoid metabolism, and decreased immune responsiveness [99].

C CALCIUM

As noted previously, a number of studies that have examined the relationship of dairy product consumption to prostate cancer risk found a positive association. Dairy products could be a marker of exposure to calcium, although this food group is also a major source of saturated or animal fat in the Western diet. The WCRF/AICR report concluded that a diet high in calcium is a probable cause of prostate cancer. In the SLR, a meta-analysis of eight cohort studies yielded a summary relative risk estimate of 1.27 (95% CI: 1.09, 1.48) for total prostate cancer and 1.32 (95% CI: 1.05, 1.64) for advanced or aggressive tumors, whereas the meta-analysis of case—control studies showed no significant increased risk. Since that SLR, six cohort studies [55,75,76,78,80,129] have reported statistically significant positive associations for this nutrient, especially with advanced or metastatic cancer. However, one case—control study [74] and five cohort studies [60,77,79,81,82], along with two others that examined prediagnostic blood calcium [130,131], did not show an effect of calcium on prostate cancer risk. In view of the fact that the findings from the recent studies are conflicting, but that several of them continue to show a positive association, the conclusion of the WCRF/AICR report seems somewhat weakened, although it cannot be discounted.

A mechanism for an adverse effect of calcium on prostate carcinogenesis has been proposed based on the observation that a high intake of calcium decreases the circulating levels of $1,25(OH)_2$ vitamin D, which may inhibit cell proliferation and promote differentiation in prostatic tissue [132,133]. The role of vitamin D in prostatic carcinogenesis is discussed later.

D ZINC AND CADMIUM

The trace elements zinc and cadmium are considered together because they act as antagonists in biological systems. Due to limited evidence, the WCRF/AICR report reached no firm conclusion regarding zinc in the diet or supplements. Since that SLR, a positive association for zinc was reported in two case—control studies [134,135]. One cohort study found no association of supplemental zinc with total prostate cancer, although a decreased risk was found for advanced tumors [136].

The frequent association of prostate cancer risk with high intake of red meat (discussed previously) could also be explained by a higher intake of zinc, rather than animal fat, because meat, especially red meat, is an important source of zinc in the American diet (other sources are shellfish, whole grain cereals, nuts, and legumes) [137]. Reports based on zinc levels in blood or prostatic tissue of patients with cancer and controls have not been consistent [138—140], but such studies are unreliable because the levels of zinc measured after diagnosis in the cases may reflect physiologic changes in the prostate as a result of the cancer ("reverse causation"). One study measured prediagnostic toenail zinc

in prostate cancer patients and in controls; no association was found [141].

As a major constituent of prostatic fluid [142—144], zinc is essential for normal prostate function. Zinc is also essential for normal testicular function, and high levels of zinc have been proposed to increase the production of testosterone, leading to enhanced tissue growth in the prostate. Blood levels of zinc have been positively correlated with testosterone and dihydrotestosterone levels in men [145,146]. Furthermore, in the rat prostate, zinc has been shown to increase 5α-reductase activity [147] and to potentiate androgen receptor binding [148]. Thus, one might speculate that higher intake of zinc could partially offset the normal decline in testosterone levels with age [149—151], thereby contributing to prostate cancer risk. However, an epidemiologic study that analyzed prediagnostic zinc levels in serum in relation to prostate cancer risk reported no clear association [152]. Thus, evidence to support a role of zinc in prostate cancer is still limited, and no firm conclusion can be reached.

Epidemiologic evidence for cadmium as a risk factor for prostate cancer is also limited [153]. The WCRF/AICR SLR found only four case—control studies that assessed cadmium exposure in relation to prostate cancer risk, and all showed no significant association. Since that SLR, a hospital-based case—control study found some evidence that higher levels of cadmium in blood and urine (measured after diagnosis) were associated with higher risk of advanced prostate cancer [154]. Another hospital-based case—control study found a positive association between toenail cadmium and prostate cancer risk [155]. With so few studies and a lack of data from cohorts in particular, no firm conclusion can be reached regarding the association of cadmium exposure with prostate cancer risk.

Cadmium is a competitive inhibitor of zinc in enzyme systems and accumulates in the body throughout life because no mechanism exists for excreting it. Thus, the hypothesis that cadmium may be carcinogenic for the prostate has biologic plausibility. This hypothesis is further supported by studies showing that cadmium is carcinogenic in animals, and that the effect can be blocked by simultaneous injection of zinc [156,157].

4 Diet-Associated Risk Factors

A OBESITY, WEIGHT, AND HEIGHT

Prostate cancer is sometimes considered a male counterpart to breast cancer in women, for which there is clear evidence of a positive association with obesity, especially in postmenopausal cases. However, evidence for a similar association of adult obesity with prostate cancer is much less clear. Due to insufficient data, the

WCRF/AICR panel reached no firm conclusion on body fatness, abdominal fatness, and birth weight. The meta-analyses in the SLR yielded no statistically significant risk for body mass index and prostate cancer risk; summary estimates were 1.00 (95% CI: 0.99, 1.01) from 28 cohort studies, 1.00 (95% CI: 0.99, 1.00) from 11 population-based case—control studies, and 1.00 (95% CI: 0.99, 1.01) from 18 hospital-based case—control studies. Since that SLR, a few epidemiological studies, including 3 cohort studies [158—160] and 1 case—control study [161], reported a significant positive association of obesity with prostate cancer risk. However, the majority of recent epidemiologic studies have found no clear relationship between measures of obesity and prostate cancer risk, including both cohort [162—166] and case—control [87,167,168] studies. Indeed, 1 case—control study [169] even reported inverse associations. Three studies reported reversals of effect: In two, obesity increased the risk of high-grade but decreased the risk of low-grade prostate cancer [170,171]; in the other, obesity was associated with decreased prostate cancer incidence but with increased prostate cancer mortality [172]. Some studies examined obesity in early adulthood or at birth, but the meta-analyses of these studies in the WCRF/AICR SLR showed no significant overall association. Since then, one study found that heavier birth weight was associated with an increased risk of prostate cancer in later life [173].

In the WCRF/AICR SLR, the meta-analysis yielded no significant association between height and prostate cancer risk; summary risk estimates were 1.02 (95% CI: 0.97, 1.08) per 10 cm based on 23 cohort studies, 1.03 (95% CI: 0.97, 1.09) from 15 population-based case—control studies, and 1.01 (95% CI: 0.91, 1.12) from 9 hospital-based case—control studies. Since that SLR, several studies reported a direct association [160,165,167,170,174,175], whereas others found no relationship [159,163,164,168]. Thus, taken together, the newer studies since the WCRF/AICR report do not provide clear evidence to support a positive association of obesity, weight, or height with prostate cancer risk.

The basis for an association between obesity and prostate cancer could involve endocrine factors because adult obesity in men has been associated with decreased circulating levels of testosterone and increased levels of estrogen [176,177]. However, this mechanism would suggest an inverse rather than a direct association between obesity and this cancer. Other possible mechanisms entail pathways that involve insulin, leptin, adipokines, IGF-I, and chronic inflammation [178]. For example, leptin is a hormone produced by adipocytes. Obese men have more and larger adipocytes, and they have been shown to have higher serum levels of leptin [179]. In *in vitro* studies,

leptin promoted proliferation of androgen-independent prostate cancer [180].

C Dietary Factors that Decrease Risk

1 Dietary Patterns

The three case—control [45—47] and three cohort studies [48—50] that investigated dietary patterns and prostate cancer risk identified healthful eating patterns, generally characterized by high intakes of fruits, vegetables, and/or whole grains (referred to as a fruit/vegetable, prudent, health-conscious, or healthy living diet). However, none of the studies found a significant relationship of the healthful dietary pattern to prostate cancer risk.

2 Foods and Beverages

A VEGETABLES

Intake of vegetables has been inversely associated with cancer risk at many sites. This has led to strong recommendations to consume significant quantities of these foods as part of a healthful diet. However, the evidence for a beneficial effect of vegetables on prostate cancer risk is not overwhelming. The WCRF/AICR report reached no firm conclusion on vegetables because of limited evidence. The meta-analyses for all vegetables in the SLR yielded summary estimates of 0.98 (95% CI: 0.92, 1.04) based on six cohort studies, 0.95 (95% CI: 0.93, 0.97) based on seven population based case—control studies, and 0.96 (95% CI: 0.83, 1.10) based on five hospital-based case—control studies. When restricted to green leafy, yellow-orange, or cruciferous vegetables, summary estimates were not statistically significant. Since that SLR, two case—control studies showed inverse associations [87,181], but two others did not [182,183]. Two prospective cohort studies observed no relation [184,185]. Thus, the limited number of new studies since the WCRF/AICR report are inconsistent and do not provide evidence for an effect of vegetable consumption overall on prostate cancer risk. The findings for legumes, a vegetable subgroup, are considered separately (discussed later), and the findings for tomatoes are included in the later discussion of carotenoids.

Because vegetables contain numerous compounds that can act through a variety of mechanisms to inhibit carcinogenesis [186,187], an inverse association between vegetables and prostate cancer is plausible. Some of these mechanisms are discussed later with respect to specific food constituents.

B FRUITS

The WCRF/AICR report reached no firm conclusion on fruit consumption and prostate cancer risk. The meta-analysis in the SLR yielded no significant association: The summary relative risk estimate was 1.03 (95% CI: 0.98, 1.10) based on nine cohort studies. Since that SLR, three case–control [87,181,188] and three cohort [184,185,189] studies reported no association.

Fruits contain many of the same compounds with anticarcinogenic properties that are found in vegetables, such as various carotenoids and vitamin C [190]. Because most of the findings for this food group have been null, it does appear that fruit intake has no particular benefit with regard to the risk of prostate cancer.

C LEGUMES, INCLUDING SOY PRODUCTS

Prostate cancer rates have traditionally been low in populations, such as those of Japan and China, in which the intake of soy products is relatively high. The WCRF/AICR report concluded that the evidence, mostly from case–control studies, was too limited for a firm conclusion regarding a role of legumes in increasing or decreasing the risk of prostate cancer. The meta-analyses in the SLR yielded summary estimates of 0.96 (95% CI: 0.95, 0.98) for legumes from four population-based case–control studies and 0.97 (95% CI: 0.95, 0.99) for soybean products from two population-based case–control studies. Since that SLR, one case–control study [191] and one cohort study [192] reported inverse associations between intake of legumes and prostate cancer risk, including soy products specifically. In addition, a later meta-analysis of five cohort and nine case–control studies supported an overall inverse association between soyfood consumption and prostate cancer risk (Figure 36.2) [193].

In the past, legumes were of interest in nutritional epidemiology primarily because of their important contribution to fiber intake. However, these foods also contain phytoestrogens, plant constituents that have mild estrogenic properties. Because estrogens are associated with lower risk of prostate cancer and are used in prostate cancer therapy, there is a good rationale for the hypothesis that phytoestrogen intake can protect against prostate cancer. Soybeans and many products made from soy, such as tofu, are rich in a class of phytoestrogens known as isoflavones (other classes of phytoestrogens include the coumestans and lignans). The main isoflavones found in soy include genistein, daidzein, and glycetein [206]. Several epidemiologic studies assessed the intake of dietary phytoestrogens, particularly isoflavones, and found inverse associations with prostate cancer risk [105,182,197,202,207,208]. Indeed, a meta-analysis of two cohort and six case–control studies suggested that isoflavone consumption was related to a reduction in prostate cancer risk [193]. Furthermore, an analysis of urinary isoflavone excretion within a large cohort study showed inverse associations, suggesting that high intake of isoflavones may

be protective against prostate cancer risk [209], although another nested case–control study did not confirm this result [210]. Taking into account the recent reports on legumes, particularly soy products, and prostate cancer risk, the evidence in support of a protective effect on prostate cancer risk appears to have strengthened.

The mechanism for a benefit of soy products on prostate carcinogenesis could entail the estrogenic effects of isoflavones, although other actions of these compounds, such as inhibition of protein tyrosine phosphorylation, induction of apoptosis, and suppression of angiogenesis, have also been proposed [211]. Laboratory data, based on human tissue as well as animal models, offer support for the hypothesis that soy products may protect against prostate cancer [212–215].

Although soy products and isoflavones are of particular interest, legumes contain other bioactive microconstituents, including saponins, protease inhibitors, inositol hexaphosphate, γ-tocopherol, and phytosterols. Mechanisms by which each of these compounds can inhibit carcinogenesis have been proposed [211,212,216].

D TEA

Due to limited evidence, the WCRF/AICR report reached no firm conclusion on tea consumption. The meta-analyses in the SLR found no support for an association based on one cohort and six case–control studies. Since that SLR, a cohort study in Japan [217] showed an inverse relationship between daily tea consumption and prostate cancer risk, but another cohort study in Japan did not [218]. A meta-analysis of three cohort and three case–control studies in an Asian population suggested that green tea may have a protective effect on prostate cancer risk (summary risk estimate = 0.62; 95% CI: 0.38, 1.01) [219]. However, the evidence is still insufficient to draw firm conclusions regarding the effect of tea consumption on this cancer.

Tea contains polyphenols that are potentially anticarcinogenic because of their antioxidant properties, effects on signal transduction pathways, inhibition of cell proliferation, and other actions in the body [220,221].

3 Nutrients and Other Food Constituents

A VITAMIN D

Evidence for a protective effect of vitamin D against prostate cancer is not convincing. The WCRF/AICR report reached no firm conclusion on vitamin D. The meta-analyses in the SLR showed no significant association based on four cohort and three case–control studies. Since that SLR, one cohort study [82] and one

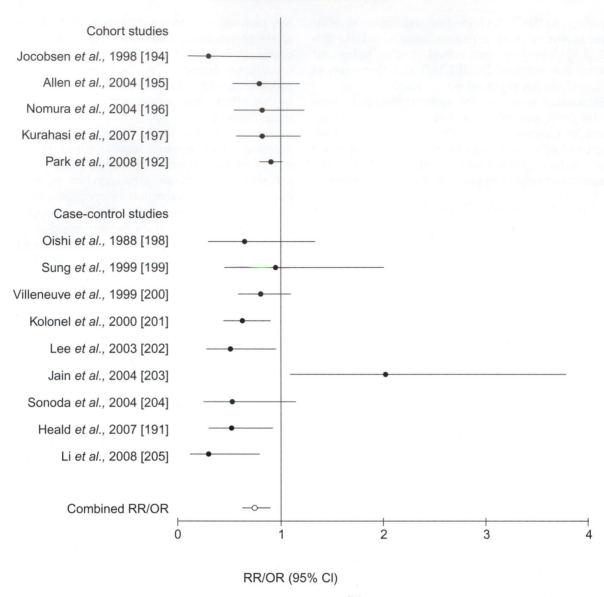

FIGURE 36.2 Soy food intake and prostate cancer. OR, odds ratio, comparing highest with lowest intake; RR, relative risk; error bars indicate 95% confidence intervals. *Source: Adapted, with permission of the American Society for Nutrition, from Yan, L., and Spitznagel, E. L. (2009). Soy consumption and prostate cancer risk in men: A revisit of a meta-analysis. Am. J. Clin. Nutr. **89**, 1155–1163 [193].*

case–control study [105] found no association of estimated dietary intake of vitamin D, whether from foods or supplements, with prostate cancer risk. Furthermore, a meta-analysis of six cohort and five case–control studies also did not support a role of dietary vitamin D in preventing prostate cancer [222]. However, because circulating vitamin D levels are substantially determined by the conversion of 7-dehydrocholesterol in the skin in response to solar UVB radiation, studies based on dietary vitamin D intake alone may be misleading [223,224].

Several cohort studies have examined the relationship of prediagnostic blood levels of 25-hydroxyvitamin D (25(OH)D), the most abundant circulating form of the vitamin, to subsequent development of prostate cancer. A meta-analysis in the WCRF/AICR SLR showed no significant association: The summary risk estimate was 1.01 (95% CI: 0.94, 1.10) based on 6 prospective studies. Studies since that SLR found either no association [225–228] or an unexpected direct association with higher blood levels of 25(OH)D [229], especially for aggressive tumors [230,231]. Furthermore, two meta-analyses of prospective studies did not find evidence of an inverse relation for circulating vitamin D [222,232]. One of them reported a summary risk estimate of 0.99 (95% CI: 0.95, 1.03) per

10 ng/ml increase in 25(OH)D based on 11 studies [232], and the other found a borderline increase in risk (summary risk estimate = 1.04; 95% CI: 0.99, 1.10) based on 14 studies (Figure 36.3) [222]. Thus, there is little epidemiologic data to support the hypothesis of a protective effect of vitamin D against prostate cancer, with some evidence even suggesting an adverse effect at high circulating levels of 25(OH)D.

The hormonal form of vitamin D, 1,25(OH)$_2$D, reduces cell proliferation in the prostate (and other tissues) and enhances cell differentiation, both of which would be expected to lower the risk of cancer [132,241].

B VITAMIN E

The WCRF/AICR report concluded that there was limited evidence suggesting that foods containing vitamin E decrease the risk of prostate cancer. The SLR found two cohort and 13 case–control studies that investigated dietary vitamin E and prostate cancer. In the meta-analyses, summary risk estimates were 0.91 (95% CI: 0.82, 1.02) based on two cohort studies, 1.04 (95% CI: 0.99, 1.11) based on 7 population-based case–control studies, and 0.66 (95% CI: 0.10, 4.29) based on 3 hospital-based case–control studies. Since that SLR, 1 case–control study [105] and three cohort studies [184,242,243] found no association with prostate cancer risk, whereas 3 other case–control studies found an inverse association [182,244] and one cohort study reported a positive association [245]. Several cohort studies have reported findings for vitamin E and prostate cancer based on prediagnostic blood levels. A meta-analysis in the WCRF/AICR SLR yielded summary estimates of 0.99 (95% CI: 0.97, 1.00) for α-tocopherol in blood based on seven cohort studies and 0.90 (95% CI: 0.81, 0.996) for γ-tocopherol in blood based on six cohort studies. Since that SLR, one study [243] found an inverse association for vitamin E in blood and two others did not [246,247].

The WCRF/AICR report also concluded that there was limited evidence that α-tocopherol supplements protect against prostate cancer in smokers, mainly based on one intervention trial among male heavy smokers in Finland [248]. However, protection against prostate cancer was not a prespecified hypothesis in the trial. A later intervention trial of vitamins E (400 IU/alternate days) and C (500 mg/day) in 14,641 male physicians conducted in the United States provided no support for a benefit of vitamin E supplements in the prevention of prostate cancer (relative risk = 0.97; 95% CI: 0.85–1.09) [249]. In another intervention trial of vitamin E (400 IU/day) and selenium (200 μg/day) among 35,533 healthy men, there was a statistically significant increase in risk (relative risk = 1.17; 95% CI: 1.004–1.36) in the vitamin E group, suggesting that vitamin E supplementation actually

increases the risk of prostate cancer among healthy men [250]. One cohort study of vitamin E supplement use reported no overall effect, although long-term use was associated with a reduced risk for advanced cancers [251]. Thus, the weight of the existing epidemiological evidence does not support a protective effect of vitamin E, either dietary or through supplementation, against prostate cancer. Indeed, one intervention trial suggested that vitamin E supplementation may actually be harmful.

Vitamin E inhibits prostate carcinogenesis in rats and mice [252,253] and the growth of human prostate cancer cells in nude mice [254–256]. Possible cancer prevention mechanisms include antioxidative and anti-inflammatory activities, modulation of nuclear receptors, inhibition of cell growth, and induction of apoptosis [257].

C CAROTENOIDS (β-CAROTENE AND LYCOPENE)

The epidemiologic evidence related to carotenoids and prostate cancer is inconsistent. The WCRF/AICR report concluded that a substantial effect of β-carotene or of foods containing β-carotene on the risk of prostate cancer was unlikely. The meta-analyses in the SLR showed no significant association for β-carotene in diet; summary risk estimates were 1.00 (95% CI: 0.99–1.01) from six cohort studies, 0.99 (95% CI: 0.98, 1.00) from nine population-based case–control studies, and 0.975 (95% CI: 0.94, 1.01) from six hospital-based case–control studies. In addition, the SLR included three intervention trials on β-carotene supplements, none of which reported a significant effect on prostate cancer risk. The meta-analysis in the SLR also showed no significant association of β-carotene in prediagnostic blood with prostate cancer (summary risk estimate = 1.00; 95% CI: 0.91, 1.09) based on seven prospective studies.

Since that SLR, one case–control [182] and two cohort [184,242] studies offered no support for a protective effect of dietary carotenoids. Recent studies based on prediagnostic blood have reported both an increased risk [258] and no association [246,247] with higher β-carotene levels. Overall, the recent studies add to the previous conclusion that there is no association between β-carotene and prostate cancer risk.

A carotenoid of particular interest with regard to prostate cancer is lycopene, found primarily in tomatoes and tomato products (other food sources include watermelon, grapefruit, and guava). The WCRF/AICR report concluded that foods containing lycopene probably protect against prostate cancer. The SLR identified 17 studies that investigated tomatoes, 17 that investigated dietary lycopene, and 8 that investigated blood lycopene; most of the studies showed a decreased risk with increasing intake. The meta-analysis in the SLR

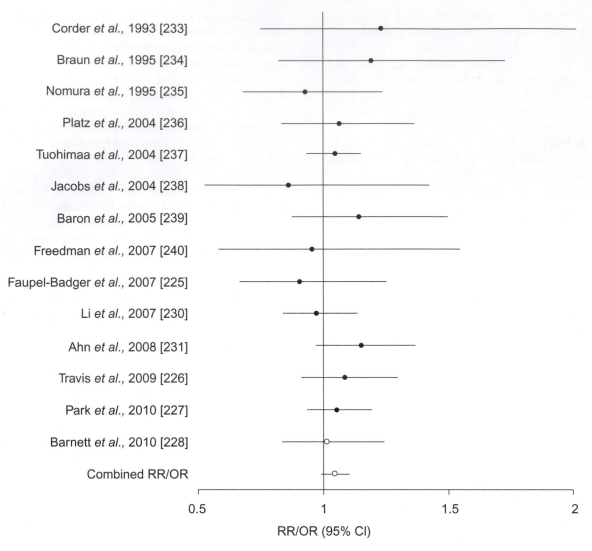

FIGURE 36.3 Circulating 25-hydroxyvitamin D and prostate cancer in prospective studies. OR, odds ratio, comparing highest with lowest intake; RR, relative risk; error bars indicate 95% confidence intervals. Source: *Adapted, with permission of Springer, from Gilbert, R., Martin, R. M., Beynon, R., Harris, R., Savovic, J., Zuccolo, L., Bekkering, G. E., Fraser, W. D., Sterne, J. A., and Metcalfe, C. (2011). Associations of circulating and dietary vitamin D with prostate cancer risk: A systematic review and dose–response meta-analysis. Cancer Causes Control **22**, 319–340 [222].*

yielded a nonstatistically significant summary relative risk estimate of 0.69 (95% CI: 0.43, 1.08) for tomato consumption based on 4 cohort studies. In addition, a summary risk estimate based on 4 cohort studies that measured lycopene in blood was 0.962 (95% CI: 0.926, 0.999) [259–261].

Since that SLR, one case–control study of dietary lycopene intake found no association for lycopene per se [182], although another study found an inverse association [262]. Two cohort studies also found no association [184,263]. For tomato product consumption, two cohort studies [184,263] found no association with prostate cancer risk. The results of investigations based on prediagnostic circulating levels of lycopene were mostly null. One study showed an inverse relationship

for advanced tumors but not with total prostate cancer [246]. Four others [247,258,264,265], two of which [258,265] were able to exclude screening bias, found no association. Thus, the data obtained since the WCRF/AICR report seem to weaken the overall evidence for a beneficial effect of lycopene on prostate cancer risk. Results of the analyses of prediagnostic blood lycopene in relation to prostate cancer risk are summarized in Table 36.3.

β-Carotene, lycopene, and other carotenoids are widely distributed in human tissues, including the prostate [266,267], where, as potent antioxidants, they help protect cell membranes, DNA, and other macromolecules from damage by reactive oxygen species. Other biological activities of carotenoids, such as the

TABLE 36.3 Blood Lycopene and Prostate Cancer Risk in Nested Case–Control Studies

Reference	Cases/controls	Odds ratio (95% confidence interval)[a]
Gann et al., 1999 [259]	578/1294	0.75 (0.54, 1.06)
Goodman et al., 2003 [260]	205/205	1.04 (0.61, 1.77)
Huang et al., 2003 [261]	182/364	0.83 (0.46, 1.48)
Huang et al., 2003 [261]	142/284	0.79 (0.41, 1.54)
Key et al., 2007 [246]	966/1064	0.97 (0.70, 1.34)
Peters et al., 2007 [258]	692/844	1.14 (0.82, 1.58)
Gill et al., 2009 [247]	372/765	0.78 (0.53, 1.14)
Beilby et al., 2010 [264]	96/225	0.77 (0.40, 1.47)
Kristal et al., 2011 [265]	735/1008	0.99 (0.74, 1.32)[b]
	204/1008	1.16 (0.74, 1.81)[c]

[a]Highest vs. lowest category.
[b]Low-grade tumors.
[c]High-grade tumors.

upregulation of gap-junctional communication [268], may also contribute to their anticarcinogenic effects. In three human prostate cancer cell lines (PC-3, DU 145, and LNCaP), β-carotene and lycopene significantly inhibited in vitro growth rates [269,270].

D FRUCTOSE

Intake of fructose was inversely associated with the risk of prostate cancer in one cohort study [271], which found a similar relationship for the intake of fruit, a major source of fructose in the diet. However, two other cohort studies found no association [272,273]. Although few epidemiologic studies have assessed fructose intake per se, several, as noted previously, examined the relationship of fruit intake to prostate cancer and most did not find an inverse association. However, the metabolism of calcium, phosphorus, fructose, and vitamin D is interrelated, and unless all components are considered simultaneously in an analysis, their individual effects could be missed [271].

The hypothesis for the protective effect of fructose is that it reduces plasma phosphate levels, resulting in increased levels of circulating $1,25(OH)_2$ vitamin D, which in turn may reduce the risk of prostate cancer [271,274] (discussed previously).

E SELENIUM

The WCRF/AICR report concluded that foods containing selenium probably protect against prostate cancer. There was also very good evidence from a randomized intervention trial and from several cohort studies at the time indicating that selenium

supplementation probably protects against prostate cancer. In meta-analyses of cohort studies in the SLR, summary risk estimates for selenium in blood were 0.947 (95% CI: 0.892, 1.000) for total prostate cancer based on nine cohort studies and 0.873 (95% CI: 0.790, 0.965) for advanced or aggressive cancer based on two cohort studies. Two studies based on selenium content of toenails also showed an inverse association for advanced or aggressive prostate cancer (summary risk estimate = 0.795; 95% CI: 0.693, 0.912). In a randomized intervention trial of a daily selenium supplement (200 μg) for men with a history of skin cancers, an incidental finding was a lower incidence of prostate cancer in the men who received the intervention [275].

Since that SLR, one case–control study [105] found no association between estimated selenium intake and prostate cancer risk, and baseline selenium intake was not associated with subsequent development of prostate cancer in a cohort study [184]. Furthermore, pre-diagnostic blood selenium was not related to prostate cancer in three prospective cohort studies [247,276,277]. Of particular significance, the findings of a large prostate cancer randomized intervention trial using supplemental selenium (200 μg/day) and vitamin E (400 IU/day) were reported. The results provided no evidence in support of a beneficial effect of selenium on prostate cancer risk [278]. A second randomized intervention trial of supplemental selenium (200 μg/day) in men at high risk of prostate cancer failed to support the hypothesis that selenium protects against prostate cancer [279]. Thus, the basis for the previous WCRF/AICR conclusion has been weakened in the interval, and there is now no basis for recommending selenium supplementation to reduce prostate cancer risk.

Selenium is a component of glutathione peroxidase, an important enzyme in certain antioxidative pathways. In in vitro experiments, selenium was shown to inhibit the growth of human prostate carcinoma cells [280,281]. Selenium may exert its anticancer effects through any of several proposed mechanisms, such as antioxidation, enhanced immune function, inhibition of cell proliferation, and induction of apoptosis [281].

F ISOFLAVONOIDS

The potential role of isoflavonoids in prostate carcinogenesis was discussed in the section on legumes.

4 Diet-Associated Protective Factors

A PHYSICAL ACTIVITY

The role of physical activity in human prostate carcinogenesis is quite unclear. Due to limited evidence, no conclusion on physical activity was reached in the WCRF/AICR report. Since that SLR, several studies have been reported. Some of these, including 3 cohort

[282−284] and 2 case−control [87,285] studies, found an inverse association with prostate cancer risk, whereas others, including 2 cohort studies [286,287] and 1 case−control study [288], found no association. Despite these inconsistencies, a meta-analysis of 19 cohort and 24 case−control studies found that total physical activity was inversely associated with prostate cancer risk [23]. This meta-analysis also suggested that occupational physical activity and physical activity in the 20−45 and 45−65 age groups was more beneficial than was recreational activity or physical activity in the older than 65 age group. The discrepancies in the findings among physical activity studies may be resolved, in part, if future studies can distinguish better between different types of physical activity (e.g., occupational, recreational, or household activity) and can establish the time of life (e.g., young adulthood vs. older ages) that may be most relevant. Indeed, one study found inconsistent associations depending on the types of activity, age period of life, and intensity of physical activity [289]. Another study observed that physical activity during young adulthood among black, but not white, men was related to a decreased risk of prostate cancer, whereas activity at older ages was not related to risk in either race [290]. Thus, the inconsistent findings from the studies performed since the WCRF/AICR report do not make possible any firm conclusion regarding the effects of physical activity on prostate cancer risk.

Because exercise influences androgen levels in the body, an effect of physical activity on prostate cancer risk is biologically plausible. Exercise lowers testosterone in the blood, and it also raises the level of sex hormone-binding globulin, which reduces the circulating free testosterone levels; both effects would be expected to lower prostate cancer risk [291−293].

IV GENETICS AND GENE−ENVIRONMENT INTERACTIONS

As noted previously, prostate cancer has a tendency to aggregate in families, and men whose fathers or brothers have had prostate cancer are at a two- or threefold increased risk of getting the disease compared to men without such a family history. The mapping by linkage studies of rare highly penetrant genes that could explain at least part of this familial aggregation identified a number of regions, including several loci on chromosome 1, but the results were not definitive [294].

Because diet (and other behaviors, such as physical activity [295]) can influence androgen, vitamin D, and IGF-I levels in the body, interactions may occur between dietary exposures and inherited susceptibilities in determining the actual risk for prostate cancer. During the past several years, many studies of single nucleotide polymorphisms (SNPs) in candidate genes have been reported, with largely disappointing results with regard to both the main effects of the genes and interactions between the genes and other exposures ("gene−environment interactions"). Recently, the research focus has been on genome-wide association studies (GWAS), which take an agnostic approach and require large consortial efforts to obtain sufficient numbers of cases. To date, the latter studies have identified more than 40 distinct prostate cancer susceptibility loci associated with small differences in the risk of this disease [296]. One particular region on chromosome 8 (8q24) has been the source of considerable current research activity [297]. Unfortunately, overall, the GWAS-identified loci explain only a small portion of the variability in prostate cancer susceptibility [298].

V CONCLUSIONS AND IMPLICATIONS FOR PREVENTION AND TREATMENT

Considering the combined evidence from descriptive epidemiologic studies (especially the remarkable changes in migrant populations), analytic epidemiologic studies in widely varying populations, experimental studies in animals, and in vitro studies, the likelihood that certain dietary components or general patterns of eating influence the risk of prostate cancer remains high. However, no specific relationships have been established conclusively. Research on this topic should be continued because diet is a modifiable risk factor and because prostate cancer incidence is extremely high in many populations. In addition, further research on genetic polymorphisms that affect susceptibility to prostate cancer, and their possible interactions with dietary risk factors, may help identify high-risk subgroups of men who can be targeted for future preventive programs.

Currently, the primary treatment modalities for prostate cancer consist of surgery, radiation, and hormonal therapy. The fact that the findings for some dietary factors (e.g., fat) were stronger in advanced or metastatic cases of prostate cancer implies that dietary effects can occur very late in the disease process. This suggests that dietary interventions have the potential not only to reduce the incidence but also to improve the survival rates of the disease, providing another possible treatment modality. Indeed, one study of prostate cancer patients showed significantly worse survival for men in the upper tertile of saturated fat intake (>13.2% of calories) compared with men in the lowest tertile (<10.8% of calories) [299], whereas another study found that survival was improved in patients who consumed higher amounts of tomato products [300]. Explanations for such observations might be a beneficial effect of lower fat intake on circulating androgen levels [301] or an inhibitory effect of lycopene on tumor growth rates [270].

Based on current knowledge, it is not prudent to make very specific dietary recommendations to prevent or treat prostate cancer. However, taken as a whole, the evidence is consistent with a diet that emphasizes vegetables, including legumes, and is moderate or low in the consumption of processed meat and milk and other dairy products.

References

[1] D.G. Bostwick, M.B. Amin, Prostate and seminal vesicles, in: tenth ed., I. Damjanov, J. Linder (Eds.), Anderson's Pathology, vol. 2, Mosby, St. Louis, MO, 1996, pp. 2197—2230.

[2] A.W. Partin, D.S. Coffey, The molecular biology, endocrinology and physiology of the prostate and seminal vesicles, in: P.C. Walsh, A.B. Retik, E.D. Vaughan Jr., A.J. Wein (Eds.), Campbell's Urology, seventh ed., vol. 2, Saunders, Philadelphia, 1998, pp. 1381—1428.

[3] M.J. Barry, PSA screening for prostate cancer: the current controversy—A viewpoint. Patient Outcomes Research Team for Prostatic Diseases, Ann. Oncol. 9 (1998) 1279—1282.

[4] J.M. Croswell, B.S. Kramer, E.D. Crawford, Screening for prostate cancer with PSA testing: current status and future directions, Oncology 25 (2011) 452—460463

[5] R. Chou, J.M. Croswell, T. Dana, C. Bougatsos, I. Blazina, R. Fu, et al., Screening for prostate cancer: a review of the evidence for the U.S. Preventive Services Task Force, Ann. Intern. Med. 155 (2011) 762—771.

[6] M.P. Curado, B. Edwards, H.R. Shin, H. Storm, J. Ferlay, M. Heanue, et al., Cancer Incidence in Five Continents, vol. 9, IARC, Lyon, France, 2007 (IARC Sci. Pub. No. 160).

[7] American Cancer Society, Cancer Facts and Figures 2011, American Cancer Society, Atlanta, GA, 2011.

[8] B.F. Hankey, E.J. Feuer, L.X. Clegg, R.B. Hayes, J.M. Legler, P.C. Prorok, et al., Cancer surveillance series: interpreting trends in prostate cancer—Part I: evidence of the effects of screening in recent prostate cancer incidence, mortality, and survival rates, J. Natl. Cancer Inst. 91 (1999) 1017—1024.

[9] A.V. Sarma, D. Schottenfeld, Prostate cancer incidence, mortality, and survival trends in the United States: 1981—2001, Semin. Urol. Oncol. 20 (2002) 3—9.

[10] National Cancer Institute, Cancer Trends Progress Report—2009/2010 Update, National Cancer Institute, Bethesda, MD, 2010.

[11] B.A. Miller, L.N. Kolonel, L. Bernstein, J.L.J. Young, G.M. Swanson, D.W. West, C.R. Key, J.M. Liff, C.S. Glover, G.A. Alexander (Eds.), Racial/Ethnic Patterns of Cancer in the United States, 1988—1992, National Cancer Institute, Bethesda, MD, 1996 (NIH Pub. No. 96-4104).

[12] I.J. Powell, Epidemiology and pathophysiology of prostate cancer in African-American men, J. Urol. 177 (2007) 444—449.

[13] L.N. Kolonel, Racial and geographic variations in prostate cancer and the effect of migration, in: J.G. Fortner, P.A. Sharp (Eds.), Accomplishments in Cancer Research 1996, Lippincott—Raven, Philadelphia, 1997, pp. 221—230.

[14] Foundation for Promotion of Cancer Research, Cancer Statistics in Japan 2010, Foundation for Promotion of Cancer Research, Tokyo, 2010.

[15] A.M. Nomura, L.N. Kolonel, Prostate cancer: a current perspective, Epidemiol. Rev. 13 (1991) 200—227.

[16] A.S. Whittemore, A.H. Wu, L.N. Kolonel, E.M. John, R.P. Gallagher, G.R. Howe, et al., Family history and prostate cancer risk in black, white, and Asian men in the United States and Canada, Am. J. Epidemiol. 141 (1995) 732—740.

[17] L.E. Johns, R.S. Houlston, A systematic review and meta-analysis of familial prostate cancer risk, BJU Int. 91 (2003) 789—794.

[18] M.E. Parent, J. Siemiatycki, Occupation and prostate cancer, Epidemiol. Rev. 23 (2001) 138—143.

[19] M.L. Taylor, A.G. Mainous III, B.J. Wells, Prostate cancer and sexually transmitted diseases: a meta-analysis, Fam. Med. 37 (2005) 506—512.

[20] K. Hickey, K.A. Do, A. Green, Smoking and prostate cancer, Epidemiol. Rev. 23 (2001) 115—125.

[21] L.K. Dennis, R.B. Hayes, Alcohol and prostate cancer, Epidemiol. Rev. 23 (2001) 110—114.

[22] L.K. Dennis, D.V. Dawson, M.I. Resnick, Vasectomy and the risk of prostate cancer: a meta-analysis examining vasectomy status, age at vasectomy, and time since vasectomy, Prostate Cancer Prostatic Dis 5 (2002) 193—203.

[23] Y. Liu, F. Hu, D. Li, F. Wang, L. Zhu, W. Chen, et al., Does physical activity reduce the risk of prostate cancer? A systematic review and meta-analysis, Eur. Urol. 60 (2011) 1029—1044.

[24] D.G. Bostwick, H.B. Burke, D. Djakiew, S. Euling, S.M. Ho, J. Landolph, et al., Human prostate cancer risk factors, Cancer 101 (2004) 2371—2490.

[25] G. Wilding, Endocrine control of prostate cancer, Cancer Surv. 23 (1995) 43—62.

[26] P.H. Gann, Androgenic hormones and prostate cancer risk: status and prospects, IARC Sci. Publ 156 (2002) 283—288.

[27] A. Nomura, L.K. Heilbrun, G.N. Stemmermann, H.L. Judd, Prediagnostic serum hormones and the risk of prostate cancer, Cancer Res. 48 (1988) 3515—3517.

[28] A.W. Hsing, G.W. Comstock, Serological precursors of cancer: serum hormones and risk of subsequent prostate cancer, Cancer Epidemiol. Biomarkers Prev. 2 (1993) 27—32.

[29] P.H. Gann, C.H. Hennekens, J. Ma, C. Longcope, M.J. Stampfer, Prospective study of sex hormone levels and risk of prostate cancer, J. Natl. Cancer Inst. 88 (1996) 1118—1126.

[30] N.A. Daniels, C.M. Nielson, A.R. Hoffman, D.C. Bauer, Sex hormones and the risk of incident prostate cancer, Urology 76 (2010) 1034—1040.

[31] J.K. Gill, L.R. Wilkens, M.N. Pollak, F.Z. Stanczyk, L.N. Kolonel, Androgens, growth factors, and risk of prostate cancer: the Multiethnic Cohort, Prostate 70 (2010) 906—915.

[32] G. Severi, H.A. Morris, R.J. MacInnis, D.R. English, W. Tilley, J.L. Hopper, et al., Circulating steroid hormones and the risk of prostate cancer, Cancer Epidemiol. Biomarkers Prev. 15 (2006) 86—91.

[33] B.A. Mohr, H.A. Feldman, L.A. Kalish, C. Longcope, J.B. McKinlay, Are serum hormones associated with the risk of prostate cancer? Prospective results from the Massachusetts Male Aging Study, Urology 57 (2001) 930—935.

[34] C. Chen, N.S. Weiss, F.Z. Stanczyk, S.K. Lewis, D. DiTommaso, R. Etzioni, et al., Endogenous sex hormones and prostate cancer risk: a case—control study nested within the carotene and retinol efficacy trial, Cancer Epidemiol. Biomarkers Prev. 12 (2003) 1410—1416.

[35] R.C. Travis, T.J. Key, N.E. Allen, P.N. Appleby, A.W. Roddam, S. Rinaldi, et al., Serum androgens and prostate cancer among 643 cases and 643 controls in the European Prospective

Investigation into Cancer and Nutrition, Int. J. Cancer 121 (2007) 1331–1338.

[36] J.M. Weiss, W.Y. Huang, S. Rinaldi, T.R. Fears, N. Chatterjee, A.W. Hsing, et al., Endogenous sex hormones and the risk of prostate cancer: a prospective study, Int. J. Cancer 122 (2008) 2345–2350.

[37] A.W. Roddam, N.E. Allen, P. Appleby, T.J. Key, E.H.P. Canc, Endogenous sex hormones and prostate cancer: a collaborative analysis of 18 prospective studies, J. Natl. Cancer Inst. 100 (2008) 170–183.

[38] A.W. Hsing, L.W. Chu, F.Z. Stanczyk, Androgen and prostate cancer: Is the hypothesis dead? Cancer Epidemiol. Biomarkers Prev. 17 (2008) 2525–2530.

[39] World Cancer Research Fund/American Institute for Cancer Research, Food, Nutrition, Physical Activity, and the Prevention of Cancer: A Global Perspective, American Institute for Cancer Research, Washington, DC, 2007.

[40] A.S. Morisset, K. Blouin, A. Tchernof, Impact of diet and adiposity on circulating levels of sex hormone-binding globulin and androgens, Nutr. Rev. 66 (2008) 506–516.

[41] World Cancer Research Fund/American Institute for Cancer Research (2006). Systematic Literature Review Report. The Associations between Food, Nutrition, Physical Activity and the Risk of Prostate Cancer and Underlying Mechanisms. (Available at <http://www.dietandcancerreport.org/expert_report/view_slrs.php>).

[42] M.L. Slattery, K.M. Boucher, B.J. Caan, J.D. Potter, K.N. Ma, Eating patterns and risk of colon cancer, Am. J. Epidemiol. 148 (1998) 4–16.

[43] A.K. Kant, Dietary patterns and health outcomes, J. Am. Diet. Assoc. 104 (2004) 615–635.

[44] P.K. Newby, K.L. Tucker, Empirically derived eating patterns using factor or cluster analysis: a review, Nutr. Rev. 62 (2004) 177–203.

[45] M. Walker, K.J. Aronson, W. King, J.W. Wilson, W. Fan, J.P. Heaton, et al., Dietary patterns and risk of prostate cancer in Ontario, Canada, Int. J. Cancer 116 (2005) 592–598.

[46] G.L. Ambrosini, L. Fritschi, N.H. de Klerk, D. Mackerras, J. Leavy, Dietary patterns identified using factor analysis and prostate cancer risk: a case–control study in Western Australia, Ann. Epidemiol. 18 (2008) 364–370.

[47] E. De Stefani, A.L. Ronco, H. Deneo-Pellegrini, P. Boffetta, D. Aune, G. Acosta, et al., Dietary patterns and risk of advanced prostate cancer: a principal component analysis in Uruguay, Cancer Causes Control 21 (2010) 1009–1016.

[48] K. Wu, F.B. Hu, W.C. Willett, E. Giovannucci, Dietary patterns and risk of prostate cancer in U.S. men, Cancer Epidemiol. Biomarkers Prev. 15 (2006) 167–171.

[49] M. Tseng, R.A. Breslow, R.F. DeVellis, R.G. Ziegler, Dietary patterns and prostate cancer risk in the National Health and Nutrition Examination Survey Epidemiological Follow-up Study cohort, Cancer Epidemiol. Biomarkers Prev. 13 (2004) 71–77.

[50] D.C. Muller, G. Severi, L. Baglietto, K. Krishnan, D.R. English, J.L. Hopper, et al., Dietary patterns and prostate cancer risk, Cancer Epidemiol. Biomarkers Prev. 18 (2009) 3126–3129.

[51] C. Rodriguez, M.L. McCullough, A.M. Mondul, E.J. Jacobs, A. Chao, A.V. Patel, et al., Meat consumption among black and white men and risk of prostate cancer in the Cancer Prevention Study II Nutrition Cohort, Cancer Epidemiol. Biomarkers Prev. 15 (2006) 211–216.

[52] R. Sinha, Y. Park, B.I. Graubard, M.F. Leitzmann, A. Hollenbeck, A. Schatzkin, et al., Meat and meat-related compounds and risk of prostate cancer in a large prospective cohort study in the United States, Am. J. Epidemiol. 170 (2009) 1165–1177.

[53] S.Y. Park, S.P. Murphy, L.R. Wilkens, B.E. Henderson, L.N. Kolonel, Fat and meat intake and prostate cancer risk: the Multiethnic Cohort Study, Int. J. Cancer 121 (2007) 1339–1345.

[54] S. Koutros, A.J. Cross, D.P. Sandler, J.A. Hoppin, X. Ma, T. Zheng, et al., Meat and meat mutagens and risk of prostate cancer in the Agricultural Health Study, Cancer Epidemiol. Biomarkers Prev. 17 (2008) 80–87.

[55] N.E. Allen, T.J. Key, P.N. Appleby, R.C. Travis, A.W. Roddam, A. Tjonneland, et al., Animal foods, protein, calcium and prostate cancer risk: the European Prospective Investigation into Cancer and Nutrition, Br. J. Cancer 98 (2008) 1574–1581.

[56] J. Hu, C. La Vecchia, M. DesMeules, E. Negri, L. Mery, Meat and fish consumption and cancer in Canada, Nutr. Cancer 60 (2008) 313–324.

[57] E.M. John, M.C. Stern, R. Sinha, J. Koo, Meat consumption, cooking practices, meat mutagens, and risk of prostate cancer, Nutr. Cancer 63 (2011) 525–537.

[58] D. Aune, E. De Stefani, A. Ronco, P. Boffetta, H. Deneo-Pellegrini, G. Acosta, et al., Meat consumption and cancer risk: a case–control study in Uruguay, Asian Pacific J. Cancer Prev. 10 (2009) 429–436.

[59] J.L. Wright, M.L. Neuhouser, D.W. Lin, E.M. Kwon, Z. Feng, E.A. Ostrander, et al., AMACR polymorphisms, dietary intake of red meat and dairy and prostate cancer risk, Prostate 71 (2011) 498–506.

[60] S. Rohrmann, E.A. Platz, C.J. Kavanaugh, L. Thuita, S.C. Hoffman, K.J. Helzlsouer, Meat and dairy consumption and subsequent risk of prostate cancer in a U.S. cohort study, Cancer Causes Control 18 (2007) 41–50.

[61] M.L. Neuhouser, M.J. Barnett, A.R. Kristal, C.B. Ambrosone, I. King, M. Thornquist, et al., (n-6) PUFA increase and dairy foods decrease prostate cancer risk in heavy smokers, J. Nutr. 137 (2007) 1821–1827.

[62] D.D. Alexander, P.J. Mink, C.A. Cushing, B. Sceurman, A review and meta-analysis of prospective studies of red and processed meat intake and prostate cancer, Nutr. J. 9 (2010) 50.

[63] A. Tappel, Heme of consumed red meat can act as a catalyst of oxidative damage and could initiate colon, breast and prostate cancers, heart disease and other diseases, Med. Hypotheses 68 (2007) 562–564.

[64] R. Goldman, P.G. Shields, Food mutagens, J. Nutr. 133 (Suppl. 3) (2003) 965S–973S.

[65] T. Shirai, M. Sano, S. Tamano, S. Takahashi, M. Hirose, M. Futakuchi, et al., The prostate: a target for carcinogenicity of 2-amino-1-methyl-6-phenylimidazo[4,5-*b*]pyridine (PhIP) derived from cooked foods, Cancer Res. 57 (1997) 195–198.

[66] T. Sugimura, K. Wakabayashi, H. Nakagama, M. Nagao, Heterocyclic amines: Mutagens/carcinogens produced during cooking of meat and fish, Cancer Sci. 95 (2004) 290–299.

[67] D.H. Phillips, Polycyclic aromatic hydrocarbons in the diet, Mutat. Res. 443 (1999) 139–147.

[68] A.J. Cross, U. Peters, V.A. Kirsh, G.L. Andriole, D. Reding, R.B. Hayes, et al., A prospective study of meat and meat mutagens and prostate cancer risk, Cancer Res. 65 (2005) 11779–11784.

[69] S. Sharma, X. Cao, L.R. Wilkens, J. Yamamoto, A. Lum-Jones, B.E. Henderson, et al., Well-done meat consumption, NAT1 and NAT2 acetylator genotypes and prostate cancer risk: the multiethnic cohort study, Cancer Epidemiol. Biomarkers Prev. 19 (2010) 1866–1870.

[70] A.E. Norrish, L.R. Ferguson, M.G. Knize, J.S. Felton, S.J. Sharpe, R.T. Jackson, Heterocyclic amine content of cooked meat and risk of prostate cancer, J. Natl. Cancer Inst. 91 (1999) 2038–2044.

[71] A. Sander, J. Linseisen, S. Rohrmann, Intake of heterocyclic aromatic amines and the risk of prostate cancer in the EPIC-Heidelberg cohort, Cancer Causes Control 22 (2011) 109–114.

[72] D.A. Snowdon, R.L. Phillips, W. Choi, Diet, obesity, and risk of fatal prostate cancer, Am. J. Epidemiol. 120 (1984) 244–250.

[73] S. Torniainen, M. Hedelin, V. Autio, H. Rasinpera, K.A. Balter, A. Klint, et al., Lactase persistence, dietary intake of milk, and the risk for prostate cancer in Sweden and Finland, Cancer Epidemiol. Biomarkers Prev. 16 (2007) 956–961.

[74] S. Raimondi, J.B. Mabrouk, B. Shatenstein, P. Maisonneuve, P. Ghadirian, Diet and prostate cancer risk with specific focus on dairy products and dietary calcium: a case–control study, Prostate 70 (2010) 1054–1065.

[75] E. Kesse, S. Bertrais, P. Astorg, A. Jaouen, N. Arnault, P. Galan, et al., Dairy products, calcium and phosphorus intake, and the risk of prostate cancer: results of the French prospective SU. VI.MAX (Supplementation en Vitamines et Mineraux Antioxydants) study, Br. J. Nutr. 95 (2006) 539–545.

[76] J. Ahn, D. Albanes, U. Peters, A. Schatzkin, U. Lim, M. Freedman, et al., Dairy products, calcium intake, and risk of prostate cancer in the Prostate, Lung, Colorectal, and Ovarian Cancer Screening Trial, Cancer Epidemiol. Biomarkers Prev. 16 (2007) 2623–2630.

[77] Y. Park, P.N. Mitrou, V. Kipnis, A. Hollenbeck, A. Schatzkin, M.F. Leitzmann, Calcium, dairy foods, and risk of incident and fatal prostate cancer: The NIH-AARP Diet and Health Study, Am. J. Epidemiol. 166 (2007) 1270–1279.

[78] P.N. Mitrou, D. Albanes, S.J. Weinstein, P. Pietinen, P.R. Taylor, J. Virtamo, et al., A prospective study of dietary calcium, dairy products and prostate cancer risk (Finland), Int. J. Cancer 120 (2007) 2466–2473.

[79] N. Kurahashi, M. Inoue, M. Iwasaki, S. Sasazuki, A.S. Tsugane, Dairy product, saturated fatty acid, and calcium intake and prostate cancer in a prospective cohort of Japanese men, Cancer Epidemiol. Biomarkers Prev. 17 (2008) 930–937.

[80] E. Giovannucci, Y. Liu, M.J. Stampfer, W.C. Willett, A prospective study of calcium intake and incident and fatal prostate cancer, Cancer Epidemiol. Biomarkers Prev. 15 (2006) 203–210.

[81] K.A. Koh, H.D. Sesso, R.S. Paffenbarger Jr., I.M. Lee, Dairy products, calcium and prostate cancer risk, Br. J. Cancer 95 (2006) 1582–1585.

[82] S.Y. Park, S.P. Murphy, L.R. Wilkens, D.O. Stram, B.E. Henderson, L.N. Kolonel, Calcium, vitamin D, and dairy product intake and prostate cancer risk: the Multiethnic Cohort Study, Am. J. Epidemiol. 166 (2007) 1259–1269.

[83] M. Huncharek, J. Muscat, B. Kupelnick, Dairy products, dietary calcium and vitamin D intake as risk factors for prostate cancer: a meta-analysis of 26,769 cases from 45 observational studies, Nutr. Cancer 60 (2008) 421–441.

[84] L.Q. Qin, K. He, J.Y. Xu, Milk consumption and circulating insulin-like growth factor-I level: a systematic literature review, Int. J. Food Sci. Nutr. 60 (Suppl. 7) (2009) 330–340.

[85] A. Benedetti, M.E. Parent, J. Siemiatycki, Lifetime consumption of alcoholic beverages and risk of 13 types of cancer in men: results from a case–control study in Montreal, Cancer Detect. Prev. 32 (2009) 352–362.

[86] J. Hu, C. La Vecchia, L. Gibbons, E. Negri, L. Mery, Nutrients and risk of prostate cancer, Nutr. Cancer 62 (2010) 710–718.

[87] S. Gallus, R. Foschi, R. Talamini, A. Altieri, E. Negri, S. Franceschi, et al., Risk factors for prostate cancer in men aged less than 60 years: a case–control study from Italy, Urology 70 (2007) 1121–1126.

[88] J.L. Watters, Y. Park, A. Hollenbeck, A. Schatzkin, D. Albanes, Alcoholic beverages and prostate cancer in a prospective U.S. cohort study, Am. J. Epidemiol. 172 (2010) 773–780.

[89] L. Baglietto, G. Severi, D.R. English, J.L. Hopper, G.G. Giles, Alcohol consumption and prostate cancer risk: results from the Melbourne collaborative cohort study, Int. J. Cancer 119 (2006) 1501–1504.

[90] S.J. Weinstein, R. Stolzenberg-Solomon, P. Pietinen, P.R. Taylor, J. Virtamo, D. Albanes, Dietary factors of one-carbon metabolism and prostate cancer risk, Am. J. Clin. Nutr. 84 (2006) 929–935.

[91] S. Sutcliffe, E. Giovannucci, M.F. Leitzmann, E.B. Rimm, M.J. Stampfer, W.C. Willett, et al., A prospective cohort study of red wine consumption and risk of prostate cancer, Int. J. Cancer 120 (2007) 1529–1535.

[92] S. Rohrmann, J. Linseisen, T.J. Key, M.K. Jensen, K. Overvad, N.F. Johnsen, et al., Alcohol consumption and the risk for prostate cancer in the European Prospective Investigation into Cancer and Nutrition, Cancer Epidemiol. Biomarkers Prev. 17 (2008) 1282–1287.

[93] C. Chao, R. Haque, S.K. Van Den Eeden, B.J. Caan, K.Y. Poon, V.P. Quinn, Red wine consumption and risk of prostate cancer: the California men's health study, Int. J. Cancer 126 (2010) 171–179.

[94] K. Middleton Fillmore, T. Chikritzhs, T. Stockwell, A. Bostrom, R. Pascal, Alcohol use and prostate cancer: a meta-analysis, Mol. Nutr. Food Res. 53 (2009) 240–255.

[95] R.B. Hayes, L.M. Brown, J.B. Schoenberg, R.S. Greenberg, D.T. Silverman, A.G. Schwartz, et al., Alcohol use and prostate cancer risk in U.S. blacks and whites, Am. J. Epidemiol. 143 (1996) 692–697.

[96] A.G. Schuurman, R.A. Goldbohm, P.A. van den Brandt, A prospective cohort study on consumption of alcoholic beverages in relation to prostate cancer incidence (The Netherlands), Cancer Causes Control 10 (1999) 597–605.

[97] P. Boffetta, M. Hashibe, Alcohol and cancer, Lancet Oncol. 7 (2006) 149–156.

[98] P. Mukherjee, A.V. Sotnikov, H.J. Mangian, J.R. Zhou, W.J. Visek, S.K. Clinton, Energy intake and prostate tumor growth, angiogenesis, and vascular endothelial growth factor expression, J. Natl. Cancer Inst. 91 (1999) 512–523.

[99] L.N. Kolonel, A.M. Nomura, R.V. Cooney, Dietary fat and prostate cancer: current status, J. Natl. Cancer Inst. 91 (1999) 414–428.

[100] L.N. Kolonel, Fat, meat, and prostate cancer, Epidemiol. Rev. 23 (2001) 72–81.

[101] L. Kushi, E. Giovannucci, Dietary fat and cancer, Am. J. Med. 113 (Suppl. 9B) (2002) 63S–70S.

[102] A. Lophatananon, J. Archer, D. Easton, R. Pocock, D. Dearnaley, M. Guy, et al., Dietary fat and early-onset prostate cancer risk, Br. J. Nutr. 103 (2010) 1375–1380.

[103] P. Wallstrom, A. Bjartell, B. Gullberg, H. Olsson, E. Wirfalt, A prospective study on dietary fat and incidence of prostate cancer (Malmo, Sweden), Cancer Causes Control 18 (2007) 1107–1121.

[104] F.L. Crowe, T.J. Key, P.N. Appleby, R.C. Travis, K. Overvad, M.U. Jakobsen, et al., Dietary fat intake and risk of prostate cancer in the European Prospective Investigation into Cancer and Nutrition, Am. J. Clin. Nutr. 87 (2008) 1405–1413.

[105] Y. Nagata, T. Sonoda, M. Mori, N. Miyanaga, K. Okumura, K. Goto, et al., Dietary isoflavones may protect against prostate cancer in Japanese men, J. Nutr. 137 (2007) 1974–1979.

[106] A.G. Schuurman, P.A. van den Brandt, E. Dorant, H.A. Brants, R.A. Goldbohm, Association of energy and fat intake with prostate carcinoma risk: results from The Netherlands Cohort Study, Cancer 86 (1999) 1019–1027.

[107] A.E. Norrish, C.M. Skeaff, G.L. Arribas, S.J. Sharpe, R.T. Jackson, Prostate cancer risk and consumption of fish oils: a dietary biomarker-based case–control study, Br. J. Cancer 81 (1999) 1238–1242.

[108] M.F. Leitzmann, M.J. Stampfer, D.S. Michaud, K. Augustsson, G.C. Colditz, W.C. Willett, et al., Dietary intake of n-3 and n-6 fatty acids and the risk of prostate cancer, Am. J. Clin. Nutr. 80 (2004) 204–216.

[109] J.E. Chavarro, M.J. Stampfer, H. Li, H. Campos, T. Kurth, J. Ma, A prospective study of polyunsaturated fatty acid levels in blood and prostate cancer risk, Cancer Epidemiol. Biomarkers Prev. 16 (2007) 1364–1370.

[110] V. Fradet, I. Cheng, G. Casey, J.S. Witte, Dietary omega-3 fatty acids, cyclooxygenase-2 genetic variation, and aggressive prostate cancer risk, Clin. Cancer Res. 15 (2009) 2559–2566.

[111] L.M. Newcomer, I.B. King, K.G. Wicklund, J.L. Stanford, The association of fatty acids with prostate cancer risk, Prostate 47 (2001) 262–268.

[112] S. Mannisto, P. Pietinen, M.J. Virtanen, I. Salminen, D. Albanes, E. Giovannucci, et al., Fatty acids and risk of prostate cancer in a nested case–control study in male smokers, Cancer Epidemiol. Biomarkers Prev. 12 (2003) 1422–1428.

[113] J.E. Chavarro, M.J. Stampfer, M.N. Hall, H.D. Sesso, J. Ma, A 22-y prospective study of fish intake in relation to prostate cancer incidence and mortality, Am. J. Clin. Nutr. 88 (2008) 1297–1303.

[114] P. Terry, P. Lichtenstein, M. Feychting, A. Ahlbom, A. Wolk, Fatty fish consumption and risk of prostate cancer, Lancet 357 (2001) 1764–1766.

[115] K. Augustsson, D.S. Michaud, E.B. Rimm, M.F. Leitzmann, M.J. Stampfer, W.C. Willett, et al., A prospective study of intake of fish and marine fatty acids and prostate cancer, Cancer Epidemiol. Biomarkers Prev. 12 (2003) 64–67.

[116] P.D. Terry, J.B. Terry, T.E. Rohan, Long-chain (n-3) fatty acid intake and risk of cancers of the breast and the prostate: recent epidemiological studies, biological mechanisms, and directions for future research, J. Nutr. 134 (2004) 3412S–3420S.

[117] P. Astorg, Dietary N-6 and N-3 polyunsaturated fatty acids and prostate cancer risk: a review of epidemiological and experimental evidence, Cancer Causes Control 15 (2004) 367–386.

[118] E. De Stefani, H. Deneo-Pellegrini, P. Boffetta, A. Ronco, M. Mendilaharsu, Alpha-linolenic acid and risk of prostate cancer: a case–control study in Uruguay, Cancer Epidemiol. Biomarkers Prev. 9 (2000) 335–338.

[119] D.O. Koralek, U. Peters, G. Andriole, D. Reding, V. Kirsh, A. Subar, A. Schatzkin, R. Hayes, M.F. Leitzmann, A prospective study of dietary alpha-linolenic acid and the risk of prostate cancer (United States), Cancer Causes Control 17 (2006) 783–791.

[120] J.A. Simon, Y.H. Chen, S. Bent, The relation of alpha-linolenic acid to the risk of prostate cancer: a systematic review and meta-analysis, Am. J. Clin. Nutr. 89 (2009) 1558S–1564S.

[121] I.B. King, A.R. Kristal, S. Schaffer, M. Thornquist, G.E. Goodman, Serum trans-fatty acids are associated with risk of prostate cancer in beta-Carotene and Retinol Efficacy Trial, Cancer Epidemiol. Biomarkers Prev. 14 (2005) 988–992.

[122] J.E. Chavarro, M.J. Stampfer, H. Campos, T. Kurth, W.C. Willett, J. Ma, A prospective study of trans-fatty acid levels in blood and risk of prostate cancer, Cancer Epidemiol. Biomarkers Prev. 17 (2008) 95–101.

[123] M. Pollard, P.H. Luckert, Promotional effects of testosterone and high fat diet on the development of autochthonous prostate cancer in rats, Cancer Lett 32 (1986) 223–227.

[124] S.K. Clinton, S.S. Palmer, C.E. Spriggs, W.J. Visek, Growth of Dunning transplantable prostate adenocarcinomas in rats fed diets with various fat contents, J. Nutr. 118 (1988) 908–914.

[125] Y. Wang, J.G. Corr, H.T. Thaler, Y. Tao, W.R. Fair, W.D. Heston, Decreased growth of established human prostate LNCaP tumors in nude mice fed a low-fat diet, J. Natl. Cancer Inst. 87 (1995) 1456–1462.

[126] T.H. Ngo, R.J. Barnard, T. Anton, C. Tran, D. Elashoff, D. Heber, et al., Effect of isocaloric low-fat diet on prostate cancer xenograft progression to androgen independence, Cancer Res. 64 (2004) 1252–1254.

[127] P.K. Pandalai, M.J. Pilat, K. Yamazaki, H. Naik, K.J. Pienta, The effects of omega-3 and omega-6 fatty acids on in vitro prostate cancer growth, Anticancer Res. 16 (1996) 815–820.

[128] R.A. Karmali, P. Reichel, L.A. Cohen, T. Terano, A. Hirai, Y. Tamura, et al., The effects of dietary omega-3 fatty acids on the DU-145 transplantable human prostatic tumor, Anticancer Res. 7 (1987) 1173–1179.

[129] L.M. Butler, A.S. Wong, W.P. Koh, R. Wang, J.M. Yuan, M.C. Yu, Calcium intake increases risk of prostate cancer among Singapore Chinese, Cancer Res. 70 (2010) 4941–4948.

[130] H.G. Skinner, G.G. Schwartz, Serum calcium and incident and fatal prostate cancer in the National Health and Nutrition Examination Survey, Cancer Epidemiol. Biomarkers Prev. 17 (2008) 2302–2305.

[131] C. Halthur, A.L. Johansson, M. Almquist, J. Malm, H. Gronberg, J. Manjer, et al., Serum calcium and the risk of prostate cancer, Cancer Causes Control 20 (2009) 1205–1214.

[132] D. Feldman, X.Y. Zhao, A.V. Krishnan, Vitamin D and prostate cancer, Endocrinology 141 (2000) 5–9.

[133] J.P. Bonjour, T. Chevalley, P. Fardellone, Calcium intake and vitamin D metabolism and action, in healthy conditions and in prostate cancer, Br. J. Nutr. 97 (2007) 611–616.

[134] S. Gallus, R. Foschi, E. Negri, R. Talamini, S. Franceschi, M. Montella, et al., Dietary zinc and prostate cancer risk: a case–control study from Italy, Eur. Urol. 52 (2007) 1052–1056.

[135] Y. Zhang, P. Coogan, J.R. Palmer, B.L. Strom, L. Rosenberg, Vitamin and mineral use and risk of prostate cancer: the case–control surveillance study, Cancer Causes Control 20 (2009) 691–698.

[136] A. Gonzalez, U. Peters, J.W. Lampe, E. White, Zinc intake from supplements and diet and prostate cancer, Nutr. Cancer 61 (2009) 206–215.

[137] M.E. Shils, J.A. Olson, M. Shike, Modern Nutrition in Health and Disease, eighth ed., Lea & Febiger, Philadelphia, 1994.

[138] A. Feustel, R. Wennrich, Zinc and cadmium plasma and erythrocyte levels in prostatic carcinoma, BPH, urological malignancies, and inflammations, Prostate 8 (1986) 75–79.

[139] P. Whelan, B.E. Walker, J. Kelleher, Zinc, vitamin A and prostatic cancer, Br. J. Urol. 55 (1983) 525–528.

[140] L.C. Costello, R.B. Franklin, P. Feng, M. Tan, O. Bagasra, Zinc and prostate cancer: a critical scientific, medical, and public interest issue (United States), Cancer Causes Control 16 (2005) 901–915.

[141] E.A. Platz, K.J. Helzlsouer, S.C. Hoffman, J.S. Morris, C.K. Baskett, G.W. Comstock, Prediagnostic toenail cadmium and zinc and subsequent prostate cancer risk, Prostate 52 (2002) 288–296.

[142] L.E. Tisell, B. Fjelkegard, K.H. Leissner, Zinc concentration and content of the dorsal, lateral and medical prostatic lobes and of periurethral adenomas in man, J. Urol 128 (1982) 403–405.

[143] A. Feustel, R. Wennrich, Determination of the distribution of zinc and cadmium in cellular fractions of BPH, normal prostate and prostatic cancers of different histologies by atomic and laser absorption spectrometry in tissue slices, Urol. Res. 12 (1984) 253–256.

[144] L.C. Costello, R.B. Franklin, P. Feng, M. Tan, O. Bagasra, Zinc and prostate cancer: a critical scientific, medical, and public

interest issue (United States), Cancer Causes Control 16 (2005) 901–915.

[145] F.K. Habib, M.K. Mason, P.H. Smith, S.R. Stitch, Cancer of the prostate: Early diagnosis by zinc and hormone analysis? Br. J. Cancer 39 (1979) 700–704.

[146] T.R. Hartoma, K. Nahoul, A. Netter, Zinc, plasma androgens and male sterility, Lancet 2 (1977) 1125–1126.

[147] A.S. Om, K.W. Chung, Dietary zinc deficiency alters 5 alpha-reduction and aromatization of testosterone and androgen and estrogen receptors in rat liver, J. Nutr. 126 (1996) 842–848.

[148] D.S. Colvard, E.M. Wilson, Zinc potentiation of androgen receptor binding to nuclei *in vitro*, Biochemistry 23 (1984) 3471–3478.

[149] A. Vermeulen, J.M. Kaufman, V.A. Giagulli, Influence of some biological indexes on sex hormone-binding globulin and andro-gen levels in aging or obese males, J. Clin. Endocrinol. Metab. 81 (1996) 1821–1826.

[150] A.H. Wu, A.S. Whittemore, L.N. Kolonel, E.M. John, R.P. Gallagher, D.W. West, et al., Serum androgens and sex hor-mone-binding globulins in relation to lifestyle factors in older African-American, white, and Asian men in the United States and Canada, Cancer Epidemiol. Biomarkers Prev. 4 (1995) 735–741.

[151] A. Gray, H.A. Feldman, J.B. McKinlay, C. Longcope, Age, dis-ease, and changing sex hormone levels in middle-aged men: results of the Massachusetts Male Aging Study, J. Clin. Endocrinol. Metab. 73 (1991) 1016–1025.

[152] S.Y. Park, L. Kolonel, Serum Zinc and Prostate Cancer Risk in the Multiethnic Cohort study, Epidemiology 20 (2009) S131 (S131)

[153] A.E. Sahmoun, L.D. Case, S.A. Jackson, G.G. Schwartz, Cadmium and prostate cancer: a critical epidemiologic analysis, Cancer Invest. 23 (2005) 256–263.

[154] Y.C. Chen, Y.S. Pu, H.C. Wu, T.T. Wu, M.K. Lai, C.Y. Yang, et al., Cadmium burden and the risk and phenotype of prostate cancer, BMC Cancer 9 (2009) 429.

[155] M. Vinceti, M. Venturelli, C. Sighinolfi, P. Trerotoli, F. Bonvicini, A. Ferrari, et al., Case–control study of toenail cad-mium and prostate cancer risk in Italy, Sci. Total Environ. 373 (2007) 77–81.

[156] D. Beyersmann, A. Hartwig, Carcinogenic metal compounds: recent insight into molecular and cellular mechanisms, Arch. Toxicol. 82 (2008) 493–512.

[157] M.M. Brzoska, J. Moniuszko-Jakoniuk, Interactions between cadmium and zinc in the organism, Food Chem. Toxicol. 39 (2001) 967–980.

[158] T. Pischon, H. Boeing, S. Weikert, N. Allen, T. Key, N.F. Johnsen, et al., Body size and risk of prostate cancer in the European Prospective Investigation into Cancer and Nutrition, Cancer Epidemiol. Biomarkers Prev. 17 (2008) 3252–3261.

[159] B.Y. Hernandez, S.Y. Park, L.R. Wilkens, B.E. Henderson, L.N. Kolonel, Relationship of body mass, height, and weight gain to prostate cancer risk in the multiethnic cohort, Cancer Epidemiol. Biomarkers Prev. 18 (2009) 2413–2421.

[160] T. Stocks, M.P. Hergens, A. Englund, W. Ye, P. Stattin, Blood pressure, body size and prostate cancer risk in the Swedish Construction Workers cohort, Int. J. Cancer 127 (2010) 1660–1668.

[161] M.D. Jackson, S.P. Walker, C.M. Simpson, N. McFarlane-Anderson, F.I. Bennett, K.C. Coard, et al., Body size and risk of prostate cancer in Jamaican men, Cancer Causes Control 21 (2010) 909–917.

[162] J. Baillargeon, E.A. Platz, D.P. Rose, B.H. Pollock, D.P. Ankerst, S. Haffner, et al., Obesity, adipokines, and prostate cancer in a prospective population-based study, Cancer Epidemiol. Biomarkers Prev. 15 (2006) 1331–1335.

[163] N. Kurahashi, M. Iwasaki, S. Sasazuki, T. Otani, M. Inoue, S. Tsugane, Association of body mass index and height with risk of prostate cancer among middle-aged Japanese men, Br. J. Cancer 94 (2006) 740–742.

[164] E. Lundqvist, J. Kaprio, P.K. Verkasalo, E. Pukkala, M. Koskenvuo, K.C. Soderberg, et al., Co-twin control and cohort analyses of body mass index and height in relation to breast, prostate, ovarian, corpus uteri, colon and rectal cancer among Swedish and Finnish twins, Int. J. Cancer 121 (2007) 810–818.

[165] P. Wallstrom, A. Bjartell, B. Gullberg, H. Olsson, E. Wirfalt, A prospective Swedish study on body size, body composition, diabetes, and prostate cancer risk, Br. J. Cancer 100 (2009) 1799–1805.

[166] C. Chamberlain, P. Romundstad, L. Vatten, D. Gunnell, R.M. Martin, The association of weight gain during adulthood with prostate cancer incidence and survival: a population-based cohort, Int. J. Cancer 129 (2011) 1199–1206.

[167] B. Cox, M.J. Sneyd, C. Paul, D.C. Skegg, Risk factors for pros-tate cancer: a national case–control study, Int. J. Cancer 119 (2006) 1690–1694.

[168] S. Weinmann, J.A. Shapiro, B.A. Rybicki, S.M. Enger, S.K. Van Den Eeden, K.E. Richert-Boe, et al., Medical history, body size, and cigarette smoking in relation to fatal prostate cancer, Cancer Causes Control 21 (2010) 117–125.

[169] P. Dimitropoulou, R.M. Martin, E.L. Turner, J.A. Lane, R. Gilbert, M. Davis, et al., Association of obesity with prostate cancer: a case–control study within the population-based PSA testing phase of the ProtecT study, Br. J. Cancer 104 (2011) 875–881.

[170] Z. Gong, M.L. Neuhouser, P.J. Goodman, D. Albanes, C. Chi, A.W. Hsing, et al., Obesity, diabetes, and risk of pros-tate cancer: results from the Prostate Cancer Prevention Trial, Cancer Epidemiol. Biomarkers Prev. 15 (2006) 1977–1983.

[171] C. Rodriguez, S.J. Freedland, A. Deka, E.J. Jacobs, M.L. McCullough, A.V. Patel, et al., Body mass index, weight change, and risk of prostate cancer in the Cancer Prevention Study II Nutrition Cohort, Cancer Epidemiol. Biomarkers Prev. 16 (2007) 63–69.

[172] M.E. Wright, S.C. Chang, A. Schatzkin, D. Albanes, V. Kipnis, T. Mouw, et al., Prospective study of adiposity and weight change in relation to prostate cancer incidence and mortality, Cancer 109 (2007) 675–684.

[173] M. Eriksson, H. Wedel, M.A. Wallander, I. Krakau, J. Hugosson, S. Carlsson, et al., The impact of birth weight on prostate cancer incidence and mortality in a population-based study of men born in 1913 and followed up from 50 to 85 years of age, Prostate 67 (2007) 1247–1254.

[174] L. Zuccolo, R. Harris, D. Gunnell, S. Oliver, J.A. Lane, M. Davis, et al., Height and prostate cancer risk: a large nested case–control study (ProtecT) and meta-analysis, Cancer Epidemiol. Biomarkers Prev. 17 (2008) 2325–2336.

[175] J. Ahn, S.C. Moore, D. Albanes, W.Y. Huang, M.F. Leitzmann, R.B. Hayes, Height and risk of prostate cancer in the prostate, lung, colorectal, and ovarian cancer screening trial, Br. J. Cancer 101 (2009) 522–525.

[176] R. Pasquali, F. Casimirri, S. Cantobelli, N. Melchionda, A.M. Morselli Labate, R. Fabbri, et al., Effect of obesity and body fat distribution on sex hormones and insulin in men, Metabolism 40 (1991) 101–104.

[177] C.L. Amling, Relationship between obesity and prostate cancer, Curr. Opin. Urol. 15 (2005) 167–171.

[178] A.W. Hsing, L.C. Sakoda, S. Chua Jr., Obesity, metabolic syndrome, and prostate cancer, Am. J. Clin. Nutr. 86 (2007) s843–s857.

[179] S.J. Freedland, E.A. Platz, Obesity and prostate cancer: making sense out of apparently conflicting data, Epidemiol. Rev. 29 (2007) 88–97.

[180] R. Ribeiro, C. Lopes, R. Medeiros, The link between obesity and prostate cancer: the leptin pathway and therapeutic perspectives, Prostate Cancer Prostatic Dis. 9 (2006) 19–24.

[181] J. Hardin, I. Cheng, J.S. Witte, Impact of consumption of vegetable, fruit, grain, and high glycemic index foods on aggressive prostate cancer risk, Nutr. Cancer 63 (2011) 860–872.

[182] J.E. Lewis, H. Soler-Vila, P.E. Clark, L.A. Kresty, G.O. Allen, J.J. Hu, Intake of plant foods and associated nutrients in prostate cancer risk, Nutr. Cancer 61 (2009) 216–224.

[183] D. Aune, E. De Stefani, A. Ronco, P. Boffetta, H. Deneo-Pellegrini, G. Acosta, et al., Fruits, vegetables and the risk of cancer: a multisite case–control study in Uruguay, Asian Pacific J. Cancer Prev. 10 (2009) 419–428.

[184] D.O. Stram, J.H. Hankin, L.R. Wilkens, S. Park, B.E. Henderson, A.M. Nomura, et al., Prostate cancer incidence and intake of fruits, vegetables and related micronutrients: the Multiethnic Cohort Study (United States), Cancer Causes Control 17 (2006) 1193–1207.

[185] R. Takachi, M. Inoue, N. Sawada, M. Iwasaki, S. Sasazuki, J. Ishihara, et al., Fruits and vegetables in relation to prostate cancer in Japanese men: the Japan Public Health Center-Based Prospective Study, Nutr. Cancer 62 (2010) 30–39.

[186] P. Terry, J.B. Terry, A. Wolk, Fruit and vegetable consumption in the prevention of cancer: an update, J. Intern. Med. 250 (2001) 280–290.

[187] R. Chan, K. Lok, J. Woo, Prostate cancer and vegetable consumption, Mol. Nutr. Food Res. 53 (2009) 201–216.

[188] R. Foschi, C. Pelucchi, L. Dal Maso, M. Rossi, F. Levi, R. Talamini, et al., Citrus fruit and cancer risk in a network of case–control studies, Cancer Causes Control 21 (2010) 237–242.

[189] V.A. Kirsh, U. Peters, S.T. Mayne, A.F. Subar, N. Chatterjee, C.C. Johnson, et al., Prospective study of fruit and vegetable intake and risk of prostate cancer, J. Natl. Cancer Inst. 99 (2007) 1200–1209.

[190] J.M. Chan, E.L. Giovannucci, Vegetables, fruits, associated micronutrients, and risk of prostate cancer, Epidemiol. Rev. 23 (2001) 82–86.

[191] C.L. Heald, M.R. Ritchie, C. Bolton-Smith, M.S. Morton, F.E. Alexander, Phyto-oestrogens and risk of prostate cancer in Scottish men, Br. J. Nutr. 98 (2007) 388–396.

[192] S.Y. Park, S.P. Murphy, L.R. Wilkens, B.E. Henderson, L.N. Kolonel, Legume and isoflavone intake and prostate cancer risk: the Multiethnic Cohort Study, Int. J. Cancer 123 (2008) 927–932.

[193] L. Yan, E.L. Spitznagel, Soy consumption and prostate cancer risk in men: a revisit of a meta-analysis, Am. J. Clin. Nutr. 89 (2009) 1155–1163.

[194] B.K. Jacobsen, S.F. Knutsen, G.E. Fraser, Does high soy milk intake reduce prostate cancer incidence? The Adventist Health Study (United States), Cancer Causes Control 9 (1998) 553–557.

[195] N.E. Allen, C. Sauvaget, A.W. Roddam, P. Appleby, J. Nagano, G. Suzuki, et al., A prospective study of diet and prostate cancer in Japanese men, Cancer Causes Control 15 (2004) 911–920.

[196] A.M. Nomura, J.H. Hankin, J. Lee, G.N. Stemmermann, Cohort study of tofu intake and prostate cancer: no apparent association, Cancer Epidemiol. Biomarkers Prev. 13 (2004) 2277–2279.

[197] N. Kurahashi, M. Iwasaki, S. Sasazuki, T. Otani, M. Inoue, S. Tsugane, Soy product and isoflavone consumption in relation to prostate cancer in Japanese men, Cancer Epidemiol. Biomarkers Prev. 16 (2007) 538–545.

[198] K. Oishi, K. Okada, O. Yoshida, H. Yamabe, Y. Ohno, R.B. Hayes, et al., A case–control study of prostatic cancer with reference to dietary habits, Prostate 12 (1988) 179–190.

[199] J.F. Sung, R.S. Lin, Y.S. Pu, Y.C. Chen, H.C. Chang, M.K. Lai, Risk factors for prostate carcinoma in Taiwan: a case–control study in a Chinese population, Cancer 86 (1999) 484–491.

[200] P.J. Villeneuve, K.C. Johnson, N. Kreiger, Y. Mao, Risk factors for prostate cancer: results from the Canadian National Enhanced Cancer Surveillance System. The Canadian Cancer Registries Epidemiology Research Group, Cancer Causes Control 10 (1999) 355–367.

[201] L.N. Kolonel, J.H. Hankin, A.S. Whittemore, A.H. Wu, R.P. Gallagher, L.R. Wilkens, et al., Vegetables, fruits, legumes and prostate cancer: a multiethnic case–control study, Cancer Epidemiol. Biomarkers Prev. 9 (2000) 795–804.

[202] M.M. Lee, S.L. Gomez, J.S. Chang, M. Wey, R.T. Wang, A.W. Hsing, Soy and isoflavone consumption in relation to prostate cancer risk in China, Cancer Epidemiol. Biomarkers Prev. 12 (2003) 665–668.

[203] L. Jian, D.H. Zhang, A.H. Lee, C.W. Binns, Do preserved foods increase prostate cancer risk? Br. J. Cancer 90 (2004) 1792–1795.

[204] T. Sonoda, Y. Nagata, M. Mori, N. Miyanaga, N. Takashima, K. Okumura, et al., A case–control study of diet and prostate cancer in Japan: possible protective effect of traditional Japanese diet, Cancer Sci. 95 (2004) 238–242.

[205] X.M. Li, J. Li, I. Tsuji, N. Nakaya, Y. Nishino, X.J. Zhao, Mass screening-based case–control study of diet and prostate cancer in Changchun, China, Asian J. Androl. 10 (2008) 551–560.

[206] L. Jian, Soy, isoflavones, and prostate cancer, Mol. Nutr. Food Res. 53 (2009) 217–226.

[207] S.S. Strom, Y. Yamamura, C.M. Duphorne, M.R. Spitz, R.J. Babaian, P.C. Pillow, et al., Phytoestrogen intake and prostate cancer: a case–control study using a new database, Nutr. Cancer 33 (1999) 20–25.

[208] S.E. McCann, C.B. Ambrosone, K.B. Moysich, J. Brasure, J.R. Marshall, J.L. Freudenheim, et al., Intakes of selected nutrients, foods, and phytochemicals and prostate cancer risk in western New York, Nutr. Cancer 53 (2005) 33–41.

[209] S.Y. Park, L.R. Wilkens, A.A. Franke, L. Le Marchand, K.K. Kakazu, M.T. Goodman, et al., Urinary phytoestrogen excretion and prostate cancer risk: a nested case–control study in the Multiethnic Cohort, Br. J. Cancer 101 (2009) 185–191.

[210] H. Ward, G. Chapelais, G.G. Kuhnle, R. Luben, K.T. Khaw, S. Bingham, Lack of prospective associations between plasma and urinary phytoestrogens and risk of prostate or colorectal cancer in the European Prospective into Cancer-Norfolk study, Cancer Epidemiol. Biomarkers Prev. 17 (2008) 2891–2894.

[211] M.J. Messina, Emerging evidence on the role of soy in reducing prostate cancer risk, Nutr. Rev. 61 (2003) 117–131.

[212] D.B. Fournier, J.W. Erdman Jr., G.B. Gordon, Soy, its components, and cancer prevention: a review of the *in vitro*, animal, and human data, Cancer Epidemiol. Biomarkers Prev. 7 (1998) 1055–1065.

[213] W.J. Aronson, C.N. Tymchuk, R.M. Elashoff, W.H. McBride, C. McLean, H. Wang, et al., Decreased growth of human prostate LNCaP tumors in SCID mice fed a low-fat, soy protein diet with isoflavones, Nutr. Cancer 35 (1999) 130–136.

[214] K. Suzuki, H. Koike, H. Matsui, Y. Ono, M. Hasumi, H. Nakazato, et al., Genistein, a soy isoflavone, induces glutathione peroxidase in the human prostate cancer cell lines LNCaP and PC-3, Int. J. Cancer 99 (2002) 846–852.

[215] L. Rice, R. Handayani, Y. Cui, T. Medrano, V. Samedi, H. Baker, et al., Soy isoflavones exert differential effects on androgen responsive genes in LNCaP human prostate cancer cells, J. Nutr. 137 (2007) 964–972.

[216] M.J. Messina, Legumes and soybeans: overview of their nutritional profiles and health effects, Am. J. Clin. Nutr. 70 (1999) 439S–450S.

[217] N. Kurahashi, S. Sasazuki, M. Iwasaki, M. Inoue, S. Tsugane, Green tea consumption and prostate cancer risk in Japanese men: a prospective study, Am. J. Epidemiol. 167 (2008) 71–77.

[218] N. Kikuchi, K. Ohmori, T. Shimazu, N. Nakaya, S. Kuriyama, Y. Nishino, et al., No association between green tea and prostate cancer risk in Japanese men: the Ohsaki Cohort Study, Br. J. Cancer 95 (2006) 371–373.

[219] J. Zheng, B. Yang, T. Huang, Y. Yu, J. Yang, D. Li, Green tea and black tea consumption and prostate cancer risk: an exploratory meta-analysis of observational studies, Nutr. Cancer 63 (2011) 663–672.

[220] C.S. Yang, J.Y. Chung, G. Yang, S.K. Chhabra, M.J. Lee, Tea and tea polyphenols in cancer prevention, J. Nutr. 130 (2000) 472S–478S.

[221] J.J. Johnson, H.H. Bailey, H. Mukhtar, Green tea polyphenols for prostate cancer chemoprevention: a translational perspective, Phytomedicine 17 (2010) 3–13.

[222] R. Gilbert, R.M. Martin, R. Beynon, R. Harris, J. Savovic, L. Zuccolo, et al., Associations of circulating and dietary vitamin D with prostate cancer risk: a systematic review and dose–response meta-analysis, Cancer Causes Control 22 (2011) 319–340.

[223] M.F. Holick, The vitamin D epidemic and its health consequences, J. Nutr. 135 (2005) 2739S–2748S.

[224] E. Giovannucci, The epidemiology of vitamin D and cancer incidence and mortality: a review (United States), Cancer Causes Control 16 (2005) 83–95.

[225] J.M. Faupel-Badger, L. Diaw, D. Albanes, J. Virtamo, K. Woodson, J.A. Tangrea, Lack of association between serum levels of 25-hydroxyvitamin D and the subsequent risk of prostate cancer in Finnish men, Cancer Epidemiol. Biomarkers Prev. 16 (2007) 2784–2786.

[226] R.C. Travis, F.L. Crowe, N.E. Allen, P.N. Appleby, A.W. Roddam, A. Tjonneland, et al.,). Serum vitamin D and risk of prostate cancer in a case–control analysis nested within the European Prospective Investigation into Cancer and Nutrition (EPIC), Am. J. Epidemiol. 169 (2009) 1223–1232.

[227] S.Y. Park, R.V. Cooney, L.R. Wilkens, S.P. Murphy, B.E. Henderson, L.N. Kolonel, Plasma 25-hydroxyvitamin D and prostate cancer risk: the multiethnic cohort, Eur. J. Cancer 46 (2010) 932–936.

[228] C.M. Barnett, C.M. Nielson, J. Shannon, J.M. Chan, J.M. Shikany, D.C. Bauer, et al., Serum 25-OH vitamin D levels and risk of developing prostate cancer in older men, Cancer Causes Control 21 (2010) 1297–1303.

[229] D. Albanes, A.M. Mondul, K. Yu, D. Parisi, R. Horst, J. Virtamo, et al., Serum 25-hydroxyvitamin D and prostate cancer risk in a large nested case–control study, Cancer Epidemiol. Biomarkers Prev. 20 (2011) 1850–1860.

[230] H. Li, M.J. Stampfer, J.B. Hollis, L.A. Mucci, J.M. Gaziano, D. Hunter, et al., A prospective study of plasma vitamin D metabolites, vitamin D receptor polymorphisms, and prostate cancer, PLoS Med. 4 (2007) e103.

[231] J. Ahn, U. Peters, D. Albanes, M.P. Purdue, C.C. Abnet, N. Chatterjee, et al., Serum vitamin D concentration and prostate cancer risk: a nested case–control study, J. Natl. Cancer Inst. 100 (2008) 796–804.

[232] S. Gandini, M. Boniol, J. Haukka, G. Byrnes, B. Cox, M.J. Sneyd, et al., Meta-analysis of observational studies of serum 25-hydroxyvitamin D levels and colorectal, breast and prostate cancer and colorectal adenoma, Int. J. Cancer 128 (2011) 1414–1424.

[233] E.H. Corder, H.A. Guess, B.S. Hulka, G.D. Friedman, M. Sadler, R.T. Vollmer, et al., Vitamin D and prostate cancer: a prediagnostic study with stored sera, Cancer Epidemiol. Biomarkers Prev. 2 (1993) 467–472.

[234] M.M. Braun, K.J. Helzlsouer, B.W. Hollis, G.W. Comstock, Prostate cancer and prediagnostic levels of serum vitamin D metabolites (Maryland, United States), Cancer Causes Control 6 (1995) 235–239.

[235] A.M. Nomura, G.N. Stemmermann, J. Lee, L.N. Kolonel, T.C. Chen, A. Turner, et al., Serum vitamin D metabolite levels and the subsequent development of prostate cancer (Hawaii, United States), Cancer Causes Control 9 (1998) 425–432.

[236] E.A. Platz, M.F. Leitzmann, B.W. Hollis, W.C. Willett, E. Giovannucci, Plasma 1,25-dihydroxy- and 25-hydroxyvitamin D and subsequent risk of prostate cancer, Cancer Causes Control 15 (2004) 255–265.

[237] P. Tuohimaa, L. Tenkanen, M. Ahonen, S. Lumme, E. Jellum, G. Hallmans, et al., Both high and low levels of blood vitamin D are associated with a higher prostate cancer risk: a longitudinal, nested case–control study in the Nordic countries, Int. J. Cancer 108 (2004) 104–108.

[238] E.T. Jacobs, A.R. Giuliano, M.E. Martinez, B.W. Hollis, M.E. Reid, J.R. Marshall, Plasma levels of 25-hydroxyvitamin D, 1,25-dihydroxyvitamin D and the risk of prostate cancer, J. Steroid Biochem. Mol. Biol. 89–90 (2004) 533–537.

[239] J.A. Baron, M. Beach, K. Wallace, M.V. Grau, R.S. Sandler, J.S. Mandel, et al., Risk of prostate cancer in a randomized clinical trial of calcium supplementation, Cancer Epidemiol. Biomarkers Prev. 14 (2005) 586–589.

[240] D.M. Freedman, A.C. Looker, S.C. Chang, B.I. Graubard, Prospective study of serum vitamin D and cancer mortality in the United States, J. Natl. Cancer Inst. 99 (2007) 1594–1602.

[241] J. Moreno, A.V. Krishnan, D. Feldman, Molecular mechanisms mediating the anti-proliferative effects of vitamin D in prostate cancer, J. Steroid Biochem. Mol. Biol. 97 (2005) 31–36.

[242] V.A. Kirsh, R.B. Hayes, S.T. Mayne, N. Chatterjee, A.F. Subar, L.B. Dixon, et al., Supplemental and dietary vitamin E, beta-carotene, and vitamin C intakes and prostate cancer risk, J. Natl. Cancer Inst. 98 (2006) 245–254.

[243] S.J. Weinstein, M.E. Wright, K.A. Lawson, K. Snyder, S. Mannisto, P.R. Taylor, et al., Serum and dietary vitamin E in relation to prostate cancer risk, Cancer Epidemiol. Biomarkers Prev. 16 (2007) 1253–1259.

[244] E. Bidoli, R. Talamini, A. Zucchetto, C. Bosetti, E. Negri, O. Lenardon, et al., Dietary vitamins E and C and prostate cancer risk, Acta Oncol. 48 (2009) 890–894.

[245] M.E. Wright, S.J. Weinstein, K.A. Lawson, D. Albanes, A.F. Subar, L.B. Dixon, et al., Supplemental and dietary vitamin E intakes and risk of prostate cancer in a large prospective study, Cancer Epidemiol. Biomarkers Prev. 16 (2007) 1128–1135.

[246] T.J. Key, P.N. Appleby, N.E. Allen, R.C. Travis, A.W. Roddam, M. Jenab, et al., Plasma carotenoids, retinol, and tocopherols and the risk of prostate cancer in the European Prospective Investigation into Cancer and Nutrition study, Am. J. Clin. Nutr. 86 (2007) 672–681.

[247] J.K. Gill, A.A. Franke, J. Steven Morris, R.V. Cooney, L.R. Wilkens, L. Le Marchand, et al., Association of selenium, tocopherols, carotenoids, retinol, and 15-isoprostane F(2t) in serum

or urine with prostate cancer risk: the multiethnic cohort, Cancer Causes Control 20 (2009) 1161–1171.

[248] J. Virtamo, P. Pietinen, J.K. Huttunen, P. Korhonen, N. Malila, M.J. Virtanen, et al., Incidence of cancer and mortality following alpha-tocopherol and beta-carotene supplementation: a postintervention follow-up, JAMA 290 (2003) 476–485.

[249] J.M. Gaziano, R.J. Glynn, W.G. Christen, T. Kurth, C. Belanger, J. MacFadyen, et al., Vitamins E and C in the prevention of prostate and total cancer in men: the Physicians' Health Study II randomized controlled trial, JAMA 301 (2009) 52–62.

[250] E.A. Klein, I.M. Thompson Jr., C.M. Tangen, J.J. Crowley, M.S. Lucia, P.J. Goodman, et al., Vitamin E and the risk of prostate cancer: the Selenium and Vitamin E Cancer Prevention Trial (SELECT), JAMA 306 (2011) 1549–1556.

[251] U. Peters, A.J. Littman, A.R. Kristal, R.E. Patterson, J.D. Potter, E. White, Vitamin E and selenium supplementation and risk of prostate cancer in the Vitamins and Lifestyle (VITAL) study cohort, Cancer Causes Control 19 (2008) 75–87.

[252] D.L. McCormick, K.V. Rao, Chemoprevention of hormone-dependent prostate cancer in the Wistar–Unilever rat, Eur. Urol. 35 (1999) 464–467.

[253] V. Venkateswaran, N.E. Fleshner, L.M. Sugar, L.H. Klotz, Antioxidants block prostate cancer in lady transgenic mice, Cancer Res. 64 (2004) 5891–5896.

[254] N. Fleshner, W.R. Fair, R. Huryk, W.D. Heston, Vitamin E inhibits the high-fat diet promoted growth of established human prostate LNCaP tumors in nude mice, J. Urol. 161 (1999) 1651–1654.

[255] J. Limpens, F.H. Schroder, C.M. de Ridder, C.A. Bolder, M.F. Wildhagen, U.C. Obermuller-Jevic, et al., Combined lycopene and vitamin E treatment suppresses the growth of PC-346C human prostate cancer cells in nude mice, J. Nutr. 136 (2006) 1287–1293.

[256] A. Basu, B. Grossie, M. Bennett, N. Mills, V. Imrhan, Alpha-tocopheryl succinate (alpha-TOS) modulates human prostate LNCaP xenograft growth and gene expression in BALB/c nude mice fed two levels of dietary soybean oil, Eur. J. Nutr. 46 (2007) 34–43.

[257] J. Ju, S.C. Picinich, Z. Yang, Y. Zhao, N. Suh, A.N. Kong, et al., Cancer-preventive activities of tocopherols and tocotrienols, Carcinogenesis 31 (2010) 533–542.

[258] U. Peters, M.F. Leitzmann, N. Chatterjee, Y. Wang, D. Albanes, E.P. Gelmann, et al., Serum lycopene, other carotenoids, and prostate cancer risk: a nested case–control study in the prostate, lung, colorectal, and ovarian cancer screening trial, Cancer Epidemiol. Biomarkers Prev. 16 (2007) 962–968.

[259] P.H. Gann, J. Ma, E. Giovannucci, W. Willett, F.M. Sacks, C.H. Hennekens, et al., Lower prostate cancer risk in men with elevated plasma lycopene levels: results of a prospective analysis, Cancer Res. 59 (1999) 1225–1230.

[260] G.E. Goodman, S. Schaffer, G.S. Omenn, C. Chen, I. King, The association between lung and prostate cancer risk, and serum micronutrients: results and lessons learned from beta-carotene and retinol efficacy trial, Cancer Epidemiol. Biomarkers Prev. 12 (2003) 518–526.

[261] H.Y. Huang, A.J. Alberg, E.P. Norkus, S.C. Hoffman, G.W. Comstock, K.J. Helzlsouer, Prospective study of antioxidant micronutrients in the blood and the risk of developing prostate cancer, Am. J. Epidemiol. 157 (2003) 335–344.

[262] M. Goodman, R.M. Bostick, K.C. Ward, P.D. Terry, C.H. van Gils, J.A. Taylor, et al., Lycopene intake and prostate cancer risk: effect modification by plasma antioxidants and the XRCC1 genotype, Nutr. Cancer 55 (2006) 13–20.

[263] V.A. Kirsh, S.T. Mayne, U. Peters, N. Chatterjee, M.F. Leitzmann, L.B. Dixon, et al., A prospective study of lycopene

and tomato product intake and risk of prostate cancer, Cancer Epidemiol. Biomarkers Prev. 15 (2006) 92–98.

[264] J. Beilby, G.L. Ambrosini, E. Rossi, N.H. de Klerk, A.W. Musk, Serum levels of folate, lycopene, beta-carotene, retinol and vitamin E and prostate cancer risk, Eur. J. Clin. Nutr. 64 (2010) 1235–1238.

[265] A.R. Kristal, C. Till, E.A. Platz, X. Song, I.B. King, M.L. Neuhouser, et al., Serum lycopene concentration and prostate cancer risk: results from the Prostate Cancer Prevention Trial, Cancer Epidemiol. Biomarkers Prev. 20 (2011) 638–646.

[266] S.K. Clinton, C. Emenhiser, S.J. Schwartz, D.G. Bostwick, A.W. Williams, B.J. Moore, et al., cis-trans lycopene isomers, carotenoids, and retinol in the human prostate, Cancer Epidemiol. Biomarkers Prev. 5 (1996) 823–833.

[267] V.L. Freeman, M. Meydani, S. Yong, J. Pyle, Y. Wan, R. Arvizu-Durazo, et al., Prostatic levels of tocopherols, carotenoids, and retinol in relation to plasma levels and self-reported usual dietary intake, Am. J. Epidemiol. 151 (2000) 109–118.

[268] C.Y. Young, H.Q. Yuan, M.L. He, J.Y. Zhang, Carotenoids and prostate cancer risk, Mini Rev. Med. Chem. 8 (2008) 529–537.

[269] A.W. Williams, T.W. Boileau, J.R. Zhou, S.K. Clinton, J.W. Erdman Jr., Beta-carotene modulates human prostate cancer cell growth and may undergo intracellular metabolism to retinol, J. Nutr. 130 (2000) 728–732.

[270] L. Tang, T. Jin, X. Zeng, J.S. Wang, Lycopene inhibits the growth of human androgen-independent prostate cancer cells in vitro and in BALB/c nude mice, J. Nutr. 135 (2005) 287–290.

[271] E. Giovannucci, E.B. Rimm, A. Wolk, A. Ascherio, M.J. Stampfer, G.A. Colditz, et al., Calcium and fructose intake in relation to risk of prostate cancer, Cancer Res. 58 (1998) 442–447.

[272] J.M. Chan, P. Pietinen, M. Virtanen, N. Malila, J. Tangrea, D. Albanes, et al., Diet and prostate cancer risk in a cohort of smokers, with a specific focus on calcium and phosphorus (Finland), Cancer Causes Control 11 (2000) 859–867.

[273] S.I. Berndt, H.B. Carter, P.K. Landis, K.L. Tucker, L.J. Hsieh, E. J. Metter, et al., Calcium intake and prostate cancer risk in a long-term aging study: the Baltimore Longitudinal Study of Aging, Urology 60 (2002) 1118–1123.

[274] E. Giovannucci, Dietary influences of 1,25(OH)2 vitamin D in relation to prostate cancer: a hypothesis, Cancer Causes Control 9 (1998) 567–582.

[275] A.J. Duffield-Lillico, B.L. Dalkin, M.E. Reid, B.W. Turnbull, E. H. Slate, E.T. Jacobs, et al., Selenium supplementation, baseline plasma selenium status and incidence of prostate cancer: an analysis of the complete treatment period of the Nutritional Prevention of Cancer Trial, BJU Int. 91 (2003) 608–612.

[276] U. Peters, C.B. Foster, N. Chatterjee, A. Schatzkin, D. Reding, G.L. Andriole, et al., Serum selenium and risk of prostate cancer: a nested case–control study, Am. J. Clin. Nutr. 85 (2007) 209–217.

[277] N.E. Allen, P.N. Appleby, A.W. Roddam, A. Tjonneland, N.F. Johnsen, K. Overvad, et al.,). Plasma selenium concentration and prostate cancer risk: results from the European Prospective Investigation into Cancer and Nutrition (EPIC), Am. J. Clin. Nutr. 88 (2008) 1567–1575.

[278] S.M. Lippman, E.A. Klein, P.J. Goodman, M.S. Lucia, I.M. Thompson, L.G. Ford, et al., Effect of selenium and vitamin E on risk of prostate cancer and other cancers: the Selenium and Vitamin E Cancer Prevention Trial (SELECT), JAMA 301 (2009) 39–51.

[279] J.R. Marshall, C.M. Tangen, W.A. Sakr, D.P. Wood Jr., D.L. Berry, E.A. Klein, et al., Phase III trial of selenium to prevent

prostate cancer in men with high-grade prostatic intraepithelial neoplasia: SWOG S9917, Cancer Prev. Res. 4 (2011) 1761–1769.

[280] D.G. Menter, A.L. Sabichi, S.M. Lippman, Selenium effects on prostate cell growth, Cancer Epidemiol. Biomarkers Prev. 9 (2000) 1171–1182.

[281] N. Nadiminty, A.C. Gao, Mechanisms of selenium chemoprevention and therapy in prostate cancer, Mol. Nutr. Food Res. 52 (2008) 1247–1260.

[282] T.I. Nilsen, P.R. Romundstad, L.J. Vatten, Recreational physical activity and risk of prostate cancer: a prospective population-based study in Norway (the HUNT study), Int. J. Cancer 119 (2006) 2943–2947.

[283] N.F. Johnsen, A. Tjonneland, B.L. Thomsen, J. Christensen, S. Loft, C. Friedenreich, et al., Physical activity and risk of prostate cancer in the European Prospective Investigation into Cancer and Nutrition (EPIC) cohort, Int. J. Cancer 125 (2009) 902–908.

[284] N. Orsini, R. Bellocco, M. Bottai, M. Pagano, S.O. Andersson, J.E. Johansson, et al., A prospective study of lifetime physical activity and prostate cancer incidence and mortality, Br. J. Cancer 101 (2009) 1932–1938.

[285] M.E. Parent, M.C. Rousseau, M. El-Zein, B. Latreille, M. Desy, J. Siemiatycki, Occupational and recreational physical activity during adult life and the risk of cancer among men, Cancer Epidemiol 35 (2011) 151–159.

[286] A.J. Littman, A.R. Kristal, E. White, Recreational physical activity and prostate cancer risk (United States), Cancer Causes Control 17 (2006) 831–841.

[287] S.C. Moore, T.M. Peters, J. Ahn, Y. Park, A. Schatzkin, D. Albanes, et al., Physical activity in relation to total, advanced, and fatal prostate cancer, Cancer Epidemiol. Biomarkers Prev. 17 (2008) 2458–2466.

[288] F. Wiklund, Y.T. Lageros, E. Chang, K. Balter, J.E. Johansson, H.O. Adami, et al., Lifetime total physical activity and prostate cancer risk: a population-based case–control study in Sweden, Eur. J. Epidemiol. 23 (2008) 739–746.

[289] C.M. Friedenreich, S.E. McGregor, K.S. Courneya, S.J. Angyalfi, F.G. Elliott, Case–control study of lifetime total physical activity and prostate cancer risk, Am. J. Epidemiol. 159 (2004) 740–749.

[290] S.C. Moore, T.M. Peters, J. Ahn, Y. Park, A. Schatzkin, D. Albanes, et al., Age-specific physical activity and prostate cancer risk among white men and black men, Cancer 115 (2009) 5060–5070.

[291] I.M. Lee, H.D. Sesso, J.J. Chen, R.S. Paffenbarger Jr., Does physical activity play a role in the prevention of prostate cancer? Epidemiol. Rev. 23 (2001) 132–137.

[292] C.M. Friedenreich, M.R. Orenstein, Physical activity and cancer prevention: Etiologic evidence and biological mechanisms, J. Nutr. 132 (2002) 3456S–3464S.

[293] R.U. Newton, D.A. Galvao, Exercise in prevention and management of cancer, Curr. Treat Options Oncol. 9 (2008) 135–146.

[294] D.J. Schaid, The complex genetic epidemiology of prostate cancer, Hum. Mol. Genet. 13 (Spec. No. 1) (2004) R103–R121.

[295] C.N. Tymchuk, S.B. Tessler, W.J. Aronson, R.J. Barnard, Effects of diet and exercise on insulin, sex hormone-binding globulin, and prostate-specific antigen, Nutr. Cancer 31 (1998) 127–131.

[296] Z. Kote-Jarai, A.A. Olama, G.G. Giles, G. Severi, J. Schleutker, M. Weischer, et al., Seven prostate cancer susceptibility loci identified by a multi-stage genome-wide association study, Nat. Genet. 43 (2011) 785–791.

[297] C.A. Haiman, N. Patterson, M.L. Freedman, S.R. Myers, M.C. Pike, A. Waliszewska, et al., Multiple regions within 8q24 independently affect risk for prostate cancer, Nat. Genet. 39 (2007) 638–644.

[298] J.P. Ioannidis, P. Castaldi, E. Evangelou, A compendium of genome-wide associations for cancer: critical synopsis and reappraisal, J. Natl. Cancer Inst. 102 (2010) 846–858.

[299] F. Meyer, I. Bairati, R. Shadmani, Y. Fradet, L. Moore, Dietary fat and prostate cancer survival, Cancer Causes Control 10 (1999) 245–251.

[300] J.M. Chan, C.N. Holick, M.F. Leitzmann, E.B. Rimm, W.C. Willett, M.J. Stampfer, et al., Diet after diagnosis and the risk of prostate cancer progression, recurrence, and death (United States), Cancer Causes Control 17 (2006) 199–208.

[301] C. Wang, D.H. Catlin, B. Starcevic, D. Heber, C. Ambler, N. Berman, et al., Low-fat high-fiber diet decreased serum and urine androgens in men, J. Clin. Endocrinol. Metab. 90 (2005) 3550–3559.

37

Nutrition and Colon Cancer

Daniel D. Gallaher, Sabrina P. Trudo

University of Minnesota, St. Paul, Minnesota

I INTRODUCTION

Colorectal cancer is the third most common cancer and third leading cause of cancer death in both men and women in the United States [1]. Affecting approximately 141,000 people each year, 72% of new cases arise in the colon and 28% in the rectum [1]. Epidemiologic evidence from migrant populations suggests there are some modifiable environmental risk factors, such as diet, in the etiology of colorectal cancer [2]. Hence, extensive research has probed the relationship between dietary components and altered colorectal cancer risk. Given that the majority of cases arise in the colon and evidence suggests some differences in etiology between colon and rectal cancers [3–5], this chapter focuses on the emerging evidence of dietary impacts on the risk of colon cancer.

Many approaches have been developed to examine how diet influences risk of colon cancer. Broadly, these include case–control studies, prospective cohort studies, intervention trials using putative intermediate markers of colon cancer risk, animal studies, and cell culture studies. Each approach has advantages and limitations. Epidemiologic studies such as case–control and cohort studies can only demonstrate associations between a particular dietary component or dietary pattern and colon cancer risk and thus are most useful to generate hypotheses or provide support to findings from intervention or animal studies. However, because they directly examine humans consuming their normal diets, epidemiologic studies are invaluable in identifying potentially beneficial or harmful foods or dietary patterns.

Another approach for examining the role of nutrition in the etiology of colon cancer is the intervention trial. The advantages of these studies are that foods or dietary patterns being studied are well controlled and

there is no question about applicability to humans. However, this approach requires an outcome measure other than the development of cancer because trials are necessarily of shorter time than the induction period for colon cancer. Currently, there is no unequivocally validated intermediate marker for colon cancer. Recurrence of colon adenomas (polyps) after their removal has been used, but studies of polyp recurrence are long and expensive. Furthermore, even polyps are not completely validated as a marker of colon cancer risk. However, there is reason for optimism because studies suggest the possibility that molecular markers collected from either rectal swabs [6] or fecal samples [7] may provide the long-sought validated marker of elevated risk of colon cancer.

Animal studies represent a complementary approach that allows a more mechanistic examination to the study of diet and colon cancer. Although questions about the applicability of findings from animals to the human situation must continually be considered, there is no doubt that findings from animal studies provide insight into colon cancer in humans. Animal studies are often the best approach to examine how consuming different dietary components influences initiation events such as biotransformation of carcinogens, DNA adduct formation, DNA repair, and apoptosis, as well as post-initiation events such as changes in signaling pathways and eventual tumor formation.

Cell culture studies are frequently employed for the study of how isolated compounds influence cancer cell growth and signaling pathways, in addition to other aspects of carcinogenesis. Nonetheless, they are severely limited in that whole foods requiring digestion cannot be examined nor can food components that are normally metabolized after consumption. Consequently, for the purposes of this chapter, we focus on only animal, case–control, prospective

Nutrition in the Prevention and Treatment of Disease, Third Edition.
DOI: http://dx.doi.org/10.1016/B978-0-12-391884-0.00037-8

cohort, and intervention studies related to nutrition and cancer. In discussion of the animal studies, we focus on studies using whole foods and their effect on morphological end points of colon cancer: adenomas (benign tumors that may progress to cancer), adenocarcinomas (cancerous tumors), or aberrant crypt foci (ACF), believed to be precancerous lesions. For discussion of human studies, we similarly focus on studies using colon cancer as the end point, with the exception of intervention trials. Emphasis is likewise on studies of whole foods, with a few exceptions.

The majority of these studies have investigated diet components that can be grouped into five categories: fruits, vegetables, and legumes; meats; milk and dairy foods; whole grains; and beverages. For each category, we summarize the proposed impact on colon cancer risk, including putative biological mechanisms for influencing cancer risk, and review the relevant animal and human data.

II FRUITS, VEGETABLES, AND LEGUMES

A Proposed Mechanisms for Influencing Cancer Risk

It has been hypothesized that plant foods protect against cancers such as colon cancer [8]. Thousands of phytochemicals have been identified in fruits, vegetables, and legumes, many of which are capable of modulating various processes related to colon cancer development. For example, apoptosis (or programmed cell death) is a means by which cells with DNA damage can be safely eliminated instead of becoming cancerous. Flavonoids that are found in many fruits and vegetables induce apoptosis in a variety of models [9,10]. Other phytochemicals that induce apoptosis include proanthocyanidins (apples, chocolate, grapes, berries, and other fruits), resveratrol (grape skins and peanuts), isothiocyanates (derived from cruciferous vegetables such as broccoli and cabbage), and limonene (citrus fruits and cherries) (reviewed in [10,11]).

Second, many of the naturally occurring compounds in plant foods also interfere with oxidative processes by acting as antioxidants or increasing antioxidant activity. Antioxidants inhibit or mitigate the damage to cells from reactive oxygen species that can lead to carcinogenesis. Compounds shown to be antioxidants or to increase antioxidative activities include vitamin C, vitamin E, provitamin A and other carotenoids, flavonoids, proanthocyanidins, isoflavonoids (soy), isothiocyanates and indoles (cruciferous vegetables), and resveratrol (see reviews [10–12]).

A third major process modulated by phytochemicals is the metabolism of carcinogens. Several groups of biotransformation enzymes metabolize carcinogens by typically first exposing functional groups on the parent compound and, second, conjugating the metabolite with another molecule. The net effect is usually a more safe and water-soluble product that can be safely excreted. The cytochrome P450s (CYPs) are generally involved in the first step, and the second step is mediated by conjugating enzymes such as glutathione S-transferases (GSTs), UDP-glucuronosyltransferases (UGTs), and sulfotransferases (SULTs). However, carcinogen metabolism by these collective enzymes is complex in that the enzymes have broad substrate specificities and in some instances actually toxify the substrate instead of detoxifying it by the chemistry they mediate (i.e., activate procarcinogens). Given the number of phytochemicals that modulate biotransformation enzyme expression and activity, a widely investigated hypothesis is that diet could optimize biotransformation activity toward net detoxification of carcinogens. For example, isothiocyanates, furanocoumarins, and phenolic compounds influence CYP activity [13,14]; isothiocyanates and cruciferous vegetables modulate GST activity [14–16]; many flavonoids, isoflavonoids, polyphenols, and some carotenes modulate UGT activity [17]; and evidence indicates that flavonoids and isoflavonoids inhibit several SULTs [18].

A fourth cancer-related process that is modulated by phytochemicals is inflammation. During promotion, cytokines and chemokines can serve as tumor growth factors and tumor survivor factors; pro-inflammatory cytokines can also regulate epithelial–mesenchymal transition and thus influence invasion and metastasis [19]. Flavonoids, proanthocyanidins, isothiocyanates, and resveratrol have demonstrated anti-inflammatory activity [11,19].

In addition, many plant foods are rich in folate, a water-soluble B vitamin. Folate aids in methylation of DNA and methylation patterns are key in epigenetic regulation of gene expression. Finally, fruits, vegetables, and legumes provide fiber, which may prevent colon cancer by increasing bulk of stool, decreasing transit time through the gut, and diluting carcinogens [20].

However, whereas in vitro studies, animal studies, and many human intervention trials suggest mechanisms that are biologically plausible, cohort and case–control studies have been inconsistent regarding protection against colon cancer by plant foods. Most studies through the 1990s reported 30–40% reduction in risk in those with the highest vegetable intake relative to those with the lowest intake [8,21–25]. Accordingly, the World Cancer Research Fund/American Institute for Cancer Research (WCRF/AICR) reported in 1997 that the evidence for protection against colon cancer by diets rich in vegetables "is convincing" [26]. Subsequent studies, however, were less supportive; thus, in the second report released in 2007 by WCRF/AICR, the reassessment indicated limited suggestive evidence for risk reduction by fruits and nonstarchy vegetables. The inconsistencies could be related to study design differences in population-based studies such as inconsistent discrimination between effects on proximal versus distal colon, low sample size and case numbers, low or narrow range of intake of plant-based foods in the population studied, types of plant foods consumed in different populations studied, and error in measuring dietary intake. In addition, a possible explanation for existing discrepancies between animal data and population-based data is that animal studies frequently use purified phytochemicals as the interventions and there may be differences in net effects between phytochemical treatment and treatment with the intact food source (see review [27]).

B Animal Studies

Few studies have examined the effect of whole fruits on colon carcinogenesis. Carcinogen-treated rats fed freeze-dried blueberries, blackberries, plums, or mangos at 5% of the diet had large reductions in ACF compared to the control group [28]. A similar finding was reported with freeze-dried black raspberries [29] and with whole apples [30]. In contrast, feeding dried plum powder, produced by air drying, did not result in a reduction of ACF [31]. Thus, studies of fruit feeding have been mostly consistent in showing a reduction in colon cancer risk, although the manner of preparation of the fruit may be important.

Of the vegetables, cruciferous (*Brassica*) vegetables such as cabbage, broccoli, Brussels sprouts, and cauliflower have received the most attention for their chemopreventive properties. Cruciferous vegetables contain glucosinolates, which are hydrolyzed by the plant enzyme myrosinase after tissue damage, such as by chopping or chewing, to isothiocyanates and indoles, which evidence suggests are the active agents. Cruciferous vegetables fed to carcinogen-treated animals result in significant reductions in ACF [32]. Furthermore, a tendency for reduction in ACF has been found with juices of garden cress [33] and Brussels sprouts [34] but not red cabbage [34]. Finally, carcinogen-treated mice that were fed cabbage had fewer adenomas, a benign tumor that can progress to a cancerous tumor [35]. Allium vegetables, such as garlic and onion, have also been examined. This family of vegetables is notable for high concentrations of organosulfur constituents, such as diallyl disulfide and *S*-allyl-cysteine. Studies of carcinogen-treated rats given garlic have shown a reduction in either ACF [36] or

mucin-depleted foci [37] (subset of ACF that are thought to more likely progress to tumors), as well as a reduction in tumor incidence [38]. Dried onions also reduced ACF in carcinogen-treated rats [39]. Thus, vegetables from different botanical families, containing very different profiles of phytochemicals, appear to be chemopreventive in animal models.

Legumes commonly consumed by humans include soy, beans, peas, lentils, and peanuts. Of these, soy has received the most attention for colon cancer prevention due to evidence that isoflavones present in soy, which have phytoestrogenic activity, may be chemopreventive. Soy, however, is essentially never consumed as the whole bean. It is consumed as a myriad of processed products, including soy flour or protein isolates, tofu, and fermented forms such as tempeh and miso. Soy protein isolate fed to carcinogen-treated rats has reduced tumor incidence [40] and ACF number [41,42]. Soy flour has also reduced ACF number [43]. Interestingly, miso had no effect on ACF number or tumor incidence [44]. Few other legumes have been examined. In carcinogen-treated rats, garbanzo bean flour [43] and lentils [42] reduced ACF number, whereas cooked navy beans had no effect on tumor incidence [45]. Thus, the evidence suggests that soy, as either a protein isolate or whole flour, is chemopreventive in animal models; too few studies have been reported to be confident about the effect of other legumes.

C Human Studies

Case—control studies have taken differing approaches but generally suggest a protective association between fruit and vegetable intake or specific groups of phytochemicals and colon cancer. Utilizing the expansion of dietary databases to include flavonoid data, the association was investigated between six groups of flavonoids and colorectal cancer in Scotland [46]. The six groups were flavonols, flavones, flavan-3-ols or catechins, procyanidins, flavanones, and phytoestrogens. For colon cancer, individual inverse relationships were observed between increasing intake of quercetin, catechin, and epicatechin (p-trends <0.05) across quartiles of intake. Also in Scotland, four different subclasses of flavonoids (flavonols, procyanidins, flavan-3-ols, and flavanones) were investigated with regard to colorectal cancer [47]. A weak negative trend was observed for flavanones (p-trend = 0.07), whereas quercetin specifically was associated with a reduced colon cancer risk with increasing intake (odds ratio and 95% confidence interval (OR (95% CI)) = 0.50 (0.3, 0.8) for highest vs. lowest intake quartile; p-trend = 0.01). Proanthocyanidins were the focus of an Italian study of colorectal cancer; whereas decreased risk for colorectal cancer was observed with increased proanthocyanidin intakes, the inverse associations were apparently stronger for rectal cancer than for colon cancer [48]. A study in the United States (North Carolina) investigating risk modification of colon cancer identified three distinct dietary patterns and compared their associations with colon cancer [49]. The three dietary patterns were "Western—Southern" (high loadings for red meats, fried foods, cheese dishes, and sweets), "fruit—vegetable" (high loadings for fruits, vegetables, and legumes), and "metropolitan" (salad, seafood, pastas, Mexican foods, turkey, chicken, veal, lamb, cruciferous vegetables, and alfalfa sprouts). The "fruit—vegetable" pattern was significantly inversely associated with colon cancer risk in whites (OR (95% CI) = 0.40 (0.30, 0.60)) but not in African Americans. In the population-based Western Australian Bowel Health Study, the association of fruit and vegetable intake with colorectal cancer was assessed by subsite (proximal colon, distal colon, and rectum) [50]. Cruciferous vegetable intake was inversely associated with proximal colon cancer (OR (95% CI) = 0.62 (0.41, 0.93) for highest vs. lowest intake quartile), whereas for distal colon cancer there were significant negative trends for total fruit and vegetable intake and total vegetable intake. Furthermore, risk for distal colon cancer significantly decreased with increased intake specifically of dark yellow vegetables and apples; however, no associations were found with legumes at any of the subsites. Case—control studies, in general, have fairly consistently found an inverse association between cruciferous vegetable intake and colon cancer (reviewed in [51]).

Prospective cohort studies are typically considered stronger than case—control studies due to less susceptibility to recall and selection bias. Cohort studies have been less consistent with regard to fruit, vegetable, and legumes decreasing colon cancer risk. In the Multiethnic Cohort Study, inverse associations were seen only in men and mostly for vegetables: relative risk and 95% confidence interval (RR (95% CI)) = 0.72 (0.55, 0.94), p-trend = 0.037 for vegetables and fruit combined; RR (95% CI) = 0.80 (0.63, 1.03), p-trend = 0.039 for vegetables only; and RR (95% CI) = 0.75 (0.58, 0.97), p-trend = 0.108 for fruit only [52]. The European Prospective Investigation into Cancer and Nutrition study observed an inverse association for usual combined fruit and vegetable intake; however, with adjustment for total fiber, the risk estimate for colon cancer lost significance when comparing the highest with the lowest quintile of intake [53]. Dietary flavonol, flavones, and catechin were assessed in the Netherlands Cohort Study, and no association was observed with colon cancer [54]. In one meta-analysis, the data from 14 cohort studies were pooled and no associations were found for total fruit and vegetable intake, total fruit intake, or

total vegetable intake with colon cancer [55]. However, when analyzed by colon subsite and comparing total fruit and vegetable intake of 800 g/day or more versus less than 200 g/day, an inverse association was observed for distal colon cancer (RR (95% CI) = 0.74 (0.57, 0.95), p-trend = 0.02) but not for proximal colon cancer. For total fruits and total vegetables, similar site-specific associations were observed [55]. The data were further examined for associations by intake of botanically defined food groups. There was a modest risk reduction associated with intake of Umbelliferae (i.e., Apiaceae, carrot or parsley family) but no additional associations for any other botanically defined food group such as cruciferous vegetables [55]. In another meta-analysis, assessments were made for high versus low, dose—response, and nonlinear reduction in colon cancer risk [56]. Inverse associations were observed when comparing high versus low intake of combined fruit and vegetables, high and low intake of fruit, and high and low intake of vegetables. However, none of the risk estimates were less than 0.90, suggesting a weak effect. Lastly, a meta-analysis of case—control and cohort studies was conducted to determine the relationship between soy intake and colorectal, colon, and rectal cancers [57]. There was no association for colorectal, colon, or rectal cancers when men and women were combined. When analyzing by gender, there was a 21% reduction in risk of colorectal cancer in women only; the authors did not indicate if this varied by subsite. In a 12-month randomized intervention trial, 50- to 80-year-old men diagnosed with adenomatous polyps supplemented their diets with soy protein containing isoflavones to assess the effect on colorectal epithelial proliferation, an intermediate end point biomarker for neoplasia [58]. There was no reduction in epithelial cell proliferation or the average height of proliferating cells in the cecum or sigmoid colon.

In summary, the human data on fruit, vegetable, and legume intake reducing colon cancer risk are inconsistent. Plant foods contain thousands of bioactive constituents that may interact or counteract each other as normally consumed in whole foods and complex diet patterns. Nonetheless, that individual phytochemicals show promise mechanistically in animal and *in vitro* studies gives impetus for continued work in identifying the role of plant foods in colon cancer prevention.

III MEAT

A Proposed Mechanisms for Influencing Cancer Risk

There are several components of meat whose consumption can plausibly be linked to enhancing the risk of colon cancer. Cooking meat at high temperature causes formation of heterocyclic aromatic amines (HAAs), which are known carcinogens in rodents [59]. However, the failure to detect differences in colon cancer risk between populations consuming well-done meat versus normal meat [60] has caused some to question the role of HAAs in human colon carcinogenesis. A second meat component is heme—present in myoglobin, hemoglobin, and various heme proteins—which is suggested to act as a colon cancer promoter by an uncertain mechanism [61]. Nitrite and N-nitroso compounds represent yet another class of compounds that are present in primarily certain processed meats (e.g., grilled bacon) and smoked fish and have been shown to be carcinogenic in animal studies [62]. Finally, animal sources of dietary fat, primarily saturated fat, are implicated as a risk factor in epidemiologic studies [63,64]. Why saturated fat may promote colon carcinogenesis remains uncertain. However, carcinogen-treated rats fed beef tallow were reported to have greater expression of β-catenin (part of the WNT signaling pathway) and decreased apoptosis in the colonic mucosa [65], both of which are associated with greater colon cancer risk. Thus, saturated fat may shift intracellular signaling pathways toward a condition of greater cancer risk.

B Animal Studies

A large number of animal studies on the effect of red meat on colon carcinogenesis have been conducted. These include studies in which the end points were either colonic tumors [66–68] or ACF [69] and in which either carcinogen-treated animals or genetic models [70] of colon carcinogenesis were used. Overall, these studies do not support an effect of red meat on promoting colon carcinogenesis, and in some cases beef was protective [67,68,70]. For example, diets containing either 30 or 60% of freeze-dried beef, chicken, or bacon were fed to carcinogen-treated rats and ACF number was determined after 100 days of feeding. These diets were compared to casein-based control diets that used either olive oil or lard as fat sources in order to approximate the fat content of the meat diets. There were no differences in the number of ACF among any of the diets [69]. Pence et al. [67] examined the effect of lean beef versus casein at two levels of dietary fat (5 vs. 20%) and two types of dietary fat (corn oil vs. tallow) on tumor development in carcinogen-treated rats. After 27 weeks of feeding, total incidence and the number of tumors were lower in the beef-fed rats than in the casein-fed rats.

To explain why animal studies do not support a promotional effect of red meat, whereas epidemiologic studies largely do (discussed later), Pierre et al. [71] proposed that high-calcium diets may protect against the promotional effect of red meat. This was based on observations that most rodent diets are relatively high in calcium, that heme added to the diets of rats promoted colonic epithelial proliferation [72], and that this heme-induced proliferation was inhibited by high calcium [73]. This hypothesis was examined in carcinogen-treated rats fed diets containing 60% beef in the context of either a low- or a high-calcium diet. A casein-based diet served as the control. Both ACF and mucin-depleted foci (MDF) were increased in the low-calcium beef diet compared to the low-calcium casein diet. However, the high-calcium beef diet did not differ in ACF or MDF from the low-calcium casein group, supporting the hypothesis that calcium suppresses the promotional effect of red meat. Unfortunately, complicating the interpretation of these results was the finding that the high-calcium casein diet had ACF and MDF numbers equivalent to those of the low-calcium beef diet. The authors suggested that this unexpected finding may be due to the phosphate component of the calcium phosphate used as the calcium source in the diet. Furthermore, a diet of 60% beef represents a concentration of beef in the diet well beyond what would be consumed by humans. However, this work suggests an important interaction between dietary red meat and calcium in terms of colon cancer risk that warrants further study.

C Human Studies

In the 2007 WCRF/AICR report, the evidence was assessed as "convincing" for intake of red meat and processed meat (smoked, cured, salted, etc.) increasing the risk of colon and rectal cancer [20]. Additional studies have been published since the report; a meta-analysis of only prospective studies, including the additional studies published since the 2007 report, similarly concluded that red meat and processed meat (assessed separately) were both associated with increased risk of colon cancer [74]. However, some investigators critically reviewing the prospective epidemiologic data contradictorily conclude that the data show weak associations; lack a clear dose–response trend; vary by gender; and are susceptible to the colinearity of meat intake with other dietary and behavioral factors, which limits isolation of the independent effects of meat [75]. They also suggest that the lack of an established mechanism by which meat causes colon cancer underscores the insufficiency of the evidence for a positive association between meat intake and colon cancer risk. The 2007 WCRF/AICR report also concluded that there was insufficient evidence for the mechanism by which meats cause cancer. One group investigated potential mechanisms in a large prospective cohort [76]. Whereas heme iron was positively associated with colorectal and rectal cancer, it was not associated with colon cancer. For the highest quintile of intake of nitrate from processed meat compared to the lowest quintile, the hazard ratio (HR) and 95% CI were 1.13 (0.97, 1.32), p-trend = 0.009 for colon cancer. An even higher elevated risk was observed for two HAAs: HR (95% CI) = 1.26 (1.09, 1.45), p-trend < 0.001 for MeIQx, and HR (95% CI) = 1.23 (1.10, 1.39), p-trend < 0.001 for DiMeIQx. In a meta-analysis that included five prospective cohort studies, a positive association was found for heme iron with colon cancer (summary RR (95% CI) = 1.18 (1.06, 1.32)) [77]. Potential challenges to finding consistency across human studies of meat and colon cancer may include accuracy in assessing cooking or processing methods of meats and level of doneness of meats (thus HAA exposure). In addition, genetic polymorphisms, such as in genes involved in metabolism of HAA or DNA repair, could modify the risk related to a putative mechanism [78–80].

IV MILK AND DAIRY FOODS

A Proposed Mechanisms for Influencing Cancer Risk

A number of constituents in dairy foods have been investigated for their chemopreventive potential. Calcium and vitamin D have received the most attention. However, lipid components found in dairy fat, such as conjugated linoleic acid and sphingolipids, as well as dairy proteins, particularly the whey proteins, have also been studied.

Perhaps the earliest suggestion for the chemopreventive action of dietary calcium was put forth by Newmark et al. [81], who suggested that calcium would precipitate fatty acids and bile acids within the colonic lumen, thereby reducing their ability to irritate the colonic epithelium. This irritation was suggested to be the manner in which they act as cancer promoters. This hypothesis received experimental support from studies showing that dietary calcium decreased the solubility of fatty acids and bile acids in the large intestine [82] and thereby reduced the cytotoxicity of the fecal water [83]. Another potential mechanism involves the calcium sensing receptor, which is involved in controlling differentiation of colonic epithelial cells. In cell culture studies, calcium increased transcriptional activity of the calcium sensing receptor and induced a less malignant phenotype in colon cancer cells—an effect also noted with 1,25(OH)D$_3$, the active form of vitamin D [84].

Because the active form of vitamin D functions as a steroid hormone, it is understandable that the proposed mechanisms of action of vitamin D would involve effects on gene expression, functioning as a transcription factor bound to the vitamin D receptor (VDR). Because many sporadic colon cancers show mutations in the adenomatous polyposis coli gene (Apc) [85], several studies have examined the role of the active form of vitamin D on pathways related to Apc. Inactivation of Apc results in activation of the WNT pathway and accumulation of β-catenin in the nucleus that, through a complex series of events [86], leads to constitutive activation of target genes promoting proliferation of epithelial cells. Subsequent mutations are thought to lead to tumor development. In mice with mutations in Apc, those also carrying a mutation in VDR accumulated more nuclear β-catenin [87], suggesting that 1,25(OH)D$_3$ acts to modulate the WNT pathway.

Conjugated linoleic acid (CLA) is a term for a group of isomers of linoleic acid that contain a conjugated double-bond system. Dairy products represent a major dietary source of CLA, with the two major forms being cis-9,trans-11 CLA and trans-10,cis-12 CLA. Almost all studies examining the chemopreventive mechanisms of CLA have used purified CLA in cell culture studies. No clear mechanism has emerged from these studies. There is evidence that cis-9,trans-11 CLA decreases cyclooxygenase-2 expression in breast cancer cell lines [88]—a change associated with reduced cancer risk in the colon. Increased rates of apoptosis are associated with decreased colon cancer risk, and several studies showed induction of apoptosis with CLA [89,90]. However, additional studies are necessary to establish the chemopreventive mechanism of CLA.

Sphingolipids are a category of structurally diverse lipids having a sphingoid base with long-chain fatty acids attached in an amide linkage and containing polar head groups. They are present in small amounts in most foods and, along with their digestion products (ceramides and sphingosines), are highly bioactive. A mechanism of chemoprevention by sphingolipids has not been conclusively identified, but ceramides are involved in cancer cell growth, differentiation, and apoptosis [91]; supplementing the diet with sphingolipid increases apoptosis in the colonic epithelium in carcinogen-treated mice [92]. Thus, sphingolipid-induced changes in differentiation and apoptosis are likely to be involved in the chemopreventive action of sphingolipids.

Dairy proteins have several distinct properties that make them plausible dietary chemopreventive agents. Caseins, the most abundant group of dairy proteins at 80% of the total, have been shown to bind HAAs [93], which are known carcinogens. A casein hydrolysate was shown to inhibit β-glucuronidase activity [94]. Decreased β-glucuronidase activity has the potential to reduce colon cancer risk because carcinogens can be inactivated by glucuronidation in the liver and excreted in the bile. However, colonic bacteria express β-glucuronidase activity, which hydrolyzes the glucuronide, releasing the active carcinogen. Inhibiting this bacterial β-glucuronidase activity could reduce carcinogen release in the colon. Whey proteins, the second most abundant group of dairy proteins at 20% of the total, are notable as a rich source of the sulfur amino acid cysteine. Feeding whey proteins to rats increases tissue levels of the cysteine-containing tripeptide glutathione [95]. This is significant for two reasons. First, glutathione is a potent intracellular antioxidant and can participate in the elimination of reactive oxygen species (ROS), either directly or as a co-substrate for glutathione peroxidase, which reduces lipid peroxides. ROS can damage cellular macromolecules including DNA, and high levels of ROS are believed to promote cancer. Second, glutathione is a co-substrate for GST, an enzyme involved in detoxification of xenobiotics, including carcinogens. Animal studies show an inverse relationship between liver glutathione concentration and colon tumor incidence [66], suggesting that increasing tissue glutathione may be chemopreventive.

B Animal Studies

Tavan et al. [96] reported that carcinogen-treated rats given a diet containing 30% skim milk had a significant reduction in ACF relative to the control group. However, almost no additional studies have been conducted on milk and colon cancer risk in animal models. The focus has been almost exclusively on milk components, both major and minor. Whey proteins, which constitute approximately 20% of milk proteins, reduce tumor formation in carcinogen-treated rats [97], and partially hydrolyzed whey proteins reduce ACF number compared to casein-fed animals [98].

Another major milk component, milk fat, has been examined as two different fractions—the anhydrous milk fat and the milk fat globule membrane. This latter fraction is a protein–lipid complex, rich in sphingolipids, that surrounds the milk fat globules. In carcinogen-treated rats, the milk fat globule membrane, but not the anhydrous milk fat, reduced ACF number [99], pointing to the potential of sphingolipids as an important chemopreventive compound in milk. This is plausible because a number of animal studies have demonstrated that sphingolipids show chemopreventive effects [100].

A large number of animal studies have examined the potential for calcium to reduce tumorigenesis.

A meta-analysis of studies through 2005 concluded that high-calcium diets reduced tumor incidence in carcinogen-treated animals (RR = 0.91, $p = 0.03$) [100]. Animal studies conducted since 2005 continue to support a role for high-calcium diets reducing carcinogenesis. A high-calcium diet (5.2 g/kg diet) reduced ACF number in both mice and rats compared to a low-calcium diet (1.4 g/kg diet) [101]. A relatively new animal model of colon carcinogenesis is the so-called "new Western diet," which is low in calcium and vitamin D and high in fat and also has relatively low levels of folic acid, cysteine, and choline bitartrate. Long-term feeding (e.g., 18 months) of the new Western diet resulted in intestinal tumor formation, primarily in the large intestine [102]. Using this model, 2 years of feeding the new Western diet with added calcium and vitamin D resulted in no colon tumors compared to 27% of mice fed the new Western diet [103]. Because both calcium and vitamin D were added, this study cannot determine if either one alone would have had a comparable effect. Regardless, overall, animal studies strongly support a chemopreventive effect of dietary calcium.

Relatively few animal studies have reported the influence of vitamin D, independent of calcium (i.e., when dietary calcium was adequate), on tumorigenesis or precancerous lesion. In rats given the direct-acting colon carcinogen N-methyl-N-nitrosourea and lithocholic acid (which acts as a tumor promoter), there were fewer tumors when 1-(OH)-D$_3$ was also administered [104]. In the Apc^{min} mouse, a genetic model of colon cancer, intraperitoneal injection of 1,25-(OH)$_2$-D$_3$, the active form of the vitamin, did not reduce the number of intestinal polyps. However, the total tumor load was significantly reduced compared to that of the control group, which was not administered 1,25-(OH)$_2$-D$_3$ [105]. In carcinogen-treated rats, administration of 1,25-(OH)$_2$-D$_3$ prior to administration of the carcinogen reduced tumor formation by 50% [106]. The previously described studies examined supplemental vitamin D. In a study using carcinogen-treated rats, it was found that animals fed a high-calcium diet had fewer colonic tumors per rat (tumor multiplicity) compared to animals fed a normal calcium diet. However, feeding a high-calcium diet that was also vitamin D deficient resulted in the loss of the protective effect of the high-calcium diet [107]. These few studies suggest that supplemental vitamin D may reduce colon cancer risk, and that vitamin D is necessary for the chemopreventive effect of high dietary calcium. However, in a study using both rats and mice with a defective Apc gene (Pirc rat and Apc^{min} mouse), supplemental vitamin D did not alter either tumor number or tumor multiplicity compared to those of animals of the same species given a normal amount of vitamin D [108]. Thus, the results from animal studies are inconsistent and do not provide strong support for a chemopreventive effect of supplemental vitamin D.

C Human Studies

Unlike animal studies, there have been several investigations of the effects of actual milk and other dairy items on colon cancer in humans, in addition to the effects of milk components. The most recent meta-analysis pooled data from 26 cohort studies and 34 case–control studies to examine the relationship between milk and dairy, calcium, and vitamin D intakes with colon cancer [109]. The summary RR (95% CI) for high milk intake was 0.78 (0.67, 0.92), and for high dairy intake it was 0.84 (0.75, 0.95). The same meta-analysis also showed that high intake of dietary/total calcium had a stronger protective effect on distal colon cancer versus proximal colon cancer. The association of dietary vitamin D with reduced risk was not statistically significant, but the authors speculated that this might be due to the relatively low levels of intake across the studies [109]. Other meta-analyses examining only vitamin D have been published since but with inconsistent results. A marginal nonsignificant risk reduction was reported with increased serum 25-hydroxyvitamin D (integrated measure of vitamin D from diet, supplements, and skin production) [110]. However, a meta-analysis showed an inverse association with 25-hydroxyvitamin D status as well as supplemental vitamin D and total vitamin D [111]. Although Lee et al. [112] reported an inverse association between 25-hydroxyvitamin D and colorectal cancer, their meta-analysis also indicated that the association was stronger for rectal, not colon, cancer (OR for top vs. bottom quantile (95% CI) = 0.50 (0.28, 0.88) for rectal and 0.77 (0.56, 1.07) for colon). In recent cohort studies on milk, an inverse association was observed in the Shanghai Women's Health Study [113] and an inverse association was observed for adolescent and midlife intake in the NIH-AARP Diet and Health Study [114], but no association was observed in the Netherlands Cohort Study [115].

Although not conclusive, the evidence is somewhat consistent for a protective effect from milk and dairy and possibly calcium intake. The human data on vitamin D are not as consistent, and the relationship to colon cancer warrants further investigation.

V WHOLE GRAINS

A Proposed Mechanisms for Influencing Cancer Risk

Whole grains include a heterogeneous collection of cereals, including wheat, corn, barley, oats, rye, and rice, as well as less commonly consumed cereals such as sorghum, millet, and triticale. Whole grains represent the intact grain, containing the endosperm, germ, and bran. The endosperm is largely composed of starch with some protein, whereas the bran contains most of the dietary fiber and many compounds thought to be highly bioactive, including phenolic acids, flavonoids, and vitamin E. The germ is rich in vitamins, minerals, and oil, and it also contains a variety of antioxidants, including vitamin E.

Unsurprisingly, cereals show great variation in their composition of components thought to have health benefits. For example, oats and barley contain substantial amounts of β-glucans, a viscous and highly fermentable type of dietary fiber, whereas wheat, corn, and rice have little β-glucans. There are similar wide variations in antioxidant capacity among the whole grains. Nevertheless, there are sufficient commonalities among the cereals that it is still useful to consider them as a group in terms of colon cancer prevention.

The dietary fiber from whole grains has long been postulated as providing protection from colon cancer by several different mechanisms. One long-standing hypothesis is that dietary fiber reduces contact of potential carcinogens or procarcinogens with the colon, either by dilution of potential carcinogens or procarcinogens due to fecal bulking or by reducing exposure due to a decreased colonic transit time. Another potential mechanism involves the increased production of short-chain fatty acids within the colon due to greater quantities of fermentable substrate for colonic bacteria. Of the short-chain fatty acids, butyrate has been of particular interest due to many *in vitro* studies showing that butyrate inhibits growth of cancer cells, causing normalization of cancer cells, or increases cancer cell elimination by increased apoptosis [116]. Another potential dietary fiber mechanism is the promotion of the growth of probiotic bacteria (e.g., bifidobacteria) by fructans (e.g., inulin). Although increasing probiotic bacteria in the colon by feeding prebiotics reduces colon cancer risk in animal models [117,118], it appears unlikely that humans consuming a normal cereal-containing diet could consume a sufficient quantity of fructans to significantly increase the colonic bifidobacteria population [119]. Therefore, this particular mechanism of chemoprevention may not be relevant to humans not consuming supplements of fructans.

Another oft-discussed potential mechanism of chemoprevention by whole grains is the delivery of antioxidants from whole grains. There are two issues with regard to this mechanism. First, the ability of antioxidants to reduce colon cancer risk is still in doubt. Trials in humans and animal models of colon cancer do not provide strong support for a reduction in risk by α-tocopherol, the form of vitamin E commonly found in supplements, although a mixture of tocopherols shows some promise [120]. For most other natural compounds present in foods, it is uncertain whether the chemopreventive benefit they provide is due to their antioxidant effect or some other property. The second issue is the often poor bioavailability of compounds in cereals with antioxidant activity. For example, ferulic acid, the major phenolic acid in cereals, displays antioxidant activity *in vitro* [121] but is almost entirely bound within the cereal matrix [122] and therefore poorly available for absorption. Consistent with this is the finding in diabetic rats, which exhibit elevated levels of oxidative stress, that feeding cereal-based diets had no effect on markers of oxidative stress [123].

A number of other compounds found in cereals have been shown, in purified form, to reduce colon cancer risk, including phytic acid [124,125], sphingolipids [92], and lignans [126] (compounds with a diphenolic ring structure that have phytoestrogen activity). However, whether these compounds, either alone or in combination, contribute significantly to chemoprevention by cereals is difficult to ascertain, in part due to questions about bioavailability.

Thus, cereals contain a plethora of bioactive compounds that could explain any observed chemopreventive effects. As with other whole foods, determining which compound or combination of compounds is responsible for chemoprevention is a difficult task.

B Animal Studies

Very few studies have examined the effect of whole versus refined grains on colon cancer risk in animal models. Maziya-Dixon *et al.* [127] fed red and white flour, in both whole and refined forms, to mice given a chemical carcinogen. After 40 weeks, mice fed the wheat-containing diets did not differ from those fed the wheat-free control diet with regard to tumor incidence. Interestingly, however, mice fed the red wheat diets, regardless of refining state, had significantly lower tumor incidence than mice fed white flour, again regardless of refining state. In other words, it was wheat color, not the state of refinement, that influenced tumor incidence. In another study, whole and refined wheat were fed to rats given HAA as a carcinogen. No difference was found between the groups fed whole and refined wheat in the number of colonic ACF [128], although the number of ACF per animal was extremely small.

Given the paucity of studies in which whole and refined grains have been directly compared, an alternative is to examine studies in which bran feeding has been investigated. This is an imperfect comparison because whole grains differ from refined grains by the inclusion of both bran and germ in the whole grain. However, because germ represents only approximately 2.5% of the whole grain, in the case of wheat, this is likely a useful approach.

The vast majority of studies that used cereal bran examined wheat bran, usually at dietary concentrations of 15–20%. Using carcinogen-treated rats, most have found a reduction in colon tumor incidence [129–137]. A study using Min (multiple intestinal neoplasia) mice, which have a mutated *Apc* gene, similar to the mutation in familial adenomatous polyposis patients, and thus spontaneously develop intestinal tumors, reported fewer tumors after feeding brans of several wheat varieties. The efficacy of tumor number reduction inversely correlated with the orthophenolic content (e.g., ferulic acid) of the wheat from which the bran was derived [138]. In addition, several studies have reported a decrease in ACF in carcinogen-treated rats fed wheat bran relative to rats fed a fiber-free or low-fiber diet [136,139]. A study in carcinogen-treated mice found that a diet of 20% wheat bran reduced adenomas relative to a fiber-free control diet but had no effect on adenocarcinoma incidence [140]. Several studies have even reported an enhancement in tumor incidence in carcinogen-treated rodents fed wheat bran. Carcinogen-treated mice fed 20% wheat bran, from either soft winter white or hard spring wheat, had a much higher incidence of colon tumors than animals fed a fiber-free diet [141]. Similarly, carcinogen-treated rats fed a 20% wheat bran diet also had a greater number of colonic tumors compared to animals fed fiber-free diet, but this was only observed when the wheat bran was fed during carcinogen administration [142]. Overall, however, studies in carcinogen-treated rodents support a reduction in tumor development with feeding of wheat bran.

Fewer studies have been carried out with the bran of cereals other than wheat. Oat bran fed to carcinogen-treated rats resulted in a greater number of colonic tumors in the proximal colon, but not the distal colon, compared to a fiber-free control [143]. In Min mice, however, oat bran feeding had no effect on the development of intestinal tumors [144]. Feeding rye bran to carcinogen-treated rats resulted in fewer colon tumors and fewer ACF compared to those in the cellulose-fed control group [145]. However, rye bran fed to Min mice resulted in either no effect [144,146] or an increase in intestinal tumors [147]. Barley bran was shown to reduce tumor incidence in carcinogen-treated rats compared to cellulose-fed control group [137], whereas corn bran increased colon tumor incidence in carcinogen-treated rats [132,148]. Finally, rice bran at 30%, but not 10%, of the diet reduced intestinal tumor number in Min mice compared to a cellulose-fed control group [149], but it had no effect in carcinogen-treated rats [132].

Thus, animal studies provide considerable support for protection against colon cancer by whole wheat, primarily based on studies of wheat bran. For other cereals, studies are highly inconsistent and are too few to ascertain whether the cereals have a chemopreventive effect or may even promote colon cancer.

C Human Studies

According the 2007 WCRF/AICR report, the evidence for an association between whole grains and colon cancer is limited [20]. However, several encouraging studies showed that whole grain products reduce the risk of colon cancer [22,150–153], but in some instances the protective association was only observed in men [52,154]. Further evidence that grains may influence risk of colon cancer includes studies in which an increased risk was observed with intake of refined grains [155–157].

Using putative intermediary biomarkers of colorectal cancer, a few intervention trials have been conducted [158–161]. However, they typically used an isolated grain fraction such as the bran or fiber instead of actual whole grain foods, or they combined high intake of whole grain foods with other practices that may have an independent effect (e.g., low fat and high vegetable intakes) and thus make it difficult to assess effects attributable to whole grain intake.

VI BEVERAGES

A Proposed Mechanisms for Influencing Cancer Risk

Three types of non-nutritive beverages have been studied extensively for potential protective effects against colon cancer (coffee and tea) and harmful effects (alcoholic beverages). The interest in coffee stems from evidence that coffee components such as diterpenes (cafestol and kahweol) mitigate the genotoxicity of HAA [162–164], increase the activities of enzymes that generally detoxify carcinogens (UGTs and GSTs), decrease the activity of some carcinogen-activating enzymes (N-acetyltransferase and SULTs), and decrease HAA-mediated genotoxicity [162–167]. In addition, cafestol and kahweol have antioxidant properties and induce γ-glutamylcysteine synthetase (the rate-limiting enzyme in glutathione synthesis) [168,169]. Human consumption of Italian-style coffee (or espresso) increases plasma glutathione and unfiltered French press coffee increases glutathione content in colorectal mucosa [170,171]. Moreover, coffee is rich in phenolic acids, flavonoids, and melanoidins, many of which have demonstrated antioxidant properties

that can depend on degree of roasting [172–174]. In vitro studies suggest that chlorogenic and caffeic acids found in coffee may decrease cell proliferation, cell invasion, angiogenesis, and metastasis, further supporting the hypothesized chemopreventive potential of coffee [175–179].

Both green tea and black tea have also interested cancer prevention researchers. Theaflavin-2 (black tea polyphenol) exhibits anti-inflammatory and proapoptotic activities [180]. Green tea polyphenols inhibit proliferation and invasiveness of colon cancer cells [181], induce apoptosis and demonstrate antioxidant activity [11,16], modulate GST activity [16], and are anti-inflammatory [19].

Alcohol, on the other hand, may have detrimental effects. For example, it may enhance penetration of carcinogens by functioning as a solvent; be metabolized to reactive metabolites such as acetaldehyde; produce prostaglandins, lipid peroxidation, and free radical oxygen species; and/or alter folate metabolism [20,182,183].

B Animal Studies

Very few studies have examined the effect of coffee on colon cancer in animal models. Mori and Hirono [184] examined the effect of coffee in rats treated with cycasin, a compound derived from the cycad sago palm that is metabolized to the colon carcinogen methylazoxymethanol. In their study, neither coffee nor cycasin alone induced a significant number of tumors. However, coffee and cycasin combined resulted in a high incidence of tumors, indicating that coffee promoted the carcinogenicity of cycasin. In another study, the influence of organic and conventional coffees, each at three different dietary levels (5, 10, and 20%), as well as 4% powdered coffee (eight coffee groups total) was examined in carcinogen-treated rats [185]. The authors reported no significant effect of the coffee on ACF number. However, every coffee group had a greater number of ACF than the coffee-free control group, in most cases twice as many, raising the question as to whether further statistical analysis might have led to a different conclusion. In contrast, in a study in which 1% coffee was fed to carcinogen-treated rats, no difference in ACF number was found in the coffee group compared to the control group [186]. Because caffeine alone has been shown to increase tumor number and decrease long-term survival in rats treated with an HAA [187], it may be that the caffeine in coffee promotes carcinogenesis but that phytochemicals within coffee counteract this effect when the quantity of caffeine is low.

Considerably more attention has been focused on the potential chemopreventive effects of tea, both green and black. In a study using an HAA as the carcinogen, green tea, but not black tea, was found to reduce ACF in rats [188]. However, in rats treated with azoxymethane as a carcinogen, the group fed black tea, but not green tea, had fewer adenomas [189]. There were also fewer cancers in the black tea group, but this reduction was not statistically significant. A second study using azoxymethane reported that green tea did not reduce the number of ACF [190]. Furthermore, Weisburger *et al.* [191] reported that extracts of black or green tea given to azoxymethane-treated rats had no influence on tumor development. White tea, which is the least processed type of tea and therefore has the greatest quantity of the putative chemopreventive catechins, was found to greatly reduce ACF in rats administered an HAA as the carcinogen [192]. However, in a second study by the same investigators, white tea was found to promote the formation of colon tumors in rats administered an HAA [187]. Clearly, the results from animal studies on tea and colon carcinogenesis are highly inconsistent, and no conclusions can yet be drawn as to whether tea, in any form, is chemopreventive.

Few animal studies examining the effect of fermented beverages such as beer and wine have been performed. Feeding beer to carcinogen-treated rats led to a significant reduction in gastrointestinal tumor incidence but not colon tumor incidence [193]. This finding is consistent with those of two studies in which colonic tumor incidence was unaltered by beer consumption, although it led to a shift in tumor incidence from the right and transverse colon to the left colon [194,195]. However, in another study, feeding freeze-dried beer, which contains no ethanol or the volatile components of beer, reduced ACF formation when fed in both initiation and promotion phases of carcinogenesis [196]. When the freeze-dried beer was fed only in the promotion phase, the effect was somewhat attenuated. Ethanol alone had no effect on ACF formation. In contrast to the situation with beer, in which there are studies of feeding the beverage itself, there appear to be no studies in which wine was fed to carcinogen-treated animals. Studies with extracts from wine have been inconsistent. In one study, feeding an extract of complex polyphenols and tannins from wine did not reduce the number of ACF in carcinogen-treated rats [197]. Interestingly, in two subsequent studies by the same investigators, a polyphenolic extract of red wine reduced adenoma incidence in carcinogen-treated rats [198,199]. Given that the polyphenolic extract differs from wine, and that the results with the extracts were inconsistent, no conclusion can be drawn regarding the influence of wine consumption on colon carcinogenicity from animal studies.

C Human Studies

Lee *et al.* [200] reported a protective association for coffee intake, particularly for invasive disease and in women (RR (95% CI) = 0.44 (0.19, 1.04), *p*-trend = 0.04), but not men, in the Japanese Public Health-based Prospective Study. A meta-analysis of 12 prospective studies resulted in somewhat similar assessments of the risk association: A "slight suggestion of an inverse association" was indicated for women (RR (95% CI) = 0.79 (0.60, 1.04) when comparing the highest to the lowest intake group [201]. This is in contrast to a subsequent meta-analysis of prospective cohort studies that indicated no association [202]. For the highest coffee drinkers in a meta-analysis of 24 case−control studies, the OR (95% CI) = 0.75 (0.64, 0.88), but the authors noted the association could reflect actual protection or be largely due to reverse causation [203]. Published the same year as the latter two meta-analyses, the findings of three cohort studies were inconsistent. No association was found for colorectal cancer in a Swedish cohort [204] and no association was found for colon cancer in a Dutch cohort [115], but in analysis by subsite and stage restricted to ever smokers, a statistically significant coffee−colon cancer association was observed for advanced disease in Singapore Chinese (*p*-trend = 0.01) [205]. In the Singapore cohort, the HR (95% CI) was 0.56 (0.35, 0.90) for advanced colon cancer in drinkers of two or more cups per day compared with those who drank no coffee or less than one cup per day [205]. Perhaps subgroups of populations are more responsive to the effects of coffee, or perhaps another issue in clearly assessing the relationship between coffee and colon cancer is insufficient measurement of the method of coffee preparation or type of coffee. Instant, filtered, and percolated coffees have negligible amounts of cafestol and kahweol (paper filters significantly trap cafestal and kahweol) [206,207]; espresso has intermediate amounts; and Turkish, cafetière, and Scandinavian-type boiled coffees have large amounts [208].

The majority of studies on tea have primarily focused on green tea and have frequently indicated a protective effect, but an assessment of the evidence was deemed limited and inconclusive in the 2007 WCRF/AICR report [20]. For example, results of a meta-analysis published in 2006 indicated reduced risk of colon cancer with green tea intake based on case−control studies (OR (95% CI) = 0.74 (0.60, 0.93)); however, results from cohort studies were compatible with the null hypothesis (OR (95% CI) = 0.99 (0.79, 1.24)), leading the authors to conclude that there was insufficient data to indicate a protective effect from green tea [209]. In addition, they also found no association between black tea intake and colon cancer, regardless of study design. Studies since 2007 have more consistently reported a protective association. Examples include an inverse relationship reported between green tea intake and colon cancer (RR (95% CI) = 0.66 (0.43, 1.01)) in a cohort of Chinese women [210]. Also, in a randomized control trial of 136 colorectal adenoma patients, adenomas were removed and patients randomized to 1.5 g green tea extract per day or no supplement for 1 year; there were fewer patients with metachronous adenomas in the supplement group ($p < 0.05$) and the size of relapsed adenomas was smaller in patients in the supplement group compared to the control group ($p < 0.001$) [211]. However, in a Singapore cohort there was suggestion of an actual increased risk with green tea for advanced colon cancer in men and no association with black tea [212]. Using urinary biomarkers of tea polyphenols, Yuan et al. [213] observed that in comparing the highest tertile of urinary epigallocatechin to undetected epigallocatechin, the OR (95% CI) = 0.40 (0.19, 0.83), p-trend = 0.002; there was a similar inverse relation seen for 4'-O-methyl-epigallocatechin, and the strongest protective effect was observed for regular tea drinkers with high levels of both urinary polyphenols. Lastly, in a cohort of Chinese men, green tea intake was associated with reduced risk of colon cancer in male non-smokers (HR (95% CI) = 0.51 (0.28,0.93)) [214].

Alcohol is one of a few dietary exposures with some of the most convincing human evidence for increasing risk of colon cancer [20]. For instance, results of a meta-analysis of 16 cohort studies indicated that high intake of alcohol increased risk of colon cancer (RR (95% CI) = 1.50 (1.25, 1.79)) when the highest intake group was compared to the lowest; this was equivalent to a 15% increased risk of colon cancer for an increase of 100 g of alcohol per week [215]. A subsequent meta-analysis sought to clarify the dose—risk relation of alcohol to colorectal cancer and found a positive association with more than one drink per day, and the association of alcohol drinking with colorectal cancer did not differ by colon and rectal subsites [216].

VII SUMMARY

With regard to fruit, vegetable, and legume intake, there is some indication from animal studies of protection against colon cancer by fruit and soy but not other legumes. The animal-based evidence for protective effects from vegetables is stronger. Evidence from human studies is inconsistent. Whereas animal data are not supportive of meat increasing colon cancer risk, human studies are more consistent, although confirmation of the exact mechanism is lacking. Strong data from animal studies are supportive of a protective effect from calcium, but the animal data are inconsistent for vitamin D and virtually absent for milk and dairy. There is some consistency in the human data regarding milk and dairy intake, and possibly calcium, but not regarding vitamin D. Relatively few studies with whole grains have been conducted in animals, but effects from isolated wheat bran are supportive of a chemopreventive potential. Evidence in humans is limited with regard to whole grains but is generally encouraging of potential protection. Finally, with regard to non-nutritive beverages, few animal studies have been done on coffee, and the tea and alcohol data are inconsistent. Likewise, human data are inconsistent for coffee and somewhat inconsistent for tea but strong or convincing for alcohol increasing risk of colon cancer.

There is a general paucity of whole food studies in the body of literature on nutrition and colon cancer, which represents a severe limitation in diet and cancer research. People eat food as opposed to individual constituents or fractions, and a presumption that there are no differences between pure individual constituents and intact foods is clearly false in some cases [27]. A greater use of foods in animal and human studies is needed to move us closer to developing appropriate dietary recommendations regarding cancer prevention. In addition, there are relatively few feeding intervention trials in humans. Although of necessity they rely on intermediary markers of colon cancer, they could prove valuable in testing or confirming hypotheses and findings from population-based studies and animal studies [217]. Furthermore, future human studies may need to better account for genetic variation among individuals that can not only impact metabolism of carcinogens (as briefly mentioned previously) but also may impact tolerance, absorption, and metabolism of the putative chemopreventive constituents in the diet [218].

References

[1] American Cancer Society, Colorectal cancer facts & figures, American Cancer Society, Atlanta, GA, 2011.

[2] A.E. Grulich, M. McCredie, M. Coates, Cancer incidence in Asian migrants to New South Wales, Australia, Br. J. Cancer 71 (1995) 400—408.

[3] D. Schottenfeld, J.F. Fraumeni, Cancer Epidemiology and Prevention, Oxford University Press, New York, 2006.

[4] P. Gervaz, P. Bucher, P. Morel, Two colons—two cancers: paradigm shift and clinical implications, J. Surg. Oncol. 88 (2004) 261—266.

[5] E.K. Wei, E. Giovannucci, K. Wu, B. Rosner, C.S. Fuchs, W.C. Willett, et al., Comparison of risk factors for colon and rectal cancer, Int. J. Cancer 108 (2004) 433—442.

[6] S. Lu, Y.S. Chiu, A.P. Smith, D. Moore, N.M. Lee, Biomarkers correlate with colon cancer and risks: a preliminary study, Dis. Colon Rectum 52 (2009) 715—724.

[7] C. Zhao, I. Ivanov, E.R. Dougherty, T.J. Hartman, E. Lanza, G. Bobe, et al., Noninvasive detection of candidate molecular biomarkers in subjects with a history of insulin resistance and colorectal adenomas, Cancer Prev. Res. 2 (2009) 590−597.

[8] K.A. Steinmetz, J.D. Potter, Vegetables, fruit, and cancer: I. Epidemiology, Cancer Causes Control 2 (1991) 325−357.

[9] S. Ramos, Effects of dietary flavonoids on apoptotic pathways related to cancer chemoprevention, J. Nutr. Biochem. 18 (2007) 427−442.

[10] M.H. Pan, C.S. Lai, J.C. Wu, C.T. Ho, Molecular mechanisms for chemoprevention of colorectal cancer by natural dietary compounds, Mol. Nutr. Food Res. 55 (2011) 32−45.

[11] M.H. Pan, C.T. Ho, Chemopreventive effects of natural dietary compounds on cancer development, Chem. Soc. Rev. 37 (2008) 2558−2574.

[12] J.M. Mates, J.A. Segura, F.J. Alonso, J. Marquez, Anticancer antioxidant regulatory functions of phytochemicals, Curr. Med. Chem. 18 (2011) 2315−2338.

[13] W.W. Johnson, Cytochrome P450 inactivation by pharmaceuticals and phytochemicals: therapeutic relevance, Drug Metab. Rev. 40 (2008) 101−147.

[14] H. Steinkellner, S. Rabot, C. Freywald, E. Nobis, G. Scharf, M. Chabicovsky, et al., Effects of cruciferous vegetables and their constituents on drug metabolizing enzymes involved in the bioactivation of DNA-reactive dietary carcinogens, Mutat. Res. 480−481 (2001) 285−297.

[15] B. Pool-Zobel, S. Veeriah, F.D. Bohmer, Modulation of xenobiotic metabolising enzymes by anticarcinogens: focus on glutathione S-transferases and their role as targets of dietary chemoprevention in colorectal carcinogenesis, Mutat. Res. 591 (2005) 74−92.

[16] A.C. Tan, I. Konczak, D.M. Sze, I. Ramzan, Molecular pathways for cancer chemoprevention by dietary phytochemicals, Nutr. Cancer 63 (2011) 495−505.

[17] M.R. Saracino, J.W. Lampe, Phytochemical regulation of UDP-glucuronosyltransferases: implications for cancer prevention, Nutr. Cancer 59 (2007) 121−141.

[18] R.M. Harris, R.H. Waring, Sulfotransferase inhibition: potential impact of diet and environmental chemicals on steroid metabolism and drug detoxification, Curr. Drug Metab. 9 (2008) 269−275.

[19] J. Terzic, S. Grivennikov, E. Karin, M. Karin, Inflammation and colon cancer, Gastroenterology 138 (2010) 2101−2114.e5.

[20] World Cancer Research Fund/American Institute for Cancer Research, Food, Nutrition, Physical Activity and the Prevention of Cancer: A Global Perspective, American Institute for Cancer Research, Washington, DC, 2007.

[21] G.R. Howe, E. Benito, R. Castelleto, J. Cornee, J. Esteve, R.P. Gallagher, et al., Dietary intake of fiber and decreased risk of cancers of the colon and rectum: evidence from the combined analysis of 13 case−control studies, J. Natl. Cancer Inst. 84 (1992) 1887−1896.

[22] M.L. Slattery, J.D. Potter, A. Coates, K.N. Ma, T.D. Berry, D.M. Duncan, et al., Plant foods and colon cancer: an assessment of specific foods and their related nutrients (United States), Cancer Causes Control 8 (1997) 575−590.

[23] J. Shannon, E. White, A.L. Shattuck, J.D. Potter, Relationship of food groups and water intake to colon cancer risk, Cancer Epidemiol. Biomarkers Prev. 5 (1996) 495−502.

[24] P. Terry, E. Giovannucci, K.B. Michels, L. Bergkvist, H. Hansen, L. Holmberg, et al., Fruit, vegetables, dietary fiber, and risk of colorectal cancer, J. Natl. Cancer Inst. 93 (2001) 525−533.

[25] Y. Park, A.F. Subar, V. Kipnis, F.E. Thompson, T. Mouw, A. Hollenbeck, et al., Fruit and vegetable intakes and risk of colorectal cancer in the NIH-AARP diet and health study, Am. J. Epidemiol. 166 (2007) 170−180.

[26] World Cancer Research Fund, Food, Nutrition and the Prevention of Cancer: A Global Perspective, American Institute for Cancer Research, Washington, DC, 1997.

[27] R.H. Liu, Potential synergy of phytochemicals in cancer prevention: mechanism of action, J. Nutr. 134 (2004) 3479S−3485S.

[28] J. Boateng, M. Verghese, L. Shackelford, L.T. Walker, J. Khatiwada, S. Ogutu, et al., Selected fruits reduce azoxymethane (AOM)-induced aberrant crypt foci (ACF) in Fisher 344 male rats, Food Chem. Toxicol. 45 (2007) 725−732.

[29] G.K. Harris, A. Gupta, R.G. Nines, L.A. Kresty, S.G. Habib, W.L. Frankel, et al., Effects of lyophilized black raspberries on azoxymethane-induced colon cancer and 8-hydroxy-2'-deoxyguanosine levels in the Fischer 344 rat, Nutr. Cancer 40 (2001) 125−133.

[30] M. Poulsen, A. Mortensen, M.L. Binderup, S. Langkilde, J. Markowski, L.O. Dragsted, The effect of apple feeding on markers of colon carcinogenesis, Nutr. Cancer 63 (2011) 402−409.

[31] Y. Yang, D.D. Gallaher, Effect of dried plums on colon cancer risk factors in rats, Nutr. Cancer 53 (2005) 117−125.

[32] A.Y. Arikawa, D.D. Gallaher, Cruciferous vegetables reduce morphological markers of colon cancer risk in dimethylhydrazine-treated rats, J. Nutr. 138 (2008) 526−532.

[33] F. Kassie, S. Rabot, M. Uhl, W. Huber, H.M. Qin, C. Helma, et al., Chemoprotective effects of garden cress (*Lepidium sativum*) and its constituents towards 2-amino-3-methyl-imidazo[4,5-f] quinoline (IQ)-induced genotoxic effects and colonic preneoplastic lesions, Carcinogenesis 23 (2002) 1155−1161.

[34] F. Kassie, M. Uhl, S. Rabot, B. Grasl-Kraupp, R. Verkerk, M. Kundi, et al., Chemoprevention of 2-amino-3-methylimidazo [4,5-f]quinoline (IQ)-induced colonic and hepatic preneoplastic lesions in the F344 rat by cruciferous vegetables administered simultaneously with the carcinogen, Carcinogenesis 24 (2003) 255−261.

[35] N.J. Temple, T.K. Basu, Selenium and cabbage and colon carcinogenesis in mice, J. Natl. Cancer Inst. 79 (1987) 1131−1134.

[36] A. Sengupta, S. Ghosh, S. Das, Tomato and garlic can modulate azoxymethane-induced colon carcinogenesis in rats, Eur. J. Cancer Prev. 12 (2003) 195−200.

[37] T. Chihara, K. Shimpo, T. Kaneko, H. Beppu, K. Mizutani, T. Higashiguchi, et al., Inhibition of 1,2-dimethylhydrazine-induced mucin-depleted foci and O-methylguanine DNA adducts in the rat colorectum by boiled garlic powder, Asian Pacific J. Cancer Prev. 11 (2010) 1301−1304.

[38] J.Y. Cheng, C.L. Meng, C.C. Tzeng, J.C. Lin, Optimal dose of garlic to inhibit dimethylhydrazine-induced colon cancer, World J. Surg. 19 (1995) 621−626.

[39] S. Tache, A. Ladam, D.E. Corpet, Chemoprevention of aberrant crypt foci in the colon of rats by dietary onion, Eur. J. Cancer 43 (2007) 454−458.

[40] R. Hakkak, S. Korourian, M.J. Ronis, J.M. Johnston, T.M. Badger, Soy protein isolate consumption protects against azoxymethane-induced colon tumors in male rats, Cancer Lett. 166 (2001) 27−32.

[41] T.M. Badger, M.J. Ronis, R.C. Simmen, F.A. Simmen, Soy protein isolate and protection against cancer, J. Am. Coll. Nutr. 24 (2005) 146S−149S.

[42] M.A. Faris, H.R. Takruri, M.S. Shomaf, Y.K. Bustanji, Chemopreventive effect of raw and cooked lentils (*Lens culinaris* L) and soybeans (*Glycine max*) against azoxymethane-induced aberrant crypt foci, Nutr. Res. 29 (2009) 355−362.

[43] G. Murillo, J.K. Choi, O. Pan, A.I. Constantinou, R.G. Mehta, Efficacy of garbanzo and soybean flour in suppression of aberrant crypt foci in the colons of CF-1 mice, Anticancer Res. 24 (2004) 3049−3055.

[44] Y. Ohuchi, Y. Myojin, F. Shimamoto, N. Kashimoto, K. Kamiya, H. Watanabe, Decrease in size of azoxymethane induced colon carcinoma in F344 rats by 180-day fermented miso, Oncol. Rep. 14 (2005) 1559–1564.

[45] G. Bobe, K.G. Barrett, R.A. Mentor-Marcel, U. Saffiotti, M.R. Young, N.H. Colburn, et al., Dietary cooked navy beans and their fractions attenuate colon carcinogenesis in azoxymethane-induced ob/ob mice, Nutr. Cancer 60 (2008) 373–381.

[46] E. Theodoratou, J. Kyle, R. Cetnarskyj, S.M. Farrington, A. Tenesa, R. Barnetson, et al., Dietary flavonoids and the risk of colorectal cancer, Cancer Epidemiol. Biomarkers Prev. 16 (2007) 684–693.

[47] J.A. Kyle, L. Sharp, J. Little, G.G. Duthie, G. McNeill, Dietary flavonoid intake and colorectal cancer: a case–control study, Br. J. Nutr. 103 (2010) 429–436.

[48] M. Rossi, E. Negri, M. Parpinel, P. Lagiou, C. Bosetti, R. Talamini, et al., Proanthocyanidins and the risk of colorectal cancer in Italy, Cancer Causes Control 21 (2010) 243–250.

[49] J.A. Satia, M. Tseng, J.A. Galanko, C. Martin, R.S. Sandler, Dietary patterns and colon cancer risk in whites and African Americans in the North Carolina Colon Cancer Study, Nutr. Cancer 61 (2009) 179–193.

[50] N. Annema, J.S. Heyworth, S.A. McNaughton, B. Iacopetta, L. Fritschi, Fruit and vegetable consumption and the risk of proximal colon, distal colon, and rectal cancers in a case–control study in Western Australia, J. Am. Diet. Assoc. 111 (2011) 1479–1490.

[51] M.K. Kim, J.H. Park, Conference on "Multidisciplinary Approaches to Nutritional Problems": Symposium on "Nutrition and Health." Cruciferous vegetable intake and the risk of human cancer: epidemiological evidence, Proc. Nutr. Soc. 68 (2009) 103–110.

[52] A.M. Nomura, L.R. Wilkens, S.P. Murphy, J.H. Hankin, B.E. Henderson, M.C. Pike, et al., Association of vegetable, fruit, and grain intakes with colorectal cancer: the Multiethnic Cohort Study, Am. J. Clin. Nutr. 88 (2008) 730–737.

[53] F.J. van Duijnhoven, H.B. Bueno-De-Mesquita, P. Ferrari, M. Jenab, H.C. Boshuizen, M.M. Ros, et al., Fruit, vegetables, and colorectal cancer risk: the European Prospective Investigation into Cancer and Nutrition, Am. J. Clin. Nutr. 89 (2009) 1441–1452.

[54] C.C. Simons, L.A. Hughes, I.C. Arts, R.A. Goldbohm, P.A. van den Brandt, M.P. Weijenberg, Dietary flavonol, flavone and catechin intake and risk of colorectal cancer in the Netherlands Cohort Study, Int. J. Cancer 125 (2009) 2945–2952.

[55] A. Koushik, D.J. Hunter, D. Spiegelman, W.L. Beeson, P.A. van den Brandt, J.E. Buring, et al., Fruits, vegetables, and colon cancer risk in a pooled analysis of 14 cohort studies, J. Natl. Cancer Inst. 99 (2007) 1471–1483.

[56] D. Aune, R. Lau, D.S. Chan, R. Vieira, D.C. Greenwood, E. Kampman, et al., Nonlinear reduction in risk for colorectal cancer by fruit and vegetable intake based on meta-analysis of prospective studies, Gastroenterology 141 (2011) 106–118.

[57] L. Yan, E.L. Spitznagel, M.C. Bosland, Soy consumption and colorectal cancer risk in humans: a meta-analysis, Cancer Epidemiol. Biomarkers Prev. 19 (2010) 148–158.

[58] K.F. Adams, P.D. Lampe, K.M. Newton, J.T. Ylvisaker, A. Feld, D. Myerson, et al., Soy protein containing isoflavones does not decrease colorectal epithelial cell proliferation in a randomized controlled trial, Am. J. Clin. Nutr. 82 (2005) 620–626.

[59] R.J. Turesky, Formation and biochemistry of carcinogenic heterocyclic aromatic amines in cooked meats, Toxicol. Lett. 168 (2007) 219–227.

[60] J.H. Barrett, G. Smith, R. Waxman, N. Gooderham, T. Lightfoot, R.C. Garner, et al., Investigation of interaction between N-acetyltransferase 2 and heterocyclic amines as potential risk factors for colorectal cancer, Carcinogenesis 24 (2003) 275–282.

[61] R.L. Santarelli, F. Pierre, D.E. Corpet, Processed meat and colorectal cancer: a review of epidemiologic and experimental evidence, Nutr. Cancer 60 (2008) 131–144.

[62] T.M. de Kok, J.M. van Maanen, Evaluation of fecal mutagenicity and colorectal cancer risk, Mutat. Res. 463 (2000) 53–101.

[63] A.S. Whittemore, A.H. Wu-Williams, M. Lee, S. Zheng, R.P. Gallagher, D.A. Jiao, et al., Diet, physical activity, and colorectal cancer among Chinese in North America and China, J. Natl. Cancer Inst. 82 (1990) 915–926.

[64] G.A. Kune, S. Kune, The nutritional causes of colorectal cancer: an introduction to the Melbourne study, Nutr. Cancer 9 (1987) 1–4.

[65] T. Fujise, R. Iwakiri, T. Kakimoto, R. Shiraishi, Y. Sakata, B. Wu, et al., Long-term feeding of various fat diets modulates azoxymethane-induced colon carcinogenesis through Wnt/beta-catenin signaling in rats, Am. J. Physiol. Gastrointest. Liver Physiol. 292 (2007) G1150–G1156.

[66] G.H. McIntosh, G.O. Regester, R.K. Le Leu, P.J. Royle, G.W. Smithers, Dairy proteins protect against dimethylhydrazine-induced intestinal cancers in rats, J. Nutr. 125 (1995) 809–816.

[67] B.C. Pence, M.J. Butler, D.M. Dunn, M.F. Miller, C. Zhao, M. Landers, Non-promoting effects of lean beef in the rat colon carcinogenesis model, Carcinogenesis 16 (1995) 1157–1160.

[68] R.L. Nutter, D.S. Gridley, J.D. Kettering, A.G. Goude, J.M. Slater, BALB/c mice fed milk or beef protein: differences in response to 1,2-dimethylhydrazine carcinogenesis, J. Natl. Cancer Inst. 71 (1983) 867–874.

[69] G. Parnaud, G. Peiffer, S. Tache, D.E. Corpet, Effect of meat (beef, chicken, and bacon) on rat colon carcinogenesis, Nutr. Cancer 32 (1998) 165–173.

[70] H.L. Kettunen, A.S. Kettunen, N.E. Rautonen, Intestinal immune responses in wild-type and Apcmin/+ mouse, a model for colon cancer, Cancer Res. 63 (2003) 5136–5142.

[71] F. Pierre, A. Freeman, S. Tache, R. Van der Meer, D.E. Corpet, Beef meat and blood sausage promote the formation of azoxymethane-induced mucin-depleted foci and aberrant crypt foci in rat colons, J. Nutr. 134 (2004) 2711–2716.

[72] A.L. Sesink, D.S. Termont, J.H. Kleibeuker, R. Van Der Meer, Red meat and colon cancer: dietary haem, but not fat, has cytotoxic and hyperproliferative effects on rat colonic epithelium, Carcinogenesis 21 (2000) 1909–1915.

[73] A.L. Sesink, D.S. Termont, J.H. Kleibeuker, R. Van der Meer, Red meat and colon cancer: dietary haem-induced colonic cytotoxicity and epithelial hyperproliferation are inhibited by calcium, Carcinogenesis 22 (2001) 1653–1659.

[74] D.S. Chan, R. Lau, D. Aune, R. Vieira, D.C. Greenwood, E. Kampman, et al., Red and processed meat and colorectal cancer incidence: meta-analysis of prospective studies, PloS One 6 (2011) e20456.

[75] D.D. Alexander, C.A. Cushing, Red meat and colorectal cancer: a critical summary of prospective epidemiologic studies, Obes. Rev. 12 (2011) e472–e493.

[76] A.J. Cross, L.M. Ferrucci, A. Risch, B.I. Graubard, M.H. Ward, Y. Park, et al., A large prospective study of meat consumption and colorectal cancer risk: an investigation of potential mechanisms underlying this association, Cancer Res. 70 (2010) 2406–2414.

[77] N.M. Bastide, F.H. Pierre, D.E. Corpet, Heme iron from meat and risk of colorectal cancer: a meta-analysis and a review of the mechanisms involved, Cancer Prev. Res. 4 (2011) 177–184.

[78] A.D. Joshi, R. Corral, K.D. Siegmund, R.W. Haile, L. Le Marchand, M.E. Martinez, et al., Red meat and poultry intake, polymorphisms in the nucleotide excision repair and mismatch repair pathways and colorectal cancer risk, Carcinogenesis 30 (2009) 472–479.

[79] H. Girard, L.M. Butler, L. Villeneuve, R.C. Millikan, R. Sinha, R.S. Sandler, et al., UGT1A1 and UGT1A9 functional variants, meat intake, and colon cancer, among Caucasians and African-Americans, Mutat. Res. 644 (2008) 56–63.

[80] L.M. Butler, R.C. Millikan, R. Sinha, T.O. Keku, S. Winkel, B. Harlan, et al., Modification by N-acetyltransferase 1 genotype on the association between dietary heterocyclic amines and colon cancer in a multiethnic study, Mutat. Res. 638 (2008) 162–174.

[81] H.L. Newmark, M.J. Wargovich, W.R. Bruce, Colon cancer and dietary fat, phosphate, and calcium: a hypothesis, J. Natl. Cancer Inst. 72 (1984) 1323–1325.

[82] M.J. Govers, R. Van der Meet, Effects of dietary calcium and phosphate on the intestinal interactions between calcium, phosphate, fatty acids, and bile acids, Gut 34 (1993) 365–370.

[83] M.J. Govers, D.S. Termont, J.A. Lapre, J.H. Kleibeuker, R.J. Vonk, R. Van der Meer, Calcium in milk products precipitates intestinal fatty acids and secondary bile acids and thus inhibits colonic cytotoxicity in humans, Cancer Res. 56 (1996) 3270–3275.

[84] S. Chakrabarty, H. Wang, L. Canaff, G.N. Hendy, H. Appelman, J. Varani, Calcium sensing receptor in human colon carcinoma: interaction with Ca(2+) and 1,25-dihydroxyvitamin D(3), Cancer Res. 65 (2005) 493–498.

[85] S.M. Powell, N. Zilz, Y. Beazer-Barclay, T.M. Bryan, S.R. Hamilton, S.N. Thibodeau, et al., APC mutations occur early during colorectal tumorigenesis, Nature 359 (1992) 235–237.

[86] K.M. Cadigan, M. Peifer, Wnt signaling from development to disease: insights from model systems., Cold Spring Harbor Perspect Biol. 1 (2009) a002881–a002881.

[87] M.J. Larriba, P. Ordonez-Moran, I. Chicote, G. Martin-Fernandez, I. Puig, A. Munoz, et al., Vitamin D receptor deficiency enhances Wnt/beta-catenin signaling and tumor burden in colon cancer, PLoS One 6 (2011) e23524.

[88] N.S. Kelley, N.E. Hubbard, K.L. Erickson, Conjugated linoleic acid isomers and cancer, J. Nutr. 137 (2007) 2599–2607.

[89] F. Beppu, M. Hosokawa, L. Tanaka, H. Kohno, T. Tanaka, K. Miyashita, Potent inhibitory effect of trans9, trans11 isomer of conjugated linoleic acid on the growth of human colon cancer cells, J. Nutr. Biochem. 17 (2006) 830–836.

[90] H.J. Cho, W.K. Kim, J.I. Jung, E.J. Kim, S.S. Lim, D.Y. Kwon, et al., Trans-10,cis-12, not cis-9,trans-11, conjugated linoleic acid decreases ErbB3 expression in HT-29 human colon cancer cells, World J. Gastroenterol. 11 (2005) 5142–5150.

[91] Y.A. Hannun, L.M. Obeid, The ceramide-centric universe of lipid-mediated cell regulation: stress encounters of the lipid kind, J. Biol. Chem. 277 (2002) 25847–25850.

[92] L.A. Lemonnier, D.L. Dillehay, M.J. Vespremi, J. Abrams, E. Brody, E.M. Schmelz, Sphingomyelin in the suppression of colon tumors: prevention versus intervention, Arch. Biochem. Biophys. 419 (2003) 129–138.

[93] S. Yoshida, X. Ye, The binding ability of bovine milk caseins to mutagenic heterocyclic amines, J. Dairy Sci. 75 (1992) 958–961.

[94] G.R. Gourley, B.L. Kreamer, M. Cohnen, Inhibition of beta-glucuronidase by casein hydrolysate formula, J. Pediatr. Gastroenterol. Nutr. 25 (1997) 267–272.

[95] G. Bounous, F. Gervais, V. Amer, G. Batist, P. Gold, The influence of dietary whey protein on tissue glutathione and the diseases of aging, Clin. Invest. Med. 12 (1989) 343–349.

[96] E. Tavan, C. Cayuela, J.M. Antoine, G. Trugnan, C. Chaugier, P. Cassand, Effects of dairy products on heterocyclic aromatic amine-induced rat colon carcinogenesis, Carcinogenesis 23 (2002) 477–483.

[97] R. Hakkak, S. Korourian, M.J. Ronis, J.M. Johnston, T.M. Badger, Dietary whey protein protects against azoxymethane-induced colon tumors in male rats, Cancer Epidemiol. Biomarkers Prev. 10 (2001) 555–558.

[98] R. Xiao, J.A. Carter, A.L. Linz, M. Ferguson, T.M. Badger, F.A. Simmen, Dietary whey protein lowers serum C-peptide concentration and duodenal SREBP-1c mRNA abundance, and reduces occurrence of duodenal tumors and colon aberrant crypt foci in azoxymethane-treated male rats, J. Nutr. Biochem. 17 (2006) 626–634.

[99] D.R. Snow, R. Jimenez-Flores, R.E. Ward, J. Cambell, M.J. Young, I. Nemere, et al., Dietary milk fat globule membrane reduces the incidence of aberrant crypt foci in Fischer-344 rats, J. Agric. Food Chem. 58 (2010) 2157–2163.

[100] D.E. Corpet, F. Pierre, How good are rodent models of carcinogenesis in predicting efficacy in humans? A systematic review and meta-analysis of colon chemoprevention in rats, mice and men, Eur. J. Cancer 41 (2005) 1911–1922.

[101] Y. Liu, J. Ju, H. Xiao, B. Simi, X. Hao, B.S. Reddy, et al., Effects of combination of calcium and aspirin on azoxymethane-induced aberrant crypt foci formation in the colons of mice and rats, Nutr. Cancer 60 (2008) 660–665.

[102] H.L. Newmark, K. Yang, M. Lipkin, L. Kopelovich, Y. Liu, K. Fan, et al., A Western-style diet induces benign and malignant neoplasms in the colon of normal C57Bl/6 mice, Carcinogenesis 22 (2001) 1871–1875.

[103] H.L. Newmark, K. Yang, N. Kurihara, K. Fan, L.H. Augenlicht, M. Lipkin, Western-style diet-induced colonic tumors and their modulation by calcium and vitamin D in C57Bl/6 mice: a preclinical model for human sporadic colon cancer, Carcinogenesis 30 (2009) 88–92.

[104] A. Kawaura, N. Tanida, K. Sawada, M. Oda, T. Shimoyama, Supplemental administration of 1 alpha-hydroxyvitamin D_3 inhibits promotion by intrarectal instillation of lithocholic acid in N-methyl-N-nitrosourea-induced colonic tumorigenesis in rats, Carcinogenesis 10 (1989) 647–649.

[105] S. Huerta, R.W. Irwin, D. Heber, V.L. Go, H.P. Koeffler, M.R. Uskokovic, et al., 1α,25-(OH)(2)-D(3) and its synthetic analogue decrease tumor load in the Apc(min) mouse, Cancer Res. 62 (2002) 741–746.

[106] A. Belleli, S. Shany, J. Levy, R. Guberman, S.A. Lamprecht, A protective role of 1,25-dihydroxyvitamin D_3 in chemically induced rat colon carcinogenesis, Carcinogenesis 13 (1992) 2293–2298.

[107] M.D. Sitrin, A.G. Halline, C. Abrahams, T.A. Brasitus, Dietary calcium and vitamin D modulate 1,2-dimethylhydrazine-induced colonic carcinogenesis in the rat, Cancer Res. 51 (1991) 5608–5613.

[108] A.A. Irving, R.B. Halberg, D.M. Albrecht, L.A. Plum, K.J. Krentz, L. Clipson, et al., Supplementation by vitamin D compounds does not affect colonic tumor development in vitamin D sufficient murine models, Arch. Biochem. Biophys. 515 (2011) 64–71.

[109] M. Huncharek, J. Muscat, B. Kupelnick, Colorectal cancer risk and dietary intake of calcium, vitamin D, and dairy products: a meta-analysis of 26,335 cases from 60 observational studies, Nutr. Cancer 61 (2009) 47–69.

[110] L. Yin, N. Grandi, E. Raum, U. Haug, V. Arndt, H. Brenner, Meta-analysis: longitudinal studies of serum vitamin D and colorectal cancer risk, Aliment. Pharmacol. Ther. 30 (2009) 113–125.

[111] M. Touvier, D.S. Chan, R. Lau, D. Aune, R. Vieira, D.C. Greenwood, et al., Meta-analyses of vitamin D intake, 25-hydroxyvitamin D status, vitamin D receptor polymorphisms, and colorectal cancer risk, Cancer Epidemiol. Biomarkers Prev. 20 (2011) 1003–1016.

[112] J.E. Lee, H. Li, A.T. Chan, B.W. Hollis, I.M. Lee, M.J. Stampfer, et al., Circulating levels of vitamin D and colon and rectal cancer: the Physicians' Health Study and a meta-analysis of prospective studies, Cancer Prev. Res. 4 (2011) 735–743.

[113] S.A. Lee, X.O. Shu, G. Yang, H. Li, Y.T. Gao, W. Zheng, Animal origin foods and colorectal cancer risk: a report from the Shanghai Women's Health Study, Nutr. Cancer 61 (2009) 194–205.

[114] E.H. Ruder, A.C. Thiebaut, F.E. Thompson, N. Potischman, A.F. Subar, Y. Park, et al., Adolescent and mid-life diet: risk of colorectal cancer in the NIH-AARP Diet and Health Study, Am. J. Clin. Nutr. 94 (2011) 1607–1619.

[115] C.C. Simons, L.J. Leurs, M.P. Weijenberg, L.J. Schouten, R.A. Goldbohm, P.A. van den Brandt, Fluid intake and colorectal cancer risk in the Netherlands Cohort Study, Nutr. Cancer 62 (2010) 307–321.

[116] D. Scharlau, A. Borowicki, N. Habermann, T. Hofmann, S. Klenow, C. Miene, et al., Mechanisms of primary cancer prevention by butyrate and other products formed during gut flora-mediated fermentation of dietary fibre, Mutat. Res. 682 (2009) 39–53.

[117] B.L. Pool-Zobel, Inulin-type fructans and reduction in colon cancer risk: review of experimental and human data, Br. J. Nutr. 93 (Suppl. 1) (2005) S73–S90.

[118] D.D. Gallaher, J. Khil, The effect of synbiotics on colon carcinogenesis in rats, J. Nutr. 129 (1999) 1483S–1487S.

[119] T.S. Manning, G.R. Gibson, Microbial–gut interactions in health and disease: prebiotics, Best Pract. Res. Clin. Gastroenterol. 18 (2004) 287–298.

[120] J. Ju, S.C. Picinich, Z. Yang, Y. Zhao, N. Suh, A.N. Kong, et al., Cancer-preventive activities of tocopherols and tocotrienols, Carcinogenesis 31 (2010) 533–542.

[121] M. Srinivasan, A.R. Sudheer, V.P. Menon, Ferulic acid: therapeutic potential through its antioxidant property, J. Clin. Biochem. Nutr. 40 (2007) 92–100.

[122] A. Adam, V. Crespy, M.A. Levrat-Verny, F. Leenhardt, M. Leuillet, C. Demigne, et al., The bioavailability of ferulic acid is governed primarily by the food matrix rather than its metabolism in intestine and liver in rats, J. Nutr. 132 (2002) 1962–1968.

[123] M. Youn, A. Saari Csallany, D.D. Gallaher, Whole grain consumption has a modest effect on the development of diabetes in the Goto–Kakisaki rat, Br. J. Nutr. 107 (2012) 192–201.

[124] S. Norazalina, M.E. Norhaizan, I. Hairuszah, M.S. Norashareena, Anticarcinogenic efficacy of phytic acid extracted from rice bran on azoxymethane-induced colon carcinogenesis in rats, Exp. Toxicol. Pathol. 62 (2010) 259–268.

[125] M. Jenab, L.U. Thompson, The influence of phytic acid in wheat bran on early biomarkers of colon carcinogenesis, Carcinogenesis 19 (1998) 1087–1092.

[126] A.L. Webb, M.L. McCullough, Dietary lignans: potential role in cancer prevention, Nutr. Cancer 51 (2005) 117–131.

[127] B.B. Maziya-Dixon, C.F. Klopfenstein, H.W. Leipold, Protective effects of hard red versus hard white winter wheats in chemically induced colon cancer in CF1 mice, Cereal Chem. 71 (1994) 359–363.

[128] Z. Yu, M. Xu, G. Santana-Rios, R. Shen, M. Izquierdo-Pulido, D.E. Williams, et al., A comparison of whole wheat, refined wheat and wheat bran as inhibitors of heterocyclic amines in the Salmonella mutagenicity assay and in the rat colonic aberrant crypt focus assay, Food Chem. Toxicol. 39 (2001) 655–665.

[129] R.B. Wilson, D.P. Hutcheson, L. Wideman, Dimethylhydrazine-induced colon tumors in rats fed diets containing beef fat or corn oil with and without wheat bran, Am. J. Clin. Nutr. 30 (1977) 176–181.

[130] B.S. Reddy, H. Mori, M. Nicolais, Effect of dietary wheat bran and dehydrated citrus fiber on azoxymethane-induced intestinal carcinogenesis in Fischer 344 rats, J. Natl. Cancer Inst. 66 (1981) 553–557.

[131] K. Watanabe, B.S. Reddy, J.H. Weisburger, D. Kritchevsky, Effect of dietary alfalfa, pectin, and wheat bran on azoxymethane- or methylnitrosourea-induced colon carcinogenesis in F344 rats, J. Natl. Cancer Inst. 63 (1979) 141–145.

[132] D.S. Barnes, N.K. Clapp, D.A. Scott, D.L. Oberst, S.G. Berry, Effects of wheat, rice, corn, and soybean bran on 1,2-dimethyl-hydrazine-induced large bowel tumorigenesis in F344 rats, Nutr. Cancer 5 (1983) 1–9.

[133] R.J. Calvert, D.M. Klurfeld, S. Subramaniam, G.V. Vahouny, D. Kritchevsky, Reduction of colonic carcinogenesis by wheat bran independent of fecal bile acid concentration, J. Natl. Cancer Inst. 79 (1987) 875–880.

[134] O. Alabaster, Z.C. Tang, A. Frost, N. Shivapurkar, Potential synergism between wheat bran and psyllium: enhanced inhibition of colon cancer, Cancer Lett. 75 (1993) 53–58.

[135] O. Alabaster, Z. Tang, A. Frost, N. Shivapurkar, Effect of beta-carotene and wheat bran fiber on colonic aberrant crypt and tumor formation in rats exposed to azoxymethane and high dietary fat, Carcinogenesis 16 (1995) 127–132.

[136] G.P. Young, A. McIntyre, V. Albert, M. Folino, J.G. Muir, P.R. Gibson, Wheat bran suppresses potato starch-potentiated colorectal tumorigenesis at the aberrant crypt stage in a rat model, Gastroenterology 110 (1996) 508–514.

[137] G.H. McIntosh, R.K. Le Leu, P.J. Royle, G.P. Young, A comparative study of the influence of differing barley brans on DMH-induced intestinal tumours in male Sprague–Dawley rats, J. Gastroenterol. Hepatol. 11 (1996) 113–119.

[138] K. Drankhan, J. Carter, R. Madl, C. Klopfenstein, F. Padula, Y. Lu, et al., Antitumor activity of wheats with high orthophenolic content, Nutr. Cancer 47 (2003) 188–194.

[139] C.W. Compher, W.L. Frankel, J. Tazelaar, J.A. Lawson, S. McKinney, S. Segall, et al., Wheat bran decreases aberrant crypt foci, preserves normal proliferation, and increases intraluminal butyrate levels in experimental colon cancer, J. Parenter. Enteral. Nutr. 23 (1999) 269–278.

[140] T. Takahashi, M. Satou, N. Watanabe, Y. Sakaitani, A. Takagi, K. Uchida, et al., Inhibitory effect of microfibril wheat bran on azoxymethane-induced colon carcinogenesis in CF1 mice, Cancer Lett. 141 (1999) 139–146.

[141] N.K. Clapp, M.A. Henke, J.F. London, T.L. Shock, Enhancement of 1,2-dimethylhydrazine-induced large bowel tumorigenesis in Balb/c mice by corn, soybean, and wheat brans, Nutr. Cancer 6 (1984) 77–85.

[142] L.R. Jacobs, Enhancement of rat colon carcinogenesis by wheat bran consumption during the stage of 1,2-dimethylhydrazine administration, Cancer Res. 43 (1983) 4057–4061.

[143] L.R. Jacobs, J.R. Lupton, Relationship between colonic luminal pH, cell proliferation, and colon carcinogenesis in 1,2-dimethyl-hydrazine treated rats fed high fiber diets, Cancer Res. 46 (1986) 1727–1734.

[144] M. Mutanen, A.M. Pajari, S.I. Oikarinen, Beef induces and rye bran prevents the formation of intestinal polyps in Apc(Min) mice: relation to beta-catenin and PKC isozymes, Carcinogenesis 21 (2000) 1167–1173.

[145] M.J. Davies, E.A. Bowey, H. Adlercreutz, I.R. Rowland, P.C. Rumsby, Effects of soy or rye supplementation of high-fat diets on colon tumour development in azoxymethane-treated rats, Carcinogenesis 20 (1999) 927–931.

[146] S. Oikarinen, S. Heinonen, S. Karppinen, J. Matto, H. Adlercreutz, K. Poutanen, et al., Plasma enterolactone or intestinal Bifidobacterium levels do not explain adenoma formation

in multiple intestinal neoplasia (Min) mice fed with two different types of rye–bran fractions, Br. J. Nutr. 90 (2003) 119–125.

[147] H.J. van Kranen, A. Mortensen, I.K. Sorensen, J. van den Berg-Wijnands, R. Beems, T. Nurmi, et al., Lignan precursors from flaxseed or rye bran do not protect against the development of intestinal neoplasia in ApcMin mice, Nutr. Cancer 45 (2003) 203–210.

[148] B.S. Reddy, Y. Maeura, M. Wayman, Effect of dietary corn bran and autohydrolyzed lignin on 3,2′-dimethyl-4-aminobiphenyl-induced intestinal carcinogenesis in male F344 rats, J. Natl. Cancer Inst. 71 (1983) 419–423.

[149] R.D. Verschoyle, P. Greaves, H. Cai, R.E. Edwards, W.P. Steward, A.J. Gescher, Evaluation of the cancer chemopreventive efficacy of rice bran in genetic mouse models of breast, prostate and intestinal carcinogenesis, Br. J. Cancer 96 (2007) 248–254.

[150] M. Lipkin, B. Reddy, H. Newmark, S.A. Lamprecht, Dietary factors in human colorectal cancer, Annu. Rev. Nutr. 19 (1999) 545–586.

[151] D.R. Jacobs Jr., J. Slavin, L. Marquart, Whole grain intake and cancer: a review of the literature, Nutr. Cancer 24 (1995) 221–229.

[152] S.C. Larsson, E. Giovannucci, L. Bergkvist, A. Wolk, Whole grain consumption and risk of colorectal cancer: a population-based cohort of 60,000 women, Br. J. Cancer 92 (2005) 1803–1807.

[153] A. Schatzkin, T. Mouw, Y. Park, A.F. Subar, V. Kipnis, A. Hollenbeck, et al., Dietary fiber and whole-grain consumption in relation to colorectal cancer in the NIH-AARP Diet and Health Study, Am. J. Clin. Nutr. 85 (2007) 1353–1360.

[154] R. Egeberg, A. Olsen, S. Loft, J. Christensen, N.F. Johnsen, K. Overvad, et al., Intake of whole grain products and risk of colorectal cancers in the Diet, Cancer and Health cohort study, Br. J. Cancer 103 (2010) 730–734.

[155] F. Levi, C. Pasche, C. La Vecchia, F. Lucchini, S. Franceschi, Food groups and colorectal cancer risk, Br. J. Cancer 79 (1999) 1283–1287.

[156] M.C. Boutron-Ruault, P. Senesse, J. Faivre, N. Chatelain, C. Belghiti, S. Meance, Foods as risk factors for colorectal cancer: a case–control study in Burgundy (France), Eur. J. Cancer Prev. 8 (1999) 229–235.

[157] L. Chatenoud, C. La Vecchia, S. Franceschi, A. Tavani, D.R. Jacobs Jr., M.T. Parpinel, et al., Refined-cereal intake and risk of selected cancers in Italy, Am. J. Clin. Nutr. 70 (1999) 1107–1110.

[158] S.A. Beresford, K.C. Johnson, C. Ritenbaugh, N.L. Lasser, L.G. Snetselaar, H.R. Black, et al., Low-fat dietary pattern and risk of colorectal cancer: the Women's Health Initiative Randomized Controlled Dietary Modification Trial, JAMA 295 (2006) 643–654.

[159] D.S. Alberts, M.E. Martinez, D.J. Roe, J.M. Guillen-Rodriguez, J.R. Marshall, J.B. van Leeuwen, et al., Lack of effect of a high-fiber cereal supplement on the recurrence of colorectal adenomas: Phoenix Colon Cancer Prevention Physicians' Network, N. Engl. J. Med. 342 (2000) 1156–1162.

[160] F. Macrae, Wheat bran fiber and development of adenomatous polyps: evidence from randomized, controlled clinical trials, Am. J. Med. 106 (1999) 38S–42S.

[161] J.W. Lampe, J.L. Slavin, E.A. Melcher, J.D. Potter, Effects of cereal and vegetable fiber feeding on potential risk factors for colon cancer, Cancer Epidemiol. Biomarkers Prev. 1 (1992) 207–211.

[162] R. Edenharder, J.W. Sager, H. Glatt, E. Muckel, K.L. Platt, Protection by beverages, fruits, vegetables, herbs, and flavonoids against genotoxicity of 2-acetylaminofluorene and 2-amino-1-methyl-6-phenylimidazo[4,5-b]pyridine (PhIP) in metabolically competent V79 cells, Mutat. Res. 521 (2002) 57–72.

[163] B.J. Majer, E. Hofer, C. Cavin, E. Lhoste, M. Uhl, H.R. Glatt, et al., Coffee diterpenes prevent the genotoxic effects of 2-amino-1-methyl-6-phenylimidazo[4,5-b]pyridine (PhIP) and N-nitrosodimethylamine in a human derived liver cell line (HepG2), Food Chem. Toxicol. 43 (2005) 433–441.

[164] W.W. Huber, L.P. McDaniel, K.R. Kaderlik, C.H. Teitel, N.P. Lang, F.F. Kadlubar, Chemoprotection against the formation of colon DNA adducts from the food-borne carcinogen 2-amino-1-methyl-6-phenylimidazo[4,5-b]pyridine (PhIP) in the rat, Mutat. Res. 376 (1997) 115–122.

[165] W.W. Huber, S. Prustomersky, E. Delbanco, M. Uhl, G. Scharf, R.J. Turesky, et al., Enhancement of the chemoprotective enzymes glucuronosyl transferase and glutathione transferase in specific organs of the rat by the coffee components kahweol and cafestol, Arch. Toxicol. 76 (2002) 209–217.

[166] W.W. Huber, C.H. Teitel, B.F. Coles, R.S. King, F.W. Wiese, K.R. Kaderlik, et al., Potential chemoprotective effects of the coffee components kahweol and cafestol palmitates via modification of hepatic N-acetyltransferase and glutathione S-transferase activities, Environ. Mol. Mutagen. 44 (2004) 265–276.

[167] R.J. Turesky, J. Richoz, A. Constable, K.D. Curtis, K.H. Dingley, K.W. Turteltaub, The effects of coffee on enzymes involved in metabolism of the dietary carcinogen 2-amino-1-methyl-6-phenylimidazo[4,5-b]pyridine in rats, Chem.–Biol. Interact. 145 (2003) 251–265.

[168] K.J. Lee, H.G. Jeong, Protective effects of kahweol and cafestol against hydrogen peroxide-induced oxidative stress and DNA damage, Toxicol. Lett. 173 (2007) 80–87.

[169] W.W. Huber, G. Scharf, W. Rossmanith, S. Prustomersky, B. Grasl-Kraupp, B. Peter, et al., The coffee components kahweol and cafestol induce gamma-glutamylcysteine synthetase, the rate limiting enzyme of chemoprotective glutathione synthesis, in several organs of the rat, Arch. Toxicol. 75 (2002) 685–694.

[170] F. Esposito, F. Morisco, V. Verde, A. Ritieni, A. Alezio, N. Caporaso, V. Fogliano, Moderate coffee consumption increases plasma glutathione but not homocysteine in healthy subjects, Aliment. Pharmacol. Ther. 17 (2003) 595–601.

[171] M.J. Grubben, C.C. Van Den Braak, R. Broekhuizen, R. De Jong, L. Van Rijt, E. De Ruijter, et al., The effect of unfiltered coffee on potential biomarkers for colonic cancer risk in healthy volunteers: a randomized trial, Aliment. Pharmacol. Ther. 14 (2000) 1181–1190.

[172] K. Yanagimoto, H. Ochi, K.G. Lee, T. Shibamoto, Antioxidative activities of fractions obtained from brewed coffee, J. Agric. Food Chem. 52 (2004) 592–596.

[173] R.C. Borrelli, A. Visconti, C. Mennella, M. Anese, V. Fogliano, Chemical characterization and antioxidant properties of coffee melanoidins, J. Agric. Food Chem. 50 (2002) 6527–6533.

[174] M.D. del Castillo, J.M. Ames, M.H. Gordon, Effect of roasting on the antioxidant activity of coffee brews, J. Agric. Food Chem. 50 (2002) 3698–3703.

[175] H. Mori, K. Kawabata, K. Matsunaga, J. Ushida, K. Fujii, A. Hara, et al., Chemopreventive effects of coffee bean and rice constituents on colorectal carcinogenesis, Biofactors 12 (2000) 101–105.

[176] U.H. Jin, J.Y. Lee, S.K. Kang, J.K. Kim, W.H. Park, J.G. Kim, et al., A phenolic compound, 5-caffeoylquinic acid (chlorogenic acid), is a new type and strong matrix metalloproteinase-9 inhibitor: isolation and identification from methanol extract of Euonymus alatus, Life Sci. 77 (2005) 2760–2769.

[177] A. Belkaid, J.C. Currie, J. Desgagnes, B. Annabi, The chemopreventive properties of chlorogenic acid reveal a potential

new role for the microsomal glucose-6-phosphate translocase in brain tumor progression, Cancer Cell Int. 6 (2006) 7.

[178] J.E. Jung, H.S. Kim, C.S. Lee, D.H. Park, Y.N. Kim, M.J. Lee, et al., Caffeic acid and its synthetic derivative CADPE suppress tumor angiogenesis by blocking STAT3-mediated VEGF expression in human renal carcinoma cells, Carcinogenesis 28 (2007) 1780–1787.

[179] N.J. Kang, K.W. Lee, B.H. Kim, A.M. Bode, H.J. Lee, Y.S. Heo, et al., Coffee phenolic phytochemicals suppress colon cancer metastasis by targeting MEK and TOPK, Carcinogenesis 32 (2011) 921–928.

[180] A. Gosslau, D.L. En Jao, M.T. Huang, C.T. Ho, D. Evans, N.E. Rawson, et al., Effects of the black tea polyphenol theaflavin-2 on apoptotic and inflammatory pathways *in vitro* and *in vivo*, Mol. Nutr. Food Res. 55 (2011) 198–208.

[181] C.A. Larsen, R.H. Dashwood, (−)-Epigallocatechin-3-gallate inhibits Met signaling, proliferation, and invasiveness in human colon cancer cells, Arch. Biochem. Biophys. 501 (2010) 52–57.

[182] P. Boffetta, M. Hashibe, Alcohol and cancer, Lancet Oncol. 7 (2006) 149–156.

[183] A. Hamid, N.A. Wani, J. Kaur, New perspectives on folate transport in relation to alcoholism-induced folate malabsorption: association with epigenome stability and cancer development, FEBS J. 276 (2009) 2175–2191.

[184] H. Mori, I. Hirono, Effect of coffee on carcinogenicity of cycasin, Br. J. Cancer 35 (1977) 369–371.

[185] C. Carvalho Ddo, M.R. Brigagao, M.H. dos Santos, F.B. de Paula, A. Giusti-Paiva, L. Azevedo, Organic and conventional *Coffea arabica* L.: a comparative study of the chemical composition and physiological, biochemical and toxicological effects in Wistar rats, Plant Foods Hum. Nutr. 66 (2011) 114–121.

[186] C.V. Rao, D. Chou, B. Simi, H. Ku, B.S. Reddy, Prevention of colonic aberrant crypt foci and modulation of large bowel microbial activity by dietary coffee fiber, inulin and pectin, Carcinogenesis 19 (1998) 1815–1819.

[187] R. Wang, W.M. Dashwood, C.V. Lohr, K.A. Fischer, C.B. Pereira, M. Louderback, et al., Protective versus promotional effects of white tea and caffeine on PhIP-induced tumorigenesis and beta-catenin expression in the rat, Carcinogenesis 29 (2008) 834–839.

[188] M. Xu, A.C. Bailey, J.F. Hernaez, C.R. Taoka, H.A. Schut, R.H. Dashwood, Protection by green tea, black tea, and indole-3-carbinol against 2-amino-3-methylimidazo[4,5-f]quinoline-induced DNA adducts and colonic aberrant crypts in the F344 rat, Carcinogenesis 17 (1996) 1429–1434.

[189] G. Caderni, C. De Filippo, C. Luceri, M. Salvadori, A. Giannini, A. Biggeri, et al., Effects of black tea, green tea and wine extracts on intestinal carcinogenesis induced by azoxymethane in F344 rats, Carcinogenesis 21 (2000) 1965–1969.

[190] A. Challa, D.R. Rao, B.S. Reddy, Interactive suppression of aberrant crypt foci induced by azoxymethane in rat colon by phytic acid and green tea, Carcinogenesis 18 (1997) 2023–2026.

[191] J.H. Weisburger, A. Rivenson, C. Aliaga, J. Reinhardt, G.J. Kelloff, C.W. Boone, et al., Effect of tea extracts, polyphenols, and epigallocatechin gallate on azoxymethane-induced colon cancer, Proc. Soc. Exp. Biol. Med. 217 (1998) 104–108.

[192] G. Santana-Rios, G.A. Orner, M. Xu, M. Izquierdo-Pulido, R.H. Dashwood, Inhibition by white tea of 2-amino-1-methyl-6-phenylimidazo[4,5-*b*]pyridine-induced colonic aberrant crypts in the F344 rat, Nutr. Cancer 41 (2001) 98–103.

[193] R.L. Nelson, S.L. Samelson, Neither dietary ethanol nor beer augments experimental colon carcinogenesis in rats, Dis. Colon Rectum 28 (1985) 460–462.

[194] S.R. Hamilton, J. Hyland, D. McAvinchey, Y. Chaudhry, L. Hartka, H.T. Kim, et al., Effects of chronic dietary beer and ethanol consumption on experimental colonic carcinogenesis by azoxymethane in rats, Cancer Res. 47 (1987) 1551–1559.

[195] A.E. Howarth, E. Pihl, High-fat diet promotes and causes distal shift of experimental rat colonic cancer—beer and alcohol do not, Nutr. Cancer 6 (1984) 229–235.

[196] H. Nozawa, A. Yoshida, O. Tajima, M. Katayama, H. Sonobe, K. Wakabayashi, et al., Intake of beer inhibits azoxymethane-induced colonic carcinogenesis in male Fischer 344 rats, Int. J. Cancer 108 (2004) 404–411.

[197] G. Caderni, S. Remy, V. Cheynier, G. Morozzi, P. Dolara, Effect of complex polyphenols on colon carcinogenesis, Eur. J. Nutr. 38 (1999) 126–132.

[198] P. Dolara, C. Luceri, C. De Filippo, A.P. Femia, L. Giovannelli, G. Caderni, et al., Red wine polyphenols influence carcinogenesis, intestinal microflora, oxidative damage and gene expression profiles of colonic mucosa in F344 rats, Mutat. Res. 591 (2005) 237–246.

[199] A.P. Femia, G. Caderni, F. Vignali, M. Salvadori, A. Giannini, A. Biggeri, et al., Effect of polyphenolic extracts from red wine and 4-OH-coumaric acid on 1,2-dimethylhydrazine-induced colon carcinogenesis in rats, Eur. J. Nutr. 44 (2005) 79–84.

[200] K.J. Lee, M. Inoue, T. Otani, M. Iwasaki, S. Sasazuki, S. Tsugane, Coffee consumption and risk of colorectal cancer in a population-based prospective cohort of Japanese men and women, Int. J. Cancer 121 (2007) 1312–1318.

[201] Y. Je, W. Liu, E. Giovannucci, Coffee consumption and risk of colorectal cancer: a systematic review and meta-analysis of prospective cohort studies, Int. J. Cancer 124 (2009) 1662–1668.

[202] X. Zhang, D. Albanes, W.L. Beeson, P.A. van den Brandt, J.E. Buring, A. Flood, et al., Risk of colon cancer and coffee, tea, and sugar-sweetened soft drink intake: Pooled analysis of prospective cohort studies, J. Natl. Cancer Inst. 102 (2010) 771–783.

[203] C. Galeone, F. Turati, C. La Vecchia, A. Tavani, Coffee consumption and risk of colorectal cancer: a meta-analysis of case–control studies, Cancer Causes Control 21 (2010) 1949–1959.

[204] L.M. Nilsson, I. Johansson, P. Lenner, B. Lindahl, B. Van Guelpen, Consumption of filtered and boiled coffee and the risk of incident cancer: a prospective cohort study, Cancer Causes Control 21 (2010) 1533–1544.

[205] S. Peterson, J.M. Yuan, W.P. Koh, C.L. Sun, R. Wang, R.J. Turesky, et al., Coffee intake and risk of colorectal cancer among Chinese in Singapore: the Singapore Chinese Health Study, Nutr. Cancer 62 (2010) 21–29.

[206] W.M. Ratnayake, R. Hollywood, E. O'Grady, B. Stavric, Lipid content and composition of coffee brews prepared by different methods, Food Chem. Toxicol. 31 (1993) 263–269.

[207] G. Gross, E. Jaccaud, A.C. Huggett, Analysis of the content of the diterpenes cafestol and kahweol in coffee brews, Food Chem. Toxicol. 35 (1997) 547–554.

[208] R. Urgert, G. Van der Weg, T.G. Kosmeiher-Schuil, P. Van Bovenkamp, R. Hovenier, M.B. Katan, Levels of the cholesterol-elevating diterpenes cafestol and kahweol in various coffee brews, J. Agric. Food Chem. 43 (1995) 2167–2172.

[209] C.L. Sun, J.M. Yuan, W.P. Koh, M.C. Yu, Green tea, black tea and colorectal cancer risk: a meta-analysis of epidemiologic studies, Carcinogenesis 27 (2006) 1301–1309.

[210] G. Yang, X.O. Shu, H. Li, W.H. Chow, B.T. Ji, X. Zhang, et al., Prospective cohort study of green tea consumption and colorectal cancer risk in women, Cancer Epidemiol. Biomarkers Prev. 16 (2007) 1219–1223.

[211] M. Shimizu, Y. Fukutomi, M. Ninomiya, K. Nagura, T. Kato, H. Araki, et al., Green tea extracts for the prevention of

metachronous colorectal adenomas: a pilot study, Cancer Epidemiol. Biomarkers Prev. 17 (2008) 3020–3025.

[212] C.L. Sun, J.M. Yuan, W.P. Koh, H.P. Lee, M.C. Yu, Green tea and black tea consumption in relation to colorectal cancer risk: the Singapore Chinese Health Study, Carcinogenesis 28 (2007) 2143–2148.

[213] J.M. Yuan, Y.T. Gao, C.S. Yang, M.C. Yu, Urinary biomarkers of tea polyphenols and risk of colorectal cancer in the Shanghai Cohort Study, Int. J. Cancer 120 (2007) 1344–1350.

[214] G. Yang, W. Zheng, Y.B. Xiang, J. Gao, H.L. Li, X. Zhang, et al., Green tea consumption and colorectal cancer risk: a report from the Shanghai Men's Health Study, Carcinogenesis 32 (2011) 1684–1688.

[215] A. Moskal, T. Norat, P. Ferrari, E. Riboli, Alcohol intake and colorectal cancer risk: a dose–response meta-analysis of published cohort studies, Int. J. Cancer 120 (2007) 664–671.

[216] V. Fedirko, I. Tramacere, V. Bagnardi, M. Rota, L. Scotti, F. Islami, et al., Alcohol drinking and colorectal cancer risk: an overall and dose–response meta-analysis of published studies, Ann. Oncol. 22 (2011) 1958–1972.

[217] J.W. Lampe, Nutrition and cancer prevention: small-scale human studies for the 21st century, Cancer Epidemiol. Biomarkers Prev. 13 (2004) 1987–1988.

[218] J.W. Lampe, Interindividual differences in response to plant-based diets: implications for cancer risk, Am. J. Clin. Nutr. 89 (2009) 1553S–1557S.

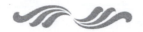

GASTROINTESTINAL HEALTH AND DISEASE

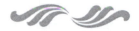

Intestinal Microflora and Diet in Health

Merlin W. Ariefdjohan, Onikia N. Brown-Esters, Dennis A. Savaiano

Purdue University, West Lafayette, Indiana

I INTRODUCTION

The human gastrointestinal (GI) tract contains bacterial communities that are diverse and complex. This intestinal microflora plays an important role in digestion and production of essential vitamins and protects the GI tract from pathogen colonization. Although the intestinal microflora appears to be relatively stable, it can be altered by environmental factors such as disease, antibiotics, and diet. Furthermore, it has been postulated that dominant bacterial groups influence the well-being of their host by forming close interactions with the mammalian cells.

For approximately the past 35 years, there has been relatively little progress in understanding the GI microbe—host relationship, primarily because of methodological limitations. Consequently, the mechanisms by which the intestinal microflora influences human health and disease are not well understood. Traditional plating methods are both time-consuming and insensitive. Advances in molecular techniques can overcome these limitations and pave the way for a better understanding of the complex GI tract ecosystem. Scientific breakthroughs in this field will permit researchers to move from observation to the prediction of disease using biomarkers based on the metabolic capabilities of intestinal microflora. Dietary intervention strategies including the consumption of prebiotics, probiotics, and synbiotics may also be developed to enhance overall health and reduce disease incidence. Therefore, understanding the intricate relationship between GI tract microflora and health is an important item on the research agenda.

This chapter serves to provide a comprehensive review of the following: (1) the concept of intestinal microflora, (2) the methodology used to investigate the intestinal microflora and their limitations, (3) the influence of diet on intestinal microflora, and (4) future directions in the field.

II DISTRIBUTION AND DIVERSITY OF THE HUMAN INTESTINAL MICROFLORA

When the word *ecosystem* comes to mind, most people conjure up images of the rain forest with its myriads of animals, plants, and insects or the oceans teeming with fish, algae, and phytoplankton. Rarely do we think of the ecosystem on our body in the form of bacterial communities residing on the skin, oral cavity, genitals, and GI tract. On average, the human GI tract (i.e., small intestine and large intestine (colon)) is 27 feet long. Its surface area is greatly enhanced by the formation of microvilli on the surface of each intestinal villus (Figure 38.1). Because of this anatomical folding, the GI tract creates a large surface area for bacterial colonization (approximately $150-200$ m^2 or $1614-2153$ ft^2) [1]. As a comparison, the human skin covers only approximately 2 m^2 (21.5 ft^2). The adult GI tract is estimated to harbor up to 10^{14} bacteria/g of intestinal contents. This number easily exceeds the population size of other microbial communities associated with the human body. Remarkably, the microbial population in the GI tract is approximately 10 times greater than the total number of cells in the human body [2].

The intestinal microflora of the adult GI tract is composed of all three domains of life—Bacteria, Archaea, and Eukarya, with Bacteria having the highest cell densities [3]. The flora is distributed along the entire GI tract from the esophagus to the rectum (Figure 38.2). The intestinal microflora is also distributed in a vertical gradient within a specific part of the GI tract. Four microhabitats have been described (Figure 38.3): the intestinal lumen, the unstirred water layer, the mucous layer at the surface of the mucosal epithelial cells, and the mucus layer in the intestinal crypts [4].

The population size and diversity of the intestinal microflora are influenced by intrinsic factors such as pH, secretion of intestinal fluids, and transit time. The stomach and duodenum create a harsh environment for bacterial colonization. The former has low pH (ranging from 2.5 to 3.5) due to secretions of intestinal fluids (e.g., hydrochloric acid), and the latter has a short transit time. Consequently, approximately only 10^1 to 10^3 bacteria/ml of intestinal content reside in the stomach and duodenum, with a majority of them being transient. As the environment becomes less acidic and transit time gradually increases toward the distal end of the GI tract, the microflora community flourishes both in number and in diversity (Figure 38.2).

In comparison to the other parts of the GI tract, the colon has the slowest cell turnover rate, the lowest redox potential, and the longest transit time. Hence, the colon harbors the most diverse and the highest number of bacteria (Figure 38.2). The colon is the major site for bacterial fermentation of nondigestible food components. Approximately $10^{10}-10^{12}$ bacteria/ml of intestinal contents reside in the colon. This microbial population includes more than 500 species belonging to more than 190 genera [5]. Because of the complexity of collecting samples from within the GI tract, most studies investigating the intestinal microflora have been based on fecal sample analyses. Thus, our current understanding of the population size may not accurately reflect "true" species abundance and their relative importance in metabolic processes [6].

A few major groups of strict anaerobes dominate the colonic microflora community, including *Bacteroides* spp., *Eubacterium* spp., and *Bifidobacterium* spp. [7]. Facultative aerobes such as *Enterobacter* spp., *Streptococcus* spp., and *Lactobacillus* spp. are also present as subdominant flora. Minor groups of pathogenic and opportunistic microflora (e.g., *Clostridium* spp. and *Vibrio* spp.) are also present in low numbers [8]. The metabolic functions of many of the dominant bacterial species in the GI tract are not well understood. However, several studies indicate that *Bifidobacterium* spp. and *Lactobacillus* spp. are intestinal bacterial species that directly contribute to health [9] (Figure 38.4).

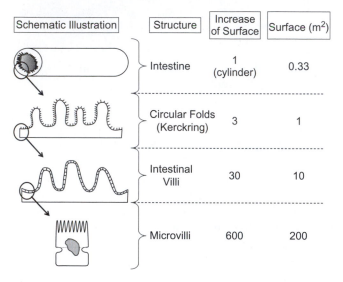

Schematic Illustration	Structure	Increase of Surface	Surface (m²)
	Intestine	1 (cylinder)	0.33
	Circular Folds (Kerckring)	3	1
	Intestinal Villi	30	10
	Microvilli	600	200

FIGURE 38.1 Folding on the intestinal mucosa significantly increased the surface area of the GI tract, providing a large surface area for bacterial colonization. Source: *Modified from Waldeck [221].*

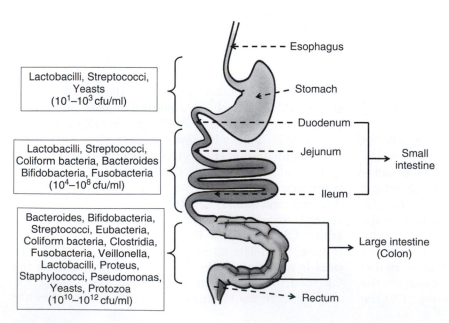

Lactobacilli, Streptococci, Yeasts (10^1-10^3 cfu/ml)

Lactobacilli, Streptococci, Coliform bacteria, Bacteroides Bifidobacteria, Fusobacteria (10^4-10^8 cfu/ml)

Bacteroides, Bifidobacteria, Streptococci, Eubacteria, Coliform bacteria, Clostridia, Fusobacteria, Veillonella, Lactobacilli, Proteus, Staphylococci, Pseudomonas, Yeasts, Protozoa ($10^{10}-10^{12}$ cfu/ml)

Esophagus — Stomach — Duodenum — Jejunum — Ileum — Small intestine — Large intestine (Colon) — Rectum

FIGURE 38.2 The human GI tract and the distribution of the intestinal microflora. Source: *Modified from Simon and Gorbach [222].*

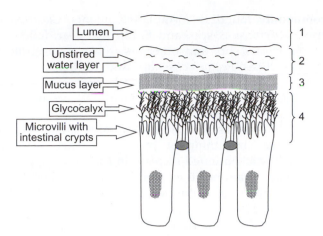

FIGURE 38.3 The four microhabitats within the GI tract representing the vertical distribution of the intestinal microflora: (1) the intestinal lumen, (2) the unstirred water layer, (3) the mucus layer at the surface of the mucosal epithelial cells, and (4) the mucus layer in the intestinal crypts.

III BACTERIAL COLONIZATION, SUCCESSION, AND METABOLISM

A Colonization and Succession

The GI tract of a fetus is apparently sterile [10,11]. Bacterial colonization occurs immediately at delivery and gradually becomes more extensive as the newborn is introduced to the living environment and various foods [6,10–14]. Bacterial colonization of the GI tract occurs in four phases [15,16]. Phase I, the initial acquisition phase, occurs between birth and 1 or 2 weeks. Phase II is considered a transitional period that takes place during lactation with either breast milk or formula. This event typically starts at the end of the second week after birth and ends when supplementary feeding begins. Phase III is initiated with the introduction of other food sources, especially at weaning (e.g., when breast milk or formula is

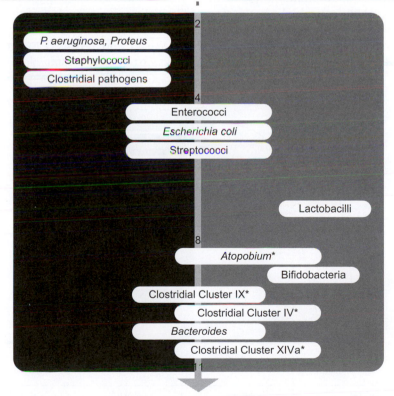

FIGURE 38.4 Dominant intestinal microflora as categorized into potentially harmful or health-promoting groups. Source: *Reprinted with permission from Thomas and Flower [223].*

supplemented with solid foods). Phase IV follows once weaning is completed and the child is introduced to an adult diet.

In phase I, *Enterobacter* and *Streptococcus* appear to colonize the infant GI tract within 48 hours of birth. *Escherichia coli* follows soon after. These bacteria are thought to create a favorable environment for subsequent colonization by anaerobic bacteria including *Bacteroides* spp., *Bifidobacterium* spp., and *Clostridium* spp. This secondary colonization usually occurs within 4–7 days [6,17,18]. During later stages of phase I, a marked reduction in the levels of *E. coli* and *Streptococcus* was observed in the stools of exclusively breast-fed infants. This event was followed by a decrease in the levels of *Clostridium* and *Bacteroides* spp., whereas *Bifidobacterium* spp. gradually dominate. It appears that these trends are not as distinct in formula-fed infants [15].

In phase II, *Bifidobacterium* spp. remain at high levels and become the dominant bacterial group in the intestinal microflora of breast-fed infants [15]. Apparently, this is different from the intestinal microflora profile of formula-fed infants, in whom relatively high numbers of *Bacteroides* spp., *Clostridium* spp., and *Streptococcus* spp. are present and *Bifidobacterium* spp. is no longer the dominant group [15].

The introduction of new foods to infants in phase III results in a major shift in microbial succession [12,13,15,18]. This shift is more significant in breast-fed infants. Following weaning, the intestinal microflora of breast-fed infants gradually changes to resemble the community found in formula-fed infants. *Clostridium* spp., *Streptococcus* spp. and *E. coli* reappear, followed by *Bacteroides* spp. and other anaerobic gram-positive cocci such as *Peptococcus* spp. and *Peptostreptococcus* spp. [18]. At the end of phase III, differences in the intestinal microflora of breast-fed and formula-fed infants are no longer observed.

Bacterial succession continues until weaning is completed (i.e., beginning of phase IV). This phase is denoted by a continued increase in *Bacteroides* spp. and anaerobic gram-positive cocci. Colonic levels of *Bifidobacterium* spp. continue to remain high. At this time, *Bifidobacterium* spp. is found in all individuals regardless of their starting diet [15]. *Escherichia coli* and *Streptococcus* spp. gradually decline to a typical adult level (i.e., approximately 10^6–10^8 bacteria/g of feces) [19]. *Clostridium* spp. is also present [19]. At the end of phase IV, the infant intestinal microflora begins to resemble the bacterial community profile of an adult, which is typically diverse but relatively stable [12,13,18] (Figure 38.5). Phase IV is usually attained by 2 years of age [12,13,18].

During adulthood, the intestinal microflora can be modified by external factors including diet, environment, and medication. Due to reasons that are still unclear, the number of bacterial species residing in the GI tract declines with age [20–22] (Figure 38.5). Typically, the population levels (in terms of $\log_{10}$ CFU1g) of *Bifidobacterium* spp. are markedly decreased and reduced to one or two dominant species, particularly *B. adolescentis* and *B. longum*[20,23].

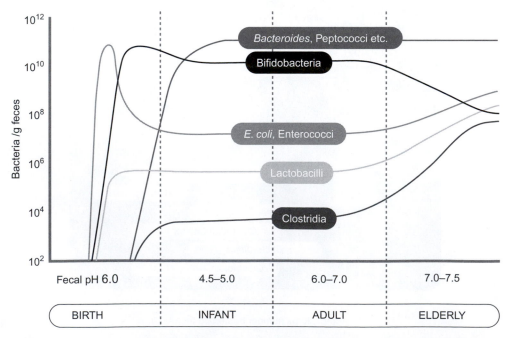

FIGURE 38.5 Bacterial succession throughout the lifetime. Source: *Reprinted with permission from Thomas and Flower [223].*

In contrast, *Enterococcus* spp., *Lactobacillus* spp., *Bacteroides* spp., and *Clostridium* spp. are increased in GI tracts of the elderly [21,22].

B Metabolic Consequences of Bacterial Colonization and Succession

Changes in the intestinal microflora of infants due to bacterial colonization and succession are reflected metabolically, especially in terms of fecal short-chain fatty acid (SCFA) profiles [24]. During the period when *Bifidobacterium* spp. predominate in the GI tract of breast-fed infants, acetic acid is the major SCFA detected [25,26]. Accumulation of acetic acid decreases the stool pH from values originally observed at birth. This trend is expected because *Bifidobacterium* spp. are a major producer of acetic acid. In formula-fed infants, however, lower levels of acetic acid are present and the stool pH tends to rise slightly. Therefore, changes in the fecal SCFA profile of breast-fed infants appear to be more profound than those in formula-fed infants [15,26]. Breast-fed infants are also observed to exhibit a gradual increase in total SCFA. Concurrently, lactic acid decreases while acetic and propionic acid increase. At later stages of weaning, butyric acid production gradually increases as well. In contrast, changes in the fecal SCFA profile of formula-fed infants are less profound [15,26,27]. This may be attributed to fewer fluctuations in the GI microflora in these infants.

The ability to ferment complex carbohydrates from diet may also reflect the variability in bacterial succession rate in breast-fed and formula-fed infants. Although variations exist among individual infants, fermentation capability appears to develop faster in formula-fed infants than in breast-fed infants [27]. This is expected because the colons of formula-fed infants are inhabited by more diverse bacterial strains and a greater population of gram-negative anaerobes, many of which are involved in the fermentation of complex carbohydrates. Unlike breast-fed infants, the colonic fermentation capacity of formula-fed infants does not vary significantly through weaning stages [27]. This observation suggests that the colonic microflora of formula-fed infants matures faster than that of breast-fed infants and does not experience major shifts in composition [26–28].

C Factors Influencing Bacterial Colonization and Succession

In phase I of colonization, environmental factors introduce bacteria to the infant GI tract. With infants born by vaginal delivery, the length of the birthing process significantly influences the chance of detecting viable bacteria from the mouth and stomach of the newborn [29]. Infants born by cesarean section may also acquire the mother's microflora. However, initial exposure is most likely from the environment (e.g., hospital condition, nursing staff, and other infants in the nursery) [30–33]. In addition to mode of delivery, hygiene practices may influence the bacterial species introduced to the infant GI tract. For example, bacterial colonization of the GI tract of Pakistani infants born in poor areas with minimal sanitation occurred significantly earlier than in Swedish infants delivered in more sanitary conditions, regardless of delivery method [14].

There are numerous external and internal factors that shape the composition of the microbial community in the GI tract (Figure 38.6). External factors include mode of birth, composition of the diet, sanitation of the living environment, and the use of medicines, especially antibiotics. Internal factors include changes in the physiological condition of the host (e.g., stress, health status, and aging) and conditions in the GI tract (e.g., pH, substrate availability, redox potential, transit time, flow of enteric fluid, and IgA secretions) [6]. A disruption of the "normal" intestinal bacteria may lead to the growth of those that are potentially harmful and physiologically manifest as a disease. Studies show that changes in diet, climate, aging, medication, illness, stress, and/or infection generally lead to an increase in anaerobes and *E. coli* in the small intestine and to an increase of *Enterobacter* and streptococci in the colon, with a concurrent decrease of *Bifidobacterium* spp. [34]. Although predicting the occurrence of a disease based on intestinal microflora profile is currently not possible, it is hypothesized that a marked decline in intestinal bacteria that are

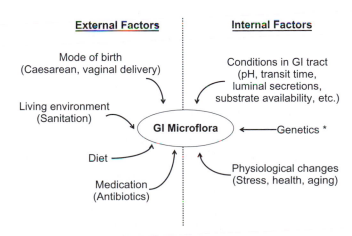

FIGURE 38.6 External and internal factors influencing bacterial succession in the GI tract. *Genetics has been speculated to play a role in intestinal microflora succession, but the current body of literature has not provided strong evidence for it.

beneficial to health, such as *Bifidobacterium* spp., will ultimately influence the health of the host.

IV FUNCTIONS OF THE GASTROINTESTINAL TRACT MICROFLORA

A Production of Vitamin K

Prothrombin, which is involved in blood clotting, is activated by vitamin K. Food sources of vitamin K are liver, eggs, milk, and spinach. However, this vitamin can also be synthesized by bacteria in the GI tract. Administration of antibiotics eradicates intestinal bacteria and consequently may diminish *de novo* vitamin K production. Newborn infants, whose GI tracts are typically devoid of bacteria, may be given an injection of vitamin K at birth to counter deficiency until their vitamin K-producing bacteria are established [35]. Another vitamin that is exclusively synthesized by bacteria is vitamin B_{12} (cobalamin) [36], which is important for the formation of red blood cells.

B Protection against Pathogens

Colonization of the GI tract by the intestinal microflora confers protection on the human host. A fully established GI tract microflora community can "outcompete" pathogens for carbon and other energy sources, as well as for adhesion sites on the intestinal mucosa. Consequently, pathogens are less able to establish themselves on the intestinal mucosa and thus are prevented from causing physiological damage to the host [37]. Some species of indigenous intestinal microflora may also produce bacteriocins that kill pathogens [38].

C Enhanced Histological and Physiological Development of the Gastrointestinal Tract and the Immune System

Intestinal microflora plays a role in the development of intestinal mucosa and gut-associated lymphoid tissue (GALT). Evidence for this role was provided by comparative assessments of histological and physiological data from germ-free (GF) mice and conventionally raised (CONV-R) mice. GF mice are devoid of intestinal microflora because they are delivered by cesarean and raised in a sterile environment. On the other hand, CONV-R mice are delivered and raised in a standard environment in order to acquire a "normal" intestinal microflora. Histological data show that CONV-R mice have a higher epithelial cell turnover rate than that of GF mice (i.e., 2 days in CONV-R vs. 4 days in GF).

In addition, the secondary lymphatic organs of GF mice (e.g., GALT and spleen) are significantly less developed than those of CONV-R mice [3]. The intestinal microflora has also been found to stimulate the development of immune tissues in the GI tract such as the lamina propria, Peyer's patches, and mesenteric lymph nodes [39]. In the absence of the intestinal microflora, these tissues do not fully develop and become less "primed" to fight infection. The serum of GF mice contains lower concentrations of immunoglobulins than that of CONV-R mice; GF mice have a reduced immune function, are more susceptible to severe infection, and usually have poorer survival.

In humans, differences in the composition of intestinal microflora have also been suggested to influence immune function. Evidence for this is derived from comparing the prevalence of allergies and atopic diseases in infants [40]. GI tracts of infants born and raised in developing countries (i.e., assumed to have a low level of sanitation) appear to be colonized at an early stage by gram-negative bacteria and variable enterobacterial strains. On the other hand, infants in developed countries (i.e., assumed to have a high level of sanitation) acquired gram-negative bacteria later and more stable enterobacterial strains. Such differences in the intestinal microflora composition have been associated with a higher prevalence of allergies and atopic diseases in infants born and raised in developed countries than those in developing countries [40]. A study that compared the intestinal microflora profiles of children in Europe observed that Swedish and Estonian toddlers with low counts of *Lactobacillus* spp., *Bifidobacterium* spp., *Bacteroides* spp., and *Enterococcus* spp., but having higher levels of clostridia and *Staphylococcus aureus*, were more prone to allergies than were healthy infants [41,42]. Much remains to be learned about intestinal colonization, immune function, and disease in humans.

D Production of Short-Chain Fatty Acids

Food components that are not digested in the small intestine travel to the colon. These nondigestible elements are substrates for fermentation by the intestinal microflora. By-products of fermentation include carbon dioxide, hydrogen, and methane gases. Nongaseous by-products include SCFAs such as acetate, propionate, and butyrate (Figure 38.7). Butyrate is mainly produced by *Clostridium* spp. and *Eubacterium* spp. [43]. *Roseburia intestinalis*, *Eubacterium rectale*, and *Faecalibacterium prausnitzii* have also been identified as butyrate producers [44,45]. Acetate is produced by *Lactobacillus* spp. and *Bifidobacterium* spp. [43].

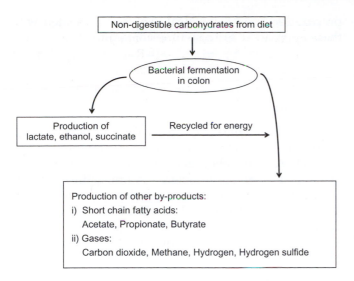

FIGURE 38.7 Bacterial fermentation of nondigestible food components.

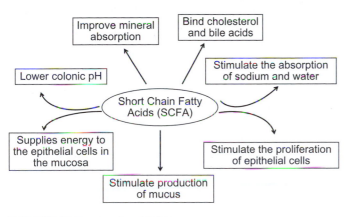

FIGURE 38.8 Benefits of SCFA.

Approximately 40—50% of the available energy from carbohydrate in the diet is converted into SCFAs by the colonic microflora [46]. These volatile fatty acids provide energy for cellular maintenance and metabolism by being passively absorbed by the colonic epithelium (butyrate), liver (propionate), and muscle (acetate) [43,47,48]. Studies suggest that butyrate plays an important role in cellular differentiation and proliferation in the colonic mucosa by inducing apoptosis and may confer protection against colitis and colorectal cancer by modulating oncogene expression [49,50]. Production of SCFAs also lowers intestinal pH, which increases the solubility of minerals such as calcium and magnesium [51,52] and consequently enhances absorption [53]. Furthermore, reduction of colonic pH by accumulation of SCFAs has been hypothesized to protect the intestinal mucosa from being colonized by pathogens that are less tolerant of an acidic

environment (e.g., *Helicobacter pylori*) [54]. Additional benefits of SCFAs are outlined in Figure 38.8.

E Utilization of Nutrients

Absorption of nutrients from food is largely dependent on the action of various digestive enzymes. However, numerous food components cannot be digested. For example, stachyose (a tetrasaccharide) and raffinose (a trisaccharide) are long-chain carbohydrates (i.e., commonly termed oligosaccharides) found in soy. The unique α-(1—6) galactose linkage present in stachyose and raffinose can be broken down by α-galactosidase, which is not secreted by the human intestinal mucosa. As a result, these oligosaccharides (and other nondigestible food components) pass to the large intestine, where they become fermentation substrates for the colonic microflora. Fructo-oligosaccharides (FOS), transgalacto-oligosaccharides, and galacto-oligosaccharides (GOS) are other types of nondigestible oligosaccharides that can be fermented by the colonic microflora. Thus, the intestinal microflora salvages a significant amount of energy from an otherwise nonavailable source [43,46—48].

Evidence that the intestinal microflora plays an important role in fermenting nondigestible foodstuffs is based on studies using GF and CONV-R mice [3,55]. The latter were more efficient in nutrient absorption than GF mice because they had acquired "normal" intestinal microflora. CONV-R mice gained more body weight, grew faster, and had as much as 40% more body fat than their GF counterparts even though they were maintained on the same diet. This growth difference was present even though CONV-R mice consumed less chow per day [3]. In order for GF mice to achieve the body weight of the CONV-R counterparts, they had to consume approximately 30% more calories [55]. However, following inoculation of GF mice with the intestinal microflora of CONV-R mice, GF mice quickly gained body fat to levels equivalent to those of CONV-R mice without having to consume additional chow [55].

F Conversion of Isoflavones

Soy isoflavones, which may be classified as "other non-nutritive components," are phytochemicals found in soy beans. Currently, soy is the only recognized nutritionally relevant source of isoflavones. The primary isoflavones in soy are genistin and daidzin. Following ingestion, these glycosides are hydrolyzed by intestinal glucosidases and converted to the aglycone form of genistein and daidzein. These aglycones are further converted by certain intestinal microflora into specific metabolites, such as equol. Chemically, equol is similar to the hormone estradiol. Results of *in vitro* animal studies indicate that equol has a higher estrogenic effect than its precursor, daidzein [56]. Hence, equol has garnered much attention for its potential in the prevention and/or treatment of chronic diseases or conditions associated with estrogen levels (e.g., breast cancer, osteoporosis, and menopause) [57].

In humans, the conversion of soy isoflavones (genistein and daidzein) to the more potent metabolite (equol) appears to be dependent on intestinal microflora. Evidence for this conversion comes from animal and clinical studies. First, all rodents are equol producers, except those that are bred germ-free. Second, infants fed soy-based formulas do not form a substantial amount of equol for the first 4 months of life, coinciding with intestinal microflora development. In addition, individuals who are known to be equol producers have significantly lower equol excretion after antibiotic treatment [58]. It appears that the large interindividual variability in the intestinal microflora composition results in only 30−40% of individuals producing equol after soy consumption [56,59−61]. In 2000, Hur and colleagues [62] identified two strains of bacteria from human feces that can produce primary and secondary metabolites from the natural isoflavone glycosides daidzein and genistin, but it is still unclear whether the ability to convert daidzein to equol can be induced in nonproducers [63].

V METHODOLOGY FOR STUDYING INTESTINAL MICROFLORA

A Conventional Methodology and Its Limitations

Our knowledge of intestinal microflora is largely based on classical approaches of cultivation, direct microscopic observation, and biochemical analysis [64]. Results obtained using these conventional methodologies have improved our understanding of the intestinal microflora. However, many intestinal bacteria are difficult to culture because the media may not be specific (i.e., causing overestimation) or may be too selective (i.e., resulting in underestimation or absence of growth) for culturing the particular bacteria of interest [65]. It is estimated that only 20−40% [66−68] of the total intestinal microflora can be cultured and identified using conventional microbiological methods. Thus, evaluating intestinal microflora using conventional methods will bias our knowledge in favor of those genera that are most easily grown under laboratory conditions [69]. In addition, media

preparation and biochemical analyses associated with these approaches are also time-consuming.

B Molecular Analysis of the Human Intestinal Microflora

In approximately the past two decades, novel analytical approaches based on the manipulation of 16S rDNA and other genetic materials have been developed to analyze bacterial communities in environmental samples (e.g., soil, lakes, oceans, and hydrothermal vents). These methods have been adapted to evaluate bacterial communities in the GI tract [9,70]. Molecular techniques do not require the presence of viable bacteria [9,71]. Furthermore, the use of genetic materials (e.g., DNA and RNA) allows species that cannot be cultured using current standard laboratory protocols to be detected. Thus, data derived from molecular techniques depict a more complete and real picture of the bacterial community. These "new" molecular methods have shown a great potential to overcome the limitations associated with conventional techniques and have become increasingly favored [71]. Many molecular techniques, especially after being optimized, are now being developed as rapid assays, allowing large-scale studies with high-throughput analyses. Biological samples can now be frozen at the site of collection and then transported to laboratories for analyses. However, because RNA is degraded more easily than DNA, sample storage and handling largely depend on the choice of method and outcome measures.

Molecular techniques can be categorized as follows:

1. Direct molecular detection and/or enumeration: dot blot hybridization, fluorescent *in situ* hybridization (FISH), and real-time polymerase chain reaction (RT-PCR)
2. Molecular fingerprinting techniques to monitor changes in the composition of bacterial community: terminal restriction fragment length polymorphism (T-RFLP) and denaturing gradient gel electrophoresis (DGGE)
3. Genotyping: rapid amplification polymorphic DNA−polymerase chain reaction (RAPD-PCR) and enterobacterial repetitive intergenic consensus−polymerase chain reaction (ERIC-PCR)
4. Other novel molecular methods under development: microarray, magnetic-immuno PCR, and *recA* gene analysis.

Other molecular techniques have been developed to study microbial communities in the environment. Figure 38.9 outlines several common methods of analysis.

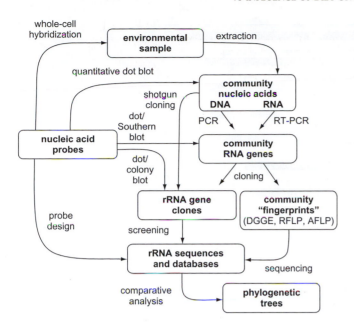

FIGURE 38.9 Various molecular methods and analytical approaches that are applicable for studying the intestinal microflora communities. Source: *Reprinted with permission from Lawson [224].*

C Limitations Associated with Molecular Techniques

Despite their superiority to conventional microbiological approaches, molecular techniques do have limitations. The main drawback of molecular techniques, which significantly influences downstream analytical processes, is their reliance on cell lysis efficiency and the quality of DNA recovered from the environmental samples. DNA isolation methods that contribute to insufficient cell lysis or shearing of DNA bias PCR amplification [72–75]. Inhibitors in feces, such as bile salts and complex polysaccharides, will create similar problems [72,76,77]. Furthermore, special equipment and reagents are needed for sample processing and analyses (e.g., thermal cycler, RT-PCR unit, DGGE setup, bead-beating equipment for lysing cells, and DNA or RNA extraction kits). Thus, initial laboratory setup may be costly, especially for novice researchers. However, research in this field has advanced rapidly in approximately the past decade. Technological progress has significantly reduced costs as well as improved quality and performance of equipment and reagents. Note that some molecular techniques are semiquantitative (DGGE and TGGE) and may lack sensitivity (e.g., dot blot hybridization and FISH). Primer bias may also occur in PCR reactions. In addition, almost all of these molecular techniques rely on primers and oligonucleotide probes to detect bacteria. Hence, the choice of primers and probes in analyses is crucial for detecting the bacteria

of interest. Although primer and probe availability may be limited, their numbers are steadily increasing as interest in this field grows. Despite these limitations, molecular techniques are continually being developed and modified to increase efficiency and sensitivity in analyzing the diverse bacterial community in environmental samples, including those found in the GI tract and feces.

VI INFLUENCE OF DIET ON INTESTINAL MICROFLORA

Several bacterial genera make up a large majority of the intestinal microflora (Figures 38.2 and 38.4). However, external and internal factors can modify the overall number and dominant species within the community (i.e., the concept of microbial succession; Figure 38.6). One of the most studied external factors that influences microbial succession is diet.

A Can Diet Alter the Intestinal Microflora?

Comparative analyses of fecal samples from breast-fed and formula-fed infants have shown differences in the composition of their intestinal microflora as a response to the diet (Figures 38.10 and 38.11). The intestinal microflora of adults is more diverse and stable than that of infants; however, it can still be modified by diet. In 1974, Finegold *et al.* [78] compared the fecal flora of subjects who consumed a traditional Japanese diet to that of those who consumed a Western diet. In this study, a significantly higher number of *Clostridium* spp., *Eubacterium* spp., and *E. coli* were recovered in the feces of subjects on the traditional Japanese diet than in those on the Western diet. On the other hand, *Bacteroides* spp. (especially *B. infantis* and *B. putredinis*) and *Bifidobacterium* spp. were more prevalent in the fecal samples of subjects on the Western diet. In addition, differences in intestinal bacterial profiles were also found to vary by ethnicity (e.g., Asians, North Americans, and Europeans), implicating regional dietary habits [34]. Hence, from these observational studies, it appears that dietary patterns influence intestinal microflora communities.

Intervention studies provide more direct evidence of the ability of diet to modify intestinal microflora. We conducted unpublished experiments in which diet was strictly controlled and modified from basal, free-living diet. Asian adolescents participated in two 3-week sessions of supervised clinical camp. The "camp" diet comprised food items such as peanut butter-and-jelly sandwiches, pasta, and pizza, but without the addition of probiotics, prebiotics, and other high-fiber food.

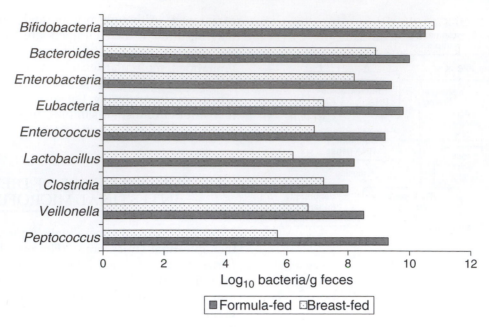

FIGURE 38.10   Comparison of bacterial populations in breast-fed versus formula-fed infants. Source: *Data adapted from Benno et al. [225].*

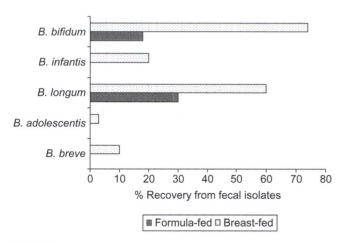

FIGURE 38.11   Differences in the *Bifidobacterium* spp. isolated from fecal samples of breast-fed versus formula-fed infants. Source: *Data adapted from Beerens et al. [226].*

Meals were given such that all subjects consumed the same types of food at any given meal time (i.e., controlled diet). Changes in intestinal microflora profile were assessed based on fecal samples using the DGGE method. It was observed that the bacterial community shifts to a different profile within 2—4 days of consuming the new diet and the profile is maintained as long as the diet remains largely unchanged. The intestinal microflora profiles of these subjects changed from "basal" profile to "camp" profile in the first session of camp, reverted to "basal" profile during the wash-out period, and then slipped back to "camp" profile in the second session of camp [79]. However, intersubject

variability remained high, indicating that regardless of dietary changes, each individual maintains his or her unique intestinal microflora profile [79,80]. Intestinal microflora profile can also be altered when one type of food is consumed at a higher than usual intake [81,82]. The number of *Bacteroides* spp. and *Staphylococcus* spp. was elevated during periods of high meat consumption, whereas the number of these bacteria decreased when the diet was devoid of meat. In addition, the number of *Eubacterium* spp., *Bifidobacterium* spp., and *Lactobacillus* spp. was much lower following a high-meat diet compared to a meat-free diet [81]. A high intake of cruciferous vegetables has also been shown to cause a major shift in the intestinal microflora composition compared to the intestinal microflora profile of subjects maintained on a fruit- and vegetable-free diet [82].

B Altering the Intestinal Microflora Using Food Supplements

1 Probiotics

Probiotics contain viable microorganisms that are proposed to improve the health of the host primarily by altering its intestinal microbial communities. Various probiotic bacterial strains are available, but the genera *Lactobacillus* spp., *Bifidobacterium* spp., and *Streptococcus* spp. are the most commonly used. Yogurt, kefir, and capsules containing freeze-dried probiotic bacteria are examples of commercially available probiotics.

The beneficial effects of consuming probiotics, which include improvement in lactose tolerance and a reduction in the risk and severity of diarrheal symptoms (i.e., as a side effect to antibiotics, traveler's diarrhea, or induced by rotavirus as in the case of gastroenteritis), have been observed in clinical studies. Inflammatory bowel disease (IBD), which is characterized by chronic or recurring intestinal inflammation, has been postulated to be caused by abnormal host immune responses to certain members of the intestinal microflora and/or from a defective mucosal barrier [83]. Some clinical studies have indicated that probiotics can treat IBD (e.g., ulcerative colitis, Crohn's disease, and pouchitis; Table 38.1). Probiotics

TABLE 38.1 Clinical Studies Investigating Various Applications of Probiotics

Intestinal condition	Probiotic	References
Lactose intolerance	*Lactobacillus acidophilus*	[91]
	Lactobacillus acidophilus *Lactobacillus casei*	[92]
	Lactobacillus acidophilus	[93]
	Bifidobacterium longum	[94]
	Lactobacillus bulgaricus *Streptococcus thermophilus*	[95]
	Lactobacillus bulgaricus	[96]
	Lactobacillus bulgaricus	[97]
Diarrhea associated with the use of antibiotics	*Saccharomyces boulardii*	[98]
	Lactobacillus acidophilus *Lactobacillus bulgaricus*	[99]
	Streptococcus faecium	[100]
	Lactobacillus acidophilus *Lactobacillus bulgaricus*	[101]
	Bifidobacterium longum	[102]
	Saccharomyces boulardii	[103]
	Enterococcus faecium SF68	[104]
	Lactobacillus GG	[105]
	Bifidobacterium longum *Lactobacillus acidophilus*	[106]
	Saccharomyces boulardii	[107]
	Lactobacillus acidophilus	[108]
	Lactobacillus GG	[109]
	Lactobacillus GG	[110]
	Lactobacillus GG	[111]
	Saccharomyces boulardii	[112]

(Continued)

TABLE 38.1 *(Continued)*

Intestinal condition	Probiotic	References
Rotavirus-induced diarrhea and/or pediatric diarrhea, including gastroenteritis	*Enterococcus faecium* SF68	[113]
	Lactobacillus acidophilus	[114]
	Saccharomyces boulardii	[115]
	Lactobacillus GG	[116]
	Lactobacillus GG	[117]
	Bifidobacterium bifidum *Streptococcus thermophilus*	[118]
	Lactobacillus spp.	[119]
	Lactobacillus GG	[120]
	Lactobacillus GG	[121]
	Lactobacillus GG	[122]
	Enterococcus faecium SF68	[123]
	Lactobacillus GG	[124]
	Lactobacillus GG	[125]
	Lactobacillus reuteri, *Lactobacillus* GG	[126,127]
	Lactobacillus GG	[128]
	Lactobacillus casei DN-114001	[129]
	Bifidobacterium sp. Bb12 *Streptococcus thermophilus*	[130]
	Lactobacillus GG	[131]
	Lactobacillus casei	[132]
	Lactobacillus GG	[133]
	Lactobacillus GG	[134]
	Lactobacillus sporogenes	[135]
	Lactobacillus rhamnosus 19070-2 *Lactobacillus reuteri* DSM 12246	[136,137]
	Lactobacillus casei	[138]
	Saccharomyces boulardii	[139]
Traveler's diarrhea	*Lactobacillus acidophilus* *Lactobacillus bulgaricus*	[140]
	A mixture of Lactobacilli, Bifidobacteria, and Streptococci	[141]
	Lactobacillus GG	[142]
	Saccharomyces boulardii	[143]
	Lactobacillus GG	[144]
Diarrhea induced by tube feeding	*Saccharomyces boulardii*	[145]
	Saccharomyces boulardii	[146]

(Continued)

TABLE 38.1   *(Continued)*

Intestinal condition	Probiotic	References
	Saccharomyces boulardii	[147]
	Lactobacillus sp.	[148]
Diarrhea in immunocompromised individuals	*Lactobacillus acidophilus*	[149]
	Bifidobacterium sp.	[150]
	Saccharomyces boulardii	[151]
	Lactobacillus reuteri	[152]
	Lactobacillus rhamnosus[a]	[153]
	VSL#3[b]	[154]
Small bowel bacterial overgrowth	*Lactobacillus acidophilus*	[155]
	Lactobacillus acidophilus	[156]
	Lactobacillus plantarum 299 V *Lactobacillus* GG	[157]
	Lactobacillus casei Lactobacillus acidophilus Cerela	[158]
Allergic dermatitis	*Lactobacillus* GG	[159]
	Bifidobacterium lactis Bb-12 or *Lactobacillus* GG	[160]
	Lactobacillus GG	[161]
	Lactobacillus rhamnosus GG	[162]
Necrotizing enterocolitis, irritable bowel syndrome	*Lactobacillus acidophilus Bifidobacterium infantis*	[163]
	Saccharomyces boulardii	[164]
	Lactobacillus acidophilus	[165]
	Enterococcus faecium M74	[166]
	Lactobacillus acidophilus[c]	[167]
	Enterococcus faecium PRSS	[168]
	Lactobacillus plantarum	[169]
	Lactobacillus helveticus Lactobacillus acidophilus	[170]
	Escherichia coli[d]	
	Lactobacillus plantarum	[171]
	Propionibacterium freudenreichii	[172]
	Lactobacillus plantarum	[173]
	VSL#3[b]	[174]
	VSL#3[b] *Enterococcus faecium* SF68[e]	[175]
	Lactobacillus plantarum 299 V	[176]
	Bifidobacterium animalis DN-173010	[177]

TABLE 38.1   *(Continued)*

Intestinal condition	Probiotic	References
	Lactobacillus plantarum 299 V	[178]
	VSL#3[b]	[179]
	Bifidobacterium infantis 35624	[180]
Inflammatory bowel disease (e.g., ulcerative colitis, pouchitis, and Crohn's disease)	*Saccharomyces boulardii*	[181]
	Lactobacillus GG	[182]
	Escherichia coli	[183]
	Escherichia coli	[184]
	Escherichia coli	[185]
	VSL#3[b]	[186]
	Saccharomyces boulardii 5-aminosalicylic acid	[187]
	Lactobacillus GG	[188]
	Saccharomyces boulardii	[189]
	VSL#3[b]	[190]
	Lactobacillus GG	[191]
	Lactobacillus GG	[192]
	Escherichia coli Nissle 1917	[193]
	Lactobacillus GG	[194]
	Lactobacillus GG	[195]
Intestinal infection caused by pathogens: *Clostridium difficile*	*Lactobacillus* GG	[196]
	Saccharomyces boulardii	[197]
	Saccharomyces boulardii	[198]
	Saccharomyces boulardii	[199]
	Saccharomyces boulardii	[200]
	Lactobacillus GG	[201]
	Lactobacillus GG	[202]
	Lactobacillus plantarum 299 v	[203]
Intestinal infection caused by pathogens: *Helicobacter pylori*	*Lactobacillus acidophilus (Johnsonii)* La1	[204]
	Lactobacillus acidophilus	[205]
	Lactobacillus gasseri 2716 (LG21)	[206]

[a]*Antibiophilus.*
[b]*VSL#3 contains four strains of lactobacilli (L. casei, L. plantarum, L. acidophilus, and* L. delbruekii *subsp.* bulgaricus), *three strains of bifidobacteria* (B. longum, B. breve, *and* B. infantis), *and one strain of* Streptococcus salivarius *subsp.* thermophilus.
[c]*Lacteol Forte.*
[d]*Hylac N and Hylac N Forte.*
[e]*Bioflorin.*

(Continued)

may also be a treatment for intestinal infection caused by pathogens (e.g., *Clostridium difficile* and *H. pylori*) (Table 38.1). Furthermore, it is hypothesized that regular consumption of probiotics may reduce the levels of secondary bile acids and other mutagens that are involved in colon carcinogenesis [84]. Other studies outlining the efficacy of probiotics in various clinical applications are summarized in Table 38.1.

The efficacy of probiotics remains unproven. Mixed results raise concerns regarding the suitability of the strains, effective dosage, toxicity levels, and the viability of the bacteria in the product. Furthermore, mechanisms by which these bacteria colonize the intestinal tract have not been described [85—87]. Colonization success of the ingested probiotic bacteria is questionable because probiotic bacteria typically are not able to permanently colonize the GI tract. Hence, colonization and benefits are usually transient in nature [88,89].

2 Prebiotics

Prebiotics are defined as nondigestible and fermentable food components that selectively stimulate the growth and/or activity of certain colonic bacteria that bring beneficial health effects to the host. Unlike probiotics, where one attempts to introduce beneficial bacteria into the GI tract, prebiotics attempt to stimulate the growth of endogenous beneficial bacteria by providing specific fermentable substrate(s). Examples of prebiotics are inulin, FOS, GOS, and lactulose.

It has been proposed that a food component has to satisfy the following criteria to be recognized as a prebiotic: (1) resistant to the acidic condition of the stomach, (2) unable to be broken down in the small intestine, (3) transferable to the colon as a fermentable substrate, and (4) able to stimulate the growth of a selective group of beneficial colonic bacteria (e.g., *Bifidobacterium* spp. and *Lactobacillus* spp.) [90]. Clinical studies investigating the effects of prebiotics such as inulin, FOS, GOS, and lactulose are listed in Table 38.2. Although most of these studies resulted in the enhancement of *Bifidobacterium* spp., few of them were able to correlate bacterial data with health-related biomarkers. It is speculated that increases in the colonic levels of *Bifidobacterium* spp. modulate immune function, inhibit pathogen

TABLE 38.2   Clinical Studies Investigating Alterations in Intestinal Microflora as a Response to Prebiotics

Prebiotic	Dose and duration	Microflora modulation	Reference
Inulin	8 g/day, 14 days	Increase in bifidobacteria, slight increase in clostridia	[207]
Inulin	Up to 34 g/day, 64 days	Increase in bifidobacteria	[208]
Inulin	15 g/day, 15 days	Increase in bifidobacteria	[209]
Inulin	20 g/day, 19 days	Increase in bifidobacteria, decrease in enterococci and enterobacteria	[210]
FOS	15 g/day, 15 days	Increase in bifidobacteria, decrease in *Bacteroides*, clostridia, and fusobacteria	[209]
FOS and PHGG	6.6 g/day FOS, 3.4 g/day PHGG, 21 days	Increase in bifidobacteria	[208]
FOS	0—20 g/day, 7 days	Increase in bifidobacteria	[211]
FOS	4 g/day, 42 days	Increase in bifidobacteria	[212]
FOS + GOS	0.04 g/l, 0.08 g/l, 28 days	Increase in bifidobacteria and lactobacilli	[213]
FOS + GOS	10 g/l, 28 days	Increase in bifidobacteria	[214]
Lactulose	10 g/day, 26 days	Increase in bifidobacteria	[215]
Lactulose	3 g/day, 14 days	Increase in bifidobacteria, decrease in lactobacilli	[216]
Lactulose	2 × 10 g/day, 4 weeks	Increase in bifidobacteria and lactobacilli	[217]
Lactulose	5 g/l and 10 g/l, 3 weeks	Increase in bifidobacteria, decrease in coliforms	[218]
GOS	0—10 g/day, 8 weeks	Increase in bifidobacteria and lactobacilli	[219]
GOS	2.5 g/day, 3 weeks	Increase in bifidobacteria, decrease in *Bacteroides* and clostridia	[220]

FOS, fructo-oligosaccharides; GOS, galacto-oligosaccharides; PHGG, partially hydrolyzed guar gum.
Source: *Reprinted with permission from Tuohy et al. [90].*

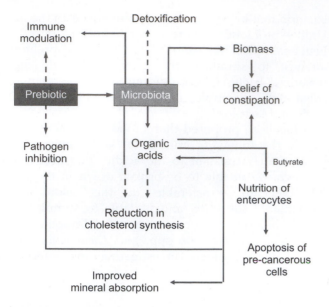

FIGURE 38.12 Possible mechanisms of prebiotic action. Solid lines indicate well-established modes of action, and dotted lines indicate speculative mechanisms. *Source: Modified from Ouwehand et al. [227].*

colonization, and augment the production of SCFA (Figure 38.12).

VII CHALLENGES IN THE FIELD

The study of the human intestinal microflora is a relatively new field. Interest in this field has been stimulated by the active marketing of probiotics and prebiotics for intestinal health. In addition, concerns about the effects of antibiotics (i.e., due to a medical treatment or residues in animal products) have focused research on the GI microflora.

Given the unknown role that the GI tract plays in maintaining overall health, efforts to advance our knowledge of the complex interaction between host and microflora are needed. As a first goal, the diversity of the intestinal microflora needs to be characterized. With better basic knowledge, we can move toward elucidating microbe–microbe and host–microbe interactions. Investigations of the effects of age, gender, host genotype, various components of diet, and the environment on intestinal microbial community are additional goals. Reliable methods to detect alterations in the composition of the intestinal microflora are required to meet these objectives. Molecular methods hold much promise in this regard [64,65].

References

[1] J. van Dijk, Morphology of the gut barrier, Eur. J. Compar. Gastroenterol. 2 (1997) 23–27.

[2] T. Luckey, M. Floch, Introduction to intestinal microecology, Am. J. Clin. Nutr. 25 (1972) 1291–1295.

[3] F. Backhed, R.E. Ley, J.L. Sonnenburg, D.A. Peterson, J.I. Gordon, Host-bacterial mutualism in the human intestine, Science 307 (2005) 1915–1920.

[4] R.D. Berg, The indigenous gastrointestinal microflora, Trends Microbiol. 4 (1996) 430–435.

[5] D.S. Savage, Microbial ecology of the human large intestine, Annu. Rev. Microbiol. 31 (1977) 107–133.

[6] R.I. Mackie, A. Sghir, H.R. Gaskins, Developmental microbial ecology of the neonatal gastrointestinal tract, Am. J. Clin. Nutr. 69 (1999) 1035–1045.

[7] W.H. Holzapfel, P. Haberer, J. Snel, U. Schillinger, J.H.J. Huis in't Veld, Overview of gut flora and probiotics, Int. J. Food Microbiol. 41 (1998) 85–101.

[8] B. Gedek, Darmflora: physiologie und okologie, Chemother. J (Suppl. 1) (1993) 2–6.

[9] G.W. Tannock, Molecular methods for exploring the intestinal ecosystem, Br. J. Nutr. 87 (2002) 199–201.

[10] G.W. Tannock, R. Fuller, S. Smith, M. Hall, Plasmid profiling of members of the family enterobacteriaceae, lactobacilli and bifidobacteria to study the transmission of bacteria from mother to infant, J. Clin. Microbiol. 28 (1990) 1225–1228.

[11] R. Zetterstrom, R. Bennet, K. Nord, Early infant feeding and microecology of the gut, Acta Pediatr. Japonica 36 (1994) 562–571.

[12] C. Edwards, A. Parrett, Intestinal flora during the first months of life: new perspectives, Br. J. Nutr. 88 (2002) S11–S18.

[13] C.F. Favier, E.E. Vaughan, W.M. De Vos, A.D.L. Akkermans, Molecular monitoring of succession of bacterial communities in human neonates, Appl. Environ. Microbiol. 68 (2002) 219–226.

[14] I. Adlerberth, B. Carlsson, P. de Man, F. Jalil, S.R. Khan, P. Larsson, et al., Intestinal colonization with enterobacteriaceae in Pakistani and Swedish hospital-delivered infants, Acta Paediatr. Scand. 80 (1991) 602–610.

[15] M.S. Cooperstock, A.J. Zedd, Intestinal flora of infants, in: D.J. Hentges (Ed.), Human Intestinal Microflora in Health and Disease, Academic Press, New York, 1983, pp. 79–99.

[16] K. Orrhage, C. Nord, Factors controlling the bacterial colonization of the intestine in breastfed infants, Acta Paediatr. 88 (1999) 47–57.

[17] D. Dai, W.A. Walker, Protective nutrients and bacterial colonization in the immature human gut, Adv. Pediatr. 46 (1999) 353–382.

[18] P.L. Stark, A. Lee, The microbial ecology of the large bowel of breast-fed and formula-fed infants during the first year of life, J. Med. Microbiol. 15 (1982) 189–203.

[19] R. Ellis-Pegler, C. Crabtree, H. Lambert, The faecal flora of children in the United Kingdom, J. Hyg. 75 (1975) 135–142.

[20] F. Gavini, C. Cayuela, J.-M. Antoine, C. Lecoq, B. Lefebvre, J.-M. Membre, et al., Differences in the distribution of bifidobacterial and enterobacterial species in human faecal microflora of three different (children, adults, elderly) age groups, Microb. Ecol. Health Dis. 13 (2001) 40–45.

[21] M.J. Hopkins, G.T. Macfarlane, Changes in predominant bacterial populations in human faeces with age and with *Clostridium difficile* infection, J. Med. Microbiol. 51 (2002) 448–454.

[22] E.J. Woodmansey, Intestinal bacteria and ageing, J. Appl. Microbiol. 102 (2007) 1178–1186.

[23] F. He, A. Ouwehand, E. Isolauri, M. Hosoda, Y. Benno, S. Salminen, Differences in composition and mucosal adhesion of bifidobacteria isolated from healthy adults and healthy seniors, Curr. Microbiol. 43 (2001) 351–354.

[24] A.C. Midtvedt, T. Midtvedt, Production of short-chain fatty acids by the intestinal microflora during the first two years of human life, J. Pediatr. Gastroenterol. Nutr. 18 (1992) 321–326.

[25] C. Bullen, P. Tearle, M. Stewart, The effect of "humanised" milks and supplemented breast feeding on the faecal flora of infants, J. Med. Microbiol. 10 (1977) 403–413.

[26] A. Parrett, K. Farley, A. Fletcher, C. Edwards, Comparison of faecal short chain fatty acids in breast-fed, formula-fed and mixed-fed neonates, Proc. Nutr. Soc. 60 (2001) 48A.

[27] A. Parrett, Development of colonic fermentation in early life, Glasgow University, Glasgow, UK, 2001.

[28] S. Sakata, T. Tonooka, S. Ishizeki, M. Takada, M. Sakamoto, M. Fukuyama, et al., Culture-independent analysis of fecal microbiota in infants, with special reference to *Bifidobacterium* species, FEMS Microbiol. Lett. 243 (2005) 417–423.

[29] I. Brook, C. Barett, C. Brinkman, W. Martin, S. Finegold, Aerobic and anaerobic bacterial flora of the maternal cervix and newborn gastric fluid and conjunctiva: a prospective study, Pediatrics 63 (1979) 451–455.

[30] S. Lennox-King, S. O'Farrell, K. Bettelheim, R. Shooter, Colonization of caesarean section babies by *Escherichia coli*, Infection 4 (1976) 134–138.

[31] S. Lennox-King, S. O'Farrol, K. Bettelheim, R. Shooter, *Escherichia coli* isolated from babies delivered by caesarean section and their environment, Infection 4 (1976) 439–445.

[32] M. Gronlund, O. Lehtonen, E. Eerola, P. Kero, Fecal microflora in healthy infants born by different methods of delivery: permanent changes in intestinal flora after cesarean delivery, J. Pediatr. Gastroenterol. Nutr. 28 (1999) 19–25.

[33] J. Penders, C. Thijs, C. Vink, F.F. Stelma, B. Snijders, I. Kummeling, et al., Factors influencing the composition of the intestinal microbiota in early infancy, Pediatrics 118 (2006) 511–521.

[34] T. Mitsuoka, Intestinal flora and aging, Nutr. Rev. 50 (1992) 438–446.

[35] E. Whitney, S. Rolfes, The fat soluble vitamins: A, D, E, and K, Understanding Nutrition, Wadsworth, Belmont, CA, 2002, pp. 370–372

[36] G. Wardlaw, J. Hampl, The water-soluble vitamins, Perspectives in Nutrition, 7th ed., McGraw-Hill, New York, 2006, pp. 335–378.

[37] P. Raibaud, Bacterial interactions in the gut, in: R. Fuller (Ed.), Probiotics, Chapman & Hall, London, 1992, pp. 9–28.

[38] G.W. Tannock, Invisible forces: the influence of the normal microflora on host characteristics, Normal Microflora: An Introduction to Microbes Inhabiting the Human Body, Chapman & Hall, London, 1995, pp. 63–84

[39] H. Gordon, L. Pesti, The gnotobiotic animal as a tool in the study of host-microbial relationship, Bacteriol. Rev. 35 (1971) 390–429.

[40] M. Wills-Karp, J. Santeliz, C.L. Karp, The germless theory of allergic disease: revisiting the hygiene hypothesis, Nat. Rev. Immunol. 1 (2001) 69–75.

[41] B. Bjorksten, P. Naaber, E. Sepp, M. Mikelaar, The intestinal microflora in allergic Estonian and Swedish 2-year-old children, Clin. Exp. Allergy 29 (1999) 342–346.

[42] B. Bjorksten, E. Sepp, K. Julge, T. Voor, M. Mikelsaar, Allergy development and the intestinal microflora during the first year of life, J. Allergy Clin. Immunol. 108 (2001) 516–520.

[43] J.H. Cummings, G.T. Macfarlane, A review: the control and consequences of bacterial fermentation in the colon, J. Appl. Microbiol. 70 (1991) 443–459.

[44] S. Duncan, G. Hold, A. Barcenilla, C. Stewart, H. Flint, *Roseburia intestinalis* spp. nov., a novel saccharolytic, butyrate-producing bacterium from human faeces, Int. J. Syst. Evol. Microbiol. 52 (2002) 1–6.

[45] S.H. Duncan, P. Louis, H.J. Flint, Lactate-utilizing bacteria, isolated from human feces, that produce butyrate as a major fermentation product, Appl. Environ. Microbiol. 70 (2004) 5810–5817.

[46] W.E.W. Roediger, The effect of bacterial metabolites on nutrition and function of the colonic mucosa: symbiosis between men and bacteria, in: H. Kasper, H. Goebell (Eds.), Colon and Nutrition, Plenum, New York, 1982, pp. 11–24.

[47] T. Hoverstad, The normal microflora and short-chain fatty acids, in: R. Grubb, T. Midtvedt, E. Norin (Eds.), The Regulatory and Protective Role of the Normal Microflora, Macmillan, London, 1989, pp. 89–108.

[48] S.E. Pryde, S.H. Duncan, G.L. Hold, C.S. Stewart, H.J. Flint, The microbiology of butyrate formation in the human colon, FEMS Microbiol. Lett. 217 (2002) 133–139.

[49] A. McIntyre, P. Gibson, G.P. Young, Butyrate production from dietary fiber and protection against large bowel cancer in a rat model, Gut 34 (1993) 386–391.

[50] C. Demigne, C. Remesy, C. Morand, Short chain fatty acids, in: G.R. Gibson, M.B. Gibson (Eds.), Colonic Microbiota, Nutrition and Health, Kluwer, Dordrecht, The Netherlands, 1999, pp. 55–70.

[51] H. Younes, C. Coudray, J. Bellanger, C. Demigne, Y. Rayssiguier, C. Remesy, Effects of two fermentable carbohydrates (inulin and resistant starch) and their combination on calcium and magnesium balance in rats, Br. J. Nutr. 86 (2001) 479–485.

[52] C. Coudray, J.C. Tressol, E. Gueux, Y. Rayssiguier, Effects of inulin-type fructans of different chain length and type of branching on intestinal absorption and balance of calcium and magnesium in rats, Eur. J. Nutr. 42 (2003) 91–98.

[53] E.G. van den Heuvel, T. Muys, W. van Dokkum, G. Schaafsma, Oligofructose stimulates calcium absorption in adolescents, Am. J. Clin. Nutr. 69 (1999) 544–548.

[54] J.H. Cummings, Dietary carbohydrates and the colonic microflora, Curr. Opin. Clin. Nutr. Metab. Care 1 (1998) 409–414.

[55] L.V. Hooper, J.I. Gordon, Commensal host–bacterial relationships in the gut, Science 292 (2001) 1115–1118.

[56] K.D.R. Setchell, N.M. Brown, E. Lydeking-Olsen, The clinical importance of the metabolite equol: a clue to the effectiveness of soy and its isoflavones, J. Nutr. 132 (2002) 3577–3584.

[57] A.M. Duncan, B.E. Merz-Demlow, X. Xu, W.R. Phipps, M.S. Kurzer, Premenopausal equol excretors show plasma hormone profiles associated with lowered risk of breast cancer, Cancer Epidemiol. Biomarkers Prev. 9 (2000) 581–586.

[58] K.D.R. Setchell, A. Cassidy, Dietary isoflavones: biological effects and relevance to human health, J. Nutr. 129 (1999) 758S–767S.

[59] A. Cassidy, J.E. Brown, A. Hawdon, M.S. Faughnan, L.J. King, J. Millward, et al., Factors affecting the bioavailability of soy isoflavones in humans after ingestion of physiologically relevant levels from different soy foods, J. Nutr. 136 (2006) 45–51.

[60] S. Karr, J. Lampe, A. Hutchins, J. Slavin, Urinary isoflavonoid excretion in humans is dose dependent at low to moderate levels of soy–protein consumption, Am. J. Clin. Nutr. 66 (1997) 46–51.

[61] K. Decroos, S. Vanhemmens, S. Cattoir, N. Boon, W. Verstraete, Isolation and characterization of an equol-producing mixed microbial culture from a human faecal sample and its activity under gastrointestinal conditions, Arch. Microbiol 183 (2005) 45–55.

[62] H.G. Hur, J.O. Lay, R.D. Beger, J.P. Freeman, F. Rafii, Isolation of human intestinal bacteria metabolizing the natural isoflavone glycosides daidzin and genistin, Arch. Microbiol. 174 (2000) 422–428.

[63] N. Vedrine, J. Mathey, C. Morand, M. Brandolini, M.-J. Davicco, L. Guy, et al., One-month exposure to soy isoflavones did not induce the ability to produce equol in postmenopausal women, Eur. J. Clin. Nutr. 60 (2006) 1039–1045.

[64] D. O'Sullivan, Methods for analysis of the intestinal microflora, Curr. Issues Intest. Microbiol. 1 (2000) 39—50.

[65] A.H. Franks, H.J.M. Harmsen, G.C. Raangs, G.J. Jansen, F. Schut, G.W. Welling, Variations of bacterial populations in human feces measured by fluorescent *in situ* hybridization with group-specific 16S rRNA-targeted oligonucleotide probes, Appl. Environ. Microbiol. 64 (1998) 3336—3345.

[66] K. Wilson, R. Blitchington, Human colonic biota studied by ribosomal DNA sequence analysis, Appl. Environ. Microbiol. 62 (1996) 2273—2278.

[67] A. Sghir, G. Gramet, A. Suau, V. Rochet, P. Pochart, J. Dore, Quantification of bacterial groups within human fecal flora by oligonucleotide probe hybridization, Appl. Environ. Microbiol. 66 (2000) 2263—2266.

[68] J.H.A. Apajalahti, A. Kettunen, P.H. Nurminen, H. Jatila, W.E. Holben, Selective plating underestimates abundance and shows differential recovery of bifidobacterial species from human feces, Appl. Environ. Microbiol. 69 (2003) 5731—5735.

[69] R.M. Satokari, E.E. Vaughan, A.D.L. Akkermans, M. Saarela, W. M. de Vos, Bifidobacterial diversity in human feces detected by genus-specific PCR and denaturing gradient gel electrophoresis, Appl. Environ. Microbiol. 67 (2001) 504—513.

[70] M. Blaut, M.D. Collins, G.W. Welling, J. Dore, J. van Loo, W. de Vos, Molecular biological methods for studying the gut microbiota: the EU human gut flora project, Br. J. Nutr. 8 (2002) S203—S211.

[71] E. Vaughan, F. Schut, H. Heilig, E. Zoetendal, W. de Vos, A. Akkermans, A molecular view of the intestinal ecosystem, Curr. Issues Intest. Microbiol. 1 (2000) 1—12.

[72] J.L. Holland, L. Louie, A.E. Simor, M. Louie, PCR detection of *Escherichia coli* O157:H7 directly from stools: evaluation of commercial extraction methods for purifying fecal DNA, J. Clin. Microbiol. 38 (2000) 4108—4113.

[73] E. Zoetendal, K. Ben-Amor, A. Akkermans, T. Abee, W. de Vos, DNA isolation protocols affect the detection limit of PCR approaches of bacteria in samples from the human gastrointestinal tract, Syst. Appl. Microbiol. 24 (2001) 405—410.

[74] A.L. McOrist, M. Jackson, A.R. Bird, A comparison of five methods for extraction of bacterial DNA from human faecal samples, J. Microbiol. Methods 50 (2002) 131—139.

[75] M. Li, J. Gong, M. Cottrill, H. Yu, C. de Lange, J. Burton, et al., Evaluation of QIAamp DNA Stool Mini Kit for ecological studies of gut microbiota, J. Microbiol. Methods 54 (2003) 13—20.

[76] L. Monteiro, D. Bonnemaison, A. Vekris, K.G. Petry, J. Bonnet, R. Vidal, et al., Complex polysaccharides as PCR inhibitors in feces: *Helicobacter pylori* model, J. Clin. Microbiol. 35 (1997) 995—998.

[77] A. Cavallini, M. Notarnicola, P. Berloco, A. Lippolis, A. Di Leo, Use of macroporous polypropylene filter to allow identification of bacteria by PCR in human fecal samples, J. Microbiol. Methods 39 (2000) 265—270.

[78] S. Finegold, H. Attebery, V. Sutter, Effect of diet on human fecal flora: comparison of Japanese and American diets, Am. J. Clin. Nutr. 27 (1974) 1456—1469.

[79] M.W. Ariefdjohan, D. Savaiano, C.H. Nakatsu, Dietary changes may influence the stability of the bacterial community in the human gut, poster no. N-221 (Abstract 206-GM-A-1530-ASM), Presented at the 106th General Meeting of the American Society for Microbiology, Orlando, FL, 2006.

[80] E.G. Zoetendal, A.D.L. Akkermans, W.M. De Vos, Temperature gradient gel electrophoresis analysis of 16S rRNA from human fecal samples reveals stable and host-specific communities of active bacteria, Appl. Environ. Microbiol. 64 (1998) 3854—3859.

[81] B.R. Maier, M.A. Flynn, G.C. Burton, R.K. Tsutakawa, D.J. Hentges, Effects of a high-beef diet on bowel flora: a preliminary report, Am. J. Clin. Nutr. 27 (1974) 1470—1474.

[82] F. Li, M.A.J. Hullar, J.W. Lampe, Human gut bacterial community change due to cruciferous vegetables in a controlled feeding study, poster no. N-16 (session 264/N), Presented at the 107th General Meeting of the American Society for Microbiology, Toronto, Canada, 2007.

[83] F. Shanahan, Inflammatory bowel disease: immunodiagnostics, immunotherapeutics, and ecotherapeutics, Gastroenterology 120 (2001) 622—635.

[84] I. Wollowski, G. Rechkemmer, B.L. Pool-Zobel, Protective role of probiotics and prebiotics in colon cancer, Am. J. Clin. Nutr. 73 (2001) 451S—455S.

[85] M.E. Sanders, J. Huis in't Veld, Bringing a probiotic-containing functional food to the market: microbiological, product, regulatory and labeling issues, Antonie Van Leeuwenhoek 76 (1999) 293—315.

[86] S. Fasoli, M. Marzotto, L. Rizzotti, F. Rossi, F. Dellaglio, S. Torriani, Bacterial composition of commercial probiotic products as evaluated by PCR-DGGE analysis, Int. J. Food Microbiol. 82 (2003) 59—70.

[87] M. Saxelin, S. Tynkkynen, T. Mattila-Sandholm, W.M. de Vos, Probiotic and other functional microbes: from markets to mechanisms, Curr. Opin. Biotechnol. 16 (2005) 204—211.

[88] M. Alander, R. Satokari, R. Korpela, M. Saxelin, T. Vilpponen-Salmela, T. Mattila-Sandholm, et al., Persistence of colonization of human colonic mucosa by a probiotic strain, *Lactobacillus rhamnosus* G. G., after oral consumption, Appl. Environ. Microbiol. 65 (1999) 351—354.

[89] G.W. Tannock, K. Munro, H.J.M. Harmsen, G.W. Welling, J. Smart, P.K. Gopal, Analysis of the fecal microflora of human subjects consuming a probiotic product containing *Lactobacillus rhamnosus* DR20, Appl. Environ. Microbiol. 66 (2000) 2578—2588.

[90] K.M. Tuohy, G.C.M. Rouzaud, W.M. Bruck, G.R. Gibson, Modulation of the human gut microflora towards improved health using prebiotics: assessment of efficacy, Curr. Pharm. Des. 11 (2005) 75—90.

[91] D. Savaiano, A. Abou ElAnouar, D. Smith, M. Levitt, Lactose malabsorption from yogurt, pasteurized yogurt, sweet acidophilus milk, and cultured milk in lactase-deficient individuals, Am. J. Clin. Nutr. 40 (1984) 1219—1223.

[92] D. Gaon, Y. Doweck, A. Zavaglia, A. Holgado, G. Oliver, Lactose digestion of a milk fermented by *Lactobacillus acidophilus* and *Lactobacillus casei* of human origin [in Spanish], Medicina (B. Aires) 55 (1995) 237—242.

[93] R.G. Montes, T.M. Bayless, J.M. Saavedra, J.A. Perman, Effect of milks inoculated with *Lactobacillus acidophilus* or a yogurt starter culture in lactose-maldigesting children, J. Dairy Sci. 78 (1995) 1657—1664.

[94] T. Jiang, A. Mustapha, D.A. Savaiano, Improvement of lactose digestion in humans by ingestion of unfermented milk containing *Bifidobacterium longum*, J. Dairy Sci 79 (1996) 750—757.

[95] M. Shermak, J. Saavedra, T. Jackson, S. Huang, T. Bayless, J. Perman, Effect of yogurt on symptoms and kinetics of hydrogen production in lactose-malabsorbing children, Am. J. Clin. Nutr. 62 (1995) 1003—1006.

[96] M.-Y. Lin, C.-L. Yen, S.-H. Chen, Management of lactose maldigestion by consuming milk containing Lactobacilli, Dig. Dis. Sci. 43 (1998) 133—137.

[97] M. de Vrese, A. Stegelmann, B. Richter, S. Fenselau, C. Laue, J. Schrezenmeir, Probiotics: compensation for lactase insufficiency, Am. J. Clin. Nutr. 73 (2001) 421S—429S.

[98] G. Ligny, *Saccharomyces boulardii* as a treatment for antibiotic associated disorders: a double blind study [in French], Rev. Française Gastroenteérologie 114 (1975) 45–50.

[99] V. Gotz, J. Romankiewicz, J. Moss, H. Murray, Prophylaxis against ampicillin-associated diarrhea with a *Lactobacillus* preparation, Am. J. Hosp. Pharm. 36 (1979) 754–757.

[100] M. Borgia, N. Sepe, V. Brancato, et al., A controlled clinical study on *Streptococcus faecium* preparation for the prevention of side reactions during long-term antibiotic treatments, Curr. Ther. Res. 31 (1982) 265–271.

[101] M. Clements, M. Levine, P. Ristaino, V. Daya, T. Hughes, Exogenous lactobacilli fed to man: their fate and ability to prevent diarrheal disease, Prog. Food Nutr. Sci. 7 (1983) 29–37.

[102] J. Colombel, A. Cortot, C. Neut, C. Romond, Yoghurt with *Bifidobacterium longum* reduces erythromcyin-induced gastrointestinal effects, Lancet 2 (1987) 43.

[103] C. Surawicz, G. Elmer, P. Speelman, L. McFarland, J. Chinn, G. van Belle, Prevention of antibiotic-associated diarrhea by *Saccharomyces boulardii*: a prospective study, Gastroenterology 96 (1989) 981–988.

[104] P. Wunderlich, L. Braun, I. Fumagalli, V. D'Apuzzo, F. Heim, M. Karly, et al., Double-blind report on the efficacy of lactic acid-producing *Enterococcus* SF68 in the prevention of antibiotic-associated diarrhoea and in the treatment of acute diarrhoea, J. Int. Med. Res. 17 (1989) 333–338.

[105] S. Siitonen, H. Vapaatalo, S. Salminen, A. Gordin, M. Saxelin, R. Wikberg, et al., Effect of *Lactobacillus* GG yoghurt in prevention of antibiotic associated diarrhoea, Ann. Med. 22 (1990) 57–59.

[106] K. Orrhage, B. Brismar, C. Nord, Effects of supplements of *Bifidobacterium longum* and *Lactobacillus acidophilus* on the intestinal microbiota during administration of clindamycin, Microb. Ecol. Health Dis. 7 (1994) 17–25.

[107] L.V. McFarland, C.M. Surawicz, R.N. Greenberg, G.W. Elmer, K.A. Moyer, S.A. Melcher, et al., Prevention of beta-lactam-associated diarrhea by *Saccharomyces boulardii* compared with placebo, Am. J. Gastroenterol. 90 (1995) 439–448.

[108] D. Witsell, C. Garrett, W. Yarbrough, S. Dorrestein, A. Drake, M. Weissler, Effect of *Lactobacillus acidophilus* on antibiotic-associated gastrointestinal morbidity: a prospective randomized trial, J. Otolaryngol. 24 (1995) 230–233.

[109] T. Arvola, K. Laiho, S. Torkkeli, H. Mykk, S. Salminen, L. Maunula, et al., Prophylactic *Lactobacillus* GG reduces antibiotic-associated diarrhea in children with respiratory infections: a randomized study, Pediatrics 104 (1999) 64–68.

[110] J. Vanderhoof, D. Whitney, D. Antonson, T. Hanner, J. Lupo, R. Young, *Lactobacillus* GG in the prevention of antibiotic-associated diarrhea in children, J. Pediatr. 135 (1999) 564–568.

[111] A. Armuzzi, F. Cremonini, F. Bartolozzi, F. Canducci, M. Candelli, V. Ojetti, et al., The effect of oral administration of *Lactobacillus* GG on antibiotic-associated gastrointestinal side-effects during *Helicobacter pylori* eradication therapy, Aliment. Pharmacol. Ther. 15 (2001) 163–169.

[112] M. Kotowska, P. Albrecht, H. Szajewska, *Saccharomyces boulardii* in the prevention of antibiotic-associated diarrhoea in children: a randomized double-blind placebo-controlled trial, Aliment. Pharmacol. Ther. 21 (2005) 583–590.

[113] G. Bellomo, A. Mangiagle, L. Nicastro, G. Frigerio, A controlled double blind study of SF68 strain as a new biological preparation for the treatment of diarrhea in pediatrics, Curr. Ther. Res. 28 (1980) 927–936.

[114] J. Bodilis, Lacteol versus placebo in acute adult diarrhea: a controlled study [in French], Médecine Actuelle 10 (1983) 232–235.

[115] P. Chapoy, Treatment of acute diarrhea in children: a controlled trial with *Saccharomyces boulardii* [in French], Ann. Pediatr. (Paris) 32 (1985).

[116] E. Isolauri, T. Rautanen, M. Juntunen, P. Sillanaukee, T. Koivula, A human *Lactobacillus* strain (*Lactobacillus casei* spp. strain GG) promotes recovery from acute diarrhea in children, Pediatrics 88 (1991) 90–97.

[117] E. Isolauri, M. Kaila, H. Mykkanen, W. Ling, S. Salminen, Oral bacteriotherapy for viral gastroenteritis, Dig. Dis. Sci. 39 (1994) 2595–2600.

[118] J.M. Saavedra, N.A. Bauman, I. Oung, J.A. Perman, R.H. Yolken, Feeding of *Bifidobacterium bifidum* and *Streptococcus thermophilus* to infants in hospital for prevention of diarrhea and shedding of rotavirus, Lancet 344 (1994) 1046–1049.

[119] T. Sugita, M. Togawa, Efficacy of lactobacillus preparation bio-lactis powder in children with rotavirus enteritis [in Japanese], Jpn. Pediatr. 47 (1994) 2755–2762.

[120] M. Kaila, E. Isolauri, M. Saxelin, H. Arvilommi, T. Vesikari, Viable versus inactivated lactobacillus strain GG in acute rotavirus diarrhoea, Arch. Dis. Child. 72 (1995) 51–53.

[121] H. Majamaa, E. Isolauri, M. Saxelin, T. Vesikari, Lactic acid bacteria in the treatment of acute rotavirus gastroenteritis, J. Pediatr. Gastroenterol. Nutr. 20 (1995) 333–338.

[122] S. Raza, S. Graham, S. Allen, S. Sultana, L. Cuevas, C. Hart, *Lactobacillus* GG promotes recovery from acute nonbloody diarrhea in Pakistan, Pediatr. Infect. Dis. J. 14 (1995) 107–111.

[123] P. Buydens, S. Debeuckelaere, Efficacy of SF68 in the treatment of acute diarrhea: a placebo-controlled trial, Scand. J. Gastroenterol. 31 (1996) 887–891.

[124] A.R. Pant, S.M. Graham, S.J. Allen, S. Harikul, A. Sabchareon, L. Cuevas, et al., Lactobacillus GG and acute diarrhoea in young children in the tropics, J. Trop. Pediatr. 42 (1996) 162–165.

[125] A. Guarino, R. Canani, M. Spagnuolo, F. Albano, L. DiBenedetto, Oral bacterial therapy reduces the duration of symptoms and of viral excretion in children with mild diarrhea, J. Pediatr. Gastroenterol. Nutr. 25 (1997) 516–519.

[126] A. Shornikova, I. Casas, H. Mykkanen, E. Salo, T. Vesikari, Bacteriotherapy with *Lactobacillus reuteri* in rotavirus gastroenteritis, Pediatr. Infect. Dis. J. 16 (1997) 1103–1107.

[127] A. Shornikova, E. Isolauri, L. Burkanova, S. Lukovnikova, T. Vesikari, A trial in the Karelian Republic of oral rehydration and *Lactobacillus* GG for treatment of acute diarrhoea, Acta Paediatr. 86 (1997) 460–465.

[128] R. Oberhelman, R. Gilman, P. Sheen, D.N. Taylor, R.E. Black, L. Cabrera, et al., A placebo-controlled trial of *Lactobacillus* GG to prevent diarrhea in undernourished Peruvian children, J. Pediatr. 134 (1999) 15–20.

[129] C. Pedone, A. Bernabeu, E. Postaire, C. Bouley, P. Reinert, The effect of supplementation with milk fermented by *Lactobacillus casei* (strain DN-114001) on acute diarrhoea in children attending day care centres, Int. J. Clin. Pract. 53 (1999) 179–184.

[130] P. Phuapradit, W. Varavithya, K. Vathanophas, R. Sangchai, A. Podhipak, U. Suthutvoravut, et al., Reduction of rotavirus infection in children receiving bifidobacteria-supplemented formula, J. Med. Assoc. Thai. 82 (1999) S43–S48.

[131] S. Guandalini, I. Pensabene, M. Zikri, J.A. Dias, L.G. Casali, H. Hoekstra, et al., *Lactobacillus* GG administered in oral rehydration solution to children with acute diarrhea: a multicenter European trial, J. Pediatr. Gastroenterol. Nutr. 30 (2000) 54–60.

[132] C. Pedone, C. Arnaud, E. Postaire, C. Bouley, P. Reinert, Multicentric study of the effect of milk fermented by *Lactobacillus casei* on the incidence of diarrhoea, Int. J. Clin. Pract. 54 (2000) 568–571.

[133] K. Hatakka, E. Savilahti, A. Ponka, J.H. Meurman, T. Poussa, L. Nase, et al., Effect of long term consumption of probiotic milk on infections in children attending day care centres: double blind, randomised, Br. Med. J. 322 (2001) 1327–1330.

[134] H. Szajewska, M. Kotowska, J.Z. Mrukowics, M. Armanska, W. Mikolajczyk, Efficacy of Lactobacillus GG in prevention of nosocomial diarrhea in infants, J. Pediatr. 138 (2001) 361–365.

[135] R. Chandra, Effect of Lactobacillus on the incidence and severity of acute rotavirus diarrhea in infants: a prospective placebo-controlled double-blind study, Nutr. Res. 22 (2002) 65–69.

[136] V. Rosenfeldt, K. Michaelsen, M. Jakobsen, C.N. Larsen, P.L. Moller, P. Pedersen, et al., Effect of probiotic Lactobacillus strains in young children hospitalized with acute diarrhea, Pediatr. Infect. Dis. J. 21 (2002) 411–416.

[137] V. Rosenfeldt, K. Michaelsen, M. Jakobsen, C.N. Larsen, P.L. Moller, M. Tvede, et al., Effect of probiotic Lactobacillus strains on acute diarrhea in a cohort of nonhospitalized children attending day-care centers, Pediatr. Infect. Dis. J. 21 (2002) 417–419.

[138] D. Pereg, O. Kimhi, A. Tirosh, N. Orr, R. Kayouf, M. Lishner, The effect of fermented yogurt on the prevention of diarrhea in a healthy adult population, Am. J. Infect. Control 33 (2005) 122–125.

[139] A. Billoo, M. Memon, S. Khaskheli, G. Murtaza, K. Iqbal, M. Saeed Shekhani, et al., Role of a probiotic (Saccharomyces boulardii) in management and prevention of diarrhoea, World J. Gastroenterol. 12 (2006) 4557–4560.

[140] J. De Dios-Pozo-Alano, J. Warram, R. Gomez, M. Cavazos, Effect of a Lactobacilli preparation on traveler's diarrhea: a randomized double-blind clinical trial, Gastroenterology 74 (1978) 829–830.

[141] F. Black, P. Anderson, J. Orskow, F. Orskow, K. Gaarslev, S. Laudlund, Prophylactic efficacy of lactobacilli on travellers diarrhea, Travel Med. 7 (1989) 333–335.

[142] P.J. Oksanen, S. Salminen, M. Saxelin, P. Hamalainen, A. Ihantolavormisto, L. Muurasniemiisoviita, et al., Prevention of traveler's diarrhea by Lactobacillus GG, Ann. Med. 22 (1990) 53–56.

[143] v.H. Kollaritsch, H. Holst, P. Grobara, G. Wiedermann, Prevention of travelers' diarrhea by Saccharomyces boulardi [in French], Fortischritte Medizin 111 (1993) 153–156.

[144] E. Hilton, P. Kolakowski, C. Singer, M. Smith, Efficacy of Lactobacillus GG as a diarrheal preventive in travelers, J. Travel Med. 4 (1997) 41–43.

[145] J. Tempé, A. Steidel, H. Bléhaut, M. Hasselmann, P. Lutun, F. Maurier, Prevention of tube feeding-induced diarrhea by Saccharomyces boulardii [in French], Semaine Hópitaux Paris 59 (1983) 1409–1412.

[146] M. Schlotterer, P. Bernasconi, F. Lebreton, D. Wassermann, Effect of Saccharomyces boulardii on the digestive tolerance of enteral nutrition in burn [in French], Nutr. Clin. Métabolisme 1 (1987) 31–34.

[147] G. Bleichner, H. Bléhaut, H. Mentec, D. Moyse, Saccharomyces boulardii prevents diarrhea in critically ill tube-fed patients: a multicenter, randomized, double-blind placebo-controlled trial, Intens. Care Med. 23 (1997) 517–523.

[148] D. Heimburger, D. Sockwell, W. Geels, Diarrhea with enteral feeding: prospective reappraisal of putative causes, Nutrition 10 (1994) 392–396.

[149] E. Salminen, I. Elomaa, J. Minkkinen, H. Vapaatalo, S. Salminen, Preservation of intestinal integrity during radiotherapy using live Lactobacillus acidophilus cultures, Clin. Radiol. 39 (1988) 435–437.

[150] T. Tomoda, Y. Nakano, T. Kageyama, Intestinal Candida overgrowth and Candida infection in patients with leukemia: effect of Bifidobacterium administration, Bifidobacteria Microflora 7 (1988) 71–74.

[151] G. Elmer, K. Moyer, C. Surawicz, A. Collier, T. Hooton, L. McFarland, Evaluation of Saccharomyces boulardii for patients with HIV-related chronic diarrhoea and healthy volunteers receiving antifungals, Microecol. Ther. 25 (1995) 23–31.

[152] B. Wolf, K. Wheeler, D. Ataya, K. Garleb, Safety and tolerance of Lactobacillus reuteri supplementation to a population infected with the human immunodeficiency virus, Food Chem. Toxicol. 36 (1998) 1085–1094.

[153] H. Urbancsek, T. Kazar, I. Mezes, K. Neumann, Results of a double-blind, randomized study to evaluate the efficacy and safety of antibiophilus in patients with radiation-induced diarrhoea, Eur. J. Gastroenterol. Hepatol. 13 (2001) 391–396.

[154] P. Delia, G. Sansotta, V. Donato, G. Messina, P. Frosina, S. Pergolizzi, et al., Prevention of radiation-induced diarrhea with the use of VSL#3, a new high-potency probiotic preparation, Am. J. Gastroenterol. 97 (2002) 2150–2152.

[155] M.L. Simenhoff, S.R. Dunn, G.P. Zollner, M.E. Fitzpatrick, S.M. Emery, W.E. Sandine, et al., Biomodulation of the toxic and nutritional effects of small bowel bacterial overgrowth in end-stage kidney disease using freeze-dried Lactobacillus acidophilus, Miner. Electrolyte Metab. 22 (1996) 92–96.

[156] S. Dunn, M. Simenhoff, K. Ahmed, W.J. Gaughan, B.O. Eltayeb, M.-E.D. Fitzpatrick, et al., Effect of oral administration of freeze-dried Lactobacillus acidophilus on small bowel bacterial overgrowth in patients with end stage kidney disease: reducing uremic toxins and improving nutrition, Int. Dairy J. 8 (1998) 545–553.

[157] J. Vanderhoof, R. Young, N. Murray, S. Kaufman, Treatment strategies for small bowel bacterial overgrowth in short bowel syndrome, J. Pediatr. Gastroenterol. Nutr. 27 (1998) 155–160.

[158] D. Gaon, C. Garmendia, N. Murrielo, A. de Cucco Games, A. Cerchio, R. Quintas, et al., Effect of Lactobacillus strains (L. casei and L. acidophilus strains CERELA) on bacterial overgrowth-related chronic diarrhea, Medicina (Buenos Aires) 62 (2002) 159–163.

[159] H. Majamaa, E. Isolauri, M. Saxelin, T. Vesikari, Probiotics: a novel approach in the management of food allergy, J. Allergy Clin. Immunol. 99 (1997) 179–185.

[160] E. Isolauri, T. Arvola, Y. Sutas, E. Moilanen, E. Salminen, Probiotics in the management of atopic eczema, Clin. Exp. Allergy 30 (2000) 1604–1610.

[161] M. Kalliomaki, S. Salminen, H. Arvilommi, P. Kero, P. Koskinen, E. Isolauri, Probiotics in primary prevention of atopic disease: a randomised placebo-controlled trial, Lancet 357 (2001) 1076–1079.

[162] M. Kalliomaki, S. Salminen, T. Poussa, H. Arvilommi, E. Isolauri, Probiotics and prevention of atopic disease: 4-year follow-up of a randomised placebo-controlled trial, Lancet 361 (2003) 1869–1871.

[163] A. Hoyos, Reduced incidence of necrotizing enterocolitis associated with enteral administration of Lactobacillus acidophilus and Bifidobacterium infantis to neonates in an intensive care unit, Int. J. Infect. Dis. 3 (1999) 197–202.

[164] J. Maupas, P. Champemont, M. Delforge, Treatment of irritable bowel syndrome with Saccharomyces boulardii: a double-blind, placebo controlled study [in French], Med. Chirurg. Dig. 12 (1983) 77–79.

[165] A. Newcomer, H. Park, P. O'Brien, D. McGill, Response of patients with irritable bowel syndrome and lactase deficiency

using unfermented acidophilus milk, Am. J. Clin. Nutr. 38 (1983) 257–263.

[166] J. Gade, P. Thorn, Paraghurt for patients with irritable bowel syndrome: a controlled clinical investigation from general practice, Scand. J. Primary Health Care 7 (1989) 23–26.

[167] G. Halpern, T. Prindiville, M. Blankenburg, T. Hsia, M. Gershwin, Treatment of irritable bowel syndrome with Lacteol Fort: a randomized, double-blind, crossover trial, Am. J. Gastroenterol. 91 (1996) 1579–1584.

[168] J. Hunter, A. Lee, T. King, M. Barratt, M. Linggood, J. Blades, Enterococcus faecium strain PR88: An effective probiotic, Gut 38 (Suppl.) (1996) A62.

[169] R. Young, J. Vanderhoof, Successful probiotic therapy of chronic recurrent abdominal pain in children, Gastroenterology 112 (1997) A856.

[170] C. Hentschel, J. Bauer, N. Dill, Complementary medicine in non-ulcer-dyspepsia: is alternative medicine a real alternative? a randomised placebo-controlled double-blind clinical trial with two probiotic agents (Hylac N and Hylac N Forte), Gastroenterology 112 (1997) A146.

[171] H. Kordecki, K. Niedzielin, New possibility in the treatment of irritable bowel syndrome: probiotics as a modification of the microflora of the colon, Gastroenterology 114 (1998) A402.

[172] D. Bougle, N. Roland, F. Lebeurrier, P. Arhan, Effect of propionibacteria supplementation on fecal bifidobacteria and segmental colonic transit time in healthy human subjects, Scand. J. Gastroenterol. 34 (1999) 144–148.

[173] S. Nobaek, M.-L. Johansson, G. Molin, S. Ahrne, B. Jeppsson, Alteration of intestinal microflora is associated with reduction in abdominal bloating and pain in patients with irritable bowel syndrome, Am. J. Gastroenterol. 95 (2000) 1231–1238.

[174] P. Brigidi, B. Vitali, E. Swennen, G. Bazzocchi, D. Matteuzzi, Effects of probiotic administration upon the composition and enzymatic activity of human fecal microbiota in patients with irritable bowel syndrome or functional diarrhea, Res. Microbiol. 152 (2001) 735–741.

[175] C. De Simone, G. Famularo, B. Salvadori, S. Moretti, S. Marcellini, V. Trinchieri, et al., Treatment of irritable bowel syndrome (IBS) with the newer probiotic VSL#3: a multicenter trial, Am. J. Clin. Nutr. 73 (2001) 491S.

[176] K. Niedzielin, H. Kordecki, B. Birkenfeld, A controlled, double-blind, randomized study on the efficacy of Lactobacillus plantarum 299 V in patients with irritable bowel syndrome, Eur. J. Gastroenterol. Hepatol. 13 (2001) 1143–1147.

[177] P. Marteau, E. Cuillerier, S. Meance, M.F. Gerhardt, A. Myara, M. Bouvier, et al., Bifidobacterium animalis strain DN-173 010 shortens the colonic transit time in healthy women: a double-blind, randomized, controlled study, Aliment. Pharmacol. Ther. 16 (2002) 587–593.

[178] S. Sen, M. Mullan, T. Parker, J. Woolner, S. Tarry, J. Hunter, Effect of Lactobacillus plantarum 299 v on colonic fermentation and symptoms of irritable bowel syndrome, Dig. Liver Dis. 47 (2002) 2615–2620.

[179] H. Kim, M. Vazquez Roque, M. Camilleri, D. Stephens, D. Burton, K. Baxter, et al., A randomized controlled trial of a probiotic combination VSL#3 and placebo in irritable bowel syndrome with bloating, Neurogastroenterol. Motil. 17 (2005) 687–696.

[180] P.J. Whorwell, L. Altringer, J. Morel, Y. Bond, D. Charbonneau, L. O'Mahony, et al., Efficacy of an encapsulated probiotic Bifidobacterium infantis 35624 in women with irritable bowel syndrome, Am. J. Gastroenterol. 101 (2006) 1581–1590.

[181] K. Plein, J. Hotz, Therapeutic effects of Saccharomyces boulardii on mild residual symptoms in a stable phase of Crohn's disease with special respect to chronic diarrhea: a pilot study. Z, Gastroenterol. 31 (1993) 129–134.

[182] M. Malin, H. Suomalainen, M. Saxelin, E. Isolauri, Promotion of IgA immune response in patients with Crohn's disease by oral bacteriotherapy with Lactobacillus GG, Ann. Nutr. Metab. 40 (1996) 137–145.

[183] W. Kruis, E. Schutz, P. Fric, B. Fixa, G. Judmaier, M. Stolte, Double-blind comparison of an oral Escherichia coli preparation and mesalazine in maintaining remission of ulcerative colitis, Aliment. Pharmacol. Ther. 11 (1997) 853–858.

[184] H. Malchow, Crohn's disease and Escherichia coli: a new approach in therapy to maintain remission of colonic Crohn's disease? J. Clin. Gastroenterol. 25 (1997) 653–658.

[185] B. Rembacken, A. Snelling, P. Hawkey, D. Chalmers, A. Axon, Non-pathogenic Escherichia coli versus mesalazine for the treatment of ulcerative colitis: a randomised trial, Lancet 354 (1999) 635–639.

[186] M. Campieri, F. Rizzello, A. Venturi, G. Poggioli, F. Ugolini, U. Helwig, et al., Combination of antibiotic and probiotic treatment is efficacious in prophylaxis of post-operative recurrence of Crohn's disease: a randomized controlled study vs. mesalamine [Abstract], Gastroenterology 118 (2000) G4179.

[187] I. Copaci, L. Micu, C. Chira, I. Rovinaru, Maintenance of remission of ulcerative colitis (UC): mesalamine, dietary fiber, S. boulardii [Abstract], Gut 47 (Suppl. 3) (2000) A240–P929.

[188] P. Gupta, H. Andrew, B. Kirschner, S. Guandalini, Is Lactobacillus GG helpful in children with Crohn' s disease? results of a preliminary, open-label study, J. Pediatr. Gastroenterol. Nutr. 31 (2000) 453–457.

[189] M. Guslandi, G. Mezzi, M. Sorghi, P.A. Testoni, Saccharomyces boulardii in maintenance treatment of Crohn's disease, Dig. Dis. Sci. 45 (2000) 1462–1464.

[190] P. Gionchetti, F. Rizzello, A. Venturi, P. Brigidi, D. Matteuzzi, G. Bazzochi, et al., Oral bacteriotherapy as maintenance treatment in patients with chronic pouchitis: a double-blind, placebo-controlled trial, Gastroenterology 119 (2000) 305–309.

[191] S. Guandalini, Use of Lactobacillus-GG in paediatric Crohn's disease, Dig. Liver Dis. 34 (2002) S63–S65.

[192] C. Prantera, M.L. Scribano, G. Falasco, A. Andreoli, C. Luzi, Ineffectiveness of probiotics in preventing recurrence after curative resection for Crohn's disease: a randomised controlled trial with Lactobacillus GG, Gut 51 (2002) 405–409.

[193] W. Kruis, P. Fric, J. Pokrotnieks, M. Lukas, B. Fixa, M. Kascak, et al., Maintaining remission of ulcerative colitis with the probiotic Escherichia coli Nissle 1917 is as effective as with standard mesalazine, Gut 53 (2004) 1617–1623.

[194] M. Schultz, A. Timmer, H. Herfarth, R. Balfour Sartor, J. Vanderhoof, H. Rath, Lactobacillus GG in inducing and maintaining remission of Crohn's disease, BMC Gastroenterol. 4 (2004) 5–8.

[195] A. Bousvaros, S. Guandalini, R. Baldassano, C. Botelho, J. Evans, G.D. Ferry, et al., A randomized, double-blind trial of Lactobacillus GG versus placebo in addition to standard maintenance therapy for children with Crohn's disease, Inflamm. Bowel Dis. 11 (2005) 833–839.

[196] S. Gorbach, T. Chang, B. Goldin, Successful treatment of relapsing Clostridium difficile colitis with Lactobacillus GG, Lancet 2 (1987) 1519.

[197] C. Surawicz, L. McFarland, G. Elmer, J. Chinn, Treatment of recurrent Clostridium difficile colitis with vancomycin and Saccharomyces boulardii, Am. J. Gastroenterol. 84 (1989) 1285–1287.

[198] M. Kimmey, G. Elmer, C. Surawicz, L. McFarland, Prevention of further recurrence of Clostridium difficile colitis with Saccharomyces boulardii, Dig. Dis. Sci. 35 (1990) 897–901.

[199] J. Buts, G. Corthier, M. Delmée, *Saccharomyces boulardii* for *Clostridium difficile* associated enteropathies in infants, J. Pediatr. Gastroenterol. Nutr. 16 (1993) 419−425.

[200] L.V. McFarland, C.M. Surawicz, R.N. Greenberg, R. Fekety, G. W. Elmer, K.A. Moyer, et al., A randomized placebo-controlled trial of *Saccharomyces boulardii* in combination with standard antibiotics for *Clostridium difficile* disease, JAMA 271 (1994) 1913−1918.

[201] J. Biller, A. Katz, A. Flores, T. Buie, S. Gorbach, Treatment of recurrent *Clostridium difficile* colitis with *Lactobacillus* GG, J. Pediatr. Gastroenterol. Nutr. 21 (1995) 224−226.

[202] R.G. Bennet, S.L. Gorbach, B.R. Goldin, T.W. Chang, B.E. Laughon, W.B. Greenough, et al., Treatment of relapsing *C. difficile* diarrhea with *Lactobacillus* GG 31 (Suppl.) (1996) 35S−38S.

[203] J. Levy, Experience with live *Lactobacillus plantarum* 299 v: a promising adjunct in the management of recurrent *Clostridium difficile* infection [Abstract], J. Gastroenterol. 112 (1997) A379.

[204] P. Michetti, G. Dorta, P. Wiesel, D. Brassart, E. Verdu, M. Herranz, et al., Effect of whey-based culture supernatant of *Lactobacillus acidophilus* (*johnsonii*) la1 on *Helicobacter pylori* infection in humans, Digestion 60 (1999) 203−209.

[205] F. Canducci, A. Armuzzi, F. Cremonini, G. Cammarota, F. Bartolozzi, P. Pola, et al., A lyophilized and inactivated culture of *Lactobacillus acidophilus* increases *Helicobacter pylori* eradication rates, Aliment. Pharmacol. Ther. 14 (2000) 1625−1629.

[206] I. Sakamoto, M. Igarashi, S. Kimura, A. Takagi, T. Miwa, Y. Koga, Suppressive effect of *Lactobacillus gasseri* OLL 2716 (LG21) on *Helicobacter pylori* infection in humans, J. Antimicrob. Chemother. 47 (2001) 709−710.

[207] K. Tuohy, S. Kolida, A. Lustenberger, G. Gibson, The prebiotic effects of biscuits containing partially hydrolysed guar gum and fructo-oligosaccharides: a human volunteer study, Br. J. Nutr. 86 (2001) 341−348.

[208] H. Kruse, B. Kleesen, M. Blaut, Effect of inulin on faecal bifidobacteria in human subjects, Br. J. Nutr. 82 (1999) 375−382.

[209] G. Gibson, E. Beatty, X. Wang, J. Cummings, Selective stimulation of bifidobacteria in the human colon by oligofructose and inulin, Gastroenterology 108 (1995) 975−982.

[210] B. Kleessen, B. Sykura, H. Zunft, M. Blaut, Effects of inulin and lactose on fecal microflora, microbial activity, and bowel habit in elderly constipated persons, Am. J. Clin. Nutr. 65 (1997) 1397−1402.

[211] Y. Bouhnik, K. Vahedi, L. Achour, A. Attar, J. Salfati, P. Pochart, et al., Short-chain fructo-oligosaccharide administration dose-dependently increases fecal bifidobacteria in healthy humans, J. Nutr. 129 (1999) 113−116.

[212] R. Buddington, C. Williams, S. Chen, S. Witherly, Dietary supplement of neosugar alters the fecal flora and decreases activities of some reductive enzymes in human subjects, Am. J. Clin. Nutr. 63 (1996) 709−716.

[213] G. Moro, I. Minoli, M. Mosca, S. Fanaro, J. Jelinek, B. Stahl, et al., Dosage-related bifidogenic effects of galacto- and fructooligosaccharides in formula-fed term infants, J. Pediatr. Gastroenterol. Nutr. 34 (2002) 291−295.

[214] G. Boehm, M. Lidestri, P. Casetta, J. Jelinek, F. Negretti, B. Stahl, et al., Supplementation of a bovine milk formula with an oligosaccharide mixture increases counts of faecal bifidobacteria in preterm infants, Arch. Dis. Child. Fetal Neonatal 86 (2002) F178−F181.

[215] K. Tuohy, C. Ziemer, A.Y.K. Klinder, B.L. Pool-Zobel, G.R. Gibson, A human volunteer study to determine the prebiotic effects of lactulose powder on human colonic microbiota, Microb. Ecol. Health Dis. 14 (2002) 165−173.

[216] A. Terada, H. Hara, M. Kataoka, T. Mitsuoka, Effect of lactulose on the composition and metabolic activity of the human faecal flora, Microb. Ecol. Health Dis. 5 (1992) 43−50.

[217] J. Ballongue, C. Schumann, P. Quignon, Effects of lactulose and lactitol on colonic microbiota and enzymatic activity, Scand. J. Gastroenterol. 32 (1997) 41−44.

[218] R. Nagendra, S. Viswanatha, S. Arun Kumar, Effect of feeding milk formula containing lactulose to infants on faecal bifidobacterial flora, Nutr. Res. 15 (1995) 15−24.

[219] M. Ito, Y. Deguchi, A. Miyamori, K. Matsumoto, H. Kikuchi, K. Matsumoto, et al., Effects of administration of galactooligosaccharides on the human faecal microflora, stool weight and abdominal sensation, Microb. Ecol. Health Dis. 3 (1990) 285−292.

[220] M. Ito, Y. Deguchi, K. Matsumoto, M. Kimura, N. Onodera, T. Yajima, Influence of galactooligosaccharides on the human fecal microflora, J. Nutr. Sci. Vitaminol. 39 (1993) 635−640.

[221] F. Waldeck, Funktionen des magen-darm-kanals, in: R. Schmidt, G. Thews (Eds.), Physiologie des Menschen, Springer, Berlin, 1990, p. 24.

[222] G. Simon, S. Gorbach, Intestinal microflora, Med. Clin. North Am. 66 (1982) 557−574.

[223] L. Thomas, M. Flower, A Guide for Healthcare Professionals: *Lactobacillus casei* Shirota and Yakult, Science for Health, Yakult, UK, 2006.

[224] P. Lawson, Taxonomy and systematics of predominant gut anaerobes in: G.R. Gibson, M.B. Roberfroid (Eds.), Colonic Microbiota, Nutrition and Health, Kluwer, Dordrecht, The Netherlands, 1999, pp. 149−166.

[225] Y. Benno, K. Sawada, T. Mitsuoka, The intestinal microflora of infants: composition of fecal flora in breast-fed and bottle-fed infants, Microbiol. Immunol. 28 (1984) 975−986.

[226] H. Beerens, C. Romond, C. Neut, Influence of breast-feeding on the bifid flora of the newborn intestine, Am. J. Clin. Nutr. 33 (1980) 2434−2439.

[227] A.C. Ouwehand, M. Derrien, W. de Vos, K. Tiihonen, N. Rautonen, Prebiotics and other microbial substrates for gut functionality, Curr. Opin. Biotechnol. 16 (2005) 212−217.

Nutritional Management of Inflammatory Bowel Disease and Short Bowel Syndrome

Jennifer L. Barnes, Kelly A. Tappenden

University of Illinois at Urbana-Champaign, Urbana, Illinois

I INFLAMMATORY BOWEL DISEASE

Crohn's disease and ulcerative colitis are the two most common forms of inflammatory bowel disease (IBD). Although the precise etiology is not known, evidence suggests that the body launches an immune response to a healthy, normal intestinal environment, resulting in inflammation. Inflammatory episodes range from mild to very severe and are often relapsing. During the past several decades, the prevalence of IBD, particularly Crohn's disease (CD), has been on the rise, indicating an environmental contribution, although the genetic component cannot be disputed. It has been suggested in the literature that people in Western countries are more likely to develop IBD, but perhaps not coincidentally; this is also where the greatest number of population-based studies are performed. Nevertheless, worldwide incidence estimates range from 0.5 to 24.5 cases for ulcerative colitis (UC) and from 0.1 to 16 cases for CD per 100,000 people per year [1,2], usually presenting in adolescence or young adulthood. Caucasians and individuals of Jewish descent show a greater incidence of IBD, females are at increased risk of CD compared to males, whereas no difference is observed in UC [3].

The cause of IBD is yet to be elucidated, but it is likely due to an unusually aggressive innate and adaptive immune response. This immune response is thought to be in response to intestinal bacteria and has a genetic component [4–6]. The microbiota, diet, and environment all deliver antigens to the gastrointestinal (GI) tract that can activate a potentially abnormal immune response, thereby initiating an IBD episode. These interactions are an active area of research. IBD significantly impacts the patient's health, quality of life, and, of course, nutritional status and relationship with food. Medications and other therapies employed in treating IBD can further compromise dietary intake and nutritional status.

Nutrition is a key component of any IBD care plan. Food choices can trigger or exacerbate, and even reduce, the symptoms of IBD. During active disease and following surgery, adequate nutrition provided in an absorbable form is critical to prevent deficiencies. This chapter reviews IBD and short bowel syndrome (SBS). Items covered for each include variants of the diagnosis, etiology, medical management, and medical nutrition therapy.

A Characteristics of IBD

CD and UC both result from a robust, cytokine-driven inflammation of the intestinal tract [5]. Several symptoms are shared by the two inflammatory conditions, but others are unique to either CD or UC. Individuals with CD or UC often experience weight loss and/or growth failure in children, abdominal pain, diarrhea, and an increased risk of colon cancer long-term [7,8]. Malabsorption results in macro- and micronutrient deficiencies with consequences such as anemia and metabolic bone disease. Some CD and UC patients experience arthritis and dermatologic manifestations due to the widespread inflammation. Table 39.1 presents common disease characteristics.

The key differences in CD are that inflammation can occur through the length of the GI tract and is not limited to the mucosa. Indeed, inflammation in CD is transmural, affecting the full thickness of the tissue. The anatomical location of the disease may change

Nutrition in the Prevention and Treatment of Disease, Third Edition.
DOI: http://dx.doi.org/10.1016/B978-0-12-391884-0.00039-1

TABLE 39.1   Characteristics of Crohn's Disease and Ulcerative Colitis

Crohn's disease	Ulcerative colitis	Both
Can occur in length of GI tract	Bloody diarrhea	Relapse and remission
Transmural	Anemia	Abdominal pain
Healthy mucosa interrupted with diseased mucosa	Limited to the colon	Diarrhea
Fistulas	Mucosal ulceration	Tenesmus
Strictures		Weight loss, growth failure
		Systemic inflammation
		Fever
		Increased risk of colorectal cancer

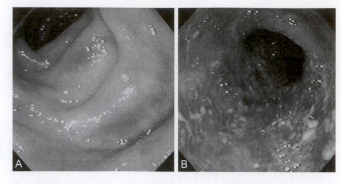

FIGURE 39.2   (A) Mild ulcerative colitis with some evidence of hemorrhage; (B) severe ulcerative colitis with extensive hemorrhage. Source: *Reprinted from* Sleisenger and Fordtran's Gastrointestinal and Liver Disease, *7th ed. Saunders W., Sleisenger M., Feldman M., 2002, with permission from Elsevier.* See color plate.

cases, and in both ileum and colon in 21% of cases [4]. Diseased tissue is often intermittent and surrounded by healthy tissue. Malabsorption, mucosal thickening, strictures, obstruction, abscess and fistula formation, and kidney stones are also more common with CD (Figure 39.1). On the other hand, UC is confined to the colon, and inflammation affects the mucosa only. Progression of UC differs from that of CD in that it characteristically begins at the most distal tissue and extends proximally in a continuous manner. The hallmark of UC is bloody diarrhea and mucus (Figure 39.2) [4,9,10]. Unlike CD, obstruction is rarely seen. Surgical resection of diseased tissues resulting in a colectomy cures UC, and approximately one-third of patients eventually require the procedure.

B Inflammatory Response in IBD

The normal inflammatory response is a protective action for the host and is generated to stimuli such as microbial invasion, trauma, or toxins. This initiates a cascade of events wherein leukocytes are recruited and proliferate [11,12]. Proinflammatory and regulatory cytokines, eicosanoids, proteases, and oxygen radicals are released. Clotting mechanisms, production of granular matrix, and fibrous tissue all serve to contain the new injury, microbial invasion, or toxin. Apoptosis, phagocytosis, and destruction of pathogens aid in resolution of the inflammatory trigger. Anti-inflammatory cytokines and eicosanoids are also important. If the inflammatory response is too robust, damage and ultimately dysfunction of tissue and organs can result.

IBD and its associated symptoms can be attributed to the prolonged and dysfunctional inflammatory response. Changes in intestinal mucosal architecture, strictures, bowel thickening, ulcerations, altered motility, and malabsorption are all examples of the

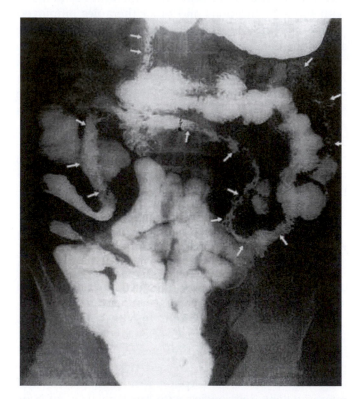

FIGURE 39.1   Radiologic image of patient with Crohn's disease. White arrows indicate areas of narrowed small intestine. Source: *Reprinted from* Sleisenger and Fordtran's Gastrointestinal and Liver Disease, *7th ed. Saunders W., Sleisenger M., Feldman M., 2002, with permission from Elsevier.*

over time, but it is most commonly found in the distal small intestine. Specifically, at diagnosis, CD is located in the ileum in 47% of cases, in the colon in 28% of consequences of the heightened inflammatory response [4,5,12]. Symptoms of fatigue, intestinal and extraintestinal pain, bloating, diarrhea, steatorrhea, weight loss, and malnutrition are manifestations of increased local and circulating levels of cytokines and other products of inflammation. Impaired intestinal permeability, local edema, ulceration, and damage to the intestinal structures may occur. Secretions, digestion, absorption, and motility may be abnormal, especially in active stages, and the normal barrier function may be compromised [4,5].

C What May Trigger the Onset or Exacerbation of IBD?

IBD is often an intermittent disease characterized by relapse and remission. Environmental factors can trigger relapse or help maintain remission, and knowledge of these factors is important for clinical management of these individuals. However, the potential triggers are many, including genetic and environmental contributions, and often difficult to predict. In addition, a number of years may elapse between histologic onset, symptoms, and IBD diagnosis. Microscopic or endoscopic evidence of the disease may occur long before clinical symptoms become apparent. Normal reactions to dietary indiscretions may cause GI symptoms (gas, bloating, pain, cramping, and diarrhea) and may be confused with active disease. Dietary factors considered to provoke active disease include high sugar intake, specific lipids, lack of dietary fiber (fruits and vegetables) [9,13–16], abnormal metabolism of sulfur-containing amino acids as in hyperhomocysteinemia [15,17], inadequate micronutrient intake such as folate [17,18] and vitamin D [19], and individual food intolerances or food allergies [4,13,15,16]. Breast-feeding and consumption of fruits, vegetables, dietary fiber, and n-3 lipids are considered protective [4,9,16,20].

D Medical Management of IBD

Several classes of medications are utilized to treat IBD. The most common categories of medications include anti-inflammatory agents, immunomodulator or immunosuppressive compounds, biologic agents, and antibiotics. These medicinal classes are used to induce and/or maintain remission and help to control complications of IBD. Drugs are also prescribed or recommended to treat specific symptoms, including antidiarrheal or antiemetic medications and antibiotics [21–23]. Although often helpful in managing IBD, in some cases, medications are not effective at inducing or maintaining remission even at high doses and for

TABLE 39.2 Medical Management of Inflammatory Bowel Disease

5-Aminosalicylic acid (anti-inflammatory)
Mesalamine, sulfasalazine
Corticosteroids
Prednisone, prednisolone
Immunosuppressives
Azathioprine, 6-mercaptopurine, methotrexate
Biologicals
Infiximab, adalimumab, etanercept, certolizumab
Antibiotics
Antimycobacterial, metronidazole

prolonged periods of time. Medications carry additional costs and short- and long-term side effects. A nutrition professional must always be aware of medications prescribed to patients and any potential drug–nutrient interactions. Table 39.2 lists medications commonly used in IBD.

E Surgical Treatment of IBD

Surgical intervention is often used to control CD and/or cure UC. Specific indications for surgery include severe, unrelenting disease; strictures; obstruction; hemorrhage; increasing risk of cancer; repair of fistulas; and failure of other medical therapy [9,10,24]. Because UC is restricted to the colon, a complete colectomy eliminates any further relapse and is considered curative. It is estimated that approximately 25–30% of patients with UC have surgery during their lifetime [25–27]. The most common surgical intervention is colectomy with the creation of an ileoanal pouch. An ileoanal pouch is created using folds of ileum that are pulled into the rectal canal and anastomosed to the ileum. This pouch develops a microbiota and serves to some degree as a colonic/rectal reservoir.

Unlike UC, surgical resection of severely involved segments of small or large bowel in CD does not bring resolution of the disease, and duration of clinical remission varies greatly. In fact, many patients experience relapse that may occur in months, whereas other patients appear to remain in remission for years. Approximately 70–80% of patients with CD eventually have at least one surgery during their lifetime [27]. Strictureplasty is a procedure to relieve narrowed segments of bowel generally caused by fibrous tissue. This procedure may be preferable because it helps to preserve intestinal tissue [28]. However, in some cases, patients with prolonged or severe episodes of CD have multiple resections resulting in SBS and the host of new nutritional considerations associated with that diagnosis (discussed later).

F Nutrition-Related Considerations in IBD

1 Macronutrients

Patients with IBD often experience anorexia and malabsorption as a consequence of the widespread inflammation [29–33]. Individuals may also avoid food due to unpleasant symptoms and perceived food intolerances, negatively influencing the amount and quality of food consumed. Weight loss, muscle wasting, growth failure, and delayed maturation are some of the most common problems in adults and children with IBD, particularly CD. Evidence of protein–energy malnutrition may include decreased levels of transport proteins such as albumin, transferrin, or prealbumin [34]. Decreased intake is further confounded by increased fecal loss of macronutrients during IBD flares.

Growth failure is observed in approximately 30% of pediatric CD patients and 5–10% of UC pediatric patients [35,36]. Permanent growth impairment is seen in 19–35% of children with CD but is rare in UC [37–39]. Indeed, an estimated 7–30% of pediatric patients with CD remain at less than the fifth percentile for height upon adulthood [40]. The etiology of growth failure is similar to that of weight loss and wasting in adults where anorexia and malabsorption are the primary causes [41].

2 Fluid and Electrolytes

Diarrhea is one of the most common symptoms exhibited in IBD [4,9]. Dehydration and electrolyte imbalances may occur in flares of IBD and after significant small bowel resections in CD. Several dietary factors, including specific carbohydrates and lipids, magnesium salts, and pre- and probiotics, may worsen or attenuate diarrhea and fluid losses [42–45].

3 Micronutrients

Micronutrient deficiencies including vitamin B_{12}, folate, zinc, calcium, iron, magnesium, selenium, copper, and vitamins A, D, and E have all been reported in IBD [34,46–49]. Anemia often results from lack of one or several micronutrients resulting from inadequate intake, malabsorption, increased requirements, and drug–nutrient interactions. Up to 70% of children and 40% of adults with IBD have anemia [46]. One of the most common symptoms of UC is blood in the feces. The bleeding colonic ulcerations may be responsible for iron-deficiency anemia rather than poor iron intake or malabsorption. CD patients who have undergone intestinal resection are at increased risk of micronutrient deficiencies. Vitamin B_{12} is exclusively absorbed in the distal ileum. Patients with ileal resections will likely require B_{12} supplementation. Micronutrient deficiencies may be more profound in CD patients, especially those who have undergone surgical resection [50,51].

G Nutrition Assessment in IBD

A comprehensive assessment is required when evaluating nutrition risk and considering nutritional interventions in IBD. Standard anthropometric measurements, including growth rate for age in children, weight and history of weight changes, body mass index, and skinfold thickness, are also important in IBD. Biochemical laboratory data reflect protein–energy and micronutrient status, as outlined in the previous section. Evaluation of the patient's medical and surgical history, including duration and severity of the disease, presence of strictures, fistulas, resections, and ostomies, is necessary to identify nutritional risk. Symptoms including diarrhea (stool volume, frequency, and duration) or malabsorption (increased fecal fat, very low serum cholesterol, abdominal cramping, bloating, or distention) also affect nutritional status. A careful diet history of typical food intake, quantity and quality of food choices, intolerance and aversions to various foods, and food allergies provides insight into macro- and micronutrient intake. IBD patients may utilize herbal or other nutrition supplements and alternative therapies, prescriptions, and over-the-counter medications, which may or may not influence the management of the disease. The nutrition assessment should also include an evaluation of the patient's knowledge and understanding of his or her nutritional status, needs, problems, and therapeutic options.

H Medical Nutrition Therapy in IBD

1 Goals of Medical Nutrition Therapy

The primary nutrition goals in IBD are to restore and maintain nutrition status, help control symptoms, and decrease inflammation. Nutrition counseling can also aid the patient in identifying and avoiding foods that exacerbate symptoms. Inadequate intake of protein, energy, and micronutrients may create changes in gastrointestinal barrier function and digestive functions and may also alter immune mechanisms. Individual dietary components may act as antioxidants, serve as precursors to inflammatory mediators, and alter the relative types of microbes existing in the GI tract. Nutritional rehabilitation may be required after acute or prolonged reduction in the quantity or quality of dietary intake. Special diets and supplements may be needed to provide adequate nourishment with complications such as SBS, strictures, or fistulas. Refeeding protocols may be appropriate after severe malnutrition, particularly aggressive bouts of the disease, or after surgical procedures. Nutrition may also have some role in the regulation of the inflammatory response and inducing or maintaining remission.

Nutrition counseling can also aid the patient in identifying and avoiding foods that exacerbate symptoms. Foods that may worsen symptoms in active disease or remission include but are not limited to lactose, gluten, alcohol, spices, and salt, particularly in patients being treated with corticosteroids. Intolerances are highly individualized and should be treated on a case-by-case basis. In addition, patients may choose to avoid foods they perceive as responsible for adverse symptoms such as diarrhea, abdominal pain, nausea, and bloating. Medications can also influence appetite and gastrointestinal-related symptoms, resulting in decreased intake, increased malabsorption, and/or altered requirement for nutrients. Restoration of nutritional status may include a carefully considered oral diet, any combination of vitamin and mineral supplements, and enteral and/or parenteral nutrition.

2 Energy and Protein Requirements

The energy requirements of persons with IBD are not generally increased compared to those of the average person. However, under conditions of further stress such as sepsis and fever, requirements are elevated. Other scenarios wherein increased energy is indicated include weight restoration, return to normal growth velocity in children, and to compensate for malnutrition. Regardless, the presence of active disease alone does not appear to raise energy requirements appreciably [52,53]. Protein needs may be increased significantly because of gastrointestinal nitrogen losses, the inflammatory response, and the need for new tissue for weight gain and growth.

3 Parenteral Nutrition during Active IBD

In previous years, parenteral nutrition (PN) was a primary therapy in IBD, particularly CD. PN aids in restoration of nutritional status by providing sufficient nutrition for growth and weight gain. It was observed that patients on PN appeared to enter remission. This initiated a protocol wherein PN was provided as a means of "bowel rest" [54–57]. However, the concept of bowel rest is no longer in favor. According to the 2009 European Society of Parenteral and Enteral Nutrition (ESPEN) guidelines on PN in gastroenterology, PN is not indicated as a primary therapy in the treatment of CD or UC [40,58]. PN is indicated in patients with obstruction, perforation, complicated fistula, SBS, or a nonfunctioning GI tract that precludes adequate enteral nutrition. Withholding oral/enteral nutrition can also be considered undesirable because it may compromise gut integrity, including atrophy of the intestinal mucosa [59,60]. In addition, PN does not contain the phytonutrients found in a complex, whole food diet.

4 Enteral Nutrition during Active IBD

Enteral nutrition is the route of choice for nutrition support whenever possible. In almost all studies, CD appears to be more amenable to enteral treatment than UC, although different forms of nutrition interventions (other than standard enteral formulas) may be of value in UC. Guidelines from ESPEN [61] cite that enteral feeding is first-line therapy in CD and should be used as sole therapy in adults when treatment with steroids is not feasible. Undernourished patients with CD or UC should receive oral or tube-fed supplements.

The most robust evidence based reviews of the CD literature [61,62] indicate that medicinal corticosteroid treatment is more effective than enteral nutrition for the acute phase of UC and CD. However, when considering enteral nutrition alone, a clear superior choice among elemental and polymeric formulas is not seen. Exclusive enteral feeding appears to be more effective than partial enteral nutrition, whereas lower fat formulas are more favorable. Remission rates in the individual studies ranged from 20 to 84%. Overall, enteral diets have the advantage of providing/restoring nutritional status and reducing the risks of medications. The majority of reports indicate that mucosal healing is more likely to occur with enteral feeding than with steroids. The possible mechanisms for these benefits include an altered antigen load and positive alterations in the gastrointestinal microbiota resulting in improved structure and function of the mucosal layer. Enteral nutrition is not generally recommended for UC patients during active disease; however, patients with poor oral intake or deficiencies may be candidates [61]. Most enteral feedings are based on one or two protein sources compared to hundreds of potential proteins consumed during even a simple daily diet. Enteral feedings are typically sterile and well-fortified with vitamins, minerals, and trace elements. They are normally relatively low in fat, contain at least small amounts of n-3 fatty acids, but lack the phytochemicals provided by a complex, whole food diet.

5 Emerging Nutrients Therapies and Bioactives

Specific nutrients and other dietary interventions may aid in managing IBD flares and inducing and maintaining remission. This is an emerging area of research, with probiotics, prebiotics, short-chain fatty acids (SCFA), and omega-3 fatty acids being the most commonly investigated. In each instance, the mechanism of action is believed to be a reduction in the regulatory response.

A PROBIOTICS

Probiotics are traditionally defined as live microorganisms that when ingested in adequate amounts, confer health benefits on the host. Probiotics are of interest to modify the microbiota population; modulate intestinal immunity and inflammation; and for their ability to influence antigen tolerance, cytokine levels, and adhesion mechanisms [63–66]. UC and probiotics have been more thoroughly investigated compared to CD. VSL#3, a probiotic supplement containing *Bifidobacterium breve*, *Bifidobacterium longum*, *Bifidobacterium infantis*, *Lactobacillus acidophilus*, *Lactobacillus plantarum*, *Lactobacillus paracasei*, *Lactobacillus bulgaricus*, and *Streptococcus thermophilus*, has shown efficacy in decreasing evidence and symptoms of active disease and inducing remission [67,68]. Similar effects, including decreased markers of inflammation, are reported with *Lactobacillus delbrukeii* and *Lactobacillus fermentum* in UC [69]. A meta-analysis concluded that probiotics are better at maintaining remission of UC compared to placebo [70]. Probiotics in the meta-analysis included VSL#3, *Bifidobacterium* species, *Lactobacillus* species, and *Escherichia coli* Nissle 1917. It is important to note that probiotic supplementation often occurs in tandem with traditional medicinal therapy. Unlike UC, results of the human intervention trials with probiotics for treating CD have not been very successful [71,72]. Probiotics, including VSL#3, *Lactobacillus rhamnosus*, and *Bifidobacterium*, also have considerable evidence of effectiveness in maintaining remission from pouchitis, the inflammatory state that occurs in the "pouch" surgically created from distal loops of ileum after colectomy [73–76].

B PREBIOTICS AND SCFA

Prebiotics are functional fibers that selectively stimulate grow of beneficial gut microbiota and are fermented to SCFA. SCFA, specifically butyrate, have been shown to decrease markers of inflammation, primarily through decreasing NF-κB [77–80]. However, a study investigating the efficacy of fructo-oligosaccharides, a prebiotic, on active CD found no benefit compared to placebo [81]. Synbiotics, the combination of pre- and probiotics, have exhibited benefit in both CD and UC [82,83].

C OMEGA-3 FATTY ACIDS

Fatty acids are unique in their ability not only to provide energy but also to influence the inflammatory state in IBD and other inflammatory diseases. The Western diet greatly favors n-6 polyunsaturated fatty acids compared to n-3 fatty acids. Omega-6 and omega-3 fatty acids are incorporated into cell membranes and affect the physical, chemical, and functional properties of the cell and cell wall [84–86]. The lipids also serve as precursors for potent mediators in many physiologic reactions, including the immune and inflammatory response. The n-6 and n-3 polyunsaturated fatty acids are metabolized to eicosanoids, which are important in regulating the inflammatory state. Eicosanoids produced from n-6 fatty acids, including arachidonic and linoleic acids, are proinflammatory and encourage blood clotting and thrombosis. Conversely, eicosanoids produced from n-3 fatty acids are anti-inflammatory and decrease cellular adherence. Data from animal and human studies show that consumption of a high n-6:n-3 fatty acid ratio results in increased peripheral proinflammatory cytokines tumor necrosis factor-α, interleukin (IL)-6 and IL-1 concentrations, membrane permeability, edema, and increased reactive oxygen species—all consistent with an increased inflammatory state. Similarly, diets containing n-3 fatty acids have been shown to decrease gene expression of inflammatory cytokines, increase anti-inflammatory resolvins, and alter signaling pathways in the inflammatory response, with the majority of the data from cardiovascular disease.

Clinical trial evidence for n-3 fatty acids in the management of IBD is conflicting. Cochrane evidence-based reviews concluded that omega-3 fatty acids in both CD and UC did not improve maintenance of remission [87,88]. A trial by Nielsen and colleagues [89] reported a decrease in proinflammatory cytokines after omega-3 supplementation compared to omega-6 during active CD. Turner *et al.* [88] recommend that future investigations utilize enteric coated capsules to ensure intact delivery to the inflamed tissue.

I Nutrition in IBD Remission

The majority of patients with IBD can achieve a full oral diet during disease remission. Individuals with extreme short bowel after surgical resection secondary to CD are the primary examples of who may require additional support to maintain nutritional status (see Section II). Characteristics of a healthy diet during IBD remission are similar to those of an individual without IBD. Fruits and vegetables are excellent sources of antioxidant nutrients that help to reduce oxidative stress. A low omega-6:omega-3 fatty acid ratio encourages production of anti-inflammatory eicosanoids. Consuming sources of fermentable fiber will increase fermentation and therefore butyrate production in the large intestine. Foods that are not well tolerated should be identified on an individual basis. The nutrition professional can not only help identify food items that increase symptoms but also offer suggestions on alternatives and label reading. Pre- and/or probiotics may be indicated for some patients. Small frequent meals can also help to increase tolerance. Individuals continuing to suffer from malabsorption or who are unable to consume and/or absorb adequate nutrients from food in their diet may require supplementation of macro- and micronutrients.

II SHORT BOWEL SYNDROME

A Definition

Short bowel syndrome is best defined functionally rather than by anatomical length of residual intestine.

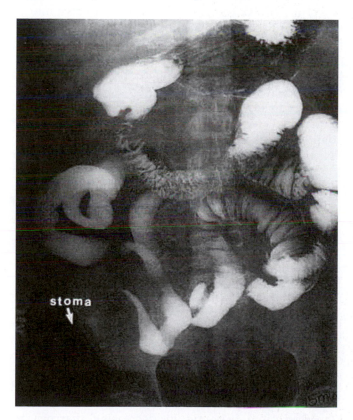

FIGURE 39.3 Radiologic image of patient following intestinal resection. *Source: Reprinted from* Sleisenger and Fordtran's Gastrointestinal and Liver Disease, *7th ed. Saunders W., Sleisenger M., Feldman M., 2002, with permission from Elsevier.*

SBS is due to surgical resection of intestinal tissue resulting in a decrease in functional surface area and malabsorption [90—92]. Intestinal failure (IF) is defined as a decrease in functional intestinal mass below the amount required for digestion and absorption to meet the body's needs, be it growth in pediatric patients or maintenance in adult patients, and results in dependence on PN [93,94]. SBS is a common cause of IF wherein the individual's previously normal enteral nutrient intake is not enough to support growth and/or maintain weight due to malabsorption of macronutrients, micronutrients, fluid, electrolytes, and endogenous secretions. Deficiencies are common, with the severity of such depending on the amount and location of resection, age, and disease activity in the remaining intestinal tissue. Complications due to SBS include weight loss, growth retardation, diarrhea, dehydration, electrolyte disturbances, bone loss, renal oxalate stones, gallstones, lactic acidosis, and bacterial overgrowth, depending on the anatomical nature of the resection, function of the residual intestine, and age/growth status of the patient (Figure 39.3) [95,96].

B Causes

In adults, the most common causes of SBS are mesenteric infarction, small intestine volvulus, CD, obstruction, trauma, and radiation [97—99]. Causes of pediatric SBS can be prenatal, neonatal, or postnatal and include atresia, volvulus, Hirschsprung's disease, necrotizing enterocolitis, and IBD [93,94]. Table 39.3 presents the causes of pediatric SBS.

TABLE 39.3 Etiologies of Pediatric Short Bowel Syndrome

Prenatal	Neonatal	Postnatal
Atresia (unique or multiple)	Midgut volvulus (midgut or segmental)	Midgut volvulus (malrotation, bands, or tumor)
Apple peel syndrome	Necrotizing enterocolitis	Complicated intussusceptions
Midgut volvulus (malrotation)	Arterial thrombosis	Arterial thrombosis
Segmental volvulus (with omphalomesenteric duct or intra-abdominal bands)	Venous thrombosis	Inflammatory bowel disease
Abdominal wall defects		
Gastroschisis omphalocele		
Extensive Hirschsprung's disease		

Source: Reprinted from Gastroenterology, *Vol. 130, No. 2 Suppl. 1, Goulet O., Ruemmele F., Causes and management of intestinal failure in children, pp. S116—S128, 2006, with permission from Elsevier.*

C Predictors of the Severity and Prognosis in SBS

The prognosis for SBS can range from a temporary condition with less extreme intestinal resections to permanent in instances in which little functional intestinal tissue remains. Symptoms appear immediately after resection and continue until sufficient adaptation occurs and/or medical, nutritional, or surgical interventions are successful. The length, location, and function of the remaining intestinal tissue and overall health of the patient greatly impact the need for nutrition support, the severity and duration of symptoms, and survival. Patients who survive without PN tend to have fewer adverse symptoms and are at decreased nutritional risk. It is well-established that the ileum maintains a greater compensatory capacity compared to the jejunum [100–102]. In addition, the ileocecal valve plays an integral role in releasing chyme from the small intestine to the large intestine and keeping bacteria in the colon [103]. Therefore, patients who are very young, have remaining distal ileum and ileocecal valve, have colon-in-continuity, and are otherwise healthy and well-nourished have the best prognosis. Alternatively, qualities of a poor prognosis include loss of terminal ileum and ileocecal valve, advanced age at resection, loss of the colon in addition to small bowel, and the presence of residual gastrointestinal disease [95,104]. These patient attributes often result in dependence on large volumes of PN support, increased nutritional risk, and decreased quality of life.

D Intestinal Adaptation

Following intestinal resection, the remaining intestine undergoes dynamic structural and functional adaptation to compensate for the loss in tissue. Much of the data detailing intestinal adaptation are from

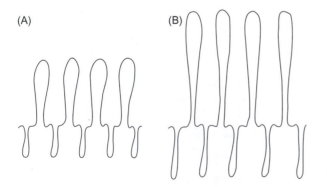

FIGURE 39.4 (A) Normal epithelium; (B) adapted epithelium with increased villus height and crypt depth following small bowel resection. *Source: Reprinted from* Gastroenterology, *Vol. 113, No. 5, Vanderhoof J. A., Langnas A. N., Short-bowel syndrome in children and adults, pp. 1767–1778, 1997, with permission from Elsevier.*

animal models and include lengthening and dilation of the residual bowel and increased proliferation [105–107]. This results in greater absorptive surface area through increased villus height and crypt depth (Figure 39.4). Importantly, nutrient transport is also upregulated. These adaptations are also observed in humans [101,108,109]. As mentioned previously, the ileum has the greatest potential for adaptation, although adaptation does occur through the length of the residual intestine [100,102].

E Massive Intestinal Resections in Infants

The same risk factors for increased morbidity apply in infants, including loss of ileum, ileocecal valve, and colon, except that infants adapt significantly better after resections than do adults. Healthy infants and children experience incredible intestinal growth from *in utero* until early adulthood. According to Weaver and colleagues [110], the small intestine doubles in length from 20 to 40 weeks of gestation and nearly doubles again from term (275 cm) to age 10 years (500 cm). Infants are reported to survive independent of PN with as little as approximately 30–60 cm of small bowel if they have retained the ileocecal valve and as little as 30–100 cm without the ileocecal valve [110,111]. When the ileocecal valve is lost, retained colon becomes more important for maintenance of electrolyte balance and adequate hydration and to salvage malabsorbed substrates.

For pediatric patients with extremely short lengths of residual functional intestine, who cannot fully adapt, several options remain. They can remain on PN, undergo small bowel lengthening procedures, or submit to small bowel transplantation. PN, although lifesaving, imposes on the quality of life for the patient and caretakers and carries increased risk of infection, cholestasis and hepatic failure, gallstone formation, and nutrient deficiencies.

F Medical Management of SBS

Patients with SBS may also be treated with several medications to improve symptoms, decrease GI secretions, delay gastric emptying, slow intestinal transit, and/or bind bile acids. Antisecretory drugs such as proton pump inhibitors or histamine-2 receptor blockers are used in the initial stages of gastric acid hypersecretion that follows intestinal resection. Cholestyramine may aid in decreasing diarrhea by binding bile acids within the intestinal lumen and reduce the osmotic load present within the distal intestine [94]. Antimotility agents are utilized to slow transit time and extend the window of absorption.

Conversely, prokinetic agents may be necessary to relieve symptoms such as abdominal distention and vomiting. Small intestine bacterial overgrowth is most commonly managed with antibiotic therapy. Table 39.4 provides a list of common medications utilized in SBS.

Glucagon-like peptide-2 (GLP-2) is an intestinotrophic hormone secreted from the distal intestine. Animal models indicate that GLP-2 enhances intestinal adaptation following experimental resection [112–116]. A GLP-2 analog, teduglutide, is currently in phase III clinical trials. GLP-2 or teduglutide has shown efficacy by decreasing stomal energy output, increasing urine output, increasing wet weight absorption, and increasing body weight and lean body mass [117,118]. Increased villus height and crypt depth and decreased PN volume were reported in a study that included 83 patients who received teduglutide for 24 weeks [119,120]. Depending on the outcome of additional studies, GLP-2 may become an important component of SBS care by stimulating the adaptation of the residual intestine.

G Surgical Interventions in SBS

Although total PN is a lifesaving measure and has improved the prognosis for SBS and IF patients, serious complications exist, including catheter sepsis and PN-associated liver disease. Currently, there are several surgical procedures performed to lengthen the residual intestine. In longitudinal intestinal lengthening and tailoring or the Bianchi procedure, the dilated bowel is divided in half longitudinally, creating two loops of bowel, which are anastamosed together, doubling the intestinal length [121]. The serial transverse enteroplasty (STEP), first reported in a porcine model in 2003, is another lengthening procedure. STEP involves stapling the dilated bowel in a zigzag pattern

to increase absorptive surface area [122]. Small intestinal and multivisceral transplants have now become more successful for patients with IF and are indicated when complications of long-term PN arise, such as PN-associated liver disease [123–125]. There are several forms of small bowel transplant, including small intestinal segments alone, small intestine with colon, and intestine with liver and/or pancreatic transplant. Transplant procedures and immunosuppressive therapies continue to improve and with time may provide more viable options for more patients with severe SBS.

H Nutrition-Related Considerations in SBS

Careful consideration of the anatomical location of resection, if known, and corresponding digestive and absorptive function is necessary for optimal nutrition therapy in SBS (Figure 39.5). SBS can be classified based on resected tissue, which aids in predicting the severity and nutritional risk.

1 Jejunal Resections with Intact Ileum and Colon

The jejunum is the primary site of absorption for lipids, monosaccharides, peptides, and amino acids as well as a host of vitamins and minerals. As mentioned previously, the ileum has the capacity to adapt and restore much of the lost functionality over time. With this in mind, pediatric and adult jejunal resection patients experience relatively mild malabsorption as long as the patient and the remaining GI tract are healthy. PN may initially be required, but small,

TABLE 39.4 Medical Management of Short Bowel Syndrome

Antimotility
Loperamide
Prokinetic
Metoclopramide, erythromycin, cisapride
Immunosuppressive
Azathioprine, 6-mercaptopurine, methotrexate
Antisecretory
Octreotide, cholestyramine
Antibiotics
Metronidazole

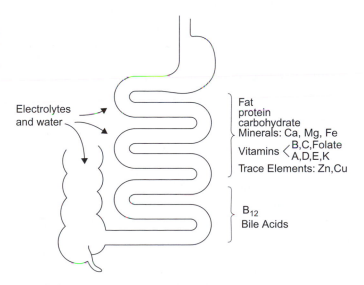

FIGURE 39.5 Sites of nutrient absorption in the healthy gastrointestinal tract. Source: *Reprinted from* Sleisenger and Fordtran's Gastrointestinal and Liver Disease, *7th ed. Saunders W., Sleisenger M., Feldman M., 2002, with permission from Elsevier.*

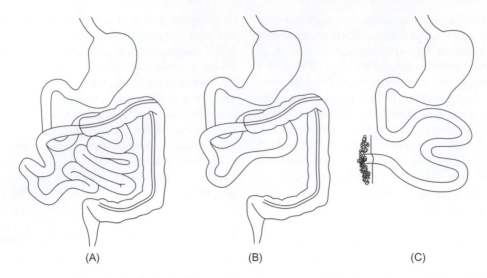

FIGURE 39.6 Common types of intestinal resection include (A) jejunal resections, (B) ileal resections, and (C) end jejunostomy with resection of the ileum and colon. Source: *Reprinted from* Sleisenger and Fordtran's Gastrointestinal and Liver Disease, *7th ed. Saunders W., Sleisenger M., Feldman M., 2002, with permission from Elsevier.*

frequent snacks and beverages may also be provided. Enteral nutrients encourage adaptation of the remaining intestine that will begin immediately and occur for the next several months to years. Ultimately, the patient should be able to consume oral meals with limited restrictions and minimal compromise in digestive and absorptive capacity. Food items containing lactose may be problematic for patients without a jejunum because lactase is primarily located in the proximal small intestine. Many patients with SBS experience decreased transit time wherein the digesta moves more rapidly through the GI tract, resulting in limited tolerance of large quantities of hyperosmolar or highly concentrated foods and beverages. In most cases, macronutrient, micronutrient, and fluid balance are not substantially disrupted, although these should be monitored. Iron, calcium, magnesium, and lipid-soluble nutrients may be slightly compromised (Figure 39.6).

2 Ileal Resections

Although the ileum is not the major site of digestion and absorption of most nutrients, it is critical for vitamin B_{12}, remaining fat-soluble vitamins, bile salts, and acids. The jejunum does not exhibit the level of adaptation achieved by the ileum, resulting in malabsorption of ileum-exclusive nutrients. Whereas adults consume approximately 2 liters of fluid daily, the proximal small intestine secretes a much greater volume of 7−9 liters per day. The healthy intestine is capable of reabsorbing the majority of these secretions with only 1−1.5 liters entering the colon, where approximately 100 ml is lost to the feces. The ileum is the primary location of fluid reabsorption. Following ileal resection, the jejunum

and colon are challenged to compensate for the lost functional tissue.

The distal ileum is the sole absorption site for several important nutrients and digestive secretions. First, the distal ileum is the primary location for vitamin B_{12} absorption. Depending on the site of ileal resection, it is common for patients to require vitamin B_{12} injections. Second, the distal ileum is the sole site of bile acid reabsorption. Bile salts serve as emulsifiers, breaking up lipid droplets, increasing surface area for lipases, and facilitating formation of micelles. After ileal resection, unabsorbed bile acids result in a significant malabsorption cascade. Normally, bile acids are absorbed and reused through enterohepatic circulation. Without enterohepatic circulation, the liver cannot fully compensate with *de novo* synthesis, resulting in malabsorption of lipid and lipid-soluble nutrients. In addition, unabsorbed bile acids stimulate secretion within the colonic mucosa. This confounds the already burdened colon with the additional fluid needing absorption and exacerbates diarrhea. The unabsorbed lipid-containing molecules can also decrease bioavailability of calcium, magnesium, and zinc.

Patients with ileal resections are at increased risk of developing kidney stones. Under normal conditions, dietary oxalate binds calcium and other divalent cations, forming insoluble complexes. Following surgery, free oxalate becomes available for absorption in the colon. In the case of SBS, kidney stones occur when the concentrations of calcium and oxalate increase in the urine. Supplemental calcium and dietary oxalate restriction is often indicated to reduce absorption of oxalate and improve colonic fluid and electrolyte absorption [95,126]. Dietary sources of oxalate include berries, chocolate, coffee, tea, nuts, and green leafy vegetables such as kale and spinach.

Loss of the ileum, and especially the ileocecal valve, puts individuals with SBS at risk of small bacterial overgrowth. The ileocecal valve or sphincter provides a one-way outlet from the small intestine to the colon and is responsible for keeping colonic contents in the large intestine. However, resection of the ileocecal valve increases the likelihood of large intestine bacteria entering the small intestine. Small intestine bacterial overgrowth is an increase or alteration in the number and/or type of bacteria in the small intestine [127]. Bacterial overgrowth is usually treated with antibiotics, but pre- and probiotics may also be efficacious [128]. D-Lactic acidosis can also occur, especially in SBS patients with ileal resections and colon-in-continuity. As carbohydrates are malabsorbed and reach the colon in larger quantities, the production of D-lactate increases and it enters the bloodstream [129], resulting in metabolic acidosis and neurologic symptoms. This can be exacerbated when small intestine bacterial overgrowth is also present.

3 End Jejunostomy (Loss of Ileum and Colon)

The loss of both the ileum and the colon renders hydration maintenance difficult. Electrolytes, magnesium, and energy balance are all impaired. These patients are left with only a jejunum and consequently present with poor fluid absorption, not only of consumed but also of endogenously secreted fluids. Evidence of decreased absorptive capability is seen in jejunostomies, exceeding 3–5 liters daily in some cases. The fecal output contains large amounts of sodium and other electrolytes, resulting in increased risk of hypovolemia, hypokalemia, and hypomagnesemia and other forms of nutrient depletion [95,98,126].

The distal intestine is integral not only to the absorption of nutrients but also to endocrine function. The presence of chyme in the distal ileum and colon is responsible for stimulating release of neuropeptide hormones with vast physiologic consequences. These hormones modulate gene expression, immunologic and neurologic activity, endocrine secretions, transport mechanisms, and muscular activity [130,131]. Examples of these hormones are GLP-1, GLP-2, and peptide YY. These regulatory mechanisms, such as the ileal brake regulated by peptide YY, are severely compromised in SBS.

The colon is the site of bacterial fermentation of non-digestible carbohydrates and other substrates. This fermentation is of great benefit to the host by salvaging the energy that would otherwise be lost to feces. SBS results in a much greater portion of macronutrients reaching the colon compared to a healthy GI tract.

Healthy persons receive approximately 5–10% of energy from colonic fermentation [118]. Nordgaard and colleagues [132] compared fecal energy loses in patients with and without a colon via bomb calorimetry and reported that the amount of energy salvage was dependent on the residual small intestine. Individuals with 150–200 cm of remaining small intestine but no colon excreted 0.8 MJ/day (110 kcal) more than those with an intact colon. When patients had 100 cm or less residual small bowel, preservation of the colon for energy salvage from malabsorbed substrates clearly became more important. Colectomy resulted in loss of 4.9 MJ/day (~1150 kcal). Overall, end jejunostomy (loss of the ileum and colon) results in severely impaired fluid and electrolyte absorption, energy imbalance, nutrient deficiencies, decreased transit time, and a loss of energy salvage.

I Nutrition Assessment in SBS

Nutrition assessment in the SBS patient involves accurate measurement of current weight and weight history, height, and body composition by measuring skin folds or other available methods. For pediatric patients, anthropometrics should be compared to standardized growth charts. Surgical history and radiologic examination aid in determining the anatomical location and length of residual bowel, which will influence individual nutrition concerns. Hydration status evaluation includes stoma or stool output, serum electrolytes, and urine sodium content [95,133]. Serum proteins such as albumin, transferrin, prealbumin, and hematological assessment can also help establish nutrition status. Vitamin- and mineral-specific laboratory tests are also available.

Determining the level of intestinal function in the residual tissue is a challenge in the clinical setting. Steatorrhea and fecal levels of macronutrients are the current gold standard [134]. A relatively new proposed measure of intestinal functional mass is plasma concentration of the amino acid citrulline, a metabolite not inserted into proteins and produced almost exclusively by the enterocytes. Studies indicate a strong correlation between plasma citrulline concentration and residual intestine length [135–138]; however, the evidence is conflicting with regard to the use of citrulline to predict function [136–138].

J Medical Nutrition Therapy in SBS

The majority of SBS patients require PN following surgical resection, especially individuals with an end jejunostomy. The ultimate goal of nutrition support in the immediate postoperative phase is to restore and maintain hydration status. Depending on the stability of the patient and the amount of residual intestine, small amounts of oral nutrients may be provided [40]. During this time, urine volume, urine sodium content, and blood glucose should be monitored closely [139]. Enteral and/or oral nutrition should be initiated as soon as they are tolerated, with continued parenteral support as needed. Although there is no clearly superior formula in the literature, elemental enteral formulas may be beneficial in patients with rapid transit and severe malabsorption [61,140,141]. As oral nutrients are introduced, patients at greatest risk of dehydration, including jejunostomy patients, should be encouraged to sip on oral rehydration solutions. Electrolytes including sodium, potassium, and magnesium should be closely monitored.

Many patients, particularly those with an intact colon, progress to a fully oral diet. Weaning from PN should not be considered until all other aspects of care are stabilized, including medications and fluid management [142]. DiBaise and colleagues [142] recommend patients achieve 80% of energy needs orally before complete PN weaning is initiated. Educational counseling with goal setting should occur before weaning is attempted. Individuals with colon-in-continuity are more likely to achieve independence from PN, although patients without a colon may also be successful [143]. However, the colon does help in maintaining fluid balance and salvaging energy via fermentation. These patients with colon-in-continuity are generally more successful on a high-carbohydrate, low-fat diet [144]. Depending on location of resection, micronutrients may need to be supplemented and should be closely monitored. Certain micronutrients, such as magnesium and vitamin B_{12}, may need to be administered intravenously if absorption is not adequate. Oral nutrition solutions or enteral feedings may be recommended if oral whole food intake is inadequate [61]. Adaptive hyperphagia, or oral consumption at least 1.5 times greater than calculated energy needs, occurs in most patients with SBS and may be helpful in the adaptive process and for maintaining energy balance [145]. This biologic compensatory action should be encouraged, based on tolerance.

K Nutrients for Intestinal Adaptation

There is great interest in strategically formulating the diet in SBS patients to maximize intestinal adaptation. Beginning soon after resection and continuing for months to several years, intestinal adaptation is a dynamic process that can be influenced by nutrition. Much of the data for specific interventions are from animal models and include adaptations such as increased bowel length and dilation, enhanced mucosal architecture including villus height and crypt depth yielding increased absorptive surface area, as well as increased nutrient transport [105−107]. There is also a body of evidence supporting these adaptations in humans [101,108,109].

1 Monomeric Versus Polymeric Enteral Formulas

Monomeric formulas consist of hydrolyzed amino acids, whereas polymeric formulas contain whole proteins. An intermediate, semi-elemental formula is composed of oligopeptides averaging four or five amino acids in length. When considering monomeric and polymeric enteral formulas, the optimal enteral composition is controversial [93] and the data are conflicting. Elemental formula has been reported to aid in weaning from PN in a small sample size of 4 pediatric SBS patients [146]; however, a randomized, crossover double-blind trial of 10 pediatric SBS patients failed to detect a difference between a hydrolyzed and an intact nutrient formula [147]. No clear choice between monomeric and polymeric emerges from the current literature.

2 Glutamine and Growth Hormone

Glutamine is an important energy source for enterocytes and has been investigated for inducing adaptation in SBS; however, glutamine alone does not seem to be efficacious [148]. Glutamine is often supplemented in combination with growth hormone, and benefits such as increased remnant bowel length and improved architecture are reported in animal models [149,150]. Human studies indicate an increase in plasma proteins, weaning from PN in a portion of studied patients, and increased macronutrient and electrolyte absorption [151−154]. Studies reporting no beneficial effect [155,156] and/or a return to baseline following treatment cessation also exist in the literature [152,157]. Adverse events attributable to growth hormone are also commonly reported [154−157]. In all, the evidence from an intestinal adaptation perspective is not promising and difficult to interpret. In fact, a commercial growth hormone pharmaceutical targeted for SBS, Zorbtive, has seen limited success [158].

3 Fish Oil

Linolenic acid is an essential omega-3 fatty acid found in fish oil and is necessary to synthesize eicosapentaenoic acid (EPA) and docosahexenoic acid (DHA). EPA serves as a precursor to eicosanoids including thromboxanes, prostaglandins, and leukotrienes, which modulate inflammation and thrombosis, as discussed previously. Pediatric intestinal failure-associated liver disease is a life-threatening complication associated with PN; however, promising evidence suggests that fish oil lipid emulsions may reduce the risk and even reverse the disease [159−161]. Fish oil, delivered enterally or systemically, is also being investigated for its potential intestinotrophic properties. Studies utilizing intestinal resection rat models demonstrate an increase in structural and functional adaptation [162−164]. Fish oil as an intestinal adaptation modulator is a new concept; thus, well-designed human trials are lacking, with most studies being observational.

4 Butyrate

Acetate, propionate, and butyrate are the primary SCFA produced in the human intestine through fermentation of nondigestible carbohydrates by anaerobic bacteria. Butyrate is an energy source for colonocytes, is absorbed with sodium and water, and has intestinotrophic properties. Human studies are lacking, but strong animal data suggest that butyrate stimulates structural and functional adaptations of the residual intestine [165−168]. Although the mechanism remains to be determined, it is hypothesized that GLP-2 may be involved.

5 Pre- and Probiotics

Pre- and probiotics are used alone or in combination in SBS, specifically for use in adaptation and managing small intestine bacterial overgrowth. Probiotic supplementation in rats including a mixture of *L. acidophilus*, *Bifidobacteria*, and *S. thermophilus* and also *L. rhamnosus* GG (LGG) alone resulted in increased indices of intestinal architecture such as villus height and crypt depth [169,170]. Few intervention trials have been completed in humans with SBS; however, a double-blind, placebo-controlled, crossover clinical trial in pediatric SBS patients observed no effect of LGG on intestinal permeability [171]. A pediatric case study reported successful treatment of small intestine bacterial overgrowth with the synbiotic combination of *B. breve*, *Lactobacillus casei*, and the prebiotic, galacto-oligosaccharides [128]. Interestingly, two other studies utilizing the same synbiotic treatment reported decreased pathogenic bacteria in the feces, increased fecal SCFA, accelerated weight gain, and decreased nutrition support [172,173].

III CONCLUSIONS

IBD and SBS are gastrointestinal diseases with profound nutritional consequences. CD and UC are inflammatory conditions with an etiology yet to be determined, whereas SBS is a functional disorder resulting from intestinal resection. Continued scientific advances in medicine and nutritional science provide a rich and ever-evolving body of knowledge that continues to improve the prognosis for individuals with IBD and SBS. In both IBD and SBS, medical and surgical treatments are often necessary and can impact nutritional status. Medical nutrition therapy often takes the form of parenteral and/or enteral nutrition but in most cases is temporary. Emerging research suggests that nutrients can aid in decreasing inflammation in IBD and increase adaptation in SBS. It is imperative that clinicians carefully follow the nutrition intervention research in IBD and SBS to stay up-to-date on the most effective treatments.

References

[1] C.S. Gismera, B.S. Aladren, Inflammatory bowel diseases: a disease(s) of modern times? is incidence still increasing? World J. Gastroenterol. 14 (2008) 5491−5498.

[2] P.L. Lakatos, Recent trends in the epidemiology of inflammatory bowel diseases: up or down? World J. Gastroenterol. 12 (2006) 6102−6108.

[3] E. Langholz, Current trends in inflammatory bowel disease: the natural history, Therap. Adv. Gastroenterol. 3 (2010) 77−86.

[4] D.C. Baumgart, W.J. Sandborn, Inflammatory bowel disease: clinical aspects and established and evolving therapies, Lancet 369 (2007) 1641−1657.

[5] W. Strober, I. Fuss, P. Mannon, The fundamental basis of inflammatory bowel disease, J. Clin. Invest. 117 (2007) 514−521.

[6] K.J. Maloy, F. Powrie, Intestinal homeostasis and its breakdown in inflammatory bowel disease, Nature 474 (2011) 298−306.

[7] D. Burger, S. Travis, Conventional medical management of inflammatory bowel disease, Gastroenterology 140 (2011) 1827−1837.

[8] T.A. Ullman, S.H. Itzkowitz, Intestinal inflammation and cancer, Gastroenterology 140 (2011) 1807−1816.

[9] R.M. Beattie, N.M. Croft, J.M. Fell, N.A. Afzal, R.B. Heuschkel, Inflammatory bowel disease, Arch. Dis. Child. 91 (2006) 426−432.

[10] R.R. Cima, J.H. Pemberton, Medical and surgical management of chronic ulcerative colitis, Arch. Surg. 140 (2005) 300−310.

[11] T. Lawrence, D.W. Gilroy, Chronic inflammation: a failure of resolution? Int. J. Exp. Pathol. 88 (2007) 85−94.

[12] A. Meneghin, C.M. Hogaboam, Infectious disease, the innate immune response, and fibrosis, J. Clin. Invest. 117 (2007) 530−538.

[13] E.V. Loftus Jr., Clinical epidemiology of inflammatory bowel disease: Incidence, prevalence, and environmental influences, Gastroenterology 126 (2004) 1504−1517.

[14] S. Danese, C. Fiocchi, Etiopathogenesis of inflammatory bowel diseases, World J. Gastroenterol. 12 (2006) 4807−4812.

[15] J.R. Korzenik, Past and current theories of etiology of IBD: toothpaste, worms, and refrigerators, J. Clin. Gastroenterol. 39 (2005) S59−S65.

[16] K.D. Cashman, F. Shanahan, Is nutrition an aetiological factor for inflammatory bowel disease? Eur. J. Gastroenterol. Hepatol. 15 (2003) 607−613.

[17] D.G. Burrin, B. Stoll, Emerging aspects of gut sulfur amino acid metabolism, Curr. Opin. Clin. Nutr. Metab. Care 10 (2007) 63−68.

[18] S. Danese, A. Sgambato, A. Papa, F. Scaldaferri, R. Pola, M. Sans, et al., Homocysteine triggers mucosal microvascular activation in inflammatory bowel disease, Am. J. Gastroenterol. 100 (2005) 886−895.

[19] M. Stio, M. Martinesi, S. Bruni, C. Treves, G. d'Albasio, S. Bagnoli, et al., Interaction among vitamin D(3) analogue KH 1060, TNF-alpha, and vitamin D receptor protein in peripheral blood mononuclear cells of inflammatory bowel disease patients, Int. Immunopharmacol. 6 (2006) 1083–1092.

[20] D.J. Rose, M.T. DeMeo, A. Keshavarzian, B.R. Hamaker, Influence of dietary fiber on inflammatory bowel disease and colon cancer: importance of fermentation pattern, Nutr. Rev. 65 (2007) 51–62.

[21] E.V. Loftus, B.G. Feagan, J.F. Colombel, D.T. Rubin, E.Q. Wu, A. P. Yu, et al., Effects of adalimumab maintenance therapy on health-related quality of life of patients with Crohn's disease: patient-reported outcomes of the CHARM trial, Am. J. Gastroenterol. 103 (2008) 3132–3141.

[22] B.G. Feagan, W.J. Sandborn, S. Hass, T. Niecko, J. White, Health-related quality of life during natalizumab maintenance therapy for Crohn's disease, Am. J. Gastroenterol. 102 (2007) 2737–2746.

[23] N.J. Talley, M.T. Abreu, J.P. Achkar, C.N. Bernstein, M.C. Dubinsky, S.B. Hanauer, et al. American College of Gastroenterology IBD Task Force, An evidence-based systematic review on medical therapies for inflammatory bowel disease, Am. J. Gastroenterol. 106 (Suppl. 1) (2011) S2–S26.

[24] S.C. Truelove, L.J. Witts, Cortisone in ulcerative colitis; Final report on a therapeutic trial, Br. Med. J. 2 (1955) 1041–1048.

[25] S.P. Bach, N.J. Mortensen, Ileal pouch surgery for ulcerative colitis, World J. Gastroenterol. 13 (2007) 3288–3300.

[26] P. Collins, J. Rhodes, Ulcerative colitis: diagnosis and management, Br. Med. J. 333 (2006) 340–343.

[27] C. Mowat, A. Cole, A. Windsor, T. Ahmad, I. Arnott, R. Driscoll, , et al.IBD Section of the British Society of Gastroenterology, Guidelines for the management of inflammatory bowel disease in adults, Gut 60 (2011) 571–607.

[28] R. Ambe, L. Campbell, B. Cagir, A comprehensive review of strictureplasty techniques in Crohn's disease: types, indications, comparisons, and safety, J. Gastrointest. Surg. 16 (2011) 209–217.

[29] D. Rigaud, L.A. Angel, M. Cerf, M.J. Carduner, J.C. Melchior, C. Sautier, et al., Mechanisms of decreased food intake during weight loss in adult Crohn's disease patients without obvious malabsorption, Am. J. Clin. Nutr. 60 (1994) 775–781.

[30] P. Hodges, M. Gee, M. Grace, R.W. Sherbaniuk, R.H. Wensel, A. B. Thomson, Protein–energy intake and malnutrition in Crohn's disease, J. Am. Diet. Assoc. 84 (1984) 1460–1464.

[31] J.M. Reimund, Y. Arondel, G. Escalin, G. Finck, R. Baumann, B. Duclos, Immune activation and nutritional status in adult Crohn's disease patients, Dig. Liver Dis. 37 (2005) 424–431.

[32] N. Vaisman, I. Dotan, A. Halack, E. Niv, Malabsorption is a major contributor to underweight in Crohn's disease patients in remission, Nutrition 22 (2006) 855–859.

[33] S.H. Murch, Local and systemic effects of macrophage cytokines in intestinal inflammation, Nutrition 14 (1998) 780–783.

[34] K. Vagianos, S. Bector, J. McConnell, C.N. Bernstein, Nutrition assessment of patients with inflammatory bowel disease, J. Parenter. Enteral Nutr. 31 (2007) 311–319.

[35] K.J. Motil, R.J. Grand, L. Davis-Kraft, L.L. Ferlic, E.O. Smith, Growth failure in children with inflammatory bowel disease: a prospective study, Gastroenterology 105 (1993) 681–691.

[36] S.R. Rosenthal, J.D. Snyder, K.M. Hendricks, W.A. Walker, Growth failure and inflammatory bowel disease: approach to treatment of a complicated adolescent problem, Pediatrics 72 (1983) 481–490.

[37] J. Markowitz, K. Grancher, J. Rosa, H. Aiges, F. Daum, Growth failure in pediatric inflammatory bowel disease, J. Pediatr. Gastroenterol. Nutr. 16 (1993) 373–380.

[38] R.G. Castile, R.L. Telander, D.R. Cooney, D.M. Ilstrup, J. Perrault, J. van Heerden, et al., Crohn's disease in children: assessment of the progression of disease, growth, and prognosis, J. Pediatr. Surg. 15 (1980) 462–469.

[39] T.A. Sentongo, E.J. Semeao, D.A. Piccoli, V.A. Stallings, B.S. Zemel, Growth, body composition, and nutritional status in children and adolescents with Crohn's disease, J. Pediatr. Gastroenterol. Nutr. 31 (2000) 33–40.

[40] A. Van Gossum, E. Cabre, X. Hebuterne, P. Jeppesen, Z. Krznaric, B. Messing, , et al.ESPEN, ESPEN guidelines on parenteral nutrition, Gastroenterology. Clin. Nutr. 28 (2009) 415–427.

[41] D.P. Mallon, D.L. Suskind, Nutrition in pediatric inflammatory bowel disease, Nutr. Clin. Pract. 25 (2010) 335–339.

[42] V.K. Sabol, K.K. Carlson, Diarrhea: applying research to bedside practice, AACN Adv. Crit. Care 18 (2007) 32–44.

[43] L.R. Schiller, Nutrition management of chronic diarrhea and malabsorption, Nutr. Clin. Pract. 21 (2006) 34–39.

[44] R. Spiller, Role of motility in chronic diarrhoea, Neurogastroenterol. Motil. 18 (2006) 1045–1055.

[45] F. Yan, D.B. Polk, Probiotics as functional food in the treatment of diarrhea, Curr. Opin. Clin. Nutr. Metab. Care 9 (2006) 717–721.

[46] J.R. Goodhand, N. Kamperidis, A. Rao, F. Laskaratos, A. McDermott, M. Wahed, et al., Prevalence and management of anemia in children, adolescents, and adults with inflammatory bowel disease, Inflamm. Bowel Dis. 18 (2011) 513–519.

[47] A. Ulitsky, A.N. Ananthakrishnan, A. Naik, S. Skaros, Y. Zadvornova, D.G. Binion, et al., Vitamin D deficiency in patients with inflammatory bowel disease: association with disease activity and quality of life, J. Parenter. Enteral Nutr 35 (2011) 308–316.

[48] J. Goh, C.A. O'Morain, Nutrition and adult inflammatory bowel disease, Aliment. Pharmacol. Ther. 17 (2003) 307–320.

[49] R.E. Kleinman, R.N. Baldassano, A. Caplan, A.M. Griffiths, M.B. Heyman, R.M. Issenman, et al. North American Society for Pediatric Gastroenterology, Hepatology and Nutrition, Nutrition support for pediatric patients with inflammatory bowel disease: a clinical report of the North American society for pediatric gastroenterology, hepatology and nutrition, J. Pediatr. Gastroenterol. Nutr. 39 (2004) 15–27.

[50] D.R. Duerksen, G. Fallows, C.N. Bernstein, Vitamin B_{12} malabsorption in patients with limited ileal resection, Nutrition 22 (2006) 1210–1213.

[51] S. Saibeni, M. Cattaneo, M. Vecchi, M.L. Zighetti, A. Lecchi, R. Lombardi, et al., Low vitamin B(6) plasma levels, a risk factor for thrombosis, in inflammatory bowel disease: role of inflammation and correlation with acute phase reactants, Am. J. Gastroenterol. 98 (2003) 112–117.

[52] N. Barak, E. Wall-Alonso, M.D. Sitrin, Evaluation of stress factors and body weight adjustments currently used to estimate energy expenditure in hospitalized patients, J. Parenter. Enteral Nutr 26 (2002) 231–238.

[53] R.F. Kushner, D.A. Schoeller, Resting and total energy expenditure in patients with inflammatory bowel disease, Am. J. Clin. Nutr. 53 (1991) 161–165.

[54] J.E. Fischer, G.S. Foster, R.M. Abel, W.M. Abbott, J.A. Ryan, Hyperalimentation as primary therapy for inflammatory bowel disease, Am. J. Surg. 125 (1973) 165–175.

[55] J. Reilly, J.A. Ryan, W. Strole, J.E. Fischer, Hyperalimentation in inflammatory bowel disease, Am. J. Surg. 131 (1976) 192–200.

[56] V.F. Zurita, D.E. Rawls, W.P. Dyck, Nutritional support in inflammatory bowel disease, Dig. Dis. 13 (1995) 92–107.

[57] G.E. Wild, L. Drozdowski, C. Tartaglia, M.T. Clandinin, A.B. Thomson, Nutritional modulation of the inflammatory response

in inflammatory bowel disease—from the molecular to the integrative to the clinical, World J. Gastroenterol. 13 (2007) 1—7.

[58] N. Alemzadeh, L.T. Rekers-Mombarg, M.L. Mearin, J.M. Wit, C.B. Lamers, R.A. van Hogezand, Adult height in patients with early onset of Crohn's disease, Gut 51 (2002) 26—29.

[59] Y. Inoue, N.J. Espat, D.J. Frohnapple, H. Epstein, E.M. Copeland, W.W. Souba, Effect of total parenteral nutrition on amino acid and glucose transport by the human small intestine, Ann. Surg. 217 (1993) 604—614.

[60] T.M. Rossi, P.C. Lee, C. Young, A. Tjota, Small intestinal mucosa changes, including epithelial cell proliferative activity, of children receiving total parenteral nutrition (TPN), Dig. Dis. Sci. 38 (1993) 1608—1613.

[61] H. Lochs, C. Dejong, F. Hammarqvist, X. Hebuterne, M. Leon-Sanz, T. Schütz, et al., ESPEN guidelines on enteral nutrition: gastroenterology, Clin. Nutr. 25 (2006) 260—274.

[62] M. Zachos, M. Tondeur, A.M. Griffiths, Enteral nutritional therapy for induction of remission in Crohn's disease, Cochrane Database Syst. Rev. (1) (2007) CD000542.

[63] C. Su, J.D. Lewis, B. Goldberg, C. Brensinger, G.R. Lichtenstein, A meta-analysis of the placebo rates of remission and response in clinical trials of active ulcerative colitis, Gastroenterology 132 (2007) 516—526.

[64] J.B. Ewaschuk, L.A. Dieleman, Probiotics and prebiotics in chronic inflammatory bowel diseases, World J. Gastroenterol. 12 (2006) 5941—5950.

[65] K.P. Rioux, R.N. Fedorak, Probiotics in the treatment of inflammatory bowel disease, J. Clin. Gastroenterol. 40 (2006) 260—263.

[66] J.L. Jones, A.E. Foxx-Orenstein, The role of probiotics in inflammatory bowel disease, Dig. Dis. Sci. 52 (2007) 607—611.

[67] R. Bibiloni, R.N. Fedorak, G.W. Tannock, K.L. Madsen, P. Gionchetti, M. Campieri, et al., VSL#3 probiotic-mixture induces remission in patients with active ulcerative colitis, Am. J. Gastroenterol. 100 (2005) 1539—1546.

[68] A. Tursi, G. Brandimarte, A. Papa, A. Giglio, W. Elisei, G.M. Giorgetti, et al., Treatment of relapsing mild-to-moderate ulcerative colitis with the probiotic VSL#3 as adjunctive to a standard pharmaceutical treatment: a double-blind, randomized, placebo-controlled study, Am. J. Gastroenterol. 105 (2010) 2218—2227.

[69] S.K. Hegazy, M.M. El-Bedewy, Effect of probiotics on proinflammatory cytokines and NF-κB activation in ulcerative colitis, World J. Gastroenterol. 16 (2010) 4145—4151.

[70] L.X. Sang, B. Chang, W.L. Zhang, X.M. Wu, X.H. Li, M. Jiang, Remission induction and maintenance effect of probiotics on ulcerative colitis: a meta-analysis, World J. Gastroenterol. 16 (2010) 1908—1915.

[71] R. Rahimi, S. Nikfar, F. Rahimi, B. Elahi, S. Derakhshani, M. Vafaie, et al., A meta-analysis on the efficacy of probiotics for maintenance of remission and prevention of clinical and endoscopic relapse in Crohn's disease, Dig. Dis. Sci. 53 (2008) 2524—2531.

[72] J. Shen, H.Z. Ran, M.H. Yin, T.X. Zhou, D.S. Xiao, Meta-analysis: the effect and adverse events of lactobacilli versus placebo in maintenance therapy for Crohn disease, Intern. Med. J. 39 (2009) 103—109.

[73] P. Gionchetti, F. Rizzello, U. Helwig, A. Venturi, K.M. Lammers, P. Brigidi, et al., Prophylaxis of pouchitis onset with probiotic therapy: a double-blind, placebo-controlled trial, Gastroenterology 124 (2003) 1202—1209.

[74] T. Mimura, F. Rizzello, U. Helwig, G. Poggioli, S. Schreiber, I.C. Talbot, et al., Once daily high dose probiotic therapy (VSL#3) for maintaining remission in recurrent or refractory pouchitis, Gut 53 (2004) 108—114.

[75] J. Kuisma, S. Mentula, H. Jarvinen, A. Kahri, M. Saxelin, M. Farkkila, Effect of lactobacillus rhamnosus GG on ileal pouch inflammation and microbial flora, Aliment. Pharmacol. Ther. 17 (2003) 509—515.

[76] K.O. Laake, A. Bjorneklett, G. Aamodt, L. Aabakken, M. Jacobsen, A. Bakka, et al., Outcome of four weeks' intervention with probiotics on symptoms and endoscopic appearance after surgical reconstruction with a J-configurated ileal-pouch—anal-anastomosis in ulcerative colitis, Scand. J. Gastroenterol. 40 (2005) 43—51.

[77] M.S. Inan, R.J. Rasoulpour, L. Yin, A.K. Hubbard, D.W. Rosenberg, C. Giardina, The luminal short-chain fatty acid butyrate modulates NF-kappaB activity in a human colonic epithelial cell line, Gastroenterology 118 (2000) 724—734.

[78] J.P. Segain, D. Raingeard de la Bletiere, A. Bourreille, V. Leray, N. Gervois, C. Rosales, et al., Butyrate inhibits inflammatory responses through NF-κB inhibition: implications for Crohn's disease, Gut 47 (2000) 397—403.

[79] M. Schwab, V. Reynders, S. Loitsch, D. Steinhilber, J. Stein, O. Schroder, Involvement of different nuclear hormone receptors in butyrate-mediated inhibition of inducible NF kappa B signalling, Mol. Immunol. 44 (2007) 3625—3632.

[80] L. Klampfer, J. Huang, T. Sasazuki, S. Shirasawa, L. Augenlicht, Inhibition of interferon gamma signaling by the short chain fatty acid butyrate, Mol. Cancer Res. 1 (2003) 855—862.

[81] J.L. Benjamin, C.R. Hedin, A. Koutsoumpas, S.C. Ng, N.E. McCarthy, A.L. Hart, et al., Randomised, double-blind, placebo-controlled trial of fructo-oligosaccharides in active Crohn's disease, Gut 60 (2011) 923—929.

[82] H. Steed, G.T. Macfarlane, K.L. Blackett, B. Bahrami, N. Reynolds, S.V. Walsh, et al., Clinical trial: the microbiological and immunological effects of synbiotic consumption? A randomized double-blind placebo-controlled study in active Crohn's disease, Aliment. Pharmacol. Ther. 32 (2010) 872—883.

[83] S. Fujimori, K. Gudis, K. Mitsui, T. Seo, M. Yonezawa, S. Tanaka, et al., A randomized controlled trial on the efficacy of synbiotic versus probiotic or prebiotic treatment to improve the quality of life in patients with ulcerative colitis, Nutrition 25 (2009) 520—525.

[84] U.N. Das, Essential fatty acids: biochemistry, physiology and pathology, Biotechnol. J. 1 (2006) 420—439.

[85] A.P. Simopoulos, Essential fatty acids in health and chronic disease, Am. J. Clin. Nutr. 70 (1999) 560S—569S.

[86] S.R. Shaikh, M. Edidin, Polyunsaturated fatty acids, membrane organization, T cells, and antigen presentation, Am. J. Clin. Nutr. 84 (2006) 1277—1289.

[87] D. Turner, S.H. Zlotkin, P.S. Shah, A.M. Griffiths, Omega 3 fatty acids (fish oil) for maintenance of remission in Crohn's disease, Cochrane Database Syst. Rev. (1)) (2009) CD006320.

[88] D. Turner, A.H. Steinhart, A.M. Griffiths, Omega 3 fatty acids (fish oil) for maintenance of remission in ulcerative colitis, Cochrane Database Syst. Rev. (3) (2007) CD006443.

[89] A.A. Nielsen, L.G. Jorgensen, J.N. Nielsen, M. Eivindson, H. Gronbaek, I. Vind, et al., Omega-3 fatty acids inhibit an increase of proinflammatory cytokines in patients with active Crohn's disease compared with omega-6 fatty acids, Aliment. Pharmacol. Ther. 22 (2005) 1121—1128.

[90] J.S. Scolapio, Short bowel syndrome, J. Parenter. Enteral Nutr 26 (2002) S11—S16.

[91] J.A. Vanderhoof, A.N. Langnas, Short-bowel syndrome in children and adults, Gastroenterology 113 (1997) 1767—1778.

[92] D.W. Wilmore, M.K. Robinson, Short bowel syndrome, World J. Surg. 24 (2000) 1486—1492.

[93] O. Goulet, F. Ruemmele, F. Lacaille, V. Colomb, Irreversible intestinal failure, J. Pediatr. Gastroenterol. Nutr. 38 (2004) 250–269.

[94] Y.A. Ching, K. Gura, B. Modi, T. Jaksic, Pediatric intestinal failure: nutrition, pharmacologic, and surgical approaches, Nutr. Clin. Pract. 22 (2007) 653–663.

[95] J. Nightingale, J.M. Woodward, Small Bowel and Nutrition Committee of the British Society of Gastroenterology, Guidelines for management of patients with a short bowel, Gut 55 (Suppl. 4) (2006) iv1–12.

[96] G.L. Gupte, S.V. Beath, D.A. Kelly, A.J. Millar, I.W. Booth, Current issues in the management of intestinal failure, Arch. Dis. Child. 91 (2006) 259–264.

[97] P.B. Jeppesen, P.B. Mortensen, Significance of a preserved colon for parenteral energy requirements in patients receiving home parenteral nutrition, Scand. J. Gastroenterol 33 (1998) 1175–1179.

[98] B. Messing, P. Crenn, P. Beau, M.C. Boutron-Ruault, J.C. Rambaud, C. Matuchansky, Long-term survival and parenteral nutrition dependence in adult patients with the short bowel syndrome, Gastroenterology 117 (1999) 1043–1050.

[99] J.S. Thompson, Inflammatory disease and outcome of short bowel syndrome, Am. J. Surg. 180 (2000) 551–555.

[100] R.H. Dowling, C.C. Booth, Structural and functional changes following small intestinal resection in the rat, Clin. Sci. 32 (1967) 139–149.

[101] R.H. Dowling, C.C. Booth, Functional compensation after small-bowel resection in man. Demonstration by direct measurement, Lancet 2 (1966) 146–147.

[102] J.S. Thompson, D.C. Ferguson, Effect of the distal remnant on ileal adaptation, J. Gastrointest. Surg. 4 (2000) 430–434.

[103] S.F. Phillips, E.M. Quigley, D. Kumar, P.S. Kamath, Motility of the ileocolonic junction, Gut 29 (1988) 390–406.

[104] F. Carbonnel, J. Cosnes, S. Chevret, L. Beaugerie, Y. Ngo, M. Malafosse, et al., The role of anatomic factors in nutritional autonomy after extensive small bowel resection, J. Parenter. Enteral Nutr 20 (1996) 275–280.

[105] A.I. Sacks, G.J. Warwick, J.A. Barnard, Early proliferative events following intestinal resection in the rat, J. Pediatr. Gastroenterol. Nutr. 21 (1995) 158–164.

[106] E.E. Whang, J.C. Dunn, H. Joffe, H. Mahanty, M.J. Zinner, D.W. McFadden, et al., Enterocyte functional adaptation following intestinal resection, J. Surg. Res. 60 (1996) 370–374.

[107] T.P. O'Connor, M.M. Lam, J. Diamond, Magnitude of functional adaptation after intestinal resection, Am. J. Physiol. 276 (1999) R1265–R1275.

[108] J.H. Solhaug, S. Tvete, Adaptative changes in the small intestine following bypass operation for obesity. A radioglocal and histological study, Scand. J. Gastroenterol 13 (1978) 401–408.

[109] L.D. Weinstein, C.P. Shoemaker, T. Hersh, H.K. Wright, Enhanced intestinal absorption after small bowel resection in man, Arch. Surg. 99 (1969) 560–562.

[110] L.T. Weaver, S. Austin, T.J. Cole, Small intestinal length: a factor essential for gut adaptation, Gut 32 (1991) 1321–1323.

[111] O. Goulet, Short bowel syndrome in pediatric patients, Nutrition 14 (1998) 784–787.

[112] D.J. Drucker, P. Erlich, S.L. Asa, P.L. Brubaker, Induction of intestinal epithelial proliferation by glucagon-like peptide 2, Proc. Natl. Acad. Sci. USA 93 (1996) 7911–7916.

[113] G.R. Martin, L.E. Wallace, D.L. Sigalet, Glucagon-like peptide-2 induces intestinal adaptation in parenterally fed rats with short bowel syndrome, Am. J. Physiol. Gastrointest. Liver Physiol. 286 (2004) G964–G972.

[114] D.L. Sigalet, O. Bawazir, G.R. Martin, L.E. Wallace, G. Zaharko, A. Miller, et al., Glucagon-like peptide-2 induces a specific pattern of adaptation in remnant jejunum, Dig. Dis. Sci. 51 (2006) 1557–1566.

[115] X. Liu, D.W. Nelson, J.J. Holst, D.M. Ney, Synergistic effect of supplemental enteral nutrients and exogenous glucagon-like peptide 2 on intestinal adaptation in a rat model of short bowel syndrome, Am. J. Clin. Nutr. 84 (2006) 1142–1150.

[116] P.T. Sangild, K.A. Tappenden, C. Malo, Y.M. Petersen, J. Elnif, A.L. Bartholome, et al., Glucagon-like peptide 2 stimulates intestinal nutrient absorption in parenterally fed newborn pigs, J. Pediatr. Gastroenterol. Nutr. 43 (2006) 160–167.

[117] P.B. Jeppesen, B. Hartmann, J. Thulesen, J. Graff, J. Lohmann, B.S. Hansen, et al., Glucagon-like peptide 2 improves nutrient absorption and nutritional status in short-bowel patients with no colon, Gastroenterology 120 (2001) 806–815.

[118] P.B. Jeppesen, E.L. Sanguinetti, A. Buchman, L. Howard, J.S. Scolapio, T.R. Ziegler, et al., Teduglutide (ALX-0600), a dipeptidyl peptidase IV resistant glucagon-like peptide 2 analogue, improves intestinal function in short bowel syndrome patients, Gut 54 (2005) 1224–1231.

[119] P.B. Jeppesen, P. Lund, I.B. Gottschalck, H.B. Nielsen, J.J. Holst, J. Mortensen, et al., Short bowel patients treated for two years with glucagon-like peptide 2 (GLP-2): compliance, safety, and effects on quality of life, Gastroenterol. Res. Pract. 2009 (2009) 425759.

[120] P.B. Jeppesen, R. Gilroy, M. Pertkiewicz, J.P. Allard, B. Messing, S.J. O'Keefe, Randomised placebo-controlled trial of teduglutide in reducing parenteral nutrition and/or intravenous fluid requirements in patients with short bowel syndrome, Gut 60 (2011) 902–914.

[121] A. Bianchi, Intestinal loop lengthening—a technique for increasing small intestinal length, J. Pediatr. Surg. 15 (1980) 145–151.

[122] H.B. Kim, D. Fauza, J. Garza, J.T. Oh, S. Nurko, T. Jaksic, Serial transverse enteroplasty (STEP): a novel bowel lengthening procedure, J. Pediatr. Surg. 38 (2003) 425–429.

[123] M. DeLegge, M.M. Alsolaiman, E. Barbour, S. Bassas, M.F. Siddiqi, N.M. Moore, Short bowel syndrome: parenteral nutrition versus intestinal transplantation. Where are we today? Dig. Dis. Sci. 52 (2007) 876–892.

[124] G. Selvaggi, A.G. Tzakis, Intestinal and multivisceral transplantation: future perspectives, Front. Biosci. 12 (2007) 4742–4754.

[125] T. Ueno, M. Fukuzawa, Current status of intestinal transplantation, Surg. Today 40 (2010) 1112–1122.

[126] L.E. Matarese, E. Steiger, Dietary and medical management of short bowel syndrome in adult patients, J. Clin. Gastroenterol. 40 (Suppl. 2) (2006) S85–S93.

[127] P.P. Toskes, Bacterial overgrowth of the gastrointestinal tract, Adv. Intern. Med. 38 (1993) 387–407.

[128] Y. Kanamori, K. Hashizume, M. Sugiyama, M. Morotomi, N. Yuki, Combination therapy with bifidobacterium breve, lactobacillus casei, and galactooligosaccharides dramatically improved the intestinal function in a girl with short bowel syndrome: a novel synbiotics therapy for intestinal failure, Dig. Dis. Sci 46 (2001) 2010–2016.

[129] C. Petersen, D-Lactic acidosis, Nutr. Clin. Pract. 20 (2005) 634–645.

[130] L. Drozdowski, A.B. Thomson, Intestinal mucosal adaptation, World J. Gastroenterol. 12 (2006) 4614–4627.

[131] T.R. Ziegler, M.E. Evans, C. Fernandez-Estivariz, D.P. Jones, Trophic and cytoprotective nutrition for intestinal adaptation, mucosal repair, and barrier function, Annu. Rev. Nutr. 23 (2003) 229–261.

[132] I. Nordgaard, B.S. Hansen, P.B. Mortensen, Importance of colonic support for energy absorption as small-bowel failure proceeds, Am. J. Clin. Nutr. 64 (1996) 222–231.

[133] J.S. Soden, Clinical assessment of the child with intestinal failure, Semin. Pediatr. Surg 19 (2010) 10–19.

[134] P. Crenn, B. Messing, L. Cynober, Citrulline as a biomarker of intestinal failure due to enterocyte mass reduction, Clin. Nutr. 27 (2008) 328–339.

[135] A.M. Pita, Y. Wakabayashi, M.A. Fernandez-Bustos, N. Virgili, E. Riudor, J. Soler, et al., Plasma urea-cycle-related amino acids, ammonium levels, and urinary orotic acid excretion in short-bowel patients managed with an oral diet, Clin. Nutr. 22 (2003) 93–98.

[136] J.M. Rhoads, E. Plunkett, J. Galanko, S. Lichtman, L. Taylor, A. Maynor, et al., Serum citrulline levels correlate with enteral tolerance and bowel length in infants with short bowel syndrome, J. Pediatr. 146 (2005) 542–547.

[137] P. Crenn, C. Coudray-Lucas, F. Thuillier, L. Cynober, B. Messing, Postabsorptive plasma citrulline concentration is a marker of absorptive enterocyte mass and intestinal failure in humans, Gastroenterology 119 (2000) 1496–1505.

[138] M. Luo, C. Fernandez-Estivariz, A.K. Manatunga, N. Bazargan, L.H. Gu, D.P. Jones, et al., Are plasma citrulline and glutamine biomarkers of intestinal absorptive function in patients with short bowel syndrome? J. Parenter. Enteral Nutr 31 (2007) 1–7.

[139] J.M. Nightingale, J.E. Lennard-Jones, D.J. Gertner, S.R. Wood, C.I. Bartram, Colonic preservation reduces need for parenteral therapy, increases incidence of renal stones, but does not change high prevalence of gall stones in patients with a short bowel, Gut 33 (1992) 1493–1497.

[140] G.E. Griffin, E.F. Fagan, H.J. Hodgson, V.S. Chadwick, Enteral therapy in the management of massive gut resection complicated by chronic fluid and electrolyte depletion, Dig. Dis. Sci. 27 (1982) 902–908.

[141] J.E. Lennard-Jones, Review article: practical management of the short bowel, Aliment. Pharmacol. Ther. 8 (1994) 563–577.

[142] J.K. DiBaise, L.E. Matarese, B. Messing, E. Steiger, Strategies for parenteral nutrition weaning in adult patients with short bowel syndrome, J. Clin. Gastroenterol. 40 (Suppl. 2) (2006) S94–S98.

[143] E. Weser, Nutritional aspects of malabsorption: short gut adaptation, Clin. Gastroenterol. 12 (1983) 443–461.

[144] I. Nordgaard, B.S. Hansen, P.B. Mortensen, Colon as a digestive organ in patients with short bowel, Lancet 343 (1994) 373–376.

[145] P. Crenn, M.C. Morin, F. Joly, S. Penven, F. Thuillier, B. Messing, Net digestive absorption and adaptive hyperphagia in adult short bowel patients, Gut 53 (2004) 1279–1286.

[146] J. Bines, D. Francis, D. Hill, Reducing parenteral requirement in children with short bowel syndrome: impact of an amino acid-based complete infant formula, J. Pediatr. Gastroenterol. Nutr. 26 (1998) 123–128.

[147] J. Ksiazyk, M. Piena, J. Kierkus, M. Lyszkowska, Hydrolyzed versus nonhydrolyzed protein diet in short bowel syndrome in children, J. Pediatr. Gastroenterol. Nutr. 35 (2002) 615–618.

[148] J.S. Scolapio, K. McGreevy, G.S. Tennyson, O.L. Burnett, Effect of glutamine in short-bowel syndrome, Clin. Nutr. 20 (2001) 319–323.

[149] P.H. Benhamou, J.P. Canarelli, C. Cordonnier, J.P. Postel, E. Grenier, A. Leke, et al., Human recombinant growth hormone increases small bowel lengthening after massive small bowel resection in piglets, J. Pediatr. Surg. 32 (1997) 1332–1336.

[150] Y. Gu, Z.H. Wu, J.X. Xie, D.Y. Jin, H.C. Zhuo, Effects of growth hormone (rhGH) and glutamine supplemented parenteral nutrition on intestinal adaptation in short bowel rats, Clin. Nutr. 20 (2001) 159–166.

[151] T.A. Byrne, R.L. Persinger, L.S. Young, T.R. Ziegler, D.W. Wilmore, A new treatment for patients with short-bowel syndrome: growth hormone, glutamine, and a modified diet, Ann. Surg. 222 (1995) 243–255.

[152] G.H. Wu, Z.H. Wu, Z.G. Wu, Effects of bowel rehabilitation and combined trophic therapy on intestinal adaptation in short bowel patients, World J. Gastroenterol. 9 (2003) 2601–2604.

[153] T.A. Byrne, T.B. Morrissey, T.V. Nattakom, T.R. Ziegler, D.W. Wilmore, Growth hormone, glutamine, and a modified diet enhance nutrient absorption in patients with severe short bowel syndrome, J. Parenter. Enteral Nutr. 19 (1995) 296–302.

[154] J.S. Scolapio, M. Camilleri, C.R. Fleming, L.V. Oenning, D.D. Burton, T.J. Sebo, et al., Effect of growth hormone, glutamine, and diet on adaptation in short-bowel syndrome: a randomized, controlled study, Gastroenterology 113 (1997) 1074–1081.

[155] J. Szkudlarek, P.B. Jeppesen, P.B. Mortensen, Effect of high dose growth hormone with glutamine and no change in diet on intestinal absorption in short bowel patients: a randomised, double blind, crossover, placebo controlled study, Gut 47 (2000) 199–205.

[156] P.B. Jeppesen, J. Szkudlarek, C.E. Hoy, P.B. Mortensen, Effect of high-dose growth hormone and glutamine on body composition, urine creatinine excretion, fatty acid absorption, and essential fatty acids status in short bowel patients: a randomized, double-blind, crossover, placebo-controlled study, Scand. J. Gastroenterol. 36 (2001) 48–54.

[157] J.S. Scolapio, Effect of growth hormone, glutamine, and diet on body composition in short bowel syndrome: a randomized, controlled study, J. Parenter. Enteral Nutr. 23 (1999) 309–313.

[158] E. Steiger, J.K. DiBaise, B. Messing, L.E. Matarese, S. Blethen, Indications and recommendations for the use of recombinant human growth hormone in adult short bowel syndrome patients dependent on parenteral nutrition, J. Clin. Gastroenterol. 40 (Suppl. 2) (2006) S99–S106.

[159] M. Puder, C. Valim, J.A. Meisel, H.D. Le, V.E. de Meijer, E.M. Robinson, et al., Parenteral fish oil improves outcomes in patients with parenteral nutrition-associated liver injury, Ann. Surg. 250 (2009) 395–402.

[160] H.M. Cheung, H.S. Lam, Y.H. Tam, K.H. Lee, P.C. Ng, Rescue treatment of infants with intestinal failure and parenteral nutrition-associated cholestasis (PNAC) using a parenteral fish-oil-based lipid, Clin. Nutr. 28 (2009) 209–212.

[161] I.R. Diamond, A. Sterescu, P.B. Pencharz, J.H. Kim, P.W. Wales, Changing the paradigm: omegaven for the treatment of liver failure in pediatric short bowel syndrome, J. Pediatr. Gastroenterol. Nutr. 48 (2009) 209–215.

[162] K.A. Kollman, E.L. Lien, J.A. Vanderhoof, Dietary lipids influence intestinal adaptation after massive bowel resection, J. Pediatr. Gastroenterol. Nutr. 28 (1999) 41–45.

[163] I. Sukhotnik, A. Shany, Y. Bashenko, L. Hayari, E. Chemodanov, J. Mogilner, et al., Parenteral but not enteral omega-3 fatty acids (omegaven) modulate intestinal regrowth after massive small bowel resection in rats, J. Parenter. Enteral Nutr 34 (2010) 503–512.

[164] Q. Yang, N.D. Kock, Effects of dietary fish oil on intestinal adaptation in 20-day-old weanling rats after massive ileocecal resection, Pediatr. Res 68 (2010) 183–187.

[165] K.A. Tappenden, A.B. Thomson, G.E. Wild, M.I. McBurney, Short-chain fatty acids increase proglucagon and ornithine decarboxylase messenger RNAs after intestinal resection in rats, J. Parenter. Enteral Nutr. 20 (1996) 357–362.

[166] K.A. Tappenden, L.A. Drozdowski, A.B. Thomson, M.I. McBurney, Short-chain fatty acid-supplemented total parenteral nutrition alters intestinal structure, glucose transporter 2 (GLUT2) mRNA and protein, and proglucagon mRNA abundance in normal rats, Am. J. Clin. Nutr. 68 (1998) 118–125.

[167] A.L. Bartholome, D.M. Albin, D.H. Baker, J.J. Holst, K.A. Tappenden, Supplementation of total parenteral nutrition with butyrate acutely increases structural aspects of intestinal

adaptation after an 80% jejunoileal resection in neonatal piglets, J. Parenter. Enteral Nutr. 28 (2004) 210–223.

[168] K.A. Tappenden, A.B. Thomson, G.E. Wild, M.I. McBurney, Short-chain fatty acid-supplemented total parenteral nutrition enhances functional adaptation to intestinal resection in rats, Gastroenterology 112 (1997) 792–802.

[169] M.A. Tolga Muftuoglu, T. Civak, S. Cetin, L. Civak, O. Gungor, A. Saglam, Effects of probiotics on experimental short-bowel syndrome, Am. J. Surg. 202 (2011) 461–468.

[170] J.G. Mogilner, I. Srugo, M. Lurie, R. Shaoul, A.G. Coran, E. Shiloni, et al., Effect of probiotics on intestinal regrowth and bacterial translocation after massive small bowel resection in a rat, J. Pediatr. Surg. 42 (2007) 1365–1371.

[171] T.A. Sentongo, V. Cohran, S. Korff, C. Sullivan, K. Iyer, X. Zheng, Intestinal permeability and effects of lactobacillus rhamnosus therapy in children with short bowel syndrome, J. Pediatr. Gastroenterol. Nutr. 46 (2008) 41–47.

[172] K. Uchida, T. Takahashi, M. Inoue, M. Morotomi, K. Otake, M. Nakazawa, et al., Immunonutritional effects during synbiotics therapy in pediatric patients with short bowel syndrome, Pediatr. Surg. Int. 23 (2007) 243–248.

[173] Y. Kanamori, M. Sugiyama, K. Hashizume, N. Yuki, M. Morotomi, R. Tanaka, Experience of long-term synbiotic therapy in seven short bowel patients with refractory enterocolitis, J. Pediatr. Surg. 39 (2004) 1686–1692.

CHAPTER

40

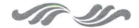

Nutrient Considerations in Lactose Intolerance

Steve Hertzler*, *Dennis A. Savaiano*†, *Karry A. Jackson*†, *Sinead Ni Bhriain*‡, *Fabrizis L. Suarez**

*Abbott Laboratories, Ross Products Division, Columbus, Ohio, †Purdue University, West Lafayette, Indiana, ‡Trinity College, University of Dublin, and Dublin Institute of Technology, Dublin, Ireland

I INTRODUCTION

Ingestion of a large single dose of lactose (e.g., 50 g, the quantity in a quart of milk) by lactose maldigesters commonly results in diarrhea, bloating, and flatulence [1]. The wide dissemination of this information has led some of the lay population and a fraction of the medical community to attribute common gastrointestinal symptoms to lactose intolerance, independent of the dose of lactose ingested. As a result, a segment of the population avoids dairy products in the belief that even trivial doses of lactose will induce diarrhea or gas. However, multiple factors affect the ability of lactose to induce perceptible symptoms, including residual lactase activity [2], gastrointestinal transit time [3], lactose consumed with other foods [4], lactose load [5], and colonic fermentation [6]. The estimated 25% of adults in the United States who maldigest lactose are composed mainly of the Hispanic, Asian, and African American populations (Table 40.1). These race/ethnic groups are rapidly growing segments of the population. Thus, the overall number of lactose maldigesters will grow in the United States in coming years. A major challenge for diet therapy of lactose maldigesters is to ensure adequate intakes of calcium, vitamin D, and other nutrients found largely in dairy products while at the same time minimizing the occurrence of lactose intolerance symptoms that would tend to limit milk consumption.

This chapter (1) reviews the pathophysiology of lactose maldigestion, (2) attempts to correct common misconceptions concerning the frequency and severity of lactose intolerance symptoms, and (3) provides dietary strategies to minimize symptoms of intolerance.

II LACTOSE IN THE DIET

Lactose is the primary disaccharide in virtually all mammalian milks. It is unique among the major dietary sugars because of the $\beta\text{-}1 \rightarrow 4$ linkage between its component monosaccharides, galactose and glucose. Lactose production in nature is limited to the mammalian breast, which contains the enzyme system (lactose synthase) necessary to create this linkage [7]. Human milk contains approximately 7% lactose by weight, which is among the highest lactose concentrations of all mammalian milks [5]. Cow's milk contains 4 or 5% lactose. Lactose, being water soluble, is associated with the whey portion of dairy foods. Thus, hard cheeses (with the whey removed from the curds) contain very little lactose compared with fluid milk (Table 40.2 shows the lactose content of selected foods).

In addition to food sources of lactose, small amounts of lactose are found in a wide variety of medications because of the excellent tablet-forming properties of lactose [5]. However, lactose is usually present in milligram, rather than gram, quantities in most medications, and the amount is biologically insignificant for lactose maldigesters.

Nutrition in the Prevention and Treatment of Disease, Third Edition.
DOI: http://dx.doi.org/10.1016/B978-0-12-391884-0.00040-8

TABLE 40.1   Prevalence of Lactase Nonpersistence in Various Populations

Group	Prevalence (%)
Northern European	2–15
American white	6–22
Central European	9–23
Indian (Indian subcontinent)	
Northern	20–30
Southern	60–70
Hispanic	50–80
Ashkenazi Jew	60–80
Black	60–80
American Indian	80–100
Asian	95–100

Source: *Used with permission from Swagerty, D. L., Walling, A. D., and Klein, R. M. (2002). Lactose intolerance.* Am. Fam. Physician *65, 1845–1850.*

TABLE 40.2   Lactose Content of Selected Foods

Product	Portion size	Lactose content (g/portion)
Milk, full fat	1 c. (244 g)	11
Milk, reduced fat (2%)	1 c. (244 g)	9–13
Milk, nonfat	1 c. (244 g)	12–14
Milk, chocolate	1 c. (244 g)	10–12
Buttermilk, fluid	1 c. (245 g)	9–11
Half and half	1 T. (15 g)	0.6
Yogurt, low-fat	8 fl. oz. (227–258 g)	11–15
Cheese (blue, Camembert, cheddar, Colby, cream, Gouda, Limburger, grated Parmesan)	1 oz. (28 g)	0.1–0.8
Cheese, pasteurized processed (American, pimento, Swiss)	1 oz. (28 g)	0.4–1.7
Cottage cheese, whole	1 c. (210 g)	5–6
Cottage cheese, 2% fat	1 c. (226 g)	7–8
Butter	2 pats (10 g)	0.1
Ice cream, vanilla, regular	1 c. (133 g)	9
Ice milk, vanilla	1 c. (131 g)	10
Sherbet, orange	1 c. (193 g)	4

Source: *Adapted with permission from Welsh, J. D. (1978). Diet therapy in adult lactose malabsorption: Present practices.* Am. J. Clin. Nutr. *31, 592–596.*

III DIGESTION OF LACTOSE

The small intestine is normally impermeable to lactose. Lactose must first be hydrolyzed to glucose and galactose, which are subsequently absorbed. Inability to digest lactose is referred to as *lactose maldigestion*. Lactose digestion is dependent on the enzyme lactase-phlorizin hydrolase (LPH), a microvillar protein that has at least three enzyme activities: β-galactosidase, phlorizin hydrolase, and glycosylceramidase [8,9]. Synthesis of LPH occurs in enterocytes, with the highest and most uniform synthesis being in the jejunum in humans [10]. The LPH gene is located on chromosome 2 and directs the synthesis of a pre-proLPH that is processed intracellularly (and possibly by pancreatic proteases) into the mature form that is anchored in the cell membrane at the brush border [11,12]. Lactase activity develops late in gestation compared to other disaccharidases. Lactase activity in a fetus at 34 weeks is only 30% that of a full-term infant, rising to 70% of the full-term activity by 35–38 weeks [13].

IV LOSS OF LACTASE ACTIVITY

Full-term infants possess high lactase activity, except for *congenital lactase deficiency*, in which lactase is completely absent at birth. Holzel *et al.* [14] first described congenital lactase deficiency in 1959. It is a very rare condition, such that even in Finland, where it is most common, only 42 cases were diagnosed from 1966 to 1998 [11]. Lactase activity in jejunal biopsy specimens from infants with congenital lactase deficiency is reduced to 0–10 IU/g protein, and severe diarrhea results from unabsorbed lactose [11]. Treatment with a lactose-free formula eliminates symptoms and promotes normal growth and development [15].

Primary acquired hypolactasia, in which there is up to a 90–95% reduction in lactase activity, is much more common than congenital lactase deficiency (alactasia) [16]. The preferred term for this type of hypolactasia is *lactase nonpersistence* (LNP). It is estimated that approximately 75% of the world's population are LNP (see Table 40.1), with the exception of northern Europeans and a few pastoral tribes in Africa and the Middle East that maintain infantile levels of lactase throughout life [17]. Thus, LNP is not a "lactase deficiency" disease but is the normal pattern in human physiology, similar to the physiology of other mammalian species. This permanent loss of lactase occurs sometime after 3–5 years of age [9,18].

Lactase persistence is inherited as a highly penetrant, autosomal-dominant characteristic [17]. It has been hypothesized that individuals with a genetic mutation coding for lactase persistence would have gained a selective evolutionary advantage over LNP individuals in areas where dairy farming developed several thousand years ago [19,20]. Under marginal nutritional conditions, the individual with lactase persistence would be able to comfortably consume dairy products, deriving greater nutritional benefit. A key question has been whether the lactase persistence mutation in humans occurred before (the reverse cause hypothesis) or after (the cultural–historical hypothesis) the advent of dairying. DNA studies on the skeletal remains of pre-dairy farming Neolithic Europeans [21] indicate that the most common allele for lactase persistence in Europeans (−13910*T) was not present, arguing for the cultural–historical hypothesis (this mutation is discussed in more detail in the following section). In addition, Tishkoff *et al.* [22] have identified three single-nucleotide polymorphisms (SNPs) for lactase persistence that developed in African populations as few as 3000 years ago. This date corresponds well with archeological data suggesting that cattle domestication came to different areas of Africa 3300–9000 years ago. These SNPs developed independently of the European mutation, providing striking evidence of both convergent evolution and the strong and relatively recent impact of a cultural practice such as dairy farming on the genome.

The genetic regulation of LPH has been studied extensively. Most evidence supports reduced levels of lactase mRNA in lactose maldigesters, suggesting that regulation is primarily at the level of transcription [23–26]. However, hypolactasia is sometimes present even when lactase mRNA is abundant, suggesting that post-transcriptional factors play a role [10,27,28]. One potential reason for conflicting results is the intestinal segment examined (duodenum vs. jejunum). Lactase expression is higher and more uniform in the jejunum compared to the duodenum [29,30]. Another potential discrepancy is the age of the subjects studied. A poor correlation between lactase mRNA and lactase activity was reported in intestinal biopsies from children, although the biopsy specimens in this study were from duodenal sites [28]. Lactase activity in the jejunal enterocytes is found in a "mosaic"-type pattern [31]. In hypolactasic individuals, some jejunal enterocytes produce high amounts of lactase, whereas others, even those sharing the same villus, do not produce lactase [10]. Thus, rather than a uniform reduction in lactase production among all enterocytes, a hypolactasic individual may have a "patchy" distribution of lactose-producing enterocytes that are low in number relative to the non-lactase-producing enterocytes. In lactase-persistent individuals, all villus enterocytes may produce lactase. Current evidence suggests that the regulation of lactase is accomplished primarily at the

level of transcription, although post-transcriptional factors (e.g., degradation of mRNA and post-translational processing of the LPH protein) could be important in some individuals.

Secondary hypolactasia occurs as the result of damage to the enterocytes via disease, medications, surgery, or radiation to the gastrointestinal tract (Table 40.3) [5,32,33]. For example, the prevalence of microsporidiosis, which is associated with hypolactasia, can be as high as 50% in HIV-infected patients [34]. Seventy percent of HIV-infected patients showed evidence of lactose maldigestion compared to only 34% of controls [35]. In addition, the severity of lactose maldigestion increases in the more advanced stages of the disease. In general, secondary hypolactasia is reversible once the underlying cause is treated, but this reversal may require 6 months or more of diet therapy [5].

V DIAGNOSIS OF LACTOSE MALDIGESTION

A Genetic Testing

Historically, biochemical and/or symptom tests (described in Sections V.B and V.C) have been used to

TABLE 40.3 Potential Causes of Secondary Hypolactasia

Disease		
Small bowel	**Multisystem**	**Iatrogenic**
HIV enteropathy	Carcinoid syndrome	Chemotherapy
Regional enteritis (e.g., Crohn's disease)	Cystic fibrosis	Radiation enteritis
Sprue (celiac and tropical)	Diabetic gastropathy	Surgical resection of intestine
Whipple's disease (intestinal lipodystrophy)	Protein energy malnutrition	Medications
Ascaris lumbricoides infection	Zollinger–Ellison syndrome	Colchicine (antigout)
Blind loop syndrome	Alcoholism	Neomycin (antibiotic)
Giardiasis	Iron deficiency	Kanamycin (antibiotic)
Infectious diarrhea	Aminosalicylic acid (antibiotic)	
Short gut		

Sources: *Adapted with permission from Srinivasan, R., and Minocha, A. (1998). When to suspect lactose intolerance: Symptomatic, ethnic, and laboratory issues. Postgrad. Med.* **104**(3), 109–123; Scrimshaw, N. S., and Murray, E. B. (1998). The acceptability of milk and milk products in populations with a high prevalence of lactose intolerance. Am. J. Clin. Nutr. **48**, 1083–1159; and Savaiano, D. A., and Levitt, M. D. (1987). Milk intolerance and microbe-containing dairy foods. J. Dairy Sci. **70**, 397–406.

diagnosis lactose maldigestion. In approximately the past 5−10 years, however, the focus has been the development of genetic tests to identify markers of lactose maldigestion. These types of tests have several advantages over present methods. First, the measurements can be done on buccal cell samples, which are rapidly and easily obtained and require little or no preparation on the part of the individual being tested. Second, because the symptoms of lactose intolerance may often be confused with other gastrointestinal disorders, such as irritable bowel syndrome or Crohn's disease, genetic testing would allow for the ready differentiation of lactose maldigestion (resulting from LNP) from other gastrointestinal conditions. Enattah et al. [36] isolated two SNPs that are strongly associated with LNP in a primarily Finnish population. Both of these SNPs are located in a region adjacent to the lactase gene (LCT) on chromosome 2q21. The first, a substitution of cytosine for thymine 13,910 base pairs upstream of the 5′ end of LCT (termed C/T_{-13910}), was completely associated with biochemical evidence of LNP in 236 individuals. The second, g/A_{-22018}, was found in 229 of 236 cases. A subsequent study of intestinal biopsy samples showed that these SNPs coincided with low levels of mRNA for LPH consistent with transcriptional regulation [37]. It is likely that the C/T_{-13910} mutation impairs the binding of transcription factor Oct-1 [38]. The association between C/T_{-13910} and LNP was also observed in a study of children [39]. The presence of C/T_{-13910} had 100% specificity and 93% sensitivity in children older than 12 years compared with intestinal biopsy. Although these findings caused a great deal of excitement regarding the possibility of widespread genetic testing for LNP, other researchers have argued that genetic testing for LNP, based on C/T_{-13910}, is premature. In two reports of genetic testing of LNP among sub-Saharan African subjects, the C/T_{-13910} variant was extremely rare, and the authors suggested that other SNPs may be responsible for the LNP found in these populations [38,40]. The DNA regions encompassing the C/T_{-13910} LP/LNP variant have become the obvious targets in the search for additional lactose persistent variants in such populations. T/G_{-13915} and G/C_{-14010} have been associated with lactose persistence in African populations [41,42], and Oct-1 has been shown to interact with T/G_{-13915}[43]. Novel substitutions are being continually found, and further studies are required to confirm the possible relationships of these substitutions to the lactose persistent trait [44,42]. The fact that individuals who are digesters have been found to carry no recognized causative allele is indicative of the fact that many more unidentified variants are in existence [45]. More research is required to determine the appropriate genetic markers of LNP in different populations before genetic testing becomes commonplace.

B Direct Assessment of Lactase Activity

Lactose digestion can be assessed directly or indirectly. The direct method involves obtaining a biopsy specimen of intestinal tissue and assaying for lactase activity or by intestinal perfusion studies [46]. Although these tests can accurately measure lactase activity, they are invasive and seldom used clinically.

C Indirect Assessment Methods for Lactose Maldigestion

The metabolic basis for different indirect tests of lactose maldigestion is shown in Figure 40.1. Several indirect methods for assessing lactose digestion are available, including blood, urine, stool, and breath tests. Blood tests involve feeding a standard 50 g lactose dose and measurement of plasma glucose every 15−30 minutes over a period of 30 minutes to 2 hours. A rise in blood glucose of at least 25−30 mg/dl (1.5−1.7 mmol/l) is indicative of normal lactose digestion [41]. Unfortunately, blood glucose levels are subject to a variety of hormonal influences, reducing the reliability of this test. A blood test for galactose has been developed to correct this problem. The lactose dose is administered with a 500 mg/kg dose of ethanol (to prevent conversion of galactose to glucose in the liver) [46]. The galactose test is more reliable than the glucose test, but the ethanol exposure and somewhat invasive blood sampling are disadvantages.

A test has been devised to simultaneously measure intestinal lactose digestion (lactose digestion index [LDI]) and intestinal permeability (sugar absorption test [SAT]) [47]. The LDI/SAT test consists of the oral administration of a 250-ml solution containing 25 g ^{13}C-lactose, 0.5 g ^{2}H-glucose, 5 g lactulose (a nonabsorbable disaccharide of galactose and fructose), and 1 g L-rhamnose. For the LDI test, the blood levels of ^{13}C-glucose and ^{2}H-glucose are measured before and at several time intervals after the LDI solution, and a low ^{13}C glucose:^{2}H-glucose ratio (< 0.60) indicates significant failure to hydrolyze lactose. Urine collections more than 10 hours after the solution are obtained for measurements of the lactulose:rhamnose ratio, with a higher ratio indicating increased intestinal permeability. The LDI test was shown to outperform other measures of lactose digestion in one study [48] and it is less invasive than an intestinal biopsy, but it still has a number of limitations. The test requires the use of expensive isotopes and analytical equipment, involves both blood and urine collection, and has not been evaluated in persons with mucosal damage that might increase intestinal permeability.

A sometimes-used urine test involves the measurement of galactose in the urine, rather than the blood,

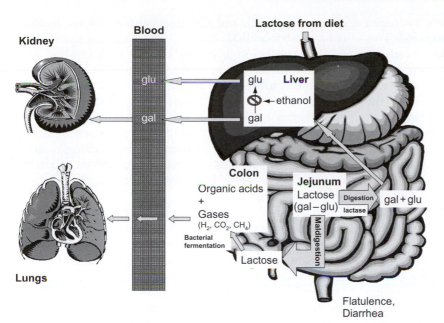

FIGURE 40.1 Metabolic background for understanding the diagnosis of lactose maldigestion and intolerance. gal, galactose; glu, glucose. Source: *Adapted with permission from Arola, H. (1994). Diagnosis of hypolactasia and lactose malabsorption.* Scand. J. Gastroenterol. **29**(Suppl. 202), 26−35.

during the lactose tolerance test with ethanol. Another urine test is conducted by simultaneously administering lactose and lactulose [46]. Small amounts of lactose (up to 1% of the ingested dose) and lactulose diffuse unmediated across the intestinal mucosa and are excreted in the urine. The ratio of lactose to lactulose in the urine (collected over 10 hours) is determined by the hydrolysis of lactose. A value of less than 0.3 indicates normal lactose digestion, and a ratio approaching 1.0 is observed in hypolactasia [46].

The measurement of stool pH and reducing substances in the stool has been used to assess lactose digestion in children. The analyses are easy to perform and convenient for the individuals being tested. However, stool pH has been shown to be unreliable in the diagnosis of hypolactasia in children and adults [46]. Furthermore, changes in gut motility and water excretion can alter the level of reducing substances in the stool. Thus, diagnosis of hypolactasia should not be based on stool tests alone [46].

Breath tests are the most widely used method for diagnosing carbohydrate maldigestion/malabsorption. The principle behind breath tests is that lactose, which escapes digestion in the small intestine, is fermented by bacteria in the colon, producing short-chain fatty acids (SCFA) and hydrogen, carbon dioxide, and methane (in some individuals). One breath test measures the amount of $^{13}CO_2$ excreted in the breath following administration of ^{13}C-lactose [46]. This stable isotope test has a safety advantage over older tests employing radioactive ^{14}C-lactose, but the high cost of the equipment prohibits widespread use of this method.

The current "gold standard" for diagnosis of carbohydrate maldigestion/malabsorption is the breath hydrogen test. Bacterial fermentation is the only source of hydrogen gas in the body. A portion of the hydrogen gas produced in the colon diffuses into the blood, with ultimate pulmonary excretion [49]. The hydrogen breath test is widely used because it is noninvasive and easy to perform. Typically, a subject is given an oral dose of lactose following an overnight (~12 hours) fast. Breath samples are collected at regular intervals for a period of 3−8 hours. In early studies, 50 g of lactose was used as a challenge dose. Almost all lactose maldigesters will experience intolerance symptoms following a dose of lactose this large [32], and yet many will be able to tolerate smaller, more physiologic doses of lactose. Doses of lactose that are in the range of 1 or 2 cups (240−480 ml) of milk (12−24 g lactose) have been more frequently used in recent years [50]. The dose of lactose used in the breath hydrogen test influences the diagnostic criterion for lactose maldigestion. Early studies with 50 g lactose showed perfect separation of lactose digesters from maldigesters using a rise in breath hydrogen of greater than 20 parts per million (ppm) above the fasting level [51]. Strocchi *et al.* [52] evaluated different criteria for diagnosis of carbohydrate maldigestion, using small doses of carbohydrate (10 g lactulose). Using a cut point of a 10-ppm or greater rise in breath hydrogen above fasting over an 8-hour period resulted in improved sensitivity (93 vs. 76%) and only a slight decrease in specificity (95 vs. 100%) compared to the 20-ppm cutoff. Furthermore, it was shown that using a sum of breath hydrogen values from hours 5, 6, and 7 and a 15-ppm or greater rise above fasting cut point resulted in 100% sensitivity and specificity.

Despite the advantages of breath hydrogen testing, care must be taken to ensure an accurate test. First, it is important to establish a low baseline breath hydrogen value, to which subsequent values are compared. This is accomplished by fasting before and after consumption of the lactose dose. In addition, it has been shown that a meal low in nondigestible carbohydrate (e.g., white rice and ground meat) the evening before the test results in lower baseline hydrogen [53]. Second, it is possible that some individuals may have a colonic microflora that is incapable of producing hydrogen. However, these individuals are rare, and the possibility of a non-hydrogen-producing flora can be ruled out by the administration of lactulose [52]. Third, approximately 40% of adults harbor significant numbers of methane-producing bacteria in the colon [49]. Because methanogenic bacteria consume four parts of hydrogen to produce one part methane [54], some authors have suggested that simultaneous measurement of methane will improve the accuracy of breath hydrogen testing in methane-producing subjects [55]. The availability of gas chromatographs that can analyze both hydrogen and methane in breath samples eliminates this potential problem. Finally, a number of factors (sleep, antibiotics, smoking, bacterial overgrowth of the small intestine, and exercise) may complicate the interpretation of breath hydrogen tests [46]. Therefore, standardization of the breath test protocol and appropriate controls are important.

Breath testing has been employed as a comparison to assess the clinical value of genetic testing. Positive breath tests have been correlated with both the C/T$_{-13910}$[56] and the g/A$_{-22018}$ polymorphisms [57]. However, better correlation has been identified between the lactase persistent genotype and a negative breath test [58]. Genetic testing does not provide information on actual patient symptoms, and the current usefulness of this test in populations with unestablished LP/LNP variants is questionable.

VI LACTOSE MALDIGESTION AND INTOLERANCE SYMPTOMS

A positive breath hydrogen test is indicative of lactose maldigestion. However, reduced lactase levels do not necessarily lead to intolerance symptoms. Symptoms of intolerance occur when the amount of lactose consumed exceeds the ability of both the small intestine and the colon to effectively metabolize the dose. Unhydrolyzed lactose passes from the small intestine to the large intestine, where it is fermented by enteric bacteria, producing the gases that are partially responsible for causing intolerance symptoms. The intensity of symptoms varies with the amount of lactose consumed [33,59—61], the degree of colonic

adaptation [6,62], and the physical form of the lactose-containing food [63].

The correlation between lactose maldigestion and reported intolerance symptoms is unclear. Most maldigesters can tolerate the amount of lactose in up to 1 or 2 cups of milk without experiencing severe symptoms. However, some lactose maldigesters believe that small amounts of lactose, such as the amount used with coffee or cereal, cause gastrointestinal distress [64]. Individual differences observed in symptom reporting may reflect learned behaviors, cultural attitudes, or other social issues.

Lactose maldigesters, unselected for their degree of lactose intolerance, tolerated a cup of milk without experiencing appreciable symptoms [65—67]. However, the results of these studies did not gain general acceptance, in part because of failure to enlist subjects with "severe" lactose intolerance. In 1995, Suarez et al. [64] conducted a study of 30 self-described "severely lactose intolerant individuals." Initial breath hydrogen test measurements indicated that approximately 30% (9 of 30) of the subjects claiming severe lactose intolerance were digesters and, thus, had no physiological basis for intolerance symptoms. These findings further demonstrate how strongly behavioral and psychological factors influence symptom reporting. Additional research is necessary to evaluate the psychological component of symptom reporting in lactose maldigesters.

VII LACTOSE DIGESTION, CALCIUM, AND OSTEOPOROSIS

Individuals who are lactose intolerant can generally tolerate moderate amounts of lactose with minimal or no gastrointestinal discomfort [64,68]. However, some lactose maldigesting individuals may unnecessarily restrict their intake of lactose-containing, calcium-rich dairy foods, thus compromising calcium intake. Milk and milk products contribute 73% of the calcium to the U.S. food supply [69]. Lactose maldigestion is associated with lower calcium intakes and is more frequent in osteoporotic cases than in controls [70—73]. For example, Newcomer et al. [70] found that 8 of 30 women with osteoporosis were lactose maldigesters compared to only 1 of 30 controls. In addition, calcium intakes of postmenopausal women positive for LNP in this study were significantly lower than in the lactase-persistent women (530 vs. 811 mg/day). Interestingly, in this report, and another by Horowitz et al. [71], few of the LNP subjects reported a history of milk intolerance and yet they still restricted milk intake. The lower milk intakes in these subjects may have been due to factors other than lactose intolerance. However, it is also possible that these subjects restricted their milk intakes because of lactose intolerance in childhood, forgot that they had done so, and simply maintained that pattern of milk intake throughout life.

Another potential explanation for the increased prevalence of osteoporosis among lactose maldigesters is that maldigestion of lactose might decrease the absorption of calcium. Human and animal studies suggest that lactose stimulates the intestinal absorption of calcium [69]. However, there is considerable disagreement regarding the influence of lactose and lactose maldigestion on calcium absorption in adults. This disagreement results from a number of factors, including the dose of lactose given, the choice of method for assessing calcium absorption (single isotope, double isotope, and balance methods), prior calcium intake of the subjects, and the form in which the calcium is given (milk vs. water).

Kocian *et al.* [74], using a single-isotope (^{47}Ca) method, demonstrated improved absorption of a 972-mg calcium dose from lactose-hydrolyzed milk compared to milk containing lactose in lactose maldigesters. Conversely, the regular milk resulted in increased calcium absorption versus the lactose-hydrolyzed milk in lactose digesters. Another study—using dual-isotope methods, a 50 g lactose load, and 500 mg of calcium chloride in water—found similar results [75]. Total fractional calcium absorption was decreased in maldigesters and increased in digesters with lactose feeding. However, the doses of lactose given in these studies (39—50 g or the equivalent of 3 or 4 cups of milk) were unphysiologic and may have resulted in more rapid intestinal transit than would be observed with more physiologic amounts of lactose.

Several studies have been conducted with physiologic doses of lactose. Griessen *et al.* [76], using dual-isotope methods, found that lactose maldigesters (*n* = 7) had a slightly, but not statistically significant, greater total fractional calcium absorption from 500 ml of milk compared to 500 ml of lactose-free milk. They also observed a nonsignificant decline in fractional calcium absorption in normal subjects (*n* = 8) when comparing lactose-free milk with regular milk. In another dual-isotope study, lactose maldigesters absorbed more calcium from a 240 ml dose of milk than did digesters (∼35 vs. 25%), which was thought to be due to lower calcium intakes in the lactose maldigesting group [77]. Most important, however, no difference was observed in fractional calcium absorption between lactose-hydrolyzed and regular milk in either group of subjects. Calcium absorption from milk and yogurt, each containing 270 mg of calcium, was studied using a single-isotope method [78]. No significant differences were observed in calcium absorption between milk and yogurt in either the lactose maldigesting or digesting subjects. Interestingly, yogurt resulted in slightly, but

significantly ($p < 0.05$), greater calcium absorption in lactose maldigesters compared to lactose digesters.

Differences in study methodology (milk vs. water, dose of lactose, and the choice of method for determining calcium absorption) may explain contrasting results. Physiologic doses of lactose (e.g., amounts provided by up to 2 cups of milk) are not likely to have a significant impact on calcium absorption. The increased prevalence of osteoporosis in lactose maldigesters is most likely related to inadequate calcium intake rather than impaired intestinal calcium absorption.

VIII DIETARY MANAGEMENT FOR LACTOSE MALDIGESTION

It is difficult for lactose maldigesters to consume adequate amounts of calcium if dairy products are eliminated from the diet. Fortunately, lactose intolerance is easily managed. Dietary management approaches that effectively reduce or eliminate intolerance symptoms are discussed next and shown in Table 40.4.

A Dose—Response to Lactose

There is a clear relationship between the dose of lactose consumed and the symptomatic response. Small doses (up to 12 g of lactose) yield no symptoms [1,64,66—68], whereas high doses (>20—50 g of lactose) produce appreciable symptoms in most individuals [1,79—81]. In a well-controlled trial, Newcomer *et al.* [1] demonstrated that more than 85% of lactose maldigesters developed intolerance symptoms after consuming 50 g of lactose (the approximate amount of lactose in 1 quart of milk) as a single dose. The frequency of reported symptoms may be attributed to the nonphysiologic nature of the lactose dose and the physical form of lactose load administered. A lactose dose of 15—25 g produces appreciable symptoms in some subjects [30,74]. The incidence of symptom reporting generally remains higher than 50% with intermediate doses. However, the frequency varies from less than 40% to greater than 90% [32]. In a double-blind protocol, Suarez *et al.* [64] demonstrated that feeding 12 g of lactose with a meal resulted in minimal to no symptoms in maldigesters. Interestingly, in unblinded studies [82,83], lactose maldigesters more frequently reported intolerance symptoms after consuming lactose loads similar to those given by Suarez *et al.* Subsequently, Suarez *et al.* [68] provided further evidence that individuals who are lactose intolerant can consume lactose-containing foods without experiencing appreciable symptoms by feeding lactose maldigesters 2 cups of milk daily. One cup of milk was given

TABLE 40.4 Dietary Strategies for Lactose Intolerance

Factors affecting lactose digestion	Dietary strategy	References
Dose of lactose	Consume a cup of milk or less at a time, containing up to 12 g lactose.	Suarez et al. [64] Hertzler et al. [6] Suarez et al. [68]
Intestinal transit	Consume milk with other foods, rather than alone, to slow the intestinal transit of lactose.	Solomons et al. [85] Martini and Savaiano [4] Dehkordi et al. [86]
Yogurt	Consume yogurt containing active bacteria cultures. One serving, or even two, should be well tolerated. Lactose in yogurts is better digested than the lactose in milk. Pasteurized yogurt does not improve lactose digestion; however, these products, when consumed, produce few to no symptoms.	Kolars et al. [93] Gilliland and Kim [99] Savaiano et al. [63] Shermak et al. [98] Savaiano et al. [63] Kolars et al. [93] Gilliland and Kim [99]
Digestive aids	Over-the-counter lactase supplements (pills, capsules, and drops) may be used when large doses of lactose (>12 g) are consumed at once. Lactose-hydrolyzed milk is also well tolerated.	Moskovitz et al. [116] Lin et al. [111] Ramirez et al. [117] Nielsen et al. [123] Biller et al. [128] Rosado et al. [125] Brand and Holt [121]
Colon adaptation	Consume lactose-containing foods daily to increase the ability of the colonic bacteria to metabolize undigested lactose.	Perman et al. [135] Florent et al. [62] Hertzler et al. [6]

with breakfast, and the second was given with the evening meal. The symptoms reported by maldigesters after consumption of 2 cups of milk a day were trivial.

Symptoms from excessive lactose in the intestine may increase out of proportion to dose, which raises the possibility that the absorption efficiency decreases with increased loads. Fractional lactose absorption is most likely influenced by dose, with more effective absorption of small loads and less effective utilization of larger doses. Hertzler et al. [60], using breath hydrogen as an indicator, suggested that 2 g of lactose is almost completely absorbed, whereas there was some

degree of maldigestion when a 6 g load was ingested. The only study directly measuring the lactose absorption efficiency in lactose maldigesting subjects is that of Bond and Levitt [84], who intubated the terminal ileum and then fed the subjects ^{14}C-lactose mixed with polyethylene glycol, a nonabsorbable volumetric marker. Analysis of the ratio of ^{14}C-lactose to polyethylene glycol passing through the terminal ileum allowed researchers to calculate the percentage of lactose absorbed. On average, maldigesters absorbed approximately 40% of a 12.5 g lactose load, whereas the other 60% passed to the terminal ileum. However, sizable differences were seen in absorption efficiency among lactose maldigesters. These differences may represent differences in residual lactase efficiency and/or gastric emptying and intestinal transit time.

B Factors Affecting Gastrointestinal Transit of Lactose

Consuming milk with other foods can minimize symptoms from lactose maldigestion [4,85,86]. A probable explanation for these findings is that the presence of additional foods slows the intestinal transit of lactose. Slowed transit allows more contact between ingested lactose and residual lactase in the small intestine, thus improving lactose digestion. It is also possible that additional foods may simply slow the rate at which lactose arrives in the colon because a delay in peak breath hydrogen production, rather than a significant decrease in total hydrogen production, has been reported [4]. The slower fermentation of lactose might allow for more efficient disposal of fermentation gases, reducing the potential for symptoms.

The energy content, fat content, and added components such as chocolate may influence gastrointestinal transit of lactose and subsequent lactose digestion. Leichter [87] showed that 50 g of lactose from whole milk (1050 ml) resulted in fewer symptoms (abdominal discomfort, bloating, and flatulence) compared to 50 g of lactose from either skim milk (1050 ml) or an aqueous solution (330 ml). However, only blood glucose was measured to determine lactose digestion, and no statistical evaluation of symptoms was done in this study. Other studies have demonstrated that higher fat milk may slightly decrease breath hydrogen relative to skim milk [86] but not improve tolerance [86,88,89]. Furthermore, increasing the energy content or viscosity of milk has not been effective in improving lactose digestion or tolerance [90,91].

Chocolate milk has been recommended for individuals who are lactose intolerant. Apparently, chocolate milk empties from the stomach more slowly than unflavored milk, possibly because of its higher osmolality or energy content [3]. Two reports [86,92] have demonstrated improved lactose digestion (i.e., reduced breath hydrogen) following consumption of chocolate milk. One of these studies [92] documented fewer symptoms in subjects.

Clearly, consumption of milk with other foods results in improved tolerance compared to consumption of milk alone. Therefore, consuming small amounts of milk routinely with meals is a recommended approach for individuals who are lactose intolerant to obtain sufficient calcium from dairy products. These individuals may also try chocolate milk to improve tolerance.

C Yogurt

The lactose in yogurt with live cultures is digested better than lactose in milk and is well tolerated by those who are lactose intolerant [93]. Prior to fermentation, most commercially produced yogurt is nearly 6% lactose because of the addition of milk solids to milk during yogurt production. However, as the lactic acid bacteria (*Lactobacillus delbrueckii* subsp. *bulgaricus* and *Streptococcus salivarius* subsp. *thermophilus*) multiply to nearly 100 million organisms per milliliter, 20–30% of the lactose is utilized, decreasing the lactose content of yogurt to approximately 4% [94]. During fermentation, the activity of the β-galactosidase (lactase) enzyme substantially increases. Casein, calcium phosphate, and lactate in yogurt act as buffers in the acidic environment of the stomach, thus protecting a portion of the microbial lactase from degradation and allowing the delivery of intact cells to the small intestine [95,96]. In the duodenum, once the intact bacterial cells interact with bile acids, they are disrupted, allowing substrate access to enzyme activity.

Yogurt consumption results in enhanced digestion of lactose and improved tolerance [63,93,97–99]. In 1984, Kolars *et al.* [93] and Gilliland and Kim [99] reported enhanced lactose digestion from yogurt in lactose maldigesters. In both studies, breath hydrogen excretion was significantly reduced with the consumption of live culture yogurt. Furthermore, Kolars *et al.* found that an 18-g load of lactose in yogurt resulted in significantly fewer intolerance symptoms reported by subjects compared to the other forms of lactose given. Also in 1984, Savaiano *et al.* [63] demonstrated that yogurt feeding resulted in one-third to one-fifth less hydrogen excretion compared to other lactose-containing dairy foods with no symptoms. Shermak *et al.* [98] reported that a 12 g load of lactose in yogurt resulted in lower peak hydrogen in children with a delay in the time for breath hydrogen to rise compared to a similar lactose load given in milk. These children experienced significantly fewer intolerance symptoms with yogurt consumption.

Yogurt pasteurization following fermentation has been somewhat controversial [99]. One advantage of pasteurizing yogurt is a longer shelf life. However, removing the active cultures that are partly responsible for improved lactose digestion may increase intolerance symptoms and cause lactose maldigesters to avoid yogurt products. Pasteurizing yogurt increases the maldigestion of lactose [63,98,99]. However, pasteurized yogurt is moderately well tolerated, producing minimal symptoms [63,97,98]. Because pasteurized yogurt is relatively well tolerated, other factors such as the physical form, or gelling, and the energy density of yogurt may play a role in tolerance. The level of the β-galactosidase enzyme in yogurt may not be the limiting factor for improving lactose digestion because not all yogurts have the same level of lactase activity [100]. Martini *et al.* [100] fed yogurts with varying levels of microbial β-galactosidase. The remaining characteristics of the test yogurts (pH, cell counts, and lactose concentrations) were similar. Despite the different levels of β-galactosidase activity, all yogurts improved lactose digestion and minimized intolerance symptoms.

D Kefir

Kefir is a fermented dairy beverage that originated in Eastern Europe and has been made for centuries. Unlike yogurt, it is drinkable, and the kefir grains used to culture the milk contain a wider variety of starter culture microorganisms. Hertzler and Clancy [101] investigated the effect of kefir ingestion on lactose maldigestion and intolerance symptoms in a group of lactose maldigesters. The kefir used in the study contained *Streptococcus lactis, Lactobacillus plantarum, Streptococcus cremoris, Lactobacillus casei, Streptococcus diacetylactis, Saccharomyces florentinus*, and *Leuconostoc cremoris* (as per label information) as the starter cultures. Feeding a 20 g lactose load as plain kefir reduced breath hydrogen excretion (8-hour area under the curve) by nearly threefold and decreased flatulence symptoms by 50% compared with the same amount of lactose from milk. The response to yogurt was similar to that observed with kefir.

E Unfermented Acidophilus Milk

Individuals who are lactose maldigesters may consume unfermented milk containing cultures of *Lactobacillus acidophilus* in an effort to consume adequate amounts of calcium and avoid intolerance symptoms [102–104]. Various strains of *L. acidophilus* exist; however, strain NCFM has been most extensively studied and used in commercial products. Unfermented acidophilus milk tastes identical to unaltered milk because the NCFM strain does not multiply in the product, provided that the storage temperature is below 40°F (5°C) [102,103,105]. *Lactobacillus acidophilus* strain NCFM is derived from human fecal samples [95] and contains β-galactosidase. The effectiveness of acidophilus milk on improving lactose digestion and intolerance symptoms has been evaluated. Most evidence suggests that unfermented acidophilus milk does not enhance lactose digestion or reduce intolerance symptoms [63,106—108], primarily because of the low concentration of the species in the milk. Improved lactose digestion has been observed by some [108]; however, the test milk in this study contained a much higher concentration of *L. acidophilus* than is normally used to produce commercial acidophilus milks.

Furthermore, the microbial lactase from *L. acidophilus* may not be available to hydrolyze the lactose *in vivo* [100,103,107]. *Lactobacillus acidophilus* is not a bile-sensitive organism [95,105]. Therefore, once the intact bacterial cells reach the small intestine, bile acids may not disrupt the cell membrane to allow the release of the microbial lactase. However, sonicated acidophilus milk improved lactose digestion by reducing breath hydrogen [109]. Thus, if less bile-resistant strains were developed and used in adequate amounts, these strains may allow the β-galactosidase to be released, possibly yielding an effective approach to the dietary management of lactose maldigestion.

Finally, fermented and unfermented milks containing bifidobacteria may also be useful in the management of lactose intolerance. Studies of milks treated with *Bifidobacterium bifidus* GD428 [100] and *B. longum* (strains B6 and 15708) [110] lower breath hydrogen excretion and flatulence symptoms compared with milk in lactose maldigesters. However, the beneficial effects, as with acidophilus milk, were still less than those observed with yogurt.

F Lactase Supplements and Lactose-Reduced Milk

Lactase pills, capsules, and drops contain lactase derived from yeast (*Kluyveromyces lactis*) or fungal (*Aspergillus niger and A. oryzae*) sources. Common brands include Lactaid and Lacteeze. Dosages of lactase per pill or caplet vary from 4000 to 9000 FCC (Food Chemical Codex) units [111—113]. Since 1984, these over-the-counter preparations have been given GRAS (generally recognized as safe) status by the U.S. Food and Drug Administration [114]. Lactase pretreated milks (100% lactose hydrolysis) are available from Lactaid and Dairy Ease [112,115].

A number of studies have evaluated the effectiveness of these products. Doses of 3000—6000 FCC units of lactase administered just prior to milk consumption decrease both breath hydrogen and symptom responses to lactose loads ranging from 17 to 20 g [111,116,117]. The decrease in breath hydrogen and symptoms is generally dose dependent. Doses up to 9900 FCC units may be needed for digestion of a large lactose load, such as 50 g of lactose [111,118,119].

Lactose-hydrolyzed milks also improve lactose intolerance symptoms in both children and adults [80,81,120—130]. A by-product of lactose-hydrolyzed milk is increased sweetness due to the presence of free glucose [64]. This increased sweetness may increase its acceptability in children [123].

G Colonic Fermentation and Colonic Bacterial Adaptation of Lactose

The colonic bacteria ferment undigested lactose and produce SCFA and gases. Historically, this fermentation process was viewed negatively as a cause of lactose intolerance symptoms. However, it is now recognized that the fermentation of lactose, as well as other nonabsorbed carbohydrates, plays an important role in the health of the colon and affects the nutritional status of the individual.

The loss of intestinal lactase activity in lactose maldigesters is permanent. Studies from Israel, India, and Thailand have reported that feeding 50 g of lactose or more per day for periods of 1—14 months has no impact on jejunal lactase activity [17,131,132]. Despite this observation, milk has been used successfully in the treatment of malnourished children in areas of the world where lactose maldigestion is common. In Ethiopia, for example, 100 schoolchildren, aged 6—10 years, were fed 250 ml of milk per day for a period of 4 weeks [133]. Although the children initially experienced some degree of gastrointestinal symptoms, the symptoms rapidly abated and returned to pretrial levels within 4 weeks. Similar results were observed with schoolchildren in India [131]. Finally, a study of African American males and females aged 13—39 years who were lactose maldigesters and lactose intolerant showed that 77% of the subjects could ultimately tolerate 12 g or more of lactose if lactose was increased gradually and fed daily over a period of 6—12 weeks [134]. Approximately 80% of the subjects (18 of 22) had rises in breath hydrogen of at least 10 ppm above baseline at the maximum dose of lactose tolerated, suggesting that improved digestion of lactose in the small intestine was not responsible for the increased tolerance. Therefore, the authors proposed that colonic bacterial adaptation was a likely explanation for these findings.

Evidence for colonic bacterial adaptation to disaccharides (lactulose and lactose) is substantial. Perman *et al.* [135] fed adults 0.3 g/kg lactulose per day for 7 days and observed a decrease in fecal pH from 7.1 ± 0.3 to 5.8 ± 0.6. The breath hydrogen response to a challenge dose of lactose (0.3 g/kg) fell significantly after lactulose adaptation. Employing the same experimental design and doses of lactulose, Florent *et al.* [62] measured fecal β-galactosidase, colonic pH, breath hydrogen, fecal carbohydrates, SCFA, and ^{14}C-lactulose catabolism in subjects before and after the 7-day lactulose maintenance period. Fecal β-galactosidase was six times greater after lactulose feeding, and breath hydrogen fell significantly. Breath $^{14}CO_2$ (indicating catabolism of ^{14}C-lactulose) increased and fecal outputs of lactulose and total hexose units were low after the lactulose feeding. Symptoms were not measured; however, a follow-up study showed that adaptation to lactulose (40 g/day for 8 days) reduced symptoms of diarrhea induced by a large dose (60 g) of lactulose [136]. Breath hydrogen decreased significantly, and fecal β-galactosidase activity increased as in the previous study.

Two feeding trials directed to adapting lactose maldigesters to lactose have been reported. The first was a blinded, crossover study conducted at the University of Minnesota [6]. Feeding increasing doses of lactose (from 0.3 to 1.0 g/kg/day) for 16 days resulted in a threefold increase in fecal β-galactosidase activity, which returned to baseline levels within 48 hours after substitution of dextrose for lactose. Furthermore, 10 days of lactose feeding (from 0.6 to 1.0 g/kg/day), compared to dextrose feeding, dramatically decreased the breath hydrogen response to a lactose challenge dose (0.35 g/kg; Figure 40.2). After lactose adaptation, the subjects no longer appeared to be lactose maldigesters, based on a 20-ppm rise in breath hydrogen above fasting. The large doses of lactose fed during the adaptation period (averaging 42–70 g/day) resulted in only minor symptoms. In addition, the severity and frequency of flatus symptoms in response to the lactose challenge dose were reduced by 50%.

The second study was a double-blind, placebo-controlled trial conducted in France with a group of 46 subjects who were lactose intolerant [137]. Following a baseline lactose challenge with 50 g of lactose, subjects were randomly assigned to either a lactose-fed group ($n=24$) or a sucrose-fed control group ($n = 22$). Subjects were fed 34 g of either lactose or sucrose per day for 15 days. Fecal β-galactosidase increased and breath hydrogen decreased as a result of lactose feeding. Clinical symptoms (except diarrhea) were 50% less severe after lactose feeding. However, the sucrose-fed control group also experienced a comparable decrease in symptoms, despite no evidence of metabolic adaptation. Thus, these

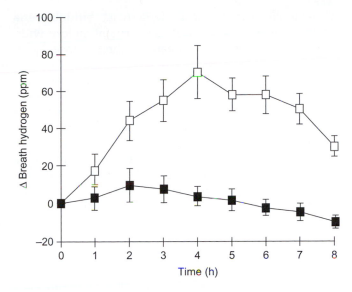

FIGURE 40.2 **Breath hydrogen response to a lactose challenge after lactose (□) or dextrose (■) feeding periods.** Data are the means ± SEM, $n = 20$. Source: *Reprinted with permission from Hertzler, S. R., and Savaiano, D. A. (1996). Colonic adaptation to daily lactose feeding in lactose maldigesters reduces lactose intolerance. Am. J. Clin. Nutr.* **64***, 232–236.*

authors concluded that the improvements in symptoms resulted from familiarization with the test protocol rather than from metabolic adaptation.

Colonic bacteria develop an increased ability to ferment lactose (indicated by increased fecal β-galactosidase) following prolonged lactose feeding. Because hydrogen gas is an end product of fermentation, it might be expected that the increased ability to ferment lactose would result in an increase, rather than the observed decrease, in breath hydrogen. However, breath hydrogen excretion represents the net of bacterial hydrogen production and consumption in the colon [54]. A decrease in net production of hydrogen could result from either decreased bacterial production or increased consumption. To examine the mechanism for decreased breath hydrogen after lactose adaptation, Hertzler *et al.* [138] employed metabolic inhibitors of bacterial hydrogen consumption (methanogenesis, sulfate reduction, and acetogenesis) to obtain measures of absolute hydrogen production. Subjects were fed increasing amounts of lactose or dextrose in a manner similar to previous studies. Fecal samples were assayed *in vitro* for absolute hydrogen production and hydrogen consumption. Absolute hydrogen production after 3 hours of incubation with lactose was threefold lower after lactose adaptation (242 ± 54 ml) compared to the dextrose feeding period (680 ± 7 ml, $p = 0.006$). Fecal hydrogen consumption was unaffected by either feeding period. These findings tend to support the hypothesis that prolonged lactose feeding favors the growth or metabolic activity of bacteria (e.g., bifidobacteria and lactic acid bacteria) that can ferment lactose without the production of hydrogen. Feeding lactose, lactulose, and nonabsorbable oligosaccharides stimulates the proliferation of lactic acid bacteria in the colon [139–141]. In addition, high populations of bifidobacteria inhibit the growth of known hydrogen-producing organisms, such as clostridia or *Escherichia coli* [142].

Colonic bacterial adaptation to lactose does occur. Although the role of colonic adaptation in improving symptoms is not firmly established, it is clear that many individuals who are lactose intolerant can develop a tolerance to milk if they consume it regularly. This may represent a simpler and less expensive solution than the use of lactose digestive aids. A product called Lactagen has been marketed as a therapy for lactose intolerance, largely based on the colonic adaptation hypothesis. Lactagen is a powder containing lactose, *L. acidophilus*, fructo-oligosaccharides, and small amounts of calcium and phosphorus. It is recommended by the manufacturer that the product be taken for a 38-day period, which is said to be sufficient to permanently "recondition" the intestinal microflora for lactose tolerance. One double-blind study of this product, published only as an abstract [143], reported that 80% of lactose-intolerant subjects had reductions in lactose intolerance symptoms compared with 19% in the placebo group. However, objective evidence of improved lactose digestion or altered colonic bacterial fermentation of lactose (e.g., decreased breath hydrogen) was not obtained in this study. Furthermore, longer term follow-up studies to assess the permanence of the symptom reductions were not conducted.

IX GENE THERAPY FOR LACTOSE INTOLERANCE

Although conventional dietary therapies for lactose intolerance exist, the possibility of gene therapy for lactase nonpersistence was examined by During *et al.* [144]. An adeno-associated virus vector was orally administered to hypolactasic rats to increase lactase mRNA. The adeno-associated virus vector is a defective, helper-dependent virus, and the wild type is non-pathogenic in humans and other species. Following a single administration of a recombinant adeno-associated virus vector expressing β-galactosidase, all rats treated with this vector ($n = 4$) were positive for *lacZ* mRNA in the proximal intestine within 3 days. There was no lactase mRNA in the rats treated with the control vector. On day 7, following vector administration, the rats were challenged with a lactose solution. The treated rats had a rise in blood glucose from 114 ± 4 to 130 ± 3 mg/dl after 30 minutes, whereas the control

rats had a flat blood glucose curve. Furthermore, the treated rats still displayed similar lactase activity when challenged with lactose 6 months later. Thus, the potential of gene therapy for lactose intolerance is an interesting prospect, but this has not been studied in humans.

X SUMMARY

A majority of the world's population and approximately 25% of the U.S. population are lactose maldigesters. Milk and milk products not only contain lactose but also are important sources of calcium, riboflavin, and high-quality protein. Some maldigesters may avoid dairy products because of the perception that intolerance symptoms will inevitably follow dairy food consumption. Avoiding dairy products may limit calcium intake and bone density, thus increasing the risk for osteoporosis. Avoidance of milk and milk products is unnecessary because moderate lactose consumption does not usually produce a symptomatic response in maldigesters. In addition, various dietary strategies effectively manage lactose intolerance by reducing or eliminating gastrointestinal symptoms. Dairy food consumption is possible for individuals who are lactose intolerant if simple dietary management strategies are incorporated into daily living.

References

[1] A.D. Newcomer, D.B. McGill, P.J. Thomas, A.F. Hofmann, Tolerance to lactose among lactase deficient American Indians, Gastroenterology 74 (1978) 44–46.

[2] W.J. Ravich, T.M. Bayless, Carbohydrate absorption and malabsorption, Clin. Gastroenterol. 12 (1983) 335–356.

[3] J.D. Welsh, W.H. Hall, Gastric emptying of lactose and milk in subjects with lactose malabsorption, Am. J. Dig. Dis. 22 (1977) 1060–1063.

[4] M.C. Martini, D.A. Savaiano, Reduced intolerance symptoms from lactose consumed with a meal, Am. J. Clin. Nutr. 47 (1988) 57–60.

[5] N.S. Scrimshaw, E.B. Murray, The acceptability of milk and milk products in populations with a high prevalence of lactose intolerance, Am. J. Clin. Nutr. 48 (1988) 1083–1159.

[6] S.R. Hertzler, D.A. Savaiano, Colonic adaptation to the daily lactose feeding in lactose maldigesters reduces lactose tolerance, Am. J. Clin. Nutr. 64 (1996) 1232–1236.

[7] N. Kretchmer, P. Sunshine, Intestinal disaccharidase deficiency in the sea lion, Gastroenterology 53 (1967) 123–129.

[8] L. Zeccha, J.E. Mesonero, A. Stutz, J.-C. Poiree, J. Giudicelli, R. Cursio, et al., Intestinal lactase-phlorizin hydrolase (LPH): the two catalytic sites; the role of the pancreas in pro-LPH maturation, FEBS Lett. 435 (1998) 225–228.

[9] R.K. Montgomery, H. Buller, E.H.H.M. Rings, R.J. Grand, Lactose intolerance and the genetic regulation of intestinal lactase phlorizin hydrolase, FASEB J. 5 (1991) 2824–2832.

[10] M. Rossi, L. Maiuri, M.I. Fusco, V.M. Salvati, A. Fuccio, S. Aurrichio, et al., Lactase persistence versus decline in human

adults: multifactorial events are involved in downregulation after weaning, Gastroenterology 112 (1997) 1506—1514.

[11] I. Järvelä, N.S. Enattah, J. Kokkonen, T. Varilo, E. Sahvilahti, L. Peltonen, Assignment of the locus for congenital lactase deficiency to 2q21, in the vicinity of but separate from the lactase-phlorizin hydrolase gene, Am. J. Hum. Genet. 63 (1998) 1078—1085.

[12] E.E. Sterchi, P.R. Mills, J.A.M. Fransen, H.-P. Hauri, M.J. Lentze, H.Y. Naim, et al., Biogenesis of intestinal lactase-phlorizin hydrolase in adults with lactose intolerance: evidence for reduced biosynthesis and slowed-down maturation in enterocytes, J. Clin. Invest. 86 (1990) 1329—1337.

[13] C.L. Kien, L.A. Heitlinger, U. Li, R.D. Murray, Digestion, absorption, and fermentation of carbohydrates, Semin. Perinatol. 13 (1989) 78—87.

[14] A. Holzel, V. Schwarz, K.W. Sutcliffe, Defective lactose absorption causing malnutrition in infancy, Lancet 1 (1959) 1126—1128.

[15] E. Sahvilahti, K. Launiala, P. Kuitunen, Congenital lactase deficiency, Arch. Dis. Child. 58 (1983) 246—252.

[16] A.D. Newcomer, D.B. McGill, Clinical consequences of lactase deficiency, Clin. Nutr. 3 (1984) 53—58.

[17] T. Sahi, Genetics and epidemiology of adult-type hypolactasia, Scand. J. Gastroenterol. 29 (1994) 7—20.

[18] T. Gilat, S. Russo, E. Gelman-Malachi, T.A.M. Aldor, Lactase in man: a nonadaptable enzyme, Gastroenterology 62 (1972) 1125—1127.

[19] F.J Simoons, The geographic hypothesis and lactose malabsorption—A weighing of the evidence, Am. J. Dig. Dis. 23 (1978) 963—980.

[20] R.D. McCracken, Adult lactose tolerance [letter], JAMA 213 (1970) 2257—2260.

[21] J. Burger, M. Kirchner, B. Bramanti, W. Haak, M.G. Thomas, Absence of the lactose-persistence-associated allele in early Neolithic Europeans, Proc. Natl. Acad. Sci. USA 104 (2007) 3736—3741.

[22] S.A. Tishkoff, F.A. Reed, A. Ranciaro, B.F. Voight, C.C. Babbitt, J.S. Silverman, et al., Convergent adaptation of human lactase persistence in Africa and Europe, Nat. Genet. 39 (2007) 31—40.

[23] M.-F. Lee, S.D. Krasinski, Human adult-onset lactase decline: an update, Nutr. Rev. 56 (1998) 1—8.

[24] M. Lloyd, G. Mevissen, M. Fischer, W. Olsen, D. Goodspeed, M. Genini, et al., Regulation of intestinal lactase in adult hypolactasia, J. Clin. Invest. 89 (1992) 524—529.

[25] O. Fajardo, H.Y. Naim, S.W. Lacey, The polymorphic expression of lactase in adults is regulated at the messenger RNA level, Gastroenterology 106 (1994) 1233—1241.

[26] J.C. Eschler, N. de Koning, C.G.J. van Engen, S. Arora, H.A. Buller, R.K. Montgomery, et al., Molecular basis of lactase levels in adult humans, J. Clin. Invest. 89 (1992) 480—483.

[27] G. Sebastio, M. Villa, R. Sartorio, V. Guzetta, V. Poggi, S. Aurrichio, et al., Control of lactase in human adult-type hypolactasia and in weaning rabbits and rats, Am. J. Hum. Genet. 45 (1989) 489—497.

[28] W.A. Olsen, B.U. Li, M. Lloyd, H. Korsmo, Heterogeneity of intestinal lactase activity in children: relationship to lactase-phlorizin hydrolase messenger RNA abundance, Pediatr. Res. 39 (1996) 877—881.

[29] A.D. Newcomer, D.B. McGill, Distribution of disaccharidase activity in the small bowel of normal and lactase-deficient subjects, Gastroenterology 51 (1966) 481—488.

[30] N. Triadou, J. Bataille, J. Schmitz, Longitudinal study of the human intestinal brush border membrane proteins, Gastroenterology 85 (1983) 1326—1332.

[31] L. Maiuri, M. Rossi, V. Raia, V. Garipoli, L.A. Hughes, D. Swallow, et al., Mosaic regulation of lactase in human adult-type hypolactasia, Gastroenterology 107 (1994) 54—60.

[32] D.A. Savaiano, M.D. Levitt, Milk intolerance and microbe-containing dairy foods, J. Dairy Sci. 70 (1987) 397—406.

[33] R. Srinivasan, A. Minocha, When to suspect lactose intolerance: symptomatic, ethnic, and laboratory clues, Postgrad. Med. 104 (1998) 109—123.

[34] W. Schmidt, T. Schneider, W. Heise, J.-D. Schulze, T. Weinke, R. Ignatius, et al., Mucosal abnormalities in microsporidiosis, AIDS 11 (1997) 1589—1594.

[35] G.R. Corazza, L. Ginaldi, N. Furia, G. Marani-Toro, D. Di Giammartino, D. Quaglino, The impact of HIV infection on lactose absorptive capacity, J. Infect. 35 (1997) 31—35.

[36] N.S. Enattah, T. Sahi, E. Savilahti, J.D. Terwilliger, L. Peltonen, I. Jarvella, Identification of a variant associated with adult-type hypolactasia, Nat. Genet. 30 (2002) 233—237.

[37] M. Kuokkanen, N.S. Enattah, A. Okasanen, E. Savilahti, A. Orpana, I. Järvelä, Transcriptional regulation of the lactase-phlorizin hydrolase gene by polymorphisms associated with adult-type hypolactasia, Gut 52 (2003) 647—652.

[38] C.J.E. Ingram, M.F. Elamin, C.A. Mulcare, M.E. Weale, A. Tarekegn, T.O. Raga, et al., A novel polymorphism associated with lactose tolerance in Africa: multiple causes for lactase persistence? Hum. Genet. 120 (2007) 779—788.

[39] H. Rasinpera, E. Savilahti, N.S. Enattah, M. Kuokkanen, N. Tötterman, H. Lindahl, et al., A genetic test which can be used to diagnose adult-type hypolactasia in children, Gut 53 (2004) 1571—1576.

[40] C.A. Mulcare, M.E. Weale, A.L. Jones, B. Connell, D. Zeitlyn, A. Tarekegn, et al., The T allele of a single-nucleotide polymorphism 13.9 kb upstream of the lactase gene (LCT) (C-13.9kbT) does not predict or cause the lactase-persistence phenotype in Africans, Am. J. Hum. Genet. 74 (2004) 1102—1110.

[41] N.S. Enattah, T.G.K. Jensen, M. Nielsen, R. Lewinski, M. Kuokkanen, H. Rasinpera, et al., Independent introduction of two lactase-persistence alleles into human populations reflects different history of adaptation to milk culture, Am. J. Hum. Genet. 82 (2008) 57—72.

[42] S. Torniainen, M.I. Parker, V. Holmberg, E. Lahtela, C. Dandara, I. Jarvela, Screening of variants for lactase persistence/non-persistence in populations from South Africa and Ghana, BMC Genet. 10 (2009) 31.

[43] L.C. Olds, J.K. Ahn, E. Sibley, 13915*G DNA polymorphism associated with lactase persistence in Africa interacts with Oct-1, Hum. Genet. 129 (2011) 111—113.

[44] C.J. Ingram, T.O. Raga, A. Tarekegn, S.L. Browning, M.F. Elamin, E. Bekele, et al., Multiple rare variants as a cause of a common phenotype: several different lactase persistence associated alleles in a single ethnic group, J. Mol. Evol. 69 (2009) 579—588.

[45] C.J. Ingram, C.A. Mulcare, Y. Itan, M.G. Thomas, D.M. Swallow, Lactose digestion and the evolutionary genetics of lactase persistence, Hum. Genet. 124 (2009) 579—591.

[46] H. Arola, Diagnosis of hypolactasia and lactose malabsorption, Scand. J. Gastroenterol. 29 (1994) 26—35.

[47] H.A. Koetse, D. Klaassen, A.R.H. van der Molen, H. Elzinga, K. Bijsterveld, R. Boverhof, et al., Combined LDI/SAT test to evaluate intestinal lactose digestion and mucosa permeability, Eur. J. Clin. Invest. 36 (2006) 730—736.

[48] R.J. Vonk, F. Stellarrd, M.G. Priebe, H.A. Koetse, R.E. Hagedoorn, S. de Bruijn, et al., The $^{13}Cy^{2}H$-glucose test for determination of small intestinal lactase activity, Eur. J. Clin. Invest. 31 (2001) 226—233.

[49] M.D. Levitt, R.M. Donaldson, Use of respiratory hydrogen (H$_2$) excretion to detect carbohydrate malabsorption, J. Lab. Clin. Med. 75 (1970) 937−945.

[50] N.W. Solomons, Evaluation of carbohydrate absorption: the hydrogen breath test in clinical practice, Clin. Nutr. 3 (1984) 71−78.

[51] G. Metz, D.J. Jenkins, J.J. Peters, A. Newman, L.M. Blendis, Breath hydrogen as a diagnostic method for hypolactasia, Lancet 1 (1975) 1155−1157.

[52] A. Strocchi, G. Corazza, C.J. Ellis, G. Gasbarrini, M.D. Levitt, Detection of malabsorption of low doses of carbohydrate: accuracy of various breath hydrogen criteria, Gastroenterology 105 (1993) 1404−1410.

[53] I.H. Anderson, A.S. Levine, M.D. Levitt, Incomplete absorption of the carbohydrate in all-purpose wheat flour, N. Engl. J. Med. 304 (1981) 891−892.

[54] M.D. Levitt, G.R. Gibson, S.U. Christl, Gas metabolism in the large intestine, in: G.R. Gibson, G.T. Macfarlane (Eds.), Human Colonic Bacteria: Role in Nutrition, Physiology, and Disease, CRC Press, Boca Raton, FL, 1995, pp. 131−154.

[55] A. Bjorneklett, E. Jenssen, Relationships between hydrogen (H$_2$) and methane (CH$_4$) production in man, Scand. J. Gastroenterol. 17 (1982) 985−992.

[56] M. Krawczyk, M. Wolska, S. Schwartz, F. Gruenhage, B. Terjung, P. Portincasa, et al., Concordance of genetic and breath tests for lactose intolerance in a tertiary referral centre, J. Gastrointestin. Liver Dis. 17 (2008) 135−139.

[57] M. Di Stefano, V. Terulla, P. Tana, S. Mazzocchi, E. Romero, G.R. Corazza, Genetic test for lactase non-persistence and hydrogen breath test: is genotype better than phenotype to diagnose lactose malabsorption? Dig. Liver Dis. 41 (2009) 474−479.

[58] D. Nagy, E. Bogacsi-Szabo, A. Varkonyi, B. Csanyi, A. Czibula, O. Bede, et al., Prevalence of adult-type hypolactasia as diagnosed with genetic and lactose hydrogen breath tests in Hungarians, Eur. J. Clin. Nutr. 63 (2009) 909−912.

[59] E. Gudmand Høyer, The clinical significance of disaccharide maldigestion, Am. J. Clin. Nutr. 59 (1994) 735S−741S.

[60] S.R. Hertzler, B. Huynh, D.A. Savaiano, How much lactose is "low lactose"? J. Am. Diet. Assoc. 96 (1996) 243−246.

[61] T.H. Vesa, R.A. Korpela, T. Sahi, Tolerance to small amounts of lactose in lactose maldigesters, Am. J. Clin. Nutr. 64 (1996) 197−201.

[62] C. Florent, B. Flourie, A. Leblond, M. Rautureau, J.-J. Bernier, J.-C. Rambaud, Influence of chronic lactulose ingestion on the colonic metabolism of lactulose in man (an in vivo study), J. Clin. Invest. 75 (1985) 608−613.

[63] D.A. Savaiano, A. Abou El Anouar, D.E. Smith, M.D. Levitt, Lactose malabsorption from yogurt, pasteurized yogurt, sweet acidophilus milk, and cultured milk in lactase-deficient individuals, Am. J. Clin. Nutr. 40 (1984) 1219−1223.

[64] F.L. Suarez, D.A. Savaiano, M.D. Levitt, A comparison of symptoms after the consumption of milk or lactose-hydrolyzed milk by people with self-reported severe lactose intolerance, N. Engl. J. Med. 333 (1995) 1−4.

[65] M.H. Rorick, N.S. Scrimshaw, Comparative tolerance of elderly from differing ethnic background to lactose-containing and lactose-free daily drinks: a double-blind study, J. Gerontol. 34 (1979) 191−196.

[66] L. Haverberg, P.H. Kwon, N.S. Scrimshaw, Comparative tolerance of adolescents of differing ethnic backgrounds to lactose-containing and lactose-free dairy drinks. I. Initial experience with a double-blind procedure, Am. J. Clin. Nutr. 33 (1980) 17−21.

[67] M. Unger, N.S. Scrimshaw, Comparative tolerance of adults of differing ethnic backgrounds to lactose-free and lactose-containing dairy drinks, Nutr. Res. 1 (1981) 1227−1233.

[68] F.L. Suarez, D.A. Savaiano, P. Arbisi, M.D. Levitt, Tolerance to the daily ingestion of two cups of milk by individuals claiming lactose intolerance, Am. J. Clin. Nutr. 65 (1997) 1502−1506.

[69] G.D. Miller, J.K. Jarvis, L.D. McBean, Handbook of Dairy Foods and Nutrition, second ed., CRC Press, Boca Raton, FL, 2000, pp. 311−354.

[70] A.D. Newcomer, S.F. Hodgson, D.B. McGill, P.J. Thomas, Lactase deficiency: prevalence in osteoporosis, Ann. Intern. Med. 89 (1978) 218−220.

[71] M. Horowitz, J. Wishart, L. Mundy, B.E.C. Nordin, Lactose and calcium absorption in postmenopausal osteoporosis, Arch. Intern. Med. 147 (1987) 534−536.

[72] G. Finkenstedt, F. Skrabal, R.W. Gasser, H. Braunsteiner, Lactose absorption, milk consumption, and fasting blood glucose concentrations in women with idiopathic osteoporosis, Br. Med. J. 292 (1986) 161−162.

[73] G.R. Corazza, G. Benati, A. DiSario, C. Tarozzi, A. Strocchi, M. Passeri, et al., Lactose intolerance and bone mass in postmenopausal Italian women, Br. J. Nutr. 73 (1995) 479−487.

[74] J. Kocian, I. Skala, K. Bakos, Calcium absorption from milk and lactose-free milk in healthy subjects and patients with lactose intolerance, Digestion 9 (1973) 317−324.

[75] B. Cochet, A. Jung, M. Griessen, P. Bartholdi, P. Schaller, A. Donath, Effects of lactose on intestinal calcium absorption in normal and lactase-deficient subjects, Gastroenterology 84 (1983) 935−940.

[76] M. Griessen, B. Cochet, F. Infante, A. Jung, P. Bartholdi, A. Donath, et al., Calcium absorption from milk in lactase-deficient subjects, Am. J. Clin. Nutr. 49 (1989) 377−384.

[77] W.J. Tremaine, A.D. Newcomer, L. Riggs, D.B. McGill, Calcium absorption from milk in lactase-deficient and lactase-sufficient adults, Dig. Dis. Sci. 31 (1986) 376−378.

[78] T.M. Smith, J.C. Kolars, D.A. Savaiano, M.D. Levitt, Absorption of calcium from milk and yogurt, Am. J. Clin. Nutr. 42 (1985) 1197−1200.

[79] A.O. Johnson, J.G. Semenya, M.S. Buchowski, C.O. Enwonwu, N.S. Scrimshaw, Correlation of lactose maldigestion, lactose intolerance, and milk intolerance, Am. J. Clin. Nutr. 57 (1993) 399−401.

[80] J. Reasoner, T.P. Maculan, A.G. Rand, W.R. Thayer Jr., Clinical studies with low-lactose milk, Am. J. Clin. Nutr. 34 (1981) 54−60.

[81] E.R. Pedersen, B.H. Jensen, H.J. Jensen, I.L. Keldsbo, E.H. Moller, S.N. Rasmussen, Lactose malabsorption and tolerance of lactose-hydrolyzed milk: a double-blind controlled crossover trial, Scand. J. Gastroenterol. 17 (1982) 861−864.

[82] T.M. Bayless, B. Rothfeld, C. Masser, L. Wise, D. Paige, M.S. Bedine, Lactose and milk intolerance: clinical implications, N. Engl. J. Med. 292 (1975) 1156−1159.

[83] J.L. Rosado, C. Gonzales, M.E. Valencia, B. Lopez, L. Mejia, M. Del Carmen Baez, Lactose maldigestion and milk intolerance: a study in rural and urban Mexico using physiological doses of milk, J. Nutr. 124 (1994) 1052−1059.

[84] J.H. Bond, M.D. Levitt, Quantitative measurement of lactose absorption, Gastroenterology 70 (1976) 1058−1062.

[85] N.W. Solomons, A.-M. Guerrero, B. Torun, Dietary manipulation of postprandial colonic lactose fermentation: I. Effect of solid foods in a meal, Am. J. Clin. Nutr. 41 (1985) 199−208.

[86] N. Dehkordi, D.R. Rao, A.P. Warren, C.B. Chawan, Lactose malabsorption as influenced by chocolate milk, skim milk, sucrose, whole milk, and lactic cultures, J. Am. Diet. Assoc. 95 (1995) 484−486.

[87] J.L. Leichter, Comparison of whole milk and skim milk with aqueous lactose solution in lactose tolerance testing, Am. J. Clin. Nutr. 26 (1973) 393−396.

[88] T.H. Vesa, M. Lember, R. Korpela, Milk fat does not affect the symptoms of lactose intolerance, Eur. J. Clin. Nutr. 51 (1997) 633—636.

[89] L.T. Cavalli-Sforza, A. Strata, Double-blind study on the tolerance of four types of milk in lactose malabsorbers and absorbers, Hum. Nutr. Clin. Nutr. 40C (1986) 19—30.

[90] T.H. Ves, P.R. Marteau, F.B. Briet, M.-C. Boutron-Ruault, J.-C. Rambaud, Raising milk energy content retards gastric emptying of lactose in lactose-intolerant humans with little effect on lactose digestion, J. Nutr. 127 (1997) 2316—2320.

[91] T.H. Vesa, P.R. Marteau, F.B. Briet, B. Flourie, A. Briend, J.-C. Rambaud, Effects of milk viscosity on gastric emptying and lactose intolerance in lactose maldigesters, Am. J. Clin. Nutr. 66 (1997) 123—126.

[92] C.M. Lee, C.M. Hardy, Cocoa feeding and human lactose intolerance, Am. J. Clin. Nutr. 49 (1989) 840—844.

[93] J.C. Kolars, M.D. Levitt, M. Aouji, D.A. Savaiano, Yogurt—An autodigesting source of lactose, N. Engl. J. Med. 310 (1984) 1—3.

[94] J. Räsic, J.A. Kurmans, The nutritional—physiological value of yoghurt, Yogurt; Scientific Grounds, Technology, Manufacture and Preparations, Tech. Dairy Pub. House, Copenhagen, Denmark, 1978, pp. 99—137.

[95] D.A. Savaiano, C. Kotz, Recent advances in the management of lactose intolerance, Contemp. Nutr. 13 (1988) 9—10.

[96] P. Pochart, O. Dewit, J.-H. Desjeux, P. Bourlioux, Viable starter culture, β-galactosidase activity, and lactose in duodenum after yogurt ingestion in lactase-deficient humans, Am. J. Clin. Nutr. 49 (1989) 828—831.

[97] E. Lerebours, C. N'Djitoyap Ndam, A. Lavoine, M.F. Hellot, J.M. Antoine, R. Colin, Yogurt and fermented—then-pasteurized milk: effects of short-term and long-term ingestion on lactose absorption and mucosal lactase activity in lactase-deficient subjects, Am. J. Clin. Nutr. 49 (1989) 823—827.

[98] M.A. Shermak, J.M. Saavedra, T.L. Jackson, S.S. Huang, T.M. Bayless, J.A. Perman, Effect of yogurt on symptoms and kinetics of hydrogen production in lactose-malabsorbing children, Am. J. Clin. Nutr. 62 (1995) 1003—1006.

[99] S.E. Gilliland, H.S. Kim, Effect of viable starter culture bacteria in yogurt on lactose utilization in humans, J. Dairy Sci. 67 (1984) 1—6.

[100] M.C. Martini, E.C. Lerebours, W.-J. Lin, S.K. Harlander, N.M. Berrada, J.M. Antoine, et al., Strains and species of lactic acid bacteria in fermented milks (yogurts): effect on in vivo lactose digestion, Am. J. Clin. Nutr. 54 (1991) 1041—1046.

[101] S.R. Hertzler, S.M. Clancy, Kefir improves lactose digestion and tolerance in adults with lactose maldigestion, J. Am. Diet. Assoc. 103 (2003) 582—587.

[102] M.-Y. Lin, D. Savaiano, S. Harlander, Influence of nonfermented dairy products containing bacterial starter cultures on lactose maldigestion in humans, J. Dairy Sci. 74 (1991) 87—95.

[103] H. Hove, H. Nørgaard, P.B. Mortensen, Lactic acid bacteria and the human gastrointestinal tract, Eur. J. Clin. Nutr. 53 (1999) 339—350.

[104] S.E. Gilliland, Acidophilus milk products: a review of potential benefits to consumers, J. Dairy Sci. 72 (1989) 2483—2494.

[105] A.D. Newcomer, H.S. Park, P.C. O'Brien, D.B. McGill, Response of patients with irritable bowel syndrome and lactase deficiency using unfermented acidophilus milk, Am. J. Clin. Nutr. 38 (1983) 257—263.

[106] D.L. Payne, J.D. Welsh, C.V. Manion, A. Tsegaye, L.D. Herd, Effectiveness of milk products in dietary management of lactose malabsorption, Am. J. Clin. Nutr. 34 (1981) 2711—2715.

[107] C.I. Onwulata, D.R. Rao, P. Vankineni, Relative efficiency of yogurt, sweet acidophilus milk, hydrolyzed lactose milk, and a commercial lactase tablet in alleviating lactose maldigestion, Am. J. Clin. Nutr. 49 (1989) 1233—1237.

[108] H.S. Kim, S.E. Gilliland, Lactobacillus acidophilus as a dietary adjunct for milk to aid lactose digestion in humans, J. Dairy Sci. 66 (1984) 959—966.

[109] F.E. McDonough, A.D. Hitchins, N.P. Wong, P. Wells, C.E. Bodwell, Modification of sweet acidophilus milk to improve utilization by lactose-intolerant persons, Am. J. Clin. Nutr. 45 (1987) 570—574.

[110] T. Jiang., A. Mustapha, D.A. Savaiano, Improvement of lactose digestion in humans by ingestion of unfermented milk containing, Bifidobacterium longum. J. Dairy Sci. 79 (1996) 750—757.

[111] M.-Y. Lin, J.A. DiPalma, M.C. Martini, C.J. Gross, S.K. Harlander, D.A. Savaiano, Comparative effects of exogenous lactase (β-galactosidase) preparations on in vivo lactose digestion, Dig. Dis. Sci. 38 (1993) 2022—2027.

[112] P. P. C.McNeil, About lactaid and lactaid ultra. Available at <http://www.lactaid.com>. Accessed April 2007.

[113] digestMILK.com. Lacteeze Enzyme Drops and Tablets. Available at <http://www.digestmilk.com>. Accessed April, 2007.

[114] Lactase preparation from K. lactis affirmed as GRAS (1984, December 10). Food Chem. News, p. 30.

[115] Land O' Lakes. Dairy Ease Products. Available at <http://www.dairyease.com>. Accessed April 2007.

[116] M. Moskovitz, C. Curtis, J. Gavaler, Does oral enzyme replacement therapy reverse intestinal lactose malabsorption? Am. J. Gastroenterol. 82 (1987) 632—635.

[117] F.C. Ramirez, K. Lee, D.Y. Graham, All lactase preparations are not the same: results of a prospective, randomized, placebo-controlled trial, Am. J. Gastroenterol. 89 (1994) 566—570.

[118] J.A. DiPalma, M.S. Collins, Enzyme replacement for lactose malabsorption using a beta-D-galactosidase, J. Clin. Gastroenterol. 11 (1989) 290—293.

[119] S.W. Sanders, K.G. Tolman, D.P. Reitberg, Effect of a single dose of lactase on symptoms and expired hydrogen after lactose challenge in lactose-intolerant adults, Clin. Pharm. 11 (1992) 533—538.

[120] A.H. Cheng, O. Brunser, J. Espinoza, H.L. Fones, F. Monckeberg, C.O. Chichester, et al., Long-term acceptance of low-lactose milk, Am. J. Clin. Nutr. 32 (1979) 1989—1993.

[121] J.C. Brand, S. Holt, Relative effectiveness of milks with reduced amounts of lactose in alleviating milk intolerance, Am. J. Clin. Nutr. 54 (1991) 148—151.

[122] S.J. Turner, T. Daly, J.A. Hourigan, A.J. Rand, W.R. Thayer Jr., Utilization of a low-lactose milk, Am. J. Clin. Nutr. 29 (1976) 739—744.

[123] O.H. Nielsen, P.O. Schiotz, S.N. Rasmussen, P.A. Krasilnikoff, Calcium absorption and acceptance of low-lactose milk among children with lactase deficiency, J. Pediatr. Gastroenterol. 3 (1984) 219—223.

[124] D.M. Paige, T.M. Bayless, E.D. Mellits, L. Davis, W.S. Dellinger Jr., M. Kreitner, Effects of age and lactose tolerance on blood glucose rise with whole cow and lactose-hydrolyzed milk, J. Agric. Food Chem. 27 (1979) 677—680.

[125] J.L. Rosado, M. Morales, A. Pasquetti, Lactose digestion and clinical tolerance to milk, lactose-prehydrolyzed milk, and enzyme-added milk: a study in undernourished continuously enteral-fed patients, J. Parenter. Enteral Nutr. 13 (1989) 157—161.

[126] L. Nagy, G. Mozsik, M. Garamszegi, E. Sasreti, C. Ruzsa, T. Javor, Lactose-poor milk in adult lactose intolerance, Acta Med. Hung. 40 (1983) 239—245.

[127] D.L. Payne, J.D. Welsh, C.V. Manion, A. Tsegaye, L.D. Herd, Effectiveness of milk products in dietary management of lactose malabsorption, Am. J. Clin. Nutr. 34 (1981) 2711—2715.

G. GASTROINTESTINAL HEALTH AND DISEASE

[128] J.A. Biller, S. King, A. Rosenthal, R.J. Grand, Efficacy of lactase-treated milk for lactose-intolerant pediatric patients, J. Pediatr. 111 (1987) 91–94.

[129] J.L. Rosado, M. Morales, A. Pasquetti, R. Nobara, L. Hernandez, Nutritional evaluation of a lactose-hydrolyzed milk-based enteral formula diet: I. A comparative study of carbohydrate digestion and clinical tolerance, Rev. Invest. Clin. 40 (1988) 141–147.

[130] D. Payne-Bose, J.D. Welsh, H.L. Gearhart, R.D. Morrison, Milk and lactose-hydrolyzed milk, Am. J. Clin. Nutr. 30 (1977) 695–697.

[131] V. Reddy, J. Pershad, Lactase deficiency in Indians, Am. J. Clin. Nutr. 25 (1972) 114–119.

[132] G.T. Keusch, F.J. Troncale, B. Thavaramara, P. Prinyanot, P.R. Anderson, N. Bhamarapravthi, Lactase deficiency in Thailand: effect of prolonged lactose feeding, Am. J. Clin. Nutr. 22 (1969) 638–641.

[133] D. Habte, G. Sterky, B. Hjalmarsson, Lactose malabsorption in Ethiopian children, Acta Pediatr. Scand. 62 (1973) 649–654.

[134] A.O. Johnson, J.G. Semenya, M.S. Buchowski, C.O. Enwonwu, N.S. Scrimshaw, Adaptation of lactose maldigesters to continued milk intakes, Am. J. Clin. Nutr. 58 (1993) 879–881.

[135] J.A. Perman, S. Modler, A.C. Olson, Role of pH in production of hydrogen from carbohydrates by colonic bacterial flora: studies in vivo and in vitro, J. Clin. Invest. 67 (1981) 643–650.

[136] B. Flourie, F. Briet, C. Florent, P. Pellier, M. Maurel, J.-C. Rambaud, Can diarrhea induced by lactulose be reduced by prolonged ingestion of lactulose? Am. J. Clin. Nutr. 58 (1993) 369–375.

[137] F. Briet, P. Pochart, P. Marteau, B. Flourie, E. Arrigoni, J.C. Rambaud, Improved clinical tolerance to chronic lactose ingestion in subjects with lactose intolerance: a placebo effect? Gut 41 (1997) 632–635.

[138] S.R. Hertzler, D.A. Savaiano, M.D. Levitt, Fecal hydrogen production and consumption measurements: response to daily lactose ingestion by lactose maldigesters, Dig. Dis. Sci. 42 (1997) 348–353.

[139] A. Terada, H. Hara, M. Kataoka, T. Mitsuoka, Effect of lactulose on the composition and metabolic activity of the human fecal flora, Microb. Ecol. Health Dis. 5 (1992) 43–50.

[140] G.R. Gibson, E.R. Beatty, X. Wang, J.H. Cummings, Selective stimulation of bifidobacteria in the human colon by oligofructose and insulin, Gastroenterology 108 (1995) 975–982.

[141] M. Ito, M. Kimura, Influence of lactose on faecal microflora in lactose maldigesters, Microb. Ecol. Health Dis. 6 (1993) 73–76.

[142] G.R. Gibson, X. Wang, Regulatory effects of bifidobacteria on the growth of other colonic bacteria, J. Appl. Bacteriol. 77 (1994) 412–420.

[143] C. Landon, T. Tran, D.B. Connell, A randomized trial of a pre- and probiotic formula to reduce symptoms of dairy products in patients with dairy intolerance, FASEB J. 20 (2006) Abstract A1053.

[144] M.J. During, R. Xu, D. Young, M.G. Kaplitt, R.S. Sherwin, P. Leone, Peroral gene therapy of lactose intolerance using an adeno-associated virus vector, Nat. Med. 4 (1998) 1131–1135.

41

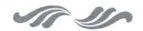

Nutritional Considerations in the Management of Celiac Disease

Michelle Pietzak

University of Southern California Keck School of Medicine, Los Angeles, California

I INTRODUCTION

Celiac disease (also spelled coeliac disease in the European literature) has been known by many names in the medical literature in the past, including gluten-sensitive enteropathy, gliadin-sensitive enteropathy, and celiac sprue (to differentiate it from tropical sprue). Celiac disease occurs in genetically predisposed individuals who develop a permanent immunologic reaction to gluten, found in wheat, rye, and barley. When individuals with celiac disease ingest gluten, the result is malabsorption of sugars, proteins, fats, vitamins, and other minerals. Individuals with celiac disease have a permanent intolerance to the gliadin fraction of wheat protein and related alcohol-soluble proteins (called prolamins) found in rye and barley. Susceptible individuals who ingest these proteins develop an immune-mediated enteropathy, which self-perpetuates as long as these gluten-containing grains are in the diet. Removal of gluten from the diet, in the majority of people with celiac disease, leads to both resolution of symptoms and improvement in the intestinal damage. However, in individuals with long-standing disease, there may not be a response to the gluten-free diet (called "refractory sprue"), and intense nutritional support and immune-suppressing medications may be required.

Classic symptoms of celiac disease in childhood include diarrhea, short stature, anemia, and obvious physical signs of protein-calorie malnutrition. In the United States, and worldwide, more individuals are being diagnosed with celiac disease as adults. They may present with gastrointestinal symptoms, such as gastroesophageal reflux, irritable bowel syndrome, and diarrhea or constipation. Adults may also present with symptoms outside the gastrointestinal tract; these may include complaints of the joints, skin, reproductive, hematologic, musculoskeletal, and neurologic systems. Individuals with celiac disease, and their family members, often have other autoimmune diseases, such as type 1 diabetes, inflammatory bowel disease, and thyroid disease. The diagnosis of celiac disease is often delayed for years because its symptoms are often attributed to these other autoimmune conditions.

Serum antibodies are useful as a screening method for celiac disease. However, a small-intestinal biopsy, done by endoscopy, and a patient's clinical response to a gluten-free diet are used to confirm a diagnosis. Individuals with long-standing disease are at risk for complications, such as iron-deficiency anemia, vitamin deficiencies, osteoporosis, infertility, and gastrointestinal cancers. The long-term maintenance of a gluten-free lifestyle is challenging. Individuals diagnosed with celiac disease benefit most from a team approach, which includes regular supervision by a physician, nutritional counseling by a dietitian, and access to support groups knowledgeable about celiac disease and the gluten-free diet.

II SYMPTOMS OF CELIAC DISEASE

The clinician must have a high index of suspicion for celiac disease because its symptoms can affect almost every organ system of the body, and its clinical features can be highly variable. The disease may present at any age, with the "classic" presentation occurring after the introduction of gluten in the diet during infancy and the toddler years. However, many adolescents, young adults, and even the elderly are now being diagnosed. Likewise, the severity of the

Nutrition in the Prevention and Treatment of Disease, Third Edition.
DOI: http://dx.doi.org/10.1016/B978-0-12-391884-0.00041-X

presentation of celiac disease can be highly variable, with some patients experiencing severe diarrhea and weight loss, and others having no gastrointestinal symptoms whatsoever. Because celiac disease is a multisystemic disease, it can affect not only the gastrointestinal tract but also the neurologic, endocrine, orthopedic, reproductive, and hematologic systems. Thus, it is not uncommon that a patient with celiac disease may be seen by multiple physicians over many years before the disorder is correctly identified.

The presentations of celiac disease can be classified into the following six categories based on symptomatology: a classic gastrointestinal form, a late-onset gastrointestinal form, an extraintestinal form, a form presenting with associated conditions, an asymptomatic form, and a latent form. The patients diagnosed with celiac disease who have the "classic" gastrointestinal form in childhood are thought to represent the "tip of the iceberg," in that they are the obvious, visible patients [1]. The point in using this iceberg model is that the majority of patients with celiac disease are "submerged"; that is, many patients are not presenting in childhood with "classic" disease. Therefore, what has historically been considered the "classic" presentation is now a misnomer [2]. Many individuals with undiagnosed celiac disease will fall into the other five classifications ("nonclassic") and therefore may experience chronic ill health and multiple complications of the disease, without ever being correctly diagnosed.

A Classic Gastrointestinal Form

The "classic" gastrointestinal form of celiac disease occurs in infants or toddlers usually between the ages of 6 and 18 months, after the introduction of gluten-containing foods into the diet. The onset is usually insidious, with "failure to thrive" and obvious physical signs of wasting over a period of weeks to months. The "classic" symptoms are those of diarrhea, weight loss, abdominal distention, gassiness, and foul-smelling stools due to carbohydrate (primarily lactose) and fat malabsorption. Parents will often report that the child becomes irritable after meals, and the child may also develop a secondary anorexia due to the pain associated with the diarrhea and abdominal distention. These children exhibit classic signs on physical exam of protein-calorie malnutrition: hypotonia, poor muscle bulk, peripheral edema, decreased subcutaneous fat stores, abdominal distention, and ascites in severe cases. Anemia is common. The anemia is usually microcytic, due to iron malabsorption. However, if the disease is long-standing, and small bowel involvement is severe, a macrocytic anemia can develop as a result of folate malabsorption. Radiographs can show osteopenia due to vitamin D and

calcium malabsorption in prolonged, severe cases. As opposed to cases that present in adulthood, these children are usually referred to a gastroenterologist because of their poor nutritional status, and the diagnosis is prompt because of the "classic" presentation that most clinicians were taught to look for in medical school. However, as discussed later, most patients are now presenting outside of the "classic" age range with varied symptoms both within and outside the gastrointestinal tract, making the category of "classic" a misnomer.

B Late-Onset Gastrointestinal Form

As in the "classic" gastrointestinal form, the late-onset gastrointestinal form also includes gastrointestinal symptoms, but at an age range outside of the infant and toddler years. School-age children, adolescents, young adults, and even the elderly often complain of mild to intermittent diarrhea, gassiness, urgency, and abdominal distention and cramping. A presenting patient may also complain of chronic abdominal pain; constipation rather than diarrhea; and upper gastrointestinal tract symptoms such as nausea, dyspepsia, indigestion, gastroesophageal reflux, and chronic vomiting. Rather than being examined for celiac disease, these patients often are labeled as having irritable bowel syndrome (IBS), lactose intolerance, recurrent abdominal pain of childhood, or even an inflammatory bowel disease such as Crohn's disease. Patients are therefore treated with lactose-free or high-fiber diets, medications to treat constipation or IBS, or medications to suppress gastric acid or the immune system. Not surprisingly, the celiac patient will not get relief from these treatments. Some of these therapies, such as a high-fiber diet, which often contains a great deal of gluten, may increase symptomatology. Many patients will have upper and lower endoscopies performed by a gastroenterologist, and the results may look visually normal without obvious ulcers or cancers; thus, biopsies for celiac disease will not be taken. Because of this, the diagnosis of celiac disease is often missed.

C Extraintestinal Form

Because celiac disease is a multisystemic immune-mediated disorder, it can present with signs and symptoms outside the gastrointestinal tract. Organ systems affected can include the musculoskeletal system, skin and mucous membranes, reproductive system, hematologic system, hepatic system, and central nervous system.

1 Musculoskeletal System

One of the most common presenting features in childhood in the musculoskeletal system is idiopathic short stature. In European studies [3–5], it is estimated that approximately 1 of 10 children whose height is far below his or her genetic predisposition for unclear reasons is short because of celiac disease. Short stature can be an isolated feature of this condition. The children often have delayed onset of puberty, and stimulation testing may reveal growth hormone deficiency [6]. The potential to achieve normal stature and bone mineralization is good if these patients are diagnosed with celiac disease before puberty and placed on a gluten-free diet in a timely fashion [7]. However, after the growth plates have closed, individuals will have short stature for life.

Dental enamel defects are common in children affected by celiac disease during the toddler years. They may experience caries at an early age and in atypical locations. One report has noted that up to 30% of older patients with celiac disease have enamel hypoplasia [8]. If gluten is in the diet, these enamel defects affect only the permanent (secondary) dentition that is forming before the age of 7 years. The primary dentition or "baby teeth" are formed *in utero*, which is a gluten-free environment, and thus the primary dentition is unaffected. The dental enamel defects are linear and occur symmetrically in all four quadrants [9]. The precise cause of these defects is unknown.

Joint pain is a common complaint among both adolescents and adults with undiagnosed celiac disease. The joints are often only painful, and not red, hot, or visibly swollen. The pain often resolves with the implementation of a gluten-free diet. Clubbing of the fingers and toes (broad digits with abnormally curved nails) has also been reported. Interestingly, and to confuse the issue further, celiac disease is also seen in higher incidence in patients with rheumatologic disorders such as systemic lupus erythematosus and rheumatoid arthritis [10–12]. In an adolescent, arthritis may be the only presenting symptom [13].

One of the most serious causes of morbidity in older individuals diagnosed with celiac disease is fractures associated with osteoporosis. The potential health implications are grave and include vertebral fractures, kyphosis, hip fractures, and Colles' fracture of the lower radius in the arm [14]. These problems can begin in childhood, when radiographs may reveal delayed bone age, rickets, or osteomalacia, which left untreated may lead to osteoporosis. It is believed that early interventional therapy with a gluten-free diet may prevent progression and may even reverse bone loss [15]. However, severe osteoporosis associated with celiac disease diagnosed very late in life will not revert on the glucose-free diet after a critical point in time [16].

2 Skin and Mucous Membranes

Often overlooked, the skin and mucous membranes can be obvious sites for the expression of symptoms from celiac disease. The classic skin manifestation of celiac disease is a skin rash called dermatitis herpetiformis, often abbreviated DH. It occurs primarily in adults and is rarely seen in children before puberty. This skin rash is classically pruritic (itchy) and symmetrical and does not respond to topical creams and medications. The rash begins as flat, red lesions, which then progress to erythematous, fluid-filled blisters. They usually occur on the face, elbows, back, buttocks, and knees. The lesions initially can be confused with urticaria (hives) or varicella (chickenpox). Patients will often scratch and pick at the lesions, so that the skin will then develop an eczematous appearance. A biopsy of the normal-appearing skin next to the affected area demonstrates the characteristic histology of granular IgA deposits [17]. DH is now known to be the pathognomonic skin rash for celiac disease, and once a skin biopsy has proven the diagnosis of DH, an intestinal biopsy for celiac disease is unnecessary. If a patient with DH does have a small-intestinal biopsy, the majority of the time there will be intestinal damage [18]. For complete resolution of DH, a gluten-free diet is required. Some patients with DH also require an anti-inflammatory antibiotic, in addition to a gluten-free diet, during acute onset of DH. The skin lesions, or just the pruritis of DH, may appear when gluten is intentionally or inadvertently ingested. This should alert the affected individual to scrutinize the diet for gluten contamination.

Celiac disease can have many other manifestations in the skin and mucous membranes, including urticaria, psoriasis, and oral aphthous stomatitis [18–20]. Oral aphthous stomatitis ("fever sores" or "canker sores"), which can appear on the cheeks, tongue, gums, and lips, usually correlates with histologic changes in the small intestine. However, because aphthous ulcers are also seen with common viral infections (such as herpes viruses) and other types of autoimmune and inflammatory diseases of the gastrointestinal tract (particularly Crohn's disease), they are not pathognomonic for celiac disease.

3 Reproductive System

The reproductive systems of both women and men can be affected by celiac disease. Compared to the general population, women with undiagnosed celiac disease have greater difficulty becoming pregnant [21] and a higher risk for spontaneous abortions [22,23]. Men with undiagnosed celiac disease may also experience infertility due to gonadal dysfunction [24]. Adult patients with undiagnosed celiac disease may often undergo exhaustive and expensive infertility studies, without discovery of an etiology. Many of these infertile women will also give a history of delayed menarche, anemia, and IBS symptoms, similar to the pediatric patients described previously with short stature and delayed puberty. Women with undiagnosed and diagnosed celiac disease have infants with higher rates of neural tube defects because of folic acid deficiency, as well as more infants with intrauterine growth retardation [25—27]. Whether these individuals experience reproductive challenges because of nutritional factors, or having an undiagnosed autoimmune disease, or a combination of both is unclear.

4 Hematologic System

Iron-deficiency anemia is one of the most common micronutrient deficiencies in the undiagnosed celiac patient. In addition to anemia, leukopenia (low white blood cell count) and thrombocytopenia (low platelet count) have also been reported. The anemia in celiac disease is usually microcytic and hypochromic, due to iron deficiency [28]. However, a macrocytic anemia should warrant an investigation into gut malabsorption of vitamin B_{12} or folic acid. Because fat-soluble vitamins are also malabsorbed in this disorder, vitamin K deficiency may occur, resulting in an increased risk for bruising and bleeding. Vitamin E deficiency may also occur, resulting in a hemolytic anemia and jaundice.

5 Liver

In children and adults with celiac disease, diseases of the liver, such as autoimmune hepatitis and chronic transaminasemia (liver enzymes), have been reported [28—31]. In children initially diagnosed with celiac disease with elevated aspartate transaminase (AST) and alanine transaminase (ALT) liver enzymes at presentation, these biochemical markers of hepatocyte damage returned to normal with strict adherence to a gluten-free diet [32]. Autoimmune liver diseases, such as autoimmune hepatitis, sclerosing cholangitis, and primary biliary cirrhosis, are all more likely to occur in the individual with celiac disease [33]. Patients with celiac disease who have evidence of chronic liver disease that has not responded to a gluten-free diet require an evaluation for these autoimmune liver diseases.

6 Central Nervous System

There is evidence that patients with celiac disease have increased rates of both neurologic and psychiatric disorders. Their associations are not always clear: Some symptoms can be attributed to nutritional deficiencies; others perhaps related to autoimmunity; and many are hypothesized to be due to yet-unproven pathways by which gluten may cross the blood—brain barrier and interact with endogenous neurotransmitter receptors. It is unclear whether these patients truly have immune-mediated phenomena associated with celiac disease or suffer from a type of "gluten sensitivity." Neurological complications have been reported in association with established celiac disease for decades [34], and gluten sensitivity can present with neurological dysfunction as its sole symptom [35].

In the neurologic system, patients with celiac disease are 20 times more likely than the general population to have epilepsy and have been reported with associated cerebral and cerebellar calcifications imaged by both computed tomography (CT) and magnetic resonance imaging (MRI) [36]. In children with celiac disease, focal white matter lesions in the brain have been reported and are thought to be either ischemic in origin as a result of vasculitis or caused by inflammatory demyelination [37].

Gluten-associated ataxia is the most common neurological manifestation of gluten sensitivity [38] and presents as difficulty with speech, movement, and balance due to atrophy of the cerebellum. It rarely occurs before puberty, has a mean age of onset in the late 40s, and has a paucity of gastrointestinal symptoms [39]. Emerging evidence indicates that early initiation of a gluten-free diet is beneficial for treating the symptoms of both ataxia and peripheral neuropathy, even in the absence of intestinal damage [40].

In both treated and untreated persons with celiac disease, psychiatric co-morbidities, such as depression, dementia, and schizophrenia, are common. In children, behavioral changes such as irritability, increased separation anxiety, emotional withdrawal, and autistic behaviors have improved, by parental report, on a gluten-free diet [41]. Although not scientifically validated, the gluten-free diet, along with a casein-free diet, is now also being advocated by several groups for children with autism [42—44]. Whether children with autism are at a higher risk for celiac disease, or celiac children have a higher incidence of autism, remains to be proven. However, children with Down syndrome, who often have autistic behaviors, are at higher risk for celiac disease [45]. It has been hypothesized that gluten may be broken down into small peptides that may cross the blood—brain barrier and interact with morphine receptors, leading to alterations in conduct and perceptions of reality [35]. It is important to note that only a proportion of patients presenting with neurological dysfunction associated with a gluten sensitivity will also have biopsy-proven intestinal damage [46].

D Associated Conditions

There are several groups of patients who are at substantially increased risk of having celiac disease: those with another autoimmune disorder, those with certain syndromes, and relatives of biopsy-diagnosed patients. These associated conditions are further described in Table 41.1. Patients with other autoimmune diseases,

TABLE 41.1 Conditions and Syndromes at Increased Risk for Celiac Disease (CD)

Condition	% Diagnosed with CD	Increased risk	References
Arthritis	1.5–7.5	3- to 10-fold	[10,66,113,114]
Cardiomyopathy (idiopathic dilated)	5.7		[115]
Dental enamel defects	19–30	19-fold	[8,9,116]
Dermatitis herpetiformis	100		[17,78,117]
Diabetes type 1	3.5–10	4- to 10-fold	[118–122]
Down syndrome	4–20	17- to 50-fold	[49,66,123,124]
Epilepsy	2		[36,125]
IgA deficiency	7	31-fold	[126]
Infertility (idiopathic)	6.3		[66]
Iron-deficiency anemia	4.2	16-fold	[28,66]
Osteoporosis	2.6		[66]
Primary biliary cirrhosis	6		[33]
Relatives, first- or second-degree	2.6–20	18-fold	[64–66]
Short stature (idiopathic)	4–10	23-fold	[3–5,66]
Sjögren's syndrome	2–3		[66,127]
Thyroid disease (autoimmune)	4		[128]
Turner syndrome	4–8		[129–131]
Williams syndrome	9.5		[132]

such as type 1 diabetes, as well as relatives of persons with biopsy-diagnosed celiac disease, are more likely to carry the HLA (human leukocyte antigen) haplotypes that put them at risk for the disease. It has been demonstrated that patients diagnosed with celiac disease early in life, and treated early with a gluten-free diet, have a significantly lower risk of developing other autoimmune disorders than do individuals diagnosed later in life [47].

Persons with both Down and Turner syndromes classically have short stature and are at increased risk for skeletal and other autoimmune diseases such as diabetes mellitus, Crohn's disease, and thyroid disease [48], which makes the diagnosis in this population exceptionally difficult. A multicenter study from Italy strongly suggested the need for screening all children with Down syndrome, regardless of the presence or absence of gastrointestinal symptomatology [49]. It is unclear why individuals with certain syndromes are at higher risk for celiac disease. However, because several of these syndromes have as part of their constellation poor growth and short stature, anthropometric measures are poor screening tools for malabsorption in these populations. The NIH Consensus Development Conference on Celiac Disease, held in June 2004, recommended that patients with Down, Turner, or Williams syndrome should be offered screening for celiac disease at least once [50].

E Asymptomatic Form

It can be debated whether or not there is truly an "asymptomatic" form of celiac disease, as historically, *asymptomatic* meant not fitting into the definition of the "classic" presentation, with severe diarrhea and protein-calorie malnutrition. As described in the previous sections, patients who present with gastrointestinal symptoms outside of the pediatric age range, with extra-intestinal symptoms or associated conditions, may have previously been described as "asymptomatic." The medical literature describes patients lacking the signs and symptoms occurring in the gastrointestinal tract or extra-intestinal systems as "asymptomatic." With a more detailed history, physical exam, and laboratory investigations, these "asymptomatics" may have revealed evidence of trace mineral deficiencies, anemia, short stature, low bone density, and low serum fat-soluble vitamin levels. These patients may be identified through mass serologic screenings and are often first- and second-degree relatives of a patient with biopsy-diagnosed disease. A family history of gastrointestinal cancers or other autoimmune disorders is often elicited [51–54].

F Latent Form

Patients with the latent form of celiac disease have positive antibodies for the condition but an initial normal intestinal biopsy. It is believed that over time, with further ingestion of gluten, individuals with the latent form will develop celiac disease with subsequent abnormal histology of the small bowel. These small intestinal changes will then revert to normal with the initiation of a gluten-free diet [53–55].

III DIAGNOSIS OF CELIAC DISEASE

A Serologic and Genetic Screening Tests

The tests of choice to screen for celiac disease are serum immunological markers with high sensitivity and specificity. The classic screening tests that are used for other gastrointestinal malabsorption disorders, such as fecal fat, glucose tolerance tests, D-xylose uptake, serum carotene levels, and permeability tests (e.g., lactulose/mannitol ratios), are poorly specific for celiac disease and should not be used in place of the serologic markers that are discussed hereafter. The clinician must remember, however, that no screening test is perfect, and that the current "gold standard" to confirm the diagnosis of celiac disease remains a small-intestinal biopsy and the patient's clinical response to a gluten-free diet. Any patient with suggestive symptoms should have a small-bowel biopsy, even if the serology is negative.

There are three frequently used commercially available serologic tests (antibodies): anti-gliadin (AGA), anti-endomysial or anti-endomysium (EMA or AEA), and anti-tissue transglutaminase (tTG). Sensitivity, specificity, and positive and negative predictive values can vary widely for each antibody, depending on the age of the patient, the population being studied, the substrates and laboratory kits being used to run the assays, and the proficiency of the laboratory performing the test [56]. Conditions that may yield false negative antibody results include a patient who makes low levels of or no immunoglobulin A (IgA), young children who may not manufacture autoimmune antibodies, an inexperienced lab, and testing while the patient is already on a gluten-free diet. False positive tests can also be seen with these antibody tests, as delineated later, in normal individuals with other gastrointestinal disorders and in other autoimmune disorders.

1 Anti-Gliadin Antibodies

The anti-gliadin antibodies were the first serologic tests available to screen for celiac disease during the late 1970s and were the first step toward recognizing this condition as an immune-mediated disorder. The anti-gliadin antibodies IgG and IgA recognize a small antigenic portion of the gluten protein called gliadin [57]. AGA IgG has good sensitivity, whereas AGA IgA has good specificity, and therefore their combined use provided the first reliable screening test. Unfortunately, many normal individuals can have an elevated AGA IgG, causing much confusion among general practitioners. AGA IgG is useful in screening IgA-deficient individuals because the other antibodies used for routine screening are usually of the IgA class. Whereas only 0.2–0.4% of the general population has selective IgA deficiency, as many as 2 or 3% of people with celiac disease are IgA deficient, complicating the screening procedure [58]. Other conditions under which an elevated AGA IgG can be seen include enteropathies where the gut is more permeable to gluten, such as parasitic infections, Crohn's disease, allergic gastroenteropathy, and autoimmune enteropathy. A strength of the AGA antibodies is that they are enzyme-linked immunosorbent assay (ELISA) tests, and the results are independent of observer variability.

2 Anti-Endomysium Antibodies

The serologic test currently commercially available with the highest sensitivity and specificity is the anti-endomysium IgA immunofluorescent antibody (EMA). The EMA was discovered in the early 1980s and rapidly gained use as part of a screening "celiac panel" by commercial labs in combination with AGA IgG and AGA IgA. False negative EMA can be seen in young children, those with IgA deficiency, and in the hands of an inexperienced laboratory because of the subjective nature of the test [56]. Also, the substrate for this antibody was initially monkey esophagus, making it expensive and unsuitable for screening large numbers of people. Human umbilical cord is now used as an alternative to monkey esophagus in most commercial laboratories [59].

3 Tissue Transglutaminase Antibodies

Tissue transglutaminase (tTG) was described in 1997 as the autoantigen of EMA [60]. The initial tTG ELISA was guinea pig IgA, with a lower sensitivity and specificity than EMA [61,62]. However, most commercial labs now use human recombinant tTG, which has improved sensitivity and specificity and correlates better with EMA IgA and intestinal biopsy results [60–63]. The tTG IgA ELISA represents an improvement over the EMA IgA assay because it is less expensive, is less time-consuming, is not a subjective test, and can be performed on a single drop of blood using a dot-blot technique, making this an ideal test for mass serologic screenings. Positive tTG results may be seen in other autoimmune diseases, such as type 1 diabetes, autoimmune liver disease, autoimmune thyroid disease, and inflammatory bowel disease.

4 Genetic Testing

Although celiac disease is the only autoimmune disease for which we know the environmental trigger, gluten, we also know that there is a strong genetic influence. For example, as discussed under "associated conditions," in first- and second-degree relatives, there can be up to a 20% disease prevalence [64–66]. Also, identical twins have a 75% concordance rate for celiac disease (one of the highest rates reported for any disease), whereas nonidentical twins do not differ from siblings [67]. This again indicates a genetic, in addition to an environmental, component.

Celiac disease is a complex genetic disorder, but the actual "celiac genes" have not yet been identified. The strongest genetic determinant of risk for celiac disease appears to be the presence of certain HLA alleles. The presence of these HLA alleles, DQ2 and DQ8, is thought to account for up to 40% of the genetic load of the familial risk for celiac disease [68]. The HLA are markers that help identify cells as "self" versus "nonself." The HLA prevent the immune system from attacking "self." HLA DQ2 or DQ8 are found in 95% of celiac patients. It is extremely rare for a celiac patient to have neither of these genes. However, if an individual has these HLA alleles, it does not mean that the individual has celiac disease because these alleles are found in 39.5% of the general population [69–71]. This is a great source of confusion for patients and physicians because it is counterintuitive to other types of genetic testing, where the presence of the gene confirms the disease.

The value of genetic testing is that it has a high negative predictive value to rule out celiac disease for a patient's lifetime. Negativity for HLA DQ2 and DQ8 excludes the diagnosis of celiac disease with 99% confidence. However, positivity for DQ2 or DQ8 has limited diagnostic value because of the high prevalence of these genotypes in the general population. The strength of genetic testing is that the patient does not need to be on a gluten-containing diet to be tested because the presence of these genes is not affected by diet. Therefore, genetic testing can evaluate

- Infants not yet exposed to gluten
- Young children who may not make all of the antibodies
- Patients who have self-imposed a gluten-free diet
- Patients with serology or biopsies that were not conclusive
- Relatives of biopsy-diagnosed individuals with celiac disease.

5 Current Guidelines on the Use of Serologic and Genetic Testing to Screen for Celiac Disease

As described previously, the IgA class human anti-tTG antibody, coupled with a determination of total serum IgA to rule out deficiency, currently seems to be the most cost-effective way to screen for celiac disease in an otherwise healthy adult. EMA should be used as a confirmatory, pre-biopsy test, whereas AGA determinations should be restricted to the diagnostic workup of younger children and patients with IgA deficiency. Given the high prevalence of the HLA haplotypes associated with celiac disease in the general population, genetic testing is not recommended as a routine screening test for celiac disease. The practitioner should remember that serologic tests are screens and that to confirm the diagnosis of celiac disease, a small bowel biopsy must be performed, as discussed next.

B The Intestinal Biopsy

Confirmation of either a clinical suspicion of celiac disease or a positive serologic screen requires a small intestinal biopsy. Before the advent of fiberoptic and chip technology for endoscopes, biopsies of the jejunum were obtained using a Crosby spring-loaded capsule, passed orally under fluoroscopic guidance. Most biopsies are performed today using a flexible endoscope, passed orally under either conscious sedation or general anesthesia. This has the advantages of allowing direct visualization of the mucosa with a camera to look for changes suggestive of small bowel damage, such as notching or scalloping of the small bowel folds or lymphonodular hyperplasia [72]. Endoscopy also allows the endoscopist to look for other lesions, such as ulcers, esophagitis, or gastritis, which may help explain the patient's symptomatology.

The detailed description of the characteristic small bowel changes seen in celiac disease that was given by Marsh in 1988 has become accepted as the standard [73]. The Marsh criteria describe four patterns of mucosal pathology: type 0 (pre-infiltrative), which is without detectable inflammation or changes in the crypt/villous architecture; type 1 (infiltrative), with an increase in the intraepithelial lymphocytes but without detectable changes in the crypt/villous architecture; type 2 (hyperplastic), with inflammation, villous blunting, and an increased crypt/villous height ratio; and type 3 (destructive), with severe inflammation, flat villi, and hyperplastic crypts. The clinician, however, needs to be aware that villous atrophy (shortening of the finger-like projections in the small bowel, which increase absorptive surface area) can be caused by a wide variety of gastrointestinal diseases and infections, and that correlation with serology and the patient's response to a gluten-free diet is imperative to confirm the diagnosis. In rare instances, a gluten challenge may be necessary to confirm that the villous atrophy was due to celiac disease and not a concomitant gastrointestinal infection. In cases in which serology is suggestive, the biopsy is confirmative, and the patient has had a clinical response to the gluten-free diet, a gluten challenge and repeat small bowel biopsy are no longer required [74].

IV TREATMENT OF CELIAC DISEASE WITH A GLUTEN-FREE DIET

The only known treatment for celiac disease is a gluten-free diet. This was first discovered after World War II in children with celiac disease when the toxicity of wheat proteins was established after the bread shortages resolved in Europe [75,76]. Gluten is important in baked goods because it plays an important role in leavening, in forming the structure of the dough, and in holding the baked product together [57]. Removal of gluten from the diet of a biopsy-diagnosed person with celiac disease results in complete symptomatic and histologic resolution of the disease in the majority of patients. The identified agents responsible for the immune-mediated response and intestinal damage are prolamins, storage proteins located in the seeds of different grains. Gluten is the general name for the prolamins found in wheat (gliadin), rye (secalin), barley (hordein), and oats (avenin) [57].

The prolamin of oats, avenin, accounts for only 5–15% of the total seed protein, as opposed to gliadin, which comprises approximately 50% of wheat proteins [77]. This oat prolamin is thought not to elicit the same immune response as gliadin and is thought by some to be safe for patients with celiac disease to ingest [78]. The risk that oats are contaminated with wheat in the United States is great because oats are often crop-rotated, harvested, and milled with wheat. A study in the United States in newly diagnosed children with celiac disease who were allowed to eat oats found that these children had symptomatic and histologic resolution of the disease comparable to children who were denied oats [79]. Prolamins are also found in corn and rice, but they likewise do not elicit an immune reaction in the intestines of individuals with celiac disease [57].

Table 41.2 provides some basic dietary guidelines for persons following a gluten-free diet. Although not all-inclusive, it is meant to serve as a starting point for discussion between patients and health care practitioners. Many newly diagnosed individuals are not aware that "gluten-free" does not mean just eliminating bread and pastries from the diet, because gluten

TABLE 41.2 Basic Dietary Guidelines for Individuals Following a Gluten-Free Diet

Not allowed	Allowed	Questionable
Barley	Amaranth	Dextrin[a]
Bran	Beans	Flavorings[b]
Bulgur	Buckwheat	Hydrolyzed plant protein (HPP)
Cereal binding	Cheese[c]	Hydrolyzed vegetable protein (HVP)
Couscous	Corn (maize)	Modified food starch
Einkorn wheat	Egg	Oats[d]
Emmer wheat	Fish	Seasonings[e]
Farro	Fruit	Spices[f]
Farina	Kasha	Starch[g]
Filler	Meat[h]	
Graham flour	Milk[c]	
Kamut	Millet	
Malt	Nuts	
Rye	Potato	
Semolina	Peas	
Spelt	Quinoa	
Triticale	Rice, wild rice	
	Sorghum	
	Soybean	
	Teff	
	Tapioca	

[a]In North America, usually derived from corn or tapioca.
[b]In North America, gluten-containing grains are almost never used as flavorings, with the exception of barley malt, which is usually indicated on the label.
[c]Many individuals with celiac disease are lactose intolerant, and the coating of some cheeses may contain gluten.
[d]See text for detailed explanation on oats.
[e]A blend of flavoring agents, often using a carrier such as cereal flour or starch.
[f]Pure spices do not contain gluten, but imitation spices may have fillers.
[g]Corn, potato, tapioca, and rice are the usual sources of modified food starch in North America; however, food starch can be made from wheat.
[h]Without breading or gluten-containing seasonings.
Sources: Hardman et al. [78], Case [57], Forssell and Weiser [80], Ellis et al. [81].

(especially wheat) can be identified on food labels and in restaurants by many other names. For example, triticale (a combination of wheat and rye), kamut, and spelt are all forms of wheat and are considered toxic [80]. Other forms of wheat, such as bulgur, couscous, einkorn, farina, and semolina (durum), are also not permitted on the gluten-free diet. Any food product that contains rye, barley, or malt (a partial hydrolysate of barley) has prolamins that are considered harmful [81]. In general, a food product that includes wheat in its name (e.g., cracked wheat, wheat bran, wheat grass, wheat germ, or whole wheat) or malt in its name (barley malt, malt extract, malt flavoring, or malt syrup) is considered to contain gluten. One notable exception, however, is buckwheat, which is not directly related to *Triticum* and is considered safe to consume. Distilled ingredients (e.g., vinegar and alcohol) are allowed because gluten does not pass into the distillate. However, beverages made with barley (e.g., beer, ale, lager, and some rice and soy drinks) are not allowed [57].

Food labeling in the United States has undergone some changes. The Food Allergen Labeling and Consumer Protection Act was signed into law in August 2004. It requires food labels to clearly state if a product contains any of the top eight food allergens: milk, eggs, fish, crustacean shellfish, tree nuts, peanuts, soybeans, and wheat. All food products manufactured in the United States after January 1, 2006, are required to have updated labels declaring the presence of any of the top eight food allergens in the product. The Food Allergen Labeling and Consumer Protection Act of 2004 was primarily passed to benefit individuals with food allergies. However, it is also of tremendous value to those with celiac disease because wheat is often hidden on ingredient labels as "starch," "flavorings," "seasonings," "couscous," "farro," "farina," or "hydrolyzed vegetable protein" (Table 41.2). Because wheat is the most commonly used grain in the United States, by clarifying the source of ingredients and identifying "wheat," approximately 90% of labeling concerns are resolved for celiac and gluten-sensitive patients. The law also calls for the Food and Drug Administration (FDA) to issue rules, by 2008, detailing what it means when a product is labeled "gluten-free." Unlike Europe, Canada, and Australia, the United States does not have a defined standard for "gluten-free" foods, causing a great deal of confusion over what it means when an American manufacturer puts "gluten-free'" on a product's label. The FDA rules will establish a standard that will make it even easier for those with celiac disease to readily identify products that are safe.

Because of current food-labeling practices in the United States, it still may not be obvious whether or not an item contains gluten. Products to question include those labeled "wheat-free" (which may contain other harmful grains, such as rye or barley) and ingredients that do not state their sources (e.g., flavorings, spices, starch, or hydrolyzed vegetable protein). Gluten is often used as a flavoring in candy, sauces, seasonings, soups, and salad dressings and as a filler in vitamins and medications [57,82]. Often, the only way for persons with celiac disease to be certain that a specific product is gluten-free is to call the manufacturer directly and often because ingredients in products commonly change without warning. Toiletries, such as shampoos, conditioners, and skin care products, are

thought not harmful as long as they are not ingested. Patients with open skin lesions, such as with dermatitis herpetiformis, may have reactions on the skin or systemically if gluten gets into an open wound.

The education of the person newly diagnosed with celiac disease should consist of a team approach between the patient (or parents), the gastroenterologist, the primary care physician, the dietitian, and local branches of national support groups. Medical management primarily consists of monitoring for compliance with the gluten-free diet and screening for the well-known complications to be discussed later. After the gastroenterologist who performed the biopsy confirms the diagnosis, the patient should be immediately referred to a knowledgeable dietitian for medical nutrition therapy [83]. Physicians and dietitians should encourage the patient to join local chapters of national support organizations, which can aid in finding local resources, such as supermarkets, food manufacturers, literature, and restaurants, that are familiar with the gluten-free diet.

Lifelong compliance with the gluten-free diet is challenging. The most important factors in achieving compliance are patient education, close supervision by an interested physician, and regular nutritional counseling by a registered dietitian with expertise in this area [65,83]. Compliance can be improved even in adolescents if they are seen by a physician on a regular basis [84,85]. One of the best and least expensive markers for dietary compliance is assessment by a trained interviewer (either a physician or a dietitian) because of the low cost and noninvasive nature of dietary assessment. There is a strong correlation between self-reported intake of foods containing gluten and intestinal damage [85].

V MANAGEMENT OF THE COMPLICATIONS OF CELIAC DISEASE

Patients with undiagnosed and untreated celiac disease, as well as those diagnosed later in life, have increased morbidity and mortality due to associated conditions, including osteoporosis, nutritional deficiencies, other autoimmune diseases, and some cancers. These patients also incur increased health care costs because of being chronically ill, the need to see multiple subspecialists, and the tests performed on them until the correct diagnosis is obtained [86]. Corrao and other investigators of the Club del Tenue Study Group formed a prospective cohort study that included 1072 adults with diagnosed celiac disease and 3384 first-degree relatives. These individuals were followed for 32 years. The number of deaths between the two groups were compared and expressed as the standardized mortality ratio (SMR) and relative survival ratio. Two times the number of persons with celiac disease died compared to the relatives (SMR, 2.0; 95% confidence interval, 1.5–2.7). The greatest excess of deaths occurred during the first 3 years after diagnosis. These results suggest that prompt and strict dietary treatment may decrease premature mortality among persons with celiac disease [87].

The primary reason for the increased mortality is the association with gastrointestinal malignancies, primarily intestinal lymphoma, which has been reported in up to 10–15% of adult patients who have been noncompliant with the diet [88]. The odds ratio overall for non-Hodgkin's lymphoma associated with celiac disease compared to first-degree relatives was reported to be 3.1, with odds ratios of 16.9 for gut lymphoma and 19.2 for T cell lymphoma, respectively [89]. The good news is that the reported risk for lymphoma decreases to that of the general population on the gluten-free diet [90].

In a minority of patients with biopsy-diagnosed celiac disease, there will continue to be gastrointestinal symptoms and failure of normalization of intestinal damage, despite vigorous adherence to the gluten-free diet. Despite this, the majority of patients who are not better on the diet should not immediately be labeled as "refractory" to the diet. Given the challenges of living a gluten-free lifestyle, a thorough dietary history should first be taken to exclude inadvertent (or intentional) ingestion of gluten. Compliance can also be assessed by measuring the immunological markers (antibodies) for the disease. Also, in any celiac patient with persistent symptomatology, one should consider a repeat intestinal biopsy [91].

Histologic evidence of villous atrophy, despite rigorous adherence to the gluten-free diet for more than 1 year, should provoke a workup for gastrointestinal infections (e.g., viruses, bacteria, and parasites) and noninfectious diseases (e.g., other autoimmune and allergic diseases). Additional reasons for nonresponsiveness to the gluten-free diet include pancreatic insufficiency and T cell lymphoma, both of which are complications of long-standing celiac disease [92,93]. As many as 75% of adults with refractory sprue may have an aberrant clonal intraepithelial T cell population associated with a condition classified as "cryptic enteropathy-associated T cell lymphoma" [94]. These patients frequently require immunosuppressing medications, such as steroids, azathioprine, and cyclosporine [95–99], in addition to a gluten-free diet. For more information regarding refractory sprue, comprehensive reviews have been published [100,101].

All patients with celiac disease, whether it be long- or short-standing, are at risk for nutritional deficiencies. Children should be examined for protein-calorie malnutrition, linear growth failure, and delayed puberty. All patients should be screened for the nutritional deficiencies that can accompany this malabsorptive disorder, such as iron deficiency anemia and fat-soluble vitamin deficiencies (vitamins A, E, 25-hydroxy-D, and a prothrombin time to check vitamin K status). Adult patients should also be monitored for the common extraintestinal complications, including osteoporosis, neurologic complaints, and the development of other autoimmune diseases, especially of the thyroid and liver [102,103]. Bone density should be measured in the newly diagnosed celiac patient because numerous studies have documented low bone density in both children and adults at the time of initial diagnosis of celiac disease. Osteopenia can improve with the gluten-free diet, and progression of osteoporosis can be halted with appropriate supplementation [104–107]. Osteopenic patients should be evaluated for deficient intake and absorption of vitamin D and calcium and the development of secondary hyperparathyroidism [108].

Special considerations need to be given to patients who have both celiac disease and type 1 diabetes because many of the well-known complications of type 1 diabetes can be exacerbated by nutritional deficiencies. Nocturnal hypoglycemia with seizures and recurrent, unexplained hypoglycemia with a reduction in insulin requirements should prompt the physician to investigate for celiac disease [50,109,110]. In the young child, growth failure and delayed sexual maturation may be seen. Vitamin A deficiency may aggravate retinopathy; deficiencies of vitamins E and B_{12} may cause peripheral neuropathy; iron and folic acid deficiencies may lead to complications of fertility and pregnancy; and vitamin D can complicate dental disease, limit joint mobility, and cause osteopenia and osteoporosis. There is also an increased incidence of other autoimmune diseases in type 1 diabetics who have "silent" celiac disease [111,112]. The gluten-free diet presents additional challenges to the diabetic patient, who may see acute hyperglycemia and a steady rise in hemoglobin A1c on initiation of this diet. This can be due to intestinal healing and better absorption, as well as gluten-free food substitutes, which can be corn-, rice-, or potato-based and have a higher glycemic index.

Once the patient has undergone initial counseling, the primary care physician (or gastroenterologist) and dietitian should follow up with the patient in 3–6 months to discuss compliance with the diet and reinforce its importance. If the patient has been able to adjust to the lifestyle and has had no complications of the disorder, he or she can be seen annually. At the annual visit, a detailed dietary history should be elicited, and serum antibodies should be measured to gauge adherence. First- and second-degree relatives should be offered serologic screening. The primary care physician should perform a detailed history and physical aimed at screening for nutritional deficiencies and searching for signs and symptoms of other autoimmune disorders, gastrointestinal cancers, and refractory sprue. If the patient is doing well without clinical symptoms and has normal antibody titers, he or she should continue to be followed annually. If the patient is doing poorly, indicated by symptoms, nutritional deficiencies, or elevated antibodies, more extensive medical nutritional therapy should be given by a knowledgeable dietitian [83]. This patient will also require closer monitoring for the development of the aforementioned nutritional, autoimmune, and possibly malignant complications.

The reader is invited to review separate chapters in this book about additional nutritional considerations in colon cancer, type 1 diabetes, gastroesophageal reflux disease, diarrhea, constipation, lactose intolerance, liver disease, food allergy, osteomalacia, and osteoporosis, all of which can complicate celiac disease.

VI SUMMARY

The astute clinician must have a high index of suspicion to make the diagnosis of celiac disease. Although this condition is very common, it is underdiagnosed because of its protean manifestations. Although classically thought to present in childhood with diarrhea and protein-calorie malnutrition, we now know this disease can present outside of the pediatric age range with a variety of symptoms ranging from joint pain to infertility and anemia. Serum antibodies are an excellent screening tool for this disease. However, confirmation requires a small bowel biopsy performed by a gastroenterologist via an upper endoscopy. Celiac disease is the only autoimmune disease for which we know the trigger: gluten. Removal of gluten from the diet results in a complete histologic and symptomatic recovery in the majority of patients. Not uncommon complications of celiac disease can include vitamin and mineral deficiencies, the development of other autoimmune diseases, and a higher risk for osteoporosis and gastrointestinal cancers. Living a gluten-free lifestyle is challenging because the potential for contamination of foods by wheat, rye, and barley is great, and food labeling is not ideal. The patient benefits best from the involvement of a physician, a dietitian, and a support group who are up-to-date about the diet as well as the latest literature and advances in the understanding of the complex interactions between gluten and the immune system.

References

[1] R.F. Logan, Descriptive epidemiology of celiac disease, in: D. Branski, P. Rozen, M.F. Kagnoff (Eds.), Gluten-Sensitive Enteropathy (Frontiers of Gastrointestinal Research), Karger, Basel, 1991, pp. 1–14.

[2] C. Catassi, E. Fabiani, I.M. Ratsch, G.V. Coppa, P.L. Giorgi, R. Pierdomenico, et al., The coeliac iceberg in Italy: a multicentre antigliadin antibodies screening for coeliac disease in school-age subjects, Acta Paediatr. (Suppl. 412) (1996) 29–35.

[3] A. Groll, D.C. Candy, M.A. Preece, J.M. Tanner, J.T. Harries, Short stature as the primary manifestation of coeliac disease, Lancet 2 (1980) 1097–1099.

[4] E. Cacciari, S. Salardi, R. Lazzari, A. Cicignani, A. Collina, P. Pirazzoli, et al., Short stature and celiac disease: a relationship to consider even in patients with no gastrointestinal tract symptoms, J. Pediatr. 103 (1983) 708–711.

[5] L. Stenhammar, S.P. Fallstrom, G. Jansson, U. Jansson, T. Lindberg, Coeliac disease in children of short stature without gastrointestinal symptoms, Eur. J. Pediatr. 145 (1986) 185–186.

[6] M. Verkasalo, P. Kuitunen, S. Leisti, J. Perheentupa, Growth failure from symptomless celiac disease, Helv. Paediatr. Acta 33 (1978) 489–495.

[7] D.G. Barr, D.H. Shmerling, A. Prader, Catch-up growth in malnutrition, studied in celiac disease after institution of a gluten-free diet, Pediatr. Res. 6 (1972) 521–527.

[8] D.M. Smith, J. Miller, Gastroenteritis, coeliac disease and enamel hypoplasia, Br. Dent. J. 147 (1979) 91–95.

[9] L. Aine, Dental enamel defects and dental maturity in children and adolescents with celiac disease, Proc. Finn. Dent. Soc. 3 (Suppl.) (1986) 1–71.

[10] E.K. George, R. Hertzberger-ten Cate, L.W. van Suijekom-Smit, B.M. von Blomberg, S.O. Stapel, R.M. van Elburg, et al., Juvenile chronic arthritis and coeliac disease in the Netherlands, Clin. Exp. Rheumatol. 14 (1996) 571–575.

[11] L. Lepore, S. Martelossi, M. Pennesi, F. Falcini, M.L. Ermini, S. Perticarari, et al., Prevalence of celiac disease in patients with juvenile chronic arthritis, J. Pediatr. 129 (1996) 111–113.

[12] C. O'Farrelly, D. Marten, D. Melcher, B. McDougall, R. Price, A.J. Goldstein, et al., Association between villous atrophy in rheumatoid arthritis and rheumatoid factor and gliadin-specific IgG, Lancet 2 (1988) 819–822.

[13] M. Maki, O. Hallstrom, P. Verronen, T. Reunala, M.L. Lahdeaho, K. Holm, et al., Reticulin antibody, arthritis, and coeliac disease in children, Lancet 1 (1988) 479–480.

[14] T. Valdimarsson, O. Lofmano, G. Toss, M. Strom, Reversal of osteopenia with diet in adult coeliac disease, Gut 38 (1996) 322–327.

[15] S. Mora, G. Barera, S. Beccio, M.C. Proverbio, G. Weber, C. Bianchi, et al., Bone density and bone metabolism are normal after long-term gluten-free diet in young celiac patients, Am. J. Gastroenterol. 94 (1999) 398–403.

[16] D. Meyer, S. Stavropolous, B. Diamond, E. Shane, P.H. Green, Osteoporosis in North American adult population with celiac disease, Am. J. Gastroenterol. 96 (2001) 112–119.

[17] L. Fry, Dermatitis herpetiformis, Bailliere's Clin. Gastroenterol. 9 (1995) 371–393.

[18] J. Zone, Skin manifestations of celiac disease, Gastroenterology 128 (2005) S87–S91.

[19] E. Scala, M. Giani, L. Pirrotta, E.C. Guerra, O. DePita, P. Pudda, Urticaria and adult celiac disease, Allergy 54 (1999) 1008–1009.

[20] G. Michaelsson, B. Gerden, E. Hagforsen, B. Nilsson, I. Pihl-Ludin, W. Kraaz, et al., Psoriasis patients with antibodies to gliadin can be improved by gluten-free diet, Br. J. Dermatol. 142 (2000) 44–51.

[21] S. Auricchio, L. Greco, R. Troncone, Gluten-sensitive enteropathy in childhood, Pediatr. Clin. North Am. 35 (1988) 157−187.

[22] A. Gasbarrini, E. Torre, C. Trivellini, S. DeCarolis, A. Carso, G. Gasbarrini, Recurrent spontaneous abortion and intrauterine fetal growth retardation as symptoms of coeliac disease, Lancet 356 (2000) 399−400.

[23] C. Ciacci, M. Cirillo, G. Auriemma, G. DiDato, F. Sabbatini, G. Mazzacca, Celiac disease and pregnancy outcome, Obstet. Gynecol. Surv. 51 (1996) 643−644.

[24] M.J. Farthing, L.H. Rees, C.R. Edwards, A.M. Dawson, Male gonadal function in coeliac disease: 2. Sex hormones, Gut 24 (1983) 127−135.

[25] P. Collin, S. Vilska, P.K. Heinonen, O. Hallstrom, P. Pikkarainen, Infertility and coeliac disease, Gut 39 (1996) 382−384.

[26] K.L. Kolho, A. Tiitinen, M. Tulppala, L. Unkila-kallio, E. Savilahti, Screening for coeliac disease in women with a history of recurrent miscarriage or infertility, Br. J. Obstet. Gynaecol. 106 (1999) 171−173.

[27] K.S. Sher, J.F. Mayberry, Female fertility, obstetric and gynaecological history in coeliac disease, Digestion 55 (1994) 243−246.

[28] A. Carroccio, E. Iannitto, F. Cavataio, G. Montalto, M. Tumminello, P. Campagna, et al., Sideropenic anemia and celiac disease: one study, two points of view, Dig. Dis. Sci. 43 (1998) 673−678.

[29] G. Maggiore, C. De Giacomo, M.S. Scotta, F. Sessa, Coeliac disease presenting as chronic hepatitis in a girl, J. Pediatr. Gastroenterol. Nutr. 5 (1986) 501−503.

[30] S. Loenardi, G. Bottaro, R. Patane, S. Musumeci, Hypertransaminasemia as first symptom in infant coeliac disease, J. Pediatr. Gastroenterol. Nutr. 11 (1990) 404−406.

[31] S. Davison, Coeliac disease and liver dysfunction, Arch. Dis. Child. 87 (2002) 293−296.

[32] A. Fontanella, P. Vajro, E. Ardia, L. Greco, Danno epatico in corso di malattia celiaca: studio retrospettivo in 123 bambini, Riv. Ital. Pediatr. 5 (1987) 80−85.

[33] J.G.C. Kingham, D.R. Parker, The association between biliary cirrhosis and coeliac disease: a study of relative prevalences, Gut 42 (1998) 120−122.

[34] W.T. Cooke, W.T. Smith, Neurological disorders associated with adult coeliac disease, Brain 89 (1966) 683−722.

[35] M. Hadjivassiliou, A. Gibson, G.A. Davies-Jones, A.J. Lobo, T.J. Stephenson, A. Milford-Ward, Does cryptic gluten sensitivity play a part in neurological illness? Lancet 347 (1996) 371.

[36] G. Gobbi, F. Bouquet, L. Greco, A. Lambertini, C.A. Tassinari, A. Ventura, et al., Coeliac disease, epilepsy, and cerebral calcifications, Lancet 340 (1992) 439−443.

[37] M. Kieslich, G. Errazuriz, H.G. Posselt, W. Moeller-Hartmann, F. Zanella, H. Boehles, Brain white-matter lesions in celiac disease: a prospective study of 75 diet-treated patients, Pediatrics 108 (2001) e21.

[38] M. Hadjivassiliou, R.A. Grunewald, A.K. Chattopadhyay, G.A. Davies-Jones, A. Gibson, J.A. Jarratt, et al., Clinical, radiological, neurophysiological and neuropathological characteristics of gluten ataxia, Lancet 352 (1998) 1582−1585.

[39] M. Hadjivassiliou, R. Grunewald, B. Sharrack, D. Sanders, A. Lobo, C. Williamson, et al., Gluten ataxia in perspective: Epidemiology, genetic susceptibility and clinical characteristics, Brain 126 (2003) 685−691.

[40] M. Hadjivassiliou, R.A. Grunewald, G.A. Davies-Jones, Gluten sensitivity as a neurological illness, J. Neurol. Neurosurg. Psychiatry 72 (2002) 560−563.

[41] E. Fabiani, C. Catassi, A. Villari, P. Gismondi, R. Pierdomenico, I.M. Ratsch, G.V. Coppa, P.L. Giorgi, Dietary compliance in screening-detected coeliac disease adolescents, Acta Paediatr. Acta Paediatr (Suppl. 412) (1996) 65−67.

[42] A.M. Knivsberg, K.L. Reichelt, M. Nodland, H. Torleiv, Autistic syndromes and diet: A follow-up study, Scand. J. Educ. Res. 39 (1995) 223−236.

[43] Autism Network for Dietary Intervention. Retrieved September 2007 from <http://www.autismndi.com/> 2007.

[44] The gluten free casein free diet. Retrieved September 2007 from <http://www.gfcfdiet.com/> 2007.

[45] L. Book, A. Hart, J. Black, M. Feolo, J.J. Zone, S.L. Neuhausen, Prevalence and clinical characteristics of celiac disease in Down's syndrome in a U.S. study, Am. J. Med. Genet. 98 (2001) 70−74.

[46] M. Hadjivassiliou, R.A. Grunewald, G.A. Davies-Jones, Gluten sensitivity: a many headed hydra, BMJ 318 (1999) 1710−1711.

[47] A. Ventura, G. Maazzu, L. Greco, Duration of exposure to gluten and risk for autoimmune disorders in patients with celiac disease, Gastroenterology 117 (1999) 297−303.

[48] D.W. Smith, Recognizable patterns of Malformation, Saunders, Philadelphia, 1988, pp. 10, 12, 74, 75

[49] M. Bonamico, P. Mariani, H.M. Danesi, M. Crisogianni, P. Faill, G. Gemme, et al., Prevalence and clinical picture of celiac disease in Italian Down syndrome patients: a multicenter study, J. Pediatr. Gastroenterol. Nutr. 33 (2001) 139−143.

[50] The NIH Consensus Development Conference on Celiac Disease. Retrieved September 2007 from <http://consensus.nih.gov/2004/2004CeliacDisease118html.htm/> June 28−30, 2004.

[51] S. Auricchio, G. Mazzacca, R. Toi, J. Visakorpi, M. Maki, E. Polanco, Coeliac disease as a familial condition: identification of asymptomatic coeliac patients within family groups, Gastroenterol. Int 1 (1988) 25−31.

[52] J. Hed, G. Leiden, E. Ottosson, M. Strom, A. Walan, O. Groth, et al., IgA antigliadin antibodies and jejunal mucosal lesions in healthy blood donors, Lancet 2 (1986) 215.

[53] A. Ferguson, E. Arran, S. O'Mahony, Clinical and pathological spectrum of coeliac disease—Active, silent, latent, potential, Gut 34 (1993) 150−151.

[54] R. Troncone, L. Greco, M. Mayer, F. Paparo, N. Caputo, M. Micillo, et al., Latent and potential coeliac disease, Acta Paediatr. Acta Paediatr (Suppl. 412) (1996) 10−14.

[55] P. Collin, K. Kaukinen, M. Maki, Clinical features of celiac disease today, Dig. Dis. 17 (1999) 100−106.

[56] J.A. Murray, J. Herlein, F. Mitros, J.A. Goeken, Serologic testing for celiac disease in the United States: results of a multilaboratory comparison study, Clin. Diagn. Lab. Immunol. 7 (2000) 584−587.

[57] S. Case, The gluten-free diet, Gluten-Free Diet: A Comprehensive Resource Guide, Centax Books, Saskatchewan, Canada, 2001, pp. 9-43

[58] F. Cataldo, V. Marino, A. Ventura, G. Botarro, G.R. Corazza, Prevalence and clinical features of selective immunoglobulin a deficiency in coeliac disease: an Italian multicenter study, Gut 42 (1998) 362−365.

[59] T. Not, K. Horvath, I.D. Hill, J. Partanen, A. Hammed, G. Magazzu, et al., Celiac disease risk in the USA: high prevalence of antiendomysium antibodies in healthy blood donors, Scand. J. Gastroenterol. 33 (1997) 494−498.

[60] W. Dieterich, T. Ehnis, M. Bauer, P. Donner, U. Volta, E.O. Riecken, et al., Identification of tissue transglutaminase as the autoantigen of celiac disease, Nat. Med 3 (1997) 797−801.

[61] S. Sulkanen, T. Halttunen, K. Laurila, K.L. Kolho, I.R. Korponay-Szabo, A. Sarnesto, et al., Tissue transglutaminase autoantibody enzyme-linked immunosorbent assay in detecting celiac disease, Gastroenterology 115 (1998) 1322−1328.

[62] R. Troncone, F. Maurano, M. Rossi, M. Micillo, L. Greco, R. Auricchio, et al., IgA antibodies to tissue transglutaminase: an effective diagnostic test for celiac disease, J. Pediatr. 134 (1999) 166−171.

[63] A. Fasano, Tissue transglutaminase: the holy grail for the diagnosis of celiac disease, at last, J. Pediatr. 134 (1999) 134−135.

[64] M. Mylotte, B. Egan-Mitchel, P.F. Fottrell, B. McNicholl, C.F. Carthy, Family studies in coeliac disease, Gut 16 (1975) 598−602.

[65] F.M. Stevens, R. Lloyd, B. Egan-Mitchel, M.J. Mylott, P.F. Fottrell, R. Write, B. McNicholl, C.F. McCarthy, Reticulin antibodies in patients with coeliac disease and their relatives, Gut 16 (1975) 598−602.

[66] A. Fasano, I. Berti, T. Gerarduzzi, T. Not, R.B. Colletti, S. Drago, et al., Prevalence of celiac disease in at-risk and not at-risk groups in the United States: alarge multicenter study, Arch. Intern. Med. 163 (2003) 286−292.

[67] L. Greco, R. Romino, I. Coto, N. Di Cosmo, S. Percopo, M. Maglio, et al., The first large population based twin study of coeliac disease, Gut 50 (2002) 624−628.

[68] S. Bevan, S. Popat, C.P. Braegger, A. Busch, D. O'Donoghue, K. Falth-Magnusson, et al., Contribution of the MHC region to the familial risk of coeliac disease, J. Med. Genet. 36 (1999) 687−690.

[69] L. Hogberg, K. Falth-Magnusson, E. Grodzinsky, L. Stenhammer, Familial prevalence of coeliac disease: a twenty-year follow-up study, Scand. J. Gastroenterol. 38 (2003) 61−65.

[70] A.H. Gudjonsdottir, S. Nilsson, J. Ek, B. Kristiansson, H. Ascher, The risk of celiac disease in 107 families with at least two affected siblings, J. Pediatr. Gastroenterol. Nutr. 38 (2004) 338−342.

[71] L. Brook, J.J. Zone, S.L. Neuhausen, Prevalence of celiac disease among relatives of sib pairs with celiac disease in U.S. families, Am. J. Gastroenterol. 98 (2003) 377−381.

[72] M. Jabbari, G. Wild, A.C. Goresky, D.S. Daly, J.O. Lough, D.P. Cleland, D.G. Kinnear, Scalloped valvulae connivenetes: an endoscopic marker of celiac sprue, Gastroenterology 95 (1988) 1518−1522.

[73] M.N. Marsh, Studies on intestinal lymphoid tissue: XI. The immunopathology of the cell-mediated reactions in gluten sensitivity and other enteropathies, Scanning Microsc 2 (1988) 1663−1665.

[74] J.A. Walker-Smith, B.K. Sandhu, E. Isolauri, G. Banchini, C. Van, M. Bertrand, et al., Guidelines prepared by the ESPGAN working group on acute Diarrhoea. Recommendations for feeding in childhood gastroenteritis. European Society of Pediatric Gastroenterology and Nutrition, J. Pediatr. Gastroenterol. Nutr. 24 (1997) 619−620.

[75] W. Dicke, Coeliac Disease: Investigation of Harmful Effects of Certain Types of Cereal on Patients with Coeliac Disease, University of Utrecht, Utrecht, The Netherlands, 1950.

[76] J.H. Van de Kamer, H.A. Weijers, W.K. Dicke, Coeliac disease: IV. An investigation into the injurious constituents of wheat in connection with their action in patients with coeliac disease, Acta Paediatr. 42 (1953) 223−231.

[77] G. Holmes, C. Catassi, Pathophysiology, Coeliac Disease, Health Press, Oxford, 2000, pp. 18-20

[78] C.M. Hardman, J.J. Garioch, J.N. Leonard, H.J.W. Thomas, M.M. Walker, J.E. Lortan, et al., Absence of toxicity of oats in patients with dermatitis herpetiformis, N. Engl. J. Med. 337 (1997) 1884−1887.

[79] E.J. Hoffenberg, J. Haas, A. Drescher, R. Barnhurst, I. Osberg, F. Bao, et al., A trial of oats in children with newly diagnosed celiac disease, J. Pediatr. 137 (2000) 361−366.

[80] F. Forssell, H. Weiser, Spelt wheat and celiac disease, Z. Lebens. Untersuch. Forsch. 201 (1995) 35−39.

[81] H.J. Ellis, A.P. Doyle, P. Day, H. Wieser, P.J. Ciclitira, Demonstration of the presence of coeliac-activating gliadin-like epitopes in malted barley, Int. Arch. Allergy Immunol. 104 (1994) 308−310.

[82] J.P. Crowe, N.P. Falini, Gluten in pharmaceutical products, Am. J. Health Syst. Pharmacy 58 (2001) 396−401.

[83] M. Pietzak, The follow-up of patients with celiac disease—achieving compliance with treatment, Gastroenterology 128 (2005) S135−S141.

[84] G. Ljungman, U. Myrdal, Compliance in teenagers with coeliac disease—a Swedish follow-up study, Acta Paediatr. 82 (1993) 238.

[85] M. Maki, M.L. Lahdeaho, O. Hallstrom, M. Viander, J.K. Visokorpi, Postpubertal gluten challenge in coeliac disease, Arch. Dis. Child. 64 (1989) 1604−1607.

[86] G.L. Hankey, G.K. Holmes, Coeliac disease in the elderly, Gut 35 (1994) 65−67.

[87] G. Corrao, G.R. Corazza, V. Bagnardi, G. Brusco, C. Ciacci, M. Cottone, et al., Club del Tenue Study Group, Mortality in patients with coeliac disease and their relatives: A cohort study, Lancet 358 (2001) 356−361.

[88] C.M. Swimson, G. Slavin, E.C. Coles, C.C. Booth, Coeliac disease and malignancy, Lancet 1 (1983) 111−115.

[89] C. Catassi, E. Fabiani, G. Corrao, M. Barbato, A. De Renzo, A.M. Carella, et al., Risk of non-Hodgkin lymphoma in celiac disease, JAMA 287 (2002) 1413−1419.

[90] G.K. Holmes, P. Prior, M.R. Lane, D. Pope, R.N. Allan, Malignancy in coeliac disease: effect on gluten-free diet, Gut 30 (1989) 333−338.

[91] S.K. Lee, W. Lo, L. Memeo, H. Rotterdam, P.H. Green, Duodenal histology in patients with celiac disease after treatment with gluten-free diet, Gastrointest. Endosc. 57 (2003) 187−191.

[92] A. Carroccio, G. Iacono, P. Lerro, F. Cavataio, E. Malorgio, M. Soresi, et al., Role of pancreatic impairment in growth recovery during gluten-free diet in childhood celiac disease, Gastroenterology 112 (1997) 1839−1844.

[93] I.J. Pink, B. Creamer, Response to a gluten-free diet of patients with the coeliac syndrome, Lancet 1 (1967) 300−304.

[94] C. Cellier, E. Delabesse, C. Helmer, N. Patey, C. Matuchansky, B. Jalori, et al., Refractory sprue, coeliac disease, and enteropathy-associated T-cell lymphoma, Lancet 356 (2000) 203−208.

[95] B.M. Stuart, A.E. Gent, Atrophy of the coeliac mucosa, Eur. J. Gastroenterol. Hepatol. 10 (1998) 523−525.

[96] H.C. Mitchison, H. al Mardini, S. Gillespie, M. Laker, A. Zaitoun, C.O. Record, A pilot study of fluticasone propionate in untreated coeliac disease, Gut 32 (1991) 260−265.

[97] A. Viadya, J. Bolanos, C. Berkelhammer, Azathioprine in refractory sprue, Am. J. Gastroenterol. 94 (1999) 1967−1969.

[98] P. Rolny, H.A. Sigurjonsdottir, H. Remotti, L.A. Nilsson, H. Ascher, H. Tlaskalova-Hogenova, et al., Role of immunosuppressive therapy in refractory sprue-like disease, Am. J. Gastroenterol. 94 (1999) 219−225.

[99] S. O'Mahony, P.D. Howdle, S.M. Losowsky, Management of patients with non-responsive coeliac disease, Aliment. Pharmacol. Ther. 10 (1996) 671−680.

[100] B.M. Ryan, D. Kelleher, Refractory celiac disease, Gastroenterology 119 (2000) 243−251.

[101] S. Daum, C. Cellier, C. Mulder, Refractory coeliac disease, Best Pract. Res. Clin. Gastroenterol. 19 (2005) 413−424.

[102] C. Sategna-Guidetti, U. Volta, C. Ciacci, P. Usai, A. Carlino, L. Franceschi, et al., Prevalence of thyroid disorders in untreated adult celiac disease patients and effect of gluten withdrawal: an Italian multicenter study, Am. J. Gastroenterol. 96 (2001) 751−757.

[103] K. Kaukinen, L. Halme, P. Collin, M. Farkkila, M. Maki, P. Vehmanen, et al., Celiac disease in patients with severe liver disease: gluten-free diet may reverse hepatic failure, Gastroenterology 122 (2002) 881−888.

[104] C. Sategna-Guidetti, S.B. Grosso, S. Grosso, G. Mengozzi, G. Aimo, T. Zaccaria, et al., The effects of a 1-year gluten withdrawal on bone mass, bone metabolism and nutritional status in newly diagnosed adult coeliac patients, Aliment. Pharmacol. Ther. 14 (2000) 35–43.

[105] S. Mora, G. Barera, S. Beccio, L. Menni, M.C. Proverbio, C. Bianchi, et al., A prospective, longitudinal study of the long-term effect of treatment on bone density in children with celiac disease, J. Pediatr. 139 (2001) 516–521.

[106] T. Kemppainen, H. Kroger, E. Janatuinen, I. Arnala, C. Lamberg-Allardt, M. Karkkainen, et al., Bone recovery after a gluten-free diet: a 5-year follow-up study, Bone 25 (1999) 355–360.

[107] T. Kemppainen, H. Kroger, E. Janatuinen, I. Arnala, V.-M. Kosma, P. Pikkarainen, et al., Osteoporosis in adult patients with celiac disease, Bone 24 (1999) 249–255.

[108] T. Valdimarsson, G. Toss, O. Lofman, M. Strom, Three years' follow-up of bone density in adult coeliac disease: significance of secondary hyperparathyroidism, Scand. J. Gastroenterol. 35 (2000) 274–280.

[109] C.M. Smith, C.F. Clarke, L.E. Porteous, H. Elsori, D.J.S. Cameron, Prevalence of celiac disease and longitudinal follow-up of antigliadin antibody status in children and adolescents with type 1 diabetes mellitus, Pediatr. Diabetes 1 (2000) 199–203.

[110] A. Mohn, M. Cerruto, D. Iafusco, F. Prisco, S. Tumini, O. Stoppoloni, et al., Celiac disease in children and adolescents with type 1 diabetes: importance of hypoglycemia, J. Pediatr. Gastroenterol. Nutr. 32 (2001) 37–40.

[111] T. Not, A. Tommasini, G. Tonini, E. Buratti, M. Pocecco, C. Tortul, et al., Undiagnosed coeliac disease and risk of autoimmune disorders in subjects with type 1 diabetes mellitus, Diabetologia 44 (2001) 151–155.

[112] C. Jaeger, E. Hatziagelaki, R. Petzoldt, R. Bretzel, Comparative analysis of organ-specific autoantibodies and celiac disease-associated antibodies in type 1 diabetic patients, their first-degree relatives, and healthy control subjects, Diabetes Care 24 (2001) 27–32.

[113] E. Lubrano, C. Ciacci, P.R.J. Ames, G. Mazzacca, P. Ordente, R. Scarpa, The arthritis of coeliac disease: prevalence and pattern in 200 adult patients, Br. J. Rheumatol. 35 (1996) 1314–1318.

[114] L. Paimela, P. Kurki, M. Leirisalo-Repo, H. Piirainen, Gliadin immune reactivity in patients with rheumatoid arthritis, Clin. Exp. Rheumatol. 13 (1995) 603–607.

[115] M. Curione, M. Barbato, L. De Biase, F. Viola, L. LoRusso, E. Cardi, Prevalence of celiac disease in idiopathic dilated cardiomyopathy, Lancet 354 (1999) 222–223.

[116] S. Martelossi, E. Zanatta, E. Del Santo, P. Clarich, P. Radovich, A. Ventura, Dental enamel defects and screening for coeliac disease, Acta Paediatr. Acta Paediatr. (Suppl. 412) (1996) 47–48.

[117] T. Ruenala, P. Collin, Diseases associated with dermatitis herpetiformis, Br. J. Dermatol. 136 (1997) 315–318.

[118] P. Collin, T. Reunala, E. Pukkala, P. Laippala, O. Keyrilainen, A. Pasternak, Celiac disease-associated disorders and survival, Gut 35 (1994) 1215–1218.

[119] M.E. Thain, J.R. Hamilton, R.M. Erlich, Coexistence of diabetes mellitus and celiac disease, J. Pediatr. 85 (1974) 527–529.

[120] E. Savilahti, O. Simell, S. Koskimies, A. Rilva, H.K. Akerblom, Celiac disease in insulin-dependent diabetes mellitus, J. Pediatr. 108 (1986) 690–693.

[121] P. Collin, J. Salmi, O. Hallstrom, H. Oksa, H. Oksala, M. Maki, et al., High frequency of coeliac disease in adult patients with type-I diabetes, Scand. J. Gastroenterol. 24 (1989) 81–84.

[122] A.H. Talal, J.A. Murray, J.A. Goeken, W.F. Sivitz, Celiac disease in an adult population with insulin-dependent diabetes mellitus: use of endomysial antibody testing, Am. J. Gastroenterol. 92 (1997) 1280–1284.

[123] I. Hill, A. Fasano, R. Schwartz, D. Counts, M. Glock, K. Hovath, The prevalence of celiac disease in at-risk groups of children in the United States, J. Pediatr. 136 (2000) 86–90.

[124] A. Carlsson, I. Axelsson, S. Borulf, A. Bredberg, M. Forslund, B. Lindberg, et al., Prevalence of IgA-antigliadin antibodies and IgA-antiendomysium antibodies related to celiac disease in children with Down syndrome, Pediatrics 101 (1998) 272–275.

[125] C.C. Cronin, L.M. Jackson, C. Feighery, F. Shanahan, M. Abuzakouk, D.Q. Ryder, et al., Coeliac disease and epilepsy, Q. J. Med. 71 (1998) 359–369.

[126] P. Collin, M. Maki, O. Keyrilainen, O. Hallstrom, T. Reunala, A. Pasternak, Selective IgA deficiency and celiac disease, Scand. J. Gastroenterol. 27 (1992) 367–371.

[127] P. Collin, M. Korpela, O. Hallstrom, M. Viander, O. Keyrilainen, M. Maki, Rheumatic complaints as a presenting symptom in patients with celiac disease, Scand. J. Rheumatol. 21 (1992) 20–23.

[128] P. Collin, J. Salmi, O. Hallstrom, T. Reunala, A. Pasternak, Autoimmune thyroid disorders and coeliac disease, Eur. J. Endocrinol. 130 (1994) 140.

[129] J. Rujner, A. Wisniewicz, H. Gregorere, B. Wozniewicz, W. Mynarski, H.W. Witas, Coeliac disease and HLA-DQ2 (DQA1*0501 and DQB1*0201) in patients with Turner syndrome, J. Pediatr. Gastroenterol. Nutr. 32 (2001) 114–115.

[130] M. Bonamico, G. Bottaro, A.M. Pasquino, M. Caruso-Nicoletti, P. Mariani, G. Gemme, et al., Celiac disease and Turner syndrome, J. Pediatr. Gastroenterol. Nutr. 26 (1998) 496–499.

[131] S.A. Ivarsson, A. Carlsson, A. Bredberg, J. Alm, S. Aronsson, J. Gustafsson, et al., Prevalence of coeliac disease in Turner syndrome, Acta Paediatr. 88 (1999) 933–936.

[132] A. Giannotti, G. Tiberio, M. Castro, F. Virgilii, F. Colistro, F. Ferretti, et al., Celiac disease in Williams syndrome, J. Med. Genet. 38 (2001) 767–768.

42

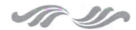

Nutrition and Cystic Fibrosis

Zhumin Zhang, HuiChuan J. Lai
University of Wisconsin, Madison, Wisconsin

I OVERVIEW OF CYSTIC FIBROSIS

Cystic fibrosis (CF) is one of the most common, life-shortening autosomal recessive disorders, with estimated incidences of approximately 1 in 3000 white live births, 1 in 17,000 black live births, and 1 in 90,000 Oriental live births [1,2]. CF was recognized as a distinct clinical entity in 1938. It is a generalized disease of the exocrine glands characterized by abnormal sodium and chloride transport, leading to elevated electrolyte levels in sweat [3,4]. Dysfunction of the other exocrine glands occurs, producing viscid secretions of low water content. This results in pancreatic insufficiency (PI), which leads to malabsorption and failure to gain weight, as well as airway obstruction, which leads to increased susceptibility to recurrent bronchial infection, progressive lung damage, and eventual respiratory failure.

A Clinical Presentation

There are three categories of major clinical abnormalities in CF: (1) gastrointestinal tract involvement, characterized by PI leading to malabsorption and malnutrition; (2) respiratory tract involvement, characterized by recurrent infections and chronic obstructive pulmonary disease; and (3) salt loss in sweat that can lead to severe hyponatremic dehydration. The pancreatic disturbance begins prenatally and can cause intestinal obstruction in newborns with CF, a problem referred to as meconium ileus (MI). It has been estimated that 85–90% of CF patients have PI [5] and 15–20% have MI [6].

Studies have shown that PI develops during the first year of life such that approximately half the patients who develop this problem show intestinal malabsorption by approximately 1 month of age, two-thirds by 6 months, and the remainder by 1 year [7]. Unlike PI, pulmonary status of patients with CF often appears normal at birth [8]; however, it inevitably shows obstruction and infection. The onset and rate of progression of CF lung disease are not well understood but appear to vary widely among individuals [9–12]. Other complications may occur as the disease progresses. For example, glucose intolerance and diabetes mellitus may develop [13,14]. The prevalence of CF-related diabetes (CFRD) is reported to be between 5 and 15% in children younger than 18 years and up to 50% in adults with CF [15–19]. Because of focal biliary cirrhosis, up to 11% of CF patients develop overt liver disease in adolescence or adulthood [15]. Due to an absent vas deferens at birth (presumably resulting from ductal obstruction with dehydrated secretions), infertility in males with CF is virtually universal [20]. Approximately 10% of patients reported in 2009 CF Foundation Patient Registry had bone disease [15].

B Pathogenesis

On the basis of molecular genetics research [21], CF fundamentally can be attributed to mutations occurring in the long arm of chromosome 7. With cloning of the CF gene, it has been demonstrated that the most common mutation is a 3-base pair (bp) deletion; this results in the loss of a phenylalanine residue at amino acid position 508 of the predicted gene product, namely the cystic fibrosis transmembrane conductance regulator (CFTR) [22–24]. The 3-bp deletion mutant, commonly referred to as F508del, occurs in approximately 70% of the CF chromosomes [22], and more than 85% of CF patients in the United States have at least one F508del allele [25]. However, more than 1800 other DNA mutations in the CFTR gene have been identified (http://www.genet.sickkids.on.ca/cftr/app), and more are still being found. Most mutations occur infrequently, and only approximately 10% are common enough to be

Nutrition in the Prevention and Treatment of Disease, Third Edition.
DOI: http://dx.doi.org/10.1016/B978-0-12-391884-0.00042-1

well characterized (http://www.cftr2.org). Among these gene mutations, some are disease causing, some are sequence variations that do not cause CF, some are associated with single or milder organ system involvement than is typically seen in CF (sometimes called "CFTR-associated disorders" or "CFTR-related metabolic syndrome"), and some have variable or unknown consequences [26–29]. Approximately half the CF patients are homozygous for F508del, and nearly 40% more have at least one such mutation; however, in the latter circumstance, it is the second mutation that determines genotype–phenotype implications [27,30].

The abnormal CFTR protein is the underlying pathogenic factor in the disease process due to its role in regulating ion transport across the apical membrane of epithelial cells, particularly chloride conductance, which is invariably defective in CF [2,4]. This defect leads to abnormally high chloride concentration in the sweat, which constitutes the classical diagnostic test for CF [31]. Research suggests that the CFTR protein is a structural component of the chloride channel and may itself account for the channel core [4,32].

C Diagnosis and Treatment

Traditionally, the diagnosis of CF has been made because of (1) a positive family history; (2) the presence of MI; or (3) symptoms of malabsorption or pulmonary disease with infection, which occur at variable ages [33,34]. Once the characteristic signs and symptoms become evident, the diagnosis of CF can be readily established by performing a sweat test using pilocarpine iontophoresis [28,31]. Traditional diagnosis by signs or symptoms of CF often leads to delays in diagnosis and referral to a CF center. These delays are associated with severe malnutrition in approximately half the patients [28], but this can be prevented with early diagnosis and treatment [35–38]. Consequently, there has been considerable interest in establishing newborn screening (NBS) methods for detection of presymptomatic cases for the purpose of instituting early treatment and preventing ameliorating symptoms.

In 1979, Crossley et al. first described the use of dry-blood specimens obtained from newborns to measure immunoreactive trypsinogen (IRT) level, which was shown to be highly elevated in patients with CF [39,40]. The discovery of the CFTR gene in 1989 [6] has promoted the development of new screening methods in which the IRT test is coupled with detection of the most common mutant allele (F508del) or with a multipanel CFTR mutation analysis [41,42]. Various NBS protocols are used to screen newborns for CF [43]. All protocols begin with a first-tier phenotypic test that measures IRT in dried blood spots. Infants who have an elevated IRT are then referred for further testing—either a repeat IRT test at 2 weeks of age or DNA analysis for CFTR mutations. Infants with a second positive screening result are referred for sweat testing to establish the diagnosis of CF. It is important to understand that a positive IRT test alone is not equivalent to a diagnosis of CF. In fact, only approximately 1% of newborns with positive IRT have CF [44], In addition, not all CF cases are detected by screening for IRT; approximately 5% of CF patients show false-negative IRT in their dry-blood specimens obtained at birth [44].

In the United States, CF NBS began in Colorado [45] and Wisconsin [41,42] in the mid-1980s. The potential benefits and risks associated with CF NBS programs have been under investigation in various regions of the world [42,46–50]. In many reports [37–42], clear evidence of nutritional benefits attributable to early diagnosis has been demonstrated by anthropometric indexes. The most convincing evidence was obtained from a randomized clinical trial in Wisconsin after 10 years of investigation [36–38]. This trial and other studies [51,52] led the Centers for Disease Control and Prevention (CDC) to recommend universal screening in a report published in 2004 [53]. Currently, almost all infants in the United States and more than 8 million newborns worldwide are screened annually for CF. In the United States, approximately 90% of infants are evaluated with the IRT/DNA two-tiered strategy.

Clinical management of CF involves treatment programs with three principal objectives: (1) improve nutritional status, (2) promote clearance of respiratory secretions, and (3) control bronchopulmonary infections. Care programs for CF patients in North America and many European countries are organized in specialized regional centers. These centers have placed particular emphasis on enhancing nutrition and using aggressive strategies to prevent progressive pulmonary disease [54]. Although CF lung disease cannot be cured, treatment programs have been generally effective, as evidenced by the increasing longevity of CF patients in the United States during the past three decades from less than 20 years to approximately 36 years [15,55]. The primary causes of death in patients with CF are cardiorespiratory complications, accounting for approximately 80% of deaths. For this reason, most CF centers in the United States place a great deal of emphasis on respiratory management for patients with CF. In addition, with diagnosis through NBS, an increased emphasis has been placed on preventing malnutrition in recent years.

D Consequences of Malnutrition

Evidence has accumulated from longitudinal studies that the consequences of malnutrition in CF are more severe than previously appreciated from clinic-based cross-sectional observations. Long-term adverse consequences of malnutrition include (1) permanently stunted growth [36–38], (2) cognitive dysfunction [56,57], and (3) greater susceptibility to lung disease [58–61]. Research is underway to address whether early nutritional intervention could alter long-term pulmonary disease progression.

II MALNUTRITION IN CYSTIC FIBROSIS

CF is associated with an increased risk of protein-calorie malnutrition, as well as deficiencies in fat-soluble vitamins and other micronutrients. Malnutrition associated with CF is characterized by its early onset and is often present at the time of CF diagnosis. At the mild end of the malnutrition spectrum, CF patients may have depleted stores or low circulating concentrations of a given nutrient but no associated signs or symptoms. More pronounced nutritional deficiencies lead to metabolic abnormalities, structural changes, functional disturbances, growth failure, developmental delay, and a variety of other characteristics of malnutrition. Malnutrition is most likely to occur during periods of rapid growth when nutritional requirements are high, during pulmonary exacerbations, and with increased severity of lung disease.

Growth impairment, abnormalities in the biochemical markers of nutritional status, as well as clinical symptoms of malnutrition all have been reported in patients with CF. Historically, malnutrition in patients with CF was thought to represent either an inherent consequence of disease process or a physiologic adaptation to advanced pulmonary disease. However, it is now recognized that the causes of malnutrition in CF are multiple and can be attributed to three primary mechanisms [62–64]: increased energy and nutrient losses, increased energy expenditure, as well as decreased energy and nutrient intakes. Table 42.1 lists the major risk factors for malnutrition associated with CF.

A Causes of Malnutrition

1 Increased Losses

Loss of nutrients from maldigestion and malabsorption as a result PI is the primary factor contributing to energy and nutrient deficiencies in patients with CF [65]. The ductular cells of the pancreas respond to stimulation with secretin by producing a high-volume, bicarbonate-rich secretion. This secretion functions to neutralize gastric acid, thus enabling the pancreatic digestive enzymes to function at their pH optimum. The abnormal chloride transport caused by the defected CFTR protein leads to

TABLE 42.1 Factors Contributing to Malnutrition in Cystic Fibrosis

Disease factors

Presence of pancreatic insufficiency (PI)

Severity of PI (the degree of steatorrhea and azotorrhea)

Partial intestinal resection secondary to bowel obstruction (caused by meconium ileus)

Severity of respiratory disease

Loss of bile salts associated with steatorrhea

Cholestatic liver disease

Diabetes mellitus

Nutritional factors

Growth rate (of particular concern in young children and adolescents with CF)

Energy and macronutrient intakes (e.g., the quantity and quality of food consumed)

Micronutrient deficiencies (e.g., fat-soluble vitamins)

Energy expenditure

Eating behaviors

thickened secretions that obstruct the pancreatic ducts and prevent the secretion of enzymes and bicarbonate. In CF, PI is defined by the presence of measurable steatorrhea. This does not occur until 1 or 2% of pancreatic enzymatic capacity remains [66]. Therefore, CF patients with PI have severe, irreversible loss of pancreatic function. It is also important to understand that CF patients with pancreatic sufficiency (PS) do not have normal pancreatic function [67]. They have decreased volume of bicarbonate-rich secretion but continue to produce enough pancreatic enzymes to avoid steatorrhea.

Maldigestion and malabsorption caused by PI can be attributed to three major abnormalities: lack of digestive enzymes, inadequate bicarbonate secretion, and loss of bile salts and bile acids. Inadequate bicarbonate secretion results in impaired capacity to neutralize gastric acid in the duodenum and a lower intestinal pH until well into the jejunium, which often reduces the effectiveness of pancreatic enzyme replacement therapy (PERT) [65–67] (see Section IV.A.2). Loss of bile salts and bile acids often exacerbates maldigestion and malabsorption. Bile acids are readily precipitated in an acid milieu, and duodenal bile acid concentration may fall below the critical micellar concentration, thereby exacerbating fat maldigestion. Precipitated bile salts also appear to be lost from the enterohepatic circulation in greater quantities, thus reducing the total bile acid pool and altering the glycocholate:taurocholate ratio. Oral taurine supplements have been reported to benefit some CF patients [68].

Other factors also contribute to energy and nutrient losses in CF. Patients presenting with MI, particularly those who have undergone intestinal resection, have further reduction in intestinal absorptive capabilities. Viscid, thick intestinal mucus, with altered physical properties, may affect the thickness of the intestinal unstirred layer, further limiting nutrient absorption. CFRD may increase caloric losses due to glycosuria if not adequately controlled. Advanced liver disease and biliary cirrhosis may result in reduced bile salt synthesis and secretion, which may lead to severe fat malabsorption.

2 Increased Requirement

Energy requirements in patients with CF are highly variable. Several studies have reported that patients with CF have increased energy expenditure compared with non-CF patients [69–72]. A variety of explanations have been proposed to explain the increased energy expenditure observed in CF patients, including chronic respiratory infection, increase in work of breathing, genetic and cellular defects, and changes in body composition.

Chronic respiratory infections, particularly with *Pseudomonas aeruginosa*, have been shown to be associated with a 25–80% increase in metabolic rate and energy requirements [73]. The link between CF genotype and energy requirement was reported in a study by Tomezsko *et al.* [72], who demonstrated that energy expenditure was increased by 23% in CF patients with homozygous F508del mutations compared with non-CF controls. Therefore, a patient with advanced lung disease might not be able to ingest sufficient calories to meet energy needs.

The hypothesis that a basic cellular defect may increase energy requirement was supported by *in vitro* studies showing that mitochondria from cultured fibroblasts obtained from CF patients had higher rates of oxygen consumption compared with control tissues [74,75]. When F508del was identified, it was proposed that the defected CFTR protein may affect cellular energy metabolism through its involvement in the regulation of ion transport across membranes because CFTR is a cAMP-regulated chloride channel [4].

3 Decreased Consumption

The appetite or caloric intake of CF patients may be limited due to a variety of disease complications. Acute pulmonary exacerbations are a common cause of anorexia, and respiratory infections often give rise to nausea and vomiting, which may further reduce caloric intake [63]. The biochemical causes of anorexia associated with acute infection are unclear, but elevated circulating levels of tumor necrosis factor may play a role [76].

In addition to pulmonary complications, a variety of gastrointestinal complications also contribute to anorexia and inadequate caloric intake [62]. Increased

occurrence of gastroesophageal reflux disease (GERD) and esophagitis are observed in patients with CF. Distal intestinal obstruction syndrome (DIOS), a form of subacute or chronic partial bowel obstruction, usually occurs in older patients with PI. Large fecal masses, palpable in the abdomen, give rise to intermittent abdominal distention and cramping accompanied by reduced appetite. Constipation in the absence of DIOS is another cause of anorexia and abdominal discomfort in older patients with CF.

A number of dietary surveys indicate that CF patients often eat less than normal. This was particularly the case during the 1970s and early 1980s, when CF patients were commonly prescribed fat-restricted diets based on the assumption that a reduction in dietary fat intake might improve bowel symptoms [77]. The observation of better growth and survival in CF patients who received unrestricted-fat, high-calorie diet in combination with PERT compared with those who received low-fat diet in the early 1980s has changed dietary practices in most CF centers [78,79]. Nutritionists recommend energy intakes 110% or greater of the estimated energy requirement (ER) for patients with CF, with 35–40% of energy from fat [80,81]. However, CF patients often fail to consume such high quantities of calories and/or fat because of their disease manifestation. In several cross-sectional or short-term studies [82–86] and a small prospective 3-year study of 25 patients [87], energy and fat intakes of CF patients were reported to be much lower than the previously mentioned recommendations. A longitudinal study evaluating dietary intake patterns in children with CF from the time of diagnosis to age 10 years revealed mean energy intake was approximately 110% of ER, with fat consisting of approximately 37% of energy [37].

B Common Nutritional Deficiencies

1 Energy and Macronutrients

As discussed previously, patients with CF are at high risk of energy deficiency due to their increased requirement and decreased consumption. Protein poses less of a nutritional problem than does fat in the CF population. The major risk of protein deficiency in CF patients occurs during the first year of life, when the average requirement is at least three times as great as that in adulthood. Low serum markers of protein (e.g., albumin, prealbumin, and retinol binding protein) are commonly found in infants and young children with newly diagnosed CF. One-third to one-half of infants diagnosed using CF NBS were reported to be hypoalbuminemic [88–90]. Normalization of serum albumin level often occurs following comprehensive nutrition therapy [91].

Energy deficiency leads to impaired growth in children with CF. Weight retardation and linear growth failure are the most common observations documented in CF clinics [92,93], although their severity and prevalence vary greatly. Accurate estimates of the prevalence of malnutrition in the CF population have been difficult to obtain in the past due to lack of sufficient data. In recent years, comprehensive national databases known as CF patient registries have been compiled by the U.S. Cystic Fibrosis and Canadian Cystic Fibrosis Foundations, as well as the European Cystic Fibrosis Society, making it possible to determine population estimates of the prevalence of malnutrition associated with CF. Analysis of 13,000 pediatric CF patients documented in the 1993 U.S. CF Patient Registry revealed that CF children grew substantially below normal at all ages [35]. Malnutrition was particularly prevalent in infants (47%) and adolescents (34%) compared with children at other ages (22%), and it was also prevalent in patients with newly diagnosed, untreated CF (44%). Underweight is also prevalent in adults with CF; approximately 35% of the 7200 adults with CF documented in the 1992−1994 U.S. and Canadian CF patient registries were found to be underweight [94]. The prevalence of malnutrition in pediatric CF patients has decreased steadily from approximately 25% in 1995 to approximately 15% in 2005 [95].

2 Essential Fatty Acids

Essential fatty acid deficiency (EFAD) has been reported to occur in CF patients [88,94,96,97]. During infancy, particularly before diagnosis, EFAD can occur with desquamating skin lesions, increased susceptibility to infection, poor wound healing, thrombocytopenia, and growth retardation. In patients who are adequately treated, clinical evidence of EFAD is rare, although biochemical abnormalities of EFA status remain common [98−100]. The major fatty acid abnormalities found in patients with CF are low levels of linoleic acid (18:2, n-6) and docosahexaenoic acids (22:6, n-3); a normal or mildly decreased level of arachidonic acid (20:4, n-6); and elevated levels of palmitoleic, oleic (18:1, n-9), and eicosatrienoic (20:3, n-9) acid. In EFAD, oleic acid is converted to eicosatrienoic acid, which is commonly referred to as the "pathologic triene" because its increase in EFAD couples to the usual decrease in arachidonic acid, leading to a high triene:tetraene ratio [91,101,102]. Multiple hypotheses have been proposed to explain the underlying mechanisms of abnormal EFA status associated with CF. Fat malabsorption secondary to PI is the most common explanation for EFA. However, some investigators have postulated a primary metabolic defect in fatty acid metabolism [98−104].

Many studies have reported a clear association between better EFA status and better growth in children with CF. Plasma linoleic acid was shown to be positively correlated with growth in children whose CF was diagnosed before 3 months and followed up to 12 years of age [88]. van Egmond et al. [105] showed better growth among CF infants who consumed a predigested formula that contained high linoleic acid (12% of energy) compared with those who consumed a comparable formula with lower linoleic acid (7% of energy), despite a lower total energy intake in the former group. Shoff et al. [106] demonstrated that in children who experienced longer and more severe malnutrition due to delayed diagnosis, maintaining normal plasma linoleic acid (i.e., >26% of total plasma fatty acids) in addition to sustaining a high caloric intake (i.e., >120% of ER) is a critical determinant in promoting catch-up weight gain.

Despite the previously discussed evidence, EFA supplementation for CF patients remains controversial for several reasons. First, not all patients respond to EFA supplementation; normalizing plasma linoleic acid is particularly difficult in patients with MI [64,72]. Second, n-6 fatty acids, including linoleic acid and its metabolite arachidonic acid, have been proposed to play a role in CF inflammation [107−111]. In the 2009 CF Foundation infant care guidelines [112], clinical trials to "answer questions related to EFA supplementation in infants" are recommended as a priority of research to resolve this controversy.

3 Fat-Soluble Vitamins

Deficiencies of fat-soluble vitamins in the CF population have been demonstrated in many studies [87,89,110,111,113−120]. Vitamins A and E are of the greatest concern, particularly in patients with severe malabsorption or liver disease. However, studies show that deficiencies in vitamin D or vitamin K are also common, especially in CF patients with advanced cholestatic liver disease. Abnormalities in fat-soluble vitamins are particularly prevalent in newly diagnosed infants with CF. Studies of infants diagnosed through NBS showed that 20−40% had low serum retinol, 35% had low serum 25-hydoxyvitamin D, and 40−70% had low serum α-tocopherol [88,89,113].

Vitamin A deficiency was the first micronutrient deficit demonstrated in patients with CF. Clinical symptoms of vitamin A deficiency reported in CF patients include keratinizing metaplasia of the bronchial epithelium, xerophthalmia, and night blindness. Pancreatic lipase is required to digest retinyl esters prior to absorption. Other mechanisms for vitamin A deficiency in CF have been proposed, ranging from a defect in the mobilizing hepatic storage of vitamin A due to liver disease to low levels of retinol binding protein, which is responsible for transporting vitamin A in the circulation [113,114].

Vitamin E deficiency in CF is most commonly evidenced by low plasma levels of α-tocopherol and has been associated with hemolytic anemia [115]. Low α-tocopherol levels are prevalent in infants with CF identified with NBS programs [88,113]. Those with early, prolonged severe deficiency may also show cognitive dysfunction [56].

Evidence also indicates that vitamin D deficiency is prevalent in both children and adults with CF [117–119]. Suboptimal vitamin D status has been directly linked to poor bone mineralization in CF patients, although the cause of CF bone disease is multifactorial and not completely understood [117].

Vitamin K deficiency has not been routinely demonstrated in patients with CF. However, vitamin K deficiency is likely to develop in CF patients with severe cholestatic liver disease, short bowel syndrome, and lung disease requiring frequent antibiotic use [120–122]. Low levels of vitamin K are also seen in patients with CF not taking appropriate vitamin supplementation. Vitamin k status can be evaluated by prothrombin time or the more sensitive PIVKA (proteins inducted in vitamin K absence) measurement.

4 Minerals

Minerals of concern in CF include sodium, calcium, and phosphorus. Sodium is of concern in CF patients because of its abnormally high content in the sweat. Salt depletion can be catastrophic, leading to severe hyponatremic dehydration and shock [123,124]. Therefore, sodium requirement may be considerably higher for CF patients than for normal individuals. Although routine sodium supplements may not be necessary because the average American diet contains an overabundance of sodium, sodium supplements are definitely needed in conditions that may cause prolonged sweat loss. In addition, there has been concern that marginal or low body sodium may limit the growth of children with CF [125].

Low calcium intake and suboptimal bone density accrual are of concerns even in the general pediatric population [126]. Children with CF have a higher risk of bone diseases because of poor growth and delayed puberty, malabsorption of nutrients needed for bone health (e.g., calcium and vitamins D and K), reduced physical activity, pulmonary inflammation with increased cytokines, and medication such as glucocorticoid therapy [117]. The relative contribution of these factors to the development of bone disease in patients with CF remains to be elucidated. Few data are available regarding calcium supplementation for improving bone health in the CF population. A double-blind, crossover, randomized trial with 15 CF children aged 7–13 years showed that supplementation with calcium (1000 mg), vitamin D_3 (2000 IU), or both for 6 months did not change serum calcium and 25-hydroxy-D

concentrations and bone mineral gain compared to the placebo (400 IU of vitamin D_3) group [127].

Stable isotope studies have reported increased fecal zinc losses and decreased zinc absorption in infants and children with CF [128,129]. Zinc deficiency affects growth and vitamin A status but is difficult to identify because serum zinc is not an adequate measure for zinc status. Therefore, current CF foundation guidelines recommend a trial of zinc supplementation, 1 mg/kg/day elemental zinc for 6 month, for CF children experiencing poor growth despite adequate caloric intake and pancreatic enzyme supplementation [80,112].

Anemia in CF has been reported with varying prevalence as high as 33%, with iron deficiency proposed to be the main cause [130]. Chronic lung inflammation may also alter iron metabolism. CF patients with advanced pulmonary disease have been shown to have low serum ferritin levels [130,131]. The importance of diagnosis and prevention of iron deficiency in the general pediatric population has been emphasized based on newer evidence showing the adverse, long-term, and irreversible effect on neurodevelopment and behavior caused by iron deficiency [132]. In children with CF, chronic lung inflammation poses additional risk for iron deficiency and anemia. In patients with CF, serum transferrin receptor is a more sensitive indicator of iron status than serum ferritin because the latter is an acute phase reactant to inflammation, which may be artificially elevated in the presence of lung disease.

III NUTRITION ASSESSMENT

Frequent monitoring of the nutritional status of patients with CF is essential to ensure early detection of any deterioration and prompt initiation of nutrition intervention. Patients with CF are most vulnerable to experience malnutrition due to delayed diagnosis, during times of rapid growth (e.g., infancy and adolescence), and during pulmonary exacerbations. During these periods, close monitoring and intervention are critical to prevent nutritional decline. It should be emphasized that with comprehensive nutrition assessment and intervention, children with CF who are diagnosed early through NBS can achieve normal growth throughout childhood [38,39], and adults with CF can maintain normal weight status. In addition, optimizing growth and nutritional status is critical for CF patients because malnutrition worsens lung disease, affects quality of life, and reduces survival [92,133].

Assessment of nutritional status for patients with CF must include anthropometric, biochemical, clinical, and dietary assessments. The frequencies of measurement for the different indices of nutritional status monitoring are given in Table 42.2.

TABLE 42.2 Nutritional Assessment and Monitoring in CF

Age at visit	At diagnosis	Early infancy (0–6 months)						Late infancy (7–12 months)			Second year of life		Age 2–20 years		Age 20 + years	
	1 month	2 months	3 months	4 months	5 months	6 months	8 months	10 months	12 months	Every 2–3 months	24 months	Every 3 months	Annually	Every 3 months	Annually	
Anthropometric assessment																
Weight, length/height	x	x	x	x	x	x	x	x	x	x	x	x	x		x	
Head circumference (up to age 3 years)	x	x	x	x	x	x	x	x	x	x	x	x	x			
Body mass index (ages >2 years)										x	x	x	x		x	
Skinfold measures														x		
Pubertal status (Tanner stages)														x[a]		
Biochemical assessment																
Complete blood count			x[b]							x		x		x		
Albumin			x[b]							x		x		x		
Essential fatty acids (EFA)[c]			x[b]							x		x				
Vitamin A, D, and E, iron[d]			x[b]							x		x		x		
Vitamin K,[e] zinc,[f] and sodium[g]																
Calcium and bone status[h]																
Clinical assessment																
Pancreatic functional status[i]	x															
Dietary assessment																
Energy and nutrient intake[j]	x		x	x	x	x	x	x	x	x	x	x	x			
Feeding/eating behavior					x					x				x		

[a]Starting at age 9 years for girls and 10 years for boys until sexual maturation completes; annual pubertal self-assessment (patients, or parent and patient) or physician assessment using Tanner stage system [172,173]; annual question as to menarchal status for girls.

[b]At one of the visits between 1 and 3 months.

[c]The 2002 guidelines recommended checking EFA status in children with failure to thrive [80]. Based on abundant literature (see text) and recent findings [106], we recommend routine monitoring of EFA status at ages 2–4 months, 1 year, and 2 years.

[d]Consider checking serum transferrin receptor levels for iron status.

[e]In patients with liver disease or if patient has hemoptysis or hematemesis [80]; recommended tests include PIVKA-II (preferred) or prothrombin time.

[f]In children with poor growth despite adequate caloric intake and pancreatic enzyme replacement therapy [80,112]; no recommended test because serum zinc does not reflect zinc sufficiency. Instead, a trial of zinc supplementation should be given (see text).

[g]In patients exposed to heat stress and who become dehydrated; recommended tests include serum sodium and spot urine sodium [80].

[h]In patients older than 8 years of age if risk factors are present (see text); recommended tests include serum calcium, phosphorus, ionized PTH, and DEXA.

[i]Recheck a measure of pancreatic function if PS patients have weight loss or gastrointestinal symptoms.

[j]A review of enzymes, vitamins, minerals, oral or enteral formulas, and herbal, botanical, and other complementary and alternative medicine.

Source: Adapted from Borowitz et al. [80], Borowitz et al. [112], and Yankaskas et al. [183].

A Anthropometric Assessment

Anthropometric assessment, with an emphasis on physical growth in children and body weight in adults, is an important component of nutritional assessment in patients with CF. For children with CF, accurate and sequential measurements of head circumference (ages 0–3 years), recumbent length (ages 0–2 years), height (ages 2–20 years), weight (ages 0–20 years), and body mass index (BMI; ages 2–20 years) should be obtained at each clinic visit using standardized techniques. For adults with CF, body weight should be measured at each clinic visit. Growth measurements should be plotted on the 2000 CDC growth charts [134] and converted to sex- and age-specific percentiles. Mid-arm circumference and triceps skinfold thickness measurements provide additional information about lean body mass and subcutaneous fat stores.

1 Evaluation of Stature

In addition to evaluating whether an individual CF patient's stature is appropriate for his or her age, it is useful to determine whether the patient is growing to his or her genetic potential. Therefore, the genetic potential for height/length for each CF patient should be determined. According to the 2005 CF foundation guidelines (Table 42.3), CF children who are below their genetic potential for stature are considered at nutritional risk [80,81]. However, the target height method to estimate genetic potential suggested by CF foundation guidelines has flaws [135] and should be used with caution.

2 Evaluation of Weight-for-Stature

The 1992 and 2002 CF consensus reports [80,136] recommend using two weight-for-stature indexes to evaluate the relative proportion of weight for stature, namely percentage of ideal body weight (%IBW) based on the Moore method [137] and BMI. However, recent studies and clinical applications demonstrated that use of the %IBW method is methodologically flawed [138–140]. Specifically, %IBW underestimates the severity of underweight in short children and overestimates it in tall children [139,140]. In adults with CF, %IBW based on the Metropolitan Life Insurance reference weights for medium/large frames overestimates the severity of underweight [139]. Consequently, use of %IBW leads to misclassification of nutritional status [139,140]. The %IBW method has additional disadvantages in that its calculation is time-consuming and there is no readily available clinical resource to track its progress over time, making longitudinal monitoring difficult [141]. The Cystic Fibrosis Foundation (CFF) recognized the drawback associated with the use of %IBW and recommended the discontinuation of its use in 2008 [81].

Guidelines for classifying nutritional status based on stature and weight-for-stature indexes are summarized in Table 42.3. The CFF made a major shift to broaden the screening of malnutrition from "nutritional failure" in the 2002 guidelines [80] to "nutritional risk" in the 2005 guidelines [81]. The new BMI indicators to identify nutritional risk—that is, <50th percentile for children, <22 for females, and <23 for males—were established based on their associations to lung function parameter forced expiratory volume in 1 second (FEV1) to replace the arbitrarily chosen 10th percentile cutoff that was recommended to define "nutritional failure" in the 2002 guidelines [80].

B Biochemical Assessment

Monitoring biochemical indices of nutritional status is essential in patients with CF [80]. Current guidelines (Table 42.2) recommend routine, annual measurements of serum protein (albumin), vitamin A (retinol), vitamin D (25-hydroxycholecalciferol), vitamin E (α-tocopherol), and iron (hemoglobin and hematocrit).

Assessment of EFA is not routinely performed but, rather, only as indicated. However, findings on the relationships between abnormal EFA status and growth in children with CF [88,89,106], particularly those with MI, warrant the consideration of routine monitoring of EFA status, at least annually, in patients with CF. Similarly, routine measurements of vitamin K, calcium, zinc, and sodium are not regarded as necessary in current guidelines [80,112] but may be needed in individual patients.

C Clinical Assessment

Clinical assessment of nutritional status in children with CF focuses on evaluation of the severity of

TABLE 42.3 Classification of Height and Weight-for-height Status in Patients with CF

	Children with CF		Adults with CF
	Stature	Weight-for-stature	Weight-for-stature
US Consensus Reports:[a]			
At risk	Stature-for-age percentile not at genetic potential	Weight-for-length <50th %tile (age 0–2) BMI <50th %tile (age 2–20)	BMI <23 (males) BMI <22 (females)
European Consensus Report:[b]			
Malnutrition	Stature <0.4 %tile or % Stature <90%	%IBW <90%[c]	BMI <18.5

[a] Adapted from Borowitz et al. [80], Stallings et al. [81] and Yankakas et al. [183]
[b] Adapted from Sinaasappel et al. [184]
[c] IBW: ideal body weight; %IBW method was discontinued by Stallings et al. [81].

maldigestion and malabsorption caused by PI. A total of 85–90% of CF patients have PI. Pancreatic functional status not only has a direct influence on nutritional status but also is a strong predictor of long-term outcome [67,142]. Data from the 1990–1995 U.S. CF patient registry demonstrated that patients with PS have an approximately 20-year longer life span than PI patients [67].

The clinical signs and symptoms of PI include abdominal discomfort (bloating, flatus, and pain), steatorrhea (frequent, malodorous, greasy stools), and the presence of MI or DIOS. Objective tests for PI include (1) duodenal measurement of pancreatic enzymes and bicarbonate, (2) 72-hour fecal fat balance study, and (3) fecal elastase-1 in spot stool samples. Among these, 72-hour fecal fat balance study has been the gold standard historically. A high-fat diet is ingested for 72 hours, and stool is collected and analyzed for fat excreted. For the most precise results, oral dye markers are used to indicate the period of high-fat ingestion, and the stool that follows the first marker, up to and including the second marker, represents the stool produced during the period of high-fat intake. In clinical practice, diet is often measured for 3 days and stool collected simultaneously. A coefficient of fat absorption—that is, (fat intake − fecal fat loss)/fat intake × 100%—is calculated. In CF, PI is defined by a coefficient of fat absorption less than 93% [80].

Because 72-hour fecal fat balance study is cumbersome and not well accepted by CF patients and care providers, measurement of fecal elastase-1 in a small stool sample has gained wide acceptance and is becoming the standard method of care in most CF centers [67]. Elastase is one of the 20+ enzymes secreted by the pancreas. It has the physical property of being stable as it transits the intestinal tract, unlike other enzymes that may be degraded by intraluminal proteases. As water is withdrawn from the intestinal contents in the colon, elastase concentrations increase, making it easy to measure in stool. This protein is stable through a wide range of pH and temperature, making it ideal to collect at home. Levels greater than 100–200 μg fecal elastase-1 per gram of stool generally indicate PS [67,143].

It is important to assess pancreatic functional status as soon as CF diagnosis is made. Approximately half of CF patients whose initial tests indicate PS become PI later [4]. Therefore, PS patients should be re-evaluated at least annually to determine if they have changed to PI, especially if genotype studies reveal mutations that are generally associated with PI. For patients diagnosed with PI, PERT and vitamin supplementation should be started. It is important to understand that although PI can be treated with PERT, it cannot be completely corrected; many patients continue to have steatorrhea when they receive PERT [144]. In addition, response to PERT varies greatly among individual patients.

D Dietary Assessment

Assessments of energy requirement and dietary intakes are important ways of determining whether the patient is at negative energy balance. Evaluation of dietary intakes is best performed by dietitians/nutritionists specializing in the care of patients with CF. For patients with good nutritional status, a 24-hour dietary recall may be used to assess dietary habits and the quality of dietary intake. However, for patients with suboptimal nutritional status, a 3-day prospective food record is the best way to obtain quantitative estimates of energy and nutrient intakes. This assessment can then be used as the basis for initiating appropriate nutrition intervention.

Assessment of energy requirement for patients with CF is best determined by estimating the basal metabolic rate, the degree of malabsorption, and the severity of pulmonary disease. For patients older than 2 years of age, current CFF guidelines [81] recommend energy intakes at 110–200% of ER for the general population [145,146] to support weight maintenance in adults and weight gain at an age-appropriate rate in children. Alternatively, the 2002 CFF guidelines [80] provide a method to calculate energy requirement for individual patients based on their pancreatic functional status and the severity of lung disease, as outlined in Table 42.4.

IV NUTRITION MANAGEMENT

Nutrition management for patients with CF varies and depends on the stage of diagnosis (newly diagnosed CF vs. routine management), patient's age (infancy, early childhood, adolescence, and adulthood), and disease severity. Nutrition management begins at the time of CF diagnosis. The first 6 months after the diagnosis of CF is a crucial period for establishing therapeutic interventions, dietary counseling, and nutritional education. Nutrition management for patients with stable CF focuses on maintaining optimal nutritional status and preventing malnutrition, and for patients experiencing malnutrition it focuses on achieving catch-up growth (for children) and weight gain (for adults). In addition, PERT and vitamin supplementation are essential for all categories of nutrition management.

The multidisciplinary CF care team should monitor growth, provide anticipatory counseling, and plan intervention strategies for each individual CF patient. Achieving and maintaining normal growth and nutritional status require management of gastrointestinal and pulmonary symptoms, dietary intakes and eating behaviors, and psychosocial and financial issues. Guidelines for nutritional management for patients with CF were established by the CFF in 1992 [136] and

TABLE 42.4   Method for Estimating Energy Requirement for CF Patients

Step 1: Estimate basal metabolic rate (BMR) by using the WHO equations[a]

	Males	Females
0–3 years	$60.9 \times \text{wt} - 54$	$61.0 \times \text{wt} - 51$
3–10 years	$22.7 \times \text{wt} + 495$	$22.5 \times \text{wt} + 499$
10–18 years	$17.5 \times \text{wt} + 651$	$12.2 \times \text{wt} + 476$
18–30 years	$15.3 \times \text{wt} + 679$	$14.7 \times \text{wt} + 496$
>30 years	$11.6 \times \text{wt} + 879$	$8.7 \times \text{wt} + 829$

Step 2: Estimate energy expenditure (EE) using the following equation

EE = BMR × (activity coefficient + disease coefficient)

Where activity coefficient = 1.3 (confine to bed)

1.5 (sedentary)

1.7 (active)

Disease coefficient = 0 (normal lung function; i.e., $FEV_1 > 80\%$)

0.2 (moderate lung disease; i.e., $FEV_1 = 40-79\%$)

0.3 (severe lung disease; i.e., $FEV_1 < 40\%$)

Step 3: Estimate total energy requirement (ER), taking into account pancreatic functional status

a. For PS patients; i.e., coefficient of fat absorption (CFA) ≥ 93%

ER = EE

b. For PI patients with a CFA < 93%

ER = EE × (0.93÷CFA)

c. For PI patients whose CFA has not been determined, use 0.85 as an approximate for CFA

ER = EE × (0.93÷0.85)

[a]*World Health Organization (1985). "Energy and Protein Requirements," WHO Tech Rep Ser, No. 724, p. 924. World Health Organization, Geneva.*
Source: *Adapted from Borowitz* et al. *[80].*

were revised in 2002 [80] and 2008 [81] to incorporate more evidence-based recommendations. Guidelines for lung disease therapy are also available in Flume *et al.* [147–149]. Guidelines for the care of infants diagnosed early through NBS were published in 2009 by Borowitz *et al.* [112]; key components of early care are summarized in Table 42.5. The core objectives of CF treatment after early diagnosis through NBS are to prevent malnutrition, control respiratory infections, and promote mucus clearance [112].

A Diagnosis and Treatment of Malabsorption

1 Diagnosis of Pancreatic Insufficiency

Exocrine pancreatic function should be assessed in the following situations: (1) at or soon after diagnosis to provide objective evaluation of pancreatic status before enzyme therapy is initiated and (2) to monitor PS patients for evidence of developing fat maldigestion,

particularly when frequent bulky bowel movements or unexplained weight loss occur. The preferred test for assessment of pancreatic functional status is fecal elastase-1, as described previously. Fecal elastase-1 level is not diagnostic by itself but aids in defining PS ($>200 \, \mu g/g$) or PI ($<100 \, \mu g/g$).

2 Pancreatic Enzyme Replacement Therapy

There is a strong association between genotype and pancreatic phenotype [27,30,150]. PERT should be started if the patient is known to have two CFTR mutations associated with PI or objective evidence of PI [112]. PERT should not be started in infants with a CFTR mutation known to be associated with PS, unless there are unequivocal signs or symptoms of malabsorption [112].

Regarding young infants diagnosed through NBS, PI is not present in some infants at the time of diagnosis but develops later in infancy or even early childhood [7].

TABLE 42.5 Important Aspects of Early Care for Newly Diagnosed Infants and Young Children with CF

Pancreatic enzyme replacement therapy (for pancreatic insufficiency)

High-calorie and high-fat diet (after human milk)

Fat-soluble vitamin supplementation (vitamins A, D, E, and K)

Salt supplements (essential to prevent fatalities)

Infection control (prevent all risky exposures)

Respiratory cultures (by vigorous oralpharyngeal technique)

Antibiotic therapy as needed (goal: eradicate pseudomonas)

Airway clearance teaching and recommendations

CF education with genetic counseling (CFTR genotype)

Lifestyle counseling (promote normal/quality life)

Source: *Adapted from Borowitz et al. [112].*

Therefore, it is important to repeat fecal elastase-1 measurement in infants who are initially PS, especially when gastrointestinal symptoms appear or poor weight gain occurs. CF children with laboratory evidence of PI should be started on PERT even in the absence of signs or symptoms of fat malabsorption.

Pancreatic enzymes are extracts of porcine origin containing amylase, proteases, and lipase. In the past, a large variety of enzyme products were available. However, many were marketed without formal testing. In 2004, the U.S. Food and Drug Administration (FDA) issued a notice requiring that manufacturers submit a new drug application for pancreatic enzyme products. As of 2010, there were three FDA-approved products. The actual activity of these enzymes varies considerably according to specific batches and the commercial manufacturer. Enzyme potency is based on the content of amylase, protease, and lipase in each capsule. However, many caregivers use lipase content to determine enzyme dosing to treat fat maldigestion. Commercial products are sold in capsules with varying lipase activity, ranging from 4200 to 24,000 lipase units/capsule.

The enteric coated forms of pancreatic enzymes vary considerably in their biochemical coating, biophysical dissolution properties, and size of microspheres or microtablets [151,152]. There are few carefully performed clinical studies comparing the different formulations, and few *in vivo* data are available that demonstrate the superiority of a single product. In fact, all currently available enzyme products fail to completely correct nutrient maldigestion in all patients with CF [153]. The reasons are multiple, are likely to vary from patient to patient, and in some cases may be due to factors unrelated to failed pancreatic digestion [154]. The enteric coating of enzyme microspheres or microtablets requires a pH > 5.2−6.0 for dissolution to occur in the proximal intestine, which may be acidic in the CF patient. Patients with CF and PI have gastric acid hypersecretion and a relative deficiency of bicarbonate secretion from the pancreaticobiliary tree. This may result in a more acidic proximal intestinal environment, which may be below the ideal optimal pH for maximal pancreatic enzyme activity and may hasten the inactivation of enzymes, especially lipase, within the small intestine. Histamine antagonists or proton pump inhibitors may be used to improve the intestinal milieu, but studies have reported mixed results [155,156]. Even if nutrient digestion is achieved, malabsorption of nutrients may occur because of thick intestinal mucus, which may affect the unstirred water layer, reducing absorption of fatty acids in the small intestinal epithelium [157]. Nevertheless, enzymes do improve nutrient digestion and absorption in CF patients, but the caregiver must be aware of the less than ideal efficacy of these products in individual patients.

a DOSING GUIDELINES

To date, no studies have been performed in infants to determine the optimal dose of PERT. Data are insufficient with regard to the association of enzyme dose to macronutrient content, coefficient of fat absorption, or growth [81]. Dosing is based on consensus recommendations established by the CFF and the FDA, pending reliable data [80,81,158]. These include 500−2500 units lipase per kilogram body weight per meal, or <10,000 units lipase per kilogram body weight per day, or <4000 units lipase per gram dietary fat per day. These guidelines were established when it was recognized that many CF centers were giving excessive doses of enzymes, which is strongly associated with a severe intestinal complication termed fibrosing colonopathy [158,159].

Response to PERT by individual patients will vary considerably, as will their required dosing schedule. Although dosing is best calculated using lipase units per gram fat ingested, it is perhaps more practical to use a dosing schedule with weight-adjusted guidelines [80,81,112]. Use of weight-adjusted guidelines, with a limit of 4000 U lipase/g fat or 2500 U lipase/kg/meal after 1 year of age, would avoid overdosing.

b ENZYME ADMINISTRATION

There are no convincing data concerning timing of enzyme dosing with meals, but for practical reasons, we recommend that enzymes be taken in two or three divided doses before and during meals [160]. Theoretically, this will result in more even mixing and gastric emptying of enzymes, although this has not been clinically proven. Enzymes are not required with simple carbohydrates (i.e., hard candy, popsicles, pop, and Jell-O) but are needed for foods containing fat, protein, and starch (rice, potatoes, etc.).

c ADJUNCTIVE THERAPY

Histamine (H_2) antagonists and proton pump inhibitors inhibit gastric acid and in some cases may improve enzyme activity either by decreasing gastric acidity, resulting in less destruction of unprotected conventional powder enzymes in the stomach, or by increasing pH in the upper intestine, allowing for more rapid dissolution of the enteric coating dissolution and optimal conditions for enzymes to catalyze nutrients. As mentioned previously, efficacy of this treatment is not clear because results in one study proved proton pump inhibitors to be helpful [155], whereas another found no benefit [156]. The CF caregiver should be cautioned that there are no safety data on the long-term use of these medications in children.

B Newly Diagnosed Infants and Young Children Up to 2 Years of Age

1 Initial Visits and Coordination with Primary Care Physician

The majority of young infants diagnosed through NBS appear to be totally healthy to the parents, and the diagnosis of CF is largely unexpected. Therefore, the psychosocial impact on the family must be carefully addressed at the initial visits [112]. Newly diagnosed infants with CF should be treated at an accredited CF center, ideally within 24−72 hours of diagnosis. At the first visit, adequate time for the family to receive comprehensive education and counseling is very important. Disbelief, anger, or anxiety about the new diagnosis is likely to be present, which affects the retention of information. Giving basic information in the clearest of terms and conveying the information in a sensitive, empathetic, and positive manner are key components of the visit. A variety of formats should be used to provide information, including verbal, written, and audiovisual.

Introduction of other CF clinicians, namely the nurse, dietitian, respiratory therapist, and social worker, should occur during the first two visits [112]. This allows key components of nutrition and airway clearance to be taught, and it facilitates the development of relationships with team members. A genetic counselor should meet with the family within 2 months of diagnosis to discuss in greater depth how mutations in the CFTR gene cause CF and the implications for other family members [112]. Equally important, the positive outlook for newly diagnosed infants should be reinforced and a sense of hope instilled.

The pivotal role that both parents and primary care provider play as part of the CF team should be emphasized during the early visits [112]. Coordination with the primary care physician is essential because families will be making numerous visits to their primary care provider and CF center during the first 2 years of life. Therefore, regular and open trilateral communications among the family, the primary care physician, and the CF center should be established. Communication between the primary care physician and the CF center is critical to ensure parents do not get conflicting messages because many CF care goals are different from those of standard pediatric care (e.g., an emphasis on the need for the CF child to be chubby versus concerns about obesity in the general pediatric population).

2 Types of Feeding

Special attention to growth and nutrition early in life is essential because it is a time of extraordinary metabolic need; healthy infants double their birth weight by 4−6 months of age and triple it by 1 year [134]. The first 6 months of life represent a unique window of opportunity to promote optimal growth, whereas poor growth during this critical period may be irreversible [37]. The CFF recommends that children reach a weight-for-length status of the 50th percentile by 2 years of age, with an emphasis on achieving this goal early in infancy [81,112]. However, optimal nutritional care to achieve this goal has not been defined.

a HUMAN MILK VERSUS FORMULA

The basic principles of infant feeding for healthy term babies apply to feeding infants with CF. However, optimal feeding (i.e., breast milk, formula, or a combination) to meet the increased nutritional requirement for infants with CF is unknown. The benefits of breast-feeding for healthy infants are widely recognized [161]. However, breast milk may be nutritionally inadequate in caloric density, protein, EFA, and sodium to meet the increased requirements of CF infants, especially for those with MI or PI, who are at greater risks of poor growth and malnutrition [7,88,89,162−165]. On the other hand, breast milk's antimicrobial constituents are likely to offer protection against respiratory infections [166−169]. The breast-feeding issue was less relevant before nationwide implementation of NBS, when CF infants were diagnosed at a median age of 8 or 9 months [170]—an age when most infants would no longer be breast-fed; now, the breast-feeding issue is of prime importance.

Breast-feeding was historically discouraged for CF infants because of concerns about protein energy malnutrition, which is manifested by hypoproteinemia, hyponatremia, edema, and anemia [7,89,162−165]. Despite these reports, a 1990 survey showed that 77% of CF centers encouraged breast-feeding, with nearly 37% of CF centers recommending exclusive breast-feeding [171]. Similar trends were confirmed by a 2004 survey [172]. The 2009 CFF infant care guidelines [112] continued its 2002 recommendation [80] to suggest breast milk as the initial type of feeding for CF infants, on the basis of surprisingly little evidence from only one U.S. [172] and two European studies [173,174]. Of utmost importance, the CFF guidelines [112] do not specify the exclusiveness or the duration of breast-feeding. Therefore, whether exclusive breast-feeding promotes optimal growth and provides respiratory benefits for CF infants remains to be elucidated. A study from Wisconsin revealed that exclusive breast-feeding for less than 2 months was associated with adequate growth and protected against *P. aeruginosa* infections during the first 2 years of life [175]. On the other hand, exclusive breast-feeding longer than 2 months was associated with attenuated growth without additional reduction in respiratory infections [175]. More studies are needed to evaluate the long-term risks on growth faltering associated with prolonged exclusive breast-feeding (i.e., whether attenuated growth persists or catch-up growth occurs after 2 years of age) and to investigate whether the respiratory infection benefit associated with breast-feeding leads to better pulmonary function later in life in children with CF.

b STANDARD FORMULA VERSUS SPECIAL FORMULA

There is limited evidence to address whether formula-fed infants with CF and PI should consume special formula (e.g., predigested formula containing protein hydrolysates and/or medium-chain triglycerides). Among the three studies conducted in the 1980s and 1990s, one reported similar nutritional status for CF infants fed hydrolyzed and those fed standard formulas [176], another showed better anthropometric measures in infants fed hydrolysates [177], and the other study found improved fat and nitrogen absorption in infants fed semi-elemental formula when PERT was not given [178]. These conflicting results led the CFF to conclude that there is insufficient evidence to recommend special formula for formula-fed infants with CF [112].

It is also unclear whether, for the purpose of sustaining normal growth or preventing growth faltering, breast milk and standard formula should be routinely fortified to increase caloric and nutrient densities for feeding infants with CF who are growing adequately. This is another urgent nutritional issue recommended by the CFF for future research [112].

c COMPLIMENTARY FOODS

Infants with CF should be introduced to solid foods at the same age as healthy children (i.e., 4−6 months of life), according to recommendations from the American Academy of Pediatrics. Nutrient- and caloric-dense foods, such as meat, that will enhance weight gain and provide a good source of iron and zinc [132] are ideal as first foods for infants with CF. Breast milk or formula should continue through the first year of life; thereafter, whole cow's milk can be used in the thriving child.

As infants are introduced to table foods, it is important that families and primary care physicians understand that most children with CF need a balanced diet that is moderately high in fat to meet their nutritional requirement, which is different from the usual nutritional education given to families with healthy children for overweight and obesity prevention. For example, families should buy whole milk for the child with CF and lower fat milk for other children. During the second year of life, children establish self-feeding skills, food preferences, and dietary habits. Dietitians caring for children with CF should inquire about feeding behaviors to promote positive interactions and to prevent negative behaviors.

3 Enzyme Dose and Administration

PERT should be given with breast milk and formulas, including elemental and medium-chain triglycerides-containing formulas and all foods. An initial dose of 2000−5000 lipase units for each 120-ml feeding is recommended [112]. As the infant grows and the volume of intake increases, adjust the dose to up to 2500 lipase units per kilogram body weight per feeding, but do not exceed a maximal daily dose of 10,000 lipase units per kilogram body weight per day [112]. Enzyme dose in relation to caloric/fat intake and weight gain should be evaluated at each visit. The goal is to prescribe enzyme doses that are sufficient but not excessive to support optimal weight gain while minimizing the risk of fibrosing colonopathy. Nevertheless, caution to avoid fibrosing colonopathy may lead to excessive conservatism in enzyme dosing, as revealed from the CFF registry data that average enzyme dose tended to be at the low end of weight-based dosing early in life.

In infants with CF, PERT should be offered before feeding, mixed with 2 or 3 ml ($^1/_2$ tsp) applesauce, and given by spoon [112]. Other strained fruit can be tried if applesauce is not taken, but parents should be encouraged to use only one type of food to avoid problems with potential food refusal if many different types of food are used as the vehicle for enzyme delivery.

After 1 year of age, children can be offered enteric-coated products mixed with one food. Swallowing of capsules is encouraged as soon as parents believe the child is ready. This varies considerably from patient to patient but occurs usually at approximately 4 or 5 years of age. If children continue to experience difficulties swallowing capsules, parents should open the capsule and sprinkle the beads in the mouth, which can then be ingested by drinking a liquid. Children should be discouraged from chewing the capsules because this will destroy the protective coating of enzymes.

4 Energy Intake and Nutrient Supplementation

Sufficient calories are critical in infants with CF, and the best indicators that energy requirement is met are maintenance of normal growth or achievement of catch-up growth. In addition to energy intake, adequate intakes of EFA and micronutrients such as zinc and sodium are needed to promote normal growth.

All infants with CF should receive standard, age-appropriate non-fat-soluble vitamins plus fat-soluble vitamins A, D, E, and K as recommended by the CFF guidelines (Table 42.6). Because of increased risk of hyponatremia, sodium supplementation is especially important in infants with CF [112], particularly in those fed human milk, which contains a very low amount of sodium. Older infants receiving solid foods are likely to have low sodium intake because baby foods contain no added salt. CF infants younger than 6 months should receive a daily dose of $1/8$ teaspoon of table salt, which should be increased to $1/4$ teaspoon for older infants aged 6–12 months [112].

C Routine Management for Patients Older Than 2 Years of Age

1 Energy Intake and Nutrient Supplementation

To obtain adequate energy intake and compensate for fat malabsorption, CF patients typically require a greater fat intake (35–40% of calories) than that normally recommended for the general population (25–35%). Fat restriction is not recommended because fat is the most energy-dense macronutrient and provides EFA. Medium-chain triglyceride supplements may be utilized as a good source of fat because they require less lipase activity, less bile salt for solubilization, and can be transported as free fatty acids through the portal system.

In CF patients, vitamin supplementation is necessary to prevent the occurrence of deficiencies. A standard, age-appropriate multivitamin supplement should be given to all CF patients. Additional supplementation with fat-soluble vitamins is needed (Table 42.6).

CF patients are at risk of hyponatremia because of salt loss through the skin. Children and adults are advised to consume a high-salt diet, especially during summer months and for those who live in hot climates.

2 Age-Specific Recommendations

a PRESCHOOL AGE (2–4 YEARS)

Children in this age group have developed self-feeding skills, food preferences, and dietary habits. Food intake and physical activity vary from day to day. For these reasons, close monitoring of dietary habits, caloric intake, and growth velocity is important. Routinely adding calories to table foods may help to maintain optimal growth at this stage. The importance of serving calorie-dense foods (e.g., whole milk rather than low-fat milk) and establishing positive mealtime interactions should be emphasized.

Studies have shown that toddlers with CF have longer mealtimes than their peers without CF but still do not meet the CFF's dietary recommendations for increased energy intake [179]. As the duration of mealtimes increases, difficult behaviors also occur more frequently [180]. Therefore, dietary counseling should include assessment of eating behaviors. One strategy to address behavioral problems is to limit mealtimes to 15 minutes for toddlers and use snack times as mini-meals. Another strategy is to teach parents alternative ways of responding to their child who eats slowly or negotiates what he or she will eat.

b SCHOOL AGE (4–10 YEARS)

Children in this age group are at risk of declining growth for various reasons. They typically participate in a variety of activities, leading to limited time for meals and snacks. They are also exposed to peer pressure and challenged to begin self-managing their disease. These may affect compliance with prescribed medications such as pancreatic enzymes and fat-soluble vitamins. In addition, acceptance and understanding by teachers and fellow students may be lacking, further stressing a child with CF. Encouraging

TABLE 42.6 Recommendations for Daily Fat-Soluble Vitamin Supplementation[a]

	Vitamin A (IU)	Vitamin E (IU)	Vitamin D (IU)	Vitamin K (mg) [b]
0–12 months	1,500	40–50	400	0.3–0.5
1–3 years	5,000	80–150	400–800	0.3–0.5
4–8 years	5,000–10,000	100–200	400–800	0.3–0.5
>8 years	10,000	200–400	400–800	0.3–0.5

[a]Currently, commercially available products do not have ideal doses for supplementation.
[b]Prothrombin time or, ideally, PIVKA-II levels should be checked in patients with liver disease, and vitamin K dose should be titrated as indicated.
Source: Adapted from Borowitz et al. [80] and Borowitz et al. [112].

children to help in meal planning and preparation may be helpful in improving food intake.

It is important to begin monitoring bone health at this age [117]. Bone health can be evaluated by history (atraumatic bone fracture), physical examination (poor growth and back pain), and radiologic and laboratory assessment. According to current guidelines [117], CF children age 8 years or older who are at risk for poor bone health (i.e., poor growth, poor lung function, history of bone fracture, delayed puberty, or chronic use of glucocorticoids) should be screened by dual-energy x-ray absorptiometry to assess their bone mass. In addition, serum calcium, phosphorus, 25-hydroxyvitamin D, and parathyroid hormone should be measured annually [117].

c ADOLESCENCE (10–18 YEARS)

This stage represents another vulnerable period of developing malnutrition because of increased nutritional requirement associated with accelerated growth, endocrine development, and high levels of physical activity. In addition, pulmonary disease often becomes more severe in this period, increasing energy requirement. This is also the age when other complications, such as CFRD, begin to occur more frequently, which further increases the risk of poor growth and malnutrition.

Puberty is often delayed in adolescents with CF; it is usually related to growth failure and poor nutritional status rather than to a primary endocrine disorder. Assessment of puberty should be performed annually at age 9 years in girls and age 10 years in boys by a standardize self-assessment or physician examination [181,182]. In addition to plotting growth on the growth charts, evaluating height and weight velocity [181] in association with Tanner stages can be very useful in identifying delayed or attenuated pubertal growth.

Nutritional counseling should be directed toward the patient rather than the parents. Teenagers may be more receptive to efforts to improve muscular strength and body image as a justification for better nutrition than to an emphasis on weight gain and improved disease status.

d ADULTHOOD

CF patients reaching adulthood are usually responsible for the entire management of their disease, as well as for the financial burden of a chronic illness [183,184]. While in college or working, adults with CF are constantly adapting to new schedules and stresses. The goal of nutrition management is to maintain optimal BMI and to prevent unintentional weight loss. Nutritional counseling must be practical and pragmatic to help adults with CF adjust to these changes. A minimum of one comprehensive evaluation per year is recommended [183]. However, more specific recommendations are needed for adult CF clinical care.

e PREGNANCY AND LACTATION

Widespread experience in recent years has demonstrated that pregnancy and lactation can be accomplished successfully by some women with CF. Pregnant women with CF should follow the guidelines from the Dietary Reference Intakes [146] for nutrient intakes. Special attention should be given to appropriate weight gain, particularly during the last trimester of pregnancy. In addition to the usual multivitamin supplementation for CF, one prenatal vitamin should be consumed daily. During lactation, marked increase in caloric intake is necessary to meet the high energy requirement during this period.

D Nutrition Intervention for Poor Growth and Malnutrition

For CF patients who are experiencing poor growth and malnutrition, nutritional intervention beyond the level of routine management is required. Nutrition support can be delivered at various levels, ranging from behavioral intervention to dietary modification, oral supplementation, and enteral or parenteral supplementation. In addition, the presence of co-morbid medical conditions that are likely to affect growth and nutritional status, such as GERD, DIOS, and CFRD, should be evaluated.

1 Behavioral Intervention

In an effort to increase dietary intakes, caregivers of young children with CF may be engaged in ineffective feeding practices such as coaxing, commanding, physical prompts, and parental feeding. Adolescents with CF may intentionally skip pancreatic enzymes in order to achieve a certain body image. An in-depth assessment of eating behavior, feeding patterns, and family interactions at mealtimes should be performed for CF patients at risk or experiencing malnutrition. If negative behaviors are present, behavioral intervention should be used in conjunction with dietary intervention to improve intake. For example, one behavioral strategy is to gradually increase calories by working on one meal at a time. Another strategy is to teach parents alternative ways of responding to their child who eats slowly or negotiates what he or she will eat. Referral for more in-depth behavioral therapy is also encouraged.

2 Dietary Intervention
a ORAL SUPPLEMENTS

For infants experiencing inadequate weight gain, increasing caloric density of the feedings is the first step. This can be achieved by fortifying breast milk or by concentrating formula. For infants who are taking solids, additional calories can be added to infant cereal with the addition of carbohydrate polymers (e.g., Polucose) and/or fats (e.g., vegetable oil, MCT oil, or Microlipids).

Dietary intervention should begin with dietary modification to increase caloric density of the diet—that is, addition of high-calorie foods to the patient's regular diet without dramatically increasing the amount of food consumed. For example, margarine or butter may be added to many foods, and half-and-half can be used in place of skim milk or water when preparing canned soup. More examples of how to maximize the caloric density of the diet are given in Table 42.7. If dietary modification is ineffective, use of energy supplement may be introduced. However, it is important to ensure that the energy supplement is not used as a substitute for normal food intake.

b ENTERAL FEEDINGS

Enteral feeding can be initiated when oral supplementation does not improve growth and nutritional status significantly. The goals of enteral feeding should be explained to the patient and family—that is, as a supportive therapy to improve quality of life and outcome—and their acceptance and commitment to this intervention should be realistically assessed.

Enteral feeding can be delivered via nasogastric tubes, gastrostomy tubes, and jejunostomy tubes. The choice of enterostomy tube and technique for its placement should be based on the expertise of the CF center. Nasogastric tubes are appropriate for short-term nutritional support in highly motivated patients. Gastrostomy tubes are more appropriate for patients who need long-term enteral nutrition. Jejunostomy tubes may be indicated in patients with severe GERD; use of predigested or elemental formula may be needed with jejunostomy feeding.

Standard enteral feeding formulas (complete protein and long-chain fat) are typically well tolerated. Calorically dense formulas (1.5–2.0 kcal/ml) are usually required to provide adequate energy. Nocturnal infusion is encouraged to promote normal eating patterns during the day. Initially, 30–50% of estimated energy requirement may be provided overnight. Pancreatic enzymes should be given with enteral feeding. However, optimal dosing regimen is unclear with overnight feeding.

3 Evaluation of Co-Morbid Medical Conditions

a SEVERE MALABSORPTION

A large number of patients with CF continue to have malabsorption despite adequate dosing with potent pancreatic enzymes [152]. Subjective symptoms such as abdominal bloating or cramps or bulky stools cannot reliably assess the severity of malabsorption [67]. Instead, objective assessment is advocated by a 72-hour fat collection (while eating a regular diet) and the prescribed dose of enzymes. If severe fat malabsorption is identified (fecal fat losses exceeding 20% of intake) and is clearly contributing to abdominal symptoms or malnutrition, the dose of enzymes could be increased up to the maximum recommended amount. Alternatively, inhibition of gastric acid secretion with a histamine antagonist or a proton pump inhibitor may raise intestinal pH and improve the efficacy of enzyme therapy. Several weeks after the adjustment to therapy has been made, the individual patient should be reassessed by a repeat 72-hour fecal fat collection.

b GASTROESOPHAGEAL REFLUX DISEASE

GERD is quite common in CF infants [185], particularly in those with respiratory disease. Drugs to suppress gastric acid may be indicated if reflux is severe.

TABLE 42.7 Maximizing Calories for Healthy Patients with CF

Adding calories to foods	High-calorie foods and snacks[a]
• Add fats such as butter, gravy, cheese, or dressings to starches, fruits, and vegetables • Use whipped cream on fruits and desserts • Makes "super" milk: ½ cup whole milk + ½ cup half-and-half • Flavor milk with syrups or powders (chocolate, strawberry, etc.) or add whole milk yogurt to milk • Add eggs to hamburger meat or casseroles (never serve raw eggs) • Use extra salad dressing; avoid low-calorie or reduced-calorie dressings • Serve gravies and cheese sauces	• Full-fat ice cream, puddings • Cookies and milk • Cheese or peanut butter crackers • Muffins or bagels with cream cheese or butter • Cheese breadsticks • Chips and dip • French fries • Whole milk yogurt • Egg salad, tuna salad, cheese or avocado slices with crackers • Trail mixes, nuts, and granola (after the age of 2 years) • Cold cuts, pizza • Fresh vegetables with salad dressing or dip

[a]*Assess age appropriateness, especially with respect to choking risk in young children, before recommending.*
Source: *Adapted from Borowitz et al. [80].*

A predigested formula offers no advantage and should only be considered for individuals who have had significant bowel resection following complicated MI [176].

c DISTAL INTESTINAL OBSTRUCTION SYNDROME

DIOS is unique to CF [186]. It is characterized by cramping abdominal pain, which may be periumbilical or in the right lower quadrant. A mass is usually palpable in the ileocecal area. It should be emphasized that simple constipation is a common problem in individuals with CF. Consequently, a careful history, abdominal examination, and abdominal x-ray are indicated when abdominal pain due to DIOS is suspected in order to distinguish it from constipation and other CF-associated complications, such as intussusception and appendiceal abscess.

DIOS is treated using several different approaches. If DIOS is severe, a balanced electrolyte solution (used for cleansing the bowel prior to colonoscopy) is very effective in relieving the subacute obstruction. Complete bowel obstruction is an absolute contraindication to the use of these solutions. Volumes of 4–8 l, delivered at 1 l/hour, are usually required for a complete clean out in children older than age 10 years. In younger children, the electrolyte solution should be administered at a rate of 10–40 ml/kg body weight/ hour for 4–6 hours until the stools no longer have any solid material. N-acetylcysteine and, in severe cases, large-volume enemas with hyperosmolar contrast agents are also used. A polyethylene glycol solution without electrolytes has been used by some practitioners to help with the management of DIOS and/or constipation in CF. Anecdotal reports suggest that this solution, a powder mixed with any choice of beverage, at doses of approximately 17–34 g once or twice per day is effective in children with CF. Most patients who have an episode of DIOS are prone to have recurrent episodes, and it is logical for these patients to maintain a bowel regimen using polyethylene glycol, although there are no published studies [185].

d CF-RELATED DIABETES

Adolescents and adults with CF and PI are at increased risk of developing CFRD. The prevalence of CFRD is reported to be between 5 and 15% in children younger than 18 years and up to 50% in adults with CF [16–19]. In many instances, patients exhibit no clear-cut signs and symptoms of diabetes. Furthermore, determination of hemoglobin A1c is not a reliable test for the diagnosis of CFRD. The diagnosis should be considered in any patient who is exhibiting weight loss or poor weight gain. In 2010, the CFF recommended annual screening for CFRD by a modified oral glucose tolerance test after the age of 10 years [18,19]. In the patient who has CFRD, high-energy meals and snacks are encouraged, but energy needs and insulin requirements must be carefully balanced. Foods high in simple sugars may be limited according to insulin needs. Multidisciplinary care and the support of an endocrinologist are essential. For individuals who have impaired glucose tolerance, close monitoring by both the CF and endocrine teams is required because these patients are at increased risk of developing CFRD.

V CONCLUSIONS

The clear associations between nutritional status and clinical outcomes in CF mandate careful nutritional assessment, management, and monitoring of all patients with CF. In recent years, with new knowledge arising from NBS research [43], there has been a shift away from the idea that malnutrition is inevitable for most CF patients toward the more optimistic view that normal nutrition and growth are possible if early diagnosis is made and aggressive nutritional monitoring and therapy are undertaken for each patient. This task is best accomplished by involving a multidisciplinary team that includes dietitians in the care and management of CF patients. In this way, the goals of normal growth and prevention of malnutrition can be attained, which will improve the prognosis and quality of life for patients with CF.

References

[1] M.R. Kosorok, W.H. Wei, P.M. Farrell, The incidence of cystic fibrosis, Stat. Med. 15 (1996) 449–462.

[2] T.F. Boat, M.J. Welsh, A.L. Beaudet, Cystic fibrosis, in: C.R. Scriver, A.L. Beaudet, W.S. Sly, D. Valle (Eds.), The metabolic basis of inherited disease, McGraw-Hill, New York, 1989, pp. 2649–2680.

[3] P.A. di Sant'Agnese, P.B. Davis, Research in cystic fibrosis, N. Engl. J. Med. 295 (1976) 481.

[4] S.M. Rowe, S. Miller, E.J. Sorscher, Mechanisms of cystic fibrosis, N. Engl. J. Med. 352 (2005) 1992–2001.

[5] D.L. Waters, S.F.A. Dorney, K.J. Gaskin, M.A. Gruca, M. O'Halloran, B. Wilcken, Pancreatic function in infants identified as having cystic fibrosis in a neonatal screening program, N. Engl. J. Med. 322 (1990) 303–308.

[6] E. Kerem, M. Corey, B. Kerem, P. Durie, L.-C. Tsui, H. Levison, Clinical and genetic comparisons of patients with cystic fibrosis, with or without meconium ileus, J. Pediatr. 114 (1989) 767–773.

[7] M.N. Bronstein, R.J. Sokol, S.H. Abman, B.A. Chatfield, K.B. Hammond, K.M. Hambidge, et al., PI, growth, and nutrition in infants identified by newborn screening as having cystic fibrosis, J. Pediatr. 120 (1992) 533–540.

[8] C.W.M. Bedrossian, S.C. Greenberg, D.B. Singer, J. Hansen, H. Rosenberg, The lung in CF: a quantitative study including prevalence of pathologic findings among different age groups, Hum. Pathol. 7 (1976) 195–204.

[9] M.L. Corey, Longitudinal studies in cystic fibrosis, in: J.M. Sturgess (Ed.), Perspectives in Cystic Fibrosis: Proceedings of the 8th International Cystic Fibrosis Congress, Canadian Cystic Fibrosis Foundation, Toronto, 1980, pp. 246−261.

[10] J.N. Katz, R.I. Horwitz, T.F. Dolan, E.D. Shapiro, Clinical features as predictors of functional status in children with cystic fibrosis, Pediatrics 108 (1986) 352−358.

[11] C.W.M. Bedrossian, S.C. Greenberg, D.B. Singer, J. Hansen, H. Rosenberg, The lung in CF: a quantitative study including prevalence of pathologic findings among different age groups, Hum. Pathol. 7 (1976) 195−204.

[12] P.M. Farrell, Z. Li, M.R. Kosorok, A. Laxova, C.G. Green, J. Collins, et al., Longitudinal evaluation of bronchopulmonary disease in children with cystic fibrosis, Pediatr. Pulmonol. 36 (2003) 230−240.

[13] D.S. Hardin, A. Moran, Diabetes mellitus in cystic fibrosis, Endocrinol. Metabol. Clin. North Am. 28 (1999) 787−800.

[14] A.D.R. Mackie, S.J. Thornton, F.P. Edenborough, Cystic fibrosis-related diabetes, Diabet. Med. 20 (2003) 425−436.

[15] Cystic Fibrosis Foundation, National Cystic Fibrosis Patient Registry Annual Data Report 2009, Cystic Fibrosis Foundation, Bethesda, MD, 2009.

[16] S. Lanng, B. Thorsteinsson, C. Lund-Andersen, J. Nerup, P.O. Schiotz, C. Koch, Diabetes mellitus in Danish cystic fibrosis patients: prevalence and late diabetic complications, Acta Paediatr. 83 (1) (1994) 72−77.

[17] M.P. Solomon, D.C. Wilson, M. Corey, D. Kalnins, J. Zielenski, L.C. Tsui, Glucose intolerance in children with cystic fibrosis, J. Pediatr. 142 (2) (2003) 128−132.

[18] T.A. Laguna, B.M. Nathan, A. Moran, Managing diabetes in cystic fibrosis, Diabetes Obes. Metab. 12 (10) (2010) 858−864.

[19] A. Moran, D. Becker, S.J. Casella, P.A. Gottlieb, M.S. Kirkman, B.C. Marshall, et al., Epidemiology, pathophysiology, and prognostic implications of cystic fibrosis-related diabetes: a technical review, Diabetes Care 33 (12) (2010) 2677−2683.

[20] R.Z. Sokol, Infertility in men with cystic fibrosis, Curr. Opin. Pulm. Med. 7 (2001) 421−426.

[21] B.S. Kerem, J.M. Rommens, J.A. Buchanan, D. Markiewicz, T.K. Cox, A. Chakravarti, et al., Identification of the cystic fibrosis gene: genetic analysis, Science 245 (1989) 1073−1080.

[22] F.S. Collins, Cystic fibrosis: molecular biology and therapeutic implications, Science 256 (1992) 29−33.

[23] L.C. Tsui, M. Buchwald, Biochemical and molecular genetics of cystic fibrosis, in: H. Harris, K. Hirschhorn (Eds.), Advances in Human Genetics, Plenum, New York, 1991, pp. 153−266.

[24] R.G. Gregg, A. Simantel, P.M. Farrell, et al., Newborn screening for cystic fibrosis in Wisconsin: comparison of biochemical and molecular methods, Pediatrics 99 (1997) 819−824.

[25] Cystic Fibrosis Genotype−Phenotype Consortium, Correlation between genotype and phenotype in patients with cystic fibrosis, N. Engl. J. Med. 329 (1993) 1308−1313.

[26] K. De Boeck, M. Wilschanski, C. Castellani, C. Taylor, H. Cuppens, J. Dodge, et al., Cystic fibrosis: terminology and diagnostic algorithms, Thorax 61 (7) (2006) 627−635.

[27] C. Castellani, H. Cuppens, M. Macek Jr., J.J. Cassiman, E. Kerem, P. Durie, et al., Consensus on the use and interpretation of cystic fibrosis mutation analysis in clinical practice, J. Cyst. Fibros. 7 (2008) 179−196.

[28] P.M. Farrell, B.J. Rosenstein, T.B. White, F.J. Accurso, C. Castellani, G.R. Cutting, et al., Cystic Fibrosis Foundation guidelines for diagnosis of cystic fibrosis in newborns through older adults: cystic Fibrosis Foundation consensus report, J. Pediatr. 153 (2008) S4−S14.

[29] D. Borowitz, R.B. Parad, J.K. Sharp, K.A. Sabadosa, K.A. Robinson, M.J. Rock, et al., Cystic Fibrosis Foundation practice guidelines for the management of infants with cystic fibrosis transmembrane conductance regulator-related metabolic syndrome during the first two years of life and beyond, J. Pediatr. 155 (2009) S106−S116.

[30] P. Kristidis, D. Bozon, M. Corey, D. Markiewicz, J. Rommens, L.C. Tsui, et al., Genetic determination of exocrine pancreatic function in cystic fibrosis, Am. J. Hum. Genet. 50 (6) (1992) 1178−1184.

[31] L.E. Gibson, R.E. Cooke, A test for the concentration of electrolytes in sweat in cystic fibrosis of the pancreas utilizing pilocarpine iontophoresis, Pediatrics 23 (1959) 545−549.

[32] M.P. Anderson, D.P. Rich, R.J. Gregory, A.E. Smith, M.J. Welsh, Generation of cAMP-activated chloride currents by expression of CFT, Science 251 (1991) 679−682.

[33] S.A. Blythe, P.M. Farrell, Advances in the diagnosis and management of cystic fibrosis, Clin. Biochem. 17 (1984) 277−283.

[34] B.J. Rosenstein, G.R. Cutting, The diagnosis of cystic fibrosis: a consensus statement, J. Pediatr. 132 (1998) 589−595.

[35] H.C. Lai, M.R. Kosorok, S.A. Sondel, S.T. Chen, S.C. FitzSimmons, C. Green, et al., Growth status in children with cystic fibrosis based on National Cystic Fibrosis Patient Registry data: evaluation of various criteria to identify malnutrition, J. Pediatr. 132 (1998) 478−485.

[36] P.M. Farrell, M.R. Kosorok, A. Laxova, et al., Nutritional benefits of neonatal screening for cystic fibrosis, N. Engl. J. Med. 337 (1997) 963−969.

[37] P.M. Farrell, M.R. Kosorok, M.J. Rock, A. Laxova, L. Zeng, H.C. Lai, the Wisconsin Cystic Fibrosis Neonatal Screening Study Group, et al., Early diagnosis of cystic fibrosis through neonatal screening prevents severe malnutrition and improves long-term growth, Pediatrics 107 (2001) 1−13.

[38] P.M. Farrell, H.J. Lai, Z. Li, M.R. Kosorok, A. Laxova, C.G. Green, et al., Evidence on improved outcomes with early diagnosis of cystic fibrosis through neonatal screening: enough is enough!, J. Pediatr. 147 (2005) S30−S36.

[39] J.R. Crossley, R.B. Elliot, R.A. Smith, Dried blood spot screening for cystic fibrosis in the newborn, Lancet 1 (1979) 472−474.

[40] A.F. Heely, M.E. Heely, D.N. King, J.A. Kuzemko, M.P. Walsh, Screening for cystic fibrosis by dried blood spot trypsin assay, Arch. Dis. Child. 57 (1981) 18.

[41] P.M. Farrell, E.H. Mischler, N.C. Fost, B.S. Wilfond, A. Tluczek, R.G. Gregg, et al., Current issues in neonatal screening for cystic fibrosis and implications of the CF gene discovery, Pediatr. Pulmonol. 57 (1991) 11−18.

[42] P.M. Farrell, E.H. Mischler, Newborn screening for cystic fibrosis, Adv. Pediatr. 39 (1992) 31−64.

[43] Centers for Disease Control and Prevention, Newborn screening for cystic fibrosis: evaluation of benefits and risks and recommendations for state newborn screening programs, MMWR 53 (RR-13) (2004) 1−36.

[44] M.J. Rock, G. Hoffman, R.H. Laessig, G.J. Kopish, T.J. Litshem, P.M. Farrell, Newborn screening for cystic fibrosis in Wisconsin: nine-year experience with routine trypsinogen/DNA testing, J. Pediatr. 147 (2005) S73−S77.

[45] K.B. Hammond, S.H. Abman, R.J. Sokol, F.J. Accurso, Efficacy of statewide neonatal screening for cystic fibrosis by assay of trypsinogen concentrations, N. Engl. J. Med. 325 (1991) 769−774.

[46] G. Mastella, E.G. Barlocco, B. Antonacci, G. Borgo, C. Braggion, G. Cazzola, et al., Is neonatal screening for cystic fibrosis advantageous? The answer of a wide 15 years follow-up study, Mucoviscidose: Depistage Neonatal et Prise en Charge Precoce Caen, CHRU de Caen, Caen, France, 1988, pp. 127−143.

[47] B. Wilcken, Newborn screening for cystic fibrosis: its evolution and a review of the current situation, Screening 2 (1993) 43−62.

[48] J.E. Dankert-Roelse, G.J. te Meerman, A. Martin, L.P. ten Kate, K. Knol, Survival and clinical outcome in patients with cystic

fibrosis, with or without neonatal screening, J. Pediatr. 114 (1989) 362–367.

[49] D.L. Waters, B. Wilcken, L. Irwing, P. van Asperen, C. Mellis, J.M. Simpson, et al., Clinical outcomes of newborn screening for cystic fibrosis, Arch. Dis. Child. 80 (1999) F1–F7.

[50] S. Ghosal, C.J. Taylor, M. Pickering, J. McGaw, Head growth in cystic fibrosis following early diagnosis by neonatal screening, Arch. Dis. Child. 75 (1996) 191–193.

[51] H.J. Lai, Y. Cheng, P.M. Farrell, The survival advantage of cystic fibrosis patients diagnosed through neonatal screening: evidence from the U.S. Cystic Fibrosis Patient Registry data, J. Pediatr. 147 (2005) S57–S63.

[52] J.E. Dankert-Roelse, M.E. Merelle, Review of outcomes of neonatal screening for cystic fibrosis versus non-screening in Europe, J. Pediatr. 147 (2005) S15–S21.

[53] S.D. Grosse, C.A. Boyle, J.R. Botkin, A.M. Comeau, M. Kharrazi, M. Rosenfeld, et al., Newborn screening for cystic fibrosis: evaluation of benefits and risks and recommendations for state newborn screening programs, MMWR 53 (RR-13) (2004) 1–36.

[54] Cystic Fibrosis Foundation, Clinical Practice Guidelines for Cystic Fibrosis, Cystic Fibrosis Foundation, Bethesda, MD, 1997.

[55] S.C. FitzSimmons, The changing epidemiology of cystic fibrosis, J. Pediatr. 122 (1993) 1–9.

[56] R.L. Koscik, P.M. Farrell, M.R. Kosorok, K.M. Zaremba, A. Laxova, H.C. Lai, et al., Cognitive function of children with cystic fibrosis: deleterious effect of early malnutrition, Pediatrics 113 (2004) 1549–1558.

[57] R.L. Koscik, H.J. Lai, A. Laxova, K. Zaremba, M.R. Kosorok, J.A. Douglas, et al., Preventing early, prolonged vitamin E deficiency: an opportunity for better cognitive outcomes via early diagnosis through neonatal screening, J. Pediatr. 147 (2005) S51–S56.

[58] M. Rosenfeld, Overview of published evidence on outcomes with early diagnosis from large U.S. observational studies, J. Pediatr. 147 (2005) S11–S14.

[59] R. Sharma, V.G. Florea, A.P. Bolger, Q. Doehner, N.D. Florea, A.J.S. Coats, et al., Wasting as an independent predictor of mortality in patients with cystic fibrosis, Thorax 56 (2001) 746–750.

[60] M.W. Konstan, S.M. Butler, M.E.B. Wohl, M. Stoddard, R. Matouse, J.S. Wagner, et al., Growth and nutritional indexes in early life predict pulmonary function in cystic fibrosis, J. Pediatr. 142 (2003) 624–630.

[61] B.S. Zemel, A.F. Jawad, S. FitzSimmons, V.A. Stallings, Longitudinal relationship among growth, nutritional status, and pulmonary function in children with cystic fibrosis: analysis of the Cystic Fibrosis Foundation National CF Patient Registry, J. Pediatr. 137 (2000) 374–380.

[62] P.R. Durie, P.B. Pencharz, Nutrition in cystic fibrosis, Br. Med. Bull. 48 (1992) 823–847.

[63] P.B. Pencharz, P.R. Durie, Nutritional management of cystic fibrosis, Annu. Rev. Nutr. 13 (1993) 111–136.

[64] V.A. Stallings, Nutritional deficiencies in cystic fibrosis: causes and consequences, New Insights Cystic Fibrosis 2 (1994) 1–5.

[65] P.B. Pencharz, P.R. Durie, Nutritional management of cystic fibrosis, Annu. Rev. Nutr. 13 (1993) 111–136.

[66] K.J. Gaskin, P.R. Durie, L. Lee, R. Hill, G.G. Forstner, Colipase and lipase secretion in childhood-onset pancreatic insufficiency: delineation of patients with steatorrhea secondary to relative colipase deficiency, Gastroenterology 86 (1984) 1–7.

[67] D. Borowitz, Update on the evaluation of pancreatic exocrine status in cystic fibrosis, Curr. Opin. Pulm. Med. 11 (2005) 524–527.

[68] D.C. Belli, E. Levy, P. Darling, C. Leroy, G. Lepage, Taurine improves the absorption of a fat meal in patients with cystic fibrosis, Pediatrics 80 (1987) 517–523.

[69] N. Vaisman, P.B. Pencharz, M. Corey, G.J. Canny, E. Hahn, Energy expenditure of patients with cystic fibrosis, J. Pediatr. 111 (1987) 496–500.

[70] R.M. Buchdahl, M. Cox, C. Fulleylove, J.L. Marchant, A.M. Tomkins, M.J. Brueton, et al., Increased resting energy expenditure in cystic fibrosis, J. Appl. Physiol. 64 (1988) 1810–1816.

[71] H. Anthony, J. Bines, P. Phelan, S. Paxton, Relation between dietary intake and nutritional status in cystic fibrosis, Arch. Dis. Child. 78 (1998) 443–447.

[72] J.L. Tomezsko, V.A. Stallings, D.A. Kawchak, J.E. Goin, G. Diamond, T.F. Scanlin, Energy expenditure and genotype of children with cystic fibrosis, Pediatr. Res. 35 (4 Pt 1) (1994) 451–460.

[73] P. Pencharz, R. Hill, E. Archibald, L. Levy, C. Newth, Energy needs and nutritional rehabilitation in undernourished adolescents and young adult patients with cystic fibrosis, J. Pediatr. Gastroenterol. Nutr. 3 (1984) S147–S153.

[74] R.J. Feigal, B.L. Shapiro, Mitochondrial calcium uptake and oxygen consumption in cystic fibrosis, Nature 278 (1979) 276–277.

[75] M.J. Stutts, M.R. Knowles, J.T. Gatzy, R.C. Boucher, Oxygen consumption and ouabain binding sites in cystic fibrosis nasal epithelium, Pediatr. Res. 20 (1986) 1316–1320.

[76] D. Norman, J.S. Elborn, S.M. Cordon, R.J. Rayner, M.S. Wiseman, E.J. Hiller, et al., Plasma tumour necrosis factor alpha in cystic fibrosis, Thorax 46 (1991) 91–95.

[77] J.A. Dodge, J.G. Yassa, Food intake and supplemental feeding programs, in: J.M. Sturgess (Ed.), Perspectives in Cystic Fibrosis: Proceedings of the 8th International Cystic Fibrosis Congress, Canadian cystic Fibrosis Foundation, Toronto, 1980, pp. 125–136.

[78] M. Corey, F.J. McLaughlin, M. Williams, et al., A comparison of survival, growth, and pulmonary function in patients with cystic fibrosis in Boston and Toronto, J. Clin. Epidemiol. 41 (1988) 583–591.

[79] P.B. Pencharz, Energy intakes and low-fat diets in children with cystic fibrosis, J. Pediatr. Gastroenterol. Nutr. 2 (1983) 400–402.

[80] D. Borowitz, R.D. Baker, V. Stallings, Consensus report on nutrition for pediatric patients with cystic fibrosis, J. Pediatr. Gastroenterol. Nutr. 35 (2002) 246–259.

[81] V.A. Stallings, L.J. Stark, K.A. Robinson, A.P. Feranchak, H. Quinton, Clinical Practice Guidelines on Growth and Nutrition Subcommittee, Evidence-based practice recommendations for nutrition-related management of children and adults with cystic fibrosis and pancreatic insufficiency: results of a systematic review, J. Am. Diet. Assoc. 108 (2008) 832–839.

[82] D. Bell, P. Durie, G.G. Forstner, What do children with cystic fibrosis eat? J. Paediatr. Gastroenterol. Nutr. 3 (Suppl. 1) (1984) S137–S146.

[83] R.M. Buchdahl, C. Fulleylov, J.L. Matchant, J.O. Warner, M.J. Brueton, Energy and nutrient intakes in cystic fibrosis, Arch. Dis. Child. 64 (1989) 373–378.

[84] P. Hodges, D. Sauriol, S.F. Man, A. Reichert, M. Grace, T.W. Talbot, et al., Nutrient intake of patients with cystic fibrosis, J. Am. Diet. Assoc. 84 (1984) 664–669.

[85] J.D. Lloyd-Still, A.E. Smith, H.U. Wessel, Fat intake is low in cystic fibrosis despite unrestricted dietary practices, J. Perenter. Enteral Nutr. 13 (1989) 296–298.

[86] J.L. Tomezsko, V.A. Stallings, T.F. Scanlin, Dietary intake of healthy children with cystic fibrosis compared with normal control children, Pediatrics 90 (1992) 547–553.

[87] D.A. Kawchak, H. Zhao, T.F. Scanlin, J.L. Tomezsko, A. Cnaan, V.A. Stallings, Longitudinal, prospective analysis of dietary intake in children with cystic fibrosis, J. Pediatr. 129 (1996) 119–129.

[88] H.C. Lai, M.R. Kosorok, A. Laxova, L.A. Davis, S. FitzSimmons, P.M. Farrell, Nutritional status of patients with cystic fibrosis

with meconium ileus: a comparison with patients without meconium ileus and diagnosed early through neonatal screening, Pediatrics 105 (2000) 53−61.

[89] R.J. Sokol, M.C. Reardon, F.J. Accurso, C. Stall, M. Narkewicz, S.H. Abman, et al., Fat-soluble vitamin status during the first year of life in infants with cystic fibrosis identified by screening of newborns, Am. J. Clin. Nutr. 50 (1989) 1064−1071.

[90] H. Benabdeslam, I. Garcia, G. Bellon, R. Gilly, A. Revol, Biochemical assessment of the nutritional status of cystic fibrosis patients treated with pancreatic enzyme extracts, Am. J. Clin. Nutr. 67 (1998) 912−918.

[91] M.S. Marcus, S.A. Sondel, P.M. Farrell, A. Laxova, P.M. Carey, R. Langhough, et al., Nutritional status of infants with cystic fibrosis associated with early diagnosis and intervention, Am. J. Clin. Nutr. 54 (1991) 578−585.

[92] R. Kraemer, A. Rudeberg, B. Hadorn, et al., Relative underweight in cystic fibrosis and its prognostic value, Acta Paediatr. Scand. 67 (1978) 33−37.

[93] V.L. Soutter, P. Kristidis, M.A. Gruca, et al., Chronic undernutrition/growth retardation in cystic fibrosis, Clin. Gastroenterol. 15 (1986) 137−154.

[94] H.C. Lai, M. Corey, S.C. FitzSimmons, M.R. Kosorok, P.M. Farrell, Comparison of growth status in patients with cystic fibrosis in the United States and Canada, Am. J. Clin. Nutr. 69 (1999) 531−538.

[95] Cystic Fibrosis Foundation, National Cystic Fibrosis Patient Registry Annual Data Report 2005, Cystic Fibrosis Foundation, Bethesda, MD, 2006.

[96] P.M. Farrell, E.H. Mischler, M.J. Engle, D.J. Brown, S. Lau, Fatty acid abnormalities in cystic fibrosis, Pediatr. Res. 19 (1985) 104−109.

[97] M. Roulet, P. Frascarolo, I. Rappaz, M. Pilet, Essential fatty acid deficiency in well-nourished young cystic fibrosis patients, Eur. J. Pediatr. 156 (1997) 952−956.

[98] S. Ozsoylu, Clinical importance of essential fatty acid deficiency, Eur. J. Pediatr. 157 (1998) 779.

[99] J.D. Lloyd-Still, D.M. Bibus, C.A. Powers, S.B. Johnson, R.T. Holman, Essential fatty acid deficiency and predisposition to lung disease in cystic fibrosis, Acta Paediatr. 85 (1996) 1426−1432.

[100] V.S. Hubbard, D.G. Dunn, P.A. di Sant Agnese, Abnormal fatty acid composition of plasma lipids in cystic fibrosis: a primary or secondary effect? Lancet 2 (1977) 1302−1304.

[101] B. Strandvik, Fatty acid metabolism in cystic fibrosis, N. Engl. J. Med. 350 (2004) 605−607.

[102] A. Maqbool, J.I. Schall, J.F. Garcia-Espana, B.S. Zemel, B. Strandvik, V.A. Stallings, Serum linoleic acid status as a clinical indicator of essential fatty acid status in children with cystic fibrosis, J. Perenter. Enteral Nutr. 47 (2008) 635−644.

[103] F.N. Bhura-Bandali, M. Suh, S.F.P. Man, M.T. Clandinin, The F508del mutation in the CFTR alters control of essential fatty acid utilization in epithelial cells, J. Nutr. 130 (2000) 2870−2875.

[104] B. Strandvik, E. Gronowitz, F. Enlund, T. Martinsson, J. Wahlstrom, Essential fatty acid deficiency in relation to genotype in patients with cystic fibrosis, J. Pediatr. 139 (2001) 650−655.

[105] A.W. van Egmond, M.R. Kosorok, R. Koscik, R. Laxova, P.M. Farrell, Effect of linoleic acid intake on growth of infants with cystic fibrosis, Am. J. Clin. Nutr. 63 (1996) 746−752.

[106] S.M. Shoff, H. Ahn, L.A. Davis, H.J. Lai, the Wisconsin CF Neonatal Screening Group, Temporal associations among energy intake, plasma linoleic acid, and growth improvement in response to treatment initiation after diagnosis of cystic fibrosis, Pediatrics 117 (2006) 391−400.

[107] S.D. Freedman, P.G. Blanco, M.M. Zaman, et al., Association of cystic fibrosis with abnormalities in fatty acid metabolism, N. Engl. J. Med. 350 (2004) 560−569.

[108] S. Beharry, C. Ackerley, M. Corey, G. Kent, Y.M. Heng, H. Christensen, et al., Long-term docosahexaenoic acid therapy in a congenic murine model of cystic fibrosis, Am. J. Physiol. Gastrointest. Liver Physiol. 292 (2007) G839−G848.

[109] A. Werner, M.E.J. Bongers, M.J. Bijvelds, H.R. de Jonge, H.J. Verkade, No indications for altered essential fatty acid metabolism in two murine models for cystic fibrosis, J. Lipid Res. 45 (2004) 2277−2286.

[110] C. Andersson, M.R. Al-Turkmani, J.E. Savaille, R. Alturkmani, W. Katrangi, J.E. Cluette-Brown, et al., Cell culture models demonstrate that CFTR dysfunction leads to defective fatty acid composition and metabolism, J. Lipid Res. 49 (2008) 1692−1700.

[111] M.R. Al-Turkmani, C. Andersson, R. Alturkmani, W. Katrangi, J.E. Cluette-Brown, S.D. Freedman, et al., A mechanism accounting for the low cellular level of linoleic acid in cystic fibrosis and its reversal by DHA, J. Lipid Res. 49 (2008) 1946−1954.

[112] D. Borowitz, K.A. Robinson, M. Rosenfeld, S.D. Davis, K.A. Sabadosa, S.L. Spear, et al., Cystic Fibrosis Foundation evidence-based guidelines for management of infants with cystic fibrosis, J. Pediatr. 155 (2009) S73−S93.

[113] A.P. Feranchak, M.K. Sontag, J.S. Wagener, K.B. Hammond, F.J. Accurso, R.J. Sokol, Prospective, long-term study of fat-soluble vitamin status in children with cystic fibrosis identified by newborn screen, J. Pediatr. 1355 (1999) 601−610.

[114] F. Ahmed, J. Ellis, J. Murphy, S. Wootton, A.A. Jackson, Excessive faecal losses of vitamin A (retinol) in cystic fibrosis, Arch. Dis. Child. 65 (1990) 589−593.

[115] B.S. Wilfond, P.M. Farrell, A. Laxova, E. Mischler, Severe hemolytic anemia associated with vitamin E deficiency in infants with cystic fibrosis: implications for neonatal screening, Clin. Pediatr. 33 (1994) 2−7.

[116] L. Lancellotti, C. D'Orazio, G. Mastella, G. Mazzi, U. Lippi, Deficiency of vitamins E and A in cystic fibrosis is independent of pancreatic function and current enzyme and vitamin supplementation, Eur. J. Pediatr. 155 (1996) 281−285.

[117] R.M. Aris, P.A. Merkel, L.K. Bachrach, D.S. Borowitz, M.P. Boyle, S.L. Elkin, et al., Consensus statement: guide to bone health and disease in cystic fibrosis, J. Clin. Endocrinol. Metab. 90 (2005) 1888−1896.

[118] R.J. Chavasse, J. Francis, I. Balfour-Lynn, M. Rosenthal, A. Bush, Serum vitamin D levels in children with cystic fibrosis, Pediatr. Pulmonol. 38 (2004) 119−122.

[119] A. Stepheson, M. Brotherwood, R. Robert, E. Atenafu, M. Corey, E. Tullis, Cholecalciferol significantly increases 25-hydroxyvitamin D concentrations in adults with cystic fibrosis, Am. J. Clin. Nutr. 85 (2007) 1307−1311.

[120] P.R. Durie, Vitamin K and the management of patients with cystic fibrosis, Can. Med. Assoc. J. 15 (1994) 933−936.

[121] J.H. van Hoorn, J.J. Hendriks, C. Vermeer, P.P. Forget, Vitamins K supplementation in cystic fibrosis, Arch. Dis. Child. 88 (2003) 974−975.

[122] S.P. Conway, S.P. Wolfe, K.G. Brownlee, H. White, B. Oldroyd, J.G. Truscott, et al., Vitamin K status among children with cystic fibrosis and its relationship to bone mineral density and bone turnover, Pediatrics 115 (2005) 1325−1331.

[123] A. Sojo, J. Rodriguez-Soriano, J.C. Vitoria, C. Vazquez, G. Ariceta, A. Villate, Chloride deficiency as a presentation or complication of cystic fibrosis, Eur. J. Pediatr. 153 (1994) 825−828.

[124] H.M. Corneli, C.J. Gormley, R.C. Baker, Hyponatremia and seizures presenting in the first two years of life, Pediatr. Emerg. Care 1 (1985) 190−193.

[125] U. Ozcelik, A. Gocmen, N. Kiper, T. Coskun, E. Yilmaz, M. Ozguc, Sodium chloride deficiency in cystic fibrosis patients, Eur. J. Pediatr. 153 (1994) 829–831.

[126] F.R. Greer, N.F. Krebs, the Committee on Nutrition, Optimizing bone health and calcium intakes of infants, children and adolescents, Pediatrics 117 (2006) 578–585.

[127] L.S. Hillman, J.T. Cassidy, M.F. Popescu, J.E. Hewett, J. Kyger, J.D. Robertson, Percent true calcium absorption, mineral metabolism, and bone mineralization in children with cystic fibrosis: effect of supplementation with vitamin D and calcium, Pediatr. Pulmonol. 43 (2008) 772–780.

[128] D. Easley, N. Krebs, M. Jefferson, L. Miller, J. Erskine, F. Accurso, Effect of pancreatic enzymes on zinc absorption in cystic fibrosis, J. Pediatr. Gastroenterol. Nutr. 26 (1998) 136–139.

[129] N.F. Krebs, J.E. Westcott, T.D. Arnold, B.M. Kluger, F.J. Accurso, L.V. Miller, Abnormalities in zinc homeostasis in young infants with cystic fibrosis, Pediatr. Res. 48 (2000) 256–261.

[130] A. von Drygalski, J. Biller, Anemia in cystic fibrosis: incidence, mechanisms, and association with pulmonary function and vitamin deficiency, Nutr. Clin. Prac. 23 (2008) 557–563.

[131] M.N. Pond, A.M. Morton, S.P. Conway, Functional iron deficiency in adults with cystic fibrosis, Resp. Med. 90 (1996) 409–413.

[132] R.D. Baker, F.R. Greer, the Committee on Nutrition, Clinical report: diagnosis and prevention of iron deficiency and iron-deficiency anemia in infants and young children (0–3 years of age), Pediatrics 126 (2010) 1040–1050.

[133] C.E. Milla, Association of nutritional status and pulmonary function in children with cystic fibrosis, Curr. Opin. Pulm. Med. 10 (2004) 505–509.

[134] R.J. Kuczmarski, C.L. Ogden, L.M. Grummer-Strawn, et al., CDC Growth Charts: United States. Advanced Data from Vital and Health Statistics, National Center for Health Statistics, Hyattsville, MD, 2000, No. 314

[135] Z. Zhang, S.M. Shoff, H.C.J. Lai, Incorporating genetic potential when evaluating stature in children with cystic fibrosis, J. Cystic Fibrosis 9 (2010) 135–142.

[136] B.W. Ramsey, P.M. Farrell, P. Pencharz, Nutritional assessment and management in cystic fibrosis: a consensus reportthe Consensus Committee Am. J. Clin. Nutr. 55 (1992) 108–116.

[137] D.J. Moore, P.R. Durie, G.G. Forstner, P.B. Pencharz, The assessment of nutritional status in children, Nutr. Res. 5 (1985) 797–799.

[138] Z. Zhang, H.J. Lai, Comparison of the use of body mass index percentiles and percentage of ideal body weight to screen for malnutrition in children with cystic fibrosis, Am. J. Clin. Nutr. 80 (2004) 982–991.

[139] H.J. Lai, Classification of nutritional status in cystic fibrosis, Curr. Opin. Pulm. Med. 12 (2006) 422–427.

[140] H.J. Lai, S.M. Shoff, Classification of malnutrition in cystic fibrosis: implications for evaluating and benchmarking clinical practice performance, Am. J. Clin. Nutr. 88 (2008) 161–166.

[141] V.J. Poustie, R.M. Watling, D. Ashby, R.L. Smyth, Reliability of percentage ideal weight for height, Arch. Dis. Child. 83 (2000) 183–184.

[142] K. Gaskin, D. Gurwitz, P. Durie, et al., Improved respiratory prognosis in patients with cystic fibrosis with normal fat absorption, J. Pediatr. 100 (1982) 857–862.

[143] D. Kalnins, P.R. Durie, P. Pencharz, Nutritional management of cystic fibrosis, Curr. Opin. Clin. Nutr. Metab. Care 10 (2007) 348–354.

[144] E.J. Mischler, S. Parrell, P.M. Farrell, G.B. Odell, Effectiveness of enteric coated pancreatic enzymes compared to a conventional enzymes in males with cystic fibrosis, Am. J. Dis. Child. 136 (1982) 1060–1063.

[145] National Research Council, Recommended Dietary Allowances, tenth ed, National Academy Press, Washington, DC, 1989.

[146] National Academy of Sciences, Dietary Reference Intakes for Energy, Carbohydrate, Fiber, Fat, Fatty Acids, Cholesterol, Protein, and Amino Acids (Macronutrients), National Academies Press, Washington, DC, 2002.

[147] P.A. Flume, B.P. O'Sullivan, K.A. Robinson, C.H. Goss, P.J. Mogayzel Jr., D.B. Willey-Courand, et al., Cystic fibrosis pulmonary guidelines: chronic medications for maintenance of lung health, Am. J. Respir. Crit. Care Med. 176 (2007) 957–969.

[148] P.A. Flume, K.A. Robinson, B.P. O'Sullivan, J.D. Finder, R.L. Vender, D.B. Willey-Courand, et al., Cystic fibrosis pulmonary guidelines: airway clearance therapies, Respir. Care 54 (2009) 522–537.

[149] P.A. Flume, P.J. Mogayzel Jr., K.A. Robinson, C.H. Goss, R.L. Rosenblatt, R.J. Kuhn, et al., Cystic fibrosis pulmonary guidelines: treatment of pulmonary exacerbations, Am. J. Respir. Crit. Care Med. 180 (2009) 802–808.

[150] E. Kerem, M. Corey, B.S. Kerem, J. Rommens, D. Markiewicz, H. Levison, et al., The relation between genotype and phenotype in cystic fibrosis: analysis of the most common mutation (delta F508), N. Engl. J. Med. 323 (22) (1990) 1517–1522.

[151] A. Carroccio, F. Pardo, G. Montalto, L. Japichino, G. Iacono, M. Collura, et al., Effectiveness of enteric-coated preparations on nutritional parameters in cystic fibrosis: a long-term study, Digestion 41 (4) (1988) 201–206.

[152] P. Durie, D. Kalnins, L. Ellis, Uses and abuses of enzyme therapy in cystic fibrosis, J. R. Soc. Med. 91 (Suppl. 34) (1998) 2–13.

[153] D. Kalnins, M. Corey, L. Ellis, P.R. Durie, P.B. Pencharz, Combining unprotected pancreatic enzymes with pH-sensitive enteric-coated microspheres does not improve nutrient digestion in patients with cystic fibrosis, J. Pediatr. 146 (4) (2005) 489–493.

[154] D.S. Borowitz, P.R. Durie, L.L. Clarke, S.L. Werlin, C.J. Taylor, J. Semler, et al., Gastrointestinal outcomes and confounders in cystic fibrosis, J. Pediatr. Gastroenterol. Nutr. 41 (3) (2005) 273–285.

[155] H.G. Heijerman, C.B. Lamers, W. Bakker, Omeprazole enhances the efficacy of pancreatin (pancrease) in cystic fibrosis, Ann. Intern. Med. 114 (3) (1991) 200–201.

[156] M.P. Francisco, M.H. Wagner, J.M. Sherman, D. Theriaque, E. Bowser, D.A. Novak, Ranitidine and omeprazole as adjuvant therapy to pancrelipase to improve fat absorption in patients with cystic fibrosis, J. Pediatr. Gastroenterol. Nutr. 35 (2002) 79–83.

[157] K.M. Laiho, J. Gavin, J.L. Murphy, G.J. Connett, S.A. Wootton, Maldigestion and malabsorption of ^{13}C labelled tripalmitin in gastrostomy-fed patients with cystic fibrosis, Clin. Nutr. 23 (3) (2004) 347–353.

[158] D.S. Borowitz, R.J. Grand, P.R. Durie, Use of pancreatic enzyme supplements for patients with cystic fibrosis in the context of fibrosing colonopathy: Consensus Committee, J. Pediatr. 127 (5) (1995) 681–684.

[159] S.C. FitzSimmons, G.A. Burkhart, D. Borowitz, R.J. Grand, T. Hammerstrom, P.R. Durie, et al., High-dose pancreatic-enzyme supplements and fibrosing colonopathy in children with cystic fibrosis, N. Engl. J. Med. 336 (18) (1997) 1283–1289.

[160] M.S. Brady, K. Rickard, P.L. Yu, H. Eigen, Effectiveness of enteric coated pancreatic enzymes given before meals in reducing steatorrhea in children with cystic fibrosis, J. Am. Diet. Assoc. 92 (7) (1992) 813–817.

[161] American Academy of Pediatrics, Policy statement: breastfeeding and the use of human milk, Pediatrics 115 (2005) 496–506.

[162] D.S. Fleisher, A.M. DiGeorge, L.A. Barness, D. Cornfeld, Hypoproteinemia and edema in infants with cystic fibrosis of the pancreas, J. Pediatr. 64 (1964) 341–348.

[163] P.A. Lee, D.W. Roloff, W.F. Howatt, Hypoproteinemia and anemia in infants with cystic fibrosis: a presenting symptom complex often misdiagnosed, JAMA 228 (1974) 585–588.

[164] O.H. Nielsen, B.F. Larsen, The incidence of anemia, hypoproteinemia, and edema in infants as presenting symptoms of cystic fibrosis: a retrospective survey of the frequency of this symptom complex in 130 patients with cystic fibrosis, J. Pediatr. Gastroenterol. Nutr. 1 (1982) 355–359.

[165] S. Fustik, T. Jacovska, L. Spirevska, S. Koceva, Protein-energy malnutrition as the first manifestation of cystic fibrosis in infancy, Pediatr. Int. 51 (2009) 678–683.

[166] A.L. Wright, C.J. Holberg, F.D. Martinez, W.J. Morgan, L.M. Taussig, Breast feeding and lower respiratory tract illness in the first year of life: Group Health Medical Associates, BMJ 299 (1989) 946–949.

[167] M.J. Heinig, Host defense benefits of breastfeeding for the infant: effect of breastfeeding duration and exclusivity, Pediatr. Clin. North Am. 48 (2001) 105–123.

[168] F. Ietta, R. Romagnoli, S. Liberatori, V. Pallini, L. Bini, S.A. Tripodi, et al., Presence of macrophage migration inhibitory factor in human milk: evidence in the aqueous phase and milk fat globules, Pediatr. Res. 51 (2002) 619–624.

[169] W.H. Oddy, P.D. Sly, N.H. de Klerk, L.I. Landau, G.E. Kendall, P.G. Holt, et al., Breast feeding and respiratory morbidity in infancy: a birth cohort study, Arch. Dis. Child. 88 (2003) 224–228.

[170] F.J. Accurso, M.K. Sontag, J.S. Wagener, Complications associated with symptomatic diagnosis in infants with cystic fibrosis, J. Pediatr. 147 (2005) S37–S41.

[171] E. Luder, M. Kattan, G. Tanzer-Torres, R.J. Bonforte, Current recommendations for breast-feeding in cystic fibrosis centers, Am. J. Dis. Child. 144 (1990) 1153–1156.

[172] E.M. Parker, B.P. O'Sullivan, J.C. Shea, M.M. Regan, S.D. Freedman, Survey of breast-feeding practices and outcomes in the cystic fibrosis population, Pediatr. Pulmonol. 37 (2004) 362–367.

[173] K.E. Holiday, J.R. Allen, D.L. Waters, M.A. Gruca, S.M. Thompson, K.J. Gaskin, Growth of human milk-fed and formula-fed infants with cystic fibrosis, J. Pediatr. 118 (1991) 77–79.

[174] C. Colombo, D. Costantini, L. Zazzeron, N. Faelli, M.C. Russo, D. Ghisleni, et al., Benefits of breastfeeding in cystic fibrosis: a single-centre follow-up survey, Acta Paediatr. 96 (2007) 1228–1232.

[175] S. Jadin, G.S. Wu, Z. Zhang, S.M. Shoff, B.M. Tippets, P.M. Farrell, et al., Growth and pulmonary outcomes during the first two years of life of breastfed and formula-fed infants diagnosed through the Wisconsin routine cystic fibrosis newborn screening program, Am. J. Clin. Nutr. 93 (2011) 1037–1047.

[176] L. Ellis, D. Kalnins, M. Corey, J. Brennan, P. Pencharz, P. Durie, Do infants with cystic fibrosis need a protein hydrolysate formula? A prospective, randomized comparative trial, J. Pediatr. 132 (1998) 270–276.

[177] P.M. Farrell, E.H. Mischler, S.A. Sondel, M. Palta, Predigested formula for infants with cystic fibrosis, J. Am. Diet. Assoc. 87 (1987) 1353–1356.

[178] M. Canciani, G. Mastella, Absorption of a new demielemental diet in infants with cystic fibrosis, J. Pediatr. Gastroenterol. Nutr. 4 (1985) 735–740.

[179] S.W. Powers, S.R. Patton, K.C. Byars, M.J. Mitchell, E. Jelalian, M.M. Mulvihill, Caloric intake and eating behavior in infants and toddlers with cystic fibrosis, Pediatrics 109 (2002) E75–E85.

[180] L.J. Stark, L. Opipari-Arrigan, A.L. Quittner, J. Bean, S.W. Powers, The effects of an intensive behavior and nutrition intervention compared to standard of care on weight outcomes in CF, Pediatr. Pulmonol. 46 (1) (2011) 31–35.

[181] J.M. Tanner, R.H. Whitehouse, Clinical longitudinal standards for height, weight, height velocity, weight velocity, and stages of puberty, Arch. Dis. Child. 51 (1976) 170–179.

[182] N.M. Morris, J.R. Udry, Validation of a self-administered instrument to assess stage of adolescent development, J. Youth Adol. 9 (1980) 271–280.

[183] J.R. Yankaskas, B.C. Marshall, B. Sufian, R.H. Simon, D. Rodman, Cystic fibrosis adult care: Consensus conference report, Chest 125 (2004) 1S–39S.

[184] M. Sinaasappel, M. Stern, J. Littlewood, S. Wolfe, G. Steinkamp, H.G. Heijerman, et al., Nutrition in patients with cystic fibrosis: a European consensus, J. Cystic Fibrosis 1 (2002) 51–75.

[185] R.G. Heine, B.M. Button, A. Olinsky, P.D. Phelan, A.G. Catto-Smith, Gastro-oesophageal reflux in infants under 6 months with cystic fibrosis, Arch. Dis. Child. 78 (1) (1998) 44–48.

[186] H.P. van der Doef, F.T.M. Kokke, C.K. van der Ent, R.H. Houwen, Intestinal obstruction syndromes in cystic fibrosis: meconium ileus, distal intestinal obstruction syndrome, and constipation, Curr. Gastroenterol. Rep. 13 (2011) 265–270.

BONE HEALTH AND DISEASE

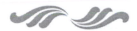

Current Understanding of Vitamin D Metabolism, Nutritional Status, and Role in Disease Prevention[1]

Susan J. Whiting[*], *Mona S. Calvo*[†]

[*]University of Saskatchewan, Saskatoon, Saskatchewan, Canada, [†]Center for Food Safety and Applied Nutrition, U.S. Food and Drug Administration, Laurel, Maryland

I INTRODUCTION

Vitamin D is a nutrient that, until recently, was neglected by the nutrition community. Although recognized in the early 20th century as an essential nutrient, recommendations for intake were often qualified as being needed only in the absence of sunlight. In theory (and in ancient times when early humans all lived closer to the equator), all vitamin D needs could be met by exposure to sunlight that provided ultraviolet (UV) B radiation, but only recently have we come to understand how UVB acts and what other factors—particularly environmental—mitigate cutaneous vitamin D synthesis. Studying vitamin D requirements is difficult. Early dietary recommendations for vitamin D, such as the 1989 Recommended Dietary Allowance [1], indicated a "relative paucity of recent controlled studies [and] . . . lack of data" on which to base requirements." It further stated that "[c]linical osteomalacia appears to be rare in the United States." What is known today, however, is that vitamin D deficiency and insufficiency are widespread [2], which was not identified when the Dietary Reference Intakes (DRIs) for vitamin D were first published in 1997 [3]. In 2011, new DRIs for vitamin D reflected the need for more dietary vitamin D [4]. Although the 2011 DRI report did not set recommendations based on functions other than bone

health, there remains a growing body of evidence for vitamin D's many roles in the body [5–7].

The role of vitamin D in preventing rickets was discovered early in the 19th century, but it was not until the 1970s that the sequence of steps from skin precursors to active metabolite was understood. Despite the interest generated in solving the puzzle of how vitamin D increased intestinal calcium absorption, there were several reasons why progress toward a better understanding of vitamin D requirements was not made. There were technical challenges in analyzing vitamin D and its metabolites. There was, beginning in the 1980s, a greater focus on dietary calcium as the major "bone" nutrient, leaving vitamin D with only a minor role in osteoporosis research. Finally, the important contribution of sun exposure to vitamin D status was not fully realized until recently. Indeed, dietary intake recommendations for situations of complete year-round absence of sun exposure give values that are five to eight times higher than those recommended to maintain vitamin D status only through the winter. It has been shown that globally there is a greater prevalence of chronic diseases such as cancer and immune disorders at extremes of latitudes where sun exposure for skin synthesis of vitamin D is limited [5].

Vitamin D affects people starting with fetal development and continuing to old age, functioning at both the

---

[1]**FDA Disclaimer**: The findings and conclusions presented in this chapter are those of the authors and do not necessarily represent the views or opinions of the U.S. Food and Drug Administration. Mention of trade names, product labels or food manufacturers does not constitute endorsement or recommendation for use by the United States Food and Drug Administration.

Nutrition in the Prevention and Treatment of Disease, Third Edition.
DOI: http://dx.doi.org/10.1016/B978-0-12-391884-0.00043-3

genomic and the nongenomic level in the regulation of key protein synthesis or in the intracellular metabolic pathways in virtually all tissues [5–7]. Growth, development, and maintenance of health are all affected, and in many regards, quality of life is as well. This chapter, while acknowledging vitamin D's contribution through the life span, focuses on vitamin D needs for maintenance of health and on vitamin D's specific actions in selected clinical conditions. Because research is ongoing, the reader can expect to learn enough about vitamin D's roles to be able to understand and apply the research as it unfolds.

II METABOLISM OF VITAMIN D

A Overview of Vitamin D Synthesis and Conversion to Its Active Metabolite

1 Vitamin D is a Family of Compounds

To understand vitamin D is to appreciate the functions of the numerous metabolites that arise during its metabolism. Figure 43.1 shows how vitamin D is provided, either through skin synthesis or from diet, and undergoes successive hydroxylations to form the active metabolite, 1,25-dihydroxyvitamin D. There are several natural occurring forms of vitamin D and many metabolites, and these are outlined in Table 43.1. The term "vitamin D" really represents all compounds having or potentially having the activity that we associate with the active metabolite of vitamin D. However, in nutrition we also refer to the precursor molecules provided in the diet or in supplements, which are cholecalciferol (for vitamin D_3) and ergocalciferol (for vitamin D_2), as "vitamin D." Generic use of the term "vitamin D" is a source of great confusion. In this chapter, an attempt has been made to use the exact term for each metabolite in order to prevent confusion. Table 43.1 can be used as a guide for this purpose. When vitamins D_2 and D_3 can contribute to the same function, then "vitamin D" with no subscript is used.

2 Vitamin D_3 Synthesis in Skin

In the skin, there is 7-dehydrocholesterol (also called "provitamin D_3") in the epidermis and the dermis, which reacts, when UVB radiation in the wavelength range of 280–315 nm passes through these skin layers, to form previtamin D_3. Previtamin D_3 forms rapidly; however, skin pigmentation (melanin) competes with 7-dehydrocholesterol for the UVB photons and therefore reduces the amount of UVB that can act on 7-dehydrocholesterol to form previtamin D_3. With prolonged exposure to UVB, inactive compounds are formed instead of previtamin D_3. Over a prolonged period of time, the previtamin D_3 that is formed is changed due

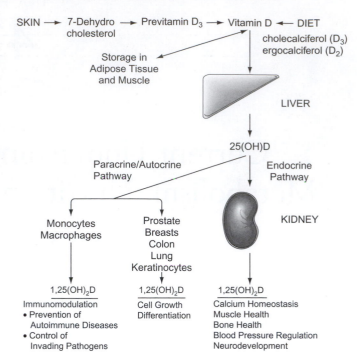

FIGURE 43.1   Overview of vitamin D metabolism, from synthesis (or provision in the diet) through to synthesis of active form. Once vitamin D_3 is made in skin, or provided from the diet (and some of this could be as vitamin D_2), it is converted in the liver to 25-hydroxyvitamin D [25(OH)D], which is the major circulating form of vitamin D. This 25(OH)D is now the substrate for production of the active form, 1,25-dihydroxyvitamin D, via two pathways. In the endocrine pathway, 1,25-dihydroxyvitamin D is made in the kidney under tight regulatory control; this 1,25-dihydroxyvitamin D circulates in the blood and acts to promote active calcium and phosphate absorption; working with parathyroid hormone, it affects bone metabolism and kidney reabsorption of calcium. In the paracrine/autocrine pathway, 1,25-dihydroxyvitamin D is made and used locally by a variety of cells, including those of the immune system. Source: *Modified from Hollis, B. W., and Wagner, C. L. (2006). Nutritional vitamin D status during pregnancy: Reasons for concern.* Can. Med. Assoc. J.*174, 1287–1290.*

to thermal isomerization to vitamin D_3 (more appropriately called "cholecalciferol" or, less commonly, "calciol"). The reaction to form previtamin D_3 takes little time, but the reaction converting previtamin D_3 to cholecalciferol takes hours to occur [7] and is a rate-limiting step. Should more UVB photons reach the epidermis and dermis, previtamin D_3 is converted to inactive compounds with no vitamin D activity (tachysterol and luminsterol). Thus, excess exposure to UVB does not result in excess vitamin D production [7].

In addition to the skin pigment melanin, other factors reduce skin synthesis of cholecalciferol, including the following: clothing (although some loosely woven clothing does permit UVB to pass through); window glass; sun screens formulated to block UVB, particularly when the sun protection factor (SPF) is higher than 8 [7]; being indoors; tall buildings creating urban

TABLE 43.1   A Glossary of Vitamin D Compounds and Metabolites

Vitamin D metabolite	Alternate name	Function	Clinical utility of measurement
"Vitamin D" (often used as synonym for vitamin D_3 or all dietary sources)	N/A	Term used to describe actions of the active metabolites of vitamins D_2 and D_3	N/A
7-Dehydrocholesterol	Provitamin D_3	Precursor to cholecalciferol found in skin; is acted upon by UVB	Not measured
Previtamin D_3	NA	Intermediate in synthesis of cholecalciferol from 7-dehydrocholesterol	Not measured
Vitamin D_3	Cholecalciferol; calciol	Form of vitamin synthesized by animals in the presence of UVB light	Provides information of recent sun exposure or ingestion of vitamin D_3
Vitamin D_2	Ergocalciferol	Form of vitamin synthesized by animals in the presence of UVB light	Provides information of ingestion of vitamin D_2
25-Hydroxyvitamin D_3 [25(OH)D_3]	25-Hydroxycholecalciferol; calcidiol	Circulating form of vitamin D_3, made from cholecalciferol	Measure of vitamin D_3 status
25-Hydroxyvitamin D_2 [25(OH)D_3]	25-Hydroxyergocalciferol	Circulating form of vitamin D_2, made from ergocalciferol	Measure of vitamin D_2 status
1,25-Dihydroxyvitamin D_3 [1,25-DHD]	1,25-Dihydroxycholecalciferol; calcitriol	Active metabolite of vitamin D_3	Measured to determine if active form can be made or to monitor treatment; not useful for vitamin D status
1,25-Dihydroxyvitamin D_2	1,25-Dihydroxyergocalciferol	Active metabolite of vitamin D_2	Measured to determine if active form can be made or to monitor treatment; not useful for vitamin D status
24,25-Dihydroxyvitamin D	24,25-Dihydroxycholecalciferol (or −ergocalciferol)	Inactive; made instead of 1,25 metabolite if 1-hydroxylase not stimulated	Not measured
1,24,25-Trihydroxyvitamin D	Calcitroic acid	Inactive; made from 1,25 metabolite as mechanism for inactivation	Not measured

canyons; cloudy days; smog and light-blocking air pollution; and winter, when the sun does not rise far enough above the horizon to allow sufficient UVB irradiation to stimulate dermal vitamin D_3 synthesis. Thus, the term "vitamin D winter" refers to the time of year when UVB radiation is not sufficient for cholecalciferol synthesis in the skin.

Latitude is the major determining factor for intensity of UVB irradiation—whether in the Southern or Northern Hemisphere. At the equator, vitamin D can be made year-round even in darker pigmented skin. Above latitude 37°, there are 4 months of vitamin D winter; at latitude 42°, there are 5 months, and close to the poles there is no time during the year when vitamin D synthesis in the skin occurs [7,8]. Yet not all analyses of vitamin D status and latitude show the expected relationship [9,10]. For example, there is now considerable vitamin D deficiency and insufficiency in people living near the equator in countries of the Middle East, southern Europe [10], and in India [11]. This suggests that many factors are determining skin synthesis so that lack of UVB (e.g., "vitamin D winter") affects some countries, whereas clothing and customs such as time spent outdoors determine vitamin D in other countries. Age is another factor decreasing skin synthesis of cholecalciferol, as described later.

3 Conversion of Cholecalciferol and Ergocalciferol to 25-Hydroxyvitamin D

The cholecalciferol made from skin synthesis is released from the epidermis into the blood, where it is bound to vitamin D binding protein. Cholecalciferol and ergocalciferol (vitamin D_2) in the diet are absorbed and carried to the liver in chylomicrons. Intestinal absorption is not a limiting factor except when there is fat malabsorption (e.g., cystic fibrosis and Crohn's disease). Generally, fat-soluble vitamins are better absorbed with dietary fat, but vitamin D_3 added to orange juice is well absorbed [12]. Cholecalciferol and ergocalciferol circulate for only 1 or 2 days. This quick turnover is due to rapid hepatic conversion and uptake by fat and muscle cells [7,13].

There are two steps leading to the active form of vitamin D, which is 1,25-dihydroxyvitamin D (see Table 43.1). The first step is converting cholecalciferol or ergocalciferol to the major circulating form. This pathway involves four hepatic cytochrome P450 enzymes (CYP2R1, CYP27A1, CYP3A4, and CYP2J3) [7] that hydroxylate cholecalciferol or ergocalciferol at carbon 25. The resulting metabolites, 25-hydroxyvitamin D_3 and 25-hydroxyvitamin D_2 (together denoted as 25(OH)D), are released into circulation. The amount of 25(OH)D that circulates is determined by the availability of its substrate, cholecalciferol or ergocalciferol [13,14]. With increasing levels of cholecalciferol made in skin or of dietary cholecalciferol and ergocalciferol, levels of 25(OH)D increase [14]. It is important to appreciate that 25(OH)D is the key metabolite indicating vitamin D status [7]. It is not the metabolically most active form, but it is the form that most accurately reflects deficiency or excess and is therefore used as a measure of vitamin D nutritional status [13].

Availability of serum 25(OH) is required for vitamin D activity. Figure 43.2 illustrates the changes in 25(OH) D over a year, demonstrating how sun exposure impacts vitamin D status in light-skinned individuals living at approximately 50° N latitude [15]. One can see the impact of "vitamin D winter" in these subjects. This figure also demonstrates how an oral supplement of cholecalciferol can maintain the summer level of 25 (OH)D through the winter months [15]. Studies indicate that whereas the molecule 25(OH)D has a half-life of 2 or 3 weeks [5], the amount in blood has an effective half-life of 2 months due to contribution from stores [16]. This means that in the absence of both sun and adequate dietary source of cholecalciferol, serum levels of 25(OH)D will decline throughout the winter months. Controversy surrounds the equivalency of the two precursors in the liver conversion to 25(OH)D, and this has been interpreted by some to reflect the inappropriateness of vitamin D_2 as a dietary supplement or food fortificant [17]. When a single dose of either vitamin D_2 or vitamin D_3 was administered, 25(OH)D_2 was shown to remain in blood for a much shorter time than a comparable dose of 25(OH)D_3, declining after 1 week [18]. Nevertheless, when equal doses (1000 IU) of vitamin D_2 or vitamin D_3 were given daily to subjects, levels of 25(OH)D rose to the same extent, suggesting that physiologic amounts of either vitamin D form work similarly [19] when used on a daily basis, as is typical of most dietary supplement use.

A study examining whether provision of the substrate for synthesis of 25(OH)D was rate limiting reported a

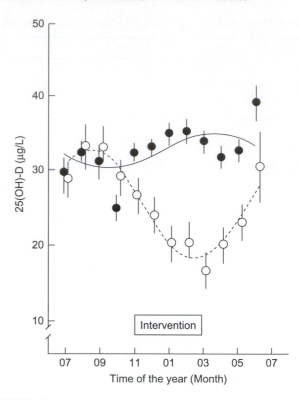

FIGURE 43.2 The data for this graph were derived from a randomized control trial conducted in Germany (latitude 50°N). Open circles represent mean levels of serum 25(OH)D of subjects throughout the year. Closed circles are mean levels of serum 25(OH) in subjects who received the treatment regimen of 12.5 μg (500 IU) cholecalciferol and 500 mg calcium. Note that the units for 25(OH)D are expressed as μg/L (to convert to nmol/l, multiply by 2.5).
Source: *Reproduced with permission from Meier, C., Woitge, H. W., Witte, K., Lemmer, B., and Seibel, M. J. (2004). Supplementation with oral vitamin D_3 and calcium during winter prevents seasonal bone loss: A randomized controlled open-label prospective trial.* J. Bone Miner. Res. **19**, 1221–1230.

wide range of substrate levels in subjects given high doses of cholecalciferol or those living in a sunny near-equatorial region [13]. As shown in Figure 43.3, high doses of cholecalciferol from supplements (as much as 6400 IU) or from sun exposure in Hawaii affected serum 25(OH)D levels similarly. The relationship is not linear, indicating a controlled, saturable reaction. Unless cholecalciferol is provided in sufficient amounts, the production of 25(OH)D is limited by its substrate.

4 Renal Conversion to the Active Metabolite: Endocrine Pathway of 1,25-Dihydroxyvitamin D Synthesis and Use

There are two pathways for conversion of 25-hydroxyvitamin D to the active form of vitamin D, which is 1,25-dihydroxyvitamin D (Figure 43.1). The first to be described is the better known and understood pathway, now referred to as the endocrine pathway. In the endocrine pathway, 1,25-dihydroxyvitamin D [1,25(OH)$_2$D] is synthesized

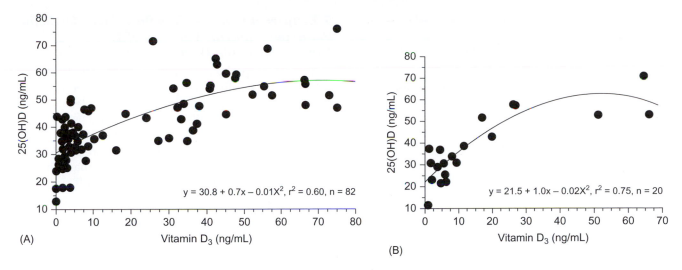

FIGURE 43.3 These graphs illustrate how either a high dose of cholecalciferol from a supplement of 150 μg (6000 IU) in panel A or sun exposure in Hawaii in panel B affect serum 25(OH)D. The authors of the study concluded that vitamin D status, as measured by serum 25(OH) D, is affected equally by diet and sun exposure. Furthermore, unless cholecalciferol is provided in sufficient amounts, the production of 25 (OH)D is limited by its substrate. Source: *Reproduced with permission from Hollis, B. W. (2007). Circulating vitamin D_3 and 25-hydroxyvitamin D in humans: An important tool to define adequate nutritional vitamin D status. J. Steroid. Biochem. Mol. Biol.* **103**, *631−634.*

in one tissue but acts elsewhere, thus fulfilling the definition of a "hormone."

In proximal renal epithelial cells, 1,25-dihydroxyvitamin D is made when the enzyme 1-α hydroxylase (also called CYP27B1) is stimulated by parathyroid hormone (which had previously been stimulated by a low circulating plasma calcium level) or by a fall in intracellular phosphate levels [7,20]. This is a tightly controlled endocrine system and considered to be the major contributor to the circulating levels of the active metabolite of vitamin D. Plasma levels of 1,25-dihydroxyvitamin D rise only when needed, as a result of synthesis in the kidney. The "need" for vitamin D action relates to its primary role (endocrine function) of providing the building blocks of bone—calcium and phosphate. A need for calcium, expressed as hypocalcemia, acts as the trigger for synthesis and release of parathyroid hormone (PTH). An increase in PTH has three actions relating to calcium metabolism: (1) increased resorption of bone in order to provide immediate calcium to the blood, (2) more efficient reabsorption of calcium in the renal tubule in order to conserve blood calcium, and (3) increased activity of the 1-hydroxylase in the proximal renal tubule to increase levels of 1,25-dihydroxyvitamin D [21]. This third action, therefore, increases the concentration of 1,25-dihydroxyvitamin D in the blood that can travel to the small intestine and promote active absorption of calcium. The increase in plasma 1,25-dihydroxyvitamin D is also a way to provide this metabolite to other cells, such as bone, parathyroid gland, and kidney, where it acts in concert with PTH to increase blood calcium levels. To complete the cycle, a rise in serum 1,25-dihydroxycholecalciferol

acts to suppress PTH secretion. This type of regulation is a classical endocrine negative feedback mechanism.

The main action of circulating 1,25-dihydroxyvitamin D is to increase calcium (and phosphate) absorption [22]. This occurs in the duodenum, in enterocytes, where active calcium (and phosphate) absorption is promoted through genomic and nongenomic actions. The genomic mechanism of action of 1,25-dihydroxyvitamin D operates through receptors in the membrane of the cell nucleus, similar to that of other steroid hormones, whereas the nongenomic receptor is thought to operate through the cell's plasma membrane receptors. In either case, there is binding to a specific receptor called the vitamin D receptor (VDR) at the cell membrane of the enterocyte. In the nucleus, this complex, along with other co-activators, binds to a vitamin D response element (VDRE) to promote transcription of specific gene products. It has been long assumed that one protein product, a calcium binding protein called calbindin 9K, was required for translocation of calcium through the enterocyte during active transport of calcium (otherwise calcium absorption is passive, via paracellular channels) [5]. However, studies of a knockout mouse having no gene for calbindin 9K showed that 1,25-dihydroxyvitamin D-mediated calcium absorption was normal in this mouse, thus leaving the exact gene products for active calcium translocation in doubt [23].

Without active absorption, the amount of calcium that can be absorbed is limited to approximately 15% of calcium intake [24]. The dependency of calcium absorption on vitamin D is illustrated in Figure 43.4.

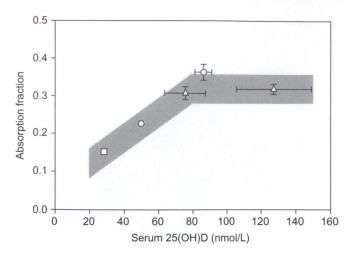

FIGURE 43.4 The dependency of calcium absorption on vitamin D status, as measured by serum 25(OH)D. Source: *Reproduced with permission from Heaney, R. P. (2007). The case for improving vitamin D status.* J. Steroid Biochem. Mol. Biol.*103*, 635–641.

When levels of 25(OH)D are low, calcium absorption proceeds by passive absorption only—that is, only 15% is absorbed. This occurs as paracellular absorption, dependent on the lumen concentration of calcium. As vitamin D status improves, as indicated by increasing 25(OH)D, calcium absorption rises and then reaches a threshold level. The data in the study described in Figure 43.4 were collected from healthy adults, and 30% absorption of calcium is all one would expect in an adult who has no urgent need for calcium. In growth and pregnancy, calcium absorption can rise to levels of 80%, but only if vitamin D status is adequate; hormones, such as growth hormone and prolactin (respectively), are important for this high absorption value [3,5].

A second important action of circulating 1,25-dihydroxyvitamin D is to promote synthesis of mature osteoclasts [7]. Here, 1,25-dihydroxyvitamin D stimulates the osteoblasts to synthesize a specific receptor ligand, known as RANKL (receptor activator of the nuclear factor kappa–B ligand; NF-κB). These osteoblasts have the VDRs, and the action of 1,25-dihydroxyvitamin D is genomic, stimulating the RANKL protein synthesis. Once the RANKL is made, it exits the osteoblast and binds to a receptor (RANK) on preosteoclasts. This binding induces maturation of the cells into osteoclasts, which function to resorb bone. The net result is release of calcium and phosphate into circulation. Thus, having been made in the kidney in response to a need for calcium or phosphate, 1,25-dihydroxyvitamin D's actions in the intestine and bone result in an increase of blood levels of both calcium and phosphorus.

5 Extrarenal Conversion to the Active Metabolite: Paracrine/Autocrine Pathway of 1,25-Dihydroxyvitamin D Synthesis and Use

The other pathway for conversion of 25(OH)D to 1,25(OH)$_2$D is called the paracrine/autocrine pathway because these terms denote that the molecule is used locally in adjacent cells or used in the same cell in which it is made, respectively (Figure 43.1). Less is known about this, but researchers found the 1-hydroxylase enzyme in many tissues other than the renal proximal tubule, and those working in cell culture systems were able to measure 1,25(OH)$_2$D production [25]. Furthermore, the vitamin D receptor has been identified in most tissues, including brain, prostate, breast, gonads, colon, pancreas, heart, monocytes, and lymphocytes. Extrarenal 1,25(OH)$_2$D production is not regulated by serum calcium, phosphate, PTH, or other hormones such as fibroblast growth factor (FGF-23) released from bone [7]. Many actions have been proposed, but the modulation of immune function through actions on lymphocytes and macrophages is the most developed and has the greatest impact on chronic disease risk.

Studies also demonstrate that cells of the immune system can produce 1,25(OH)$_2$D that acts in a paracrine manner to modulate the immune response [25–27]. For example, macrophages are an important part of the host defense against a variety of pathogenic organisms, including *Mycobacterium tuberculosis*, the etiologic agent of tuberculosis. Macrophages are activated to kill such pathogens because pattern-recognition receptors, such as toll-like receptor (TLR) 1 and TLR2, recognize molecular patterns associated with microorganisms that are not found in mammalian cells. In the case of tuberculosis, macrophages are activated via recognition of *M. tuberculosis* lipopeptides by a TLR2/1 dimer. This interaction triggers antibacterial mechanisms of the macrophage, including the production of the antibacterial peptide cathelicidin, which can kill susceptible pathogens [26]. Cathelicidin transcription is enhanced by 1,25(OH)$_2$D acting via the VDR to increase gene transcription. This TLR2/1 interaction also stimulates the expression of the 1-hydroxylase enzyme, which catalyzes 1,25(OH)$_2$D synthesis, suggesting that vitamin D deficiency may impair protection against tuberculosis by limiting 1,25(OH)$_2$D production by macrophages; however, human intervention trials are needed to test this hypothesis [26]. In addition to vitamin D stimulation of antimicrobial peptides, it functions in the modulation of pro-inflammatory and anti-inflammatory cytokines and chemokines secreted in response to bacterial endotoxins and viral and parasitic agents [25].

Vitamin D also regulates aspects of adaptive immunity. Adaptive immunity refers to the acquired immune response that develops to infections (and vaccinations). This process not only disables infectious agents but also provides "memory" that subsequently prevents a person from getting most infections a second time. T lymphocytes are an important component of adaptive immunity, acting to function as helper cells that promote antibody production by B cells. T lymphocytes (natural killer cells) also act as effector cells to kill virus-infected host cells or to promote macrophage-mediated responses, such as the one described in the previous paragraph against *M. tuberculosis*. Studies indicate that 1,25-dihydroxyvitamin D is also a modulator of the adaptive immune system, thus having a role in infectious and autoimmune disease beyond its well-characterized control of the innate immune response [25,27].

6 Mechanism of Action of the Active Metabolite

The active form of vitamin D, $1,25(OH)_2D$, whether synthesized in the kidneys and released to the circulation or originating from extrarenal 1-α-hydroxylase activity, is thought to operate through two distinctly different mechanisms: the classical genomic action and the rapid membrane-initiated action or nongenomic action [28].

A GENOMIC ACTION

The classical genomic action of $1,25(OH)_2D$ involves the binding of this steroid hormone to its nuclear receptor, which is a stereo-specific interaction. The vitamin D nuclear receptor is a member of the superfamily of steroid hormone nuclear receptors. Ligand nuclear receptor binding initiates the cell's transcriptional machinery to regulate gene transcription. In the currently accepted model of $1,25(OH)_2D$ and vitamin D receptor (VDR_{nuc}) activation of gene transcription, when the ligand or $1,25(OH)D$ binds the nuclear receptor, it forms a heterodimer with the nuclear retinoid-X receptor. This heterodimer-DNA complex then interacts with the appropriate VDRE on the promoter genes of specific target cells, which are up- or downregulated. The heterodimer-DNA complex then recruits necessary co-activator proteins to form a competent transcriptional complex capable of modulating mRNA production [28,29]. The discovery of the presence of the VDR_{nuc} in more than 30 human tissues led to our new understanding of vitamin D's role in the regulation of B and T lymphocytes of the immune system, hair follicles, muscle, adipose tissue, bone marrow, and cancer cells through the mechanism of nuclear VDR regulation of gene transcription [29].

B NONGENOMIC ACTION

A $1,25(OH)_2D$-mediated response that was observed to occur within minutes to an hour was discovered to be too rapid to be explained by nuclear VDR regulating gene transcription. Such rapid responses included secretion of insulin by pancreatic β cells; rapid migration of endothelial cells; Ca^{2+} influx in skeletal muscle cells as modulated by phospholipase C, protein kinase C, and tyrosine kinase; and activation of mitogen-activated kinase [28,29]. $1,25(OH)_2D$ can rapidly activate signal transduction pathways in addition to activating the slower classical genomic mechanism of gene transcriptional regulation [30]. Studies show that $1,25(OH)_2D$ can rapidly stimulate ion fluxes and activate protein kinases after binding to a unique receptor in the caveolae of the plasma membrane [31]. The plasma membrane receptor, termed membrane-associated rapid response steroid binding protein (MARRS), does not behave as traditional membrane spanning receptors and can be found in the endoplasmic reticulum or relocated in the nucleus [31]. Specific VDRs have been identified within the plasma membrane caveolae in a variety of different cell types, including intestine, kidney, lungs, and osteoblast-like cells [29,31,32]. As emphasized by Fleet [31], many important questions remain to be resolved concerning membrane-initiated vitamin D action. Foremost among these unknowns is the need to better understand whether rapid vitamin D actions significantly influence physiologic processes unique to certain cell types.

B Inactivation and Excretion of Vitamin D

Vitamin D metabolites turnover and are excreted. When 25(OH)D is extracted by renal cells and there is no need for increasing calcium or phosphate levels in the body, 25(OH)D is hydroxylated at carbon 24 to form 24,25-dihydroxyvitamin D. This is catalyzed by 24-hydroxylase (also called CYP24) [20,33], an enzyme located in the kidney that plays an important role in preventing unwanted buildup of 1,25-dihydroxyvitamin D by inactivating its precursor. This enzyme may also be induced in other tissues to inactivate locally produced (autocrine) 1,25-dihydroxyvitamin D, and the resulting metabolite, with a hydroxyl group at carbon 24, will be further metabolized and excreted. The metabolite formed when 1,25-dihydroxyvitamin D is hydroxylated by the 24-hydroxyase enzyme to form 1,24,25-trihydroxyvitamin D is also called calcitroic acid. This compound is the first step in the inactivation of 1,25-dihydroxyvitamin D (Table 43.1). Many other hydroxylations of vitamin D metabolites have been observed [7], but the exact roles of these compounds are not known. Similar to other steroid hormones, most vitamin D metabolites are conjugated with gluconate or sulfate and excreted into the bile.

III SOURCES OF VITAMIN D

A Food Sources of Cholecalciferol and Ergocalciferol

Vitamin D content in foods and supplements for either ergocalciferol or cholecalciferol is expressed in international units (IU) and in micrograms (μg), where $1\,\mu g = 40\,IU$. Most food and supplement sources continue to use IU as the way to express content, so this convention is presented in this chapter. There are only a few foods that naturally contain vitamin D as ergocalciferol or cholecalciferol [34] (Table 43.2). In the wild, fish are part of a food chain that allows for concentration of vitamin D in the flesh of fatty fish (e.g., salmon, sardines, and mackerel), whereas in lean fish, vitamin D is concentrated in liver (e.g., cod liver oil). With fish farming, levels of cholecalciferol in fish raised in aquaculture cannot be assumed to be equivalent to those of wild species. Furthermore, it is now recognized that levels in fish are much more variable than previously recognized [35]; therefore, caution must be taken in using data from Table 43.2. Other concerns about overconsumption of fish or fish oils include consumption of too much mercury and vitamin A. The muscle (meat) or liver of land animals that are exposed to sunlight or have vitamin D in their feed may be a source of vitamin D. Eggs are a natural source of vitamin D that can be increased when vitamin D is added to chicken feed. Currently, in the United States, there is no mandatory labeling of the vitamin D content of foods on food labels [36].

Fortification provides approximately three-fourths of the food-derived intake of vitamin D as measured in NHANES 2003–2006 [37]. Most foods are fortified with vitamin D_3 primarily added to milk, ready-to-eat cereals, and juices. Plant foods such as mushrooms, which when briefly exposed to UVB produce significant amounts of vitamin D_2[38], and some fortified plant-based foods may contain significant levels of vitamin D_2. In accord with a 2010 U.S. Food and Drug Administration regulation, soy products and other plant-based milks can be fortified with vitamin D_2 only. Such foods can appeal to vegetarians, who may prefer to consume a plant-based form of vitamin D [39].

B Supplement Sources of Vitamin D

Supplements provide another source of intake. Vitamin D (i.e., cholecalciferol or ergocalciferol) is usually (but not always) found in multivitamin preparations at 400–1000 IU per tablet. In addition to multivitamins, there are single vitamin D supplements largely available as cholecalciferol in 400, 1000, 2000, and 5000 IU dosages. Some calcium supplements contain various amounts of cholecalciferol or ergocalciferol, in the range of 200–400 IU. These supplements are intended mainly for maintenance of status and not for repletion of vitamin D deficiency. For that purpose, higher dosage forms are available through prescription, denoted in Table 43.3 as therapeutic preparations. Not shown are cod and other fish liver oil capsules; these are available over-the-counter, but their use is discouraged due to high levels of preformed vitamin A (retinol) relative to levels of vitamin D [40]. Vitamin D metabolites (primarily the active form 1,25-dihydroxyvitamin D)

TABLE 43.2 Food Sources of Vitamin D in the United States

Food	Source of vitamin D	Vitamin D_3 IU per serving
Fluid cow's milk, 250 ml (1 cup)	Fortification	100
Orange juice with added calcium and vitamin D, 125 ml ($\frac{1}{2}$ cup)	Fortification of selected brands	50
Plant-based milks such as soy or almond, 250 ml (1 cup)[a]	Fortification of selected brands	100–120 as vitamin D_2
Yogurt, 170 g[a]	Fortification of selected brands	60–200
Cheese slice, 16 g[a]	Fortification of selected brands	60
Margarine, 10 g (2 teaspoons)[a]	Fortification of selected brands	30–200
Cereals, ready-to-eat, 1 serving ($\frac{1}{2}$ to $\frac{3}{4}$ cup)	Fortification of selected brands	40–100
Salmon, canned, 85 g (3 ounces)	Naturally occurring but variable	396–649
Sun-dried shiitake mushrooms, 36 g ($\frac{1}{4}$ cup cooked)	Naturally occurring; exposed to sun (UVB)	110 as vitamin D_2
Portobello mushrooms, 85 g[a]	Irradiated with UVB	400 IU as vitamin D_2
Bread, 100 g[a]	Fortification of selected brands	74–106

[a]*New food values shown are from product labels on U.S. products as of September 30, 2011.*
Sources: *U.S. Department of Agriculture, Agricultural Research Service (2011). "National Nutrient Database." http://www.nal.usda.gov/fnic/foodcomp/search; and Johnson, M. A., and Kimlin, M. G. (2006). Vitamin D, aging, and the 2005 Dietary Guidelines for Americans. Nutr. Rev. **64**, 410–421.*

TABLE 43.3   Vitamin D and Related Compounds Found in Commonly Used Vitamin D Medications in the United States

Brand name or type of product	Related compound	Dosage forms	
Vitamin D (supplemental)[a]			
Multivitamin	Cholecalciferol	Tablet	400—1000 IU
Calcium supplement with vitamin D	Cholecalciferol	Tablet	200—400 IU per 500—600 mg calcium
Vitamin D supplement	Cholecalciferol	Tablet, drops	400, 1000, 2000, 5000 IU
Vitamin D (therapeutic)[b]			
Drisdol	Ergocalciferol	Capsule	50,000 IU
Drisdol drops	Ergocalciferol	Solution	8288 IU/ml
1,25-Dihyroxyvitamin D (calcitriol)[b]			
Calcijex	Calcitriol	Injection	1 μg/ml
Rocaltrol	Calcitriol	Capsule	0.25 and 0.5 μg
		Solution	1 μg/ml
Vertical	Calcifediol	Ointment	3 μg

[a]*Available over-the-counter in the United States.*
[b]*Requires a prescription from a physician in the United States.*
Source: *U.S. Food and Drug Administration. http://www.accessdata.fda.gov/scripts/cder/drugsatfda/index.cfm?fuseaction = Search.Search_Drug_Name. Accessed September 2011.*

are available to treat clinical conditions, and these are also listed in Table 43.3.

The biological equivalency of the two forms of vitamin D, ergocalciferol (vitamin D_2) and cholecalciferol (vitamin D_3), in humans has been challenged [17,18,41]. Both forms of dietary vitamin D are converted to their corresponding 25(OH)D form equally well. Controversy stems from studies examining the physiological response of a single large dose of ergocalciferol compared to a comparable dose of cholecalciferol [19]. The resulting level of 25 (OH)D_2 declined more rapidly than the levels of 25(OH)D_3[19]. One positive aspect of the rapid disappearance of 25(OH)D_2 is that although it may be less effective in maintaining plasma 25(OH)D levels, it is a potentially safer form of the vitamin to use in higher doses on a daily basis. Evidence of the safe use of vitamin D2 in postmenopausal women has been reported [42,43]. Reports of toxicity of vitamin D_3 supplement use have been attributed to mistakes in the formulation and manufacturing of the dietary supplements that resulted in extreme intakes exceeding 50,000 IU daily [44]. To date, normal daily use of vitamin D_3 supplements within the DRI guidelines has not resulted in vitamin D intoxication.

C Dietary Intake of Vitamin D in the U.S. Population

Vitamin D intakes of Americans became available with analysis of NHANES III data, and subsequent surveys have been analyzed for vitamin D intakes [36,37,45–47]. The most recent data, NHANES 2005–2006, are shown in Table 43.4. Data shown are mean intake from food and mean intake from food and supplements. For all age/sex groups, intake from food averaged only 144–288 IU [47], and other studies have shown that most food-derived vitamin D is from fortified foods [37,46]. Supplement use contributed to vitamin D intake, adding as little as 32 IU for males 14–18 years old to as much as 248 IU for women 51–70 years old. When considering total intakes, the mean intake of each age group did not meet the current DRI recommendation in any age group. Because many individuals are not consuming supplements, it is clear from these data [47] that the current vitamin D content of the U.S. food supply does not provide enough vitamin D for most Americans to meet the 2011 RDAs of 600 IU (800 IU for adults older than 70 years) [4].

Intakes of vitamin D by African Americans are lower than those of white Americans, which, along with skin pigmentation blocking skin synthesis of cholecalciferol, are contributing factors to their low circulating 25(OH)D [36,37]. African Americans consume lower amounts of vitamin D (Table 43.5) than the general population (Table 43.4). Much has been written to indicate a public health concern regarding the vitamin D status of African Americans [2,39,48–50]. Their low vitamin D intake is largely attributed to limited consumption of milk, milk products, and ready-to-eat breakfast cereals [36,48–50]. As described later in the chapter, vitamin D status is much lower in the African American population, which may contribute to the higher prevalence of certain diseases shown to be significantly associated with poor vitamin D status of this group.

TABLE 43.4   Estimated Mean Usual Daily Intake of Vitamin D from Food and from Food and Supplements, NHANES 2005–2006

Sex	Age group (years)	Total food intake (IU)	Total food and supplements intake (IU)
Male	1–3	288	328
Male	4–8	256	364
Male	9–13	228	300
Male	14–18	244	276
Male	19–30	204	264
Male	31–50	216	316
Male	51–70	204	352
Male	71+	224	428
Female	1–3	276	336
Female	4–8	220	316
Female	9–13	212	308
Female	14–18	152	200
Female	19–30	144	232
Female	31–50	176	308
Female	51–70	156	404
Female	71+	180	400

Source: *Bailey, R. L., Dodd, K. W., Goldman, J. A., Gahche, J. J., Dwyer, J. T., Moshfegh, A. J., Sempos, C. T., and Picciano, M. F. (2010). Estimation of total usual calcium and vitamin D intakes in the United States.* J. Nutr.**140**, *817–822.*

TABLE 43.5   Median Usual Vitamin D Intakes among African Americans Estimated from NHANES III (1988–1994)

Subjects (years)	Intake from food alone (IU)	Intake from food and supplements (IU)
Females		
6–11	192	224
12–19	140	152
20–49	112	140
≥50	132	160
Males		
6–11	220	244
12–19	188	196
20–49	148	168
≥50	136	152

Source: *Calvo, M. S., Barton, C. N., and Whiting, S. J. (2004). Vitamin D fortification in the U.S. and Canada: Current status and data needs.* Am. J. Clin. Nutr. **80**, *1710S–1716S.*

D Sun Exposure as a Source of Vitamin D

Sunlight contributes UVB and UVA radiation, but only UVB permits cholecalciferol synthesis [51]. UVB includes the wavelength range of 280–315 nm; conversion of 7-dehydrocholsterol to provitamin D_3 is optimal at 290–315 nm [5]. Exposure to sunlight can be quantified in erythemal doses—that is, the appearance of reddening of the skin. A minimal erythemal dose (1 MED) causes reddening, and further exposure results in more severe

TABLE 43.6 Reasons for Low Sun (UVB) Exposure and Inability to Synthesize Cholecalciferol

Factor	Notes
Angle of sun in winter (November–March, inclusive at latitude 45°) not sufficient UVB	No synthesis.
Being indoors and/or behind glass windows	No synthesis.
Clothing, especially head-to-toe for cultural or environmental reasons	No synthesis if fabric blocks UVB. Some cloth is loosely woven and does permit UVB to penetrate.
Darkly pigmented skin	More sun exposure time is needed than for person with little pigment.
Impairment of skin synthesis of vitamin D with age	More sun exposure time needed compared to younger person; amount made limited by substrate availability.
Sunscreen use (SPF 8 or greater)	SPF indicates amount of UV blocked: SPF blocks at 1/SPF. For example, SPF of 8 would allow 1/8 (~12%) of UV to penetrate.

Sources: Hollis, B. W. (2005). Circulating 25-hydroxyvitamin D levels indicative of vitamin D sufficiency: Implications for establishing a new effective dietary intake recommendation for vitamin D. J. Nutr. **135**, 317–322; Holick, M. F. (2006). Resurrection of vitamin D deficiency and rickets. J. Clin. Invest.**116**, 2062–2072; Holick, M. F. (2007). Vitamin D deficiency. N. Engl. J Med. **357**(3), 266–281.

sun burning. Tanning (the induction of the synthesis of the pigment melanin in the skin) also occurs but takes longer to manifest, and it occurs with UVA as well as UVB exposure [52].

Many environmental factors affect synthesis of cholecalciferol, as listed in Table 43.6. One that impacts a huge portion of the country is latitude. Because the United States stretches from 20 °N (Puerto Rico) to more than 70 °N (Alaska), it is important to recognize how latitude can impact vitamin D status. As illustrated in Figure 43.2, there is a seasonal variation in circulating 25(OH)D levels at latitudes close to 50° where presumably casual exposure to sun in the late spring, summer, and early autumn has resulted in levels of 25 (OH)D that, on average, approach 75 nmol/l, which is the level recommended by many researchers [7] as well as the Endocrine Society [53]. However, in winter, 25(OH)D levels fall to half of this level [15], presumably because dietary intake is not sufficient to provide enough vitamin D in the absence of UVB.

Studies have shown that one full body (i.e., almost completely naked) minimal erythemal dose (1 MED) will synthesize as much as 20,000 IU of vitamin D$_3$ [51]. This intensity of sun exposure is not recommended due to concerns about skin phototoxicity, and an exposure less than 1 MED will provide maximal cholecalciferol production [52]. Accordingly, one can calculate that an exposure of one-fourth of a MED to 25% of body surface is sufficient for vitamin D$_3$ production of 1000 IU [8,54]. To achieve 25% of body surface, one needs more than hands and face exposed; exposure of arms and legs is necessary, and trunk exposure is also recommended [51]. Indeed, the "rule of nines" calculation for body surface area [55] indicates that to achieve exposure of 25% of body surface area, one would have to expose both lower arms (9%) and lower legs (18%). Exposure of the head could contribute an additional

9% of surface area. The time to achieve this exposure will vary greatly by season, latitude, skin pigmentation, and use of sun-blocking lotions or cosmetics.

One can measure skin type and the resulting amount of melanin that is produced in response to UV exposure. The Fitzpatrick skin type (also called skin phototypes [52,55]) was originally developed in the United States in 1975 to facilitate UV dosage for psoriasis photochemotherapy in subjects with "white" skin, and it classified skin types into categories I–IV; it was later expanded to categories V and VI, as shown in Table 43.7 [56]. These skin types vary in ability to burn and tan. The time to burn (i.e., 1 MED) reflects melanin production and is an approximate indicator of the relative dose of UVB needed to synthesize an equivalent amount of previtamin D$_3$ [57]. As shown in Table 43.7, skin type I needs only 40% of the time for 1 MED compared to the time required for skin type III, and skin type VI needs four times the exposure time of skin type III. The times given for $\frac{1}{4}$ MED are estimates based on exposure at 42° N (i.e., Boston) at noon in summer, and they may be used to calculate the exposure time to reach a vitamin D dose of 1000 IU when 25% of body surface is exposed [8]. Other factors related to timing, such as age, have not been considered.

Thus, there is no single answer to how much sun exposure is needed to achieve and maintain an adequate vitamin D status. Some dermatologists have advocated for no sun exposure [52]; however, the World Health Organization's [58] report on solar UV radiation indicates that it is not appropriate to strive for zero sun exposure because this would create a huge burden of skeletal disease from vitamin D deficiency. However, it is important to avoid excess exposure because this has been linked with skin cancers and skin photoaging [52]. A rational scheme to achieve skin synthesis of cholecalciferol without significant risk of

TABLE 43.7   Categorization of Skin Type Using a Traditional Dermatological System (Fitzpatrick Skin Type) and Association of These Categories with Vitamin D Synthetic Capacity of Skin

Fitzpatrick skin type	Skin color	Common geographic origins	Skin response to sun exposure[a]	Relative MED[b]	Approximate time for ¼ MED[c] (minutes)
I	White; (blue eyes, freckled, albino)	Northern European	Always burn, never tan	0.38	4
II	White (blond hair, blue or green eyes)	Northern European	Burn slightly, then tan slightly	0.75	6
III	White (brown eyes, darker complexion)	Southern European, Middle East	Rarely burn, tan moderately	1.0	7
IV	White ("Mediterranean")		Never burn, tan darkly	1.3	10
V	Brown	Asian, Native American, Pacific Islander	Never burn, tan darkly; Oriental or Hispanic skin	2.0	13
VI	Black	African	Never burn, tan darkly; black skin	3.8	21

[a]*Characteristics of previously unexposed skin after 30 minutes of direct exposure to sun, from Gilcrest reference.*
[b]*Relative minimal erythemal (MED) dose of UVB exposure derived from Fitzpatrick reference.*
[c]*Time estimated for sun exposure at 10:30 a.m. on June 21 to reach ¼ MED at 11.5 °N, 29 °N, and 42.5 °N (values for 62.5 °N would be double) from Webb and Engelsen reference.*

Sources: *Gilchrest, B. A. (2007). Sun protection and vitamin D: Three dimensions of obfuscation. J. Steroid Biochem. Mol. Biol. 103, 655−663; Webb, A. R., and Engelsen, O. (2006). Calculated ultraviolet exposure levels for a healthy vitamin D status. Photochem. Photobiol.82, 1697−1703; Fitzpatrick, T. B. (1988). The validity and practicality of sun-reactive skin types I through VI. Arch. Dermatol. 124, 869−871; Holick, M. F., and Jenkins, M. (2003). "The UV Advantage." Simon & Schuster, New York.*

overexposure has been published [8]. Although this subject remains a source of considerable controversy, the public now has access to information that will allow weighing of personal risks and benefits of sun exposure. Sensible sun exposure is most important in growing children. Estimates of how much vitamin D_3 young Americans produce from their everyday outdoor UV exposure in the north (45°N) and south (35°N) for each season have been reported [59]. The resulting estimates suggest that most American children are not getting enough sun exposure to meet either minimal (~600 IU/day) or optimal (≥2000 IU/day) vitamin D requirements [59].

IV   VITAMIN D NUTRITIONAL STATUS ASSESSMENT AND RELATION TO DISEASE RISK

A   Indicators of Vitamin D Status

1   The Main Indicator of Vitamin D Status Is 25-Hydroxyvitamin D

Vitamin D status is evaluated by measuring the circulating levels of 25(OH)D, which are related to the combined contributions of diet (including supplements) and skin synthesis. Measuring cholecalciferol and ergocalciferol is technically difficult and will only provide information on recent exposure (within the past 72 hours or less) [51]. In contrast, cholecalciferol and ergocalciferol are stored in fatty tissues (adipose, liver, and muscle) and can possibly be made available for conversion to 25(OH)D when needed. However, these stores cannot maintain 25(OH)D levels during a long period of dietary or UBV deprivation [13]. There is some uncertainty regarding whether storage of cholecalciferol in adipose is available to the body. Studies show that in obese individuals, serum levels of cholecalciferol, ergocalciferol, and 25(OH)D are lower than those in non-obese [60,61]. This may relate to cholecalciferol and ergocalciferol being sequestered in adipose without an ability to be released.

Measurement of 25(OH)D provides the best assessment of vitamin D "stores"—that is, the form of vitamin D available to tissues for synthesis of 1,25-dihydroxyvitamin D by endocrine or paracrine/autocrine pathways (Figure 43.1). This is because 25(OH)D, although not the active form of vitamin D, rises with intake and/or sun exposure and declines with combined sun avoidance and low intake. Measurement of 1,25-dihydroxyvitamin D, the active vitamin D metabolite, is not the indicator of vitamin D status but, rather, a reflection, primarily, of the need for calcium and phosphate [5], as described previously. Furthermore, the amount of 1,25-dihydroxyvitamin D in blood is influenced by renal function and other dietary and hormonal factors.

2   Classification of Vitamin D Status by Serum 25 (OH)D

Until recently [7], there was a lack of understanding of tissue needs for 25(OH)D as a precursor for cellular synthesis of 1,25(OH)2D that functioned in the paracrine/autocrine pathways. Moreover, there was a lack of appreciation that vitamin D deficiency (low serum levels of 25(OH)D) may contribute to the risk of developing many chronic conditions besides rickets and osteomalacia. The cutoff level determining vitamin D deficiency was serum 25(OH)D below 30 nmol/l because below this value, the patient has or will soon experience rickets (in children) or osteomalacia (in adults) [51].

There is disagreement regarding what the normal range of 25(OH)D should be for adequate vitamin D status. Table 43.8 outlines the various cutoff points that have been used in the two most recent guidelines for vitamin D [4,53], highlighting disagreement regarding the definition of "deficient" and "insufficient." In the 2011 DRI report [4], the level of 25(OH)D that represented adequacy for almost everyone (i.e., the RDA) was defined as a serum level of 25(OH)D at or above 50 nmol/l, deemed to provide for maximal calcium absorption, minimal risk of rickets in children, reduced fracture risk in adults, and minimal risk of osteomalacia in adults. The level of 30 nmol/l was set as the cutoff for deficiency. In strong opposition to this cutoff value for sufficiency, the Endocrine Society has set sufficiency at 75 nmol/l based on suppression of PTH levels, which reflects the amount required for calcium absorption, and it defined "deficiency" at <50 nmol/l [53].

In the 2001–2006 NHANES survey data analysis for vitamin D status, a cutoff for 25(OH)D levels of <30 nmol/l was used to define risk of vitamin D deficiency, cutoffs of 30–49 nmol/l were used to define risk of inadequacy, and a cutoff of >50 nmol/l was used to define sufficient [62]. In Table 43.9, levels of 25(OH)D for age and sex groups in the United States are shown. For the total population, two-thirds were

sufficient (i.e., >50 nmol/l), one-fourth were at risk for inadequacy, and 8% were deficient. Children ages 4—8 years showed the least insufficiency. Interestingly, older adults were no worse off than younger adults. There were marked racial/ethnic differences in the distribution of 25(OH)D levels. As shown in Figure 43.5, among white Americans, only 3% were deficient, whereas 32% of black Americans were deficient; Mexican Americans were intermediate, with 12% being deficient. Prevalence of inadequacy was similarly distributed. Based on the cumulative prevalence of deficiency and inadequacy for black Americans, white Americans, and Mexican Americans, it is apparent that black and Mexican Americans have significantly higher risk for poor vitamin D status (71 and 46%, respectively) than do white Americans (20%). Because these NHANES data were collected in the northern states during sunny seasons and the southern states during winter months, these 25(OH)D data represent optimal levels of sun exposure opportunities for participants in NHANES [63]; that is, they reflect vitamin D status when conditions are optimal for sun exposure and not under conditions of decreased skin synthesis.

Levels of 25(OH)D are influenced by exposure of skin to UVB and by dietary intakes of ergocalciferol or cholecalciferol. Based on its use in many research trials as well as in dosing studies [15], it can be estimated that 40 IU (1 μg) of cholecalciferol daily raises serum 25(OH)D by 2 nmol/l at basal levels—that is, in persons having serum levels of 25(OH)D less than 50 nmol/l. After this level is reached, 40 IU (1 μg) will raise 25(OH)D levels by 1 nmol/l [64]. As described previously, sun exposure will also impact on serum levels of 25(OH)D. Effects of dietary vitamin D and skin synthesis of cholecalciferol are additive; both contribute to

TABLE 43.8 Classification of Vitamin D Status by Serum 25(OH)D and Disease Risk

Serum 25(OH)D[a]	Category
<20 nmol/l	Vitamin D deficiency
<30 nmol/l	At risk for rickets or osteomalacia
<50 nmol/l	Not at risk for clinical rickets or osteomalacia
30–75 nmol/l	Vitamin D insufficiency defined for at-risk populations with chronic conditions
≥75 nmol/l	Vitamin D adequacy for at-risk populations
250 nmol/l	Level of 25(OH)D when 10,000 IU is ingested chronically, and level where no adverse effects are detected; potential for adverse effects above this level

[a]To convert nmol/l to ng/ml, divide by 2.5.
Sources: Institute of Medicine (2011). "Dietary Reference Intakes for Calcium, Phosphorus, Magnesium, Vitamin D, and Fluoride. National Academies Press, Washington, DC; Holick, M. F., Binkley, N. C., Bischoff-Ferrari, H. A., Gordon, C. M., Hanley, D. A., Heaney, R. P., Murad, M. H., and Weaver, C. M. (2011). Evaluation, treatment, and prevention of vitamin D deficiency: An Endocrine Society clinical practice guideline. J. Clin. Endocrinol. Metab. **96**, 1911–1930.

TABLE 43.9 Median Serum Levels of 25(OH)D[a] and Prevalence of Vitamin D Insufficiency (<50 nmol/l), NHANES 2001–2006

Sex	Age group (years)	nmol/l	% <50 nmol/l
Male	1–3	69.5	—
Male	4–8	67.3	10[b]
Male	9–13	62.1	21
Male	14–18	58.5	29
Male	19–30	55.3	36
Male	31–50	57.4	31
Male	51–70	58.1	31
Male	71+	57.2	31
Female	1–3	68.3	—
Female	4–8	67.2	12[b]
Female	9–13	57.6	27
Female	14–18	57.2	34
Female	19–30	55.9	37
Female	31–50	55.3	36
Female	51–70	54.7	37
Female	71+	55.5	38

[a]To convert nmol/l to ng/ml, divide by 2.5.
[b]Values are for ages 1–8 years.
Source: Looker, A. C., Johnson, C. L., Lacher, D. A., Pfeiffer, C. M., Schleicher, R. L., and Sempos, C. T. (2011). "Vitamin D Status: United States, 2001–2006 (Corrected)," NCHS Data Brief No. 59. National Center for Health Statistics, Hyattsville, MD.

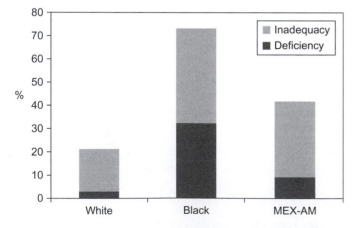

FIGURE 43.5 Age-adjusted prevalence of risk for vitamin D deficiency, defined as 25(OH)D levels < 30 nmol/l, and vitamin D inadequacy, defined as 25(OH)D between 30 and 49 nmol/l, from the National Health and Nutrition Examination Survey (NHANES) measured between 2001 and 2006. MEX-AM, Mexican Americans
Source: Looker, A. C., Johnson, C. L., Lacher, D. A., Pfeiffer, C. M., Schleicher, R. L., and Sempos, C. T. (2011). "Vitamin D Status: United States, 2001–2006," NCHS Data Brief No. 59. National Center for Health Statistics, Hyattsville, MD.

serum 25(OH)D [13]. Thus, it should be possible to predict vitamin D status in light-skinned individuals. For example, if a background of moderate sun exposure during the summer achieves a serum 25(OH)D level of 50 nmol/l, then a further 1000 IU per day of dietary cholecalciferol would be needed to reach a serum 25(OH)D level of 75 nmol/l.

Most of the studies determining dietary or solar contributions to circulating levels of 25(OH)D have been conducted in light-skinned subjects. Our current understanding of dietary intakes needed to raise serum 25(OH)D is lacking for African Americans and others with darker skin, but evidence points to significant differences that should be taken into consideration when setting dietary requirements.

3 Issues Related to 25-Hydroxyvitamin D Measurement

There are many methods for determining circulating levels of 25(OH)D. A radioimmunoassay and a competitive protein binding assay have been employed clinically. Enzyme immunoassay is now often used [65]. The accepted standard is high-performance liquid chromatography, which is not practical for general clinical use. Combination liquid chromatography—mass spectrometry is being promoted as the most accurate method, but this method has limitations: highly technical skills are required to run these assays in a clinical setting. Fortunately, all of the widely used clinical laboratory methods perform reasonably well in identifying clinically important low levels. However, all clinical laboratories performing 25(OH)D testing should take part in external quality assessment programs; particularly because some of the commercially available assays may fail to recognize and accurately measure 25(OH)D$_2$.

Measurement of blood 25(OH)D is preferably performed on fasting serum sample because lipid-rich plasma can interfere with the assay and high-fat meals should be avoided at least 12 hours before the blood draw. Otherwise, blood may be taken at any time of day because there is no observed pronounced circadian variation in serum levels. Results are reported as nanomoles per liter or nanograms per milliliter. The conversion factor between these different units is as follows: 1 ng/ml = 2.5 nmol/l.

When repleting deficient patients, one expects the serum 25(OH)D response to high-dose supplementation with cholecalciferol or ergocalciferol to reach a plateau after 3 months of continuous treatment [15]. Therefore, if a patient's response to vitamin D supplements is to be monitored by blood levels, they should be checked no sooner than 3 months after treatment has been commenced. Monitoring of routine supplementation use is not necessary, but in situations in which severe deficiency is being treated or there is reason to believe the patient may have impaired intestinal absorption, assessment of serum 25(OH)D would indicate the effectiveness of therapy.

4 Biomarkers of Vitamin Deficiency

Although it is well-established that serum 25(OH)D is the best static indicator of vitamin D status, functional indicators provide information on how the deficiency/insufficiency is impacting on the health of the person. They also confirm that a deficiency exists and may confer additional information to the diagnosis of monitoring of interventions. The most common responsive functional indicator examined to date is the suppression of secondary hyperparathyroidism, based on the endocrine function of 1,25-dihydroxyvitamin D in providing enough calcium through active intestinal absorption to suppress PTH levels that were raised with hypocalcemia [66]. Performance indicators such as the "get up and go" test vary in proportion to serum levels of 25(OH)D; they reflect muscle strength and balance, which are negatively affected in vitamin D insufficiency [67]. Pain is also associated with vitamin D deficiency, and minimal trauma fractures may also occur. These alone are not specific enough for diagnosis; however, they should be triggers to seek vitamin D testing.

B Clinical Conditions Associated with Vitamin D Deficiency and Insufficiency

1 Rickets and Osteomalacia

Vitamin D deficiency results in rickets and osteomalacia; the former term is used to describe the clinical signs observed in children, and the latter is used to describe those signs in adults. As outlined in Table 43.10, the physical signs of rickets in children result in severe bone, muscle, respiratory, and overall growth problems. Rickets is a disabling disease that usually begins in early childhood before the age of 18 months [5]. Once children can stand, gravity worsens the bone changes so that the classic picture of inward or outward bowed legs is observed. Osteomalacia is characterized by muscle atrophy (i.e., a waddling gait), bone pain, and fatigue; these signs are also seen in rickets.

The musculoskeletal effects of chronically low vitamin D—rickets in children and osteomalacia in adults—arise primarily because of a lack of calcium and phosphate for bone mineralization and muscle function. With chronic severe vitamin D deficiency, there is malabsorption of calcium and phosphate with resultant hypocalcemia, hypophosphatemia, and secondary hyperparathyroidism. These lead to impaired growth plate development and bone mineralization [5].

Not all cases of rickets are due to a primary deficiency of cholecalciferol (or ergocalciferol). Although rare, there are many other types of rickets, as shown in Table 43.11, Many of these rarer types are inherited forms of rickets due to mutations in important receptors (e.g., VDR) or enzymes (e.g., 1-hydroxylase) involved in vitamin D metabolism or action. Some forms of rickets are not due to problems with vitamin D (e.g., calcium deficiency rickets).

There are drugs that cause osteomalacia. The most common is due to anticonvulsant therapy, particularly phenytoin, barbiturate derivatives, and carbamazepine. Although the exact mechanisms require further study, it is thought that these drugs result in greater inactivation of 1,25-dihydroxyvitamin D by inducing the enzyme 24-hydroxylase in the kidney [33].

Diagnosis of osteomalacia is often missed, even when bone pain and muscle weakness are present [68]. In an examination that used iliac crest biopsies at autopsy from otherwise healthy male and female individuals (primarily accident victims), biopsies were quantified for indices of osteomalacia and related to serum 25(OH)D levels [69]. In subjects in whom 25(OH)D levels were below 75 nmol/l, more than one-third experienced mineralization defects (i.e., pathological increase in osteoid), whereas no defects were observed in individuals with 25(OH)D levels exceeding 75 nmol/l. Osteomalacia may be misdiagnosed as osteoporosis, but a rise in serum alkaline phosphatase is seen only in the former condition [68]. Osteomalacia in younger women, when the pelvis is severely malformed, can cause craniopelvic disproportion, obstructed labor, and result in the need for caesarian section in some areas of the world [70].

2 Osteoporosis

The mild, secondary hyperparathyroidism that occurs with vitamin D insufficiency (i.e., levels of 25(OH)D below 75 nmol/l) may cause increased bone turnover and bone loss—a clinical picture compatible with osteoporosis [71]. Vitamin D insufficiency is very commonly found in patients with osteoporosis and contributes to the clinical presentation of osteoporosis (low bone density, fractures, and falls), as well as the variety of conditions that have been found to have a higher incidence when associated with insufficient vitamin D.

Vitamin D insufficiency or deficiency should be considered in any patient with osteoporosis. A survey of patients attending osteoporosis clinics found that even after osteoporosis treatment had been initiated, approximately 50% of the patients had suboptimal serum 25(OH)D levels. Vitamin D insufficiency or deficiency should always be considered in patients with osteoporosis who do not appear to be responding to therapy

TABLE 43.10 Physical and Clinical Signs of Rickets

Body system affected	Physical and clinical signs
Bone	Poor mineralization
	Hypertrophy of costochondral junctions
	Rachitic rosary: involution of the ribs and protrusion of the sternum
	Tibial and femoral bowing (inward or outward)
	Chest deformation
	Delayed closing of fontanelles
	Bone pain[a]
Teeth	Delayed eruption
	Enamel hypoplasia
	Early dental caries
Muscle	Delayed motor development
	Toneless and flabby legs
	Waddling gait[a]
Heart	Myocardiopathy
Lungs	Defective ventilation
	Respiratory obstruction
	Infections
Other	Secondary hyperparathyroidism
	Low plasma phosphate
	Tenany and seizures
	Hypochromic anemia
	Fatigue[a]

[a]*Symptoms of osteomalacia.*
Source: *Holick, M. F. (2006). Resurrection of vitamin D deficiency and rickets.* J. Clin. Invest. **116**, 2062–2072.

(i.e., continuing to lose bone density or continuing to suffer fragility fractures) [71].

Several pathological conditions contribute to secondary vitamin D deficiency that may lead to osteoporosis or osteomalacia. These include gastrointestinal disease, kidney disease, and drug-induced deficiency. Several common gastrointestinal disorders cause malabsorption [53], resulting in incomplete or the absence of absorption of cholecalciferol/ergocalciferol. These include celiac disease, inflammatory bowel disease, gastrectomy, pancreatic insufficiency, and cystic fibrosis. In addition, vitamin D deficiency can be precipitated from gastrointestinal surgeries such as bariatric surgery (intestinal bypass) or small bowel resection (short gut syndrome).

Randomized controlled trials in older adults have evaluated the effect of either vitamin D_3 or D_2 on bone mineral density. A systematic review of the literature found that supplementation with 800 IU of vitamin D_3 daily, in combination with calcium, reduced fracture risk [72], supporting previous analyses of reductions of bone mineral loss in studies [73]. A major limitation has been compliance rates for consuming the supplements of less than 80% and lack of assessment of vitamin D status (i.e., no 25(OH)D levels measured). Poor compliance with vitamin D supplementation is an issue noted more often in large community-based trials. When the daily vitamin D dose was only 10 µg (400 IU), there was no reduction in fracture risk [7,74]. This finding is not unexpected because that low amount of vitamin D_3 would result in only a small rise in serum 25(OH)D, approximately 7–10 nmol/l, and the subjects receiving this likely would not have 25 (OH)D levels above even 50 nmol/l.

The risk of fracture is increased due to not only low bone density but also falls. Studies show that vitamin D reduces fracture risk in part by reducing risk of falls [75]. Here, vitamin D is acting to increase muscle

TABLE 43.11 Types and Treatment of Rickets

Type of rickets	Metabolic abnormality mechanism	Treatment
Vitamin D dependent	Insufficient cholecalciferol production from UVB exposure and lack of dietary cholecalciferol or ergocalciferol	Supplemental cholecalciferol or ergocalciferol or sun exposure (with appropriate UVB); aggressive therapy needed initially
Calcium-deficiency rickets	Low calcium intake	Provide adequate calcium and cholecalciferol or ergocalciferol
Fat malabsorption (e.g., cystic fibrosis)	Insufficient cholecalciferol production from UVB exposure and lack of dietary cholecalciferol or ergocalciferol	Subcutaneous or intramuscular injections of cholecalciferol recommended
Hereditary vitamin D-dependent rickets type 1	Inactive or absent renal 1-hydroxylase enzyme	Provide 1,25-dihydroxyvitamin D (or 1-hydroxyvitamin D)
Hereditary vitamin D-dependent rickets type 2	Mutations in VDR prevent normal actions of 1,25-dihydroxyvitamin D	Respond to high dose of either cholecalciferol or 1,25-dihydroxyvitamin D
Hereditary vitamin D-dependent rickets type 3	Abnormal hormone response element binding protein	Respond to high dose of either cholecalciferol or 1,25-dihydroxyvitamin D
Hypophosphatemic rickets	Phosphatemia (acquired and inherited) and decreased 1-hydroxylase enzyme	Intravenous phosphate; remove tumor
Tumor-induced osteomalacia	Tumor secretes phosphate factor that causes phosphatemia (acquired and inherited) and decreased 1-hydroxylase enzyme	

Source: Holick, M. F. (2006). Resurrection of vitamin D deficiency and rickets. J. Clin. Invest. **116**, 2062–2072.

strength and may thus improve balance and reduce falls. In a study of adults age 65 years or older, neuro-muscular performance tests such as chair stands and walking tests were performed and related to vitamin D status (Figure 43.6). Performance improved as vitamin D status improved, up to a cutoff for serum 25(OH)D of 50–75 nmol/l.

C Vitamin D Insufficiency as an Emerging Public Health Problem

Research is ongoing concerning how vitamin D status can impact on chronic disease. Both the endocrine pathway and the paracrine pathway are implicated as mechanisms for understanding how vitamin D is involved in chronic disease prevention. As shown in Figure 43.1, the endocrine pathway, which maintains calcium and phosphate homeostasis, impacts on bone, muscle, and cardiovascular health. The paracrine/auto-crine pathways provide 1,25-dihydroxyvitamin D for cell functioning. Systems that are affected are those involving cell differentiation, such as the immune system. These paracrine pathways may impact on a variety of diseases under investigation, such as cancer and infectious, neurological, and autoimmune diseases [76]. A summary of disease conditions under investigation as being influenced by vitamin D status is listed in Table 43.12.

1 Vitamin D and Cancer Prevention

The connection between vitamin D status and cancer becomes clearer if one considers the disruption of normal cell activities that characterize cancers. Malignancies are characterized by disregulation in cell growth and differentiation. Observational studies of sun exposure or vitamin D status in relation to cancer risk show protective relationships between sufficient vitamin D status and lower risk of cancer. A systemic review and meta-analysis was conducted for colorectal cancer by Gorham et al. [77]. Eighteen studies were included in the analysis, with 4 based on serum levels of 25(OH)D and 14 based on oral intake. Most of the studies showed that inadequate vitamin D status was significantly associated with higher risk of cancer of the colon and/or rectum. Individuals with 1000 IU per day or more of cholecalciferol intake or who had serum 25(OH)D concentrations greater than 80 nmol/l had a 50% lower incidence of colorectal cancer compared to reference values. Breast cancer has also been studied [78], and a meta-analysis of 11 eligible studies indicated that a serum 25(OH)D level of 120 nmol/l was associated with a 50% lower risk of breast cancer.

A randomized control trial of vitamin D, originally intended as an osteoporosis study, provides compelling evidence of cancer prevention [79]. Approximately 1200 white postmenopausal women living in Nebraska

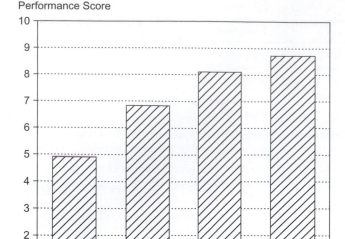

FIGURE 43.6 Improvement in physical performance of elderly residents who received graded amounts of vitamin D resulting in different serum levels of 25(OH)D. Source: *Reproduced with permission from Heaney, R. P. (2007). The case for improving vitamin D status.* J. Steroid Biochem. Mol. Biol. *103, 635–641.*

TABLE 43.12 Health Outcomes Associated with Vitamin D Justify a Public Health Concern

Skeletal diseases
   Rickets
   Osteomalacia
   Osteoporosis
Cancer
   Breast
   Prostate
   Colon
Microbial infections
   Tuberculosis
   Influenza
Autoimmune diseases
   Multiple sclerosis
   Diabetes (type 1)
   Others (e.g., irritable bowel syndrome, rheumatoid arthritis, and lupus)
Cardiovascular disease
   Hypertension
   Arteriosclerosis
Renal disease
   Chronic renal failure
   End-stage renal disease
Malabsorption disorders
   Crohn's
   Celiacs
   Cystic fibrosis
Neuromuscular disorders
   Parkinson's
   Multiple sclerosis
Neuronal disorders
   Dementia/Alzheimer's
   Depression
   Autism

Sources: *Holick, M. F., Binkley, N. C., Bischoff-Ferrari, H. A., Gordon, C. M., Hanley, D. A., Heaney, R. P., Murad, M. H., and Weaver, C. M. (2011). Evaluation, treatment, and prevention of vitamin D deficiency: An Endocrine Society clinical practice guideline.* J. Clin. Endocrinol. Metab. *96, 1911–1930; Bischoff-Ferrari, H.A., Giovannucci, E., Willett, W. C., Dietrich, T., and Dawson-Hughes, B. (2006). Estimation of optimal serum concentrations of 25-hydroxyvitamin D for multiple health outcomes.* Am. J. Clin. Nutr. *84, 18–28; Mathieu, C., Gysemans, C., Giulietti, A., and Bouillion, R. (2005). Vitamin D and diabetes.* Diabetologia *48, 1247–1257; Cannell, J. J. (2010). On the aetiology of autism.* Acta Paediatr. *99, 1128–1130; Mozaffarian, G. A. (2011). Investigating factors of decline in cognitive function or dementia.* Arch. Intern. Med. *171, 266–267; Evatt, M. L., DeLong, M. R., Kumari, M., Auinger, P., McDermott, M. P., Tangrpricha, V.; Parkisnon Study Group DATATOP Investigators (2011). High prevalence of hypovitaminosis D status in patients with early Parkinson disease.* Arch. Neurol. *68, 314–319; Dickens, A. P., Lang, I. A., Langa, K. M., Kos, K., and Llewellyn, D. J. (2011). Vitamin D, cognitive dysfunction and dementia in older adults.* CNS Drugs *25, 629–639.*

were enrolled in the 4-year study, which compared calcium alone (1400–1500 mg) with calcium plus vitamin D (1100 IU). At baseline, two-thirds of the women had 25(OH)D levels less than 80 nmol/l. Vitamin D treatment increased levels in that group by an average of 24 nmol/l, an expected amount (i.e., 40 IU vitamin D should raise 25(OH)D by 1 nmol/l) considering compliance was 85%. As shown in Figure 43.7, the relative risk for developing cancer in these older women indicates that vitamin D-supplemented women had only 40% of the risk of developing cancer compared to the placebo group; this risk decreased to less than 25% when cancer incidence beyond the first year of the study was used in the analysis. Treatment with calcium alone had no significant effect on cancer incidence, but subject numbers may have been too low for the apparent 50% reduction by this treatment. There were no patterns in the types of cancer these women developed. Thus, when vitamin D intakes were raised above an average level of 80 nmol/l, a significant reduction in cancer incidence was observed, which is in agreement with the cohort studies described previously.

Further support for the role of vitamin D insufficiency in cancer development relates to the finding that in addition to their well-documented low 25(OH)D levels as a group, black men in the United States have a 40% higher rate for total cancer mortality and black

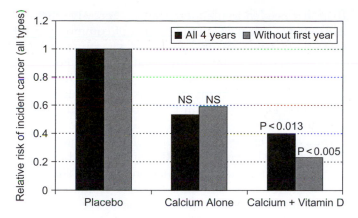

FIGURE 43.7 Relative risk (RR) of incident cancer is plotted for the first randomized controlled trial of vitamin D and cancer risk. More than 1000 postmenopausal women in Nebraska were given one of three treatments (placebo, 1400–1500 mg calcium, or 1400–1500 mg calcium and 1100 IU vitamin D_3) and followed for 4 years. *Source: Data are taken from Lappe, J. M., Travers-Gustafson, D., Davies, K. M.,Recker, R. R. and Heaney, R. P. (2007). Vitamin D and calcium supplementation reduces cancer risk: Results of a randomized trial. Am. J. Clin. Nutr.* **85**, *1586–1591.*

women have a 20% higher mortality rate compared to their white counterparts [80]. Giovannucci *et al.* [80] demonstrated significantly higher risk of total cancer incidence and total cancer mortality among black men compared to whites in a study population that was relatively homogeneous with respect to socioeconomic, education, lifestyle, and dietary factors.

There remains a debate regarding whether vitamin D status should be improved by diet or sun exposure. In a study of persons with a diagnosis of nonmelanoma skin cancer, for whom sun exposure was the likely cause of this cancer, there were lower rates of second cancers (colon, gastric, and rectal cancers) [81]. This study underscores the need for better understanding of the role of vitamin D, which for many people is obtained through sun exposure. Although sun exposure increases the risk of developing skin cancer [52], current findings suggest it has the potential to reduce the risk of developing more severe forms of cancer [81].

2 Vitamin D and Autoimmune Diseases

Other chronic diseases have been implicated, especially in relation to immunity. Vitamin D deficiency may also predispose individuals to type 1 and type 2 diabetes. Several reviews and meta-analyses of the relationship between vitamin D status and development of diabetes are available [82–84]. Epidemiological studies have suggested that high circulating levels of vitamin D are associated with a lower risk of multiple sclerosis (MS). Overall, studies support a protective effect of vitamin D, but there are some unanswered questions,

including the mechanism of action and how genetic variations modify the effect of vitamin D status [85]. Also promising is whether vitamin D can influence the course of MS progression or influence the prevention of MS.

In conditions in which there is chronic pain and disability, such as fibromyalgia or chronic muscle fatigue, vitamin D deficiency should be investigated as a cause because inadequacy of vitamin D is seen in patients with chronic pain and the use of pain-reducing opioid medications is twice as high in patients with vitamin D deficiency (<50 nmol/l) [86].

3 Vitamin D and Prevention of Chronic Kidney Disease and Cardiovascular Disease

Serum 25(OH)D levels are lower in patients with varying stages of renal function [87–93]. Although this relationship was initially shown in small studies involving few subjects, later evidence from the general U.S. population using NHANES III data demonstrated significantly lower 25(OH)D levels only in those survey participants with low estimated glomerular filtration rates (eGFR)—that is, with values <29 ml/minute/1.73 m² [92]. In contrast, patients in the general population with mild to moderate loss of renal function had relatively normal levels of 25(OH)D. These findings support the hypothesis that vitamin D status may be involved in the pathophysiology of progressive renal disease. Vitamin D status may affect the progression of renal failure through a number of mechanisms, including control of cell proliferation and differentiation, changes in the loss of podocytes, modulation of inflammation such as the suppression of pro-inflammatory cytokines, regulation of the renin—angiogenesis system to lower hypertension, and reduction of intact parathyroid hormone (iPTH) levels [93]. Secondary hyperparathyroidism is a well-recognized hallmark of low circulating levels of 25(OH)D, even in individuals with normal renal function; however, low serum 25(OH)D in chronic kidney disease (CKD) has been shown to aggravate the secondary hyperparathyroidism [93].

In 2010, the Kidney Disease Improving Global Outcomes (KDIGO) guidelines made the following recommendation regarding vitamin D: "In patients with chronic kidney disease (CKD) stages 3–5 [i.e., predialysis], we suggest that 25(OH)D might be measured ... [and] that vitamin D deficiency and insufficiency be corrected using treatment strategies recommended for the general population" [87]. The Endocrine Society [53] lists patients with CKD as an at-risk group for vitamin D deficiency. Ergocalciferol treatment corrected hypovitaminosis D and effectively decreased serum iPTH by 13% over 7.4 months, but only in patients with CKD stage 3 and not in those with stage 4 who were followed over 6.8 months [91]. Deville *et al.* [90]

examined ergocalciferol doses ranging from 800 IU/day to 100,000 IU/week over 90 days in patients with stages 3–5 CKD but none on dialysis. Serum iPTH levels decreased among CKD stages 3 and 5, but statistically significant decreases were reached only in patients with stage 4 CKD. As with the other vitamin D supplementation trial, there was a significant increase in serum levels of 25(OH)D in all CKD patients. Whether or not cholecalciferol (vitamin D_3) treatment would be more effective in CKD remains to be determined. Also, the appropriate effective dose level of vitamin D and stage of CKD for initiation of treatment are not yet known.

Kidney dysfunction is also associated with insulin resistance and glucose intolerance. Chonchol and Scragg [92], in their analyses of kidney function and vitamin D status in the NHANES III survey, also demonstrated that serum 25(OH)D and levels of kidney function (eGFR) were both inversely associated with the homeostasis model assessment of insulin resistance (HOMA-IR) but were independent of each other. Conversely, they found that survey participants with serum 25(OH)D levels in excess of 81 nmol/l had lower HOMA-IR. These findings suggest that low-serum 25(OH)D may be a risk factor in cardiovascular disease because insulin resistance is an integral part of the putative path to cardiovascular disease development.

Strategies to raise serum 25(OH)D levels may decrease the risk of cardiovascular disease [94–96]. Evidence for a role of adequate vitamin D status in slowing the development of cardiovascular disease was demonstrated in a randomized, placebo-controlled, double-blind vitamin D supplementation trial in which 2000 IU of cholecalciferol markedly improved the inflammatory cytokine profiles in patients with congestive heart failure [96]. In a review, the plausibility of vitamin D's involvement was highlighted. There are vitamin D metabolizing enzymes in the heart and blood vessels. In animal models of cardiovascular disease, vitamin D is anti-atherosclerotic, anti-inflammatory, and has direct cardioprotective actions. In epidemiologic studies of the general population, low levels of 25(OH)D are associated with increased risk of cardiovascular disease and mortality. However, there are few and inconsistent data from randomized controlled trials concerning cardiovascular disease prevention and treatment; thus, a recommendation cannot be made other than ensuring vitamin D adequacy in those at risk for cardiovascular disease [94].

D Treatment of Vitamin D Deficiency

When an individual is depleted of vitamin D, the amount of vitamin D needed for repletion is higher than that needed to maintain status; aggressive therapy is needed. Table 43.3 provides a list of commonly used vitamin D supplements, and new vitamin D-related medications are updated continuously on the Food and Drug Administration's website [97]. As indicated in Table 43.11, many forms of rickets require high doses of vitamin D. This vitamin D can be provided daily or in intermittent doses. It is not necessary to be concerned about exceeding the tolerable upper intake level for vitamin D because this DRI is not intended as a barrier for treatment under a physician's care. In situations in which rickets is determined to be a vitamin D-resistant form (Table 43.11), doses of the active metabolite 1,25-dihydroxyvitamin D or an analog with similar properties are often administered.

Historically, sunlight was prescribed for vitamin D deficiency [5]. It was common practice for children with rickets and for adults with tuberculosis [5]. For some diseases for which fat malabsorption precludes oral dosing, UVB lamps have been used, and there is a growing interest in sunlamps to treat seasonal affective disorders. A new generation of lamps are now available for which harmful UVC radiation is filtered [98]. A timing device is provided to prevent overexposure to UVB and to deliver only suberythemal doses. The subject should receive exposure at different areas of the body to avoid tanning, which is an indicator of overexposure.

V DIETARY REQUIREMENTS

A Institute of Medicine Recommended Intake Values for Vitamin D, 2011

New reference values for vitamin D that apply to Canada and the United States were announced by the Institute of Medicine (IOM) in November 2010 and published in 2011 [4]. These revised DRIs generated much discussion, some of it in support [99] and some critical of the way in which the evidence for new roles of vitamin D was dismissed in the deliberations [100]. DRIs provide the reference values for assessment and planning functions in nutrition [101]: the estimated average requirement (EAR), which is the median requirement; the recommended dietary allowance (RDA), which is the amount that meets the needs of almost all (97.5%) healthy persons in the population; the adequate intake (AI), which set for infants age 0 to 1 year; and the tolerable upper intake level (UL), which is set at a level that poses no risk for adverse effects. Since first setting DRI recommendations in 1997, evidence emerged suggesting a need to revise the initial DRI values [102]. The 2011 DRI committee used evidence-based reports and other data in its deliberations.

The challenges that the committee identified in setting the new DRIs included (1) an acknowledgment that vitamin D can be made through skin synthesis, so setting intake values must be made in the context of minimal sun exposure; (2) recognition that studies designed to provide evidence for dietary effects on bone gave both calcium and vitamin D, so isolating vitamin D's effects was a challenge; (3) complications in interpreting the impact of poor vitamin D status because bone health can be maintained with high intakes of calcium, making the link between vitamin D and bone health very dependent on usual calcium intakes; and (4) the inability to distinguish the contribution to total 25(OH)D levels of sun-induced synthesis of vitamin D from ingested vitamin D, except in studies in which 25(OH)D is measured in winter in subjects and in which other sources of exposure, such as trips to sun destinations or use of tanning beds, are not confounders [4].

The values for each age/sex group for EAR, RDA, and AI are provided in Table 43.13. The level of 25(OH)D that was defined for adequacy for almost everyone, including individuals with darkly pigmented skin (i.e., the RDA), was set at a serum level of 25(OH)D at or above 50 nmol/l. This circulating level of 25(OH)D was deemed to provide for maximal calcium absorption, minimal risk of rickets in children, reduced fracture risk in adults, and minimal risk of osteomalacia in adults [4]. Using data from studies conducted during winter or at very high latitudes where sun exposure is assumed to be minimal, the committee used simulated dose—response prediction equations to find the intake of vitamin D that would achieve a mean 25(OH)D level of 50 nmol/l in almost everyone, and this was determined to be 600 IU, irrespective of age, gender, or race/ethnicity. There was recognition that older adults demonstrated a high degree of variability in attaining 25(OH)D in studies; thus, the RDA was set at 800 IU. The level to achieve 40 nmol/l was estimated as 400 IU; this is the EAR. The vitamin D recommendation of 400 IU for infants, as an AI, is based on maintaining adequate serum 25(OH)D above 50 nmol/l. Recommended values during pregnancy and lactation are not different from those for other women in the same age group [4].

B Recommendations for at-Risk Groups

1 Recommendations of the Endocrine Society, 2011

The IOM recommendations are for healthy individuals who are free of most chronic conditions, and the

TABLE 43.13 Dietary Recommendations for Vitamin D Intake Based on Healthy and At-Risk Status

Organization and criterion	Age group (years)	Recommendation (IU)	Level of 25(OH)D achieved (nmol/l)	Notes
Healthy population				
Institute of Medicine, 2011	0—1	400	50	Recommended Dietary Allowance (RDA) for healthy Canadians and Americans to achieve a 25(OH)D level of 50 nmol/l. Infant level is an adequate intake (AI)
	1—18	600		
	19—70	600		
	71+	800		
At-risk population				
Endocrine Society, 2011	0—1	400—1000	75	Recommended intake for at-risk patients in the United States to achieve a 25(OH)D level of 75 nmol/l. At-risk includes those who have a vitamin D deficiency, kidney failure, malabsorption syndrome, hyperparathyroidism, on medications that interfere with vitamin D, are African-American or Hispanic, are pregnant or lactating, are older adults with a history of falls or nontraumatic fractures, are obese, or have granuloma-forming disorders.
	1—18	600—1000		
	18+	1500—2000		

*Sources: Institute of Medicine (2011). "Dietary Reference Intakes for Calcium and Vitamin D." National Academies Press. Washington, DC; Holick, M. F., Binkley, N. C., Bischoff-Ferrari, H. A., Gordon, C. M., Hanley, D. A., Heaney, R. P., Murad, M. H., and Weaver, C. M. (2011). Evaluation, treatment, and prevention of vitamin D deficiency: An Endocrine Society clinical practice guideline. J. Clin. Endocrinol. Metab. **96**, 1911—1930.*

target level of 25(OH)D used to determine the RDA was 50 nmol/l [4]. Subsequent to the IOM publication of the DRIs for vitamin D and calcium, the Endocrine Society published intake guidelines for individuals with chronic conditions known to influence vitamin D status [53]. The Endocrine Committee of experts defined vitamin D adequacy for those at risk as 75 nmol/l 25(OH)D [53]. The Endocrine Society focused on at-risk groups and stated that evidence is available to define "deficiency" as a level of 25(OH)D < 50 nmol/l Individuals with a designation of "at-risk" include those with rickets, osteomalacia, osteoporosis, chronic kidney disease, malabsorption syndromes, medication use that interferes with vitamin D (e.g., antiseizure medications and glucocorticoids), and granuloma-forming disorders. In addition, life-stage groups (pregnancy, lactation, and older adults with fracture or fall history) and racial/ethnic groups (African American and Hispanic children and adults) are included in the "at-risk" designation. Finally, obesity puts people more at risk for vitamin D deficiency. The dietary recommendations for at-risk groups published by the Endocrine Society are found in Table 43.13. Intakes are provided as ranges because it is not known how much cholecalciferol or ergocalciferol is needed to raise serum 25(OH)D levels over 75 nmol/l.

2 Recommendations for Older Adults

Older adults (age > 50 years) have higher vitamin D needs for several reasons. Physiologically, there are two concerns. The enzyme responsible for synthesis of 1,25(OH)2D in the kidney (the endocrine pathway) becomes more resistant to PTH stimulation with age [4]. This means that the 1-hydroxylase is not increased by PTH when there is need for calcium, inducing prolonged secondary hyperparathyroidism without increased calcium renal reabsorption or intestinal absorption, leading to increased bone loss. A low level of 25(OH)D exacerbates this hyperparathyroidism. In addition, skin cells are less able to make cholecalciferol because there are fewer molecules of 7-dehydrocholesterol (provitamin D_3) in the epidermis. When young and old subjects are exposed to the same amount of UVB, elderly subjects produce only one-third the amount of cholecalciferol [4]. Another concern is that older adults are often indoors, especially when in institutional settings [103].

There is a question of whether older adults (>65 years) need higher amounts of cholecalciferol or ergocalciferol for repletion than younger adults. An examination of repletion studies was done to document doses of vitamin D that had been used in older and younger adults from 13 published studies [104]. It was also determined whether the repletion doses

employed could achieve levels of 25(OH)D above 75 nmol/l. Most published dosing regimens failed to achieve 75 nmol/l in most subjects, whether young adults (<65 years) or older adults (>65 years). Whether administered as a daily dose or bolus oral supplementation, elderly subjects appeared to need more supplemental vitamin D_3 compared with younger adults. However, caution in the interpretation is warranted because baseline levels, end points, study duration, compliance, and other factors were different among these studies. In all the studies examined, no risks or side effects of supplemental vitamin D were reported [104].

3 Recommendations for Infants

Infants (age 0—12 months) represent a very vulnerable group. Infants do have the capacity for skin synthesis of vitamin D_3; however, dietary intakes are needed by almost all infants because they are usually kept indoors, swaddled, and/or may be born at times of the year when no skin synthesis is possible. For decades, researchers have believed that vitamin D was present in only small amounts in breast milk, and therefore supplemental vitamin D is recommended for all breast-fed infants. An apparent re-emergence of rickets in breast-fed infants has heightened this concern [105,106]. These infants were born in situations in which the mothers' vitamin D status was poor because there was poor dietary intake and there was also limited sun exposure for mother or child (due to living conditions, season, or skin pigmentation). The recommendation of 400 IU for all infants [4] will go far to prevent rickets; however, some health professional associations have called for even higher intakes. The Canadian Pediatric Society recommends 800 IU for infants who live in higher latitudes of Canada (which would also apply to Alaska) [107]; indeed, any infant deprived of sun exposure may need this higher intake.

4 Recommendations for Pregnancy and Lactation

By the third trimester of pregnancy, there is an elevation of 1,25-dihydroxyvitamin D by the mother, corresponding to the time when the fetus begins to calcify bones and the need for calcium is greatest [53]. Overall, pregnant women are at high risk for vitamin D deficiency, and complications such as preeclampsia and caesarean section are increased in those who are deficient [53]. In the 2011 IOM report, no special considerations were made for pregnancy; that is, during these times women would follow the recommendations for nonpregnant or nonlactating women. The IOM justification was that there were no data to suggest the needs of pregnant women were different; for example, fetal outcomes were compromised only when maternal 25(OH)D was below 40 nmol/l, a level that should be met if women follow RDA recommendations. IOM indicated that during lactation, small increases in maternal 25(OH)D do not appear to impact breast milk content or infant 25(OH)D levels [4].

In the 2011 Endocrine Society guidelines on vitamin D, pregnancy and lactation are classified as times when screening for 25(OH)D should occur [53]. Recommendations during pregnancy by this group are the same as for at-risk adults of the corresponding age (Table 43.13). Others believe that during pregnancy and lactation, vitamin D intakes should be higher than either the IOM or the Endocrine Society recommendations. They have shown that when intakes of vitamin D by lactating mothers are greater than 4000 IU, breast milk levels reach "physiological" levels, supplying 400 IU of vitamin D per day to the infant [108]. In a study of 350 pregnant women who continued to delivery, women who achieved 25(OH)D > 80 nmol/l were those taking 4000 IU compared to 400 IU [109]. These investigators suggest that this intake is safe and may be needed for women of different race/ethnicities to achieve 25(OH)D levels greater than 75 nmol/l [109].

VI SAFETY OF VITAMIN D

A The Tolerable Upper Intake Level for Vitamin D

The daily tolerable UL was established to discourage potentially dangerous self-medication [101]. The two main indicators of excess vitamin D are hypercalcemia, which can lead to calcification of soft tissues such as arteries (arteriosclerosis) and kidney (nephrocalcinosis), and hypercalciuria, which reflects the presence of excess serum calcium and could be damaging on its own (i.e., kidney stones). However, there are no data linking excess vitamin D to kidney stone risk [4]. In infants, retarded growth may also be present [4].

A risk assessment for vitamin D showed that based on an analysis of all published reports related to excess vitamin D ingestion up to 2007, doses of supplemental vitamin D_3 ingested at levels less than 10,000 IU/day were not associated with toxicity [110]. It is possible that intakes consistently greater than 50,000 IU/day could be linked to side effects including hypercalcemia [4].

UL values for infants 0−6 months and 6−12 months were set at 1000 and 1500 IU, respectively (Table 43.14). A no-observable-adverse-effect level of 1800 IU was used to set these ULs based on studies in which high doses of vitamin D produced hypercalcemia. An uncertainty factor (UF) of 1.8 was set for very young infants, and a smaller UF was set for older infants, indicting greater tolerance to vitamin D. For adults older than age 18 years, the committee concluded that 25(OH)D should not be greater than 125−150 nmol/l. It also

TABLE 43.14 Comparison of Safety Assessments for Vitamin D Based on Healthy and At-Risk Status

Organization and criterion	Tolerable upper intake level (UL)
Healthy population	
Institute of Medicine, 2011	0−0.5 years: 1000
	0.5−1 years: 1500
	1−3 years: 2500
	4−8 years: 3000
	9−13 years: 4000
	14 + years: 4000
At-risk population	
Endocrine Society, 2011	0−0.5 years: 2000
	0.5−1 years: 2000
	1−3 years: 4000
	4−8 years: 4000
	9−13 years: 4000
	14 + years: 10000

Sources: *Institute of Medicine* (2011). *"Dietary Reference Intakes for Calcium and Vitamin D."* National Academies Press, Washington, DC; Holick, M. F., Binkley, N. C., Bischoff-Ferrari, H. A., Gordon, C. M., Hanley, D. A., Heaney, R. P., Murad, M. H., and Weaver, C. M. (2011). *Evaluation, treatment, and prevention of vitamin D deficiency: An Endocrine Society clinical practice guideline.* J. Clin. Endocrinol. Metab. **96**, 1911−1930.

determined, using published data from a dosing study, that 4000 IU would not raise 25(OH)D levels above this threshold [4]. In that dosing study, Heaney *et al.* [16] gave cholecalciferol to subjects in doses up to 10,000 IU, and they found no adverse effects in men treated for 5 months. IOM indicated that attaining a 25 (OH)D greater than 125 nmol/l had no potential benefit and possible (unknown) risk; therefore, the UL was set at 4000 IU, which is an adjustment down from the 5000 IU that subjects ingested to reach125 nmol/l with 5 months of dosing. For children, the committee chose to "scale down" the adult UL [4].

The Endocrine Society recommends higher UL values than those recommended by IOM. The Endocrine Society uses these higher amounts, shown in Table 43.14, because they represent intakes that would be used in treatment regimens for those at high risk of vitamin D deficiency or insufficiency [53]. Unless a person is under a physician's care, it is prudent to use the IOM values for ULs as the highest safest intakes.

B Vitamin D Intoxication

Accidental poisoning or uninformed supplementation with vitamin D can occur and cause vitamin D intoxication [4,110]. Nine cases involved levels in the range of approximately 30,000—2,600,000 IU, and durations were between days and decades [110]. The signs and symptoms of vitamin D intoxication are associated with hypercalcemia and include constipation, lethargy, confusion, polyuria, and polydypsia. Generally, toxicity occurred in cases in which intake is more than 50,000 IU per day, well above the revised UL. Levels of 25(OH)D associated with these high intakes ranged between 700 and 1600 nmol/l, well above the value of 250 nmol/l considered "high."

One study indicates the need for caution in providing large one-time doses of vitamin D supplementation. In a randomized, double-blind, placebo-controlled trial of women older than 70 years, the treatment group was given 500,000 IU vitamin D_3 orally once yearly for 3—5 consecutive years [111]. The treatment group experienced significantly higher incidences of falls and fractures. What caused the increase in falls and fractures is not known, but it may have been true toxicity subsequent to ingesting this dose. Based on this study, there has been a call for caution with regard to the use of high loading doses of vitamin supplements [112].

VII CONCLUSION

Vitamin D inadequacy, whether it is defined by IOM as 25(OH)D < 50 nmol/l or by the Endocrine Society as 25(OH)D < 75 nmol/l, is of concern in the United States. Many Americans are in high-risk groups or get little sun exposure. Having a food supply that is relatively low in vitamin D exacerbates this problem. Action is needed to ensure adequate dietary intakes from food and dietary supplements and/or appropriate sun exposure. Vitamin D deficiency leads not only to rickets and osteomalacia, which are likely to go undiagnosed in the population, and to osteoporosis but also to neuromuscular disabilities, deficits in cognition, increased risk of cancer development, and other problems still under investigation. Better understanding of vitamin D metabolism and status will lead to its effective use in the prevention and treatment of a variety of chronic diseases.

References

[1] National Research Council, Recommended Dietary Allowances, 10th ed., National Academy Press, Washington, DC, 1989.
[2] M.S. Calvo, S.J. Whiting, Prevalence of vitamin D insufficiency in Canada and the United States: importance to health status and efficacy of current food fortification and dietary supplement use, Nutr. Rev. 61 (2003) 107—113.
[3] Institute of Medicine, Dietary Reference Intakes for Calcium, Phosphorus, Magnesium, Vitamin D, and Fluoride., National Academy Press, Washington, DC, 1997.
[4] Institute of Medicine, Dietary Reference Intakes for Calcium and Vitamin D, National Academies Press, Washington, DC, 2011.
[5] M.F. Holick, Resurrection of vitamin D deficiency and rickets, J. Clin. Invest. 116 (2006) 2062—2072.
[6] A. Norman, Sunlight, season, skin pigment, vitamin D, and 25-hyd[r]xy D: integral components of the vitamin D endocrine system, Am. J. Clin. Nutr. 67 (1998) 1108—1110.
[7] M.F. Holick, Vitamin D deficiency, N. Engl. J Med. 357 (3) (2007) 266—281.
[8] A.R. Webb, O. Engelsen, Calculated ultraviolet exposure levels for a healthy vitamin D status, Photochem. Photobiol. 82 (2006) 1697—1703.
[9] M.G. Kimlin, W.J. Olds, M.R. Moore, Location and vitamin D synthesis: is the hypothesis validated by geophysical data? J. Photochem. Photobiol. 86 (2007) 234—239.
[10] P. Lips, Vitamin D status and nutrition in Europe and Asia, J. Steroid. Biochem. Mol. Biol. 103 (2007) 620—625.
[11] U.S. Babu, M.S. Calvo, Modern India and the vitamin D dilemma: evidence for the need of a national food fortification program, Mol. Nutr. Food Res. 54 (2010) 1134—1147.
[12] V. Tangpricha, P. Koutkia, S.M. Rieke, T.C. Chen, A.A. Perez, M.F. Holick, Fortification of orange juice with vitamin D: a novel approach for enhancing vitamin D nutritional health, Am. J. Clin. Nutr. 77 (2003) 1478—1483.
[13] B.W. Hollis, C.L. Wagner, M.K. Drezner, N.C. Binkley, Circulating vitamin D_3 and 25-hydroxyvitamin D in humans: an important tool to define adequate nutritional vitamin D status, J. Steroid Biochem. Mol. Biol. 103 (2007) 631—634.
[14] P. Lips, Vitamin D physiology, Prog. Biophys. Mol. Biol. 92 (2006) 4—8.
[15] C. Meier, H.W. Woitge, K. Witte, B. Lemmer, M.J. Seibel, Supplementation with oral vitamin D_3 and calcium during winter prevents seasonal bone loss: a randomized controlled open-label prospective trial, J. Bone Miner. Res. 19 (2004) 1221—1230.
[16] R.P. Heaney, K.M. Davies, T.C. Chen, M.F. Holick, M.J. Barger-Lux, Human serum 25-hydroxycholecalciferol response to extended oral dosing with cholecalciferol, Am. J. Clin. Nutr. 77 (2003) 204—210.
[17] L.A. Houghton, R. Vieth, The case against ergocalciferol (vitamin D_2) as a vitamin supplement, Am. J. Clin. Nutr. 84 (2006) 694—697.
[18] A.G. Armas, B.W. Hollis, R.P. Heaney, Vitamin D_2 is much less effective than vitamin D_3 in humans, J. Clin. Endocrinol. Metab. 89 (2004) 5387—5391.
[19] M.F. Holick, R.M. Biancuzzo, T.C. Chen, E.K. Klein, A. Young, D. Bibuld, et al., Vitamin D_2 is as effective as vitamin D_3 in maintaining circulating concentrations of 25-hydroxyvitamin D, J. Clin. Endocrinol. Metab. 93 (2008) 677—681.
[20] P.H. Anderson, P.D. O'Loughlin., B.K. May, H.A. Morris, Quantification of mRNA for the vitamin D metabolizing enzymes CYP27B1 and CYP24 and vitamin D receptor in kidney using real-time reverse transcriptase-polymerase chain reaction, J. Mol. Endocrinol. 31 (2003) 123—132.
[21] A.S. Dusso, A.J. Brown, E. Slatopolsky, Vitamin D, Am. J. Physiol. Renal Physiol. 289 (2005) F8—F28.
[22] H.F. DeLuca, Overview of general physiologic features and functions of vitamin D, Am. J. Clin. Nutr. 80 (2004) 1689s—1696s.
[23] S. Akhter, G.D. Kutuzova, S. Christakos, H.F. Deluca, Calbindin D(9k) is not required for 1,25-dihydroxyvitamin D(3)-mediated Ca(2+) absorption in small intestine, Arch. Biochem. Biophys. 460 (2006) 227—232.
[24] R.P. Heaney, The case for improving vitamin D status, J. Steroid Biochem. Mol. Biol. 103 (2007) 635—641.
[25] M. Hewison, Vitamin D and the immune system, Endocrinol. Metab. Clin. North Am. 39 (2010) 365—379.

[26] P.T. Liu, S. Stenger, L. Huiying, L. Wenzel, B.H. Tan, S.R. Krutzik, et al., Toll-like receptor triggering of a vitamin D-mediated human antimicrobial response, Science 311 (2006) 1770–1773.

[27] F. Baeke, T. Takiishi, H. Korf, C. Gysemans, C. Mathieu, Vitamin D: Modulator of the immune system, Curr. Opin. Pharmacol. 10 (2010) 482–496.

[28] G. Jones, S.A. Strugnell, D.F. Deluca, Current understanding of the molecular actions of vitamin D, Physiol. Rev. 78 (1998) 1193–1231.

[29] A.W. Norman, Minireview: Vitamin D receptor: New assignments for an already busy receptor, Endocrinology 147 (2006) 5542–5548.

[30] J.C. Fleet, Genomic and proteomic approaches for probing the role of vitamin D in health, Am. J. Clin. Nutr. 80 (2004) 1730s–1734s.

[31] J.C. Fleet, Rapid, membrane-initiated actions of 1,25 dihydroxyvitamin D: what are they and what do they mean? J. Nutr. 134 (2004) 3215–3218.

[32] A.W. Norman, W.H. Okamura, J.E. Bishop, H.L. Henry, Update on biological actions of 1-alpha, 25(OH)$_2$-vitamin D$_3$ (rapid effects) and 24R,25(OH)$_2$-vitamin D$_3$, Mol. Cell. Endocrinol. 197 (2002) 1–13.

[33] C. Zhou, M. Assem, J.C. Tay, P.B. Watkins, B. Blumberg, E.G. Schuetz, et al., Steroid and xenobiotic receptor and vitamin D receptor cross-talk mediates CYP24 expression and drug-induced osteomalacia, J. Clin. Invest. 116 (2006) 1703–1712.

[34] U.S. Department of Agriculture, Agricultural Research Service (2011). "National Nutrient Database." Available at <http://www.nal.usda.gov/fnic/foodcomp/search/>, Accessed September 2011.

[35] Z. Lu, T.C. Chen, A. Zhang, K.S. Persons, N. Kohn, R. Berkowiitz, et al., An evaluation of the vitamin D$_3$ content in fish: Is the vitamin D content adequate to satisfy the dietary requirement for vitamin D?, J. Steroid Biochem. Mol. Biol. 103 (2007) 642–644.

[36] M.S. Calvo, C.N. Barton, S.J. Whiting, Vitamin D fortification in the U.S. and Canada: current status and data needs, Am. J. Clin. Nutr. 80 (2004) 1710S–1716S.

[37] V.L. Fulgoni, D.R. Keast, R.L. Bailey, J. Dwyer, Foods, fortificants, and supplements: where do Americans get their nutrients?, J. Nutr. 141 (2011) 1847–1854.

[38] M.S. Calvo, U.S. Babu, L.H. Garthoff, T.O. Woods, M. Dreher, G. Hill, et al., Vitamin D$_2$ from light exposed edible mushrooms is safe, bioavailable and effectively supports bone growth in rats, Osteoporos. Int. (2012) [Epub ahead of print]

[39] M.S. Calvo, S.J. Whiting, Public health strategies to overcome barriers to optimal vitamin D status in populations with special needs, J. Nutr. 136 (2006) 135–139.

[40] J. Cannell, H. Bischoff-Ferarri, C. Garland, E. Giovannucci, W. Grant, J. Hathcock, et al., Cod liver oil, vitamin A toxicity, frequent respiratory infections and the vitamin D deficiency epidemic [editorial], Ann. Otol. Rhinol. Laryngol. 117 (2008) 864–870.

[41] H.M. Trang, D.E. Cole, L.A. Ribin, A. Pierratos, S. Siu, R. Vieth, Evidence that vitamin D$_3$ increases serum 25-hydroxyvitamin D more efficiently than does vitamin D$_2$, Am. J. Clin. Nutr. 68 (1998) 854–858.

[42] P.B. Rapuri, J.C. Gallagher, G. Haynatzki, Effect of vitamins D$_2$ and D$_3$ supplement use on serum 25OHD concentrations in elderly women in summer and winter, Calcif. Tissue Int. 74 (2004) 150–156.

[43] S.R. Mastaglia, C.A. Mautalen, M.S. Parisi, B. Oliveri, Vitamin D$_2$ dose required to rapidly increase 25OHD levels in osteoporotic women, Eur. J. Clin. Nutr. 60 (2006) 681–687.

[44] T. Araki, M.F. Holick, B.D. Alfonso, E. Charlap, C.M. Romero, D. Rizk, et al., Vitamin D intoxication with severe hypercalcemia due to manufacturing and labeling errors of two dietary supplements made in the United States, J. Clin. Endocrinol. Metab. 96 (2011) 3603–3608.

[45] C. Moore, M.M. Murphy, D.R. Keast, M.F. Hollick, Vitamin D intake in the United States, J. Am. Diet. Assoc. 104 (2004) 980–983.

[46] S.J. Whiting, M.S. Calvo, Dietary recommendations for vitamin D: a critical need for functional end points to establish an estimated average requirement, J. Nutr. 125 (2005) 304–309.

[47] R.L. Bailey, K.W. Dodd, J.A. Goldman, J.J. Gahche, J.T. Dwyer, A.J. Moshfegh, et al., Estimation of total usual calcium and vitamin D intakes in the United States, J. Nutr. 140 (2010) 817–822.

[48] S. Nesby-O'Dell, K.S. Scanlon, M.E. Cogswell, C. Gillespie, B.W. Hollis, A.C. Looker, et al., Hypovitamininosis D prevalence and determinants among African American and white women of reproductive age: third National Health and Nutrition Examination Survey, 1988–1994, Am. J. Clin. Nutr. 76 (2002) 187–192.

[49] A. Zadshir, N. Tareen, D. Pan, K. Norris, D. Martins, The prevalence of hypovitaminosis D among U.S. adults: data from the NHANES III, Ethn. Dis. 15 (Suppl. 5) (2005) 97–101.

[50] N. Taureen, D. Martins, A. Zadshir, D. Pan, K.C. Norris, The impact of routine vitamin supplementation on serum levels of 25(OH)D$_3$ among the general adult population and patients with chronic kidney disease, Ethn. Dis. 15 (Suppl. 5) (2005) 102–106.

[51] B.W. Hollis, Circulating 25-hydroxyvitamin D levels indicative of vitamin D sufficiency: implications for establishing a new effective dietary intake recommendation for vitamin D, J. Nutr. 135 (2005) 317–322.

[52] B.A. Gilchrest, Sun protection and vitamin D: three dimensions of obfuscation, J. Steroid Biochem. Mol. Biol. 103 (2007) 655–663.

[53] M.F. Holick, N.C. Binkley, H.A. Bischoff-Ferrari, C.M. Gordon, D.A. Hanley, R.P. Heaney, et al., Evaluation, treatment, and prevention of vitamin D deficiency: an Endocrine Society clinical practice guideline, J. Clin. Endocrinol. Metab. 96 (2011) 1911–1930.

[54] Working Group of the Australian and New Zealand Bone and Mineral Society, Endocrine Society of Australia, Osteoporosis Australia, Vitamin D and adult bone health in Australia and New Zealand: a position statement, Med. J. Austr 182 (2005) 281–285.

[55] E.H. Livingston, S. Lee, Percentage of burned body surface area determination in obese and nonobese patients, J Surg. Res. 91 (2000) 106–110.

[56] T.B. Fitzpatrick, The validity and practicality of sun-reactive skin types I through VI, Arch. Dermatol. 124 (1988) 869–871.

[57] N.G. Jablonski, G. Chaplin, The evolution of human skin coloration, J. Hum. Evol. 39 (2000) 57–106.

[58] R. Lucas, T. McMichael, W. Smith, B. Armstrong, Solar Ultraviolet Radiation: Global Burden of Disease from Solar Ultraviolet Radiation, World Health Organization, Geneva, 2006Environmental Burden of Disease Series No. 13

[59] D.E. Godar, S.J. Pope, W.B. Grant, M.F. Holick, Solar UV doses of young Americans and vitamin D$_3$ production, Environ. Health Perspect. 120 (2012) 139–143.

[60] S. Arunabh, S. Pollack, J. Yeh, J.F. Aloia, Body fat content and 25-hydroxyvitamin D levels in healthy women, J. Clin. Endocrinol. Metab. 88 (2003) 157–161.

[61] J. Wortsman, L.Y. Matsuoka, T.C. Chen, Z. Lu, M.F. Holick, Decreased bioavailability of vitamin D in obesity, Am. J. Clin. Nutr. 72 (2000) 690–693.

[62] Looker, A. C., Johnson, C. L., Lacher, D. A., Pfeiffer, C. M., Schleicher, R. L., and Sempos, C. T. (2011). "Vitamin D Status: United States, 2001–2006," NCHS Data Brief No 59. National Center for Health Statistics,Hyattsville, MD. Available at <http://www.cdc.gov/nchs/data/databriefs/db59.pdf/>, Accessed September 2011.

[63] A.C. Looker, B. Dawson-Hughes, M.S. Calvo, E.W. Gunter, N. R. Sahyoun, Serum 25-hydroxyvitamin D status of adolescents and adults in two seasonal subpopulations from NHANES III, Bone 30 (2002) 771–777.

[64] H.A Bischoff-Ferrari, E. Giovannucci, W.C. Willett, T. Dietrich, B. Dawson-Hughes, Estimation of optimal serum concentrations of 25-hydroxyvitamin D for multiple health outcomes, Am. J. Clin. Nutr. 84 (2006) 18–28.

[65] B.W. Hollis, R.L. Horst, The assessment of circulating 25(OH)D and 1,25(OH)2D: where are we and where are we going? J. Steroid Biochem. Mol. Biol. 103 (2007) 473–476.

[66] P. Lips, T. Duong, A. Oleksik, D. Black, S. Cummings, D. Cox, et al., A global study of vitamin D status and parathyroid function in postmenopausal women with osteoporosis: baseline data from the Multiple Outcomes of Raloxifene Evaluation clinical trial, J. Clin. Endocrinol. Metab. 86 (2001) 1212–1221.

[67] M. Pfeifer, B. Bergow, H. Minne, Vitamin D and muscle function, Osteoporos. Int. 13 (2002) 187–194.

[68] C. Paterson, Vitamin D deficiency: A diagnosis often missed, Br. J. Hosp. Med. 72 (2011) 456–462.

[69] M. Preimel, C. von Domarcus, T.O. Klatte, S. Kessler, J. Schlie, S. Meir, et al., Bone mineralization defects and vitamin D deficiency: Histomorphometric analysis of iliac crest bone biopsies and circulating 25-hydroxyvitamin D in 675 patients, J. Bone Miner. Res. 25 (2010) 305–312.

[70] F.B. Herm, H. Killguss, A.G. Stewart, Osteomalacia in Hazara District, Pakistan, Trop. Doct. 35 (2005) 8–10.

[71] M.F. Holick, E.S. Siris, N. Binkley, M.K. Beard, A. Khan, J.T. Katzer, et al., Prevalence of vitamin D inadequacy among postmenopausal North American women receiving osteoporosis therapy, J. Clin. Endocrinol. Metab. 90 (2005) 3215–3224.

[72] A. Cranney, T. Horsley, S. O'Donnell, H. Weiler, L. Puil, D. Ooi, et al., Effectiveness and safety of vitamin D in relation to bone health, Evid. Rep. Technol. Assess. (2007) 1–235.

[73] R.M. Daly, M. Brown, S. Bass, S. Kukuljian, C. Nowson, Calcium- and vitamin D_3-fortified milk reduces bone loss at clinically relevant skeletal sites in older men: a 2-year randomized controlled trial, J. Bone Miner. Res. 21 (2006) 397–405.

[74] H.A. Bischoff-Ferrari, W.C. Willett, J.B. Wong, E. Giovannucci, T. Dietrich, B. Dawson Hughes, Fracture prevention with vitamin D supplementation: a meta-analyses of randomized controlled trials, J. Am. Med. Assoc. 293 (2005) 2257–2264.

[75] C. Jackson, S.S. Gaugris, D. Hosking, The effect of cholecalciferol (vitamin D_3) on the risk of fall and fracture: a meta-analysis, Q. J. Med. 100 (2007) 185–192.

[76] M. Holick, Vitamin D: extraskeletal health, Endocrinol. Metabol. Clin. 39 (2010) 381–400.

[77] E.D. Gorham, C.F. Garland, F.C. Garland, W.B. Grant, S.B. Mohr, M. Lipkin, et al., Vitamin D and prevention of colorectal cancer, J. Steroid. Biochem. Mol. Biol. 97 (2005) 179–194.

[78] S.B. Mohr, E.D. Gorham, J.E. Alcaraz, C.J. Kane, C.A. Macera, J.K. Parsons, et al., Serum 25-hydroxyvitamin D and prevention of breast cancer: pooled analysis, Anticancer Res. 31 (2011) 2939–2948.

[79] J.M. Lappe, D. Travers-Gustafson, K.M. Davies, R.R. Recker, R. P. Heaney, Vitamin D and calcium supplementation reduces cancer risk: results of a randomized trial, Am. J. Clin. Nutr. 85 (2007) 1586–1591.

[80] E. Giovannucci, Y. Liu, W. Willett, Cancer incidence and mortality and vitamin D in black and white male health professionals. Cancer Epidemiol, Biomarkers Prev. 15 (2006) 2467–2472.

[81] W.B. Grant, A meta-analysis of second cancers after a diagnosis of nonmelanoma skin cancer: additional evidence that solar ultraviolet-B irradiance reduces the risk of internal cancers, J. Steroid Biochem. Mol. Biol. 103 (2007) 668–674.

[82] C. Mathieu, C. Gysemans, A. Giulietti, R. Bouillon, Vitamin D and diabetes, Diabetologia 48 (2005) 1247–1257.

[83] A. Pittas, J. Lau, F. Hu, B. Dawson-Hughes, The role of vitamin D and calcium in type 2 diabetes: a systematic review and meta-analysis, J. Clin. Endocrinol. Metab. 92 (2007) 2017–2029.

[84] A.G. Pittas, S.S. Harris, P.C. Stark, B. Dawson-Hughes, Vitamin D and type 2 diabetes: a systematic review, Eur. J. Clin. Nutr. 65 (2011) 1005–1015.

[85] A. Ascherio, K.L. Munger, K.C. Simon, Vitamin D and multiple sclerosis, Lancet Neurol. 9 (2010) 599–612.

[86] M.K. Turner, W.M. Hooten, J.E. Schmidt, J.L. Kerkvliet, C.O. Townsend, B.K. Bruce, Prevalence and clinical correlates of vitamin D inadequacy among patients with chronic pain, Pain Med. 9 (2008) 979–984.

[87] J.D. Goldsmith, A. Covic, D. Fouque, F. Locatelli, K. Olgaard, M. Rodriguez, et al., Endorsement of the Kidney Disease Improving Global Outcomes (KDIGO) Chronic Kidney Disease–Mineral and Bone Disorder (CKD-MBD) Guidelines: a European Renal Best Practice (ERBP) commentary statement, Nephrol. Dial. Transplant. 25 (2010) 3823–3831.

[88] E.A. Gonzales, A. Sachdeva, D.A. Oliver, K.J. Martin, Vitamin D insufficiency and deficiency in chronic kidney disease: a single center observation study, Am. J. Nephrol. 24 (2004) 503–510.

[89] R.E. LaClair, R.N. Hellman, S.L. Karp, M. Kraus, S. Ofner, Q. Li, et al., Prevalence of calcidiol deficiency in CKD: a cross-sectional study across latitudes in the United States, Am. J. Kidney Dis. 45 (2005) 1026–1033.

[90] J. Deville, M.L. Thorp, L. Tobin, E. Gray, E.S. Johnson, D.H. Smith, Effect of ergocalciferol supplementation on serum parathyroid hormone and serum 25-hydroxyvitmain D in chronic kidney disease, Nephrology 11 (2006) 555–559.

[91] A.L. Zisman, M. Hrisrova, L.T. Ho, S.M. Sprague, Impact of ergocalciferol treatment of vitamin D deficiency on serum parathyroid hormone concentrations in chronic kidney disease, Nephrology 27 (2007) 36–43.

[92] M. Chonchol, R. Scragg, 25-Hydroxyvitamin D, insulin resistance, and kidney function in the Third National Health and Nutrition Examination Survey, Kidney Int 71 (2007) 134–139.

[93] M.F. Holick, Vitamin D for health and in chronic kidney disease, Semin. Dial. 18 (2005) 266–275.

[94] S. Pilz, A. Tomaschitz, W. März, C. Drechsler, E. Ritz, A. Zittermann, et al., Vitamin D, cardiovascular disease and mortality, Clin. Endocrinol. (Oxford). 75 (2011) 575–584.

[95] A. Zittermann, S.S. Schleitoff, R. Koerfer, Putting cardiovascular disease and vitamin D insufficiency into perspective, Br. J. Nutr. 94 (2005) 483–492.

[96] S.S. Schleithoff, A. Zitterman, G. Tenderich, H.K. Berthold, P. Stehle, R. Koerfer, Vitamin D supplementation improves cytokine profiles in patients with congestive heart failure: A double-blind, randomized, placebo-controlled trial, Am. J. Clin. Nutr. 83 (2006) 754–759.

[97] U.S. Food and Drug Administration, Center for Drug Evaluation and Research. "Drugs." Available at <http://www.fda.gov/cder/index.html/>, (2011)Accessed September 2011.

[98] R.M. Sayre, J.C. Dowdy, J.G. Shepherd, Reintroduction of a classic vitamin D ultraviolet source, J. Steroid Biochem. Mol. Biol. 103 (2007) 686–688.

[99] I. Reid, A. Avenell, Evidence-based policy on dietary calcium and vitamin D, J. Bone Miner. Res. 26 (2011) 452–454.

[100] R. Heaney, M. Holick, Why the IOM recommendations for vitamin D are deficient, J. Bone Miner. Res. 26 (2011) 455–457.

[101] J.J. Otten, J.P. Hellwig, L.D. Meyers, Dietary Reference Intakes: the Essential Guide to Nutrient Requirements, National Academies Press, Washington, DC, 2006.

[102] R. Vieth, H. Bischoff-Ferrari, B.J. Boucher, B. Dawson-Hughes, C.F. Garland, R.P. Heaney, et al., The urgent need to recommend an intake of vitamin D that is effective, Am. J. Clin. Nutr. 85 (2007) 649–650.

[103] M.A. Johnson, M.G. Kimlin, Vitamin D, aging, and the 2005 Dietary Guidelines for Americans, Nutr. Rev. 64 (2006) 410–421.

[104] S.J. Whiting, M.S. Calvo, Correcting vitamin D deficiency: do older adults need higher repletion doses of vitamin D_3 than younger adults?, Mol. Nutr. Food Res. 54 (2010) 1077–1084.

[105] P. Weisberg, K.S. Scanlon, R. Li, M.E. Cogswell, Nutritional rickets among children in the United States: review of cases reported between 1986 and 2003, Am. J. Clin. Nutr. 80 (2004) 1697S–1705S.

[106] N.F. Carvalho, R.D. Kenney, P.H. Carrington, D.E. Hall, Severe nutritional deficiencies in toddlers resulting from health food milk alternatives, Pediatrics 107 (2001) 1–7.

[107] Canadian Pediatric Society reaffirmed October 2010.Vitamin D supplementation: Recommendations for Canadian mothers and infants. Paediatr. Child Health (2007)**12**,583–589.

[108] C.L. Wagner, T.C. Hulsey, D. Fanning, M. Ebeling, B.W. Hollis, High-dose vitamin D_3 supplementation in a cohort of breast-feeding mothers and their infants: a 6-month follow-up pilot study, Breastfeeding Med. 1 (2006) 59–70.

[109] B.W. Hollis, D. Johnson, T.C. Hulsey, M. Ebeling, C.L. Wagner, Vitamin D supplementation during pregnancy: Double blind, randomized clinical trial of safety and effectiveness, J. Bone Miner. Res. 26 (2011) 2341–2357.

[110] J.N. Hathcock, A. Shao, R. Vieth, R.P. Heaney, Risk assessment for vitamin D, Am. J. Clin. Nutr. 85 (2007) 6–18.

[111] K.M. Sanders, A.L. Stuart, E.J. Williamson, J.A. Simpson, M.A. Kotowicz, D. Young, et al., Annual high-dose oral vitamin D and falls and fractures in older women: a randomized controlled trial, J. Am. Med. Assoc. 303 (2010) 1815–1822.

[112] B. Dawson-Hughes, S.S. Harris, High-dose vitamin D supplementation: too much of a good thing? J. Am. Med. Assoc. 303 (2010) 1861–1862.

Osteoporosis: The Early Years

Connie M. Weaver, Kathleen M. Hill

Purdue University, West Lafayette, Indiana

I INTRODUCTION

The risk of developing osteoporosis is largely determined by the mass and size of bone acquired by adulthood known as peak bone mass [1]. The greater the skeletal mass at its peak and the stronger the geometry, the greater the amount of loss that can occur before entering the fracture risk zone. An interplay between heritable factors and environmental factors determines peak bone mass (Figure 44.1). It is estimated that genetics contributes 60—80% and lifestyle factors contribute the remaining 20—40% [2,3]. Genes that control growth and development are thought to also largely determine bone acquisition [2].

Nutrition and physical activity are the primary lifestyle determinants of bone acquisition, and increasing evidence suggests that the interactions between these two are stronger determinants than either alone. Nutrition plays an important role in preventing osteoporosis through building optimal peak bone mass within one's genetic potential. This chapter reviews the influence of diet and nutrients on bone health and the basis of requirements for nutrients that are based on skeletal health. Nutrition likely can also play a role in fracture risk during childhood. Skeletal fragility in childhood occurs when bone mineral density (BMD), as assessed by dual-energy x-ray absorptiometry (DXA), expressed as a Z-score is less than −2.0 [4]. Skeletal fragility can arise from a lag between peak height velocity and bone mineralization during the pubertal growth spurt or as a consequence of eating disorders or disease. Less is known about the role of diet in the context of pediatric disorders, and research is needed to address these gaps.

This chapter focuses on the development of peak bone mass and the role of nutrition in bone acquisition. The reader should consult the companion chapter by Marcus (Chapter 45) for a discussion of osteoporosis and bone qualities.

II ACQUIRING PEAK BONE MASS AND BONE STRENGTH

Understanding the timing for an effective nutritional intervention can be as important as the nature of the intervention. Textbooks commonly cite that bone mass is acquired throughout the third decade of life and frequently quote a longitudinal study that averaged annual bone gains over a decade, ignoring the fact that the rate of accrual decreased over time and became trivial by age 30 years [5]. In a metabolic balance study, women older than age 21 years were not in positive calcium retention on intakes of 1300 mg calcium per day [6]. Increase in BMD with age depends on the skeletal site. For total body BMD, 95% of adult peak bone mass was achieved by age 16.2 years and 99% was achieved by age 22.1 years [7]. Peak BMD in white women occurred at age 23 years for the spine, 18.5 years for the femoral neck, 14.2 years for the greater trochanter, and 15.8 years for Ward's triangle [8] (Figure 44.2). Clearly, to markedly influence peak bone mass, lifestyle practices are more important prior to the end of puberty than post adolescence.

When there are transient periods during which diet is inadequate, some catch-up growth is possible [9]. In a calcium-supplemented controlled trial from early puberty until development of peak bone mass in girls habitually consuming on average 830 mg calcium per day, calcium supplementation increased accrual of BMD of total body (Figure 44.3) and radius through puberty compared to the placebo group [10]. However, by age 18 years, the advantage was reduced. There was an interaction with size such that girls who were taller

Nutrition in the Prevention and Treatment of Disease, Third Edition.
DOI: http://dx.doi.org/10.1016/B978-0-12-391884-0.00044-5

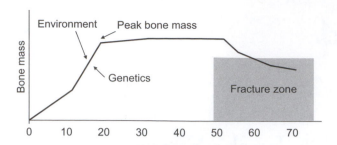

FIGURE 44.1 Bone mass throughout the life span. The influence of genetics and the environment is greatest during growth.

by age 18 years did not fully catch up. The extent of catch-up growth undoubtedly depends on the degree of inadequacy of the diet, the timing and duration of the period of inadequacy, and the degree of repletion. Regardless, the period of inadequacy is itself a period of vulnerability—that is, in this example, a higher risk of fracture.

The impact of genetics on development of peak bone mass is evident in Figure 44.3. The light gray lines show tracking of total body BMD of 15 representative individuals. Those who began the trial with lower BMD remained lower throughout development of peak bone mass. Modifications through lifestyle choices occur within one's genetic potential.

Bone geometry plays an additional role beyond bone mass in resistance to fracture. Bone geometry includes dimensions of bone such as length and cross-sectional area. The relationship of bone geometry to fracture risk in childhood and measurement by peripheral quantitative computed tomography has been described by Kalkwarf [11]. The effect of diet on bone geometry is a rather recent field of study because of the relative newness of this technique. The exercise intervention trials that have used this outcome measure have illustrated additional information gained about bone strength.

III SKELETAL FRAGILITY IN CHILDREN

Fractures in children are associated with low bone mass and density for age [12]. If low bone mass in childhood leads to lower peak bone mass in adulthood, the risk of fracture increases later in life. Relative skeletal fragility can occur naturally with growth spurts. Beyond genetically programmed qualities, bone mass and density throughout life are influenced primarily by nutrition, physical activity, and hormones. Furthermore, eating disorders, smoking, alcohol abuse, and various drugs also influence bone mass. To a large extent, these factors work independently in that one cannot compensate for inadequacy of another. However, dietary calcium and physical

activity have important interactions. Finally, some disorders are associated with low BMD.

A Relatively Low BMD during Puberty

Puberty is a period of rapid skeletal growth that is genetically programmed and hormonally driven. The rate of total body bone mass accrual throughout adolescence was determined by Bailey *et al.* in a longitudinal study of white boys and girls [13]. From this study, we know that approximately 25% of adult peak bone mass is acquired over approximately 2 years—on average this occurs from age 12 to 14 years in girls and age 13 to 15 years in boys. Peak bone mineral content velocity is higher and occurs later for boys than for girls. The timing of bone mineral acquisition is more closely linked to pubertal development than to chronological age [2,13].

During puberty, bones first elongate and then mineralization, or bone consolidation, ensues. At the age of peak height velocity, adolescents have acquired 90% of their adult height (or bone size) but only 60% of adult total body bone mineral content (BMC). Thus, early puberty is a period of relatively low BMD and, therefore, susceptibility to fracture not unlike that of age-related bone loss [14–16]. The higher incidence of fracture during this time of life corresponding to the lower BMD in the study by Bailey *et al.* [13] is shown in Figure 44.4. Approximately 51% of boys and 40% of girls experience fractures by age 18 years [16].

The dramatic increase in rates of childhood fracture in the United States during the past three decades is apparent in Figure 44.5. Fracture incidence increased 32% in males, with the greatest increase at age 11–14 years, and 56% in girls, with the greatest increase at age 8–11 years. Increased rates of childhood fracture may relate to reduced consumption of milk, change in physical activity or recreational activities, and/or increased body weight during this time period. The prevalence of excessive adiposity in children and adolescents has nearly tripled while the incidence of fracture has increased [19]. In adults, increased weight has been associated with increased bone mass [20], but overweight children and adolescents have higher rates of fracture [12,21,22]. The increased incidence in fracture with excessive body weight in children has been hypothesized to occur because of greater force being placed on bones such as the radius during falls, lower bone mass and bone strength with increasing body fat when adjusted for total body weight, and impaired mobility [21,23–28]. The interaction between calcium intake and body mass index is described later. Changes in bone geometry that accompany increases in bone size throughout childhood include increases in cortical thickness and bone diameter [29].

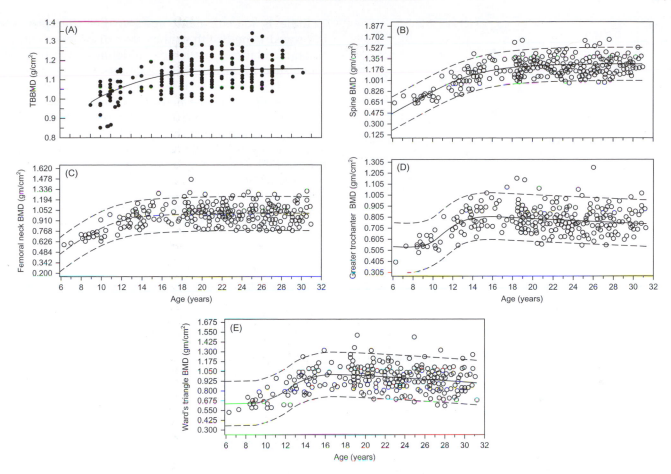

FIGURE 44.2 Bone mineral density accumulation with age in females. Gains in bone mineral density (BMD) vary with skeletal site. Almost 95% of adult peak total body BMD occurred by age 15.2 years (A), and the highest BMD of the spine occurs by age 23 years (B), by age 18.5 years for the femoral neck (C), by age 14.2 years for the greater trochanter (D), and by age 15.8 years for Ward's triangle (E). *Reproduced from Teegarden* et al.*[7] and Lin* et al.*[8].)*

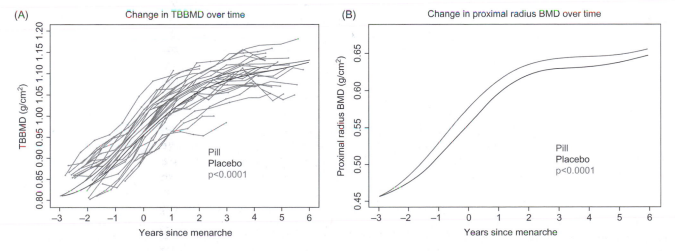

FIGURE 44.3 Total body BMD (A) and proximal radius (B) was significantly higher in prepubertal girls randomized to 1 g calcium supplement daily compared to those assigned to placebo from age 10 to 18 years [15].

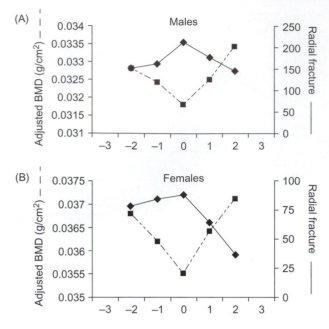

FIGURE 44.4 Distal radius fracture incidence for (A) boys and (B) girls from local hospital admissions compared with the total body BMD adjusted for body size aligned by biological age (years from peak height velocity) from the Bailey *et al.* study [13]. *Adapted from Faulkner et al. [17] with permission.*

Bone diameter and cortical thickness are less in children with excess body fat [28]. This emphasizes the need to maintain ideal body weight in children.

B Disorders Associated with Low Bone Mass

A number of disorders have been associated with low bone mass in children (Table 44.1).

Skeletal health should be evaluated with diagnosis of these disorders. If skeletal fragility develops, bone fractures can occur with minimal or no trauma, a condition known as osteoporosis. The ability to reverse bone deficits with early diagnosis and treatment remains uncertain.

Amenorrhea most often results from excessive exercise or energy intakes too low to sustain physiologic levels of estrogen. Anorexia nervosa is an eating disorder characterized by intense fear of gaining weight or becoming fat. In this condition, body weight is less than 86% of normal for height and age. Reduction in bone gains or acceleration of bone loss resulting in low BMD for age can occur with anorexia nervosa [31]. Osteoporosis that develops as a result of anorexia nervosa is more severe than with other causes of estrogen deficiency. Girls with anorexia nervosa had lower fat and energy intakes than did girls without anorexia nervosa [31]. Severity of low bone mass (i.e., osteopenia) is worse if the eating disorder is initiated in adolescence than in adulthood and worse for a longer duration [32].

Little is known about specific diet therapies and improved bone health in the other disorders. Nutrient recommendations or dietary guidelines have not been established for any of these disorders for lowering risk of low bone mass. It is logical that recovery of low body weight would be helpful to bone. Some interesting associations suggest that future research may show a benefit for nutritional therapies. For example, vitamin K deficiency is prevalent among children with cystic fibrosis [33].

IV NUTRITION AND DEVELOPMENT OF PEAK BONE MASS

The role of diet in development of peak bone mass is thought to have a great impact on risk of osteoporosis [1]. The formative years set the foundation for the skeletal reserves and for lifelong eating and exercise habits. In fact, osteoporosis has been called a pediatric disease. This chapter approaches the role of diet under two themes: diet patterns and individual nutrients. So much of the research base has focused on individual nutrients that supplementation with calcium and vitamin D has become a first-line strategy of prevention and therapy. Although calcium and vitamin D are the two nutrients important to bone most likely to be deficient, this reductionist approach to research and medical nutrition therapy aimed at building strong bones is woefully inadequate. Dietitians can play a critical role in assessing the overall diet and making recommendations that will have greater impact on body weight and health than simply recommending supplements. To understand the quality of the evidence behind public health recommendations related to bone health, a discussion of the limitations of our research designs and measures is warranted.

A Limitation in Methodology

Whether interpreting the effects of diet patterns or individual nutrients on bone, the limitations of investigation of nutritional effects on bone should be appreciated. Difficulty in assessing diet and individual nutrient consumption is not unique to studies of bone and is discussed elsewhere in this book. To quantitatively determine the effect of intake of a nutrient or diet pattern is best accomplished through controlled feeding studies. However, to control diets for sufficiently long periods for bone properties to change is not practical except in animal studies. Although changes in bone properties occur faster in pediatric studies than in studies of adults, it still requires a year or several years to evaluate the magnitude of the effect

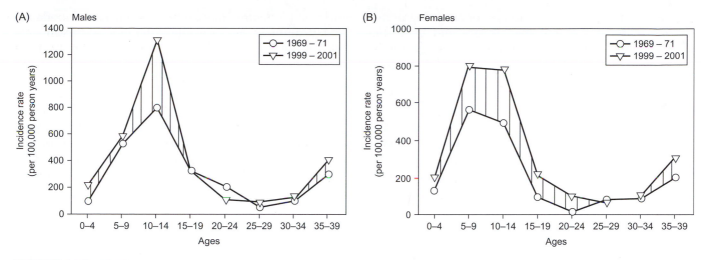

FIGURE 44.5 Childhood forearm fracture incidence in males (A) and females (B) from 1969–1971 (lower line) and 1999–2001 (upper line) in Rochester, Minnesota. *Reproduced from Heaney and Weaver [18] using data from Khosla et al.[14].*

TABLE 44.1 Pediatric Conditions Associated with Low Bone Mass[a]

Amenorrhea
Anorexia nervosa
Brain tumors (craniospinal irradiation)
Celiac disease
Congenital hypothyroidism
Cystic fibrosis
Diabetes mellitus
Epilepsy
Glucocorticoid-sensitive nephrotic syndrome
Hemophilia
HIV/antiretroviral therapy
Inflammatory bowel disease
Liver transplantation
Osteogenesis imperfecta
Renal disease and transplantation
Rheumatologic disease
Turner's syndrome

Source: Derived from Gordon [30].

of interventions on bone. During the first 6 or more months following onset of an intervention, changes in bone reflect the bone remodeling transient [34]. This is a period of adaptation through changes in bone formation rate or bone resorption rate if the intervention is effective. Longer periods are required to determine the effect of the intervention on steady-state bone balance.

In children, changes in bone are relatively rapid during periods of active growth. Often, the major challenge is to distinguish between the effects of intervention and growth [35].

The traditional outcome measures for assessing nutritional effects on bone properties—that is, BMC and BMD—may be altered by 2% or less per year as a result of a nutritional intervention. This magnitude of change is difficult to detect by DXA in short-term studies. However, this level of impact over many years can have a profound effect on risk of fracture. Other changes in bone that can indicate strength, such as bone geometry that can be assessed by three-dimensional imaging, also require substantial intervention periods and, to date, do not offer improved precision over DXA. It is preferable to use BMC rather than BMD as the primary outcome measure to assess efficacy of interventions in children. Effective dietary interventions could augment bone size rather than merely affect the mass of bone per unit volume. Thus, because BMD is calculated to adjust for size, it can miss most of the actual change in bone mass during growth. However, DXA only captures two-dimensional space, and consequently it is somewhat affected by size [36] and can correlate with changes in BMC. Interventions during growth that influence bone mass and bone size have a dramatic influence on bone strength [11]. A number of investigators have attempted to correct DXA measures for bone size, such as calculating bone mineral apparent density, BMC for height, and BMC for bone area, but there is no consensus regarding the best approach [37–39]. Currently, it is recommended to use BMC as the primary outcome, and it is also helpful to measure bone area and other indicators of bone size. Anthropometric measures can be good predictors of BMC in children [40].

Several shorter term approaches for assessing perturbations in bone are available. Serum and urine biochemical markers of bone turnover can determine qualitative changes in bone turnover, but within-subject variation is high [41]. Furthermore, biochemical markers of bone turnover do not measure bone mineral but, rather, measure fragments of collagen in connective tissue that leak into circulation when bone remodels. Thus, the units cannot be converted into units of bone.

Other short-term methods for analyzing perturbations in bone most often measure calcium as a surrogate for bone. Calcium is a good surrogate for bone because it is present in a fixed proportion of bone mineral. By multiplying bone mineral content determined from DXA by the fraction 0.31, one can derive calcium content in grams. Calcium levels in the blood are not a good indicator of calcium/bone status because they are tightly controlled within a narrow range. Short-term changes in bone balance can be estimated from calcium balance studies. During growth, bone balance is positive. The use of calcium balance studies to determine requirements and response to an intervention has been described [42]. In children, adaptation to a new calcium intake requires approximately 1 week before balance is determined. Calcium isotopic tracers can be used to measure all components of calcium metabolism [42–44]. Combining calcium balance studies and use of oral and intravenous tracers of calcium can provide the data for compartmental modeling whereby determination rates of transport of calcium in and out of pools and the mass of each pool are possible.

B Dietary Patterns and Bone Health

When formulating recommendations for food patterns for different subgroups, the 2010 Dietary Guidelines Advisory Committee for Americans considered bone health [45]. The food patterns were designed to meet nutrient recommendations including bone-related nutrients. The evidence for a relationship between milk and milk products and bone health was also reviewed in determining quantities to recommend for optimal health. In addition to getting adequate nutrients and milk products, the committee considered dietary habits detrimental to health, especially with regard to energy excess but also for bone health. Dietary patterns as they influence acid–base balance may also play a role in bone health.

1 Milk and Milk Products

The *Dietary Guidelines for Americans* includes 2 cups of milk or milk product daily for children ages 2–8 years and 3 cups after age 8 years [45]. The amount of milk was set to help meet requirements for several nutrients, including calcium, magnesium, potassium, riboflavin, and vitamin D. Milk products provide approximately 50–79% of the calcium in the diets for children in the food patterns for age and gender recommended by the Dietary Guidelines Advisory Committee. The milk group also provides more than 10% of the nutrients in the pattern for riboflavin, vitamin B_{12}, vitamin A, thiamin, vitamin B_{12}, phosphorus, magnesium, zinc, potassium, protein, and carbohydrate. If milk products are excluded from the patterns, intake for calcium falls below 64% for all children and below 33% for young children; it also falls below 88% for magnesium—as low as 33% for some age groups [45]. Alternatives to milk products given in the Dietary Guidelines Advisory Committee report were low-lactose milk products [45]. Although some fortified foods, such as calcium-fortified soy milk, have nutrient profiles similar to that of milk, it is difficult to meet calcium and potassium requirements without milk. Milk product consumption has been associated with overall diet quality. Adequacy of milk intake has been associated with adequacy of calcium, potassium, magnesium, zinc, iron, riboflavin, vitamin A, folate, and vitamin D for children [46].

Many calcium-fortified foods are on the market that could theoretically be used to provide the requirements for this nutrient. Gao *et al.* [47] evaluated the ability of dairy-free diets to meet calcium intake while meeting other nutrient requirements using diets in U.S. children aged 9–18 years for those participants in NHANES 2001–2002 who reported no intake of dairy. Calcium requirements were not met without use of calcium-fortified foods, and only one child accomplished this. Average calcium intake without dairy products was 498 mg/day for girls and 480 mg/day for boys compared to 866 and 1070 mg/day, respectively, with dairy products. At calcium intakes of approximately 400 mg/day, calcium retention was only 131 mg/day compared to almost three times that much if the adequate intake for calcium is met [48]. Milk intervention trials in children have shown increased bone mass compared to that of control groups [49,50]. Interestingly, in trials in children using milk as the intervention, the positive effects of treatment were maintained after the intervention ceased [51,52], in contrast to several trials that used calcium supplements as the intervention [53,54]. In a longitudinal study of 151 white girls, dairy product/calcium intake at age 9 years was associated with total body BMD gain from age 9 to 11 years [55]. Milk avoiders have increased risk for prepubertal bone fractures [56]. Retrospective studies have shown that the incidence of postmenopausal fracture is inversely related to drinking milk in childhood [57,58]. In the nationally representative NHANES database, the incidence of hip fracture was twice as high for those who consumed one glass of milk or less per week compared to those who consumed at least one serving per day during childhood [57].

Milk consumption in children has declined over time. In the Bogalusa Heart Study, during the two decades from 1972 to 1994, average milk consumption by 10-year-olds declined by an average of 64 g [59]. Fluid milk consumption was negatively correlated with soft drink consumption, which had a detrimental effect on bone gain in girls [60]. The displacement of milk with soft drinks removes a rich package of nutrients from the diet.

2 Plants Versus Animal-Based Diets

The mix of animal- and plant-derived foods in the diet of an individual influences two postulated determinants of bone health—acid—base balance and amount of protein. Although dietary protein is a nutrient, because the type of protein influences acid—base balance, dietary protein is discussed in this section on dietary patterns. Intake of fruits and vegetables also influences the acid—base balance.

The role of the type and amount of proteins in bone health has been studied for several decades, but little work has been done in children. Alkaline dietary salts contain the cations K^+, Ca^{2+}, and Mg^{2+}, which act as buffers for organic acids produced during metabolism and hepatic oxidation of S-containing amino acids that would otherwise lower blood pH. Increased metabolic acidosis has been associated with increased bone resorption in cell culture systems [61] and increased urinary calcium excretion in humans [62]. Bone is thought to serve as a reservoir of buffering capacity due to the carbonate and hydroxyapatite salts. Typical acid loads produced on a Western diet are on the order of 1 mEq of acid/kg/day. Investigators have attempted to estimate the renal acid load of diets as a measure of acid—base load by taking into account the mineral and protein composition of foods [63]. Thus, diets high in fruits and vegetables that contain potassium and produce an alkaline ash and those richer in plant proteins than animal proteins, which contribute more S-containing amino acids, have been promoted for better bone health through improving acid—base balance. A high ratio of dietary animal to vegetable protein intake has been associated with increased rates of bone loss and increased risk of fracture [64].

The hypothesis that increasing dietary protein or animal versus plant proteins or even acid—base balance influences bone has been challenged. Bonjour [65] argues that bone is unlikely to be the main source of buffering acid loads because bone mineral is not in direct contact with systemic circulation. Rather, buffering of acid loads is accomplished through elimination of carbon dioxide by the lungs and hydrogen ions by the kidney. The increased urinary calcium with increased protein intake generally, or S-containing amino acids specifically, is offset by, and in fact is due to, increased calcium absorption with no increase in bone resorption or net differences in calcium retention [66,67]. Increased dietary potassium does reduce urinary calcium excretion, but this did not appear to affect calcium balance because calcium absorption was also reduced as dietary potassium increased [68]. Intake of fruits, vegetables, and herbs does inhibit bone resorption, but this effect is independent of their alkali or potassium contributions [69].

There is evidence that adequate dietary protein promotes bone accrual in children. In an 18-month randomized controlled trial (RCT) in which 12-year-old girls consumed a pint of milk a day, an increase in total body BMD was associated with an increase in serum insulin-like growth factor-1 (IGF-1) [70]. The relation between protein intake and bone gains in lumbar spine and femoral neck in 193 subjects ages 9—19 years was positive, particularly in prepubertal children [71]. An interesting hypothesis has been put forth that aromatic amino acid intake may induce an increase in calcium absorption and serum IGF-1 compared with branched-chain amino acids through activation of calcium sensor receptors in the gut to increase gastric acid production [72].

A study that related biomarkers of diet over 4 years to bone strength in children indicated that both anabolic and catabolic actions influenced bone strength [73]. Urinary nitrogen reflecting protein intake was positively associated with BMD and measures of bone size. Conversely, potential renal acid load (PRAL) was negatively associated with BMC and cortical area. Dietary protein contributes to PRAL.

3 Salt

Dietary salt is the largest dietary predictor of urinary calcium excretion [74]. However, the response of adolescents to dietary salt is racially dependent. In controlled feeding studies using a crossover design with high (4 g, 172 mmol) and low (1.3 g, 5.7 mmol) sodium diets, white adolescent girls excreted more sodium on a high-salt diet than did black girls of matched weight and sexual maturity [75]. Because calcium is excreted with sodium through the shared transport proteins in the kidney, high-salt diets resulted in more calcium excretion and lower calcium retention in white girls than in black girls in the same study [76]. Thus, a high intake of dietary salt is detrimental to growing bone, but the consequences to bone are greater for white than black individuals.

C Individual Nutrients and Bone Health

Calcium is by far the most studied single nutrient related to bone health. Vitamin D is the focus of much current research. These two nutrients are the most likely ones of those important to bone health to be deficient. It should be understood that because bone is a living tissue, all essential nutrients are required for bone growth.

1 Calcium

A CURRENT RECOMMENDED REQUIREMENTS AND THEIR BASIS

Current recommended dietary allowances (RDAs) and upper levels (ULs) for calcium vitamin D, phosphorus, and magnesium are given in Table 44.2 [77].

Calcium requirements can be determined by using the factorial approach (replacement of losses through urine, stools, and skin adjusted for absorption) or by estimating the intake for maximal calcium retention. The 2010 panel used the factorial approach [77] and the 1997 panel used the intake for maximal retention approach where possible [78], but recommended intakes for most age groups by both panels were the same.

Determining calcium intakes for maximal calcium retention requires studies on a range of calcium intakes. The RCTs described next studied only two levels of calcium intake—that of the self-selected diet or one's dietary intake plus the calcium intervention source. One can assess whether calcium supplementation is effective with this study design, but it is not possible to determine an optimal intake. It would be desirable to estimate bone accretion over a range of calcium intakes in different age groups, but this would require large, expensive studies. Instead, data on calcium retention at different calcium intakes are available from short-term controlled-feeding studies in which composites of diet and complete urine and stool collections are analyzed for calcium so that calcium retention or balance (intake − loss from urine, stools, and sometimes sweat) can be calculated. As calcium intakes increase, calcium retention increases until a plateau intake is reached at which further calcium intakes are excreted. A comparison of calcium retention as a function of intake between boys and girls is shown in Figure 44.6 [79]. Although boys retained more calcium at a given level of calcium intake than did girls, the calcium intake at which retention was not further significantly increased did not differ by gender. Similarly, black girls had higher calcium retention across a range of calcium intakes without different slopes [80]. Thus, boys are more efficient than girls in using calcium, and blacks are more efficient than whites, which results in higher bone mass as adults; however, the need for calcium to produce skeletons of greater bone mass is not detectably different over short periods. Asian girls are also more efficient than white girls in retaining calcium across a range of calcium intakes [81].

B CALCIUM AND BODY MASS INDEX

There is an interaction between calcium intake and body mass index (BMI) on calcium retention. Figure 44.7 illustrates this relationship for white 12-year-old girls [82]. As BMI increases, skeletal calcium accretion increases, but only if calcium intakes are adequate to provide the necessary structural materials. Without adequate dietary calcium, insufficient calcium is retained

TABLE 44.2　Dietary Reference Intakes for Bone-Related Nutrients in Children and Adolescents

	Nutrient							
	Calcium (mg/day)		Vitamin D (µg/day)[a]		Phosphorus (mg/day)		Magnesium (mg/day)	
Life-stage group	RDA	UL	RDA	UL	RDA	UL	RDA	UL
0−6 months	200[b]	ND	10	25	100[b]	ND	30[b]	ND
7−12 months	260[b]	ND	10	37	275[a]	ND	75	ND
1−3 years	700	2500	15	62.5	460	3000	80	65[b]
4−8 years	1000	2500	15	75	500	3000	130	110[c]
9−13 years	1300	3000	15	100	1250	4000	240	
14−18 years	1300	3000	15	100	1250	4000		
Females							350[c]	350[c]
Males							350[c]	350[c]

[a] 10 µg = 400 IU.
[b] Adequate intake.
[c] Supplementary, not in food.
ND, not determined; RDA, recommended dietary allowance; UL, upper level.

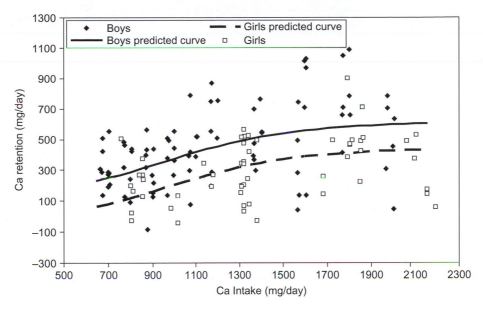

FIGURE 44.6 Calcium retention as a function of calcium intake in adolescent boys (upper curve) and girls (lower curve) [79].

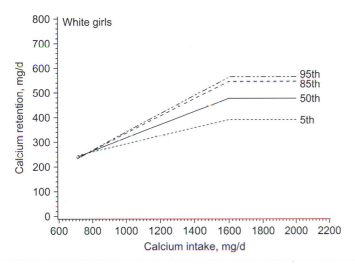

FIGURE 44.7 Influence of BMI (as percentiles of BMI-for-age) on calcium retention curve in white 12-year-old girls [82].

to build enough skeletal mass appropriate for body weight, which may explain the doubling of fractures shown in Figure 44.5.

C EVIDENCE FOR RELATIONSHIP TO BONE

There is a large body of evidence from RCTs of calcium intake in children that have reported positive effects on one or more skeletal sites (Table 44.3). Intervention studies have used calcium salts, calcium-fortified foods, and milk with a variety of bone outcomes. Cheese was more effective than calcium carbonate at increasing tibial cortical thickness [94]. A meta-analysis of 19 RCTs reported that the effect of

calcium supplementation on bone was modest and effective only on upper limbs [96]. However, this meta-analysis was criticized [97] for use of BMD as the outcome for evaluation rather than BMC for reasons already discussed. The authors rebutted that BMD correlates reasonably well with fracture risk in children [98].

Retaining a high-calcium intake during growth for optimizing peak bone mass is prudent. The limitations of our methodologies contribute to lack of clarity, but several observations support the importance of adequate dietary calcium and bone development during childhood. Retrospective studies showing a benefit of childhood consumption of milk reducing fracture incidence later in life offer one example. Also, adequate dietary calcium can have a positive interaction with exercise in young children and adolescents. In one study, the presence of both mechanical loading and adequate calcium was required for increased BMD [99]. In other studies, calcium alone increased bone size, an index of greater bone strength [50,93]. Neither the effects of dietary calcium on bone quality nor potential interactions with physical activity were usually considered in the BMD-based RCTs evaluated in the meta-analysis of Winzenberg *et al.* [96].

One hypothesis to explain the influence of dietary calcium on bone proposed that calcium alters the timing of menarche [100]. Evidence for this possibility came from the RCT of Bonjour *et al.* [50]. The initial trial was a 1-year intervention of calcium-fortified foods in 7.9-year-old girls that showed a positive effect of calcium on mean BMD changes in six skeletal sites. This cohort was followed through age 16.4 years, which allowed determination of the age of menarche

TABLE 44.3 Differences in Mean Changes in Bone Mineral Content and Bone Mineral Density in Calcium Treated Versus Placebo Groups in Randomized, Controlled Trials in Children

Source	Ref. No.	Subj. No.	Age (years)	Sex	Race/location	Length study (months)	Calcium intake, controls (mg/day)	Calcium intake, treatment (mg/day)	Site	Measure	Group mean increase Treatment (T)	Placebo (P)
Johnston et al., 1992	83	140 twins	6–14	F/M	White, IN	36	908	1612	Midshaft radius	BMD	17.7%	15.2%
									Distal radius	BMD	21.5%	18.2%
									Lumbar spine	BMD	20.1%	19.5%
									Femoral neck	BMD	15.3%	14.9%
									Ward's triangle	BMD	15.4%	14.2%
									Greater trochanter	BMD	18.1%	17.11%
Lloyd et al., 1993	84	94	11.9±0.5	F	White, PA	18	960	1314	Total body	BMC	9.6%	8.3%, p = 0.003
									Spine	BMC	2.9%, p = 0.03	4.7%, p = 0.05
Chan et al., 1995	49	48	9–13	F	White, UT	12	728	1437	Total body	BMC	14.2±7.0%	7.6±6.0%, p < 0.001
Lee et al., 1994	85	109	7	F/M	Asian, China	18	571	1363	Lumbar spine	BMD	22.8±6.9%	12.9±8.3%, p < 0.001
									Distal radius	BMC	15.92 (T) vs. 14.95% (P) gain, p = 0.53	
										Area	7.74 (T) vs. 6.00% (P) gain, p = 0.081	
									Lumbar spine	BMC	20.92 (T) vs. 16.34% (P) gain, p = 0.035	
										Area	11.16 (T) vs. 8.71% (P) gain, p = 0.049	
									Proximal femoral neck	BMC	24.19 (T) vs. 23.42% (P) gain, p = 0.37	
Cadogan et al., 1997	70	82	12.2	F	White, Sheffield, UK	18	753	1125	Total body	BMD	9.6 (T) vs. 8.5% (P), p = 0.017	
										BMC	27.0 (T) vs. 24.1% (P), p = 0.009	
Bonjour et al., 1997	50	149	7.9±0.1	F	White, Geneva, CH	12	916	1723	Radial metaphysis	BMD	16±3 (T) vs. 9±2 g/cm² (P), p < 0.08	
Nowson et al., 1997	86	87	10-17	F	White, Australia	18	692	>1600	Spine	BMD	1.62±0.84% (TisP)	

No.	Reference	n	Age	Sex	Population			Duration	Site		Result
87	Dibba et al., 2000	160	8.3–11.9	F/M	Black, Gambia	342	1056	12	Hip	BMD	NS
									Femoral neck	BMD	22±4 (T) vs. 13±4 g/cm² (P)
									Femoral diaphysis	BMD	66±3 (T) vs. 54±4 g/cm² (P), p < 0.01
									Lumbar spine	BMD	25±3 (T) vs. 23±3 g/cm² (P)
									Midshaft radius	BMC	3.0±1.4% (T-P), p = 0.034
										BMD	4.5±0.9% (T-P), p < 0.0001
88	Moyer-Mileur et al., 2003	71	12	F	White, UT	865	1524	12	pQCT of distal tibia	BMC	4.1 (T) vs. 1.6% (P), p < 0.006
										vBMD	1.0 (T) vs. −2.0% (P), p < 0.006
89	Rozen et al., 2003	100	14±0.5	F	85 Jewish/26 Arab, Haifa, Israel	480	1110	12	Total body	BMC	4.63 (T) vs. 4.65 (P), NS
										BMD	3.80 (T) vs. 3.07% (P), p < 0.05
									Lumbar spine	BMD	4.52 (T) vs. 3.95% (P), NS
										BMC	3.66±0.35 vs. 3.00±0.43% (P), p < 0.05
									Femoral neck	BMC	4.30 (T) vs. 3.00% (P), NS
										BMD	2.00 (T) vs. 1.39% (P), NS
90	Stear et al., 2003	144	17.3±0.3	F	Cambridge, UK	938	+1 g Ca supplement	15.5	Whole body	BMC	0.8±0.5% (T vs. P), p < 0.01
									Lumbar spine	BMC	0.9±0.8% (T vs. P), p < 0.001
									Hip	BMC	5.3±1.0% (T vs. P), p < 0.001
91	Cameron et al., 2004	102	10.3±1.5	F	White, Australia	715	+1200	2.4	Total body, lumbar spine, femoral neck, total hip	BMD	NS
92	Mølgaard et al., 2004	113	12–14	F	White, Denmark	2 groups, 1717/1320	2 groups, 953/660	12	Whole body	BMC	0.8% (T vs. P), p = 0.049
											0.5% (T vs. P), p = 0.08
93	Prentice et al., 2005	143	16–18	M	White, UK	1283	1858	13	Whole body	BMC	1.3% (T vs. P), p = 0.02

(Continued)

TABLE 44.3 (*Continued*)

Source	Ref. No.	Subj. No.	Age (years)	Sex	Race/location	Length study (months)	Calcium intake, controls (mg/day)	Calcium intake, treatment (mg/day)	Site	Measure	Group mean increase Treatment (T)	Placebo (P)
									Lumbar spine	BMC	2.5%	(T vs. P), $p = 0.004$
									Total lumbar spine	Bone area	1.5%	(T vs. P), $p = 0.0003$
									Total hip	BMC	23%	(T vs. P), $p = 0.01$
									Femoral neck	BMC	2.4%	(T vs. P), $p = 0.01$
									Intertrochanter	BMC	2.7%	(T vs. P), $p = 0.01$
Matkovic et al., 2005	10	354	10.9±0.9	F	White, OH	48	830	1498	Whole body	BMD	0.215 vs. 0.204 g/cm², $p < 0.0006$	
									Distal radius	BMD	0.106 vs. 0.092 g/cm², $p < 0.0026$	
						84			Whole body	BMD	0.268 vs. 0.263 g/cm², $p < 0.0006$	
									Distal radius	BMD	0.171 vs. 0.165 g/cm², $p < 0.0006$	
Cheng et al., 2005	94	195	10–12	F	White, Finland	24	1566	671	Whole body	BMC	34.7%	35.5%
									Femoral neck	BMC	24.0%	22.4%
									Total femur	BMC	33.6%	33.6%
									Spine	BMC	46.9%	47.0%
									Tibia cortical thickness	pQCT	31.7%	31.1%
Lambert et al., 2008	95	196	11–12	F	United Kingdom	18	636	1174	Whole body	BMC	25.2%	22.9%, $p < 0.001$
										BMD	0.09%	0.07%, $p < 0.001$
									Total hip	BMC	NS	
										BMD	1.14%	0.16%, $p = 0.002$
									Spine	BMC	0.37%	0.32%, $p < 0.01$
										BMD	0.16%	0.14%, $p < 0.001$

BMC, bone mineral content; BMD, bone mineral density; F, female; M, male; NS, not significant; pQCT, peripheral quantitative computed tomography.

and subsequent changes in bone. Interestingly, girls assigned to the calcium intervention for 1 year began menarche earlier than girls assigned to the placebo group [100]. The extra time of exposure to estrogen resulted in more bone gain in subsequent years even though the calcium intervention was discontinued.

D DIETARY CALCIUM

Calcium intake in most diets is predominantly from dairy products—that is, 75% of calcium intake in the early 1970s and 72% in 2000 [45]. The particular dairy product distribution varies somewhat with race and ethnicity [101]. The discrepancy between calcium intakes and recommendations becomes a large gap after age 11 years. This is a common problem. Looker [102] compiled calcium recommendations and intakes across the life span for 20 countries. The percentage of adolescents meeting country-specific recommendations was approximately 60% for males and approximately 50% for females. Most children older than age 8 years in the United States have calcium intakes below recommended levels. Only 6% of girls and 28% of boys ages 9–13 years and 9% of girls and 31% of boys ages 14–18 years have calcium intakes above the recommended intakes [103].

It is important to reach children early to establish and maintain dietary habits that will ensure lifelong adequate calcium intakes. There is a fair degree of consistency of calcium intake over time. In a 15-year longitudinal study begun as adolescents, tracking of calcium intake resulted in correlations of $r = 0.43$ for males and $r = 0.38$ for females [104]. Calcium intake is also a marker for intake of other nutrients [45]. This is not true for individuals who consume calcium in the form of supplements.

Calcium absorption from dairy products does not depend on fat content or flavoring. In fact, children who drink flavored milk have higher calcium intakes than non-milk drinkers and have similar total intakes of added sugars in diet and similar BMI as children who drink exclusively white milk [105]. A comparison of calcium bioavailability and the number of servings of various foods required to replace 1 cup of milk or yogurt on the basis of absorbed calcium is given in Table 44.4.

For children 4–8 years old, the equivalent of 2.6 cups of milk would be required to meet the RDA, and for children older than 9 years, it would be 4.3 cups. Other foods typically provide the equivalent of at least two-thirds of a cup of milk, so milk is not expected to provide all of the calcium requirements.

E SAFETY OF HIGH INTAKES

The UL for calcium is 2500–3000 mg/day [77]. The primary concern for excessive calcium intake from supplements in adults is kidney stones. Interactions with trace mineral absorption are also a concern. Dose–response safety data are not available for children 1–18 years old.

2 Vitamin D

A RECOMMENDATIONS, DIETARY SOURCES AND INTAKES, AND STATUS

The RDAs for children for vitamin D are given in Table 44.2. The American Academy of Pediatrics supports these recommendations, but it recommends supplemental vitamin D of 5 µg/day to infants not ingesting fortified formula [107]. The amount of new evidence bearing on inputs for optimal health and safety has been remarkable. However, the strength of the new evidence is largely in adults, and we have much to learn about children.

Vitamin D across the life span and dietary sources of vitamin D are described in Chapter 43. Dietary sources of vitamin D are limited and mostly consumed as fortified foods, especially milk. A summary of studies on vitamin D status in children and adolescents worldwide was compiled by El-Hajj Fuleihan [108]. The range in mean serum 25-hydroxyvitamin D levels (the best status indicator for vitamin D) was large: 13–142 nmol/l. Clinical guidelines are now available for those at risk for vitamin D deficiency [109]. For children at risk for vitamin D deficiency, recommended intakes are 600–1000 IU/day.

B EVIDENCE FOR A RELATIONSHIP TO BONE

Vitamin D deficiency in young children has long been associated with rickets. An intake of 2.5 µg (100IU)/day is thought to be adequate to prevent rickets [110,111]. This disorder is described in Chapter 43.

The vitamin D–parathyroid hormone (PTH) homeostatic regulatory axis helps regulate serum calcium levels in response to dietary calcium. Under conditions of low calcium intake, serum calcium levels fall, PTH is released, and vitamin D is converted to its active form, 1,25-dihydroxyvitamin D. Serum calcium levels rise as intestinal calcium absorption is upregulated; renal reabsorption of calcium increases, which conserves urinary excretion of calcium; and bone resorption increases. Interestingly, improving vitamin D status with supplementation of 1000 IU (25 µg) vitamin D_3 per day for 4 weeks resulted in a significant decrease in fractional calcium absorption in adolescents [112]. Apparently, vitamin D status was adequate at 4.5 nmol serum 25(OH)D and/or calcium intake of approximately 1000 mg/day was sufficiently high without supplementation to optimize fractional calcium absorption.

TABLE 44.4 Comparing Sources for Absorbable Calcium

Source	Serving size (g)	Calcium content (mg/serving)	Estimated absorption efficiency (%)	Food amount to equal calcium in 1 C milk
Milk	240	300	32.1	1.0 C
Beans, red	172	40.5	24.4	4.8 C
Beans, white	110	113	21.8	2.0 C
Bokchoy	85	79	53.8	1.2 C
Broccoli	71	35	61.3	2.3 C
Cheddar cheese	42	303	32.1	1.5 oz.
Cheese food	42	241	32.1	1.8 oz.
Chinese cabbage flower leaves	85	239	39.6	0.5 C
Chinese mustard green	85	212	40.2	0.6 C
Chinese spinach	85	347	8.36	1.7 C
Kale	85	61	49.3	1.6 C
Orange juice w/Ca citrate maleate	240	300	36.3	0.9 C
Soy milk w/calcium phosphate	240	300	24.0	1.3
Spinach	85	115	5.1	8.1 C
Tofu, calcium set	126	258	31.0	0.6 C
Whole wheat bread	28	20	82.0	5.8 slices
Wheat bran cereal	28	20	38.0	12.8 oz.
Yogurt	240	300	21.1	1.0 C

Source: *Taken from Weaver and Heaney [106]. With kind permission of Springer Science and Business Media.*

There are three RCTs of vitamin D in children with bone outcomes (Table 44.5). The results are quite varied among the studies. As with calcium absorption, vitamin D and calcium intakes would be interdependent.

In addition, response to vitamin D levels used in the RCTs would only be effective if doses were adequate and beginning vitamin D status of the subjects sufficiently inadequate so that supplementation would result in a substantial change in vitamin D status. Short-term dose–response studies of vitamin D and calcium on calcium absorption and excretion and vitamin D status in children could inform RCTs with bone outcomes. One RCT of two doses of vitamin D equivalent to 200 and 2000 IU/day in 10- to 17-year-old Lebanese girls was able to improve vitamin D status on the higher dose and improve total hip BMC and area but not other bone measures [112]. Dietary calcium intakes were low in that study. Lean mass was increased with vitamin D supplementation. Subjects in both the Cheng *et al.* [94] study and the Viljakainen *et al.* [113] study had adequate calcium together with vitamin D.

C SAFETY OF HIGH DOSES

Dose–response studies of longer duration than have been reported are needed to truly determine ULs of safety studies in which risk intoxication is unmentioned. The current ULs are given in Table 44.2.

Safety is assessed by observing no change in serum or urinary calcium levels. The 5-μg dose of vitamin D was ineffective in the Cheng *et al.* [94] study but effective for the femur in the study by Viljakainen *et al.* [113], but only when a compliance-based analysis was used. That study showed a dose–response change in vitamin D. Single oral doses of vitamin D have been given with no change in mean serum or urinary Ca:Cr ratios [114].

In the study by El Hajj Fuleihan *et al.* [114], adolescents given 14,000 IU (350 μg/week) of vitamin D_3 for 1 year showed no change in mean serum calcium level. This is equivalent on a daily dose to the UL. We do not know the safety of much higher doses in children.

TABLE 44.5 Differences in Mean Changes in Bone Mineral Content and Bone Mineral Density in Vitamin D Versus Placebo in Randomized, Controlled Trials in Children

Source	Ref. No.	Subj. No.	Age (years)	Sex	Race/location	Length study (months)	Vitamin D supplement (µg/day)	Site	Measure	Group mean increase	
										Treatment (T)	Placebo (P)
Cheng et al., 2005	94	195	10–12	F	White, Finland	24	5	Whole body	BMC	34.7	35.0, NS
								Femoral neck	BMC	24.0	22.4, NS
								Total femur	BMC	33.6	33.6, NS
								Spine	BMC	46.9	47.0, NS
								Tibia cortical thickness	pQCT	31.7	31.1, NS
El-Hajj Fuleihan et al., 2006	113	179	10–17	F	White, Lebanese	24	5	Total body	BMC	11.3	8.7, NS
								Total hip	BMC	11.2	7.8, NS
								Total hip	Area	4.0	2.4, $p = 0.05$
								Femoral neck	BMC	4.4	3.9, NS
								Femoral neck	Area	0.03	0.7, NS
								Trochanter	BMC	13.6	9.4, NS
								Trochanter	Area	6.8	4.7, NS
								Total body	BMC	12.0	8.7, NS
								Total hip	BMC	12.8	7.8, $p = 0.005$
								Total hip	Area	5.7	2.4, $p = 0.001$
								Femoral neck	BMC	5.2	3.9, NS
								Femoral neck	Area	0.8	0.7, NS
								Trochanter	BMC	14.2	9.4, NS
								Trochanter	Area	7.8	4.7, NS
Viljakainen et al., 2006[a]	114	212	11.4±0.4	F	White, Finland	12	5	Femur	BMC	14.3 (T vs. P), $p = 0.012$	
								Lumbar spine	BMC	NS	
							10	Femur	BMC	17.2 (T vs. P), $p = 0.012$	
								Lumbar spine	BMC	12.5 (T vs. P), $p = 0.039$	

[a] Analysis included only those >80% compliant.

BMC, bone mineral content; F, female; NS, not significant; pQCT, peripheral quantitative computed tomography.

3 Other Nutrients

Although many other nutrients are necessary for growing bone, there is little evidence that current intakes compromise development of peak bone mass for most individuals. Two minerals besides calcium that comprise a substantial protein of bone mineral are phosphorus and magnesium. Bone mineral is calcium phosphate, but 60% of the magnesium in the body resides in bone. RDAs and ULs for these nutrients for children are given in Table 44.2. The dietary Ca:P ratio affects bone mineralization and turnover through intestinal calcium and phosphorus transports [116]. Phosphorus is clearly essential for bone acquisition, but deficiency has not been a concern for children. Excessive intakes of phosphorus in soft drinks have been a concern. However, as discussed previously, the negative association of soft drink consumption and bone in girls is likely due to displacement of milk as a beverage.

Magnesium deficiency disrupts bone accretion. Rats fed 50% of their requirement for magnesium have structural changes that lead to reduced bone volume [117]. Obtaining recommended intakes of magnesium is not of concern for children. Iron deficiency also has a detrimental effect on bone morphology in growing animals that is exacerbated by calcium deficiency [118].

V CONCLUSION

Making wise nutritional choices during growth is a window of opportunity to build optimal peak bone mass to reduce risk of fracture later in life. If the opportunity is neglected, the consequence can be fracture. During infancy, it is not as difficult to meet requirements through breast-feeding or infant formulas. The other accelerated growth period, puberty, is much more difficult. Diets vary widely in nutrient sufficiency; peers may have more influence than caregivers. Fracture incidence in childhood is highest during the pubertal growth spurt when bones elongate before they consolidate and bone mineral density is lower. The incidence of pubertal fractures is increasing, possibly related to the increase in obesity coupled with a decline in consumption of milk as the beverage of choice. Diet patterns may be as important in building strong bones as adequacy of individual nutrients. The *Dietary Guidelines* offer a good plan. Supplements may be useful for some individuals and in some conditions.

References

[1] R.P. Heaney, S. Abrams, B. Dawson-Hughes, A. Looker, R. Marcus, V. Matkovic, et al., Peak bone mass, Osteoporos. Int. 11 (2000) 985–1009.

[2] J.-P. Bonjour, T. Chevalley, Pubertal timing, peak bone mass and fragility fracture risk, Bone Key-Osteovision 4 (2) (2007) 30–48.

[3] E.A. Krall, B. Dawson-Hughes, Heritable and lifestyle determinants of bone mineral density, J. Bone Miner. Res. 8 (1993) 1–9.

[4] E.S. Leib, Writing group for the ISCD position development conference: diagnosis of osteoporosis in men, premenopausal women and children, J. Clin. Densitom. 7 (2004) 17–26.

[5] R.R. Recker, M. Davies, S.M. Hinders, R.P. Heaney, M.R. Stegman, D.B. Kimmel, Bone gain in young adult women, JAMA 268 (1992) 2403–2408.

[6] L.A. Jackman, S.S. Millane, B.R. Martin, O.B. Wood, G.P. McCabe, M. Peacock, et al., Calcium retention in relation to calcium intake and postmenarcheal age in adolescent females, Am. J. Clin. Nutr. 66 (1997) 327–333.

[7] D. Teegarden, W.R. Proulx, B.R. Martin, J. Zhao, G.P. McCabe, R.M. Lyle, et al., Peak bone mass in young women, J. Bone Miner. Res. 10 (5) (1995) 711–715.

[8] Y.-C. Lin, R.M. Lyle, C.M. Weaver, L.D. McCabe, G.P. McCabe, C.C. Johnston, et al., Peak spine and femoral neck bone mass in young women, Bone 32 (5) (2003) 546–553.

[9] R.I. Gafni, J. Baron, Catch-up growth: Possible mechanisms, Pediatr. Nephrol. 14 (2000) 616–619.

[10] V. Matkovic, P.K. Goel, N.E. Badenkop-Stevens, et al., Calcium supplementation and bone mineral density in females from childhood to young adulthood: a randomized controlled trial, Am. J. Clin. Nutr. 81 (2005) 175–188.

[11] H.J. Kalkwarf, Forearm fractures in children and adolescents, Nutr. Today 41 (4) (2006) 171–177.

[12] A. Goulding, R. Cannan, S.M. Williams, E.J. Gold, R.W. Taylor, N.J. Lewis-Barned, Bone mineral density in girls with forearm fractures, J. Bone Miner. Res. 13 (1998) 143–148.

[13] D.A. Bailey, H.A. McKay, R.L. Mirwald, et al., A six-year longitudinal study of the relationship of physical activity to bone mineral accrual in growing children: The University of Saskatchewan Bone Mineral Accrual Study, J. Bone Miner. Res. 14 (1999) 1672–1679.

[14] S. Khosla, I.J. Melton III, M.B. Delatoski, et al., Incidence of childhood distal forearm fractures over 30 years, JAMA 290 (2003) 1479–1485.

[15] D.A. Bailey, A.D. Martin, A.A. McKay, S. Whiting, R. Miriwald, Calcium accretion in girls and boys during puberty: a longitudinal analysis, J. Bone Miner. Res. 15 (2000) 2245–2250.

[16] I.E. Jones, S.M. Williams, N. Dow, A. Goulding, How many children remain fracture-free during growth? a longitudinal study of children and adolescents participating in Dunedin Multidisciplinary Health and Development Study, Osteoporos. Int. 13 (2002) 990–995.

[17] R.A. Faulkner, K.S. Davison, D.A. Bailey, R.L. Mirwald, A.D.G. Baxter-Jones, Size-corrected BMD decreases during peak linear growth: implications for fracture incidence during adolescence, J. Bone Miner. Res. 21 (2006) 1864–1870.

[18] R.P. Heaney, C.M. Weaver, Newer perspectives on calcium and bone quality, J. Am. Coll. Nutr. 24 (6) (2005) 574S–581S.

[19] C.L. Ogden, M.D. Carroll, L.R. Curtin, M.A. McDowell, C.J. Tabak, K.M. Flegal, Prevalence of overweight and obesity in the United States, 1999–2004, JAMA 295 (2006) 1549–1555.

[20] M.B. Leonard, J. Shults, B.A. Wilson, A.M. Tershakovec, B.S. Zemel, Obesity during childhood and adolescence augments bone mass and bone dimensions, Am. J. Clin. Nutr. 80 (2004) 514–523.

[21] D.L. Skaggs, M.L. Loro, P. Pitukcheewanont, V. Tolo, V. Gilsanz, Increased body weight and decreased radial cross-sectional dimensions in girls with forearm fractures, J. Bone Miner. Res. 16 (2001) 1337–1342.

[22] A. Goulding, I.E. Jones, R.W. Taylor, S.M. Williams, P.J. Manning, Bone mineral density and body composition in boys with distal forearm fractures: a dual-energy x-ray absorptiometry study, J. Pediatr. 139 (2001) 509–515.

[23] A. Goulding, R.W. Taylor, I.E. Jones, K.A. McAuley, P.J. Manning, S.M. Williams, Overweight and obese children have low bone mass and area for their weight, Int. J. Obes. Relat. Metab. Disord. 24 (2000) 627–632.

[24] A. Goulding, I.E. Jones, R.W. Taylor, P.J. Manning, S.M. Williams, More broken bones: a 4-year double cohort study of young girls with and without distal forearm fractures, J. Bone Miner. Res. 15 (2000) 2011–2018.

[25] A. Goulding, R.W. Taylor, I.E. Jones, P.J. Manning, S.M. Williams, Spinal overload: a concern for obese children and adolescents? Osteporos. Int. 13 (2002) 835–840.

[26] A. Goulding, A.M. Grant, S.M. Williams, Bone and body composition of children and adolescents with repeated forearm fractures, J. Bone Miner. Res. 20 (2005) 2090–2096.

[27] E.D. Taylor, K.R. Theim, M.C. Mirch, S. Ghorbani, M. Tanofsky-Draff, D.C. Adler-Wailers, et al., Orthopedic complications of overweight in children and adolescents, Pediatrics 117 (2006) 2167–2174.

[28] N.K. Pollock, E.M. Laing, C.A. Baile, M.W. Hamrick, D.B. Hall, R.D. Lewis, Is adiposity advantageous for bone strength? A peripheral quantitative computed tomography study in late adolescent females, Am. J. Clin Nutr. 86 (2007) 1530–1538.

[29] E. Seeman, From density to structure growing up and growing old on the surfaces of bone, J. Bone Miner. Res. 12 (1997) 509–521.

[30] C.M. Gordon, Evaluation of bone density in children, Curr. Opin. Endocrinol. Diabetes 12 (2005) 444–451.

[31] M. Misra, P. Tsai, E.J. Anderson, et al., Nutrient intake in community-dwelling adolescent girls with anorexia nervosa in healthy adolescents, Am. J. Clin. Nutr. 84 (2006) 698–706.

[32] B.M.K. Biller, J.F. Caughlin, V. Sake, D. Schoenfeld, D.I. Spratt, A. Klitanski, Osteopenia in women with hypothalamic amenorrhea: a prospective study, Obstet. Gynecol. 78 (1991) 996–1001.

[33] S.P. Conway, S.P. Wolfe, K.G. Brownie, Vitamin K status among children with cystic fibrosis and its relationship to bone mineral density and bone turnover, Pediatrics 115 (2005) 1325–1331.

[34] R.P. Heaney, The bone remodeling transient: implications for the interpretation of clinical studies of bone mass change, J. Bone Miner. Res. 9 (1994) 1515–1523.

[35] A.J. Sawyer, L.K. Bachrach, E.B. Fung (Eds.), Bone Densitometry in Growing Patients: Guidelines for Clinical Practices., Humana Press, Totowa, NJ, 2007.

[36] E. Seeman, Editorial: growth in bone mass and size—are racial and gender differences in bone mineral density more apparent than real? J. Clin. Endocrinol. Metab. 83 (1998) 1414–1419.

[37] D.K. Katzman, L.K. Bachrach, D.R. Carter, R. Marcus, Clinical and anthropometric correlates of bone mineral acquisition in healthy adolescent girls, J. Clin. Endocrinol. Metab. 73 (1991) 1332–1339.

[38] D.R. Carter, M.L. Bouxsein, R. Marcus, New approaches for interpreting projected bone density data, J. Bone Miner. Res. 7 (1992) 137–145.

[39] M.B. Leonard, J. Shults, D.M. Elliott, V.A. Stallings, B.S. Zemel, Interpretation of whole body dual energy x-ray absorptiometry measures in children: comparison with peripheral quantitative computed tomography, Bone 34 (2004) 1044–1052.

[40] C.M. Weaver, L.D. McCabe, G.P. McCabe, R. Novotny, M. Van Loan, S. Going, , et al.the ACT research team, Bone mineral and predictors of bone mass in white, Hispanic, and Asian early pubertal girls, Calcif. Tissue Int. 81 (2007) 352–363.

[41] C.M. Gundberg, A.C. Looker, S.D. Nieman, M.S. Calvo, Patterns of osteocalcin and bone specific alkaline phosphatase by age, gender, and race or ethnicity, Bone 31 (2002) 707–708.

[42] C.M. Weaver, Clinical approaches for studying calcium metabolism and its relationship to disease, in: C.M. Weaver, R.P. Heaney (Eds.), Calcium in Human Health, Humana Press, Totowa, NJ, 2006, pp. 65–81.

[43] M.E. Wastney, Y. Zhao, C.M. Weaver, Kinetic studies, in: C.M. Weaver, R.P. Heaney (Eds.), Calcium in Human Health, Humana Press, Totowa, NJ, 2006, pp. 83–93.

[44] C.M. Weaver, A.P. Rothwell, K.V. Wood, Measuring calcium absorption and utilization in humans, Curr. Opin. Clin. Nutr. Metab. Care 9 (2006) 568–574.

[45] U.S. Department of Health and Human Services and U.S. Department of Agriculture, Dietary Guidelines for Americans, 2005, sixth ed., U.S. Government Printing Office, Washington, DC, 2005.

[46] C. Ballow, S. Kuester, C. Gillespie, Beverage choices affect adequacy of children's nutrient intakes, Arch. Pediatr. Adolesc. Med. 154 (2000) 1148–1152.

[47] X. Gao, P.E. Wilde, A.H. Lichtenstein, K.L. Tucker, Meeting adequate intake for dietary calcium without dairy foods in adolescents aged 9 to 18 years (National Health and Nutrition Examination Survey 2001–2002), J. Am. Diet. Assoc. 106 (2006) 1759–1765.

[48] S.A. Abrams, L.J. Griffin, P.D. Hicks, S.K. Gunn, Pubertal girls only partially adapt to low dietary calcium intakes, J. Bone Miner. Res. 19 (2004) 759–763.

[49] G.M. Chan, K. Hoffman, M. McMurry, Effects of dairy products on bone and body composition in pubertal girls, J. Pediatr. 126 (4) (1995) 551–556.

[50] J.P. Bonjour, A.L. Carrie, S. Ferrari, H. Clavien, D. Slosman, G. Thientz, et al., Calcium-enriched foods and bone mass growth in prepubertal girls: a randomized, double-blind, placebo-controlled trial, J. Clin. Invest. 99 (1997) 1287–1294.

[51] J.P. Bonjour, T. Chevalley, P. Aminan, D. Slosman, R. Rizzoli, Gain in bone mineral mass in prepubertal girls 3.5 y after discontinuation of calcium supplementation: a follow-up study, Lancet 358 (2001) 1208–1213.

[52] K.D. Ghatge, H.L. Lambert, M.E. Barker, R. Eastell, Bone mineral gain following calcium supplementation in teenage girls is preserved two years after withdrawal of the supplement, J. Bone Miner. Res. 16 (S1) (2001) S173.

[53] W.T.K. Lee, S.S.F. Leung, D.M.Y. Leung, J.C.Y. Cheng, A follow-up study on the effect of calcium-supplement withdrawal and puberty on bone acquisition of children, Am. J. Clin. Nutr. 64 (1996) 71–77.

[54] C.W. Slemenda, M. Peacock, S. Hui, L. Zhou, C.C. Johnston, Reduced rates of skeletal remodeling are associated with increased bone mineral density during the development of peak skeletal mass, J. Bone Min. Res. 12 (1997) 676–682.

[55] L.M. Fiorito, D.C. Mitchell, H. Smiciklas-Wright, L.L. Berch, Girls' calcium intake is associated with bone mineral content during middle childhood, J. Nutr. 136 (2006) 1281–1286.

[56] A. Goulding, J.E. Rockell, R.E. Black, A.M. Grant, I.E. Jones, S.M. Williams, Children who avoid drinking cow's milk are at increased risk for prepubertal bone fractures, J. Am. Diet. Assoc. 104 (2004) 250–253.

[57] H.J. Kalkwarf, J.C. Khoury, B.P. Lanphear, Milk intake during childhood and adolescence, adult bone density, and osteoporotic fractures in U.S. women, Am. J. Clin. Nutr. 77 (2003) 257–265.

[58] R.B. Sandler, C.W. Slemenda, R.E. LaPorter, J.A. Cauley, M.M. Schramm, M.I. Banesi, et al., Postmenopausal bone density and milk consumption in childhood and adolescence, Am. J. Clin. Nutr. 43 (1985) 270–274.

[59] T.A. Nicklas, Calcium intake trends and health consequences from childhood through adulthood, J. Am. Coll. Nutr. 22 (2003) 340—356.

[60] S.J. Whiting, H. Vatanparast, A. Baxter-Jones, R.A. Faulkner, R. Miriwald, D.A. Bailey, Factors that affect bone mineral accrual in the adolescent growth spurt, J. Nutr. 134 (2004) 696S—700S.

[61] U.S. Barzel, L.K. Massey, Excess dietary protein can adversely affect bone, J. Nutr. 128 (1998) 1051—1053.

[62] J.E. Kerstetter, L.H. Allen, Dietary protein increases urinary calcium, J. Nutr. 120 (1990) 134—136.

[63] T. Remer, T. Dimitrios, T. Manz, Dietary potential renal acid load and renal net acid excretion in healthy, free-living children and adolescents, Am. J. Clin. Nutr. 77 (2003) 1255—1260.

[64] D.E. Sellmeyer, K.L. Stone, A. Sebastian, S.R. Cummings, A high ratio of dietary animal to vegetable protein increases the rate of bone loss and the risk of fracture in postmenopausal women, Am. J. Clin. Nutr. 73 (2001) 118—122.

[65] J.P. Bonjour, Dietary protein: an essential nutrient for bone health, Am. J. Coll. Nutr. 24 (2005) 5265—5365.

[66] J.E. Kerstetter, K.O. O'Brien, D.M. Caseria, D.E. Wall, K.L. Insogna, The impact of dietary protein on calcium absorption and kinetic measures of bone turnover in women, J. Clin. Endocrinol. Metab. 90 (2005) 26—31.

[67] Z.K. Roughead, L.K. Johnson, G.I. Lykken, J.R. Hunt, Controlled high meat diets do not affect calcium retention or indices of bone status in healthy postmenopausal women, J. Nutr. 133 (2003) 1020—1026.

[68] K. Rafferty, K.M. Davies, R.P. Heaney, Potassium intake and the calcium economy, J. Am. Coll. Nutr. 24 (2005) 99—106.

[69] R.C. Muhlbauer, A. Lozano, A. Reiuli, Onion and a mixture of vegetables, salads, and herbs affect bone resorption in the rat by a mechanism independent of their base exceeds, J. Bone Miner. Res. 17 (2002) 1230—1236.

[70] J. Cadogan, R. Eastell, N. Jones, M.E. Barker, Milk intake and bone mineral acquisition in adolescent girls: randomized, controlled intervention trial, Br. Med. J. 315 (1997) 1255—1260.

[71] J.-P. Bonjour, P. Ammann, T. Chevalley, S. Ferrari, R. Rizzoli, Nutritional aspects of bone growth: an overview, in: S.A. Newand, J.-P. Bonjour (Eds.), Nutritional Aspects of Bone Health, Royal Society of Chemistry, Cambridge, UK, 2005, pp. 111—127.

[72] B. Dawson-Hughes, Protein and calcium absorption: potential role of the calcium sensor receptor, in: P. Burckhardt, R.P. Heaney, B. Dawson-Hughes (Eds.), Nutritional Aspects of Osteoporosis, Elsevier, New York, 2007, pp. 217—227. Elsevier International Congress Series, vol. 1297.

[73] T. Remer, F. Manz, V. Alexy, E. Schoenau, S.A. Wudy, L. Shi, Long-term high urinary potential renal acid load and low nitrogen excretion predict reduced diaphyseal bone mass and bone size in children, J. Clin. Endocrinol. Metab. 96 (2011) 2861—2868.

[74] V. Matkovic, J.Z. Ilich, M.B. Andon, L.C. Hsieh, M.A. Tzagournis, B.J. Lagger, et al., Urinary calcium, sodium, and bone mass of young females, Am. J. Clin. Nutr. 62 (1995) 417—425.

[75] C. Palacios, K. Wigertz, B.R. Martin, L. Jackman, J.H. Pratt, M. Peacock, et al., Sodium retention in black and white female adolescents in response to salt intake, J. Clin. Endocrinol. Metab. 89 (4) (2004) 1858—1863.

[76] K. Wigertz, C. Palacios, L.A. Jackman, B.R. Martin, L.D. McCabe, G.P. McCabe, et al., Racial differences in calcium retention in response to dietary salt in adolescent girls, Am. J. Clin. Nutr. 81 (2005) 845—850.

[77] Institute of Medicine, Dietary Reference Intakes for Calcium and Vitamin D, National Academies Press, Washington, DC, 2010.

[78] Institute of Medicine, Dietary Reference Intakes for Calcium, Phosphorus, Magnesium, Vitamin D, and Fluoride, National Academy Press, Washington, DC, 1997.

[79] M.M. Braun, B.R. Martin, M. Kern, G.P. McCabe, M. Peacock, Z. Jiang, et al., Calcium retention in adolescent boys on a range of controlled calcium intakes, Am. J. Clin. Nutr. 84 (2006) 414—418.

[80] M. Braun, C. Palacios, K. Wigertz, L.A. Jackman, R.J. Bryant, L.D. McCabe, et al., Racial differences in skeletal calcium retention in adolescent girls on a range of controlled calcium intakes, Am. J. Clin. Nutr. 85 (2007) 1657—1663.

[81] L. Wu, B.R. Martin, M.M. Braun, M.E. Wastney, G.P. McCabe, L.D. McCabe, et al., Calcium requirements and metabolism in Chinese American boys and girls, J. Bone Miner. Res. 25 (8) (2010) 1842—1849.

[82] K.M. Hill, M.M. Braun, K.A. Egan, B.R. Martin, L.D. McCabe, M. Peacock, et al., Obesity augments calcium-induced increases in skeletal calcium retention in adolescents, J. Clin. Endocrinol. Metab. 96 (2011) 2171—2177.

[83] C.C. Johnston Jr., J.Z. Miller, C.W. Slemenda, T.K. Reister, S. Hui, J.C. Christian, et al., Calcium supplementation and increases in bone mineral density in children, N. Engl. J. Med. 327 (1992) 82—87.

[84] T. Lloyd, M.B. Andon, N. Rollings, J.K. Martel, J.R. Landis, C.M. Demers, et al., Calcium supplementation and bone mineral density in adolescent girls, JAMA 270 (1993) 841—844.

[85] W.T.K. Lee, S.S.F. Leung, S.H. Wang, Y.C. Xu, W.P. Zeng, J. Lau, et al., Double-blind controlled calcium supplementation and bone mineral accretion in children accustomed to low calcium diet, Am. J. Clin. Nutr. 60 (1994) 744—752.

[86] C.A. Nowson, R.M. Green, J.L. Hopper, A.J. Sherwin, D. Young, B. Kaymakci, et al., A co-twin study of the effect of calcium supplementation on bone density in adolescence, Osteoporos. Int. 7 (1997) 219—225.

[87] B. Dibba, A. Prentice, M. Ceesay, et al., Effect of calcium supplementation on bone mineral accretion in Gambian children accustomed to a low-calcium diet, Am. J. Clin. Nutr. 71 (2) (2000) 544—549.

[88] L.J. Moyer-Mileur, B. Xie, S.D. Ball, T. Pratt, Bone mass and density response to a 12-month trial of calcium and vitamin D supplement in preadolescent girls, J. Musculoskel. Neuron. Interact. 3 (2003) 63—70.

[89] G.S. Rozen, G. Rennert, R. Dodiuk-Gad, H.S. Rennert, N. Ish-Schalom, G. Diaf, et al., Calcium supplementation provides an extended window of opportunity for bone mass accretion after menarche, Am. J. Clin. Nutr. 78 (2003) 993—998.

[90] S.J. Stear, A. Prentice, S.C. Jones, et al., Effect of a calcium and exercise intervention on the bone mineral status of 16—18 year-old adolescent girls, Am. J. Clin. Nutr. 77 (4) (2003) 985—992.

[91] M.A. Cameron, L.M. Paton, C.A. Newson, C. Margerison, M. Frame, J.D. Wark, The effect of calcium supplementation on bone density in premenarcheal females: a co-twin approach, J. Clin. Endocrinol. Metab. 89 (2004) 4916—4922.

[92] C. Mølgaard, B.L. Thomson, K.F. Michaelson, Effect of habitual dietary calcium intake on calcium supplementation in 12—14 year old girls, Am. J. Clin. Nutr. 80 (2004) 1422—1427.

[93] A. Prentice, F. Gintz, S.J. Stear, S.C. Jones, M.A. Laskey, T.J. Cole, Calcium supplementation increases stature and bone mineral mass of 16—18 year old boys, J. Clin. Endocrinol. Metab. 90 (2005) 3153—3161.

[94] S. Cheng, A. Lyytikäinen, H. Kröger, C. Lamberg-Allardt, M. Alén, A. Koisteinen, et al., Effects of calcium, dairy product, and vitamin D supplementation on bone mass accrual and body composition in 10- to 12-year old girls: 12-year randomized trial, Am. J. Clin. Nutr. 82 (2005) 1115—1126.

[95] H.L. Lambert, R. Eastell, K. Karnik, J.M. Russell, M.E. Barker, Calcium supplementation and bone mineral accretion in adolescent girls: an 18-month randomized controlled trial with 2-year follow-up, Am. J. Clin. Nutr. 87 (2008) 455−462.

[96] T. Winzenberg, K. Shaw, J. Fryer, G. Jones, Effect of calcium supplementation on bone density in health children: meta-analysis of randomized controlled trials, Br. Med. J. 333 (2006) 775−781.

[97] R.P. Heaney, C.M. Weaver. Letter to the editor. BMJ.com Rapid Response 26.09.2006.

[98] G. Jones, T. Winzenberg. In reply. BMJ.com Rapid Response 3.08.2006.

[99] B. Specker, T. Binkley, J. Wermers, Randomized trial of physical activity and calcium supplementation BMC in 3−5 year old healthy children: The South Dakota Children's Health Study, J. Bone Miner. Res. 17 (2002) S398.

[100] T. Chevalley, R. Rizzoli, D. Hans, S. Ferrari, J.-P. Bonjour, Interaction between calcium intake and menarcheal age on bone mass gain: an eight-year follow-up study from prepuberty to postmenarche, J. Clin. Endocrinol. Metab. 90 (2005) 44−51.

[101] G. Auld, C.J. Boushey, M.A. Bock, C. Bruhn, K. Gabel, D. Gustafson, et al., Perspectives on intake of calcium rich foods among Asian, Hispanic, and white preadolescent and adolescent females, J. Nutr. Educ. 34 (2002) 242−251.

[102] A.C. Looker, Dietary calcium: recommendations and intakes around the world, in: C.M. Weaver, R.P. Heaney (Eds.), Calcium in Human Health, Humana Press, Totowa, NJ, 2006, pp. 105−127.

[103] A. Moshfegh, J. Goldman, L. Cleveland, What We Eat in America, NHANES 2001−2002: Usual Nutrient Intakes from Food Compared to Dietary Reference Intakes, U.S. Department of Agriculture, Washington , DC, 2005.

[104] L.A. Lytle, S. Seifert, J. Greenstein, P. Overn, How do children's eating patterns and food choices change over time? Results from a cohort study, Am. J. Health Promot. 14 (2003) 222−228.

[105] M.M. Murphy, J.S. Douglass, R.K. Johnson, L.A. Spence, Drinking flavored or plain milk is positively associated with nutrient intake and is not associated with adverse effects on weight status in U.S. children and adolescents, J. Am. Diet. Assoc. 108 (4) (2008) 631−639.

[106] C.M. Weaver, R.P. Heaney (Eds.), Calcium in Human Health, Humana Press, Totowa, NJ, 2006.

[107] L.M. Gartner, F.R. Greer, Prevention of rickets and vitamin D deficiency: new guidelines for vitamin D intake, Pediatrics 111 (2003) 908−910.

[108] G. El-Hajj Fuleihan, R. Vieth, Vitamin D insufficiency and musculoskeletal health in children and adolescents, in: P. Burckhardt, R.P. Heaney, B. Dawson-Hughes (Eds.), Nutritional Aspects of Osteoporosis, Elsevier, New York, 2007, pp. 91−108. Elsevier International Congress Series, vol. 1297.

[109] M.F. Holick, N.C. Binkley, H.A. Birschoff-Ferrari, C.M. Gordon, D.A. Hanley, R.P. Heaney, et al., Evaluation, treatment, and prevention of vitamin D deficiency: an Endocrine Society clinical practice guideline, J. Clin. Endocrinol. Metab. 96 (2011) 1911−1930.

[110] K. Glazer, A.H. Parmelee, W.S. Hoffman, Comparative efficacy of vitamin D preparations in prophylactic treatment of premature infants, Am. J. Dis. Child. 77 (1949) 1−14.

[111] B.L. Specker, M.L. Ho, A. Oesteich, T.A. Yin, Q.M. Shui, X.C. Chen, et al., Prospective study of vitamin D supplementation and rickets in China, J. Pediatr. 120 (1992) 733−739.

[112] C.Y. Park, K.M. Hill, A.E. Elble, B.R. Martin, L.A. DiMeglio, M. Peacock, et al., Daily supplementation with 25 μg cholecalciferol does not increase calcium absorption or skeletal retention in adolescent girls with low serum 25-hydroxyvitamin D, J. Nutr. 140 (2010) 2139−2144.

[113] G. El-Hajj Fuleihan, M. Nabulsi, H. Tamim, J. Maalouf, M. Salamoun, H. Khalife, et al., Effect of vitamin D replacement on musculoskeletal parameters in schoolchildren: a randomized controlled trial, J. Clin. Endocrinol. Metab. 91 (2006) 405−412.

[114] H.T. Viljakainen, A.-M. Natri, M. Kärkkäinen, M.M. Huttenen, A. Palssa, J. Jakobsen, et al., A positive dose−response effect of vitamin D supplementation on site-specific bone mineral augmentation in adolescent girls: a double-blinded randomized placebo-controlled 1-year intervention, J. Bone Miner. Res. 21 (2006) 836−844.

[115] M.B. Oliveri, M. Ladizesky, C.A. Mautelen, A. Alouse, L. Martinez, Seasonal variations of 25-hydroxyvitamin D and parathyroid hormone in Ushuaia (Argentina), the southernmost city of the world, Bone Miner. 20 (1993) 99−108.

[116] R. Masuyama, Y. Nakaya, S. Katsumata, Y. Kajita, M. Uehara, S. Tanaka, et al., Dietary calcium and phosphorus ratio regulates bone mineralization and turnover in vitamin D receptor knockout mice by affecting intestinal calcium and phosphorus absorption, J. Bone Miner. Res. 18 (2003) 1217−1226.

[117] R.K. Rude, H.E. Gruber, H.J. Norton, L.Y. Wei, A. Fransto, J. Kilburn, Reduction of dietary magnesium by only 50% in the rat disrupts bone and mineral metabolism, Osteoporos. Int. 17 (2006) 1022−1032.

[118] D.M. Medeiros, A. Plattner, D. Jennings, B. Stoecker, Bone morphology, strength and density are comprised in iron-deficiency rats and exacerbated by calcium restriction, J. Nutr. 132 (2002) 135−3141.

45

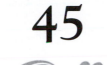
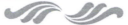

Osteoporosis in Adults

Robert Marcus

Stanford University, Stanford, California

I INTRODUCTION

Osteoporosis is a global skeletal disorder of decreased bone strength in which the only important consequence is an increased risk for fracture with minimal trauma. The term *porosis* means "spongelike," which aptly describes the appearance of that portion of the skeleton, the trabecular skeleton, which is most afflicted with this disease (Figure 45.1). Bone strength is a complex function integrating bone mineral density and bone quality. Bone mineral density (BMD) is the concept most familiar to the public, to patients, and to physicians, but it is only one determinant of bone strength, all other contributions that are not captured by a BMD measurement falling under the rubric of "bone quality." The term *quality* should more properly be considered as the plural *qualities* because it encompasses a wide variety of characteristics that are enumerated later in this chapter. Osteoporotic, or fragility, fractures traditionally have been grouped according to their location, either in the spine (vertebral) or non-spine, the latter including those of the distal radius (Colles' fractures) and the proximal femur (hip fracture). It is important to understand that because of its global nature, osteoporosis imposes an increased risk for virtually all fractures in affected individuals.

Already more common than any other generalized skeletal condition, osteoporosis continues to increase in prevalence. Based on data from the National Health and Nutrition Examination Survey III (NHANES) and from the 2000 National Census, the National Osteoporosis Foundation estimated that in 2002, 20% of postmenopausal white women in the United States had osteoporosis, and an additional 52% had low bone density at the hip [1]. In the whole population, approximately 8 million have osteoporosis, of whom approximately 1.5 million will fracture each year. One out of

every two white women will experience an osteoporotic fracture at some point in her lifetime [1—3].

Although men have a lower prevalence of osteoporosis than women, perhaps 25% as great, fragility fractures certainly occur in men, and some of these, particularly at the hip, carry a less favorable prognosis in men than for women. The most common osteoporotic fractures occur as compression deformities of the thoracic or lumbar spine. Although two-thirds of these do not acutely produce symptoms, they must not be viewed in any sense as benign events. Even mild compression fractures aggravate by four- or fivefold the short-term risk for subsequent fractures. Approximately one-third of vertebral fractures produce symptoms when they occur and are referred to as "clinical" vertebral fractures. These are more likely to be of moderate or severe degree in deformity and are the fractures most likely to result in long-term pain, deformity, and disability. In the Study of Osteoporotic Fractures (SOF), a long-term observational study of thousands of older women, clinical vertebral fractures were associated with an eightfold excess of mortality similar to that observed with hip fracture [4]. The incidence of vertebral fractures in women begins to rise early in the sixth decade, corresponding in time to the menopausal loss of endogenous estrogen. The incidence continues to increase in succeeding decades (Figure 45.2) [3].

At nonvertebral sites, forearm fractures, particularly at the distal radius, also increase during the sixth decade but stabilize thereafter, at which time the incidence of hip fracture begins exponentially to increase [3]. Both forearm and hip fractures result directly from a fall. Whether an individual fractures the arm or the hip reflects the manner of falling. Younger women with normal locomotion generally fall while walking and break a fall by arm extension. Older and more frail women often fall while transferring from a seated to a

Nutrition in the Prevention and Treatment of Disease, Third Edition.
DOI: http://dx.doi.org/10.1016/B978-0-12-391884-0.00045-7

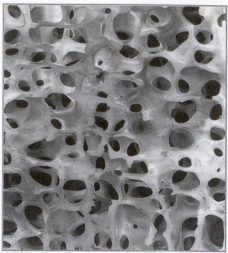

A: NORMAL TRABECULAR BONE

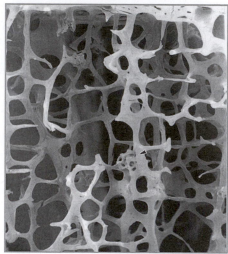

B: OSTEOPOROTIC TRABECULAR BONE

FIGURE 45.1 (A) Normal trabecular bone. Note the highly inter-connected vertical and horizontal bars, fairly homogeneous size and shape of holes, and platelike appearance of many of the trabecular units. Source: *Courtesy Dr. David Dempster. Copyright David Dempster Ph.D.* (B) Osteoporotic bone. Note substantial reduction in the amount of bone substance per unit volume compared to normal bone (A). Note the narrow rodlike appearance of vertical trabeculae com-pared to the normal platelike structures. Note the wide variation in the size of holes throughout the trabecular structure. In many regions, trabecular struts are hanging in space without connection to neighboring structures. Source: *Courtesy Dr. David Dempster. Copyright David Dempster Ph.D.*

standing position. If they fail to elevate their centers of gravity sufficiently to support an upright posture, they fall backwards or to the side, directly impacting the femoral greater trochanter and possibly leading to hip fracture [5,6].

This chapter focuses on the characteristics of a healthy skeleton, the underlying pathophysiology of osteoporo-sis, the characteristics of osteoporotic bone, approaches

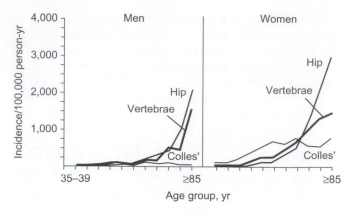

FIGURE 45.2 Age-specific incidence rates for hip, vertebral, and distal forearm fractures in men and women. Source: *Data derived from the population of Rochester, Minnesota. From Cooper, C., and Melton, L. J., III (1992). Epidemiology of osteoporosis. Trends Endocrinol. Metab.3, 224–229 (1992).*

to conserving bone throughout adult life, and therapeu-tic approaches to treating skeletal fragility. A compre-hensive discussion of the various pharmacologic agents available for patient management lies outside the scope of this chapter, and the critical role of bone acquisition during years of growth through adolescence appears in the companion chapter by Weaver and Hill (Chapter 44), which the reader is strongly urged to consult.

II THE SKELETON

Bone is a complex cellular tissue that contains, by weight, approximately 30% organic constituents and 70% mineral. The most abundant protein in the organic com-partment is type I collagen, a fibrillar structure consisting of three interweaving strands—normally two strands of alpha-1 collagen and one of alpha-2 collagen. Collagen represents 98% of the organic phase of bone, and various noncollagen proteins account for the remainder [7].

The mineral phase of bone is approximately 95% hydroxyapatite, a highly organized crystal of calcium and phosphorus. Other minerals normally found in bone mineral include sodium (indeed, approximately 30% of total body sodium can be stored in bone crys-tal), magnesium, and fluoride. Incorporation of fluo-ride and strontium into bone crystal is of particular relevance because these compounds have seen use as therapy for osteoporosis.

A Bone Cells

The processes of bone formation and breakdown (resorption) require cellular activity. Three major cell types reside in bone and conduct these processes: osteoblasts, osteocytes, and osteoclasts.

Osteoblasts are the primary bone-forming cells. They derive from stem cells in the bone marrow stroma. These stem cells are pluripotential, having the capacity to develop along multiple lineages, including fibroblasts, hematopoietic cells, smooth myocytes, adipocytes, chondrocytes, and osteoblasts. During linear growth, osteoblasts invade a temporary cartilaginous template to form primary lamellar bone. During remodeling (see later discussion), a wave of osteoblast precursors migrates to the base of a resorption cavity, acquires the characteristics of mature osteoblasts, and lays down new bone (Figure 45.3).

Osteocytes are osteoblasts that have become embedded within their own secreted matrix. Each osteocyte sits in its individual hole, or *lacuna*, connected to one another throughout the bone matrix by a highly developed network of channels, or *canaliculi*. Osteocytes appear to be the monitors and responders to a bone's mechanical environment (Figure 45.4).

Osteoclasts are multinucleated giant cells of macrophage lineage. They undertake the enzymatic destruction of bone during the resorption phase of remodeling (see later discussion). During this process, osteoclasts form a seal at the bone surface with the aid of anchoring proteins called integrins whose receptors exist in the bone matrix. This seal creates a sequestered region underneath the osteoclast into which hydrogen ion is secreted using a carbonic anhydrase-dependent pump and resulting in a highly acidic local environment. In addition, the osteoclast secretes a variety of hydrolytic enzymes, such as cathepsins, which hydrolyze bone matrix (Figure 45.5).

A fourth cell is also observed in bone. So-called *lining cells* are seen as a syncytial layer of dormant cells that covers bone surfaces. This group of cells is thought to serve a surveillance function that responds to microscopic damage by locally stimulating new remodeling activity. Lining cells also originate from osteoblasts and, although dormant, retain the capacity in certain circumstances to convert into functional osteoblasts and lay down new bone. This appears to be one mechanism through which administration of parathyroid hormone achieves a rapid increase in bone formation (see section on therapeutics).

Eighty percent of the adult skeleton consists of compact bone. This is referred to as the *cortical* or *appendicular* skeleton and comprises mostly the long bones as well as the outer shells of the central, or *axial*, skeleton, which includes the spine, pelvis, and the ends (metaphyses) of long bones. The axial skeleton has a heavy complement (perhaps 40% by weight or 80% by surface area) of a honeycomb-like series of vertical and horizontal bars, or *trabeculae*, and is therefore frequently called *trabecular* bone (in orthopedics this may also be called *cancellous* bone). In adults, the trabecular bone of the spine and pelvis constitutes the primary residence

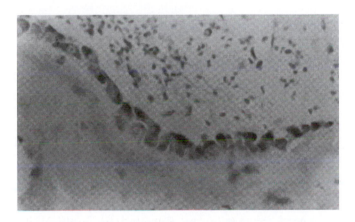

FIGURE 45.3 Low-power view of osteoblasts lining the bone surface. Source: *From Lee et al. [7], with permission.*

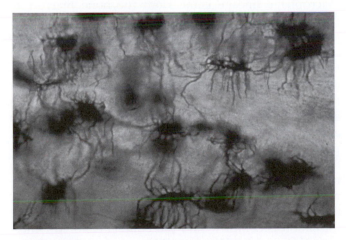

FIGURE 45.4 Osteocytes occupying individual lacunae with extensive canalicular interconnections. Source: *From Lee et al. [7], with permission.*

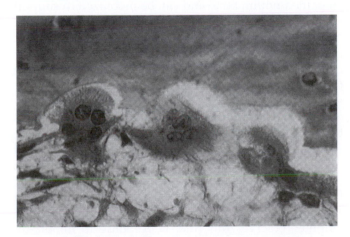

FIGURE 45.5 Low-power view of osteoclasts occupying resorption lacunae. Source: *From Lee et al. [7], with permission.*

of red bone marrow. Because the cells responsible for conducting the processes underlying adult bone loss originate in the bone marrow, and because these processes occur on the surfaces of bone, it should be no surprise that trabecular bone, with its rich complement of bone marrow and extensive surface area, should be the bone compartment that experiences the earliest and most rapid loss of bone with aging.

At any time during adult life, the amount of bone contained within the skeleton consists of that bone which was present at the end of growth, the so-called "peak bone mass," minus that which has been lost. One frequently encounters patients who report being told, following a bone density test, that they have "lost 30% of their skeleton." The problem with such conclusions is that one simply cannot determine from a single BMD measurement whether a deficit in bone mineral reflects bone loss or failure to achieve the peak bone mass that might have been predicted for that individual. In fact, the majority of young adults with low bone mass have not lost bone at all but, rather, have age-related deficits related to poor acquisition of peak bone mass. (See Chapter 44.)

B Physiologic Roles of the Skeleton

During vertebrate evolution, the skeleton acquired two fundamental but not necessarily compatible functions. By virtue of its dense mineralization, bone provides the structural rigidity necessary to withstand the effect of gravity and support terrestrial locomotion. By adapting to region-specific differences in its mechanical environment, denser, stronger bone exists where it is needed without requiring a universal increase in skeletal weight to the point that mobility is jeopardized.

Bone also constitutes the *primary* repository in the body for calcium. Indeed, 99.5% of body calcium is contained within bone and can be mobilized to support the extracellular calcium concentration at times of need. For the great majority of vertebrates, the calcium environment is extremely high, reflecting its very high concentration in ocean water ($\sim$400 mg/l). Facing the threat of calcium toxicity, ocean fish must be able to eliminate excess calcium from their bodies, which they accomplish through a calcium-dependent ATPase system in the gills. Progression of vertebrates onto land, with freshwater far more dilute in calcium, required mechanisms to promote calcium extraction from the environment and to conserve it within the body. Parathyroid hormone (PTH), the peptide secretory product of the parathyroid glands (first appearing in amphibia), serves this role. In response to minute-to-minute relatively mild reductions in extracellular calcium concentration, such as during the hours following

a meal, PTH stimulates the kidney to conserve calcium by regulating renal tubular reabsorption efficiency. When calcium deficits become sustained or severe, such as in the face of chronically inadequate dietary calcium, PTH stimulates the renal production of 1,25 $(OH)_2$ vitamin D (calcitriol), the potent hormonal form of the parent vitamin, which in turn enhances intestinal calcium absorption. In this setting, PTH also stimulates bone remodeling by initiating the formation of new remodeling units and resulting in delivery of calcium from the skeleton to the extracellular environment. Together, these actions restore plasma calcium concentrations to their normal level [8]. It must be understood that PTH action on the skeleton does not selectively remove calcium from the skeleton but is accomplished by an increase in bone remodeling (see later discussion) so that the release of mineral to the plasma compartment is accompanied by a net loss of bone.

C Remodeling: The Key to Understanding Age-Related Bone Loss

Many mammals, primates, and humans maintain skeletal integrity through a continuous process of breakdown and renewal known as *remodeling*. This process occurs lifelong, although during childhood and adolescence it is overshadowed by the events of linear growth (modeling). Once growth centers have fused and skeletal maturation is complete, remodeling becomes the dominant—and indeed, with rare exception, the only—mechanism through which bone is added to or removed from the skeleton. Each remodeling event is carried out by discrete bone multicellular units (BMUs) and consists of an initial phase of bone resorption that is coupled to a longer phase of bone formation (Figure 45.6). These are initiated when cells of macrophage lineage come from the bone marrow to points on the bone surface and fuse into multinucleated osteoclasts that dig into and remove bone. The cavity thus created reaches a depth of 60 μm within 6−8 weeks. In this manner, both mineral and matrix constituents are returned to the circulating extracellular fluid. Released from the resorbed matrix is a rich assortment of cytokines and growth factors that then attract into the base of the cavity a wave of osteoblast precursor cells from the marrow stroma. These transform into functional osteoblasts and begin to lay down new bone matrix. Once the new bone reaches a thickness of approximately 20 μm, it begins to accumulate mineral. By the end of approximately 6 months, bone formation is complete and the bone is restored almost to its basal state. However, like many biological processes, bone remodeling is not 100% efficient; that is, the amount of new bone formed does not completely

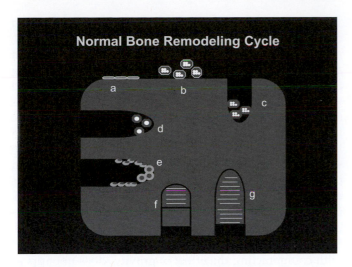

FIGURE 45.6 The bone remodeling cycle. This drawing represents a region of trabecular bone. All remodeling events occur on the bone surface. (a) 90% of bone surface is generally covered by thin layer of dormant lining cells. (b) Coalescence of osteoclast precursors at a site on the bone surface with creation of multinucleated osteoclasts. (c) Osteoclasts remove a divot of bone, reaching 60 μm in depth by 6–8 weeks. (d) Soluble factors released by osteoclastic resorption recruit a new wave of cell proliferation (preosteoblasts) into the base of the resorption cavity. (e) Preosteoblasts acquire the osteoblast phenotype. (f) Osteoblasts secrete new bone matrix, which begins to acquire mineral after a thickness of approximately 20 μm is achieved. (g) New mineralized bone almost fully replaces resorbed bone by approximately 6 months. Small deficits are left, reflecting remodeling inefficiency and accounting for the process of age-related bone loss. Source: *Copyright Robert Marcus, M.D.*

make up for the older bone removed, so a small bone deficit remains as a consequence of each remodeling event, called the "remodeling imbalance." The cumulative effect of the hundreds of thousands of remodeling units in play at any one time is the readily observable phenomenon of age-related bone loss. Consequently, anything that promotes an overall increase in whole body bone remodeling aggravates the rate of bone loss and, by contrast, interventions that slow remodeling constrain bone loss. This forms the basis for using drugs that slow remodeling as a mainstay of osteoporosis treatment, as discussed later in this chapter.

Another word should be said concerning matrix mineralization during the bone formation phase of remodeling. Mineral is rapidly laid down for the initial several weeks but thereafter changes to a slow, linear rate. Mineral is never fully saturated in bone, so it continues to accumulate as long as that particular unit of bone survives. The only thing to terminate this process would be the initiation of a new wave of osteoclastic resorption to clear out this region of older bone. Thus, if overall remodeling slows, bone survives longer and becomes more densely mineralized. The consequences of this finding are also discussed later.

If, as described, bone remodeling leads to loss (and presumably weakening) of bone, one may ask why it has evolved and what its purpose may be. It appears that the cardinal role of remodeling is to serve a scavenger function, through which fatigued or damaged bone is cleared away and replaced (albeit at the long-term price of gradual bone loss). In addition, remodeling is the means by which PTH restores normocalcemia in response to hypocalcemia.

D Intercellular Communication among Bone Cells: Triggers and Constraints on Remodeling

Because initiation of each remodeling event begins with delivery of osteoclasts or their precursors to the bone surface, it is important to have passing familiarity with the signals that control this initial event [9,10]. The key cell for controlling osteoclast production is the osteoblast. This bone-forming cell elaborates two distinct proteins, a stimulator and a repressor, that regulate osteoclast production. The osteoclast stimulator was initially called "osteoclast differentiation factor," but now that its primary target is known, it has been given the less transparent name of RANK-ligand. RANK is an abbreviation for the "receptor that activates NF-kappa β" (a gene present in osteoclasts and other cells of macrophage origin). Under stimulation by agents known to increase bone remodeling (e.g., PTH and L-thyroxine), the osteoblast synthesizes and extrudes RANK-ligand that binds to RANK located on osteoclast precursors, leading to production of new osteoclasts. The repressor molecule, also produced by osteoblasts, is a protein called osteoprotegerin (OPG). Production of this protein increases when the osteoblast binds agents that inhibit remodeling, such as estrogen. OPG exhibits high affinity for RANK-ligand and therefore acts as a false receptor, neutralizing the effect of any RANK-ligand with which it comes into contact.

The RANK–RANK-ligand–OPG complex acts in a push–pull manner to regulate osteoclast production and hence control the rate of bone remodeling. When stimuli favor greater remodeling, RANK-ligand production increases, OPG decreases, and RANK is activated. When remodeling is suppressed, RANK-ligand decreases, OPG increases, and RANK is constrained. Interference with RANK-ligand function is the basis of a recently developed therapy for osteoporosis (See Section V.B.1.f).

III ADULT BONE MAINTENANCE

For many years, scientific inquiry into the basis of adult bone loss and development of osteoporosis was highly parochial. Nutrition scientists focused on the diet, exercise physiologists and mechanical engineers focused on physical activity and the mechanical environment, and physicians whose responsibility it was to care for patients with osteoporosis focused largely on menopausal estrogen loss. It is now abundantly clear that acquisition and maintenance of a healthy skeleton is far more complex than can be explained by any of these individual spheres. One needs to view the skeleton as subject to diverse influences throughout life so that bone status at any particular time is the result of a stochastic process by which each individual insult or event over a lifetime has made its independent contribution.

A Major Influences on Age-Related Bone Loss

Successful bone maintenance requires continued attention to the same "hygienic" factors that influenced bone acquisition: physical activity, diet, and reproductive status. Bone maintenance requires sufficiency in all areas, and the others do not compensate deficiency in one. For example, amenorrheic athletes lose bone despite frequent high-intensity physical activity and supplemental calcium intake [11,12]. Successful bone maintenance is also jeopardized by known toxic exposures such as smoking, alcohol excess, immobility, systemic illnesses, and many medications.

1 Habitual Physical Activity

The skeleton's mechanical function was referred to previously. To accomplish this role in a manner that optimizes bone strength while at the same time not unduly increasing its weight, bones accommodate the loads imposed on them by undergoing alterations in mass, in external geometry, and in internal microarchitecture. The first enunciation of this principle is credited to the German scientist Julius Wolff as "Wolff's law" [13]. As a consequence of such adaptation, steady-state bone mass should reflect the mechanical environment, a concept that applies when comparing bone mass among individuals, different bones within an individual, and even different regions within a single bone. A substantial body of research has addressed this prediction. These studies are of two general types: (1) comparisons of bone mass of athletes to that of sedentary controls and (2) descriptions of associations between level of physical activity and bone mass within a general population. The first type of study generally considers only very active or sedentary individuals, and hence extreme differences in activity are represented. In the latter case, a broader range of physical activity is examined.

Considerable evidence indicates that elite athletes and chronic exercisers have higher BMD than age-matched, nonexercising subjects—a finding, not surprisingly, that applies primarily to sites that undergo loading during the exercise (reviewed in [14]). Activities associated with high load magnitude at low number of repetitions (cycles) are associated with substantial increases in bone mass. For example, world-class and recreational weight lifters have 10–35% greater lumbar spine BMD than sedentary age-matched controls. Comparing dominant to nondominant limbs in athletes whose sport involves unilateral loading represents a special case. For example, increased BMD in the playing compared to the nonplaying arm of tennis players has been repeatedly observed. By contrast, swimming, a buoyant activity not associated with counteracting the effect of gravity, does not appear to increase BMD. In one study of elite university athletes, swimmers actually had lower bone mass than gymnasts or nonathletic controls, despite increased muscle bulk and regular weight training [15]. Young athletes who spend more than 20 hours each week in a buoyant environment for many years may simply not experience sufficient gravitational stress to promote fully the expected degree of bone acquisition.

These comparisons of athletes and control subjects must be interpreted with caution. Because no measurements of bone mass are made prior to initiating the exercise program, a causal relationship between exercise and bone cannot be proven. It may be that individuals with higher bone density are more apt to succeed in athletics, and therefore they enter the "athlete" and chronic exercising groups. Conversely, elite swimmers may have excelled in buoyant activity because of a lighter skeleton. In many studies, important characteristics of the matched controls have been overlooked. Factors such as menstrual status, nutrient intake, and use of tobacco or alcohol may have confounded the results. Finally, skeletal status is most frequently expressed as the areal BMD (g/cm^2), a term that overestimates BMD in persons with large bones and underestimates it in smaller people. Thus, if exercisers and controls are not well matched for height, conclusions based on BMD may be spurious.

With respect to the impact of habitual physical activity within the general population, many studies now point to a significant skeletal effect of physical activity in children on the acquisition of bone during the second and third decades (see Chapter 44). The situation is less clear for moderately active adults, in whom no consistent relationship between current activity level and bone mass has been established. In our own work, strong relationships between estimates of daily energy expenditure and BMD were completely negated by normalizing the data for body weight or lean mass [14]. Several reports document positive relationships between lifelong physical activity and bone status.

Thus, cross-sectional studies generally support the notion that elite athletes and chronic exercisers have increased BMD, the magnitude of this difference likely depending on the type and intensity of exercise, age, sex, and hormonal status. However, data concerning moderate physical activity remain uncertain.

One approach to eliminating the selection bias of cross-sectional studies is a randomized controlled trial in which exercise is the intervention. A number of properly controlled studies of this sort have been reported. Although most indicate a positive effect of imposed exercise on BMD, the magnitude of response has been very disappointing to those who anticipated the large differences observed in cross-sectional studies. Rarely do the increases in BMD exceed 2% after 1 or 2 years of rigorous training, regardless of the type of exercise used (endurance vs. resistance training) [16–19].

Understanding the meager response to exercise interventions is related to the fact that skeletal response to mechanical loads is curvilinear in nature. Complete immobilization, as seen with high-level spinal cord injury, leads rapidly to devastating bone loss, with deficits approaching 30–40% over several months. By contrast, imposition of even substantial training regimens on normally ambulatory people or animals increases bone mass by only a few percent over a similar period. This is illustrated in Figure 45.7, in which the effect of walking on bone mass is schematized. As an individual goes from immobility to full ambulation, duration of time spent walking becomes progressively less efficient for increasing bone mass. A person who habitually walks 6 hours each day might require another 4–6 hours just to add a few more percent BMD. On the other hand, adding a more rigorous stimulus, such as high-impact loading, for even a few cycles would increase the response slope.

The worst thing that can happen to the skeleton is to be immobilized. For maintaining bone mass during adult life, a certain degree of daily weight bearing is required, and the vast majority of even sedentary individuals achieve this. Small increments in BMD can be achieved by increasing one's daily exercise schedule, but, as a consequence of Wolff's law, these will remain only so long as the added activity continues. For most individuals, particularly if they are elderly or frail, walking provides the soundest and most prudent physical activity for skeletal maintenance.

2 Nutrition

A ENERGY

Reflecting the major influence of weight-bearing activity on bone, bone mass is strongly related to body weight, so it should be no surprise that severe deficits in bone occur in states of profound malnutrition. Although frank starvation is extremely rare in developed societies, bone deficits are frequently encountered in medical conditions associated with extremely low body mass, such as anorexia nervosa, as well as various forms of intestinal malabsorption and cachexia. It may be difficult to assign responsibility for bone deficits in such patients to any specific nutrient because patients generally show profound reductions in the consumption of many nutrients. In teenagers with anorexia nervosa, skeletal deficits appear very early, and their magnitude is exacerbated because bone is lost at a time when other girls of similar age are gaining bone at an accelerated rate. Bachrach et al. [20] observed that whole body bone mass correlates linearly with body mass in normal teens, and that the bone mass of girls with anorexia nervosa lies exactly on this curve. In other words, skeletal deficits in young girls with anorexia nervosa primarily reflect their body mass. When these girls were observed over time, weight rehabilitation (a gain of at least 5 kg) was associated with a gain in bone mass.

B CALCIUM

The concept that osteoporosis is a disease of calcium deficiency was proposed more than a century ago, although a central role for calcium intake did not emerge into the scientific mainstream for many years. This largely reflected the overpowering influence of Professor Fuller Albright, who conceived of osteoporosis as a deficiency of bone matrix due to osteoblast failure, usually as a consequence of menopausal loss of estrogen [21]. Intensification of interest in calcium occurred with the publication of three independent reports. The first, by Matkovic et al. [22], demonstrated a difference in hip fracture incidence in two different regions of Croatia that were demographically very

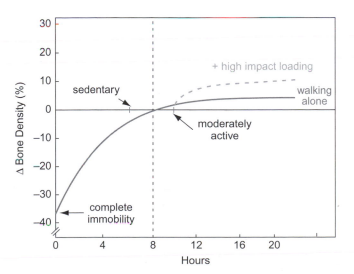

FIGURE 45.7 The curvilinear nature of skeletal response to mechanical loading. Source: *Copyright Robert Marcus, M.D.*

similar except for a substantial difference in the calcium content of local water supplies. Second was publication of NHANES II, which showed that habitual calcium intakes of American girls and women failed to meet recommended daily standards (RDAs) as early as age 11 years [23]. Third was a landmark paper by Chapuy *et al.* [24] that clearly demonstrated the ability of supplemental calcium and vitamin D to reduce the incidence of hip fracture in a highly vulnerable population.

When one considers that the skeleton is the repository for more than 99% of total body calcium, it is inconceivable that individuals whose intakes are below the amount necessary to maintain whole body calcium balance could be in negative balance without losing bone. Heaney discussed the issues surrounding the concept of a nutrient requirement (see Chapter 14) and refers to calcium as a "threshold nutrient," by which he means that below a critical value, some physiological function (e.g., calcium balance) is dependent on intake, but above that value no further benefit accrues from additional intake. Because the mineral demands for growth, early adult, and older adult maintenance differ substantially, the "threshold" value and therefore the intake requirements also differs by age [25,26]. Table 45.1 shows that recommendations for calcium intake have increased substantially over time from previous RDAs [27] and are closely allied to those derived from the literature of formal calcium balance studies [28].

In 2010, the Institute of Medicine (IOM) published updated values for dietary reference intakes for calcium and vitamin D following a comprehensive review of the literature and scientific testimony. The full report is available online (www.iom.edu/reports/2010/dietary-reference-intakes-for-calcium-and-vitamin-D.aspx). An abbreviated table appears in Table 45.2 (see the

Appendix for more detail.) In general, the IOM recommendations are reasonably close to earlier elaborations (Table 45.1). One emphasis of the IOM statement was that intakes above those shown as upper level increased the risk of adverse experiences, such as kidney stones.

Although a consensus conference on optimal calcium intake concluded that habitual calcium intakes by both men and women are inadequate for optimal bone health [25], and several clinical trials demonstrated the ability of calcium supplementation to constrain the rate of bone loss and even reduce fractures [24,29–35], there remains in the medical and research communities some resistance to reaching consensus regarding the role of calcium inadequacy in the pathogenesis of osteoporosis. In part, this reflects considerable uncertainty in estimating the amount of calcium that people habitually consume. For example, dietary histories and food frequency questionnaires carry substantial imprecision. Also, it must be remembered that calcium is not absorbed in a vacuum but, rather, in the course of eating or drinking other foods, and its availability from foods is highly influenced by other nutrients. For example, although the calcium content of spinach is quite good, it is rendered essentially nonabsorbable by the presence of oxalate and perhaps other anions to which it binds [36]. Further consideration of the roles of phosphorus, sodium, and protein appears later.

TABLE 45.1 Various Estimates of the Calcium Requirement (mg/day) in Women

Age (years)	1989 RDA[a]	NIH[b]	1997 AI[c]	Balance[d]
1–5	800	800	–	1100
6–10	800	800–1200	960	1100
11–24	1200	1200–1500	1560	1600
Pregnancy/lactation	1200	1200–1500	1200–1560	–
24–50/65	800	1000	1200	800–1000
65–	800	1500	1440	1500–1700

[a]*National Research Council [27].*
[b]*Recommendations for women as proposed by the Consensus Development Conference on Optimal Calcium Intake [25].*
[c]*The so-called adequate intakes of the new DRI values, multiplied by a factor of 1.2 to convert them into RDA format [26].*
[d]*Estimates derived from published balance studies [28].*
Source: *Adapted from Heaney [85].*

TABLE 45.2 Dietary Reference Intakes for Calcium (mg/day)

Age	Estimated average requirement	RDA	Upper level intake
Infants			
0–6 months			1000
6–12 months			1500
1–3 years	500	700	2500
4–8 years	800	1000	2500
9–18 years	1100	1300	3000
19–30 years	800	1000	2500
31–50 years	800	1000	2500
51–70 men	800	1000	2000
51–70 women	1000	1200	2000
>70 years	1000	1200	2000
Pregnant/lactating			
14–18 years	1100	1300	3000
19–50 years	800	1000	2500

Source: *Institute of Medicine (2010). Dietary Reference Intakes for Calcium and Vitamin D. Available at www.iom.edu/reports/2010/dietary-reference-intakes-for-calcium-and-vitamin-D.aspx.*

For adults, calcium intakes in the range of 1000–1500 mg/day are recommended. Note that individuals in early to middle adult life, such as 20–50 years of age, have calcium intakes within reasonable proximity to recommended values and, by virtue of being young enough to undertake regular weight-bearing activity and to maintain normal reproductive function, generally have only modest stress on skeletal balance, as shown by very low rates of bone loss. After menopause (average age, 51 years), and certainly at more advanced ages, declines in endogenous reproductive hormone concentrations and in the growth hormone–insulin-like growth factor 1 axis, coupled with overall trends toward less physical activity, make it less likely that dietary deficiency will be buffered and more likely that age-related bone loss will be aggravated.

C PHOSPHORUS

Various domestic animals respond to excessive dietary phosphorus by increasing the endogenous concentration of PTH, resulting in negative calcium balance and bone loss. In such animals, optimal dietary ratios of calcium to phosphorus approach 1.0. This has led to a popular theory that because calcium:phosphorus ratios in human diets typically are well below 1.0, phosphorus overconsumption initiates a similar process in humans.

Firm evidence to support a role for phosphorus excess in human osteoporosis has not been forthcoming. In contrast, some evidence indicates that intestinal calcium absorption and balance are fairly impervious to very wide variations in daily phosphorus consumption [37,38]. Separate mention should be made concerning the role of phosphorus-containing soft drinks. Cola drinks contain phosphoric acid as their source of effervescence, and one reads frequently in the lay press that the high content of phosphorus in colas is an important contributor to developing osteoporosis. However, although excessive soft drink consumption may well contribute to poor bone status, this is so because these beverages have been substituted for milk, thus exchanging a calcium-rich drink for one that contains essentially no calcium [39].

D PROTEIN

For many years, a concept has circulated as a subtext in osteoporosis research that consumption of excess protein, particularly from animal sources, is an important contributor to the development of osteoporosis. This is considered the consequence of the fact that protein catabolism generates ammonium ion from ammonia and sulfate from sulfur-containing amino acids. When protein intake increases, citrate and carbonate ions are released from bone to neutralize these acids,

and, because urinary calcium is closely linked to renal acid excretion, urinary calcium rises. However, plant proteins contain amounts of sulfur similar to those in eggs, milk, and meats, and therefore increased intake of protein from either animal or plant sources similarly increases urinary calcium. Furthermore, the impact of protein on calcium balance depends to a major degree on other nutrients contained in the consumed food. For example, milk calcium compensates for urinary calcium losses generated by milk protein, potassium in such plants as legumes and grains decreases calcium excretion, and the high phosphorus content of meat offsets the calciuric effect of the protein [40].

Nutritional status assessments of patients with osteoporosis do not support a view that these patients have enjoyed a life of luxurious protein consumption. Barger-Lux et al. [41] reported that women with low calcium intakes generally consumed insufficient amounts of multiple nutrients, including protein. Sellmeyer et al. [42] reported higher protein intakes to be associated with greater age-related bone loss in the SOF cohort. However, a substantial body of evidence does not sustain this view. Protein consumption was reported to be an important positive predictor of bone mass in elderly women [43]. In the Framingham cohort, Hannan et al. [44] reported bone loss over time to be inversely related to protein intake, with rates of loss in the highest quartile of protein consumption less than one-third of those in the lowest quartile. Kerstetter et al. [45] conducted a series of controlled balance studies that showed that although calciuria increased with increased protein intake, this did not come from bone but was rather a reflection of improved intestinal calcium absorption. In a randomized controlled trial, Dawson-Hughes and Harris [46] showed that the improvement in BMD in subjects supplemented with calcium and vitamin D was confined mainly to individuals whose protein intake was in the highest tertile. Delmi et al. [47] found that supplemental protein improved recovery from hip fracture, accelerated hospital discharge, and also slowed bone loss in the contralateral hip. Heaney [48] concluded that the weight of evidence shows high protein intake to be osteoprotective, but only if calcium intake is adequate, whereas the protective effect of calcium occurs only when protein intake is relatively high.

E SODIUM

Urinary excretion of calcium and that of sodium are highly linked, and increased sodium intake is known to promote calcium excretion. A similar effect occurs with most diuretic agents (with the single exception of thiazides, which uncouple the handling of these two cations). Thus, it is not unreasonable to expect that increased dietary sodium might be conducive to negative calcium balance and aggravate bone loss. In a 2-year prospective trial, Devine *et al.* [49] examined the influence of urinary sodium excretion and dietary calcium intake on bone density of postmenopausal women. Urinary sodium excretion (a robust indication of intake) correlated negatively with changes in BMD, and the data suggested that halving sodium intake had the same effect on BMD as increasing daily calcium intake by 891 mg [49].

F VITAMIN D

The importance of vitamin D to skeletal maintenance is thoroughly discussed in Chapter 43. When severe, vitamin D deficiency is associated with significant undermineralization of bone matrix, a condition known as osteomalacia [50]. At milder levels of vitamin D inadequacy, impaired calcium absorption promotes compensatory secretion of PTH, which increases bone remodeling and aggravates bone loss. Maintaining vitamin D adequacy is an important and widespread issue for the general population and for the vast majority of patients with osteoporosis. It appears that optimal vitamin D status is achieved at 25-hydroxyvitamin D concentrations of approximately 30 ng/ml (80 nmol/l). To achieve this goal, previously recommended vitamin D consumption of 400–800 units/day is not adequate, and doses of 1000–2000 units/day are preferable.

3 Reproductive Hormonal Status

Decades of studies in animals and humans support the concept that achieving and maintaining normal gonadal function is a critical determinant of bone health during pubertal bone acquisition and throughout adult life in both women and men. Indeed, the impact of menopausal loss of endogenous estrogen on skeletal balance can be so profound that many investigators have focused solely on the contribution of estrogen withdrawal to osteoporosis without regard for the other contributions described previously. We now understand that permanent loss of estrogen at menopause is not the only circumstance in which gonadal status has a skeletal impact. During earlier adult life, transient episodes of oligo- or amenorrhea may also be associated with at least transient bone loss [51].

The mechanisms by which estrogen withdrawal affects the skeleton involve multiple organs. The direct skeletal effect of the most potent circulating estrogen, 17-β estradiol, is to suppress the rate of bone remodeling. This is achieved by downregulating the formation of osteoclasts. In some rodents, this effect has been related to the suppression of an osteoclast-stimulating cytokine, interleukin-6 [52,53]. In other animal models and in humans, strong evidence has been presented for the participation of other cytokines, including interleukins and transforming growth factor-β [54]. In addition,

estrogen withdrawal reduces osteoblast production of osteoprotegerin, the decoy receptor for RANK-ligand discussed previously [55]. These cytokine effects are reversed when estrogen is replaced. The use of estrogen as pharmacologic therapy for the prevention and treatment of osteoporosis is described later.

IV DIAGNOSIS OF OSTEOPOROSIS

Because traditional radiographic techniques cannot distinguish osteoporosis until it is severe, diagnosis was, until recently, clinical, requiring a history of one or more low-trauma fractures. Although highly specific, such a grossly insensitive diagnostic criterion offered no assistance to physicians who hope to identify and treat affected individuals who have been fortunate not yet to have sustained a fracture. The focus in this section is the measurement of bone mineral density. However, one must be cognizant of a wide variety of risk factors other than bone density that may profoundly influence an individual's risk for fracture. A partial list of these factors is presented in Table 45.3.

TABLE 45.3   Partial List of Risk Factors for Osteoporosis and Related Fractures

Major factors
Personal history of fracture as an adult
History of fragility fracture in a first-degree relative
Low body weight (less than approximately 127 lb)
Current smoking
Use of oral corticosteroid therapy for more than 3 months
Additional risk factors
Impaired vision
Estrogen deficiency at an early age (<45 years)
Thyroid hormone excess
Intestinal malabsorption
Some varieties of hypercalciuria
Selected medications (cyclosporin and related agents, thiazolidinediones, possibly selective serotonin inhibitors [SSRIs])
Dementia
Poor health/frailty
Recent falls
Low calcium intake (lifelong)
Immobilization or low physical activity
Alcohol in amounts > 2 drinks per day

Source: *Adapted from the National Osteoporosis Foundation [1].*

The introduction of accurate noninvasive bone mass measurements afforded the opportunity to estimate a person's fracture risk and to make an early diagnosis of osteoporosis. Large prospective studies have shown that a reduction in BMD of 1 standard deviation (SD) from the mean value for an age-specific population confers a two- or threefold increase in long-term fracture risk [56–59]. In a manner similar to that by which serum cholesterol concentration predicts risk for heart attack or blood pressure predicts risk for stroke, BMD measurements can successfully identify subjects at risk of fracture and can help physicians select those individuals who will derive greatest benefit for initiation of therapy. Indeed, the gradient of risk associated with a 1 SD difference in BMD is even greater than those for cholesterol and heart attack.

Several factors limit the ability of BMD measurements to predict an individual's fracture risk with great accuracy. The normative data against which BMD comparisons are most often made have been determined for Caucasian men and women and do not necessarily apply to other ethnic groups. This problem is gradually being overcome as ethnic-specific BMD data have begun to penetrate the literature. BMD is clearly related to body weight, but routine clinical bone mass assessments are not weight-adjusted. Various features of bone geometry that affect bone strength and fracture risk are not considered in the clinical interpretation of bone mass measurements. These include bone size, the distribution of bone mass around its bending axis (moments of inertia), and some derivative functions such as the hip axis length [60]. Moreover, bone mass measurements cannot distinguish individuals with low mass and intact microarchitecture from those with equal mass who have trabecular disruption and cortical porosity. They also cannot distinguish other aspects of bone quality.

In 1994, a group of senior investigators in this field offered a working definition of osteoporosis based exclusively on bone mass [61]. The reasoning behind this proposal, made on behalf of the World Health Organization, was that the clinical significance of osteoporosis lies exclusively in the occurrence of fracture, that bone mass predicts long-term fracture risk, and that selection of rigorous diagnostic criteria would minimize the number of patients who are incorrectly diagnosed. The authors suggested a cutoff BMD value of 2.5 SD below the average for healthy young adult women. Using this value, approximately 30% of postmenopausal women would be designated as osteoporotic, which gives a realistic projection of lifetime fracture rates. In addition, Kanis *et al.* [61] proposed that BMD values of 1 or 2 SD below the young adult mean be designated as "osteopenic." Such values identify individuals at modestly increased risk for fracture

but for whom a diagnosis of osteoporosis would not be justified because it would mislabel far more individuals than would actually be expected ever to fracture.

This approach has proven useful for clinical management, but it has limitations. Its application to young people prior to their acquisition of peak bone mass would be inappropriate, and it remains unclear exactly what the best means to assess fracture risk in men may be. The BMD measurement is subject to several confounding factors, including bone size and geometry. Because BMD correlations among skeletal sites are not strong, designating a person "normal" based on a single site, such as the lumbar spine, necessarily overlooks individuals with low bone density elsewhere, such as the hip. It seems reasonable to suppose that adjustment of bone density readings for such factors as body size, bone geometry, and ethnic background might improve the accuracy of this technique. Finally, studies indicate that although individuals with low BMD are at greater relative risk to fracture, many fractures in the population are experienced by individuals with normal bone mass [62–64]. Knowledge of a low bone density at a particular point in time offers no information regarding the adequacy of peak bone mass attained, the amount of bone that may have been lost, or the quality of bone that remains.

The World Health Organization completed an initiative to give individuals an estimate of their absolute 10-year fracture risk. Because the goal of this initiative was to provide a useful document for all nations, it relies primarily on osteoporosis risk factors rather than on BMD. However, for areas of the world in which BMD testing is widely available, BMD scores may be added as an additional predictive variable. This initiative, called FRAX, has been published and is readily available for routine use via an online program (www.shef.ac.uk/FRAX). Separate calculation tools are provided at this website for individuals living in Asia, Europe, the Middle East and Africa, North and Latin America, and Oceania. In the United States, the National Osteoporosis Foundation (www.nof.org) makes a FRAX calculator available as software for bone densitometry providers.

A Beyond BMD: The Question of Bone Quality

As stated in the introduction to this chapter, osteoporosis is a condition of decreased bone strength, where strength is a composite function of BMD and bone quality. Several diverse qualitative characteristics have been described that directly influence bone strength. The more important factors—bone geometry, microarchitectural integrity, mineralization state, and remodeling rate—are briefly considered here. For more detailed information, the reader may consult Seeman and Delmas [65]. The first factor is overall bone geometry. A bone of greater diameter is better able than a smaller bone to withstand either a compressive or a bending force. One reason that men are relatively less susceptible to forearm fractures than are women is the fact that long bones of men are wider. A second feature, particularly in trabecular bone, is microarchitectural integrity. Normal trabecular bone is a honeycomb of highly connected vertical and horizontal trabeculae (Figure 45.1A), and the holes, or spaces between the trabeculae, are fairly uniform. By contrast, osteoporotic trabecular bone gives the appearance of Swiss cheese (Figure 45.1B). The holes are not uniform because excessive bone resorption has perforated the trabeculae, leaving confluent, sometimes extremely large holes that represent the permanent loss of entire trabecular units. A third important qualitative factor is the state of bone remodeling. It will be remembered that each remodeling event begins with the removal by osteoclasts of a divot of bone from trabecular surface. At any one time, then, there are hundreds of thousands of resorption holes, or *lacunae*, on bone surfaces. These holes are an inherent point of weakness to the bone, permitting very modest mechanical loads to overload the structure and fracture it. In mechanical engineering parlance, such points of weakness are called "stress concentrators." Mechanical stresses that are generated across an area of bone divert from their normal path of stress transmission to focus on the area of weakening, thereby overloading it. Thus, individuals with higher levels of bone remodeling activity will have more stress-concentrating lacunae on their bone surfaces, giving them a greater chance for fracture than somebody in a low remodeling state. Finally, the degree of bone mineralization is also an important feature of bone quality. Roughly speaking, except in extreme cases, the more mineralized the bone matrix, the greater its mechanical strength. Because a portion of bone continues to accumulate mineral as long as it exists, individuals with lower remodeling rates will have bone that is older, and therefore more mineralized and stronger, than individuals whose bone is remodeled more rapidly.

One message from this inquiry into bone quality is that a BMD measurement simply does not describe a sufficient amount of information about the nature of the skeleton ever to be a gold standard for the presence of osteoporosis. Unfortunately, currently, no suitable noninvasive measurements are available to assess bone quality in patients outside a research environment. Therefore, one is forced to rely on BMD measures to some degree. That being said, one also should not depend on changes in BMD over time as a true index of whether patients have improved or deteriorated in response to therapeutic interventions. One important indication of overall bone quality is whether a given person has already sustained a low-trauma fracture. Evidence has been published that individuals with such fractures have more serious disruption of qualitative measures seen on bone biopsies than individuals who have not fractured [66]. Therefore, the presence of a vertebral compression fracture on a radiograph of the spine may reasonably permit the physician to conclude that the patient has poor bone quality.

V OSTEOPOROSIS PREVENTION AND TREATMENT

A Hygienic Management

The term *hygienic* is used here in the sense of being nonpharmacologic. It refers to the appropriate attention to lifestyle factors that either protect or damage bone. These principles have universal application regardless of whether one wishes to forestall bone loss and development of osteoporosis or treat established disease.

1 Physical Activity

As described previously, the skeleton adapts to its mechanical environment so that the steady-state amount of bone reflects daily exposure to mechanical forces. Although the skeletal response to vigorous exercise, such as weight lifting (resistance activity) or running (endurance activity), may be greater than that observed with walking, the majority of middle-aged and older individuals are more likely to persist long term with a program of walking. A progressive schedule of walking 30 minutes or more several days each week provides a mechanical load to the legs and axial skeleton and should form the basis of skeletal maintenance for ambulatory persons in their middle and advanced years. Younger individuals should certainly be encouraged to pursue more vigorous activities, but it must be remembered that the effects of high-load environments persist only so long as the high loading schedule continues. If a person stops training, the bone perceives a reduction in mechanical environment and adaptive responses will lead to loss of bone until a new steady state is reached.

2 Dietary Factors

With respect to overall dietary intakes, substantial weight loss during adult life is a risk factor for fractures. Weight-loss programs are associated with measurable decreases in BMD, and the impact of so-called yo-yo weight fluctuations, although unclear, carries some skeletal risk. As discussed previously, the nutrients of most relevance to skeletal maintenance are calcium and vitamin D. A daily calcium intake of 1200–1500 mg should be the goal for most healthy adults. Consuming a quart of nonfat milk each day could approach this, but it is very unlikely that most adults, even dairy enthusiasts, will consistently accomplish that. Each quart of milk contains approximately 1100 mg calcium, although this may vary somewhat depending on its fat content. Because calcium is contained within the aqueous phase of milk, an equal volume of low-fat or skim milk has more water, and hence more calcium, than whole milk. In addition, some brands of reduced-fat milk are enriched by the addition of milk solids, which further increases calcium content.

Many segments of the population experience loss of the enzyme lactase, which is necessary for the hydrolysis of the major milk sugar lactose. Many afflicted individuals experience bloating, cramps, or other symptoms of intestinal distress if they consume lactose-containing dairy products. Several strategies can be recommended for such individuals. Lactose-free milk is readily available in markets. Lactose in this product has been prehydrolyzed to its constituent sugars, glucose and galactose, by incubation with commercial lactase. This milk has a slightly sweet taste due to the taste of its hexose sugars. For those who do not care for this taste, lactase tablets can be taken immediately prior to drinking milk. Yogurt and other products in which lactose is hydrolyzed provide an excellent substitute for milk. Many cheeses are rich in calcium (not cottage cheese, however) but have the complicating feature of high sodium content. The calcium:sodium ratio of most liquid dairy products is approximately 1.0, but the ratio is well below 1 for hard cheeses. Given the relationship between sodium intake and calciuria [49], depending on cheese for calcium consumption may not be effective.

Other reasonably good food sources of calcium include small fish (anchovies, herrings, and sardines), nuts, and some green vegetables (broccoli). However, it is quite difficult to attain calcium adequacy with these foods alone without also consuming dairy products. For example, it may require 6 cups of broccoli to provide as much calcium as would be consumed in a single 8-ounce glass of milk.

For many individuals, a calcium supplement offers the most convenient approach to reaching target levels of calcium intake. Many calcium salts are available on an over-the-counter basis. Calcium carbonate has the advantage of having the highest percentage by weight in calcium (40% of calcium carbonate is calcium) so that the fewest number of pills need be taken. Calcium citrate is a reliable calcium supplement. It has been alleged that individuals who have achlorhydria or are taking medications that reduce gastric acid secretion better absorb the citrate salt than the carbonate. However, it has been shown that when calcium carbonate is taken with food, there is sufficient acidity in the food to permit normal calcium absorption [67]. Therefore, my general recommendation for individuals who will likely not consume more than 1000 mg calcium per day through food alone is to take a 500 mg calcium supplement as calcium carbonate each morning with breakfast. For individuals with osteoporosis who are receiving pharmacological treatment, I increase that recommendation to 1000 mg calcium/day.

In 2008, Bolland et al. [68] reported on a calcium intervention trial in older women, in which consumption of calcium as supplement, but not food, was associated with an increased risk for cardiovascular complications, including myocardial infarction. Subsequently, the same group published a meta-analysis from which they concluded that "calcium supplements without vitamin D are associated with an increased risk of myocardial infarction" [69]. This publication created a storm of controversy. Although the meta-analysis was constructed from multiple clinical trials, the most cases came from the single trial reported by Bolland and colleagues [68]. Myocardial infarction was not an end point of that trial, and cases were not adjudicated. The 2-year pill compliance rate was only 55% and was lower yet in the group receiving calcium. Although the conclusions were based on an intervention in older women, a number of the studies included in the meta-analysis included both men and women, and none independently showed even a trend toward a cardiovascular adverse effect. All these factors could introduce bias into group comparisons. Moreover, some independent studies failing to support the views of Bolland et al. were not represented in the meta-analysis [70]. In particular, a well-designed and executed clinical trial in which cardiovascular end points were prespecified showed no impact of calcium supplementation on either atherosclerotic vascular mortality or first hospitalization, either during the 5-year clinical trial or during a 4.5-year follow-up period [70]. Given the importance of this topic, a committee from the American Society for Bone and Mineral Research evaluated the available data and concluded that "the weight of evidence is insufficient to conclude that calcium supplements cause adverse cardiovascular events; however, the debate continues."

B Pharmacologic Therapy

The variety of approved drugs for the prevention and treatment of osteoporosis has expanded enormously during approximately the past decade (Table 45.4). These are grouped into two general categories—antiresorptive (sometimes called anticatabolic)

TABLE 45.4 Approved Medications for the Prevention and Treatment of Osteoporosis

Antiresorptive

　Calcium/vitamin D

　Estrogens

　Bisphosphonates

　　Alendronate

　　Risedronate

　　Ibandronate

　　Zoledronatic Acid

　Calcitonin

　Strontium ranelate (not approved in United States)

Bone-forming

　Teriparatide

　PTH(1−84) (not approved in United States)

and bone-forming (or anabolic). The first category contains the great majority of registered products. Although the fundamentals of their mechanism of action differ from one product to the next, they all act ultimately to inhibit either the development of osteoclasts from their precursors or the action of mature osteoclasts. Such action confers skeletal protection in two ways, both of which are predictable consequences of slowing the remodeling rate by 30−70%, as per the previous discussion of bone quality. First, and perhaps most important, at least during the first year or so of therapy, reducing the creation of new resorption lacunae results in a major reduction in the prevalence of stress concentrators on bone surfaces. Second, because any given point on the bone surface will survive longer when the remodeling rate is low, the bone continues to gain mineral for a longer period of time and ultimately becomes relatively hypermineralized.

By contrast, only one bone-forming agent—the 1−34 fragment of human parathyroid hormone (teriparatide; see later discussion)—is currently approved in the United States for the treatment of osteoporosis, Its actions involve the direct stimulation of bone-forming osteoblasts.

Selection of appropriate therapies for individual patients is beyond the scope of this chapter. The following material briefly describes each of these approved products.

1 Antiresorptive Agents

A CALCIUM AND VITAMIN D

Strictly speaking, calcium and vitamin D have an antiresorptive activity on bone. By slightly elevating blood calcium concentrations, endogenous PTH secretion is reduced and overall bone remodeling decreases. The role of calcium and vitamin D in skeletal maintenance was described previously. Calcium administration to osteoporotic women with previous vertebral fractures has been shown to decrease the risk for subsequent fracture [33] and, when combined with a modest amount of vitamin D, has been shown to reduce the incidence of hip fracture in elderly women [24]. Suffice it to say that calcium and vitamin D adequacy are essential components of all successful therapies, and the general approach described previously must be pursued if any pharmacologic regimen is to succeed. Indeed, therapeutic failures are frequently attributable to inadequate vitamin D status. Note that all major osteoporosis trials were designed to show an effect of drug on bone turnover, BMD, and fracture incidence superior to that of the control regimens, which invariably consisted of calcium and vitamin D.

B ESTROGEN

The use of estrogen to treat postmenopausal osteoporosis has been popular for at least 50 years. The era of the 1970s and 1980s saw the publication of many small clinical trials demonstrating the effect of various estrogen and estrogen/progestin combinations in early and postmenopausal women to improve calcium balance, to suppress markers of bone turnover, to increase BMD, and in small series to protect against vertebral compression fractures [71]. Because the available studies did not demonstrate a compelling case that estrogen administration to women with established osteoporosis led to a significant reduction in fracture incidence, U.S. Food and Drug Administration (FDA) approval of estrogen was specified for prevention of osteoporosis, not for treatment. With publication of results from the Women's Health Initiative, we now have conclusive evidence for the nonvertebral fracture efficacy of estrogen, even in women who were not osteoporotic or at high risk for fracture [72]. Unfortunately, the Women's Health Initiative also established that estrogen, particularly when given in combination with progestin, increased the development of breast cancer, myocardial infarction, and other cardiovascular events and potentially contributed to cognitive decline. Thus, although estrogens remain highly effective when treating women with hot flashes, current opinion holds that they should be used at the lowest possible dose and for the shortest possible duration and are not recommended as long-term therapy for prevention or treatment of osteoporosis.

C SELECTIVE ESTRADIOL RECEPTOR MODULATORS

These compounds are neither hormones nor estrogens but, rather, molecules that interact with the estradiol receptor in multiple tissues of the body. For a comprehensive description of selective estradiol receptor modulator (SERM) physiology, the reader is referred to the review of Siris and Muchmore [73]. Briefly summarized, unlike estrogens, SERMs interact with the estradiol receptor and activate estrogen-regulated genes in a manner that is tissue specific. For example, like estrogen, tamoxifen stimulates uterine hyperplasia and suppresses bone remodeling, but unlike estrogen, it inhibits estrogen actions at the breast. On the other hand, raloxifene has no effect on the endometrium, acts like estrogen on bone, and antagonizes estrogen action at the breast. Although several such molecules were introduced into clinical medicine before their mechanisms of action were clarified (e.g., tamoxifen), recent years have seen the development of numerous molecules in this class for the intended purpose of treating osteoporosis. As of this writing, only one SERM, raloxifene (Evista), is FDA approved for prevention and treatment of osteoporosis. Raloxifene has been shown to prevent the development of frank osteoporosis in women with low bone mass and to offer substantial long-term protection against vertebral fracture in women with established osteoporosis [74]. At the approved dose of 60 mg daily, raloxifene offers significant protection against the development of estrogen receptor-positive breast cancer, for which it also has received FDA approval.

D BISPHOSPHONATES

Bisphosphonates are analogs of the naturally occurring phosphate ester pyrophosphate, in which a carbon atom has replaced the central oxygen bridge. This substitution renders the compounds nonsusceptible to hydrolysis by alkaline phosphatase, a ubiquitous enzyme that hydrolyzes pyrophosphate. Bisphosphonates are poorly absorbed from the gut, but once absorbed they are taken up by bone. The presence of two phosphate groups permits the molecule to bind avidly to hydroxyapatite so that the half-life of bisphosphonates in the skeleton may be a matter of many years. In theory, osteoclasts imbibe the bisphosphonate during the course of bone resorption, resulting in osteoclast death and a decrease in resorption. Differences in one of the two side chains underlie differences in action among agents of this class. The first generation of bisphosphonates acted to inhibit intermediary metabolism. More recent compounds that have amino groups on the side chain act in a manner similar to the statin class of antilipid drugs—that is, inhibiting the mevalonate synthesis pathway, but at a level (farnesyl diphosphate synthetase) that is further downstream, leading to interference with prenylation of plasma membrane lipids [75]. First developed and introduced for the treatment of Paget's disease of bone in the 1960s, several bisphosphonates have shown significant improvement in BMD and reductions in fracture.

Three oral bisphosphonates are currently approved for prevention and treatment of osteoporosis: alendronate (Fosamax) [76], risedronate (Actonel) [77,78], and ibandronate (Boniva) [79]. The last may also be administered by intravenous infusion. Another very potent bisphosphonate, zoledronic acid, has received FDA approval for treatment of osteoporosis. This agent is administered only once each year by intravenous infusion.

In recent years, it has become apparent that some patients receiving long-term potent bisphosphonates may experience potentially serious complications of treatment, including osteonecrosis of the jaw (ONJ) and nonclassical or "atypical" hip fractures [80]. Although the precise mechanisms by which such complications may be induced remain unsettled, it appears likely that they reflect in some manner the degree to which bone remodeling has been suppressed. For example, because of its role in chewing, the mandible receives some of the heaviest mechanical loads of any bone in the body. To maintain mandibular health and prevent fatigue damage, it is necessary to have a robust and responsive remodeling system. In the presence of potent antiresorptive therapy, remodeling might not be adequate to prevent tissue breakdown and subsequent necrosis. Similarly, a number of case reports and patient series have described the occurrence of fractures in the subtrochanteric region of the femur in patients exposed to long-term bisphosphonates. These transverse fractures show a characteristic radiographic appearance, with thickening of the bony cortex and "beaking" of the fracture fragment. In a very large population-based study, it was determined that although there is a small added risk for such atypical fractures, the overall benefit:risk ratio for bisphosphonates remained substantially positive in that the overall fracture incidence in bisphosphonate-treated patients was considerably lower than that of nontreated patients [81]. Nonetheless, a trend in treatment strategy has attended the emergence of ONJ and atypical fractures, in that many experts now recommend bisphosphonate therapy be stopped following 5 consecutive years of treatment, with subsequent monitoring of BMD so that treatment can be restarted if and when bone loss recurs.

E CALCITONIN

This 32-amino acid peptide is a natural hormone throughout the vertebrate phylum. Its primary physiological role appears to be to reduce the rate of bone remodeling by inhibiting the action of mature osteoclasts. Calcitonin obtained from salmon is considerably more potent than the human hormone and has been approved for treatment of osteoporosis [82]. Although calcitonin can be given by subcutaneous injection, most patients take the drug as a nasal spray (Miacalcin).

In approved doses, calcitonin is a relatively weak anti-resorptive drug with efficacy characteristics that are less pronounced than those of the other approved anti-resorptive agents.

F DENOSUMAB

In Section II.D, I described the role of the RANK—RANK-ligand (RANKL) system for regulating bone turnover. In 2010, the FDA approved denosumab, a human monoclonal antibody that specifically binds to RANKL, prevents the activation of RANK on the surface of osteoclasts and their precursors, and thereby inhibits osteoclast formation and function, substantially decreasing the rate of bone remodeling [83]. In its pivotal clinical trial, denosumab reduced the occurrence of all categories of fragility fracture: vertebral, hip, and nonvertebral. Based on its mechanism of action, denosumab is considered a potent antiresorptive drug. Marketed under the trade name Prolia, it is approved for treatment of men and postmenopausal women with osteoporosis at high risk of fracture. The drug is administered by vein every 6 months and is generally well tolerated. Some concern has been expressed regarding the tendency for patients to experience lower blood calcium concentrations when treated with denosumab, and hypocalcemia is considered a contraindication for its use. In addition, in clinical trials, serious infections leading to hospitalization were more frequent in the denosumab group than with placebo. These include bacterial endocarditis, skin infections, and infections in the abdomen and urinary tract. Osteonecrosis of the jaw has been reported in a few patients receiving denosumab.

G STRONTIUM RANELATE

Strontium has received approval in Europe and Asia for treatment of osteoporosis. It becomes incorporated directly into the bone mineral, which creates an artifactual increase in BMD. However, strontium does appear to be an effective antiresorptive compound and has been shown to reduce fracture risk. Because no studies of this compound have been conducted in the United States, it does not appear that strontium can ever receive FDA approval and so it is unlikely to be introduced into the U.S. market.

2 Bone Formation Therapy

A TERIPARATIDE (FORTEO AND FORSTEO IN EUROPE)

Teriparatide is the generic term for the 1—34 fragment of human PTH. It is approved as a single daily subcutaneous injection for up to 2 years at a dose of $20\,\mu g$/day. Teriparatide is the first bone anabolic agent approved for treatment of osteoporosis.

(The full-length PTH(1—84) molecule has not received approval in the United States but is marketed in Europe. Its actions are qualitatively similar to those of teriparatide.) Teriparatide directly stimulates osteoblasts to form new bone and results in considerably greater increases in BMD than are observed with antiresorptive drugs. In addition, teriparatide uniquely repairs the disrupted microarchitecture of trabecular bone to a normal pattern and also increases the thickness of cortical bone. These effects result in substantial reduction in both vertebral and nonvertebral fracture [84]. Teriparatide given very long term at high dose to Fischer 344 rats led to a high rate of osteosarcoma. Other animal models have shown no such effect, and although a relationship to human carcinogenesis seems very unlikely, one cannot be certain that no relationship exists. Because duration of therapy was a critical element for carcinogenesis in rats, teriparatide use is currently restricted to 2 years. Teriparatide is marketed for the treatment of men and postmenopausal women with osteoporosis whose physicians consider them at high risk for fracture. As opposed to several of the antiresorptive agents, it is not a drug for prevention of osteoporosis.

VI CONCLUSION

Efforts are underway to bring forth additional compounds of both the antiresorptive and bone-formation classes. Other developmental targets for antiresorptive agents include inhibitors of cathepsins, the osteoclast-derived enzymes that hydrolyze bone. With respect to bone-forming agents, new PTH analogs and modes of delivery for teriparatide are in early phase human trials, as is suppression of a bone formation-inhibiting molecule, sclerostin. Still largely in animal studies, strategies to activate a newly discovered anabolic pathway in bone, the Wnt pathway, have begun.

Thus, the future of pharmacologic therapy for osteoporosis seems reasonably bright. However, the overall outlook for this disease remains clouded. With aging of the population, trends toward increasingly sedentary life, and substandard intakes of critical nutrients, the worldwide burden of osteoporotic fractures is likely to increase dramatically. Even now, it is difficult in the United States to get appropriate diagnosis and treatment for afflicted patients, even those with multiple fractures. With growing competition from other aspects of health care and with continued threats of onerous governmental and health insurance constraints on reimbursement for osteoporosis diagnosis and treatment, it is not at all certain that an explosive increase in fragility fractures and their consequences will be avoided.

References

[1] National Osteoporosis Foundation, Physician's Guide to Prevention and Treatment of Osteoporosis, Excerpta Medica, Belle Mead, NJ, 1998.

[2] L.J. Melton III, How many women have osteoporosis now? J. Bone Miner. Res. 10 (1995) 175–177.

[3] L.J. Melton III, C. Cooper, Magnitude and impact of osteoporosis and fractures, in: R. Marcus, D. Feldman, J. Kelsey (Eds.), Osteoporosis, second ed., Academic Press, San Diego, 2001, pp. 557–567.

[4] J.A. Cauley, D.E. Thompson, K.C. Ensrud, J.C. Scott, D. Black, Risk of mortality following clinical fractures, Osteoporos. Int. 11 (2000) 556–561.

[5] S.R. Cummings, M.C. Nevitt, A hypothesis: the causes of hip fractures, J. Gerontol. 44 (1989) M107–M111.

[6] A.V. Schwartz, E. Capezuti, J.A. Grisso, Falls as risk factors for fractures, in: R. Marcus, D. Feldman, J. Kelsey (Eds.), Osteoporosis, second ed., Academic Press, San Diego, 2001, pp. 795–807.

[7] C.A. Lee, T.A. Einhorn, The bone organ system, form and function, in: R. Marcus, D. Feldman, J. Kelsey (Eds.), Osteoporosis, second ed., Academic Press, San Diego, 2001, pp. 3–20.

[8] E.M. Brown, Homeostatic mechanisms regulating extracellular and intracellular calcium metabolism, in: J.P. Bilezikian, M.A. Levine, R. Marcus (Eds.), The Parathyroids, Raven Press, New York, 1994, pp. 15–54.

[9] F.P. Ross, S.L. Teitelbaum, Osteoclast biology, in: R. Marcus, D. Feldman, J. Kelsey (Eds.), Osteoporosis, second ed., Academic Press, San Diego, 2001, pp. 73–105.

[10] M. Asagiri, H. Takayanagi, Review: the molecular understanding of osteoclast differentiation, Bone 40 (2007) 251–264.

[11] B.L. Drinkwater, K. Nilson, C.H. Chesnut, W.J. Bremner, S. Shainholtz, M.B. Southworth, Bone mineral content of amenorrheic and eumenorrheic athletes, N. Engl. J. Med. 311 (1984) 277–281.

[12] R. Marcus, C. Cann, P. Madvig, J. Minkoff, M. Goddard, M. Bayer, et al., Menstrual function and bone mass in elite women distance runners, Ann. Int. Med. 102 (1985) 158–163.

[13] J. Wolff, Das Gesetz der Transformation der Knochen, Hirschwald Verlag, Berlin, 1892.

[14] B.R. Beck, J. Shaw, C.M. Snow, Physical activity and osteoporosis, in: R. Marcus, D. Feldman, J. Kelsey (Eds.), Osteoporosis, second ed., Academic Press, San Diego, 2001, pp. 701–720.

[15] D.R. Taaffe, C. Snow-Harter, D.A. Connolly, T.L. Robinson, R. Marcus, Differential effects of swimming versus weight-bearing activity on bone mineral status of eumenorrheic athletes, J. Bone Miner. Res. 10 (1995) 586–593.

[16] C. Snow-Harter, M. Bouxsein, B.T. Lewis, D.R. Carter, R. Marcus, Effects of resistance and endurance exercise on bone mineral status of young women: a randomized exercise intervention trial, J. Bone Miner. Res. 7 (1992) 761–769.

[17] A.L. Friedlander, H.K. Genant, S. Sadowsky, N.N. Byl, C.C. Gluer, A two-year program of aerobics and weight-training enhances BMD of young women, J. Bone Miner. Res. 10 (1995) 574–585.

[18] T. Lohman, S. Going, R. Pamenter, M. Hall, T. Boyden, L. Houtkooper, et al., Effects of resistance training on regional and total bone mineral density in premenopausal women: a randomized prospective study, J. Bone Miner. Res. 10 (1995) 1015–1024.

[19] A. Heinonen, H. Sievanen, P. Kannus, P. Oja, I. Vuori, Effects of unilateral strength training and detraining on bone mineral mass and estimated mechanical characteristics of the upper limb bones in young women, J. Bone Miner. Res. 11 (1996) 490–501.

[20] L.K. Bachrach, D. Guido, D. Katzman, I.F. Litt, R. Marcus, Decreased bone density in adolescent girls with anorexia nervosa, Pediatrics 86 (1990) 440–447.

[21] F. Albright, E.C. Reifenstein Jr., The Parathyroid Glands and Metabolic Bone Disease: Selected Studies, Williams & Wilkins, Baltimore, 1948. p. 145

[22] V. Matkovic, K. Kostial, I. Simonovic, R. Buzina, A. Brodarec, B.E.C. Nordin, Bone status and fracture rates in two regions of Yugoslavia, Am. J. Clin. Nutr. 32 (1979) 540–549.

[23] K. Alaimo, M.A. McDowell, R.R. Briefel, A.M. Bischof, C.R. Caughman, C.M. Loria, et al., Dietary intake of vitamins, minerals, and fiber of persons ages 2 months and over in the United States: third National Health and Nutrition Examination Survey, Phase 1, 1988–1991, Adv. Data. 258 (1994) 1–28.

[24] M.C. Chapuy, M.E. Arlot, F. Duboeuf, J. Brun, B. Crouzet, S. Arnaud, et al., Vitamin D_3 and calcium to prevent hip fractures in elderly women, N. Engl. J. Med. 327 (1992) 1637–1642.

[25] National Institutes of Health Consensus Conference, Optimal calcium intake, JAMA 272 (1994) 1942–1948.

[26] Food and Nutrition Board, Institute of Medicine, Dietary Reference Intakes for Calcium, Magnesium, Phosphorus, Vitamin D, and Fluoride, National Academy Press, Washington, DC, 1997.

[27] National Research Council, Recommended Dietary Allowances, tenth ed., National Academy Press, Washington, DC, 1989.

[28] V. Matkovic, R.P. Heaney, Calcium balance during human growth: Evidence for threshold behavior, Am. J. Clin. Nutr. 55 (2002) 992–996.

[29] B. Dawson-Hughes, G.E. Dallal, E.A. Krall, L. Sadowski, N. Sahyoun, S. Tannenbaum, A controlled trial of the effect of calcium supplementation on bone density in postmenopausal women, N. Engl. J. Med. 323 (1990) 878–883.

[30] I.R. Reid, R.W. Ames, M.C. Evans, G.D. Gamble, S.J. Sharpe, Effect of calcium supplementation on bone loss in postmenopausal women, N. Engl. J. Med. 328 (1993) 460–464.

[31] I.R. Reid, R.W. Ames, M.C. Evans, S.J. Sharpe, G.D. Gamble, Determinants of the rate of bone loss in normal postmenopausal women, J. Clin. Endocrinol. Metab. 79 (1994) 950–954.

[32] T. Chevalley, R. Rizzoli, V. Nydegger, D. Slosman, C.-H. Rapin, J.-P. Michel, et al., Effects of calcium supplements on femoral bone mineral density and vertebral fracture rate in vitamin D-replete elderly patients, Osteoporos. Int. 4 (1994) 245–252.

[33] R.R. Recker, S. Hinders, K.M. Davies, R.P. Heaney, M.R. Stegman, D.B. Kimmel, et al., Correcting calcium nutritional deficiency prevents spine fractures in elderly women, J. Bone Miner. Res. 11 (1996) 1961–1966.

[34] B. Dawson-Hughes, S.S. Harris, E.A. Krall, G.E. Dallal, Effect of calcium and vitamin D supplementation on bone density in men and women 65 years of age or older, N Engl. J. Med. 337 (1997) 670–676.

[35] J.F. Aloia, A. Vaswani, J.K. Yeh, P.L. Ross, E. Flaster, F.A. Dilmanian, Calcium supplementation with and without hormone replacement therapy to prevent postmenopausal bone loss, Ann. Intern. Med. 120 (1994) 97–103.

[36] R.P. Heaney, C.M. Weaver, R.R. Recker, Calcium absorbability from spinach, Am. J. Clin. Nutr. 47 (1988) 707–709.

[37] H. Spencer, L. Kramer, D. Osis, C. Norris, Effect of phosphorus on the absorption of calcium and on the calcium balance in man, J. Nutr. 108 (1978) 447–457.

[38] R.P. Heaney, R.R. Recker, Effects of nitrogen, phosphorus, and caffeine on calcium balance in women, J. Lab. Clin. Med. 99 (1982) 46–55.

[39] R.P. Heaney, K. Rafferty, Carbonated beverages and urinary calcium excretion, Am. J. Clin. Nutr. 74 (2001) 343–347.

[40] L.K. Massey, Dietary animal and plant protein and human bone health: a whole foods approach, J. Nutr. 133 (2003) 862S–865S.

[41] M.J. Barger-Lux, R.P. Heaney, P.T. Packard, J.M. Lappe, R.R. Recker, Nutritional correlates of low calcium intake, Clin. Appl. Nutr. 2 (1992) 39–44.

[42] D.E. Sellmeyer, K.L. Stone, A. Sebastian, S.R. Cummings, A high ratio of dietary animal to vegetable protein increases the rate of bone loss and the risk of fracture in postmenopausal women: Study of Osteoporotic Fractures Research Group, Am. J. Clin. Nutr. 73 (2001) 118–122.

[43] A. Devine, I.M. Dick, A.F. Islam, S.S. Dhaliwal, R.L. Prince, Protein consumption is an important predictor of lower limb bone mass in elderly women, Am. J. Clin. Nutr. 81 (2005) 1423–1428.

[44] M.T. Hannan, K.L. Tucker, B. Dawson-Hughes, L.A. Cupples, D.T. Felson, D.P. Kiel, Effect of dietary protein on bone loss in elderly men and women: the Framingham Osteoporosis Study, J. Bone Miner. Res. 15 (2000) 2504–2512.

[45] J.E. Kerstetter, K.O. O'Brien, D.M. Caseria, D.E. Wall, K.L. Insogna, The impact of dietary protein on calcium absorption and kinetic measures of bone turnover in women, J. Clin. Endocrinol. Metab. 90 (2005) 26–31.

[46] B. Dawson-Hughes, S.S. Harris, Calcium intake influences the association of protein intake with rates of bone loss in elderly men and women, Am. J. Clin. Nutr. 75 (2002) 773–779.

[47] M. Delmi, C.H. Rapin, J.M. Bengoa, P.D. Delmas, H. Vasey, J.P. Bonjour, Dietary supplementation in elderly patients with fractured neck of the femur, Lancet 335 (1990) 1013–1016.

[48] R.P. Heaney, Effects of protein on the calcium economy, in: B. Dawson-Hughes, R.P. Henry (Eds.), Nutritional Aspects of Osteoporosis 2006, Elsevier, Amsterdam, 2007, pp. 191–197.

[49] A. Devine, R.A. Criddle, I.M. Dick, D.A. Kerr, R.L. Prince, A longitudinal study of the effect of sodium and calcium intakes on regional bone density in postmenopausal women, Am. J. Clin. Nutr. 62 (1995) 740–745.

[50] R. Marcus, Osteomalacia, in: A.M. Coulston, C.L. Rock, E.R. Monsen (Eds.), Nutrition in the Prevention and Treatment of Disease, Academic Press, San Diego, 2001, pp. 729–740.

[51] M.F. Sowers, Premenopausal reproductive and hormonal characteristics and the risk for osteoporosis, in: R. Marcus, D. Feldman, J. Kelsey (Eds.), Osteoporosis, second ed., Academic Press, San Diego, 2001, pp. 721–740.

[52] R.L. Jilka, G. Hangoc, G. Girasole, G. Passeri, D.C. Williams, J.S. Abrams, et al., Increased osteoclast development after estrogen loss: mediation by interleukin-6, Science 3 (1992) 88–91.

[53] G. Girasole, R.L. Jilka, G. Passeri, S. Boswell, G. Boder, D.C. Williams, et al., 17-β-Estradiol inhibits interleukin-6 production by bone marrow-derived stromal cells and osteoblasts in vitro: a potential mechanism for the antiosteoporotic effect of estrogens, J. Clin. Invest. 89 (1992) 883–891.

[54] M.N. Weitzmann, R. Pacifici, Estrogen deficiency and bone loss: An inflammatory tale, J. Clin. Invest. 116 (2006) 1186–1194.

[55] A. Zallone, Direct and indirect estrogen actions on osteoblasts and osteoclasts, Ann. N. Y. Acad. Sci. 1068 (2006) 173–179.

[56] S. Hui, C. Slemenda, C.J. Johnston, Baseline measurement of bone mass predicts fracture in white women, Ann. Intern. Med. 111 (1989) 355–361.

[57] L. Melton, E. Atkinson, W. O'Fallon, H. Wahner, B. Riggs, Long-term fracture prediction by bone mineral assessed at different skeletal sites, J. Bone Miner. Res. 8 (1993) 1227–1233.

[58] S.R. Cummings, D.M. Black, M.C. Nevitt, W. Browner, J. Cauley, K. Ensrud, et al., Bone density at various sites for prediction of hip fractures: the Study of Osteoporotic Fractures Research Group, Lancet 341 (8837) (1993) 72–75.

[59] O. Johnell, J.A. Kanis, A. Oden, H. Johansson, C. De Laet, P. Delmas, et al., Predictive value of BMD for hip and other fractures, J. Bone Miner. Res. 20 (2005) 1185–1194.

[60] K.G. Faulkner, Improving femoral bone density measurements, J. Clin. Densitom. 6 (2003) 353–358.

[61] J.A. Kanis, L.J. Melton 3rd, C. Christiansen, C.C. Johnston, N. Khaltaev, The diagnosis of osteoporosis, J. Bone Miner. Res. 9 (1994) 1137–1141.

[62] E.S. Siris, Y.T. Chen, T.A. Abbott, E. Barrett-Connor, P.D. Miller, L.E. Wehren, et al., Bone mineral density thresholds for pharmacological intervention to prevent fractures, Arch. Intern. Med. 164 (2004) 1108–1112.

[63] E. Sornay-Rendu, F. Munoz, P. Garnero, F. Duboeuf, P.D. Delmas, Identification of osteopenic women at high risk of fracture: the OFELY study, J. Bone Miner. Res. 20 (2005) 1813–1819.

[64] S.A. Wainwright, L.M. Marshall, K.E. Ensrud, J.A. Cauley, D.M. Black, T.A. Hillier, et al., Hip fracture in women without osteoporosis, J. Clin. Endocrinol. Metab. 90 (2005) 2787–2793.

[65] E. Seeman, P.D. Delmas, Bone quality—The material and structural basis of bone strength and fragility, N. Engl. J. Med. 354 (2006) 2250–2261.

[66] H.K. Genant, P.D. Delmas, P. Chen, Y. Jiang, E.F. Eriksen, G.P. Dalsky, et al., Severity of vertebral fracture reflects deterioration of bone microarchitecture, Osteoporos. Int. 18 (2007) 69–76.

[67] R.P. Heaney, M.S. Dowell, M.J. Barger-Lux, Absorption of calcium as the carbonate and citrate salts, with some observations on method, Osteoporos. Int. 9 (1999) 19–23.

[68] M.J. Bolland, P.A. Barber, R.N. Doughty, B. Mason, A. Horne, R. Ames, et al., Vascular events in healthy older women receiving calcium supplementation: randomised controlled trial, BMJ 336 (2008) 262–266.

[69] M.J. Bolland, A. Avenell, J.A. Baron, A. Grey, G.S. MacLennan, G.D. Gamble, et al., Effect of calcium supplements on risk of myocardial infarction and cardiovascular events: meta-analysis, BMJ 341 (2010) c3691.

[70] J.R. Lewis, J. Calver, K. Zhu, L. Flicker, R.L. Prince, Calcium supplementation and the risks of atherosclerotic vascular disease in older women: results of a 5 year RCT and a 4.5 year follow-up, J Bone MinerRes 26 (2010) 35–41.

[71] R. Lindsay, D.M. Hart, C. Forrest, C. Baird, Prevention of spinal osteoporosis in oophorectomized women, Lancet 2 (1980) 1151–1153.

[72] Women's Health Initiative Investigators, R.D. Jackson, A.Z. LaCroix, M. Gass, R.B. Wallace, J. Robbins, C.E. Lewis, et al., Calcium plus vitamin D supplementation and the risk of fractures, N. Engl. J. Med. 354 (2006) 669–683 [Erratum in N. Engl. J. Med. (2006), 354, 1102].

[73] E.S. Siris, D.B. Muchmore, Selective estrogen receptor modulators (SERMS), in: R. Marcus, D. Feldman, J. Kelsey (Eds.), Osteoporosis, second ed., Academic Press, San Diego, 2001, pp. 603–620.

[74] B. Ettinger, D.M. Black, B. Mitlak, Reduction of vertebral fracture risk in postmenopausal women with osteoporosis treated with raloxifene: results from a 3-year randomized clinical trial, JAMA 282 (1999) 637–645.

[75] K.I. Kavanagh, K. Guo, J.E. Dunford, X. Wu, S. Knapp, F.H. Ebetino, The molecular mechanism of nitrogen-containing bisphosphonates as antiosteoporosis drugs, Proc. Natl. Acad. Sci. USA 103 (2006) 7829–7834.

[76] D.M. Black, S.R. Cummings, D.B. Karpf, J.A. Cauley, D.E. Thompson, M.C. Nevitt, et al., Randomised trial of effect of

alendronate on risk of fracture in women with existing vertebral fractures: Fracture Intervention Trial Research Group, Lancet 348 (1996) 1535−1541.

[77] S.T. Harris, N.B. Watts, H.K. Genant, C.D. McKeever, T. Hangartner, M. Keller, et al., Effects of risedronate treatment on vertebral and nonvertebral fractures in women with postmenopausal osteoporosis: a randomized controlled trial. Vertebral Efficacy with Risedronate Therapy (VERT) Study Group, JAMA 282 (1999) 1344−1352.

[78] M.R. McClung, P. Geusens, P.D. Miller, H. Zippel, W.G. Bensen, C. Roux, et al., Hip Intervention Program Study Group: effect of risedronate on the risk of hip fracture in elderly womenHip Intervention Program Study Group N. Engl. J. Med. 344 (2001) 333−340.

[79] P.D. Delmas, R.R. Recker, C.H. Chesnut 3rd, A. Skag, J.A. Stakkestad, R. Emkey, et al., Daily and intermittent oral ibandronate normalize bone turnover and provide significant reduction in vertebral fracture risk: results from the BONE study, Osteoporos. Int. 15 (2004) 792−798.

[80] E.M. Lewiecki, Safety of long-term bisphosphonate therapy for the management of osteoporosis, Drugs 71 (2011) 791−814.

[81] L.Y. Park-Wylie, M.M. Mamdani, D.N. Juurlink, C.A. Hawker, N. Cunraj, P.C. Austin, et al., Bisphosphonate use and the risk of subtrochanteric or femoral shaft fractures in older women, JAMA 305 (2011) 783−789.

[82] C.H. Chesnut, S. Silverman, K. Andriano, H. Genant, A. Gimona, S. Harris, et al., A randomized trial of nasal spray salmon calcitonin in postmenopausal women with established osteoporosis: The Prevent Recurrence of Osteoporotic Fractures Study Group, Am. J. Med. 109 (2000) 267−276.

[83] S.R. Cummings, J.S. Martin, M.R. McClung, E.S. Siris, R. Eastell, I.R. Reid, et al., Denosumab for prevention of fratures in postmenopausal women with osteoporosis, N. Engl. Med. J. 361 (2009) 756−765.

[84] R.M. Neer, C.D. Arnaud, J.R. Zanchetta, R. Prince, G.A. Gaich, J.Y. Reginster, et al., Effect of parathyroid hormone (1−34) on fractures and bone mineral density in postmenopausal women with osteoporosis, N. Engl. J. Med. 344 (2001) 1434−1441.

[85] R.P. Heaney, Nutrition and risk for osteoporosis, in: R. Marcus, D. Feldman, D.A. Nelson, C.J. Rosen (Eds.), Osteoporosis, third ed., Academic Press, San Diego, 2007, pp. 799−828.

Appendix:
Dietary Reference Intakes (DRIs)

Dietary Reference Intakes (DRIs): Recommended Dietary Allowances and Adequate Intakes, Vitamins
Food and Nutrition Board, Institute of Medicine, National Academies (http://www.iom.edu/Activities/Nutrition/SummaryDRIs/DRI-Tables.
aspx)

Life stage group	Vitamin A (μg/d)[a]	Vitamin C (mg/d)	Vitamin D (μg/d)[b,c]	Vitamin E (mg/d)[d]	Vitamin K (μg/d)	Thiamin (mg/d)	Riboflavin (mg/d)	Niacin (mg/d)[e]	Vitamin B6 (mg/d)	Folate (μg/d)[f]	Vitamin B12 (μg/d)	Pantothenic acid (mg/d)	Biotin (μg/d)	Choline (mg/d)[g]
Infants[h]														
0 to 6 mo	400*	40*	10	4*	2.0*	0.2*	0.3*	2*	0.1*	65*	0.4*	1.7*	5*	125*
6 to 12 mo	500*	50*	10	5*	2.5*	0.3*	0.4*	4*	0.3**	80*	0.5*	1.8*	6*	150*
Children														
1–3 y	300	15	15	6	30*	0.5	0.5	6	0.5	150	0.9	2*	8*	200*
4–8 y	400	25	15	7	55*	0.6	0.6	8	0.6	200	1.2	3*	12*	250*
Males														
9–13 y	600	45	15	11	60*	0.9	0.9	12	1.0	300	1.8	4*	20*	375*
14–18 y	900	75	15	15	75*	1.2	1.3	16	1.3	400	2.4	5*	25*	550*
19–30 y	900	90	15	15	120*	1.2	1.3	16	1.3	400	2.4	5*	30*	550*
31–50 y	900	90	15	15	120*	1.2	1.3	16	1.3	400	2.4	5*	30*	550*
51–70 y	900	90	15	15	120*	1.2	1.3	16	1.7	400	2.4[h]	5*	30*	550*
>70 y	900	90	20	15	120*	1.2	1.3	16	1.7	400	2.4[h]	5*	30*	550*
Females														
9–13 y	600	45	15	11	60*	0.9	0.9	12	1.0	300	1.8	4*	20*	375*
14–18 y	700	65	15	15	75*	1.0	1.0	14	1.2	400[i]	2.4	5*	25*	400*
19–30 y	700	75	15	15	90*	1.1	1.1	14	1.3	400[i]	2.4	5*	30*	425*
31–50 y	700	75	15	15	90*	1.1	1.1	14	1.3	400[i]	2.4	5*	30*	425*
51–70 y	700	75	15	15	90*	1.1	1.1	14	1.5	400	2.4[h]	5*	30*	425*
>70 y	700	75	20	15	90*	1.1	1.1	14	1.5	400	2.4[h]	5*	30*	425*
Pregnancy														
14–18 y	750	80	15	15	75*	1.4	1.4	18	1.9	600[j]	2.6	6*	30*	450*
19–30 y	770	85	15	15	90*	1.4	1.4	18	1.9	600[j]	2.6	6*	30*	450*
31–50 y	770	85	15	15	90*	1.4	1.4	18	1.9	600[j]	2.6	6*	30*	450*

(Continued)

(Continued)

Life stage group	Vitamin A (µg/d)[a]	Vitamin C (mg/d)	Vitamin D (µg/d)[b,c]	Vitamin E (mg/d)[d]	Vitamin K (µg/d)	Thiamin (mg/d)	Riboflavin (mg/d)	Niacin (mg/d)[e]	Vitamin B6 (mg/d)	Folate (µg/d)[f]	Vitamin B12 (µg/d)	Pantothenic acid (mg/d)	Biotin (µg/d)	Choline (mg/d)[g]
Lactation														
14–18 y	**1,200**	**115**	**15**	**19**	75*	**1.4**	**1.6**	**17**	**2.0**	**500**	**2.8**	7*	35*	550*
19–30 y	**1,300**	**120**	**15**	**19**	90*	**1.4**	**1.6**	**17**	**2.0**	**500**	**2.8**	7*	35*	550*
31–50 y	**1,300**	**120**	**15**	**19**	90*	**1.4**	**1.6**	**17**	**2.0**	**500**	**2.8**	7*	35*	550*

[a] *As retinol activity equivalents (RAEs). 1 RAE = 1 µg retinol, 12 µg β-carotene, 24 µg α-carotene, or 24 µg β-cryptoxanthin. The RAE for dietary provitamin A carotenoids is twofold greater than retinol equivalents (RE), whereas the RAE for preformed vitamin A is the same as RE.*

[b] *As cholecalciferol. 1 µg cholecalciferol = 40 IU vitamin D.*

[c] *Under the assumption of minimal sunlight.*

[d] *As α-tocopherol. α-Tocopherol includes RRR-α-tocopherol, the only form of α-tocopherol that occurs naturally in foods, and the 2 R-stereoisomeric forms of α-tocopherol (RRR-, RSR-, RRS-, and RSS-α-tocopherol) that occur in fortified foods and supplements. It does not include the 2 S-stereoisomeric forms of α-tocopherol (SRR-, SSR-, SRS-, and SSS-α-tocopherol), also found in fortified foods and supplements.*

[e] *As niacin equivalents (NE). 1 mg of niacin = 60 mg of tryptophan; 0–6 months = preformed niacin (not NE).*

[f] *As dietary folate equivalents (DFE). 1 DFE = 1 µg food folate = 0.6 µg of folic acid from fortified food or as a supplement consumed with food = 0.5 µg of a supplement taken on an empty stomach.*

[g] *Although AIs have been set for choline, there are few data to assess whether a dietary supply of choline is needed at all stages of the life cycle, and it may be that the choline requirement can be met by endogenous synthesis at some of these stages.*

[h] *Because 10–30% of older people may malabsorb food-bound B_{12}, it is advisable for those older than 50 years to meet their RDA mainly by consuming foods fortified with B_{12} or a supplement containing B_{12}.*

[i] *In view of evidence linking folate intake with neural tube defects in the fetus, it is recommended that all women capable of becoming pregnant consume 400 µg from supplements or fortified foods in addition to intake of food folate from a varied diet.*

[j] *It is assumed that women will continue consuming 400 µg from supplements or fortified food until their pregnancy is confirmed and they enter prenatal care, which ordinarily occurs after the end of the periconceptional period—the critical time for formation of the neural tube.*

Note: This table (taken from the DRI reports, see www.nap.edu) presents Recommended Dietary Allowances (RDAs) in **bold type** and adequate intakes (AIs) in ordinary type followed by an asterisk (*). An RDA is the average daily dietary intake level; sufficient to meet the nutrient requirements of nearly all (97–98%) healthy individuals in a group. It is calculated from an estimated average requirement (EAR). If sufficient scientific evidence is not available to establish an EAR, and thus calculate an RDA, an AI is usually developed. For healthy breast-fed infants, an AI is the mean intake. The AI for other life stage and gender groups is believed to cover the needs of all healthy individuals in the groups, but lack of data or uncertainty in the data prevent being able to specify with confidence the percentage of individuals covered by this intake.

Sources: *Dietary Reference Intakes for Calcium, Phosphorous, Magnesium, Vitamin D, and Fluoride (1997); Dietary Reference Intakes for Thiamin, Riboflavin, Niacin, Vitamin B_6, Folate, Vitamin B_{12}, Pantothenic Acid, Biotin, and Choline (1998); Dietary Reference Intakes for Vitamin C, Vitamin E, Selenium, and Carotenoids (2000); Dietary Reference Intakes for Vitamin A, Vitamin K, Arsenic, Boron, Chromium, Copper, Iodine, Iron, Manganese, Molybdenum, Nickel, Silicon, Vanadium, and Zinc (2001); Dietary Reference Intakes for Water, Potassium, Sodium, Chloride, and Sulfate (2005); and Dietary Reference Intakes for Calcium and Vitamin D (2011). These reports may be accessed via www.nap.edu.*

Dietary Reference Intakes (DRIs): Recommended Dietary Allowances and Adequate Intakes, Elements
Food and Nutrition Board, Institute of Medicine, National Academies (http://www.iom.edu/Activities/Nutrition/SummaryDRIs/DRI-Tables.aspx)

Life stage group	Calcium (mg/d)	Chromium (µg/d)	Copper (µg/d)	Fluoride (mg/d)	Iodine (µg/d)	Iron (mg/d)	Magnesium (mg/d)	Manganese (mg/d)	Molybdenum (µg/d)	Phosphorus (mg/d)	Selenium (µg/d)	Zinc (mg/d)	Potassium (g/d)	Sodium (g/d)	Chloride (g/d)
Infants															
0 to 6 mo	200*	0.2*	200*	0.01*	110*	0.27*	30*	0.003*	2*	100*	15*	2*	0.4*	0.12*	0.18*
6 to 12 mo	260*	5.5*	220*	0.5*	130*	11	75*	0.6*	3*	275*	20*	3	0.7*	0.37*	0.57*
Children															
1–3 y	700	11*	340	0.7*	90	7	80	1.2*	17	460	20	3	3.0*	1.0*	1.5*
4–8 y	1,000	15*	440	1*	90	10	130	1.5*	22	500	30	5	3.8*	1.2*	1.9*
Males															
9–13 y	1,300	25*	700	2*	120	8	240	1.9*	34	1,250	40	8	4.5*	1.5*	2.3*
14–18 y	1,300	35*	890	3*	150	11	410	2.2*	43	1,250	55	11	4.7*	1.5*	2.3*
19–30 y	1,000	35*	900	4*	150	8	400	2.3*	45	700	55	11	4.7*	1.5*	2.3*
31–50 y	1,000	35*	900	4*	150	8	420	2.3*	45	700	55	11	4.7*	1.5*	2.3*
51–70 y	1,000	30*	900	4*	150	8	420	2.3*	45	700	55	11	4.7*	1.3*	2.0*
>70 y	1,200	30*	900	4*	150	8	420	2.3*	45	700	55	11	4.7*	1.2*	1.8*
Females															
9–13 y	1,300	21*	700	2*	120	8	240	1.6*	34	1,250	40	8	4.5*	1.5*	2.3*
14–18 y	1,300	24*	890	3*	150	15	360	1.6*	43	1,250	55	9	4.7*	1.5*	2.3*
19–30 y	1,000	25*	900	3*	150	18	310	1.8*	45	700	55	8	4.7*	1.5*	2.3*
31–50 y	1,000	25*	900	3*	150	18	320	1.8*	45	700	55	8	4.7*	1.5*	2.3*
51–70 y	1,200	20*	900	3*	150	8	320	1.8*	45	700	55	8	4.7*	1.3*	2.0*
>70 y	1,200	20*	900	3*	150	8	320	1.8*	45	700	55	8	4.7*	1.2*	1.8*
Pregnancy															
14–18 y	1,300	29*	1,000	3*	220	27	400	2.0*	50	1,250	60	12	4.7*	1.5*	2.3*
19–30 y	1,000	30*	1,000	3*	220	27	350	2.0*	50	700	60	11	4.7*	1.5*	2.3*
31–50 y	1,000	30*	1,000	3*	220	27	360	2.0*	50	700	60	11	4.7*	1.5*	2.3*
Lactation															
14–18 y	1,300	44*	1,300	3*	290	10	360	2.6*	50	1,250	70	13	5.1*	1.5*	2.3*
19–30 y	1,000	45*	1,300	3*	290	9	310	2.6*	50	700	70	12	5.1*	1.5*	2.3*
31–50 y	1,000	45*	1,300	3*	290	9	320	2.6*	50	700	70	12	5.1*	1.5*	2.3*

Note: This table (taken from the DRI reports, see www.nap.edu) presents Recommended Dietary Allowances (RDAs) in **bold type** and adequate intakes (AIs) in ordinary type followed by an asterisk (*). An RDA is the average daily dietary intake level; sufficient to meet the nutrient requirements of nearly all (97–98%) healthy individuals in a group. It is calculated from an estimated average requirement (EAR). If sufficient scientific evidence is not available to establish an EAR, and thus calculate an RDA, an AI is usually developed. For healthy breast-fed infants, an AI is the mean intake. The AI for other life stage and gender groups is believed to cover the needs of all healthy individuals in the groups, but lack of data or uncertainty in the data prevent being able to specify with confidence the percentage of individuals covered by this intake.

Sources: *Dietary Reference Intakes for Calcium, Phosphorous, Magnesium, Vitamin D, and Fluoride (1997); Dietary Reference Intakes for Thiamin, Riboflavin, Niacin, Vitamin B₆, Folate, Vitamin B₁₂, Pantothenic Acid, Biotin, and Choline (1998); Dietary Reference Intakes for Vitamin C, Vitamin E, Selenium, and Carotenoids (2000); Dietary Reference Intakes for Vitamin A, Vitamin K, Arsenic, Boron, Chromium, Copper, Iodine, Iron, Manganese, Molybdenum, Nickel, Silicon, Vanadium, and Zinc (2001); Dietary Reference Intakes for Water, Potassium, Sodium, Chloride, and Sulfate (2005); and Dietary Reference Intakes for Calcium and Vitamin D (2011). These reports may be accessed via www.nap.edu.*

Dietary Reference Intakes (DRIs): Recommended Dietary Allowances and Adequate Intakes, Total Water and Macronutrients
Food and Nutrition Board, Institute of Medicine, National Academies
(http://www.iom.edu/Activities/Nutrition/SummaryDRIs/DRI-Tables.aspx)

Life stage group	Total water[a] (l/d)	Carbohydrate (g/d)	Total fiber (g/d)	Fat (g/d)	Linoleic acid (g/d)	α-Linolenic acid (g/d)	Protein[b] (g/d)
Infants							
0 to 6 mo	0.7*	60*	ND	31*	4.4*	0.5*	9.1*
6 to 12 mo	0.8*	95*	ND	30*	4.6*	0.5*	**11.0**
Children							
1–3 y	1.3*	**130**	19*	ND[c]	7*	0.7*	**13**
4–8 y	1.7*	**130**	25*	ND	10*	0.9*	**19**
Males							
9–13 y	2.4*	**130**	31*	ND	12*	1.2*	**34**
14–18 y	3.3*	**130**	38*	ND	16*	1.6*	**52**
19–30 y	3.7*	**130**	38*	ND	17*	1.6*	**56**
31–50 y	3.7*	**130**	38*	ND	17*	1.6*	**56**
51–70 y	3.7*	**130**	30*	ND	14*	1.6*	**56**
>70 y	3.7*	**130**	30*	ND	14*	1.6*	**56**
Females							
9–13 y	2.1*	**130**	26*	ND	10*	1.0*	**34**
14–18 y	2.3*	**130**	26*	ND	11*	1.1*	**46**
19–30 y	2.7*	**130**	25*	ND	12*	1.1*	**46**
31–50 y	2.7*	**130**	25*	ND	12*	1.1*	**46**
51–70 y	2.7*	**130**	21*	ND	11*	1.1*	**46**
> 70 y	2.7*	**130**	21*	ND	11*	1.1*	**46**
Pregnancy							
14–18 y	3.0*	**175**	28*	ND	13*	1.4*	**71**
19–30 y	3.0*	**175**	28*	ND	13*	1.4*	**71**
31–50 y	3.0*	**175**	28*	ND	13*	1.4*	**71**
Lactation							
14–18	3.8*	**210**	29*	ND	13*	1.3*	**71**
19–30 y	3.8*	**210**	29*	ND	13*	1.3*	**71**
31–50 y	3.8*	**210**	29*	ND	13*	1.3*	**71**

[a]*Total water includes all water contained in food, beverages, and drinking water.*

[b]*Based on g protein per kg of body weight for the reference body weight; for example, for adults 0.8 g/kg body weight for the reference body weight.*

[c]*Not determined.*

Note: This table (take from the DRI reports, see www.nap.edu) presents Recommended Dietary Allowances (RDA) in **bold type** and adequate intakes (AI) in ordinary type followed by an asterisk (*). An RDA is the average daily dietary intake level; sufficient to meet the nutrient requirements of nearly all (97–98%) healthy individuals in a group. It is calculated from an estimated average requirement (EAR). If sufficient scientific evidence is not available to establish an EAR, and thus calculate an RDA, an AI is usually developed. For healthy breast-fed infants, an AI is the mean intake. The AI for other life stage and gender groups is believed to cover the needs of all healthy individuals in the groups, but lack of data or uncertainty in the data prevent being able to specify with confidence the percentage of individuals covered by this intake.

Source: *Dietary Reference Intakes for Energy, Carbohydrate, Fiber, Fat, Fatty Acids, Cholesterol, Protein, and Amino Acids (2002/2005) and Dietary Reference Intakes for Water, Potassium, Sodium, Chloride, and Sulfate (2005). These reports may be accessed via www.nap.edu.*

Dietary Reference Intakes (DRIs): Acceptable Macronutrient Distribution Ranges Food and Nutrition Board, Institute of Medicine, National Academies (http://www.iom.edu/Activities/Nutrition/SummaryDRIs/DRI-Tables.aspx)

Macronutrient	Range (percent of energy)		
	Children, 1–3 y	Children, 4–18 y	Adults
Fat	30–40	25–35	20–35
n-6 polyunsaturated fatty acids[a] (linoleic acid)	5–10	5–10	5–10
n-3 polyunsaturated fatty acids[a] (α-linolenic acid)	0.6–1.2	0.6–1.2	0.6–1.2
Carbohydrate	45–65	45–65	45–65
Protein	5–20	10–30	10–35

[a]*Approximately 10% of the total can come from longer chain n-3 or n-6 fatty acids.*
Source: *Dietary Reference Intakes for Energy, Carbohydrate, Fiber, Fat, Fatty Acids, Cholesterol, Protein, and Amino Acids (2002/2005). The report may be accessed via www.nap.edu.*

Dietary Reference Intakes (DRIs): Acceptable Macronutrient Distribution Ranges Food and Nutrition Board, Institute of Medicine, National Academies (http://www.iom.edu/Activities/Nutrition/SummaryDRIs/DRI-Tables.aspx)

Macronutrient	Recommendation
Dietary cholesterol	As low as possible while consuming a nutritionally adequate diet
Trans fatty acids	As low as possible while consuming a nutritionally adequate diet
Saturated fatty acids	As low as possible while consuming a nutritionally adequate diet
Added sugars[a]	Limit to no more than 25% of total energy

[a]*Not a recommended intake. A daily intake of added sugars that individuals should aim for to achieve a healthful diet was not set.*
Source: *Dietary Reference Intakes for Energy, Carbohydrate, Fiber, Fat, Fatty Acids, Cholesterol, Protein, and Amino Acids (2002/2005). The report may be accessed via www.nap.edu.*

Dietary Reference Intakes (DRIs): Tolerable Upper Intake Levels, Vitamins Food and Nutrition Board, Institute of Medicine, National Academies (http://www.iom.edu/Activities/Nutrition/SummaryDRIs/DRI-Tables.aspx)

Life stage group	Vitamin A (µg/d)[a]	Vitamin C (mg/d)	Vitamin D (µg/d)	Vitamin E (mg/d)[b,c]	Vitamin K	Thiamin	Riboflavin	Niacin (mg/d)[c]	Vitamin B6 (mg/d)	Folate (µg/d)[c]	Vitamin B12	Pantothenic acid	Biotin	Choline (g/d)	Carotenoids[d]
Infants															
0 to 6 mo	600	ND[e]	25	ND	ND	ND	ND	ND	ND	ND	ND	ND	ND	ND	ND
6 to 12 mo	600	ND	38	ND	ND	ND	ND	ND	ND	ND	ND	ND	ND	ND	ND
Children															
1–3 y	600	400	63	200	ND	ND	ND	10	30	300	ND	ND	ND	1.0	ND
4–8 y	900	650	75	300	ND	ND	ND	15	40	400	ND	ND	ND	1.0	ND
Males															
9–13 y	1,700	1,200	100	600	ND	ND	ND	20	60	600	ND	ND	ND	2.0	ND
14–18 y	2,800	1,800	100	800	ND	ND	ND	30	80	800	ND	ND	ND	3.0	ND
19–30 y	3,000	2,000	100	1,000	ND	ND	ND	35	100	1,000	ND	ND	ND	3.5	ND
31–50 y	3,000	2,000	100	1,000	ND	ND	ND	35	100	1,000	ND	ND	ND	3.5	ND
51–70 y	3,000	2,000	100	1,000	ND	ND	ND	35	100	1,000	ND	ND	ND	3.5	ND
>70 y	3,000	2,000	100	1,000	ND	ND	ND	35	100	1,000	ND	ND	ND	3.5	ND
Females															
9–13 y	1,700	1,200	100	600	ND	ND	ND	20	60	600	ND	ND	ND	2.0	ND
14–18 y	2,800	1,800	100	800	ND	ND	ND	30	80	800	ND	ND	ND	3.0	ND
19–30 y	3,000	2,000	100	1,000	ND	ND	ND	35	100	1,000	ND	ND	ND	3.5	ND
31–50 y	3,000	2,000	100	1,000	ND	ND	ND	35	100	1,000	ND	ND	ND	3.5	ND
51–70 y	3,000	2,000	100	1,000	ND	ND	ND	35	100	1,000	ND	ND	ND	3.5	ND
>70 y	3,000	2,000	100	1,000	ND	ND	ND	35	100	1,000	ND	ND	ND	3.5	ND

Pregnancy

14–18 y	2,800	1,800	100	800	ND	ND	ND	30	80	800	ND	ND	ND	3.0	ND
19–30 y	3,000	2,000	100	1,000	ND	ND	ND	35	100	1,000	ND	ND	ND	3.5	ND
31–50 y	3,000	2,000	100	1,000	ND	ND	ND	35	100	1,000	ND	ND	ND	3.5	ND

Lactation

14–18 y	2,800	1,800	100	800	ND	ND	ND	30	80	800	ND	ND	ND	3.0	ND
19–30 y	3,000	2,000	100	1,000	ND	ND	ND	35	100	1,000	ND	ND	ND	3.5	ND
31–50 y	3,000	2,000	100	1,000	ND	ND	ND	35	100	1,000	ND	ND	ND	3.5	ND

[a] *As preformed vitamin A only.*

[b] *As α-tocopherol; applies to any form of supplemental α-tocopherol.*

[c] *The ULs for vitamin E, niacin, and folate apply to synthetic forms obtained from supplements, fortified foods, or a combination of the two.*

[d] *β-Carotene supplements are advised only to serve as a provitamin A source for individuals at risk of vitamin A deficiency.*

[e] *ND = not determinable due to lack of data of adverse effects in this age group and concern with regard to lack of ability to handle excess amounts. Source of intake should be from food only to prevent high levels of intake.*

Note: A tolerable upper intake level (UL) is the highest level of daily nutrient intake that is likely to pose no risk of adverse health effects to almost all individuals in the general population. Unless otherwise specified, the UL represents total intake from food, water, and supplements. Due to a lack of suitable data, ULs could not be established for vitamin K, thiamin, riboflavin, vitamin B_{12}, pantothenic acid, biotin, and carotenoids. In the absence of a UL, extra caution may be warranted in consuming levels above recommended intakes. Members of the general population should be advised not to routinely exceed the UL. The UL is not meant to apply to individuals who are treated with the nutrient under medical supervision or to individuals with predisposing conditions that modify their sensitivity to the nutrient.

Sources: Dietary Reference Intakes for Calcium, Phosphorous, Magnesium, Vitamin D, and Fluoride (1997); Dietary Reference Intakes for Thiamin, Riboflavin, Niacin, Vitamin B_6, Folate, Vitamin B_{12}, Pantothenic Acid, Biotin, and Choline (1998); Dietary Reference Intakes for Vitamin C, Vitamin E, Selenium, and Carotenoids (2000); Dietary Reference Intakes for Vitamin A, Vitamin K, Arsenic, Boron, Chromium, Copper, Iodine, Iron, Manganese, Molybdenum, Nickel, Silicon, Vanadium, and Zinc (2001); and Dietary Reference Intakes for Calcium and Vitamin D (2011). These reports may be accessed via www.nap.edu.

Dietary Reference Intakes (DRIs): Tolerable Upper Intake Levels, Elements Food and Nutrition Board, Institute of Medicine, National Academies (http://www.iom.edu/Activities/Nutrition/SummaryDRIs/DRI-Tables.aspx)

Life stage group	Arsenic[a]	Boron (mg/d)	Calcium (mg/d)	Chromium	Copper (µg/d)	Fluoride (mg/d)	Iodine (µg/d)	Iron (mg/d)	Magnesium (mg/d)[b]	Manganese (mg/d)	Molybdenum (µg/d)	Nickel (mg/d)	Phosphorus (g/d)	Selenium (µg/d)	Silicon[c]	Vanadium (mg/d)[d]	Zinc (mg/d)	Sodium (g/d)	Chloride (g/d)
Infants																			
0 to 6 mo	ND[e]	ND	1,000	ND	ND	0.7	ND	40	ND	ND	ND	ND	ND	45	ND	ND	4	ND	ND
6 to 12 mo	ND	ND	1,500	ND	ND	0.9	ND	40	ND	ND	ND	ND	ND	60	ND	ND	5	ND	ND
Children																			
1–3 y	ND	3	2,500	ND	1,000	1.3	200	40	65	2	300	0.2	3	90	ND	ND	7	1.5	2.3
4–8 y	ND	6	2,500	ND	3,000	2.2	300	40	110	3	600	0.3	3	150	ND	ND	12	1.9	2.9
Males																			
9–13 y	ND	11	3,000	ND	5,000	10	600	40	350	6	1,100	0.6	4	280	ND	ND	23	2.2	3.4
14–18 y	ND	17	3,000	ND	8,000	10	900	45	350	9	1,700	1.0	4	400	ND	ND	34	2.3	3.6
19–30 y	ND	20	2,500	ND	10,000	10	1,100	45	350	11	2,000	1.0	4	400	ND	1.8	40	2.3	3.6
31–50 y	ND	20	2,500	ND	10,000	10	1,100	45	350	11	2,000	1.0	4	400	ND	1.8	40	2.3	3.6
51–70 y	ND	20	2,000	ND	10,000	10	1,100	45	350	11	2,000	1.0	4	400	ND	1.8	40	2.3	3.6
>70 y	ND	20	2,000	ND	10,000	10	1,100	45	350	11	2,000	1.0	3	400	ND	1.8	40	2.3	3.6
Females																			
9–13 y	ND	11	3,000	ND	5,000	10	600	40	350	6	1,100	0.6	4	280	ND	ND	23	2.2	3.4
14–18 y	ND	17	3,000	ND	8,000	10	900	45	350	9	1,700	1.0	4	400	ND	ND	34	2.3	3.6
19–30 y	ND	20	2,500	ND	10,000	10	1,100	45	350	11	2,000	1.0	4	400	ND	1.8	40	2.3	3.6
31–50 y	ND	20	2,500	ND	10,000	10	1,100	45	350	11	2,000	1.0	4	400	ND	1.8	40	2.3	3.6
51–70 y	ND	20	2,000	ND	10,000	10	1,100	45	350	11	2,000	1.0	4	400	ND	1.8	40	2.3	3.6
>70 y	ND	20	2,000	ND	10,000	10	1,100	45	350	11	2,000	1.0	3	400	ND	1.8	40	2.3	3.6
Pregnancy																			
14–18 y	ND	17	3,000	ND	8,000	10	900	45	350	9 1,700	1.0	3.5	400	ND	ND	34	2.3	3.6	
19–30 y	ND	20	2,500	ND	10,000	10	1,100	45	350	11	2,000	1.0	3.5	400	ND	ND	40	2.3	3.6
61–50 y	ND	20	2,500	ND	10,000	10	1,100	45	350	11	2,000	1.0	3.5	400	ND	ND	40	2.3	3.6

Lactation

14–18 y	ND	17	3,000	ND	8,000	10	900	45	350	9	1,700	1.0	4	400	ND	34	2.3	3.6
19–30 y	ND	20	2,500	ND	10,000	10	1,100	45	350	11	2,000	1.0	4	400	ND	40	2.3	3.6
31–50 y	ND	20	2,500	ND	10,000	10	1,100	45	350	11	2,000	1.0	4	400	ND	40	2.3	3.6

[a] Although the UL was not determined for arsenic, there is no justification for adding arsenic to food or supplements.

[b] The ULs for magnesium represent intake from a pharmacological agent only and do not include intake from food and water.

[c] Although silicon has not been shown to cause adverse effects in humans, there is no justification for adding silicon to supplements.

[d] Although vanadium in food has not been shown to cause adverse effects in humans, there is no justification for adding vanadium to food and vanadium supplements should be used with caution. The UL is based on adverse effects in laboratory animals and this data could be used to set a UL for adults but not children and adolescents.

[e] ND = not determinable due to lack of data of adverse effects in this age group and concern with regard to lack of ability to handle excess amounts. Source of intake should be from food only to prevent high levels of intake.

Note: A tolerable upper intake level (UL) is the highest level of daily nutrient intake that is likely to pose no risk of adverse health effects to almost all individuals in the general population. Unless otherwise specified, the UL represents total intake from food, water, and supplements. Due to a lack of suitable data, ULs could not be established for vitamin K, thiamin, riboflavin, vitamin B_{12}, pantothenic acid, biotin, and carotenoids. In the absence of a UL, extra caution may be warranted in consuming levels above recommended intakes. Members of the general population should be advised not to routinely exceed the UL. The UL is not meant to apply to individuals who are treated with the nutrient under medical supervision or to individuals with predisposing conditions that modify their sensitivity to the nutrient.

Sources: *Dietary Reference Intakes for Calcium, Phosphorous, Magnesium, Vitamin D, and Fluoride (1997); Dietary Reference Intakes for Thiamin, Riboflavin, Niacin, Vitamin B_6, Folate, Vitamin B_{12}, Pantothenic Acid, Biotin, and Choline (1998); Dietary Reference Intakes for Vitamin C, Vitamin E, Selenium, and Carotenoids (2000); Dietary Reference Intakes for Vitamin A, Vitamin K, Arsenic, Boron, Chromium, Copper, Iodine, Iron, Manganese, Molybdenum, Nickel, Silicon, Vanadium, and Zinc (2001); Dietary Reference Intakes for Water, Potassium, Sodium, Chloride, and Sulfate (2005); and Dietary Reference Intakes for Calcium and Vitamin D (2011). These reports may be accessed via www.nap.edu.*

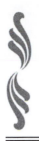

Index

Note: Page numbers suffixed by "*t*" refer to tables.

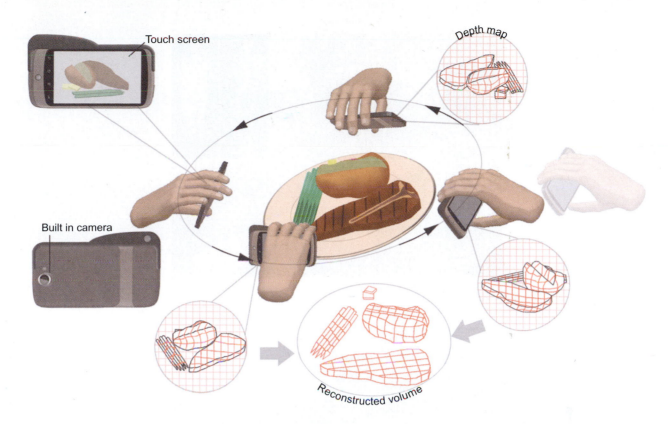

FIGURE 11.1 Volume estimation concept map for DDR. As the phone is rotated around the food items, the DDR system collects a short video, which is enough to ascertain multiple video angles for depth image generation and volume calculation. Through a series of automated queries, users can also provide additional information pertaining to the preparation, location, or time of consumption.

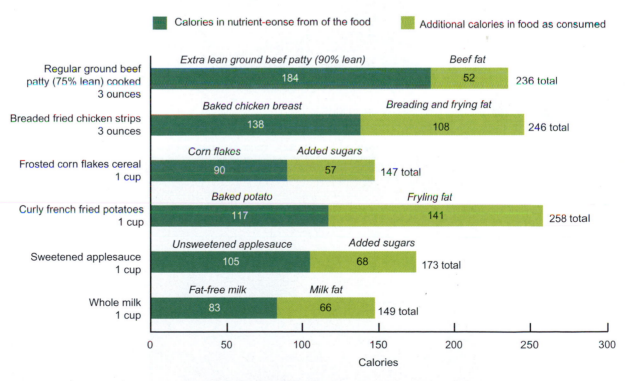

FIGURE 13.1 Examples of the calories in food choices that are not in nutrient-dense forms and the calories in nutrient-dense forms of these foods. Based on data from the U.S. Department of Agriculture, Agricultural Research Service, Food and Nutrient Database for Dietary Studies 4.1 (http://www.ars.usda.gov/Services/docs.htm?docid = 20511) and the National Nutrient Database for Standard Reference, Release 23 (http://www.nal.usda.gov/fnic/foodcomp/search). Source: *National Research Council [8], Figure 5-2, p. 47*.

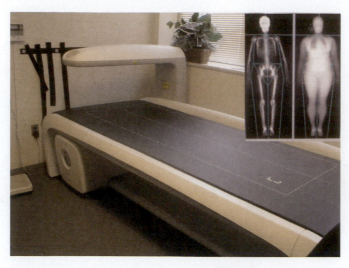

FIGURE 4.2   Dual energy x-ray absorptiometer for body composition.

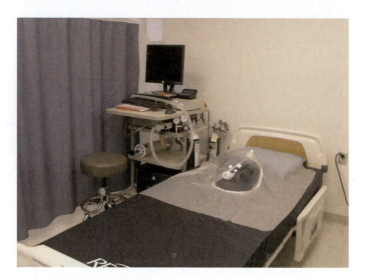

FIGURE 4.4   Indirect calorimetry system for measurement of RMR.

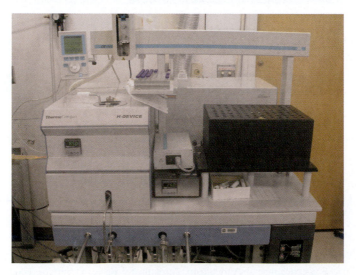

FIGURE 4.5   Mass spectrometry system used for the analysis of isotope enrichments for the DLW method.

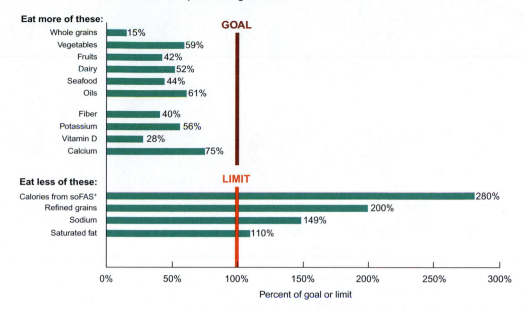

Usual intake as a percent of goal or limit

FIGURE 13.2 A comparison of typical American diets to selected recommended intake levels (goals) or limits. Bars show average intakes for all individuals (ages 1 or 2 years or older, depending on the data source) as a percentage of the recommended intake level or limit. Recommended intakes for food groups and limits for refined grains and solid fats and added sugars are based on amounts in the USDA 2000-calorie food pattern. Recommended intakes for fiber, potassium, vitamin D, and calcium are based on the highest adequate intake or Recommended Dietary Allowance for ages 14–70 years. Limits for sodium are based on the tolerable upper intake level and for saturated fat on 10A% of calories. The protein foods group is not shown here because, on average, intake is close to recommended levels. *SoFAS, solid fats and added sugars. Based on data from the U.S. Department of Agriculture, Agricultural Research Service, and the U.S. Department of Health and Human Services, Centers for Disease Control and Prevention. What We Eat in America, NHANES 2001–2004 or 2005–2006. Source: *National Research Council [8], Figure 5-1, p. 46.*

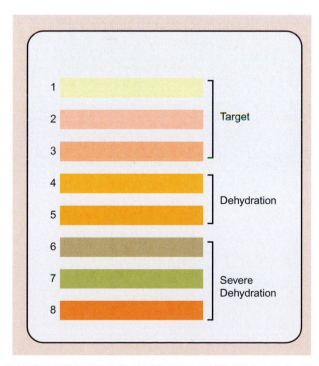

FIGURE 16.9 Urine color hydration chart. Scientific validation for this chart can be found in the *International Journal of Sport Nutrition,* Volume 4, 1994, pp. 265–279 and Volume 8, 1998, pp. 345–355.

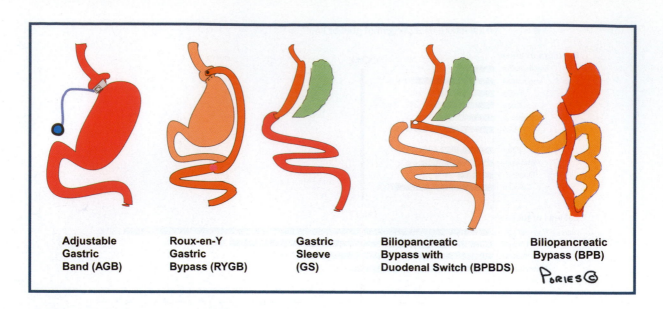

Adjustable Gastric Band (AGB)

Roux-en-Y Gastric Bypass (RYGB)

Gastric Sleeve (GS)

Biliopancreatic Bypass with Duodenal Switch (BPBDS)

Biliopancreatic Bypass (BPB)

PoRiES©

Doctor Robert Kushner has unlimited use of this drawing rendered by me and may publish it with his articles. I retain the copyright. October 11, 2011

Walter J. Pories

FIGURE 25.1 The four commonly accepted bariatric operations: laparoscopic adjustable gastric banding (AGB), Roux-en-Y gastric bypass (RYGB), laparoscopic gastric sleeve (GS), biliopancreatic bypass with duodenal switch (BPBDS), and biliopancreatic bypass (BPB). Source: *Reproduced with permission from Walter D. Pories.*

A. RWJF POLICY PRIORITIES TO REVERSE THE CHILDHOOD OBESITY EPIDEMIC

As part of its efforts to reverse the childhood obesity epidemic by 2015, the Robert Wood Johnson Foundation has outlined six broad policy priorities that evidence suggests will have the greatest and longest-lasting impact on our nation's children. There are likely a variety of policy pathways to achieve each priority. Some of these approaches, as recommended by the Centers for Disease Control, Institute of Medicine and other key governmental and research organizations, are listed below.

1. **Ensure that all foods and beverages served and sold in schools meet or exceed the most recent Dietary Guidelines for Americans.**

- Finalize and implement updated nutrition standards for all food and beverages served and sold in schools.
- Increase federal reimbursement for the National School Lunch Program.
- Expand access to the School Breakfast Program.
- Ensure schools have the resources they need to train cafeteria employees and replace outdated and broken kitchen equipment.

2. **Increase access to affordable foods through new or improved grocery stores and healthier corner stores and bodegas.**

- Create incentive programs to attract supermarkets and grocery stores to underserved neighborhoods. These may include tax credits, grant and loan programs, and small business/economic development programs.
- Introduce or modify land use policies and zoning regulations to promote, expand and protect potential sites for community gardens, mobile markets and farmers' markets. Potential sites may include vacant city-owned land or unused parking lots.

3. **Increase the time, intensity and duration of physical activity, in both schools and out-of-school programs.**

- Require physical education (PE) in schools.
- Implement a minimum standard of 150 minutes per week of PE in elementary schools and 225 minutes per week in middle schools and high schools.
- Increase opportunities for physical activity in schools outside of PE, such as classroom activity breaks, intramural and inter-scholastic sports.

4. **Increase physical activity by improving the built environment in communities.**

- Establish joint use agreements that will allow community residents to use school playing fields, playgrounds and recreation centers when schools are closed. If necessary, adopt regulatory and legislative policies to address liability issues that might block implementation.
- Build and maintain parks and playgrounds that are safe and attractive for playing, and located close to residential areas.
- Adopt community policing strategies that improve safety and security for park use, especially in higher-crime neighborhoods.
- Plan, build, and maintain a network of sidewalks and street crossings that creates a safe and comfortable walking environment that connects to schools, parks, and other destinations.

5. **Use pricing strategies – both incentives and disincentives – to promote the purchase of healthier foods.**

- Implement fiscal policies and local ordinances (e.g., taxes, incentives, land use and zoning regulations) that discourage the consumption of foods and beverages that are high in calories but low in nutrients.
- Provide incentives through federal food assistance programs to help families purchase healthier options. Examples may include "double bucks" programs that match Supplemental Nutrition Assistance Program dollars spent on healthy foods.

6. **Reduce youths' exposure to the marketing of unhealthy foods through regulation, policy, and effective industry self-regulation.**

- Adopt voluntary, industry-wide nutrition standards developed by the federal Interagency Working Group on food marketing and ensure that the definition of "marketing" includes marketing via social media (e.g., text messaging, Facebook, Twitter, etc.).
- Adopt a research-based, industry-wide, front-of-package labeling system.
- Eliminate advertising and marketing of calorie-dense, nutrient-poor foods and beverages near school grounds and public places frequently visited by youths.
- Use zoning policies to limit the number of fast-food outlets near schools and other settings frequented by youths.
- Set nutritional standards for children's meals that include a toy or other incentive item.
- Limit advertising that directly appeals to children (e.g., celebrities, cartoon characters, toys, gifts, games, food packaging).

FIGURE 26.1   RWJF Policy Policy Priorities to Reverse the Childhood Obesity Epidemic. Source: *http://healthyamericans.org/reports/obesity2011/Obesity2011Report.pdf.*

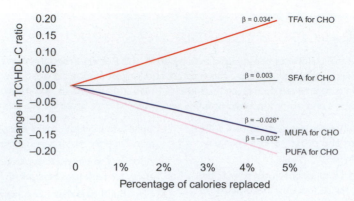

FIGURE 29.1 Changes in the TC/HDL-C ratio when carbohydrates are replaced isocalorically with SFA, MUFA, PUFA, and TFA β reflects the change for each 1% energy replacement. $*p < 0.05$. Source: *Adapted from Micha and Mozaffarian [229].*

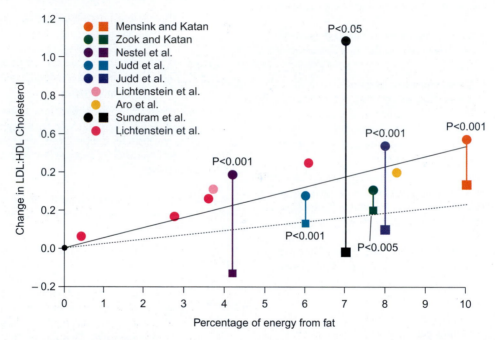

FIGURE 29.2 Results of randomized studies of the effects of a diet high in *trans* fatty acids (circles) or saturated fatty acids (squares) on the ratio of LDL cholesterol to HDL cholesterol. A diet with isocaloric amounts of *cis* fatty acids was used as the comparison group. The solid line indicates the best-fit regression for *trans* fatty acids. The dashed line indicates the best-fit regression for saturated fatty acids [100].

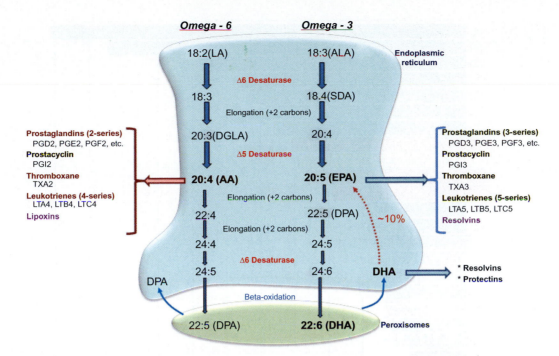

FIGURE 29.3 Biochemical pathway for the interconversion of n-6 and n-3 fatty acids. AA, arachidonic acid; ALA, α-linolenic acid; DGLA, dihomo-γ-linolenic acid; DHA, docosahexaenoic acid; DPA, docosapentaenoic acid; EPA, eicosapentaenoic acid; GLA, γ-linolenic acid; LA, linoleic acid; SDA, stearidonic acid [117].

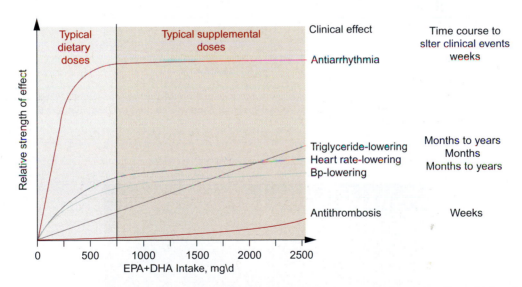

FIGURE 29.4 Schema of potential dose responses and time courses for altering clinical events of physiologic effects of fish or fish oil intake [142].

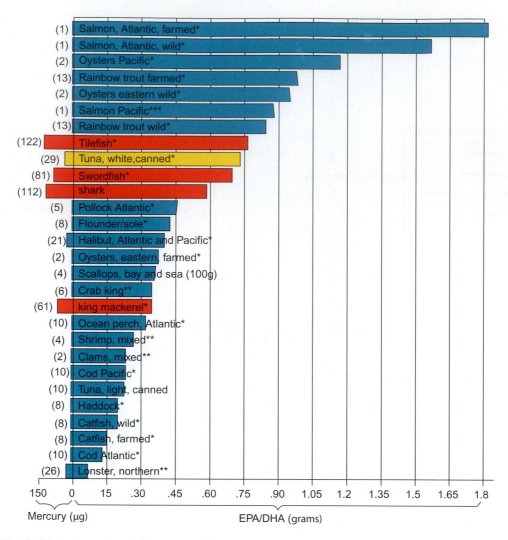

FIGURE 29.5 EPA/DHA intake and methylmercury intake exposure from one 3-ounce portion of seafood. *Cooked, dry heat; **cooked, moist heat; ***the EPA and DHA content in Pacific salmon is a composite from chum, Coho, and sockeye. Source: *Reprinted from Institute of Medicine [230] with permission by the National Academies of Sciences.*

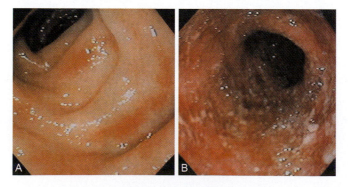

FIGURE 39.2 (A) Mild ulcerative colitis with some evidence of hemorrhage; (B) severe ulcerative colitis with extensive hemorrhage. Source: *Reprinted from* Sleisenger and Fordtran's Gastrointestinal and Liver Disease, *7th ed. Saunders W., Sleisenger M., Feldman M., 2002, with permission from Elsevier.*